Biochemical, Physiological, & Molecular Aspects *of* Human Nutrition

Biochemical, Physiological, & Molecular Aspects *of* Human Nutrition

MARTHA H. STIPANUK, PhD
Professor
Division of Nutritional Sciences
Colleges of Human Ecology and
Agriculture and Life Sciences
Cornell University
Ithaca, New York

SECOND EDITION

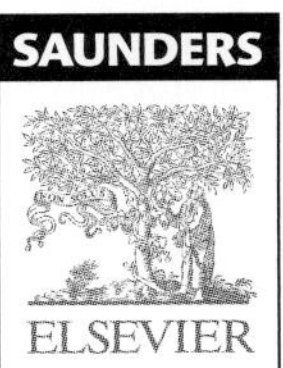

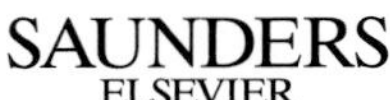

11830 Westline Industrial Drive
St. Louis, Missouri 63146

BIOCHEMICAL, PHYSIOLOGICAL, & MOLECULAR ASPECTS OF HUMAN NUTRITION

ISBN-13: 978-1-4160-0209-3
ISBN-10: 1-4160-0209-X

Notice

Knowledge and best practice in this field are constantly changing. As new research and experience broaden our knowledge, changes in practice, treatment and drug therapy may become necessary or appropriate. Readers are advised to check the most current information provided (i) on procedures featured or (ii) by the manufacturer of each product to be administered, to verify the recommended dose or formula, the method and duration of administration, and contraindications. It is the responsibility of the practitioner, relying on their own experience and knowledge of the patient, to make diagnoses, to determine dosages and the best treatment for each individual patient, and to take all appropriate safety precautions. To the fullest extent of the law, neither the Publisher nor the [Editors/Authors] [delete as appropriate] assumes any liability for any injury and/or damage to persons or property arising out or related to any use of the material contained in this book.

The Publisher

Previous edition copyrighted 2000

ISBN-13: 978-1-4160-0209-3
ISBN-10: 1-4160-0209-X

Senior Editor: Yvonne Alexopolous
Developmental Editor: Kristin Hebberd
Editorial Assistant: Sarah Vales
Publishing Services Manager: John Rogers
Senior Project Manager: Beth Hayes
Design Direction: Mark A. Oberkrom

Printed in the United States of America

Last digit is the print number: 9 8 7 6 5 4 3 2 1

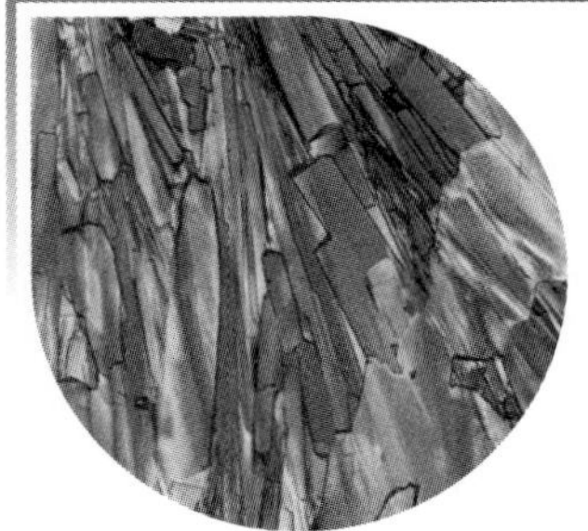

Contributors

Tracy G. Anthony, PhD
Assistant Scientist and Professor
Department of Biochemistry and Molecular Biology
Center for Medical Education
School of Medicine
Indiana University
Evansville, Indiana

J. Thomas Brenna, PhD
Professor
Division of Nutritional Sciences
Cornell University
Ithaca, New York

Qi Chen, PhD, Research Fellow
National Institute of Diabetes & Digestive & Kidney Diseases
National Institutes of Health
Bethesda, Maryland

Christopher P. Corpe, PhD
Research Fellow
National Institute of Diabetes and Digestive & Kidney Diseases
National Institutes of Health
Bethesda, Maryland

Robert R. Crichton, PhD, FRSC
Professor
Unité Biochimie
Université Catholique de Louvain
Belgium

Karen Crissinger, MD, PhD
Professor
Pediatric Gastroenterology
University of South Alabama
Mobile, Alabama

William T. Donahoo, MD
Assistant Professor
Department of Medicine
Section of Endocrinology, Diabetes, and Metabolism
University of Vermont
Burlington, Vermont

Hedley C. Freake, PhD
Professor
Department of Nutritional Sciences
College of Agriculture and Natural Resources
University of Connecticut
Storrs, Connecticut

Arthur Grider, PhD
Assistant Professor
Department of Foods and Nutrition
College of Family and Consumer Sciences
University of Georgia
Athens, Georgia

Michael F. Holick, MD, PhD
Professor, Department of Medicine
Director, General Clinical Research Center
School of Medicine
Boston University
Boston, Massachusetts

Susan M. Hutson, PhD
Professor
Department of Biochemistry
School of Medicine
Wake Forest University
Winston-Salem, North Carolina

Ronald J. Jandacek, PhD
Adjunct Professor
Department of Pathology
University of Cincinnati Medical Center
Cincinnati, Ohio

Elizabeth H. Jeffery, PhD
Professor of Nutritional Toxicology
Department of Food Science and Human Nutrition
College of Agricultural, Consumer, & Environmental Sciences
University of Illinois at Urbana-Champaign
Urbana, Illinois

Anna-Sigrid Keck, PhD
Visiting Assistant Professor
Department of Food Science and Human Nutrition
College of Agricultural, Consumer, & Environmental Sciences
University of Illinois at Urbana-Champaign
Urbana, Illinois

Martin Konrad, MD
Department of Pediatric Nephrology
University Children's Hospital
Inselspital Academic Health Centre
Bern, Switzerland

Taru Kosonen, PhD
Senior Medical Writer
Schering Oy
Helsinki, Finland

Susan M. Kundrat, RD, MS
Adjunct Lecturer
Department of Food Science and Human Nutrition
College of Agricultural, Consumer, & Environmental Sciences
University of Illinois at Urbana-Champaign
Urbana, Illinois

Je-hyuk Lee, PhD, Research Fellow
National Institute of Diabetes & Digestive & Kidney Diseases
National Institutes of Health
Bethesda, Maryland

James A. Levine, MD, PhD
Professor of Medicine
Endocrine Research Unit
Mayo Clinic College of Medicine
Rochester, Minnesota

Mark Levine, MD
Chief, Molecular and Clinical Nutrition Section
Senior Staff Physician
National Institutes of Health
Bethesda, Maryland

Betty A. Lewis, PhD
Associate Professor
Division of Nutritional Sciences
Cornell University
Ithaca, New York

Joanne R. Lupton, PhD
Regent's Professor of Nutritional Sciences, Food Science and Technology, and Veterinary Integrated Biosciences
University Faculty Fellow
William W. Allen Endowed Chair in Nutrition
Department of Nutrition and Food Science
College of Agriculture and Life Sciences
Texas A&M University
College Station, Texas

Donald B. McCormick, PhD
Professor Emeritus
Department of Biochemistry
Emory University
Atlanta, Georgia

Mary M. McGrane, PhD
Associate Professor
Department of Nutritional Sciences
University of Connecticut
Storrs, Connecticut

Margaret A. McNurlan, PhD
Associate Professor
Department of Surgery
School of Medicine
State University of New York
Stony Brook, New York

Edward L. Melanson, PhD
Assistant Professor
Division of Endocrinology, Diabetes, and Metabolism
Center for Human Nutrition
University of Colorado Health Sciences Center
Denver, Colorado

Buford L. Nichols, MD
Professor
Baylor College of Medicine
Texas Medical Center
Houston, Texas

Forrest H. Nielsen, PhD
Research Nutritionist
Grand Forks Human Nutrition Resource Center
Agricultural Research Service
U.S. Department of Agriculture
Grand Forks, North Dakota

Noa Noy, PhD
Professor
Division of Nutritional Sciences
Cornell University
Ithaca, New York

Sebastian J. Padayatty, MD, PhD, FFARCS, MRCP
Staff Clinician
National Institute of Diabetes & Digestive & Kidney Diseases
National Institutes of Health
Bethesda, Maryland

Robert S. Parker, PhD
Associate Professor
Division of Nutritional Sciences
Cornell University
Ithaca, New York

John C. Peters, PhD
Section Head
The Procter & Gamble Company
Cincinnati, Ohio

Roberto Quezada-Calvillo, MD
Visiting Professor
Baylor College of Medicine
USDA/ARS-Children's Nutrition Research Center
Houston, Texas
Facultad de Ciencias Quimicas
Universidad Autonoma de San Luis Potosi
San Luis Potosi, Mexico

Claudia C. Robayo, MD
Research Postdoctorate Fellow
Baylor College of Medicine
Children's Nutrition Research Center
Houston, Texas

Robert B. Rucker, PhD
Professor and Vice Chair
Department of Nutrition
University of California, Davis
Davis, California

Gavin L. Sacks, PhD
Research Associate
Division of Nutritional Sciences
Cornell University
Ithaca, New York

Karl-Peter Schlingmann, MD
University Children's Hospital
Philipps University
Marburg, Germany

Barry Shane, PhD
Professor
Department of Nutritional Sciences
University of California Berkeley
Berkeley, California

Hwai-Ping Sheng, PhD
Senior Lecturer and Associate Professor
Department of Physiology
The University of Hong Kong
Hong Kong

Arthur A. Spector, MD
University of Iowa Foundation Distinguished Professor
Biochemistry Department
The University of Iowa
Iowa City, Iowa

Christina Stark, MS, RD, CDN
Extension Associate
Division of Nutritional Sciences
Cornell University
Ithaca, New York

Bruce R. Stevens, PhD
Professor
Department of Physiology and Functional Genomics
College of Medicine
University of Florida
Gainesville, Florida

Judith Storch, PhD
Professor
Department of Nutritional Sciences
Cook College
Rutgers University
New Brunswick, New Jersey

Hei Sook Sul, PhD
Professor
Department of Nutritional Sciences and Toxicology
University of California Berkeley
Berkeley, California

Roger A. Sunde, PhD
Department Chairperson and Professor
Department of Nutritional Sciences
College of Agricultural and Life Sciences
University of Wisconsin–Madison
Madison, Wisconsin

Lawrence Sweetman, PhD
Professor, Institute of Biomedical Studies
Baylor University
Waco, Texas;
Director, Mass Spectrometry
Institute of Metabolic Disease
Baylor University Medical Center
Dallas, Texas

Patrick P. Tso, PhD
Professor
Department of Pathology and Laboratory Medicine
College of Medicine
University of Cincinnati
Cincinnati, Ohio

Nancy D. Turner, PhD
Associate Professor
Department of Animal Science
Texas A&M University
College Station, Texas

Reidar Wallin, PhD
Research Associate Professor
Section on Rheumatology
School of Medicine
Wake Forest University
Winston-Salem, North Carolina

Jin Wang, PhD, Research Fellow
National Institute of Diabetes & Digestive & Kidney Diseases
National Institutes of Health
Bethesda, Maryland

Yaohui Wang, MD
Biologist
National Institute of Diabetes & Digestive & Kidney Diseases
National Institutes of Health
Bethesda, Maryland

Malcolm Watford, DPhil
Associate Professor
Department of Nutritional Sciences
Cook College
Rutgers University
New Brunswick, New Jersey

Gary M. Whitford, PhD, DMD
Regents' Professor
Oral Biology and Maxillofacial Pathology
Associate Professor
Physiology and Graduate Studies
Medical College of Georgia
Augusta, Georgia

Richard J. Wood, PhD
Director, Minerals Bioavailability Laboratory
USDA Human Nutrition Research Center
Tufts University
Boston, Massachusetts

Liqun Zhang, MD, PhD, Research Fellow
National Institute of Diabetes & Digestive & Kidney Diseases
National Institutes of Health
Bethesda, Maryland

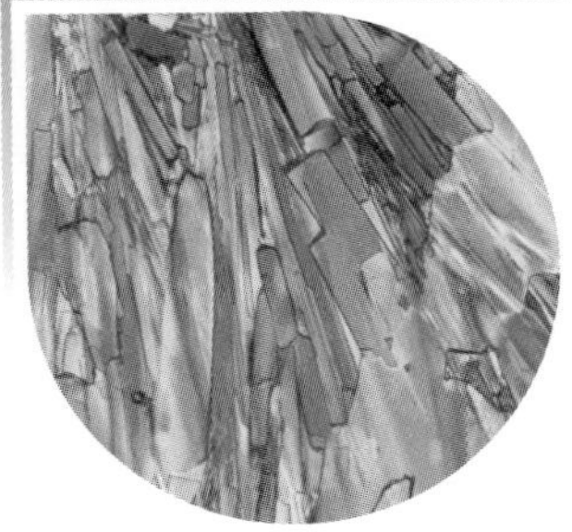

Preface

Biochemical, Physiological, & Molecular Aspects of Human Nutrition in its second edition has been revised and updated in an effort to continue to provide a book that covers the biological bases of human nutrition at the molecular, cellular, tissue, and whole-body levels. The text focuses on information from studies of human metabolism to the extent possible, but also relies on information obtained for other mammalian species. This is a book that can be used equally well as either a textbook or a reference book by students and professionals in various areas of nutrition and other life and biomedical sciences.

The second edition of *Biochemical, Physiological, & Molecular Aspects of Human Nutrition* reflects the contributions of more than 50 researchers and teachers who represent a diverse range of expertise. Authors have included the most up-to-date information and also identified areas of active research and controversy. At the same time, efforts have been made to ensure the consistency of content and approach so that the individual chapters and units work together as a whole for those who use the text as an introduction to the science of nutrition.

The study of human nutrition integrates many disciplines, and knowledge and understanding of each of these basic disciplines are essential to the understanding of nutrition. This book is intended largely for upper-level undergraduate students, graduate students, and professionals who have completed studies in organic chemistry, biochemistry, molecular biology, and physiology. Hence, topics are covered at an advanced level. Nevertheless, an effort has been made to present material in a manner that allows a reader who is unfamiliar with a particular topic to obtain a clear, concise, and thorough understanding of the essential concepts. Particular attention has been given to the design of figures and choice of tabular material to ensure that illustrations and tables clarify, extend, and enrich the text.

The text consists of six units that encompass a traditional coverage of nutrients by classification (carbohydrates, proteins, lipids, vitamins, and minerals) but that also allow for discussion of the integrated metabolism and utilization of these nutrients. In addition, in recognition of new paradigms in thinking about nutrition, a seventh unit begins the second edition, providing a discussion of the historical foundations of nutrition, the changes in how nutrients are being defined and in how dietary recommendations are being made, and of a wide variety of potentially beneficial food components. The macronutrients or energy-yielding nutrients (carbohydrates, proteins, and lipids) are discussed in Units II through V. Unit II provides an overview of the structure and properties of the macronutrients. The digestion and absorption of the macronutrients are discussed in Unit III, and the metabolism of the macronutrients is the topic of Unit IV. Finally, the relation of these macronutrients to energy is discussed in Unit V.

The vitamins are discussed in Unit VI. B vitamins have been grouped and discussed in three chapters in a manner that facilitates an understanding of their functions in macronutrient metabolism. The unique functions of vitamins C, K, E, A, and D are described in individual chapters. The minerals and water are the subjects of Unit VII; those with well-characterized nutritional or health-related roles are discussed in detail. Significant disease-related aspects of nutrition are incorporated into the individual chapters and are also highlighted in many of the feature boxes scattered throughout the book.

The text is designed so that it can easily be used for a comprehensive advanced nutrition and metabolism course in which all nutrients are covered. Alternatively, sections of the text could easily be used for courses that focus specifically on the macronutrients, energy, vitamins, or minerals. The depth and breadth of coverage given to the macronutrients make this text somewhat unique among advanced nutrition texts and make it an especially good choice for courses on macronutrient metabolism.

Each chapter begins with an outline and, when appropriate, a listing of common abbreviations. The text includes many figures drawn specifically for this book. Illustrations have been carefully selected to enhance the text and designed to provide insight and to facilitate understanding. References to the research literature and recommended readings, as well as related websites, are provided for each chapter. Also included within the text are a number of feature boxes—*Nutrition Insights, Clinical Correlations, Food Sources, RDAs/AIs Across the Life Cycle,* and *Life Cycle Considerations*—to highlight particular aspects of basic science and everyday nutrition, help readers make connections between abnormalities and their effects on normal metabolism, summarize cumbersome data pertinent to that discussion, or highlight particular nutritional processes or concepts applicable to various stages of the life span. In addition, "Thinking Critically" sections included in the *Nutrition Insight* and *Clinical Correlation* boxes encourage readers to apply the content to clinical situations.

For Instructors

An Evolve website has been created to accompany this book (http://evolve.elsevier.com/Stipanuk/nutrition/). Included within this resource are a Test Bank with approximately 850 multiple-choice examination questions and an Image Collection with nearly 400 illustrations from the textbook. Access to these materials is available free to adopting instructors through their Elsevier sales representative.

Martha H. Stipanuk

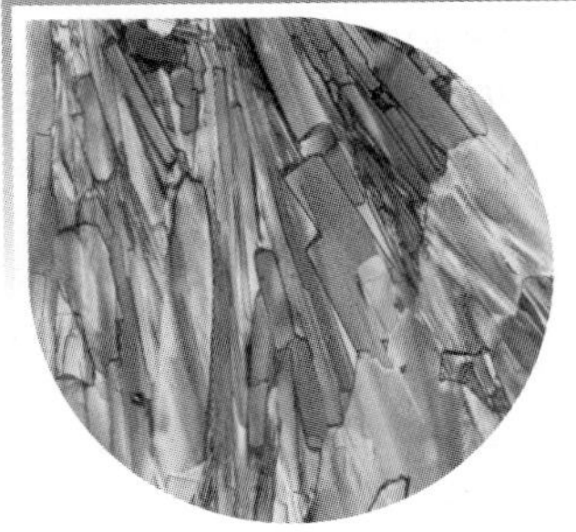

Acknowledgments

My deep appreciation goes to each of the contributors to *Biochemical, Physiological, & Molecular Aspects of Human Nutrition*. The target, as for the first edition, was "to obtain the best possible author" for each chapter, and the text is much enriched by the contributions of so many talented researchers and teachers. The commitment of the chapter contributors to education and sharing of knowledge is clear from the willingness of these busy individuals to accept the challenge and commit the time and effort required to see their chapters through the entire process. Their willingness to respond to queries, to discuss and resolve apparent differences of opinion among authors, and to allow the editorial flexibility needed to turn individual chapters into a coherent and integrated text was superb.

It has been a delight to work with the superb staff at Elsevier who handled the publication process. Senior Editor Yvonne Alexopoulos and Developmental Editor Kristin Hebberd kept the process running smoothly and efficiently and made my job much easier in so many ways. The support and efforts of Senior Project Manager Beth Hayes, who capably handled the book's production process, are greatly appreciated as well.

During the time I worked on this book, my colleagues in the Division of Nutritional Sciences at Cornell University supported my efforts in many ways, especially by serving as sources of expertise and in contributing several of the chapters. A special thanks to Charles McCormick, who assumed some of my teaching load during this past year so that I could take a semester of sabbatical leave to devote to getting the copy ready for publication. I also wish to especially acknowledge the superb efforts of Lawrence Hirschberger, Chad Simmons, John Dominy, Jr., Jeong-In Lee, and Relicardo Coloso in keeping my research program moving forward full-force during the course of my work on this book.

Finally, a special note of appreciation goes to my family and friends, who enrich each day of my life and who challenge me to a life of faith and purpose.

Working on the second edition of *Biochemical, Physiological, & Molecular Aspects of Human Nutrition* has been fun and educational. Those with whom I have worked on this project contributed to my enjoyment of this work. My thanks to each of you for your many contributions and support.

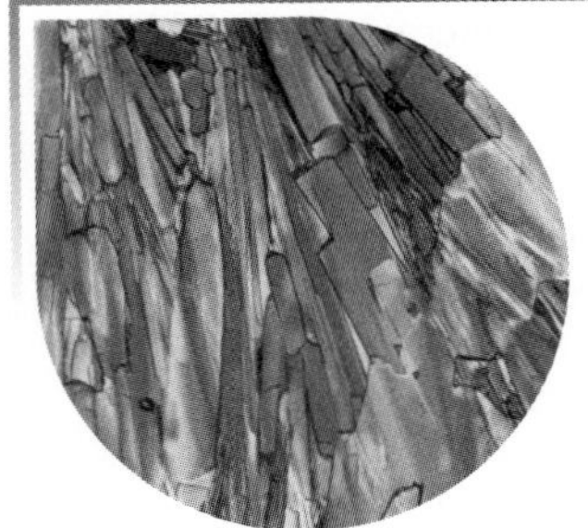

Contents

Unit I

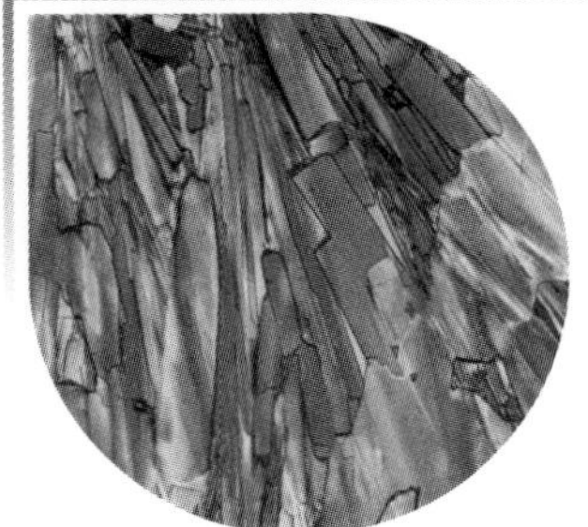

Nutrients: Essential and Nonessential

Nutrition may be defined simply as the utilization of foods by living organisms for normal growth, reproduction, and maintenance of health. Nutrients can be divided into two broad groups: (1) organic and (2) inorganic.

Inorganic nutrients include minerals and water. Those nutrients that can be used in inorganic form do not need to come from living sources such as plants or animals. Minerals are present in the earth's crust and are taken up from soil or water by plants and microorganisms, thereby making their way into the food chain. The amount of some minerals in foods can vary substantially depending on the concentration of that mineral in the soil or water in which the food was grown. Humans require more than a dozen different minerals in their diets. These include calcium and phosphorus that we need to make bones and teeth, iodine that we need to make thyroid hormone, and iron that we need as part of certain proteins including the hemoglobin in red blood cells. Much of our mineral intake comes from the foods we eat, but we also obtain minerals from water sources, salts, and food additives.

Nutrients in the organic or carbon-containing group make up the bulk of our diets and provide us with energy as well as many essential organic compounds. Organic nutrients include proteins, carbohydrates (sugars and starches), fats, and vitamins. These organic compounds are synthesized by living cells from simpler compounds. Green plants and photoplankton (such as algae and a special group of photosynthetic bacteria) form the base of the organic nutrient chain. These chlorophyll-containing forms of life use energy from sunlight to combine carbon dioxide from the atmosphere and water to make carbohydrates by a process we call photosynthesis. Therefore, plants and photoplankton are able to make organic compounds (such as sugars and carbohydrates) from inorganic compounds (CO_2 and H_2O) in the environment. Animals and most microorganisms, however, cannot carry out photosynthesis and must have preformed organic material in their diets. These species obtain organic nutrients by eating other organisms. Bacteria generally have simple nutrient needs. Most bacteria need a simple organic carbon source, usually decaying plant or animal life. Conversely, animals and humans have complex nutritional needs and require a number of different organic compounds in their diets. We obtain organic nutrients—protein, carbohydrates, fats, including some essential fatty acids, and 13 essential vitamins—by consuming a variety of plant and animal foods.

This first unit contains three chapters. Chapter 1 explores the scientific efforts that resulted in the identification and definition of essential nutrients. Much of this work took place during the first half of the twentieth century, with the goals of preventing nutrient deficiency disease and determining the actual amount of each nutrient that was required to prevent deficiency symptoms. Much more attention was given during the latter decades of the twentieth century to the role of nutrition in the maintenance or enhancement of health and in the reduction of risk of certain chronic diseases, such as heart disease and cancer. This latter focus will likely continue during the twenty-first century as much remains to be understood about the relationships of nutrition, diet, and health, and about beneficial or harmful nonnutrient components of foods. In Chapter 2, various groups of compounds that are actively being studied for their health effects and the current state of this research are presented. How we put the knowledge of the science of nutrition into practice is of only academic interest unless it is applied to improvement of the health and well-being of individuals and populations. Chapter 3 presents various means by which the understanding of biological needs and functions of nutrients is translated into information that allows consumers to make healthy dietary choices.

Martha H. Stipanuk

Chapter 1

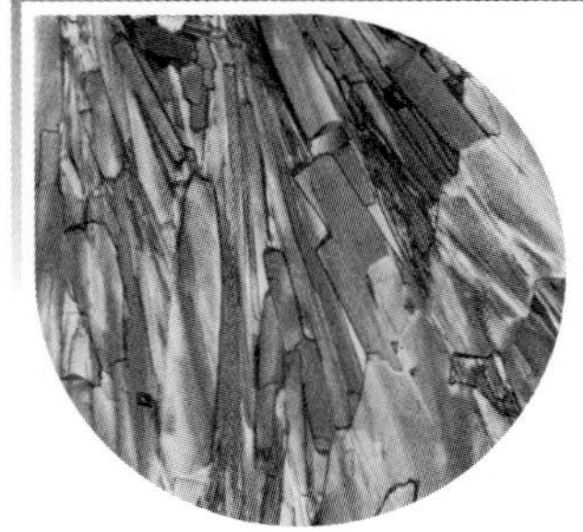

Nutrients: History and Definitions

Martha H. Stipanuk, PhD

OUTLINE

Nutrients are defined as chemical substances found in foods that are necessary for human life and growth, maintenance, and repair of body tissues. It is now commonly accepted that proteins, fats, carbohydrates, vitamins, minerals, and water are the major nutritional constituents of foods.

DISCOVERY OF THE NUTRIENTS

ALIMENT

Before the chemical nature of food was understood, food was believed to be made up of nutriment, medicines, and poisons. In ancient Greece (~500-300 BC), differences in the physical properties of foods and in their contents of medicinal and toxic substances were recognized. The role of diet in the causation and treatment of disease was recognized, as evidenced by the use of liver to treat night blindness. However, the physicians of this era had no understanding of the chemical nature of foods and believed that foods contained only a single nutritional principle that was called aliment.

The belief that foods contained a single nutritional principle persisted for more than two millennia up until the nineteenth century and impeded progress in understanding nutrition. Some recorded observations made during the seventeenth and eighteenth centuries, however, hinted at scientific progress to come. For example, during the 1670s Thomas Sydenham, a British physician, observed that a tonic of iron filings in wine produced a clinical response in patients with chlorosis, a condition now recognized as hypochromic or iron-deficiency anemia (McCollum, 1957). In 1747, James Lind of Scotland, while serving as a naval surgeon, conducted a clinical trial of various proposed treatments of sailors who were ill with scurvy. He observed that consumption of citrus fruits (oranges and lemons), but not other typical foods and medicines, cured the disease (Carpenter, 1986). Nevertheless, chlorosis and scurvy were not viewed as nutritional diseases, and the concept that a disease might be caused by a deficit of a substance that was nutritionally essential did not exist. By 1900, toxins, heredity, and infections, but not yet nutrition, were recognized as causes of disease.

PROXIMATE COMPOSITION OF FOOD

During the later part of the eighteenth century (~1770-1794), Antoine Lavoisier and Pierre-Simon Laplace conducted their studies of respiration and, in the process, made the first connection between food and chemical functions. They concluded that the oxidation of carbon compounds was the source of energy for activity and other bodily functions of animals (Lusk, 1922). This was followed by the observation by Francois Magendie in Paris that a specific organic food component was essential. In 1816, Magendie observed that dogs fed only carbohydrate or fat lost considerable body protein and weight within a few weeks, whereas dogs fed foods that contained nitrogen (protein) remained healthy. In 1827, William Prout, a physician and scientist in London, proposed that the nutrition of higher animals could be explained by their need for proteins, carbohydrates, and fats, and this explanation was widely accepted. During the next two decades, the need of animals for several mineral elements was demonstrated, and at least six mineral elements (Ca, P, Na, K, Cl, and Fe) had been established as essential for higher animals by 1850 (Harper, 1999; Carpenter et al., 1997).

The nineteenth-century German chemist Justus von Liebig postulated that energy-yielding substances (carbohydrates and fats) and proteins, together with a few minerals, represented the essentials of a nutritionally adequate diet, and he proposed that the nutritive value of foods and feeds could be predicted from knowledge of their gross chemical composition. Liebig prepared tables of food values based on this concept—work that was facilitated by the work of Wilhelm Henneberg, who devised the Weende system, known as proximate analysis, for analyzing foods and feeds for protein, fat, fiber, nitrogen-free extract (carbohydrate), and ash (McCollum, 1957). Throughout the remainder of the nineteenth century, nutrition continued to be dominated by the belief that sources of energy, protein, and a few minerals were the sole principles of a nutritionally adequate diet.

Despite the dominance of Liebig's views during the mid-to-late nineteenth century, it should be noted that the validity of his assumptions were challenged during the nineteenth century (McCollum, 1957). In 1847, J. Pereira in England stated that diets containing a wide variety of foods were essential for human well-being, whereas diets containing only a few foods were associated with the acquisition of diseases such as scurvy. Jean Baptist Dumas, based on his observation that an artificial milk containing all of the known dietary constituents failed to prevent deterioration of health of children during the siege of Paris (1870-1871), also questioned the validity of Liebig's assumptions. In addition, Ivanovich Lunin (~1881) and C. A. Socin (~1891), who both worked in Gustav von Bunge's laboratory in Basel conducting studies with mice in an effort to identify inadequacies in the mineral component of purified diets, demonstrated that mice fed a diet composed of purified proteins, fats, carbohydrates, and a mineral mixture survived less than 5 weeks, whereas mice that received milk or egg yolk in addition to the purified components remained healthy throughout the experiment. However, rather than attribute these observations to the presence of other essential nutrients in foods, the inadequacies of the purified diets were attributed to mineral imbalances, failure to supply minerals as organic complexes, or lack of palatability.

Also of significance were the studies of beriberi that were conducted during the nineteenth century. Kanehiro Takaki was concerned during the 1880s with the devastating effects of beriberi on sailors in the Japanese navy. Because of the superior health of British sailors, he compared the food supplies of the two navies and was struck by the higher protein content of the British rations. He, therefore, included evaporated milk and meat in the diet and substituted barley for part of the polished rice in the Japanese rations. These changes eradicated beriberi. He attributed this to the additional protein. In retrospect, we know that this was incorrect, but his conclusion does imply that he correctly considered beriberi to be a disease caused by a nutritional inadequacy (Takaki, 1906). Christiaan Eijkman, an army physician in the Dutch East Indies, began his investigations of beriberi in the 1890s (Jansen, 1956). He had observed a high incidence of beriberi in the prisons in Java in which polished rice was a staple. He assumed it was caused by chronic consumption of a diet consisting largely of polished rice. He noted during his experimental studies that chickens fed on a military hospital diet comprised mainly of polished rice developed a neurological disease resembling beriberi, but when the birds were fed rice with the pericarp intact they remained healthy. He concluded that ingestion of the high starch diet resulted in formation in the intestine of a substance that acted as a nerve poison and that rice hulls contained an antidote. Eijkman's conclusion illustrates the fact that a connection between nutrient deficiency and disease was still a foreign concept at the end of the nineteenth century.

DIET AND DISEASE

In 1901, Gerrit Grijns, who took over Eijkman's research in the Dutch East Indies in 1896, showed through feeding trials that Eijkman's active substance was present in other foods (Carpenter, 1995; Jansen, 1956). After demonstrating that beriberi could be prevented by including rice polishings or beans or water extracts of these foods in the diet, he proposed that beriberi was a dietary deficiency disease caused by the absence of an essential nutrient present in rice hulls. Grijns, thus, interpreted Eijkman's results correctly and provided for the first time a clear concept of a dietary deficiency disease. The broad implications of Grijns' interpretation of his investigation of beriberi were not appreciated for some years, however. In 1907, Alex Holst and Theodore Fröhlich in Norway reported that guinea pigs fed dry diets with no fresh vegetables developed a disease resembling scurvy; supplying them with fresh vegetables cured the disease—giving rise to a second example of a dietary deficiency disease (Carpenter, 1986). Interestingly, Holst and Fröhlich had been looking for a mammal to test a diet that had earlier produced beriberi in pigeons; they were surprised that scurvy resulted instead because, up until that time, scurvy had not been considered to occur in any species other than humans.

ESSENTIAL AMINO ACIDS

The first evidence of essentiality of a specific organic molecule was the discovery by Edith Willcock and Fredrick G. Hopkins (1906) that a supplement of the amino acid tryptophan, which had been discovered in 1900, prolonged survival of mice fed a zein-based diet. Zein is the major storage protein in corn endosperm and it contains only a small proportion of tryptophan.

The failure of acid hydrolysates of protein to support growth, contrasted with the ability of enzyme hydrolysates of protein to support adequate rates of growth, was attributed to a deficiency of tryptophan due to the destruction of tryptophan by acid digestion (Henriques and Hansen, 1905). Further work on amino acid requirements was delayed until the problem of failure to obtain satisfactory growth of rats fed on purified diets was solved. The work of Elmer V. McCollum and colleagues in Wisconsin and of Thomas Osborne and Lafayette Mendel in Connecticut in developing rodent models and the use of long-term growth of rats as a measure of nutritional adequacy soon opened up a new approach to the search for vitamins as well as the discovery of additional essential amino acids (Osborne and Mendel, 1914, 1911). Using purified diets supplemented with a protein-free milk extract, Osborne and Mendel demonstrated that proteins from different sources differed in nutritive value and discovered that lysine, sulfur-containing amino acids, and histidine were essential amino acids for the rat (Block and Mitchell, 1946). With gliadin as the protein source in place of casein, Osborne and Mendel (~1915) showed that rats required lysine for growth (Munro, 1964).

TESTING LIEBIG'S HYPOTHESIS

The validity of Liebig's hypothesis—that the nutritive value of foods and feeds could be predicted from measurements of their gross composition—was directly tested at the University of Wisconsin in 1907 to 1911 in what has become known as the Wisconsin single grain experiment (Carpenter et al., 1997; Hart et al., 1911). This study was suggested to E.B. Hart by his predecessor at the University of Wisconsin, Stephen M. Babcock, who had observed that milk production by cows consuming rations composed of different feedstuffs differed considerably, even when the rations were formulated to have the same gross composition and energy content. Hart and colleagues compared the performance of four groups of heifers fed rations composed entirely of the corn (corn meal, corn gluten, and corn stover), wheat (ground wheat, wheat gluten, and wheat straw), or oats (oat meal and oat straw), all formulated to be closely similar in gross composition and energy content, or a mixed ration consisting of equal parts of the three plants. Six-month-old heifers were fed the assigned rations to maturity and through two reproductive periods. Differences between performance of the corn and wheat groups was marked, with other groups being intermediate. Calves born to cows consuming the corn ration were strong and vigorous and all lived, but cows consuming the wheat ration all delivered 3 to 4 weeks prematurely and none of the calves lived beyond 12 days. Cows fed the corn ration produced almost double the amount of milk produced by those fed the wheat ration. Thus Hart and colleagues demonstrated that the nutritive value of a ration could not be predicted solely from measurements of its content of protein, energy, and a few minerals. In hindsight, the signs of inadequacy in the wheat and oat groups resembled those of vitamin A deficiency, which would have been prevented by the carotene in the ration that contained corn.

THE ANIMAL GROWTH MODEL: DISCOVERY OF FAT-SOLUBLE A AND WATER-SOLUBLE B

In the early 1900s investigators were beginning to conduct nutritional studies with rodents fed purified diets. They soon found difficulties in maintaining growth in rats using starch, lard, and mineral mixes, even with casein as the protein source. This problem was overcome by addition of a protein-free extract of milk to these diets (Block and Mitchell, 1946; Willcock and Hopkins, 1906). In 1912, F.G. Hopkins suggested that an organic complex that animals cannot synthesize was absent from the purified diets. In 1912, Casimir Funk, a young Polish chemist who had been trying to purify the anti-beriberi principle from rice polishings, expressed the opinion that beriberi as well as scurvy and pellagra were dietary deficiency diseases. Funk believed these diseases were caused by a lack in the diet of "special substances which are in the nature of organic bases, which we will call vitamines" (McCollum, 1957). Within a short time from 1912, the concept that foods contained small quantities of organic substances that were essential nutrients was generally accepted.

Between 1909 and 1913, E.V. McCollum and Margaret Davis noted that growth of rats was satisfactory if the fat was supplied as butterfat, but not if butterfat was replaced by lard or olive oil. Meanwhile, Osborne and Mendel observed that if they purified the protein-free milk included in their diets, growth failure of rats again occurred, but if they substituted milk fat for the lard in their diets, growth was restored. Both groups concluded that butterfat contained an unidentified substance essential for growth. McCollum and Davis proceeded to extract an active substance from butterfat and transferred it to olive oil, which then promoted growth. They called this substance fat-soluble A. When they further tested this substance in a polished rice diet of the type used by Eijkman and Grijns in their studies of beriberi, they found that even though the diet contained the fat-soluble A, it still failed to support growth. A water extract of wheat germ or boiled eggs provided the missing factor, which was designated water-soluble B.

ESTABLISHMENT OF CRITERIA FOR ESSENTIALITY

The emergence of the use of the animal growth model was extremely important to the identification of *essential nutrients*. By 1915, six minerals, four amino acids, and three vitamins—A, B, and the antiscorbutic factor—had been identified as essential nutrients. By 1918 the concept of the presence of "accessory factors" or "minor constituents of foods" that are essential for health was established. Also, the importance of consuming a wide variety of foods to ensure that diets provided adequate quantities of these substances was being emphasized in health programs for the public in the United States and Great Britain and by the League of Nations; this was followed by a decline in the incidence of dietary deficiency diseases during the next three decades. Acceptance of the new paradigm was followed by a period of unparalleled discovery in nutritional science from about 1915 to the 1950s. By 1950, most of the essential nutrients had been identified and characterized and their functions explored. These essential nutrients included essential fatty acids, 9 amino acids, 12 vitamins, and 11 minerals (Box 1-1). Three other trace elements—molybdenum, selenium and chromium—were identified as essential nutrients during the 1950s.

In the late 1950s, after rats were maintained successfully through four generations on diets composed of constituents of known chemical structures (Schultze, 1957), it was generally accepted that all of the essential nutrients had been discovered. Later, when human subjects were maintained for long periods on intravenous fluids containing only highly purified

Box 1-1

LIST OF ESSENTIAL NUTRIENTS FOR HUMANS

Water

Amino acids

- Histidine
- Isoleucine
- Leucine
- Lysine
- Methionine
- Phenylalanine
- Threonine
- Tryptophan
- Valine

Vitamins

- Ascorbic acid
- Vitamin A
- Vitamin D
- Vitamin E
- Vitamin K
- Thiamin
- Riboflavin
- Niacin
- Vitamin B_6
- Pantothenic acid
- Folate
- Biotin
- Vitamin B_{12}

Energy sources (carbohydrate, fat, or protein)

Fatty acids

- Linoleic
- α-Linolenic

Minerals

- Calcium
- Phosphorus
- Magnesium
- Iron
- Sodium
- Potassium
- Chloride
- Zinc
- Copper
- Manganese
- Iodine
- Selenium
- Molybdenum
- Chromium (probably)
- Boron (probably)

constituents, it was accepted that the conclusion also applied to humans. Nevertheless, an avid search for additional essential nutrients continued for some years. Over the course of studies to identify nutrients, specific criteria were established for declaring a food constituent to be an essential nutrient. Alfred E. Harper (1999, p. 5) summarized the following criteria of essentiality that had evolved by ~1950:

- The substance is required in the diet for growth, health, and survival.
- The absence of the substance from the diet or inadequate intake results in characteristic signs of a deficiency disease and, ultimately, death.
- Growth failure and characteristic signs of deficiency are prevented only by the nutrient or a specific precursor of it, not by other substances.
- Below some critical level of intake of the nutrient, growth response and severity of signs of deficiency are proportional to the amount consumed.
- The substance is not synthesized in the body and is, therefore, required for some critical function throughout life.

Harper also emphasized that nutritional essentiality is characteristic of the species, not the nutrient. For example, ascorbic acid is required by humans and guinea pigs but not by most other species that can synthesize the nutrient from glucose. During the1960s and 1970s, the concept of essentiality was modified for the mineral elements that could not be fed at dietary concentrations sufficiently low to interfere with growth, development, maturation, or reproduction—some of the ultratrace elements. The most consistently applied criterion was that a dietary deficiency must consistently and adversely change a biological function from optimal, and this change must be preventable or reversible by physiological amounts of the element (Nielsen, 2000). However, this latter basis for establishing essentiality of minerals ultimately was not very satisfactory for the ultratrace elements because it was impossible to determine whether some of the changes were really the result of low intakes causing suboptimal functions or of the mineral supplements having pharmacological actions in the body. Today, most scientists do not consider an element essential unless it has a defined biochemical function. Nevertheless, there is no universally accepted list of ultratrace elements that are considered essential. Forest Nielsen suggests that a nutritionally beneficial element be defined as "one with health restorative effects in response to an apparent deficient intake of that element, at intakes that are found with normal diets; these health restorative effects can be amplified or inhibited by nutritional, physiological, hormonal, or metabolic stressors" (Nielsen, 2000, p. 116). Nielsen (2000) gives the following examples of nutritionally beneficial elements:

- Boron, the effects of which can be amplified by a marginal vitamin D deficiency,
- Vanadium, the effects of which can be amplified by deficient or luxuriant dietary iodine, and
- Nickel, the beneficial effects of which are inhibited by vitamin B_{12}, pyridoxine, or folic acid deficiency.

Nielsen (2000, pp. 116-117) suggests the following four categories of evidence that may support the contention that a trace element is nutritionally essential:

1. A dietary deprivation in some animal model consistently results in a changed biological function, body structure, or tissue composition that is preventable or reversible by an intake of an apparent physiological amount of the element in question.
2. The element fills the need at physiological concentrations for a known in vivo biochemical action to proceed in vitro.
3. The element is a component of known biologically important molecules in some life form.
4. The element has an essential function in lower forms of life.

Using these criteria, there is strong circumstantial evidence for the essentiality of arsenic, boron, chromium, nickel, silicon, and vanadium, and limited circumstantial evidence for essentiality of aluminum, bromine, cadmium, fluorine, germanium, lead, lithium, rubidium, and tin. The strongest evidence for essentiality exists for boron and chromium,

Nutrition Insight

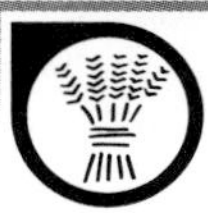

The History of American Food Composition Tables

The U.S. Department of Agriculture (USDA) has been compiling food composition data for well more than 100 years. The food composition data they maintain is widely used by nutritionists, researchers, and individuals. Tabulation of food composition data began with the work of Wilbour Olin Atwater scarcely 50 years after the classical studies of Justus von Liebig in Germany. Atwater received his Ph.D. from Yale in 1869 and then studied in Germany, where he became familiar with the work of Carl von Voit, Max Rubner, and Nathan Zuntz. In 1896 Atwater and A.P. Bryant published the proximate composition of 2,600 American foodstuffs in a bulletin called *The Chemical Composition of American Food Materials.* Within 4 years, an additional 4,000 new foods had been analyzed and a revised edition of the bulletin was published; about a quarter of these new analyses were performed by Atwater and his associates in the chemical laboratory at Wesleyan College (Middletown, CT). A 1906 reprinting of the bulletin stood until 1940 when the USDA Circular No. 549, *Proximate Composition of American Food Materials,* was published.

The first extensive revision of Atwater's work was in 1950 with the publication of the USDA Agriculture Handbook No. 8, *Composition of Foods—Raw, Processed, Prepared,* which contained values for 11 nutrients. Agriculture Handbook No. 8 was subsequently revised in 1963 and then expanded into a series of publications in 1976 to 1992. The *USDA Nutrient Database for Standard Reference* is the current form of the food composition tables. It has been maintained electronically since 1980, with frequent updates, and can be downloaded from the USDA's Nutrient Data Laboratory Home Page: http://www.ars.usda.gov/ba/bhnrc/ndl.

and these two elements likely belong in the category of established essential nutrients for higher animals including humans.

CONCERNS ABOUT EXCESSIVE INTAKES

With the successive discoveries of essential nutrients between 1915 and 1950 and the virtual disappearance of dietary deficiency diseases in developed countries, emphasis in nutrition changed to ensuring that diets would provide adequate quantities of all essential nutrients to prevent impairment of growth and development. In 1940, the Food and Nutrition Board of the National Research Council was organized in the United States with the function of advising on problems of nutrition in connection with national defense. This committee recognized the need for standards or allowances for intake of nutrients needed for maintenance of good health. The Food and Nutrition Board formulated the first set of Recommended Dietary Allowances (RDAs) for Americans in 1941. This committee has subsequently published nine revisions of the RDAs up through the 10th edition in 1989 and now has established the more extensive Dietary Reference Intakes.

During the first half of the twentieth century, relatively little attention was given to total food intake and its effects on health. An exception during this time was the work of Clive McCay (1934-1939) at Cornell (McCay et al., 1939). McCay argued that short-term trials with an emphasis on rapid growth did not provide an adequate test of the most desirable nutritional state throughout life. His studies showed that rats fed restricted amounts of a nutritionally adequate diet grew slower and survived longer than those allowed to eat freely. Concern about total food intake and health, however, increased during the second half of the twentieth century, as evidenced by the introduction of dietary guidelines for Americans in 1977 and by the growing concerns about obesity, metabolic syndrome, and chronic disease. Various editions of dietary guidelines for Americans have addressed concerns about excessive intakes of fat, saturated fat, cholesterol, salt and sodium, sugar, alcohol, and total energy.

NUTRIENTS THAT DO NOT MEET THE CRITERIA FOR ESSENTIALITY

CONDITIONALLY ESSENTIAL NUTRIENTS

As knowledge of nutritional needs grew, it became clear that there were conditions under which individuals required the presence of dispensable (nonessential) nutrients in the diet. During the 1970s, young children and certain groups of patients were found not to synthesize some of the nutritionally dispensable amino acids in amounts sufficient to meet their needs. These normally "nonessential" amino acids, therefore, had to be provided in the diet. These discoveries expanded the concept of "nutritional essentiality." Daniel Rudman and associates proposed the term *conditionally essential* for nutrients not ordinarily required in the diet but which must be supplied exogenously to specific populations that do not synthesize them in adequate amounts. The term was initially applied to dispensable nutrients needed by seriously ill patients maintained on total parenteral nutrition, but the term has been expanded to apply to similar needs that result from developmental immaturity, pathological states, or genetic defects. Rudman and A.G. Feller (1986) proposed the following three criteria that must be met to establish unequivocally that a nutrient is conditionally essential:

1. Decline in the plasma level of the nutrient into the subnormal range
2. Appearance of chemical, structural, or functional abnormalities
3. Correction of both of these by a dietary supplement of the nutrient

Harper (1999) stressed that conditional essentiality represents a qualitative change in requirements, that is, the need for a nutrient that is ordinarily dispensable. He further stressed that this term should not be used for alterations in the need for an essential nutrient, for health benefits from consumption of nonnutrients, or for health benefits from consumption of dispensable nutrients or essential nutrients in excess of amounts needed for normal physiological function. Examples of conditionally essential nutrients include a requirement of premature infants for cysteine and tyrosine, which cannot yet be synthesized in adequate amounts from their precursor amino acids; a possible requirement of long chain ω-3 fatty acids in preterm infants, because preterm infants are not able to synthesize these from α-linolenic acid at a rate that meets the infant's need; a requirement of some patients with cirrhosis of the liver for cysteine, tyrosine, and taurine owing to decreased hepatic capacity for synthesis of these amino acids from their precursors; and requirements for carnitine or tetrahydrobiopterin by individuals with genetic defects preventing the synthesis of these compounds.

MODIFICATION OF REQUIREMENTS FOR ESSENTIAL NUTRIENTS

Requirements for essential nutrients may be influenced by the presence in the diet of substances for which the nutrient is a precursor, that are precursors of the nutrient; substances that interfere with the absorption or utilization of the nutrient; imbalances and disproportions of other related nutrients; malabsorptive conditions; some genetic defects; and use of drugs that impair utilization of nutrients. These conditions do not alter basic requirements, but rather increase or decrease the amounts that must be consumed to meet requirements. Examples include the ability of tryptophan to serve as a precursor of niacin, the ability of β-carotene to serve as a precursor of vitamin A, the ability of phytic acid to impair absorption of zinc and other cations, the ability of thiomolybdate to complex copper and prevent its absorption, the interference of anticonvulsant medications with folate utilization, an increase in the vitamin B_{12} requirement resulting from malabsorption associated with atrophic gastritis, or high biotin requirements resulting from genetic defects in the enzyme responsible for reutilization of biotin in the body. Many more examples will be discussed throughout the other chapters of this book.

TOTAL HEALTH EFFECTS OF NUTRIENTS AND NONNUTRIENT COMPONENTS OF FOOD

In recent years diet-disease relationships have become major areas of investigation in nutrition. A new paradigm is emerging in which the dominating role of the concept of deficiency in determination of nutritional requirements is complemented by concern for the total health effects of nutrients (Mertz, 1993). Individual food constituents that may confer health benefits that are different from those of physiologically required quantities of essential nutrients, whether they are nonnutrients, dispensable nutrients, or essential nutrients in quantities exceeding those obtainable from the diet, are appropriately included in guidelines for health. This new paradigm includes the determination of upper safe levels of intake for nutrients as well as nonnutrients that may have harmful effects on health. This leads us to a new class of substances to consider in terms of nutrition: nonnutritional components of foods that are beneficial to health. The contribution of both fluoride and fiber to health has resulted in their inclusion in the list of nutrients for which the Institute of Medicine has now established Dietary Reference Intakes. Fluoride, in low doses, acts as a prophylactic agent in protecting teeth against the action of bacteria, but whether fluoride is essential for tooth and bone development is controversial. Fiber, in moderate amounts, is recognized to be beneficial for gastrointestinal function, and some forms of fiber may be fermented into products that can be absorbed and oxidized to yield energy, but there is no basis for classifying fiber as an essential nutrient. Numerous food constituents including certain fatty acids, fiber, carotenoids, and various nonnutrient substances in plants have been associated with lower incidences of chronic or degenerative diseases such as heart disease and cancer.

Health benefits of essential nutrients have also been given greater weight in making nutritional recommendations. Higher intakes of some essential nutrients (especially vitamins E and C, which may function as antioxidants) have been shown to be associated with lower risk of chronic disease or with enhanced immune system function. Recommendations for folic acid intake for women of child-bearing age have taken into account the ability of folic acid to reduce the incidence of neutral tube defects. Obviously, any health benefits of nonnutritive food constituents or higher intakes of essential nutrients may depend upon genetic differences among individuals, differences in lifestyle, and diet–genetic interactions that influence expression of genetic traits. With increasing knowledge of differences in genetic makeup of persons and population groups, more attention will likely be given to making nutritional recommendations relative to genetically determined metabolic differences.

USE OF NUTRIENTS AS PHARMACOLOGICAL AGENTS

Some nutrients or food components, in large doses, may function as drugs. The use of nutrients as pharmacological agents should not be considered under the category of nutrients. Nicotinic acid in large doses (up to 9 g daily) is used to lower serum cholesterol. Tryptophan has been used to induce sleep. The continuous intravenous infusion of magnesium is used in the treatment of preeclampsia and myocardial infarction. Many herbal and natural remedies are based on the use of food components as pharmacological agents.

The ancient Greeks believed that foods contain nutriment, medicines, and poisons. In some ways this ancient understanding is still appropriate in that foods do contain nutrients, substances beneficial to health, and substances that have adverse effects on health. Thus we have come full-circle to the ancient paradigm with the knowledge that each of the three principles in fact includes many different chemical compounds.

REFERENCES

Block RJ, Mitchell HH (1946) The correlation of the amino-acid composition of proteins with their nutritive value. Nutr Abstr Rev 16:249-278.

Carpenter KJ (1986) The History of Scurvy and Vitamin C. Cambridge University Press, New York.

Carpenter KJ, Sutherland B (1995) Eijkman's contribution to the discovery of vitamins. J Nutr 125:155-163.

Carpenter KJ, Harper AE, Olson RE (1997) Experiments that changed nutritional thinking. J Nutr 127:1017S-1053S.

Harper AE (1999) Defining the essentiality of nutrients. In: Shils ME, Olson JA, Shike M, Ross AC (eds) Modern Nutrition in Health and Disease, 9th ed. Williams & Wilkins, Baltimore, pp 3-10.

Hart EB, McCollum EV, Steenbock H, Humphrey GC (1911) Physiological effect on growth and reproduction of rations balanced from restricted sources. Univ Wis Agric Exp Stn Res Bull 17:131-205.

Henriques V, Hansen C (1905) Uber Eiwessynthese im Tierkorper. Hoppe-Seyler's Z. Physiol Chem 43:417-446.

Jansen BCP (1956) Early nutrition researches on beri-beri leading to the discovery of vitamin B1. Nutr Abstr Rev 26:1-14.

Lusk G (1922) A history of metabolism. Endocr Metab 3:3-78.

McCay CM, Maynard LA, Sperling G, Barnes LL (1939) Retarded growth, life span, ultimate body size and age changes in the albino rat after feeding diets restricted in calories. J Nutr 18:1-13.

McCollum EV (1957) A History of Nutrition. The Sequence of Ideas in Nutrition Investigations. Houghton-Mifflin, Boston.

Mertz W (1993) Essential trace metals: new definitions based on new paradigms. Nutr Rev 51:287-295.

Munro HN (1964) Historical introduction: the origin and growth of our present concepts of protein metabolism. In: Munro HN, Allison JB (eds) Mammalian Protein Metabolism Academic Press, New York, pp 1-29.

Nielsen FH (2000) Importance of making dietary recommendations for elements designated as nutritionally beneficial, pharmacologically beneficial, or conditionally essential. J Trace Elem Exp Med 13:113-129.

Osborne T, Mendel LB (1911) Feeding experiments with isolated food substances. Carnegie Inst. Washington. Publ 156.

Osborne T, Mendel LB (1914) Amino-acids in nutrition and growth. J Biol Chem 17:325-349.

Rudman D, Feller A (1986) Evidence for deficiencies of conditionally essential nutrients during total parenteral nutrition. J Am Coll Nutr 5:101-106.

Schultze MO (1957) Nutrition of rats with compounds of known chemical structure. J Nutr 61:585-595.

Takaki K (1906) Three lectures on the preservation of health amongst the personnel of the Japanese navy and army. Lancet 1:1369, 1451, 1520.

Willcock EG, Hopkins FG (1906) The importance of individual amino acids in metabolism. J Physiol (London) 35:88-102.

RECOMMENDED READING

Carpenter KJ, Harper AE, Olson RE (1997) Experiments that changed nutritional thinking. J Nutr 127:1017S-1053S.

Chapter 2

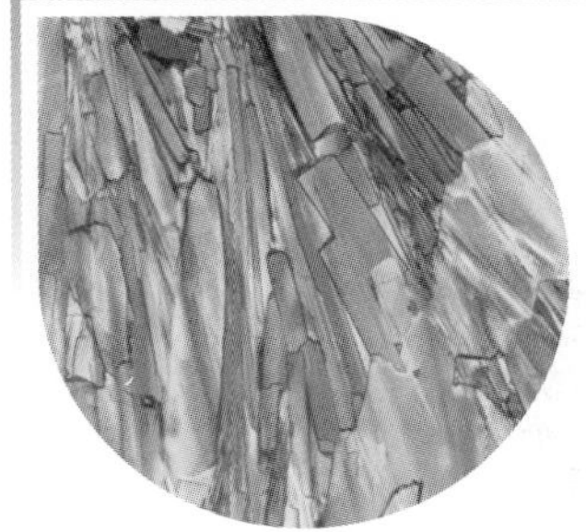

Nonessential Food Components With Health Benefits

Elizabeth H. Jeffery, PhD, Susan M. Kundrat, RD, MS, and Anna-Sigrid Keck, PhD

OUTLINE

COMMON ABBREVIATIONS

ALA α-linolenic acid
CLA conjugated linoleic acid
CVD cardiovascular disease
DHA docosahexaenoic acid
EPA eicosapentaenoic acid
FDA U.S. Food and Drug Administration
GRAS generally recognized as safe
MUFA monounsaturated fatty acid
PUFA polyunsaturated fatty acid
ROS reactive oxygen species
SCFA short-chain fatty acid
USDA U.S. Department of Agriculture

BIOACTIVE DIETARY COMPONENTS, NUTRACEUTICALS, AND FUNCTIONAL FOODS

One of the most rapidly moving, exciting areas in nutrition research today is the study of nonessential components in the diet that are associated with decreased risk for chronic diseases, including cardiovascular disease (CVD) and cancer. Because they are found naturally in the diet at levels that exert a physiological effect, foods that provide these components can be identified through epidemiological studies that relate diet to disease incidence. Unlike vitamins and minerals, these components are not essential for growth and development. It has been suggested that discovery of nonessential food components that provide health benefits, also called *bioactive food components*, may prove to be as important to good nutrition as the discovery of vitamins and minerals that occurred during the last century. Many of these compounds have been purified and characterized chemically (Figure 2-1). When studied in purified form, most have specific biochemical actions, giving rise to the term *nutraceutical*, which derives from the idea of a "drug-like" nutrient or dietary component. Whereas this reductionist approach is proving useful in the study of mechanism, studies carried out using purified components do not always reflect the full physiological effect of a whole food within the diet. Seldom is there only one bioactive component in a food, and frequently several components have interactive or synergistic effects. Furthermore, bioavailability can be very different between a purified component and the same component within its original food matrix. A substantial research literature is evolving that attempts to link the physiological effect of the whole food to the mechanisms of action shown for purified bioactive food components.

Foods rich in bioactive food components have been termed functional foods and include fruits, vegetables, and whole grains. Although there is no universally accepted definition of a functional food, the International Food Information Council defines functional foods as those foods that provide health benefits beyond basic nutrition. The American Dietetic Association states that "functional foods, including whole foods and fortified, enriched, or enhanced foods, are foods that have a potentially beneficial effect on health when consumed as part of a varied diet on a regular basis, at effective levels" (Hasler et al., 2004, p. 814). Many bioactive food components are plant secondary metabolites (phytonutrients), but these components may also be found in foods of animal origin (zoonutrients) as well as in fungal and bacterial products. The exact concentration of bioactive components in a given food can be determined only by analysis because, as with vitamins, content varies with the genotype of the plant or animal, growing conditions, and processing methods. Unlike whole foods, extracts or concentrates sold as dietary supplements may have specific analytical

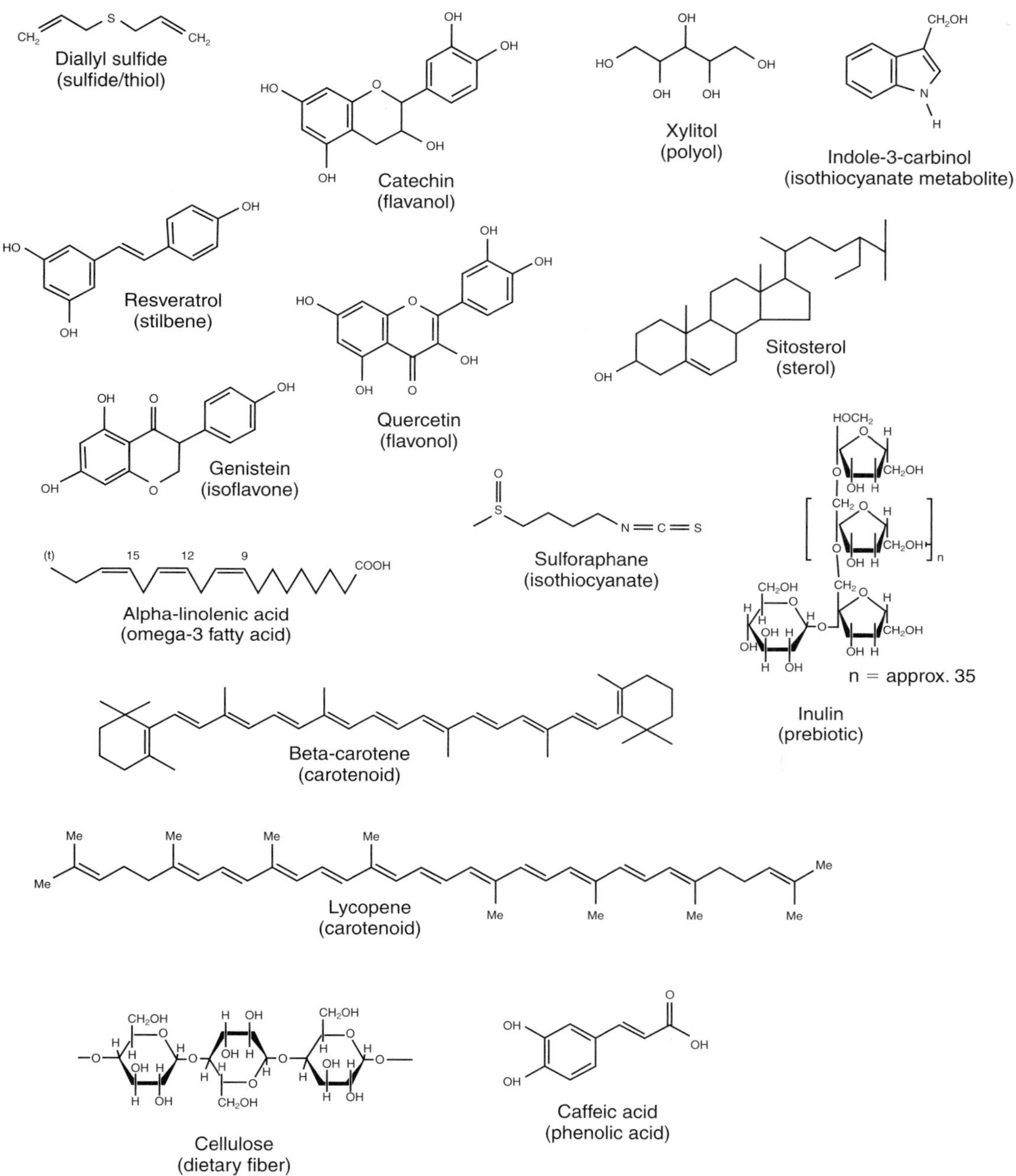

Figure 2-1 Examples of nonessential bioactive food components.

information, but such labeling is not currently required. The U.S. Department of Agriculture (USDA) recently initiated development of databases that provide typical ranges of bioactive components in foods available in the United States today.

This chapter reviews the chemical characterization and scientific basis for bioactivity of the major categories of bioactive food components. Whereas many of these may be termed "nonessential" in that they are not required for full growth and development, it should be

Nutrition Insight

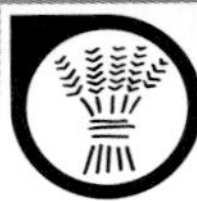

Synergy

It is common to study a single compound derived from a food to test its bioactivity and mechanism(s) of action. However, a single food contains many nonessential bioactive food components that are consumed as a mixture held within the food matrix. To add to this complexity, our diet is made up of many different kinds of foods, which are often ingested simultaneously. These different dietary factors may result in different bioavailabilities and bioactivities compared to that of the individual purified component. Frequently, when the whole food is incorporated into the diet, it does not have the same effect as the sum of the individual recognized bioactive components within that food. Some components may have additive effects, whereas others may act to enhance, inhibit, mask, or even antagonize the bioactivity of another component.

Synergy occurs when two or more components have a greater effect when given together than can be accounted for by the sum of their individual activities. Synergistic effects may occur between components present in the same food or in different foods or even between a food component and a drug. For example, vitamin C and isoflavones synergistically inhibit LDL-cholesterol oxidation in vitro; green tea and capsicum synergistically exert anticancer effects; and quercetin and catechin synergistically inhibit platelet aggregation (Morre and Morre, 2003; Pignatelli et al., 2000; Hwang et al., 2000). The overall effect of a combination of whole foods that contain these components, such as orange juice with a soy breakfast bar or green tea with a stir-fry containing peppers, has not been evaluated. One example of two bioactive components within a single food that have a synergistic effect is the glucosinolate hydrolysis products crambene and indole-3-carbinol from brussels sprouts. These individually and synergistically increased the activity of the anticancer biomarker quinone reductase when given in the diet to rodents, which may explain the larger-than-expected effect of Brussels sprouts, which are rich in both of these components (Nho and Jeffery, 2001). A recent paper evaluating inulin-soy isoflavone interactions showed that the probiotic inulin slowed intestinal microbial production of equol from the isoflavone daidzein (Zafar et al., 2004). It would be interesting to know if Jerusalem artichokes, rich in inulin, interrupt the health benefits of soy, thought to be associated with intestinal equol production from soy protein.

The potential benefits in determining synergistic effects are enormous, and more research needs to focus on the integrated effects of whole foods, or combinations of different foods, and not only on the mechanism of action of single components. The idea of synergy between components in a food not only provides a reason to test the bioactivity of the whole food in addition to that of the individual components, but provides a rationale for promotion of the consumption of whole foods as the sources of bioactive components. Foods are more available to the general public than are dietary supplements, and foods are less likely to be associated with adverse effects caused by excess intake.

noted that some well-recognized essential nutrients, at elevated levels, may also play a bioactive (nonnutritional) role in prevention of chronic disease. For example, there is a growing body of literature on the potential for excess calcium/vitamin D to prevent colon cancer, particularly in women (Slattery et al., 2004). Also, niacin has long been used as a drug for lowering plasma triglycerides and low density lipoprotein (LDL) cholesterol, for which it has undergone complete efficacy and safety evaluation (McKenney, 2004). The bulk of scientific evidence supports consuming a varied diet rich in plant foods as the optimal approach for achieving health benefits from foods. However, as our knowledge increases, we may find that some people at high risk for specific diseases should include more of certain foods and/or less of others.

DIETARY SUPPLEMENTS

The Dietary Supplement Health and Education Act (DSHEA), passed by the U.S. Congress in 1994, defined dietary supplements as products that are intended to supplement the diet, and that contain one or more of the following: vitamins, minerals, herbs or other botanicals, amino acids, or other dietary substance for use by man to supplement the diet by increasing the total dietary intake, or concentrates, metabolites, constituents, extracts, or combinations of these ingredients. The DSHEA regulates dietary supplements as foods. In so doing, this distinguishes dietary supplements, which are to "supplement one's diet," from drugs, which are to "treat, mitigate or prevent a disease." Therefore, there is a fine legal line between the "physiological" activity of a bioactive food component within a whole food or dietary supplement and the "pharmacological" activity of a drug. A key practical difference between drugs and bioactive food components is the fact that drugs must pass through safety and efficacy evaluation, tightly regulated by the U.S. Food and Drug Administration (FDA), before appearing on the market, whereas dietary supplements must undergo no formal safety or efficacy evaluation. The FDA does, however, regulate the safety of dietary supplements after they have entered the market.

In the United States, foods (including dietary supplements) and food additives that are a traditional part of the diet are "generally recognized as safe" (GRAS) for their intended use. New food additives must pass through strict premarket safety evaluation, as outlined in the FDA "Redbook II," to meet a standard of "reasonable certainty of no harm." However, safety of dietary supplements is regulated to a different standard compared to food additives. As outlined in DSHEA, a dietary supplement is adulterated only if it presents "a significant or unreasonable risk of illness or injury" under normal conditions of use. Because the safety of dietary supplements does not need to be approved prior to their being marketed, the FDA must take a postmarket initiative to identify and ban dietary supplements that do not meet this standard, as they did for ephedra.

HEALTH CLAIMS

Constantly being updated as research evolves, the list of food components that have FDA-approved health benefits includes plant sterol and stanol esters, soy, β-glucan in whole oats, and psyllium for lowering total and LDL cholesterol. Other bioactive food components for which the science supporting a role in health is encouraging are ω3 fatty acids in fatty fish, which may lower plasma triglycerides and decrease risk for CVD, and resveratrol in grape juice and red wine, which may inhibit platelet aggregation. Many other foods and food components are under study and are discussed in this chapter. Because dietary supplements may carry "structure/function" claims under the DSHEA of 1994, some foods are also marketed as dietary supplements, although the FDA will not permit this if the dietary supplement is substituting for a food in a meal rather than being used to supplement the diet. The regulation of health claims that may be used in conjunction with functional foods and dietary supplements has recently been reviewed (Taylor, 2004).

BIOMARKERS AND TOOLS FOR EVALUATING BIOACTIVITY

There is a strong scientific basis for a protective effect of a number of foods and bioactive food components in the prevention of CVD but little definitive proof for cancer prevention. This situation may well reflect the state of the art in evaluation of reversible, early signs of disease, rather than the range of efficacy of bioactivity of foods. The use of blood cholesterol as a reversible measure of cardiovascular health has provided an excellent tool both for scientists and the consumer in determining the bioefficacy of a change in diet. Early, reversible biomarkers for cancer risk are needed. There are programs available for early detection of cancer, particularly colon, breast, and prostate, but not for assessment of the risk for cancer. Maybe because of this the many mechanistic studies of dietary cancer prevention using cell culture studies, or even those using animal models of cancer, have rarely been translated to clinical trials or public health recommendations. One such marker that is under development is the pattern of urinary estrogen metabolites, which can be altered by the bioactive food component indole-3-carbinol, coming from cruciferous vegetables such as broccoli and cabbage.

Nutrition Insight

Safety of Dietary Supplements

Many bioactive components are present in herbs, spices, and botanical supplements. Because the concentrations of bioactive components in these products are often much higher than in fruits or vegetables, even small servings of these items may have profound physiologic effects. Examples are flavonoids in echinacea, isoflavones in red clover, and bergamottins in grapefruit. Information on health benefits of herbs, spices, and botanical supplements can be found in various review articles (Craig, 1999; Bent and Ko, 2004; Lampe, 2003; Sparreboom et al., 2004; Wargovich et al., 2001).

Interest in non-Western medicine, including herbal dietary supplements and other forms of complementary and alternative medicine, has greatly increased in recent years (Sparreboom et al., 2004). The top-selling herbal supplements in the United States are gingko, echinacea, garlic, ginseng, St. John's wort, soy, and saw palmetto; the total retail of these seven top selling herbs in the United States was approximately 190 million dollars in 2002 (Blumenthal, 2003). This high demand for herbal products may be influenced by an aging population, increased health care costs, a growing interest in self-medication and taking charge of one's own health, and changes in food regulation that have provided ready access to herbal supplements without a prescription. The lack of data showing efficacy or safety of a product appears to be of low importance to today's consumer. This may be based on loss of trust in the pharmaceutical industry as well as an unfounded assumption that "natural" products are safer than industrial products.

Safety of a bioactive component, a supplement, or even a traditional food is based on dose. Examples of common foods associated with toxicity if the dose is exceeded are cassava and almonds, which are rich in cyanoglycosides that release cyanide. Dietary supplements are regulated as foods, based on their use as dietary supplements. However, consumers are consistently using herbal supplements to treat disease instead of using them to promote and maintain a healthy lifestyle as an addition to a healthy diet and regular exercise. It is easier to ingest a toxic amount of a bioactive component from supplements than from foods. The FDA, in its regulatory role, may ban any product that is shown to pose a "significant or unreasonable risk of illness or injury," but proof of risk for harm from ingestion of a product is difficult to obtain because the manufacturer is not required to disclose details of any safety evaluations and the FDA's budget does not support basic research into safety. It took many years and a report contracted by the National Institutes of Health before sufficient data were accumulated for the FDA to successfully ban ephedra-containing products, even though circumstantial evidence had long connected the use of such supplements to a number of deaths (Shekelle et al., 2003). Almost immediately after the ban was instituted, a new group of supplements came onto the market containing *Citrus aurantium* (bitter orange). The safety of this herbal product is not known in detail, but it has been proposed to be similar to ephedra because the active principal, synephrine, is closely related to ephedrine, which is the active ingredient in ephedra (Fugh-Berman and Myers, 2004).

A second area of safety concern is the interaction between prescription drugs and herbal products, which may enhance or decrease the therapeutic effect of the prescription drug or even cause new side effects (Sparreboom et al., 2004). Of a cohort of cancer patients undergoing therapy, 54% to 77% reported using complementary medicines, including herbal dietary supplements, but only 28% informed their oncologist about the use of these supplements (Klepser et al., 2000). Combined use of herbs and drugs may produce pharmacodynamic and/or pharmacokinetic interactions. The former constitutes additive or inhibitory action at the site of action of the drug, whereas pharmacokinetic changes could be associated with changes in absorption, distribution, metabolism, and/or excretion of the drug. The most common interactions are related to changed levels of phase I cytochrome P450 enzymes, particularly cytochrome P450 3A4, which is responsible for

Nutrition Insight

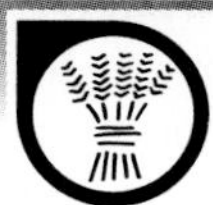

Safety of Dietary Supplements—cont'd

metabolism of most cancer drugs (Sparreboom et al., 2004). Elevated cytochrome P450 activities can lead to more rapid clearance of drugs, hence lowering the therapeutic effects. Lowered cytochrome P450 activities can lead to slower clearance and, hence, accumulation of prescription drugs, potentially to toxic levels. For example, echinacea taken for 8 days increased clearance of midazolam, a substrate for cytochrome P450 3A4 and 3A5, by 42%. However, echinacea also increased the bioavailability of midazolam from 24% to 36%, demonstrating that interactions between drugs and herbal supplements may be complex. Significant interactions of St. John's wort, a supplement used to improve mood, with drugs has been demonstrated in many clinical and animal studies. Increases in cytochrome P450 3A4 and P-glycoprotein activities are two mechanisms that have been identified as responsible for the interactions between St. John's wort and prescribed drugs. In a recent review of clinical trials on interactions between St. John's wort and drugs, 17 of 19 studies showed that plasma levels of the drug were decreased in subjects taking St. John's wort (Mills et al., 2004). This field of research has come far in the last few years but more research is needed, and patients need to inform their physicians about their supplement use to avoid dangerous interactions that could possibly contribute to the statistics of 100,000 deaths per year in the United States due to drug interactions (Lazarou et al., 1998).

A third very important issue associated with safety of herbal supplements is that the content and the profile of bioactive components in herbal supplements are not controlled. Regulations for good manufacturing practices now ensure consistency in processing, but this does not regulate the content of the starting material, which can change substantially with genotype of the plant, growing conditions, harvesting procedures, and storage conditions. This results in large variations in the efficacy and toxicity of the supplements and also confounds prediction of interactions of supplements with drugs. Recently a study of ginseng products revealed that different preparations, or "lots," can contain variable amounts of two steroid alcohols, one of which supports and one of which inhibits angiogenesis (Sengupta et al., 2004).

In rats, this change accompanies a lowering of the risk for breast cancer. Reversible biomarkers of risk for chronic diseases, such as cancer, Alzheimer's disease, and macular degeneration, and for obesity-related diseases, such as diabetes, need to be developed before dietary modulation of disease can be readily evaluated for efficacy. Biomarkers can also play an important role in providing consumers with the tools to determine that a change in diet is effective in helping them maintain a healthy, disease-free body.

CAROTENOIDS

CHEMICAL AND BIOCHEMICAL CHARACTERIZATION

The family of tetraterpenes known as carotenoids contains both vitamin A precursors (α- and β-carotene and β-cryptoxanthin) of which β-carotene is predominant) and a number of plant, algal, fungal, and bacterial products that are considered to have potential for prevention of chronic disease but lack provitamin A activity (e.g., lycopene, lutein, and zeaxanthin). Vitamin A (retinol and related metabolites) is not found as such in the plant kingdom, but it can be produced from certain plant precursors, such as β-carotene, by the action of 15,15′-mono-oxygenase in gut mucosal cells. Retinol and other retinoids, including an increasing number of synthetic vitamin A analogs used as chemotherapeutics, can interact with a family of nuclear receptors (i.e., RAR and the RXR) that act as transcription factors to regulate cellular proliferation, differentiation, and apoptosis. Recently a mucosal carotene mono-oxygenase was found to oxidize some of the carotenoids that are not vitamin A precursors, such as lycopene, to produce metabolites that may have receptor-binding activity (Nagao, 2004).

DIETARY EXPOSURE

A diet containing five servings of fruits and vegetables a day is calculated to contain roughly 5 or 6 mg of carotenoids (Ghiselli et al., 1997), which is considered sufficient to provide any possible carotenoid-related health benefits in preventing chronic disease. Whereas the typical Western diet does contain ~6 mg/day of carotenoids, only ~40% of this amount is presently derived from fruits and vegetables, with the remainder coming from animal sources such as meats, eggs, and dairy products. The lower percentage of total carotenoids from fruits and vegetables results in a different mix of carotenoids (e.g., lower lutein and zeaxanthin) than is present in fruits and vegetables alone, and the lower intake of fruits and vegetables also results in lower intake of other potentially bioactive components. Good dietary sources of carotenoids are yellow/orange fruits and vegetables and dark green leafy vegetables. Specifically, tomatoes and watermelon are good sources of lycopene; spinach is a good source of lutein and zeaxanthin as are marigold petals, which are a source of these carotenoids for dietary supplements.

Although carrots are probably the primary dietary source of β-carotene in the United States, bioavailability is better from sweet potatoes and the yellow/orange fruits such as peaches and papayas. Bioavailability of all carotenoids is enhanced by the presence of fat in the diet because carotenoids are fat soluble. Natural carotenoids are mostly in the all-*trans* form. Heating can convert *trans*-forms of lycopene to *cis*-forms, and the resulting *cis*-forms of lycopene are more completely absorbed (Miller et al., 2002). However, all-*trans* β-carotene appears more bioavailable than some *cis*-products formed during heating (Deming et al., 2002). For several reasons, including stability, toxicity, and color, β-carotene is frequently used in food fortification, in place of preformed vitamin A (e.g., retinyl palmitate or retinyl acetate). Carotenoids are absorbed through simple diffusion into the mucosal cell, followed by inclusion into chylomicrons and systemic transport via the lymphatic system to the bloodstream. There, α- and β-carotene and lycopene are found mostly in association with LDL cholesterol, whereas lutein and zeaxanthin are roughly equally distributed between high density lipoproteins (HDLs) and LDLs. Lycopene is the predominant plasma carotenoid.

EFFICACY AND MECHANISMS OF DISEASE PREVENTION

Health Effects of β-Carotene

Plasma β-carotene is commonly used as a reliable measure of dietary fruit and vegetable intake, giving support to the possibility that β-carotene might be causative in the decrease in CVD, cancer incidence, and all causes of age-related deaths, which has been reported for diets high in fruits and vegetables (Doll and Peto, 1981). Epidemiologic studies consistently support this association. For example, a recent study on prostate cancer in younger men found that diets rich in β-carotene were associated with a lower incidence of prostate cancer (Wu et al., 2004). The potential prevention of chronic diseases associated with oxidative damage by β-carotene was supported by the finding that plasma β-carotene is decreased in smokers (Fukao et al., 1996). Because of its multiple conjugated double bonds, β-carotene is an excellent antioxidant. Unfortunately, after many studies of the antioxidant effects of β-carotene in cell culture and in animals and humans following dietary exposure, the findings are inconclusive. Furthermore, of three key clinical trials evaluating a role for supplemental β-carotene (20 or 30 mg/day or 50 mg on alternate days) in prevention of lung cancer, two were halted early because smokers in the β-carotene arm had a greater incidence of cancer. The third (Physicians Health Study) showed no effect of β-carotene on lung cancer (Clarke and Armitage, 2002). The positive side to these findings has been the insight that a reevaluation is needed in the way in which epidemiologic relationships between whole-food diets and disease incidence are translated into dietary intervention studies (Greenwald, 2002).

Although trials of β-carotene supplementation and CVD have proved negative (Clarke and Armitage, 2002), there is a strong relationship between plasma carotenoids, when used as a marker for fruit and vegetable intake, and reduced risk for CVD (Hak et al., 2004). It remains to be determined if this is due to the presence of carotenoids, or whether carotenoids, as a marker for a plant-based diet, also act as a marker for exposure to fiber or other plant-based bioactive components.

Lycopene and Prostate Cancer

Evidence is accumulating that tomatoes and tomato products rich in lycopene may slow or prevent prostate cancer (Miller et al., 2002). Lycopene bioavailability is greatly enhanced by heating tomato products with oil, and lycopene appears to accumulate preferentially in a few tissues, including prostate. However, even with five prospective studies that examined the relationship between plasma lycopene and prostate cancer incidence, and several case reports, there is insufficient evidence to support a protective role for lycopene. It remains to be determined if lycopene is effective, alone or possibly together with other components from tomato (Kristal, 2004). Regardless, considering the many health benefits of a diet high in vegetables and the fact that both plasma lycopene and prostate cancer are inversely associated with age, the recommendation of five servings of a tomato product per week for improved prostate health among older men is reasonable (Miller et al., 2002).

Lutein, Zeaxanthin, and Age-Related Macular Degeneration

Lutein and zeaxanthin, but not other carotenoids, accumulate in the macula lutea region of the retina, where they may act as photoprotectors, inhibiting ultraviolet (UV)–induced oxidative damage. This appears to be a unique role for lutein and zeaxanthin among carotenoids, although other dietary carotenoids, including lycopene and β-carotene, may act as photoprotectors in skin. A few epidemiologic studies have found profound effects. For example, one study found a greater than 80% decrease in macular degeneration in those individuals in the highest quartile of plasma lutein/zeaxanthin levels (Bone et al., 2001). However, for the time being, it may be wise to learn caution from the β-carotene story. Including foods rich in these components, such as spinach and corn, may provide a safer alternative to taking a purified dietary supplement.

ADVERSE EFFECTS

Concerns that high intake of β-carotene would adversely affect intake of other lipid-soluble nutrients have not been realized. Plasma lycopene, lutein, xeaxanthin, retinol, and α-tocopherol were unaffected by a tenfold increase in plasma β-carotene to 2 μmol/L (Mayne et al., 1998). More seriously, the finding that β-carotene was associated with increased risk for cancer in two clinical trials has significantly dampened enthusiasm for research in this area. If one reviews the plasma levels reached in these two clinical trials, the β-Carotene and Retinol Efficacy Trial (CARET) reported plasma β-carotene levels of ~2 to 6 μmol/L and the Alpha-Tocopherol, Beta-Carotene Cancer Prevention (ATBC) Trial produced levels of ~4 to 8 μmol/L. In contrast, two large studies that did not show adverse effects were the Linxian Trial and the Physicians Health Study, which yielded plasma β-carotene levels of ~2 μmol/L or less. Nonsupplemented individuals typically have plasma β-carotene levels of less than 1 μmol/L. One is reminded that all things can be toxic; it is only the dose that separates a nutrient from a toxin—and very high plasma β-carotene levels may indicate that a toxicity threshold has been exceeded.

FATTY ACIDS

CHEMICAL AND BIOCHEMICAL CHARACTERIZATION

Fatty acids include both essential and nonessential nutrients in our diet, and a few fatty acids have been identified recently as possibly possessing the ability to lower the risk for chronic disease (Horrocks and Yeo, 1999). These potentially bioactive fatty acids are mostly found among the monounsaturated fatty acids (MUFAs) and ω3 (or n-3) polyunsaturated fatty acids (PUFAs). (See Chapters 6 and 18 for more information about fatty acid nomenclature.) Use of olive oil, which is rich in MUFAs, has been associated with decreased chronic disease. Virgin, or "first press" olive oil is also high in vitamin E and polyphenolics such as hydroxytyrosol, which prevent oxidation of the oils during storage and which may be partly responsible for the health effects. The ω3 fatty acids, so named because the last double bond is three carbons away from the omega carbon, include the very long-chain ω3 fatty acids, α-linolenic acid (C18:3 n-3 or ALA), docosahexaenoic acid (C22:6 n-3 or DHA), and eicosapentaenoic acid (C20:5 n-3 or EPA). Conjugated linoleic acids (CLAs) are isomeric forms of linoleic acid (C18:2 n-6) with the double bonds separated by a single bond, which adds unique physical and chemical properties to the molecule. The most abundant CLA is the *cis* 9, *trans* 11 isomer.

DIETARY EXPOSURE

α-Linolenic acid, which can serve as a precursor to EPA and DHA, is present in plant-based food products such as canola oil, olive oil, flaxseed, and nuts including walnuts, as well as in animal fats. Humans metabolize about 10% of dietary ALA to EPA and DHA. Normally DHA levels are much higher than EPA levels in human tissues, unless the diet is supplemented with fish oil. Docosahexaenoic acid and EPA are present mainly in oily fish and fish products such as salmon, tuna, herring, cod, and fish oil capsules, as shown in Table 2-1. Cow's milk may also contain EPA and DHA, although the content varies considerably with both the genetics and dietary environment of the cow. In Iceland, where cows are fed diets that include fish oils, cow's milk is an excellent source of EPA (Thorsdottir et al., 2004). In the United States, food products high in ω3 fatty acids may have a qualified health claim on the packaging for ω3 fatty acids and CVD. The Institute of Medicine (IOM, 2002) established a recommended adequate intake (AI) for ω3 fatty acids based on the median intakes of ALA by various age-groups; the AI is 1.1 g/day for women and 1.6 g/day for men. Currently, Health Canada recommends a daily intake of

Table 2-1
Abundant Dietary Sources of the ω3 Fatty Acids ALA, DHA, and EPA

Food	ALA (g/Tbsp)	EPA and DHA (g/3 oz or g/Tbsp oil)	Amount Containing ~1 g ω3 Fatty Acids
Tuna, light, canned in water, drained		0.23	12 oz
Tuna, white, canned in water, drained		0.73	4 oz
Salmon, pink		0.86	3.5 oz
Salmon, Atlantic, farmed		1.62-1.83	1.5-2 oz
Salmon, Atlantic, wild		1.22-1.56	2-2.5 oz
Herring, Pacific		1.41-1.81	1.5-2 oz
Trout, rainbow, farmed		0.79-0.98	3-4 oz
Cod, Pacific		0.18-0.24	12.5-16.5 oz
Shrimp, mixed species		0.46	6 oz
Fish oil, cod liver		2.43	5.6 oz
Fish oil, salmon		4.25	3.2 oz
Canola oil	1.30		10.6 g
Flaxseeds	2.18		5.5 g
Flaxseed oil	7.25		1.9 g
Olive oil, salad or cooking	0.11		126.3 g
Soybean oil, salad or cooking	0.93		14.7 g
Walnuts, English	0.71		11.0 g
Walnuts, black	0.16		50.0 g

Data from U.S. Department of Agriculture, Agriculture Research Sevice. USDA National Nutrient Database for Standard Reference, Release 18. Nutrient Data Laboratory Home Page, www.ars.usda.gov/ba/bhnrc/ndl (accessed Nov. 2005).
ALA, α-Linolenic acid; *DHA*, docosahexanoic acid; *EPA*, eicosapentaenoic acid.

ω3 fatty acids equal to 0.5% of total energy intake. For an adult eating 2000 kcal/day, this would be ~1 g ω3 fatty acids/day, which could be obtained from 2.5 oz pink salmon, 1.9 g flaxseed oil, or 10.6 g canola oil (see Table 2-1). Major dietary sources of CLA are dairy products and beef fat. CLAs are produced both in the rumen of ruminant animals and in the mammary gland from unsaturated C18 precursor fatty acids; CLAs constitute ~0.5 % of the fatty acid content of foods of ruminant origin.

EFFICACY AND MECHANISMS OF DISEASE PREVENTION

Consumption of fish and fish products rich in ω3 fatty acids has been proposed to provide protection against CVD, cataracts, depression, immune function diseases, and cancer. However, concerns over the wisdom of advising inclusion of more fat in the diet and about heavy metal contamination of fish cautions against recommending an increased intake of fish. Further research is needed to reach significant scientific agreement about the balance of positive and negative health effects from increasing ω3 fatty acids in the diet. The strongest association between disease prevention and dietary ω3 fatty acids is for reduction in risk for CVD. A 30-year-long study of middle-aged men reported a significant inverse relationship between fish consumption and death from CVD (Daviglus et al., 1997). The Lyon Diet Heart study compared adults consuming a normal American diet with others consuming a "Mediterranean" diet high in canola and olive oils. They found that the intervention group had significantly lower blood cholesterol and triglycerides, higher HDL cholesterol, and a 70% reduction in coronary events and cardiac deaths compared to the control group that consumed a normal American diet low in ALA (de Lorgeril et al., 1999). Some studies indicate that DHA is the principal active component in fish oil for protection against CVD, but this is still not conclusive. The FDA has approved the use of a qualified health claim for dietary supplements of ω3 fatty acids, relating them to reduced risk for heart disease. The American Heart Association also recommends consumption of fish rich in ω3 fatty acids twice a week (Kris-Etherton et al., 2003).

The ω3 fatty acids may also protect against a number of other chronic diseases. For example, a study of older men (69-89 years) showed that high ω3 PUFA intake through fish consumption was inversely associated with cognitive impairment and cognitive decline (Kalmijn et al., 1997). Inflammatory conditions, including asthma, may be ablated or prevented by consumption of fish, as shown by a study in which children who ate fresh, oily fish more than once a week were found to have a significantly ($p<0.01$) lower occurrence of asthma than children not consuming oily fish (Hodge et al., 1996). In cell culture studies, ω3 fatty acids appear to protect at various phases of the cancer process, through decreased tumor proliferation, increased apoptosis, increased differentiation, and slowed angiogenesis (Roynette et al., 2004; Nkondjock et al., 2003).

The health benefit of dietary ω3 fatty acids may depend not only on the amount in the diet but also on the ratio of ω6 to ω3 fatty acids. Between a 5:1 and 1.8:1 ratio of ω6 to ω3 fatty acids was associated with a decreased risk for colon cancer (Roynette et al., 2004; Simonsen et al., 1998). A typical American diet provides more ω6 and insufficient ω3 fatty acids, with a typical ratio greater than 10, owing to the high ratio of animal fat to vegetable and fish fat in the diet (Horrocks and Yeo, 1999). Whereas research continues in this area, one possible explanation for the importance of this ratio is competition between substrates for enzymes involved in prostaglandin synthesis. As precursors to arachidonic acid, ω6 fatty acids support prostaglandin E2 synthesis, which has been associated with stimulation of tumor growth. In contrast, EPA is metabolized by cyclooxygenase to prostaglandin E3, a compound shown to lower tumor growth in vitro.

Less well established is the suggestion that CLA may protect against CVD and certain cancers, although mechanisms are not well understood. Conjugated linoleic acid is reported to lower the risk for atherosclerosis, possibly by altering the metabolism of very low density lipoprotein (VLDL) cholesterol (McLeod et al. 2004). Protection against cancer by CLA has been reported in animal models (Belury, 2002). Unfortunately, it is unclear how to interpret the cancer protective results, since a weak positive association has also been found between CLA intake and the incidence of breast cancer (Voorrips et al., 2002).

ADVERSE EFFECTS

Excessive intake of any fats, and a ratio of 1.8:1 or less of ω6 to ω3 fatty acids, may have negative effects on health (Yamada et al., 1997). Negative effects include disturbed membrane permeability and enzyme activities and, without sufficient antioxidants, accumulation of lipid peroxides (Horrocks and Yeo, 1999). Furthermore, some species of fish may contain high levels of environmental contaminations including methyl mercury, dioxins, and polychlorinatedbiphenyls. Levels of these substances are low in fresh waters and oceans, but they have the ability to accumulate in the food chain; hence bigger and older fish contain the highest levels. There are two federal agencies in the United States, the Environmental Protection Agency and the FDA, that are responsible for sport-caught fish and commercial fish, respectively, which provide consumer information regarding mercury levels in fish.

The most recent safety issue concerns hydrogenated oils. Fatty acid structures typically exist in foods as *cis* isomers; however, *trans* isomers are found in the diet largely as a result of hydrogenation or partial hydrogenation of vegetable oils. Although there are limited data in humans, the intake of *trans* fatty acids has been suggested to increase LDL cholesterol, decrease HDL cholesterol, and promote both CVD and cancer growth (de Roos et al., 2003; Bakker et al., 1997).

PLANT STANOLS/STEROLS

CHEMICAL AND BIOCHEMICAL CHARACTERIZATION

Cholesterol is the most abundant sterol in animals but cholesterol is not synthesized in plants. In plants, more than 200 sterols and stanols have been identified, with β-sitosterol, stigmasterol, and campesterol being the most abundant sterols and sitostanol and campestanol being the most abundant stanols (Moreau et al., 2002). Structurally, the most abundant phytosterols, like cholesterol, are 4-desmethyl sterols sharing identical ring structures. The different phytosterols have varied side chains (see Fig. 2-1). Phytostanols are the saturated forms of phytosterols that lack the carbon–carbon double bonds found in cholesterol and phytosterols. Although approximately 50% of dietary cholesterol is absorbed from the intestinal tract, phytosterol absorption is considerably less, being ~10% to 15% for campesterol and campestanol, 4% to 7% for sitosterol, and ~1% for sitostanol (Katan et al., 2003).

DIETARY EXPOSURE

In Western populations, the typical diet provides ~150 to 400 mg of phytosterols and phytostanols, mostly from vegetable oils, cereals, vegetables, and fruits. The intake of these plant sterols is ~150 to 350 mg/day, and that of stanols is ~15 to 50 mg/day. A serving of cholesterol-lowering spread contains 1.7 g stanol ester. Incorporation of free stanols or sterols into food is difficult because of their low lipid solubility. Esters, which are much more easily incorporated into foods than free sterols or stanols, provide 0.6 g fatty acid together with every 1 g of sterol or stanol.

EFFICACY AND MECHANISMS OF DISEASE PREVENTION

The cholesterol-lowering effect of plant sterols was first identified in the 1950s. Large amounts (10-20 g/day) of plant sterols from vegetable fats/oils and pine trees were analyzed for their effectiveness in decreasing blood cholesterol levels. In 2000, the FDA authorized the use of health claims for the association between plant sterol/stanol esters and reduced risks for CVD. According to the FDA ruling, foods bearing the health claim should contain at least 0.65 g of plant sterol esters or 1.7 g stanol esters per serving,with the assumption that 2 servings a day would provide an effective amount (e.g., a total of 3.4 g stanol esters/day).

Plant stanol and sterol esters lower plasma cholesterol by slowing intestinal cholesterol absorption. The free stanols and sterols are structurally similar to cholesterol; hence they have the ability to interfere with cholesterol loading into the mixed micelles. In a review of more than 50 trials in adults that tested daily intake of stanol and sterol esters of 1.5 g/day or more, an average decrease in LDL cholesterol of 10% was noted (Katan et al., 2003). The cholesterol-lowering effect tapered off at intakes of 2 g/day or more, so there appears to be little additional advantage from ingesting amounts greater than 1.5 g/day.

The addition of stanol or sterol esters to diets of patients already on a heart-healthy diet or of those taking cholesterol-lowering medications can also be effective. In one study, the addition of 2.3 g/day of stanol esters to the diets of patients following the National Cholesterol Education Program (NCEP) Step I diet produced an 8% to 11% greater decrease in total cholesterol levels and a 9% to 14% greater decrease in LDL cholesterol levels than were observed in control patients treated with the NCEP diet alone (Hallikainen and Uusitupa, 1999). Many studies have shown that in hypercholesterolemic persons who are taking statin medication, stanols and sterols can provide further efficacy. In one such study, intake of 3 g/day of stanol esters resulted in an additional 10% reduction in LDL cholesterol compared to that found in subjects on statins alone (Blair et al., 2000). This was substantially better than doubling the statin dose, which would be expected to decrease plasma LDL cholesterol by an additional 6%.

ADVERSE EFFECTS

Stanol and sterol esters are considered to be GRAS by the FDA. In addition, the Scientific Committee on Foods of the European Union has concluded that phytosterol ester margarine is safe for human use. Given the FDA-approved health claims for the use of sterols and stanols in free or esterified forms for essentially any low-fat food form, including supplements, the safety of stanol and sterol esters has been reviewed extensively. In a detailed review of the efficacy and safety of plant stanols and sterols in the management of blood cholesterol, workshop participants concluded that current evidence provides a sufficient basis for promotion of the use of sterols and stanols in treatment of persons with elevated cholesterol who are at risk for CVD (Katan et al., 2003). However, Ostlund (2004) suggests that some caution still needs to be exercised.

POLYPHENOLICS

CHEMICAL AND BIOCHEMICAL CHARACTERIZATION

Polyphenolics constitute a very broad category of secondary plant compounds that includes simple phenolics as well as highly polymerized compounds, such as tannins, with molecular masses greater than 30 kDa (Fig. 2-2). Typically polyphenolics are present in their free, aglycone form or as *O*-glycosides (Bravo,1998). The biologic character that brings this broad group together (>8,000 different compounds) is the possibility that the hydroxyl groups might provide reducing power, or "antioxidant potential," which might protect the body from oxidative damage due to reactive oxygen species (ROS). This has led to the chemical evaluation of the radical "quenching power" of purified polyphenolics and plant extracts. The oxygen radical absorbance capacity (ORAC) assay evaluates the effect of polyphenol-rich samples (shown below as P-OH) from plant tissue, purified compounds, or even plasma from animals fed polyphenolic-rich diets to inhibit peroxyl radical oxidization of the fluorescent probe, fluorescein (FL) (Prior et al., 2003). Relative activity is compared to that of trolox, a water-soluble analog of α-tocopherol.

$$\text{FL-H (reduced; fluorescent)} + \text{ROO}^{\bullet} \longrightarrow \text{ROOH} + \text{FL (oxidized; no fluorescence)}$$

$$\text{FL-H (reduced; fluorescent)} + \text{P-OH} + \text{ROO}^{\bullet} \longrightarrow \text{ROOH} + \text{PO}^{\bullet} + \text{FL-H (reduced, fluorescent)}$$

A second chemical characteristic of polyphenols is their ability to reduce and/or chelate metals, particularly iron, and thereby inhibit the Fenton reaction that uses reducing power from iron to produce hydroxyl radicals from peroxide.

$$H_2O_2 + Fe^{2+} \longrightarrow OH + OH + Fe^{3+}$$

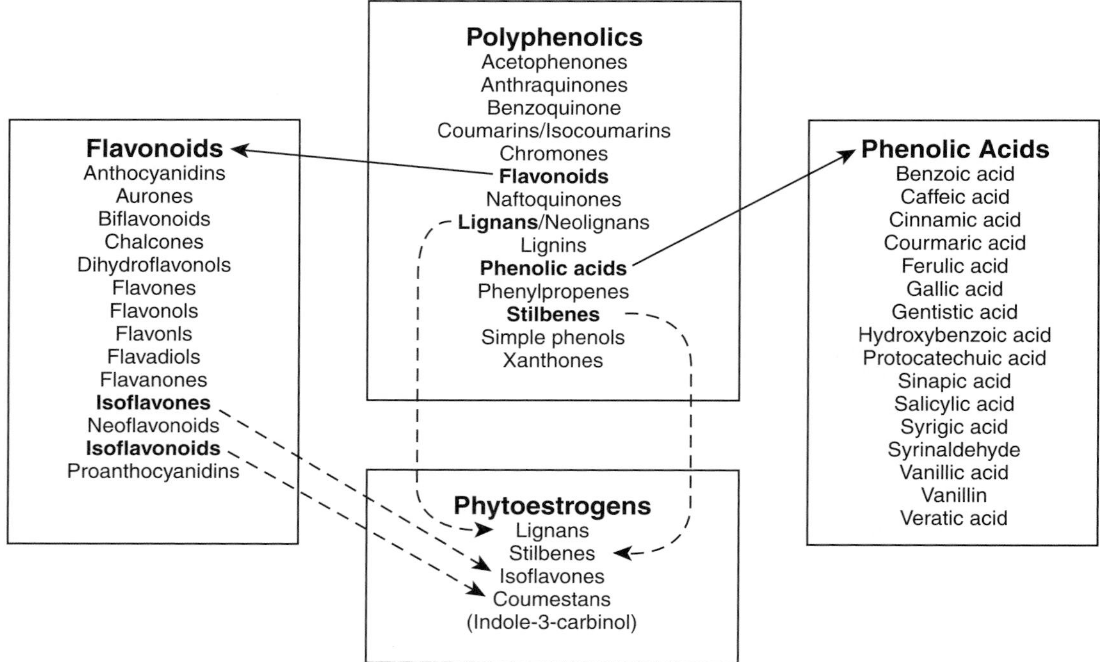

Figure 2-2 Polyphenolics and key subclasses. Flavonoids and phenolic acids are the two major subclasses, making up greater than 90% of polyphenolics. Solid lines indicate further classification of a group member. Dotted lines show secondary classification of compounds as phytoestrogens. Most phytoestrogens are polyphenolics; indole-3-carbinol is not a polyphenolic and has therefore been placed in parentheses.

The capacity to chelate iron is also often estimated in vitro, through the ferric-reducing antioxidant power (FRAP) assay. Several other related assays have been developed, notably the trolox equivalent antioxidant capacity (TEAC) assay. This is commonly used in research from European laboratories and is very similar to the ORAC, except that values are on a very different scale (Aruoma, 2003). Because values for individual bioactive components vary among the assays, they cannot be directly compared, although trends are similar (Proteggente et al., 2002).

The basis for the interest in the potential for polyphenolic compounds to act as antioxidants is that a large number of chronic diseases, including CVD, cancer, diabetes, macular degeneration, Alzheimer's disease, arthritis, Parkinson's disease, and multiple sclerosis are considered to be initiated, aggravated, or promoted by ROS and oxidative damage. Epidemiologic data show that a diet rich in fruits, vegetables, and whole grains is both rich in polyphenolics and associated with a lower incidence of many of these chronic diseases (Hirvonen et al., 2001; Hollman and Katan, 1999). However, the role of polyphenolics as antioxidants is not yet well defined, and clinical trial data are inconclusive. Chemical measurements of antioxidant potential do not correlate well with measurement of antioxidant activity within cultured cells (Kurilich et al., 2003). There are data showing that the antioxidant capacity of plasma is increased in individuals consuming a diet rich in polyphenolics, but plasma antioxidant capacity has not been consistently correlated with decreases in plasma LDL cholesterol or platelet aggregation (Kris-Etherton et al., 2002). For at least some polyphenolics there may be additional mechanisms associated with cancer prevention, such as alterations in cell signaling (Yang, 2001). The USDA is constructing a database of polyphenolic content of common foods, which should greatly enhance the ability of epidemiologists to relate polyphenolic intake to disease risk.

Many mechanistic studies of polyphenolic action are carried out as the action of purified, aglycone polyphenols in cultured cells. These are frequently difficult to interpret because most polyphenolics are found in the body not as aglycones, but as glucuronide- and sulfate-conjugates, often with the catechol moieties methylated (Kroon et al., 2004). These metabolites may have very different bioactivity than the aglycones. One specific bioactivity of polyphenolics is the protection from bacterial adhesion in the urinary bladder by proanthocyanidins isolated from cranberries, providing protection against urinary tract infection (Howell, 2002).

FLAVONOIDS

Chemical and Biochemical Characterization

Flavonoids are the most prominent subclass of dietary polyphenolics (Beecher, 2003). Chemically, the flavonoids are low-molecular-weight diphenylpropanes consisting of two aromatic rings (A and B) joined by a 3-carbon chain that most frequently incorporates oxygen into a cyclic arrangement to form a C ring (see Fig. 2-1). Common flavonoid subclasses are flavones (e.g., apigenin and luteolin), flavonols (e.g., quercetin, kaempferol, and myricetin), isoflavones (e.g., genistein and daidzein), flavanols (e.g., catechins, gallocatechin, and epigallocatechingallate), flavanones (e.g., naringenin), anthocyanidins (e.g., cyanidin and petunidin), and their glycosides (Bravo, 1998). Another common subclass is the proanthocyanidins, sometimes called *condensed tannins,* which are oligomers or polymers of flavanol units. There are three prominent proanthocyanidin groups in plants: (1) procyanidins ([epi]catechin polymers); (2) prodelephinidins ([epi]gallocatechin polymers), and (3) propelargonidins ([epi]afzelechin polymers).

Dietary Exposure

Intake of total flavonoids ranges from ~20 mg/day in the United States, Denmark, and Finland to ~70 mg/day in Holland and Japan (Beecher, 2003). Flavonoids are present in most plant-based foods, with the majority of dietary flavonoids being derived from tea, berries, other colored fruit (including red wine), and dark chocolate. In addition, flavonoids may be key bioactive components in several herbs used as dietary supplements, such as licorice, ginseng, kavakava, ginkgo biloba, and St. John's wort. Whereas flavonoid aglycones can be absorbed across the small intestinal muscosa (Manach et al., 1997), glycosides require hydrolysis by digestive enzymes and/or the colonic microflora to release the aglycone before it can be absorbed (Hollman and Katan, 1997). After absorption, flavonoids undergo methylation and/or conjugation to glucuronic acid or sulfate in the liver before being excreted in the urine or bile. If they are excreted in the bile, they can undergo deconjugation by the microflora and may be reabsorbed (enterohepatic recirculation) or fully metabolized to simple phenolic acids (Manach et al., 1997). Many published studies indicate that flavonoids are only partially absorbed, depending both on the compound and on the food matrix. For example, as much as 52% of total quercetin glycoside was absorbed from an onion meal, whereas only 24% of a purified quercetin serving was absorbed (Hollman and Katan, 1999). Disposition and excretion depend not only on the form of the compound under study but also upon other components in the ingesta. For example, tea catechins reached maximum blood levels 2 hours after ingestion of either black or green tea, but they were eliminated more rapidly when the source was green tea; the half-life for elimination of catechins from green tea was 4.8 hours, compared to 6.9 hours for those from black tea (van het Hof et al., 1998).

Efficacy and Mechanisms of Disease Prevention

Flavonoids have been proposed to exert a great variety of biologic activities in humans, including antiinflammatory, antioxidative, antiallergic, and anticarcinogenic activities (Kostyuk and Potapovich, 1998). Epidemiological studies support a role for flavonoids in prevention of both CVD and cancer (Hertog et al., 1995). Flavonoids may offer protection against LDL cholesterol oxidation, platelet aggregation, and lipid oxidation (Reed, 2002). Both clinical and animal studies have suggested an inverse relationship between intake of flavonoids and the incidence of a number of cancers. For example, in a cohort study of ~10,000 Finish men and women, diets that were high in flavonoids (e.g., apples and onions) were associated with a 20% lower incidence of cancer at all sites and a 46% decrease in incidence of lung cancer in particular (Knekt et al., 1997). Dietary quercetin is reported to inhibit chemically induced oral cancer in hamsters and mammary cancer in rats; tea rich in catechins is reported to inhibit a number of cancers, including lung cancer in A/J mice (Ren et al., 2003). Licorice extracts rich in flavonoids may provide protection against peptic ulcer or gastric cancer by inhibiting growth of *Helicobacter pylori* in humans (Fukai et al., 2002). Using gene array technology followed by functional assays, 5 μM quercetin has been shown to alter the expression of multiple genes associated with cell-cycle regulation and tumor suppression, thereby causing phenotypic changes consistent with an anticarcinogenic role for quercetin (Van Erk et al., 2004). As with the study of so many other flavonoids, this work was carried out in cultured cells and needs to be repeated in whole animals fed whole foods containing reasonable dietary levels of quercetin before the effects are confirmed. Similarly, there are numerous exciting studies suggesting a role for epigallocatechin-3-gallate (EGCG) in cancer prevention. The majority of these are cell culture studies using more than 10 μM EGCG, whereas dietary tea seldom provides a plasma level of more than 1 μM (Lambert et al., 2004). There are several whole animal studies showing cancer prevention with EGCG. Clinical studies with reliable biomarkers of efficacy are needed before the benefits of tea drinking can be fully evaluated (Higdon and Frei, 2003).

Adverse Effects

As with β-carotene, flavonoids that are known to act as antioxidants at one dose may become prooxidant at higher doses. Bioactive food components that are potentially anticarcinogenic in adults may be associated with adverse effects in the developing fetus. For example, inhibitors of topoisomerase may reverse cancer in adults but may also have a small chance of initiating cancer during fetal development. Pregnant women taking chemotherapeutic drugs and/or ingesting foods containing bioactive food components that can inhibit topoisomerase II, which includes soy, coffee, wine, tea, and cocoa, may have a greater risk for giving birth to a child with acute myeloid leukemia (Ross, 1998). Further studies are needed in this area.

PHENOLIC ACIDS

Chemical and Biochemical Characterization

Phenolic acid is a general chemical term for phenols that contain one carboxylic acid as a functional group, but the term is also used to describe a distinct type of plant metabolite: organic acids that are a subgroup of polyphenolics. These plant phenolic acids are placed into one of two groups based on the R group on the carbon ring: hydroxycinnamic acids (cinnamic acid, courmaric acid, ferulic acid, sinapic acid, and caffeic acid) or hydroxybenzoic acids (benzoic acid, salicylic acid, hydroxybenzoic acid, vanillic acid, syrigic acid, gallic acid, protocatechuic acid, gentistic acid, and veratric acid). Sometimes the aldehyde analogs (vanillin and syrinealdehyde) are included under the latter heading (Robbins, 2003).

Dietary Exposure

Major dietary sources of phenolic acids include fruits, vegetables, and grains. Coffee is a rich source of caffeic and chlorogenic acids. Human consumption of phenolic acids ranges from 25 mg to 1 g per day, depending on dietary habits (Clifford, 1999). Approximately one third of total dietary polyphenolics are phenolic acids. Little is known about the bioavailability and metabolism of the phenolic acids. Chlorogenic acid is metabolized by the colonic microflora (Gonthier et al., 2003), whereas 11% to 25% of dietary ferulic acid is excreted in the urine as free ferulic acid or as the glucuronide (Bourne and Rice-Evans, 1998).

Efficacy and Mechanisms of Disease Prevention

The primary health benefit of dietary phenolic acids is to provide "antioxidant capacity" as described for polyphenolics in general (Morton et al. 2000; Nardini et al., 1997). In addition, hydroxycinnamic acid esters may inhibit 5′-lipoxygenases, and, thus, inhibit the immune response, including inflammation, and protect against carcinogenesis (Rao et al., 1993). Natural caffeic acid derivatives, such as dicaffeoylquinic and dicaffeoyltartaric acids have been reported to inhibit human immunodeficiency virus type 1 (HIV-1) integrase, the enzyme responsible for integration of viral deoxyribonucleic acid (DNA) into the host DNA (Reinke et al., 2004).

Adverse Effects

There are few reports of adverse effects of phenolic acids in the literature. However, studies of bioactive components are sufficiently incomplete that lack of reported adverse effects cannot be interpreted to mean lack of actual adverse effects. Until sufficient research has been carried out, we cannot know the extent to which these compounds, at various doses, are healthful and/or unsafe.

PHYTOESTROGENS

CHEMICAL AND BIOCHEMICAL CHARACTERIZATION

Dietary phytoestrogens are plant-derived dietary components that structurally and functionally mimic the effects of the hormone estrogen and its metabolites. The major dietary phytoestrogens belong to four subclasses of polyphenolics: isoflavonoid coumestans (e.g., coumestrol and 4′-methoxycoumestrol), isoflavones (e.g., daidzein and genistein), lignans (e.g., secoisolariciresinol and enterolactone), and stilbenes (e.g., resveratrol) (see Figs. 2-1 and 2-2.) A chemically, mechanistically, and phylogenetically separate phytoestrogen is indole-3-carbinol from cruciferous vegetables. Phytoestrogens are present in many common botanicals sold as dietary supplements, and include flavonoids in licorice, isoflavones and lignans in kudzu and soy, isoflavones and coumestans in red clover, and unidentified phytoestrogens in saw palmetto and bloodroot (Ososki and Kennelly, 2003). These polyphenolic compounds, like estrogen, are composed of a planar aromatic ring system (1 to 3 rings) with one or more hydroxyl groups. The biologic activity of phytoestrogens varies, but overall they have lower potency compared to mammalian estrogens.

DIETARY EXPOSURE

Legume-containing foods, especially soy products, are high in isoflavones (e.g., up to ~68 mg/100 g wet weight tofu) and coumestans (e.g., up to ~7 mg/100g dry weight soybean sprouts) (Cornwell et al., 2004). Wine, grapes, and peanuts are the major dietary sources of resveratrol (30 to 1,450 μg/100 mL, 3 to 980 μg/100 g and 16 to 300 μg/100 g wet weight, respectively), and flax seed, whole grain products, vegetables, and tea are major dietary sources of lignans (up to 370 mg/100 g dry weight). In 1999, with more than 30 clinical trials as supporting material, the FDA reviewed and approved a health claim for maintenance of cardiovascular health from foods containing 6.25 g soy flour per serving, with the understanding that 4 servings per day would reach an effective dose of 25 g soy flour.

EFFICACY AND MECHANISMS OF DISEASE PREVENTION

The normal roles of estrogens in the body include growth and function of female and male reproductive tissues, maintenance of the integrity of the skeleton and central nervous system, and many other functions (Ososki and Kennelly, 2003). Because phytoestrogens mimic the effect of estrogens but have decreased potency in the body, they are proposed to affect hormone-dependent cancers, CVD, menopausal symptoms, and osteoporosis. However, particularly with regard to cancer, whether the effect is to diminish or enhance cancer growth is controversial. One possibility is that the effect will vary, depending upon the estrogenic status of the woman. Phytoestrogens might competitively inhibit estrogenic activity in the presence of estrogens but exert an estrogenic effect of their own in the postmenopausal woman who lacks endogenous estrogens. The strongest evidence for breast cancer prevention by soy isoflavones is related to consumption in adolescents, in whom endogenous estrogen production is high, and in postmenopausal women, in whom efficacy is limited to those with extremely high intake (Peeters et al. 2003).

Some studies suggest that individuals who support a gut microbial population that metabolizes daidzein to the more estrogenic metabolite equol enjoy greater cancer prevention than nonequol producers, although more data are needed to establish this (Setchell et al., 2002). Some research supports the possibility that, whereas genistein alone may support cancer growth, whole soy flour may protect against cancer (Allred et al., 2004).

Commonly, phytoestrogens are recommended as an alternative to hormone replacement therapy based on the idea that these less potent estrogens may decrease menopausal symptoms, such as hot flashes, while exerting fewer side effects. To date there is little evidence of efficacy or safety. Because bone turnover is under the control of estrogen, phytoestrogens have also been proposed to decrease the bone loss that typically accompanies menopause, but this remains controversial. After menopause, a woman's risk for CVD increases, again because of the reduction of estrogen levels in the body. Phytoestrogens are proposed to lower risk for CVD and osteoporosis through decreasing plasma LDL cholesterol, thrombus formation, and platelet aggregation, but the data are not conclusive (Cornwell et al., 2004).

Mechanistically, phytoestrogens may interact with the estrogen receptor, typically having greater affinity for the β-receptor than the α-receptor. Phytoestrogens may act as either estrogen agonists or antagonists. As an agonist, the phytoestrogen is thought to bind to the estrogen receptor in the absence of sufficient estrogen and cause an additive effect to any estrogen present. Alternatively, potency may be so low that binding acts as almost a pure antagonist in the presence or absence of estrogen. Receptor-independent activities of phytoestrogens have yet to be evaluated to any extent.

The "phytoestrogen" indole-3-carbinol interacts with the estrogen receptor in a different manner. Some data suggest that indole-3-carbinol can interfere with phosphorylation of the estrogen receptor, lowering the estrogenic response, whereas other data suggest that an indole-3-carbinol derivative may be a potent "estrogen-independent estrogen receptor agonist," causing inhibition of endometrial turmor cell growth (Kim and Milner, 2005). More recognized is indole-3-carbinol's ability to form derivatives that potently bind to the aryl hydrocarbon receptor, which then travels to the nucleus to upregulate cytochrome P450 1A1/2, an enzyme intricately involved in endogenous estrogen metabolism. The result is a shift in urinary estrogen metabolites, to more 2-hydroxy and less 16α-hydroxy estradiol and estrone. Knowing that 2-hydroxy metabolites are less estrogenic, and because both animal and clinical trials show a decrease in precancerous lesions with intake of 200 or 400 mg per day of indole-3-carbinol, it is proposed that an elevated urinary 2- to 16α-hydroxy estradiol ratio is indicative of cancer prevention associated with decreased estrogenicity of the 2-hydroxy metabolites (Bradlow et al., 1999). The effects of indole-3-carbinol and its derivatives may be further complicated by cross-talk between the aryl hydrocarbon and the estrogen receptors (Kim and Milner, 2005).

ADVERSE EFFECTS

Some animal studies indicate that pure phytoestrogens may have very different effects in the body compared to those of the whole food. When tumor-bearing mice were given soy protein isolates enriched in phytoestrogens or purified phytoestrogens, the mice exhibited increased tumor growth, whereas dietary whole soy flour did not promote growth of these mammary tumors (Allred et al., 2004). Extracts, concentrates, and semipurified phytoestrogens from a wide variety of herbs are now on the market, targeted toward postmenopausal women, with no safety information available. In addition, there is the potential for dietary isoflavones to interact with current breast cancer therapies. For example, dietary genistein negates the beneficial effects of tamoxifen on growth of estrogen-dependent breast tumors in vivo (Ju et al., 2002). Concentrates and extracts may contain unnaturally high levels of these bioactive compounds. Furthermore, it is known that growth of many cancers may be stimulated by steroid hormones. It is, therefore, imperative that more studies be done, using a variety of animal models, to determine the safety of these products.

ISOTHIOCYANATES

CHEMICAL AND BIOCHEMICAL CHARACTERIZATION

In cruciferous vegetables and a few other related plant species, isothiocyanates are found as inactive thioglycosides, termed glucosinolates. The basic chemical structure of a glucosinolate consists of a β-D-thioglucose group, a sulfonated aldoxime group, and a side chain made up of one of several different modified amino acids. More than 120 glucosinolates have been identified, although commonly there are no more than three or four major glucosinolates in each plant. When the plant cell is disrupted, through chopping or chewing, the endogenous enzyme myrosinase, a thioglucohydrolase, comes into contact with the glucosinolate and hydrolyzes it, releasing an isothiocyanate, a thiocyanate, or a nitrile. Commonly the isothiocyanate is most bioactive, with potent cancer preventative properties. In broccoli, the isothiocyanate sulforaphane (see Fig. 2-1) is formed from the glucosinolate glucoraphanin. Phenethyl isothiocyanate is formed from gluconasturtiin, rich in watercress; allyl isothiocyanate from sinigrin rich in cabbage and Brussels sprouts; and indole-3-carbinol from glucobrassicin present in all cruciferous vegetables. Isothiocyanates are electrophiles, and this property is thought to be required for their bioactivity.

DIETARY EXPOSURE

The source and amount of dietary isothiocyanates and/or their parent glucosinolates varies among cultures and countries. The primary dietary sources in North America include cabbage and broccoli. Based on USDA data, the total per capita consumption of crucifers in the United States was 19.7 lb in 2001, that is, approximately ⅓ cup or 24 g per person per day or approximately 13 mg of glucosinolates. A recent study of Shanghai women revealed an average crucifer consumption of 98 g/day, primarily as bok choy, which provided an average daily intake of glucosinolates of approximately 53 mg per person (Fowke et al., 2003).

Estimation of urinary isothiocyanates (as *N*-acetylcysteine conjugates) has been used as an indirect measure of isothiocyanate absorption. A substantially greater fraction (~30% of intake) is found in the urine following ingestion of raw vegetables than is found following ingestion of cooked vegetables (~10% of intake), suggesting higher bioavailabity of isothiocyanates from raw vegetables (Rouzaud et al., 2004; Conaway et al., 2000; Getahun and Chung, 1999). Unless very brief, cooking destroys the myrosinase, and the hydrolysis products of glucosinolates are much less available. Whereas it appears that the gut microflora can hydrolyze glucosinolates, the extent to which this occurs and the impact that this has on bioavailability are not known.

EFFICACY AND MECHANISMS OF DISEASE PREVENTION

Epidemiologic, mechanistic, animal, and clinical studies all suggest that dietary isothiocyanates help to slow or prevent many common cancers (Verhoeven et al., 1997). Clinical studies have found that as little as three to five servings of crucifers (~1.5 to 2.5 cups) each week may significantly lower risk for developing cancer. In a prospective study, three or more servings per week, as compared to one or fewer, decreased risk for prostate cancer by 41% (Cohen et al., 2000). In two other studies, five or more servings per week, compared to one or fewer servings, lowered bladder cancer risk by 51% (Michaud et al., 1999), and compared to two or fewer servings, lowered risk for non-Hodgkin's lymphoma by 33% (Zhang et al., 2000). These data suggest that the amount of isothiocyanates needed for crucifers to lower cancer risk by 30% to 50% may be achievable in a normal healthy diet. Whether a mix of isothiocyanates is more effective than a single type, and whether more frequent servings can provide greater protection, remains to be determined.

Increased detoxification of carcinogens and prevention of activation of procarcinogens are suggested as major mechanisms by which isothiocyanates protect against cancer. Dietary isothiocyanates upregulate phase II detoxification enzymes (Verhoeven et al., 1997). This increased detoxification and subsequent clearance of carcinogens in animals consuming isothiocyanates translates to similar findings clinically. For example, daily intake of 300 g of Brussels sprouts increased glutathione-*S*-transferases by 1.4-fold ($p = 0.002$) (Bogaards et al., 1994). Furthermore, many carcinogens are consumed in their precarcinogenic form, so that cytochrome P450–dependent bioactivation is needed before the carcinogen can act. In cell culture, phenethyl isothiocyanate and sulforaphane inhibited several phase I detoxification enzymes, including cytochrome P450 1A1, 2B1/2, 3A4, and 2E1 (Maheo et al., 1997; Rose et al., 2000). This inhibition would slow bioactivation of environmental carcinogens such as benz(a)pyrene and aflatoxin. Recent studies report that isothiocyanates also have the ability to protect against cancer promotion and progression by slowing the growth of tumor cells, arresting the cell cycle, and increasing apoptosis (Conaway et al., 2002). Genetic makeup may play an important role in cancer prevention by isothiocyanates. Individuals with glutathione-*S*-transferase polymorphisms expressed as null (mutated) for glutathione-*S*-transferase M1 and/or T1, are at higher risk for a number of cancers, including breast and colon cancer. Interestingly, when these individuals consume crucifers, they have a greater reduction in cancer risk than individuals with the wild-type enzymes. This may be because these individuals exhibit a longer than normal half-life for elimination of isothiocyanates as a result of their slower metabolism. However, not all studies find that the extent of prevention varies with glutathione *S*-transferase polymorphisms, and more research is needed to reach significant scientific agreement (Vogl et al., 2004).

Dietary indole-3-carbinol has the ability to upregulate cytochrome P450 1A, 1B1, and 2B1/2 (Horn et al., 2002; Bonnesen et al., 2001) as well as phase II detoxification enzymes. Because the cytochrome P450s are associated with activation of procarcinogens to carcinogens, a controversy has arisen about the benefits of indole-3-carbinol. It may be that induction of phase II enzymes balances any adverse effects of cytochrome P450 induction, because studies show that indole-3-carbinol, like the isothiocyanates, inhibits initiation of cancer (Xu et al., 1996). Furthermore, the increase in cytochrome P450 caused by indole-3-carbinol has been shown to have some beneficial effects. Indole-3-carbinol upregulation of cytochrome P450 results in an altered metabolism of estrogens, which may be associated with decreased risk for estrogen-dependent cancers (Ashok et al., 2001).

Few studies have evaluated the effect of a crucifer meal on prevention of chronic diseases other than cancer. In one study, sulforaphane was shown to arrest the growth of *Helicobacter pylori* in vitro (Fahey et al., 2002). A human study that did not include a control group reported the eradication of *H. pylori* in 3 of 9 patients who ate broccoli sprouts (Galan et al., 2004). In another recent study, a spontaneously hypertensive strain of rats was fed 200 mg dried broccoli sprouts daily for 14 weeks. Comparing the sprout-fed group to those on a control diet, cardiovascular and renal tissues exhibited less oxidative stress, as shown by increased total glutathione, decreased oxidized glutathione, and increased glutathione reductase and glutathione peroxidase activities. Interestingly, normotensive rats did not show changes in these parameters in response to ingesting the sprouts (Wu et al., 2004). These data suggest that, as with protection against cancer, people benefiting the most from consuming a diet rich in isothiocyanates may be those who have a polymorphism placing them at high risk for hypertension. This individual difference in response to a nutrient may be indicative of the fact that such individuals are missing the functional redundancy of multiple pathways that provide for metabolic integrity, but that nutrients, essential or nonessential, may at times be able to overcome this loss and thereby provide normal function.

ADVERSE EFFECTS

In humans, no toxic effects of isothiocyanates from vegetables have been reported. Crucifers may contain goiter-promoting, thyroid-enlarging compounds such as the cyclized isothiocyanate goitrin (5-vinyloxazolidine-2-thione) formed from hydrolysis of progoitrin (Fenwick et al., 1983). Reduced growth and pancreatic, liver, and kidney damage were observed in animals that consumed very large amounts of rapeseed, mustard, or crambe oilseeds, which all contain progoitrin. Purified isothiocyanates can be irritants. For example, a single oral dose of purified iberin caused irritation of the gastrointestinal tract of rats even at a dose of 0.3 to 2 nmol/kg body weight (Kore and Wallig, 1993). Possibly because of the release of isothiocyanates from the *N*-acetyl conjugate, the urinary bladder appears more sensitive to isothiocyanates than many other organs. Rats consuming a diet with 0.1% phenethyl isothiocyanate (~75 mg/kg/day) or benzyl isothiocyanate (~80 mg/kg/day) for 2 weeks had early precancerous changes in the morphology of the bladder (Akagi et al., 2003), and this treatment resulted in bladder cancer when the length of the dietary treatment period was extended (Hirose et al., 1998).

ORGANOSULFURS

CHEMICAL AND BIOCHEMICAL CHARACTERIZATION

Organosulfur or thiol-containing compounds, including diallyl sulfide (DAS), diallyl disulfide (DADS), and diallyl trisulfide (DATS) are present in allium vegetables, and a few dithiole thiones are found in cruciferous vegetables. When allium vegetables are crushed, alliin comes into contact with the enzyme alliinase to produce a lipid soluble, unstable intermediate called allicin (diallyl thiosulfinate). This decomposes to produce several lipid-soluble allyl sulfides including DAS, DADS and DATS; in addition, ajoene (4,5,9-trithiadodeca-1,6,11-triene-9-oxide) is formed from allicin when allium vegetables are crushed in oil. Garlic products on the market include oil extracts rich in sulfides, water extracts rich in sulfoxides, and aged garlic that is particularly rich in *S*-allyl cysteine (SAC) and *S*-allylmethyl cysteine (SAMC).

DIETARY EXPOSURE

Common dietary sources of organosulfurs are onion, leaks, chives, scallions, garlic, and broccoli, and other cruciferous vegetables. The richest dietary source of organosulfurs is garlic, *Allium sativum*. Garlic has been cultivated for more than 5,000 years for use as a culinary and medicinal herb and still enjoys substantial popularity today. In 2002, garlic sales exceeded that of any other single botanical supplement, with retail sales estimated at $34 million. The key water-soluble organosulfur component alliin constitutes about 1% of garlic by dry weight. However, commercial garlic products differ substantially in their composition and bioactivity depending on the way the product is prepared.

EFFICACY AND MECHANISMS OF DISEASE PREVENTION

The bioactivity of allium vegetables is considered to rest in the action of thiols and thiol metabolites. Garlic, the richest dietary source of thiols and the most studied allium, is proposed to exert antibacterial, anticancer, antithrombotic, and hypoglycemic action. The strongest clinical support is for a lipid-lowering and antithrombotic role in patients with CVD (Agarwal, 1996; Warshafsky et al., 1993). In contrast, five recent clinical studies found no lipid-lowering effect, possibly because of differences in formulation and/or serving size (many of the earlier studies provided more than 7 cloves/day of raw garlic). Even though further research is needed, using more carefully defined garlic preparations, garlic does appear to exert an antithrombotic effect via inhibition of platelet aggregation and enhanced fibrinolysis (Rahman, 2001). The antiplatelet action of ajoene has been studied in vitro and may be a result of inhibition of cyclooxygenase/prostaglandin synthesis, inhibition of mobilization of platelet calcium, or disruption of fibrinogen binding to the platelet glycoprotein IIb/IIIa receptor (integrin).

SAC and SAMC, found mostly in aged garlic preparations, have been shown to exhibit excellent radical scavenging activity (Thomson and Ali, 2003). DAS also increases apoptosis of human bladder cancer cells by a caspase 3-dependent pathway (Lu et al., 2004). An interesting study showed DAS may reverse multidrug resistance in cultured leukemia cells, but very high levels of DAS (8.75 mM) were used. It remains to be seen whether dietary garlic can counter multidrug resistance in a clinical setting.

Epidemiological studies have provided a link between dietary allium species and decreased risk for a number of cancers (Sengupta et al., 2004; Milner, 2001). Possible mechanisms have been identified from cell culture studies, and a few have been taken through to whole animal studies, but clinical studies are lacking. Rats given purified DADS and DATS (0.1 mmol/kg body weight by intraperitoneal injection) exhibited significantly increased hepatic phase II detoxification enzyme activity, supporting results found in cell culture (Fukao et al., 2004). Prevention of DNA oxidation and inhibition of DNA binding and mutagenesis have also been seen in both cell culture and in animal models (Song and Milner, 2001). More recently, many cell-culture studies have shown specific alteration of cell-signaling pathways, leading to inhibition of proliferation and enhanced apoptosis of tumor cells grown in vitro. Many of these effects have yet to be evaluated in whole animals. More research is required before a causal link between dietary allium species and cancer risk can be concluded.

ADVERSE EFFECTS

Garlic and its bioactive thiols have been studied extensively for drug interactions. The di- and trisulfides have acute inhibitory effects on cytochrome P450 2E1, whereas chronic exposure upregulates cytochrome P450 2E1. Sulfones act as irreversible inhibitors of cytochrome P450 2E1. It is important to note that clinical studies of the pharmacokinetics of drugs metabolized by cytochrome P450 3A4 suggest that there is no effect of dietary garlic on cytochrome P450 3A4, the detoxification enzyme responsible for metabolism of the majority of drugs (Markowitz et al., 2003). In addition, there is no effect on cytochrome P450 2D6, which is responsible for metabolism of some cancer chemotherapeutic drugs. In a few instances, dietary garlic has been associated with gastrointestinal distress and even anaphylactic shock, although a more common concern with high dietary garlic is red blood cell hemolysis (de Roos et al., 2003).

POLYOLS

CHEMICAL AND BIOCHEMICAL CHARACTERIZATION

Polyols, or sugar alcohols, are a class of compounds that are used as sweeteners in foods, gum, candy, and beverages. Commonly used sugar alcohols are xylitol (see Fig. 2-1), sorbitol, mannitol, and lactitol. The sugar alcohols include alcohol forms of monosaccharides (e.g., sorbitol, mannitol, xylitol, and erythritol), disaccharides (e.g., isomaltitol, lactitol, and maltitol), and polysaccharides (e.g., maltitol syrup and hydrogenated starch hydrolysates) (Van Loveren, 2004). Natural sugar alcohols are present in many fruits and vegetables, but commercial products may contain synthetically produced polyols. Products containing sugar alcohols in place of sweeteners such as sucrose or corn syrup can be labeled as sugar-free. If there is a claim on the product containing sugar alcohols, a declaration of content is required on the nutrition label.

DIETARY EXPOSURE

Sugar alcohols provide fewer calories than sugars (1.5 to 3 kcal/g compared to 4 kcal/g). This is partly due to slower absorption, which occurs by passive diffusion from the gut, and results in some of the sugar alcohol bypassing absorption and becoming substrate for fermentation by the colonic microflora (American Dietetic Association, 2004; Makinen et al., 1985). The slower absorption results in a lower glycemic response than from sugar sweeteners. Many low-calorie foods contain sugar alcohols, and the amounts can vary greatly, depending on the product and manufacturer. For example, sugarless chewing gum often contains 1 g sugar alcohol per piece, 1 serving (¼ cup) of low-calorie maple syrup may contain 6 g of sugar alcohols, and a low-carbohydrate cookie (28 g) may contain as much as 8 g of sugar alcohols.

EFFICACY AND MECHANISMS OF DISEASE PREVENTION

The potential health benefits from consuming sugar alcohols are a reduced glycemic response, a decreased risk for caries, and a prebiotic effect (Van Loveren, 2004; Makinen et al., 1985).

Evidence strongly suggests that, in people who chew gum, use of gums containing sugar alcohols in place of sugar can significantly protect against caries (Van Loveren, 2004). There is an FDA-approved health claim stating that sugar alcohols do not promote tooth decay. Use of gum containing sugar alcohols limits acid production by plaque bacteria, reduces plaque, and decreases levels of the caries-producing mutans streptococci in plaque and saliva (Makinen et al., 1989). In a Finnish study, children who used gum containing sugar alcohols during 1982 had significantly fewer caries during 1988 than children not using gum (Isokangas et al., 1991). This effect of low-caloric sweeteners may be due to more than simply elimination of sugar; sugar alcohols may stimulate saliva flow and possibly even have a direct antimicrobial effect (Van Loveren, 2004). The preventative effects depend on frequency of chewing (three to five pieces of gum per day are considered effective) as well as the type and amount of sugar alcohol present in the gum; xylitol and sorbitol have shown the strongest preventive effects (Soderling et al., 1989).

ADVERSE EFFECTS

Excessive consumption of sugar alcohols may lead to an osmotic diarrhea owing to their slow absorption from the gut. Amounts greater than 50 g sorbitol or 20 g mannitol per day can cause diarrhea (Van Loveren, 2004). Because of the risk for diarrhea and malabsorption, all products containing either of these polyols must have a label stating, "excess consumption may have a laxative effect."

DIETARY FIBER

CHEMICAL AND BIOCHEMICAL CHARACTERIZATION

The definition of fiber has varied over the years, in large part as our understanding has increased. Recently the IOM (2002, p. 2) defined dietary fiber as "non digestible carbohydrates and lignins that are intrinsic and intact in plants" and defined added fiber as "isolated, non-digestible carbohydrates that have beneficial physiological effects in humans." Total fiber is the sum of dietary and added fiber. Therefore, fiber has no single chemical structure, being made up of many nondigestible compounds including carbohydrate polymers, such as cellulose, with β-linkages. Fiber can be further divided and characterized as soluble or insoluble, fermentable or nonfermentable, and viscous or nonviscous. Fermentable fibers may be hydrolyzed by bacteria in the colon, but not by human cells, to short-chain fatty acids (SCFAs) including acetate, propionate, and butyrate. These SCFAs are important fuels for the human colon. A commonly available form of fermentable fiber is psyllium, which contains β-glucan.

DIETARY EXPOSURE

Fruits, vegetables, and whole grains are all good sources of fiber. In addition, some processed food products, such as psyllium cellulose (see Fig. 2-1) are sold specifically as good sources of fiber. The USDA nutrient database includes fiber content of common foods. High fiber foods are apples and broccoli; both contain 3 to 5 g per serving. The IOM (2002) recommends a fiber intake of 14 g for each 1,000 kcal of energy consumed, which translates to approximately 25 g/day for women (1,800 kcal/day) and 38 g/day for men (2,700 kcal/day).

EFFICACY AND MECHANISMS OF DISEASE PREVENTION

A high fiber diet may protect against CVD and certain cancers, particularly colon cancer (Giovannucci and Willett, 1994). Health claims have been approved for the beneficial effect of dietary fiber for both cardiovascular health and cancer prevention and are based on the content of the soluble fiber β-glucan. The data on cholesterol-lowering effects of soluble dietary fiber provide a strong and consistent basis for the health claims of oats and psyllium. In addition, numerous studies support a beneficial role for whole grain fiber, including a metaanalysis of 12 studies that showed that persons who consume approximately three servings daily of whole grain fiber had a 26% decrease in risk for CVD (Anderson et al., 2000). The claim for lowering of cholesterol levels by fruits and vegetables may, at least in part, be due to the presence of fiber in these foods. It is possible that fiber may adsorb cholesterol, aiding cardiovascular health by decreasing cholesterol absorption. The claim for lowering of cholesterol by soy protein (25 g/day) may also be in part due to its fiber content (~5%) although it is likely also due to other components such as estrogenic isoflavones (Erdman, 2000).

Dietary fiber has been proposed to protect against colon cancer and certain other cancers such as hormone-dependent breast cancer. Early studies on colon cancer prevention that led to the health claim have not been consistently reproduced. Mechanisms that might be involved include binding of toxic and carcinogenic components of the diet, leading to lowered exposure to these items. For example, some components of fiber, including lignins, may chelate both essential metals such as iron and contaminant carcinogenic or toxic metals such as cadmium. Studies using colon cancer cells in culture suggest that the SCFA butyrate may inhibit proliferation and promote differentiation and enhanced apoptosis of these cancer cells. For example, gluconic acid is metabolized by lactic acid bacteria to lactate and acetate, which are then further metabolized to butyrate by acid-utilizing bacteria. Animals fed sodium gluconate (50 g/kg) plus azoxymethane exhibited increased cecal butyrate and significantly fewer tumors than animals receiving this colon carcinogen and no prebiotic (Kameue et al., 2004). Furthermore, patients with colonic cancer or adenomas produce less butyrate than healthy individuals (Clausen et al., 1991). Prevention of breast cancer by fiber, possibly related to decreased estrogen bioavailability, has been found in some studies but not others (Holmes et al., 2004; Rock et al., 2004). At present there is insufficient information to reach significant scientific agreement about the effect of dietary fiber on cancer risk.

It has been suggested that fiber may have antiobesity and antidiabetic actions. This may be in part because fiber dilutes the nutrient content of a food by adding bulk to the diet while contributing relatively little energy, and in part because dietary fiber prolongs chewing time, potentially enhancing satiety and decreasing energy intake. Separately, viscous fiber is thought to add bulk to chyme, slowing stomach emptying and further affecting satiety. A slower rate of glucose absorption following a meal results in a lower glycemic index for intake of a given amount of sugar. This added bulk might also provide for more rapid transfer of chyme through the colon, which is less irritating to the epithelial tissue and musculature, leading to prevention of diverticulosis. The extent to which these actions play a significant role in health has yet to be established.

Fermentable fiber is hydrolyzed to SCFA by gut bacteria, mostly in the upper colon. Some bacterial populations, including bifidobacteria, are supported better than others by a high fiber diet, leading to a change in colonic microbiota (Gorbach and Goldin,1990). The release of acetate and propionate provides an energy source for the cells lining the colon. Butyrate has attracted significant attention as a bioactive food component because of its apparent ability to act as a cell-signaling molecule. The release of butyrate is associated with a number of physiological activities that may vary with the luminal environment. Cell-culture studies show that butyrate supports differentiation and apoptosis of human HT29 colon cells, consistent with protection against colon cancer (Cai et al., 2004). In contrast, resection studies in neonatal piglets showed that butyrate promoted proliferation and villus growth and inhibited apoptosis in this model of short bowel syndrome (Bartholome et al., 2004). Given the opposing actions of butyrate in colon cancer cells and in the resected neonatal piglet colon, a case could be made that butyrate would either promote or inhibit proliferation in cancerous colonic mucosa. Clearly more research is needed on the effects of fiber-derived SCFA on intestinal physiology.

ADVERSE EFFECTS AND CONTROVERSIES

Health claims, based on either substantial published data or significant scientific agreement within the field, are not infallible. Yet the public may choose to change their diet in place of consulting a physician, based on a health claim, even though this is not the intent of the FDA. Whereas there are substantial animal data to support a role for fiber in prevention of colon cancer, recent epidemiological data have not supported this claim (Alberts et al., 2000). This has led to uncertainty about the health benefit of fiber within the scientific community, even though a lack of dietary fiber is associated with increased colon cancer (Erhardt et al., 1997). Several reasons have been proposed to explain why recent epidemiological studies do not show fiber to protect against colon cancer (Lawlor and Ness, 2003; Mai et al., 2003). Estimation of dietary fiber intake is uncertain. Dietary fiber intake is usually based on food frequency questionnaires and does not distinguish between soluble and insoluble fiber. Furthermore, the definitions used for fiber may vary between studies, and analytical methods are not reliable. Often the population under study shows too small a range in intake between the lowest and highest intake groups to provide statistical power for the analysis. In addition, because fermentation does not occur homogeneously across the colon (most occurs in the upper colon), studies need to evaluate different sites separately to determine if prevention is limited to certain portions of the gut. Another concern is that much of the earlier data were based on an African population, which may differ in many ways, including lifestyle and genetic makeup, from populations in other parts of the world. Furthermore, common problems with prospective cancer studies in general is that most studies focus on polyp recurrence rather than on the initial cancer, are relatively short-term studies (i.e., 5 years or less), and frequently monitor a single source of fiber within the complex matrix of the diet (Alberts et al., 2000). Certainly, inconsistent data point to the need not only for more studies but also for improved experimental designs that will provide more definitive answers.

PREBIOTICS/PROBIOTICS

CHEMICAL AND BIOCHEMICAL CHARACTERIZATION

Prebiotics are nondigestible dietary substances that encourage the growth and activity of favorable intestinal bacteria, thereby improving the host health. They may include inulin, fructooligosaccharides (FOS), oligofructose, resistant starch, and other indigestible fibers and oligosaccharides (Madley, 2001). Inulin and FOS consist of linear chains of fructose units, frequently terminated by a glucose unit. Short-chain FOS is a specific, defined mixture of glucose-terminated fructose chains with a chain length of 2 to 7 units, whereas inulin may contain up to 60 units. Probiotics are live, microbial food supplements taken to improve the intestinal microbial balance of the host (Kopp-Hoolihan, 2001).

DIETARY EXPOSURE

Probiotics and prebiotics are gaining in popularity and interest in the scientific community and with consumers. They may be sold as components within conventional foods or as dietary supplements, making consumption difficult to estimate. Foods considered to be particularly good sources of prebiotics include Jerusalem artichokes, bananas, onions, garlic, honey, and leeks. Commercially used probiotic bacteria include certain species of lactobacilli, bifidobacteria, and streptococci. Probiotics are often found in yogurt, yogurt drinks, kefir, and dietary supplements. In some countries such as Japan, both probiotics and prebiotics are included in hundreds of products. The recommended amount per day to confer health benefits is estimated at 3 to 10 g/day for prebiotics and 1 to 2 billion colony-forming units (cfu) per day for probiotics (Hasler et al., 2004).

EFFICACY AND MECHANISMS OF DISEASE PREVENTION

It is estimated that there are more than 400 different types of bacteria and approximately 10^{14} bacterial cells in the human intestine. Types of bacteria most often found include bacteroides, eubacteria, peptostreptococci, bifidobacteria, enterobacteria, streptococci, lactobacilli, clostridia, and staphylococci (Kopp-Hoolihan, 2001). Loss of optimal bacterial composition in the gut may play a role in many disease states.

The primary benefits of prebiotics such as inulin are thought to be multiple: support of beneficial microflora such as bifidobacteria, with concomitant reduction of harmful bacteria such as *Escherichia coli*, which may reduce the risk for infectious diarrhea; increased large bowel motility and decreased transit time, which may improve stool quality and bowel regularity; and maintenance of healthy intestinal function and enhanced immunity. Many prebiotics, such as inulin, also improve mineral uptake (i.e., uptake of calcium and magnesium) in the body.

Fermentation of prebiotics by colonic bacteria produces SCFA, which lowers the intestinal pH, providing an environment that is more resistant to harmful bacteria and more conducive to mineral absorption. Probiotics are considered to have a wide range of health benefits including: improving intestinal health, enhancing immunity, synthesizing and enhancing the bioavailability of nutrients, reducing symptoms of lactose intolerance, decreasing the prevalence of allergy in susceptible individuals, and reducing the risk for certain cancers (Kopp-Hoolihan, 2001). Although the mechanisms by which probiotics exert these beneficial effects are not fully elucidated, several roles have been proposed in addition to modifying gut pH. Probiotics may antagonize pathogens through production of antimicrobial and antibacterial compounds; they may compete for pathogen binding at receptor sites and for available nutrients and growth factors; and they may stimulate cells involved in the immune response (Kopp-Hoolihan, 2001; Fedorak and Madsen, 2004). Probiotics, including *Lactobacillus rhamnosus, Lactobacillus reuteri, Lactobacillus casei,* and *Bifidobacterium lactis,* may shorten the duration of acute retroviral diarrhea in children (Fedorak and Madsen, 2004). In a recent study with 50 patients with irritable bowel syndrome (IBS), patients who received a probiotic preparation containing *Lactobacillus plantarum* LP 01 and *Bifidobacterium breve* BRO for 28 days had less abdominal pain (scores decreased by 52% compared to 11% for the placebo group) and fewer IBS symptoms (a decrease of 44.4% for the treatment group compared to 8.5% for the placebo group) (Saggioro, 2004).

ADVERSE EFFECTS

Cases of infection caused by probiotics such as lactobacilli and bifidobacteria organisms are rare, but have been estimated at 0.05% to 0.4% of cases of infective endocarditis and bacteremia (Borriello et al., 2003). The occasional reports of bacteremia and endocarditis associated with lactobacilli have been noted to most likely occur in immunocompromised individuals (Kopp-Hoolihan, 2001).

KEEPING UP WITH RESEARCH AND RECOMMENDATIONS

A large group of naturally occurring components in our diet, while not being essential for growth and development, exert beneficial effects on our health. Many of the key bioactive food components identified to date, their dietary sources, and the scientific basis for determining efficacy and safety have been summarized in this chapter. These nonessential food components may decrease risk for chronic diseases of aging, including CVD, chronic inflammatory diseases, and cancer. Epidemiologic studies comparing diet and disease incidence have identified foods, including certain fruits and vegetables, whole grains, and fatty fish that provide these health benefits. Therefore, food choices can greatly influence our risk for chronic disease. Interdisciplinary teams of scientists, including food chemists, nutritional scientists, and plant and health scientists, are working together to identify these components and determine their bioactivity and bioavailability. Such studies provide the information necessary to determine efficacy and potency, allowing development of FDA-approved health claims based on significant scientific agreement. Health claims describe how much of a food rich in a specific component needs to be included in the diet to gain a specific health benefit. Although it is still difficult to assess the specific amounts of foods or bioactive food components recommended for consumption on a daily or weekly basis, we are coming closer to providing sound consumption information for consumers.

REFERENCES

Agarwal KC (1996) Therapeutic actions of garlic constituents. Med Res Rev 16:111-124.

Akagi K, Sano M, Ogawa K, Hirose M, Goshima H, Shirai T (2003) Involvement of toxicity as an early event in urinary bladder carcinogenesis induced by phenethyl isothiocyanate, benzyl isothiocyanate, and analogues in F344 rats. Toxicol Pathol 31:388-396.

Alberts DS, Martinez ME, Roe DJ, Guillen-Rodriguez JM, Marshall JR, van Leeuwen JB, Reid ME, Ritenbaugh C, Vargas PA, Bhattacharyya AB, Earnest DL, Sampliner RE (2000) Lack of effect of a high-fiber cereal supplement on the recurrence of colorectal adenomas. Phoenix Colon Cancer Prevention Physicians' Network. N Engl J Med 342: 1156-1162.

Allred CD, Allred KF, Ju YH, Clausen LM, Doerge DR, Schantz SL, Korol DL, Wallig MA, Helferich WG (2004) Dietary genistein results in larger MNU-induced, estrogen-dependent mammary tumors following ovariectomy of Sprague-Dawley rats. Carcinogenesis 25:211-118.

American Dietetic Association (2004) Position of the American Dietetic Association: use of nutritive and nonnutritive sweeteners. J Am Diet Assoc 104:255-275.

Anderson JW, Hanna TJ, Peng X, Kryscio RJ (2000) Whole grain foods and heart disease risk. J Am Coll Nutr 19:291S-299S.

Aruoma OI (2003) Methodological considerations for characterizing potential antioxidant actions of bioactive components in plant foods. Mutat Res 523-524:9-20.

Ashok BT, Chen Y, Liu X, Bradlow HL, Mittelman A, Tiwari RK (2001) Abrogation of estrogen-mediated cellular and biochemical effects by indole-3-carbinol. Nutr Cancer 41:180-187.

Bakker N, Van't Veer P, Zock PL (1997) Adipose fatty acids and cancers of the breast, prostate and colon: an ecological study. EURAMIC Study Group. Int J Cancer 72:587-591.

Bartholome AL, Albin DM, Baker DH, Holst JJ, Tappenden KA (2004) Supplementation of total parenteral nutrition with butyrate acutely increases structural aspects of intestinal adaptation after an 80% jejunoileal resection in neonatal piglets. JPEN J Parenter Enteral Nutr 28:210-222; discussion 222-223.

Beecher GR (2003) Overview of dietary flavonoids: nomenclature, occurrence and intake. J Nutr 133:3248S-32254S.

Belury MA (2002) Inhibition of carcinogenesis by conjugated linoleic acid: potential mechanisms of action. J Nutr 132:2995-2998.

Bent S, Ko R (2004) Commonly used herbal medicines in the United States: a review. Am J Med 116:478-485.

Blair SN, Capuzzi DM, Gottlieb SO, Nguyen T, Morgan JM, Cater NB (2000) Incremental reduction of serum total cholesterol and low-density lipoprotein cholesterol with the addition of plant stanol ester-containing spread to statin therapy. Am J Cardiol 86:46-52.

Blumenthal M (2003) Herbs continue slide in mainstream market: sales down 14 percent. HerbalGram 58:71.

Bogaards JJ, Verhagen H, Willems MI, van Poppel G, van Bladeren PJ (1994) Consumption of Brussels sprouts results in elevated alpha-class glutathione S-transferase levels in human blood plasma. Carcinogenesis 15:1073-1075.

Bone RA, Landrum JT, Mayne ST, Gomez CM, Tibor SE, Twaroska EE (2001) Macular pigment in donor eyes with and without AMD: a case-control study. Invest Ophthalmol Vis Sci 42:235-240.

Bonnesen C, Eggleston IM, Hayes JD (2001) Dietary indoles and isothiocyanates that are generated from cruciferous vegetables can both stimulate apoptosis and confer protection against DNA damage in human colon cell lines. Cancer Res 61:6120-6130.

Borriello SP, Hammes WP, Holzapfel W, Marteau P, Schrezenmeir J, Vaara M, Valtonen V (2003) Safety of probiotics that contain lactobacilli or bifidobacteria. Clin Infect Dis 36:775-780.

Bourne LC, Rice-Evans C (1998) Bioavailability of ferulic acid. Res Commun 253:222-227.

Bradlow HL, Sepkovic DW, Telang NT, Osborne MP (1999) Multifunctional aspects of the action of indole-3-carbinol as an antitumor agent. Ann NY Acad Sci 889:204-213.

Bravo L (1998) Polyphenols: chemistry, dietary sources, metabolism, and nutritional significance. Nutr Rev 56:317-333.

Cai J, Chen Y, Murphy TJ, Jones DP, Sartorelli AC (2004) Role of caspase activation in butyrate-induced terminal differentiation of HT29 colon carcinoma cells. Arch Biochem Biophys 424:119-127.

Clarke R, Armitage J (2002) Antioxidant vitamins and risk of cardiovascular disease. Review of large-scale randomised trials. Cardiovasc Drugs Ther 16:411-415.

Clausen MR, Bonnen H, Mortensen PB (1991) Colonic fermentation of dietary fibre to short chain fatty acids in patients with adenomatous polyps and colonic cancer. Gut 32:923-928.

Clifford MN (1999) Chlorogenic acids and other cinnamates-nature, occurrence, and dietary burden. J Sci Food Agric 79:362-372.

Cohen JH, Kristal AR, Stanford JL (2000) Fruit and vegetable intakes and prostate cancer risk. J Natl Cancer Inst 92:61-68.

Conaway CC, Getahun SM, Liebes LL, Pusateri DJ, Topham DK, Botero-Omary M, Chung FL (2000)

Disposition of glucosinolates and sulforaphane in humans after ingestion of steamed and fresh broccoli. Nutr Cancer 38:168-178.

Conaway CC, Yang YM, Chung FL (2002) Isothiocyanates as cancer chemopreventive agents: their biological activities and metabolism in rodents and humans. Curr Drug Metab 3:233-255.

Cornwell T, Cohick W, Raskin I (2004) Dietary phytoestrogens and health. Phytochemistry 65:995-1016.

Craig WJ (1999) Health-promoting properties of common herbs. Am J Clin Nutr 70:491S-499S.

Daviglus ML, Stamler J, Orencia AJ, Dyer AR, Liu K, Greenland P, Walsh MK, Morris D, Shekelle RB (1997) Fish consumption and the 30-year risk of fatal myocardial infarction. N Engl J Med 336:1046-1053.

de Lorgeril M, Salen P, Martin JL, Monjaud I, Delaye J, Mamelle N (1999) Mediterranean diet, traditional risk factors, and the rate of cardiovascular complications after myocardial infarction: final report of the Lyon Diet Heart Study. Circulation 99:779-785.

de Roos NM, Schouten EG, Katan MB (2003) Trans fatty acids, HDL-cholesterol, and cardiovascular disease. Effects of dietary changes on vascular reactivity. Eur J Med Res 8:355-357.

Deming DM, Teixeira SR, Erdman JW, Jr. (2002) All-trans beta-carotene appears to be more bioavailable than 9-cis or 13-cis beta-carotene in gerbils given single oral doses of each isomer. J Nutr 132:2700-2708.

Doll R, Peto R (1981) The causes of cancer: quantitative estimates of avoidable risks of cancer in the United States today. J Natl Cancer Inst 66:1191-1308.

Erdman JW, Jr. (2000) AHA Science Advisory: Soy protein and cardiovascular disease: a statement for healthcare professionals from the Nutrition Committee of the AHA. Circulation 102:2555-2559.

Erhardt JG, Lim SS, Bode JC, Bode C (1997) A diet rich in fat and poor in dietary fiber increases the in vitro formation of reactive oxygen species in human feces. J Nutr 127:706-709.

Fahey JW, Haristoy X, Dolan PM, Kensler TW, Scholtus I, Stephenson KK, Talalay P, Lozniewski A (2002) Sulforaphane inhibits extracellular, intracellular, and antibiotic-resistant strains of Helicobacter pylori and prevents benzo[a]pyrene-induced stomach tumors. Proc Natl Acad Sci USA 99:7610-7615.

Fedorak RN, Madsen KL (2004) Probiotics and prebiotics in gastrointestinal disorders. Curr Opin Gastroenterol 20:146-155.

Fenwick GR, Heaney RK, Mullin WJ (1983) Glucosinolates and their breakdown products in food and food plants. Crit Rev Food Sci Nutr 18:123-201.

Fowke JH, Shu XO, Dai Q, Shintani A, Conaway CC, Chung FL, Cai Q, Gao YT, Zheng W (2003) Urinary isothiocyanate excretion, Brassica consumption, and gene polymorphisms among women living in Shanghai, China. Cancer Epidemiol Biomarkers Prev 12:1536-1539.

Fugh-Berman A, Myers A (2004) Citrus aurantium, an ingredient of dietary supplements marketed for weight loss: current status of clinical and basic research. Exp Biol Med 229:698-704.

Fukai T, Marumo A, Kaitou K, Kanda T, Terada S, Nomura T (2002) Anti-Helicobacter pylori flavonoids from licorice extract. Life Sci 71:1449-1463.

Fukao A, Tsubono Y, Kawamura M, Ido T, Akazawa N, Tsuji I, Komatsu S, Minami Y, Hisamichi S (1996) The independent association of smoking and drinking with serum beta-carotene levels among males in Miyagi, Japan. Int J Epidemiol 25:300-306.

Fukao T, Hosono T, Misawa S, Seki T, Ariga T (2004) The effects of allyl sulfides on the induction of phase II detoxification enzymes and liver injury by carbon tetrachloride. Food Chem Toxicol 42:743-749.

Galan MV, Kishan AA, Silverman AL (2004) Oral broccoli sprouts for the treatment of Helicobacter pylori infection: a preliminary report. Dig Dis Sci 49:1088-1090.

Getahun SM, Chung FL (1999) Conversion of glucosinolates to isothiocyanates in humans after ingestion of cooked watercress. Cancer Epidemiol Biomarkers Prev 8:447-451.

Ghiselli A, D'Amicis A, Giacosa A (1997) The antioxidant potential of the Mediterranean diet. Eur J Cancer Prev 6:S15-S19.

Giovannucci E, Willett WC (1994) Dietary factors and risk of colon cancer. Ann Med 26:443-452.

Gonthier M-P, Verny M-A, Besson C, Rémésy C, Scalbert A (2003) Chlorogenic acid bioavailability largely depends on its metabolism by the gut microflora in rats. J Nutr 133:1853-1859.

Gorbach SL, Goldin BR (1990) The intestinal microflora and the colon cancer connection. Rev Infect Dis 12:S252-S261.

Greenwald P (2002) Cancer prevention clinical trials. J Clin Oncol 20:14S-22S.

Hak AE, Ma J, Powell CB, Campos H, Gaziano JM, Willett WC, Stampfer MJ (2004) Prospective study of plasma carotenoids and tocopherols in relation to risk of ischemic stroke. Stroke 35:1584-1588.

Hallikainen MA, Uusitupa MI (1999) Effects of 2 low-fat stanol ester-containing margarines on serum cholesterol concentrations as part of a low-fat diet in hypercholesterolemic subjects. Am J Clin Nutr 69:403-410.

Hasler CM, Bloch AS, Thomson CA, Enrione E, Manning C (2004) Position of the American Dietetic Association: functional foods. J Am Diet Assoc 104:814-826.

Hertog MG, Kromhout D, Aravanis C, Blackburn H, Buzina R, Fidanza F, Giampaoli S, Jansen A, Menotti A, Nedeljkovic S (1995) Flavonoid intake and long-term risk of coronary heart disease and cancer in the seven countries study. Arch Intern Med 155:381-386.

Higdon JV, Frei B (2003) Tea catechins and polyphenols: health effects, metabolism, and antioxidant functions. Crit Rev Food Sci Nutr 43:89-143.

Hirose M, Yamaguchi T, Kimoto N, Ogawa K, Futakuchi M, Sano M, Shirai T (1998) Strong promoting activity of phenylethyl isothiocyanate and benzyl isothiocyanate on urinary bladder carcinogenesis in F344 male rats. Int J Cancer 77:773-777.

Hirvonen T, Pietinen P, Virtanen M, Ovaskainen ML, Hakkinen S, Albanes D, Virtamo J (2001) Intake of flavonols and flavones and risk of coronary heart disease in male smokers. Epidemiology 12:62-67.

Hodge L, Salome CM, Peat JK, Haby MM, Xuan W, Woolcock AJ (1996) Consumption of oily fish and childhood asthma risk. Med J Aust 164:137-140.

Hollman PC, Katan MB (1997) Absorption, metabolism and health effects of dietary flavonoids in man. Biomed Pharmacother 51:305-310.

Hollman PC, Katan MB (1999) Dietary flavonoids: intake, health effects and bioavailability. Food Chem Toxicol 37:937-942.

Holmes MD, Liu S, Hankinson SE, Colditz GA, Hunter DJ, Willett WC (2004) Dietary carbohydrates, fiber, and breast cancer risk. Am J Epidemiol 159:732-739.

Horn TL, Reichert MA, Bliss RL, Malejka-Giganti D (2002) Modulations of P450 mRNA in liver and mammary gland and P450 activities and metabolism of estrogen in liver by treatment of rats with indole-3-carbinol. Biochem Pharmacol 64:393-404.

Horrocks LA, Yeo YK (1999) Health benefits of docosahexaenoic acid (DHA). Pharmacol Res 40:211-225.

Howell AB (2002) Cranberry proanthocyanidins and the maintenance of urinary tract health. Crit Rev Food Sci Nutr 42:273-278.

Hwang J, Sevanian A, Hodis HN, Ursini F (2000) Synergistic inhibition of LDL oxidation by phytoestrogens and ascorbic acid. Free Radic Biol Med 29:79-89.

Institute of Medicine (2002) Dietary Reference Intakes: Energy, Carbohydrate, Fiber, Fat, Fatty Acids, Cholesterol, Protein, and Amino Acids. Part 2. National Academy Press, Washington, DC.

Isokangas P, Tenovuo J, Soderling E, Mannisto H, Makinen KK (1991) Dental caries and mutans streptococci in the proximal areas of molars affected by the habitual use of xylitol chewing gum. Caries Res 25:444-448.

Ju YH, Doerge DR, Allred KF, Allred CD, Helferich WG (2002) Dietary genistein negates the inhibitory effect of tamoxifen on growth of estrogen-dependent human breast cancer (MCF-7) cells implanted in athymic mice. Cancer Res 62:2474-2477.

Kalmijn S, Feskens EJ, Launer LJ, Kromhout D (1997) Polyunsaturated fatty acids, antioxidants, and cognitive function in very old men. Am J Epidemiol 145:33-41.

Kameue C, Tsukahara T, Yamada K, Koyama H, Iwasaki Y, Nakayama K, Ushida K (2004) Dietary sodium gluconate protects rats from large bowel cancer by stimulating butyrate production. J Nutr 134:940-944.

Katan MB, Grundy SM, Jones P, Law M, Miettinen T, Paoletti R (2003) Efficacy and safety of plant stanols and sterols in the management of blood cholesterol levels. Mayo Clin Proc 78:965-978.

Kim YS, Milner JA (2005) Targets for indole-3-carbinol in cancer prevention. J Nutr Biochem 16:65-73.

Klepser TB, Doucette WR, Horton MR, Buys LM, Ernst ME, Ford JK, Hoehns JD, Kautzman HA, Logemann CD, Swegle JM, Ritho M, Klepser ME (2000) Assessment of patients' perceptions and beliefs regarding herbal therapies. Pharmacotherapy 20:83-87.

Knekt P, Jarvinen R, Seppanen R, Hellovaara M, Teppo L, Pukkala E, Aromaa A (1997) Dietary flavonoids and the risk of lung cancer and other malignant neoplasms. Am J Epidemiol 146:223-230.

Kopp-Hoolihan L (2001) Prophylactic and therapeutic uses of probiotics: a review. J Am Diet Assoc 101:229-238.

Kore AM, Wallig MA (1993) Histological and serum biochemical effects of 1-isothiocyanato-3- (methylsulphinyl)-propane in the F344 rat. Food Chem Toxicol 31:549-559.

Kostyuk VA, Potapovich AI (1998) Antiradical and chelating effects in flavonoid protection against silica-induced cell injury. Arch Biochem Biophys 355:43-48.

Kris-Etherton PM, Harris WS, Appel LJ (2003) Omega-3 fatty acids and cardiovascular disease: new recommendations from the American Heart Association. Arterioscler Thromb Vasc Biol 23:151-152.

Kris-Etherton PM, Hecker KD, Bonanome A, Coval SM, Binkoski AE, Hilpert KF, Griel AE, Etherton TD (2002) Bioactive compounds in foods: their role in the prevention of cardiovascular disease and cancer. Am J Med 113:71S-88S.

Kristal AR (2004) Vitamin A, retinoids and carotenoids as chemopreventive agents for prostate cancer. J Urol 171:S54-S58.

Kroon PA, Clifford MN, Crozier A, Day AJ, Donovan JL, Manach C, Williamson G (2004) How should we assess the effects of exposure to dietary polyphenols in vitro? Am J Clin Nutr 80:15-21.

Kurilich AC, Jeffery EH, Juvik JA, Wallig MA, Klein BP (2003) Broccoli extracts protect against reactive oxygen species in HepG2 cells. J Nutra Func Med Foods 4:5-16.

Lambert JD, Hong J, Kim DH, Mishin VM, Yang CS (2004) Piperine enhances the bioavailability of the tea polyphenol (-)-epigallocatechin-3-gallate in mice. J Nutr 134:1948-1952.

Lampe JW (2003) Spicing up a vegetarian diet: chemopreventive effects of phytochemicals. Am J Clin Nutr 78:579S-583S.

Lawlor DA, Ness AR (2003) Commentary: the rough world of nutritional epidemiology: does dietary fibre prevent large bowel cancer? Int J Epidemiol 32:239-243.

Lazarou J, Pomeranz BH, Corey PN (1998) Incidence of adverse drug reactions in hospitalized patients: a meta-analysis of prospective studies. JAMA 279:1200-1205.

Lu HF, Sue CC, Yu CS, Chen SC, Chen GW, Chung JG (2004) Diallyl disulfide (DADS) induced apoptosis undergo caspase-3 activity in human bladder cancer T24 cells. Food Chem Toxicol 42:1543-1552.

Madley R (2001) Probiotics, prebiotics, & synbiotics. Nutraceuticals World 4:50-76.

Maheo K, Morel F, Langouet S, Kramer H, Le Ferrec E, Ketterer B, Guillouzo A (1997) Inhibition of cytochromes P-450 and induction of glutathione S-transferases by sulforaphane in primary human and rat hepatocytes. Cancer Res 57:3649-3652.

Mai V, Flood A, Peters U, Lacey JV, Jr., Schairer C, Schatzkin A (2003) Dietary fibre and risk of colorectal cancer in the Breast Cancer Detection Demonstration Project (BCDDP) follow-up cohort. Int J Epidemiol 32:234-239.

Makinen KK, Soderling E, Hurttia H, Lehtonen OP, Luukkala E (1985) Biochemical, microbiologic, and clinical comparisons between two dentifrices that contain different mixtures of sugar alcohols. J Am Dent Assoc 111:745-751.

Makinen KK, Soderling E, Isokangas P, Tenovuo J, Tiekso J (1989) Oral biochemical status and depression of Streptococcus mutans in children during 24- to 36-month use of xylitol chewing gum. Caries Res 23:261-267.

Manach C, Morand C, Demigne C, Texier O, Regerat F, Remesy C (1997) Bioavailability of rutin and quercetin in rats. FEBS Lett 409:12-16.

Markowitz JS, Devane CL, Chavin KD, Taylor RM, Ruan Y, Donovan JL (2003) Effects of garlic (Allium sativum L.) supplementation on cytochrome P450 2D6 and 3A4 activity in healthy volunteers. Clin Pharmacol Ther 74:170-177.

Mayne ST, Cartmel B, Silva F, Kim CS, Fallon BG, Briskin K, Zheng T, Baum M, Shor-Posner G, Goodwin WJ, Jr. (1998) Effect of supplemental beta-carotene on plasma concentrations of carotenoids, retinol, and alpha-tocopherol in humans. Am J Clin Nutr 68:642-647.

McKenney J (2004) New perspectives on the use of niacin in the treatment of lipid disorders. Arch Intern Med 164:697-705.

McLeod RS, LeBlanc AM, Langille MA, Mitchell PL, Currie DL (2004) Conjugated linoleic acids, atherosclerosis, and hepatic very-low-density lipoprotein metabolism. Am J Clin Nutr 79:1169S-1174S.

Michaud DS, Spiegelman D, Clinton SK, Rimm EB, Willett WC, Giovannucci EL (1999) Fruit and vegetable intake and incidence of bladder cancer in a male prospective cohort. J Natl Cancer Inst 91:605-613.

Miller EC, Giovannucci E, Erdman JW, Jr., Bahnson R, Schwartz SJ, Clinton SK (2002) Tomato products, lycopene, and prostate cancer risk. Urol Clin North Am 29:83-93.

Mills E, Montori VM, Wu P, Gallicano K, Clarke M, Guyatt G (2004) Interaction of St John's wort with conventional drugs: systematic review of clinical trials. BMJ 329:27-30.

Milner JA (2001) A historical perspective on garlic and cancer. J Nutr 131:1027S-1031S.

Moreau RA, Whitaker BD, Hicks KB (2002) Phytosterols, phytostanols, and their conjugates in foods: structural diversity, quantitative analysis, and health-promoting uses. Prog Lipid Res 41:457-500.

Morre DJ, Morre DM (2003) Synergistic Capsicum-tea mixtures with anticancer activity. J Pharm Pharmacol 55:987-994.

Morton LW, Croft KD, Puddey IB, Byrne L (2000) Phenolic acids protect low density lipoproteins from peroxynitrite-mediated modification in vitro. Redox Rep 5:124-125.

Nagao A (2004) Oxidative conversion of carotenoids to retinoids and other products. J Nutr 134:237S-240S.

Nardini M, Natella F, Gentili V, Di Felice M, Scaccini C (1997) Effect of caffeic acid dietary supplementation on the antioxidant defense system in rat: an in vivo study. Arch Biochem Biophys 342:157-160.

Nho CW, Jeffery E (2001) The synergistic upregulation of phase II detoxification enzymes by glucosinolate breakdown products in cruciferous vegetables. Toxicol Appl Pharmacol 174:146-152.

Nkondjock A, Shatenstein B, Maisonneuve P, Ghadirian P (2003) Specific fatty acids and human colorectal cancer: an overview. Cancer Detect Prev 27:55-66.

Ososki AL, Kennelly EJ (2003) Phytoestrogens: a review of the present state of research. Phytother Res 17:845-869.

Ostlund RE, Jr. (2004) Phytosterols and cholesterol metabolism. Curr Opin Lipidol 15:37-41.

Peeters PH, Keinan-Boker L, van der Schouw YT, Grobbee DE (2003) Phytoestrogens and breast cancer risk. Review of the epidemiological evidence. Breast Cancer Res Treat 77:171-183.

Pignatelli P, Pulcinelli FM, Celestini A, Lenti L, Ghiselli A, Gazzaniga PP, Violi F (2000) The flavonoids quercetin and catechin synergistically inhibit platelet function by antagonizing the intracellular production of hydrogen peroxide. Am J Clin Nutr 72:1150-1155.

Prior RL, Hoang H, Gu L, Wu X, Bacchiocca M, Howard L, Hampsch-Woodill M, Huang D, Ou B, Jacob R (2003) Assays for hydrophilic and lipophilic antioxidant capacity [oxygen radical absorbance capacity (ORAC(FL))] of plasma and other biological and food samples. J Agric Food Chem 51:3273-3279.

Proteggente AR, Pannala AS, Paganga G, Van Buren L, Wagner E, Wiseman S, Van De Put F, Dacombe C, Rice-Evans CA (2002) The antioxidant activity of regularly consumed fruit and vegetables reflects their phenolic and vitamin C composition. Free Radic Res 36:217-233.

Rahman K (2001) Historical perspective on garlic and cardiovascular disease. J Nutr 131: 977S-979S.

Rao CV, Desai D, Simi B, Kulkarni N, Amin S, Reddy BS (1993) Inhibitory effect of caffeic acid esters on azoxymethane-induced biochemical changes and aberrant crypt foci formation in rat colon. Cancer Res 53:4182-4188.

Reed J (2002) Cranberry flavonoids, atherosclerosis and cardiovascular health. Crit Rev Food Sci Nutr 42:301-316.

Reinke RA, Lee DJ, McDougall BR, King PJ, Victoria J, Mao Y, Lei X, Reinecke MG, Robinson WE, Jr. (2004) L-chicoric acid inhibits human immunodeficiency virus type 1 integration in vivo and is a noncompetitive but reversible inhibitor of HIV-1 integrase in vitro. Virology 326:203-219.

Ren W, Qiao Z, Wang H, Zhu L, Zhang L (2003) Flavonoids: promising anticancer agents. Med Res Rev 23:519-534.

Robbins RJ (2003) Phenolic acids in foods: an overview of analytical methodology. J Agric Food Chem 51:2866-2887.

Rock CL, Flatt SW, Thomson CA, Stefanick ML, Newman VA, Jones LA, Natarajan L, Ritenbaugh C, Hollenbach KA, Pierce JP, Chang RJ (2004) Effects of a high-fiber, low-fat diet intervention on serum concentrations of reproductive steroid hormones in women with a history of breast cancer. J Clin Oncol 22: 2379-2387.

Rose P, Faulkner K, Williamson G, Mithen R (2000) 7-Methylsulfinylheptyl and 8-methylsulfinyloctyl isothiocyanates from watercress are potent inducers of phase II enzymes. Carcinogenesis 21:1983-1988.

Ross JA (1998) Maternal diet and infant leukemia: a role for DNA topoisomerase II inhibitors? Int J Cancer Suppl 11:26-28.

Rouzaud G, Young SA, Duncan AJ (2004) Hydrolysis of glucosinolates to isothiocyanates after ingestion of raw or microwaved cabbage by human volunteers. Cancer Epidemiol Biomarkers Prev 13:125-131.

Roynette CE, Calder PC, Dupertuis YM, Pichard C (2004) n-3 polyunsaturated fatty acids and colon cancer prevention. Clin Nutr 23:139-151.

Saggioro A (2004) Probiotics in the treatment of irritable bowel syndrome. J Clin Gastroenterol 38:S104-S106.

Sengupta A, Ghosh S, Das S (2004) Modulatory influence of garlic and tomato on cyclooxygenase-2 activity, cell proliferation and apoptosis during azoxymethane induced colon carcinogenesis in rat. Cancer Lett 208:127-136.

Sengupta S, Toh SA, Sellers LA, Skepper JN, Koolwijk P, Leung HW, Yeung HW, Wong RN,

Sasisekharan R, Fan TP (2004) Modulating angiogenesis: the yin and the yang in ginseng. Circulation 110:1219-1225.

Setchell KD, Brown NM, Lydeking-Olsen E (2002) The clinical importance of the metabolite equol: a clue to the effectiveness of soy and its isoflavones. J Nutr 132:3577-3584.

Shekelle PG, Hardy ML, Morton SC, Maglione M, Mojica WA, Suttorp MJ, Rhodes SL, Jungvig L, Gagne J (2003) Efficacy and safety of ephedra and ephedrine for weight loss and athletic performance: a meta-analysis. JAMA 289:1537-1545.

Simonsen N, van't Veer P, Strain JJ, Martin-Moreno JM, Huttunen JK, Navajas JF, Martin BC, Thamm M, Kardinaal AF, Kok FJ, Kohlmeier L (1998) Adipose tissue omega-3 and omega-6 fatty acid content and breast cancer in the EURAMIC study. European Community Multicenter Study on Antioxidants, Myocardial Infarction, and Breast Cancer. Am J Epidemiol 147:342-352.

Slattery ML, Neuhausen SL, Hoffman M, Caan B, Curtin K, Ma KN, Samowitz W (2004) Dietary calcium, vitamin D, VDR genotypes and colorectal cancer. Int J Cancer 111:750-756.

Soderling E, Makinen KK, Chen CY, Pape HR, Jr., Loesche W, Makinen PL (1989) Effect of sorbitol, xylitol, and xylitol/sorbitol chewing gums on dental plaque. Caries Res 23:378-384.

Song K, Milner JA (2001) The influence of heating on the anticancer properties of garlic. J Nutr 131:1054S-1057S.

Sparreboom A, Cox MC, Acharya MR, Figg WD (2004) Herbal remedies in the United States: potential adverse interactions with anticancer agents. J Clin Oncol 22:2489-2503.

Taylor CL (2004) Regulatory frameworks for functional foods and dietary supplements. Nutr Rev 62:55-59.

Thomson M, Ali M (2003) Garlic [Allium sativum]: a review of its potential use as an anti-cancer agent. Curr Cancer Drug Targets 3:67-81.

Thorsdottir I, Hill J, Ramel A (2004) Omega-3 fatty acid supply from milk associates with lower type 2 diabetes in men and coronary heart disease in women. Prev Med 39:630-634.

Van Erk MJ, Roepman P, Van Der Lende TR, Stierum RH, Aarts JM, Van Bladeren PJ, Van Ommen B (2004) Integrated assessment by multiple gene expression analysis of quercetin bioactivity on anticancer-related mechanisms in colon cancer cells in vitro. Eur J Nutr 44:143-156.

Van het Hof KH, Kivits GA, Weststrate JA, Tijburg LB (1998) Bioavailability of catechins from tea: the effect of milk. Eur J Clin Nutr 52:356-359.

Van Loveren C (2004) Sugar alcohols: what is the evidence for caries-preventive and caries-therapeutic effects? Caries Res 38:286-293.

Verhoeven DT, Verhagen H, Goldbohm RA, van den Brandt PA, van Poppel G (1997) A review of mechanisms underlying anticarcinogenicity by Brassica vegetables. Chem Biol Interact 103:79-129.

Vogl FD, Taioli E, Maugard C, Zheng W, Pinto LF, Ambrosone C, Parl FF, Nedelcheva-Kristensen V, Rebbeck TR, Brennan P, Boffetta P (2004) Glutathione S-transferases M1, T1, and P1 and breast cancer: a pooled analysis. Cancer Epidemiol Biomarkers Prev 13:1473-1479.

Voorrips LE, Brants HA, Kardinaal AF, Hiddink GJ, van den Brandt PA, Goldbohm RA (2002) Intake of conjugated linoleic acid, fat, and other fatty acids in relation to postmenopausal breast cancer: The Netherlands Cohort Study on Diet and Cancer. Am J Clin Nutr 76:873-882.

Wargovich MJ, Woods C, Hollis DM, Zander ME (2001) Herbals, cancer prevention and health. J Nutr 131:3034S-3036S.

Warshafsky S, Kamer RS, Sivak SL (1993) Effect of garlic on total serum cholesterol. A meta-analysis. Ann Intern Med 119:599-605.

Wu K, Erdman JW, Jr., Schwartz SJ, Platz EA, Leitzmann M, Clinton SK, DeGroff V, Willett WC, Giovannucci E (2004) Plasma and dietary carotenoids, and the risk of prostate cancer: a nested case-control study. Cancer Epidemiol Biomarkers Prev 13:260-269.

Wu L, Ashraf MH, Facci M, Wang R, Paterson PG, Ferrie A, Juurlink BH (2004) Dietary approach to attenuate oxidative stress, hypertension, and inflammation in the cardiovascular system. Proc Natl Acad Sci USA 101:7094-7099.

Xu M, Bailey AC, Hernaez JF, Taoka CR, Schut HA, Dashwood RH (1996) Protection by green tea, black tea, and indole-3-carbinol against 2- amino-3-methylimidazo[4,5-f]quinoline-induced DNA adducts and colonic aberrant crypts in the F344 rat. Carcinogenesis 17:1429-1434.

Yamada N, Kobatake Y, Ikegami S, Takita T, Wada M, Shimizu J, Kanke Y, Innami S (1997) Changes in blood coagulation, platelet aggregation, and lipid metabolism in rats given lipids containing docosahexaenoic acid. Biosci Biotechnol Biochem 61:1454-1458.

Yang CS (2001) Inhibition of carcinogenesis by dietary polyphenolic compounds. Annu Rev Nutr 21:381-406.

Zafar TA, Weaver CM, Jones K, Moore DR, 2nd, Barnes S (2004) Inulin effects on bioavailability of soy isoflavones and their calcium absorption enhancing ability. J Agric Food Chem 52: 2827-2831.

Zhang SM, Hunter DJ, Rosner BA, Giovannucci EL, Colditz GA, Speizer FE, Willett WC (2000) Intakes of fruits, vegetables, and related nutrients and the risk of non-Hodgkin's lymphoma among women. Cancer Epidemiol Biomarkers Prev 9:477-485.

RECOMMENDED READINGS

Hasler CM, Bloch AS, Thomson CA (2004) Position of the American Dietetic Association: Functional foods. J Am Diet Assoc 104: 814-826.

Kris-Etherton PM, Hecker KD, Bonanome A, Coval SM, Binkoski AE, Hilpert KF, Griel AE, Etherton TD (2002) Bioactive compounds in foods: their role in the prevention of cardiovascular disease and cancer. Am J Med 113:71S-88S.

RECOMMENDED WEBSITES

National Archives and Records Administration
List of substances generally recognized as safe
www.access.gpo.gov/nara/cfr/waisidx_02/21cfr182_02.html

United States Department of Agriculture, Nutrient Data Laboratory
Links to data on bioactive compound (flavonoids) content of American foods
www.ars.usda.gov/ba/bhnrc/ndl

United States Food and Drug Administration

Food Labeling and Nutrition
www.cfsan.fda.gov/label.html

Center for Food Safety and Applied Nutrition
www.cfsan.fda.gov/~dms/lab-hlth.html

Qualified Health Claims
www.cfsan.fda.gov/~dms/lab-qhc.html

Regulation of Dietary Supplements
vm.cfsan.fda.gov/~dms/supplmnt.html

Chapter 3

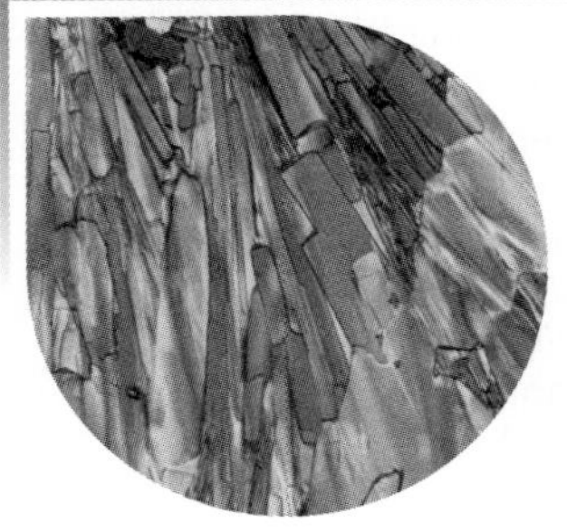

Guidelines for Food and Nutrient Intake

Christina Stark, MS, RD, CDN

OUTLINE

COMMON ABBREVIATIONS

Nutrient Standards

AI Adequate Intake
DRI Dietary Reference Intake
DRV Daily Reference Value
DV Daily Value
EAR Estimated Average Requirement
RDA Recommended Dietary Allowance
RDI Reference Daily Intake
RNI Recommended Nutrient Intake
UL Tolerable Upper Intake Level

Agencies/Organizations

FAO Food and Agriculture Organization
FDA U.S. Food and Drug Administration
IOM Institute of Medicine
NRC National Research Council
USDA U.S. Department of Agriculture
USDHHS U.S. Department of Health and Human Services
WHO World Health Organization

FOOD AS A SOURCE OF NUTRIENTS

When people sit down to a meal, they eat food, not nutrients. Most people don't think about the individual nutrients they are consuming, but instead focus on the flavor, texture, and aroma of the food. Although consumers do indicate that nutrition is an important factor when making food selections, other factors such as taste, cost, and convenience may outweigh any nutritional considerations. The challenge is to translate the biochemical and physiological requirements for nutrients into practical guidelines so that people can make healthful food choices. Simply knowing nutrient requirements does not ensure that someone will consume an adequate diet.

Food is also made up of more than just nutrients. Some of these nonnutritive components, referred to as phytochemicals from plant sources and zoochemicals from animal sources, may have important implications in terms of their health benefits (American Dietetic Association, 2004). For example, tomatoes contain lycopene, which may reduce the risk of prostate cancer, and cranberry juice contains proanthocyanidins, which may reduce urinary tract infections. Other plant compounds are being studied for their ability to lower cholesterol levels, reduce the risk of macular degeneration, or improve gastrointestinal health. Researchers are actively investigating the health benefits and risks of these naturally occurring substances, which are found in commonly consumed fruits, vegetables, and grains, as well as in less frequently consumed foods such as licorice and green tea. Understanding the importance of both nutritive and nonnutritive components in foods is critical to providing sound dietary advice.

This chapter explores various types of dietary recommendations, ranging from those focused on specific nutrients to those based on entire food groups. In the United States, these include the *Dietary Reference Intakes*, the *Dietary Guidelines for Americans,* and the *MyPyramid* food guidance system. Many other countries, including Canada, Australia, New Zealand, some in Latin America and Asia, and many in Europe, have developed their own sets of recommended dietary intakes, dietary guidelines and/or food guides (FAO/WHO, 1996; Painter et al., 2002). Both professionals and consumers can use these recommendations and guidelines in the promotion and selection of healthful diets.

DIETARY REFERENCE INTAKES

DEFINITIONS

In the United States, the Dietary Reference Intakes (DRIs) are the current standards for measuring nutritional adequacy. The term DRI was introduced in 1997 and replaced the former term Recommended Dietary Allowance (RDA), which had been the standard since 1941. The DRIs were developed jointly by the National Academy of Sciences' Institute of Medicine (IOM) and the Canadian government and have also replaced Canada's previous reference values known as Recommended Nutrient Intakes (RNIs) (IOM, 2003a).

DRIs refer to four different reference values that can be used for planning and assessing diets of individuals and groups. The DRIs were developed to address some of the limitations of having only a single set of reference values—the former RDAs. DRI is not merely a new term; the establishment of DRIs represents a new approach supported by a growing understanding that different types of reference values are needed to apply dietary recommendations to individuals and groups.

The DRIs, which have replaced all the former RDAs and RNIs, have been issued as a series of reports, with each report covering a group of related nutrients (IOM, 1997, 1998, 2000a, 2001, 2002, 2004). The reports, published in this order, group the nutrients as follows:

- Calcium, phosphorus, magnesium, vitamin D, and fluoride
- Thiamin, riboflavin, niacin, vitamin B_6, folate, vitamin B_{12}, pantothenic acid, biotin, and choline
- Vitamin C, vitamin E, selenium, and carotenoids
- Vitamin A, vitamin K, arsenic, boron, chromium, copper, iodine, iron, manganese, molybdenum, nickel, silicon, vanadium, and zinc
- Energy, carbohydrate, fiber, fat, fatty acids, cholesterol, protein, and amino acids
- Water, potassium, sodium, chloride, and sulfate

The DRIs consist of the following reference values: Estimated Average Requirement (EAR), Recommended Dietary Allowance (RDA), Adequate Intake (AI), and Tolerable Upper Intake Level (UL). The scientific data for developing DRIs consist of clinical trials; dose–response, balance, depletion/repletion, prospective observation, and case–control studies; and clinical observations in humans. The EARs, RDAs, AIs, and ULs refer to average daily intakes over 1 or more weeks. The Institute of Medicine's Food and Nutrition Board describes each value in the following way:

- EAR: the average daily nutrient intake level estimated to meet the requirement of half the healthy individuals in a particular life stage and gender group (IOM, 2004, p. 3).

This value is used as the basis for developing the RDA and can be used by nutrition policy makers in assessing the adequacy of nutrient intakes of the group and for planning how much the group should consume.

- RDA: the average daily dietary nutrient intake level sufficient to meet the nutrient requirement of nearly all (97% to 98%) healthy individuals in a particular life stage and gender group (IOM, 2004, p. 3).

The RDA should be used in guiding individuals to achieve adequate nutrient intake aimed at decreasing the risk of chronic disease. It is based on an estimate of the average requirement plus an increase to account for the variation within a particular group.

- AI: The recommended average daily nutrient intake level based on observed or experimentally determined approximations or estimates of nutrient intake by a group (or groups) of healthy people that are assumed to be adequate—used when an RDA cannot be determined (IOM, 2004, p. 3).

Individuals should use the AI as a goal for intake of a nutrient for which no RDA exists. The AI is derived through experimental or observational data that show a mean intake that appears to sustain a desired indicator of health, such as calcium retention in bone, for most members of a population group.

- UL: the highest average daily nutrient intake level likely to pose no risk of adverse health effects to almost all individuals in the general population. As intake increases above the UL, the potential risk of adverse effects may increase (IOM, 2004, p. 3).

This value is not intended to be a recommended level of intake, and there is no established benefit for individuals to consume nutrients at levels above the RDA or AI. For most nutrients, this value refers to total intakes from food, fortified food, and nutrient supplements.

In contrast to the DRIs, the former RDAs were defined as "the levels of intake of essential nutrients that, on the basis of scientific knowledge, are judged by the Food and Nutrition Board of the National Research Council (NRC) to be adequate to meet the known nutrient needs of practically all healthy persons" (NRC, 1989a, p. 1). Key aspects of the definition are that the former RDAs were only defined for essential nutrients, the amounts were adequate, and the RDAs met the needs of healthy persons. They were not intended for those with special nutritional needs.

In the DRIs, which represent a new paradigm, "three of the reference values are defined by a specific indicator of nutrient adequacy, which may relate to the reduction of the risk of chronic disease or disorders; the fourth is defined by a specific indicator of excess where one is available. In the previous paradigm, the indicator of adequacy was usually limited to a classical deficiency state" (IOM, 1997, p. 8). Figure 3-1 shows how the DRI values relate to the risks of either inadequacy or adverse effects. Like the former RDAs, the DRIs apply to the healthy general population.

The former RDAs were developed specifically for the United States. The DRIs provide for the first time one set of reference values for 12 life-stage groups for the United States and Canada. Similar sets of recommendations, typically called recommended dietary intakes, exist for other countries or in some cases for a worldwide audience (FAO/WHO, 2002). The use of professional judgment and interpretation to set an RDA, DRI, or other recommended intake is illustrated by the range of values for some nutrients in sets of standards in different countries. An FAO/WHO Expert Consultation did an analysis of the ranges of values for recommended dietary intakes around the world, based on the mean for active male adults. The ratios of the highest value to the lowest value were found to range from 1.3:1 for energy to 50:1 for vitamin K (Helsing, 1990). Although different standards may be due in part to biology, much of the difference can be explained by the varied approaches used in setting the standards.

CRITERIA FOR SETTING DIETARY RECOMMENDATIONS

The first edition of the *Recommended Dietary Allowances,* published by the National Academy of Sciences in 1943, provided recommended intakes for energy and nine essential nutrients. The RDAs were revised periodically based on new scientific knowledge and interpretations. With each revision there were changes in the numbers of nutrients considered and the levels recommended, but the basic philosophy was to define RDAs as levels sufficient to cover individual variations and provide a margin of safety above minimum requirements

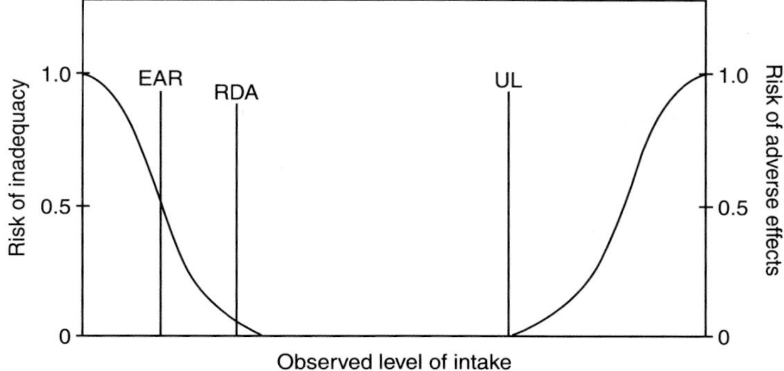

Figure 3-1 Dietary reference intakes. This figure shows that the Estimated Average Requirement (EAR) is the intake at which the risk of inadequacy is 0.5 (50%) to an individual. The Recommended Dietary Allowance (RDA) is the intake at which the risk of inadequacy is very small—only 0.02 to 0.03 (2% to 3%). The Adequate Intake (AI) does not bear a consistent relationship to the EAR or the RDA because it is set without the estimate of the requirement. At intakes between the RDA and the Tolerable Upper Intake Level (UL), the risks of inadequacy and of excess are both close to 0. At intakes above the UL, the risk of adverse effects may increase. *(From IOM [2004] Dietary References Intakes for Water, Potassium, Sodium, Chloride and Sulfate. National Academy Press, Washington, DC, pp 1-3. Retrieved November 7, 2005, from www.print.nap.edu/pdf/0309091691/pdf_image/23.pdf.)*

(IOM, 1994). In contrast, the concept of reduction in risk of chronic disease has been incorporated into formulating the new DRIs.

Other countries with recommended dietary intakes have also debated how to define their levels—should they use a minimalist amount that prevents deficiency disease in all healthy people, an intermediate amount that allows for a large margin of safety, or a level that supports optimal nutrition? For example, when setting their recommended dietary intake for vitamin C, Australia considered the following four criteria:

1. The amount to prevent scurvy
2. The amount to provide tissue saturation
3. The amount to maximize absorption of nonheme iron
4. The amount that may minimize risk of gastric cancer

The final recommended dietary intake was based on the amount required to prevent scurvy in smokers and to provide "reasonable" stores in most people but not to ensure tissue saturation (Truswell, 1990).

HOW DRIs ARE USED

The former RDAs were meant to be applied to groups of people, namely "practically all healthy people," and not any single individual. In fact, except for energy, the levels are set higher than the requirements of most individuals to account for the wide range of individual variation. Even so, the former RDAs often have been inappropriately interpreted as the amounts of essential nutrients a healthy individual needs over time. Over the years, the RDAs have also been used for several other purposes, including establishing nutrient standards for food assistance programs such as the National School Lunch Program and School Breakfast Program, evaluating dietary survey data, designing nutrition education programs, developing and fortifying food products, and setting standards for food labels (IOM, 1994).

The DRIs were purposely developed to address some of these inappropriate applications of the former RDAs. In general, the newly defined RDAs should be used by individuals as a target intake, but these values should not be used to assess or plan intakes of groups. AIs can be used as a target value for individuals if no RDAs exist. EARs are particularly useful for both assessing and planning nutrient intakes of groups. The IOM has issued two separate reports describing in more detail how the DRIs can be applied to dietary assessment and planning (IOM, 2000b, 2003b). The boxes on page 50 summarize how these applications differ between individuals and groups.

Although the DRIs can be used for dietary planning, they are not a practical guide for use

Box 3-1

USES OF DRIs FOR ASSESSING INTAKES OF INDIVIDUAL AND GROUPS

For an Individual

EAR: Use to examine the probability that usual intake is inadequate.
RDA: Usual intake at or above this level has a low probability of inadequacy.
AI: Usual intake at or above this level has a low probability of inadequacy.
UL: Usual intake above this level may place an individual at risk of adverse effects from excessive nutrient intake.

For a Group

EAR: Use to estimate the prevalence of inadequate intakes within a group.
RDA: Do not use to assess intakes of groups.
AI: Mean usual intake at or above this level implies a low prevalence of inadequate intakes.
UL: Use to estimate the percentage of the population at potential risk of adverse effects from excessive nutrient intake.

From IOM (2000b) Dietary Reference Intakes: Applications in Dietary Assessment. National Academy Press, Washington, DC.
DRI, Dietary Reference Intake; *EAR,* Estimated Average Requirement; *RDA,* Recommended Dietary Allowance; *AI,* Adequate Intake; *UL,* Tolerable Upper Intake Level.

Box 3-2

USES OF DRIs FOR PLANNING INTAKES OF APPARENTLY HEALTHY INDIVIDUALS AND GROUPS

For an Individual

EAR: Do not use as an intake goal for the individual.
RDA: Plan for this intake; usual intake at or above this level has a low probability of inadequacy.
AI: Plan for this intake; usual intake at or above this level has a low probability of inadequacy.
UL: Plan for usual intake below this level to avoid potential risk of adverse effects from excessive nutrient intake.

For a Group

EAR: Use to plan for an acceptably low prevalence of inadequate intakes within a group.
RDA: Do not use to plan intakes of groups.
AI: Plan for mean intake at this level; mean usual intake at or above this level implies a low prevalence of inadequate intakes.
UL: Use in planning to minimize the proportion of the population at potential risk of excessive nutrient intake.

From IOM (2003b) Dietary Reference Intakes: Applications in Dietary Planning. National Academy Press, Washington, DC, p 4.

by consumers in selecting a healthful diet. The DRIs focus on specific nutrients, whereas people make food selections based on individual foods and food groups. Dietary advice for consumers needs to focus on recommended food selections in the context of the total diet.

DIETARY ADVICE: GOALS AND GUIDELINES

DEVELOPMENT OF DIETARY GUIDELINES

As the relationship between diet and health has become clearer, a new type of dietary

Nutrition Insight

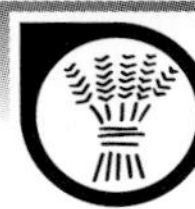

Food Fortification With Folic Acid

In developing the Dietary Reference Intakes (DRIs), the role a nutrient plays in providing optimal health, rather than just preventing a deficiency disease, is considered. For example, folate's role in reducing the risk of cardiovascular disease or preventing certain birth defects was considered in setting the DRIs for folate. The folate intake of women of child-bearing age is of concern, and the new RDA for folate for this subgroup was increased to reflect new research. (The 1989 RDA for women was 0.18 mg; the new RDA for women is 0.4 mg.)

Simply changing an RDA value, however, does not mean people will change their consumption of that nutrient. Another strategy for ensuring that a population group meets their need for a specific nutrient is to fortify certain foods. Earlier last century, American manufacturers started fortifying salt with iodine; milk with vitamin D; and bread and flour with thiamin, niacin, riboflavin, and iron. Based on studies of folic acid and birth defects, the U.S. Public Health Service recommended in 1992 that all women of child-bearing age consume 0.4 mg of folic acid daily to reduce their risk of giving birth to children with neural tube defects. The Food and Drug Administration issued a regulation in 1996 which stated that, as of 1998, American manufacturers will be required to fortify certain grain products with folic acid in an effort to reduce the risk of neural tube birth defects (USDHHS, 1996). These products include most enriched breads, flours, corn meals, pastas, and rice. Required fortification levels range from 0.43 to 1.4 mg per pound of product.

The fortification levels chosen were designed to keep total daily intake of folic acid below 1 mg; intakes higher than that may mask symptoms of pernicious anemia, a form of vitamin B_{12} deficiency that primarily affects older people. Some have suggested that foods fortified with folic acid should also be fortified with vitamin B_{12} in order to address this concern. Food fortification policies must take into account how increased consumption of one nutrient may affect other nutrients. Policy makers must also determine whether the fortified foods are likely to be consumed by the target audience (e.g., women of child-bearing age) and whether that level is safe for other populations (e.g, elderly people).

---

advice has emerged in the form of dietary goals and guidelines. Unlike the former RDAs, which focused on obtaining adequate amounts of essential nutrients, these guidelines emphasize the need to increase or decrease consumption of those food components that have been shown to affect the risk of certain chronic diseases. Another difference is that RDAs/DRIs state the amounts (weights) of intake recommended on a daily basis for various nutrients with no indication of whether typical intake is high or low, whereas dietary guidelines often start with the estimated national diet and express desired changes, generally in terms of recommending increases or decreases in various dietary components.

In the United States, this shift in focus from obtaining adequate intakes to minimizing excessive intakes began in 1977 when a United States Senate Select Committee on Nutrition and Human Needs issued a set of recommendations known as the *Dietary Goals for the United States* (United States Senate, 1977). These goals provided quantitative recommendations on the amounts of complex carbohydrates, sugar, fat, saturated fat, cholesterol, and sodium that should be consumed. The Dietary Goals were controversial, in part because the diet plans developed to meet the goals were so different from the food patterns of typical Americans.

Subsequently, a new publication, *Nutrition and Your Health: Dietary Guidelines for Americans*, was jointly issued in 1980 by the U.S. Department of Agriculture (USDA) and the Department of Health, Education, and Welfare (now Health and Human Services [USDHHS]). This publication was has been revised five times since 1980. The 1995 revision was the first one to be mandated by the government as a result of the National Nutrition Monitoring and Related Research Act, which requires the Secretaries of Agriculture and Health and Human Services to review and jointly issue the guidelines every 5 years (McMurry, 2003).

Based on the latest scientific evidence, the sixth edition of the guidelines—*Dietary Guidelines for Americans 2005*—provides information and advice for choosing a nutritious diet, maintaining a healthy weight, achieving adequate exercise, and keeping foods safe to avoid food-borne illness (USDA/USDHHS, 2005). The report identifies 41 key recommendations, of which 23 are for the general population and 18 for specific populations. For example, one key recommendation is "Consume a variety of nutrient-dense foods and beverages within and among the basic food groups while choosing foods that limit the intake of saturated and *trans* fats, cholesterol, added sugars, salt, and alcohol" (USDA/USDHHS, 2005, p. vii).

These recommendations are grouped into nine interrelated topic areas: adequate nutrients within calorie needs, weight management, physical activity, food groups to encourage, fats, carbohydrates, sodium and potassium, alcoholic beverages, and food safety. Unlike previous versions of the Dietary Guidelines, the 2005 version contains more technical information and is oriented toward policy makers, nutrition educators, nutritionists, and healthcare providers.

Like the DRIs, the Dietary Guidelines for Americans is intended for *healthy* Americans, in this case those over 2 years of age. The Guidelines are not intended for younger children and infants, whose dietary needs differ.

SOURCES OF DIETARY GUIDELINES

The Dietary Guidelines for Americans form the base of federal nutrition policy in the United States, but it is not the only set of dietary advice. Other agencies, organizations, and countries have also issued dietary goals or guidelines. In the United States, two authoritative reviews on the relationship between diet and health were published in the late 1980s. *The Surgeon General's Report on Nutrition and Health,* issued in 1988, contains advice similar to the Dietary Guidelines but also includes advice about fluoride (USDHHS, 1988). In 1989, the Committee on Diet and Health of the National Academy of Sciences issued *Diet and Health: Implications for Reducing Chronic Disease Risk* (NRC, 1989b). This publication provides quantitative targets for intake of fat, saturated fat, cholesterol, sodium, and alcohol and a recommended number of servings of fruits and vegetables and complex carbohydrates, as well as more general advice for the intake of energy, protein, calcium, fluoride, and dietary supplements. Dietary goals are also included in the U.S. Department of Health and Human Services' report *Healthy People 2010: Understanding and Improving Health,* which identifies 467 specific health objectives in 28 focus areas including nutrition and overweight (USDHHS, 2000a). Specific objectives under the nutrition focus relate to decreasing the prevalence of obesity; increasing intake of fruits, vegetables and whole grains; decreasing intakes of saturated fat, total fat and sodium; increasing calcium; and decreasing iron deficiency.

Various health organizations and expert panels have also issued dietary guidelines, often to reduce the risk of a specific disease (Hogbin et al., 2003). For example, guidelines from the American Heart Association and the American Cancer Society are aimed at reducing the risk of heart disease and cancer, respectively. Dietary recommendations developed by a WHO/FAO Expert Consultation are aimed at reducing the risk of six nutrition-related chronic diseases considered to be the greatest public health burden worldwide: obesity, diabetes, cardiovascular diseases, cancer, osteoporosis, and dental diseases (WHO/FAO, 2003).

FOOD GUIDES

DEVELOPMENT OF FOOD GUIDES

The key recommendations in the Dietary Guidelines provide general goals for how Americans should eat, but there is still a need for more specific food-related advice if the guidelines are to be implemented. Advising someone to choose a diet that is low in saturated fats and *trans* fats and rich in calcium is not helpful if the person does not know which foods are sources of fats or calcium. Food guides are designed to translate recommendations on nutrient intake into recommendations on food intake.

Over the years, the U.S. government has published various food guides (USDA, 1993). The first federal food guide, based on five food groups, was issued in 1916. The five groups (namely milk and meat, cereals, vegetables and fruits, fats and fatty foods, and sugars and sugary foods) were chosen based on the knowledge at that time of food composition and nutritional needs. During the Depression in the 1930s, there was an increased need for advice on how to select foods economically, so family food plans were developed to serve as buying guides. These food plans still exist today, adjusted for inflation, and serve as the basis for food stamp allotments.

In 1943 a food guide known as the "Basic Seven" was issued; this food guide recommended a certain number of daily servings from each of seven food groups. This guide was simplified and modified in 1956 to what became known as the "Basic Four." The Basic Four defined daily serving sizes and recommended a 2-2-4-4 pattern. This meant two servings from the milk and milk products group; two servings from the meat, fish, poultry, eggs, dry beans, and nuts group; four servings from the fruit and vegetable group; and four servings from the grain products group. The Basic Four guide was meant to represent a foundation diet that would supply a major portion of the RDAs for nutrients but only part of the energy needs. It was expected that people would eat additional foods to fulfill their needs for additional energy and nutrients.

Because the Basic Four and previous food guides were developed in the context of preventing deficiency diseases, the primary focus was on getting enough nutrients from a variety of foods. This advice complemented USDA's goal of promoting the consumption of various agricultural products.

In 1979, following the publication of the Dietary Goals, the USDA published the *Hassle-Free Guide to a Better Diet*. This food guide included the same foundation diet as recommended in the Basic Four, but identified a fifth group of fats, sweets, and alcohol for which moderation was advised. This was a significant change from previous food guides, as the government had now identified a food group for which there was no recommended number of daily servings. Instead, consumers were simply being urged to eat sparingly from this group.

After publication of the Hassle-Free Guide, the first edition of the Dietary Guidelines was issued, and it became clear that a new food guide was needed to help consumers translate the advice in the Guidelines into actual food choices. In developing the new food guide, the USDA first identified several philosophical goals for the guide: it should promote overall health, focus on the total diet, be useful to the target audience, and allow flexibility. Five steps were then used to develop the actual guide (USDA, 1993). These steps included establishing nutritional goals, defining food groups, assigning servings sizes, determining nutrient profiles for each food group, and determining the number of servings.

This new food guide was published in several USDA publications released in the mid-1980s and was also included in the third edition of the Dietary Guidelines published in 1990. Despite the release of a new food guide, many consumers and even some professionals still assumed the USDA was using the Basic Four food guide. To improve the visibility and usefulness of the new food guide, the Food Guide Pyramid was developed as a graphic representation of the guide. The USDA released the graphic and a consumer brochure, *The Food Guide Pyramid*, in 1992 (USDA, 1992). The Pyramid was designed to help Americans choose a diet that was nutritionally adequate, but also moderate in energy and limited in food components often consumed in excess.

The pyramid-shaped graphic may be familiar to many consumers, but the daily food intake patterns (i.e., the what and how much to eat) are what form the scientific foundation behind the Pyramid. In 2000, the USDA initiated a comprehensive review of the Food Guide Pyramid to make sure its recommendations continue to meet current nutritional standards and that consumers can use and apply its messages (USDA, 2003). Before revising the actual graphic, the daily food intake patterns were updated to reflect the latest nutritional standards as well as current food consumption choices in determining nutrient sources. The process involved the following five steps (Dietary Guidelines Advisory Committee, 2005, p. 23), which were similar to those used to develop the original Pyramid food patterns:

1. *Establishing nutritional goals.* Goals were obtained from the DRI reports released between 1997 and 2004 for various vitamins, minerals, macronutrients, and electrolytes.

2. *Establishing energy levels.* The food pattern was developed for caloric levels from 1,000 to 3,200 calories per day in 200-calorie increments.

3. *Assigning nutritional goals to each specific food intake pattern.* The specific nutritional goals

assigned to each food intake pattern were the goals of age/gender groups with sedentary energy requirements that most closely matched the calorie level. The sedentary level was selected so as not to overestimate energy needs when developing intake patterns to meet nutrient needs.

4. *Assigning a nutrient content to each food group and subgroup.* Foods included in each of the commodity food groups or subgroups (fruits, milk, meats and beans, whole grains, enriched grains, dark green vegetables, orange vegetables, legumes, starchy vegetables, and other vegetables) are based on the food consumption of Americans, with any food that represents 1% or more of the consumption from that group or subgroup included in the development of a nutrient profile. The nutrient profiles of each commodity group are the weighted averages of the nutrient content of foods in each food group based on consumption. Foods in their lowest fat form and with no added sugar were selected for determining the nutrient profile of each food group.

5. *Determining the daily intake amounts for each food group or subgroup.* Starting from the original Pyramid food pattern, the amounts of each food group or subgroup were increased or decreased in an iterative manner until the pattern for each calorie level achieved its nutritional goal or came within a reasonable range. After nutrient needs were met using foods in their lowest fat and no-added-sugar forms, the remaining calories needed to meet estimated energy needs were identified as "discretionary calories." These calories can be used to increase the amount of food from each group; to consume higher fat or added-sugar forms of foods; to add oil, fat, and sugars to foods; or to consume alcohol.

As a result of this process, new daily food intake patterns were created that meet the DRIs for almost all nutrients at all calorie-intake levels. The updated food intake patterns were released as part of *Dietary Guidelines for Americans* in 2005 (USDHHS/USDA, 2005). Table 3-1 shows the suggested daily amounts of food from each food group for three of the 12 calorie levels: (1) 1,600, (2) 2,000, and (3) 2,400. Table 3-2 identifies what counts as an equivalent amount of food for different food choices within each food group.

The food intake patterns (Table 3-1) list food group recommendations as total amounts in

Table 3-1
Food Intake Patterns

	Daily Amount of Food From Each Group (vegetable subgroup amounts are per week)		
Food Group	**1,600 Calories**	**2,000 Calories**	**2,400 Calories**
Fruits	1.5 cups	2 cups	2 cups
Vegetables	2 cups	2.5 cups	3 cups
Dark-green	2 cups/week	3 cups/week	3 cups/week
Orange	1.5 cups/week	2 cups/week	2 cups/week
Legumes	2.5 cups/week	3 cups/week	3 cups/week
Starchy	2.5 cups/week	3 cups/week	6 cups/week
Other	5.5 cups/week	6.5 cups/week	7 cups/week
Grains	5 oz-eq	6 oz-eq	8 oz-eq
Whole grains	3 oz-eq	3 oz-eq	4 oz-eq
Other	2 oz-eq	3 oz-eq	4 oz-eq
Lean meat and beans	5 oz-eq	5.5 oz-eq	6.5 oz-eq
Milk	3 cups	3 cups	3 cups
Oils	22 g	27 g	31 g
Discretionary calorie allowance	132 kcal	267 kcal	362 kcal

Condensed from U.S. Department of Agriculture/U.S. Department of Health and Human Services (USDHHS/USDA) (2005) Dietary Guidelines for Americans 2005, 6th ed. U.S. Government Printing Office, Washington, DC. Retrieved March 30, 2005, from *www.healthierus.gov/dietaryguidelines/*.
oz-eq, Ounce equivalent.
Note: The suggested amounts of food to consume from the basic food groups, subgroups, and oils to meet recommended nutrient intakes at three different calorie levels. Nutrient and energy contributions from each group are calculated according to the nutrient-dense forms of foods in each group (e.g., lean meats and fat-free milk). The table also shows the discretionary calorie allowance that can be accommodated within each calorie level, in addition to the suggested amounts of nutrient-dense forms of foods in each group.

Table 3-2
Equivalent Amounts for Foods Within Each Food Group

Food Group	Equivalent Amounts
Fruits	1/2 cup equivalent is: • 1/2 cup fresh, frozen, or canned fruit • 1 medium fruit • 1/4 cup dried fruit • 1/2 cup fruit juice
Vegetables	1/2 cup equivalent is: • 1/2 cup cut-up raw or cooked vegetable • 1 cup raw leafy vegetable • 1/2 cup vegetable juice
Grains	1 ounce-equivalent is: • 1 slice bread • 1 cup dry cereal • 1/2 cup cooked rice, pasta, cereal
Meat and beans	1 ounce-equivalent is: • 1 ounce cooked lean meats, poultry, fish • 1 egg • 1/4 cup cooked dry beans or tofu • 1 Tbsp peanut butter • 1/2 oz nuts or seeds
Milk	1 cup equivalent is: • 1 cup low-fat/fat-free milk, yogurt • 1/2 oz low-fat or fat-free natural cheese • 2 oz low-fat or fat-free processed cheese
Oils	1 tsp equivalent is: • 1 Tbsp low-fat mayo • 2 Tbsp light salad dressing • 1 tsp vegetable oil

Condensed from U.S. Department of Agriculture/U.S. Department of Health and Human Services (USDHHS/USDA) (2005) Dietary Guidelines for Americans 2005, 6th ed. U.S. Government Printing Office, Washington, DC. Retrieved March 30, 2005, from www.healthierus.gov/dietaryguidelines/.

household measures (e.g., cups or ounces), rather than in number of servings. USDA made this change to help address some of the confusion about what constitutes a "serving." In addition, the "portion" of a food someone chooses to eat may not equal what the government previously identified as a serving in the original Food Guide Pyramid. Care must be taken not to use how many portions someone eats as a way to assess how well his or her diet meets the recommendations. In fact, studies have shown the typical portion sizes eaten at home and away from home have increased over the years. It has been suggested that these larger portion sizes are contributing to the obesity epidemic (Rolls, 2003).

To help consumers put the new food intake patterns into practice in order to improve their food choices, a new symbol and interactive food guidance system called MyPyramid was developed and released shortly after the *Dietary Guidelines* in 2005 (USDA, 2005a). MyPyramid, with its slogan "Steps to a Healthier You," (Figure 3-2); emphasizes the need for a more individualized approach to improving diet and lifestyle. MyPyramid replaces the original Food Guide Pyramid, and, like its predecessor, it is not intended as a stand-alone educational tool. In fact, rather than trying to reflect the increased complexity of the new food intake patterns by adding more information to a visual image, the MyPyramid symbol has been made deliberately simple as a quick reminder to consumers to make healthful food choices and be active every day. The symbol was designed to illustrate personalization, gradual improvement, physical activity, variety, moderation, and proportionality.

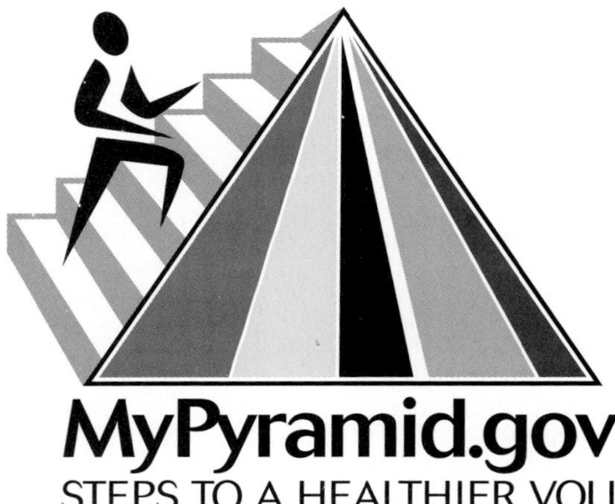

Figure 3-2 USDA'S MyPyramid. *(From USDA [2005] MyPyramid. Retrieved August 2, 2005 from www.mypyramid.gov.)*

Consumers can get more in-depth information and individualized guidance from the MyPyramid website (www.mypyramid.gov). The food guidance system also includes an education framework that explains *what* changes most Americans need to make in their eating and activity choices, *how* they can make these changes, and *why* these changes are important for health. Professionals can use the key concepts in this education framework to develop educational materials for various target audiences.

LIMITATIONS OF FOOD GUIDES

Despite the extensive research process used to develop the food intake patterns, this approach has several limitations (Dietary Guidelines Advisory Committee, 2005). As is true with all food guides, the adequacy of the diet still depends upon the food choices within food groups. Within each food group, foods vary in nutrient density (nutrients provided per kilocalorie). A poor diet could be selected consisting primarily of foods with low nutrient density that still satisfies the recommended quantities from each food group. Consumers also need to account for fats contained in milk products and meat, fats and sugars that are added when foods are processed or prepared, and calories from alcohol. These can add up to intakes of calories and saturated fats above amounts allowed. The "discretionary calorie" allowance provides for some additional fats and sugars, and for alcohol, but many consumers do not recognize the "extra" fats and sugars within their food choices.

Another limitation is that the food intake patterns are based on Americans' current consumption of foods within that group, and so the nutrient profile for a group may be relatively low in certain nutrients based on the typical choices within a group (e.g., meat over nuts). In addition, foods representative of diverse cultures and eating styles are not pictured. To address this, nutrition educators have adapted food guides to feature different foods so they can be used by culturally diverse audiences or by those who eat a vegetarian diet (Messina et al., 2003; Achterberg et al., 1994). In addition, food guides have been adapted to be more relevant for different age-groups, such as young children (USDA, 2005b) and older adults (Russell et al., 1999).

FOOD LABELS

NUTRITION INFORMATION ON FOOD LABELS

The MyPyramid food guidance system is only one tool to help Americans implement the *Dietary Guidelines;* food labels are another tool. Many consumers make food choices at the point of purchase, typically in a grocery store. The food label, which includes the "Nutrition Facts" panel, provides consumers with information about the ingredients and nutrients contained in individual foods. This information can be used to compare products and to assess how a particular food fits into the context of the total diet.

Nutrition information has been required on most packaged foods since 1994, although the government has been involved in the regulation of food labels since 1906 with the passage of the Federal Food and Drugs Act and the Federal Meat Inspection Act (USDHHS, 1993a). These laws gave the federal government the authority to regulate the safety and quality of food. The 1906 Federal Food and Drugs Act was replaced in 1938 with the Federal Food, Drug and Cosmetic Act, which prohibited any labeling that was false or misleading. In 1973, the Food and Drug Administration (FDA) issued regulations that required nutrition labeling on any food that made a claim about its nutritional properties or that contained any added nutrients. Nutrition information appeared on other foods as well, but it was done on a voluntary basis.

Following the publication of the *Surgeon General's Report on Nutrition and Health* (USDHHS, 1988) and the National Research Council's *Diet and Health* report (NRC, 1989b), the FDA and the USDA's Food Safety and Inspection Service (which regulates meat and poultry products) asked the Food and Nutrition Board of the National Research Council to make recommendations on how to improve food labels so they could be used to select healthful diets. Based on these and other recommendations, the FDA proposed new food labeling regulations in 1990, which required, among other things, mandatory nutrition labeling on most foods and standard rules for the use of health claims. In the same year, the Nutrition Labeling and Education Act (1990) was passed, which also required several changes in the food label, including mandatory nutrition labeling.

The FDA issued the final regulations implementing the Nutrition Labeling and Education Act in 1993 (USDHHS, 1993b). Although not required to do so by law, USDA's Food Safety and Inspection Service also issued new regulations at the same time mandating nutrition labeling on processed meat and poultry products and providing for voluntary nutrition information for raw meat and poultry products. Both sets of regulations went into effect in 1994.

The latest labeling regulations not only require that nutrition information be provided for more foods than in the past, but the required information has been modified to reflect current concerns about diet and health. In addition to information on total Calories (kilocalories), protein, carbohydrate, and fat, which was required on the former food label, information on calories from fat and the amounts of saturated fat, cholesterol, and dietary fiber are now required as part of the Nutrition Facts panel. More recent evidence about the health effects of *trans* fatty acids has led to a new requirement that *trans* fatty acid content must also be listed on the label as of January 2006 (USDHHS, 2003a). Figure 3-3 shows an example of a revised Nutrition Facts panel listing *trans* fat. The former label also required information on vitamin A, vitamin C, thiamin, riboflavin, niacin, calcium, and iron. The current food label makes the listing of thiamin, riboflavin, and niacin optional because there is less concern about getting adequate amounts of these three vitamins than in the past. Other values that are optional include Calories (kilocalories) from saturated fat, and the amounts of polyunsaturated fat, monounsaturated fat, potassium, soluble fiber, insoluble fiber, sugar alcohol, β-carotene, and other essential vitamins and minerals.

Nutrition Facts

Serving Size 1 cup (228g)
Servings Per Container 2

Amount Per Serving

Calories 260	Calories from Fat 120
	% Daily Value*
Total Fat 13g	**20%**
Saturated Fat 5g	**25%**
Trans Fat 2g	
Cholesterol 30mg	**10%**
Sodium 660mg	**28%**
Total Carbohydrate 31g	**10%**
Dietary Fiber 0g	**0%**
Sugars 5g	
Protein 5g	

Vitamin A 4% • Vitamin C 2%
Calcium 15% • Iron 4%

* Percent Daily Values are based on a 2,000 calorie diet. Your Daily Values may be higher or lower depending on your calorie needs:

	Calories:	2,000	2,500
Total Fat	Less than	65g	80g
Sat Fat	Less than	20g	25g
Cholesterol	Less than	300mg	300mg
Sodium	Less than	2,400mg	2,400mg
Total Carbohydrate		300g	375g
Dietary Fiber		25g	30g

Calories per gram:
Fat 9 • Carbohydrate 4 • Protein 4

Figure 3-3 Required format for nutrition information on food labels: The Nutrition Facts Panel. *(From USDHHS/FDA [2003] Examples of Revised Nutrition Facts Panel Listing Trans Fat. FDA/CFSAN, Rockville, MD. Retrieved February 1, 2005, from www.cfsan.fda.gov/~dms/labtr.html.)*

DAILY VALUES ON FOOD LABELS

As required by law, the nutrition information on the food label must be presented in a way that enables consumers to put the information into the context of the total daily diet. To meet this objective, nutrients are listed in terms of the percentage of Daily Value (DV) they provide. The DVs are based on two sets of reference values for nutrients: the Daily Reference Values (DRVs) and the Reference Daily Intakes (RDIs).

The DRVs were developed for nutrients, such as fat, carbohydrate, cholesterol, and fiber, for which no previous standards existed. The DRVs for the energy-providing nutrients are calculated based on the caloric content of the daily diet, which for labeling purposes was chosen as 2,000 kilocalories (Table 3-3). Reference Daily Intakes, which replaced the term U.S. Recommended Daily Allowances (U.S. RDA), provide reference values for certain vitamins and minerals (Table 3-4). The term Daily Value, which encompasses both DRVs and RDIs, is used on current food labels. The terms RDI and DV were chosen, in part, to eliminate the use of the term U.S. RDA, which was easily confused with the term RDA.

U.S. RDAs were the standard chosen in 1973 as a reference for the previous food label. The U.S. RDAs, which consisted of a single value for each nutrient to simplify their use on a food label, were based on the former RDAs, which consist of several values for each nutrient based on age and gender. The FDA used the 1968 RDAs as a basis for the U.S. RDAs and, in most cases, simply chose the highest value from the age/sex categories to cover those with the greatest need.

One of the purposes for developing the DRIs was to have a new set of reference values that could serve as the basis for nutrition labeling. An IOM committee was appointed by the USDA, USDHHS, and Health Canada to identify approaches on how the DRIs might be used for this purpose. In 2003 the committee issued a report containing 12 guiding principles for use in selecting reference values for nutrition

Table 3-3
Daily Reference Values (DRVs)*

Food Component	DRV
Fat	65 g
Saturated fatty acids	20 g
Cholesterol	300 mg
Total carbohydrate	300 g
Fiber	25 g
Sodium	2,400 mg
Potassium	3,500 mg
Protein†	50 g

From USDHHS (1993) Focus on Food Labeling. FDA Consumer Special Report. DHHS Publication No. [FDA] 93-2262. U.S. Government Printing Office, Washington, DC.
*Based on 2,000 kcal a day for adults and children older than 4 years only.
†DRV for protein does not apply to certain populations; Reference Daily Intake (RDI) for protein has been established for the following groups:

- Children 1 to 4 years: 16 g
- Infants under 1 year: 14 g
- Pregnant women: 60 g
- Nursing mothers: 65 g

Table 3-4
Reference Daily Intakes (RDIs)*

Nutrient	Amount
Vitamin A†	5,000 IU
Vitamin C	60 mg
Thiamin	1.5 mg
Riboflavin	1.7 mg
Niacin	20 mg
Calcium	1.0 g
Iron	18 mg
Vitamin D†	400 IU
Vitamin E†	30 IU
Vitamin B_6	2.0 mg
Folic acid	0.4 mg
Vitamin B_{12}	6 μg
Phosphorus	1.0 g
Iodine	150 μg
Magnesium	400 mg
Zinc	15 mg
Copper	2 mg
Biotin	0.3 mg
Pantothenic acid	10 mg

From USDHHS (1993) Focus on Food Labeling. FDA Consumer Special Report. DHHS Publication No. [FDA] 93-2262. U.S. Government Printing Office, Washington, DC.
*Based on The National Academy of Sciences' 1968 Recommended Dietary Allowances.
†To convert IU (International Units) to units in current use for other purposes, 1 IU of vitamin A = 0.30 μg of retinol equivalent; 1 IU of vitamin D = 0.025 μg of vitamin D_3; and 1 IU of vitamin E = 0.67 mg of α-tocopherol equivalents.

labeling. The guiding principles include the recommendations that nutrition information on food labels should continue to be expressed as percent Daily Value (%DV), that the DVs should be based on a population-weighted reference value, and that a population-weighted EAR should be the basis for DVs, or if no EAR has been set then a population-weighted AI should be used (IOM, 2003a). The U.S. and Canadian governments will be considering these principles in any revision of reference values for food labels.

SERVING SIZES ON FOOD LABELS

The nutrition information on a food label is based on a specified serving size. In the past, food manufacturers determined the serving size; under the current labeling regulations, serving sizes are more uniform and reflect the amount of that food customarily eaten at one time. The serving size does not necessarily represent the amount any given individual eats. Someone who eats more or less than the specified serving size of a given food will need to adjust the nutrition information accordingly.

The uniformity in serving sizes makes it easier for consumers to compare nutritional qualities of similar products than in the past. It also provides a consistent reference for nutrient content claims, such as "low fat" and "high fiber." The 1993 food labeling regulations provide standardized definitions for certain terms (USDHHS, 1993b). For example, a "low-fat" food must have 3 g or less of fat per serving, a "fat-free" food must have less than 0.5 g of fat per serving, a "low-sodium" food must have 140 mg or less of sodium per serving, and a "high-fiber" food must have 5 g or more of fiber per serving.

HEALTH CLAIMS ON FOOD LABELS

In addition to nutrient content claims, food labels may also carry certain health claims. These are claims that link the consumption of a food or nutrient with the prevention or reduction in risk of a certain disease. For years health claims were explicitly prohibited by federal regulations because any claim that a substance could affect the course of a disease was considered equivalent to a drug claim. That meant a food carrying a health claim on the label could be considered an unapproved new drug and technically could be seized. As the relationship between diet and disease became more established, the FDA modified its policy, as reflected in the 1993 regulations that allow specific health claims on food packages under certain conditions (USDHHS, 1993b). One condition is that the health claim must be based on significant scientific agreement by qualified experts. As of August 2005, the FDA has authorized the following health claims for food labels as meeting this criteria (USDHHS, 2000b):

- Calcium and osteoporosis
- Sodium and hypertension
- Dietary fat and cancer
- Dietary saturated fat and cholesterol and risk of coronary heart disease
- Fiber-containing grain products, fruits, and vegetables and cancer
- Fruits, vegetables, and grain products that contain fiber, particularly soluble fiber, and risk of coronary heart disease
- Fruits and vegetables and cancer
- Folate and neural tube defects
- Dietary sugar alcohol and dental caries
- Soluble fiber from certain foods (e.g., whole oats and psyllium seed husk) and risk of coronary heart disease
- Soy protein and risk of coronary heart disease
- Plant sterol/stanol esters and risk of coronary heart disease

The Food and Drug Administration Modernization Act (1997) provided a second way for health claims to be approved. In this case, health claims have to be based on "authoritative statements" from federal scientific bodies. Claims allowed under this category include the following (USDHHS, 2000b):

- Whole grain foods and risk of heart disease and certain cancers
- Potassium and the risk of high blood pressure and stroke

In 2002, the FDA allowed for another type of health claim to be used on food labels when there is only emerging evidence to suggest a relationship between a substance and a health-related condition (USDHHS, 2002). These are known as qualified health claims because a qualifying statement regarding the strength of the evidence is required on the label to prevent the claim from being misleading. For example, a qualified health claim about walnuts and heart disease requires the following statement (USDHHS, 2003b):

> Supportive but not conclusive research shows that eating 1.5 ounces per day of walnuts, as part of a low saturated fat and low cholesterol diet and not resulting in increased caloric intake, may reduce the risk of coronary heart disease. See nutrition information for fat [and calorie] content.

To help consumers better understand the level of evidence supporting a claim, the FDA has developed an interim evidence-based ranking system in order to systematically evaluate and rank the evidence. This ranking system assigns a rank, such as a letter grade, to every proposed qualified health claim. Claims earning the highest or "A" ranking would not need to be qualified, since they would meet the standard for significant scientific agreement. A "B" rank would mean there is good scientific evidence to support the claim, but that it is not conclusive. A "C" rank would mean the evidence is limited and not conclusive. Finally, a "D" rank would mean there is little scientific evidence to support the claim. The FDA is using this interim procedure until it can promulgate final regulations (USDHHS, 2003c).

LABELING OF DIETARY SUPPLEMENTS

The Nutrition Labeling and Education Act (1990) was originally intended to apply to both foods and dietary supplements, including vitamins, minerals, amino acids, herbs, and similar products. Controversy over the proposed rules on health claims affecting supplements led to the Dietary Supplement Act (1992), which exempted dietary supplements from any new labeling requirements for 1 year to allow for further discussion. Eventually the FDA issued regulations on January 4, 1994, stating that dietary supplements have to provide the same basic nutrition information as is found on labels of other foods (USDHHS, 1994). These regulations also state that health claims on dietary supplements are subject to the same approval process as is required for health claims on conventional food.

Dietary supplements are also permitted to carry qualified health claims, as described in the preceding text for foods. For example, a qualified health claim about selenium and cancer permitted on a dietary supplement label would require the following statement (USDHHS, 2003b):

> Selenium may reduce the risk of certain cancers. Some scientific evidence suggests that consumption of selenium may reduce the risk of certain forms of cancer. However, FDA has determined that this evidence is limited and not conclusive.

Other types of label claims, known as structure/function claims, are also allowed on dietary supplements. The Dietary Supplement Health and Education Act (1994) defines dietary supplement and allows manufacturers to make claims about a product's ability to affect the structure or function of the body or to affect a person's general well-being. "Calcium builds strong bones," and "fiber maintains bowel regularity" are examples of structure/function claims. Unlike health claims, structure/function claims do not need to be preapproved by the FDA, although they must still be truthful and not misleading. They must contain a "disclaimer" that the FDA has not evaluated the claim, and the manufacturer is required to notify the FDA about the statement no later than 30 days after the product is first marketed. The act also allows the FDA to remove unsafe supplements from the market, but it puts the burden of proof on the government to demonstrate that a supplement or its ingredients are unsafe. This policy is significantly different from the standards required of food additive and drug manufacturers, who must demonstrate the safety of their products *before* new products are allowed on the market.

REFERENCES

Achterberg C, McDonnell E, Bagby R (1994) How to put the Food Guide Pyramid into practice. J Am Diet Assoc 94:1030-1035.

American Dietetic Association (2004) Position of the American Dietetic Association: functional foods. J Am Diet Assoc 104:814-826.

Dietary Guidelines Advisory Committee (2005) Report of the Dietary Guidelines Advisory

Committee on the Dietary Guidelines for Americans, 2005. U.S. Department of Agriculture, Agricultural Research Service, Washington, DC. Retrieved March 28, 2005, from www.health.gov/dietaryguidelines/dga2005/report/.

Dietary Supplement Act of 1992, Public Law 102-571. 102nd Congress, 2nd session. October 29, 1992.

Dietary Supplement Health and Education Act of 1994, Public Law 103-417. 103rd Congress, 2nd session. October 25, 1994.

Food and Agriculture Organization/World Health Organization (FAO/WHO) Consultation (1996) Preparation and Use of Food-Based Dietary Guidelines. Nutrition Programme, WHO, Geneva. Retrieved August 3, 2005, from www.fao.org/docrep/x0243e/x0243e00.htm.

Food and Agriculture Organization/World Health Organization (FAO/WHO) Expert Consultation (2002) Human Vitamin and Mineral Requirements. FAO/WHO, Bangkok, Thailand. Retrieved March 28, 2005, from www.fao.org/docrep/004/y2809e/y2809e00.htm.

Food and Drug Administration Modernization Act of 1997, Public Law Public Law 105-115. 105th Congress. November 21, 1997.

Helsing E (1990) Problems in the process of formulating an RDI. Eur J Clin Nutr 44(Suppl 2): 33-36.

Hogbin M, Lyon J, Davis C (2003) Comparison of dietary recommendations using the Dietary Guidelines for Americans as a framework. Nutr Today 38(6):204-217.

Institute of Medicine (IOM) (1994) How Should the Recommended Dietary Allowances Be Revised? National Academy Press, Washington, DC.

Institute of Medicine (IOM) (1997) Dietary Reference Intakes for Calcium, Phosphorus, Magnesium, Vitamin D, and Fluoride. National Academy Press, Washington, DC.

Institute of Medicine (IOM) (1998) Dietary Reference Intakes for Thiamin, Riboflavin, Niacin, Vitamin B_6, Folate, Vitamin B_{12}, Pantothenic Acid, Biotin, and Choline. National Academy Press, Washington, DC.

Institute of Medicine (IOM) (2000a) Dietary Reference Intakes for Vitamin C, Vitamin E, Selenium and Carotenoids. National Academy Press, Washington, DC.

Institute of Medicine (IOM) (2000b) Dietary Reference Intakes: Applications in Dietary Assessment. National Academy Press, Washington, DC.

Institute of Medicine (IOM) (2001) Dietary Reference Intakes for Vitamin A, Vitamin K, Arsenic, Boron, Chromium, Copper, Iodine, Iron, Manganese, Molybdenum, Nickel, Silicon, Vanadium, and Zinc. National Academy Press, Washington, DC.

Institute of Medicine (IOM) (2002) Dietary Reference Intakes for Energy, Carbohydrate, Fiber, Fat, Fatty Acids, Cholesterol, Protein, and Amino Acids. National Academy Press, Washington, DC.

Institute of Medicine (IOM) (2003a) Dietary Reference Intakes: Guiding Principles for Nutrition Labeling and Fortification. National Academy Press, Washington, DC.

Institute of Medicine (IOM) (2003b) Dietary Reference Intakes: Applications in Dietary Planning. National Academy Press, Washington, DC.

Institute of Medicine (IOM) (2004) Dietary References Intakes for Water, Potassium, Sodium, Chloride, and Sulfate. National Academy Press, Washington, DC.

McMurry KY (2003) Setting dietary guidelines: the US process. J Am Diet Assoc 103(Suppl 2): S10-S16.

Messina V, Melina V, Mangels AR (2003) A new food guide for North American vegetarians. J Am Diet Assoc 103(6):771-775.

National Research Council (NRC) (1989a) Recommended Dietary Allowances, 10th ed. National Academy Press, Washington, DC.

National Research Council (NRC) (1989b) Diet and Health: Implications for Reducing Chronic Disease Risk. National Academy Press, Washington, DC.

Nutrition Labeling and Education Act of 1990, Public Law 101-535. 101st Congress, 2nd session. November 8, 1990.

Painter J, Rah J-H, Lee Y-K (2002) Comparison of international food guide pictorial representations. J Am Diet Assoc 102(4):483-489.

Rolls BJ (2003) The supersizing of America: portion size and the obesity epidemic. Nutr Today 38(2):42-53.

Russell RM, Rasmussen H, Lichtenstein AH (1999). Modified food guide pyramid for people over 70 years of age. J Nutr 129(3): 751-753.

Truswell AS (1990) The philosophy behind Recommended Dietary Intakes: can they be harmonized? Eur J Clin Nutr 44(Suppl 2):3-11.

U.S. Department of Agriculture (USDA) (1992) The Food Guide Pyramid. USDA Home and Garden Bulletin 252. U.S. Government Printing

Office, Washington, DC. Retrieved March 28, 2005, from www.usda.gov/cnpp/pyrabklt.pdf

U.S. Department of Agriculture (USDA) (1993) USDA's Food Guide: Background and Development. USDA Miscellaneous Publication No. 1514. U.S. Government Printing Office, Washington, DC. Retrieved March 28, 2005, from www.usda.gov/cnpp/Pubs/Pyramid/FoodGuideDevt.pdf

U.S. Department of Agriculture (USDA) (2003) Backgrounder for revision of Food Guide Pyramid. September 10, 2003. USDA, Washington, DC. Retrieved March 28, 2005, from www.usda.gov/cnpp/pyramid-update/FGP%20docs/FGPBackgrounder%20revised.pdf

U.S. Department of Agriculture (USDA) (2005a) Johanns reveals USDA's Steps to a Healthier You. USDA press release, April 19, 2005, Retrived August 3, 2005 from www.mypyramid.gov/global_nav/media_press_release.html

U.S. Department of Agriculture (USDA) (2005b). Johanns unveils MyPyramid for kids. USDA press release, September 28, 2005. Retrieved November 7, 2005 from www.mypyramid.gov/global_nav/media_kids_press_release.html

U.S. Department of Health and Human Services (USDHHS) (1988) The Surgeon General's Report on Nutrition and Health. DHHS Publication No. (PHS) 88-50210. U.S. Government Printing Office, Washington, DC.

U.S. Department of Health and Human Services (USDHHS) (1993a) Focus on Food Labeling. FDA Consumer Special Report. DHHS Publication No. (FDA) 93-2262. U.S. Government Printing Office, Washington, DC. Retrieved March 28, 2005, from www.fda.gov/fdac/special/foodlabel/food_toc.html

U.S. Department of Health and Human Services (USDHHS) (1993b). Food labeling; General provisions; Nutrition labeling; Label format; Nutrient content claims; Health claims; Ingredient labeling; State and local requirements and exemptions; Final rules. Fed Reg 58:2066-2941.

U.S. Department of Health and Human Services (USDHHS) (1994) Dietary supplements; Establishment of date of application. Fed Reg 61:350-437.

U.S. Department of Health and Human Services (USDHHS) (1996) Food Standards: Amendment of standards of identity for enriched grain products to require addition of folic acid. Fed Reg 61:8781-8797.

U.S. Department of Health and Human Services (USDHHS) (2000a) Healthy People 2010: Understanding and Improving Health, 2nd ed. U.S. Government Printing Office, Washington, DC. Retrieved March 28, 2005, from www.healthypeople.gov/

U.S. Department of Health and Human Services (USDHHS) (2000b). A Food Labeling Guide: Appendix C—Health Claims. Food and Drug Administration, Rockville, MD. Retrieved March 28, 2005, from www.cfsan.fda.gov/~dms/flg-6c.html

U.S. Department of Health and Human Services (USDHHS) (2002) Qualified Health Claims in the Labeling of Conventional Foods and Dietary Supplements. Food and Drug Administration, Rockville, MD. Retrieved March 28, 2005, from www.cfsan.fda.gov/~dms/hclmgui2.html

U.S. Department of Health and Human Services (USDHHS) (2003a) Food Labeling; Trans fatty acids in nutrition labeling; Consumer research to consider nutrient content and health claims and possible footnote or disclosure statements; Final rule and proposed rule. Fed Reg 68:41433-41506.

U.S. Department of Health and Human Services (USDHHS) (2003b) Summary of Qualified Health Claims Permitted. Food and Drug Administration, Rockville, MD. Retrieved March 28, 2005, from www.cfsan.fda.gov/~dms/qhc-sum.html

U.S. Department of Health and Human Services (USDHHS) (2003c) Interim Procedures for Qualified Health Claims in the Labeling of Conventional Human Food and Human Dietary Supplements. Food and Drug Administration, Rockville, MD. Retrieved March 28, 2005, from www.cfsan.fda.gov/~dms/hclmgui3.html

U.S. Department of Health and Human Services/U.S. Department of Agriculture (USDHHS/USDA) (2005) Dietary Guidelines for Americans 2005, 6th ed. U.S. Government Printing Office, Washington, DC. Retrieved March 28, 2005, from www.healthierus.gov/dietaryguidelines

United States Senate Select Committee on Nutrition and Human Needs (1977) Dietary Goals for the United States, 2nd ed. U.S. Government Printing Office, Washington, DC.

World Health Organization/Food and Agriculture Organization (WHO/FAO) Expert Consultation (2003) Diet, Nutrition and the Prevention of

Chronic Diseases. WHO Technical Report Series 916. WHO, Geneva. Retrieved March 28, 2005, from www.who.int/nut/documents/trs_916.pdf.

RECOMMENDED READINGS

Anderson GH, Black R, Harris, E (eds) (2003) Dietary Guidelines: past experiences and new approaches. J Am Diet Assoc 103(Suppl 2):S1-S59.

Dietary Guidelines Advisory Committee (2000) Report of the Dietary Guidelines Advisory Committee on the Dietary Guidelines for Americans, 2000. U.S. Department of Agriculture, Agricultural Research Service, National Technical Information Service, Springfield, VA. Retrieved March 28, 2005, from www.usda.gov/cnpp/Pubs/DG2000/Full%20Report.pdf.

Goldberg JP, Belury MA, Elam P, Calvert Finn S, Hayes D, Lyle R, St. Jeor S, Warren M, Hellwig JP (2004) The obesity crisis: don't blame it on the Pyramid. J Am Diet Assoc 104(7):1141-1147.

RECOMMENDED WEBSITES

National Academy of Sciences, Institute of Medicine, Food and Nutrition Board

Links to information about the Dietary Reference Intakes

www.iom.edu/project.asp?id=4574

U.S. Department of Agriculture, Center for Nutrition Policy and Promotion

Links to information about the Dietary Guidelines and MyPyramid

www.cnpp.usda.gov/

U.S. Department of Health and Human Services, Food and Drug Administration, Food Labeling and Nutrition

Links to information about labeling of foods and dietary supplements

www.cfsan.fda.gov/label.html

Unit II

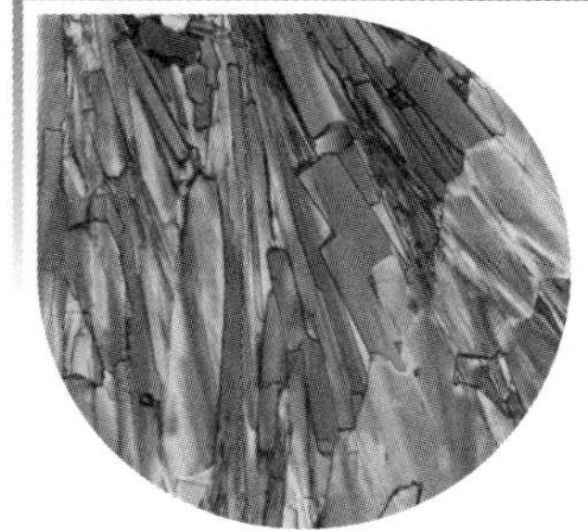

Structure and Properties of the Macronutrients

The organic macronutrients are carbon compounds synthesized by living organisms. They include carbohydrates, proteins or amino acids, and lipids. In the individual chapters in this unit on the structure and properties of the organic macronutrients, specific compounds in each class are described, both from the viewpoint of dietary macronutrients and of organic compounds formed in the human body during metabolism of carbohydrates, proteins and amino acids, and lipids. Compounds in the fourth group of organic nutrients, the vitamins, are micronutrients and are considered in Unit VI. Organic macronutrients are required in large amounts and are sources of energy for the body.

Like all organic compounds, proteins, carbohydrates, and lipids are made up largely of six elements: (1) hydrogen, (2) oxygen, (3) carbon, and (4) nitrogen along with some (5) phosphorus and (6) sulfur. These six relatively small elements with atomic weights less than or equal to 32, make up the structure of proteins, carbohydrates, lipids, and vitamins, as well as nucleic acids and intermediates of metabolism. If water (H_2O), which makes up approximately 63% of the human body, is not considered, carbon, oxygen, hydrogen, and nitrogen (in organic compounds) make up 88.5% of the "dry weight" of the human body; these elements are present in about 11 kg of protein, 10 kg of fat, and 0.6 kg of carbohydrate (mainly glycogen) in a 65-kg man.

The ability of carbon to form carbon-to-carbon bonds, extended carbon chains, and cyclic compounds permits the formation of a myriad of organic compounds; the structures of a number of these compounds are considered in this unit. In organic molecules, the atoms of carbon, hydrogen, oxygen, phosphorus, and sulfur are held together by covalent bonds, which are formed when two atoms share a pair of outer orbital electrons. Each covalent bond of every molecule represents a small amount of stored energy, thereby allowing organic molecules to serve as a source of energy to the body. Units III, IV, and V describe the processes involved in the assimilation of dietary organic macronutrients, how these are used by the body for growth and maintenance via synthesis of the structural and functional components of the human body, and how these macronutrients are used as fuels with conversion of excess substrate to stored fuels for subsequent use.

Martha H. Stipanuk

Chapter 4

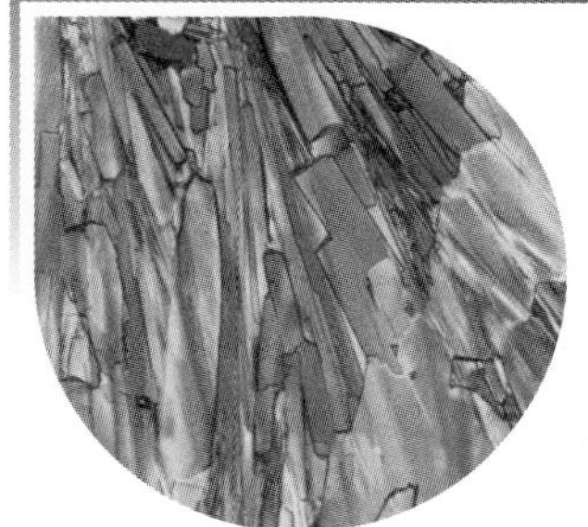

Structure, Nomenclature, and Properties of Carbohydrates

Betty A. Lewis, PhD, and Martha H. Stipanuk, PhD

OUTLINE

CLASSIFICATION, STRUCTURES, AND NOMENCLATURE OF THE MONOSACCHARIDES

Carbohydrates are the most abundant organic components in most fruits, vegetables, legumes, and cereal grains, and they provide texture and flavor in many processed foods. They are the major energy source for humans by digestion and absorption in the small intestine and, to a lesser extent, by microbial fermentation in the large intestine. Food carbohydrates are often classified as available or unavailable carbohydrates. Available carbohydrates are those that are hydrolyzed by enzymes of the human gastrointestinal tract to monosaccharides that are absorbed in the small intestine and enter the pathways of carbohydrate metabolism. Unavailable carbohydrates are not hydrolyzed by human digestive enzymes, but they may be fermented by bacteria in the large intestine to varying extents, forming short-chain fatty acids that may be absorbed and contribute to the body's energy needs. Glucose is an essential energy source for human tissues; some types of cells such as red blood cells are not able to use other fuels. Glucose for the body's use may be derived from dietary starch, sucrose, and lactose; from glycogen stores in the body; or from synthesis in vivo from gluconeogenic precursors such as amino acid carbon skeletons. Glucose also serves as a precursor for synthesis of all other carbohydrates including lactose produced by the mammary gland; the ribose needed for nucleic acid synthesis; and the sugar residues that are found as covalently bound constituents of glycoproteins, glycolipids, and proteoglycans in the body.

CLASSIFICATION

Carbohydrates are defined as polyhydroxy aldehydes (the aldoses) and ketones (the ketoses) and derivatives of these sugars. This definition emphasizes the hydrophilic nature of most carbohydrates and allows inclusion of sugar alcohols (alditols), sugar acids (uronic, aldonic, and aldaric acids), glycosides, and polymerized products (oligosaccharides and polysaccharides having linkages of the acetal type) among the classes of carbohydrates. The hydroxyl groups of carbohydrates may be modified by substitution with other groups to give esters and ethers or replaced to give deoxy and amino sugars. Carbohydrates are also covalently bound to many proteins and lipids. These glycoconjugates include the glycoproteins, proteoglycans, and glycolipids.

Aldoses and ketoses are monosaccharides (also called sugars). Monosaccharides are further classified by the number of carbon atoms in their structures (the trioses, tetroses, pentoses, hexoses, heptoses, octoses, and nonoses), by their stereochemistry (D or L), and by the degree to which they may be polymerized (disaccharides, oligosaccharides, and polysaccharides). The nutritionally important glucose is a D-aldohexose monosaccharide.

STRUCTURES OF THE ALDOSES AND KETOSES

D-Aldoses are related to D-glyceraldehyde, as can be illustrated by their chemical synthesis from D-glyceraldehyde (Fig. 4-1). L-Aldoses are similarly related to L-glyceraldehyde. In this synthetic scheme, a nucleophilic cyanide ion (:CN) adds to the carbonyl double bond (C-1) of glyceraldehyde, giving two cyanohydrin products. Selective reduction and hydrolysis of the CN group to an aldehyde completes the conversion of the triose D-glyceraldehyde to the pair of aldotetroses having a new chiral carbon at C-2. A chiral carbon atom is one that is bonded to four different groups. Accordingly, this reaction scheme lengthens the carbon chain from the carbonyl end, giving two new aldoses the last three carbons of which derive from glyceraldehyde. Therefore, the configuration of the hydroxyl on the highest numbered chiral carbon of an aldose or ketose determines D or L status. For a D-sugar, this hydroxyl is to the right of the carbon chain in the Fischer formula. Each cycle of the synthesis creates a new chiral center at C-2 and a pair of stereoisomers. Accordingly, there are two tetroses, four pentoses, and eight hexoses in the D- (see Fig. 4-1) and also in the L-series; not all of these occur commonly in nature. L-Sugars are mirror images (enantiomers) of the D-sugars, with the configuration of all chiral carbons reversed (e.g., D-glucose and L-glucose). Sugars that vary in their configuration at only one carbon are epimers. Thus, glucose and galactose are C-4 epimers, and enzymes that catalyze epimer formation are called epimerases.

In the common ketoses (Fig. 4-2), the carbonyl group is usually at C-2, but other ketoses occur as well. A few ketoses, such as fructose, are known by their trivial names, but ketoses also are named systematically with the suffix "-ulose" denoting a ketose sugar. In this nomenclature, a group of up to four consecutive chiral carbons is named after the aldose (e.g., triose, tetrose, pentose, or hexose) possessing this chiral group, and the number of carbon atoms is designated also. D-Fructose is the most common ketose, and its systematic name is D-*arabino*-hexulose, showing that the three chiral carbons in D-fructose have the same configuration as those in D-arabinose. Frequently, the names ribulose and xylulose are used for the two ketopentoses. Their correct systematic names, however, are D-*erythro*-pentulose and D-*threo*-pentulose, respectively, showing that they have only two chiral carbons.

Although the common monosaccharides are pentoses and hexoses, sugars with more than six carbon atoms also occur naturally. Some have trivial names, but most sugars having more than six carbons and possessing four or

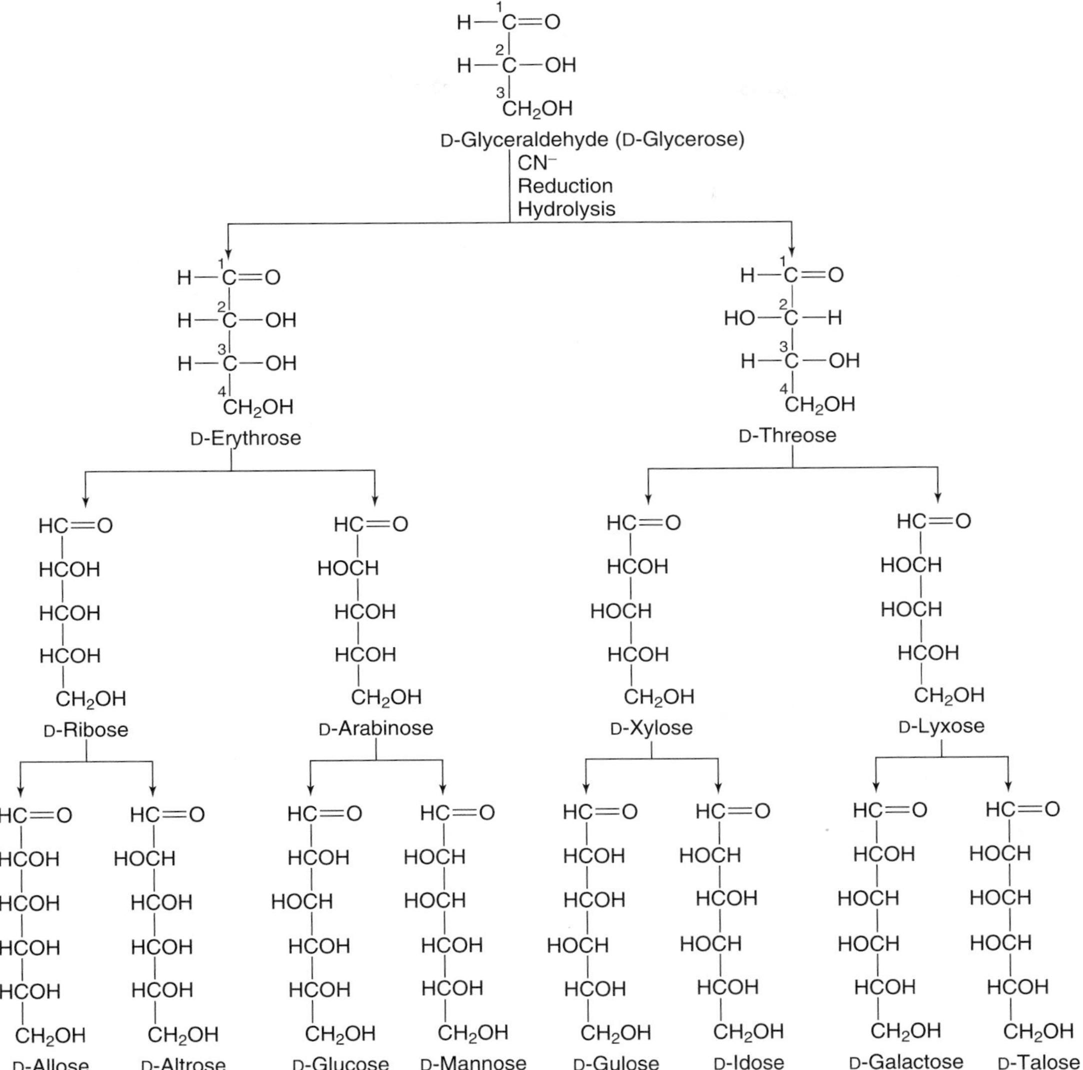

Figure 4-1 Structures of the D-aldoses (tetroses, pentoses, and hexoses) showing their derivation from D-glyceraldehyde by chemical synthesis. At each application of this reaction scheme, the :CN anion adds to the carbonyl carbon, lengthening the carbon chain by one carbon and creating a new chiral center at C-2 and a new pair of isomers. Reduction and hydrolysis of the :CN group restore the aldehyde function.

more chiral carbons are named systematically, as described in the preceding text for the ketoses. Sedoheptulose (D-*altro*-heptulose), a seven-carbon sugar, and the other ketoses shown in Figure 4-2 are involved as phosphorylated intermediates in carbohydrate metabolism. *N*-Acetylneuraminic acid, a nine-carbon acidic ketose, is an important signaling epitope in glycoproteins.

The abbreviations or symbols for the sugars usually consist of the first three letters of their names (Table 4-1). Glucose (Glc) and some ketoses are exceptions to this rule.

CYCLIC AND CONFORMATIONAL STRUCTURES

Aldoses and ketoses are more stable in their five- or six-membered cyclic hemiacetal form than in acyclic form. Cyclization of an aldose occurs via an intramolecular reaction of the nucleophilic hydroxyl group on C-4 or C-5 with the C-1 aldehyde (Fig. 4-3). This spontaneous reaction transforms the carbonyl carbon (C-1 of an aldose) into a chiral carbon (the anomeric carbon), giving new isomers: the α- and β-anomers of both the furanose and pyranose ring forms. The same type of cyclization reaction occurs with the ketoses in

CH_2OH	CH_2OH	CH_2OH	CH_2OH
C=O	C=O	C=O	C=O
HCOH	HOCH	HOCH	HOCH
HCOH	HCOH	HCOH	HCOH
CH_2OH	CH_2OH	HCOH	HCOH
		CH_2OH	HCOH
			CH_2OH
D-Ribulose	D-Xylulose	D-Fructose	D-Sedoheptulose
(D-*erythro*-pentulose)	(D-*threo*-pentulose)	(D-*arabino*-hexulose)	(D-*altro*-heptulose)

Figure 4-2 Physiologically important ketoses and their common names. Systematic names are shown in parentheses.

Nutrition Insight

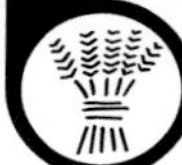

Corn Syrups: A Major Source of Dietary Sugars

The development of various types of corn syrups and maltodextrins from corn starch sources has brought about major changes in the food industry. Starch is separated from other parts of the corn kernels and is then hydrolyzed by acid- or enzyme-catalyzed processes to produce a mixture of glucose and glucose oligosaccharides. Corn syrups or maltodextrins with various degrees of hydrolysis are produced and classified according to reducing sugar content; the higher the reducing sugar value, the greater the degree of hydrolysis and the smaller the oligosaccharides.

More recently, a glucose isomerase has been used to convert some of the glucose in corn syrup to fructose to produce high-fructose corn syrups. If a higher percentage of fructose is desired, fructose is chromatographically separated and then back mixed to produce a syrup with the desired fructose concentration. High fructose corn syrup is classified according to its fructose content (e.g., 42%, 55%). High fructose corn syrup is listed as Generally Recognized as Safe (GRAS) for use by the food industry in the United States on the basis that its saccharide composition (glucose to fructose ratio) is approximately the same as that of honey, invert sugar, and the disaccharide sucrose. Several features of high-fructose corn syrup have led to its widespread use as a sweetening agent in processed foods. On a weight basis, glucose is less sweet than sucrose, whereas fructose is sweeter. Fructose is also twice as soluble as glucose at low temperatures. Thus conversion of half of the glucose to fructose produces a syrup that is more stable and sweeter than a glucose solution of the same sugar concentration. In addition, high-fructose corn syrup is less expensive than sucrose (sugar).

Because fructose is processed differently in the body than the more common sugar, glucose, and bypasses many of the regulatory sites for glucose uptake and metabolism, there is concern that high intakes of either sucrose or high-fructose corn syrup may have adverse effects in terms of obesity and diabetes beyond those associated with the intake of calories from refined products. The basis of these concerns is addressed more fully in Chapter 12.

which the C-5 or C-6 hydroxyl group reacts with the C-2 ketose carbonyl. In the Fischer formula, the hemiacetal (anomeric) –OH of the α-anomer is on the same side of the carbon chain as the D designator oxygen (e.g., C5–O– of a hexose). In aqueous solution, the acyclic and cyclic isomers are in equilibrium, with the most energetically stable isomers predominating. For most aldoses, the six-membered pyranose ring is more stable than the five-membered furanose ring. However, some sugars, including arabinose, ribose, and fructose, frequently occur in the furanose ring form in disaccharides, oligosaccharides, and polymers. The equilibrium nature of the hemiacetal reaction dictates that all hydroxyls and the carbonyl group can undergo reactions, that is, the sugar can react in acyclic or in ring form.

Sugar ring structures are depicted in several ways, as shown for glucose and fructose (Fig. 4-4). The Fischer projection formula is based on the convention that the carbons are either in the plane of the paper or in back of

Table 4-1
Abbreviated Names for Some Common Carbohydrates

Name	Abbreviation
Arabinose	Ara
Fructose	Fru
Fucose	Fuc
Galactose	Gal
Galacturonic acid	GalA
N-Acetylgalactosamine	GalNAc
Glucose	Glc
Glucuronic acid	GlcA
N-Acetylglucosamine	GlcNAc
Iduronic acid	IdoA
Mannose	Man
N-Acetylneuraminic acid	Neu5Ac
Rhamnose	Rha
Xylose	Xyl

Abbreviations for di-, oligo-, and polysaccharides often add D- or L- to indicate the enantiomeric form, *p* or *f* to indicate the pyranose or furanose ring form, α- or β- to indicate the stereochemistry of the glycosidic linkage, and carbon numbers to indicate the carbon atoms that are *O*-linked by the glycosidic bond. The designation is often omitted for the more common D-enantiomers and *p*-ring form.

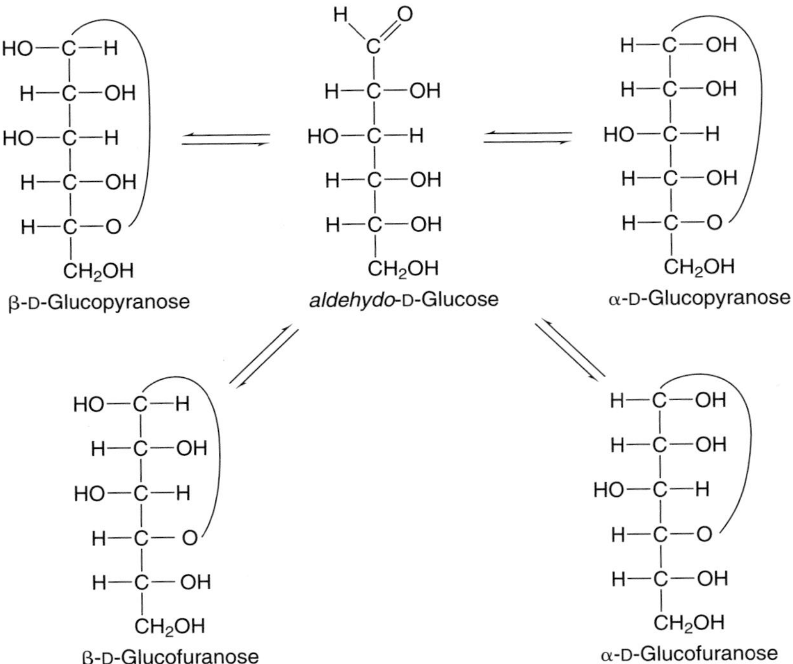

Figure 4-3 The equilibrium mixture of cyclic anomeric and acyclic forms of D-glucose in aqueous solution.

β-D-Glucopyranose:

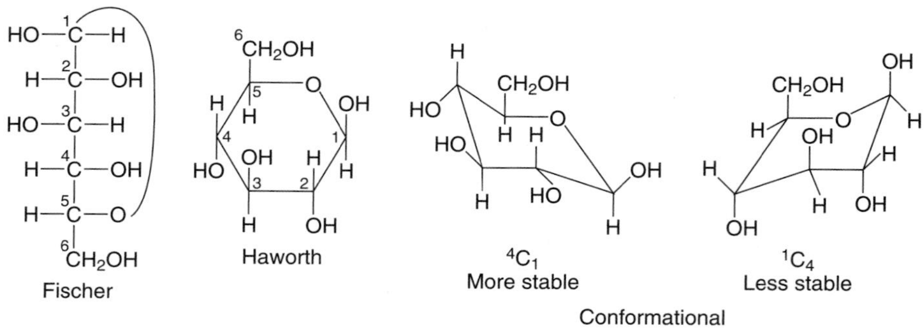

Fischer

Haworth

$^4C_1$ More stable

$^1C_4$ Less stable

Conformational

β-D-Fructofuranose:

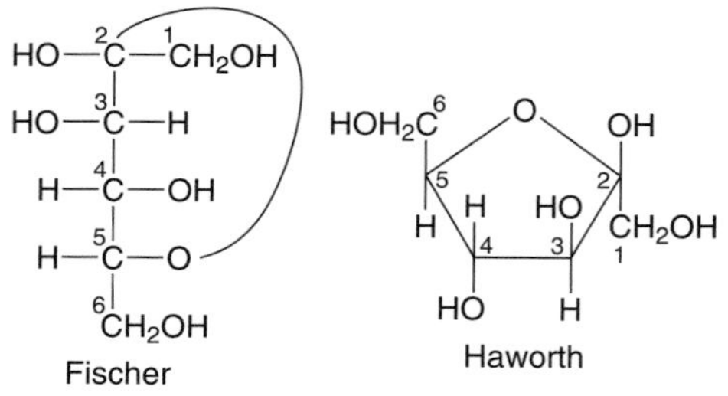

Fischer

Haworth

Figure 4-4 Representations of the cyclic structures of β-D-glucopyranose and β-D-fructofuranose. The chair conformations are designated "C" with a superscript number on the left that indicates the number of the sugar carbon that lies above the plane, and with a subscript number on the right that indicates the number of the sugar carbon that lies below the plane. The other three ring carbons and the ring oxygen lie within the plane.

the plane (never in front). The Haworth formula was introduced as a more realistic depiction of the bond lengths in the cyclic sugars. Hydroxyl groups on the right of the carbon chain in the Fischer projection are below the plane of the ring in the Haworth formula. The exocyclic group (the $-CH_2OH$ group of aldohexopyranoses, for example) is placed above or below the plane in the Haworth formula, depending on the origin of the ring oxygen (C-4 or C-5 for glucofuranose or pyranose, respectively, and C-5 for fructofuranose). If the ring connects from a hydroxyl group on the right of the carbon chain in the Fischer structure, then the exocyclic group is above the plane in the Haworth structure.

Because five- and six-membered rings are not planar, the chair conformational formula is preferred for showing spatial relationships, such as in enzyme-catalyzed reactions where fit of substrate to enzyme binding site is important.

In chair conformations, C-2, C-3, C-5, and the ring oxygen are planar, and C-1 and C-4 are out of the plane and on opposite sides of the plane. The orientations of the hydroxyls are axial or equatorial. Pyranose sugars assume a chair conformation based in part on maximizing the number of large groups (–OH and $-CH_2OH$) at equatorial positions, which are less sterically hindered than are axial positions. Thus the $^4C_1$ conformation, in which C-4 is above and C-1 is below the plane, is preferred (lower energy) for α- and β-D-glucopyranose and most of the other aldohexoses.

CHEMICAL REACTIVITY OF THE MONOSACCHARIDES

Sugars are relatively stable when pure and dry. In solution, their alcohol, aldehyde, and keto groups are involved in various reactions that are both nonenzymatic and enzymatic.

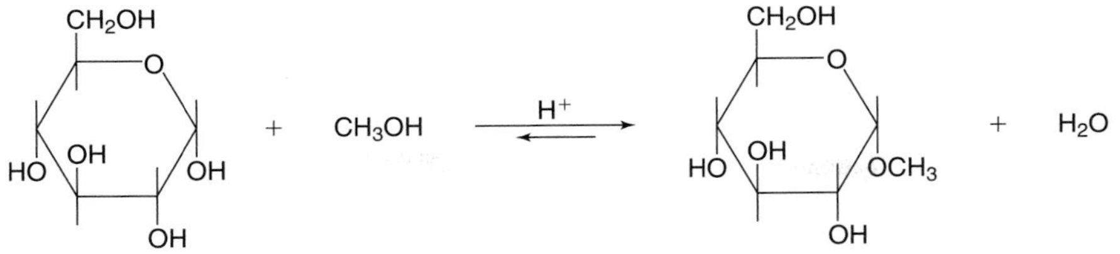

CH_2OH ... + CH_3OH $\underset{}{\overset{H^+}{\rightleftharpoons}}$ ... OCH_3 + H_2O

Methyl α-D-Glucopyranoside

Figure 4-5 Reactions of sugars with alcohols. Acid-catalyzed synthesis of the glycoside methyl α-D-glucopyranoside. This reaction is reversible. The glycosidic bond is hydrolyzed by cleavage between the anomeric carbon of the glucosyl group and the oxygen of the bond.

GENERAL REACTIVITY OF SUGARS

Aldoses are reducing agents, and the carbonyl group of an aldose is simultaneously oxidized to a carboxyl group when aldoses act as reducing agents. Ketoses are not good reducing agents because simultaneous oxidation of the carbonyl would require carbon chain cleavage. However, ketoses can isomerize to aldoses in an alkaline reducing sugar test and therefore result in a positive reducing sugar test even though they are nonreducing sugars. Formerly glucose in urine was analyzed by an assay for reducing sugars, but more specific methods are now available. In vivo, oxidation of the aldehyde group of glucose is catalyzed enzymatically by a dehydrogenase, and this reaction yields the lactone (an intramolecular ester of the newly formed carboxylic acid) as the product. An example of this type of reaction is the conversion of glucose-6-phosphate to 6-phosphoglucono-δ-lactone in the pentose phosphate pathway of metabolism (see Chapter 12, Fig. 12-20).

The carbonyl group of an aldose or ketose is readily reduced to an alcohol by chemical catalysis, giving an alditol from an aldose or an epimeric pair of alditols from a ketose. These alditols, absent the carbonyl group, are more stable than the aldoses and ketoses, and they are not reducing agents. Aldehyde reductases catalyze a similar reduction in vivo (e.g., in conversion of glucose to sorbitol [glucitol]). The carbon proton adjacent to the carbonyl (i.e., the α-carbon proton) in aldoses is acidic and easily abstracted in basic solution, leading to epimerization of the aldoses at C-2 as well as isomerization to ketoses. Thus, glucose is epimerized to mannose and isomerized to fructose. Similar reactions occur in carbohydrate metabolism, as seen in the phosphoglucose isomerase–catalyzed conversion of glucose-6-phosphate to fructose-6-phosphate (see Chapter 12, Fig. 12-3). Similar reactions occur with ketoses. Hydroxyl groups of carbohydrates are readily converted into a variety of esters, but the phosphate esters of the monosaccharides are particularly important as intermediates in metabolism. Sugar phosphates are also components of biologic polymers. This is illustrated by the nucleic acids, which have ribose and 2-deoxyribose phosphates as key constituents. Other derivatives of hydroxyls, including ethers, are also important in modification of monosaccharides in living systems and contribute to the diversity of carbohydrate structure.

FORMATION OF GLYCOSIDIC LINKAGES

Sugars react intermolecularly with alcohols under appropriate catalysis, forming α- and β-glycosides as shown in Figure 4-5 for the acid-catalyzed synthesis of methyl α-D-glucopyranoside. The alcohol may be aliphatic, aromatic, or another sugar. When properly activated, sugars react with each other to form specific oligosaccharides and polysaccharides. Thus, the sugar units in oligosaccharides and polysaccharides are linked by *O*-glycosidic bonds. Sugars also react with amines or thiols to give *N*- or *S*-glycosides, respectively. Therefore, β-D-ribose and 2-deoxy-β-D-ribose in nucleic acids are bonded to purines and pyrimidines by *N*-glycosidic bonds. In uridine diphosphate (UDP)–glucose, the β-D-ribose is linked to uracil by an *N*-glycosidic bond, and the α-D-glucose and β-D-ribose units are each ester-linked to phosphate, as shown in Figure 4-6. The sugar nucleotides are used extensively in vivo for enzymatic synthesis of carbohydrates, including lactose and glycogen. In glycoproteins, the oligosaccharide chains are linked to the β-carboxamide nitrogen of asparagine (an *N*-glycosidic bond) or to the hydroxyl of serine/threonine (an *O*-glycosidic bond). Plants use the glycosidic bond extensively in synthesizing different glycosides, many of which are physiologically active. Various hydroxylated compounds are glycosylated in the liver and excreted as glucuronic acid glycosides (β-D-glucuronides), which is a major means of detoxification and excretion.

Glycosides are more stable than aldoses and ketoses in several respects. The carbonyl/hemiacetal carbon is protected from base-catalyzed reactions and from reduction and oxidation. The pyranose and furanose ring structures and the anomeric configuration are also stabilized and do not undergo the interconversions shown in Figure 4-3. However, the glycosidic bonds can be hydrolyzed by acid or enzyme catalysis releasing the free sugar and the alcohol (with the alcohol often being another sugar molecule). Glycosidases, which catalyze hydrolysis of glycosides, have high specificity for the sugar and the anomeric linkage (α or β) but lower specificity for the alcohol unit (the aglycone).

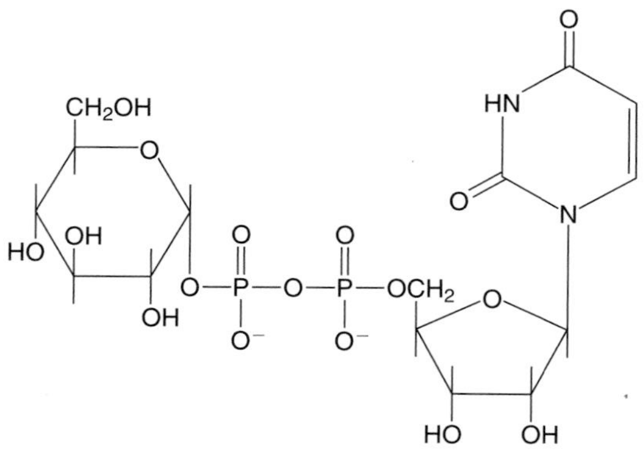

Figure 4-6 The structure of uridine diphosphate (UDP)–glucose (UDPG), an activated form of glucose and an intermediate in the synthesis of glycogen in vivo. In this structure, β-D-ribose is linked to the amine uracil by an *N*-glycosidic bond, and the α-D-glucose unit is esterified to phosphate.

MAILLARD REACTION OF REDUCING SUGARS WITH AMINES

Aldoses and ketoses react with aliphatic primary and secondary amines (including amino acids and proteins) to form *N*-glycosides, which readily dehydrate to the respective Schiff base by the Maillard reaction, as shown in Figure 4-7 (reactions *i* and *ii*). The aldose

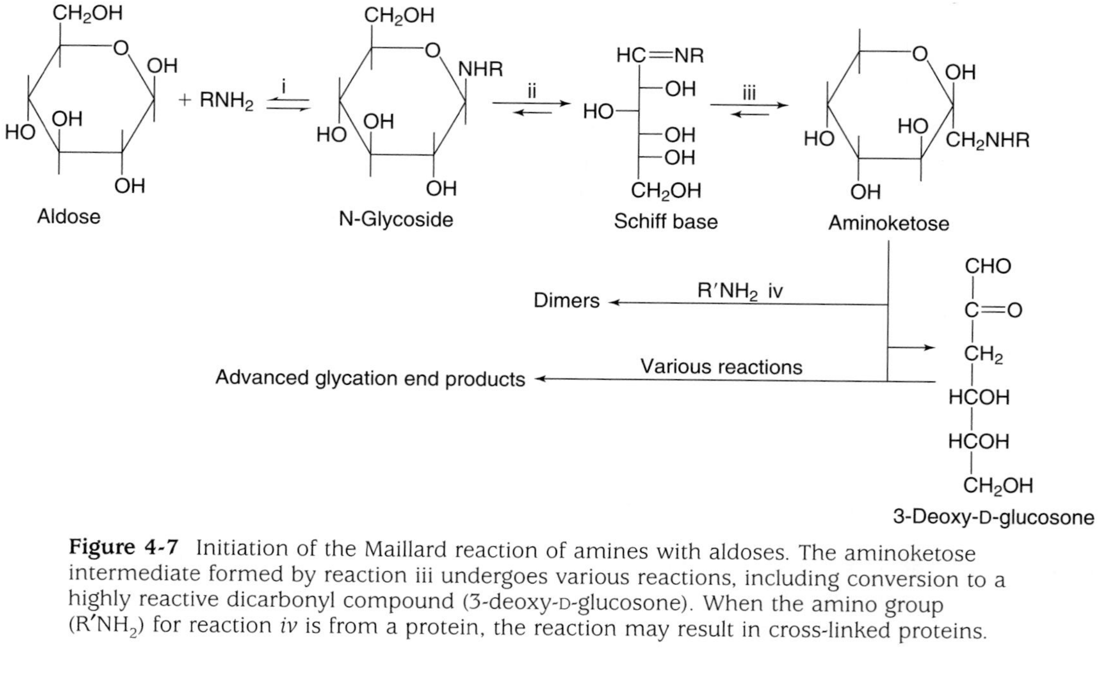

Figure 4-7 Initiation of the Maillard reaction of amines with aldoses. The aminoketose intermediate formed by reaction iii undergoes various reactions, including conversion to a highly reactive dicarbonyl compound (3-deoxy-D-glucosone). When the amino group ($R'NH_2$) for reaction *iv* is from a protein, the reaction may result in cross-linked proteins.

Schiff base spontaneously undergoes an Amadori rearrangement at C-1 and C-2, giving a substituted 1-amino-1-deoxyketose (reaction *iii*); a ketose Schiff base will rearrange to a substituted 2-amino-2-deoxyaldose. These sugar amines undergo additional very complex reactions, leading to highly reactive dicarbonyls (such as 3-deoxy-D-glucosone), cross-linking of proteins (as in reaction *iv*), fluorescent compounds and brown pigments, and to low-molecular-weight compounds, some of which are useful flavoring agents. The Maillard and subsequent reactions occur in food systems such as powdered or evaporated milk during processing or storage, giving off-white colors and decreasing the nutritive value of the proteins. Loss of lysine accounts for only part of the decrease in nutritive value. Although the Maillard complex of reactions has been studied extensively, the reactions are understood only in part. Realization that these reactions occur under physiological conditions in vivo has come more recently, and this is now an active area of research (Brownlee, 1995; Baynes and Monnier, 1989). The reaction of glucose with hemoglobin was discovered first. Plasma glucose reacts with hemoglobins via the Maillard reaction, and the modified protein, detected by gel electrophoresis, is an indicator of plasma glucose levels in diabetics over the lifespan of the erythrocytes. The term "glycated" protein is used to distinguish these Maillard-derived, carbohydrate-modified proteins from true glycosylated proteins (glycoproteins).

OTHER CLASSES OF CARBOHYDRATES

Monosaccharides or monosaccharide residues may be modified or derived in several ways. Carbonyl groups can be reduced or oxidized, and terminal $-CH_2OH$ groups can be oxidized. Hydroxyl groups on any of the carbons are subject to various modifications.

ALDITOLS

The alditols (polyols) (Fig. 4-8), which occur naturally in plants and other organisms, are reduction products of aldoses and ketoses in which the carbonyl has been reduced to an alcohol. Reduction of ketoses gives an epimeric pair of alditols unless the reaction is enzyme catalyzed and therefore stereospecific. The alditols, like the sugars, are soluble in water and vary in degree of sweetness. Xylitol, the sweetest, approaches the sweetness of sucrose. Because the alditols do not have a carbonyl group, they are considerably less reactive than the sugars. They do not undergo base-catalyzed reactions of epimerization and isomerization, the formation of glycosides (unless they are participating as the "alcohol" or aglycone), or the Maillard reaction. Alditols share the same hydrophilic character as the sugars and are used in products as humectants to prevent excessive drying. D-Glucitol (D-sorbitol) and xylitol are not readily metabolized by oral bacteria and are used in chewing gums and candies for this noncariogenic characteristic. Both D-glucitol and xylitol are passively absorbed in the small intestine and metabolized in the liver. Excessive amounts of alditols passing into the colon may induce diarrhea owing to osmotic action. (Note that xylitol, although it has three chiral carbons, is a symmetrical molecule and does not possess optical activity.)

GLYCURONIC, GLYCONIC, AND GLYCARIC ACIDS

The uronic acids are weak sugar acids that have a carboxyl group (–COOH) instead of the terminal $-CH_2OH$ (Fig. 4-9). D-Glucuronic acid is an important constituent of glycosaminoglycans in mammalian systems, and its C-5 epimer, L-iduronic acid, is present to a lesser extent. Glucuronic acid (and its 4-*O*-methyl ether), D-galacturonic acid, D-mannuronic acid, and the less common L-guluronic acid are constituents

Xylitol	D-Glucitol (D-Sorbitol)
CH_2OH	CH_2OH
HCOH	HCOH
HOCH	HOCH
HCOH	HCOH
CH_2OH	HCOH
	CH_2OH

Figure 4-8 Structures of the common sugar alcohols (alditols) xylitol and D-glucitol.

Clinical Correlation

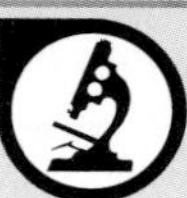

Sugar-Protein Reactions in Diabetes and Aging

The Maillard/Amadori reactions of sugars with amino acids and proteins lead to a cascade of reactions. Products of these reactions are referred to as *advanced glycation end products.* These reaction end products have been observed in collagen-rich tissues in vivo and in vitro, and they are associated with stiffening of artery walls, lung tissue, and joints and with other aging symptoms. Considerable evidence links hyperglycemia with increased formation of these end products; these products accumulate in the blood vessel wall proteins and may contribute to vascular complications of diabetes. Glycation of lens proteins increases somewhat with aging, but it is accelerated in diabetes. Incubation of lens proteins with glucose or glucose 6-phosphate in vitro results in changes in the lens proteins that mimic most of those observed with age- and cataract-related changes in the lens. Drug-induced inhibition of the reactions leading to these end products in diabetic animals prevents various disease-associated pathologies of the arteries, kidneys, nerves, and retina.

D-Gluconic acid | D-Glucono-δ-lactone | β-D-Glucuronic acid (GlcA) | β-L-Iduronic acid (IdoA)

Figure 4-9 Carboxylic acid derivatives of D-glucose and L-idose. D-Gluconic acid is shown along with its 1,5-lactone, an intramolecular ester. D-Glucuronic and L-iduronic acids are shown as their β anomers; uronic acids are important constituents of glycosaminoglycans. The acids are shown in their anionic forms (gluconate, glucuronate, and iduronate).

of the nondigestible polysaccharides of plants and algae, which contribute to dietary fiber. Glycaric acids are dicarboxylic acids in which both terminal groups of the aldose have been oxidized to carboxyls. They are much less common than the glycuronic acids. Glyconic acids are oxidation products of the aldoses in which C-1 has been oxidized to a carboxyl group. Glyconic acids lactonize easily to the neutral cyclic lactones.

DEOXY AND AMINO SUGARS

Several common sugars lack the complete complement of hydroxyl groups; examples of these are shown in Figure 4-10. Deoxy sugars, in which a hydroxyl group is replaced by a hydrogen, include 2-deoxy-D-ribose, L-fucose (6-deoxy-L-galactose), and L-rhamnose (6-deoxy-L-mannose). L-Fucose is a constituent of many glycoproteins and serves as a signaling epitope for physiological events (e.g., in the inflammatory response). The presence of fucose in crucial oligosaccharides of cell-surface glycoproteins is required for recruitment of leukocytes to sites of inflammation and injury. L-Rhamnose occurs in plant polysaccharides, and 2-deoxy-D-ribose is the sugar constituent of deoxyribonucleotides that make up DNA.

In the common amino sugars, the C-2 hydroxyl group is replaced by an amino group.

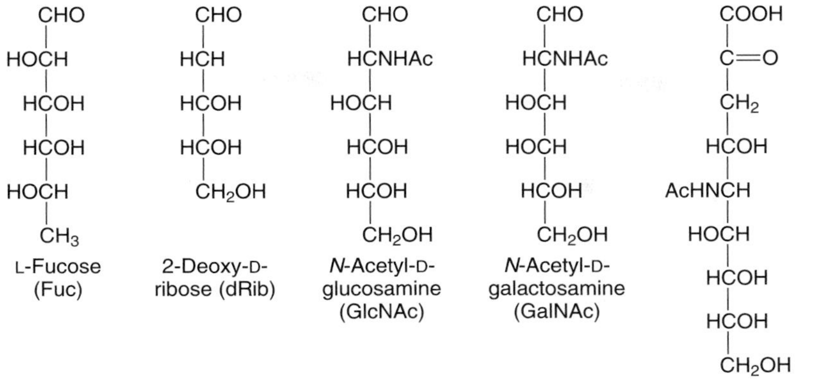

L-Fucose (Fuc)	2-Deoxy-D-ribose (dRib)	N-Acetyl-D-glucosamine (GlcNAc)	N-Acetyl-D-galactosamine (GalNAc)	N-Acetyl-neuraminic acid (NeuAc or NANA)
CHO	CHO	CHO	CHO	COOH
HOCH	HCH	HCNHAc	HCNHAc	C=O
HCOH	HCOH	HOCH	HOCH	CH_2
HCOH	HCOH	HCOH	HOCH	HCOH
HOCH	CH_2OH	HCOH	HCOH	AcHNCH
CH_3		CH_2OH	CH_2OH	HOCH
				HCOH
				HCOH
				CH_2OH

Figure 4-10 Examples of deoxy and amino sugars that are constituents of important biologic compounds such as DNA, glycoproteins, and glycoconjugates.

These common amino sugars are D-glucosamine (2-amino-2-deoxy-D-glucose) and D-galactosamine (2-amino-2-deoxy-D-galactose), which usually occur as the *N*-acetyl derivatives (*N*-acetyl-D-glucosamine and *N*-acetyl-D-galactosamine). They are constituents of glycosaminoglycans and of many glycoproteins. Glycoproteins may also contain the sialic acids, which are *N*-acyl derivatives of neuraminic acid, a unique nine-carbon amino deoxy keto sugar acid. Although the amino group of neuraminic acid is frequently acetylated in sialic acids, other acyl groups may be present in sialic acids. *N*-Acetylneuraminic acid is also an important biologic signaling epitope of glycoproteins. One role it seems to play is protection of circulating plasma proteins from degradation by proteases. Chemically, neuraminic acid is very sensitive to acid degradation, and its glycosidic linkage in glycoproteins and gangliosides is very easily hydrolyzed.

DISACCHARIDES AND OLIGOSACCHARIDES AND THEIR PROPERTIES

Oligosaccharides are composed of monosaccharides covalently linked by glycosidic bonds. They are either reducing or nonreducing. An oligosaccharide terminating with a residue that has an unsubstituted anomeric –OH is reducing. Reducing oligosaccharides undergo all the chemical reactions of the aldose sugars, including reduction, oxidation, and base-catalyzed epimerization and isomerization at their reducing end. Oligosaccharides are readily hydrolyzed to their constituent monosaccharides by acid or enzyme catalysis, with the enzymes showing strong specificity for the sugar units and their anomeric linkage. As a result of this specificity, humans digest primarily two types of oligosaccharides: those containing α-D-glucose or β-D-galactose at the nonreducing end. The structures of the three major dietary disaccharides (sucrose, lactose, and maltose) are shown in Figure 4-11.

Sucrose (table sugar), a nonreducing disaccharide, is composed of α-D-glucopyranosyl and β-D-fructofuranosyl units covalently linked through the anomeric carbon of each sugar unit to form α-D-glucopyranosyl-(1→2)-β-D-fructofuranoside. Sucrose is widely distributed in plants and produced commercially from sugar cane and sugar beets (typically called cane sugar, regardless of its source). It is easily hydrolyzed to glucose and fructose in acid solution and rapidly digested by sucrase, an α-glucosidase of the intestinal villi. Sucrose is a major caloric sweetener for commercial or home use, and the term "sugar" on food labels refers to sucrose.

Lactose
A: β-D-Galp-(1→4)-D-Glcp
B: Gal(β1-4)Glc

Maltose
A: α-D-Glcp-(1→4)-D-Glcp
B: Glc(α1-4)Glc

Sucrose
A: α-D-Glcp-(1↔2)-β-D-Fruf
B: Glc(α1-2β)Fru

Trehalose
A: α-D-Glcp-(1→1)-α-D-Glcp
B: Glc(α1-1α)Glc

Figure 4-11 Reducing (lactose and maltose) and nonreducing (sucrose and trehalose) disaccharides. The free anomeric –OH of the glucosyl unit of lactose and of maltose indicates the reducing nature of these disaccharides. In sucrose and trehalose, both anomeric carbons are involved in the glycosidic bond, and these disaccharides are nonreducing. The small arrows point to the glycosidic bonds. Two abbreviated structural notations are shown for these disaccharides. Notation A defines the complete structure, whereas B assumes the more common ring form and D-configuration for each sugar unit.

Nutrition Insight

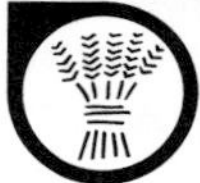

Derivatives of Sucrose Used by the Food Industry: Noncaloric Fat and Sugar Substitutes

The low cost and purity of sucrose and the 8 hydroxyl groups in its structure make sucrose an appealing starting material for chemical modification. In 1968, Procter & Gamble, while searching for a way to increase the fat intake of premature babies, created a fat substitute, sucrose polyester. Sucrose polyester, which is known as olestra or Olean, is a sucrose molecule to which as many as 8 fatty acid residues (usually 6 to 8 long-chain fatty acids) derived from vegetable oil have been esterified. It has so many fatty acid spokes around the central sucrose core that digestive enzymes and bacteria in the intestinal tract cannot find an entry point to break down the molecule. Thus it passes through the body largely unhydrolyzed. Olestra was approved by the U.S. Food and Drug Administration (FDA) in 1996 as a replacement for regular cooking oil in production of savory snack foods such as crackers, potato chips, and corn chips.

In 1976, Tate & Lyle discovered that chlorination of three hydroxyl groups on sucrose produced a modified sucrose that is about 600 times as sweet as sucrose. Use of this chlorinated sucrose derivative, which is known as sucralose or Splenda, was approved by Canada in 1991. In 1998 and 1999, the FDA granted approval for use of sucralose in certain food products. Sucralose is currently used as a sugar substitute in numerous food products, including beverages, baked goods, dairy products, canned fruits, syrups, and condiments, and is also sold to consumers, under its trade name Splenda, for use as a table and baking sugar substitute.

Clinical Correlation

Sugars and Dental Caries

Sugars are readily metabolized by oral bacteria, leading to production of organic acids in sufficient concentration to lower the pH of dental plaque. Most studies have focused on the contribution of sucrose, but monosaccharides are also readily fermented by the bacteria in the dental plaque. The acids demineralize (dissolve) the nearby tooth enamel. If the degree of demineralization exceeds remineralization over repeated cycles of acid/less acid, dissolution of the tooth enamel leads to tooth decay.

Although many studies done in the past clearly demonstrated the relationship between sucrose consumption and dental caries at the population level (e.g., association between sugar consumption and dental caries among countries) and at the individual level (e.g., persons with hereditary fructose intolerance who strictly limit sugar consumption), the apparent relationship between sugar consumption and dental caries has weakened in industrialized countries. The weakening of the observed relationship is due, at least partially, to the decreased prevalence of caries in children owing to widespread use of fluoride, which raises the threshold of sugar intake at which caries will progress to cavitation. Studies have shown that the amount of carbohydrate consumed is not as significant in the formation of dental caries as is the frequency of consumption. The form of the carbohydrate is also important because sticky carbohydrates are retained on the teeth and allow acid production to be prolonged. The American Dental Association recommends that the number of between-meal snacks eaten each day be minimized, that sweet consumption be limited to mealtime, and that infants not be allowed to sleep with bottles containing sweetened liquids, fruit juices, milk, or formula.

Lactose (β-D-galactopyranosyl-(1→4)-D-glucopyranose, milk sugar) is synthesized in the mammary glands of mammals. The concentration in milk varies with species and constitutes about 4 g/100 mL of bovine milk compared with 6.4 g/100 mL of human milk (Newburg and Neubauer, 1995). Lactose is present in dairy products and also in processed foods that contain whey products formed from the watery part of milk that remains after the manufacture of cheese. Lactose has about one third the sweetness of sucrose. It is readily digested to glucose and galactose by a β-galactosidase (lactase) of the intestinal villi. Lactose is a reducing disaccharide and therefore susceptible to reactions of the glucose carbonyl group, including the Maillard reaction. Alkaline isomerization of lactose gives lactulose, in which the glucose unit has been isomerized to fructose. This isomerization also occurs to some extent during heating of milk. Lactulose is not digested or absorbed in the body, and it appears to promote growth of bifidobacteria and lactobacilli species in the colon. Colonization by these bacteria is effective in preventing acute diarrhea. Production of short-chain fatty acids from the lactulose and dietary fiber polysaccharides leads to a decrease in colonic pH and limits potential growth of pathogenic bacteria. Lactulose is also used as a therapeutic agent in the treatment of hepatic encephalopathy.

α,α-Trehalose [α-D-glucopyranosyl-(1↔1)-α-D-glucopyranoside] is a nonreducing disaccharide found in fungi (particularly in young mushrooms), yeasts, and insects. It is digested by an intestinal α-glucosidase called trehalase. It is curious that trehalase has persisted in the brush border of the human small intestine, because trehalose is a rather insignificant dietary disaccharide.

Only small amounts of maltose [α-D-glucopyranosyl-(1→4)-D-glucopyranose] are consumed as such in the diet. Maltose occurs naturally in the seeds of starch-producing plants, and small amounts are used in processed foods. Isomaltose [α-D-glucopyranosyl-(1→6)-D-glucopyranose] probably does not occur naturally.

Both maltose and isomaltose are formed by acidic hydrolysis of starch; isomaltose results from the structural branch points of amylopectin. Digestion of starch by α-amylases in the lumen of the gastrointestinal tract yields maltose, maltotriose, and α-dextrins containing the isomaltose moiety; glucoamylase and sucrase/isomaltase also complete the digestion of these products. These α-linked glucose disaccharides are readily digested by intestinal α-glucosidases (glucoamylase, sucrase/isomaltase). Digestion of carbohydrates is discussed in detail in Chapter 8.

Although disaccharides are common components of the diet, oligosaccharides containing 3 to 10 sugar residues are not abundant. A series of α-galactosides, known as raffinose, stachyose, verbascose, and ajucose, occur in relatively large amounts in soybeans, lentils, and other legume seeds. As shown in Figure 4-12, these oligosaccharides contain a sucrose moiety to which one or more residues of α-galactose are attached by a 1→6 linkage to the glucose moiety of sucrose. Raffinose, stachyose, verbascose, and ajucose contain one, two, three or four residues of α-galactose, respectively. Multiple residues of α-galactose are attached by 1→6 linkages; for example, stachyose contains an α-D-galactopyranosyl-(1→6)-α-D-galactopyranosyl unit attached to C-6 of the glucose unit of sucrose. During plant seed development, a galactosyl derivative of inositol [i.e., α-D-galactosyl-(1→3)-D-myo-inositol, or galactinol], serves as the donor of the galactose residues in the galactosyltransferase reactions that catalyze the synthesis of raffinose family oligosaccharides. Because humans do not have a digestive α-galactosidase, these oligosaccharides pass into the lower gut to be metabolized by the anaerobic bacteria. Excessive flatulence may result from fermentation of these oligosaccharides, as well as of pectic polysaccharides.

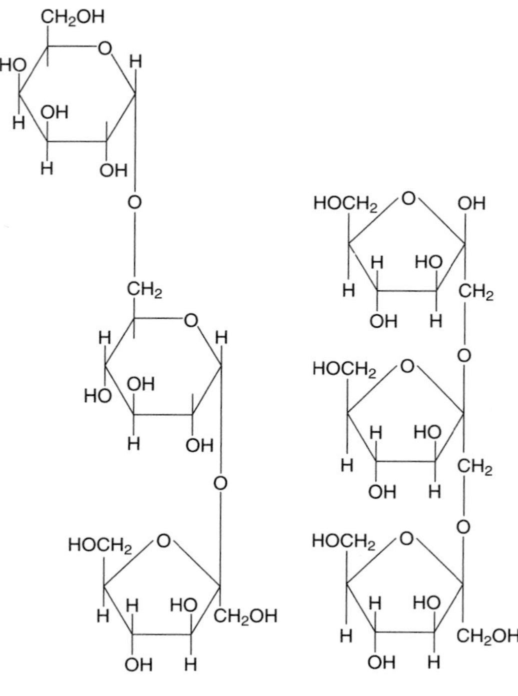

Figure 4-12 Structures of two oligosaccharides; raffinose [α-D-galactopyranosyl(1→6)α-D-glucopyranosyl(1→2)β-D-fructofuranose] and an oligofructose product of inulin hydrolysis [β-D-fructofuranosyl(2→1)β-D-fructofuranosyl-(2→1)β-D-fructofuranose].

Fructose oligosaccharides produced by hydrolysis of inulin, which is a β-fructan obtained from chicory roots. Inulin is a polymer of fructose residues with the fructose residues present as furanose rings joined by β(2→1) glycosidic linkages. The partial hydrolysate of inulin (oligofructose) is used as a food ingredient. (Although pyranose rings are more stable thermodynamically and occur more frequently in polymers than do furanose rings, furanose rings are found in inulin and in sucrose because the biosynthesis of these molecules in plants occurs via the 6-phosphate ester of fructose; in fructose 6-phosphate, the –OH on C-6 is tied up and not free to cyclize with the carbonyl carbon to form a pyranose ring.) The food industry also produces synthetic fructose oligosaccharides that are sucrose molecules to which fructose units have been added by β(2→1)-linkages. Fructose oligosaccharides are about 30% as sweet as sucrose and are used as bulking agents, emulsifiers, sugar substitutes, and prebiotics in a variety of food products. Fructose oligosaccharides are not hydrolyzed by enzymes of the digestive tract but can be fermented by bacteria in the large intestine.

POLYSACCHARIDES OF NUTRITIONAL IMPORTANCE

Polysaccharides are polymers composed of sugars linked by glycosidic bonds and they vary in size from approximately 20 to more than 10^7 sugar units (degree of polymerization). Because of the multiple hydroxyl groups in monosaccharides, which serve as linkage sites for glycosidic bonds, there is much opportunity for structural diversity in polysaccharides. The structural diversity includes molecular size, kinds and proportions of sugars, ring size (furanose or pyranose), anomeric configuration (α or β), and linkage site of the glycosidic bonds, as well as the sequence of sugars and linkages and the presence of noncarbohydrate components.

GENERAL CHARACTERISTICS

Polysaccharides may be linear or branched, and branched polysaccharides exhibit various branching modes that range from branches consisting of a single sugar unit to longer branches carrying other branches, as illustrated in Figure 4-13. In heteropolysaccharides composed of more than one kind of sugar, the sugar units may be linked in alternating sequence or in blocks of various length in which one sugar repeats itself. The physical properties of polysaccharides depend highly on their chemical and conformational structures. In general, polysaccharides that are highly branched are water soluble, whereas linear polysaccharides tend to be insoluble. However, linear polysaccharides possessing structural irregularities that hinder intermolecular hydrogen bonding may be soluble and give viscous solutions. Hyaluronic acid, a linear polysaccharide with two different sugars in alternating sequence, shows this mucilaginous characteristic. In contrast, glycogen, which is highly branched and very soluble, gives relatively nonviscous solutions. Many different polysaccharide structures are represented in the plant kingdom, whereas only a few have been identified in vertebrates. Bacteria synthesize many unusual sugars, thereby greatly increasing the diversity of their polysaccharide antigens.

Polysaccharides are designated either by a trivial name, such as starch and cellulose, or by a systematic name constructed from the constituent sugar names and the suffix "an." Thus $\alpha(1\rightarrow4)$-D-glucan is the systematic name for amylase, and $\beta(1\rightarrow4)$-D-glucan is the systematic name for cellulose.

DIGESTIBLE POLYSACCHARIDES

Starch and glycogen are digestible polysaccharides of glucose. Starch is found in plant cells, in both linear and branched forms. Glycogen has a highly branched structure and is found in animal tissues, particularly muscle and liver.

Starch

Starch is one of the most abundant polysaccharides in plants, where it is stored in the seeds, tubers, roots, and some fruits. It is composed of two families of polymers, a mostly linear amylose [$\alpha(1\rightarrow4)$-D-glucan] and the

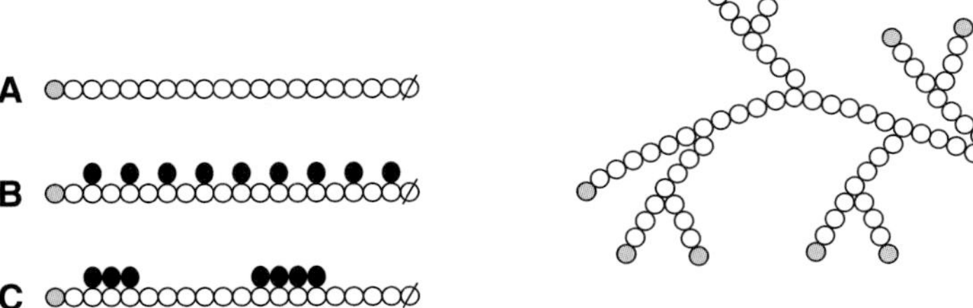

Figure 4-13 Branching structures of polysaccharides. *A,* Linear polysaccharide. Circles represent sugar units linked by glycosidic bonds. *B,* Alternating branches consisting of a single sugar unit, ●. *C,* Blocks of consecutive single sugar unit branches, ●. *D,* Ramified structure (branches on branches). Reducing end, Ø; Nonreducing end ●; ● one sugar of a sequence of sugar units.

branched amylopectin [α (1→4)-D-glucan with branches linked to C-6]. Starches from different sources vary in structure, but typically amylopectin has an average chain length between branch points of 20 to 25 glucose units. Typical starches contain 20% to 30% amylose and 70% to 80% amylopectin; however, high amylopectin (waxy corn, 98% amylopectin) and high amylose (high amylose corn, 55% to 85% amylose) starches are also available. Starches for food processing are produced from many sources. The most important sources are corn (regular, waxy, and high amylose), potato, rice, tapioca, and wheat. The physical properties and, to some extent, the digestibility of the starches vary with their fine structure and reflect their source.

Amylose and amylopectin molecules are laid down during biosynthesis in highly organized particles called granules. The more highly organized or crystalline starch granule is less susceptible to digestion by α-amylase. Therefore, certain raw (native) starch granules, particularly those in raw potatoes and green bananas, resist digestion. The hydrogen-bonded structure of the starch components renders the granules insoluble in water below approximately 55° C. However, when an aqueous suspension of granules is heated, swelling occurs and there is a transition to a disorganized structure; the starch is said to be gelatinized. Upon further heating, the granule imbibes water and undergoes further swelling and fragmentation, releasing the amylose and portions of the amylopectin to produce a viscous suspension. The gelatinization or hydration that normally occurs during cooking and food processing makes the starch more accessible, and gelatinized potato and green banana starch are readily digested by α-amylases. High-amylose maize starches have high gelatinization temperatures and typically remain resistant to digestion, even after cooking.

Cooling of starch suspensions leads to the formation of gels. Pure amylose and amylopectin have limited solubility in water, however, and there is a tendency for the amylose chains, and to a lesser extent the branched amylopectin, to realign or reaggregate through hydrogen bonding over time in a process known as retrogradation. When this occurs, liquid may be expressed from the gel, a process that is generally undesirable in food products. Amylose can be retrograded to a form that resists dispersion in water and digestion by α-amylase.

The physical structure or food matrix also affects the digestibility or availability of starch. Starch granules in whole or partly ground grains, seeds, cereals, and legumes may be resistant to digestion. Milling, grinding, and other types of food processing makes this starch available.

Gelatinized starch is hydrolyzed to glucose in the gastrointestinal tract by the combined action of salivary and pancreatic α-amylases and the intestinal mucosal α-glucosidases (glucoamylase, sucrase/α-dextrinase). The α-amylases, which cleave the α(1→4)-linkages only, catalyze hydrolysis of starch to maltose, maltotriose, and maltotetrose and to oligosaccharides called α-limit dextrins, composed of a minimum of four glucose units and including an α(1→6)-linked branch point. These disaccharides and oligosaccharides are then converted to glucose by the α-glucosidases. Figure 4-14 shows a fragment of the amylopectin structure and the α(1→4)- and α(1→6)-glucosidic linkages that can be hydrolyzed by human digestive enzymes. The human upper digestive tract does not possess an endogenous (1→4)-β-D-glucanase, and, therefore, cellulose, with its β-linkage, is not digestible.

Glycogen

Glycogen, like starch amylopectin, is an α(1→4)-D-glucan with branches on branches that are α(1→6)-linked. The average length of the α(1→4)-linked chain between branch points is 10 to 14 glucose units. Because of its greater degree of branching compared with amylopectin, glycogen is readily soluble in cold water and gives solutions of relatively low viscosity, which facilitate its use as a readily available endogenous energy source. The branching pattern interferes with intra- and intermolecular hydrogen bonding of the glycogen chains, thereby permitting rapid solvation and easy access to the enzymes. A low viscosity of the solution facilitates diffusion of the substrate to the enzymes and diffusion of products away from the enzymes that hydrolyze glycosidic bonds in glycogen.

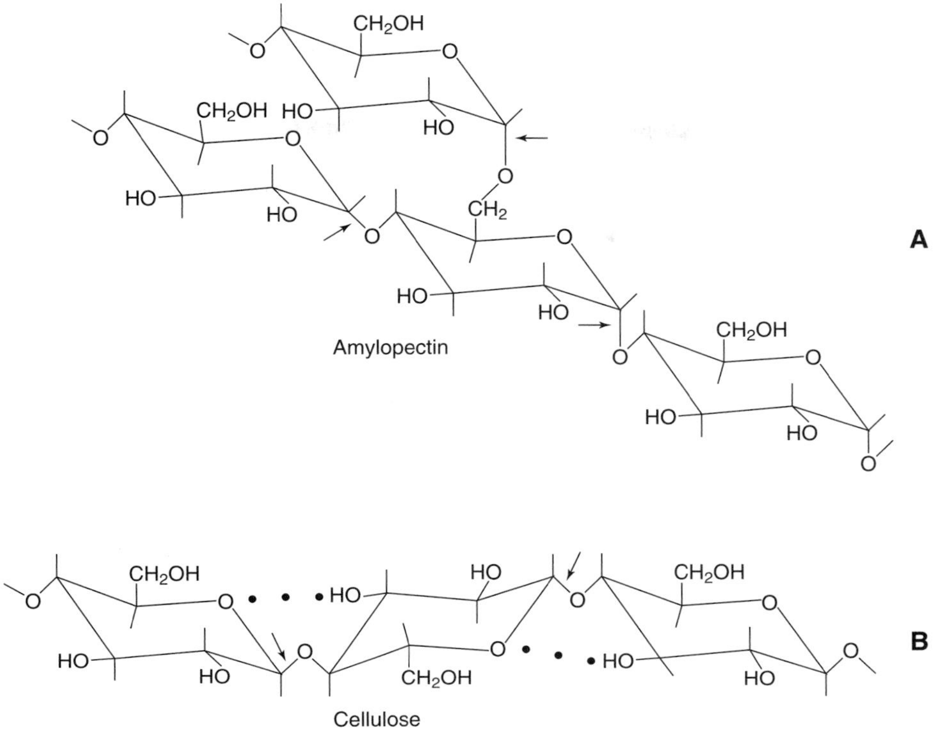

Figure 4-14 **A,** A segment of starch amylopectin structure showing the α-D-glucosidic bonds and the branch points. Glycogen has a similar structure. **B,** The conformational structure of cellulose shows that alternate β-D-glucosyl units are flipped 180 degrees, giving a flat, ribbon-like structure stabilized by hydrogen bonds (•••). The glucosidic bonds are indicated by the small arrows.

Glycogen is present in most animal tissues, with the highest content in liver and skeletal muscle. It may constitute up to 10% (wet weight) of the human liver. Mammalian tissue levels of glycogen are highly variable and affected by factors such as nutritional status and time of day. Glycogen has a high molecular mass, in the range of 10^6 to 10^9 Da.

By electron microscopy, glycogen appears as uniform spherical particles and higher molecular weight aggregates of these particles (β- and α-particles, respectively). The α-particles are composed of a few β-particle carbohydrate chains covalently linked to protein, which is aggregated by disulfide linkages.

NONDIGESTIBLE PLANT POLYSACCHARIDES

Polysaccharides represent the major components of plant cell walls and interstitial spaces. Plants also synthesize storage polysaccharides other than starch, including galactomannans, the β(1→3)(1→4)-D-glucans of cereal grains, and the fructans of grasses and some tubers. All of these nonstarch polysaccharides present in plants, as well as those added during food processing, constitute dietary fiber (Table 4-2).

Cellulose is a linear β(1→4)-D-glucan with a flat, ribbon-like conformation in which alternate glucose units are flipped 180 degrees, and hydrogen bonded intramolecularly (see Fig. 4-14). These ribbon-like chains are aligned in parallel arrays called microfibrils in which the chains are strongly hydrogen bonded to each other. The microfibrils are similarly packed together into strong fibers, which are very insoluble and which provide rigidity to the plant cell wall. Associated with cellulose in the cell wall are several other insoluble polysaccharides, the hemicelluloses. These include

Table 4-2
Nondigestible Food Polysaccharides of Plant, Algal, and Bacterial Origin

Polysaccharide	Main Chain or Repeat Unit*	Branches, Other Substituents†
PLANTS		
Cellulose	-Glc(β1–4)Glc-	none
Arabinoxylan	-Xyl(β1–4)Xyl-	L-Ara*f*(α1–2 or 1–3)-
Xyloglucan	-Glc(β1–4)Glc-	Xyl(α1–6)-β-Gal-; α-L-Ara*f* or α-L-Fuc linked to Xyl
Pectin	-[GalA(α1–4)]$_n$GalA(α1–2) L-Rha(α1–4)-	Gal- and L-Ara*f*-; methyl ester of GalA
Cereal β-glucan	-[Glc(β1–4)]$_n$Glc(β1–3)-	none
Galactomannan	-Man(β1–4)Man-	Gal(α1–6)-
Arabinogalactan	-Gal(β1–4)Gal-	L-Ara*f*(α1–5)L-Ara*f*-
ALGAE		
Alginic acid	-[ManA(β1–4)]$_n$[L-GulA(α1–4)]$_n$-	none
Carrageenan	-[Gal(β1–4)3,6-anhydroGal(α1–3]-	-SO_3^- at C–4, C–2†
BACTERIA		
Xanthan gum	-Glc(β1–4)Glc‡	4,6-Pyr-Man(β1–4)GlcA(β1–2)Man(α1-3)- Pyr = pyruvic acid $CH_3\underset{X}{C}COO$- at C–4 and C–6 of Man

*Sugars are D and pyranose from unless otherwise indicated.
†The substituent group replaces the proton of the –OH of a sugar unit in the main chain.
‡Alternating glucose units are substituted at C-3 by the trisaccharide branch. The nonreducing terminal Man carries a pyruvic acid substituent, and the other Man is substituted at C-6 by an acetyl group.

the xyloglucans, which have a cellulose-like backbone with α-D-xylose units linked to C-6 of the glucosyl unit, and arabinoxylans, in which the β(1→4)-D-xylan chain has α-L-arabinofuranose and D-glucuronic acid branches at C-2 or C-3.

Pectic polysaccharides [α (1→4)-D-galacturonans with occasional α-L-rhamnose units] and other associated polysaccharides (galactans and arabinans) are present in the cell walls of immature plant tissues and in the interstitial spaces. Native pectic galacturonan in the plant tissue is relatively insoluble, but isolated commercial pectin is soluble in hot water. Calcium ions form complexes with the galacturonic acid units of pectin, cross-linking the chains into a gel network. This is thought to account partially for the insolubility of native pectin in the plant tissue. The calcium–pectin complex is also the basis for dietary low-sugar, low-calorie fruit jams and jellies, whereas jellies prepared without calcium require a high sugar content to form a gel structure. More comprehensive descriptions of the structures and properties of the polysaccharides constituting dietary fiber, and their organization in the plant tissue, are provided in reviews by Carpita (1990) and Selvendran (1984).

NATURAL AND MODIFIED POLYSACCHARIDES FOR USE IN PROCESSED FOODS

Several natural polysaccharides are used in processed foods for their functional properties. These natural polysaccharides include starches from several sources, guar and locust bean galactomannans, alginic acid and carrageenan from seaweed, and xanthan gum. Polysaccharides are also modified physically and chemically to enhance their functionality (Table 4-3). Starch and cellulose are alkylated or esterified to convert a very small proportion of the hydroxyls into ethers or esters for increased solubility. Starches are also subjected to partial acid or enzymatic hydrolysis, resulting in starch dextrins and maltodextrins with improved solubility. Starch dextrins also are produced by a process that promotes alteration of the structure, including new linkages, increased branching, and some decrease in size. Maltodextrins are much smaller, in the oligosaccharide range, but without other

Table 4-3
Modified Polysaccharides Added to Processed Foods

Polysaccharide	Modifying Group or Treatment*	Product
Starch	$-COCH_3$	Starch acetate (ester)
	$-CH_2CHOHCH_3$	Hydroxypropyl starch (ether)
	$-PO_2^-$–	Phosphate cross-linked starch (diester)
	Acid, heat	Dextrins
	Water, heat	Cold-water–soluble starch
Cellulose	$-CH_2COOH$	Carboxymethylcellulose (CMC)
	$-CH_2CHOHCH_3$	Hydroxypropylcellulose
	$-CH_3$	Methylcellulose
	Acid, heat	Microcrystalline cellulose

*The modifying group replaces the proton of one of the three free hydroxyls of the glucose units at a degree of substitution usually less than 1 per 10 glucose units.

structural alterations. For most modified starch products, the enhanced solubility should lead to faster digestion by α-amylases. The high-amylose starches are an exception, because they tend to be more crystalline and less readily digested. In general, the modified starches are digestible and caloric, whereas the other polysaccharides added to foods contribute to dietary fiber.

GLYCOCONJUGATES OF PHYSIOLOGICAL INTEREST

Conjugates of sugars and oligosaccharides play essential physiological roles. These glycoconjugates include the glycosaminoglycans and proteoglycans, the glycoproteins, and the glycolipids.

GLYCOSAMINOGLYCANS

Glycosaminoglycans (Table 4-4) are linear polysaccharides that have a disaccharide repeat unit composed of a hexosamine and a uronic acid. They are constituents of the extracellular spaces of mammalian tissues and vary in molecular weight and in fine structure. Many are sulfated and thus more highly charged. Most glycosaminoglycans are covalently bound to proteins, and the resulting proteoglycans vary considerably in the number and types of bound glycan chains.

Hyaluronic acid (hyaluronan) is a negatively charged, soluble, high-molecular-weight, linear glycan composed of D-glucuronic acid and *N*-acetyl-D-glucosamine. It is found in the extracellular matrix, especially in soft connective tissue. Unlike most glycosaminoglycans, it is not covalently linked to protein but binds physically to receptor proteins on many different cells. Hyaluronic acid is noted for its ability to form highly viscous solutions, and some of its clinical applications depend on this rheology. The viscosity stems from the extended helical conformation, high molecular weight, and network of aggregated chains. Thus, hyaluronic acid may have a role in water and protein homeostasis in the intercellular matrix. Interaction between hyaluronic acid and its cell receptors is involved in cell locomotion and migration, as shown for lymphocytes. It may also be important in development and cell differentiation. Hyaluronic acid is synthesized by transfer of sugar units from their nucleotide diphosphate derivatives to the reducing end of the growing hyaluronic acid chain. This is in contrast to the usual mode of chain lengthening of oligo- and polysaccharides, which involves addition of sugar units to the nonreducing end of the growing chain.

Chondroitin sulfate has a disaccharide repeat unit of D-glucuronic acid and *N*-acetyl-D-galactosamine, with sulfate ester groups at C-2 of glucuronic acid and C-4 or C-6 of the galactosamine. This sulfation adds sequence heterogeneity, defined by the amount and positions of the sulfate esters along the chain. The large number of ionized sulfate groups and the weaker carboxyl groups ensure that

Table 4-4
Structural Repeating Units of the Glycosaminoglycans, Showing Sulfation Patterns and Structural Variation

Glycosaminoglycan	Repeat Unit*
Hyaluronan	[-GlcNAc(β1–4)GlcA(β1–3-]$_n$
Chondroitin 4-sulfate and 6-sulfate	[-GalNAc(β1–4)GlcA(β1–3-]$_n$ GalNAc 4 (or 6) – SO_3^-
Dermatan sulfate	[-GalNAc(β1–4)L-IdoA(α1–3)-]$_n$ GalNAc 4 – SO_3^-; IdoA 2 – R R = H or SO_3^- and [-GalNAc(β1–4)GlcA(β1–3)-]$_n$ GalNAc 4 (or 6) – SO_3^-
Keratan sulfate	[-Gal(β1–4)GlcNAc(β1–3)-]$_n$ Gal 6 – R; GlcNAc 6 – R R = H or SO_3^-
Heparan sulfate and heparin	[-GlcNR(α1–4)GlcA(β1–4)-]$_n$ GlcNR 6 – R′ R R = Ac or SO_3^- R′ R = H or SO_3^- and [-GlcNAc(α1–4)L-IdoA(α1–4)-]$_n$ IdoA 2 – R R R = H or SO_3^-

With the exception of hyaluronan and keratan sulfate, the glycosaminoglycans are glycosidically linked to the core protein chain by the sequence -4GlcA(β1-3)Gal(β1-4)Xyl(β1-3)L-serine. Keratan sulfate is glycosidically linked to core proteins by either *N*- linkage to an asparagine residue or *O*-linked to a serine/threonine residue. Hyaluronan is not covalently linked to proteins. Sugars are D unless noted as L.

*R in the abbreviated structure format refers to the proton of an –OH or an $-NH_2$ group or a subsitution for the proton. $-SO_3^-$ replaces the proton of the –OH group.

this large polysaccharide will attract counter cations and water for osmotic balance and hydration of the polysaccharide.

Dermatan sulfate is synthesized from chondroitin sulfate by intracellular C-5 epimerization of some of the D-glucuronic acid units to L-iduronic acid. The consequence of this is not only creation of a new uronic acid, but also of another element of structural diversity relative to the proportion and sequence of each acid. The other major differences between dermatan sulfate and chondroitin sulfate reside in the number of sulfate groups and their positions.

Heparin and heparan sulfate have disaccharide repeat units of D-glucuronic acid and D-glucosamine with some L-iduronic acid. The glucosamine units may be *N*-acetylated or *N*-sulfated, and all sugar residues may be *O*-sulfated. Heparin is more extensively epimerized, whereas heparan sulfate chains vary widely in extent of epimerization and sulfation, with some chains having little iduronic acid or sulfate. Heparin has a higher proportion of *N*-sulfates and total sulfate, as well as more iduronic acid. Heparin is found predominantly in the secretory granules of mast cells, whereas heparan sulfate is found linked to many cell surface proteins and as a component of matrix proteoglycans. Lipoprotein lipase in the capillaries of muscle and adipose tissue is closely associated with a heparan sulfate proteoglycan.

Keratan sulfate, composed of alternating D-galactose and *N*-acetyl-D-glucosamine units, lacks a uronic acid constituent, but it is heavily sulfated. The *N*-acetyl-D-glucosamine units carry sulfate groups at C-6, and some of the galactose units are sulfated also at C-6.

PROTEOGLYCANS

Proteoglycans are large, complex macromolecules that consist of a protein core to which glycosaminoglycans are covalently linked. These proteoglycans are found in the plasma membrane and extracellular matrices of most eukaryotic cells, where they have many functions. They may play a role in cell–cell and cell–matrix interactions and interact with a variety of ligands. The size and complexity of proteoglycans varies. A proteoglycan may carry more than one covalently linked glycosaminoglycan as well as additional oligosaccharides that are *N*- and *O*-linked to the core protein. Heparan sulfate/heparin proteoglycans contain at least one heparin sulfate chain, and usually *O*- and *N*-linked oligosaccharides in addition. The proteoglycans containing chondroitin sulfate, dermatan sulfate, and heparan sulfate frequently share a common tetrasaccharide-linkage region (GlcA-Gal-Gal-Xyl-) by which the glycosaminoglycan is covalently *O*-linked to a serine residue of the protein (see footnote, Table 4-4). Keratan sulfate is an exception and is found both *O*-linked and *N*-linked to serine/threonine or asparagine residues of core proteins. The biosynthesis of proteoglycans occurs posttranslationally and takes place in the lumen of the endoplasmic reticulum and Golgi apparatus.

GLYCOPROTEINS

Many proteins carry covalently linked oligosaccharides as minor components. The number and size of the oligosaccharide chains vary. The *N*-linked oligosaccharides tend to have a common core and are β-glycosidically linked from the *N*-acetyl-D-glucosamine unit to the nitrogen of the β-carboxamide of asparagine (Fig. 4-15). Mucin-type glycoproteins have an α-D-galactosyl unit *O*-linked to the hydroxyl group of serine or threonine. Collagen is unique in that the carbohydrate chains are *O*-linked to the C-5 of 5-hydroxylysine. The carbohydrate moieties of glycoproteins may play a role in stabilization of the proteins to denaturation and may be involved in protein folding in addition to other specific biological roles.

GLYCOLIPIDS

Glycolipids are widespread in nature but only as minor components of the lipid fraction and usually in association with proteins. The common glycolipids of mammalian systems include cerebrosides and gangliosides, which are glycosyl (glucosyl or galactosyl) derivatives of sphingolipids (Table 4-5). These glycosphingolipids contain a base such as sphingosine, which has an 18-carbon monounsaturated chain substituted with two hydroxyl groups and an amine group. The amine nitrogen of the sphingosine unit is acylated with a long-chain (14- to 26-carbon) fatty acid. A carbohydrate unit (usually glucose or galactose) is glycosidically attached to the *N*-acylsphingosine (ceramide) at its C-1 hydroxyl group to form a cerebroside (monoglycosylceramide). The sugar unit of a cerebroside may also be sulfated to form a sulfatide. Cerebrosides are neutral glycosphingolipids, whereas sulfatides are acidic glycosphingolipids. Large amounts of galactocerebroside and galactocerebroside 3-sulfate are found in the brain.

Additional sugar residues (usually glucose, galactose, L-fucose, or *N*-acetylgalactosamine) are attached to cerebrosides (usually to glucosylceramide) to form globosides and gangliosides. Neutral ceramide oligosaccharides (globosides) and acidic, sialic acid–containing ceramide oligosaccharides (gangliosides) are also sphingoglycolipids. Globosides are ceramides with two or more neutral sugar residues. The neutral diglycosylceramide, called lactosylceramide, is the precursor of other globosides and of gangliosides; lactosylceramide is also found in the membrane of red blood cells. Tetraglycosylceramides ("aminoglycolipids") are globosides

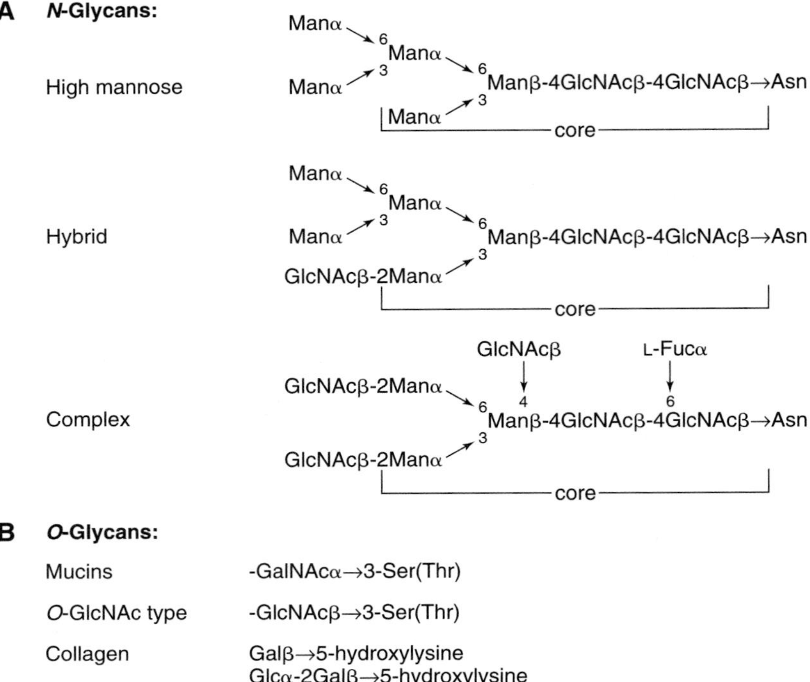

Figure 4-15 Structural variations in oligosaccharide chains of glycoproteins and their attachment site in the protein. **A,** A core of five sugar units, common to all three types of *N*-linked glycans, is linked to asparagine (Asn). High-mannose *N*-glycans contain up to nine mannose units in addition to *N*-acetylglucosamine. Other sugars, including galactose and sialic acid, also may be linked to the nonreducing ends of the antennary (branch) chains in the complex *N*-glycans. **B,** *O*-Linked oligosaccharides in the mucins and *O*-GlcNAc type in glycoproteins may be extended at the nonreducing end by addition of *N*-acetylglucosamine, galactose, L-fucose, and sialic acid. Sugars are D-enantiomers unless noted otherwise.

Table 4-5
The Major Neutral and Acidic Glycolipids of Bovine and Human Milk

Neutral Glycolipid	Acidic Glycolipid
Gal(β1-1)Cer	Neu5Ac(α2-3)Gal(β1-4)Glc(β1-1)Cer
Glc(β1-1)Cer	Neu5Ac(α2-8)Neu5Ac(α2-3)Gal(β1-4)Glc(β1-1)Cer
Gal(β1-4)Glc-(β1-1)Cer	

Cer, Ceramide. $HOCH_2$-C(H)(NHR)-C(H)(OH)-CH=CH-$C_{13}H_{27}$, with *R* representing a long-chain acyl group.

that contain an additional sugar (i.e., galactose) and an *N*-acetylhexosamine unit (i.e., *N*-acetylgalactosamine); certain globosides are antigenic determinants of blood group types.

Gangliosides are formed by the addition of sialic acid (*N*-acetylneuraminic acid) to diglycosylceramide; additional sugar residues such as galactose, *N*-acetylgalactosamine, and *N*-acetylglucosamine may also be added to form a variety of gangliosides, many containing branches formed by the addition of one or two sialic acid units to the linear portion of the oligosaccharide chain. Gangliosides are found on the surface membranes of most cells, and they make up about 6% of total brain lipids. Gangliosides are most highly concentrated in the ganglion cells of the central nervous system.

Aberrant glycosylation expressed in glycosphingolipids in tumor cells is strongly implicated as an essential mechanism in tumor progression. Abnormal accumulation of specific glycosphingolipids in specific cancers has been correlated with altered cell–cell or cell–substratum interactions, and reagents that block glycosylation have been shown to inhibit tumor cell metastasis.

Plants and microorganisms synthesize several simple glycolipids, which include fatty acid esters of the sugars and glycosides of diglycerides, hydroxy fatty acids, and *myo*-inositol phospholipids. Highly complex lipopolysaccharides of cell walls of gram-negative bacteria are both antigens and endotoxins. The lipopolysaccharides (also called endotoxins) are composed of three domains: the terminal carbohydrate chain, which defines the *O*-specific antigenicity; the lipid A, which has the endotoxin activity; and an oligosaccharide core, which is sandwiched between. These endotoxins cause some types of food poisoning (e.g., salmonellosis).

REFERENCES

Baynes JW, Monnier VM (eds) (1989) The Maillard Reaction in Aging, Diabetes, and Nutrition. Alan R. Liss, New York.

Brownlee M (1995) Advanced protein glycosylation in diabetes and aging. Annu Rev Med 46:223-234.

Carpita NC (1990) The chemical structure of the cell walls of higher plants. In: Kritchevsky D, Bonfield C, Anderson JW (eds) Dietary Fiber: Chemistry, Physiology, and Health Effects. Plenum Press, New York, pp 15-30.

Newburg DS, Neubauer SH (1995) Carbohydrates in milk. Analysis, quantities and significance. In: Jensen RG (ed) Handbook of Milk Composition. Academic Press, San Diego, pp 273-349.

Selvendran RR (1984) The plant cell wall as a source of dietary fiber: Chemistry and structure. Am J Clin Nutr 39:320-337.

RECOMMENDED READINGS

Chaplin MF, Kennedy JF (eds) (1994) Carbohydrate Analysis: A Practical Approach, 2nd ed. Oxford University Press, London.

Delzenne NM (2003) Oligosaccharides: state of the art. Proc Nutr Sco 67:177-182.

Fukuda M (1994) Cell surface carbohydrates: cell-type specific expression. In: Fukuda M, Hindsgaul O (eds) Molecular Glycobiology. Oxford University Press, London, pp 1-52.

Hall MB (2003) Challenges with nonfiber carbohydrate methods. J Anim Sci 81:3226-3232.

Kaur N, Gupta AK (2002) Applications of inulin and oligofructose in health and nutrition. J Biosci 27:703-714.

Lowe JB (1994) Carbohydrate recognition in cell-cell interaction. In: Fukuda M, Hindsgaul O (eds) Molecular Glycobiology. Oxford University Press, London, pp 163-205.

Pigman W, Horton J (eds) (1970, 1972) The Carbohydrates: Chemistry and Biochemistry. Vol. IA, IIA, IB, IIB. Academic Press, New York.

Slavin J (2003) Why whole grains are protective: biological mechanisms. Proc Nutr Soc 62:129-134.

Varki A, Marth J (1995) Oligosaccharides in vertebrate development. Semin Dev Biol 6:127-138.

RECOMMENDED WEBSITE

Nomenclature of Carbohydrates Recommendations of the International Union of Pure and Applied Chemistry (IUPAC) and the International Union of Biochemistry and Molecular Biology

www.chem.qmw.ac.uk/iupac/2carb/

Chapter 5

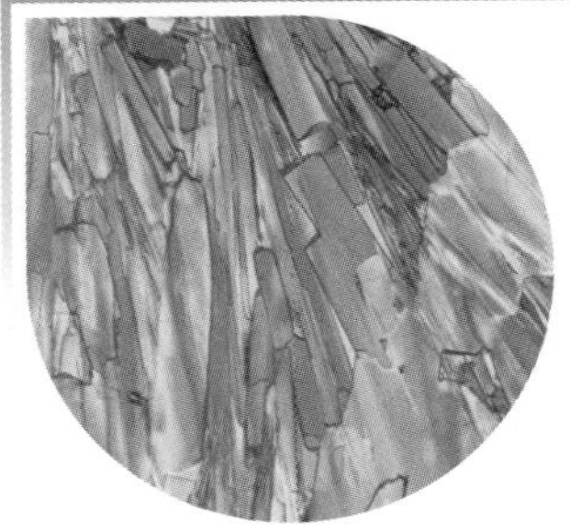

Structure and Properties of Proteins and Amino Acids

Robert B. Rucker, PhD, and Taru Kosonen, PhD

OUTLINE

AMINO ACIDS

An understanding of the chemical and structural features of amino acids, peptides, and proteins is essential from a number of perspectives. For nutritionists, there is the need to appreciate the necessity for certain dietary amino acids and other roles of amino acids, peptides, and proteins as nutrients (see Chapters 9 and 13 to 15). There is also the importance of understanding the roles of given amino acids, peptides, and proteins as informational and regulatory molecules. As an introduction, this chapter focuses on chemical characteristics of amino acids and their roles in defining properties of peptides and proteins. It is the chemical diversity of amino acids that serves in part as the basis for organisms to adapt to environments that differ substantially in polarity, water content, temperature, and pressure. Emphasis is also given to the chemical modifications that allow amino acids, peptides, and proteins to perform specific functions, such as acting as catalysts and regulatory molecules (Petsko and Ringe, 2004; Branden and Tooze, 1998;).

GENERAL FEATURES

All peptides and proteins, regardless of their origin, are constructed from a set of 20 common amino acids that are covalently linked together, usually in a linear sequence. Synthesis of a few specific proteins involve translational incorporation of either selenocysteine or pyrrolysine based on nontraditional translation of a "stop" codon; these amino acids have been referred to as the 21st and 22nd amino acid. The structures and selected chemical features of the 20 common amino acids are given in Table 5-1. Amino acids have distinctive side chains that give each amino acid a characteristic size and shape and properties that dictate solubility and electrochemical characteristics. With such diverse building blocks, it is easy to visualize

Table 5-1
Common Amino Acids

Nonpolar, Neutral R-Groups

	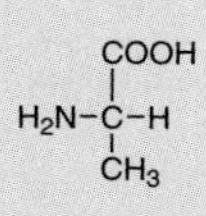	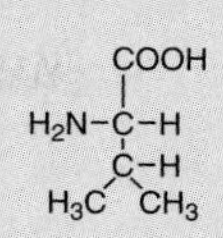	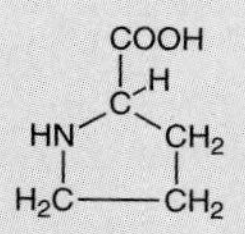	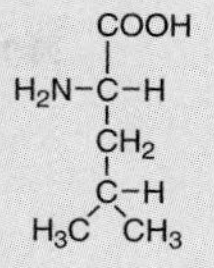	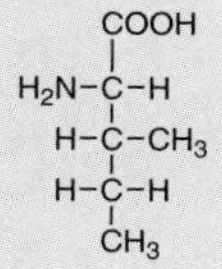
Amino acid	Alanine	Valine	Proline	Leucine	Isoleucine
Abbreviation	Ala, A	Val, V	Pro, P	Leu, L	Ile, I
Molecular weight	89	117	115	131	131
Occurrence (%)[a]	9-10	6-7	4-5	7-8	4-5
pK_a					
–COOH	2.34	2.32	1.99	2.36	2.36
$-NH_2$	9.69	9.62	10.6	9.68	9.68
–RH	—	—	—	—	—
pI	6.01	5.97	6.48	5.98	6.02
Hydropathy index (kcal/mol)[b] **and [solubility in H_2O (g/100 mL) at 25°C]**	0.5 [16.7]	1.5 [8.3]	–3.3 [162]	1.8 [2.4]	2.5 [4.1]
Nutritional essentiality[c]	—	*	—	*	*

Aromatic R-Groups **Acidic R-Groups** (Aspartate, Glutamate)

	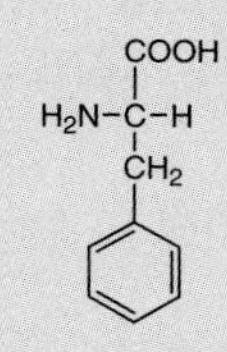	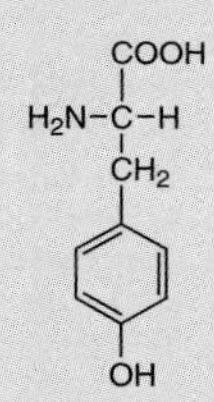	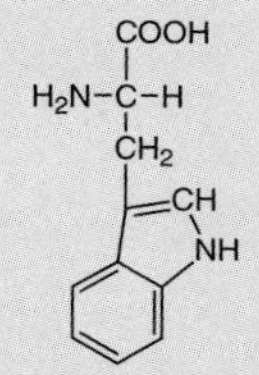	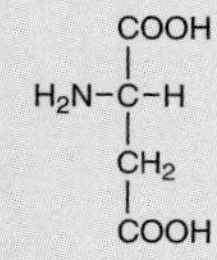	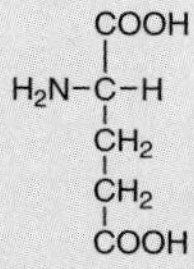
Amino acid	Phenylalanine	Tyrosine	Tryptophan	Aspartate	Glutamate
Abbreviation	Phe, F	Tyr, Y	Trp, W	Asp, D	Glu, E
Molecular weight	165	181	204	133	147
Occurrence (%)[a]	3-4	3-4	1-1.5	5-6	6-7
pK_a					
–COOH	1.83	2.20	2.38	2.09	2.19
$-NH_2$	9.13	10.07	9.39	9.82	9.67
–RH	—	9.11 (–OH)	—	3.86 (—COOH)	4.25 (—COOH)
pI	5.48	5.66	5.89	2.77	3.22
Hydropathy index (kcal/mol)[b] **and [solubility in H_2O (g/100 mL) at 25°C]**	2.5 [2.96]	2.3 [0.045]	3.4 [1.14]	–7.4 [0.5]	–9.4 [0.84]
Nutritional essentiality[c]	*	†	*	—	—

Continued

Table 5-1

Common Amino Acids—cont'd

POSITIVELY CHARGED R-GROUPS

	Lysine	Arginine	Histidine
Structure	COOH–C(H)(H$_2$N)–CH$_2$–CH$_2$–CH$_2$–CH$_2$–NH$_2$	COOH–C(H)(H$_2$N)–CH$_2$–CH$_2$–CH$_2$–NH–C(=NH)–NH$_2$	COOH–C(H)(H$_2$N)–CH$_2$–(imidazole: C=CH–NH–CH=N)
Amino acid	Lysine	Arginine	Histidine
Abbreviation	Lys, K	Arg, R	His, H
Molecular weight	146	174	154
Occurrence (%)[a]	7	4-5	2
pK_a			
–COOH	2.18	2.17	1.82
–NH_2	8.95	9.04	9.17
–RH	10.53 (–NH_2)	12.48 (–NH=CH–NH_2)	6.0 (imidazole ring)
p*I*	9.74	10.76	7.59
Hydropathy index (kcal/mol)[b] **and [solubility in H_2O (g/100 mL) at 25°C]**	–4.2 [freely soluble]	–11.2 [freely soluble]	0.5 [15]
Nutritional essentiality[c]	*	†	*

POLAR, UNCHARGED R-GROUPS

	Glycine	Serine	Threonine	Cysteine	Methionine	Asparagine	Glutamine
Structure	COOH–C(H)(H$_2$N)–H	COOH–C(H)(H$_2$N)–H$_2$C–HO	COOH–C(H)(H$_2$N)–CHOH–H$_3$C	COOH–C(H)(H$_2$N)–CH$_2$–SH	COOH–C(H)(H$_2$N)–CH$_3$–H$_2$C–S–CH$_3$	COOH–C(H)(H$_2$N)–CH$_2$–CONH$_2$	COOH–C(H)(H$_2$N)–CH$_2$–H$_2$C–CONH$_2$
Amino acid	Glycine	Serine	Threonine	Cysteine	Methionine	Asparagine	Glutamine
Abbreviation	Gly, G	Ser, S	Thr, T	Cys, C	Met, M	Asn, N	Gln, Q
Molecular weight	75	105	119	121	149	132	146
Occurrence (%)[a]	7-8	7-8	6	1-2	3-4	4-5	3-4
pK_a							
–COOH	2.34	2.21	2.63	1.71	2.28	2.04	2.17
–NH_2	9.60	9.15	10.43	10.78	9.31	9.82	9.13
–RH				8.33 (–SH)			
p*I*	5.97	5.68	5.87	5.07	6	5.41	5.65
Hydropathy index (kcal/mol)[b] **and [solubility in H_2O (g/100 mL) at 25°C]**	0 [25]	–0.3 [freely soluble]	0.4 [freely soluble]	–2.8 [freely soluble]	1.3 [18]	–0.2 [3.4]	–0.3 [4.7]
Nutritional essentiality[c]	†	—	*	†	*	—	—

[a]Distribution, expressed as a percentage of the total amino acids found in common proteins.

[b]The hydropathy index combines measures of hydrophobicity and hydrophilicity and is used to predict which amino acids will most likely be found in an aqueous environment (– values) or a nonpolar environment (+ values). Hydrophobicities are usually measured by estimating the distribution of the amino acid between a nonpolar solvent and water. Note that hydrophobicity does not relate directly to solubility in water because a number of factors related to the orientation of the R-group and its configuration (see value for proline) can directly influence how the amino acid interacts with water.

[c]The designation (*) indicates that higher order animals have a nutritional requirement for the amino acid. The designation (—) indicates that in most instances the amino acid is sufficiently synthesized at critical periods in growth or development. The designation (†) implies that for some animals there may be a conditional need (i.e., sufficient quantities may not be synthesized). For example, in the rapidly growing and feathering chick, there is a conditional need for glycine, an amino acid abundant in connective tissue proteins and feathers, because glycine is not synthesized in sufficient amounts.

why peptides and proteins can be designed for complex activities (Petsko and Ringe, 2004).

The first chemical description of an amino acid appeared in 1806 when Louis N. Vauquelin and Pierre J. Robiquet isolated asparagine from asparagus. The second amino acid to be discovered was cystine, which William H. Wollaston isolated from a bladder stone. The last of the common amino acids to be described was threonine, which was discovered by William C. Rose and coworkers in 1935 (McCoy et al., 1935). The names for amino acids are derived largely from Greek terms. For example, the designation glycine is derived from the Greek *glykos* (sweet), because glycine has a sweet taste, and the designation cystine is derived from *kystis* (bladder pouch) because cystine was discovered in bladder stones.

Although each amino acid is unique, amino acids do have a number of similar properties. As the term amino acid implies, each contains an amino group and an acid moiety, a carboxylic acid group. Both of these functional moieties are bonded directly to a central carbon atom designated as the α-carbon (Fig. 5-1). Except for glycine, the α-carbon for each of the amino acids has four different functional groups bonded to it: an amino group, a carboxylic acid group, hydrogen, and a "side chain," or "R" group.

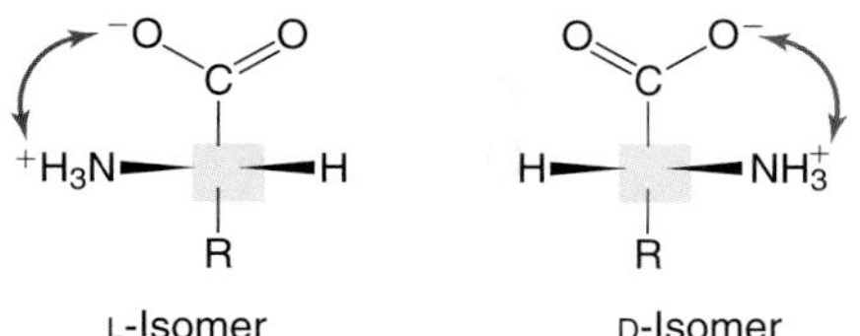

Figure 5-1 General structure for the α-amino acids. Stereoisomers are shown in their L and D forms. Note the position of the α-carbon. The four valences of carbon result in chemical bonds that may be viewed as an equilateral tetrahedron. When a carbon atom has four different substituents, two distinct spatial arrangements are possible. Fisher projections are used to depict the L and D isomers. In a Fisher projection, bonds pointing horizontally are viewed as coming out of the plane on which they are depicted, whereas those pointing vertically go below the plane. A zwitterion is also depicted, wherein the arrows designate the potential balance and interaction between the positive (+) charge of the amino group and the negative (–) charge of the carboxylate group.

Chirality and Optical Rotation

The presence of four different functional groups creates a chiral center. A chiral center exists when an arrangement around a given molecule cannot be superimposed. For all the amino acids (with the exception of glycine), there are two nonsuperimposable, mirror-image forms. These two forms are referred to as stereoisomers, designated as L- and D-isomers. This terminology comes from the Latin terms, *laevus* and *dexter* or *levo* and *dextro*, meaning left and right, respectively. The designation L or D in combination with the given name of an amino acid infers a specific spatial configuration around the amino acid's α-carbon. Another system for assigning stereochemistry, the RS system, is used most often in organic chemistry and has certain advantages. However, the L and D designations remain in common usage for most amino acids.

When an atom in a molecule is bonded to four different chemical species, it is optically active and has a tetrahedral geometry. A chiral center causes the rotation of plane-polarized light. For differing amino acids, the direction and magnitude of the rotation can differ. Furthermore, the magnitude of optical rotation is dependent on other factors, such as pH (the hydrogen ion concentration), the degree of ionization of the carboxylic acid or amine group(s), or the polarity of the solvent in which the amino acid is dissolved.

In proteins and peptides, amino acids are found almost exclusively in the L form, although D-amino acids are found in bacterial proteins and peptides (Petsko and Ringe, 2004), and D–aspartic acid is produced in brain by an enzyme that catalyzes the racemization of L–aspartic acid to D–aspartic acid. This has a number of important connotations. For example, that proteins are constructed largely of L-amino acids indicates that reactions involving amino acids are highly stereospecific. The metabolic pathways for amino acid synthesis create predominantly amino acids in their L form. Moreover, the biological machinery required for protein assembly recognizes L-amino acids almost exclusively (Petsko and Ringe, 2004; Howard & Brown, 2002).

Amphoteric Properties

Amino acids are also amphoteric, which means they can react or interact with either an acid

Nutrition Insight

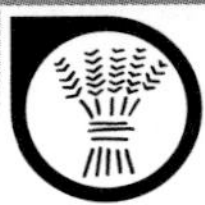

Chirality: The R-, S- System of Nomenclature

Stereoisomers are constitutional isomers (compounds that have the same molecular composition) but differ in the spatial arrangements of atoms. Those stereoisomers that are nonsuperimposable mirror images are called enantiomers, and these are often classified as D- and L- based on their structural relation to a right- or left-handed reference compound. The D-, L- nomenclature is commonly used for both sugars and amino acids. The amino acids commonly found in nature are designated L- based on their relationship to L-glyceraldehyde, and the common sugars are designated D- based on their relationship to D-glyceraldehyde.

The D-, L- system for designating the configuration of stereogenic centers proved to be inadequate and ambiguous for general application, especially to compounds with several chiral centers. In order to unambiguously distinguish between enantiomers, a set of rules, which is known as the Cahn-Ingold-Prelog system or the R-, S- system, was established by three European chemists, R.S. Cahn, C.K. Ingold, and V. Prelog. In the Cahn-Ingold-Prelog system, each stereogenic center in a molecule is assigned a prefix (R or S), according to whether its configuration is right- or left-handed. The symbol R comes from the Latin *rectus* for right, and S from the Latin *sinister* for left. In order to make the R or S assignment, relative priority values [1 (heaviest), 2, 3, or 4 (lightest)] are assigned to each of the four substituents on the chiral carbon based on the mass of the groups (heaviest to lightest) according to the following three basic rules:

1. Highest priority is given to the substituent atom with the highest mass (e.g., H<C<N<O).
2. If two substituents have the same immediate substituent atom, atoms progressively further away from the chiral center are evaluated until a difference is found (e.g., $CH_3<CH_2CH_3<CH_2CH_2Cl$).
3. If double or triple bonded groups are encountered as substituents, they are treated as if both atoms involved in the bond were present twice or three times, respectively (e.g., $CH_2CH_3<$ $CH_2{=}CH-<CH{\equiv}C-$).

Once the relative priorities of the four substituents have been determined, the molecule is oriented so that the chiral center is viewed from the side opposite the lowest priority substituent atom (i.e., so that the lightest or #4 group is pointing away from the viewer). The direction of rotation observed when moving from the highest to the lowest priority (1→2→3) will now be either clockwise (and the enantiomeric configuration at the chiral carbon will be designated R) or counterwise (and the configuration will be designated S). An amino acid is shown below as an example. For more complex molecules with multiple stereocenters, the process is repeated until all chiral centers have been given an R or S designation.

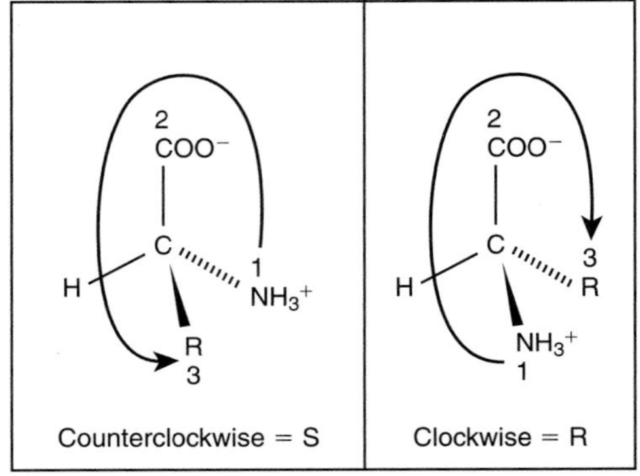

or base. In aqueous solutions, amino acids are easily ionized. Moreover, when both an amino group and carboxyl group are bonded to a common carbon atom, the combination can exist as a zwitterion. A zwitterion is an amphoteric, dipolar structure with both a positive and negative charge (see Fig. 5-1). Although the zwitterion portion of an amino acid is water soluble in the physiological pH range, it is ionically neutral because the positive charge of the amino group cancels out the negative charge associated with the carboxylate group. The zwitterionic character also causes amino acids to be held together by electrostatic forces in a crystalline lattice (i.e., analogous to the crystalline lattice of sodium chloride and other salt crystals). As a consequence, similar to many salts, thermal decomposition of amino acids usually requires a high temperature (i.e., higher than 200° C) owing to their zwitterionic characteristics and their ability to form crystalline lattices. Furthermore, in a nonhydrated state, most amino acids exist as nonvolatile crystalline solids.

AMINO ACID SIDE CHAINS

Additional physical and chemical properties of amino acids are dictated by their side chains, referred to as R-groups (Petsko and Ringe, 2004; Rucker and McGee, 1993; Rucker and Wold, 1988). A given R-group confers novel, sometimes unique, chemical properties to an amino acid. Accordingly, amino acids can be classified based on the chemical properties of their respective R-groups. For example, the relative degree of amino acid solubility is modulated by the nature of the R-group and its relative polarity or hydropathy (i.e., the tendency to interact with a polar or nonpolar solvent or environment). This property of amino acid R-groups can vary widely, ranging from totally nonpolar or hydrophobic (water-insoluble) to polar or hydrophilic (water-soluble).

Examples of nonpolar or hydrophobic R-groups are those that consist of multiple carbon units, such as the side chains of alanine, leucine, valine, proline, or isoleucine. In this group of amino acids, proline deserves special comment, because its R-group is joined both at the α-carbon and amino group to form a ring of hydrocarbon atoms. For this reason, proline is referred to as a secondary amino acid or imino acid. Its α-carbon lacks a hydrogen but remains a chiral center because a cyclic group replaces the hydrogen. The cyclization also renders proline more rigid, with no ability to rotate easily around the α-carbon. Accordingly, the presence of proline in a polypeptide segment can reduce peptide chain flexibility (Petsko and Ringe, 2004; Konig, 1993; Hamaguchi, 1992). Of the other hydrophobic amino acids, with the exception of alanine, all have bifurcated side chains. These amino acids help to define hydrophobic domains in proteins. In valine and isoleucine, the bifurcation of the side chain is adjacent to the α-carbon, which restricts conformations by steric hindrance. Note that amino acids that are hydrophobic have positive hydropathy scores (see Table 5-1). The amino acids with positive hydropathy scores tend to repel the aqueous environment and, as a consequence, reside predominantly in the interior of proteins.

The aromatic amino acids are phenylalanine, tyrosine, and tryptophan. Aromatic side chains contribute specific optical properties to proteins, such as the ability to absorb light in the ultraviolet range. Of the three, phenylalanine is the most common in proteins and enzymes with an average molar abundance of approximately 3.5 %, about double the amount of any other aromatic amino acid. In contrast, tryptophan is incorporated into proteins and enzymes at an average molar abundance of 1.1%, making it the amino acid found in least amounts in proteins. Phenylalanine serves as a precursor of tyrosine, and tyrosine plays a key role in the biosynthesis of neuroactive amines, hormones, and pigments. Tryptophan plays essential roles in the biosynthesis of NAD/NADP, the neurotransmitter serotonin, and the hormone melatonin (see Chapter 14 for details.) Aromatic amino acids are also often important components at the active sites of enzymes.

Aspartate and glutamate are examples of polar amino acids that contain a net negative charge because each of their side chains contains a carboxylate group. In contrast, lysine, arginine, and histidine are polar amino acids with functional groups capable of forming positive charges depending on the pH of the medium in which they are dissolved. Lysine, arginine, and histidine have side chains that contain amino ($-NH_2$), guanidino ($-NH_2-C=O-NH_2$), or imidazole groups ($-C_3N_2H_3$ ring) (see Table 5-1). Of the three, the imidazole side chain of histidine has the most "neutral" pK_a (~6.0), which means that relatively small shifts in cellular pH will change its charge. For this reason, this amino acid side chain is used extensively as a coordinating ligand for metals in metalloproteins and at the catalytic site of certain enzymes.

There are also amino acids with uncharged R-groups that vary in polar characteristics (e.g., threonine, serine, cysteine, asparagine, glutamine, and methionine). The polarity of threonine and serine are properties contributed by the oxygen of their respective hydroxyl groups. The polarity of cysteine and methionine is influenced by the presence of sulfur in the form of a thiol or methylthio group, respectively. The polarity of asparagine and glutamine is caused by the presence of a nitrogen- and oxygen-containing carboxamide group.

MODIFICATIONS OF AMINO ACID SIDE CHAINS

As was noted in the preceding section, the properties of the common amino acids can vary markedly depending upon their innate characteristics (e.g., charge, polarity, or hydropathy). The characteristics of some amino acids can also be altered by additional enzymatic and nonenzymatic modifications of the R-group. Such modifications can occur as co- or posttranslational events associated with or following the incorporation of the amino acid into proteins (see Chapters 13 and 14). These specific amino acid modifications are introduced to modulate or modify a given chemical property. Posttranslational modifications extend the structures and properties of amino acids in proteins well beyond those of the 20—or 21 including selenocysteine—amino acids used for protein translation in mammals.

Specific chemical properties can be modified subtly or dynamically by posttranslational modification. Consider the net change in charge (0 to 2–) that occurs when a serine residue (as a part of a peptide sequence) is phosphorylated at its hydroxyl group (Fig. 5-2). Other examples of posttranslational modifications of amino acid R-groups in proteins include the methylation of lysine and histidine residues, the hydroxylation of proline and lysine residues, and the carboxylation of glutamate residues (Fig. 5-3). These types of modifications of R-groups are essential in defining the structural and functional properties of proteins.

A number of other amino acids are derived from metabolism of the common amino acids found in proteins. Many of these amino acids are discussed in Chapter 14. Amino acids, such as ornithine, citrulline, taurine, homocysteine and certain biogenic amine compounds that act as cellular signals (e.g., dopamine, serotonin, and histamine) are derived in distinct metabolic pathways. Other examples include thyroid hormone synthesis from tyrosine as outlined in Chapter 38 and selenocysteine synthesis from serine as described in Chapter 39.

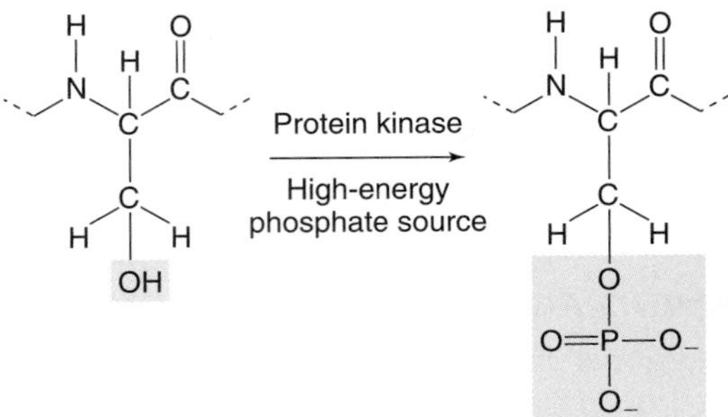

Figure 5-2 The modification of serine residues in a polypeptide to a phosphoserine residue. Some amino acids undergo chemical modifications that can significantly alter their original properties. This example emphasizes how adding a substituent such as a phosphate group can alter electrochemical properties and net charge. The reaction depicted is important to many metabolic pathways in which protein phosphorylation (addition of a phosphate group) is important for activation or inhibitions of functions. The high-energy phosphate source is usually adenosine triphosphate (ATP).

ACID AND BASE CHARACTERISTICS OF AMINO ACIDS

When an amino acid is titrated (i.e., exposed to an acid or base), the resulting reactions can be described by a titration curve. The types and number of the functional groups capable of reacting with or exchanging a hydrogen ion influence the shape of this curve. In an amino acid such as alanine, there are two titratable groups (Fig. 5-4). At a low pH (i.e., a high hydrogen ion concentration), both the amino group and the carboxylic acid group of alanine are protonated. As a result, alanine is positively charged and migrates toward the negative pole in an electrical field. If a base is added (to decrease the concentration of hydrogen ions or, alternatively, to increase the concentration of hydroxyl ions), the carboxylic acid group and then the amino group lose their protons. At the midpoint of this process when the carboxylate group is unprotonated and negatively charged and the amino group is still protonated and positively charged, alanine is neutral. The addition of more base eventually causes the amino group to lose its proton, and alanine becomes negatively charged because of the loss of the positively charged amino group. Compare the titration curve for alanine to the

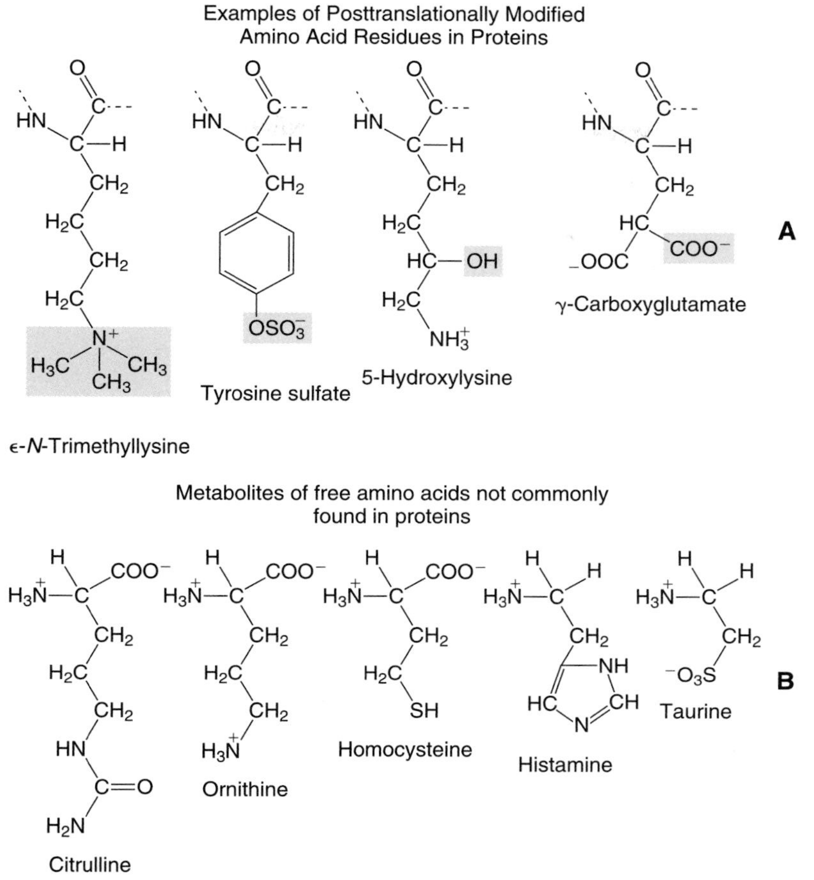

Figure 5-3 Examples of posttranslationally modified and less conventional amino acids. **A,** Some of the modifications are the result of specific enzymatic reactions wherein the amino acid to be modified is first incorporated into a given peptide or protein and then altered by an enzyme-catalyzed reaction. Examples of the products of a methylation (ε-*N*-trimethyllysine residue formation), a sulfation (tyrosine sulfate residue formation), an hydroxylation (5-hydroxylysine residue formation), and a γ-carboxylation (γ-carboxyglutamate residue formation) are shown. **B,** The structures for citrulline, ornithine, homocysteine, histamine, and taurine are also shown. These amino acids and related compounds are derived from amino acids, but in contrast to the amino acids shown in **A,** they are produced in a step-wise fashion in metabolic pathways. Arginine and glutamate are precursors of citrulline and ornithine. Homocysteine is the demethylation product of methionine. Histamine is formed by decarboxylation of histidine. Taurine is formed by oxidative catabolism of cysteine. It is the free amino acid rather than an amino acid residue in a protein that is substrate for the metabolic pathways that produce these amino acids and amino acid derivatives.

more complex titration curve for histidine, which contains three titratable functional groups (see Fig. 5-4).

As is the case with organic acids and amine compounds, amino acid titration curves can be described by constants called pK_as that help to define characteristics of the associated titratable groups. A pK_a is the negative log of the dissociation constant K_a for an acid. When the associated (protonated) and dissociated (unprotonated) species are present in equal concentrations, the pK_a is equal to the pH. The pK_as of carboxylic acid groups are relatively low, usually 2 to 4. Amino groups have pK_as that are relatively high, usually 9 to 11 (see Table 5-1). Accordingly, the classification of an amino acid as acidic or basic depends on the pK_a of a titratable group on its side chain.

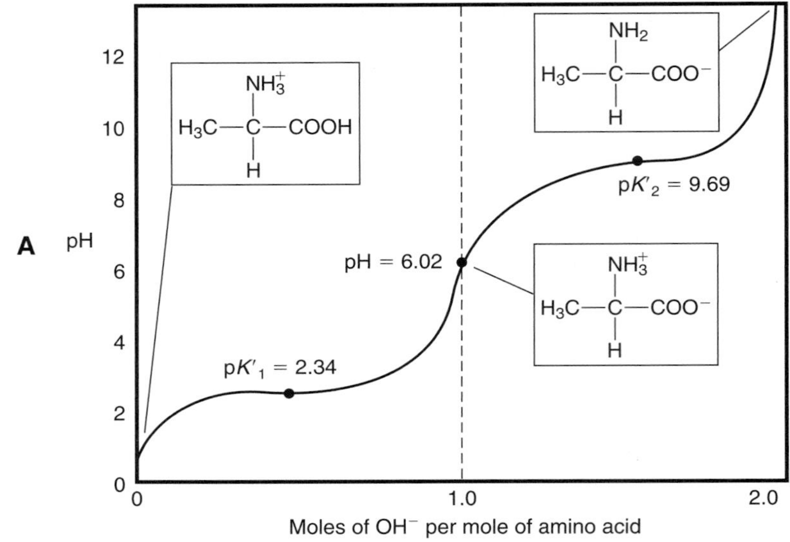

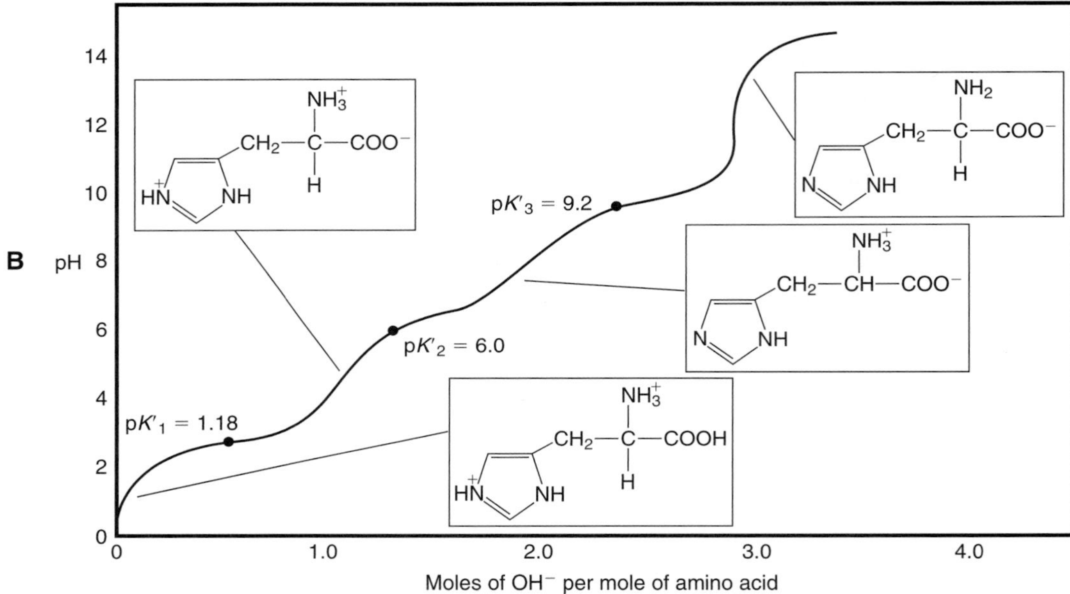

Figure 5-4 Titration curves for alanine **(A)** and histidine **(B)**. The pH equivalent to the isoelectric point (see text) for alanine is shown as the midpoint between the two pK_as.

Why is it important to know something about the titration characteristics of individual amino acids? First, intermolecular and intramolecular ionic interactions are very important to protein structure. For example, if it is essential for a protein to be electrically or ionically neutral to function, then the protein must be designed with a combination of amino acids that results in a zero or near zero net charge. In this regard, cell communication, as articulated through specific proteins, is often dependent on the ionic characteristics of given amino acids. Amino acids and proteins also have the ability to act as buffers because of their acid and base characteristics.

Information about the ionic properties of proteins also has a practical significance. When a protein is titrated to the point that corresponds to neutrality (i.e., to a pH where a protein has little/or no net charge), this pH is referred to as

Nutrition Insight

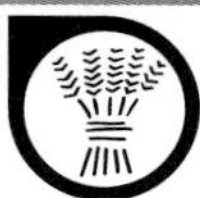

Use of Milk Proteins in Other Foods

Milk proteins are a heterogeneous mixture that includes two main groups of proteins: (1) caseins and (2) whey or serum proteins. Within these two classes of proteins are six major subclasses: α_1-casein, α_{s2}-casein, β-casein, γ-casein, β-lactoglobulin, and α-lactalbumin. In addition, a number of other proteins are present, such as albumin, immunoglobulins, and lactoferrin.

Casein makes up about 80% of milk protein, and is used in a number of food preparations. Casein may be precipitated from milk by acidification to casein's isoelectric point, a pH of approximately 6.0. This phenomenon is easily demonstrated by adding lemon to tea or coffee that contains milk or cream. The serum protein or whey fractions remain in solution, and this solution is often called whey.

The separation of casein from whey proteins is important in that both protein classes have novel properties. Casein in the presence of lipids can form micellar structures ranging in size from 30 to 300 nm. Micellar structures are responsible for the opaqueness of milk. The ability to form micelles is useful because a number of hydrophobic substances can be incorporated into casein micelles. The whey fraction in milk is also used in the preparation of fabricated foods. Whey proteins are hydrophilic and may be added to beverages to increase the protein content. Furthermore, whey proteins are highly water binding because of their hydrophilicity, which makes them well suited for addition to soups, gravies, and salad dressings. The knowledge that one can separate these two important milk fractions by acid precipitation is very useful. The separated forms differ in solubility, viscosity, and utility as thickening agents. Whey proteins are ideally suited for increasing viscosity and thickening, whereas casein is an excellent choice when emulsification is needed to add flavoring agents. Moreover, under certain processing conditions, whey or whey/casein mixtures can be formed into hydrophobic micelles. Hydrophobic micellar structures can be designed to have oily characteristics for use as fat substitutes. An example is Simplesse, a microparticulated whey protein concentrate that behaves like fat globules and is used in low-fat food products.

the isoelectric point (p*I*) of the protein. Many proteins are insoluble at their isoelectric points. Thus, protein isolation and concentration can sometimes be achieved by adjusting the pH. A good example is the use of pH to precipitate casein from milk (Darby, 1993).

PEPTIDES

Amino acids are covalently joined by peptide bonds (Fig. 5-5). Peptide bond formation is endergonic (i.e., it requires energy) with a positive free energy change of approximately 20 kJ/mol (~4.8 kcal/mol) at physiological pH. A positive free energy change of this magnitude means that combining an amino group of one amino acid with the carboxyl group of another does not occur spontaneously to any appreciable extent. Consequently, peptide synthesis requires both energy and specialized mechanisms (see Chapters 13 and 14).

PROTEINS

LEVELS OF PROTEIN STRUCTURE

It should now be apparent that altering the charge and hydrophobic or hydrophilic nature of the amino acid residues, as well as the length of polypeptide chains, can influence the function of proteins. The numerous combinations of amino acids give rise to many possibilities for primary sequence of polypeptide chains that, in turn, dictate the size, shape, charge, and function of given proteins.

Proteins differ greatly in their size. Small proteins contain 50 to 100 amino acids, and the largest known size of a protein monomer is approximately 5,000 amino acid residues. Protein and peptide molecular masses are often reported as daltons (Da) or kilodaltons (kDa). Apolipoprotein B-100, which is involved in lipid transport, is a good example of a very large protein. Apolipoprotein B-100 comprises

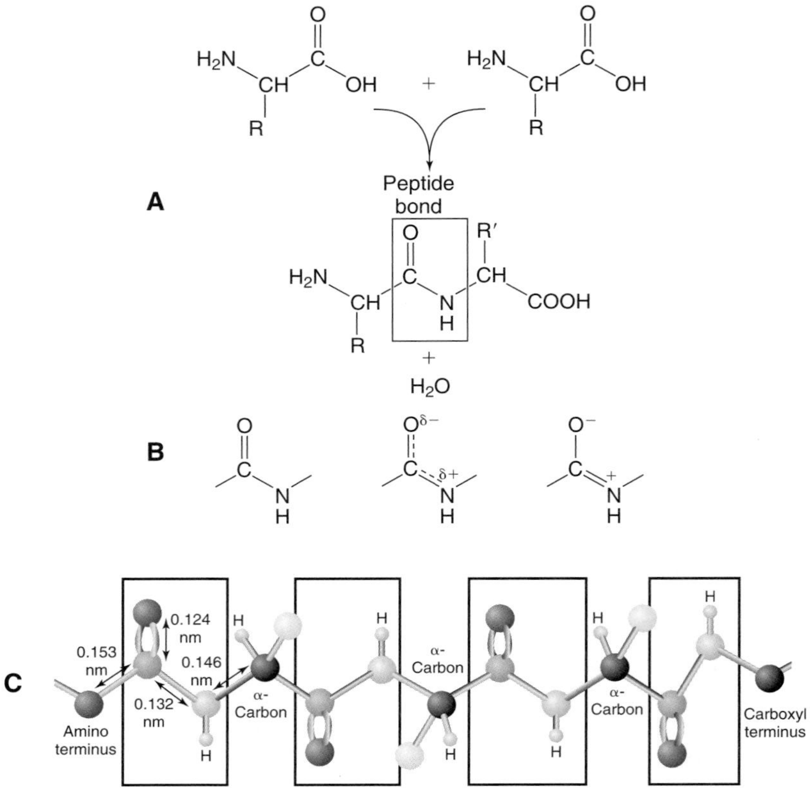

Figure 5-5 **A,** Formation of a peptide bond. The α-amino group of one amino acid displaces the hydroxyl of the carboxyl group in another. Although amino acids are good nucleophiles, the hydroxyl group is a poor leaving group. Therefore, the reaction is endergonic with a free energy change of about 20 kJ, or approximately 80 to 90 kcal per mol. As shown in **B,** the peptide bond is capable of resonance and charge separation. As indicated in **C,** the oxygen and nitrogen of the amide bond lie in a plane, and this contributes to peptide bond stabilization. The hydrogen of the amino group is usually *trans* to the oxygen in the peptide backbone. Note that the bond length between the oxygen and carbon originating from the carboxyl group is 0.124 nm, typical of a C=O double bond. The nitrogen that is attached to the C=O forming the peptide bond also has a relatively short bond length (0.132 nm), indicating some double bond character. This causes an electric dipole. Because each bond has some double bond character, there is also restricted rotation. However, the nitrogen to α-carbon bond is 0.146 nm, and the carbonyl carbon to α-carbon bond is 0.151nm, which are typical of a single bond. Rotation can occur around this bond, unless it is hindered by the presence of a bulky R-group (e.g., that of valine or isoleucine) or constrained due to the cyclic nature of a proline residue.

a single polypeptide chain of 4,536 amino acid residues and has a molecular mass of 513 kDa (Law et al., 1986). In addition, many proteins are made of multiple subunits. In some structural proteins the subunits are covalently cross-linked into larger complexes that have molecular masses in the millions of daltons.

A dalton is a relative measure of mass, named after chemist John Dalton, that is used to express atomic masses and molecular masses. One dalton is equal to $^1/_{12}$ of the mass of one atom of carbon-12; in other words, mass of an atom or molecule is calculated based on the ratio of its mass to that of carbon-12, which has 6 protons and 6 neutrons in its nucleus. Roughly:

$$\text{Mass} = \text{Number of Protons} + \text{Number of Neutrons}$$

Because atomic masses are ratios or relative values, they have no units. Avogadro's number and the mole are defined so that one mole of a substance with an atomic or molecular mass of 1 will have a mass of precisely 1 g: one mole of hydrogen atoms has a mass of 1 g; one mole of apolipoprotein B has a mass of 513 kg. That is, the mass of one mole of an atom or molecule is its atomic or molecular mass in grams.

Primary Structure

Protein structure is complex and can be described at different levels of organization. The first level is the linear sequence of amino acids. The term primary structure is used to delineate this one-dimensional linear sequence of amino acids. The amino acid sequence of a peptide or protein can be determined by sequencing the amino acids along the linear polypeptide chain. Alternatively, the sequence may be inferred from the corresponding nucleotide sequence of the protein's gene or the sequence of its corresponding messenger RNA (mRNA).

Considerable information may be inferred from knowing the primary structure. Many sequences act as specific signals for certain protein modifications that impact biological regulation. Examples include the following:

- The sequences asn-x-ser and asn-x-thr, which are commonly associated as sites for *N*-linked glycosylation in proteins (i.e., the addition of sugars at specified sites along the polypeptide chain)
- The sequence arg-gly-asp-ser, which corresponds to the cell surface–binding domain in certain proteins (e.g., fibronectin) and allows a protein to bind to a cell's surface
- The sequence lys-asp-glu-leu, which is one of the signals important for the vectoral movement of soluble proteins within the endoplasmic reticulum (ER)

The use of x in the first example indicates that a number of given amino acids can be substituted for x without affecting the functional significance of the sequence when it appears in a protein. When an amino acid sequence is associated with a definable and consistent function, the sequence is often designated as a consensus sequence, particularly if the sequence is found in proteins in a diverse array of animal, plant, or bacterial cells.

Additional information that may be obtained from a primary sequence is an indication of regions of hydrophobicity and hydrophilicity. A hydropathy plot is given in Figure 5-6. Hydropathy plots are useful in defining regions in a polypeptide or clusters of amino acids that differ in their polar or nonpolar characteristics. Protein folding is dependent on the location of hydrophobic and hydrophilic amino acids within a given segment or domain in a polypeptide chain. Moreover, hydropathy characteristics are important for the insertion of protein polypeptide sequences into cell membranes or for creation of networks of proteins that function in transmembrane communication (Davis, 2002; Hamaguchi, 1992).

Secondary Structure

Secondary structure refers to the spatial arrangement of atoms around the backbone of a given polypeptide chain. The backbone is made up of the alpha carbons of each amino acid residue along with the α-carboxyl carbon and α-amino nitrogen that are in peptide linkage. Because the C–N peptide bond shares some double bond character with the C=O bond, there is restricted rotation around the peptide bond. However, in the polypeptide main chain, Cα–C and N–Cα bonds are relatively free to rotate. The amino acid R-groups can influence the extent of rotation. For example, large, bulky groups prevent rotation around the polypeptide backbone and fix given conformations into place. As noted previously, the rotation of the R-group of the imino acid proline is restrained because the ring-structure limits its rotational freedom. Proline-containing peptide bonds tend to fold back upon themselves such that proline is often found in regions of protein that form turns. A proline residue will usually terminate a stretch of helical structure because there is no hydrogen attached to its nitrogen to take part in hydrogen bonding; the restrained rotation of proline causes a kink in the peptide chain that also disrupts the regular structure. In addition, electrostatic attractions and repulsions between amino acid residues, interactions between the amino acids at the ends of α-helix, and the electric dipole inherent to the peptide backbone contribute to secondary beta structures.

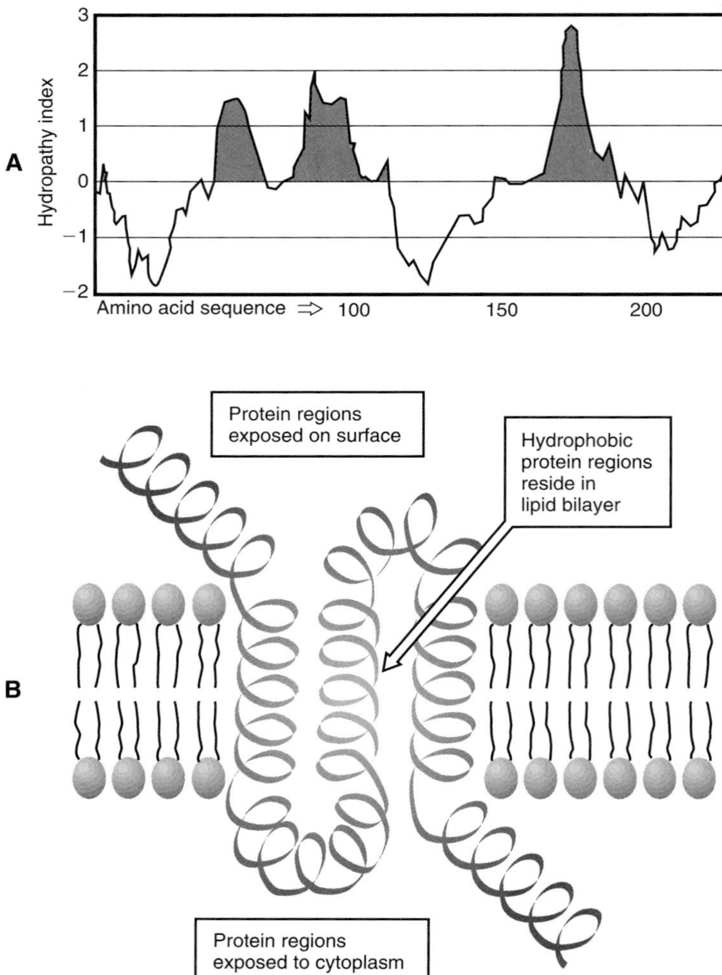

Figure 5-6 A hydropathy plot. Hydrophobic regions are usually found in the interior of proteins, whereas hydrophilic regions are likely to interact with aqueous or ionic environments. (See Table 5-1 for hydropathic indices for given amino acids.) A hydropathy plot **(A)** identifies regions of a polypeptide chain that contain amino acids that are predominantly hydrophobic *(shaded)* or, in contrast, hydrophilic *(unshaded)* in nature. The example shown could apply to a transmembrane protein **(B)**. Transmembrane proteins often cross the lipid bilayers of cell membranes. The hydrophobic regions (positive hydropathic values) are associated with the interior of the membrane, whereas the hydrophilic regions may extend into the cytoplasmic compartment or toward the exterior of the cell.

The two major classes of proteins, by shape, are fibrous proteins and globular proteins. Fibrous proteins are distinguished by their filamentous, elongated form and their extensive regions of regular secondary structure. Most fibrous proteins play structural roles in tissues. A good example of a fibrous protein in the human body is the α-keratins, which are the major proteins of hair, fingernails, and skin calluses. The secondary structure of α-keratins is composed predominantly of α-helices. Collagen, which provides much of the extracellular matrix of bone and other tissues, has a more unusual secondary structure. It is composed of chains of left-handed helical structure that are wound together with two other chains to form a right-handed helical structure. Other fibrous proteins, such as the β-keratins

Nutrition Insight

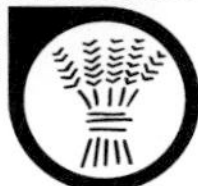

Vitamin and Mineral Prosthetic Groups Give Color to Certain Holoproteins

When some prosthetic groups associate with proteins, they lend color to the protein as a functional property. A good example is the addition of flavin adenine dinucleotide (FAD) or flavin mononucleotide (FMN) to the apoproteins that form into flavoproteins. Flavoproteins appear yellow. Proteins that contain heme as a prosthetic group have colors that range from brown to bright red, depending on the oxidation state of the iron-containing heme moiety. As an example, the amount of heme-containing myoglobin in muscle tissue imparts to meat varying amounts of color. White poultry meat contains relatively small amounts of myoglobin (0.1 to 0.4 mg/g), whereas dark poultry meat often contains five to six times that amount of myoglobin. Veal and pork contain 2 to 7 mg of myoglobin per gram, and beef usually contains 10 mg or more of myoglobin per gram. The globins of both myoglobin and hemoglobin are colorless; yet when they are complexed with heme through coordinated and synergistic interactions with histidine residues, red to pink colors are imparted.

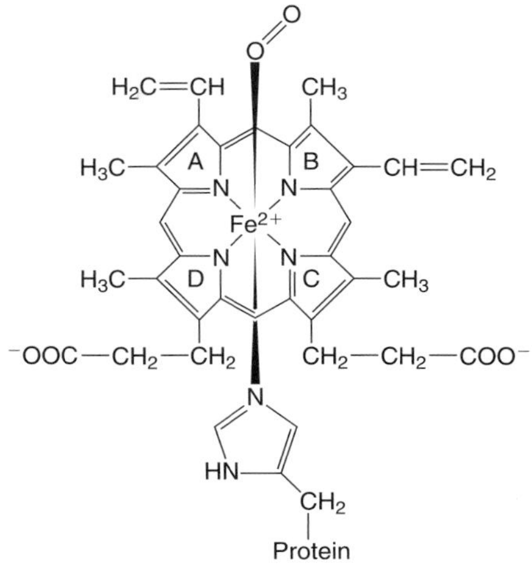

Oxymyoglobin is usually red–pink in color, whereas deoxygenated myoglobin is purple–red. Denaturation of meat protein by cooking can cause dissociation of heme and the formation of protein, iron, and imidazole (from histidine) complexes that are brown to tan. When a prosthetic group imparts color to a protein, it is referred to as a chromophore.

found in feathers and scales and the fibroin made by silkworms and spiders, contain mainly β-sheet structures. Globular proteins far outnumber fibrous proteins and perform most of the work of the cell. In general, globular proteins have many small regions of regular secondary structure rather than the extensive regions found in fibrous proteins. Globular proteins are folded into compact structures, with tertiary structure playing an important role in stabilization of the structure.

Protein secondary structure consists largely of α-helices and β-pleated sheets (Fig. 5-7). β-Turns are interruptions between secondary structures that involve hydrogen bonding between closely spaced residues of the polypeptide. Other regions of proteins may have less–well-defined structures such as irregular regions and random coils. The α-helix is a right-handed spiral conformation. In α-helical structures, the polypeptide chains are enriched in amino acids with free rotation around the polypeptide chain. This allows each main C=O and N–H group to hydrogen bond to a peptide bond four residues away to give a very regular, stable arrangement. In contrast to β-sheet structures, the hydrogen bonds in an α-helix are between amino acids that are near to each other in the linear polypeptide sequence, and all the R-groups or peptide bonds in an α-helix point in the same direction. In the polypeptides that form β-sheets, a common feature is segmental repeats of amino acids, the side chains of which restrict free rotation around the polypeptide backbone. These polypeptide regions do not form a coil but instead zig-zag in a more extended β-conformation referred to as a β-strand. These strands can associate by main-chain hydrogen bonding interactions to form a sheet. For example in a β-sheet, two or

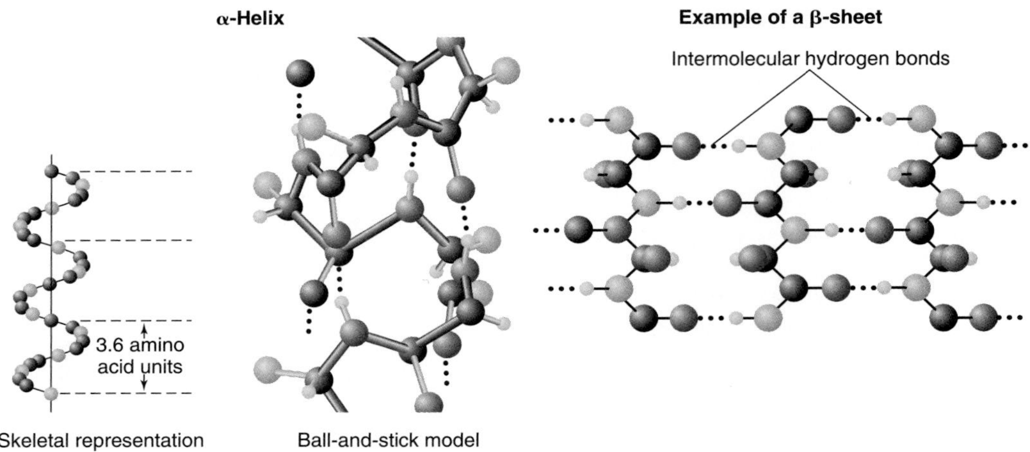

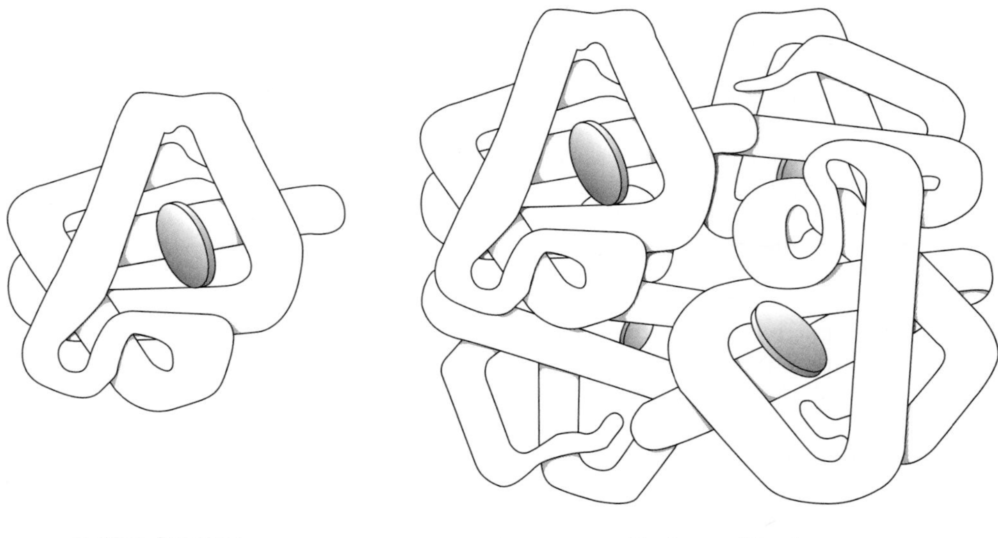

Figure 5-7 Levels of structure in proteins. The primary structure consists of a sequence of amino acids with secondary structures that often exist as α-helices or as β-sheets. These structures combine to make complex tertiary structures, which may serve as a subunit that eventually forms the quaternary structure of multimeric proteins. The example is a representation of the tertiary and quaternary structure of hemoglobin. The heme molecules are shown within the folds.

more polypeptide chains run alongside each other (in a parallel or antiparallel direction) and are linked by hydrogen bonds between the main chain C=O and N–H groups (i.e., the hydrogen bonds in a β-sheet are between different segments of the polypeptide). In the β-strand, the R-groups of adjacent residues point in opposite directions; when additional strands interact to form the β-sheet, a pleated appearance arises, which is the basis of the term "β-pleated sheet."

There are also a number of secondary features of these structures that are beyond the scope of this chapter. However, it should be appreciated that many different types of segmental polypeptide structures may exist in a single protein or polypeptide strand. Most proteins contain segments of both α-helical and β-sheet structures as well as more complex variations of these. Computer modeling programs for studies of small polypeptides, which are designed to systematically vary the rotational angle around the α-carbon with the objective of finding stable conformations, indicate that a number of β-structure variants exist. Functional proteins, such as enzymes, are very dependent upon maintenance of their "native" or intrinsic structural characteristics. When a protein is "unfolded" by various extreme conditions (e.g., low pH, high temperature, urea, or guanidinium), the consequence is denaturation, resulting in a "denatured" or less functional state.

Tertiary and Quaternary Structures

The term tertiary structure is used to describe the overall three-dimensional arrangements of amino acids within a protein. In addition to regions of secondary structure that lock the positions of some atoms relative to each other, the overall three-dimensional shape of a protein molecule is a compromise structure that has the best balance of attractive and repulsive forces between different regions of the molecule. Frequently, the tertiary structure of proteins involves the formation of two of more domains—structurally independent parts of the protein held together by a relatively thin stretch of polypeptide backbone. Complex protein structures can be determined to an atomic level by x-ray diffraction of crystallized proteins or by nuclear magnetic resonance (NMR) spectroscopy of small (less than 30 kDa) proteins in solution. Tertiary structures may also accommodate specific functional groups, such as prosthetic groups. The term prosthetic group is used to describe a unique moiety or defined chemical structure that confers a specific function or additional property to a given protein. Prosthetic groups may be covalently or noncovalently linked to the proteins they serve. Examples of prosthetic groups include the heme group in hemoglobin and myoglobin and enzyme cofactors such as lipoic acid or pyridoxal 5′-phosphate.

For proteins made up of more than one polypeptide chain, an additional term, quaternary structure, is used to describe the three-dimensional arrangement of multiple polypeptide chains in the complex. The protein may be made up of identical or different polypeptide chains, usually called subunits, that interact with each other. The subunits are held together by a variety of attractive forces such as ionic and hydrogen bonds and hydrophobic interactions; covalent interchain disulfide bonds are rarely involved. Many proteins, including many transcription factors and a number of enzymes, form homo- or heterodimers. Some examples of proteins with more than two subunits include the following:

- Hemoglobin, a heterotetramer made up of two identical α subunits and two identical β subunits
- Antibodies of the immunoglobulin G (IgG) form, which have two light chains and two heavy chains with disulfide bonds within each chain as well as between the two heavy chains
- The insulin receptor, which is a transmembrane receptor tyrosine kinase that is a disulfide-linked dimer composed of two heterodimers, each of which contains an α and a β chain
- Myosin, which is a hexamer made up of two trimers, with each trimer composed of a heavy chain, an essential light chain, and a regulatory light chain

HOW PROTEIN CONFORMATIONS ARE STABILIZED

Most protein conformations are stabilized by relatively weak interactions. Some examples of the types of interactions that stabilize proteins are given in Table 5-2. The difference in free energy between folded and unfolded states in typical proteins is in the range of 20 to 70 kJ/mol (5 to 17 kcal/mol). For comparison or perspective, 20 to 70 kJ/mol is 5 to 15 times the amount of energy needed to break covalent C–C bonds (~350 kJ/mol or 83 kcal/mol) or C–H bonds (410 kJ/mol or 98 kcal/mol). Although many conformations may be possible, a large number of weak interactions can result in a high degree of stabilization.

The stability of a given conformation is dictated by the entropy term associated with the

Table 5-2
Forces that Stabilize Protein Structures

Type of Bond or Force	Description
Ionic bond Attractive forces 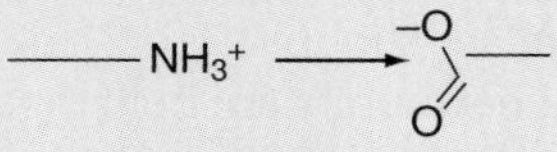 $—NH_3^+ \longrightarrow {}^-O(C=O)—$ Repulsive forces $—NH_3^+ \longleftrightarrow {}^+H_3N—$	Charged complexes that are capable of creating very strong interactions depending on the dielectric constant
Hydrogen bond 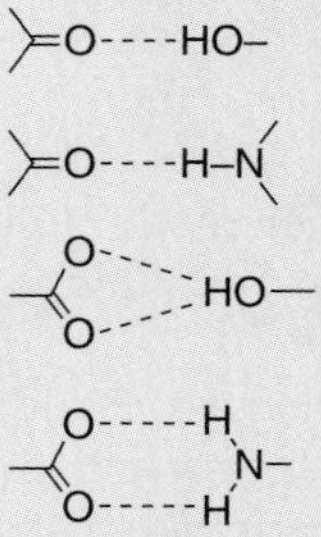 $>C=O\cdots HO—$ $>C=O\cdots H—N<$ $—C(O)(O)\cdots HO—$ $—C(O\cdots H)(O\cdots H)N—$	Noncovalent bonds that result from the association of hydrogen with atoms that are electronegative
Hydrophobic interactions 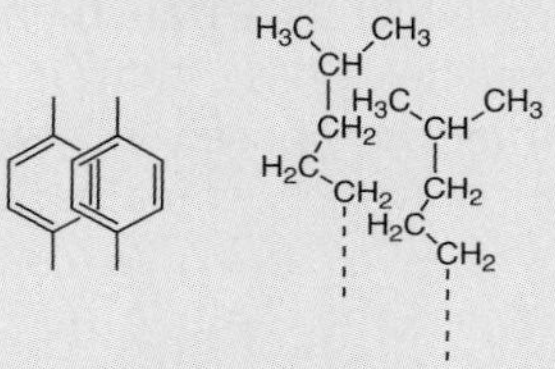	Association of hydrocarbon-rich compounds with hydrocarbon moieties in proteins or polymers; the energy required for the process comes from the reorganization of the surrounding water structure.
Van der Waals interactions	Weak electrostatic attractions

energy relationships important to the folding and unfolding of a polypeptide chain. When stabilization occurs, it is the result of the sum of the hydrophobic and ionic interactions of the various amino acid side chains. In particular, hydrophobic interactions are important for protein–protein interactions and the tertiary structure in large proteins. As proteins become smaller in size, it often becomes difficult to accommodate or appropriately place hydrophobic residues. It is for this reason that many small proteins are held together by covalent bonds, usually disulfide linkages. However, either noncovalent (hydrophobic or ionic) or covalent bonds can impose restrictions on the folding and stabilization of given structures (Hamaguchi, 1992).

The process of folding and unfolding of proteins is dynamic. For most proteins, this process results from a sequential series of events that take place in a programmed manner. When a protein is folded so that it is functional, the process is referred to as naturation (Branden and Tooze, 1998). When unfolding or inappropriate folding occurs and results in a dysfunctional state, the process is referred to as denaturation. Most commonly, proteins are denatured by substances that disrupt associated water structures, heat, and/or extremes of acid or base.

Disruption of water organization by a denaturant (e.g., urea) influences the secondary, tertiary, and quaternary structures of proteins. Extremes of heat denature proteins, because vibrational energy within the protein molecule is altered. An excessive increase in vibrational energy disrupts tertiary structures. Extremes of acid–base balance or pH cause denaturation by interfering with the organization of water or by altering the redox state of proteins. Finally, chemical modifications that change amino acid R-groups can have dramatic effects on protein structure. For example, introducing a reducing agent such as mercaptoethanol ($HSCH_2CH_2OH$) can disrupt disulfide bond formation, which in turn can cause the opening of associated polypeptide chains.

NUTRITIONAL INFLUENCES ON PROTEIN STRUCTURE, ASSEMBLY, AND FUNCTION

Protein structure or assembly is influenced when nutrition is suboptimal (Rucker and McGee, 1993). In particular, nutritional deficiencies may affect steps important to the co- and posttranslational processing of proteins, because many of the enzymatic proteins involved in protein modifications require metals or vitamin-derived cofactors to function properly. A cotranslational event occurs coincident with the actual translation (synthesis) of a protein. A posttranslational modification occurs after the protein has been synthesized. Posttranslational modifications of proteins usually occur in the Golgi or post-Golgi sites associated with the smooth ER or secretory vesicles (see Chapter 13).

Posttranslational modifications extend the range of chemical properties of the common amino acids within protein and are as important to the processing and production as any of the transcriptional and translational events involved in polypeptide synthesis. That is, a defect at any of the steps in the process of protein assembly or modification can result in a dysfunctional product. Most posttranslational modifications can be placed in one of the following three broad categories:

1. Modifications that involve peptide bond cleavage and formation
2. Modifications that involve the amino- or carboxy-terminal amino acid
3. Modifications that involve specific amino acid side chains

Modifications in the first category may already be familiar. Activation of many peptide hormones and conversion of zymogens to active enzymes are examples (Petsko and Ringe, 2004). For example, trypsinogen and other protease zymogens are converted to active proteinases by hydrolysis of an internal peptide bond to release an N-terminal segment.

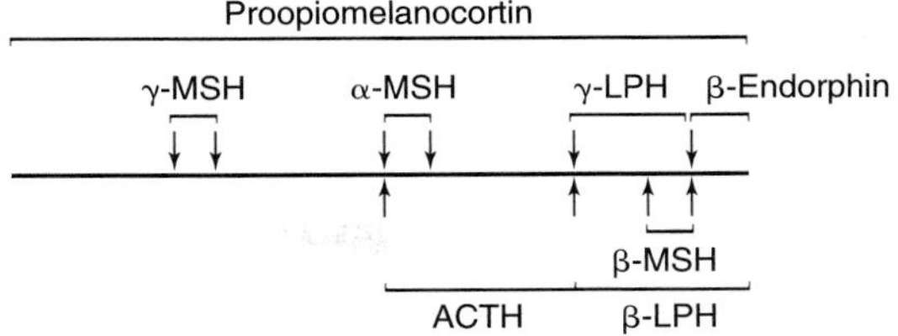

Figure 5-8 Bioactive peptides can arise by several mechanisms. As an example, the production of α-, β-, and γ-melanocyte-stimulating hormones (MSH), adrenocorticotrophic hormone (ACTH), β-endorphin, and β- and γ-lipotropin (LPH) are shown. The peptides arise from the cleavage of peptide bonds in the protein proopiomelanocortin, which acts as a precursor. *Arrows* indicate sites where enzyme proteinases cleave specific peptide bonds to give rise to the designated peptides.

Formation of the hormone insulin from its precursor polypeptide, proinsulin, occurs by proteolytic excision of an internal segment, leaving two polypeptide chains attached by disulfide bonds. Proopiomelanocortin produced by the pituitary gland can be cleaved to yield seven different polypeptide hormones as illustrated in Figure 5-8.

The second type of cotranslational or posttranslational modification, those that modify the N- or C-terminus, are important in (1) directing proteins to specific compartments within the cell, (2) protecting the amino- and carboxy-terminal sequences from proteolysis, and (3) selective activation of enzymes and hormones. For example, amidation of the carboxyl group at the C-terminus of many hormones (e.g., calcitonin) is essential for activation. The initial N-terminal methionine is removed from many newly synthesized proteins by a methionine aminopeptidase, and the new N-terminal residue may be acetylated or modified with another chemical group.

The third type of posttranslational modification, R-group or side chain modifications, provides chemical features important for cellular compartmentalization and trafficking, receptor binding, regulatory signaling, protein cross-linking, and the creation of enzymatic or functional active sites. Table 5-3 lists some examples of chemical modifications of side chains of amino acid residues in proteins that are common targets for the modifications. For example, as signals for compartmentalization, typical reactions involve acylations,

Table 5-3
Examples of Modifications Involving Amino Acid Side Chains

Selected Functions	Process or Example	Commonly Targeted Amino Acids in Proteins
Compartmentalization, receptor binding	Acylations	Asn, Cys, Gln, Lys, Ser
	Acetylations	Ala, Arg, Gly, His, Lys
	Glycosylations	Asn, Cys, Gln, Hyp, Lys, Ser, Thr, Tyr
Regulatory signaling	Acetylations	Lys
	Adenylylations	Tyr
	ADP-ribosylations	Cys, Glu, Arg, Lys, Ser
	Methylations	Arg, Asp, Glu, His, Lys, Ser, The
	Phosphorylations	Ser, Thr, Tyr, His, Lys
	Ubiquitin addition	Lys
	Sulfations	Tyr
Prosthetic group additions or formation	Biotinylations	Lys
	Flavin (FAD and FMN) additions	Cys, His
	Phosphopantetheine addition	Ser
	Pyridoxal phosphate addition	Lys
	Retinal addition	Lys
Protein cross-linking	Allysine and dehydronorleucine formation	Lys
	Cystine formation	Cys
	Glutamyllysine formation	Gln, Lys
Other	Carboxylations	Asp, Glu
	Halogen addition (iodine)	Tyr
	Hydroxylations	Asp, Lys, Pro, Asn
	Nonenzymatic glycosylations	Arg, Lys
	Sulfoxide formation	Met
	Glutamylation	Glu
	Isoprenylation	Cys

acetylations, and glycosylations. Acylation, the attachment of long-chain fatty acids, provides lipophilic "handles" that facilitate the vectoral movement of the protein from one compartment to another and creates specific sites to enhance attachments and compartmentalization within cells. The formation or incorporation of various prosthetic groups in proteins usually occurs as a posttranslational protein modification, such as the covalent addition of biotin to carboxylases or the association of pyridoxal phosphate with aminotransferases. The addition of a given prosthetic group may be essential to the creation of an enzymatic or functional active site. Hydroxylation of lysyl and prolyl side chains in collagen is essential step in their association to form the tropocollagen triple helix; and the γ-carboxylation of glutamyl residues in prothrombin is essential for its activity as a clotting factor.

For stabilization of protein structures, it is often essential to cross-link together specific polypeptide chains (Fig. 5-9). For structural proteins, such as collagen and elastin, the formation of interchain cross-links facilitates the formation of fibers and protein complexes, the molecular masses of which can range into the millions of daltons (Reiser et al., 1992). The formation of interchain cross-links also renders collagen and elastin resistant to the action of many proteinases so that these proteins can exist in a proteinase-enriched environment without significant damage or alteration.

Specific nutrient deficiencies can cause decreased enzymatic activity or protein function by a variety of mechanisms. Caloric restrictions or excesses may also alter the synthesis or degradation of amino acids and other components important to amino acid, peptide, or protein modification. Decreased cofactor

Nutrition Insight

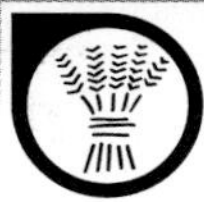

Niacin and Polyribosylation of Histone Proteins

Pellagra is a well-known deficiency disease that results from an insufficient intake of niacin and tryptophan (see Chapter 24). Niacin is a precursor for nicotinamide adenine dinucleotide (NAD) synthesis. The amount of NAD in cells is very much dependent on the amount of niacin, which is either made from tryptophan-related pathways or present in the diet as a vitamin. One of the functions of NAD is as a substrate for monoribosylation and polyribosylation reactions.

Polyribosylations change the surface property and structural conformation of some proteins (e.g., histones that are found in the nucleus of cells). Ribosylation reactions are important in many of the complex steps in enzyme regulation and also for DNA repair. In this regard, it is important to note that the skin lesions associated with pellagra may be due to the inability to carry out normal DNA repair because of an inability to alter histone structure and function via polyribosylation reactions.

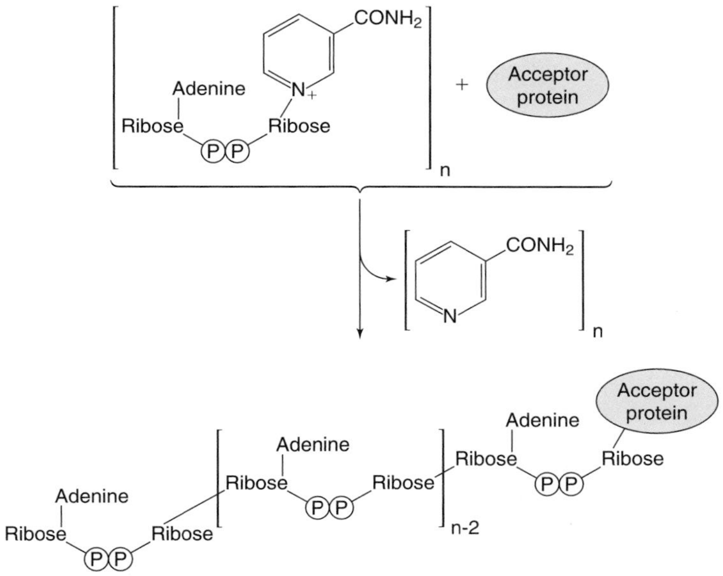

concentration, particularly if they serve as cosubstrates in posttranslational protein modifications, can result in highly specific biochemical defects and lesions. Moreover, proteins that are only partially or incompletely processed tend to be degraded more rapidly than fully processed proteins.

Much of the regulation and metabolism discussed in subsequent chapters depends on posttranslational modifications of proteins. The protein-mediated transcription of genes, translation of mRNAs into proteins, and movement of substances into, through, and out of given cells are dependent on changes in proteins brought about by enzymatic and nonenzymatic chemical modifications. In subsequent chapters, when the actions of specific nutrients are described, consider how the action or role of the nutrient may be related to some aspect of protein structure or amino acid modification.

As a final point, the range of chemical properties, the diverse conformations of peptides and proteins, and their novel chemical features have all been utilized to develop numerous approaches for the separation and quantitative and very sensitive detection of amino acids, peptides, and proteins. Use of antibodies and the growth of protein microarray technology now allow measurement of many individual proteins with both sensitivity and

Nutrition Insight

Vitamin C and Connective Tissue Protein Synthesis

The nutritional deficiency disease scurvy has a dynamic and important impact on connective tissue and extracellular matrix integrity. With respect to extracellular matrix stability, ascorbic acid serves as a cofactor for lysyl and prolyl hydroxylases. A decrease in prolyl and lysyl hydroxylase activity causes a net decrease in the production of hydroxyprolyl and hydroxylysyl residues in collagen and related proteins.

Collagen is a protein that constitutes one third of the total protein in the body and is the major protein in the extracellular matrix of the connective tissue. Under-hydroxylated collagen polypeptide chains do not associate properly and are more susceptible to degradation than normal forms of collagen; this is an underlying factor in many of the lesions associated with scurvy.

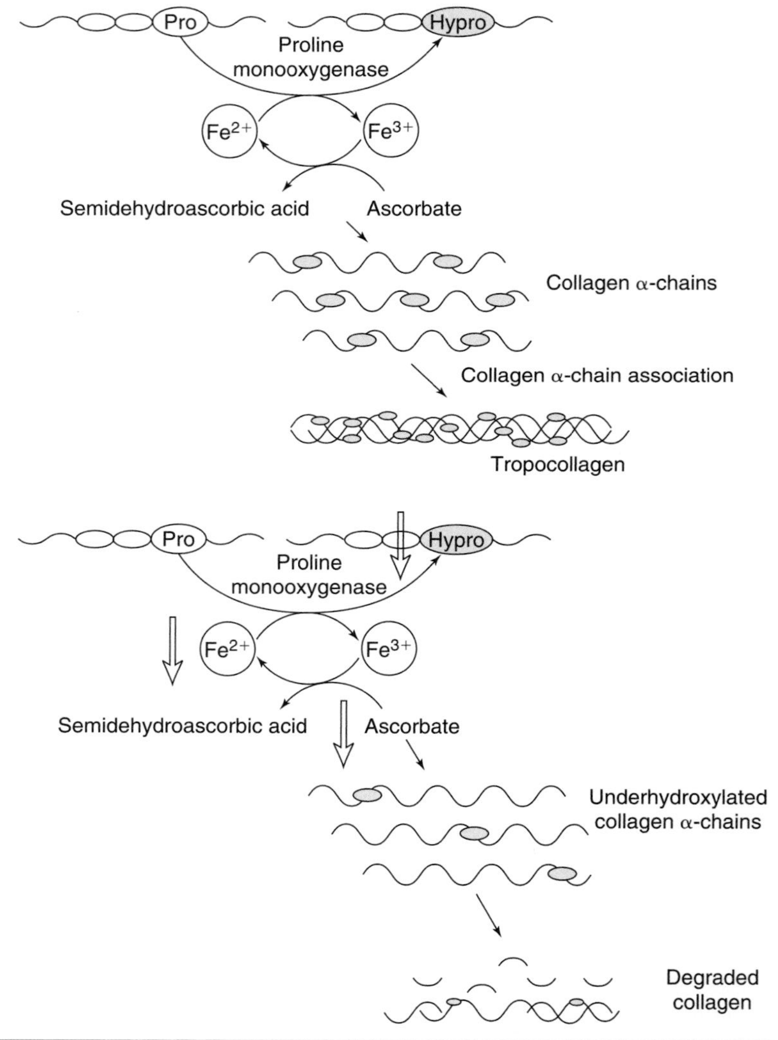

Pro, Proline; *hypro,* hydroxyproline.

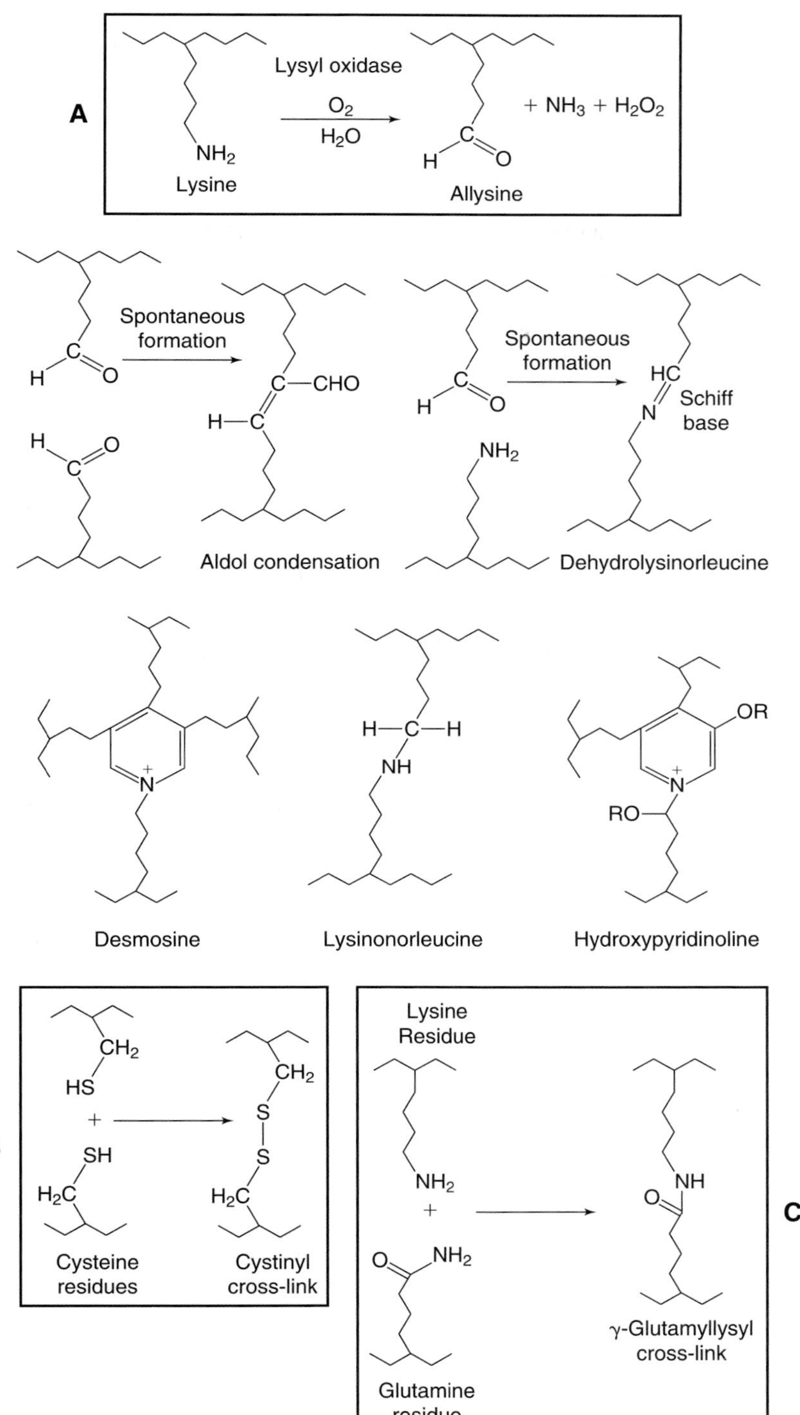

Figure 5-9 Amino acids that function to cross-link polypeptide chains. Examples include the lysine-derived cross-links **(A)**, cystine formation from cysteine **(B)**, and cross-links derived from the enzyme-catalyzed condensation of lysine and glutamine residues **(C)**. For the reactions shown in *(A)*, the first step is the oxidation and deamination of specific lysine residues in proteins such as elastin and collagen to form residues of allysine. The next steps occur nonenzymatically. Two examples are shown. An aldol condensation product is formed from condensation of two peptide-bound allysine residues.

Continued

Figure 5-9, cont'd Peptidyl dehydrolysinonorleucine occurs as a product of the Schiff-base reaction. Peptidyl allysine on a polypeptide chain reacts with peptidyl lysine on an adjacent polypeptide chain to cause cross-linking of the two chains. These products may condense further to form even more complex amino acid-derived cross-links, such as desmosine, which is found in the structural protein elastin, or hydroxypyridinoline, which occurs in collagen. Hydroxylysine residues (see Fig. 5-3) serve as lysine-derived precursors for hydroxypyridinoline. Note that the R-groups of the hydroxypyridinoline structure can also be sites for glycosylation. As shown in **B**, the formation of peptidyl cystine cross-links from peptidyl cysteine oxidation is also a common strategy for cross-linking or joining protein polypeptide chains together. Protein disulfide isomerase catalyzes the formation of disulfide bonds within or between polypeptide chains. In panel **C**, formation of another cross-linking amino acid, γ-glutamyllysine, is shown. The formation of γ-glutamyllysine from glutamine plus lysine residues in proteins such as fibrin and keratin is catalyzed by transglutaminase.

precision. In addition, advances in protein crystallography and protein NMR spectroscopy, as well as in computer modeling of protein structure, continue to provide insights into the structure and function of specific proteins. Access to genomic databases facilitates the study of sequence information for both known and unknown proteins. Some of the references in the Recommended Readings section provide more information on these methodologies.

REFERENCES

Branden C, Tooze J (eds) (1998) Introduction to Protein Structure. Garland, New York, pp 1-301.

Darby NJ (1993) Protein Structure. IRL Press/Oxford University Press, Oxford, England.

Davis BK (2002) Molecular Evolution Before the Origin of Species. Prog Biophys Mol Biol 79:77-133.

Hamaguchi K (1992) The Protein Molecule: Conformation, Stability, and Folding. Japan Scientific Societies Press, Tokyo; Springer-Verlag, New York.

Howard GC, Brown WE (2002) Modern Protein Chemistry: Practical Aspects. CRC Press, Boca Raton, FL.

Konig WS (1993) Peptide and Protein Hormones: Structure, Regulation, Activity. A Reference Manual. Weinheim VCH, New York.

Law SW, Grant SM, Higuchi K, Hospattankar A, Lackner K, Lee N, Brewer HB (1986) Human liver apolipoprotein B-100 cDNA: complete nucleic acid and derived amino acid sequence. Proc Nat Acad Sci 83:8142-8146.

McCoy RH, Meyer CE, Rose WC (1935) Feeding experiments with mixtures of highly purified amino acids. VIII. Isolation and identification of a new essential amino acid. J Biol Chem 112:283-302.

Petsko GA, Ringe D (2004) Protein Structure and Function. London, New Science; Sunderland, MA: Sinauer Associates, Oxford, Blackwell Publishing.

Reiser K, McCormick RJ, Rucker RB (1992) Enzymatic and non-enzymatic cross-linking of collagen and elastin. FASEB J 6:2439-2449.

Rucker RB, McGee C (1993) Chemical modifications of proteins in vivo: selected examples important to cellular regulation. J Nutr 123:977-990.

Rucker RB, Wold F (1988) Cofactors in and as post-translational protein modifications. FASEB J 2:2252-2261.

RECOMMENDED READINGS

Aggeli A, Boden N, Shuguang Z (eds) (2001) Self-Assembling Peptide Systems in Biology, Medicine, and Engineering. Kluwer Academic Publishers, Boston.

Howard GC, Brown WE (2002) Modern Protein Chemistry: Practical Aspects. CRC Press, Boca Raton, FL.

Karplus M, McCammon JA (1986) The dynamics of proteins. Sci Am 254:42-51.

Palzkill T (2002) Proteomics. Kluwer Academic Publishers, Boston.

Pennington SR (2001) Proteomics: From Protein Sequence to Function. BIOS, Oxford, England.

Veenstra TD (2003) Proteome Analysis of Post-Translational Modifications. Adv Protein Chem 65:161-194.

RECOMMENDED WEBSITE

Nomenclature and Symbolism for Amino Acids and Peptides
International Union of Pure and Applied Chemistry (IUPAC) and International Union of Biochemistry and Molecular Biology (IUBMB) Joint commission on Biochemical Nomenclature
www.chem.qmul.ac.uk/iupac/AminoAcid/

Chapter 6

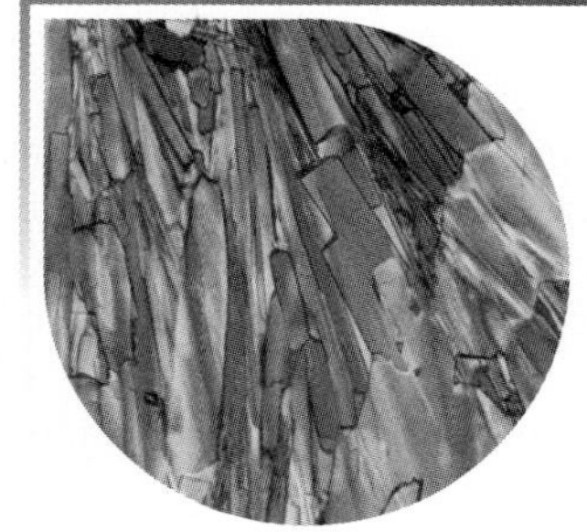

Structure, Nomenclature, and Properties of Lipids

J. Thomas Brenna, PhD, and Gavin L. Sacks, PhD

OUTLINE

COMMON ABBREVIATIONS

- CMC critical micellar concentration
- DAG diacylglycerol
- FFA free fatty acid (also called nonesterified fatty acid, NEFA)
- LT leukotriene
- LX lipoxin
- MAG monoacylglycerol
- PC phosphatidylcholine (lecithin)
- PE phosphatidylethanolamine
- PG phosphatidylglycerol
- PI phosphatidylinositol
- PS phosphatidylserine
- PUFA polyunsaturated fatty acid
- TAG triacylglycerol (also called triglyceride, TG)
- TX thromboxane

This chapter is a revision of the chapter contributed by Donald Small, MD, for the first edition.

LIPID CLASSES AND NOMENCLATURE

Lipids are a diverse set of small molecules that are unified by their solubility in nonpolar solvents. Unlike the other major components of mammalian tissue—proteins, carbohydrates, and nucleic acids and their polymers—lipids do not share any characteristic chemical structural similarity. Lipids can be categorized into classes according to structural similarities; the major classes of lipids are listed in Box 6-1. Fahy et al. (2005) recently published a comprehensive classification system for lipids that encompasses the lipids discussed in this chapter as well as more exotic lipids species, particularly nonmammalian lipids.

All mammalian biochemistry operates in aqueous solution or in a lipid environment that usually is adjacent to the aqueous phase, such as in membranes or the surfaces of oil droplets. Because the aqueous phase predominates, lipids can be thought of as the other major chemical phase in mammals. As such, the major lipids function as barriers, receptors, antigens, sensors, electrical insulators, biological detergents, membrane anchors for proteins, and as a major energy source. Phospholipids play a critical role in maintaining the integrity of all living things, plant and animal, because they form the barrier separating the living cell from the extracellular environment. This barrier is called the cell membrane or plasma membrane. It consists of a continuous bilayer of phospholipids into which other lipids, such as cholesterol and glycosphingolipids, are inserted. Into this lipid bilayer, protein channels, transporters, receptors, structural pillars such as integrins, and other functional elements are inserted to give the plasma membrane its unique characteristics. The fatty acid composition of the phospholipids and the cholesterol content regulate the chemical properties and perhaps the thickness of the membrane.

Box 6-1

CHEMICAL CLASSIFICATION OF BIOLOGICALLY IMPORTANT LIPIDS*

I. Nonesterified fatty acids
  A. Saturated fatty acids
  B. Unsaturated fatty acids
  C. *Trans* fatty acids
  D. Conjugated fatty acids
II. Glycerolipids
  A. Mono-, di-, triacylglycerols (esters of fatty acids with glycerol)
III. Glycerophospholipids
  A. Common phospholipids (PE, PS, PI, PG, PC)
  B. Lysophospholipids
  C. Ether phospholipids (platelet-activating factors, plasmalogens)
  D. Diphosphatidylglycerols (cardiolipins)
IV. Glycoglycerolipids (including sulfates)
V. Sphingolipids
  A. Sphingosine
  B. Ceramide
  C. Sphingomyelin
  D. Neutral glycosphingolipids (e.g., cerebrosides)
  E. Acidic glycosphingolipids (e.g., gangliosides)
VI. Isoprenoids (carotenoids, retinoids, prenols)
VII. Biological waxes (long-chain ester waxes and related compounds)
VIII. Steroids
  A. Sterols
  B. Steroid hormones (sex hormones and corticosteroids)
  C. Bile acids
IX. Eicosanoids
  A. Cyclooxygenase products (prostaglandins and thromboxanes)
  B. Lipoxygenase products (leukotrienes and lipoxins)
  C. Cytochrome P450 products
X. Other lipids (acyl CoA, acylcarnitine, anandamide, and lipopolysaccharides)

Modified from Small DM, Zoeller, RA (1991) Lipids. In: Encyclopedia of Human Biology, Vol. 4, Academic Press, Orlando, FL, pp 725-748.

*The chemical classification of lipids given in this table is necessarily incomplete and somewhat arbitrary. It progresses from hydrocarbons to more complex chemical structures. Simple esters and glycerol esters yield, on hydrolysis, the alcohol and/or glycerol and fatty acid. The major membrane lipids, glycerophospholipids, yield fatty acid (or alcohol), glycerol, phosphate, and the appropriate base (choline, ethanolamine, etc.). Sphingolipids yield the base sphingosine and a fatty acid on hydrolysis.

Glycosphin-golipids are present only on the external surface of the plasma membrane, where they act as receptors for toxins (e.g., ganglioside GM_1 is the receptor for cholera toxin) and probably as antigens to mark the cell as being of a certain type.

Phospholipids also are the major components of the membranes that form the functionalized barriers between compartments of the cell, for example, the membranes of the nucleus, the mitochondria, the endoplasmic reticulum (ER), the Golgi apparatus, secretory vesicles, and peroxisomes. Pure mixtures of phospholipids form bilayers that are nearly impermeable to ions and polar molecules such as water. Membranes use proteins to form selectively permeable pores to allow certain molecules or ions to pass from one side to the other. It is widely believed that the function of proteins is related to their interplay with the lipids in which they are embedded, although a detailed understanding of how this interplay operates in vivo is lacking.

Fats, oils, and waxes are stored in cytoplasmic droplets and represent a major source of cellular energy. An average human in metabolic balance may easily ingest and absorb 100 g of fat in a day. The 900 kcal derived from burning this fat would represent 35% to 45% of the total energy consumed. Components of fats (i.e., fatty acids, fatty alcohols, and glycerol) are used as building blocks for membranes during growth, maintenance, and repair. Many hormones are lipids. The steroid hormones (cortisol, estrogens, progesterones, and androgens), derived from cholesterol, and prostaglandins and leukotrienes, derived from polyunsaturated fatty acids, are examples. Low concentrations of these molecules effect important physiological changes. Cholesterol has recently been found to be essential in embryogenesis, and an absolute deficiency of this sterol leads to severe and often fatal defects. Other lipids act as regulators of intracellular processes (e.g., diacylglycerol, sphingosine, ceramides, and platelet-activating factor). Some lipids are secreted and act as pheromones that attract or repel other organisms. In higher animals, lipids are transported to and from cells in the form of small (10- to 10,000-nm diameter) aggregates called lipoproteins. Lipids in the brain, spinal cord, and nerves are ordered in a way that permits the transmission of electrical impulses without short-circuiting between nerves or tracts. Lipids also play a role in many diseases that afflict humans (e.g., atherosclerosis; obesity; gallstone disease; Reye's syndrome; the familial lipidoses such as Tay-Sachs disease, Niemann-Pick disease, and Gaucher's disease; and the familial lipoproteinemias).

The nomenclature of lipids strikes many newcomers as obtuse and difficult. This reaction is doubtless because there are many names in use that are arbitrary and reveal little in the way of chemical structure. As with all organic compounds, systematic organic chemical naming rules apply to lipids, but traditional lipid nomenclature persists for good reason. Most lipid naming conventions are convenient when viewed in the context of mammalian lipid metabolism and, to a lesser extent, are logical extensions of the traditional methods used to analyze lipids. Therefore, study of lipid nomenclature also reveals structural and metabolic relationships among lipids, and familiarity with nomenclature makes the study of lipid metabolism much clearer. That being said, lipid nomenclature is usually easiest to retain when learned in the context of specific structure–function or metabolism–function discussions. This chapter should be used as a reference because lipid nomenclature is relevant to subsequent chapters.

NONESTERIFIED OR FREE FATTY ACIDS

Fatty acyl chains are the basic units of glycerolipids that render these compounds nonpolar. They are referred to as fatty acids in part because many traditional analytical methods first hydrolyze all fatty esters into fatty acids. However, the concentration of free fatty acids (FFAs), which are also called nonesterified fatty acids (NEFAs), is very low compared to that of fatty acids esterified as glycerolipids. Fatty acids are characterized by a carboxylic acid head group and a hydrocarbon chain tail. In mammals, they may range from two carbons to as many as 40 carbons, but primarily exist as chains of 12 to 22 carbons.

Fatty acids are sometimes most conveniently classified according to chain length.

Short-chain fatty acids have 6 or fewer carbon atoms, and their chemistry is sufficiently dominated by the carboxyl group that they are soluble at least to some extent in water. Medium-chain fatty acids have 8 to 14 carbon atoms, and long-chain fatty acids have more than 14 carbons. These cutoff values are different depending on the very specific lipid subfield of interest. Fatty acids are also classified according to their degree of unsaturation, more specifically, by the number of double bonds in their hydrocarbon chains. High concentrations of FFAs are often indicative of disease states or of local cell damage. The plasma concentration of total FFAs is about 0.5 to 1.0 mmol/L, with approximately 99% of these noncovalently bound to albumin. Fatty acids have the potential to reach high local concentrations during fat catabolism. For instance, during lipolysis of chylomicron or very low density lipoprotein (VLDL) triacylglycerols by plasma lipoprotein lipase, FFAs are liberated. Sites of high lipolytic activity (e.g., the capillary beds in adipose tissue, muscle, and heart) may see very high concentrations of the FFAs.

Saturated Fatty Acids

The term "saturated" in the context of fatty acids refers specifically to carboxylic acid terminated hydrocarbon chains that are exclusively made up of sp^3 hybridized (tetrahedral geometry) carbon atoms arranged as linear $-CH_2-$ chains as shown in Figure 6-1. Without double bonds, these chains cannot add H_2 across double (or triple) bonds, and, therefore, are saturated with hydrogen (H). Saturated fatty acids in mammalian tissues are overwhelmingly of even carbon number. Fatty acids are synthesized predominantly by fatty acid synthase through the successive addition of two carbon acetyl-CoA units to a growing acyl chain within the fatty acid synthase enzyme. Chain-elongation generally ceases when the acyl chain has grown to 16 carbons so that the major fatty acid synthesized in mammals is palmitic acid, although small amounts of myristic acid (14 Cs) and stearic acid (18 Cs) are also produced. In addition, elongation enzyme systems bind to these and other fatty acids and add two carbon units. Fatty acids with an odd number of carbon atoms are present at very low concentrations under normal circumstances and typically arise as intermediates in metabolism.

Table 6-1 presents the chain lengths, systematic names, trivial names, and melting points of the most abundant saturated fatty acids in mammalian tissue. Fatty acids are referred to by either their trivial or systematic names, depending on context and specific lipid subfield.

In mammals, the majority of saturated fatty acids are configured as straight chains, but in rare cases methyl groups extend from the main chain, usually near the methyl end of the molecule. A fatty acid that terminates with a dual methyl (or isopropyl) group at the end of a hydrocarbon chain is referred to as "iso," as shown in Figure 6-2. If the chain terminates with both a methyl and an ethyl group, an isobutyl configuration, the fatty acid is said to be "anteiso." Branched-chain fatty acids in humans appear in vernix, the protective waxy, white substance that coats and protects fetuses during late gestation. They have also been detected as minor components of skin, blood, hair, and in cancer cells. They can be major components of microorganisms, as in gram-positive bacteria.

Unsaturated Fatty Acids

"Unsaturated" is used to describe fatty acids with at least one double bond, consisting of two adjacent sp^2 hybridized carbon atoms, with a trigonal, approximately planar, geometry.

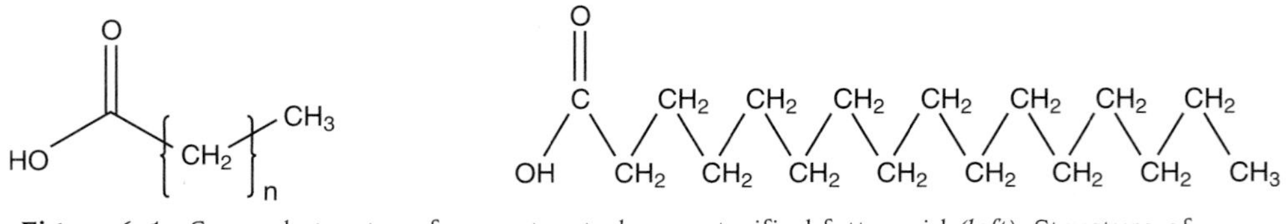

O
HO
CH_2
n
CH_3
O
C
OH
CH_2 CH_2 CH_2 CH_2 CH_2 CH_2 CH_2
CH_2 CH_2 CH_2 CH_2 CH_2 CH_2 CH_2 CH_3

Figure 6-1 General structure for a saturated nonesterified fatty acid *(left)*. Structure of hexadecanoic acid (palmitic acid) *(right)*.

They are unsaturated with respect to hydrogen, because H_2 can be covalently added across the double bond to yield sp^3 carbon atoms. Nomenclature for fatty acids is tailored to make convenient reference to their structures and basic biochemistry. The overwhelming majority of unsaturated sites in mammalian fatty acids are double bonds configured in the *cis* (Z) geometry. When two or more double bonds are present in a molecule, the fatty acid is said to be polyunsaturated. Generally, double bonds in mammalian polyunsaturated fatty acids (PUFAs) are separated by a methylene ($-CH_2-$) group ("methylene-interrupted"). This structural property of PUFAs confers special chemical properties. One important chemical property is that the double bonds are not conjugated, and thus there is free rotation about the $-CH_2-$ group. As with saturated fatty acids, trivial names dominate

Table 6-1

Naturally Occurring Straight-Chain Saturated Carboxylic Acids

Number of Carbons	Systematic Name	Trivial Name	Melting Point (° C)
2	n-Ethanoic	Acetic	17
3	n-Propanoic	Propionic	−21
4	n-Butanoic	Butyric	−8
6	n-Hexanoic	Caproic	−3
8	n-Octanoic	Caprylic	17
10	n-Decanoic	Capric	32
12	n-Dodecanoic	Lauric	44
14	n-Tetradecanoic	Myristic	54
16	n-Hexadecanoic	Palmitic	63
18	n-Octadecanoic	Stearic	70
20	n-Eicosanoic	Arachidic	75
22	n-Docosanoic	Behenic	80
24	n-Tetracosanoic	Lignoceric	84

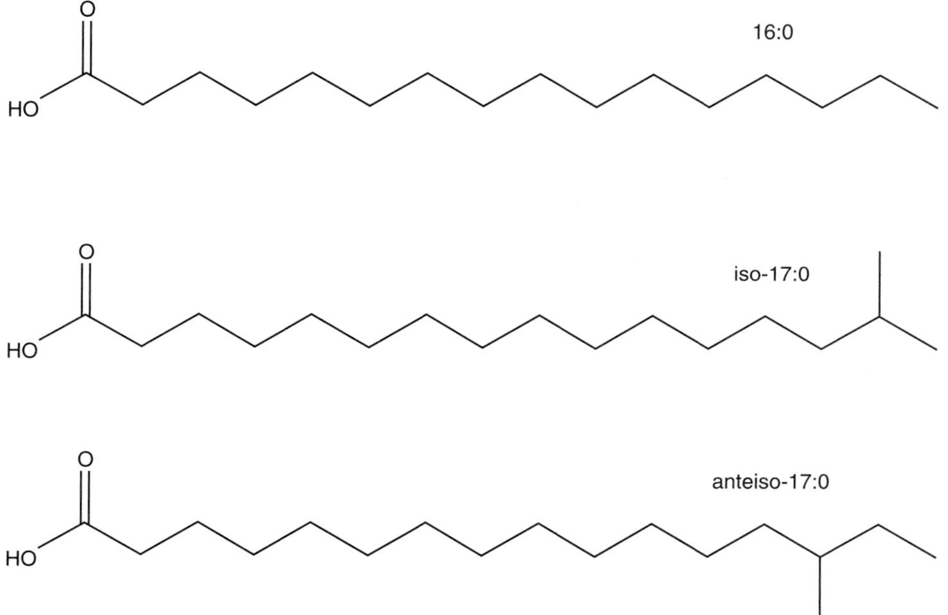

Figure 6-2 Structures of straight-chain versus branched-chain (iso and ante-iso) fatty acids.

for unsaturated fatty acids. Table 6-2 is a compilation of the systematic and trivial names for the most common unsaturated fatty acids.

Although PUFA biosynthesis will be discussed in depth in Chapter 18, a brief overview is necessary to rationalize PUFA nomenclature. The pathway for synthesis of arachidonic acid (20 Cs, 4 double bonds) from linoleic acid (18 Cs, 2 double bonds) begins with the insertion of a double bond between carbons 6 and 7 by a desaturase to make γ-linolenic acid (18 Cs, 3 double bonds). Two carbons are then added to the carboxyl end of the molecule by action of a series of enzymes known collectively as an "elongase," to make dihomo-γ-linolenic acid (20 Cs, 3 double bonds). Finally, another desaturase inserts a double bond into dihomo-γ-linolenic acid to make arachidonic acid.

Figure 6-3 shows the systematic organic chemistry names and numbering for the first

Table 6-2
Naturally Occurring Straight-Chain Unsaturated Fatty Acids

	Systematic Name	Trivial Name	Melting Point (°C)
14:1n-5	*cis*-9-tetradecenoic	Myristoleic	
16:1n-7	*cis*-9-hexadecenoic	Palmitoleic	0.5
18:1n-7	*cis*-11-octadecenoic	cis-Vaccenic	
t-18:1n-7	*trans*-11-octadecenoic	Vaccenic	
18:1n-9	*cis*-9-octadecenoic	Oleic	16.2
t-18:1n-9	*trans*-9-octadecenoic	Elaidic	46.5
20:3n-9	all-*cis*-5,8,11-eicosatrienoic	Mead	
22:1n-9	all-*cis*-13-docosenoic	Erucic	34.7
18:2n-6	all-*cis*-9,12-octadecadienoic	Linoleic (LA)	–5
18:3n-6	all-*cis*-6,9,12-octadecatrienoic	γ-Linoleic (GLA)	
20:4n-6	all-*cis*-5,8,11,14-eicosatetraenoic	Arachidonic (AA)	–49.5
22:5n-6	all-*cis*-4,7,10,13,16-docosapentaenoic	DPA	
18:3n-3	all-*cis*-9,12,15-octadecatrienoic	Linolenic (LnA)	–10
20:5n-3	all-*cis*-5,8,11,14,17-eicosapentaenoic	EPA	
22:6n-3	all-*cis*-4,7,10,13,16,19-docosahexaenoic	DHA	

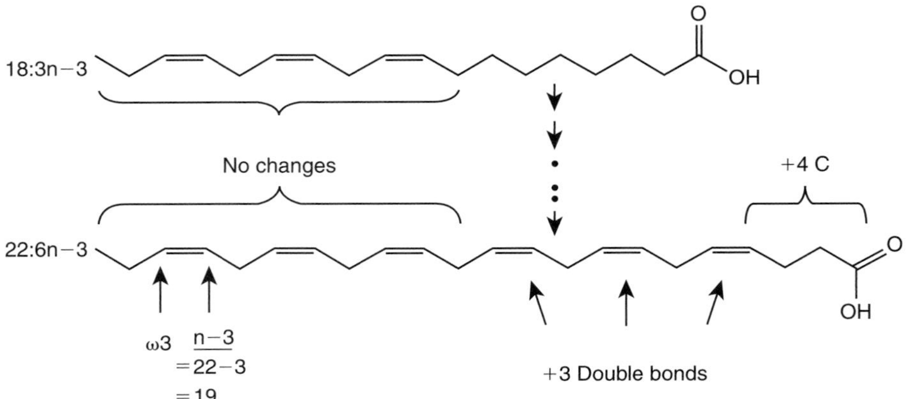

Figure 6-3 The conversion of one polyunsaturated fatty acid (PUFA) into another proceeds from the carboxyl end of the molecule in mammals, and there are no changes to the methyl end. Here, α-linolenic acid (systematic name: 9,12,15-octatrienoic acid) is converted to 4,7,10,13,16,19-docosahexaenoic acid. Numbering the first double bond from the methyl end of the molecule (using the ω numbering system) or the Miller system ("n-," where "n" is the number of C atoms in the molecule) locates the double bond closest to the methyl end of the molecule. Therefore, the naming of PUFA also reveals metabolic relationships; for example, between 18:3n-3 and 22:6n-3. Because most naturally occurring double bonds are methylene-interrupted and all-*cis*, this designation fully defines the molecular structure.

and last steps in this pathway. In the systematic system, carbon atoms are numbered from the carboxyl end (i.e., the carboxyl carbon atom is designated number 1). Thus, the systematic name of linoleic acid is 9,12-octadecadienoic acid and that of γ-linolenic acid is 6,9,12-octadecatrienoic acid, but the systematic name of arachidonic acid is 5,8,11,14-eicosatetraenoic acid because the double bonds from γ-linoleic acid that are retained in arachidonic acid were shifted to position 8 and 11 from the carboxyl end when the chain was elongated. Repeated many times for many PUFAs, these changes make it difficult to track double bonds and, more importantly, fatty acids that are derived from one another.

A solution is to effectively number double bonds from the other end of the molecule, the methyl end. Two conventions that are in routine use, and effectively are identical, are

Nutrition Insight

Vitamin F

Between 1910 and 1920, the notion of a vitamin arose—a compound that, in trace amounts, prevented disease conditions. Once this idea caught on, another very powerful principle was born, and the age of discovery of vitamins ensued. The odd list of designations we now have for vitamins (A, a series of B's, C, D, E, and K) are a remnant of the uneven but eventual progress in scientific understanding. What happened to the other letters between E and K?

Vitamin F was proposed as the name of a factor associated with fat, and this proposal appeared in several papers published in the 1920s. The discovery that fat-containing diets are essential for health is usually assigned to a 1929 paper of George and Mildred Burr (Burr and Burr, 1929), then working in the attic of the University of Minnesota Medical School (Holman, 1992). They showed that rats fed fat-free diets developed scaly and sore skin, especially on the face and tail, had hair loss, grew at approximately two thirds the normal rate, had a shortened lifespan, and were unable to reproduce. Animals that were emaciated and covered with very scaly skin were placed on a dietary regimen of 10 "drops" of lard per day. Immediately they showed signs of recovery and within 10 weeks were fully "cured." No recovery was seen when the non–fatty acid ("nonsaponifiable") fraction of lard was used, thereby indicating that the essential fat is a fatty acid. Subsequent studies established that fat of greater unsaturation improved the ability of the fat to cure eczema (Brown et al., 1938). However, the inability of scientists to reproduce these effects in humans made interest in vitamin F wane. We now know that periods greater than 6 months on fat-free diets are required to cause overt deficiency symptoms in humans.

The key structural components of polyunsaturated fatty acids (PUFAs) are the methylene-interrupted double bonds between the methyl and n-9 carbon atoms. Mammalian enzymes cannot introduce a double bond into this region, and thus mammals rely on a dietary source for these structures, derived ultimately from terrestrial plants or marine sources. Mammals can introduce double bonds into the chain starting at the n-9 position. Thus in theory, linoleic and linolenic acids can serve as precursors for the long-chain n-6 and n-3 fatty acids, respectively. Rats and other small mammals do seem to be able to meet their needs in this way, and thus 18:2n-6 and 18:3n-3 can be considered the parent or "essential" fatty acids. These compounds, at least for rats, could appropriately be considered two different components of vitamin F.

Presently, however, there is controversy about whether humans can synthesize sufficient long chain PUFA from 18:2n-6 and 18:3n-3 for optimum health. If in fact long-chain fatty acids are essential at some or all stages of the life cycle, PUFAs such as 20:4n-6, 20:5n-3, and 22:6n-3 might also be considered separate components of vitamin F. As progress continues toward defining the details of human requirements for PUFA, as well as the role of specific PUFAs in human metabolism, the concept of a series of vitamin F's may yet prove useful.

the Miller convention and the omega convention. Both notations take advantage of the fact that mammals cannot insert double bonds into PUFAs near the methyl end of the fatty acid chain. Examples of both notations are shown in Figure 6-3 for the biosynthesis of arachidonic acid.

The Miller notation retains a close connection to the systematic organic chemistry notation. The "n" represents the number of carbons in the whole molecules, 18 in the case of γ-linolenic acid; thus "n-6," pronounced "n minus six," equals 12. The 12th carbon atom counting from the carboxyl is where the last double bond in the molecule starts.

The omega notation, proposed by Ralph Holman (Holman, 1964), recognizes that the systematic organic chemistry numbering assigns the carbon next to the carboxyl the designation "α," and labels the last carbon in the acyl chain "ω." The first double bond counting from the methyl end appears at the third position, and hence is designated ω3 (pronounced "omega three"). Although the two numbering systems actually refer to different carbon atoms, they designate the equivalent fatty acids when the numeral is the same; for instance, n-6 and ω6 fatty acids are equivalent.

A simple notation can then be developed that designates the most common mammalian fatty acids. The number of carbons and number of double bonds are separated by a colon (C18:3, or simply 18:3). Recognizing that most mammalian PUFAs have *cis* double bonds arranged in methylene-interrupted positions, a designation of n-6 (ω6) fully defines the structure of the fatty acids. For instance, "18:3n-6" or "18:3ω6" completely defines the structure of γ-linolenic acid as the fatty acid with the systematic name 6,9,12-octadecatrienoic acid. In practice, these notations imply *cis* geometry and methylene interruption unless stated otherwise.

Fatty acids with *trans* or conjugated double bonds do not ordinarily appear in mammalian tissue, although they may be consumed as part of the diet. Examples of *trans* and conjugated unsaturated fatty acids are shown in Figure 6-4. These fatty acids should not be designated with the n- or ω notation, unless further specification is provided, for instance, "*trans*-18:1n-9," to specify the monounsaturated 18 carbon fatty acid with a *trans* double bond at the 9-10 position. Unlike the situation with common fatty acids, there is no universally used specialized notation. Either systematic notation or some convenient adaptation of systematic numbering are both frequently used. An example of the latter is the "Δ" (delta) notation, where a superscript Δ follows the denotation of chain length and number of double bonds; the Δ is followed by the sites of unsaturation counting from the carboxyl carbon. For instance, $18{:}3^{\Delta 6,9,12}$ designates γ-linolenic acid (all-*cis*-6,9,12-octadecatrienoic acid). This notation then lends itself to designation of isomers of γ-linolenic acid, often by adding leading "*c*" or "*t*" to specify *cis* or *trans* double bond geometry, for instance, as "*c*6,*t*8,*c*12-octadecatrienoic acid."

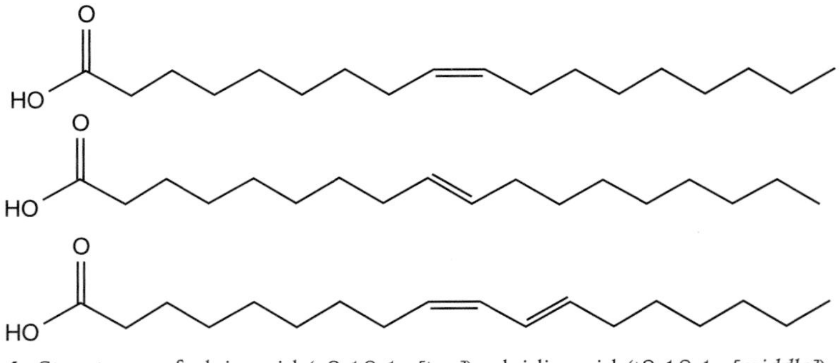

Figure 6-4 Structures of oleic acid (c9-18:1, *[top]*), elaidic acid (t9-18:1, *[middle]*), and rumenic acid (c9,t11-18:2 *[bottom]*).

Nutrition Insight

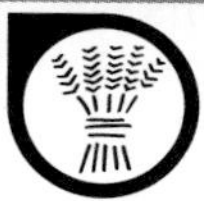

Trans Fatty Acids: The Good, the Bad, and the Ugly

Trans fatty acids are in the news because of their widespread distribution in the food supply, and scientific data point to physiological effects of these fatty acids. New food labeling rules to take effect in the United States in January 2006 specify that the content of *trans* fats must be shown on all food labels. Food producers are scrambling to remove *trans* fats from their prepared foods because of the bad reputation they have as unnatural promoters of heart disease. There are, however, some *trans* fats that have beneficial effects.

Trans fats refers to the presence of *trans* double bonds in an unsaturated fatty acid. Dietary *trans* fats arise from two sources: (1) the chemical catalytic hydrogenation of unsaturated oils and (2) as products of rumen bacterial and bovine metabolism in dairy products. The regulatory definition of *trans* fats generally refers to monoenes (1 double bond) and not to dienes. Chemical catalysis is used in the food industry to stabilize fats against oxidation and to fine tune the melting point of unsaturated fats to obtain suitable properties for fats used as components of foods, particularly baked goods. Hydrogenation lowers the cost of shortening because food companies can purchase the least expensive, high quality, deodorized/flavor-neutral oil available at a particular time, be it cottonseed, soy, corn, or another vegetable oil. Hydrogenation adjusts the melting point of oils by saturating many double bonds with H_2 and isomerizing others from *cis* to *trans*. Saturated and *trans* fatty acids in oils have higher melting points than corresponding fatty acids with *cis* double bonds. Therefore, the melting point of any oil can be finely adjusted by adding just the right amount of H_2. The resulting *trans* fatty acids are largely a series of monoenes with *trans* double bonds distributed at various positions along the hydrocarbon chain, centered at the site of an original *cis* double bond. Conjugated double bonds of various positions and geometries are also created. These *trans* fatty acids are thought to be atherogenic by promoting an increase in plasma cholesterol in a manner similar to some saturated fatty acids, especially myristic and lauric acids (Hu and Willett, 2002).

In contrast, dairy products have a very specific distribution of *trans* fatty acids. The most prominent dairy *trans* fatty acid is a monoene, *trans*-11-18:1 ("vaccenic acid") with smaller amounts of other monoenes with double bonds at various locations between C-4 and C-16. Also present at lower concentrations are dienes known as conjugated linoleic acids (CLAs). The most prominent of these is the *cis*-9, *trans*-11-18:2, named rumenic acid (Kramer et al., 1998), which constitutes about 90% of all CLAs. Rumenic acid is formed in the mammary gland by 9-desaturation of vaccenic acid that is produced in the rumen (Kay et al., 2004). Humans also convert vaccenic acid to rumenic acid (Turpeinen et al., 2002). The *trans*-7, *cis*-9 isomer of 18:2 is made in a similar way, but accounts for much less of the total. Studies in rats have shown that rumenic acid is a potent anticarcinogenic compound and that a close structural isomer, *trans*-10,*cis*-12-18:2, is an anti-obesity agent (Pariza, 2004).

A major difficulty in developing simple and effective approaches for providing *trans* fatty acid information on food labels is that the *trans* hydrogenated fats are a complex mixture of isomers that inevitably contain small quantities of "good" *trans* fat. This problem is manifest in the elaborate methods used to characterize these isomers, which are time-consuming and the subject of continuing research (Michaud and Brenna, 2005). Practically, it is impossible to capture the good and bad in one number, but it is also not yet clear how to report in a simple manner the relative contributions of the two sorts of *trans* fats to fully inform the consumer.

GLYCEROLIPIDS (ACYLGLYCEROLS)

In mammalian tissues and in most foods, more than 90% of fatty "acids" exist as esters within glycerolipids rather than as nonesterified fatty acids. Glycerolipids are based on ester and other chemical linkages between fatty acids and the three-carbon sugar, glycerol. Those linked by an ester linkage are referred to as "acyl" groups, whereas those linked by a single oxygen atom form "ethers." Other linkages, such as alkenyl, are possible, and the term "radyl" group is used to describe hydrocarbon chains linked to a glycerol without specification of the nature of the chemical linkage. In most tissues, there are hundreds of chemically distinct glycerolipids, which differ in fatty acyl groups, their positions on the glycerol backbone, the linkage (esters, ethers, and others), and the nature of polar groups esterified to specific positions.

Stereochemistry of Glycerolipids

An important property of glycerolipids is their stereochemistry. The glycerol molecule possesses a plane of symmetry such that the central carbon atom can be considered "prochiral," a chemical term referring to a carbon atom with four substituents, three of which are different. A prochiral carbon is not chiral, but substitution of one of the equivalent substituent groups with a fourth, nonequivalent group renders the central carbon chiral. This is the case for the central carbon of glycerol: when nonchemically equivalent moieties are added to the $-CH_2OH$ groups, the central carbon becomes chiral. Chirality is very important to biochemical properties and thus must be described unambiguously. Here, the systematic notation of organic chemistry, with rules for designating chiral centers as R or S, leads to even more confusing designations than in the case of fatty acid double bond position. However, a single notation that has proved remarkably robust was introduced in the 1960s that closely parallels metabolism.

As shown in Figure 6-5, glycerol can be positioned so that the –OH groups on the top and bottom carbons are extending to the right and the middle –OH is extending to the left. Then, by convention, the positions of the three carbons are referred to as *sn*-1, *sn*-2, and *sn*-3 (top to bottom), with "*sn*" short for "stereochemical numbering." In some contexts the *sn*-1 and *sn*-3 positions are metabolically equivalent, and are designated the α positions, whereas the center *sn*-2 position is designated the β position. When nonchemically equivalent groups, either different fatty acids or other groups, are added to the *sn*-1 and *sn*-3 positions, glycerol becomes chiral.

Acylglycerols

Acylglycerols are formed by the substitution of one or more of the glycerol –OH groups with a fatty acid by means of an ester linkage. A single acyl substitution to form an ester bond forms a monoacylglycerol (MAG), with general nomenclature referring to this molecule as a 1-, 2-, or 3-monoacyl-*sn*-glycerol. For example, esterification of hexadecanoic acid (palmitic acid) at the 1-position of glycerol produces 1-hexadecanoyl-*sn*-glycerol (1-palmitoyl-*sn*-glycerol). When two fatty acids are reacted with glycerol to form ester bonds, a diacylglycerol (DAG) is formed (e.g., 1,3-diacyl-*sn*-glycerol or 1,2-diacyl-*sn*-glycerol). Both mono- and diacylglycerides occur in relatively low proportion in mammals, but they are important as biochemical intermediates in many lipolytic reactions and are critical building blocks used in the synthesis of more complex phospholipids and triacylglycerols. DAGs also act as secondary messengers for some membrane-triggered reactions.

A triacylglycerol (TAG) is formed when all three hydroxyls of glycerol form ester bonds with fatty acids. TAG is the most common form of fat and energy storage in mammalian tissues. The older abbreviated term "triglyceride"

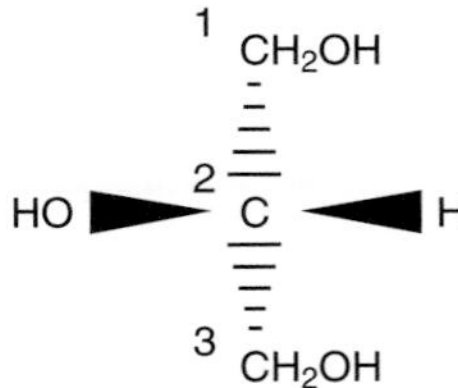

Figure 6-5 Glycerol. The carbon positions are numbered according to the *sn* convention.

is also used as a synonym for TAG. The fatty acids in a TAG may be all the same, all different, or two of a kind with one different one. If all three fatty acids are the same, the triacylglycerol is called a simple triacylglycerol (e.g., triolein). If one of the fatty acids is different, it becomes a complex triacylglycerol. If the fatty acids at the *sn*-1 and *sn*-3 positions are different, the TAG is chiral. Chirality in TAG is of less importance than in other glycerolipids because many enzymes catalyzing reactions involving TAG do not distinguish between the *sn*-1 and *sn*-3 (i.e., the two α) positions.

Examples of structure and nomenclature for mono-, di-, and triacylglycerols are shown in Figure 6-6. The *sn* nomenclature established by the International Union of Pure and Applied Chemistry and International Union of Biochemistry and Molecular Biology (IUPAC-IUBMB) is preferred in most cases, although simple acylglycerols are often reported in shorthand; 1-,2-,3-tri-*cis*-9-octadecenoyl-*sn*-glycerol

General Structure

Example

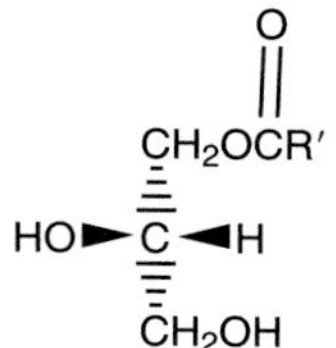

1-Monoacyl-*sn*-glycerol

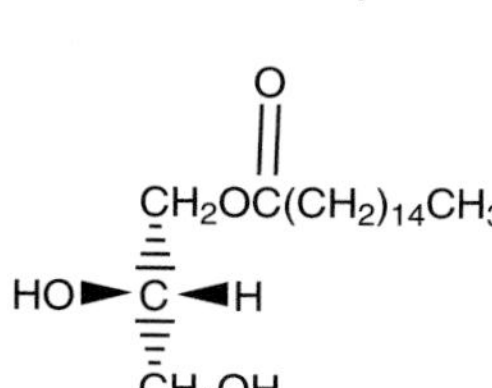

TN: 1-Palmitoyl-*sn*-glycerol
SN: 1-Hexadecanoyl-*sn*-glycerol
(1-monostearin)

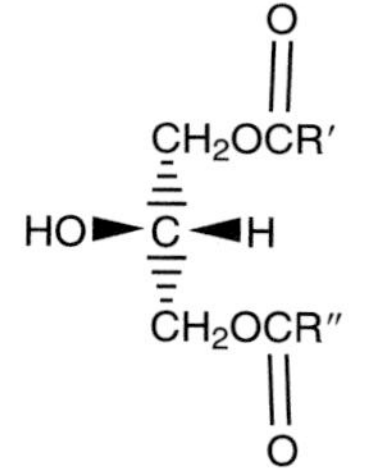

1, 3-Diacyl-*sn*-glycerol

TN: 1-Palmitoyl-3-stearoyl-*sn*-glycerol
SN: 1-Hexadecanoyl-3-octadecanoyl-*sn*-glycerol

1, 2, 3-Triacyl-*sn*-glycerol

TN: 1, 2-Dipalmitoyl-3-stearoyl-*sn*-glycerol
SN: 1, 2-Dihexadecanoyl-3-octadecanoyl-*sn*-glycerol

Figure 6-6 Examples of structures and nomenclatures for mono-, di-, and triacylglycerides. *TN,* Trivial name; *SN,* systematic name.

becomes triolein, for example. In older literature, it is not uncommon to find acylglycerols reported in R/S nomenclature. The drawback of these systems is apparent when we consider that most enzymes recognize particular positions of the acylglycerol. For example, pancreatic lipase cleaves TAG at the 1- and 3- positions. The hydrolysis of 3-myristoyl-2-palmitoyl-1-stearoyl-*sn*-glycerol at the 1-position yields 3-myristoyl-2-palmitoyl-*sn*-glycerol (Fig. 6-7). The *sn* nomenclature clearly reveals the relationship between the precursor TAG and its resulting DAG. However, the R/S stereochemistry of the lipids (i.e., the configuration at each chiral center) changes during this transformation, obscuring their biochemical relation, also shown in Figure 6-7.

Saturated fatty acids tend to be found in the *sn*-1 and *sn*-3 positions, whereas unsaturated fatty acids tend to be found in the *sn*-2 position. There are notable exceptions, for instance in lard and human milk, where 16:0 is predominantly in the *sn*-2 position with unsaturated fatty acids in the *sn*-1 and *sn*-3 positions. The three potentially unique positions of the glycerol backbone permit a tremendous number of positional and stereoisomers. For example, if a sample of fat had 10 different fatty acids, the possible number of individual TAGs would be $10^3 = 1{,}000$. This includes positional isomers and enantiomers—that is, optical isomers in which a specific fatty acid is either at the *sn*-1 or *sn*-3 position. If one simply considers racemic mixtures in which the 1- and 3- positions can be interchanged, then $N = (n^3+n^2)/2$. If one considers only the fatty acid combinations on the three positions and ignores positional isomers, then $N = (n^3+n^2+2n)/6$.

Thus if a specific sample contains only three different fatty acids (e.g., R′, R″, R‴), then the total number of isomers, including positional isomers and enantiomers, would be 27. If we exclude optical isomers, there would be 18, and if we exclude positional isomers, there would be 7. Considering that many dietary fats and oils often have 10 or more major fatty acids at concentrations greater than 1%, the number of potential individual TAGs becomes enormous. In fact, butterfat has both short- and long-chain fatty acids as well as many unsaturated ones (Breckinridge, 1978) and, therefore, probably consists of thousands of individual stereospecific TAGs. For this reason even bovine milk fat has not been completely analyzed.

The properties of acylglycerols (e.g., melting point) depend greatly on the fatty acid chains involved. TAGs are the major storage lipids of plants and higher animals. Both plant oils (olive, corn, and safflower) and animal fats (lard, suet, and tallow) are predominantly mixtures of complex TAGs. Compositions of common food fats and oils are presented in Table 6-3. A few percent (by weight) of sterols, vitamins, FFAs, carotenoids, and other fat-soluble molecules are usually present in oils and fats obtained from plants and animals. In animals, most fat is in adipose tissue, but skeletal muscle, heart, liver, skin, and bone marrow often contain appreciable amounts of TAGs in intracellular oil droplets.

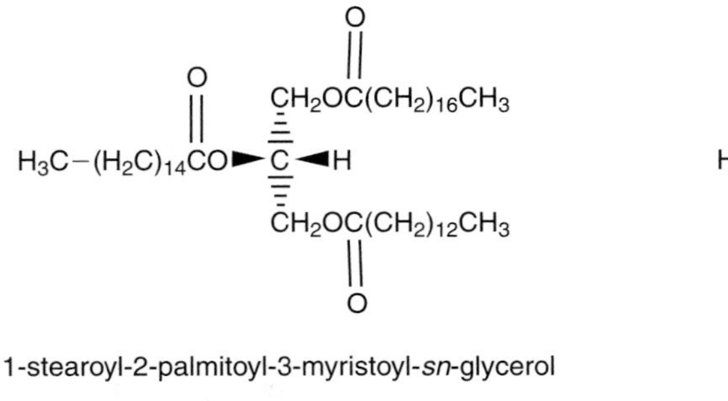

1-stearoyl-2-palmitoyl-3-myristoyl-*sn*-glycerol

R stereochemistry

2-palmitoyl-3-myristoyl-*sn*-glycerol

S stereochemistry

Figure 6-7 Demonstration of the utility of the *sn* nomenclature system. Following hydrolysis at the 1-position, the relationship between the diacylglycerol (DAG) on the right and the triacylglycerol (TAG) on the left is still clear, whereas the R/S nomenclature is reversed.

Nutrition Insight

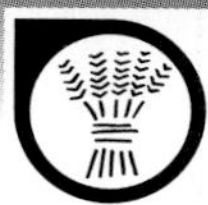

Lipidomics

Research in most fields of natural science is traditionally driven by hypothesis testing. Hypotheses, in essence, are refined explanations that reach beyond established or accepted knowledge in a field—educated guesses that guide the design of experiments. An alternative to hypothesis-driven research are studies that measure many parameters, which are chosen not to test a specific hypothesis but rather measured because the analytical techniques are available. For most of the history of biological science, this alternative "data-driven" approach has been frowned upon as inefficient because most results do not fit inside any intellectual framework and are not efficiently used.

Nevertheless, natural science research is inextricably linked to a subset of itself, the science of measurement. In recent years, there has been a surge of interest in rapid, large-scale measurements in the biological sciences, for the most part driven by rapidly improving analytical instruments and the widespread availability of fast computing. The best known prototype was the Human Genome project, which has sequenced all genes in the human genome. The data-driven approach, often called a data-driven paradigm, is identified by the suffix "-omics" appended to words denoting common scientific areas. The suffix is analogous to its use in the word economics, a social science in which the interplay of many familiar small-scale phenomena—sales, labor, currency, credit—give rise to equally familiar emergent properties like markets and industries. The biological analogy is that data from many small measurements, for example gene expression arrays, can ultimately be linked to emergent properties, such as health status and predisposition to disease. The field of bioinformatics, populated by applied mathematicians, statisticians, and computer and other information scientists, has been established to find the links between these levels of organization.

The large-scale analysis of lipids is one of the more recent data-driven fields to emerge as a definable discipline. Lipidomics is the comprehensive measurement of all lipids in a biological sample, which might be a cell, a tissue, or an organism. Because of the chemical heterogeneity of lipids, lipidomic analyses at present are limited to analysis of specific classes of lipids, some of which have been given their own names (e.g., eicosanomics). Within various subsets of lipidomics, thousands of distinct molecular species may be found. Consider, for instance, the phosphoglycerolipids, which may have any of perhaps 100 fatty acyl (radyl) groups at either of two positions and one of several headgroups at the *sn*-3 position.

The predominant analytical chemical technique driving lipidomics is tandem mass spectrometry (MS/MS). The most targeted and comprehensive developments of lipidomics focus on analysis of lipid extracts that can be directly introduced into the mass spectrometer by electrospray ionization or related techniques. Once they are transformed into ions and are in the gas phase, specific molecular ions can be chosen in a first stage of MS, collisionally dissociated, and the products analyzed in a second stage of mass spectrometry. In most cases, fragments generated by collisions reveal the number of carbons and double bonds in the acyl groups of esterified lipids, the structure of polar headgroups of phospholipids, and other structural features. Modern mass spectrometers can be set to automatically analyze for a thousand distinct lipid molecular structures in a single sample, thereby providing the platform for lipidomic analysis. Studies employing lipidomic approaches are now appearing in the scientific literature, but the field continues to develop rapidly, and it remains to be seen how the new data-driven paradigm complements and extends the hypothesis-driven approach, credited by many for most of the progress of modern science.

Table 6-3
Composition and Melting Points of Some Natural Fats and Oils*

Fat or Oil	Melting Point (°C)†	Major Triacylglycerols
Butterfat	37 to 38	PPB‡ PPC‡ POP‡
Horse fat		OOO POO LOO
Lard	46 to 49	SPO‡ OPL‡ OPO‡
Tallow (beef)	40	POO POP POS
Cocoa butter	28 to 36	POS SOS POP
Coconut oil	24 to 27	DDD CDD CDM
Palm kernel oil	24 to 29	DDD MOD ODO
Almond oil		OOO OLO OLL
Corn oil	−14	LLL LOL LLP
Cottonseed oil	5 to 11	PLL POL LLL
Egg triglycerides		POO PLO POS
Grapeseed oil	8	LLL OLL POL
Hazelnut oil		OOO OLO POO
Olive oil	−7	OOO OOP OLO
Palm oil	30 to 36	POP POO POL
Peanut oil	−8 to +12	OOL POL OLL
Rice bran oil		PLO OOL POO
Safflower oil	−15	LLL LLO LLP
Soybean oil	−14	LLL LLO LLP
Sunflower oil	−17	LLL OLL LOO
Walnut oil		LLL OLL PLL
Rapeseed oil (low Er)	5	OOO LOO OOLn
Linseed oil	−17	LnLnLn LnLnL LnLnO
Rapeseed oil (high Er)		ErOEr ErLEr ErLnEr
Mustard seed oil§		ErOEr‡ ErLEr‡ OOEr‡

From Small DM (1991) The effects of glyceride structure on absorption and metabolism. Annu Rev Nutr 11:413-434.
*Abbreviations used for acyl chains in the triacylglycerols: B = 4:0 (butyric), C = 10:0 (capric), D = 12:0 (dodecanoic), M = 14:0 (myristic), P = 16:0 (palmitic), S = 18:0 (stearic), O = 18:1 (*cis*) (oleic), E = 18:1 (*trans*) (elaidic), L = 18:2 (linoleic), Ln = 18:3 (linolenic), G = 20:1 (gogoleic), and Er = 22:1 (erucic).
†The melting points or ranges of these fats and oils are taken from references reported in Small (1991).
‡Specific triacylglycerols estimated from stereospecific fatty acid analyses, as in 1S,2P,3O-*sn*-glycerol.
§The stereospecific composition of the eight most prevalent triacylglycerols of mustard seed oil, which comprise 40% of the total, is ErOEr = 8.2%, ErLEr = 6.8%, OOEr = 5.9%, ErLnEr = 5.3%, OLEr = 4.9%, OLnEr = 3.8%, GOEr = 3.3%, and GLEr = 2.7%.

GLYCEROPHOSPHOLIPIDS (PHOSPHOLIPIDS)

The diverse phospholipids are the structural basis of all cell membranes, including internal membranes such as the ER and nuclear envelope. The general structure of phospholipids is presented in Figure 6-8, and the several classes of phospholipids and their structures are shown in Figure 6-9. The nomenclature and abbreviations of phospholipids, also called "glycerophospholipids" or "phosphoglycerides," are largely according to convention. In all cases, a phosphate group is esterified to the *sn*-3 position, and, except for phosphatidic acid, one of five common polar "headgroups" is in turn esterified to the phosphate. The simplest phospholipid is phosphatidic acid, in which phosphoric acid is esterified to the *sn*-3 position of glycerol. Although phosphatidic acid is an important intermediate in lipid metabolism, it is a very minor constituent of the phospholipid fraction. In most cases, the phosphoric acid is further esterified by one of several polar headgroups. This arrangement imparts amphipathic character to the PL so that, effectively, the head group of the molecule dissolves in aqueous solution while the fatty acyl chains congregate together. The familiar lipid bilayer of the membrane is thus stable, with the polar headgroups attracted outward via strong polar and ionic interactions with the water phase and the fatty acyl chains

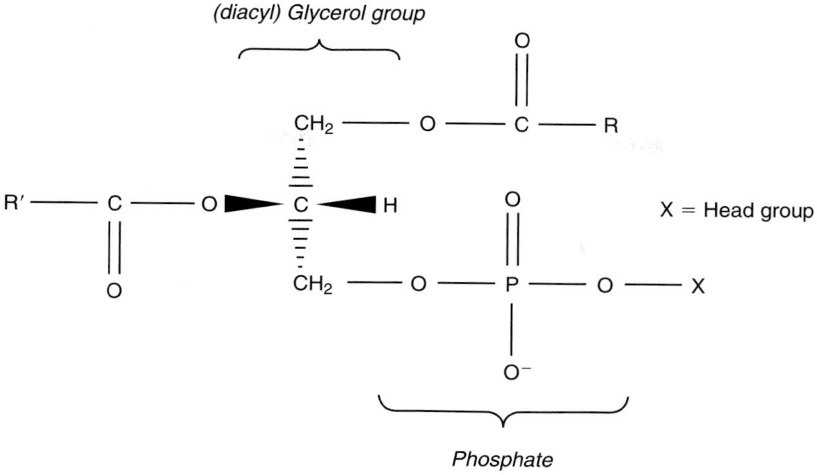

Figure 6-8 General structure of diacylphospholipids.

Common Phospholipid	Trivial Abbreviation	IUPAC Abbreviation	Structure of Head Group ("X")
Phosphatidyl choline	PC	PtdCho	$—CH_2CH_2N^+(CH_3)_3$
Phosphatidyl ethanolamine	PE	PtdEtn	$—CH_2CH_2\overset{+}{N}H_3$
Phosphatidyl serine	PS	PtdSer	$—CH_2CH(COO^-)\overset{+}{N}H_3$
Phosphatidyl inositol	PI	PtdIns	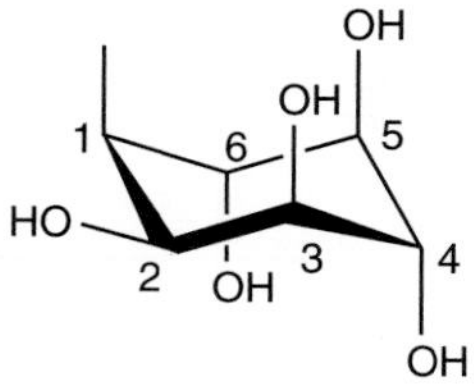
Phosphatidyl glycerol	PG	PtdGro	$—CH_2CH(OH)CH_2OH$

Figure 6-9 Common headgroups in mammalian phospholipids.

directed inward to form the nonpolar interior of the membrane.

Major Phospholipid Classes

Phospholipids are classified on the basis of their headgroup. There are five polar headgroups commonly found in phospholipids of humans (see Figure 6-9), which define the five major classes of phospholipids, as follows:

1. Phosphatidylcholine (PC, commonly called lecithin)
2. Phosphatidylethanolamine (PE)
3. Phosphatidylserine (PS)
4. Phosphatidylglycerol (PG)
5. Phosphatidylinositol (PI)

The *sn*-2 position is usually occupied by an unsaturated fatty acyl group, whereas the *sn*-1 position is occupied by a saturated acyl substituent. Again, there are notable exceptions. For instance, the major surfactant lipid of the lung has 16:0 in both positions, and some phospholipids of the retinal photoreceptors have very high concentrations of unsaturated fatty acid substituents in both positions.

The various structures of polar headgroups lead to different metabolic and structural roles. Most phospholipids are part of the main structure of membranes, but some, such as PS and PI, also have very specific functions. PS seems to be a marker for apoptotic cells. PI is a substrate for phosphorylation at the 3-, 4-, and/or 5- positions of the inositol group, and thus up to eight different phosphoinositides are possible. These are often abbreviated as "PIP" for phosphatidylinositol phosphate, followed by numbers that locate the positions of the phosphate groups. For example, phosphatidylinositol 4,5-bisphosphate is abbreviated $PI(4,5)P_2$ or PIP_2; PIP_2 is hydrolyzed to form the secondary messengers inositol triphosphate (IP_3) and diacylglycerol (DAG). Glucosyl phosphatidylinositols are a recently described class of lipid moieties that are attached to certain proteins (Englund, 1993) and act as membrane anchors for the protein (e.g., alkaline phosphatase). Such proteins may be released from the membranes by phospholipase C, which hydrolyzes the glucosyl phosphatidylinositol, releasing PI and leaving DAG in the membrane.

In addition to common phospholipids, three other classes of phospholipids are found as shown in Figure 6-10. When one of the acyl groups of a phospholipid is

PL Class	Glycerol Linkages	General Name	General Structure
Common phospholipids	*sn*-1: Ester *sn*-2: Ester	1,2-Diacyl-*sn*-phospholipids	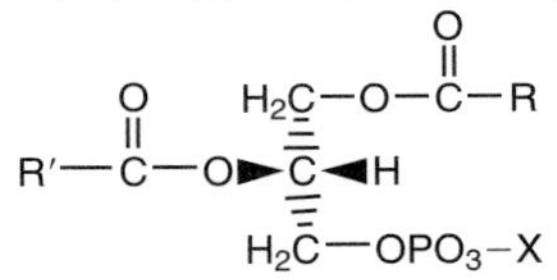 $H_2C—O—C(=O)—R$ $R'—C(=O)—O$►C◄H $H_2C—OPO_3—X$
Lysophospholipids	*sn*-1: Ester *sn*-2: none	1-Acyl-*sn*-phospholipids	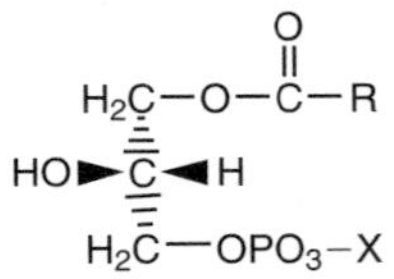 $H_2C—O—C(=O)—R$ HO►C◄H $H_2C—OPO_3—X$
Platelet activating factors	*sn*-1: Alkyl ether *sn*-2: Ester (Acetyl)	1-Acyl-2-acetyl-*sn*-Phosphatidylcholine	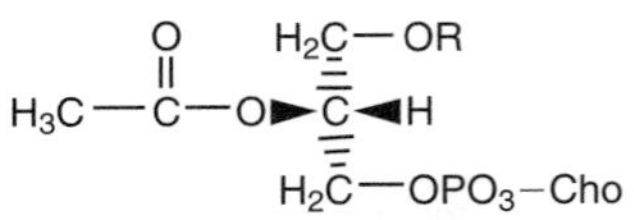 $H_2C—OR$ $H_3C—C(=O)—O$►C◄H $H_2C—OPO_3—Cho$
Plasmalogens	*sn*-1: Vinyl ether *sn*-2: Ester	1-Alkenyl-2-acyl-phospholipids (PC, PE, PS)	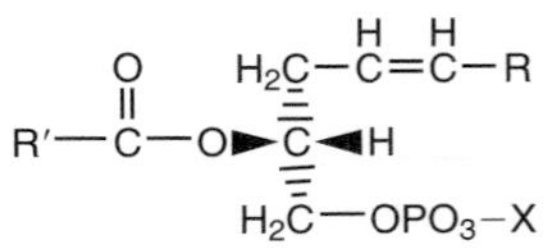 $H_2C—C(H)=C(H)—R$ $R'—C(=O)—O$►C◄H $H_2C—OPO_3—X$

Figure 6-10 Major classes of phospholipids.

removed, a phospholipid with a single hydrocarbon chain is a reaction product. These compounds are formed by the action of phospholipases that hydrolyze the fatty acyl group in the *sn*-2 or *sn*-1 positions, and the resulting phospholipid is called a lysophospholipid. Lysophospholipids are detergents because of their strong water-soluble headgroup and their lipid-soluble hydrocarbon chain. A rare genetic deficiency of the enzyme lecithin: cholesterol acyltransferase (LCAT), which transfers the fatty acid on the *sn*-2 position of PC (lecithin) to cholesterol to form a cholesterol ester and lysoPC, results in accumulation of PC (lecithin) and free cholesterol in plasma lipoproteins.

Diphosphatidylglycerols (Cardiolipins)

Diphosphatidylglycerols are very acidic phospholipids composed of two molecules of phosphatidic acid with the phosphate groups of both phosphatidic acid components linked to a glycerol headgroup. Therefore, these molecules contain three glycerol moieties. They are found in the inner mitochondrial membrane and in pulmonary surfactant. One important class of diphosphatidylglycerols is the cardiolipins, which were first isolated from heart tissue. Cardiolipins are usually observed in mammals only in the mitochondria, which is also where they are synthesized.

Ether Phospholipids

Although phospholipids typically exist as 1,2-*sn*-diacylphospholipids, in some cases alkyl chains are linked to the glycerol moiety by ether bonds (–C–O–C–) in place of acyl chains linked by ester linkages. Platelet-activating factors, which have the general formula 1-alkyl-2-acetyl-*sn*-glycerol-3-phosphocholine, are the most characterized ether-linked phospholipids. Platelet-activating factors that cause marked vasoactivity are linked to allergy, inflammation, neural functions, reproduction, and atherosclerosis. Plasmalogens have alkyl chains linked via a vinyl ether –C–O–C=C– moiety. Plasmalogens constitute 50% of choline phospholipids in the heart and are also present at significant concentration in neural tissue.

SPHINGOLIPIDS

Not all mammalian lipids rely on a glycerol backbone; the class of lipids called sphingolipids is formed by the addition of fatty acids or sugars to the long-chain amino alcohol sphingosine (Fig. 6-11). The most common sphingolipids are listed in Figure 6-12. Ceramide is formed when a fatty acid is linked to sphingosine through an amide bond at the 2 position. Substituted ceramides are important constituents of skin lipids. Elevated ceramide concentrations have been found in a disorder known as Farber's disease, which is characterized by the inability of lysosomes to catabolize ceramide. When ceramide is esterified with phosphocholine, sphingomyelin is formed. When sphingomyelin catabolic enzymes are absent, sphingomyelins accumulate in tissue, giving rise to Niemann-Pick disease.

Glycosphingolipid is a general term for any compound containing a mono- or oligosaccharide and a sphingoid base. They are often divided into two categories—(1) neutral and (2) acidic—a reflection of the extraction procedure typically used for their isolation. Neutral glycosphingolipids possess unsubstituted glycosyl groups. The simplest neutral glycosphingolipids, psychosines, have a monosaccharide (usually galactose) linked to sphingosine at C-1. The psychosines are important as biochemical intermediates, but may have some role in inhibiting cell division. Monoglycosylceramides, or cerebrosides, are formed by the linking of a monosaccharide to ceramide. In animals, galactosylcerebroside is in high concentrations in the myelin sheath of the brain, whereas glucosylcerebroside is observed in the serum. Successive linkages of hexoses to cerebrosides generate di-glycosylceramides,

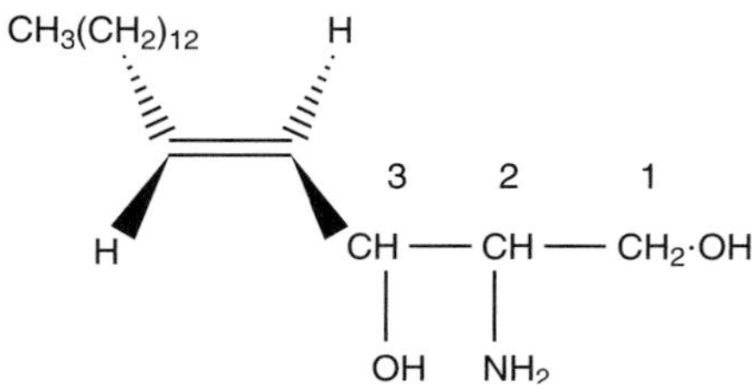

Figure 6-11 Sphingosine (2-amino-*trans*-4-octadecane-1,3-diol). C2 and C3 have S stereochemistry.

$CH_3(CH_2)_{12}$ H

H $CH-CH-CH_2-O-\mathbf{R}$

OH NH

$\mathbf{R'}$

Neutral Sphingolipid	R	R′
Ceramide	H	$-C(=O)-(CH_2)_nCH_3$
Psychosine	—Sugar	H
Sphingomyelin	—PC	$-C(=O)-(CH_2)_nCH_3$
Glycosylceramides		
Cerebroside (mono-)	—Sugar	$-C(=O)-(CH_2)_nCH_3$
Oligoglycosylceramides	$-(Sugar)_n$	

Figure 6-12 Structures of neutral sphingolipid classes. *PC,* Phosphatidyl choline.

tri-glycosylceramides, and tetraglycosylceramides. Typically, the names of the oligoglycosylceramides are written in shorthand nomenclature, with abbreviations for the sugars and the linkages. For example, the triglucosylcerebroside called globotriose has the structure: Gal(α1-4)-Gal(β1-4)-Glc-Cer.

Acidic glycosphingolipids have glycosyl groups with negatively charged substituents. In higher animals, the most important class is the gangliosides, which are formed when negatively charged sialic acid (*N*-acetylneuraminic acid, Fig. 6-13) adds to the sugars. The C-2 position of sialic acid links to the sphingolipid either through the C-3 position of one (or more) of the sugars or through the C-8 position of another sialic acid moiety.

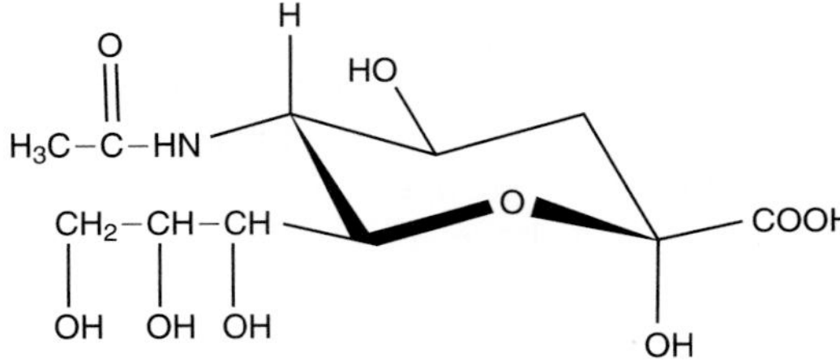

Figure 6-13 Sialic acid (*N*-acetylneuraminic acid [NANA]).

Gangliosides in low concentration are firmly anchored to the outer surfaces of many plasma membranes and appear to act as both antigens and receptors for certain toxins, antibodies, and lectins. Specific enzymes are necessary for the catabolism of each of these glycolipids;

Table 6-4
Common Terpenoid Classes and Their Respective Numbers of Monomeric Isoprene Units

Isoprene Units	Carbon Atoms	Terpenoid Class
1	5	Hemiterpenoids
2	10	Monoterpenoids
3	15	Sesquiterpenoids
4	20	Diterpenoids
5	25	Sesterterpenoids
6	30	Triterpenoids
8	40	Tetraterpenoids

NOTE: The names of the terpene classes possess an "-ene" suffix. For example, diterpenoids becomes diterpenes.

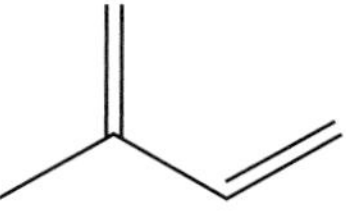

Figure 6-14 Structure of isoprene, the building block of isoprenoids.

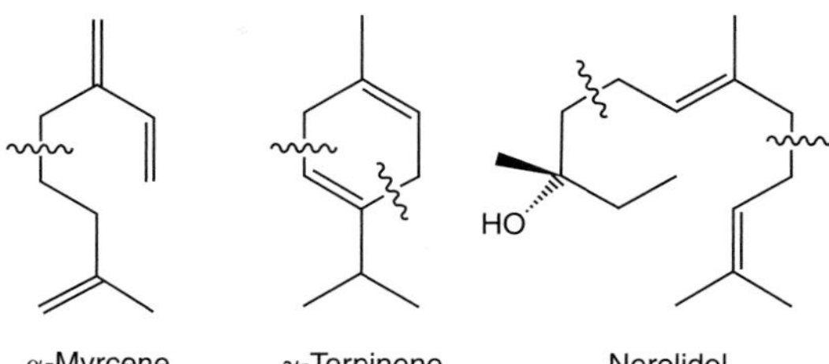

Figure 6-15 Structures of a monoterpene (γ-myrcene), a cyclic monoterpene (γ-terpinene), and a sesquiterpene (nerolidol).

when an enzyme is either absent or defective, the nonmetabolized glycolipid molecule accumulates, resulting in a lipid storage disease. Tay-Sachs disease is one such example of a ganglioside metabolic disorder.

ISOPRENOIDS

Isoprenoids are compounds that are derived from isoprene units, the skeleton of which can usually be discerned in repeated occurrence in the molecule. The 5-carbon isoprene unit is 2-methylbuta-1,3-diene (Fig. 6-14). Many of the compounds responsible for color, aroma, and chemical signaling in plants are isoprenoids, as are several important compounds in animals. The isoprenoids are occasionally further classified as terpenes if they are hydrocarbons, or as terpenoids if they contain oxygen substituents, although some texts use terpenoid and isoprenoid interchangeably. Nomenclature for the common classes of polyisoprenoids is given in Table 6-4.

Some examples of isoprenoid structures are shown in Figure 6-15, with the wavy lines showing the breakpoints between isoprene units. Typically, the smaller isoprenoids (≤25 carbons) are assembled head-to-tail, whereas the larger isoprenoids are assembled head-to-head from smaller units. The carotenoids, a class of 40-carbon isoprenoids (made of 8 isoprene units) that include lycopenes, carotenes, and xanthophylls, are synthesized from mevalonic acid in plant cells. These complex hydrocarbons are ingested by animals, and some proportion is taken up into the gut cells. One of these, β-carotene, is oxidatively cleaved to produce vitamin A, a 20-carbon polyisoprenoid alcohol, as discussed in Chapter 30. In animals, a similar pathway from mevalonic acid leads to the formation of ubiquinone (coenzyme Q), and the 30-carbon polyisoprenoid squalene, which undergoes cyclization and oxidation to form steroids, although the isoprene building blocks are difficult to discern in these compounds due to three demethylation steps. The structures of squalene and β-carotene are shown in Figure 6-16.

Head-to-tail isoprenoid alcohols called polyprenols, shown in Figure 6-17, are common constituents of essential oils. Many of these compounds and their relatives provide part of the aroma we associate with flowers, for example, geraniol with geraniums, and farnesol with lily-of-the-valley. In esterified form, they are precursors to the fat soluble vitamins A, E, and K, and they can add acyl chains to proteins. Saturated polyprenols, called isopranols, are often found in geologic sediments. Dolichols, also shown in Figure 6-17, are similar to polyprenols, except that the isoprene at the hydroxyl (α) end is saturated. They consist of 15 to 19 isoprene units (i.e., 75 to 95 carbon

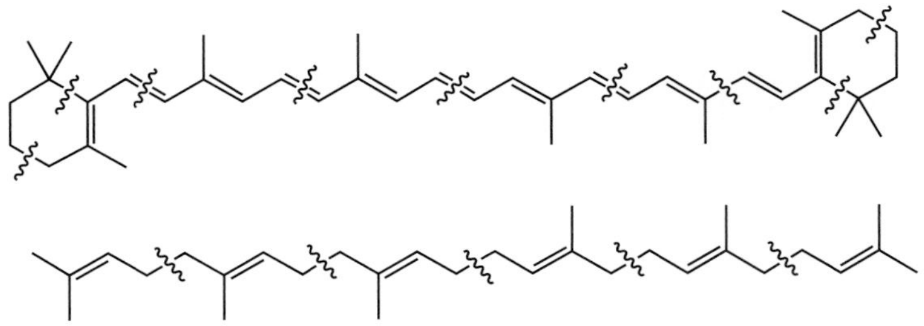

Figure 6-16 Structures of β-carotene *(top)* and squalene *(bottom)*. The wavy lines demonstrate how these isoprenoids were generated from multiple isoprene units.

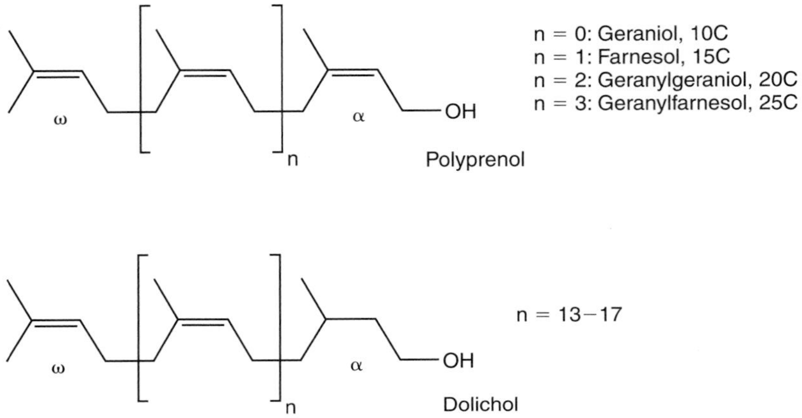

n = 0: Geraniol, 10C
n = 1: Farnesol, 15C
n = 2: Geranylgeraniol, 20C
n = 3: Geranylfarnesol, 25C

Polyprenol

n = 13–17

Dolichol

Figure 6-17 General structures for polyprenols and dolichols.

atoms) and are typically esterified to a phosphate at the terminal alcohol group. They are found in the ER and Golgi membranes and function as anchors for oligosaccharide chains being synthesized in the lumen of these organelles. Generally, these lipophilic molecules are found associated with lipid membranes or bound to specific carrier proteins.

WAXES

Waxes are long-chained, nonpolar compounds found on the surfaces of plants and animals to provide a hydrophobic barrier. Waxes tend to be solids at ambient temperature, accumulate in intracellular droplets or on surfaces of leaves or skin, and have almost no solubility in cellular membranes. Plankton and higher members of the aquatic food chain, including coral, mollusks, fish, sharks, and even whales, store large quantities of waxes for a variety of reasons, including as a food source, for buoyancy, and for insulation.

Biological waxes are heterogeneous mixtures of long-chain (~20 to 40 carbon atoms), primarily saturated, hydrocarbon compounds. The formal definition of a wax is an ester of a long chain alcohol and a long-chain fatty acid, with the general structure $R{-}COOCH_2{-}R'$. The acyl and alkyl groups are typically unbranched and saturated, although some branched or unsaturated hydrocarbons exist. For example, beeswax contains the ester triacontyl hexadecanoate as a primary component, and the primary component of spermaceti (derived from whale head oil) is hexadecyl hexadecanoate (Fig. 6-18). However, many other classes of compounds are found in biologically derived "waxes," including long-chain alkanes, sterol esters, unesterified fatty acids, triacylglycerides, aldehydes, ketones, and hydroxy fatty acids. For example, sebum (human skin lipid)

$$CH_3-(CH_3)_{14}-\overset{\displaystyle O}{\overset{\|}{C}}-O-(CH_2)_{29}-CH_3$$

Triacontyl hexadecanoate
(from beeswax)

$$CH_3-(CH_2)_{14}-\overset{\displaystyle O}{\overset{\|}{C}}-O-(CH_2)_{15}-CH_3$$

Hexadecyl hexadecanoate
(from sperm whale)

Figure 6-18 Examples of structures of ester waxes, formed from long-chain fatty alcohol and long-chain fatty acid.

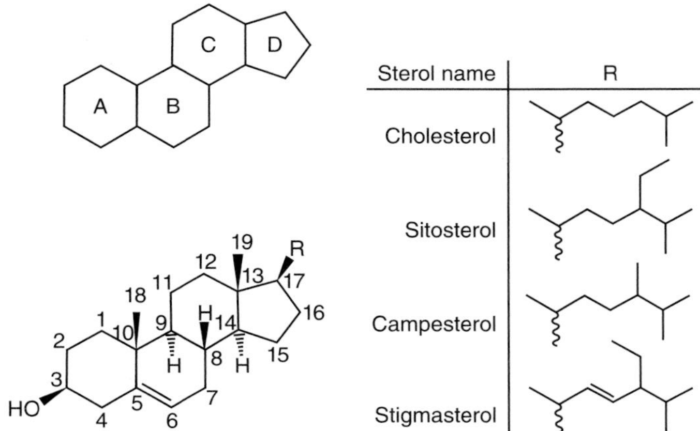

Figure 6-19 Sterane, the base structure for all sterols, showing designation of rings A, B, C, D *(top left)*. General structure for cholesterol and phytosterols, demonstrating the unique sterol numbering system *(bottom left)*. Alkyl side chains for several naturally occurring sterols are depicted on the right.

is primarily composed of squalene and triacylglycerols, with about 25% waxy esters and smaller amounts of free fatty acids, sterol esters, and ceramides.

STEROIDS

Steroids possess sterane (perhydro-1,2-cyclopentano-phenanthrene), a polycyclic hydrocarbon with four linked rings (A, B, C, D), as a common structure as shown in Figure 6-19. Most steroids fall under the category of sterols, which have a double bond between C-5 and C-6 (3β unsaturation), a hydroxyl group at C-3, methyl groups at C-10 and C-13, and an alkyl chain at C-17. The predominant sterol in higher animals is cholesterol, which may have a role in modulating membrane compressibility, permeability, fusibility, thickness, and organization. More than 200 plant sterols (phytosterols) are known to exist, including sitosterol, stigmasterol, and campesterol. They are similar to cholesterol, but contain different alkyl side chains. Structures of cholesterol and some phytosterols are shown in Figure 6-19. Normally, phytosterols are not absorbed by the intestine of humans. However, a rare genetic condition that permits their absorption leads to β-sitosterolemia, a disease in which large amounts of plant sterols are deposited in the body tissues. More complex molecules with a steroid nucleus, such as digitalis, are also found in plants. Digitalis is a strong stimulant for heart contractions and has been used for centuries to combat heart failure.

Cholesterol does not usually exist in a free form outside of the cell membrane but is instead esterified at the 3-OH group during storage and transport, often to arachidonic acid. Cholesteryl esters are stored in organs, such as the adrenal gland and the corpus luteum of the ovary, where they serve as precursors for steroid hormones. They also accumulate in certain disorders (e.g., cholesteryl ester storage disease, atherosclerosis, familial hypercholesterolemia, and Tangier disease). Cholesteryl esters form liquid crystals, which have been identified by polarizing microscopy in living tissues.

Cholesterol is the parent compound for biosynthesis of the steroid hormones that serve as long range messengers transported in the blood. There are five major classes of steroids in vertebrates: (1) androgens, (2) estrogens, (3) progestagens, (4) glucocorticoids, and (5) mineralocorticoids; examples of these structures are shown in Figure 6-20. The sex hormones (androgens, estrogens, and progestagens) are produced in the endocrine glands and help regulate biological development and processes. Androgens promote muscle development and other male secondary sex characteristics. Estrogens are responsible for regulation of the menstrual cycle and female secondary sex characteristics. The progestagens suppress ovulation and have antiestrogenic effects. Distinguishing between classes of sex hormones based only on structure can be tricky, as they are classified by their physiological role. Estrogens, such as estradiol, are characterized by a phenolic ring A and the lack of a C-19 methyl group, resulting in an 18-carbon structure. Androgens, such as testosterone, possess a 19-carbon structure and hydroxyl- or keto-groups at the C-3 and C-17 positions. Progesterone, the only natural progestagen, has a 21-carbon structure including an acetyl moiety at C-17. However, synthetic progestagens (progestins) used in oral contraceptives may lack both the acetyl group and the C-19 methyl group. The corticosteroids, produced in the adrenal gland, include the glucocorticoids, which mediate the inflammatory response, and the mineralocorticoids, which regulate Na^+/K^+ balance and water retention. Corticosteroids (both glucocorticoids and mineralocorticoids) are distinguished by

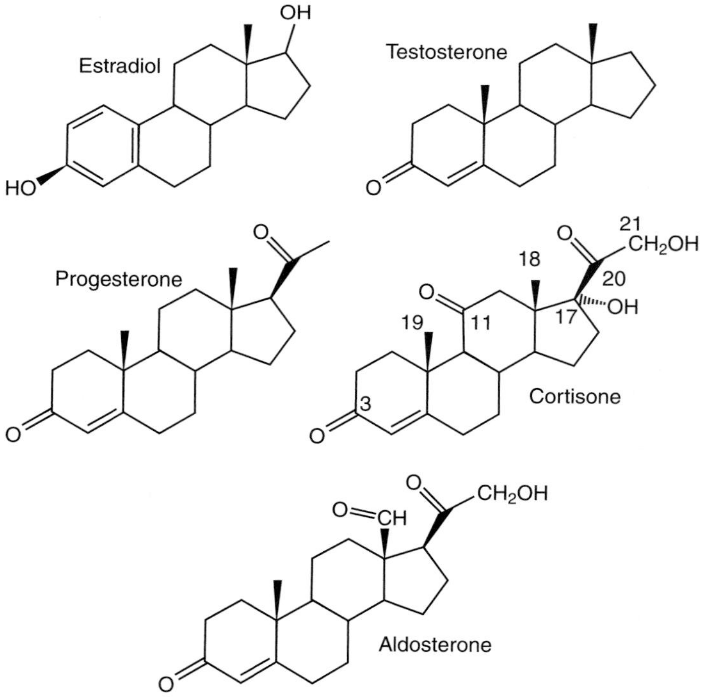

Figure 6-20 Representative structures of the five classes of steroid hormones (name of specific example given in parentheses): estrogens (estradiol), androgens (testosterone), progestagens (progesterone), glucosteroids (cortisone), and mineralosteroids (aldosterone).

Δ4 desaturation and keto groups at C-3 and C-20. The glucocorticoids, such as cortisone, also have a C-21 hydroxyl and either a hydroxyl or keto group at C-11. The primary mineralocorticoid, aldosterone, has a keto group at C-18.

Bile acids are formed by degrading the terminal side chain of cholesterol from 27 carbon atoms to 24 carbon atoms and by adding hydroxyl (–OH) groups to various positions in the ring structure. The products of mammalian bile acid biosynthesis are the so-called primary bile acids, cholic and chenodeoxycholic acids (Fig. 6-21). These primary bile acids are conjugated with taurine or glycine in the liver and are secreted in the bile. The bile acids, or their alkali metal salts, are natural detergents and act to solubilize phospholipid and cholesterol in the bile of higher animals, thereby permitting secretion of cholesterol into the gut. The excretion of both cholesterol and bile acids is the major way cholesterol is removed from the body.

Bile salts also aid in the digestion and absorption of fat and fat-soluble vitamins in the intestine. Bile salt deficiency caused by intestinal pathology (e.g., celiac disease, tropical sprue, bacterial overgrowth, or ileal resection) can cause fat malabsorption and malnutrition. This problem is especially serious in children, in whom growth may be impaired. Bile acid deficiency may also lead to cholesterol gallstone formation, because bile salt is required for cholesterol solubilization in bile. Abnormal bile acid metabolism is associated with accumulation of cholestanol (the saturated analog of cholesterol) in the disease cerebrotendinous xanthomatosis.

EICOSANOIDS

Eicosanoids are oxygenated nonesterified fatty acids principally derived from arachidonic acid (20:4n-6). Smaller amounts are generated from the other 20-carbon fatty acids, dihomo-γ-linolenic acid (20:3n-6), and eicosapentaenoic acid (20:5n-3). These derivatives are present in low concentration, are chemically unstable, have a very short lifetime, and act as autocoids to influence contractility, membrane permeability, and many other cellular functions. In contrast to endocrine hormones like the steroids, eicosanoids act on cells and tissues local to their site of production and thus have paracrine and autocrine activity. Eicosanoids are produced by three enzyme classes—cyclooxygenases, lipoxygenases, and cytochrome P450s—and their

Bile acid	R_1	R_2	R_3
Lithodeoxycholic	αOH	H	H
Deoxycholic	αOH	H	αOH
Chenodeoxycholic	αOH	αOH	H
Ursodeoxycholic	αOH	βOH	H
Cholic	αOH	αOH	αOH
Ursocholic	αOH	βOH	αOH

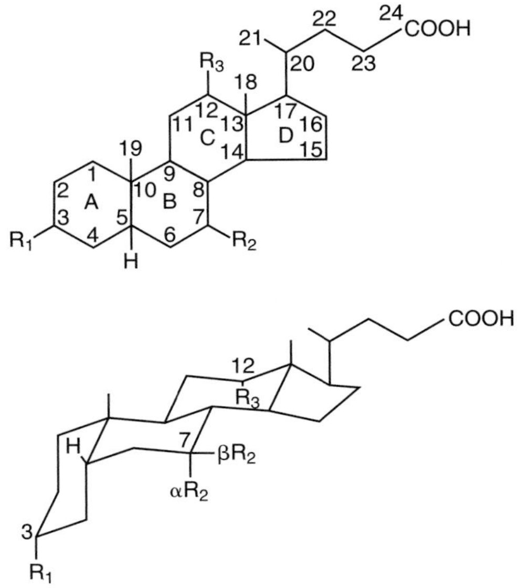

Figure 6-21 Molecular structure of common bile acids, showing the common steroid ring and side chain structure. The location and orientation of hydroxyl group(s) are given for each bile acid. NOTE: Lithodeoxycholic acid is commonly called lithocholic acid.

Figure 6-22 Prostanoic acid, the base structure for all cyclooxygenase products.

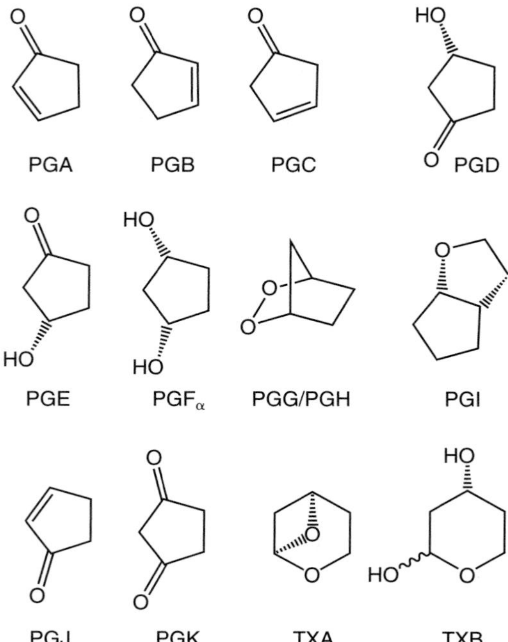

Figure 6-23 Ring structures of the prostaglandins (PGs) and thromboxanes (TXs) and nomenclature for the various prostaglandins and thromboxanes with these ring structures.

Figure 6-24 The E series of prostaglandins. The subscript corresponds to the number of double bonds in the carbon skeleton.

role and nomenclature are dependent on their biosynthetic route. In addition to these enzyme products, eicosanoids that are formed nonenzymatically have also been described and are called isoprostanes.

The cyclooxygenase products (prostaglandins and thromboxanes) have a prominent role in reproduction and in the inflammatory response, and have prostanoic acid as a general structure (Fig. 6-22). They are classified according to the nature of their ring structure. Prostaglandins (often abbreviated "PG") have a five-membered ring, and thromboxanes (TXs) have a six-membered ring, as shown in Figure 6-23. In nearly all cases, prostaglandins and TXs have a 15-hydroxyl substituent. The alphabetical nomenclature of prostaglandins (PGA, PGB, ...) is a vestige of their original classification based on solubility properties: PGA is soluble in acid, PGB soluble in base, PGE soluble in ether, and PGF in phosphate (Marks and Fürstenberger, 1999). The subscript at the end of the name corresponds to the number of double bonds in the molecule and also gives insight into the 20-carbon fatty acid precursor. Two double bonds are lost during the cyclization reaction. Thus PGE_1 derives from 20:3n-6, PGE_2 from 20:4n-6, and PGE_3 from 20:5n-3; the structures of these three PGEs are presented together in Figure 6-24. Isoprostanes are

Box 6-2

NOMENCLATURE FOR OXIDIZED DERIVATIVES OF UNSATURATED FATTY ACIDS

Number of Substituents	Substituent Name	Number of Carbons	Number of Double Bonds
1: No name	Hydroxy: H	12: D (dodeca)	1: ME (monoenoic)
2: Di	Hydroperoxy: Hp	14: T (tetradeca)	2: DE (dienoic)
3: Tri	Epoxy: Ep	15: P (pentadeca)	3: TrE (trienoic)
4: Tetra	Keto: Oxo	16: Hx (hexadeca)	4: TE (tetraenoic)
5: Penta		17: H (heptadeca)	5: PE (pentaenoic)
6: Hexa		18: O (octadeca)	6: HE (hexaenoic)
		19: N (nonadeca)	
		20: E (eicosa)	
		22: Do (docosa)	

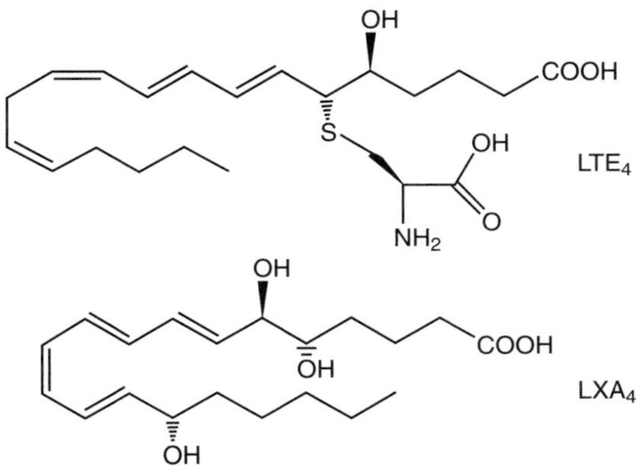

Figure 6-25 Structures of a leukotriene (LT) and a lipoxin (LX). The LT (LTE_4) possesses a partially conjugated 20-carbon skeleton, but the LX (LXA_4) is fully conjugated. The subscript corresponds to the number of double bonds.

diastereomers of prostaglandins, typically at the C-8 or C-12 chiral sites. Because they are racemic, they are known to be formed by free radical mechanisms independent of cyclooxygenase. They are frequently used as biomarkers for oxidative damage.

The major lipoxygenase products are the leukotrienes and the lipoxins. The leukotrienes (LTs) cause contraction in respiratory, vascular, and intestinal smooth muscles, in addition to other roles, and are characterized by a partially conjugated 20-carbon structure. The lipoxins (LXs) have a role in mediating cell–cell interactions and are characterized by a fully conjugated 20-carbon structure. There are five major endogenous classes of LTs (LTA, LTB, LTC, LTD, and LTE), and two classes of LXs (LXA and LXB). Analogous to the prostaglandins, the number of double bonds in LT and LX is written as a subscript. Lipoxygenases do not remove double bonds, so LTE_3 derives from 20:3n-6, LTE_4 from 20:4n-6, and LTE_5 from 20:5n-3. The structures of an example of a LT and a LX are shown in Figure 6-25.

A general nomenclature also exists for oxidized (hydroxy, hydroperoxy, epoxy, and oxo) unsaturated fatty acids that do not qualify as leukotrienes or lipoxins. This nomenclature is most commonly used for describing intermediates in the lipoxygenase pathway. Box 6-2 lists the abbreviations for substituents, carbon number, and double bond number, and examples of this nomenclature can be found in Figure 6-26. It is common practice to use shorthand and drop the double bond positions and stereochemistry; for example, (5E,8E,11E,13Z)-(15S)-15-HpETE may be written as 15-HpETE, although the full name will usually be defined at the beginning of the text. Products from the cytochrome P450 pathway, which are primarily epoxy-derivatives and dihydroxy-derivatives of arachidonic acid such as 5(6)-EpETrE, are also reported using this general nomenclature.

Docosanoids are 22-carbon analogs of eicosanoids, and often show agonistic behavior to receptors intended for their 20-carbon

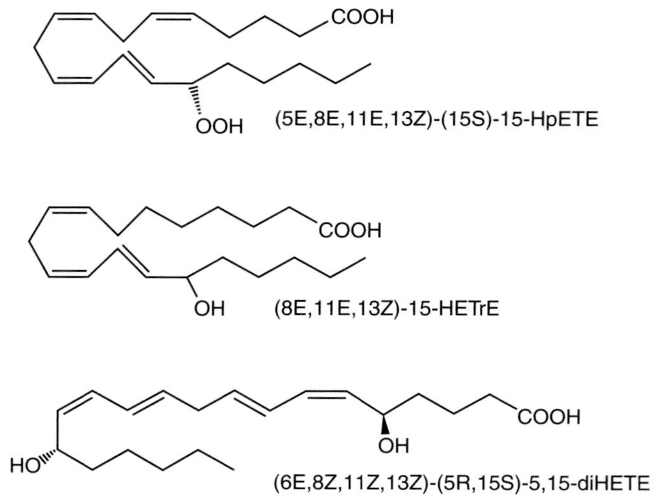

(5E,8E,11E,13Z)-(15S)-15-HpETE

(8E,11E,13Z)-15-HETrE

(6E,8Z,11Z,13Z)-(5R,15S)-5,15-diHETE

Figure 6-26 Examples of general nomenclature for oxidized unsaturated fatty acids. *HpETE*, Hydroperoxyeicosatetraenoic acid; *HETrE*, hydroxyeicosatrienoic acid; *diHETE*, dihydroxyeicosatetraenoic acid.

counterparts. For example, latanoprost and related docosanoids have been shown to lower intraocular pressure by agonistic action on the F-prostanoid receptor, and are thus effective treatments for glaucoma.

OTHER LIPIDS

Acyl coenzyme A and acylcarnitine are key intermediates in fatty acid metabolism; they are usually present in low concentrations, but under certain conditions they may accumulate and disrupt cellular functions. Cytidine diphosphate-diacylglycerol (CDP-DAG) is an intermediate in phospholipid synthesis and probably partitions into membranes.

N-Acylethanolamines have ethanolamine in place of glycerol as a backbone and are present in low concentration in human plasma. *N*-Arachidonoylethanolamine, or anandamide, has attracted special attention for its role as the neurotransmitter associated with the cannabinoid receptors. Anandamide is associated with analgesia, muscle relaxation, improvement of mood, appetite stimulation, and other effects that are generally associated with tetrahydrocannabinol (THC) and marijuana use (Grotenhermen, 2004).

Lipopolysaccharides (endotoxins) are a large, complex class of bacterial glycolipids, present in the outer leaflet of the outer membrane of gram-negative organisms. In higher animals, endotoxin is responsible for inflammation and septic shock during infection. The processes responsible for these phenomena are mediated primarily by the lipid component of endotoxin (lipid A).

α-Lipoic acid, also known as thioctic acid, contains a five-member ring with a disulfide linkage. Lipoic acid is normally bound to a lysine residue of a protein by an amide linkage. In its bound form, lipoamide, lipoic acid is a required cofactor for mitochondrial metabolism. Lipoic acid has also received attention for its function as an antioxidant and as a transcription regulator.

SOAPS AND DETERGENTS

Soaps are alkali-metal salts of long-chain fatty acids (e.g., potassium stearate). They are readily produced by treatment of TAGs (such as tallow or lard) with a strong base. Detergent is a general term for any highly amphiphilic compound that shows surfactant behavior, and includes soaps as well as the biological surfactants such as bile salts. However, the word detergent is primarily associated with synthetic detergents such as sodium dodecyl sulfate (SDS).

PHYSICAL AND STRUCTURAL PROPERTIES OF LIPIDS

Lipid structures generally fall into two categories; those that demonstrate a high degree of long-range order, or periodicity, in one or more directions; and those that possess minimal or no long-range order. Most biologically relevant lipid structures (membrane bilayers, vesicles, and micelles) fall into the second category. Well-ordered lipid structures with crystalline or crystalline-like properties are relevant to food science and processing, but are rarely, if ever, observed in vivo.

The properties of complex biological lipid structures are often extrapolated from the properties of lipids as isolated compounds. As was mentioned in the previous section, most biological fats are a mixture of many distinct compounds that are impossible to fully characterize. Glycerolipids with identical fatty acids at all positions (other than the *sn*-3 position for phospholipids) are easy to synthesize from glycerol and fatty acids, and, consequently, their properties have been carefully measured. However, organic chemical synthesis of glycerolipids with fatty acids at stereospecifically defined positions is well known but difficult, and such compounds are expensive and rare. As a result, there is a rich literature on the biochemical properties of some lipids, but not of most lipids.

More importantly, there are no situations where lipids appear in tissues in pure form in which they do not interact with other lipids and with proteins. Chemically, mixtures have drastically different properties than those of pure compounds; for instance, mixtures have complex phase change behavior that may not even have an analogy in pure systems (e.g., the segregation of like molecules as mixtures cool, leading to fractional crystallization). Within these constraints, a study of the properties of lipids is a useful exercise for understanding the role and function of lipids in biological systems.

EXTRACTION TECHNIQUES

Lipids in real samples (e.g., membranes or food matrices) are usually not studied in situ, owing to limitations of analytical techniques. Instead they are typically extracted into solvent before any analysis takes place. These extraction procedures change the lipid composition and properties significantly, sometimes in obvious ways, as for instance in destruction of the bilayer, and sometimes in less obvious ways, such as the loss of water and proteins, which can influence lipid properties. Thus it is important to consider the most commonly employed extraction techniques.

Lipids can be extracted from most any tissue with several standard methods. A classic method used since the 1950s is called the Folch method (Folch et al., 1957). A mixture of chloroform ($CHCl_3$) and methanol (CH_3OH) is added to tissue homogenate at a ratio of 20 parts solvent to 1 part tissue. The mixture is then extracted against a highly polar salt solution so that polar components dissolve into the aqueous phase, and the lipids stay behind in the nonpolar phase. Much of the methanol also dissolves into the aqueous phase as well, but enough stays in the lipid phase to dissolve amphipathic lipids, specifically phospholipids, which are not very soluble in pure chloroform.

An elegant alternative technique known as the "Bligh and Dyer" method (Bligh and Dyer, 1959) has been more popular in recent decades because it requires less solvent than the Folch method. The Bligh and Dyer technique uses a ratio of chloroform to methanol to water of approximately 2:1:0.8 to dissolve all components of the tissue homogenate into a single phase. The water component must be adjusted for the water content of every tissue to ensure that there is initially a single phase, which is essential for an efficient extraction. Salt water is then added, and polar compounds are removed while lipids remain in the organic phase. Other methods based on methylene chloride, hexane, and other solvents are in common use as well.

The results of these extractions are lipids that have been dissociated from all other noncovalently bound components of their environment. Importantly, phospholipids are removed from membranes where they existed in some complex mixture with other lipids, sugars, and, importantly, proteins. Properties of these crude lipid extracts, particularly bulk properties such as melting points and dielectric constants, bear little resemblance to those of functional, structurally intact lipids in the cell. Crude lipid mixtures derived from biological sources have thousands of distinct molecules and are never fully characterized.

SURFACE BEHAVIOR OF LIPIDS AT THE WATER INTERFACE

Lipids take on important properties at air–water or oil–water interfaces. The interaction of a specific lipid with an aqueous interface depends on the hydrophilic–lipophilic balance of the lipid (i.e., the relative strengths of the hydrocarbon and water-seeking parts). Therefore, when a lipid droplet contacts a water surface of limited area, one of the following three events will occur:

1. Very hydrophobic lipids, like mineral oil, will simply sit on the water as an intact droplet or lens.
2. Slightly hydrophilic lipids, like vegetable oils (mixtures of TAGs), will spread to form a continuous insoluble monolayer of molecules in equilibrium with the remainder of the droplet.
3. Highly hydrophilic lipids, like soap detergents or sodium cholate (a bile salt), will spread to form an unstable film from which molecules desorb into the water.

Lipids are found in almost all interfaces between cellular compartments. Between two aqueous compartments within a cell, a membrane bilayer is present. Between fat and aqueous compartments in the cytoplasm (e.g., a fat droplet in a fat cell) or plasma (e.g., a lipoprotein particle), a phospholipid monolayer forms the interface.

DETERMINANTS OF LIPID MELTING

Lipid melting is the solid to liquid phase change (e.g., the melting of butter or animal fat). The melting transition is governed by the strength of the molecular interactions of hydrocarbons, primarily of aliphatic chains and sterols. The transition is affected by chain length, polar substitution, or double bonds. This is illustrated in Figure 6-27, in which the chain-melting transition (crystal to liquid chain) is shown for lipids with increasing chain length and for a variety of molecules having different substituents. Note that as the chain length increases, the melting temperature rises. Double bonds, triple bonds, methylene branches, and halide substitutions at the end of the chain decrease the melting temperature, but polar substituents, particularly those that can form hydrogen bonds or ionic bonds, increase the temperature of the melting transition. The order of increasing melting temperatures for a given chain length is as follows: 1-olefins < alkanes < ethyl esters < normal alcohols < carboxylic or fatty acids < triacylglycerols < 1,2 diacylglycerols = 3 monoacylglycerols < dry phosphatidylcholine.

LIPID SOLUBILITY AND MICELLES

"Solubility" of lipids in aqueous phases is a more chemically complex process than what occurs when ionic or polar compounds are dissolved. True solutions are molecular dispersions in which solutes are surrounded and dynamically interact with many solvent molecules. At very low concentrations, lipids do form molecular dispersions in aqueous solution. However, at higher concentrations, lipids tend to form aggregates of various sizes defined by the composition of the lipid mixture and any amphipaths that are included in the mixture. Those aggregates that are smaller than the wavelength of visible light (400 to 700 nm) are clear and resemble true solutions in this respect, although they are not molecular dispersions and more closely resemble a dispersion of a lipid phase in an aqueous phase.

The true solubility of different types of lipids in aqueous systems is quite variable, extending from the virtually insoluble high-molecular-weight hydrocarbons and triacylglycerols to the very soluble soaps and detergents. The solubility of fatty acids is very low and decreases with increasing chain length and, thus, decreasing polarity. Fatty acid solubility also decreases as the temperature decreases.

Some of the more polar lipids, for example, K and Na soaps and bile salts, form optically clear aqueous solutions in which the apparent solubility may be as high as 60 g per 100 g of solution. These more polar lipids spontaneously form small, spherical aggregates of molecules called micelles, and such dispersions are called micellar solutions. Micellar solutions

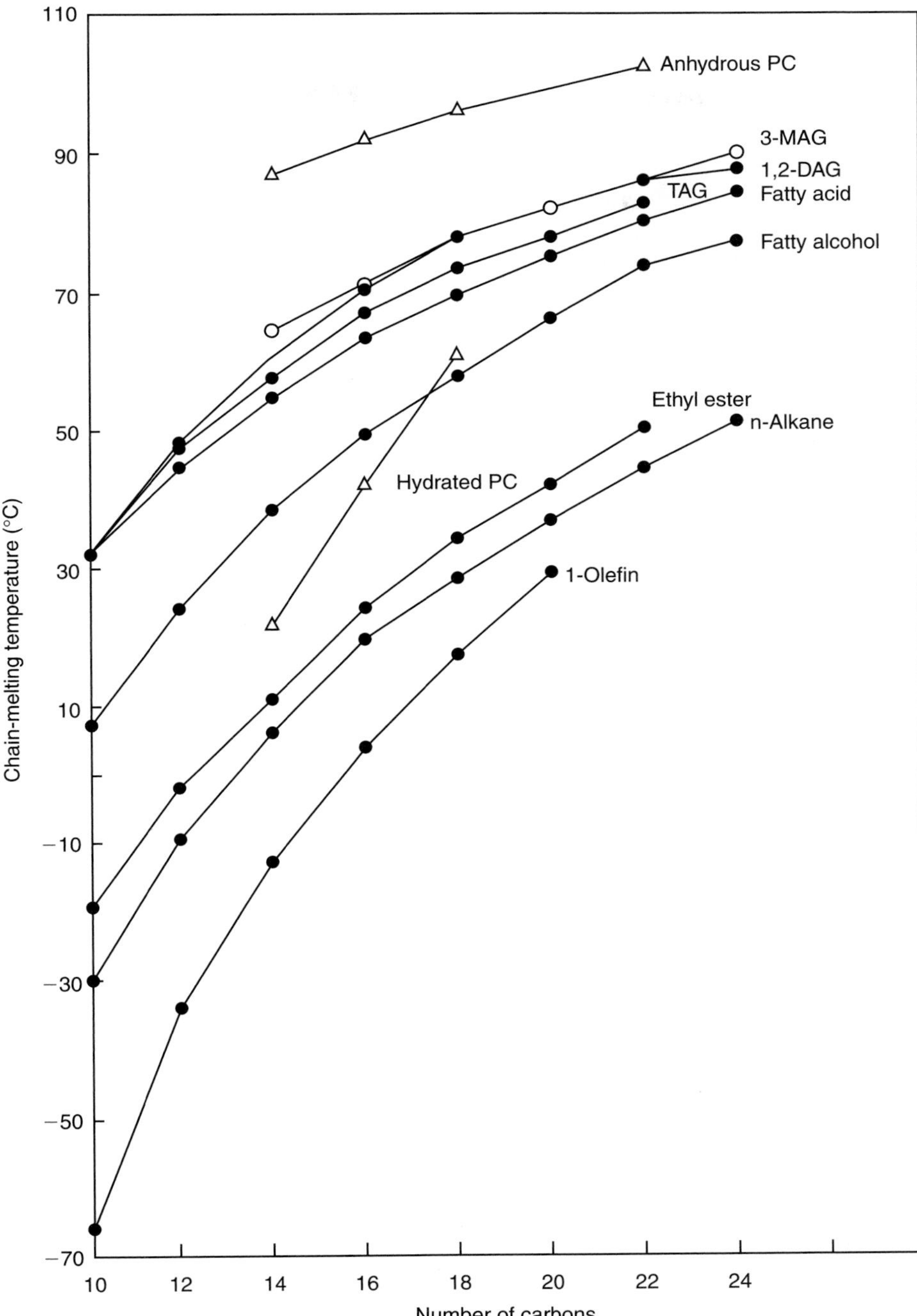

Figure 6-27 Effects of polar substituents on melting of the hydrocarbon chain for a variety of lipids. The chain-melting transition (i.e., to liquid chain) temperatures for a variety of lipids are plotted against the number of carbons in the aliphatic chain. The stronger the interactions of the polar groups with each other, the higher the melting point (MP). This is illustrated by the difference between fatty acids, which can form hydrogen bonds between the carboxyl groups, and ethyl esters of fatty acids, which cannot. The MP of the hydrogen-bonded fatty acids is 30° to 40° C higher. Note that the melting transitions increase in temperature with increasing hydrocarbon chain length, even in water. The presence of water, however, lowers the chain transition when compared with the dry lipid, as shown for phosphatidylcholine (PC). *DAG,* Diacylglycerol; *MAG,* Monoacylglycerol; *TAG,* Triacylglycerol.

are critical for fat absorption in the small intestine. Micelles in the lumen of the small intestine are made up of mono-acylglycerols and diacylglycerols, FFAs, and bile salts and can incorporate very nonpolar compounds such as fat soluble vitamins in their hydrophobic interior. A micellar solution is a thermodynamically stable system formed spontaneously by these lipids when they are present in water above a critical concentration and temperature (Fig. 6-28). The molecules of these micelles are in rapid equilibrium with a low concentration of dispersed solute molecules. The low concentration of a specific solute molecule would be considered a saturated solution of that solute in the solvent, and this concentration is called the critical micellar concentration (CMC). At concentrations higher than the CMC, the excess lipid forms micelles. Micellar solutions can solubilize other less soluble lipids to form mixed micelles. Micelles are spherical structures, about two molecular lengths in diameter in pure water, but when salt is added they often enlarge and assume cylindrical or discoid ("disk") shapes. Bile salts enhance formation of mixed micellar solutions in bile and in intestinal contents during fat absorption. Micellar solutions are necessary for the proper digestion and absorption of fat and fat-soluble vitamins.

Lipids may also be suspended in aqueous systems as emulsions, similar to an oil-water based salad dressing stabilized by amphi–pathic protein. Margarine and mayonnaise are two commonly encountered emulsions that

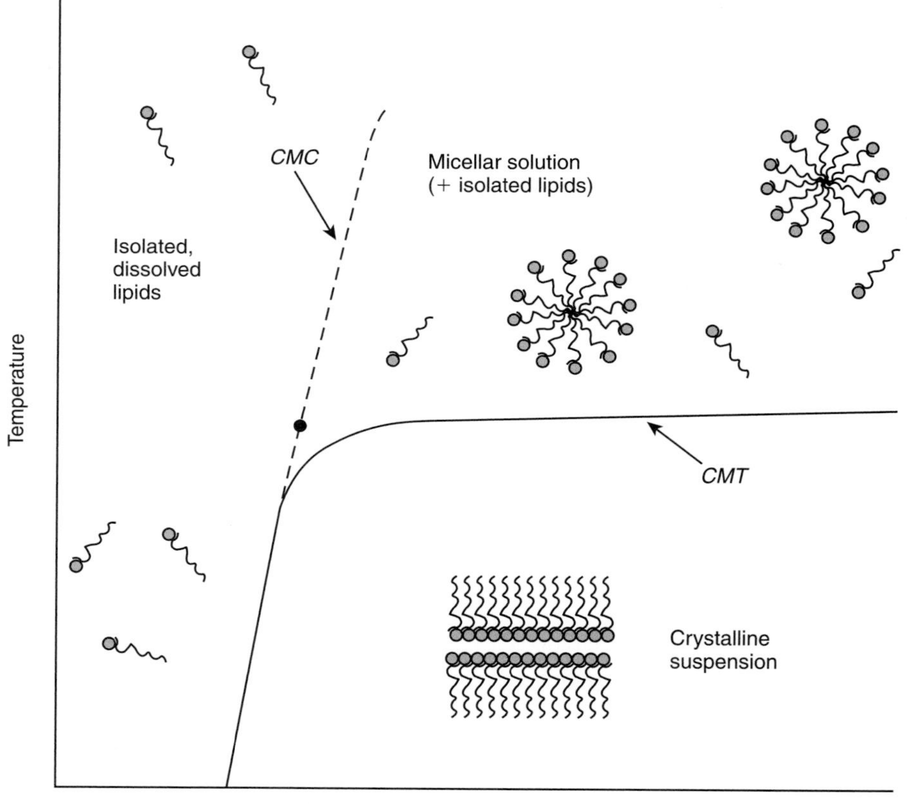

Figure 6-28 Behavior of soluble, amphiphilic lipids as a function of temperature and concentration. Micelles occur only at temperatures higher than the critical micelle temperature *(CMT)* and lipid concentrations higher than the critical micelle concentration *(CMC)*. At concentrations lower than the CMC, the detergent exists as molecularly dispersed solutes. At high lipid concentration and at temperatures lower than the CMT, the lipid forms a crystalline suspension.

are dominated by the lipid phase. Typically, emulsions have particle sizes between 10 and 100 μm and, therefore, appear opaque. Insoluble lipids such as triacylglycerols or cholesteryl esters can be made to form relatively stable aqueous-lipid emulsions by adding an emulsifier such as a phospholipid. For instance, emulsions containing particles with a core of triacylglycerol and a surface layer of an emulsifier such as PC (lecithin) can be formed in vitro by agitation. Very stable emulsions of soy oil stabilized with phospholipids are used in hospitals for intravenous (parenteral) feeding as a source of fat for individuals who are incapable of oral (enteral) feeding.

THE LIPID BILAYER

Lipids form barriers between compartments within the cell, such as for specific organelles, and between the cell and the outside chemical environment. These barriers are called membranes and are mixtures of approximately two thirds lipid and one third protein. The lipid is primarily phospholipid arranged in a bilayer that includes proteins to impart structure and function. In the phospholipid bilayer, the polar or ionic groups of the phospholipids are at the inner and outer surfaces of the bilayer, whereas the hydrocarbon chains are directed inward to form a hydrophobic barrier. The phospholipids in contact with the inside of the cell are referred to as the "inner leaflet," and the side that contacts the "outside world" is called the "outer leaflet." Particular phospholipid classes tend to be more common to one leaflet than another; for instance, phosphatidyl serine is enriched in the inner leaflet.

The favored model of the last 30 years for the cell membrane has been the "fluid mosaic" model in which the lipid bilayer is seen to be permeated by integral proteins (ion channels and integrins) and cholesterol, with glycoproteins, carbohydrates, and other molecules protruding from the leaflet surfaces. The fluid mosaic assumes that these chemical entities are distributed randomly throughout the lipid bilayer.

Treatment of membranes with mild detergents dissolves some regions but leaves others intact. The latter regions are called "detergent resistant membranes" and tend to be rich in protein, cholesterol, and sphingomyelin. These regions are frequently referred to as "lipid rafts" because they are considered to represent strongly associated functional groups of molecules drifting amid the two dimensional liquid of the membrane (Simons and Vaz, 2004). The lipid raft model is a refinement of the fluid mosaic model: the lipid raft does not float over the top of the bilayer (as the name implies) but refers to a temporary coalescence of specific proteins and lipids that operate as a unit to perform a certain task. Treatment of cells with various agents in culture causes the components of the rafts to change, presumably by exchange of material with the nondetergent resistant membrane regions, and several putative lipid raft-forming proteins have been identified. The physical presence of lipid rafts in vivo remains controversial because, if they exist, they are both small (<100 nm) and transient and, thus, particularly difficult to study in vivo. New single-particle detection techniques are being explored for this purpose (Cottingham, 2004).

In some respects, the lipid bilayer does behave like a two-dimensional fluid. For example, fluorescent and photo-bleaching studies have shown that proteins diffuse laterally through the membrane as if they were in a viscous liquid. Fluidity is defined as the reciprocal of viscosity and increases with temperature. Unfortunately, the precise chemical definition of fluidity as applied to lipids, and the related concept of "membrane fluidity" as applied to liquid crystals, is often misconstrued to explain almost any change in biochemical function that is accompanied by a change in the saturation of hydrocarbon chains in membranes. Intermolecular interactions in general, especially those in chemically complex membranes, are poorly understood chemical phenomena. Consequently, a study of pure systems is informative but is best considered a rough guide to the reality of complex interactions.

Artificial bilayers can be easily made from purified phospholipids. When a pure, very saturated phospholipid, such as dipalmitoyl phosphatidylcholine, is agitated vigorously, a spherical bilayered vesicle called a liposome can be the result. The interior of the bilayer consists of tightly packed, closely interacting hydrocarbon chains, and the bilayer tends to be rigid. As the unsaturation of the phospholipids used to form the liposomes increases, the bilayer becomes more flexible. When a mixture of cholesterol and phospholipids is used to prepare the liposomes, the cholesterol segregates to the interior of the membrane where it interacts with the hydrocarbon chains and, in general, makes them less rigid. The strength of molecular interactions in bulk phases is associated with their melting (and boiling) points. By analogy, highly interacting, rigid membranes can be thought of as having less molecular disorder than membranes that are more unsaturated and include cholesterol and other compounds.

HIGHLY ORDERED LIPIDS: TRIGLYCERIDES AND POLYMORPHISM

The most commonly encountered ordered lipids are those found in solid edible fats that are composed mostly of TAGs, such as butter, shortening, and cocoa butter. TAGs typically align along their long axes, with their hydrocarbon chains elongated, in order to maximize the Van der Waals interactions between their hydrophobic regions. The two most commonly observed orientations for TAGs in crystalline environments are the "tuning-fork" conformation and the "chair" conformation, depicted in Figure 6-29.

These conformations are capable of forming multiple solid crystalline forms (polymorphism), depending on the nature of the conformation and the packing orientation. Polymorphic solids have different lattice structures and stabilities, and, consequently, different melting points, but form the same liquid upon melting. The most common polymorphic forms are the α-, β-, and β′-states, which are depicted in Figure 6-30. The α- and β′-states are based on the tuning fork conformation, whereas the β-state is based on the chair conformation. Packing efficiency and melting point vary in the order α<β′<β. β crystals are more ordered and larger, whereas α and β′ crystals are less ordered and smaller. In general, the more disordered, lower melting-point polymorphs such as α are formed by fast cooling of fats, whereas more organized polymorphs are formed by slower cooling of fats.

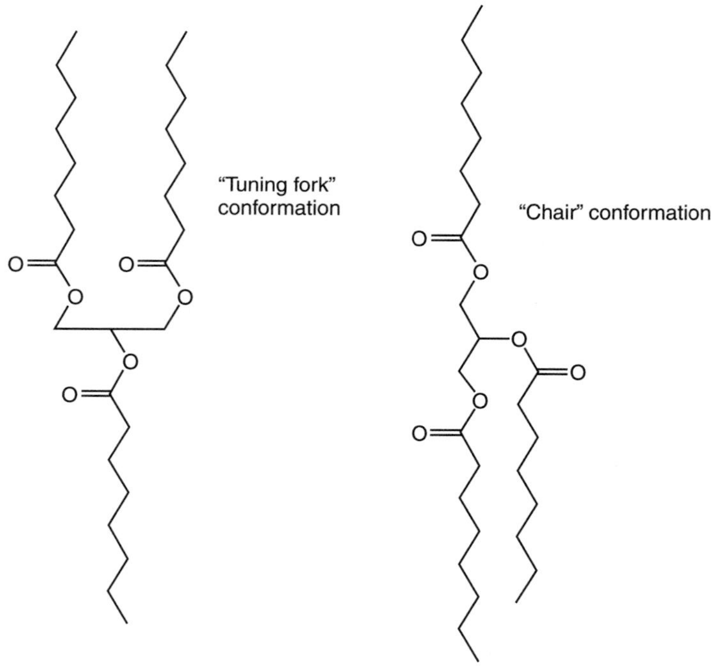

Figure 6-29 Tuning fork *(left)* and chair *(right)* conformations of crystalline triacylglycerols (TAGs).

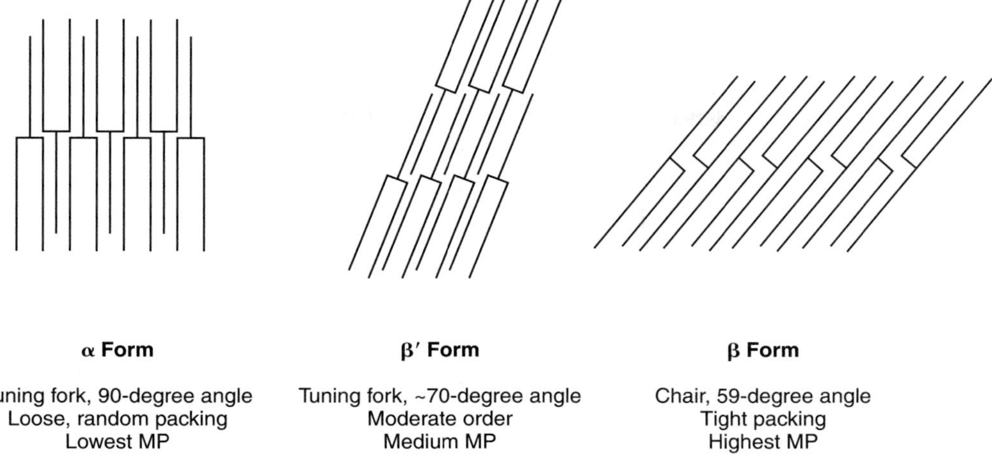

Figure 6-30 Common polymorphs of triacylglycerols. Line diagrams represent the three fatty acyl chains *(long lines)* esterified to the glycerol backbone *(short line)* for each molecule. *MP,* Melting point.

Some triacylglycerols have more complicated polymorphisms, and natural mixtures of TAGs such as oils and fats may exist as a combination of polymorphic forms and multiple TAG species of molecules in the same crystal. However, in a general sense, many natural fats and oils behave like a single species of TAG in that they show the different polymorphic forms of α, β′, and β, even though they contain multiple TAG species. Forming the correct polymorphic form is important in producing palatable and attractive foods. For example, shortening manufacturers prefer to form the β′ rather than β polymorph because it results in smaller crystals with a smoother mouth feel. Conversely, chocolate manufacturers prefer to form the β polymorph of cocoa butter, which has a melting point of 35.5° C compared to 27° C for the β′ form. Polymorphic transitions from β to β′ forms are responsible for the white, dusty layer ("bloom") sometimes seen on old chocolate. Although not toxic, bloom is unacceptable to most consumers.

DIGESTION AND ABSORPTION OF DIETARY FATS AND OILS

A single meal often contains dietary fat from a variety of sources (dairy, meat, and vegetable). These mix with digestive secretions in the stomach and small intestine and undergo digestion and absorption. Absorption from the lumen is generally quite efficient, and only approximately 4% of the ingested fat escapes into the feces (Carey et al., 1983). However, absorption of specific, highly saturated fats may be less efficient.

The triacylglycerol composition of oils, fats, and lipoproteins is usually reported as the total overall fatty acid composition of the triacylglycerol mixture. This information is widely available from various sources (Shahidi, 2005; Firestone, 1999; Gunstone et al., 1994; Sonntag, 1979; Kuksis, 1978;) and is valuable because it tells us which major fatty acids are esterified to the glycerol; however, it does not tell us the position of the fatty acid substituents on glycerol or how many specific triacylglycerol species are present in a given sample. Statistically, the number of TAGs (N) that could be present in a sample having n different fatty acids is n^3. Various methods are available to determine the position of fatty acids on the TAG molecule and even to fully characterize the molecular forms present in an oil; however, they tend to be more expensive or elaborate than analysis of overall fatty acid compositions. For this reason, and because for nutritional purposes overall absorption is very high, fatty acid compositions are typically reported without stereochemical information.

The solid–liquid phase change is important for some biological properties, for instance, for digestion, because solid fats are not well absorbed. The melting and crystallization temperatures for a variety of TAGs, DAGs, and MAGs that are present during fat metabolism have been reported (Small, 1991). The melting points of many individual dietary TAGs are higher than body temperature. For instance, the saturated TAGs tristearin (MP 73° C) and tripalmitin (MP 66° C) are not hydrolyzed by pancreatic lipase and they pass through the gut unabsorbed, still in solid form. Dietary fat is, nevertheless, well absorbed because it is a mixture of TAGs and other lipids. Unlike pure compounds, these lipids have a broad melting range in which they soften and can be emulsified sufficiently to be acted upon by components in the aqueous phase, such as acids and lipases.

TAG structure can influence absorption characteristics of some TAGs, particularly those with melting points lower than body temperature. For example, some studies indicate that if the saturated fatty acid is in the 2 position, it is more likely to be absorbed than if it is in the 1 or 3 position, at least in studies using pure fats. This relationship between stereospecific position and absorption is a function of the action of pancreatic lipases responsible for digestion in the small intestine. For example, consider the absorption of stearate contained in TAGs comprising two molecules of oleate and one of stearate; three different positional isomers are possible: OSO, OOS, or SOO in the *sn*-1, 2, and 3 positions of glycerol, respectively. OSO (MP = 25° C) and OOS (MP = 24° C) are both liquids at body temperature. In studies in rats fed OSO or OOS, approximately 94% of the stearate in OSO was absorbed, whereas only about 62% of the stearate in OOS was absorbed (Redgrave et al., 1988). When intestinal enzymes hydrolyze 1 mole of OSO, they produce 1 mole of 2-monostearin and 2 moles of oleic acid. The melting point of hydrated 2-monostearin is close to the body temperature of rats (39° C), and it can be solubilized by bile salts and thus be absorbed. However, hydrolysis of OOS gives a mole of stearic acid or its acid-soap; these products have melting points greater than 50° C and, therefore, solidify and are poorly absorbed. Overall, however, fat absorption is very efficient for normal foods, and these effects are of importance only for engineered food applications, such as the development of low calorie foods based on low absorption of fats.

REFERENCES

Bligh EG, Dyer WJ (1959) A rapid method of total lipid extraction and purification. Can J Biochem Physiol 37:911-917.

Breckinridge WC (1978) Stereospecific analysis of triacylglycerols. In: Kuksis A (ed) Handbook of Lipid Research: Fatty Acids, and Glycerides. Vol 1. Plenum Press, New York, pp. 197-232.

Brown WR, Hansen AE, Burr BO, McQuarrie I (1938) Effects of prolonged use of extremely low-fat diet in an adult human subject. J Nutr 16:511-524.

Burr GO, Burr MM (1929) A new deficiency disease produced by the rigid exclusion of fat from the diet. J Biol Chem 82:345-367.

Carey MC, Small DM, Bliss CM (1983) Lipid digestion and absorption. Annu Rev Physiol 45:651-677.

Cottingham K (2004) Do you believe in lipid rafts? Biologists are turning to several analytical techniques to find out whether lipid rafts really exist. Anal Chem 76:403A-406A.

Englund PT (1993) The structure and biosynthesis of glycosyl phosphatidylinositol. Annu Rev Biochem 62:121-138.

Fahy E, Subramaniam S, Brown HA, Glass CK, Merrill AH Jr, Murphy RC, Raetz CR, Russell DW, Seyama Y, Shaw W, Shimizu T, Spener F, van Meer G, VanNieuwenhze MS, White SH, Witztum JL, Dennis EA (2005) A comprehensive classification system for lipids. J Lipid Res 46:839-862.

Firestone D (ed) (1999) Physical and Chemical Characteristics of Oils, Fats, and Waxes. AOCS Press, Champaign, IL.

Folch J, Lees M, Sloane-Stanley GH (1957) A simple method for the isolation and purificaiton of total lipides from animal tissues. J Biol Chem 226:497-509.

Gunstone FD, Harwood JL, Padley FB (1994) The Lipid Handbook, 2nd ed. Chapman and Hall, London.

Grotenhermen F (2004) Pharmacology of cannabinoids. Neuro Endocrinol Lett 25:14-23.

Holman RT (1964) Nutritional and metabolic interrelationships between fatty acids. Fed Proc 23:1062-1067.

Holman RT (1992) A long scaly tale: the study of essential fatty acid deficiency at the University of Minnesota. Third International Congress on Essential Fatty Acids and Eicosanoids, Adelaide, Australia. AOCS Press, Champaign, IL.

Hu FB, Willett WC (2002) Optimal diets for prevention of coronary heart disease. JAMA 288:2569-2578.

Kay JK, Mackle TR, Auldist MJ, Thomson NA, Bauman DE (2004) Endogenous synthesis of cis-9, trans-11 conjugated linoleic acid in dairy cows fed fresh pasture. J Dairy Sci 87:369-378.

Kramer JK, Parodi PW, Jensen RG, Mossoba MM, Yurawecz MP, Adolf RO (1998) Rumenic acid: a proposed common name for the major conjugated linoleic acid isomer found in natural products. Lipids 33:835.

Kuksis A (1978) Fatty acids and glycerides. In: Handbook of Lipid Research. Vol 1. Plenum Press, New York.

Marks F, Fürstenberger G (eds) (1999) Prostaglandins, Leukotrienes, and Other Eicosanoids: From Biogenesis to Clinical Application. New York, Wiley-VCH.

Michaud AL, Brenna JT (2005) Structural Characterization of CLA Methyl Esters with Acetonitrile Chemical Ionization Tandem Mass Spectrometry. Advances in Conjugated Linoleic Acid Research. AOCS Press, Champaign, IL.

Redgrave TG, Kodali DR, Small DM (1988) The effect of triacyl-*sn*-glycerol structure on the metabolism of chylomicrons and triacylglycerol-rich emulsions in the rat. J Biol Chem 263: 5118-5123.

Shahidi F (ed) (2005) Bailey's Industrial Oil and Fat Products, 6th edition, 5 Volumes. John Wiley and Sons, New York.

Simons K, Vaz WL (2004) Model systems, lipid rafts, and cell membranes. Annu Rev Biophys Biomol Struct 33:269-295.

Small DM (1991) The effects of glyceride structure on absorption and metabolism. Annu Rev Nutr 11:413-434.

Sonntag NOV (1979) Composition and characteristics of individual fats and oils. In: Swern D (ed) Bailey's Industrial Oil and Fat Products. Vol. 1. John Wiley & Sons, New York, pp 289-478.

Turpeinen AM, Mutanen M, Aro A, Salminen I, Basu S, Palmquist DL, Griinari JM (2002) Bioconversion of vaccenic acid to conjugated linoleic acid in humans. Am J Clin Nutr 76:504-510.

Yurawecz MP, Pariza MW (2004) Perspective on the safety and effectiveness of conjugated linoleic acid. Am J Clin Nutr 79:1132S-1136S.

RECOMMENDED READING

Gurr MI, Frayn KN, Harwood JL (2002) Lipid Biochemistry. New York, Blackwell Publishing.

RECOMMENDED WEBSITES

The Lipid Library
Maintained by William W. Christie. Sponsored by the Lipid Analysis Unit of Mylnefield Research Services Ltd.
www.lipidlibrary.co.uk/index.html

Nomenclature of Lipids
International Union of Pure and Applied Chemistry (IUPAC) and International Union of Biochemistry and Molecular Biology (IUBMB) Commission on Biochemical Nomenclature (CBN)
www.chem.qmul.ac.uk/iupac/lipid/

Unit III

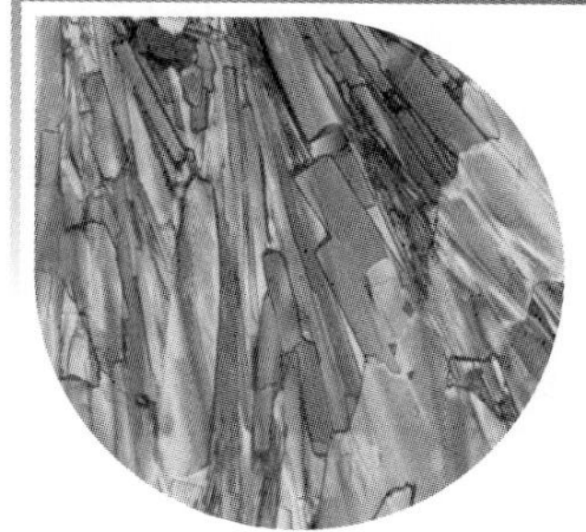

Digestion and Absorption of the Macronutrients

Earlier information regarding the biochemical and physiologic events associated with digestion was derived from the analysis of luminal fluids from the gastrointestinal tract. In 1822, William Beaumont, an American physician, studied gastric juice obtained from a gastric fistula that remained in a patient who had recovered from a gunshot wound. This led to the discovery that hydrochloric acid was secreted by the stomach. In 1836, the German anatomist and physiologist Theodor Schwann described the ability of gastric juice to break down albumin. This was the first recognition of the enzymatic breakdown of food, and Schwann coined the word *pepsin* from the Greek *pepsis* (digestion) to describe this new factor in gastric juice. In 1899 to 1902, in the laboratory of the Russian physiologist Ivan Pavlov, the observation that an intestinal factor was required for activation of pancreatic proteases was first made. Pavlov named this factor enterokinase. These processes are better understood today, and research is continuing to provide new insights into digestive, and, particularly, absorptive processes.

According to data from the Continuing Survey of Food Intakes by Individuals (CSFII, 1994-96, 1998), Americans are deriving approximately 29% of calories from fat, 15% of calories from protein, and 52% of calories from carbohydrate. The median daily intakes of carbohydrate, protein, and fat were 240 g, 71 g, and 53 g, respectively. In addition to handling the digestion and absorption of nutrients provided by the diet, the digestive system must also process a large amount of endogenous proteins (~70 g/day) and endogenous lipids (~25 g/day, mainly from bile), which are secreted into the lumen of the digestive tract in the salivary, gastric, pancreatic, biliary, and intestinal secretions, or are components of the epithelial cells shed into the lumen of the gastrointestinal tract.

Digestion largely involves the processes of enzymatic breakdown of these complex macronutrients to their smaller units (e.g., digestion of polysaccharides such as starch to monosaccharides such as glucose). Absorption of these smaller molecules across the epithelial cell layer of the intestinal mucosa into the lamina propria (the vascular layer of connective tissue beneath the epithelium) allows them to enter either the blood or lymph for circulation to the rest of the body. Release and absorption of vitamins and minerals are also essential, and these processes are described in Units VI and VII.

The gastrointestinal tract can be considered as a tubular structure extending from the mouth to the anus, and the contents in the lumen of the gastrointestinal tract can be considered as "outside" the cellular tissues of the body. Uptake of nutrients into the circulatory systems (blood and lymph), which supply the cellular tissues of the body with nutrients, depends upon the efficiency with which complex nutrients are broken down to smaller components that can be transported across the epithelial cells; the transporters located in the brush border (luminal) membrane of the mucosal epithelial cells (enterocytes), which allow their uptake from the luminal contents; further hydrolysis (e.g., peptide hydrolysis to amino acids) or processing (e.g., triacylglycerol synthesis and formation of chylomicrons) within the enterocytes; and transport out of the enterocyte across the contraluminal or basolateral membrane into the interstitium (lamina propria). In the interstitium, products of digestion and absorption enter either the capillaries (and hence the portal blood) or the lacteals (and hence the lymph and ultimately the blood). The processes involved in the entrance of nutrients into the body circulation are discussed in this unit, and the subsequent utilization of these absorbed nutrients by body tissues is discussed in Unit IV.

Certain dietary components, especially complex carbohydrates from plant cell walls, are not hydrolyzed by enzymes of the human digestive system and pass into the large intestine undigested. Some of these undigestible residues may be fermented by colonic bacteria to form short-chain fatty acids and gases, whereas others add directly to the mass of the stool or are used by the colonic bacteria for their own growth. The short-chain fatty acids may cross the colonic epithelium by diffusion, enter the portal blood, and be used as a fuel by tissues. The undigestible components of plant cells are called dietary fiber; fiber is not an essential nutrient, but it is considered to have physiologic and health benefits and to be an important component of healthy diets.

Martha H. Stipanuk

Chapter 7

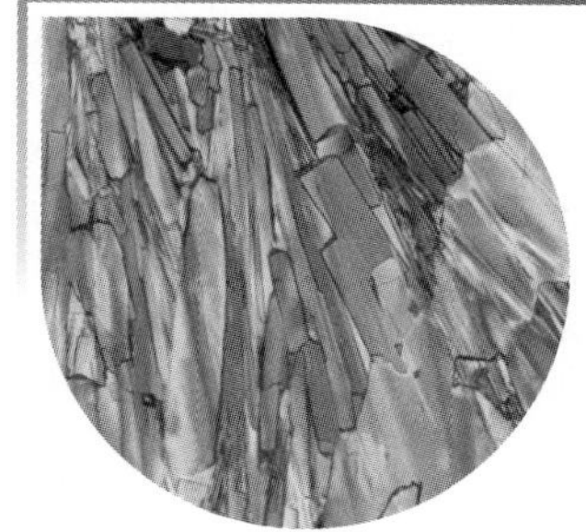

Overview of Digestion and Absorption

Patrick P. Tso, PhD, and Karen Crissinger, MD, PhD

OUTLINE

DIGESTION AND ABSORPTION IN THE GASTROINTESTINAL TRACT

Most foodstuffs are ingested in forms that are unavailable to the body and must be broken down into smaller molecules before they can be absorbed into the body fluids. The gastrointestinal tract is the system that carries out the functions of digestion and absorption. The gastrointestinal tract extends from the mouth to the anus (Fig. 7-1) and consists of a tubular structure with openings for the entry of secretions from the salivary glands, the liver, and the pancreas. The gastrointestinal system includes the mouth, esophagus, stomach, small intestine, and large intestine, as well as accessory organs (salivary glands, pancreas, liver, and gallbladder) that provide essential secretions. The major function of the gastrointestinal tract is to digest complex molecules in foods and to absorb simple nutrients, including monosaccharides, monoacylglycerols, fatty acids, amino acids, vitamins, minerals, and water. It also serves as a barrier to the entry of bacteria into the body and contains specialized cells that secrete mucus, fluids, some digestive enzymes, intrinsic factor, and some peptide hormones.

Digestion is defined as the chemical breakdown of food by enzymes secreted into the lumen of the gastrointestinal tract by glandular cells in the mouth, chief cells in the stomach, and the exocrine cells of the pancreas, and by enzymes in the brush border (luminal) membrane and in the cytoplasm of mucosal cells of the small intestine. As such, digestion occurs

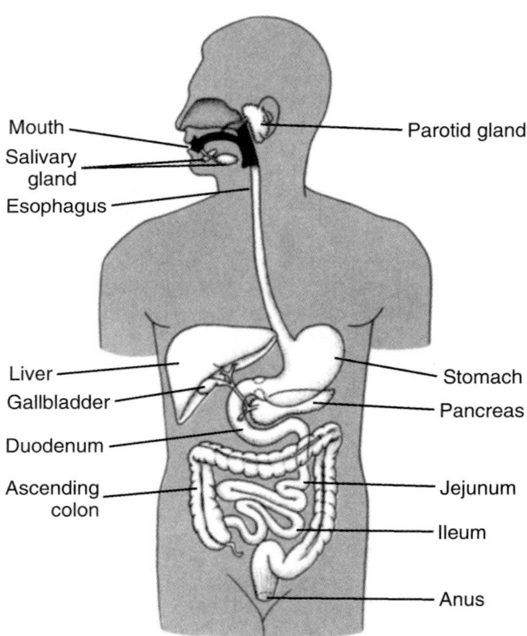

Figure 7-1 Gross anatomy of the gastrointestinal system. *(From Guyton AC, Hall JE [1997] Human Physiology and Mechanisms of Disease, 6th ed. WB Saunders, Philadelphia.)*

prior to the entrance of nutrients into the interstitial fluid and hence into the circulatory system by which nutrients are carried to all cells of the body.

Absorption is the movement of nutrients, including water and electrolytes, across the mucosal cells into the lamina propria (interstitium), where they enter the blood or lymph. Processes involved in absorption include diffusion, facilitated diffusion, active transport, solvent drag, and endocytosis. Most substances pass from the intestinal lumen into the mucosal cells and then out of the mucosal cells to the extracellular compartment, and the processes responsible for movement across the luminal or brush border membrane are often quite different from those responsible for movement across the basolateral or contraluminal cell membranes to the extracellular compartment. Once nutrients have exited from the intestinal absorptive cells into the lamina propria, they either enter the capillaries (into the blood) or lacteals (into the lymph). Water and some other molecules may be taken up by paracellular movement between cells.

THE MOUTH

Chewing involves the cutting as well as grinding of food by the teeth. The process of chewing not only ensures that the bolus of food is crushed into smaller particles but also allows the mixing of saliva with food. As food is mixed with saliva, salivary amylase may begin the digestion of starch, and, more importantly, the bolus of food is lubricated to facilitate swallowing.

Saliva has many functions, including digestion of nutrients, antibacterial activity (due to the presence of thiocyanate, lactoferrin, and lysozyme), moistening of the mouth to facilitate speech and swallowing, and buffering. The salivary glands secrete α-amylase, which is active within the food bolus until it is inactivated by the acidic secretions of the stomach. Secretion of saliva is under neural control. In some species, lingual lipase is secreted by glands in the tongue, and this enzyme is most active in the acidic environment of the gastric lumen. Secretion of lingual lipase is insignificant in humans, but the stomach of humans does secrete a lipase that has similar acid lipase activity (Abrams et al., 1988; Moreau et al., 1988).

Swallowing is a highly coordinated process, and the lower esophageal sphincter relaxes following swallowing to allow the entry of food into the stomach. Otherwise, the lower esophageal sphincter is closed to prevent the reflux of stomach acid into the esophagus. During pregnancy, the lower esophageal sphincter may not be as contracted as usual, and this may allow the reflux of acid into the esophagus to give the feeling of “heartburn.”

THE STOMACH

The major functions of the stomach are to store food and to process the swallowed food in a preliminary fashion for delivery into the small intestine. Upon entry of food into the stomach, the stomach muscles relax. This phenomenon is called adaptive relaxation. While in the stomach, the food undergoes substantial physical and chemical modifications. Although the stomach is not an important absorptive organ, some water and lipid-soluble substances are absorbed by the stomach.

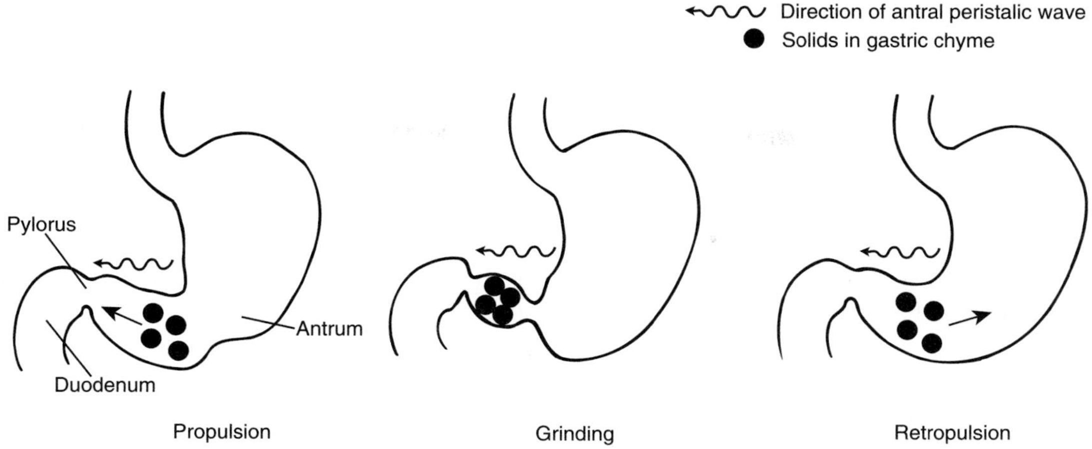

Figure 7-2 A diagram showing the consequences of antral peristalsis. *(Modified from Kelly KA [1981] Motility of the stomach and gastroduodenal junction. In: Johnson LR [ed] Physiology of the Gastrointestinal Tract. Vol. 1. Raven Press, New York, p 400.)*

For instance, ethanol and short-chain fatty acids are absorbed rapidly.

The gastric mucosa of the stomach contains many deep glands made up of chief cells, parietal cells, and mucous cells. The mixed secretions of these cells are known as gastric juice. Gastric juice contains mucin, inorganic salts, hydrochloric acid (HCl), and digestive enzymes or zymogens (gastric lipase and pepsinogens/pepsins). The parietal cells are the source of gastric HCl, with secretion of H^+ being driven by a membrane H^+, K^+-ATPase (proton pump). The gastric acidity that favors the denaturation (unfolding) of proteins is necessary for activation of pepsinogen to pepsin and for the proteolytic activity of pepsin. The gastric acidity destroys many microorganisms that enter the gastrointestinal tract via the oral cavity. The parietal cells also secrete intrinsic factor, a glycoprotein that is required for vitamin B_{12} absorption. The neck mucous cells secrete bicarbonate and mucus. The chief cells of the gastric glands secrete pepsinogens and gastric lipase. Stimulation of gastric secretions depends on neural, endocrine, and paracrine mechanisms. Protein in food is a potent stimulant of gastrin release into the bloodstream by endocrine G cells of the stomach, but vagal stimulation, calcium ions (Ca^{2+}), and alkalinization of the antrum of the stomach also promote gastrin release. Gastrin stimulates gastric HCl and pepsinogen secretion. Gastrin secretion is feedback inhibited by acid within the lumen of the antrum.

Pepsins begin the process of protein digestion in the stomach by hydrolyzing the protein into large peptide fragments and some free amino acids. Gastric lipase hydrolyzes triacylglycerol in the acidic medium to form predominantly diacylglycerol and free fatty acid. These products of fat hydrolysis may play a role in beginning the emulsification of lipids in the stomach contents.

Peristaltic contractions of the distal stomach propel the stomach contents toward the pylorus (located between the stomach and the duodenum) (Fig. 7-2). The pylorus is composed of a thickened band of circular muscle. Although it has been called the pyloric sphincter, it does not function as a true sphincter because there is not a zone of high pressure in the pyloric region. Rather, it contracts in opposition to an approaching peristalsis. As the contractions reach the terminal antrum, the pylorus closes. This results in the grinding of solids to form finer particles. In addition, the acidic chyme (semifluid mass of partially digested food) that cannot pass forward through the opening of the pylorus will be retropelled back into the body of the stomach. The retropulsion of the chyme results not only in the mixing of chyme but also in dispersion of oil droplets into very fine emulsion particles. The dispersion of oil droplets greatly facilitates the subsequent digestion of lipids in the small intestine because pancreatic lipase acts at the water–lipid interface, and emulsification significantly increases this surface area. Only liquids and small particles in chyme are allowed to pass through the pylorus into the small intestine because of the small opening that results from contraction of the pylorus.

Gastric motility and secretion are regulated by both neural and humoral mechanisms. The gastrointestinal hormone that stimulates gastric motility as well as gastric acid secretion is gastrin. The neural stimulation of gastric acid secretion and gastric motility is via the vagus nerve. The stomach regulates the amount of food presented to the duodenum so as not to exceed the absorptive capacity of the small intestine. This occurs largely as a result of the actions of hormones such as gastric inhibitory peptide and cholecystokinin, which are released by the small intestine in response to the entrance of chyme from the stomach and which inhibit gastric motility, gastric emptying, and gastric secretion.

An exciting finding in the last few years is the discovery of a hormone produced by the stomach called ghrelin (Kojima et al., 1999; Meier and Gressner, 2004). Ghrelin is synthesized by the endocrine cells situated in the fundus of the stomach. In humans, ghrelin appears to stimulate food intake by enhancing the hunger sensation. Ghrelin also stimulates gastric emptying. The release of ghrelin is stimulated by fasting and is suppressed by the ingestion of food. Ghrelin is believed to communicate to the brain the state of energy balance in the body.

THE SMALL INTESTINE

Most of the digestion and uptake of nutrients takes place in the small intestine, and the small intestine is uniquely adapted to accommodate these processes. The small intestine is quite long and is often divided into three sections. The first section is the duodenum, which is approximately 1 foot in length and ends at the ligament of Treitz. This section receives the chyme from the stomach, along with secretions from the liver or gallbladder and the pancreas. The remainder of the small intestine (~9 feet) consists of the jejunum (the upper 40% below the duodenum) and the ileum (the lower 60%).

ANATOMY

Figure 7-3 shows the general organization of the intestinal wall. Four distinct strata can be identified: mucosa, submucosa, muscularis propria, and serosa. The mucosa itself is composed of four layers: (1) a surface layer of epithelial cells, (2) a layer of basement membrane, (3) the lamina propria (containing connective tissue, blood vessels, lymphatic vessels, nerves, and various types of cells such as lymphocytes, macrophages, and mast cells), and (4) the muscularis mucosa (containing smooth muscle cells). Next to the mucosa is the submucosa, which is composed of connective tissues, blood vessels, and lymphatic vessels. The third stratum of the small intestine is the muscularis propria, which consists of a layer of circular muscle followed by a layer of neurons (myenteric plexus) and then by a layer of longitudinal muscle. The outermost stratum of the small intestine is called the serosa, composed of a layer of mesothelial cells.

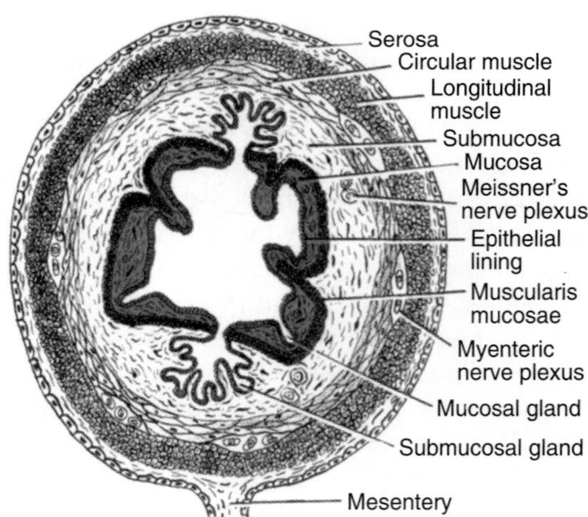

Figure 7-3 General organization of the intestinal wall. *(From Guyton AC, Hall JE [1997] Human Physiology and Mechanisms of Disease, 6th ed. WB Saunders, Philadelphia.)*

This general structural organization is preserved throughout the gastrointestinal tract in the stomach and the large intestine, but the small intestine has some additional adaptations that greatly increase its surface area.

To facilitate the surface digestion and absorption of nutrients, the small intestine is anatomically adapted to enhance greatly the epithelial digestive and absorptive surface, as illustrated in Figure 7-4. The small intestine has a surface area of approximately 200 m^2, owing to folds of the mucosa, the villi or finger-like projections of the mucosa, and the microvillar structure of the luminal or brush border membrane of the absorptive cells that make up the surface layer of the villi. Altogether, these adaptations of mucosal structure increase the surface area of the small intestine to 600 times the surface area of a cylinder of the same diameter. Each villus is supplied by its own blood and lymph vessels.

The epithelial surface of each villus is covered by absorptive cells, called enterocytes, which have a brush border apical membrane. The epithelial surface layer of the mucosa also contains a few goblet or mucus-secreting cells,

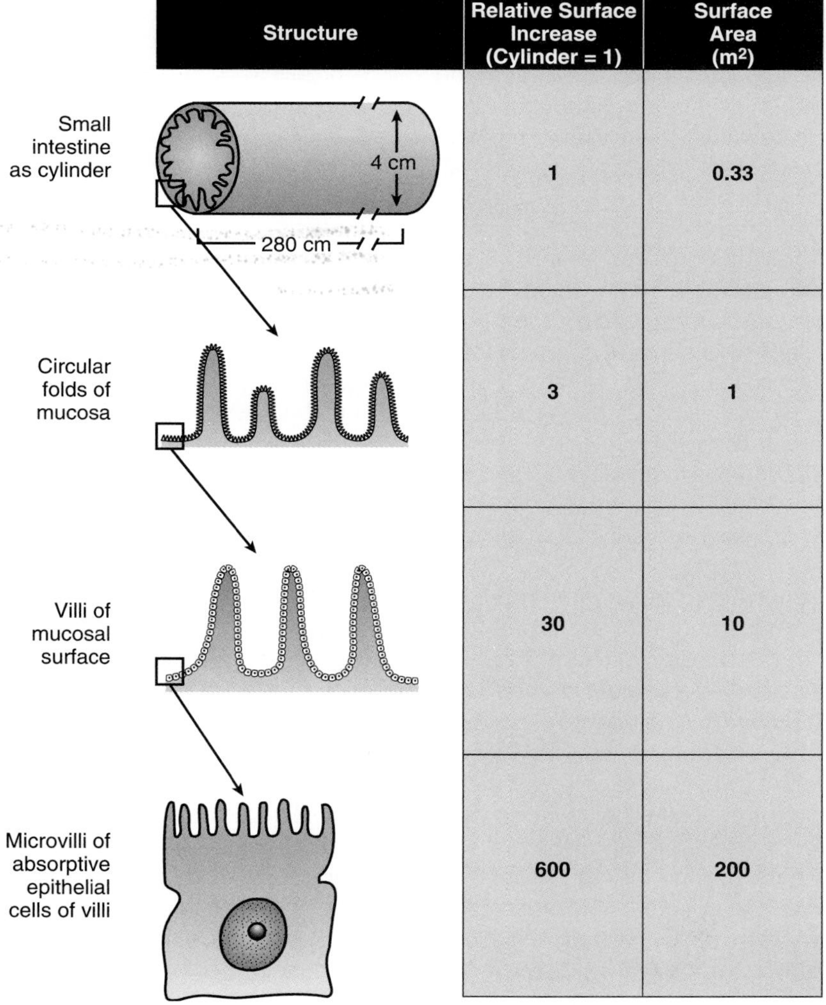

Structure
Relative Surface Increase (Cylinder = 1)
Surface Area (m2)
Small intestine as cylinder
4 cm
280 cm
1
0.33
Circular folds of mucosa
3
1
Villi of mucosal surface
30
10
Microvilli of absorptive epithelial cells of villi
600
200

Figure 7-4 The small intestinal mucosal surface is amplified by specialized features of the mucosa. *(From Waldeck F [1983] Functions of the gastrointestinal canal. In: Schmidt RF, Thews G [eds]* Human Physiology. *Springer-Verlag, New York, p 602.)*

some epithelial M cells that are associated with underlying lymphoid cells, endocrine cells that secrete gastrointestinal hormones, paneth cells at the base of the crypts that secrete antimicrobial substances such as lysozyme, and some intraepithelial lymphocytes; these nonabsorptive cells can be recognized microscopically as not having a brush border apical membrane. The epithelial cells are connected to each other by tight junctions and by desmosomes to form a mechanical seal that prevents mixing of the interstitial fluid with luminal contents.

An important characteristic of the gastrointestinal tract is that it continuously renews the cells lining its surface. Enterocytes lining the intestinal surface have an average lifespan of approximately 72 hours once they enter the villus from the crypt (simple glandular tubes at the base of the villus). Near the base of the crypts are stem cells that give rise to all epithelial cell types with the exception of the intraepithelial lymphocytes. These cells migrate up from the crypts to the tips of the villi, and, soon thereafter, are sloughed off into the intestinal lumen where they may undergo digestion. Cells in the crypts secrete a fluid called succus entericus, which contains water and electrolytes. As the epithelial cells proliferate and migrate up the villus, the activity of mucosal digestive enzymes and the capacity to absorb nutrients increases, whereas the capacity to secrete succus entericus decreases.

A single enterocyte is represented by Figure 7-5. The brush border membrane with its hundreds of microvillar projections can be observed. The brush border membrane contains many embedded glycoproteins that extend from the membrane into the lumen. The carbohydrate side chains of these membrane glycoproteins make up a glycocalyx next to the brush border membrane itself; this glycocalyx acts to "trap water" and to form an "unstirred water layer" near the absorptive surface. Many of these glycoproteins are digestive enzymes, which will be discussed in more detail in Chapters 8 and 9. Because this fluid layer next to the epithelial cell surface is poorly mixed, the major mechanism for solute movement across the unstirred water layer is diffusion down the concentration gradient.

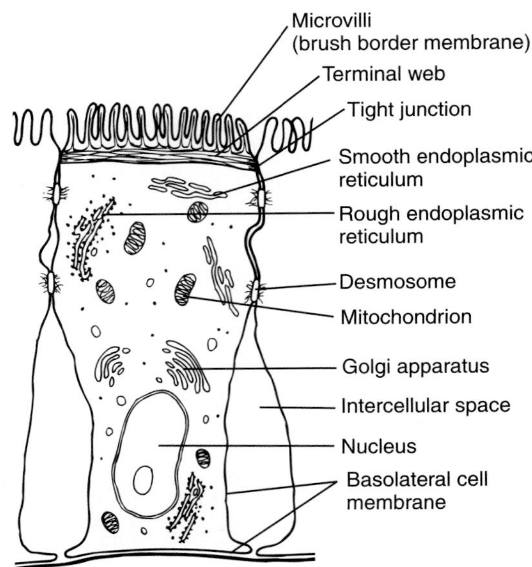

Figure 7-5 Ultrastructure of a small intestinal epithelial cell (enterocyte).

DIGESTION

Digestion in the small intestine is brought about by enzymes secreted by the pancreas, enzymes located on the luminal membranes of the enterocytes lining the small intestine, and enzymes within the enterocytes. As the acidic chyme from the stomach enters the duodenum, the acid stimulates the enteroendocrine S cells (special endocrine cells in the duodenum) to release a gastrointestinal hormone called secretin, which stimulates the pancreatic acinar cells (cells involved in the secretion of water, electrolytes, and enzymes) to secrete a bicarbonate-rich pancreatic secretion that has an alkaline pH of approximately 8. As expected, the highest densities of S cells are found in the duodenum and jejunum and lower densities are found in the ileum.

The presence of partially hydrolyzed fat (fatty acids) and protein (amino acids and peptides) in the chyme that enters the duodenum, as well as the acidic pH of the chyme, stimulates enteroendocrine I cells in the upper small intestine to release the hormone cholecystokinin (also known as pancreozymin), which causes discharge of zymogen granules from the pancreatic acinar cells and the secretion of an enzyme–zymogen-rich pancreatic juice. The pancreatic secretion contains pancreatic α-amylase, lipases (pancreatic lipase and cholesterol esterase), prophospholipase A_2, nucleolytic enzymes (ribonuclease and deoxyribonuclease), several proenzymes for proteolytic enzymes (trypsinogen, chymotrypsinogen, proelastase, and procarboxypeptidases), and a nonenzyme proprotein called procolipase. Pancreatic enzymes are most active in the neutral pH range, and the rapid neutralization of the acid in the chyme by the bicarbonate in the pancreatic juice (stimulated by secretin) in the upper duodenum facilitates digestion of nutrients by pancreatic enzymes.

The liver secretes bile into the bile duct that empties into the duodenum. Between meals, the duodenal opening of this duct is closed and bile flows into the gallbladder, a saccular organ that is attached to the hepatic bile duct and that serves to store and concentrate bile. The hormones released by the upper small intestine stimulate biliary flow. Secretin stimulates bile secretion by the liver, and cholecystokinin stimulates gallbladder contraction and the release of bile from the gallbladder into the intestine. Bile is an alkaline solution containing electrolytes, pigments, bile salts, and other substances. The pancreatic duct joins with the hepatic bile duct to form the common bile duct just prior to entering the duodenum, so the bile mixes with pancreatic secretions before they enter the duodenum. Bile salts play an important role in the normal digestion and absorption of lipids, as is discussed in more detail in Chapter 10.

Although the digestion of most nutrients in the small intestine is extensively carried out by enzymes secreted by the pancreas, enzymes located at the brush border membrane of enterocytes are responsible for the completion of this process to release molecules that can be transported across the brush border membrane. Several α-glucosidases, a β-galactosidase, and several peptidases are present; these enzymes are necessary for further digestion of oligosaccharide and peptide products of luminal hydrolysis, as well as of dietary disaccharides and other compounds. These brush border enzymes are called ectoenzymes because they are located outside the cell (i.e., on the luminal side of the membrane). In general, the hydrophobic domain of the protein is anchored to the lipid bilayer of the brush border membrane, and the bulk of the protein, including the active site domain, is exposed to the external environment.

Di- and tripeptides may be taken up by the intestinal epithelial cells, and they are further hydrolyzed to form free amino acids by intracellular peptidases. The enterocytes contain peptidases that actively catalyze the hydrolysis of these small peptides to free amino acids, as is discussed in Chapter 9. Also present in the intestinal epithelial cells are enzymes that are involved in the assimilation of lipid digestion products to form triacylglycerols, cholesteryl esters, and phospholipids for incorporation into chylomicrons. This subject is discussed in detail in Chapter 10.

SMALL INTESTINAL MOTILITY

Small intestinal motility is uniquely adapted to facilitate both digestion and uptake of nutrients by the small intestine. The rate of digestion is dependent on the exposure of nutrients to the enzymes in the lumen of the small intestine. Consequently, a major function of intestinal motility is to ensure thorough mixing of intestinal contents. Thorough mixing of the intestinal contents also ensures the efficient digestion and uptake of nutrients by the epithelial cells of the small intestine. Mixing is achieved by the presence of slow waves of contractions, followed by relaxation of different segments of the small intestine (called segmentation). Another function of the contractile activity of the small intestine is to ensure the slow migration of chyme away from the duodenum and toward the large intestine while allowing adequate time for the digestion and absorption of intestinal contents. The aboral gradient in the frequency of the slow waves along the small intestine, with approximately 12 cycles per minute in the duodenum and a gradual decrease to

Clinical Correlation

Pancreatic Insufficiency and Malabsorption in Cystic Fibrosis

Cystic fibrosis is a fatal autosomal recessive genetic disorder with an incidence of approximately 1 in 2,500 live white births. It is a systemic disorder that is caused by a dysfunction of the mucus-producing exocrine cells of the pancreas, bronchi, liver, and intestine. Symptoms of malabsorption and chronic pulmonary disease should suggest the diagnosis. However, infants and children with the disorder often present only with pancreatic insufficiency or with chronic pulmonary disease without apparent intestinal symptoms.

Diagnosis of the disease is based on the following tests:

- An abnormal sweat test with greater than 60 mEq/L of chloride
- The presence of chronic pulmonary obstruction
- Pancreatic insufficiency with evidence of steatorrhea, the presence of undigested protein in the stool, and the presence of very low concentrations of pancreatic enzymes in duodenal aspirates

Pancreatic insufficiency can be remedied by pancreatic enzyme replacement therapy.

The gene causing cystic fibrosis was identified in 1989, and the cDNA was cloned (Riordan et al., 1989). The protein product called cystic fibrosis transmembrane conductance regulator (CFTR) has been conclusively demonstrated to be a 3′,5′-cyclic adenosine monophosphate (cAMP)–regulated chloride channel (Breuer et al., 1992).

approximately 9 cycles per minute in the ileum, ensures that the chyme moves slowly, from a region of higher contractile frequency to a region of lower contractile frequency.

ABSORPTION

For nutrients to be absorbed, they must move across the mucosal cells (enterocytes) that comprise a barrier between the lumen of the gastrointestinal tract and the interstitial fluid on the other side of the mucosal cell layer. Transport processes are involved in the uptake of nutrients by the brush border or luminal membrane and also in the release of nutrients across the basolateral membrane into the extracellular fluid.

The uptake of nutrients and electrolytes by the intestinal epithelial cells is usually mediated by one of four general mechanisms. The first mechanism is mediated transport. Many compounds require a specific carrier or membrane transport protein for uptake. These carriers are located in the cell membrane. Mediated transport systems may be uniports (move only one compound), symports (move two compounds together), or antiports (exchangers that move one substance in and a different substance out of the cell).

Mediated transport systems may be passive or active. Passive transport by a carrier is also called facilitated diffusion, because passive transport, like diffusion, occurs down the electrochemical gradient from an area of high concentration to an area of low concentration. It can be bidirectional, allowing for an equalization of the concentration of a substance on both sides of the membrane. Examples of passive mediated transport are the Na^+-independent hexose transporters, which include glucose transporter 5 (GLUT5) that transports fructose across the brush border membrane into the enterocyte and GLUT2 that transports glucose, galactose, and fructose out of the enterocyte across the basolateral membrane.

Active mediated transport involves energy expenditure, and these systems can be unidirectional and concentrative. Energy is supplied via adenosine triphosphate (ATP) hydrolysis, but the energy requirement may be primary or secondary. For example, sodium (Na^+) and potassium (K^+) concentrations in cells are maintained by the Na^+,K^+-ATPase, which pumps Na^+ out of cells and K^+ into cells (against their concentration gradients) at the expense of ATP hydrolysis; this is primary active transport of Na^+ and K^+ by an antiport. The stoichiometry of the Na^+, K^+-ATPase reaction is 1 mole of ATP hydrolysis coupled to the outward pumping of 3 moles of Na^+ and the simultaneous inward pumping of 2 moles of K^+, which generates a low Na^+ concentration in the cytosol and an electrical potential of about −60 mV in the cytosol relative to the extracellular fluid. Conversely, the cotransport of Na^+ and glucose and of H^+ and dipeptides is by secondary active transport processes. In these processes the energy is directly derived from a concentration gradient or an electrical potential across the membrane rather than the chemical energy of a covalent bond change, such as ATP hydrolysis. Gradients may be established by ATP hydrolysis, as seen in the case of the Na^+,K^+-ATPase. For example, the Na^+-glucose co-transporter SGLT1 can concentrate glucose (against its concentration gradient) because of the cotransport of Na^+ down its electrochemical gradient. Therefore, it is the low intracellular Na^+ concentration and the negative electrical potential, which are maintained by the Na^+,K^+-ATPase pump, that provide the "force" for glucose uptake. Uptake of glucose by SGLT1 is an example of secondary active transport by a symport.

Mediated transport allows uptake of nutrients and other compounds to be site-specific, because only the segment of the small intestine that expresses the carrier protein is capable of taking up the substrate. The advantage of expressing the transporters in a specific segment of the small intestine is illustrated by the concentrative reuptake of bile salts by a Na^+–bile acid cotransport system in the brush border membrane of enterocytes in the lower portion of the ileum. By delaying the uptake of bile salts by the small intestine until they reach the lower ileum, the presence of adequate bile salts in the lumen of the small intestine for efficient lipid digestion is ensured.

A second mechanism for the uptake of nutrients and electrolytes by the small intestinal epithelial cells is passive diffusion. This is especially true for water, many lipid-soluble molecules such as short-chain fatty acids, and for gases such as H_2 or CO_2 because they can diffuse through the lipid bilayer of the epithelial cell membranes. These substances diffuse across membranes in both directions, with net movement occurring down the concentration gradient. Uptake of substances by diffusion may also occur in the stomach and large intestine.

A third mechanism for uptake of some large molecules is pinocytosis. Receptor-mediated endocytosis may be responsible for uptake of some proteins as well as of any smaller molecules that are trapped within endocytic vesicles. Similarly, molecules may be transported out of cells by exocytosis. Chylomicrons are exported from the enterocytes by exocytosis across the basolateral membrane.

The fourth mechanism for uptake of nutrients or of water and electrolytes by the small intestine is the paracellular pathway, which involves passage between cells through tight junctions. Osmolality plays an important role in the absorption of water and electrolytes by the small intestine via this process. The osmolality of the plasma is about 300 mOsm. When a hypotonic meal is ingested, water is rapidly absorbed by the duodenum and the jejunum paracellularly (between the cells) through the tight junctions. The tight junctions (pores between intestinal epithelial cells) of the duodenum and the jejunum have a larger diameter (8Å) than those existing in the ileum (4Å). The absorption of water facilitates the absorption of electrolytes by the small intestine via a process called solvent drag in which dissolved solutes are carried along with the water. When a hypertonic meal is ingested, water is drawn into the lumen. The accumulation of water in the lumen and the absorption of ions and nutrients by the small intestine bring the luminal contents to isotonicity. As shown in Figure 7-6, the proximal small intestine plays an important role in the absorption of water from a hypotonic meal, whereas the distal small intestine plays a more important role in the absorption of water and electrolytes following a hypertonic meal.

Pancreatic and biliary secretions enter the upper duodenum via the sphincter of Oddi, and luminal digestion may occur throughout the duodenum and jejunum. Although the entire small intestine is capable of absorbing nutrients, the jejunum is by far the major site for the uptake of nutrients, and the absorption of most nutrients is complete before the chyme reaches the ileum. If nutrients are still present in the chyme that reaches the ileum, the physiological phenomenon called "ileal brake" may occur; this phenomenon refers to the observation that the presence of nutrients in the ileum, especially long-chain fatty acids, is a potent stimulus for slowing the emptying

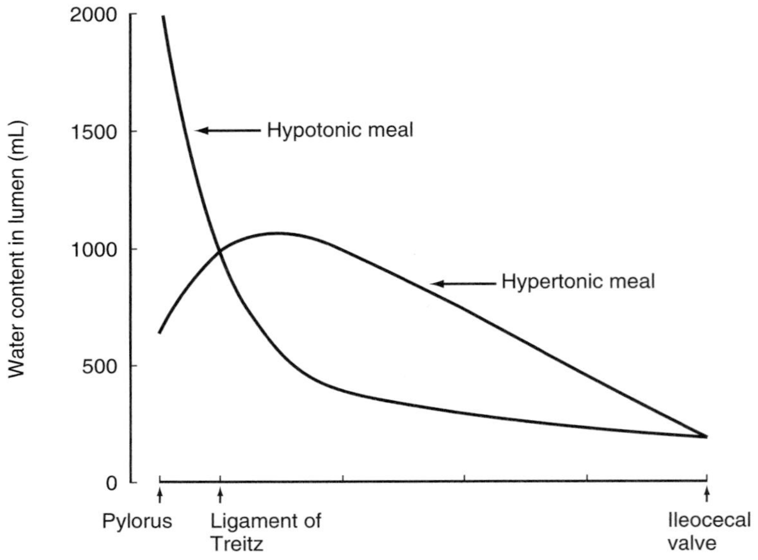

Figure 7-6 Water content in the lumen of the small intestine after a hypotonic (steak) meal and a hypertonic (doughnut and milk) meal. *(Modified from Fordtran JS, Ingelfinger FJ [1968] Absorption of water, electrolytes, and sugars from the human gut. In: Code CF, Heidel W [eds] Alimentary Canal. III: Intestinal Absorption. Williams and Wilkins, Baltimore, pp 1457-1490.)*

of chyme from the stomach as well as for reducing intestinal motility. The gastrointestinal hormone peptide YY has been implicated as a potential candidate for the factor that induces the "ileal brake response."

BILE ACIDS AND THE ENTEROHEPATIC CIRCULATION

The liver plays an important role in the digestion and uptake of lipids by the gastrointestinal tract because of its role in bile acid synthesis and secretion. Primary bile acids, cholic acid and chenodeoxycholic acid, are synthesized from cholesterol in the liver. The liver also conjugates bile acids with either taurine or glycine to form more polar compounds. The ionizable sulfonate group of taurine or the ionizable carboxyl group of glycine has a lower pK_a than the carboxyl group of the unconjugated bile acid, and conjugated bile acids exist as negatively charged sulfonate or carboxylate ions. The ratio of glycine to taurine conjugates in adult human bile is about 3:1. Because bile contains significant amounts of Na^+ and K^+ and has an alkaline pH, the bile acids and their conjugates exist in bile in a salt form and are called bile salts. The terms bile acid and bile salt may be used interchangeably. The bile salts also solubilize some cholesterol in the bile and allow cholesterol to be transported from the liver to the intestine.

Conjugated bile acids exhibit detergent properties; at neutral pH values above their pK_as (i.e., above pH 1.5 to 3.7) and at concentrations above 2 to 5 mmol/L, they reversibly form aggregates called micelles. The ability of bile salts to act as detergents and to form micelles facilitates emulsification of dietary fat to increase the surface area between the lipid and aqueous phase; the digestion of cholesteryl esters, phospholipids, and monoglycerides; and the solubilization and absorption of products of lipid digestion.

Bile salts are recovered by the body via passive diffusion along the entire small intestine and via receptor-mediated transport in the lower ileum. The recirculation of compounds such as bile salts between the small intestine and the liver is called the enterohepatic circulation. The enterohepatic circulation of bile salts is extremely efficient, with only about 1 % of the bile salts being lost via the feces per pass through the intestine. The body pool of bile salts (~4 g) is cycled through the intestine about 12 times per day (depending on the frequency of meal intake); a loss of 1% (0.04 g) per pass results in a loss of about 0.5 g of bile salts per day via the feces. This loss is compensated for by daily synthesis of an equivalent amount of bile salts by the liver. Despite the synthesis of only about 0.5 g of bile salts per day by the liver, as much as 50 g of bile salts enter the small intestinal lumen each day to participate in the digestion and uptake of lipids. The loss of a small percentage of the bile salts in the feces with each pass through the intestinal tract represents the major route for excretion of cholesterol from the body.

A portion of the primary bile acids in the intestine may be metabolized by intestinal bacteria, leading to deconjugation and 7α-dehydroxylation to produce secondary bile acids; deoxycholate is produced from cholate, and lithocholate is produced from chenodeoxycholate. These secondary bile acids, especially deoxycholate, may be reabsorbed and participate in the enterohepatic circulation along with the primary bile acids.

METABOLISM OF NUTRIENTS IN THE ENTEROCYTES

Following the uptake of digestion products into the small intestinal epithelial cells, nutrients are either assimilated into the portal blood or the lymphatic vessels for export to other parts of the body or they are utilized by the cells themselves. Because the small intestinal epithelial cells are metabolically very active and are continuously being renewed, nutrients supplied by the arterial circulation or taken up from the intestinal lumen are necessary for maintenance of the structural and functional integrity of the small intestinal mucosa. The small intestine particularly uses glutamine as a fuel, as is discussed further in Chapters 9 and 14, and glutamine also stimulates the proliferation of enterocytes. Fasting causes atrophy of the small intestinal mucosa, and this atrophy can be reversed by feeding certain amino acids such as glutamine.

Within the enterocytes, most of the products of fat digestion, particularly the monoacylglycerols and long-chain fatty acids, are reesterified to form triacylglcyerols, incorporated into chylomicrons, and exported. Chylomicrons also transport cholesteryl esters, phospholipids, and fat-soluble vitamins when they are exported from the enterocyte via exocytosis.

TRANSPORT OF NUTRIENTS IN THE CIRCULATION

Nutrients that are absorbed from the gastrointestinal tract are subsequently transported either via the portal circulation or the lymphatic system. Most of the water-soluble nutrients (amino acids, monosaccharides, glycerol, short-chain fatty acids, electrolytes, and water-soluble vitamins) are transported predominantly by the portal route. These nutrients enter the capillaries that feed into the portal vein, which carries the venous blood draining from the splanchnic bed to the liver. The liver is unusual in that its major blood supply is the venous portal blood, with the hepatic artery supplying only about one fourth of the liver's blood flow.

The lymphatic system in the gastrointestinal tract plays a pivotal role in the transport of lipophilic (lipid-soluble) substances. Chylomicrons are too large to enter the pores of the capillaries, but they can pass through the large fenestrations of the lacteals and be transported by the lymphatic system. The lymphatic vessels ultimately empty into the venous circulation (by way of the thoracic duct) prior to the point where blood enters the heart. A substance transported by the lymphatic system will thus enter the blood just before it goes to the heart and will then circulate throughout the body in the arterial blood, whereas those substances transported in the portal blood will first pass through the liver, where they may be taken up and metabolized by the hepatocytes or returned to the venous circulation via the hepatic vein.

This distinction between lymphatic versus portal transport is of great importance to the pharmaceutical industry for targeting the delivery of drugs. The lymphatic system also, of course, plays an important role in maintaining the fluid balance in the body by acting as a drainage system to return excess fluid and proteins from tissue space into the circulatory system. Although many of the molecules carried by the portal circulation can also be carried by the lymphatic circulation, the portal blood flow is many times higher than lymphatic flow, so transport by the lymphatic circulation is only of minor significance, compared with the portal circulation, for transport of most water-soluble compounds.

REGULATION OF DIGESTION AND ABSORPTION

The digestion and absorption of nutrients are both neurally and hormonally regulated. The regulation of digestive and absorptive processes involves a number of levels. In terms of the digestive process, regulation involves the modification of the rate of delivery of chyme to the small intestine for digestion, the release of gastric secretions, the release and composition of pancreatic secretions, and the release of biliary secretions. The regulation of the absorptive process involves the absorptive surface area as well as the expression of certain transporter molecules located in the brush border membrane.

NEURAL CONTROL

The gastrointestinal tract is innervated both by an intrinsic as well as an extrinsic nervous system. The intrinsic nervous system is responsible for much of the neural regulation of gastrointestinal motility and function, but it is influenced by the extrinsic nervous system, mainly the parasympathetic nervous system and to a lesser degree the sympathetic nervous system. The entire gastrointestinal tract is innervated by the vagal (parasympathetic) afferent nerve fibers (afferent refers to the fact that they are carrying information away from the gastrointestinal tract to the central nervous system). The vagal afferent system plays an important role in the regulation of gastrointestinal functions. The gastrointestinal tract is also innervated by vagal efferents (efferent refers to the fact that they are carrying information from the central nervous system to the gastrointestinal tract).

A good example of the neural control of gastrointestinal function is the regulation of salivary secretion. Salivary secretion by the salivary glands is almost exclusively controlled by neural signals. This is quite different from gastric and pancreatic secretions, which are under both neural and hormonal control. The parasympathetic nervous system is the most important physiological regulator of salivary secretion. Smell, sight, taste, and tactile stimuli excite the salivary nuclei in the central nervous system, which, in turn, increase the parasympathetic activity innervating the salivary glands. As a result of parasympathetic activation, salivary secretion can increase by as much as six- to eightfold. Although the salivary glands are also innervated by the sympathetic nervous system, the sympathetic system seems to play a minor role in the regulation of salivary secretion.

A neural mechanism is involved in the increase in gastric emptying induced by gastric distention of the stomach and in the inhibition of gastric emptying induced by the presence of a hypertonic meal in the duodenum. Neural mechanisms are also involved in the regulation of pancreatic exocrine secretion. For instance, gastric distention stimulates acetylcholine release by vagal impulses, and this, in turn, stimulates the secretion of pancreatic juice that is rich in enzymes. Vagal impulses are also involved in the release of acetylcholine in response to the presence of fat and protein digestion products in the small intestinal lumen; this, likewise, stimulates the release of an enzyme-rich pancreatic secretion.

GASTROINTESTINAL HORMONES

Gastrointestinal hormones are intimately involved in the coordinated release of secretions into the duodenum, in maintenance of the integrity and cellular homeostasis of the gastrointestinal tract, and in regulation of the motility of the gastrointestinal tract. Gut regulatory peptides are involved in a wide range of processes, and in many cases their functions overlap.

Gastrin

Gastrin is a hormone produced by the antrum of the stomach. Its major role in the gastrointestinal tract is the stimulation of gastric acid and pepsinogen secretion and gastric motility.

Gastrin also plays an important role in the proliferation of gastric mucosal cells, in particular the acid-secreting mucosa of the stomach. Gastrin is released by the gastrin (G) cells in the antrum in the presence of protein in the gastric lumen. Gastric release by the G cells is inhibited by acidification of the gastric lumen below pH 3. This feedback mechanism regulates the amount of gastrin released (and, therefore, the amount of acid secreted) in response to a meal. The circulating level of gastrin in neonates is considerably elevated compared with that of adults, and this higher level is sustained for days after birth (Christie, 1981; Euler et al., 1978). This may be due to an elevated luminal pH, because gastric acid production does not approach adult levels until an infant is about 3 months of age (Christie, 1981; Grand et al., 1976). Another possible explanation for higher levels of gastrin in neonates is that the high protein and calcium content of a milk diet stimulates gastrin release (Lichtenberger, 1984). Gastrin may contribute to both the maturation of gastrointestinal function and the acceleration of mucosal growth during the newborn period (Lucas et al., 1981).

Secretin

Secretin was the first gastrointestinal hormone discovered. Secretin is secreted by the S cells of the duodenum. Secretion by these S cells is markedly stimulated by the acidification of the duodenal lumen. The major function of secretin in the gastrointestinal tract is the stimulation of pancreatic bicarbonate secretion, which neutralizes acidic chyme and promotes intestinal digestion by pancreatic enzymes. Secretin may inhibit gastric emptying. Plasma secretin levels are higher in neonates than in adults (Lucas et al., 1980). Because secretin is considered to be a major factor in triggering the release of bicarbonate-rich secretion from the pancreas, the higher levels of circulating secretin in the neonate may be of importance in mucosal protection during the newborn period. It is notable that the postnatal surge of secretin, unlike that of the other alimentary hormones, occurs even in the absence of feeding (Lucas et al., 1982).

Cholecystokinin

Cholecystokinin is a gastrointestinal hormone secreted by the enteroendocrine cells of the duodenum and the jejunum, as well as by the neurons in the brain and the gastrointestinal tract. Cholecystokinin is responsible for postprandial pancreatic enzyme secretion and gallbladder contraction (O'Rourke et al., 1990; Liddle et al., 1985). Cholecystokinin is released in response to the presence of fat or protein in the small intestine (Liddle et al., 1985). In addition to its secretory effects, cholecystokinin can stimulate hyperplasia and hypertrophy of the pancreas (Peterson et al., 1978).

Somatostatin

Somatostatin has been found in neurons throughout the brain and spinal cord and in the D cells of the gastrointestinal tract. Somatostatin possesses powerful inhibitory effects on endogenous hormone release (growth hormone, thyroid-stimulating hormone, gastrin, glucagon, gastric inhibitory polypeptide, insulin, motilin, neurotensin, pancreatic polypeptide, secretin, calcitonin, and renin) and on gastrointestinal secretion (gastric acid, pepsin, pancreatic exocrine secretions, and small intestinal secretions). It is interesting that in the human fetus and neonate, somatostatin is the second most abundant hormone after insulin in the pancreas, but a reversal occurs postnatally so that somatostatin takes fourth place in abundance in the adult pancreas, after insulin, pancreatic polypeptide, and glucagon.

Other Peptides

In addition to those just discussed, other peptides of possible gastrointestinal significance include epidermal growth factor, transforming growth factor, insulin-like growth factor, hepatocyte growth factor, pancreatic glucagon, enteroglucagon, pancreatic polypeptide, gastric inhibitory polypeptide, motilin, vasoactive intestinal polypeptide, bombesin, neurotensin, substance P, glucagon-like polypeptide-1, peptide YY, and ghrelin. Detailed discussion of the numerous effects of these peptides is beyond the scope of this chapter.

DEVELOPMENTAL ASPECTS OF GASTROINTESTINAL PHYSIOLOGY

The development of peptic activity in the stomach is complete at birth, with term infants having pepsin levels (units per milligram of protein) similar to those of older children and adults (DiPalma et al., 1991). Premature infants weighing 1,000 g have approximately half the peptic activity of term infants (Adamson et al., 1988). Gastric lipase activity is low in premature infants younger than 26 weeks of gestation, but this activity increases from 26 to 35 weeks of gestation (Lee et al., 1993; Hamosh et al., 1981) and is similar to adult levels at birth (DiPalma et al., 1991).

Pancreatic secretory function is immature in the neonate. Although trypsin, lipase, and amylase are found in the duodenum of premature infants at 32 weeks of gestation, the concentrations of these enzymes are lower in premature infants than in term infants (Zoppi et al., 1972). During the neonatal period, the duodenal levels of pancreatic enzymes do not develop in parallel with each other. In a study of duodenal fluid of newborns, as compared with that of older children, trypsin activity was similar to that in older children, chymotrypsin activity was about 50% to 60% of the level found in older children, carboxypeptidase activity was low, lipase activity was negligible, and amylase activity was not detected (Lebenthal and Lee, 1980).

Fat malabsorption does not pose a major problem in premature and term infants despite the immature pancreatic secretion, presumably because of the action of gastric lipases as well as lipases present in milk (DeNigris et al., 1988; Hamosh and Burns, 1977; Moreau et al., 1988). In contrast to digestion of fat, however, the digestion of complex carbohydrates and starches varies (De Vizia et al., 1975). In term infants, blood glucose levels fail to rise in response to starch ingestion, and the duodenal hydrolysis of amylopectin is low (Auricchio et al., 1967). Nevertheless, formulas containing glucose polymers and corn syrup solids are generally well tolerated and support growth in infants. Salivary amylase is present early in gestation and presumably contributes to the digestion of glucose polymers (Cicco et al., 1981). Moreover, negligible amounts of carbohydrate are found in the stools of infants, presumably as a result of bacterial fermentation in the colon (Shulman et al., 1983).

Most of the luminal protein hydrolysis occurs in the duodenum and jejunum and is dependent on the presence of enteropeptidase (an intestinal enzyme) as well as pancreatic proteases. Enteropeptidase initiates the process of protein digestion by the activation of trypsinogen (see Chapter 9). Activity levels of enteropeptidase at birth are 25% of those at 1 year, and 10% of adult levels, and increase thereafter until adult levels are reached by approximately 4 years of age. The relative deficiency of enteropeptidase activity, however, is not rate-limiting for protein digestion in infants.

The activity of lactase, a brush border β-galactosidase, increases at 14 weeks of gestation but then remains at 30% of the newborn level until birth (Raul et al., 1986; Antonowicz and Lebenthal, 1977). Peak lactase activity is found during early postnatal life. Within the first few years of life, lactase activity decreases to the adult level (one tenth that at birth in most adults; see Chapter 8). In contrast, sucrase-isomaltase activity rises steadily, but at variable rates; 70% of the adult level is achieved at 34 weeks of gestation, and adult levels are achieved at birth (Raul et al., 1986). Glucoamylase (maltase) and trehalase activities have been detected at 13 weeks of gestation. Most of the activities of the brush border peptidases (peptidyl dipeptidase, aminopeptidase, dipeptidylpeptidase IV, and γ-glutamyl hydrolase) are present at 8 weeks of gestation.

Bile acid metabolism is immature in premature and term infants relative to that in adults. The rate of bile acid synthesis increases throughout gestation and with increasing postnatal age (Heubi et al., 1982; Watkins et al., 1975). The bile acid pool size in premature and term infants is approximately 3% to 4% and 10%, respectively, that of adults (Watkins et al., 1975). The pool size increases, however, with increasing postnatal age. The concentration of bile acids in the duodenum of premature infants is also less than that found in term infants and adults, and a critical micellar concentration of bile acids, sufficient to maintain adequate dispersion of the products of fat digestion, may not be achieved in premature infants (Watkins et al., 1975).

The enterohepatic pathway of bile acid absorption is also immature in the human infant. Taurine-conjugated bile acids are passively absorbed by the fetal gut (Lester et al., 1977); active ileal transport begins after birth (de Belle et al., 1979). It is likely that the immaturity of bile acid synthesis, secretion, metabolism, and enterohepatic circulation all contribute to the presence of steatorrhea in premature infants.

THE LARGE INTESTINE AND THE ROLE OF COLONIC BACTERIA

The residues from digestion and absorption in the small intestine pass through the ileocecal valve into the large intestine. The colon or large intestine is larger in diameter than the small intestine. The epithelium of the colon has folds, but no villi, and is lined mainly by goblet cells, which secrete mucus, and fewer absorptive cells, which are mainly specialized for uptake of water. The large intestine serves two general functions: The ascending colon is the location where most fermentation occurs, and the descending colon provides for water and electrolyte absorption and stool formation. It takes about 4 hours for the first part of a test meal to reach the upper large intestine, and all the undigested portion from a meal enters the large intestine within about 8 hours of eating. In contrast, transport through the large intestine is much slower, and it may take more than a week to recover all residues from a given meal in the feces.

Carbohydrates that are not absorbed in the small intestine, as well as the carbohydrate components of mucus, are transformed into acetic, propionic, and butyric acids by bacteria within the lumen of the colon. The short-chain fatty acids produced by carbohydrate fermentation account for more than 50% of the total anion content of human feces. Luminal bicarbonate neutralizes a significant fraction of the acid load generated by production of these volatile short-chain fatty acids, resulting in the formation of carbon dioxide and water. The human large intestine absorbs significant quantities of short-chain fatty acids, primarily by diffusion. Once absorbed, the fatty acids either are metabolized to ketone bodies by the colonic epithelium or are transported via the portal vein to other tissues where they can be used as an energy source. Although the nutritional importance of short-chain fatty acid absorption remains uncertain for humans, it is well recognized that some ruminants obtain 70% of their energy requirements from short-chain fatty acids produced and absorbed in the forestomach.

A variety of bacteria in the colon produce hydrogen gas, methane, and carbon dioxide through metabolism (fermentation) of unabsorbed polysaccharides and other food residues. Other bacteria consume gases produced by the bacterial gas producers. The degree of flatus passed is determined by the balance of bacterial gas production versus gas consumption.

Colonic microbes also have enzymes that can metabolize long-chain fatty acids. Up to 25% of total fecal fatty acids are hydroxylated by bacteria in the colon. Hydroxylated fatty acids such as hydroxystearic acid (a product of microbial hydration of oleic acid) can exert a profound influence on colonic electrolyte and water transport. At high luminal concentrations, these substances inhibit net absorption of water and electrolytes by the colon and induce net secretion (and diarrhea). Almost all the cholesterol entering the colon is excreted in feces. A small proportion of the cholesterol is metabolized by colonic bacteria to coprostanol and coprostanone, both of which are poorly soluble and unavailable for absorption.

The small fraction of bile acids that is not reabsorbed in the ileum enters the colon, where bile acids are extensively metabolized by the microflora. The number of bile acid metabolites produced by colonic bacteria is enormous. These degradation products are more lipid-soluble than the substrates, facilitating their passive absorption in the colon. It is estimated that the equivalent of 50 mg/day of bile acids are passively absorbed in the human colon, primarily as microbial degradation products. Both fat and fiber can sequester bile acids and their metabolites in the lumen of the colon and thereby interfere with their absorption.

Approximately 25% of the urea synthesized in the liver reaches the gastrointestinal tract by diffusion from the blood. Bacterial urease in the colon converts it to ammonia, and the ammonia diffuses readily across the colonic mucosa and enters the portal venous blood and returns to the liver, where it is used for resynthesis of urea. The absorption of ammonia from the colon is believed to contribute to the raised blood ammonia levels of patients with liver disease in whom portal-systemic shunting (the flow of blood from the gastrointestinal tract to the circulation with bypass of the liver) may occur.

REFERENCES

Abrams CK, Hamosh M, Lee TC, Ansher AF, Collen MJ, Lewis JH, Benjamin SB, Hamosh P (1988) Gastric lipase: localization in the human stomach. Gastroenterology 95:1460-1464.

Adamson I, Esangbedo A, Okolo AA, Omene JA (1988) Pepsin and its multiple forms in early life. Biol Neonate 53:267-273.

Antonowicz I, Lebenthal E (1977) Developmental pattern of small intestinal enterokinase and disaccharidase activities in the human fetus. Gastroenterology 72:1299-1303.

Auricchio S, Della-Pietra D, Vegnente A (1967) Studies on intestinal digestion of starch in man: II. Intestinal hydrolysis of amylopectin in infants and children. Pediatrics 39:853-862.

Breuer W, Kartner N, Riordan JR, Cabantchik ZI (1992) Induction of expression of the cystic fibrosis transmembrane conductance regulator. J Biol Chem 267:10465-10469.

Christie DL (1981) Development of gastric function during the first month of life. In: Lebenthal E (ed) Textbook of Gastroenterology and Nutrition in Infancy. New York, Raven Press, pp. 109-120.

Cicco R, Holzman IR, Brown DR, Becker DJ (1981) Glucose polymer tolerance in premature infants. Pediatrics 67:498-501.

de Belle RC, Vaupshas V, Vitullo BB, Haber LR, Shaffer E, Mackie GG, Owen H, Little JM, Lester R (1979) Intestinal absorption of bile salts: immature development in the neonate. J Pediatr 94:472-476.

DeNigris SJ, Hamosh M, Kasbekar DK, Lee TC, Hamosh P (1988) Lingual and gastric lipases: species differences in origin of prepancreatic digestive lipases and in the localization of gastric lipases. Biochim Biophys Acta 959:38-45.

De Vizia B, Ciccimarra F, De Cicco N, Auricchio S (1975) Digestibility of starches in infants and children. J Pediatr 86:50-55.

DiPalma JA, Kirk CL, Hamosh M, Colon AR, Benjamin SB, Hamosh P (1991) Lipase and pepsin activity in gastric mucosa in infants, children, and adults. Gastroenterology 101:116-121.

Euler AR, Ament ME, Walsh JH (1978) Human newborn hypergastrinemia: an investigation of prenatal and perinatal factors and their effects on gastrin. Pediatr Res 12:652-654.

Grand RJ, Watkins JB, Torti FM (1976) Development of the human gastrointestinal tract. Gastroenterology 70:790-810.

Hamosh M, Burns WA (1977) Lipolytic activity of human lingual glands. Lab Invest 37:603-608.

Hamosh M, Scanlon JW, Ganot D, Likel M, Scanlon KB, Hamosh P (1981) Fat digestion in the newborn: characterization of lipase in gastric aspirates of premature and term infants. J Clin Invest 67:838-846.

Heubi JE, Balistreri WF, Suchy FJ (1982) Bile salt metabolism in the first year of life. J Lab Clin Med 100:127-136.

Kojima M, Hosoda H, Date Y, Nakazato M, Matsuo H, Kangawa K (1999) Ghrelin is a growth-hormone-releasing acylated peptide from stomach. Nature 402: 656-660.

Lebenthal E, Lee PC (1980) Development of functional responses in human exocrine pancreas. Pediatrics 66:556-560.

Lee P-C, Borysewicz R, Struve M, Raab K, Werlin SL (1993) Development of lipolytic activity in gastric aspirates from premature infants. J Pediatr Gastroenterol Nutr 17:291-297.

Lester R, Smallwood RA, Little JM, Brown AS, Piasecki GJ, Jackson BT (1977) Fetal bile salt metabolism: The intestinal absorption of bile salt. J Clin Invest 59:1009-1016.

Lichtenberger L (1984) A search for the origin of neonatal hypergastrinemia. J Pediatr Gastroenterol Nutr 3:161-166.

Liddle R, Goldfine I, Rosen M, Taplitz RA, Williams JA (1985) Cholecystokinin bioactivity in human plasma: molecular forms, responses to feeding, and relationship to gallbladder contraction. J Clin Invest 75:1144-1152.

Lucas A, Adrian TE, Bloom SR, Aynsley-Green A (1980) Plasma secretin in neonates. Acta Pediatr Scand 69:205-210.

Lucas A, Aynsley-Green A, Bloom SR (1981) Gut hormones and the first meals. Clin Sci 60:349-353.

Lucas A, Bloom SR, Aynsley-Green A (1982) Postnatal surges in plasma gut hormones in term and preterm infants. Biol Neonate 41:63-67.

Meier U, Gressner AM (2004) Endocrine regulation of energy metabolism: review of pathobiochemical and clinical chemical aspects of leptin, ghrelin, adiponectin, and resistin. Clin Chem 50:1511-1525.

Moreau H, Laugier R, Gargouri Y, Ferrato F, Verger R (1988) Human preduodenal lipase is entirely of gastric fundic origin. Gastroenterology 95:1221-1226.

O'Rourke MF, Reidelberger RD, Solomon TE (1990) Effect of CCK antagonist L 364718 on meal-induced pancreatic secretion in rats. Am J Physiol 258:G179-G184.

Peterson H, Solomon T, Grossman M (1978) Effect of chronic pentagastrin, cholecystokinin, and secretin on pancreas of rats. Am J Physiol 234:E286-E293.

Raul F, Lacroix B, Aprahamian M (1986) Longitudinal distribution of brush border hydrolases and morphological maturation in the intestine of the preterm infant. Early Hum Dev 13:225-234.

Riordan JR, Rommens JM, Keren B, Alon N, Rozmahel R, Grzelczak Z, Zielenski J, Lok S, Plavsic N, Chou JL, Drumm ML, Iannuzzi MC, Collins FS, Tsui L-C (1989) Identification of the cystic fibrosis gene: Cloning and characterization of complementary DNA. Science 245:1066-1073.

Shulman RJ, Wong WW, Irving CS, Nichols BL, Klein PD (1983) Utilization of dietary cereal by young infants. J Pediatr 103:23-28.

Watkins JB, Szczepanik P, Gould JB, Klein P, Lester R (1975) Bile salt metabolism in the human premature infant. Gastroenterology 69:706-713.

Zoppi G, Andreotti G, Pajno-Ferrara F, Njai DM, Gaburro D (1972) Exocrine pancreas function in premature and full-term infants. Pediatr Res 6:880-886.

RECOMMENDED READINGS

Davenport HW (1978) A Digest of Digestion, 2nd ed. Year Book Medical Publishers, Inc., Chicago.

Hobsley M (1982) Disorders of the Digestive System. University Park Press, Baltimore.

Johnson LR, Alpers DH, Christensen J, Jacobson ED, Walsh JH (eds) (1994) Physiology of the Gastrointestinal Tract, 3rd ed. Vols. 1 and 2. Raven Press, New York.

Yamada Y, Alpers DH, Laine L, Owyang C, Powell DW (eds) (2003) Textbook of Gastroenterology, 4th ed. Lippincott Williams & Williams, Philadelphia.

Chapter 8

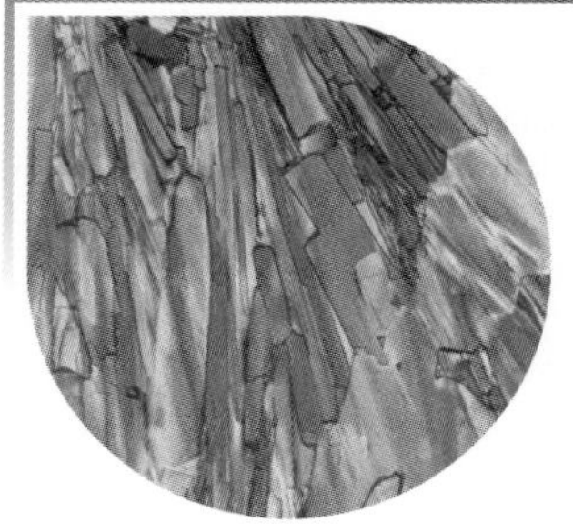

Carbohydrate Digestion and Absorption

Roberto Quezada-Calvillo, MD, Claudia C. Robayo, MD, and Buford L. Nichols, MD

OUTLINE

COMMON ABBREVIATIONS

GLUT glucose transporter
SGLT sodium–glucose transporter
K_m Michaelis constant
k_{cat} first-order rate constant corresponding to the slowest step or steps in the overall catalytic reaction

A variety of simple and complex carbohydrates are present in human diets. Food carbohydrates include the sugars, starches, and fibers found mainly in fruits, vegetables, grains, and milk products. Small amounts of digestible carbohydrates come from non-plant sources (e.g., trehalose in insects and glycogen in muscle tissues). The digestible carbohydrates give rise to monosaccharide units that are absorbed by sugar transport systems.

This chapter is a revision of the chapter contributed by Gary Gray, MD, for the first edition.

The processes involved in the digestion and absorption of the digestible carbohydrates are the focus of this chapter. The fate of the nondigestible carbohydrates, or dietary fiber, is discussed in detail in Chapter 11. Dietary fiber is made up mainly of complex nondigestible carbohydrates and resistant starches from plant foods. Although dietary fiber is not a source of glucose or other monosaccharides for the body, short-chain fatty acids produced from dietary fiber in the large intestine do supply some energy to the body.

CARBOHYDRATE COMPONENTS OF THE HUMAN DIET

Carbohydrates are the major macronutrient in most human diets. Carbohydrates are considered to include monosaccharides (glucose, fructose, and galactose), disaccharides (sucrose, lactose, maltose, and trehalose), oligosaccharides (often breakdown products of polysaccharides as found in corn syrup), polysaccharides (starches), and sugar alcohols (sorbitol and mannitol). In the United States, the median intake of total carbohydrate by adults is approximately 250 g (1,000 kcal) per day (~50% of total calories). Most of this is derived from the starch present in grains and certain vegetables (e.g., corn, tapioca, flour, cereals, popcorn, pasta, rice, and potatoes). Approximately 50 g per day of the total carbohydrate intake in the United States is from added sugars (mono- and disaccharides), with added sugars being defined as sugars and syrups (including honey and maple syrup) that are added to foods during processing or preparation. Added sugars, therefore, include those added to soft drinks, cakes, cookies, fruit-flavored drinks, ice cream, and candy, but do not include naturally occurring sugars such as lactose in milk or fructose in fruits. Lactose is the major carbohydrate in the diets of breast-fed infants (~50 g per day), but consumption of lactose declines during later childhood and adolescence as milk makes up a smaller portion of the diet.

In addition to the readily assimilated carbohydrates, nondigestible carbohydrates are present in foods. Most of these are nonstarch polysaccharides and are classified as dietary fiber; the median intake of dietary fiber by adults living in the United States is approximately 15 g/day. Nondigestible oligosaccharides, such as raffinose and stachyose, are found in small amounts in legumes. Differences in the proportions of fiber and digestible carbohydrates in foods are responsible for the differences in nutritional and energetic values of carbohydrates from various sources.

DIGESTION OF CARBOHYDRATES

Digestible carbohydrates include polymers and oligomers of glucose and dimers of glucose, galactose, or fructose that are digested efficiently as they travel down the small intestine. Digestion involves the enzymatic cleavage of the oxygen bridge, called a glycosidic bond, which links the hexose units. The released free hexoses, but not the larger sugars or oligosaccharides, are transported across the intestine into the circulation. The processes of enzymatic digestion occur mainly within the lumen of the initial segment of the small intestine (the duodenum) under the influence of secreted pancreatic amylase, and by hydrolysis on the intestinal surface membrane by the abundant constituent oligosaccharidases of the columnar epithelial enterocytes lining the small intestine. The fates of the major dietary carbohydrates within the small intestine are summarized in Table 8-1.

DIGESTION OF STARCHES

Starch digestion begins by the action of secreted α-amylase in the lumen of the gastrointestinal tract and is completed by the action of α-glucosidases that are associated with the brush-border membrane of the intestinal mucosal cells.

Luminal Digestion of Starches by α-Amylase

The first enzyme ever discovered, which was first named diastase and later amylase, caused the solubilization of starch granules in saliva. Pancreatic amylase digestion of starch was thereafter recognized. There was initial confusion about the products of amylase digestion but advances in protein purification and carbohydrate chemistry have revealed

Nutrition Insight

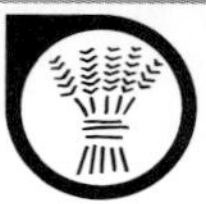

Effects of Dietary Carbohydrate on Blood Glucose: Glycemic Index and Glycemic Load

The observation that many starchy foods raise blood glucose as much as or more than comparable amounts of table sugar led David Jenkins and colleagues to propose the concept of glycemic index (GI) (Jenkins et al., 1981). GI is typically defined as the effect of ingestion of an amount of an individual food that contains a standard amount of carbohydrate (e.g., usually 50 g) on blood glucose compared with that of the same amount of glucose (or sometimes, of carbohydrate from a control food). Desserts, candies, bread, breakfast cereals, rice, and potato products have a high GI, whereas nonstarchy vegetables, fruits, legumes, and nuts generally have a low GI, reflecting the rate of their hydrolysis into glucose in the human digestive tract. Recognizing that the rise in blood glucose is influenced by the amount of carbohydrate consumed and not just by the GI of the carbohydrate within the food, Walter Willett and colleagues defined the glycemic load (GL) in 1997 as the mathematical product of GI and carbohydrate amount (Salmeron et al., 1997).

To explore the usefulness of the GL concept, Brand-Miller and colleagues conducted two feeding studies involving healthy young adults (Brand-Miller et al., 2003). Subjects were given 10 different foods, each calculated to have a GL equal to a serving of white bread, but among which GI and carbohydrate amounts varied threefold. For illustration, a few of the food portions were 34 g of white bread, 247 g of apple, 68 g of reduced-fat ice cream, and 138 g of lentils. The measured area under the glucose-over-time curve was not different from that for white bread for all but one (lentils) of the foods tested. To determine the effects of increasing GL, another group of subjects was given food portions to provide GL doses equivalent to 1, 2, 3, 4, or 6 slices of bread. The incremental increases in GL produced stepwise increases in both glycemia and insulinemia, supporting the concept of GL as a measure of overall glycemic response and insulin demand. The usefulness of the GL concept has also been supported by studies in which mixed meals were fed (Wolever and Bolognesi, 1996) and studies in which subjects were assigned to diets with different GLs due either to changes in carbohydrate amount or of the GI of foods in the diet (Wolever and Mehling, 2003). Current evidence suggests a link of the dietary GL to risk of type 2 diabetes, coronary heart disease, and obesity in the population and to blood glucose control in patients with diabetes.

Table 8-1
Digestion of Dietary Carbohydrate

Food Source	% of Dietary Carbohydrate	Products of Luminal Hydrolysis	Products of Brush-Border Membrane Hydrolysis
Starches (amylose, amylopectin)	60 to 70	Maltose, maltotriose, and α-dextrins	Glucose
Lactose	0 to 10	None	Glucose and galactose
Sucrose	30	None	Glucose and fructose

that salivary and pancreatic amylases are α(1→4) endoglucosidases that produce glucose oligomers from starch. Production and secretion of amylase is restricted to the salivary and pancreatic exocrine glands. The α-amylases are secreted as soluble proteins into the mouth or small intestine via the salivary and pancreatic ducts, respectively. The high concentration of amylase achieved within the duodenal lumen greatly exceeds that required for cleavage of the bonds joining the glucose components of the starches.

The presence of ingested carbohydrate in the intestinal lumen and the direct action of the hormone cholecystokinin on the exocrine pancreas augment the synthesis and release of amylase (Sans et al., 2004). The amylase is processed by concentration with other exocrine secretions as acidic zymogen granules, which are transported toward the apical membrane of the acinar cells by annexin IV binding on actin filaments (Tsujii-Hayashi et al., 2002; Wasle and Edwardson 2002). Amylase is discharged from the zymogen granules in response to neural or hormonal signals acting at the basal surface of acinar cells (Kalus et al., 2002; Schmidt et al., 2001). Cholecystokinin activates several mitogen activated kinase pathways, and granule discharge is mediated by a localized apical surge of ionized calcium (Wasle and Edwardson 2002; Williams et al., 2002; Williams, 2001).

Refined starches are hydrolyzed efficiently to glucose oligomers, even in patients with exocrine pancreatic insufficiency with α-amylase levels that are only about 10% of normal (Fogel and Gray, 1973). However, various inhibitory factors retard the digestion of starch in grains and legumes. Food starches are naturally present in grains and legumes in association with proteins, many of which are hydrophobic and hence hinder the luminal interaction of the secreted polar α-amylases with the polysaccharide within the interior of the starch granules. Physical processing of grains such as cracking, milling, or heating at 100° C for several minutes, changes the physical relationship of starch to the accompanying protein, making it more available to the water-soluble α-amylase. In addition, the presence of nondigestible polysaccharides (cellulose, hemicellulose, and pectin) may interfere with the efficiency of the amylase–starch interaction by blocking the physical association of amylase with its substrate. Therefore, depending upon the physical availability of starch in the prepared food, a small proportion (1% to 10%) of the ingested starch may escape α-amylase action, and this residual starch passes into the colon where is is fermented by colonic bacteria.

Digestion begins in the mouth by action of salivary α-amylase, but this ceases abruptly after the chewed food passes into the acid milieu of the stomach because of the neutral pH requirement of amylase. Although the α-amylase protein is acid labile, the presence of starch in the meal protects the enzyme from gastric degradation (Rosenblum et al., 1988), and salivary amylase may pass with the meal into the duodenum, where it may complement pancreatic α-amylase in continuing the cleavage of the starches. In newborn children, particularly in those born prematurely, the passed salivary amylase may play a functional role in the duodenum because pancreatic amylase levels are low in the early neonatal period in the premature infant. The relatively low concentration of luminal pancreatic amylase in the neonate has prompted pediatricians and nutritionists to recommend withholding starch from the diet until about 6 months of age. Nevertheless, clinical symptoms resulting from cereal feeding prior to 6 months of age are rare (Lebenthal et al., 1983).

Amylase is secreted in large quantities via the pancreatic duct into the small intestinal lumen. Most of the starch component of grains or legumes establishes contact with the α-amylases within the polar bulk phase of the intestinal luminal milieu. Indeed, the cleavage of starches to the final oligosaccharide products normally occurs in the upper part of the small intestine (the duodenum) and is virtually complete by the time the meal reaches the duodenal–jejunal junction (Fogel and Gray 1973).

It is important to consider the structure of the principal dietary starches because amylase has specificity for only the $\alpha(1 \rightarrow 4)$ linked straight-chain regions of the glucosyl polysaccharide, whereas the most abundant food starches also have $\alpha(1 \rightarrow 6)$ branching links. The simplest starch is the linear and unbranched amylose, which is a polymer of $\alpha(1 \rightarrow 4)$-linked glucosyl units (~600 glucose residues per molecule). Amylase has maximal specificity for the interior links, and its active site binds five consecutive glucose residues at specific subsites and cleaves between the second and third subsites, as shown in Figure 8-1, to form two smaller polymers. Sequential cleavage eventually leads to the production of a pentasaccharide that binds with high affinity at all five of the amylase subsites. The pentasaccharide will be hydrolyzed at the penultimate linkage from the reducing end of the pentasaccharide to release the trisaccharide maltotriose and the disaccharide maltose. Products smaller than the pentasaccharide, not being able to bind at all subsites, have very low affinity for the amylase active site; hence, productive cleavage of these smaller

Cleavage site
E D C B A
Amylase active site

Figure 8-1 Model of the active site of α-amylase. Five α(1→4)-linked glucose units indicated as O are shown positioned in subsites *A* through *E* with the reducing end glucose residue indicated as O. Each designated subsite has the appropriate conformation to accept an α(1→4)-linked glucose residue; glucose residues of amylose are shown in the figure with the potential reducing carbon on the right and the nonreducing end on the left. The cleavage site is between subsites *B* and *C*. Preference is for the interior of the α(1→4)-linked linear chain of the starch molecule. Maximal affinity (lowest K_m) and cleavage rate (highest V_{max} or k_{cat}) occurs when all subsites are occupied with glucose units. n = variable number of glucose residues in amylose; when amylopectin is the substrate, the portions of the starch in brackets also contain branches created by α(1→6) links of glucose residues as shown in Figure 8-2.

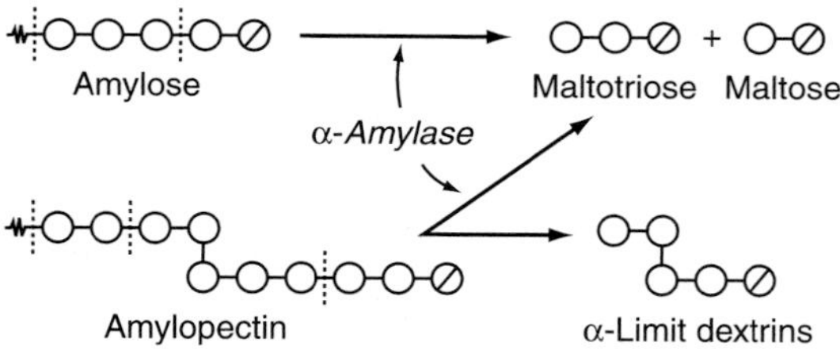

Figure 8-2 Action of salivary and pancreatic α-amylases on linear (amylose) and branched (amylopectin) forms of starch. O = Glucose units; Ø = reducing end glucose unit; horizontal links denote α(1→4) linkages; vertical links indicate α(1→6) linkages. *(From Gray GM [1981] Carbohydrate absorption and malabsorption. In: Johnson LR [ed] Physiology of the Gastrointestinal Tract. Raven Press, New York, pp 1063-1072.)*

oligosaccharides by amylase is markedly hampered. Thus, sequential actions of amylase promote the release of maltotriose and maltose as the main final products of luminal starch digestion.

Amylopectin is a more complex form of starch representing about 80% of dietary polysaccharide. Figure 8-2 depicts the action of α-amylase on amylopectin to yield the final oligosaccharide products within the distal duodenal lumen. Although its linear segments are similar to those for amylose, amylopectin is branched by virtue of α(1→6) links positioned approximately every 25 residues along the chain. Glycogen, though a minor dietary carbohydrate, has a structure analogous to that of amylopectin. Amylase is unable to cleave the α(1→6) branching link, and the structural angulation created by this linkage inhibits the enzyme from attacking some of the adjacent α(1→4) links. As a consequence, in addition to the linear maltose and maltotriose, branched oligosaccharides called α-limit dextrins (or α-dextrins) are also final products of amylopectin hydrolysis by α-amylase. Dextrins of average mass of 5 to 6 glucose units represent nearly one third the mass of the final breakdown products of amylopectin. The intraluminal hydrolysis of the starches to their final oligosaccharide products proceeds efficiently, usually providing sufficient products at the intestinal surface membrane to support optimal rates of surface digestion of the glucosyl oligosaccharides by the constituent brush-border oligosaccharidases.

Overall, the amylolytic activities of salivary and pancreatic amylases on amylose and amylopectin result in production of glucose oligosaccharides containing both α(1→4) and α(1→6) linkages, with only about 4% of the glucose residues being released as free glucose monomers (Yook and Robyt 2002).

Completion of Starch Digestion by Integral Oligosaccharides on the Outer Luminal Intestinal Surface

The luminal membrane surface of the small intestinal enterocytes that cover the villar projections of the small intestine is replete with glycoprotein oligosaccharidases. Two of these oligosaccharidases are exoglucosidases that carry out the final steps in starch digestion (Semenza and Auricchio 1991). Each one of these α-glycosidases, as synthesized, possesses two domains, each with an independent active site, and the enzyme molecules are named for the main activities of the two domains: maltase–glucoamylase and sucrase-isomaltase.

The functional differences among maltase–glucoamylase, sucrase, and isomaltase are the degree of their specificity for a particular substrate or glycosidic linkage at the nonreducing terminus of glucose oligosaccharides as illustrated in Figure 8-3, and this provides the basis for the glucosidase nomenclature. The specificity of the enzymes can be estimated from the K_m values for the various substrates (a measure of the enzyme's affinity for the substrate, or the concentration at which the enzyme is half-saturated with substrate) and from the overall rate of the reaction (k_{cat}), which is proportional to the maximal hydrolytic rate (V_{max}). Glucoamylase has high specificity for the α(1→4) link at the nonreducing terminus of straight-chain glucosyl oligosaccharides containing from two to nine glucose units. Sucrase displays high efficiency for the α(1→4) links of the smallest glucosyl oligosaccharides, maltose and maltotriose, and hence is an efficient maltase. It reinforces maltase–glucoamylase in the release of α(1→4)-linked glucose units, but its unique capacity to cleave the link between the glucose and fructose units of sucrose [α-D-glucopyranosyl(1→2′)β′-D-fructofuranoside] provides the basis for its name. Similarly, isomaltase (α-dextrinase) has appreciable specificity for the α(1→4) links in the oligosaccharide products of starch digestion, but its maximal and unique specificity is for the α(1→6) branching link of the α-dextrins. Because of its α(1→6) specificity and the use of the α(1→6) disaccharide isomaltose as substrate in in vitro assays, it is commonly called isomaltase, but isomaltose is not a natural substrate produced by α-amylase action on amylopectin. The term α-dextrinase is also used for isomaltase to more appropriately describe its capacity to cleave both α(1→4) and α(1→6) links in the oligosaccharide products (limit dextrins) of starch digestion. Maltase–glucoamylase, isomaltase (α-dextrinase), and sucrase work in a complementary

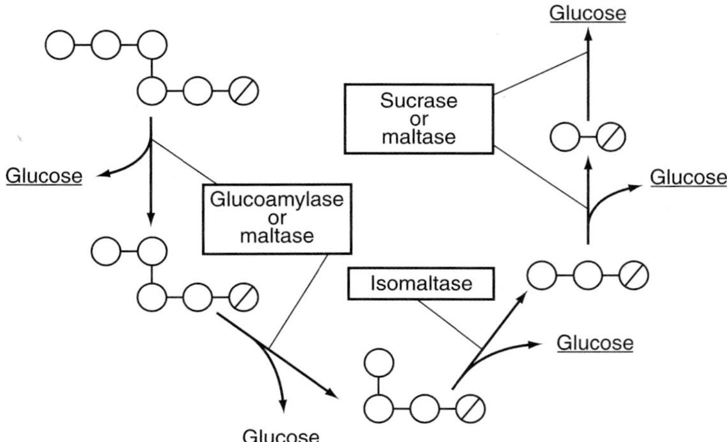

Figure 8-3 Concerted action of intestinal surface membrane oligosaccharidases on a typical α-dextrin final product of amylopectin digestion. The major active hydrolases for each removal of a glucose residue from the nonreducing terminus is shown in the boxed area. Note that only the isomaltase is capable of removing the 1-6-linked glucose "stub" from the intermediate tetrasaccharide substrate (bottom of figure). *(From Gray GM [1981] Carbohydrate absorption and malabsorption. In: Johnson LR [ed] Physiology of the Gastrointestinal Tract. Raven Press, New York, pp 1063-1072.)*

Table 8-2
Digestion of Dietary Carbohydrate

Glucose Residues	Maltase–Glucoamylase		Sucrase–Isomaltase	
N	K_m* (mmol/L)	k_{cat}† (sec^{-1})	K_m (mmol/L)	k_{cat} (sec^{-1})
2	2.1	56	14	3.2
3	1.1	149	21	3.1
4	0.4	78	24	3.5
5	0.4	63	61	3.4
6	0.7	70	57	2.1
7	1	80	120	2.2

*K_m, Substrate concentration at which the enzyme is half-saturated.
†k_{cat}, Maximal rate of overall reaction; mole of substrate hydrolyzed per second per mole of enzyme.

manner to cleave the bonds in the α-dextrins in sequence from the nonreducing end to release free glucose units. As shown in Figure 8-3, at each step in the process, one or more of these enzymes has high specificity for the α-glucosyl link closest to the nonreducing end of certain of the oligosaccharide products. These glucosidases produce free glucose for transport into the enterocyte.

These glycoprotein oligosaccharidases are synthesized in the enterocyte where they are processed in the endoplasmic reticulum (ER) and Golgi membranes with final vectorial transport to the brush-border surface. These enzymes possess a hydrophobic amino acid sequence at the N-terminus that promotes anchoring in the brush border membrane, and the orientation of these enzymes in the membrane are such that the oligosaccharidase domains, including the active catalytic sites, are on the exterior side of the brush-border membrane and available for efficient cleavage of the luminal substrates. In humans, these oligosaccharidases are acquired during the fetal period prior to birth, and newborns have a full complement of these enzymes.

The two different domains of mature maltase–glucoamylase (maltase and glucoamylase) display high homology to the respective subunits of the sucrase–isomaltase complex and contain one potential active site each (Nichols et al., 1998). These similarities have led to the suggestion that maltase–glucoamylase and sucrase–isomaltase are related proteins arising by duplication of an ancestral gene. In particular, the N-proximal subunit (glucoamylase) closer to the plasma membrane displays a high degree of amino acid homology with the isomaltase subunit of the sucrase–isomaltase complex (55% identity), which could explain the small degree of isomaltase activity that has been observed for maltase–glucoamylase.

Although maltase–glucoamylase contributes only about 20% of total intestinal maltase activity in humans, the average K_m of maltase–glucoamylase for the hydrolysis of various glucose oligomers is much lower than that for sucrase–isomaltase (Heymann et al., 1995; Heymann and Gunther 1994), which is the only other enzyme with α(1→4) hydrolytic activity against glucose oligomers (Table 8-2). Maltase–glucoamylase activity is, therefore, an efficient producer of free glucose from the products of luminal starch digestion in vivo and is limited only by branching at α(1→6) glucosidic bonds.

DIGESTION OF DIETARY DISACCHARIDES

Dietary disaccharides are hydrolyzed by α-glucosidases or the β-galactosidase associated with the brush-border membrane of enterocytes. In addition to digestion of maltose, as described for the end-products of starch breakdown, humans have the capacity to hydrolyze unique linkages present in sucrose, lactose, and trehalose. These disaccharidases are all associated with the luminal surface of the intestinal epithelial cells as illustrated in Figure 8-4.

Clinical Correlation

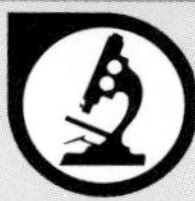

Maltase-Glucoamylase Inhibitors

Because α(1→4)-linked glucose makes up approximately 90% of the glucose linkages in dietary starches, mucosal maltase–glucoamylase activity largely determines the rate of starch digestion and glucose absorption and, hence, the quantity of starch that enters the fermentative pathway of colonic salvage. The starch digestion/glucose production gate-keeping role of maltase–glucoamylase is recognized by therapeutic use of maltase–glucoamylase inhibitors for the treatment of type 2 diabetes (Kaiser and Sawicki 2004).

The effect of acarbose is the best documented and most widely used. Acarbose is produced by a microorganism, *Actinoplanes utahensi*; it consists of a maltotriose attached to a substituted cyclohexane ring, which blocks the hydrolysis catalyzed by α-glucosidases. The effectiveness of acarbose in treatment of type 2 diabetes is added proof that maltase–glucoamylase is a gatekeeper of starch digestion. The side effects of acarbose are similar to the symptoms of maltase–glucoamylase deficiency: moderate-to-severe abdominal cramps, bloating, and, very rarely, diarrhea. Therefore, acarbose appears to reduce starch digestion, and hence glucose absorption, and to increase the amount of carbohydrate provided to bacteria in the colon for fermentation through the insulin-independent short-chain fatty acid pathway. Reducing the rate of carbohydrate digestion and absorption and/or increasing the colonic starch fermentation may be beneficial in reducing the incidence of diabetes type 2 and of cardiovascular disease (Brand-Miller, 2003).

Sucrose Digestion by Sucrase

Sucrose, which is also known as table sugar, is the most abundantly consumed natural sweetner. Table sugar is refined from sugar cane or sugar beets, and various refined forms of sucrose are used in production of various foods. Sucrose is also present in relatively large amounts in fruits, such as oranges and apples. Intestinal digestion of sucrose [α-D-glucopyranosyl(1→2′)β′-D-fructofuranoside] requires hydrolysis of the α(1→2′)β′ linkage, which involves the anomeric carbon of both hexoses, to yield glucose and fructose. In mammalian species, the hydrolysis of sucrose is performed by the sucrase activity of the sucrase–isomaltase complex of the enterocytes lining the intestine. The resulting monosaccharides are then absorbed by the intestinal epithelial cells.

Lactose Digestion by Lactase

Lactose [β-D-galactopyranosyl(1→4′)D-glucopyranoside] is a disaccharide abundant in the mammalian milk from which it takes its name ("milk sugar," from the Latin *lac* or "milk"). Milk ingestion by breast-fed infants provides approximately 70 g/L (or 55 g/day) of carbohydrates, of which approximately 60 g/L is lactose (Foda et al., 2004; Marquis et al., 2003). The remainder are oligosaccharides that are not digestible by the human gastrointestinal enzymes. The nutritional relevance of lactose is limited after infancy because of the introduction of alternate dietary carbohydrates and a decline in activity of the specific disaccharidase necessary for the digestion of lactose.

Lactose digestion in mammals requires lactase–phlorizin hydrolase activity, one of the intestinal disaccharidases present in the apical brush-border membrane of the small intestinal enterocytes. Although lactase–phlorizin hydrolase shows structural analogies with other α-glycosidases of the brush-border membrane, it has a distinctive neutral β-galactosidic activity (Montgomery et al., 1991; Buller et al., 1989). The molecule contains two independent active sites, one responsible for lactase activity and the other associated with the phlorizin hydrolase activity (Mantei et al., 1988).

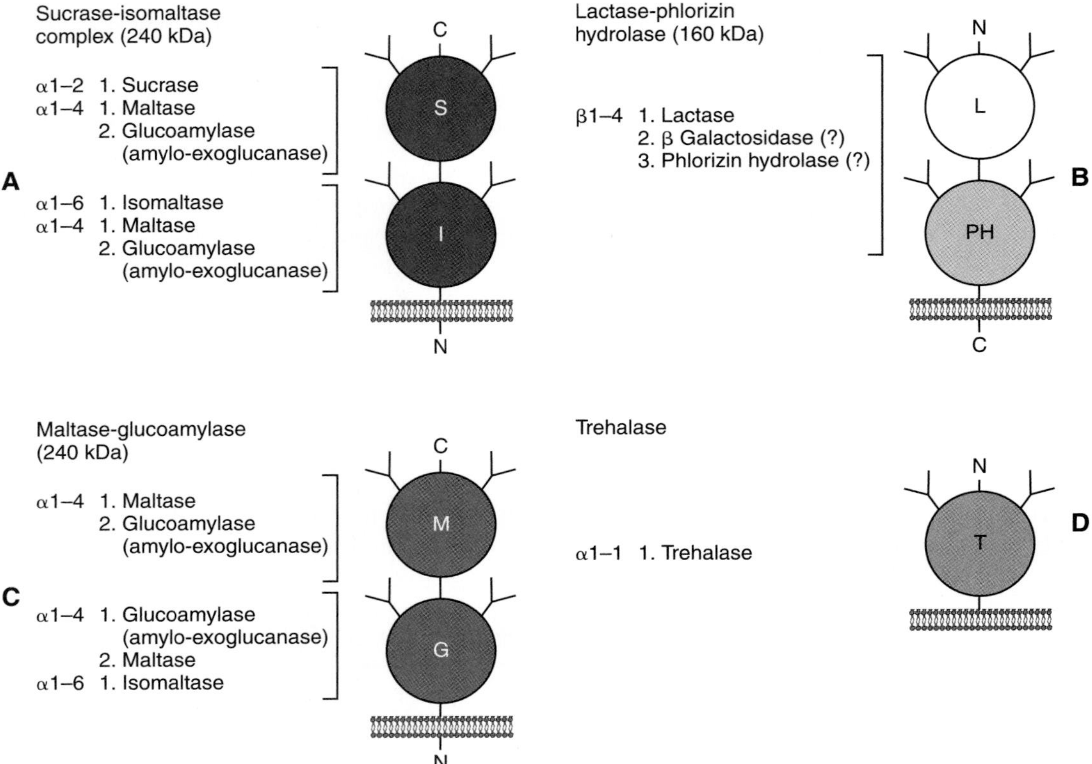

Figure 8-4 Schematic structures of human intestinal disaccharidases and their enzyme activities. The activities are ranked *(1, 2, 3)* by importance to carbohydrate nutrition. **A,** Sucrase-isomaltase is a bifunctional enzyme that hydrolyzes α(1→4) glycosidic bonds with low affinity (high K_m) and α(1→6) glycosidic bonds with high affinity (low K_m). Sucrase also hydrolyzes sucrose. **B,** Lactase-phlorizin hydrolase hydrolyzes β(1→4) glycosidic bonds such as that found in lactose. **C,** Maltase-glucoamylase has a high affinity (very low K_m) for the α(1→4) glucosidic bonds of glucose oligomers. **D,** Trehalase is anchored to the plasma membrane through a phosphatidylinositol ester and acts on trehalose.

The β-galactosidase domain has high specificity for lactose. The physiological significance of the phlorizin hydrolase domain is unknown; however, it has been proposed that this active site could be involved in hydrolysis of the glycosidic moiety of glycosylceramides and vitamins (Mackey et al., 2004; Buller et al., 1989) (Table 8-3).

Although uniformly present at birth and crucial for cleavage of lactose in maternal milk, lactase decreases appreciably either in young childhood (~age 3 to 5) or in adolescence (~age 14 to 18) in most of the world's population groups. Lactase does remain at high neonatal levels in most Caucasians of Northern European origin, but adult deficiency of this enzyme still occurs in approximately 5% to 20% of Caucasian adults. Table 8-4 shows the prevalence of adult lactase deficiency, now commonly referred to as hypolactasia, in various populations of the world.

Trehalose Digestion by Trehalase

Trehalose (α-D-glucopyranosyl-(1→1′)α′-D-glucopyranoside) is a disaccharide present in small amounts in a large variety of organisms, such as bacteria, plants, and algae (Elbein et al., 2003; Richards et al., 2002). It performs diverse functions that include energy storage and transport and protection against extreme

Table 8-3
Kinetic Properties of Intestinal Brush-Border Membrane Disaccharidases

Enzyme	Principal Substrate	K_m (mmol/L)	k_{cat} (sec^{-1})
α-Glucosidases			
Sucrase	Sucrose	18	120
Trehalase	Trehalose	3	20
β-Galactosidase			
Lactase	Lactose	2	4

Table 8-4
Prevalence of Hypolactasia in Healthy Populations*

Group	% Lactase-Deficient†
North American (white)	520
North American (black)	70-75
African Bantu	50
Puerto Rican	21
Danish	3
Asians	
Filipino	95
Indian	55
Thai	97
Chinese	87
Eskimo (Greenland)	88
Nigerian	
Yoruba	99
Fulani	58
Israeli Jews‡	61
Israeli Arabs	81
Mexican	74

Modified from Gray GM (1983) Intestinal disaccharidase deficiencies and glucose-galactose malabsorption. In: Stanbury JB, Wyngaarden JB, Fredrickson DS, Goldstein JL, Brown MS (eds) Metabolic Basis of Inherited Disease, 5th ed. Blakiston Division, McGraw-Hill, New York, pp 1729-1742.
*Based on the work of numerous authors; see Gray (1983) for primary references.
†Lactase deficiency was diagnosed based on lactase activity below 1.0 U/g tissue, or 15 U/g protein; or blood glucose rises less than 200 mg/L after ingestion of 50 g lactose accompanied by abdominal symptoms and diarrhea. One International Unit of enzyme activity is 1 μmol/min at 37° C.
‡Includes Ashkenazi, Sephardi, Iraquis, Yenemite, and Asian groups with deficiency rates of 44% to 84%.

temperatures or desiccation (Lillford and Holt 2002). Because trehalose is found in appreciable amounts only in unprocessed mushrooms, yeasts, and insects, it appears to be a carbohydrate of relatively minor importance for present day human nutrition (Richards et al., 2002; Schiraldi and Di Lernia 2002). Trehalose can be broken down by trehalase, which is present in the brush-border membrane of the intestinal epithelial cells of humans and most mammals (Semenza, 1986). Each molecule of trehalose hydrolyzed renders two molecules of free glucose. The presence of trehalase activity in the human intestine may reflect a widespread dependence of ancient humans on these foods as primary sources of nutrients.

GLYCOSIDIC BONDS NOT HYDROLYZED BY HUMAN DIGESTIVE ENZYMES

Mammals have no digestive capacity for certain oligosaccharides with α-galactosidic linkages (raffinose and stachyose) that are constituents of some legumes, particularly the kidney-shaped beans. Dietary fiber includes polysaccharide components that are homopolymers of glucose units connected by β-glycosidic linkages (e.g., cellulose and β-glucans) as well as various heteropolysaccharides (e.g., hemicelluloses, pectic substances, gums and mucilages, and algal polysaccharides) that contain a variety of sugar residues and types of linkages. Because mammalian pancreatic secretions and integral intestinal oligosaccharidases are incapable of cleaving the β-linked glucosyl and α-linked galactosyl bonds, these polysaccharides and oligosaccharidases cannot be digested. Instead, they remain intact and may have local effects on intestinal transport as they travel to lower levels of the ileum and to the colon where the resident bacteria then cleave and modify them extensively to short-chain fatty acids, hydrogen gas, carbon dioxide, and methane. Fermentation of dietary fiber produces a great increase in the concentration of osmotically active particles in the lower small intestine and colon, which results in an increase in the stool water output. Some of the potential osmotic excess is compensated for by colonic absorption of the short-chain fatty acids generated by bacterial fermentation. (See Chapter 11 for more discussion of dietary fiber.)

EXPRESSION AND POSTTRANSLATIONAL PROCESSING OF THE OLIGOSACCHARIDASES AND DISACCHARIDASES

The posttranslational processing of newly synthesized disaccharidases has been the subject of a number of studies. The general pathways, summarized in Figure 8-5, are similar for lactase–phlorizin hydrolase, sucrase–isomaltase, and maltase–glucoamylase, although each has some specific and unique characteristics. Trehalase expression and processing has little similarity to that of the other disaccharidases.

MALTASE–GLUCOAMYLASE

The human maltase–glucoamylase gene is located on chromosome 7 (Nichols et al., 2003). The encoded protein undergoes extensive *N*- and *O*-glycosylation to render a mature protein that is inserted into the plasma membrane by its N-terminal end. In contrast to sucrase–isomaltase and lactase–phlorizin hydrolase, no proteolytic processing has been documented to occur for human maltase–glucoamylase (Naim et al., 1988). Maltase–glucoamylase activity and its putative mRNA have been detected in diverse tissues such as kidney, granulocytes, mammary gland, and testis (Ben Ali et al., 1994; Pereira and Sivakami 1991), but its function in these tissues has not been studied.

In most studies done to date (Chao and Donovan 1996; Shulman, 1990; Buts et al., 1988), the activities of maltase–glucoamylase have not been clearly differentiated from those of the sucrase–isomaltase complex, hampering an accurate evaluation of the effects of feeding and hormonal stimuli on the synthesis of the maltase–glucoamylase protein. These limitations are particularly important in humans, in whom maltase–glucoamylase contributes a relatively small fraction of the maltase activity. The effects deduced from the differential changes of sucrase and maltase activities have suggested that maltase–glucoamylase expression and activity often parallel those of its complementary enzyme sucrase–isomaltase (McDonald and Henning 1992).

SUCRASE–ISOMALTASE

Sucrase–isomaltase is encoded by a gene on human chromosome 3 (Chantret et al., 1992). The molecule is synthesized as a single polypeptide, which is subjected to complex intracellular glycosylation with addition of N-linked and *O*-linked carbohydrates (Danielsen, 1982). After glycosylation, the fully active proenzyme is transported and inserted in the apical membrane of the enterocytes through its N-terminus (Hunziker et al., 1986; Sigrist et al., 1975). In the apical membrane of enterocytes, sucrase–isomaltase is subjected to extracellular processing by pancreatic proteolytic enzymes present in the intestinal lumen. The molecule is cleaved to generate a free C-terminal sucrase subunit and a membrane-bound N-terminal isomaltase subunit, which remain associated through noncovalent interactions (Saphiro et al., 1991; Hu et al., 1987; Cowell et al., 1986). Sucrase–isomaltase is normally expressed only in the intestine.

The C-terminal domain of sucrase–isomaltase is required for the protein to exit the ER and for subsequent processing of the enzyme (Fransen et al., 1991; Jacob et al., 2000a). The C-terminal sucrose domain appears to act as an intramolecular chaperone for the isomaltase domain. In the absence of the sucrase domain, isomaltase remains associated with the ER through its association with calnexin and is not processed properly (Jacob et al., 2002). The sucrase–isomaltase molecule requires *O*-glycosylation for processing to the luminal membrane (Spodsberg et al., 2001; Alfalah et al., 1999). The bifunctional enzyme is transported in lipid raft vesicles bound to actin fibers to the microvilli (Danielsen and Hansen 2003; Jacob et al., 2003; Alfalah et al., 1999). A calcium-sensitive

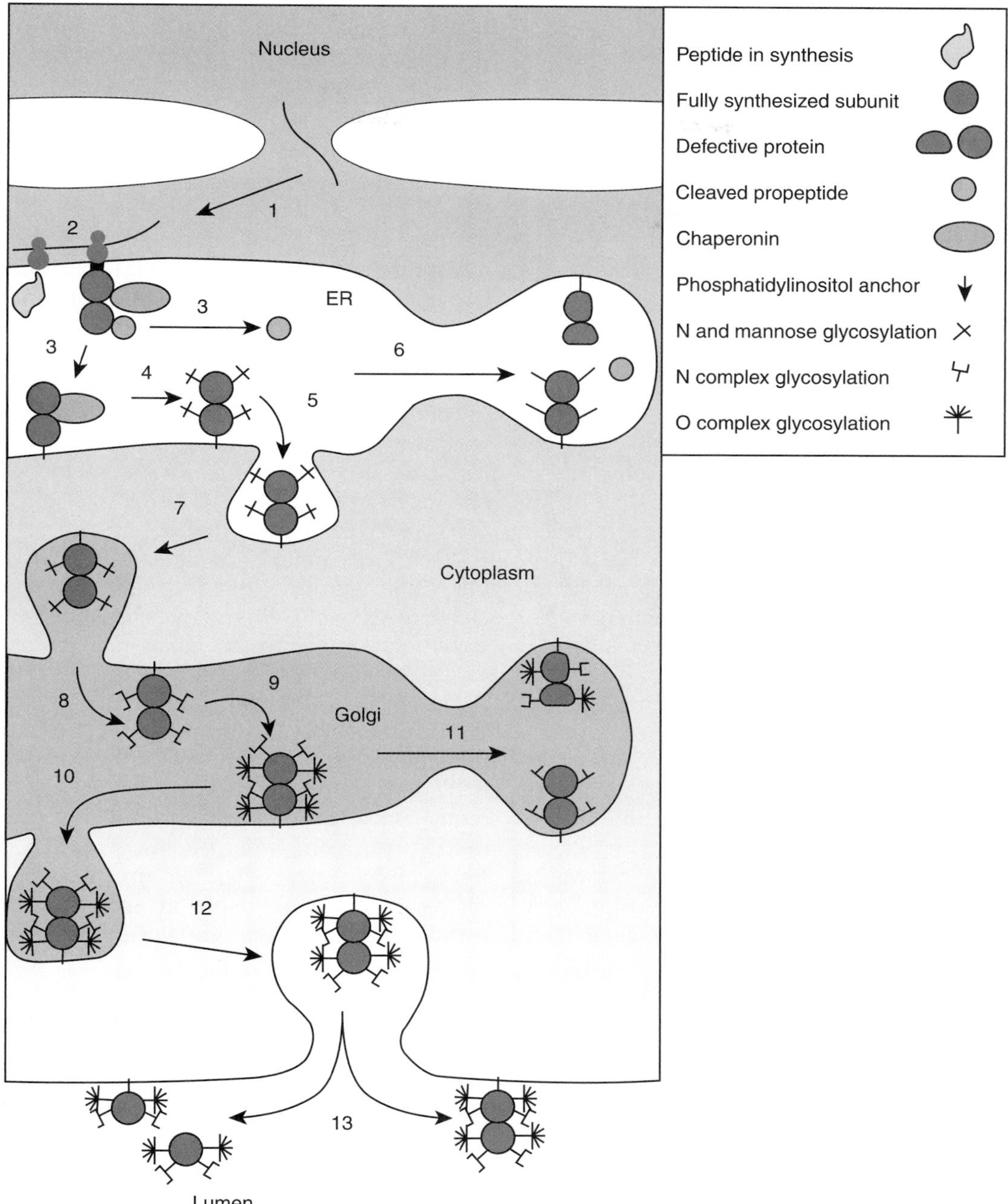

Figure 8-5 Schematic representation of pathways for synthesis and processing of brush-border membrane disaccharidases in enterocytes. *1,* Transcription and transport of messenger ribonucleic acid (mRNA) coding for disaccharidases from the nucleus to the endoplasmic reticulum *(ER)*. *2,* Ribosomal synthesis of protein with translocation and insertion into the ER membrane. *3,* Correct folding assisted by chaperonins and proteolytic processing with release of propeptide. *4,* High mannose *N*-glycosylation. *5,* Editing, evaluation of quality, and sorting of the protein. *6,* Storage, or lysosomal degradation of defective proteins. *7,* Vesicular transport into the *cis*-Golgi compartment. *8,* Editing and complex *N*-glycosylation. *9, O*-glycosylation. *10,* Evaluation of protein quality and sorting to *trans*-Golgi vesicular system. *11,* Storage, or lysosomal degradation of, defective proteins. *12,* Transport and insertion into the apical plasma membrane. *13,* Location of activity on luminal surface of the brush-border membrane and extracellular proteolytic processing.

protein, annexin II, is required for the efficient sorting of the sucrase–isomaltase complex to the luminal membrane (Jacob et al., 2004).

The activity and message levels of maltase–glucoamylase and sucrase–isomaltase are highly correlated in biopsy samples from the duodenum (Semenza et al., 2001). In most mammals, the activities of sucrase–isomaltase appear in the small intestine at the time of weaning from maternal milk to starch-based diets. In humans, however, the sucrase–isomaltase complex is present on the luminal surface of enterocytes in the small intestine from before birth. The activities of sucrase–isomaltase have been found to be increased both in subjects with uncontrolled diabetes and in subjects fed diets rich in carbohydrates, suggesting that intestinal levels of sucrase–isomaltase may be upregulated by high levels of blood glucose.

Regulation of sucrase–isomaltase activity is tightly linked to enterocyte differentiation. In mature humans, immature enterocytes developing from stem cells in crypts do not have sucrase–isomaltase activity. As enterocytes traverse to the crypt-villus junction, the sucrase–isomaltase message and activity are expressed. The level of sucrase–isomaltase mRNA reaches its peak when enterocytes are located in the lower and mid villus region and then progressively decreases as these cells move toward the tip (Traber et al., 1992). The promoter region of the sucrase–isomaltase gene has been found to bind the same transcription factors (Cdx-2, HNF-1α, and GATA factors) as the lactase–phlorizin hydrolase promoter (see following section); the GATA factors (named for the transcription element nucleotide sequence) are involved in the tissue-specific expression of these two oligosaccharidases and their crypt-villus localization (Boudreau et al., 2002; Troelsen et al., 1997).

LACTASE–PHLORIZIN HYDROLASE

The gene for human lactase–phlorizin hydrolase is located on chromosome 2 (Kruse et al., 1988). Lactase–phlorizin hydrolase is synthesized as a polypeptide of about 220 kDa, which follows a complex intracellular processing route that involves heavy glycosylation with *N*-linked and *O*-linked carbohydrates to produce intermediate forms of up to 280 kDa (Naim et al., 1987; Hauri et al., 1985; Danielsen et al., 1984; Yeh and Moog, 1974). Proteolysis is involved in production of the final mature enzyme with a molecular mass of approximately 160 kDa. The nucleotide sequence of the human lactase–phlorizin hydrolase gene indicates the presence of four domains arranged with a twofold symmetry (Kruse et al., 1988). Two of these domains are eliminated during the maturation process to render a mature protein that has two domains containing one potential active site each (Buller et al., 1989; Mantei et al., 1988). In contrast to sucrase–isomaltase and maltase–glucoamylase, mature lactase–phlorizin hydrolase is inserted into the plasma membrane of enterocytes through its C-terminus (Mantei et al., 1988; Semenza, 1986).

The N-terminal domains of lactase–phlorizin hydrolase that are intracellularly cleaved to yield the active brush-border enzyme are required as a chaperone for exit of the mature polypeptide from the ER (Jacob et al., 1996; Naim and Lentze 1992). The immunoglobulin chaperone BiP is also required (Jacob et al., 1996). *O*-Glycosylation is added in the post-Golgi region and is required for sorting of the disaccharidase to the luminal membrane (Dudley et al., 1998; Naim and Lentze 1992). The exact mechanisms of regulation of lactase–phlorizin hydrolase and sucrase–isomaltase processing are obscure. The rate of processing of lactase–phlorizin hydrolase and sucrase–isomaltase to membrane forms is reduced in fasted animals or in animals subjected to parenteral nutrition; in contrast, lactase–phlorizin hydrolase processing is accelerated by thyroid hormone, insulin, and insulin-like growth factors (Burrin et al., 2001; Dudley et al., 1998; Dudley et al., 1996; Shulman et al., 1992).

Lactase–phlorizin hydrolase mRNA is expressed only in villus enterocytes of the small intestine. Expression of lactase–phlorizin hydrolase is detected during embryonic development as early as 8 weeks of gestation in humans and reaches maximal activity at an early postnatal age (Simon-Assmann et al., 1986). Levels of lactase–phlorizin hydrolase activity remain high until weaning. After weaning, a slow and sustained loss of lactase–phlorizin hydrolase may lead to values, in young adulthood, of less than 10% those observed during infancy (Wang et al., 1998; Montgomery et al., 1991). Although a limited fraction of the human adult population retains lactase–phlorizin hydrolase activity during adulthood, lactose is a substrate for fermentation by colonic bacteria in most adults (Montgomery et al., 1991; Kien et al., 1989; Mobassaleh et al., 1985).

The direct mechanisms responsible for the expression of lactase–phlorizin hydrolase are unknown. Expression of lactase–phlorizin hydrolase activity has been observed in small intestinal epithelial embryonic cells cultured in vitro in the absence of hormonal stimuli (Simon-Assmann et al., 1986; Kendall et al., 1979) or xenotransplanted into nonintestinal organs (Choi et al., 1998; Duluc et al., 1994), suggesting that the synthesis of lactase–phlorizin hydrolase is largely a programmed event forming part of the differentiating process of enterocytes. However, hormonal control appears to participate during the perinatal age in attaining maximal levels of enzyme activity. Insulin and cortisol have been found to increase expression of lactase–phlorizin hydrolase in perinatal enterocytes, probably through the induction of cell differentiation (Buts et al., 1988). Epidermal growth factor can enhance the expression of lactase–phlorizin hydrolase, thereby potentiating the effects of steroids and insulin (Yeh et al., 1991; Menard et al., 1986; O'Loughlin et al., 1985; Malo and Menard 1982).

The expression of lactase–phlorizin hydrolase is regulated along the length of the small intestine and along the crypt–villus axis during differentiation. The distal jejunum and the proximal ileum contain the highest levels of lactase–phlorizin hydrolase mRNA (Semenza et al., 2001). *Cis*-elements with a role in lactase–phlorizin hydrolase transcription exist in genomic sequences upstream of the TATA-box in the promoter of the lactase–phlorizin hydrolase gene in the pig and other species (Kuokkanen et al., 2003; Troelsen et al., 2003a). The pig lactase–phlorizin hydrolase promoter region (position −17 to −994) is able to regulate the transcription of a reporter gene. This region contains the information for specific small intestinal expression and the postweaning downregulation of lactase–phlorizin hydrolase (Troelsen et al., 2003a; Boudreau et al., 2001).

A nuclear transcription factor NF-LPH1 (Boudreau et al., 2002; Troelsen et al., 1992) that is present exclusively in intestinal epithelium binds to a sequence that is close to a transcription initiating TATA-box in the promoter region of the lactase–phlorizin hydrolase gene. NF-LPH1 declines over the same time-period during which lactase–phlorizin hydrolase activity declines in the postweaning period. In humans, a reduction in the expression of NF-LPH1 might be the cause of adult-type hypolactasia (Kuokkanen et al., 2003; Troelsen et al., 2003a).

Cotransfection studies have shown that the human promoter of lactase–phlorizin hydrolase has greater transcriptional response to the GATA factors and hepatocyte nuclear factor HNF-1α than to the caudal-related homeodomain protein Cdx-2. The opposite occurs in the human sucrase–isomaltase promoter, where the transcriptional responses are stronger for HNF-1α and Cdx-2 than for GATA factors (Krasinski et al., 2001; Spodsberg et al., 1999). Differentiated Caco-2 cells express Cdx2 and HOXC11, a member of the homeobox-containing Hox-family of factors, which are able to bind the lactase–phlorizin hydrolase promoter (Mitchelmore et al., 1998). Cotransfection experiments in Caco-2 cells have shown that HNF-1α and HNF-1β play a competitive role in the activation of lactase–phlorizin hydrolase transcription. The forkhead-related activator (FREAC) family of proteins, which are a group of nuclear factors of the HNF-3/forkhead family, probably influence lactase–phlorizin hydrolase gene transcription during the process of enterocyte differentiation (Mitchelmore et al., 1998).

TREHALASE

Because of the apparent minor physiological significance of trehalase, its structural and catalytic characteristics have not been studied as extensively as those of the other intestinal disaccharidases. Trehalase has hydrolytic activity against the $\alpha(1\rightarrow1')\alpha'$-glucosidic linkage present in trehalose (Asano et al., 1996; Chen et al., 1987; Nakano and Sacktor, 1984). The gene coding for human intestinal trehalase is located on chromosome 11 (Ishihara et al., 1997). Trehalase is synthesized as a protein containing 583 amino acids with a molecular mass of about 66 kDa (Oesterreicher et al., 2001; Ishihara et al., 1997; Ruf et al., 1990). It is proteolytically processed intracellularly to yield a mature molecule of 63 kDa. As for the other disaccharidases, trehalase appears to be highly glycosylated during its maturation (Ruf et al., 1990). However, in contrast to the other major disaccharidases, mature trehalase is anchored to the plasma membrane via phosphatidylinositol (Ruf et al., 1990). Trehalase activity has been detected in several human tissues, particularly plasma and kidney, but the genetic and structural relationship of the responsible molecules to intestinal trehalase has not been established (Vachon et al., 1991; Baumann et al., 1981).

The ontogeny of intestinal trehalase varies among mammals. In humans and rabbits, a low level of trehalase activity has been detected in fetal intestine (Toofanian, 1984); in contrast, in mice and rats, trehalase and its coding mRNA are not detected until the postnatal period. Because trehalase activity derived from the fetal intestine and kidney can be detected in the amniotic fluid, trehalase measurement has been proposed as a diagnostic assay for detection of developmental defects (Potier et al., 1986). In mammals, adult levels of intestinal trehalase are attained during the early postnatal period (Gartner et al., 2002; Oesterreicher et al., 1998; Galand, 1989, 1986).

In the cases in which the hormonal regulation of intestinal trehalase activity has been studied, it has been found to parallel that of sucrase–isomaltase activities in developing and adult intestine and, thus, appears to be part of a preset program of intestinal development. In humans and animals, trehalase activity is increased by stimulation of growth of the intestinal epithelia as well as by signals for differentiation of enterocytes (Gartner et al., 2002; Oesterreicher et al., 1998).

ABSORPTION OF HEXOSES BY THE ENTEROCYTE: MECHANISMS AND REGULATION

The products of disaccharide digestion are the monosaccharides glucose, galactose, and fructose. Because the intestine is lined by a single layer of columnar cells that are attached by tight junctions, making it impermeable to even small solute molecules, it is necessary for one or more transporters or carriers to promote entry into and exit from the epithelial cells (enterocytes). As illustrated in Figure 8-6, transporters in the apical and basolateral membranes operate in concert to regulate the movement of the hexoses across the enterocyte layer for delivery to the capillaries within the core of the villus. First, glucose and galactose are transported into the enterocyte by the sodium–glucose cotransporter 1 (SGLT1), and fructose is transported into the enterocyte by facilitated glucose–fructose transporter 5 (GLUT5). Second, all three hexoses are transported out of the enterocyte by glucose transporter 2 (GLUT2) located in the basolateral membrane. This delivers the absorbed sugars into the core of the intestinal villi for entry into the capillaries and, hence, portal blood. (Glucose transporters are discussed further in Chapter 12).

Pentoses are naturally present in the diet as part of nucleotides, nucleosides, and nucleic acids in foods. There is little information concerning the absorption or transport of pentoses. Xylose appears to be transported by a passive mechanism that is increased when the integrity of the epithelia is compromised. Thus, xylose transport has been used as a measure of the integrity of the intestinal epithelia. Transport of free ribose appears to be very limited; however, there are several transporters involved in the recovery of nucleotides and nucleosides (salvage mechanisms). The nutritional importance of the absorption of pentose by these or other possible mechanisms has not been investigated.

HEXOSE TRANSPORTERS

Glucose and galactose, hexose isomers differing only by the position of the hydroxyl and hydrogen attached to C-4 in the ring structure,

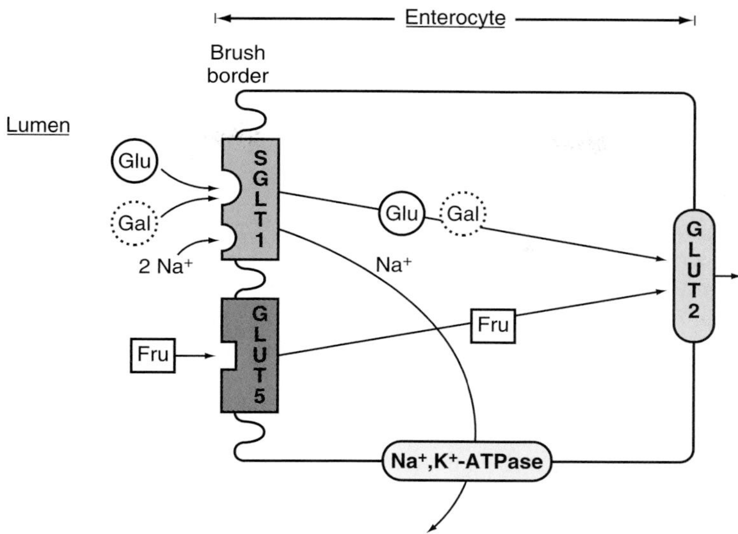

Figure 8-6 Hexose transport by the enterocyte occurs by membrane carrier proteins. Designations and positions in the brush border or basolateral membrane are shown. Energy is provided by the exit of Na^+ via the Na^+,K^+-ATPase. Glucose (Glu) and galactose (Gal), being closely related structurally, share the glucose transporter (SGLT1). Fructose (Fru) enters via GLUT5. All three hexoses exit via the high capacity GLUT2 in the basolateral membrane. See text for elaboration.

both utilize sodium–glucose cotransporter 1 (SGLT1). SGLT1 is an apical membrane imbedded protein comprised of 664 amino acids (Wright et al., 2004; Wright et al., 2003; Wright et al., 1997). SGLT1 contains 14 transmembrane domains, and both its N- and C-termini face the lumen of the small intestine. SGLT1 is an aldohexose and Na^+ co-transport protein that supports the binding and transport into the cell of two molecules of Na^+ and one molecule of glucose or galactose. SGLT1 is a high-affinity transporter with a K_t (kinetic constant of transport; analogous to the K_m for enzyme catalysis) of 0.5 mmol/L for glucose and 5 mmol/L for Na^+. Therefore, half-maximal transport rates may be observed at luminal glucose concentrations (80 mg/L, or 0.5 mmol/L) that are only one tenth of the fasting plasma glucose level and at sodium concentrations (115 mg/L, or 5 mmol/L) that are less than one twentieth of the sodium concentration of extracellular fluids in the body (Panayotova-Heiermann et al., 1996).

After glucose or galactose and its Na^+ partners have entered the enterocyte, they are released and go their separate ways. The Na^+ exits the enterocyte via the Na^+,K^+-ATPase in the basolateral membrane, an energy utilizing process that promotes glucose or galactose and Na^+ co-entry down the Na^+ concentration gradient maintained by the Na^+,K^+-ATPase. The glucose or galactose achieves relatively high intracellular concentrations to drive the low affinity, high capacity GLUT2 hexose transporter in the basolateral membrane of enterocytes, thereby facilitating the exit of glucose and other hexoses from the enterocyte for diffusion into the underlying capillaries. GLUT2 is half-saturated with glucose at an intracellular glucose concentration that is comparable to the postprandial plasma glucose concentration (K_t ~11 mmol/L, or 1,600 mg/L).

A third principal monosaccharide is fructose, a ketohexose with a structure that is distinctly different from those of glucose or galactose. Fructose is absorbed into the enterocyte by a facilitated diffusion process supported by GLUT5, a brush-border membrane protein that efficiently accommodates luminal fructose and functions independently of Na^+. Like glucose and galactose, fructose exits the enterocyte primarily via the GLUT2 transporter of the basolateral membrane. Some GLUT5 transporters also appear to be localized to the basolateral membrane, where they may complement the GLUT2 mechanism for exit of fructose from the enterocyte (Blakemore et al., 1995). In addition, the presence of high intraluminal fructose concentrations may trigger the transient transport of GLUT2 into the apical membrane, where it may assist GLUT5 in fructose absorption (Gouyon et al., 2003a).

REGULATION OF HEXOSE TRANSPORT

The mRNA abundance of all three major hexose transporters displays a diurnal variation with a marked increase just prior to feeding. On the basis of studies in rats, intraluminal glucose released from digestion of ingested poly- and oligosaccharides increases the mRNA abundance of both SGLT1 and GLUT2 (Corpe and Burant 1996). That this luminal effect is due to the hexose structure itself rather than to a metabolic product such as phosphorylated glucose is indicated by the fact that the nonmetabolizable 3-*O*-methylglucose is also capable of augmenting the mRNA levels of these transporters. Similarly, the presence of sucrose or fructose in the intestinal lumen produces a specific and abrupt increase in the GLUT5 mRNA that codes for synthesis of the fructose transporter (Shu et al., 1997). The common mechanism of enhancement of the hexose transporters appears to be an induction of their transcription by the particular transportable substrate itself. The signaling mechanism that is involved is not yet known.

Cyclic AMP (cAMP) augments the SGLT1, GLUT2, and GLUT5 transport capacity of the intestine. Both SGLT1 and GLUT2 undergo regulation at the processing level by cAMP stimulation of transporter vesicle fusion to the apical membrane and consequently increased luminal transport. In the case of SGLT1, protein kinase activation increases the transport capacity by virtue of transfer of SGLT1 units from the intracellular compartment to the apical membrane (Hirsch et al., 1996). An increase in the level of cAMP can augment glucose or galactose transport by 100-fold without changing the kinetic properties of the transporter (Wright et al., 2004). This augmentation is mediated by increased fusion of SGLT1-transporting vesicles with the apical membrane. In the cAMP-mediated upregulation

Nutrition Insight

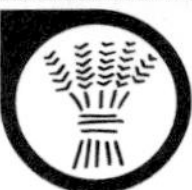

Glucose Transport via Sodium–Glucose Transporter 1 (SGLT1) Enhances Water Absorption

The absorption of NaCl and solutes is known to be accompanied by the movement of water, presumably by virtue of the osmotic gradient produced by absorption of the electrolytes, and solutes such as amino acids and monosaccharides. Although the exact mechanisms involved are still being worked out and appear to involve movement both through (*trans*-cellular) and between (*para*-cellular) the enterocytes, it is clear that glucose uptake by SGLT1 serves as a major enhancer of water absorption.

Expression of SGLT1 in *Xenopus* oocytes allowed investigators to assess the quantitative interaction of water and glucose movement. Water movement was induced by expression of the glucose/Na^+ cotransporter in the oocyte system: 260 molecules of water accompanied the transport of 2 Na^+ and a single glucose molecule by SGLT1 (Loo et al., 1996). This would amount to nearly 3 L of water accompanying the absorption of 100 g (or 400 kcal) of glucose. On the basis of this calculation, the transport of the usual quantity of glucose-containing nutrients consumed daily would support water absorption of several liters by the human intestine. Although this might seem rather amazing, we know that approximately 9 to 11 L of fluid is reabsorbed daily by the human gastrointestinal tract. The osmotic effects of glucose and amino acids are used in oral rehydration therapy; oral rehydration solutions contain these solutes to promote the absorption of water.

of hexose transport, protein kinase A and protein kinase C are critically involved (Wright et al., 1997). Cholera toxin and vasoactive intestinal peptide (VIP) are two agents in nature that regulate cAMP and, hence, alter SGLT1 function. Epidermal growth factor (EGF) has a similar effect on glucose transport (Gouyon et al., 2003b; Chung et al., 2002; Mehta et al., 1997). The activation of protein kinase C signaling can increase the presence of GLUT2 on the enterocyte apical membrane by fourfold (Helliwell et al., 2003). In contrast to the mechanism of upregulation of SGLT1 and GLUT2 by cAMP, GLUT5 is regulated at the level of its mRNA. The activation of cAMP-dependent protein kinases stabilizes the mRNA for GLUT5, resulting in enhanced transcription and GLUT5 protein synthesis. There is a suggestion that the phosphoinositide-3-kinase signaling pathway modulates GLUT5 and that this can occur without changing the mRNA abundance (Chung et al., 2002).

DISORDERS OF CARBOHYDRATE ASSIMILIATION

Digestion and absorption of dietary carbohydrate may be affected by a number of factors. The initial factor involved in carbohydrate processing is the rate of chewing and residence time in the mouth, which affect the interaction of the starch component with salivary amylase. This is usually a relatively short period, and the meal is then exposed to the low pH of the stomach, which stops the action of the salivary α-amylase. The stomach acts principally as a reservoir, and the rate of gastric emptying is dependent upon the nutrient composition of the meal. The presence of dietary fat, nondigestible carbohydrate (dietary fiber), and high osmolality (such as that present in concentrated desserts sweetened with sucrose) all will retard gastric emptying, thereby slowing the rate of overall carbohydrate assimilation. Despite these influences of ingested foods, once the stomach does empty, the intraluminal digestion of the starches is a highly efficient process that is restricted only by the physical state of the starch itself.

There is considerable variation in intestinal motility depending upon the meal composition and consequent differences in transit time through the small intestine, which may alter the rate of carbohydrate assimilation. However, in the absence of intestinal or pancreatic disease, the effect of intestinal motility on the overall assimilation of nutrients is small. Other than the physical condition of the ingested carbohydrate, particularly if it is starch, the most important factor determining the rate of carbohydrate assimilation is either enzymatic hydrolysis by the brush-border membrane oligosaccharidases or the transport of the released monosaccharides. Absorption of monosaccharide components released from starch or sucrose was as rapid as that from the same amount of carbohydrate given as the equivalent monosaccharide mixture, suggesting that the monosaccharide transporters may limit the rate of starch or sucrose assimilation. In contrast, the quantitative comparison of absorption of sugar from equimolar amounts of lactose versus glucose plus galactose by lactose-tolerant adults revealed that the assimilation of the hexoses was only about half as rapid from lactose as from the equimolar mixture of its components. This suggests that the membrane hydrolysis of lactose, rather than the transport of its products across the enterocyte, is the slowest step in the overall assimilation of lactose in lactose-tolerant adults.

PHENOTYPES OF CARBOHYDRATE AND SUGAR MALABSORPTION

The clinical phenotypes of lactase–phlorizin hydrolase and sucrase–isomaltase disaccharidase deficiencies are well understood, and progress has been made on understanding the genetic basis for these deficiencies (Treem, 1996; Buller and Grand 1990). An identical phenotype is observed if proximal defects of mucosal transport of monosaccharides are present.

Figure 8-7 depicts the consequences when lactase (or another disaccharidase or transporter) is appreciably reduced or absent from the enterocyte apical membrane surface. The proximal malabsorption of lactose (or sucrose or glucose/galactose) results in an increase in intraluminal osmolar load that delivers the undigested disaccharides and trapped fluid into the colon. In older children and adults,

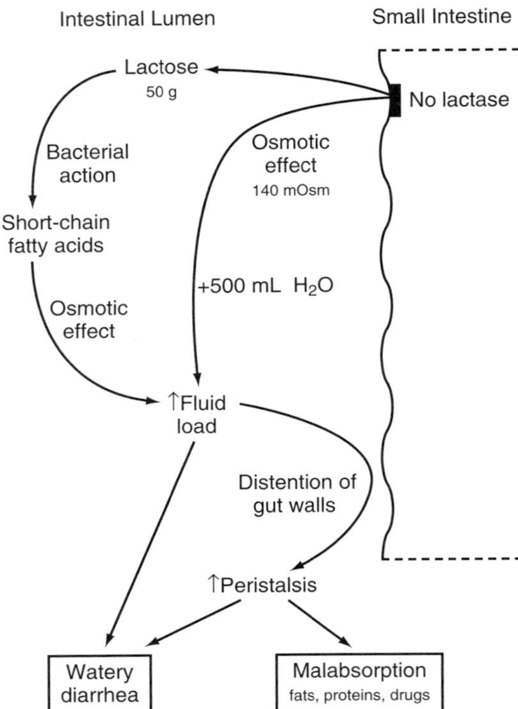

Figure 8-7 Pathogenesis of a carbohydrate malabsorption syndrome. Maldigestion of lactose allows bacteria to use it as substrate for fermentation, thereby producing short-chain fatty acids and gases. These products of fermentation increase the lumen osmolarity, which, in turn, leads to an increase in ileal and colonic water and augmentation of peristalsis of the gut, which can lead to secondary malabsorption of other nutrients. A block in any oligosaccharidase or hexose transporter would result in the same pathophysiological events. *(Modified from Gray GM [1983]) Intestinal disaccharidase deficiencies and glucose-galactose malabsorption. In: Stanbury JB, Wyngaarden JB, Fredrickson DS, Goldstein JL, Brown MS [eds] Metabolic Basis of Inherited Disease, 5th ed. Blakiston Division, McGraw Hill, New York, pp 1729-1742.)*

the colon activates a salvage pathway of carbohydrate fermentation and absorption through short-chain fatty acid products (acetate, propionate, and butyrate). This pathway requires the presence of normal bacterial flora in the colon to metabolize these disaccharides into the two- to four-carbon fatty acid products (Topping and Clifton 2001). The colonic fermentation of monosaccharides by bacteria also produces methane, carbon dioxide, and hydrogen gas. An increase in H_2 in the breath is used experimentally as evidence of increased salvage pathway digestion (i.e., fermentation). The fermentation products increase osmolarity and produce an increase in the quantity of fluid and gas in the lower small intestine and colon; this is manifested by symptoms of abdominal bloating and cramping discomfort; audible bowel sounds; and a watery, foamy diarrhea. In infants, the colonic fermentative pathway is often inadequate, and a diet-sensitive acidic osmotic diarrhea may occur with unmetabolized carbohydrate being passed in the stools. More severe symptoms, including vomiting, may develop.

The carbohydrate malabsorption phenotype is identical when a "primary" isolated disaccharidase or monosaccharide transporter deficiency is present as when mucosal damage has reduced the surface of the small intestine causing a "secondary" disaccharidase or monosaccharide transporter deficiency. The presence of mucosal inflammation can result in a "tertiary" deficiency without equivalent mucosal atrophy.

GENETIC DEFECTS IN CARBOHYDRATE DIGESTIVE OR ABSORPTIVE PROCESSES

Defects of amylase digestion of starch are rarely found. Although a small percentage of starch escapes α-amylase action, this is related to the polysaccharide's physical state rather than to a limiting quantity of the amylase. The amount of pancreatic amylase secreted in response to a meal is in great excess of the amount that is required for optimal intraluminal digestion of starch to the final oligosaccharide products. Therefore, a decrease in amylase amount or activity may not have a physiological consequence. In addition, a genetic redundancy may contribute to the rarity with which defects of amylase are found. In most humans, the genome contains two identical genes coding for salivary amylase (*AMY1A* and *AMY1B*) and two for pancreatic amylase (*AMY2A* and *AMY2B*), which are believed to be the result of gene duplication (Groot et al., 1989; Groot et al., 1988). The expression of only one of the copies or up to all four copies has been reported in different individuals (Iafrate et al., 2004).

Epidemiological studies of intestinal disaccharidase activities have revealed differences in the levels of disaccharidases among ethnic groups. For instance, among Greenland Eskimos of all ages, a relatively high number of subjects displayed a low level or total absence of both lactase–phlorizin hydrolase and sucrase–isomaltase activities (Kretchmer, 1971; Alzate et al., 1969; Gudmand-Hoyer and Jarnum 1969). Studies on normal and lactase-deficient (alactasic) subjects gave rise to a classification of the following three major phenotypes of intestinal lactase–phlorizin hydrolase activity:

1. Adult hypolactasia, corresponding to the "normal" phenotype in most of the world population, in which levels of lactase–phlorizin hydrolase activity observed at birth remain high until about 4 years of age and then fall during childhood or adolescence to about 10% of peak activity (Simoons, 1970)
2. Persistent adult lactasia, characteristic of the population of Northern European origin, in which the high lactase–phlorizin hydrolase activity present at birth persists throughout life (Kretchmer, 1985)
3. Congenital lactase–phlorizin hydrolase deficiency, in which extremely low or absent lactase–phlorizin hydrolase activity is present from birth, as found with frequency among Greenland Eskimo or Canadian Inuit populations (Montgomery et al., 1991)

After the description of congenital lactase–phlorizin hydrolase deficiencies, the search for genetic disorders of other disaccharidase activities led to discovery of deficiencies in the enzyme activities of the sucrase-isomaltase complex. Sucrase–isomaltase deficiency (asucrasia) is now one of the most frequently reported genetic intestinal disaccharidase deficiencies. The disorder may be present as an isolated sucrase deficiency, with normal levels of isomaltase activity, or as a combined sucrase and isomaltase deficiency (Jacob et al., 2000b; Moolenaar et al., 1997; Sterchi et al., 1990). Isolated deficiencies of the isomaltase subunit have not been reported, indicating that the correct processing of the sucrase–isomaltase polypeptide is dependent on the structure and function of the isomaltase subunit. The presence of an immunoreactive sucrase–isomaltase molecule has been demonstrated in all congenital sucrase–isomaltase deficiencies that have been studied. The bifunctional sucrase–isomaltase is either synthesized and transported to the apical membrane with a structurally altered and inactive sucrase subunit or contains mutations that block its movement to the apical membrane, causing it to accumulate in the cell until it undergoes degradation (Jacob et al., 2000b; Moolenaar et al., 1997; Sterchi et al., 1990).

Maltase–glucoamylase accounts for the largest activity degrading the glucose oligomers resulting from digestion of amylose and amylopectin. Despite the dependence of the last step of starch digestion on maltase–glucoamylase, no isolated genetically determined deficiency of maltase–glucoamylase (aglucoamylasia) has been clearly identified in humans. Most reported cases of maltase–glucoamylase deficiencies have been associated with other disaccharidase deficiencies (Karnsakul et al., 2002; Nichols et al., 2002; Lebenthal et al., 1994), suggesting that they may be caused by nongenetic factors or by defects in regulatory factors common to all intestinal glycohydrolases. Although polymorphisms have been found in human subjects who have maltase–glucoamylase deficiencies, no correlation has been observed between the genotype and the defective phenotype. The only recognized genetic deficiency of maltase–glucoamylase in mammals occurs in mice of the CBA/CaJ strain, which show an apparent deficiency in synthesis of the enzyme (Quezada-Calvillo et al., 1993). Interestingly, these mice, as well as maltase–glucoamylase knockout mice, do not show gross digestive disorders, although the maltase–glucoamylase knockout mice do appear to have an altered energy metabolism and a relatively low body fat content (unreported observations of authors).

Genetic trehalase deficiencies were first described among Inuit natives with a frequency of about 8% (Gudmand-Hoyer et al., 1988). However, more recent studies have shown a lower frequency of occurrence (0% to 3%) in Finnish and British subjects. The clinical symptoms observed in subjects with this disorder are similar to those of other disaccharidase deficiencies but have been found exclusively associated with the ingestion of mushrooms (Murray et al., 2000; Arola et al., 1999).

Another set of relatively rare genetic disorders involves structural defects in the glucose transporters SGLT1 and GLUT2. SGLT1 transports free glucose or galactose through the apical membrane into the cytoplasm of enterocytes in an active manner requiring cotransport of sodium (Wright et al., 2003; Brown, 2000). Mutations that cause a lack of processing and insertion of SGLT1 into the apical membrane, with its accumulation in Golgi compartments, and mutations that cause an impairment of the transport function of SGLT1 have been identified (Wright et al., 2003; Brown, 2000). Glucose–galactose malabsorption is usually identified in infancy and may be fatal unless all dietary carbohydrate is eliminated from the diet (Meeuwisse and Dahlquist 1968). Although patients with this discrete defect can absorb fructose, sucrose (which is hydrolyzed to yield both fructose and glucose) is not tolerated.

Mutations in GLUT2 do not appear to disrupt glucose and galactose absorption, and mutations of GLUT5 have not been reported for humans. The complementary roles of GLUT2 and GLUT5 in hexose transport may compensate for a loss of GLUT2 activity. GLUT2 is expressed in kidney, liver, and pancreatic β cells as well as in the enterocyte (Wright et al., 2003). GLUT2 transporters in

Clinical Correlation

Glucose and Galactose Malabsorption

Carbohydrate intolerance is a rare but very serious hereditary disorder. Cases due to lack of digestive enzyme (e.g., primary sucrase–isomaltase deficiency) and to impaired hexose transport (i.e., primary glucose–galactose malabsorption) have been reported. On the basis of experience in a Boston hospital, it was estimated that glucose–galactose malabsorption accounted for about 2% of the patients with protracted diarrhea of infancy (Lloyd-Still et al., 1988). In two reported cases of carbohydrate intolerance, the infants developed diarrhea soon after birth. Their stools contained reducing sugars and had an acidic pH. Analysis of tissue obtained by biopsy of the small intestine showed normal villi with normal disaccharidase values. Monosaccharide load tests showed a normal rise in blood glucose following a fructose load dose, which was tolerated well, in contrast to a flat glucose curve in response to a glucose load, which was accompanied by marked abdominal distention, profuse diarrhea, and the presence of reducing sugars in the stools.

Despite feeding a sugar-free formula plus fructose to these two patients with glucose–galactose malabsorption, diarrhea and the excretion of reducing sugars in the stool continued. This was due to a small amount of tapioca starch (25 g/L formula, which supplied more than 12.5 g starch per day for these patients) in the "sugar-free" formula that was being used. Rigid exclusion of all carbohydrates and sugars except for fructose resulted in cessation of diarrhea and elimination of sugars from the stools.

Thinking Critically

1. These patients were diagnosed before the hexose transporters had been identified. Which hexose transport protein was probably lacking in these patients?
2. If the plasma glucose concentration had been monitored in these two patients following a load dose of sucrose, would a rise in plasma glucose have been observed? What would be observed following a loading dose of lactose?
3. How would you expect the findings (carbohydrate tolerance, the glucose load test results, and the intestinal biopsy results) to differ in a case of secondary disaccharidase deficiency due to infective gastroenteritis (i.e., rotavirus infection) compared to those reported for these infants with hereditary carbohydrate intolerance?

the pancreas are believed to contribute to the sensing of circulating glucose levels necessary for the regulation of insulin secretion. Genetic structural alterations of this transporter are the main causative factor of the Fanconi-Bickel syndrome, a rare inherited recessive autosomal disorder consisting of hepatorenal glycogen accumulation, proximal renal tubular dysfunction, and impaired utilization of glucose and galactose (Wright et al., 2003; Brown, 2000).

ACQUIRED DEFICIENCIES OF CARBOHYDRATE DIGESTION

The most common cause of carbohydrate malabsorption syndrome is the hypolactasia that can develop in children anytime from shortly after weaning until the early teenage years. As mentioned in the preceding text, this occurs in a high proportion of the world's population groups because of a reduction in lactase expression at the enterocyte brush-border surface, and it must be considered to be the normal condition of most healthy adults worldwide. Even among Caucasians of Northern European heritage, hypolactasia develops in 5% to 20% of adult individuals. The capacity to digest lactose, even in individuals who retain high lactase activity throughout adulthood, is relatively limited compared to that for digestion of starch or sucrose.

Nutrition Insight

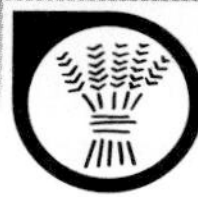

Polymorphisms and Lactase Expression in Adulthood

The genetic basis of the phenotype of lactase–phlorizin hydrolase persistence into adulthood is unknown. However, polymorphisms of C/T at −13910 and of G/A at −22018 upstream of the transcriptional start site for the human lactase–phlorizin hydrolase gene have been associated with transcriptional regulation of the gene (Mitchelmore et al., 1998). Located in introns 8 and 13 of the neighboring *MCM6* gene, the −13910C polymorphism associates 100% and the −22018G associates 97% with the lactase–phlorizin hydrolase nonpersistent phenotype of the Finnish population. In all family members who were studied, those with the nonpersistent phenotype were homozygous with respect to both −13910C and −22018G (Kuokkanen et al., 2003). The −13910 C/T polymorphism is located in a transcriptional enhancer sequence, and the −13910C variant less strongly activates the lactase–phlorizin hydrolase promoter activity than the corresponding −13910T variant. The variant −13910C is associated with the nonpersistent phenotype in both Finnish and non-Finnish populations. A consensus binding motif for the transcription factor AP-2 is present in the −13910C allele, but this binding motif is disrupted in the −13910T variant associated with lactase–phlorizin hydrolase persistence. It is possible that the AP-2 element has a long-range *cis*-transcriptional effect on developmental stage-specific regulation of lactase–phlorizin hydrolase (Olds and Sibley 2003; Troelsen et al., 2003b).

Troelsen and colleagues (2003b) proposed a model mechanism that might explain the normal downregulation of lactase–phlorizin hydrolase that results in hypolactasia in most adults. Transcription factors necessary for lactase–phlorizin hydrolase expression are present in excess during early childhood. After weaning, expression of HNF-1α and certain other transcription factors is decreased and, thus, competition of various genes for these transcriptional activators is greater. These competitive changes result in lower lactase–phlorizin hydrolase expression owing to the weak nature of the lactase–phlorizin hydrolase promoter. However, the strong enhancer effect of the −13910T variant compensates for these changes and is able to keep the lactase–phlorizin hydrolase gene active, giving the phenotype of lactase–phlorizin hydrolase persistence (Troelsen et al., 2003b). The effect of the −22018G/A polymorphism on the lactase–phlorizin hydrolase promoter activity is minimal, but the −22018G polymorphism seems to favor the enhancer activity of the −13910 region (Troelsen et al., 2003b).

The processes of starch and oligosaccharide digestion and final monosaccharide transport are usually very efficient, enabling total assimilation of ingested starch and disaccharides. Indeed, most starch is digested within the duodenal lumen. This is rapidly followed by hydrolysis at the lumen–enterocyte interface and by hexose transport within the proximal half of the small intestine. Although the ileum usually plays little role in starch digestion and absorption, the ileum can adapt to assume a more important role in carbohydrate digestion and absorption in the case of extensive jejunal disease or surgical removal of the upper small intestine.

Pathological states of the small intestine, such as celiac disease (gluten-sensitive enteropathy) and Crohn's disease, are associated with mucosal inflammation, atrophy, and deficiencies of multiple disaccharidase activities (Heitlinger et al., 1991; Horvath et al., 1983). Similarly, systemic inflammatory processes such as human immunodeficiency virus (HIV) infection can induce deficiencies of disaccharidases in the absence of mucosal atrophy (Albert and Young 1992; Bohmer, 1979). In some instances, the levels of disaccharidase deficiencies have not been correlated with morphological changes of the epithelium or with loss of other mucosal enzymes (Shulman et al., 1991; Phillips et al., 1988), suggesting that the defects can be caused by regulatory changes in enterocytes as well as to structural damage and loss of enterocytes.

The presence of low levels of disaccharidase activities is commonly observed in malnutrition. Protein- and iron-deficient diets have been found to induce a reversible deficiency of lactase–phlorizin hydrolase, sucrase–isomaltase, and maltase–glucoamylase activities, particularly during postnatal development (Fernandes et al., 1997; Jambunathan et al., 1981; Greene et al., 1975).

Other pathological conditions associated with deficiencies of intestinal disaccharidases are infections by diverse etiological agents. The deleterious effects that intestinal parasitic infections have on the activities of disaccharidases have been widely studied, in particular those caused by giardiasis (Buret et al., 1990; Belosevic et al., 1989). Nematodes *Nippostrongylus* sp. and *Trichinella spirallis* are also examples of intestinal parasites that have been observed to cause disaccharidase deficiencies (D'Inca et al., 1992; Jones, 1983). Although there are few studies examining the effects of bacterial infections on intestinal disaccharidases, toxins of bacterial origin can cause changes in the activity of intestinal disaccharidases (Chitra et al., 2002; Kohli et al., 1989). In rotaviral disease, the most common cause of diarrhea in children, there is a reduction in sucrase–isomaltase and lactase–phlorizin hydrolase activities (Martin-Latil et al., 2004; Boshuizen et al., 2003; LaMonica et al., 2001; Jourdan et al., 1998 (Collins et al., 1990; Collins et al., 1988). The effects of parasites, bacteria, and viruses on small intestinal disaccharidases may be mediated either by induction of metabolic changes in the enterocytes or by direct binding of the organisms to the carbohydrate moieties of the respective enzymes (Pothoulakis et al., 1996).

A series of other factors external to the hydrolytic ability of the gastrointestinal tract may modify the absorption of dietary carbohydrate. Physicochemical properties of the carbohydrates, such as the degree of crystallization or moisture or the presence of physical barriers, can affect the ability of the gastrointestinal tract to digest them. For instance, retrograde starch, which contains a more crystalline arrangement of molecules than natural starch, is refractory to hydrolysis by amylase and maltase–glucoamylase.

Diverse chemicals with the ability to act as inhibitors of glucohydrolytic enzymes have been used clinically or experimentally. For instance, Trizma base [2-amino-2-(hydroxymethyl)-1,3-propanediol], a low toxicity amino alcohol used on occasion to treat acidemia, is a potent reversible inhibitor of intestinal disaccharidases (Nahas et al., 1998). This compound forms part of one of the laboratory techniques used widely for the measurement of disaccharidase activities (Dahlqvist, 1984). Similarly, acarbose, a low toxicity aryl-trisaccharide analog of maltotetrose, is a strong glucosidase inhibitor. It is used therapeutically to control blood glucose levels in patients with type 1 or 2 diabetes and also it may have some potential as an aid in the control of obesity (Wolffenbuttel and Graal, 1996; Hanefeld et al., 1991;

Clissold and Edwards, 1988). Salicinol, a thiosugar with a sulfate ion–containing side chain that has a strong inhibitory effect on glucosidases, is the main active pharmacological component present in *Salacia reticulate*, a plant used in India to prepare natural antiglucemic formulations for diabetic patients (Yuasa et al., 2001; Wolffenbuttel and Graal 1996).

THERAPY FOR CARBOHYDRATE MALABSORPTION SYNDROMES

Although carbohydrates are a relatively inexpensive source of calories, they are not essential for overall nutrition. Therefore, the main approach to therapy, once a defect in carbohydrate digestion or absorption has been identified, is the elimination of the particular offending carbohydrate from the diet. Thus for individuals with hypolactasia, it is often necessary to avoid dairy products, the main source of lactose. However, because milk products are an excellent source of nutrients, it is often beneficial to add a lactose hydrolyzing enzyme, such as β-galactosidase purified from organisms, to the dairy products to promote digestion of the lactose (Lin et al., 1993). Fermented milk products may be acceptable due to their lower lactose content. Similarly, the sucrose hydrolyzing enzyme from yeast has been shown to be usable as a supplement in patients with sucrase–isomaltase deficiency (Treem et al., 1993).

REFERENCES

Albert V, Young GP (1992) Differentiation status of rat enterocytes after intestinal adaptation to jejunoileal bypass. Gut 33(12):1638-1643.

Alfalah M, Jacob R, Preuss U, Zimmer KP, Naim H, Naim HY (1999) *O*-linked glycans mediate apical sorting of human intestinal sucrase-isomaltase through association with lipid rafts. Curr Biol 9:593-596.

Alzate H, Gonzalez H, Guzman J (1969) Lactose intolerance in South American Indians. Am J Clin Nutr 22:122-123.

Arola H, Koivula T, Karvonen AL, Jokela H, Ahola T, Isokoski M (1999) Low trehalase activity is associated with abdominal symptoms caused by edible mushrooms. Scand J Gastroenterol 34:898-903.

Asano N, Kato A, Matsui K (1996) Two subsites on the active center of pig kidney trehalase. Eur J Biochem 240:692-698.

Baumann FC, Boizard-Callais F, Labat-Robert J (1981) Trehalase activity in genetically diabetic mice (serum, kidney, and liver). J Med Genet 18:418-423.

Belosevic M, Faubert GM, Maclean JD (1989) Disaccharidase activity in the small intestine of gerbils (Meriones unguiculatus) during primary and challenge infections with Giardia lamblia. Gut 30:1213-1219.

Ben Ali H, Guerin JF, Pinatel MC, Mathieu C, Boulieu D, Tritar B (1994) Relationship between semen characteristics, alpha-glucosidase and the capacity of spermatozoa to bind to the human zona pellucida. Int J Androl 17:121-126.

Blakemore SJ, Aledo JC, James J, Campbell FC, Lucocq JM, Hundal HS (1995) The GLUT5 hexose transporter is also localized to the basolateral membrane of the human jejunum. Biochem J 309(Pt 1):7-12.

Bohmer R (1979) Ligation or external fistulation of the common bile duct in the rat. II. Intestinal disaccharidase activities. Digestion 19:32-41.

Boshuizen JA, Reimerink JH, Korteland-van Male AM, van Ham VJ, Koopmans MP, Buller HA, Dekkev J, Einevhand AW (2003) Changes in small intestinal homeostasis,morphology, and gene expression during rotavirus infection of infant mice. J Virol 77:13005-13016.

Buller HA, Dekker J, Einerhand AW (2003) Changes in small intestinal homeostasis, morphology, and gene expression during rotavirus infection of infant mice. J Virol 77:13005-13016.

Boudreau F, Rings EH, van Wering HM, Kim RK, Swain GP, Krasinski SD, Moffett J, Grand RJ, Suh ER, Traber PG (2002) Hepatocyte nuclear factor-1 alpha, GATA-4, and caudal related homeodomain protein Cdx2 interact functionally to modulate intestinal gene transcription. Implication for the developmental regulation of the sucrase-isomaltase gene. J Biol Chem 277:31909-31917.

Boudreau F, Zhu Y, Traber PG (2001) Sucrase-isomaltase gene transcription requires the hepatocyte nuclear factor-1 (HNF-1) regulatory element and is regulated by the ratio of HNF-1 alpha to HNF-1 beta. J Biol Chem 276: 32122-32128.

Brand-Miller JC (2003) Glycemic load and chronic disease. Nutr Rev 61:S49-S55.

Brand-Miller JC, Thomas M, Swan V, Ahmad ZI, Petocz P, Colagiuri S (2003) Physiological validation of the concept of glycemic load in lean young adults. J Nutr 133:2728-2732.

Brown GK (2000) Glucose transporters: structure, function and consequences of deficiency. J Inherit Metab Dis 23:237-246.

Buller HA, Grand RJ (1990) Lactose intolerance. Annu Rev Med 41:141-148.

Buller HA, Van Wassenaer AG, Raghavan S, Montgomery RK, Sybicki MA, Grand RJ (1989) New insights into lactase and glycosylceramidase activities of rat lactase-phlorizin hydrolase. Am J Physiol 257:G616-G623.

Buret A, Gall DG, Nation PN, Olson ME (1990) Intestinal protozoa and epithelial cell kinetics, structure and function. Parasitology Today 6:375-380.

Burrin DG, Stoll B, Fan MZ, Dudley MA, Donovan SM, Reeds PJ (2001) Oral IGF-I alters the post-translational processing but not the activity of lactase-phlorizin hydrolase in formula-fed neonatal pigs. J Nutr 131:2235-2241.

Buts JP, De Keyser N, Dive C (1988) Intestinal development in the suckling rat: effect of insulin on the maturation of villus and crypt cell functions. Eur J Clin Invest 18:391-398.

Chantret I, Lacasa M, Chevalier G, Ruf J, Islam I, Mantei N, Edwards Y, Swallow D, Rousset M (1992) Sequence of the complete cDNA and the 5′ structure of the human sucrase-isomaltase gene. Possible homology with a yeast glucoamylase. Biochem J 285:915-923.

Chao JC, Donovan S (1996) Effects of insulin, insulin-like growth factors and epidermal growth factor on mitogenesis and disaccharidase activity in rat (IEC-6) and human (FHs 74 Int) intestinal cells. Chin J Physiol 39:253-263.

Chen CC, Guo WJ, Isselbacher KJ (1987) Rat intestinal trehalase. Studies of the active site. Biochem J 247:715-724.

Chitra, Sun P, Mahmood S (2002) Effect of Salmonella typhimurium toxin on the expression of rabbit intestinal functions. Indian J Med Res 116:186-191.

Choi RS, Riegler M, Pothoulakis C, Kim BS, Mooney D, Vacanti M, Vacanti JP (1998) Studies of brush border enzymes, basement membrane components, and electrophysiology of tissue-engineered neointestine. J Pediatr Surg 33:991-996.

Chung BM, Wallace LE, Hardin JA, Gall DG (2002) The effect of epidermal growth factor on the distribution of SGLT-1 in rabbit jejunum. Can J Physiol Pharmacol 80:872-878.

Clissold SP, Edwards C (1988) Acarbose. A preliminary review of its pharmacodynamic and pharmacokinetic properties, and therapeutic potential. Drugs 35:214-243.

Collins J, Candy DC, Starkey WG, Spencer AJ, Osborne MP, Stephen J (1990) Disaccharidase activities in small intestine of rotavirus-infected suckling mice: a histochemical study. J Pediatr Gastroenterol Nutr 11:395-403.

Collins J, Starkey WG, Wallis TS, Clarke GJ, Worton KJ, Spencer AJ, Haddon SJ, Osborne MP, Candy DC, Stephen J (1988) Intestinal enzyme profiles in normal and rotavirus-infected mice. J Pediatr Gastroenterol Nutr 7:264-272.

Corpe CP, Burant CF (1996) Hexose transporter expression in rat small intestine: effect of diet on diurnal variations. Am J Physiol 271: G211-G216.

Cowell GM, Tranum-Jensen J, Sjostrom H, Noren O (1986) Topology and quaternary structure of pro-sucrase/isomaltase and final-form sucrase/isomaltase. Biochem J 237:455-461.

Cui XL, Ananian C, Perez E, Strenger A, Beuve AV, Ferraris RP (2004a) Cyclic AMP stimulates fructose transport in neonatal rat small intestine. J Nutr 134:1697-1703.

Cui XL, Soteropoulos P, Tolias P, Ferraris RP (2004b) Fructose-responsive genes in the small intestine of neonatal rats. Physiol Genomics 18:206-217.

D'Inca R, Ernst P, Hunt RH, Perdue MH (1992) Role of T lymphocytes in intestinal mucosal injury. Inflammatory changes in athymic nude rats. Dig Dis Sci 37:33-39.

Dahlqvist A (1962) Specificity of the human intestinal disaccharidases and implications for hereditary disaccharide intolerance. J Clin Invest 41:463-469.

Dahlqvist A (1984) Assay of intestinal disaccharidases. Scand J Clin Lab Invest 44:169-172.

Danielsen EM (1982) Biosynthesis of intestinal microvillar proteins. Pulse-chase labelling studies on aminopeptidase N and sucrase-isomaltase. Biochem J 204:639-645.

Danielsen EM, Hansen GH (2003) Lipid rafts in epithelial brush borders: atypical membrane microdomains with specialized functions. Biochim Biophys Acta 1617:1-9.

Danielsen EM, Skovbjerg H, Noren O, Sjostrom H (1984) Biosynthesis of intestinal microvillar proteins. Intracellular processing of lactase-phlorizin hydrolase. Biochem Biophys Res Commun 122:82-90.

Dudley MA, Burrin DG, Quaroni A, Rosenberger J, Cook G, Nichols BL, Reeds PJ (1996)

Lactase phlorhizin hydrolase turnover in vivo in water-fed and colostrum-fed newborn pigs. Biochem J 320:735-743.

Dudley MA, Wykes LJ, Dudley AW Jr, Burrin DG, Nichols BL, Rosenberger J, Jahoor F, Heird WC, Reeds (1998) Parenteral nutrition selectively decreases protein synthesis in the small intestine. Am J Physiol 274:G131-G137.

Duluc I, Freund JN, Leberquier C, Kedinger M (1994) Fetal endoderm primarily holds the temporal and positional information required for mammalian intestinal development. J Cell Biol 126:211-221.

Elbein AD, Pan YT, Pastuszak I, Carroll D (2003) New insights on trehalose: a multifunctional molecule. Glycobiology 13:17R-27R.

Fernandes MI, Galvao LC, Bortolozzi MF, Oliveira WP, Zucoloto S, Bianchi ML (1997) Disaccharidase levels in normal epithelium of the small intestine of rats with iron-deficiency anemia. Braz.J Med Biol Res 30:849-854.

Foda MI, Kawashima T, Nakamura S, Kobayashi M, Oku T (2004) Composition of milk obtained from unmassaged versus massaged breasts of lactating mothers. J Pediatr Gastroenterol Nutr 38:484-487.

Fogel MR, Gray GM (1973) Starch hydrolysis in man: an intraluminal process not requiring membrane digestion. J Appl Physiol 35: 263-267.

Fransen JA, Hauri HP, Ginsel LA, Naim HY (1991) Naturally occurring mutations in intestinal sucrase-isomaltase provide evidence for the existence of an intracellular sorting signal in the isomaltase subunit. J Cell Biol 115:45-57.

Galand G (1984) Purification and characterization of kidney and intestinal brush-border membrane trehalases from the rabbit. Biochim Biophys Acta 789:10-19.

Galand G (1986) Maltase-glucoamylase and trehalase in the rabbit small intestine and kidney brush border membranes during postnatal development, the effects of hydrocortisone. Comp Biochem.Physiol A 85:109-115.

Galand G (1989) Brush border membrane sucrase-isomaltase, maltase-glucoamylase and trehalase in mammals. Comparative development, effects of glucocorticoids, molecular mechanisms, and phylogenetic implications. Comp Biochem Physiol B 94:1-11.

Gartner H, Shukla P, Markesich DC, Solomon NS, Oesterreicher TJ, Henning SJ (2002) Developmental expression of trehalase: role of transcriptional activation. Biochim Biophys Acta 1574:329-336.

Goda T, Koldovsky O (1985) Evidence of degradation process of sucrase-isomaltase in jejunum of adult rats. Biochem J 229:751-758.

Gouyon F, Caillaud L, Carriere V, Klein C, Dalet V, Citadelle D, Kellett GL, Thorens B, Leturque A, Brot-Laroche E (2003a) Simple-sugar meals target GLUT2 at enterocyte apical membranes to improve sugar absorption: a study in GLUT2-null mice. J Physiol 552:823-832.

Gouyon F, Onesto C, Dalet V, Pages G, Leturque A, Brot-Laroche E (2003b) Fructose modulates GLUT5 mRNA stability in differentiated Caco-2 cells: role of cAMP-signalling pathway and PABP (polyadenylated-binding protein)-interacting protein (Paip) 2. Biochem J 375:167-174.

Greene HL, McCabe DR, Merenstein GB (1975) Protracted diarrhea and malnutrition in infancy: changes in intestinal morphology and disaccharidase activities during treatment with total intravenous nutrition or oral elemental diets. J Pediatr 87:695-704.

Groot PC, Bleeker MJ, Pronk JC, Arwert F, Mager WH, Planta RJ, Eriksson (1988) Human pancreatic amylase is encoded by two different genes. Nucleic Acids Res 16:4724.

Groot PC, Bleeker MJ, Pronk JC, Arwert F, Mager WH, Planta RJ, Eriksson (1989) The human alpha-amylase multigene family consists of haplotypes with variable numbers of genes. Genomics 5:29-42.

Gudmand-Hoyer E, Fenger HJ, Skovbjerg H, Kern-Hansen P, Madsen PR (1988) Trehalase deficiency in Greenland. Scand J Gastroenterol 23:775-778.

Gudmand-Hoyer E, Jarnum S (1969) Lactose malabsorption in Greenland Eskimos. Acta Med Scand 186:235-237.

Hanefeld M, Fischer S, Schulze J, Spengler M, Wargenau M, Schollberg K, Fucker K (1991) Therapeutic potentials of acarbose as first-line drug in NIDDM insufficiently treated with diet alone. Diabetes Care 14:732-737.

Hauri HP, Sterchi EE, Bienz D, Fransen JA, Marxer A (1985) Expression and intracellular transport of microvillus membrane hydrolases in human intestinal epithelial cells. J Cell Biol 101: 838-851.

Heitlinger LA, Rossi TM, Lee PC, Lebenthal E (1991) Human intestinal disaccharidase activities: correlations with age, biopsy technique, and degree of villus atrophy. J Pediatr Gastroenterol Nutr 12:204-208.

Helliwell PA, Rumsby MG, Kellett GL (2003) Intestinal sugar absorption is regulated by phosphorylation and turnover of protein kinase

C betaII mediated by phosphatidylinositol 3-kinase- and mammalian target of rapamycin-dependent pathways. J Biol Chem 278: 28644-28650.

Heymann H, Breitmeier D, Gunther S (1995) Human small intestinal sucrase-isomaltase: different binding patterns for malto- and isomaltooligosaccharides. Biol Chem Hoppe Seyler 376:249-253.

Heymann H, Gunther S (1994) Calculation of subsite affinities of human small intestinal glucoamylase-maltase. Biol Chem Hoppe Seyler 375:451-455.

Hirsch JR, Loo DD, Wright EM (1996) Regulation of Na^+/glucose cotransporter expression by protein kinases in Xenopus laevis oocytes. J Biol Chem 271:14740-14746.

Horvath K, Horn G, Bodanszky H, Toth K, Varadi S (1983) Disaccharidases in coeliac disease. Acta Paediatr Hung. 24:131-136.

Hu CB, Spiess M, Semenza G (1987) The mode of anchoring and precursor forms of sucrase-isomaltase and maltase-glucoamylase in chicken intestinal brush-border membrane. Phylogenetic implications. Biochim Biophys Acta 896:275-286.

Hunziker W, Spiess M, Semenza G, Lodish HF (1986) The sucrase-isomaltase complex: primary structure, membrane-orientation, and evolution of a stalked, intrinsic brush border protein. Cell 46:227-234.

Iafrate AJ, Feuk L, Rivera MN, Listewnik ML, Donahoe PK, Qi Y, Scherer SW, Lee C (2004) Detection of large-scale variation in the human genome. Nat Genet 36:949-951.

Ishihara R, Taketani S, Sasai-Takedatsu M, Kino M, Tokunaga R, Kobayashi Y (1997) Molecular cloning, sequencing and expression of cDNA encoding human trehalase. Gene 202:69-74.

Jacob R, Alfalah M, Grunberg J, Obendorf M, Naim HY (2000a) Structural determinants required for apical sorting of an intestinal brush-border membrane protein. J Biol Chem 275:6566-6572.

Jacob R, Heine M, Alfalah M, Naim HY (2003) Distinct cytoskeletal tracks direct individual vesicle populations to the apical membrane of epithelial cells. Curr Biol 13:607-612.

Jacob R, Heine M, Eikemeyer J, Frerker N, Zimmer KP, Rescher U, Gerke V, Naim HY (2004) Annexin II is required for apical transport in polarized epithelial cells. J Biol Chem 279:3680-3684.

Jacob R, Purschel B, Naim HY (2002) Sucrase is an intramolecular chaperone located at the C-terminal end of the sucrase-isomaltase enzyme complex. J Biol Chem 277: 32141-32148.

Jacob R, Radebach I, Wuthrich M, Grunberg J, Sterchi EE, Naim HY (1996) Maturation of human intestinal lactase-phlorizin hydrolase: generation of the brush border form of the enzyme involves at least two proteolytic cleavage steps. Eur J Biochem 236:789-795.

Jacob R, Zimmer KP, Schmitz J, Naim HY (2000b) Congenital sucrase-isomaltase deficiency arising from cleavage and secretion of a mutant form of the enzyme. J Clin Invest 106:281-287.

Jambunathan LR, Neuhoff D, Younoszai MK (1981) Intestinal disaccharidases in malnourished infant rats. Am J Clin Nutr 34:1879-1884.

Jenkins DJ, Wolever TM, Taylor RH, Barker H, Fielden H, Baldwin JM, Bowling AC, Newman HC, Jenkins AL, Goff DV (1981) Glycemic index of foods: a physiological basis for carbohydrate exchange. Am J Clin Nutr 34: 362-366.

Jones DG (1983) Intestinal enzyme activity in lambs chronically infected with Trichostrongylus colubriformis: effect of anthelmintic treatment. Vet Parasitol 12:79-89.

Jourdan N, Brunet JP, Sapin C, Blais A, Cotte-Laffitte J, Forestier F, Quero AM, Trugnan G, Servin AL (1998) Rotavirus infection reduces sucrase-isomaltase expression in human intestinal epithelial cells by perturbing protein targeting and organization of microvillar cytoskeleton. J Virol 72:7228-7236.

Kaiser T, Sawicki PT (2004) Acarbose for prevention of diabetes, hypertension and cardiovascular events? A critical analysis of the STOP-NIDDM data. Diabetologia 47:575-580.

Kalus I, Hodel A, Koch A, Kleene R, Edwardson JM, Schrader M (2002) Interaction of syncollin with GP-2, the major membrane protein of pancreatic zymogen granules, and association with lipid microdomains. Biochem J 362: 433-442.

Karnsakul W, Luginbuehl U, Hahn D, Sterchi E, Avery S, Sen P, Swallow D, Nichols B (2002) Disaccharidase activities in dyspeptic children: biochemical and molecular investigations of maltase-glucoamylase activity. J Pediatr Gastroenterol Nutr 35:551-556.

Kast RE (2002) Acarbose related diarrhea: increased butyrate upregulates prostaglandin E. Inflamm Res 51:117-118.

Kendall K, Jumawan J, Koldovsky O (1979) Development of jejunoileal differences of activity of lactase, sucrase and acid beta-galactosidase in isografts of fetal rat intestine. Biol Neonate 36:206-214.

Kien CL, Heitlinger LA, Li BU, Murray RD (1989) Digestion, absorption, and fermentation of carbohydrates. Semin Perinatol 13:78-87.

Kohli M, Ganguly NK, Garg UC, Goyal J, Majumdar S, Walia BN (1989) Effect of heat-stable and heat-labile enterotoxins of Escherichia coli on intestinal brush border membrane enzymes of mice. Biochem Int 19:173-183.

Krasinski SD, van Wering HM, Tannemaat MR, Grand RJ (2001) Differential activation of intestinal gene promoters: functional interactions between GATA-5 and HNF-1 alpha. Am J Physiol Gastrointest Liver Physiol 281:G69-G84.

Kretchmer N (1971) Memorial Lecture: Lactose and lactase–a historical perspective. Gastroenterology 61:805-813.

Kretchmer N (1985) Weaning: enzymatic adaptation. Am J Clin Nutr 41(2 Suppl):391-398.

Kruse TA, Bolund L, Grzeschik KH, Ropers HH, Sjostrom H, Noren O, Mantei N, Semenza G (1988) The human lactase-phlorizin hydrolase gene is located on chromosome 2. FEBS Lett 240:123-126.

Kuokkanen M, Enattah NS, Oksanen A, Savilahti E, Orpana A, Jarvela I (2003) Transcriptional regulation of the lactase-phlorizin hydrolase gene by polymorphisms associated with adult-type hypolactasia. Gut 52:647-652.

LaMonica R, Kocer SS, Nazarova J, Dowling W, Geimonen E, Shaw RD, Mackow ER (2001) VP4 differentially regulates TRAF2 signaling, disengaging JNK activation while directing NF-kappa B to effect rotavirus-specific cellular responses. J Biol Chem 276:19889-19896.

Lebenthal E, Khin MU, Zheng BY, Lu RB, Lerner A (1994) Small intestinal glucoamylase deficiency and starch malabsorption: a newly recognized alpha-glucosidase deficiency in children. J Pediatr 124:541-546.

Lebenthal E, Lee PC, Heitlinger LA (1983) Impact of development of the gastrointestinal tract on infant feeding. J Pediatr 102:1-9.

Lillford PJ, Holt CB (2002) In vitro uses of biological cryoprotectants. Philos Trans R Soc Lond B Biol Sci 357:945-951.

Lin MY, DiPalma JA, Martini MC, Gross CJ, Harlander SK, Savaiano DA (1993) Comparative effects of exogenous lactase (beta-galactosidase) preparations on in vivo lactose digestion. Dig Dis Sci 38:2022-2027.

Lloyd-Still JD, Listernick R, Buentello G (1988) Complex carbohydrate intolerance: diagnostic pitfalls and approach to management. J Pediatr 112:709-713.

Loo DDF, Zeuthen T, Chandry G, Wright EM (1996) Cotransport of water by Na^+/glucose cotransporter. Proc Natl Acad Sci USA 93:13367-13370.

Mackey AD, McMahon RJ, Townsend JH, Gregory JF, III (2004) Uptake, hydrolysis, and metabolism of pyridoxine-5′-beta-D-glucoside in Caco-2 cells. J Nutr 134:842-846.

Malo C, Menard D (1982) Influence of epidermal growth factor on the development of suckling mouse intestinal mucosa. Gastroenterology 83:28-35.

Mantei N, Villa M, Enzler T, Wacker H, Boll W, James P, Hunziker W, Semenza G (1988) Complete primary structure of human and rabbit lactase-phlorizin hydrolase: implications for biosynthesis, membrane anchoring and evolution of the enzyme. EMBO J 7:2705-2713.

Marquis GS, Penny ME, Zimmer JP, Diaz JM, Marin RM (2003) An overlap of breastfeeding during late pregnancy is associated with subsequent changes in colostrum composition and morbidity rates among Peruvian infants and their mothers. J Nutr 133:2585-2591.

Martin-Latil S, Cotte-Laffitte J, Beau I, Quero AM, Geniteau-Legendre M, Servin AL (2004) A cyclic AMP protein kinase A-dependent mechanism by which rotavirus impairs the expression and enzyme activity of brush border-associated sucrase-isomaltase in differentiated intestinal Caco-2 cells. Cell Microbiol 6:719-731.

McDonald MC, Henning SJ (1992) Synergistic effects of thyroxine and dexamethasone on enzyme ontogeny in rat small intestine. Pediatr Res 32:306-311.

Meeuwisse GW, Dahlqvist A (1968) Glucose-galactose malabsorption. A study with biopsy of the small intestinal mucosa. Acta Paediatr Scand 57:273-280.

Mehta DI, Horvath K, Chanasongcram S, Hill ID, Panigrahi P (1997) Epidermal growth factor up-regulates sodium-glucose cotransport in enterocyte models in the presence of cholera toxin. J Parenter Enteral Nutr 21:185-191.

Menard D, Arsenault P, Gallo-Payet N (1986) Epidermal growth factor does not act as a primary cue for inducing developmental changes in suckling mouse jejunum. J Pediatr Gastroenterol Nutr 5:949-955.

Mitchelmore C, Troelsen JT, Sjostrom H, Noren O (1998) The HOXC11 homeodomain protein interacts with the lactase-phlorizin hydrolase promoter and stimulates HNF1alpha-dependent transcription. J Biol Chem 273:13297-13306.

Mobassaleh M, Montgomery RK, Biller JA, Grand RJ (1985) Development of carbohydrate absorption in the fetus and neonate. Pediatrics 75:160-166.
Montgomery RK, Buller HA, Rings EHHM, Grand RJ (1991) Lactose intolerance and the genetic regulation of intestinal lactase-phlorizin hydrolase. FASEB J 5:2824-2832.
Moolenaar CE, Ouwendijk J, Wittpoth M, Wisselaar HA, Hauri HP, Ginsel LA, Naim HY, Fransen JA (1997) A mutation in a highly conserved region in brush-border sucrase-isomaltase and lysosomal alpha-glucosidase results in Golgi retention. J Cell Sci 110: 557-567.
Murray IA, Coupland K, Smith JA, Ansell ID, Long RG (2000) Intestinal trehalase activity in a UK population: establishing a normal range and the effect of disease. Br J Nutr 83:241-245.
Nahas GG, Sutin KM, Fermon C, Streat S, Wiklund L, Wahlander S, Yellin P, Brasch H, Kanchuger M, Capan L, Manne J, Helwig H, Gaab M, Pfenninger E, Wetterberg T, Holmdahl M, Turndorf H (1998) Guidelines for the treatment of acidaemia with THAM. Drugs 55:191-224.
Naim HY, Lentze MJ (1992) Impact of O-glycosylation on the function of human intestinal lactase-phlorizin hydrolase. Characterization of glycoforms varying in enzyme activity and localization of O-glycoside addition. J Biol Chem 267:25494-25504.
Naim HY, Sterchi EE, Lentze MJ (1987) Biosynthesis and maturation of lactase-phlorizin hydrolase in the human small intestinal epithelial cells. Biochem J 241:427-434.
Naim HY, Sterchi EE, Lentze MJ (1988) Structure, biosynthesis, and glycosylation of human small intestinal maltase-glucoamylase. J Biol Chem 263:19709-19717.
Nakano M, Sacktor B (1984) Renal trehalase: two subsites at the substrate-binding site. Biochim Biophys Acta 791:45-49.
Nichols BL, Avery S, Sen P, Swallow DM, Hahn D, Sterchi E (2003) The maltase-glucoamylase gene: common ancestry to sucrase-isomaltase with complementary starch digestion activities. Proc Natl Acad Sci USA 100: 1432-1437.
Nichols BL, Avery SE, Karnsakul W, Jahoor F, Sen P, Swallow DM, Luginbuehl U, Hahn D, Sterchi EE (2002) Congenital maltase-glucoamylase deficiency associated with lactase and sucrase deficiencies. J Pediatr Gastroenterol Nutr 35:573-579.
Nichols BL, Eldering J, Avery S, Hahn D, Quaroni A, Sterchi E (1998) Human small intestinal maltase-glucoamylase cDNA cloning. Homology to sucrase-isomaltase. J Biol Chem 273:3076-3081.
O'Loughlin EV, Chung M, Hollenberg M, Hayden J, Zahavi I, Gall DG (1985) Effect of epidermal growth factor on ontogeny of the gastrointestinal tract. Am J Physiol 249:G674-G678.
Oesterreicher TJ, Markesich DC, Henning SJ (2001) Cloning, characterization and mapping of the mouse trehalase (Treh) gene. Gene 270:211-220.
Oesterreicher TJ, Nanthakumar NN, Winston JH, Henning SJ (1998) Rat trehalase: cDNA cloning and mRNA expression in adult rat tissues and during intestinal ontogeny. Am J Physiol 274:R1220-R1227.
Olds LC, Sibley E (2003) Lactase persistence DNA variant enhances lactase promoter activity in vitro: functional role as a cis regulatory element. Hum Mol Genet 12: 2333-2340.
Panayotova-Heiermann M, Loo DD, Kong CT, Lever JE, Wright EM (1996) Sugar binding to Na+/glucose cotransporters is determined by the carboxyl-terminal half of the protein. J Biol Chem 271:10029-10034.
Peiffer I, Bernet-Camard MF, Rousset M, Servin AL (2001) Impairments in enzyme activity and biosynthesis of brush border-associated hydrolases in human intestinal Caco-2/TC7 cells infected by members of the Afa/Dr family of diffusely adhering Escherichia coli. Cell Microbiol 3:341-357.
Pereira B, Sivakami S (1991) A comparison of the active site of maltase-glucoamylase from the brush border of rabbit small intestine and kidney by chemical modification studies. Biochem J 274:349-354.
Phillips AD, Smith MW, Walker-Smith JA (1988) Selective alteration of brush-border hydrolases in intestinal diseases in childhood. Clin Sci (Lond) 74:193-200.
Pothoulakis C, Gilbert RJ, Cladaras C, Castagliuolo I, Semenza G, Hitti Y, Montcrief JS, Linevsky J, Kelly CP, Nikulasson S, Desai HP, Wilkins TD, LaMont JT (1996) Rabbit sucrase-isomaltase contains a functional intestinal receptor for Clostridium difficile toxin Am J Clin Invest 98:641-649.
Potier M, Cousineau J, Michaud L, Zolinger M, Melancon SB, Dallaire L (1986) Fetal intestinal microvilli in human amniotic fluid. Prenat Diagn 6:429-436.

Quezada-Calvillo R, Senchyna M, Underdown BJ (1993) Characterization of intestinal gamma-glucoamylase deficiency in CBA/Ca mice. Am J Physiol 265:G1150-G1157.

Richards AB, Krakowka S, Dexter LB, Schmid H, Wolterbeek AP, Waalkens-Berendsen DH, Shigoyuki A, Kurimoto M (2002) Trehalose: a review of properties, history of use and human tolerance, and results of multiple safety studies. Food Chem Toxicol 40:871-898.

Rosenblum JL, Irwin CL, Alpers DH (1988) Starch and glucose oligosaccharides protect salivary-type amylase activity at acid pH. Am J Physiol 254:G775-G780.

Ruf J, Wacker H, James P, Maffia M, Seiler P, Galand G, von Kieckebusch A, Semenza G, Matei N (1990) Rabbit small intestinal trehalase. Purification, cDNA cloning, expression, and verification of glycosylphosphatidylinositol anchoring [published erratum appears in J Biol Chem 1990 Nov 15;265(32):20051]. J Biol Chem 265:15034-15039.

Salmeron J, Ascherio A, Rimm EB, Colditz GA, Spiegelman D, Jenkins DJ, Stampfer MJ, Wing AL, Willett WC (1997) Dietary fiber, glycemic load, and risk of NIDDM in men. Diabetes Care 20:545-550.

Sans MD, Lee SH, D'Alecy LG, Williams JA (2004) Feeding activates protein synthesis in mouse pancreas at the translational level without increase in mRNA. Am J Physiol Gastrointest Liver Physiol 287:G667-G675.

Saphiro GL, Bulow SD, Conklin KA, Scheving LA, Gray GM (1991) Postinsertional processing of sucrase-alpha-dextrinase precursor to authentic subunits: multiple steep cleavage by trypsin. Am J Physiol 24:G847-G857.

Schiraldi C, Di Lernia I, De Rosa M (2002) Trehalose production: exploiting novel approaches. Trends Biotechnol. 20:420-425.

Schmidt K, Schrader M, Kern HF, Kleene R (2001) Regulated apical secretion of zymogens in rat pancreas. Involvement of the glycosylphosphatidylinositol-anchored glycoprotein GP-2, the lectin ZG16p, and cholesterol-glycosphingolipid-enriched microdomains. J Biol Chem 276:14315-14323.

Semenza G (1986) Anchoring and biosynthesis of stalked brush border membrane proteins: Glycosidases and peptidases of enterocytes and renal tubuli. Annu Rev Cell Biol 2:255-313.

Semenza G, Auricchio S (1991) The lactase history: From physiopathology to biochemistry, molecular and cell biology—and back? In: Gracey M, Kretchmer N, Rossi E (eds) Sugars in Nutrition. Vol 25. Nestec Ltd., Vevey/Raven Press Ltd., New York.

Semenza G, Auricchio S, Mantei N (2001) Small intestinal disaccharidases. In: Scriver CR, Beaudet AL, Sly WS, Valle D (eds) The Metabolic and Molecular Basis of Inherited Disease, 8th ed. Vol 1, pp 1623-1650, McGraw-Hill, New York.

Shu R, David ES, Ferraris RP (1997) Dietary fructose enhances intestinal fructose transport and GLUT5 expression in weaning rats. Am J Physiol 272:G446-G453.

Shulman RJ (1990) Oral insulin increases small intestinal mass and disaccharidase activity in the newborn miniature pig. Pediatr Res 28: 171-175.

Shulman RJ, Langston C, Lifschitz CH (1991) Histologic findings are not correlated with disaccharidase activities in infants with protracted diarrhea. J Pediatr Gastroenterol Nutr 12:70-75.

Shulman RJ, Tivey DR, Sunitha I, Dudley MA, Henning SJ (1992) Effect of oral insulin on lactase activity, mRNA, and posttranscriptional processing in the newborn pig. J Pediatr Gastroenterol Nutr 14:166-172.

Sigrist H, Ronner P, Semenza G (1975) A hydrophobic form of the small-intestinal sucrase-isomaltase complex. Biochim Biophys Acta 406:433-446.

Simon-Assmann P, Lacroix B, Kedinger M, Haffen K (1986) Maturation of brush border hydrolases in human fetal intestine maintained in organ culture. Early Hum Dev 13:65-74.

Simoons FJ (1970) Primary adult lactose intolerance and the milking habit: a problem in biologic and cultural interrelations. II. A culture historical hypothesis. Am J Dig Dis 15:695-710.

Spodsberg N, Alfalah M, Naim HY (2001) Characteristics and structural requirements of apical sorting of the rat growth hormone through the O-glycosylated stalk region of intestinal sucrase-isomaltase. J Biol Chem 276:46597-46604.

Spodsberg N, Troelsen JT, Carlsson P, Enerback S, Sjostrom H, Noren O (1999) Transcriptional regulation of pig lactase-phlorizin hydrolase: involvement of HNF-1 and FREACs. Gastroenterology 116:842-854.

Sterchi EE, Lentze MJ, Naim HY (1990) Molecular aspects of disaccharidase deficiencies. Baillieres Clin Gastroenterol 4:79-96.

Toofanian F (1984) The fetal and postnatal development of small intestinal disaccharidases in the rabbit. Lab Anim Sci 34:268-271.

Topping DL, Clifton PM (2001) Short-chain fatty acids and human colonic function: roles of resistant starch and nonstarch polysaccharides. Physiol Rev 81:1031-1064.

Traber PG, Yu L, Wu GD, Judge TA (1992) Sucrase-isomaltase gene expression along crypt-villus axis of human small intestine is regulated at level of mRNA abundance. Am J Physiol 262:G123-G130.

Treem WR (1996) Clinical heterogeneity in congenital sucrase-isomaltase deficiency. J Pediatr 128:727-729.

Treem WR, Ahsan N, Sullivan B, Rossi T, Holmes R, Fitzgerald J, Proujansky R, Hyams J (1993) Evaluation of liquid yeast-derived sucrase enzyme replacement in patients with sucrase-isomaltase deficiency. Gastroenterology 105:1061-1068.

Troelsen JT, Mitchelmore C, Olsen J (2003a) An enhancer activates the pig lactase phlorizin hydrolase promoter in intestinal cells. Gene 305:101-111.

Troelsen JT, Mitchelmore C, Spodsberg N, Jensen AM, Noren O, Sjostrom H (1997) Regulation of lactase-phlorizin hydrolase gene expression by the caudal-related homoeodomain protein Cdx-2. Biochem J 322:833-838.

Troelsen JT, Olsen J, Moller J, Sjostrom H (2003b) An upstream polymorphism associated with lactase persistence has increased enhancer activity. Gastroenterology 125:1686-1694.

Troelsen JT, Olsen J, Noren O, Sjostrom H (1992) A novel intestinal trans-factor (NF-LPH1) interacts with the lactase-phlorizin hydrolase promoter and co-varies with the enzymatic activity. J Biol Chem 267:20407-20411.

Tsujii-Hayashi Y, Kitahara M, Yamagaki T, Kojima-Aikawa K, Matsumoto I (2002) A potential endogenous ligand of annexin IV in the exocrine pancreas. Carbohydrate structure of GP-2, a glycosylphosphatidylinositol-anchored glycoprotein of zymogen granule membranes. J Biol Chem 277:47493-47499.

Vachon V, Pouliot JF, Laprade R, Beliveau R (1991) Fractionation of renal brush border membrane proteins with Triton X-114 phase partitioning. Biochem Cell Biol 69:206-211.

Wang Y, Harvey CB, Hollox EJ, Phillips AD, Poulter M, Clay P, Walker-Smith JA, Swallow DM (1998) The genetically programmed down-regulation of lactase in children. Gastroenterology 114:1230-1236.

Wasle B, Edwardson JM (2002) The regulation of exocytosis in the pancreatic acinar cell. Cell Signal 14:191-197.

Williams JA (2001) Intracellular signaling mechanisms activated by cholecystokinin-regulating synthesis and secretion of digestive enzymes in pancreatic acinar cells. Annu Rev Physiol 63:77-97.

Williams JA, Sans MD, Tashiro M, Schafer C, Bragado MJ, Dabrowski A (2002) Cholecystokinin activates a variety of intracellular signal transduction mechanisms in rodent pancreatic acinar cells. Pharmacol Toxicol 91:297-303.

Wolffenbuttel BH, Graal MB (1996) New treatments for patients with type 2 diabetes mellitus. Postgrad Med J 72:657-662.

Wolever TM, Bolognesi C (1996) Source and amount of carbohydrate affect postprandial glucose and insulin in normal subjects. J Nutr 126:2798-2806.

Wolever TM, Mehling C (2003) Long-term effect of varying the source or amount of dietary carbohydrate on postprandial plasma glucose, insulin, triacylglycerol, and free fatty acid concentrations in subjects with impaired glucose tolerance. Am J Clin Nutr 77:612-621.

Wright EM, Hirsch JR, Loo DD, Zampighi GA (1997) Regulation of Na^+/glucose cotransporters. J Exp Biol 200:287-293.

Wright EM, Loo DD, Hirayama BA, Turk E (2004) Surprising versatility of Na^+-glucose cotransporters: SLC5. Physiology.(Bethesda.) 19:370-376.

Wright EM, Martin MG, Turk E (2003) Intestinal absorption in health and disease—sugars. Best.Pract Res Clin Gastroenterol 17:943-956.

Yeh KY, Moog F (1974) Intestinal lactase activity in the suckling rat: influence of hypophysectomy and thyroidectomy. Science 182:77-79.

Yeh KY, Yeh M, Montgomery RK, Grand RJ, Holt PR (1991) Cortisone and thyroxine modulate intestinal lactase and sucrase mRNA levels and activities in the suckling rat. Biochem Biophys Res Commun 180:174-180.

Yook C, Robyt JF (2002) Reactions of alpha amylases with starch granules in aqueous suspension giving products in solution and in a minimum amount of water giving products inside the granule. Carbohydr Res 337:1113-1117.

Yuasa H, Takada J, Hashimoto H (2001) Glycosidase inhibition by cyclic sulfonium compounds. Bioorg Med Chem Lett 11:1137-1139.

RECOMMENDED READINGS

Dalqvist A (1978) Disturbances of the digestion and absorption of carbohydrates. In: Manners DJ (ed) Biochemistry of Carbohydrates II. Vol. 16. University Park Press, Baltimore.

Semenza G, Auricchio S, Mantei N (2001) Small intestinal disaccharidases. In: Scriver CR, Beaudet AL, Sly WS, Valle D (eds) The Metabolic and Molecular Basis of Inherited Disease, 8th ed. Vol 1, pp 1623-1650, McGraw-Hill, New York.

Swallow DM (2003) Genetics of lactase persistence and lactose intolerance. Annu Rev Genet 37:197-219.

Chapter 9

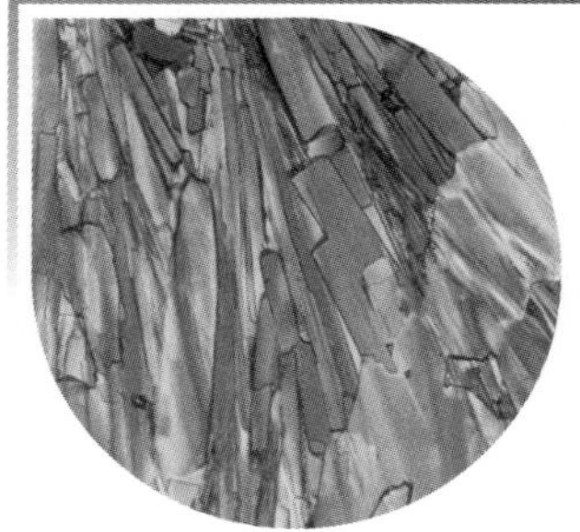

Digestion and Absorption of Protein

Bruce R. Stevens, PhD

OUTLINE

DIGESTION OF PROTEIN IN THE GASTROINTESTINAL TRACT

For the body to assimilate nutritional protein, it must be first broken down into small peptide fragments and free amino acids. This occurs to a limited extent in the stomach, with the vast majority of hydrolysis and absorption occurring in the small intestine. The digestion and absorption process ultimately supplies the circulating blood with primarily free amino acids, in addition to a very small amount of physiologically bioactive small peptide fragments. In the absorptive state, amino acids are transported via the portal blood from the small intestine directly to the liver, with subsequent transport to other organs.

The recommended dietary allowance for protein is 0.8 g dietary protein per kg body weight, or 56 g/day for the reference 70-kg man and 46 g/day for the reference 57-kg woman. The median intake of protein by 31- to 50-year-old adults in the United States is approximately 100 g/day for men and approximately 65 g/day for women. This dietary protein is rapidly and efficiently digested and absorbed. Besides food proteins, the body digests an additional 50 to 100 g of endogenous protein that is secreted into or sloughed into the lumen of the gastrointestinal tract. These sources include saliva, gastric juice, pancreatic enzymes and other secretions, sloughed intestinal cells, and proteins that leak into the intestinal lumen from the blood. Most of this mixture of exogenous and endogenous proteins (115 to 200 g/day) is efficiently digested and absorbed (as free amino acids and di- and tripeptides) with daily fecal losses from the gastrointestinal tract of only about 1.6 g nitrogen (equivalent to 10 g of protein). The nitrogen excreted in the feces represents primarily endogenous or dietary nitrogen that was not absorbed from the small intestine; this unabsorbed nitrogen was used in the large intestine by the microflora for growth and is, therefore, present in the feces as part of the bacterial mass.

An overall concept diagram of the major events of protein digestion and absorption is presented in Figure 9-1. The normal events of digestion and absorption are grouped into phases corresponding to physiological events. The major six phases covered in this chapter primarily involve the following:

1. Gastric hydrolysis of peptide linkages in the protein
2. Digestion of protein to smaller peptides by action of pancreatic proteases, which are secreted as zymogens and activated in the lumen of the small intestine where they then carry out digestion
3. Hydrolysis of peptide linkages in oligopeptides by brush-border (apical) membrane

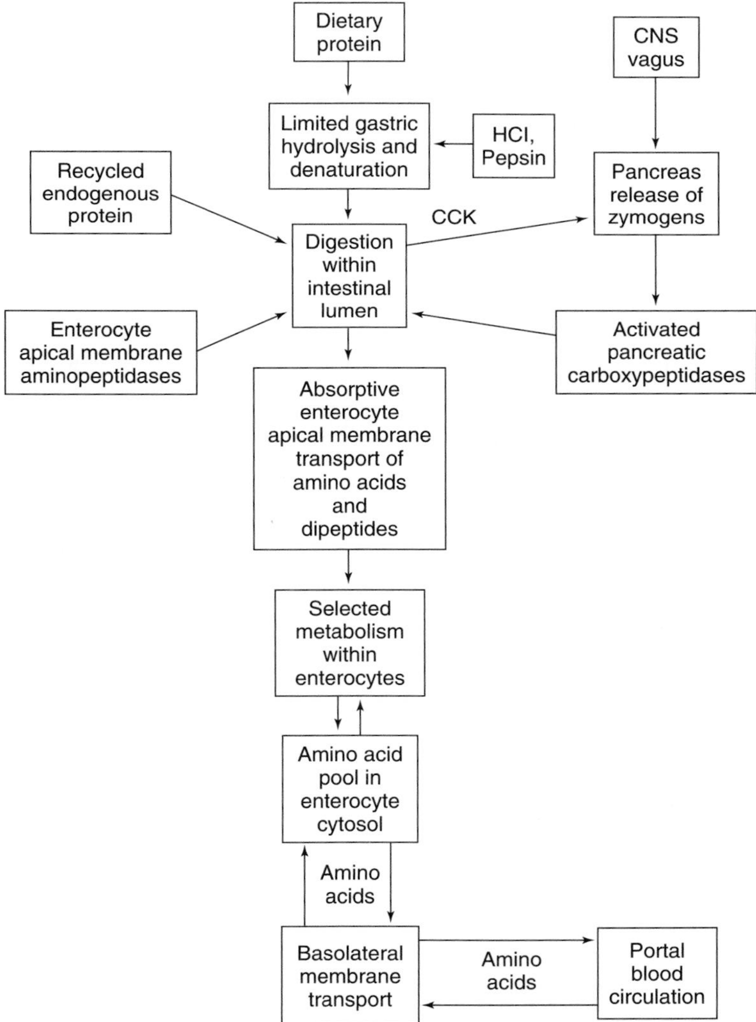

Figure 9-1 Overall "concept diagram" of the normal events of protein digestion and absorption. *CCK*, Cholecystokinin; *CNS*, central nervous system.

peptidases and transport of amino acids and di- and tripeptides across the brush-border membrane of the absorptive enterocytes
4. Further digestion of di- and tripeptides by cytoplasmic peptidases in the enterocyte
5. Metabolism of amino acids within the enterocyte
6. Transport of amino acids across the basolateral membrane of the enterocyte into the interstitial fluid from which the amino acids enter the venous capillaries and hence the portal blood.

Responding to dietary content and metabolic demands, the cells and tissues of the gastrointestinal tract adaptively regulate the digestive and absorptive processes. In addition to normal gastrointestinal physiology and biochemistry, this chapter covers some of the major pathophysiological mechanisms associated with protein digestion and absorption.

THE GASTRIC PHASE: DENATURATION AND INITIAL HYDROLYSIS OF PROTEINS

Protein digestion begins with modest processing by the stomach. Here, gastric HCl and pepsins partially denature and hydrolyze proteins. The stomach plays a minor role in the overall digestion process and serves primarily to prepare polypeptides for the main events of digestion and absorption that take place within the small intestine. Indeed, complete protein assimilation occurs even after surgical removal of the stomach.

When food is present in the stomach, or if the appropriate vagal cholinergic efferents are activated, the gastric chief cells secrete inactive pepsinogens into the stomach lumen. Several isozymes of pepsinogen are released, and each is converted to an active pepsin isozyme by cleavage of a peptide from the amino terminus. Activation occurs spontaneously at a pH of less than 5 by an intramolecular process that involves proteolytic cleavage of a highly basic amino terminal precursor segment. In the zymogen, the active site of pepsin is blocked by interaction of basic residues in the precursor segment with carboxylate side chains of residues including those of a pair of aspartyl residues at the active site. These salt bridges are broken as the carboxylates become protonated at the acidic pH of the gastric contents; this exposes the catalytic site and results in hydrolysis of the peptide bond between the precursor segment and pepsin moiety. After this autoactivation process forms some pepsin, activation of pepsinogen by active pepsin (autocatalysis) also occurs.

Pepsins are chemically categorized as endopeptidases because they attack peptide bonds within the polypeptide chain. Their catalytic mechanism involves two carboxylic acid groups at the active site of the enzyme, so pepsins are classified as carboxyl proteases. Most digestive enzymes are relatively permissive in the range of substrates they will accept, and the pepsins partially hydrolyze a broad variety of proteins to large peptide fragments and some free amino acids. Pepsins show a preference for hydrolysis of internal peptide bonds that involve the carboxyl groups of tyrosyl, phenylalanyl, or tryptophanyl residues and that do not involve a linkage to the imino group of proline.

SMALL INTESTINAL LUMINAL PHASE: ACTIVATION AND ACTION OF PANCREATIC PROTEOLYTIC ENYZMES

Following partial hydrolysis of protein in the stomach, the polypeptides and amino acids enter the lumen of the proximal small intestine where they stimulate the mucosal cells to release the hormone cholecystokinin (CCK) into the circulation. CCK subsequently reaches the pancreas, whereupon it binds to the acinar cells and stimulates the secretion of a variety of inactive precursor digestive enzymes called zymogens. Zymogens are delivered to the small intestinal lumen by way of the pancreatic duct. In addition to CCK stimulation, stomach distension or the sight and smell of food invoke parasympathetic cholinergic vagal nerve efferents, which in turn stimulate the exocrine pancreatic acinar cells to release zymogens.

Based on work that originated in the Russian laboratory of I.P. Pavlov in the late 1890s, research has established that protein digestion involves a multistep conversion of inactive zymogens to their active states within the lumen of the

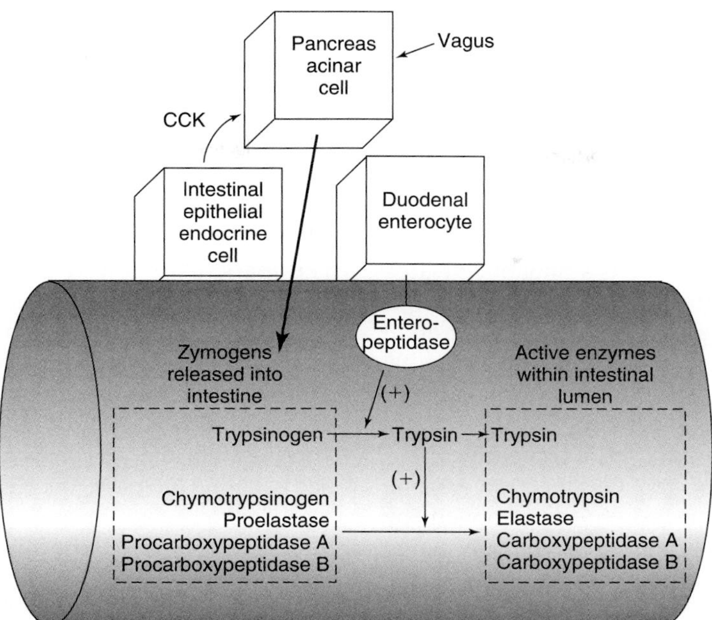

Figure 9-2 Cascade activation of pancreatic zymogens within the lumen of the small intestine. *CCK*, Cholecystokinin.

small intestine. The current understanding of the activation cascade for these pancreatic zymogens is summarized in Figure 9-2.

PANCREATIC ZYMOGENS AND THEIR ACTIVATION CASCADE

The pancreatic zymogens are released directly into the intestinal lumen via the pancreatic duct and the common bile duct. The major zymogens are trypsinogen, proelastase, chymotrypsinogen, procarboxypeptidase A, and procarboxypeptidase B. The initial step of the activation cascade is catalyzed by enteropeptidase (enterokinase), which is bound to the brush border (apical) membranes of the enterocytes that line the proximal small intestine (duodenum/upper jejunum).

The importance of enteropeptidase is emphasized by the fact that congenital deficiency of this enzyme leads to life-threatening malabsorption of nitrogen. Human enteropeptidase is structurally organized as a heavily glycosylated dimer attached to brush-border membranes of enterocytes lining the upper intestine. It is a member of the serine protease family of enzymes. The cDNA sequence for human enteropeptidase indicates that the active dimer is derived from a single-chain precursor (Kitamoto et al., 1995). In this sense, biosynthesis of the nascent enteropeptidase precursor may actually be considered the true "first" step of the cascade; it is possible that a duodenase, a serine protease formed by the mucus-secreting Brunner's glands in the duodenum, is the natural activator of the enteropeptidase zymogen (Zamolodchikova et al., 2000).

Intestinal enteropeptidase cleaves an amino terminal octapeptide from human trypsinogen, thereby forming the activated trypsin enzyme within the intestinal lumen. The specificity of enteropeptidase for trypsinogen is high; the scissile (to be cleaved) peptide bond in trypsinogen is between the carboxyl group of a lysyl residue and the amino group of an isoleucyl residue. Vertebrate trypsinogens contain a highly conserved tetra-aspartate sequence next to the scissile Lys-Ile peptide bond. Specificity of bovine trypsinogen as the substrate for bovine enteropeptidase depends upon the presence of the intact tetra-aspartate sequence, but the tetra-aspartate sequence confers only a modest catalytic improvement to enteropeptidase-mediated trypsinogen activation in humans (Nemoda and Sahin-Tóth, 2005).

Trypsin, which is also a member of the serine protease family but with very different specificity than enteropeptidase, then activates the other zymogens (chymotrypsinogen, proelastase, and carboxypeptidases A and B, as well as procolipase and prophospholipase A_2, which are required for lipid digestion) by cleaving off selected peptide sequences. The net result of this cascade is a pool of activated proteases within the lumen of the small intestine. Proteolysis is facilitated by the secretion of pancreatic bicarbonate into the intestinal lumen; the bicarbonate titrates the gastric acid in the chyme to pH 6 to 7, which is optimal for activity of pancreatic proteases.

It was formerly thought that once some trypsin was formed from trypsinogen by enteropeptidase, the active trypsin could act on trypsinogen as substrate in an autocatalytic process. However, although both trypsin and enteropeptidase cleave at scissile bonds that involve a basic (lysyl or arginyl) residue attached to an isoleucyl residue, the aspartyl-rich sequence in the activation peptide segment of trypsinogen inhibits the ability of trypsin to accept trypsinogen as a substrate. Thus enteropeptidase in the small intestine is essential for activation of trypsinogen and the subsequent zymogen activation cascade.

A benefit of synthesis of proteolytic enzymes as zymogens, with activation occurring after the proenzymes have been secreted into the intestinal lumen, is the prevention of proteolytic digestion and tissue damage within the pancreas and pancreatic duct. In addition to this protective mechanism, pancreatic juice normally contains a small peptide that acts as a trypsin inhibitor to prevent any small amount of trypsin prematurely formed within the pancreatic cells or pancreatic ducts from catalyzing proteolysis. The importance of these protective mechanisms is illustrated by the identification of mutations in the gene for trypsinogen in patients with hereditary pancreatitis. The mutations associated with this disease include those causing the substitution of a different amino acid in the tetra-aspartate sequence: D19-D20-D21-D22 preceding the K23-I24 scissile peptide bond (Chen et al., 2003a). Certain mutations (D19A, D22G, and K23R) were associated with a dramatic increase in the autoactivation of trypsinogen in vitro. Thus the tetra-aspartate sequence in mammalian trypsinogen not only serves as a unique site for cleavage/activation of trypsinogen within the intestine by enteropeptidase but also facilitates the efficient inhibition of trypsinogen autoactivation within the pancreas.

PANCREATIC DIGESTIVE ENZYMES

The pancreatic enzymes can be divided into two general types—serine proteases and carboxypeptidases. Trypsin, chymotrypsin, and elastase are all endopeptidases of the serine protease class. They are categorized as endopeptidases because they hydrolyze internal peptide bonds within the polypeptide. They are classified as serine proteases because of their catalytic mechanisms, which involve a serine residue in the catalytic site. Serine proteases, including those involved in the blood clotting cascade as will be discussed in Chapter 28, are normally synthesized in inactive zymogen or proenzyme form. Each of these serine proteases catalyzes the hydrolysis of peptide (amide) bonds but with different selectivities or preferences for the side chains flanking the scissile peptide bond. The site of hydrolysis in the polypeptide substrate is flanked by approximately four amino acid residues in both directions that can bind to the enzyme and impact on the reactivity of the peptide bond hydrolyzed; the hydrolyzable bond is designated P_1-P'_1 and adjacent amino acids are numbered P_2, P_3, and P_4 toward the amino terminus and P'_2, P'_3, and P'_4 toward the carboxyl terminus. Trypsin is most likely to cleave peptide bonds with a positively charged residue (arginine or lysine) at the P_1 site (contributing the carboxyl group to the peptide bond); chymotrypsin prefers bonds in which large hydrophobic amino acid residues such as tryptophan, phenylalanine, tyrosine, methionine, or leucine are at the P_1 site; and elastase preferentially cleaves peptide bonds that have a small neutral residue such as alanine, serine, glycine, or valine at the P_1 site. Proline at the P'_1 site inhibits cleavage by all three serine proteases. The rate at which particular bonds are cleaved also varies with the identities of the amino acid residues in the adjacent positions (P_2-P_4 and P'_2-P'_4).

The second group of proteolytic enzymes secreted by the pancreas, the carboxypeptidases, are exopeptidases that cleave off one

Nutrition Insight

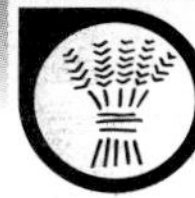

Trypsin Inhibitors

Small molecular weight proteins or polypeptides that act as protease inhibitors are naturally produced by cells in both animals and plants. In particular, pulses (peas, beans, and lentils) and cereals (wheat, buckwheat, and rice bran) contain trypsin inhibitors that can lower the nutritional quality of their proteins. These trypsin inhibitors can be inactivated to a large extent by wet heating or removed by processing techniques used during protein concentration and isolation (e.g., soy protein). Soybean trypsin inhibitors have been widely studied. Although these are inactivated by heating, animals sometimes ingest large amounts of these inhibitors by consuming raw soybeans.

The pancreas, intestinal cells, liver, and other tissues also synthesize a certain amount of trypsin inhibitors. For example, human pancreatic secretory trypsin inhibitor is secreted from pancreatic acinar cells into the pancreatic duct along with the zymogen precursors of the proteolytic digestive enzymes. The possibility that some symptoms observed in diseases such as acute pancreatitis or gastric ulcer result from an absence of normal synthesis/secretion of these inhibitors is under active investigation. The therapeutic use of trypsin inhibitors to treat pancreatitis and other inflammatory conditions is also being tested in animal models.

Thinking Critically

1. Why would the presence of trypsin inhibitors in a food decrease the nutritional quality of its protein?
2. Feeding of raw soybean flour or soybean trypsin inhibitor results in an increase in the amounts of secretory products (presumably protein synthesis) within the acinar cells and in enhanced protein secretion by the pancreas. Why might this occur?
3. Why might a lack of trypsin inhibitor result in acute pancreatitis? Why might therapeutic administration of trypsin inhibitor alleviate ulceration or inflammation of tissues?

---

amino acid at a time from the carboxyl terminus of the substrate. Exopeptidases can attack the oligopeptides formed by the endopeptidases to sequentially cleave off free amino acids, leaving a mixture of free amino acids and small peptides of two to eight residues. Carboxypeptidase A and B are both metalloenzymes that require Zn^{2+} at the active site where it functions as a Lewis acid. (See Chapter 37 for a discussion of zinc metalloenzymes.) Carboxypeptidase B preferentially cleaves C-terminal lysine or arginine residues of peptides, and carboxypeptidase A selectively hydrolyzes most C-terminal amino acids except proline, lysine, and arginine, with a preference for valine, leucine, isoleucine, and alanine. Carboxypeptidase A and B do not readily cleave C-terminal amino acids that are linked to a prolyl residue.

These pancreatic enzymes act as a team within the small intestinal lumen to hydrolyze many of the peptide bonds in proteins, resulting in efficient digestion of protein to small peptides (two to eight residues) and free amino acids.

SMALL INTESTINAL MUCOSAL PHASE: BRUSH-BORDER AND CYTOSOLIC PEPTIDASES

The products of pancreatic hydrolysis are free amino acids, tripeptides and dipeptides, and larger peptide fragments called oligopeptides. The free amino acids, dipeptides, and tripeptides are transported across the absorptive epithelial cell apical membrane by specific carriers, as described in subsequent text. Most larger oligopeptides are not transported but must be further hydrolyzed by epithelial brush-border membrane–bound enzymes.

With one known exception, the peptidases in the brush-border membrane of the enterocyte are all categorized chemically as aminopeptidases, meaning that they hydrolyze amino acids one at a time from the amino terminus. These enzymes also show specificities or preferences for the amino acid residues and peptide sequences that they hydrolyze. The apical membrane possesses a single known carboxypeptidase, which is peptidyl dipeptidase.

Both the aminopeptidases and the carboxypeptidase are classified as exopeptidases.

The enterocyte membrane-bound peptidases are dimers that extend into the lumen about 15 nm from the membrane surface. One subunit is anchored to the membrane, and the other subunit participates in the hydrolytic activity. A variety of membrane-bound aminopeptidases exist, each having a different preference for specific residues involved in the amide bonds that they hydrolyze. Some examples include aminopeptidase A, aminopeptidase N, proline iminopeptidase, and dipeptidylpeptidase IV.

For the majority of tri- and dipeptides that are transported into the enterocyte, additional cytosolic aminopeptidases act within the absorptive epithelial cells to complete the process of hydrolyzing proteins and peptides to free amino acids. Most protein nitrogen exits the basolateral membrane to the portal blood as free amino acids. As explained below, certain dipeptides such as carnosine, and a small fraction (~1%) of undigested luminal protein and peptides may enter the portal blood intact, and/or initiate antioxidant or immune responses within the intestinal wall or systemically, or serve to modulate neural and endocrine functions.

ABSORPTION OF FREE AMINO ACIDS AND SMALL PEPTIDES

The products of digestion—free amino acids, dipeptides, and tripeptides—are absorbed from the lumen by a variety of transport mechanisms. Free amino acid absorption mechanisms are presented first and are followed by a discussion of di- and tripeptide absorption.

AMINO ACID TRANSPORT SYSTEMS IN THE BRUSH-BORDER AND BASOLATERAL MEMBRANES

The free amino acids (primarily as L-stereoisomers, but D-serine and D-aspartate can be transported if present in the diet) in the intestinal lumen move across the apical membrane of villous absorptive enterocytes, are pooled within the enterocyte, and then finally exit the enterocyte via the basolateral membranes. Following basolateral membrane transport to the interstitial fluid, the amino acids are transported into mucosal capillaries and then on to the liver via the portal circulation. The intestine is highly efficient in extracting the essential and nonessential amino acids from the lumen as free amino acids. This occurs largely because of the activity of brush border and basolateral membrane transporter systems that serve specific substrates. (Enterocyte basolateral membrane transporters can also serve to take up amino acids from the blood circulation under postprandial conditions.)

A large number of transporters for the apical and basolateral membranes of enterocytes have been identified (Broer et al., 2004, 2005; Takanaga et al., 2005; Dave et al., 2004; Palacin and Kanai et al., 2004; Verrey et al., 2004; Boll et al., 2003; Chen et al., 2003b; Peral, 2002; Malliard et al., 1995; Stevens, 1992), and their expression has been localized within the intestinal tract (Terada et al., 2005). A transport "system" is a physiological functional unit formed from one or more transporter protein subunits. Each transporter subunit type is encoded by a specific gene. A transport system activity may result from the action of a single transporter protein or the multimeric arrangement of transporter proteins within the membrane bilayer. Membrane amino acid transporters composed of a monomer or single protein are listed in Table 9-1, whereas those formed by the heterodimeric interaction of two subunits are listed in Table 9-2. The genes encoding the transporter subunits have been cloned for most of the transport systems. The apical membrane pathways are generally different from those found in the basolateral membrane, as illustrated in Figure 9-3.

The primary means by which the neutral amino acids cross the apical membrane are via transport sytem B^0 (catalyzed by the B^0 AT1 transporter protein), system $B^{0,+}$ ($ATB^{0,+}$ transporter protein), system IMINO (SIT1 transporter protein), and system Iminoacid (PAT1 transporter). PAT1 is a proton-coupled secondary active transporter of proline, GABA, and taurine. Although PAT1 is H^+-dependent, its activity is also governed by Na^+ ions through energetic coupling to the activity of the apical membrane NHE3 Na^+/H^+ exchanger. System $b^{0,+}$ is a sodium-independent variant of Cl^--dependent/Na^+-dependent system $B^{0,+}$. At the basolateral membrane, neutral amino acids are served by

Table 9-1
Monomeric Amino Acid Transporters and Transport Systems in Small Intestine

Transport "System" Functional Name	Common Name of monomer (protein)	Gene	Human Gene Locus	Representative Substrate	Ion Dependency	Location in Enterocyte
A	SNAT2	*SLC38A2*	12q	Alanine, asparagine, cysteine, glutamine, glycine, histidine, methionine, proline, serine	Na^+	Basolateral
B (or B^0)	B^0AT1	*SLC6A19*	5p15	Small neutral amino acids, glutamine	Na^+	Apical
$B^{0,+}$	$ATB^{0,+}$	*SLC6A14*	Xq23-q24	Neutral and dibasic amino acids, arginine, D-serine	Na^+, Cl^-	Apical
y^+	CAT-1	*SLC7A1*	*13q12-q14*	Arginine, dibasic amino acids	None	Basolateral
X^-_{AG}	EAAT3	*SLC1A1*	9q24	L-Glutamate, D/L-aspartate	H^+, Na^+, K^+	Apical
IMINO	SIT1	*SLC6A20*	—	Proline, pipecolate	Na^+	Apical
Iminoacid	PAT1	*SLC36A1*	*5q33.1*	Proline, glycine, β-alanine, GABA, taurine, D-serine	H^+ with NHE3	Apical
GLY	GLYT1	*SLC6A9*	*1p33*	Glycine	Na^+, Cl^-	Basolateral
T	TAT1	*SLC16A10*	*6q21-q22*	Aromatic amino acids, L-DOPA	—	Basolateral
Creatine	CRTR	*SLC6A8*	Xq28	Creatine	Na^+, Cl^-	Apical
Pept1	PEPT1	*SLC15A1*	*13q33-q34*	Dipeptides and tripeptides; carnosine, β-lactam antibiotics, angiotensin-converting enzyme inhibitors	H^+ with NHE3	Apical

Table 9-2
Heterodimeric Amino Acid Transporters and Transport Systems in Small Intestine

Transport "System" Functional Name	Common Name of Heterodimer Subunit (Protein)	Gene	Human Gene Locus	Representative Substrates	Ion Dependency	Location in Enterocyte
asc	asc-1 plus 4F2hc/CD98	*SLC7A10* *SLC3A2*	19q12-13.1 11q13	Small neutral L- and D-amino acids, alanine, D-serine, cyst(e)ine, glycine	None	Basolateral
y^+L	y^+LAT1 plus 4F2hc/CD98	*SLC7A7* *SLC3A2*	14q11.2 11q13	Arginine, dibasic and neutral amino acids	None for dibasics; Na^+ for large neutrals	Basolateral
x^-_c	xCT plus 4F2hc/CD98	*SLC7A11* *SLC3A2*	4q28-q32 11q13	Cystine/glutamate exchange	None	Basolateral
L	LAT2 plus 4F2hc/CD98	*SLC7A8* *SLC3A2*	14q11.2 11q13	Branched-chain and neutral (small and large) amino acids	None	Basolateral
$b^{0,+}$	$b^{0,+}$AT plus rBAT	*SLC7A9* *SLC3A1*	19q13.1 2p16.3-p21	Dibasic amino acids, arginine, cystine, large neutral amino acids (exchanges extracellular dibasics with intracellular neutrals)	None	Apical

*The heavy chain 4F2hc subunit is synonymously called CD98.

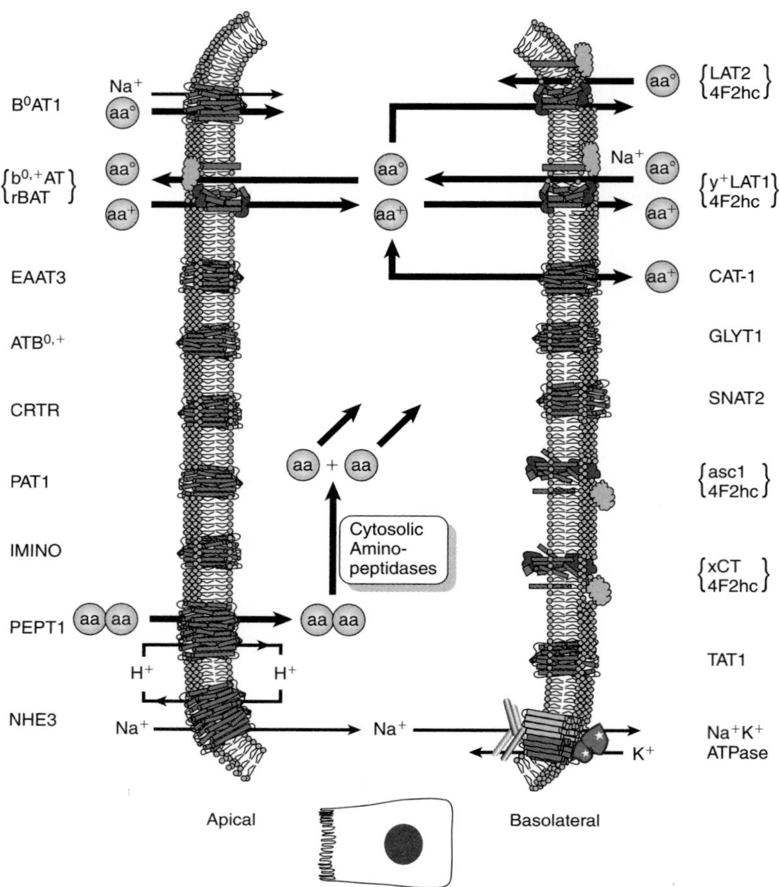

Figure 9-3 Amino acid or dipeptide transporter subunits in absorptive enterocyte membranes. Transport systems are functional units that are catalyzed by transporter proteins embedded in the plasma membrane bilayer as either monomers or heterodimers (see details in Tables 9-1 and 9-2). The monomers or subunits are denoted by their abbreviated nomenclature. Each transport system serves amino acids or dipeptides with specific structural features. The transporters are localized to either the apical (brush border) or basolateral membrane as shown. Transepithelial movement of amino acids involves interactive, concerted participation among multiple transport systems, multiple subunits, and ion electrochemical gradients. One example is shown for the interplay among neutral/zwitterionic ("aa^0") and dibasic/cationic ("aa^+") amino acid substrates. Several transport systems actively transport substrates via cotransport with Na^+ or H^+ ions. In the case of H^+-cotransport (e.g., PepT1 example shown, as well as for PAT1), energetic coupling occurs via the NHE3 Na^+/H^+ exchanger also within the membrane. The Na^+ electrochemical potential is maintained by the basolateral $3Na^+/2K^+$-ATPase.

transport systems A, asc, y^+L, L, GLY, and T. System y^+L (made up of y^+LAT1 plus 4F2hc protein subunits) serves the dibasic amino acids in a sodium-independent manner, yet it transports neutral amino acids by a Na^+-dependent mechanism. System L (comprised of LAT2 plus 4F2hc protein subunits) is Na^+-independent and handles large hydrophobic or branched substrates such as leucine, isoleucine, valine, phenylalanine, and tyrosine. The anionic substrates, L- and D-aspartate and L-glutamate are actively transported across the apical membrane through $Na^+/K^+/H^+$-dependent system X^-_{AG}, while these amino acids exit the basolateral side via Na^+-independent system x^-_c (made up of xCT plus 4F2hc protein subunits). Enterocyte cytosolic antioxidant glutathione production is governed largely by system x^-_c cystine/glutamate exchange with blood capillary free amino acids. The dibasic (cationic) substrates arginine, lysine, and ornithine are transported across the apical surface (see Fig. 9-3) via systems $b^{0,+}$ (composed of polypeptide subunits $b^{0,+}$AT plus rBAT) and $B^{0,+}$, in serial conjunction with the basolateral membrane transport systems y^+ (CAT-1 monomer) and y^+L.

The continual extraction of nutrients from the intestinal lumen results in Na^+ and amino acids moving into the enterocyte. In the absorptive state these nutrients subsequently exit the enterocyte to the interstitial fluid via the basolateral membranes. In the postabsorptive state basolateral membrane transporters can supply enterocytes with amino acids from the blood. In both states the Na^+ electrochemical potential gradient is continually maintained by the Na^+, K^+-ATPase pumps in the basolateral membrane (see Fig. 9-3). It is the Na^+ electrochemical potential that energizes the (secondary or coupled) active transport of amino acids (Gerencser and Stevens, 1994). The absorption of positively charged cationic amino acids via Na^+-independent transport systems y^+ and $b^{0,+}$ is driven by the amino acid chemical gradient plus the negative electrical potential across the enterocyte membrane. The chemical gradients of neutral amino acids are the sole driving force for absorption via transport system L.

One of the most thoroughly studied heterodimeric interactions is that of transport system $b^{0,+}$, which comprises the rBAT regulatory subunit bound to the $b^{0,+}$AT transporter catalytic subunit. (Chillaron et al., 2001; Wagner et al., 2001). As shown in Table 9-2 and Figure 9-3, the functional interaction of these two subunits gives rise to activity of transport system $b^{0,+}$. The rBAT gene (*SLC3A1*) encodes a membrane integral glycoprotein with a single transmembrane-spanning domain with most of the polypeptide chain facing the luminal or extracellular fluid. The predicted protein sequence of human rBAT is 685 amino acids long. The molecular mass is about 72 kDa, with an in vitro translation product that is glycosylated and has a mass of about 94 kDa. The predicted structure of rBAT is different from the structure of the other cloned transporter proteins, which normally contain about 12 to 14 transmembrane domains. The extracellular domain of rBAT possesses the carboxyl terminus, shows extensive homology with the α-amylases and α-glucosidases, and has six potential *N*-glycosylation sites. The main role of the SLC3 family members as part of the heteromeric amino acid transporters is to help route the holotransporter to the plasma membrane (Palacin and Kanai, 2004). A cysteinyl residue is situated near the membrane surface at the extracellular face. This cysteinyl residue forms a disulfide bridge with the $b^{0,+}$AT subunit (encoded by the *SLC7A9* gene), thereby regulating cationic and neutral amino acid uptake via Na^+-independent system $b^{0,+}$. Single point mutations in either the rBAT gene *(SLC3A1)* or $b^{0,+}$AT gene (*SLC7A9*) are responsible for the familial disease cystinuria (Palacin and Kanai, 2004; Verrey et al., 2004). Recent work (Nunes et al., 2005a, 2005b) shows that one form of cystinuria is inherited as an autosomal resessive trait characterized by mutations in the *SLC3A1* gene on chromosome 2, which encodes (heavy chain) transport activator rBAT. Another manifestation of cystinuria arises from dominant genetics, resulting from mutations in *SLC7A9* on chromosome 19 encoding the $b^{0,+}$AT (light chain) transmembrane channel subunit (see Clinical Correlation).

Transport involves cooperation at several levels. As discussed above, ion-dependent catalytic events are required for some transport systems and interactions between heterodimeric subunits are required for movement of certain amino acids across a single membrane. In addition, the transepithelial amino acid movement involves the cooperative interaction of several transport systems of both apical and basolateral membranes. For example, dibasic amino acid absorption requires serial movement of these amino acids—uptake by Na^+-independent apical system $b^{0,+}$ (heterodimer of $b^{0,+}$AT plus rBAT subunits) into the enterocyte, followed by exchange with a neutral amino acid plus Na^+ at the basolateral membrane by system y^+L (heterodimer of 4F2hc plus y^+LAT1 subunits) to release the amino acid from the enterocyte where it can then enter the bloodstream. The exchanged neutral amino acid is ultimately also transported back out of the enterocyte by one of the other basolateral systems selective for that substrate.

An intriguing transporter protein, ASCT2, is expressed in the stomach and large intestine, but not in small intestine (Terada et al., 2005). ASCT2 is encoded by the *SLC1A5* gene at human locus 19q13.3. This Na^+-dependent apical membrane protein behaves with System ASC substrate selectivity by transporting alanine, serine, cysteine, threonine, and glutamine, but likely does not contribute much to whole body nutrition of these neutral amino acids because it is not in small intestine. However, ASCT2 serves as a cell surface receptor for endogenously inherited retroviruses in humans and type-D simian retroviruses in baboons (Marin et al., 2003).

REGULATION OF INTESTINAL ABSORPTION OF AMINO ACIDS

From the perspective of the whole body, the intestinal capacity to absorb nutrients must not be the rate-limiting step that governs whole-body intermediary metabolism of amino acids. Therefore one of the major roles of the gastrointestinal tract is to maintain a net positive flow of nutrient nitrogen in the direction of diet-to-organism. To ensure this, the small intestine is able to adaptively upregulate its capacity for amino acid absorption.

As the dietary protein content and the physiological state of the body change over a period of days, the intestine adaptively regulates its capacity to absorb amino acids. The adaptations occur both at the tissue level and at the cellular level. Acting on the intestinal mucosa, various factors can nonspecifically change the absorptive surface area of the intestine. For example, in animal models mucosal hyperplasia occurs in response to corticosteroids and peptide growth factors or in response to hyperphagia associated with diabetes, hyperthyroidism, neoplasia, pregnancy and lactation, or accelerated growth.

Furthermore, in response to specific peptides, amino acids, and growth factors within the intestinal lumen, individual enterocytes upregulate expression of genes for aminopeptidases and specific membrane transporters (monomers and either one or both subunits of the dimeric transporters), resulting in increased abundance of these enzymes and transporters (Pan et al., 2002b; Pan and Stevens, 1995; Stevens, 1992). Regulation may also occur via posttranslational regulatory mechanisms as evidenced by the transmembrane stimulation of certain transporters by an increase in the intracellular concentration of one of its amino acid substrates (Pan et al., 2002a, 2002b, 2002c). Interestingly, animal studies have shown that consumption of diets supplemented with individual amino acids can activate the uptake of substrates that may be unrelated to the transporter used by the activator itself. In mice, for example, aspartate stimulates the absorption of acidic as well as basic amino acids, and orally fed arginine (but not lysine) induces aspartate uptake (Ferraris and Diamond, 1989). This pattern of interaction between substrates and transporter induction suggests that separate regulatory proteins may be involved in common regulatory processes that affect more than one transporter system, although the mechanism is unknown.

With the concerted effects of both individual cell upregulation of transporters and general mucosal hyperplasia, the small intestine can increase its absorptive capacity many-fold compared to the constitutive fasting capacity. Absorption is generally greatest in the jejunal region, and transport is upregulated to a greater extent within the jejunal mucosa than in the duodenum or ileum. The concept of regional upregulation of amino acid absorption is illustrated in Figure 9-4.

Intestinal downregulation of amino acid transport is essentially a return to the constitutive baseline absorptive capacity that occurs in the absence of stimulating agent. The downregulation occurs over a period of several days, because the absorptive cells with enhanced transport capacity are gradually sloughed off from the villus tip into the lumen and are replaced with cells possessing only constitutive transport activity (Stevens, 1992). In the absence of luminal feeding, as in the case of total parenteral nutrition (TPN), the absorptive capacity of the intestine becomes severely reduced as intestinal atrophy gradually occurs. This phenomenon underlies the importance of enteral feeding in maintaining the integrity of the gut in convalescing patients.

NONPROTEIN AMINO ACIDS

In addition to serving the amino acids that enter protein synthesis, gastrointestinal transporters also transport nonprotein amino acids from food sources (Tables 9-2 and 9-3, Fig. 9-3). For example, creatine is absorbed via

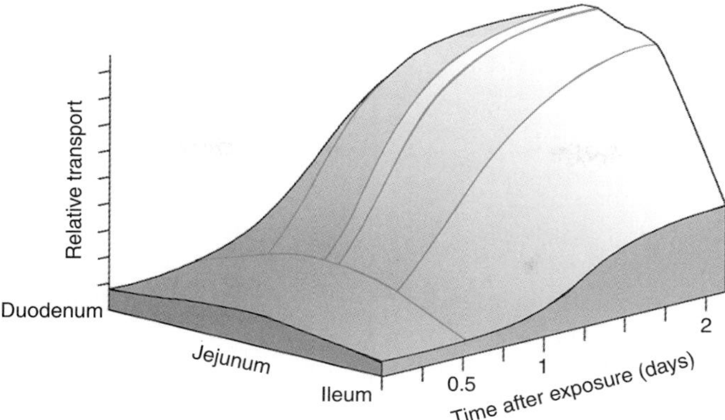

Figure 9-4 The concept of regional upregulation of amino acid transport in the small intestine. Generally, the constitutive uptake capacity and the magnitude of transport upregulation is greater in the jejunum, compared to the ileum or duodenum. Transport is upregulated over the course of hours and days as new copies of specific transporter molecules are synthesized and inserted into the membranes of enterocytes during villus maturation and hyperplasia. *(Redrawn from Stevens BR [1992] Amino acid transport in intestine. In: Kilberg MS, Haussinger D [eds] Mammalian Amino Acid Transport: Mechanisms and Control. Plenum, New York, pp 149-164.)*

the CRTR transporter (Verhoeven et al 2006; Peral et al 2002). β-Alanine and taurine are absorbed via PAT1. Neuroactive D-serine is carried by systems $B^{0,+}$, PAT1, and asc; D-aspartate is absorbed via X_{AG}^-, GABA by the IMINO (PAT1) system, and L-DOPA by the T system.

DISORDERS OF INTESTINAL AMINO ACID TRANSPORT

The absorptive epithelium of the small intestine shares many physiological and functional traits with the reabsorptive epithelium of the kidney proximal tubule. Both tissues possess aminopeptidases on their apical membranes, and both possess many of the same amino acid transport systems. Several inborn disorders of amino acid transport are associated with a defective or deleted constitutive transport system in both the intestinal and renal absorptive epithelial membranes (Mailliard et al., 1995). These are clinically observed as specific aminoacidurias, which display autosomal recessive or dominant inheritance patterns. Although specific amino acid transporters of the intestinal membrane are impaired in patients with aminoacidurias, their metabolic requirements for nutrient amino nitrogen may be met (except in the case of lysinuric protein intolerance) by other amino acid transporters with overlapping specificities or by the dipeptide/tripeptide PepT1 transporter. No genetic defects of peptide transporter proteins are known.

Cystinuria is a well-documented disease due to a genetic defect of amino acid transport. In patients with cystinuria, activity of transport system $b^{0,+}$ in both the kidney and the small intestine is impaired. The clinical signature of cystinuria is simultaneously elevated levels of lysine, ornithine, arginine, and cystine in the urine due to lack of reabsorption of these amino acids by the proximal tubular cells of the kidney. Since the intestinal apical membrane PepT1 di-peptide/tripeptide transporter gene (*SLC15A1*) is not affected in cystinuria, dibasic amino acids are absorbed sufficiently to prevent protein malnutrition.

Patients with lysinuric protein intolerance (LPI; also called hyperdibasic aminoaciduria type 2, or familial protein intolerance) show symptoms of diarrhea and vomiting following a protein meal. LPI is an autosomal recessive disease caused by a defect in the *SLC7A7* gene encoding the y^+LAT1subunit, but not in the 4F2hc subunit, of basolateral transport system y^+L (Palacin et al., 2004). Hartnup disorder involves Na^+-dependent transport system B^0 serving the neutral amino acids (Broer et al., 2004, 2005; Seow et al., 2004); this is an autosomal recessive phenotype resulting from mutations in the *SLC6A19* gene that is expressed

Clinical Correlation

Cystinuria

Cystinuria is an inherited disorder of amino acid transport that affects the epithelial cells of the small intestine as well as renal tubules. There are three cystinuria phenotypes, characterized by excretion of cystine and formation of kidney stones in the urinary tract: normal (type I), high stone-forming (type II) range, or moderate (type III) range. A urinary cystine excretion exceeding 1.2 mmol/day (compared with a normal excretion of 0.05 to 0.25 mmol/day) is usually diagnostic type II. Because cystine is very insoluble in aqueous solution, cystine stones are formed and hexagonal cystine crystals appear in the urine. Stones generally form at cystine excretion rates of greater than 300 mg cystine per gram of creatinine in acidic urine. Treatment is directed at reducing the concentration of cystine in urine by increasing urine volume, increasing cystine solubility by alkalinizing the urine, and reducing cystine excretion by use of D-penicillamine or other sulfhydryl-containing compounds to reduce the disulfide or form more soluble mixed disulfides.

Two distinct genes are involved in cystinuria. Each gene encodes a separate subunit of a heterodimeric transporter functional unit composed of rBAT plus $b^{0,+}$AT. This apical membrane transporter serves cystine, neutral amino acids, and dibasic amino acids such as lysine, arginine, and ornithine. L-Cystine is the disulfide form of L-cysteine. Cystine and dibasic amino acid transport occurs in exchange for neutral amino acids (Fig. 9-3), as driven by the enterocyte's interior negative membrane potential.

One form of cystinuria is inherited as an autosomal resessive trait characterized by mutations in the *SLC3A1* gene on chromosome 2, which encodes the rBAT subunit. rBAT is the heavy chain activator subunit of the transporter pair. Other patients with cystinuria display dominant genetics, resulting from mutations in *SLC7A9* on chromosome 19 encoding the $b^{0,+}$AT light chain transmembrane channel subunit. Homozygotes of either gene show type II traits, whereas heterozygotes of combinations of either one or both genes result in a type I, II, or III phenotype. Type I and III patients retain nutritionally significant intestinal absorption of cystine and dibasic amino acids. Several allelic variants of the subunit genes have been described as responsible for cystinuria (Nunes et al 2005a; 2005b; Palacin 1994).

Thinking Critically

1. Adequate amino acid nutrition is not a particular problem in individuals with cystinuria. Why? Discuss several factors related to diet, intestinal absorption, or renal reabsorption that could result in this defect having minimal effect on nutrition.
2. The amount of neutral amino acids excreted in the urine is not elevated in individuals with cystinuria. What are some possible reasons for this?
3. At pH values of less than 7.5, approximately 1 mmol (250 mg) of cystine per liter is the aqueous solubility limit of cystine. Cystinuric patients may excrete more than 1 g of cystine per day. What recommendations would you give a cystinuric patient with regard to water intake?

primarily in the intestine and kidney (Seow et al., 2004). In Hartup disorder, the poor absorption of the amino acid tryptophan leads to inadequate synthesis of NAD(P)/nicotinamide; this gives rise to pellagra-like clinical symptoms of rashes and cerebellar ataxia. (See Chapter 24 for more discussion of tryptophan and the niacin requirement.) In infants, the so-called blue diaper syndrome is the result of excessive, unabsorbed tryptophan reaching the large intestine, where it is converted by bacteria to blue-colored indole derivatives; this defect may be due to disruption of the aromatic amino acid transporter TAT1 encoded by gene *SLC16A10* (Kim et al., 2002). Iminoaciduria is likely attributable to the *SLC6A20* gene encoding the SIT1 proline transporter (Takanaga et al., 2005). Other less understood transport diseases include methionine malabsorptive syndrome, which leads to growth failure due to insufficient delivery and retention of the essential amino acid methionine; and dicarboxylic aminoaciduria, which is due to an impediment in the transport of glutamate and aspartate.

BRUSH-BORDER MEMBRANE TRANSPORT OF PEPTIDES

Up to this point, this chapter has considered amino nitrogen absorption only in terms of free amino acids. However, dipeptide and tripeptide products of protein hydrolysis are also transported across the brush border membrane of absorptive enterocytes, primarily via the PepT1 transporter (Daniel, 2004; Liang et al., 1995). The ability to absorb amino acids both as di- and tripeptides via PepT1 and as free amino acids via multiple amino acid transport systems ensures efficient absorption of essential and nonessential amino acids. A very small portion of the peptides originating from the diet or from digestion of dietary protein in the intestinal lumen are resistant to hydrolysis and may appear intact in the circulation via mechanisms discussed later in this chapter. Peptides that contain proline, which result from the limited ability of proteolytic enzymes to cleave amide bonds involving this imino acid, and L-carnosine (β-alanyl-histidine), a dipeptide found in food (Son et al 2004), are examples.

Di- and tripeptide transport via PepT1 (which also transports the β-lactam antibiotic drugs) is driven by the apical membrane proton (H^+) electrochemical potential, in coordination with the NHE3 Na^+/H^+ exchanger (see Fig. 9-3 and Table 9-1). In the lumen of the intestine, the acidic microenvironment (pH 5-6) near the brush-border surface establishes a pH gradient across the apical membrane and supplies H^+ for cotransport with the peptides. PepT1 energetic coupling to NHE3 Na^+/H^+ exchange activity is similar to that for the amino acid transport system PAT1.

Dipeptides and tripeptides are absorbed more efficiently across the apical surface than is the equivalent free amino acid mixture. This phenomenon has been used to rationalize the clinical feeding of partially hydrolyzed proteins in patients with pancreatic insufficiency. Once dipeptides are removed from the lumen, they are primarily hydrolyzed to the constituent free amino acids by aminopeptidases within the enterocyte cytoplasm. The free amino acids pooled in the enterocyte cytoplasm are finally transported across the basolateral membranes to the portal blood (see Fig. 9-3).

METABOLISM OF AMINO ACIDS IN INTESTINAL EPITHELIAL CELLS

Although most dietary amino acids that are taken up by enterocytes are subsequently transported across the basolateral membrane and enter the portal blood unchanged, several of the amino acids undergo considerable metabolic conversion to other compounds before exit to the portal circulation. In particular, the enterocytes metabolize glutamate, glutamine, aspartate, and arginine taken up from the luminal contents. Glutamine is extensively metabolized by enterocytes as a major energy source. The intestine partially oxidizes glutamine as a fuel, and thus spares dietary glucose and fatty acids for use by other tissues. Indeed, the intestinal requirement for glutamine is so great that, in the postabsorptive state, circulating glutamine released by muscle is avidly taken up by enterocytes via the basolateral membranes. Glutamine metabolism results in release of ammonia, lactate, alanine, proline, and citrulline into the portal circulation. (See Chapter 14 for further discussion of amino acid metabolism.)

USE OF FREE AMINO ACIDS AND PEPTIDES FOR ORAL REHYDRATION THERAPY

Intestinal absorption normally occurs across villus epithelial cells (enterocytes), while secretion of fluid and electrolytes occurs via mucosal crypt cells. When the intestine becomes infected with microorganisms that release enterotoxin (e.g., *Escherichia coli, Vibrio cholera*), excessive quantities of water and electrolytes are lost by intestinal crypt cells in the form of a secretory diarrhea. The fluid and electrolyte losses can be overcome by the use of oral rehydrating therapy (ORT) solutions. ORT exploits the coupled uptake of Na^+ ions, amino acids, glucose, and water that occurs in the absorptive villus cells. It has been experimentally demonstrated that intestinal amino acid absorption via the transport systems serving neutral and dibasic amino acids remain largely intact and functional in patients with cholera infection.

Amino acid-based ORT solutions are essentially iso-osmotic or hypo-osmotic fluids containing Na^+, Cl^-, citrate, and K^+ with free amino acids such as glutamine or alanine. Alternatively, easily digested proteins/peptides may be included to serve as the free amino acid precursors. The mechanism by which intestinal transporters couple the absorption of Na^+ ions and amino acids has been discussed above. Water absorption is subsequently osmotically coupled to the uptake of amino acids and Na^+. Enteral administration of amino acids or proteins is also beneficial in promoting the morphologic, digestive, and absorptive integrity of the mucosa. This is in contrast to long-term degradation of the absorptive capacity of the intestinal mucosa that occurs with long-term administration of total parenteral nutrition (TPN). Therefore, the use of peptide/amino acid/Na^+ rehydration should be promoted as a therapeutic aid during infection, surgery, or other trauma of the gut.

PHYSIOLOGICALLY ACTIVE DIETARY PEPTIDES

Food proteins are known to exert a variety of biologically active functions throughout the body (Wang and Gonzalez de Mejia, 2005; Bannon, 2004; Shimizu, 2004; Son et al, 2004; Sanderson, 2003; Pellegrini 2003; Zalogo and Siddiqui, 2004). A wide spectrum of peptides from plants (e.g., wheat, soy, spinach) and bovine and human milk and are know to enter the general blood circulation intact whereby they influence neural opioid receptors, immunomodulation, anti-inflammatory properties, blood vessel vasoconstriction/relaxation physiology, and sodium metabolism via angiotensin converting enzyme, as shown in Table 9-3 Within the intestinal lumen, food peptides can moduate the digestive process itself.

Virtually all proteins are completely digested and absorbed by the processes described in the preceding text. Nonetheless, a small portion (~1 % or less) of protein is only partially hydrolyzed or resists hydrolysis entirely

Table 9-3
Selected Bioactive Food-Derived Peptides

Source	Peptide Name	Amino Acid Structure	Physiological Activity
Meat	L-Carnosine	β-Alanyl-histidine	Antiinflammatory; antioxidant; prevents glycation
Wheat	Gliadorphin	YPQPQPF	Opioid agonist
Wheat	Gluten exorphin-A5	GYYPT	Peripheral inhibition of stress-induced pain; CNS opioid agonist
Milk	β-Lactorphin	ALPMHIR	ACE inhibitor
Milk	β-Casokinin-7	AVPYPQR	ACE inhibitor
Milk	β-Lactorphin dipeptide	YL	ACE inhibitor
Milk	Casoplatelin	MAIPPKKNQDK	Inhibits platelet aggregation
Milk	Lactotransferrin thrombic inhibitory peptide	KRDS	Inhibits platelet aggregation
Milk	Casoxin D	YVPFPPF	Opioid antagonist
Milk	α-Casein exorphin	RYLGYLE	Opioid agonist
Milk	β-Casomorphin-7	YPFPGPI	Opioid agonist; decreases intestinal motility; enhances NaCl absorption
Milk	Lactoferricin	FKCRRWNRMKKLGA-PSITCVRRAF	Antimicrobial; disrupts bacterial membranes
Milk	Phosphopeptide	SSSEE	Calcium/phosphate-stabilizing to enhance absorption

NOTE: Sequences use standard amino acid symbols.
ACE, Angiotensin converting enzyme.

(Wang and de Mejia 2005; Pellegrini, 2003). Many peptide fragments are generated in milligram quantities within the gastrointestinal tract by the action of peptidases from the stomach, pancreas, and intestinal membranes and enterocyte cystosol. Much of the incompletely hydrolyzed protein and peptide nitrogen passes into the large intestine where it is metabolized by colonic bacteria and excreted in the feces. However, a variety of polypeptide fragments modulate intestinal physiology even before they are excreted or absorbed. For example, phosphopeptides from milk casein enhance calcium absorption, soybean peptides inhibit cholesterol and bile acid absoption, and wheat albumin supresses luminal amylase activity. The uptake of certain intact peptide growth factors from the lumen, such as epidermal growth factor (EGF) or transforming growth factor alpha (TGFα), are especially important during development and maturation of the gastrointestinal mucosa.

Partial digestion of certain proteins found in cereal grains (gluten/gliadin), soy, or cow's milk (casein, whey, lactalbumin, β-lactoglobulin) results in incompletely hydrolyzed peptide fragments that can penetrate the mucosal barrier via a paracellular route through "leaky" tight junctions or via endocytosis/exocytosis. Central nervous system effects of dietary food peptide fragments act through opioid receptors, with physiological effects via opioid agonist as well as antagonist properties. The enterocyte aminopeptidase dipeptidyl peptidase IV (DPP-IV) is responsible for inactivating the exorphin type peptides formed from casomorphin (milk) and gluteomorphin (wheat) fragments. Thus, DPP-IV prevents these peptides from exerting opioid receptor effects in the central nervous system. It has been postulated that individuals lacking sufficient DPP-IV activity may be predisposed to certain opioid-related mood, behavior, or thought disturbances such as those experienced with depression, autism, or psychosis.

Details describing transepithelial movement of luminal peptide fragments are incompletely understood. However, a general picture has emerged regarding how partially hydrolyzed food peptides interact with the mucosal barrier. One or more of four general mechanisms are involved: (1) specific transport via PepT1, (2) paracellular movement across leaky tight junctions, (3) transcellular movement across the enterocyte via endocytosis/exocytosis, and (4) IgA/M-cell presentation to Peyer's patches/ lymphoid tissue. These fundamental mechanisms are illustrated in Figure 9-3 and Figure 9-5.

The proton-activated PepT1 transporter handles many oligopeptides, including carnosine (i.e., β-alanine-histidine), a major meat dipeptide that is absorbed as the intact dipeptide (Son et al., 2004). Interestingly, therapeutic β-lactamase antibiotics and angiotensin converting enzyme (ACE) inhibitors are also absorbed intact via the PepT1 route.

Paracellular uptake of peptides occurs by movement of peptides between the mucosal cells instead of through the mucosal cells. This can occur when the tight junctions between the mucosal epithelial cells are damaged and, thus, leaky. The leaky junctions increase the nonspecific permeability of the intestinal epithelium to all macromolecules. Pathologies associated with chronic or extensive abdominal radiation, malnutrition, or invasive microorganisms (e.g., species of salmonellae or shigellae) can include damage to the epithelial cells and to the tight-junctions of the intestinal mucosal barrier.

In the presence of a healthy mucosa with intact tight junctions, milligram amounts of intact polypeptides can be absorbed via endocytic uptake across the brush-border membrane followed by exocytosis across the basolateral membrane (van Niel and Heyman, 2002; Sanderson, 2003). In this case, the luminal free polypeptide first binds to specific receptors within clathrin-coated pits on enterocyte brush-border membranes. The brush-border membrane then invaginates to form an intracellular vesicle by the process of endocytosis. During invagination, additional molecules, other than receptor-bound polypeptide, can be simultaneously nonspecifically trapped within the vesicle fluid. Within the cell, the vesicle or endosome fuses with lysosomes, which are organelles containing acid proteases such as cathepsin B and cathepsin D. Vesicle membrane-bound macromolecules escape digestion within the lysosome, whereas unbound proteins trapped within the vesicle are digested to free amino acids and small peptide

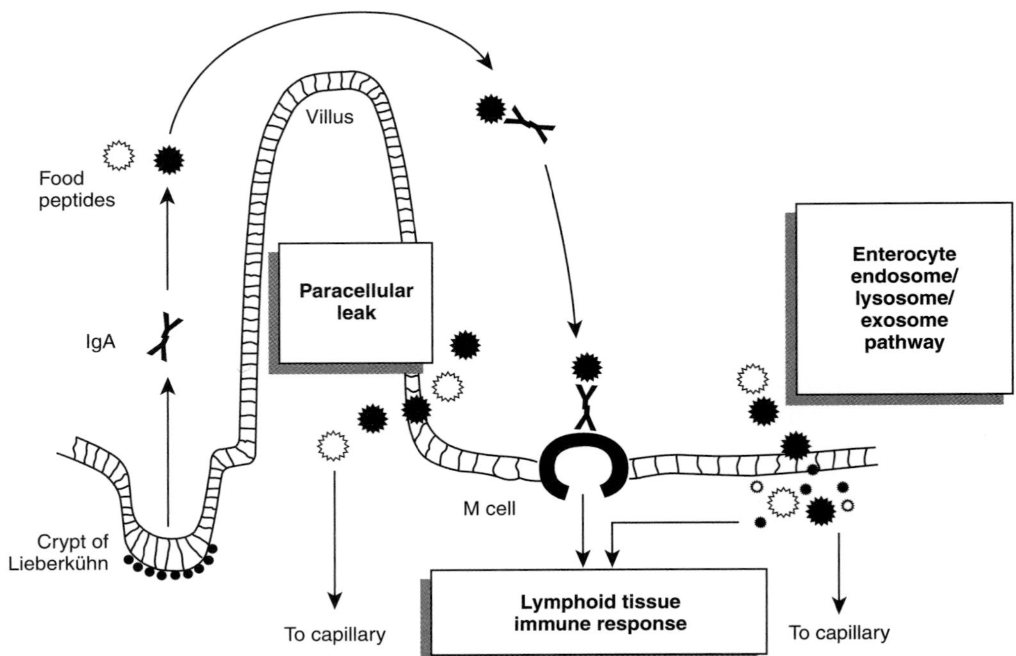

Figure 9-5 Intestinal processing of intact large peptides that escape luminal digestion. Intact large, and potentially antigenic, peptide fragments can be taken up across the epithelial barrier of the small intestine by three possible pathways: IgA/M-cell presentation to Peyer's patches; paracellular movement across leaky tight junctions; and/or transcellular movement via enterocyte endocytosis/lysosome/exocytosis processing. Dimeric IgA released from the crypt region can bind to specific epitopes of partially digested food polypeptides within the intestinal lumen. M-cells (located within the epithelium adjacent to absorptive enterocytes) are activated by the dimeric IgA/peptide complex. Activated M-cells present the food polypeptide as an antigen to lymphoid tissue within the intestinal lining, thereby initiating a local inflammatory immune response that creates leaky tight junctions and thus provides paracellular uptake pathways for additional peptide fragments. Peptide antigens can also bind the enterocyte apical membrane within clathrin-coated pits and be taken up by endocytosis. Subsequent processing by the enterocyte leads to basolateral exit of cytosolic cathepsin digest products (amino acids or smaller peptides) or intact peptides that escaped lysosomal processing. MHC II presentation of these peptides to gastrointestinal lymphoid tissues initiates inflammatory events. The food peptides that escape hydrolysis or processing by the intestinal lymphoid tissue and do enter the bloodstream via the capillaries can cause a systemic immune response.

fragments, both of which are transported out of the endosome to the cytosol. The peptide fragments of the digested proteins are eventually hydrolyzed to free amino acids by cytosolic aminopeptidases. However, the lysosomal vesicle containing the membrane-bound intact polypeptide traverses the cytosol, and the vesicle fuses with the basolateral membrane. This allows the polypeptide to exit the cell by exocytosis into the interstitial space, where it can activate the intestinal immunoglobulin A (IgA) immune response or enter the blood capillaries intact to activate systemic IgE immune responses. Simultaneously but independently, the Golgi apparatus supplies the endosome with class II major histocompatibility complex (MHC) molecules that bind to the polypeptide. The MHC-tagged peptides are also released at the basolateral membrane where they can present the peptide to lymphocytes of the gastrointestinal immune system to initiate an inflammatory response.

Immunologically important peptides are absorbed by a paracellular mechanism described in Figure 9-5. Immunoglobulin IgA, in dimeric form, is secreted across epithelial cells at the base of the intestinal crypts. Secretory IgA attaches to the mucus overlying the enterocytes, where it can neutralize pathogens or their toxins. This IgA also can bind to specific epitopes of incompletely hydrolyzed food peptides in the lumen, and present them as antigens to M cells of the epithelium. M or microfold cells are specialized epithelial cells that overlay Peyer's patches, which are lymphoid follicles similar to lymph nodes but located in the mucosa and extending into the submucosa of the small intestine. The M cells are involved in nonspecific uptake of protein and peptide antigens (Sanderson, 2003). The M cells transport the peptides into the underlying tissue and present the peptide as an antigen to dendritic cells and macrophages in the Peyer's patches to initiate a lymphoid tissue inflammatory immune response, including IgA secretion. This local immune response can create leaky tight junctions in the intestinal epithelium and thus also promote uptake of food peptides via the paracellular uptake pathway.

REFERENCES

Bannon GA (2004) What makes a food protein an allergen? Curr Allergy Asthma Rep 4:43-46.

Boll M, Foltz M, Anderson CM, Oechsler C, Kottra G, Thwaites DT, Daniel H (2003) Substrate recognition by the mammalian proton-dependent amino acid transporter PAT1. Mol Membr Biol 20:261-269.

Broer A, Klingel K, Kowalczuk S, Rasko JE, Cavanaugh J, Broer S (2004) Molecular cloning of mouse amino acid transport system B^0, a neutral amino acid transporter related to Hartnup disorder. J Biol Chem 279: 24467-24476.

Broer S, Cavanaugh JA, Rasko JE (2005) Neutral amino acid transport in epithelial cells and its malfunction in Hartnup disorder. Biochem Soc Trans 33:233-236.

Chen JM, Kukor Z, Le Marechal C, Toth M, Tsakiris L, Raguenes O, Ferec C, Sahin-Toth M (2003a) Evolution of trypsinogen activation peptides. Mol Biol Evol 20:1767-1777.

Chen Z, Fei YJ, Anderson CM, Wake KA, Miyauchi S, Huang W, Thwaites DT, Ganapathy V (2003b) Structure, function and immunolocalization of a proton-coupled amino acid transporter (hPAT1) in the human intestinal cell line Caco-2. J Physiol 546:349-361.

Chillaron J, Roca R, Valencia A, Zorzano A, Palacin M (2001) Heteromeric amino acid transporters: biochemistry, genetics, and physiology. Am J Physiol. 281:F995-F1018.

Dave MH, Schulz N, Zecevic M, Wagner CA, Verrey F (2004) Expression of heteromeric amino acid transporters along the murine intestine. J Physiol 558:597-610.

Ferraris RP, Diamond JM (1989) Specific regulation of intestinal nutrient transporters by their dietary substrates. Annu Rev Physiol 51:125-141.

Gerencser GA, Stevens BR (1994) Thermodynamics of symport and antiport catalyzed by cloned or native transporters. J Exper Biol 196:59-75.

Kim DK, Kanai Y, Matsuo H, Kim JY, Chairoungdue A., Kobayashi Y, Enomoto A, Cha SH, Goya T, Endou H (2002) The human T-type amino acid transporter-1: characterization, gene organization, and chromosomal location. Genomics 79:95-103.

Kitamoto Y, Veile RA, Donin-Keller H, Sadler JE (1995) cDNA sequence and chromosomal localization of human enterokinase, the proteolytic activator of trypsinogen. Biochemistry 34:4562-4568.

Liang R, Fei Y-J, Prasad PD, Ramamoorthy S, Han H, Yang-Feng T, Hediger MA, Ganapathy V, Leibach FH (1995) Human intestinal H^+/peptide cotransporter cloning, functional expression, and chromosomal localization. J Biol Chem 270:6456-6463.

Mailliard ME, Stevens BR, Mann GE (1995) Amino acid transport by small intestinal, hepatic, and pancreatic epithelia. Gastroenterology 108:888-910.

Marin M, Lavillette D, Kelly SM, Kabat D (2003) N-linked glycosylation and sequence changes in a critical negative control region of the ASCT1 and ASCT2 neutral amino acid transporters determine their retroviral receptor functions. J Virol 77:2936-45.

Nemoda Z, Sahin-Tóth M (2005) The tetra-aspartate motif in the activation peptide of human cationic trypsinogen is essential or autoactivation control but not for enteropeptidase recognition. J Biol Chem 280:29645-29652.

Nunes V, Font-Llitjos M, Jimenez-Vidal M, Bisceglia L, Di Perna M, de Sanctis L, Rousaud F, Zelante L, Palacin M, Nunes V (2005a) Gene symbol: SLC3A1. Disease: Cystinuria. Hum Genet May 116:541.

Nunes V, Font-Llitjos M, Jimenez-Vidal M, Bisceglia L, Di Perna M, de Sanctis L, Rousaud F, Zelante L, Palacin M (2005b) Gene symbol: SLC7A9. Disease: cystinuria, type non-I. Hum Genet 116:244.

Palacin M (1994) A new family of proteins (rBAT and 4F2hc) involved in cationic and zwitterionic amino acid transport. A tale of two proteins in search of a transport function. J Exp Biol 196:123-137.

Palacin M, Bertran J, Chillaron J, Estevez R, Zorzano A (2004) Lysinuric protein intolerance: mechanisms of pathophysiology. Mol Genet Metab 81(Suppl 1):S27-S37.

Palacin M, Kanai Y (2004) The ancillary proteins of HATs: SLC3 family of amino acid transporters. Pflugers Arch 447:490-494.

Pan M, Souba WW, Karinch AM, Lin CM, Stevens BR (2002a) Specific reversible stimulation of system y(+) L-arginine transport activity in human intestinal cells. J Gastrointest Surg 6:379-386.

Pan M, Souba WW, Karinch AM, Lin CM, Stevens BR (2002b) Epidermal growth factor regulation of system L alanine transport in undifferentiated and differentiated intestinal Caco-2 cells. J Gastrointest Surg 6:410-417.

Pan M, Souba WW, Wolfgang CL, Karinch AM, Stevens BR (2002c) Posttranslational alanine trans-stimulation of zwitterionic amino acid transport systems in human intestinal Caco-2 cells. J Surg Res104:63-69.

Pan M, Stevens BR (1995) Protein kinase C-dependent regulation of L-arginine transport activity in Caco-2 intestinal cells. Biochim Biophys Acta 1239:27-32.

Pellegrini, A (2003) Bioactive peptides from food proteins. Current Pharmaceutical Design, 9:16.

Peral MJ, Garcia-Delgado M, Calonge ML, Duran JM, De La Horra MC, Wallimann T, Speer O, Ilundain A (2002) Human, rat and chicken small intestinal Na^+- Cl^- -creatine transporter: functional, molecular characterization and localization. J Physiol 545:133-44.

Sanderson IR (2003) The innate immune system of the gastrointestinal tract. Mol Immunol 40:393-394.

Seow HF, Broer S, Broer A, Bailey CG, Potter SJ, Cavanaugh JA, Rasko JE (2004) Hartnup disorder is caused by mutations in the gene encoding the neutral amino acid transporter SLC6A19. Nat Genet 36:1003-1007.

Shimizu, M (2004) Food-derived peptides and intestinal functions. BioFactors 21:43-47.

Son DO, Satsu H, Kiso Y, Shimizu M (2004) Characterization of carnosine uptake and its physiological function in human intestinal epithelial Caco-2 cells. Biofactors 21(1-4): 395-398.

Stevens BR (1992) Amino acid transport in intestine. In: Kilberg MS, Haussinger D (eds) Mammalian Amino Acid Transport: Mechanisms and Control. Plenum, New York, pp 149-164.

Takanaga H, Mackenzie B, Suzuki Y, Hediger MA (2005) Identification of mammalian proline transporter SIT1 (SLC6A20) with characteristics of classical system imino. J Biol Chem 280:8974-8984.

Terada T, Shimada Y, Pan X, Kishimoto K, Sakurai T, Doi R, Onodera H, Katsura T, Imamura M, Inui KI (2005) Expression profiles of various transporters for oligopeptides, amino acids and organic ions along the human digestive tract. Biochem Pharmacol 70:1756-1763.

van Niel G, Heyman M (2002) The epithelial cell cytoskeleton and intracellular trafficking. II. Intestinal epithelial cell exosomes: perspectives on their structure and function. Am J Physiol Gastrointest Liver Physiol 283: G251-G255.

Verhoeven NM, Salomons GS, Jakobs C (2005) Laboratory diagnosis of defects of creatine biosynthesis and transport. Clinica Chimica Acta 361:1-9.

Verrey F, Closs EI, Wagner CA, Palacin M, Endou H, Kanai Y (2004) CATs and HATs: the SLC7 family of amino acid transporters. Pflugers Arch 47:532-542.

Wagner CA, Lang, F, Bröer S (2001). Function and structure of heterodimeric amino acid transporters. Am J Physiol Cell Physiol 281:C1077-C1093.

Wang W, Gonzalez de Mejia E (2005) A new frontier in soy bioactive peptides that may prevent age-related chronic diseases. Comp Rev Food Sci Food Safety 4:63-78.

Zaloga, GP, Siddiqui RA (2004) Biologically active dietary peptides. Mini Rev Med Chem 4:815-821.

Zamolodchikova RS, Sokolova EA, Lu D, Sadler JE (2000) Activation of recombinant proenteropeptidase by duodenase. FEBS Lett 466:295-299.

RECOMMENDED READING

Johnson LR (ed) (2001) Gastrointestinal Physiology, 6th ed. Mosby, St. Louis.

Chapter 10

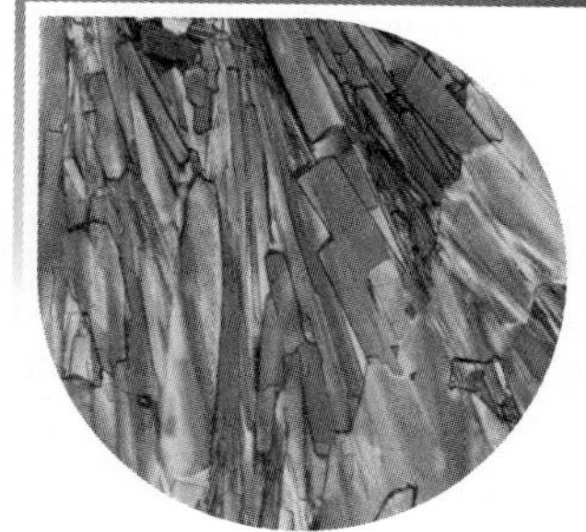

Digestion and Absorption of Lipids

Patrick P. Tso, PhD, Karen Crissinger, MD, PhD, and Ronald J. Jandacek, PhD

OUTLINE

COMMON ABBREVIATIONS

ACAT acyl CoA:cholesterol acyltransferase
FABP fatty acid–binding protein
MTP microsomal triglyceride transfer protein
SCP sterol carrier protein

DIETARY LIPIDS

Dietary lipids have been described as that part of the diet that can be extracted by organic solvents (Borgstrom, 1986). According to this definition, a variety of compounds qualify, including both nonpolar lipids such as triacylglycerols and polar lipids such as phospholipids.

Although a variety of types of lipids are consumed in the diet, by far the greatest quantity of dietary lipids is in the form of triacylglycerols (triglycerides). Furthermore, most of these dietary triacylglycerols contain predominantly long-chain fatty acids (chain lengths of 14 to 20 carbons) esterified to the glycerol backbone. According to the 1999-2000 National Health and Nutrition Examination Survey (NHANES), men in the United States eat on the average approximately 96 g of fat each day, and women eat 70 g. Fat accounts for an average of 33% of energy in both sexes. The American Heart Association and the Dietary Guidelines for Americans recommend that the intake of fat be reduced to 30% of calories to reduce the risk of atherosclerosis. Dietary triacylglycerol is a major source of energy, with a higher caloric density than the other macronutrients, and also it is a source of essential fatty acids in the ω3 and ω6 classes, mainly as linoleate (18:2ω6) and linolenate (18:3ω3). (See Chapter 18 for a discussion of essential fatty acids.)

Other dietary lipids include fat-soluble vitamins A, D, E, and K (micronutrients discussed in Chapters 28 through 31), cholesterol and cholesteryl esters, and phospholipids. The amount of cholesterol/cholesteryl ester and phospholipid in the diet is considerably less than the amount of triacylglycerol; daily intake of cholesterol is generally less than 350 mg and that of phospholipid is equal to 1 to 2 g. However, endogenous biliary lipids present additional cholesterol (1 g) and phospholipid (10 to 20 g) to the intestine over the course of a day; in the case of phospholipid, the biliary supply is much greater than that obtained from the diet, and absorbed phospholipids reflect the phospholipid content of the biliary secretions (Borgstrom, 1976; Northfield and Hofmann, 1975).

LUMINAL DIGESTION OF LIPIDS

Digestion and absorption of lipids by the intestinal tract is a complex process that requires a number of steps that occur in the lumen of the gastrointestinal tract plus further processing of absorbed lipids that occurs after digestion products have been taken up into the enterocytes of the small intestinal mucosa.

The hydrolysis of triacylglycerol (fatty acid esters) is absolutely required for it to be absorbed from the intestine. Some early electron microscopic studies of fat absorption suggested that fat might be absorbed by assimilation of emulsified oil droplets in the intestine based on the appearance of a "stream of fat droplets filtering through the striated border, entering the epithelial cell by pinocytosis" (Palay and Karlin, 1959, p. 373). However, subsequent electron microscopic studies of triacylglycerol absorption in the rat clearly demonstrated that pinocytosis of oil droplets did not contribute to normal fat digestion. Cardell and colleagues (1967) fed rats corn oil that contained suspended silver particles of dimensions of 70 to 100 Å. If oil droplets of the size that are found in the intestinal emulsion were to be taken up directly without hydrolysis, there would have been observable silver particles in the intestinal cells. The absence of these particles supported the view that pinocytosis of intact fat droplets does not take place in normal fat absorption. These electron microscopic data complemented the classic physical chemistry studies of Hofmann (1966) and Hofmann and Borgstrom (1962), who presented the concept of micellar transport of the fatty acid and monoacylglycerol products of fat digestion.

Mattson and Volpenhein (1972a, 1972b) synthesized a series of polyol oleate esters and used these as a tool for further exploration of the process of fat absorption. The oleate esters of sucrose, erythritol, and other polyols have physical properties essentially identical to those of triolein. Their melting point and lipophilicity result in the same kinds of emulsified oil droplets that triolein forms in the small intestine. In studies performed in vitro, Mattson and Volpenhein (1972a) measured the rates of hydrolysis of these oleate esters by pancreatic lipases and by bile salt–stimulated lipase (carboxyl ester lipase) and found that the oleate ester of erythritol was partially hydrolyzed, whereas that of sucrose was not hydrolyzed at all. Using rats with lymphatic cannulation, Mattson and Volpenhein (1972b) further explored the relationship of the hydrolysis of oleate esters to their absorbability. They found that erythritol tetraoleate, which was partially hydrolyzed, was partially absorbed, whereas sucrose octaoleate, which was not hydrolyzed, was not absorbed. The studies of Mattson and Volpenhein with sucrose octaoleate led to the development of olestra (Olean [Procter & Gamble, Cincinnati, OH]), which is a nondigestible fat made up of hexa-, hepta-, and octaesters of sucrose that is used in the preparation of snack foods (potato chips and crackers).

Further evidence of the requirement for hydrolysis for fat absorption has been provided in studies of orlistat (tetrahydrolipstatin, Xenical [Hoffman-La Roche, Nutley, NJ]), a drug that inactivates gastric and pancreatic lipases by covalently binding to the active site serine residue (Hadvary et al., 1991). The inhibition of pancreatic lipase by orlistat results in a significant reduction in fat absorption (~30%) as shown by markedly increased fat excretion (Hartmann et al., 1993). Orlistat has been approved for use in obesity management.

DIGESTION OF TRIACYLGLYCEROLS

The digestion of triacylglycerols begins in the stomach, with the action of gastric lipase, which is secreted by the gastric mucosa. Gastric lipase is called an acid lipase because its activity is highest in an acidic medium. Acid lipases hydrolyze triacylglycerols that contain medium-chain fatty acids faster than they hydrolyze those containing long-chain fatty acids. Acid lipase preferentially cleaves the fatty acid at the *sn*-3 position of the triacylglycerol molecule, regardless of the fatty acid esterified to this position. The 1,2-diacylglycerols (diglycerides) and fatty acids produced as a result of the action of acid lipases may promote the emulsification of dietary fat in the stomach. Grinding and mixing of the gastric contents as a result of gastric motility also contribute to dispersion of the lipid droplets. Acid lipases do not hydrolyze cholesteryl esters or phospholipids such as phosphatidylcholine. Although the optimal pH of gastric lipase is around 4, the enzyme is still quite active at pH 6 to 6.5, and probably continues to digest triacylglycerol in the upper duodenum where the pH is between 6 and 7. Human milk fat, which can include 12% of fatty acids with 10 to 14 carbon atoms, is hydrolyzed efficiently by acid lipases (Genzel-Baroviczeny et al., 1997); this probably contributes to the efficient digestion of milk fat observed in infants. Gastric lipase is particularly important in the digestion of triacylglycerols in infants because they have immature levels of pancreatic lipase (Hamosh, 1996).

The lipid emulsion leaves the stomach and enters the small intestine as fine lipid droplets less than 0.5 mm in diameter. The combined action of bile and pancreatic juice brings about a marked change in the chemical and physical form of this lipid emulsion. Most of the digestion of triacylglycerol is brought about by pancreatic lipase in the lumen of the upper part of the small intestine. Pancreatic lipase works at the interface between the oil and aqueous phases. Pancreatic lipase acts mainly on the *sn*-1 and *sn*-3 positions of the triacylglycerol molecule to release 2-monoacylglycerol and free fatty acids.

Pure pancreatic lipase works inefficiently in a bile salt–lipid mixture, and yet lipase present in pancreatic juice hydrolyzes triacylglycerols extremely efficiently. This apparent discrepancy led to the discovery of the cofactor called colipase. Colipase is a heat-stable protein required for lipase activity when bile salt is present; it is synthesized and secreted by the pancreas as procolipase and is activated to colipase in the small intestine by proteolytic cleavage by trypsin. As shown in Figure 10-1, the triacylglycerol lipid droplets covered with bile salts (*BS* in the diagram) are not accessible to pancreatic lipase. However, the binding of colipase to the triacylglycerol–aqueous interface allows the binding of lipase to the lipid–aqueous interface. Lipase binds with colipase in a 1:1 molar ratio.

DIGESTION OF PHOSPHOLIPIDS

Digestion of phospholipids occurs in the small intestine. In addition to phospholipids in the diet, a large amount of endogenous phospholipid enters the lumen of the small intestine in the bile. In bile, the phospholipid (predominantly phosphatidylcholine) is found in mixed micelles along with cholesterol and bile salts. Once in the lumen of the small intestine, the

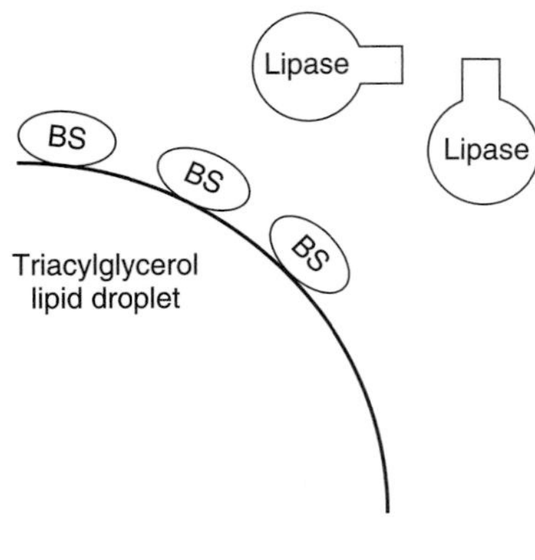

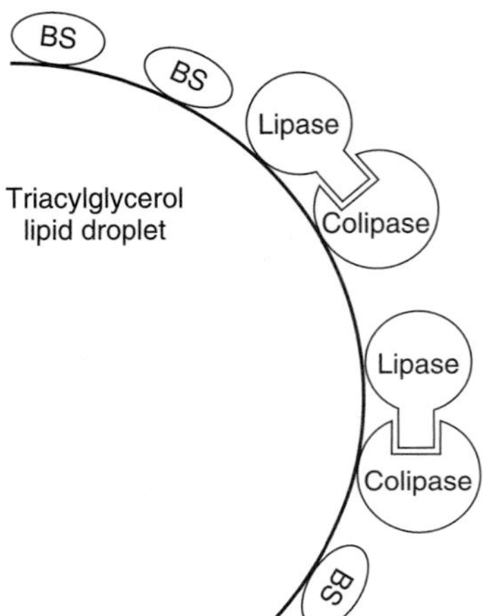

Figure 10-1 Interaction between lipase, colipase, and triacylglycerol droplets. Lipase normally binds poorly to the triacylglycerol lipid droplets. In the presence of colipase, lipase molecules bind to the lipid droplets and hydrolyze the triacylglycerol to form 2-monoacylglycerol and fatty acids. *BS*, Bile salt.

biliary phosphatidylcholine will distribute between the mixed micelles and triacylglycerol droplets, but phosphatidylcholine tends to favor the micellar phase over the oily phase. It is phospholipids in micelles that serve as substrates for hydrolysis. Hydrolysis of phospholipids is largely brought about by phospholipase A_2, which is secreted by the pancreas as prophospholipase A_2 and then activated by trypsin within the lumen of the small intestine. Phospholipase A_2 releases the fatty acid from the *sn*-2 position of phosphatidylcholine to yield a fatty acid and lysophosphatidylcholine. Although the bulk of luminal intestinal phospholipase A_2 activity is derived from pancreatic juice, there is probably some minor contribution from the intestinal mucosa, which has an intrinsic membrane enzyme that has phospholipase and retinyl ester hydrolase activity, which is known as retinyl ester hydrolase, or phospholipase B.

DIGESTION OF CHOLESTERYL ESTERS

Only free cholesterol is absorbed by the small intestine. Most dietary cholesterol is present as the free sterol, but 10% to 15% is present as the sterol ester. Biliary cholesterol is also mainly free cholesterol. Cholesteryl ester is hydrolyzed to free cholesterol in the presence of cholesterol esterase (also called carboxyl ester hydrolase, bile salt–stimulated lipase, and nonspecific esterase), which is secreted by the pancreas as an active enzyme. The human cholesterol esterase has a broad specificity, and it can hydrolyze triacylglycerols, cholesteryl esters, phosphoglycerides, sphingolipids, esters of vitamins A and D, and monoacylglycerols. Because it will hydrolyze all three ester linkages of triacylglycerols, it is sometimes called nonspecific esterase.

As is phospholipase A_2, cholesterol esterase is active against substrates that have been incorporated into bile salt micelles. Cholesterol esterase activity is stimulated by bile salts, particularly trihydroxy bile salts such as sodium taurocholate. The activation of cholesterol esterase by bile salts is mediated by changing the conformation of this protein. A unique property of cholesterol esterase is its self association; the presence of trihydroxy bile salts (taurocholate or glycocholate) promotes the self-aggregation of the enzyme into polymeric forms. The self-association of cholesterol esterase protects the enzyme from proteolytic inactivation. Purified pancreatic cholesterol esterase appears to exist mainly as dimers, especially in the presence of taurocholate.

UPTAKE OF LIPID DIGESTION PRODUCTS BY THE ENTEROCYTES

The digestion products of triacylglycerols, phospholipids, and cholesteryl esters are predominantly monoacylglycerols, fatty acids,

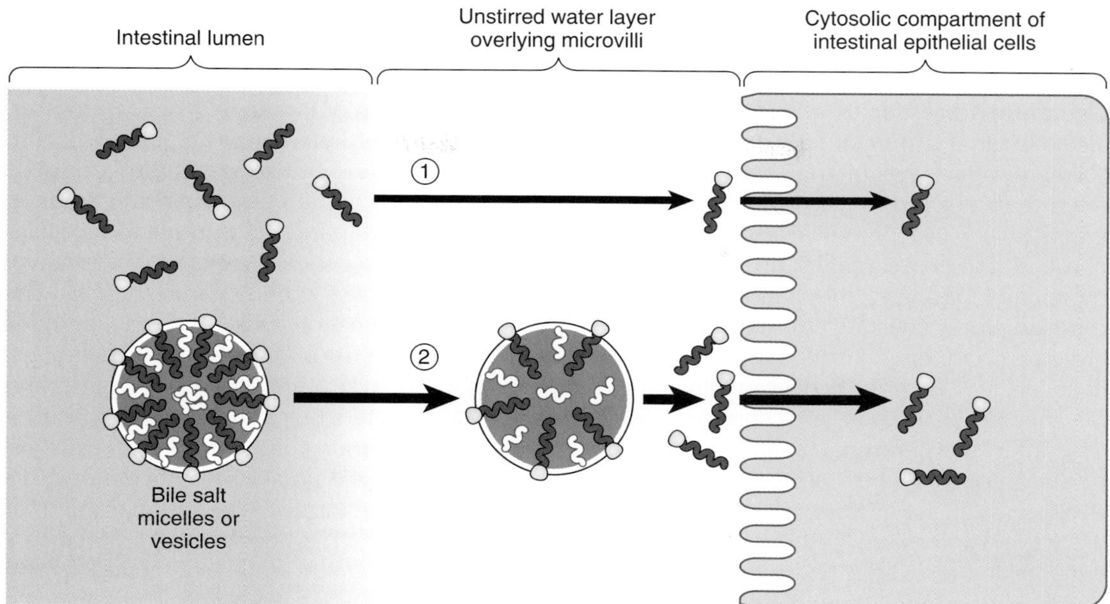

Figure 10-2 The role of bile salt micelles in overcoming the diffusion barrier associated with the unstirred water layer. In the absence of bile salts *(1)*, only a limited number of lipid molecules diffuse through the unstirred water layer to be taken up across the brush-border membrane of the enterocytes. In the presence of bile salts *(2)*, more lipid molecules can be delivered to the brush-border membrane by bile salt micelles.

lysophosphatidylcholine, and cholesterol. Although these lipid digestion products are somewhat polar, they have very limited capacity to dissolve in water. The epithelial surface of the small intestine is surrounded by a layer of water called the unstirred water layer, and the thickness of the unstirred water layer depends on how vigorously the small intestinal contents are mixed. Increased mixing reduces the thickness of the unstirred water layer. As illustrated in Figure 10-2, this unstirred water layer represents a barrier that lipids must cross before they can be absorbed by the enterocytes (small intestinal epithelial cells).

IMPORTANCE OF MICELLAR SOLUBILIZATION

As shown in Figure 10-2, the limited aqueous solubility of lipid digestion products results in only a few individual molecules crossing the unstirred water layer and being absorbed by the enterocytes. To overcome this barrier, lipid digestion products are first solubilized in mixed bile salt micelles. Bile acids (or salts) are biological detergents, and they will form micelles (aggregates) when the concentration of bile salts in the lumen is at or above the critical micellar concentration (approximately 1 to 2 mM, depending on composition of bile salts). Pure micelles contain only bile salts, whereas mixed micelles contain bile salts as well as other lipid moieties. The concentration of bile salts in the lumen is almost always greater than the critical micellar concentration. Free cholesterol and other lipid digestion products can be incorporated into the mixed micelles, thereby rendering these lipid molecules soluble in the bulk water phase. The mixed micelles containing polar lipids and cholesterol readily cross the unstirred water layer and thereby increase the aqueous concentrations of fatty acids, monoacylglycerols, cholesterol, and lysophosphatidylcholine near the epithelial absorptive surface by a factor of 100 to 1,000. This provides an efficient mechanism for diffusion across the unstirred water layer, facilitating the subsequent uptake of these lipid molecules by the enterocytes.

IMPORTANCE OF UNILAMELLAR VESICLES

When the jejunal contents of humans are sampled during digestion of a lipid meal and subjected to ultracentrifugation, one can observe a solid particulate layer on the bottom of the tube. Next, there is a mostly clear micellar phase followed by an oily phase on the top. The oily phase is composed mainly of triacylglycerols, mono- and diacylglycerols, and fatty acids. The micellar phase contains bile acids, monoacylglycerols, and fatty acids. When Porter and Saunders (1971) performed a careful analysis of the aqueous phase after ultracentrifugation and also after the intestinal contents had been passed through a series of filters with progressively smaller pores, they observed that both the ultracentrifugation and the filtering procedure yielded a micellar phase that was slightly turbid. Furthermore, they found that there was a concentration gradient of lipids in the micellar phase, an important point that was missed previously. This observation is important because it hinted to the fact that the micellar phase is not homogeneous.

The explanation for this intriguing observation came later when Carey and colleagues (1983) proposed that the lipid in the intestinal lumen following a meal contains, in addition to the fat emulsion particles, two dispersed phases: (1) a phase of large disc-like mixed bile salt micelles more or less saturated with lipids, which have hydrodynamic radii of approximately 200 Å, and (2) a phase consisting of lipid crystalline or unilamellar vesicles (liposomes) of mixed lipids saturated with bile salts, which have hydrodynamic radii of approximately 400 to 600 Å. The existence of vesicles has important pathophysiological implications. Patients with low intraluminal bile salt concentrations (Mansbach et al., 1980) and patients with bile fistulae (Porter et al., 1971) have reasonably good fat absorption. In these patients, who have elevated concentrations of lipids in the intestinal lumen, liquid crystalline vesicles may play an important role in the uptake of lipid digestion products.

PERMEATION OF DIGESTED FAT INTO ENTEROCYTES

At least two different mechanisms have been proposed for the uptake of lipid digestion products by the small intestine—passive uptake and carrier-mediated uptake. Once digested lipid is presented to the surface of the brush-border membrane of the enterocytes, the products of lipid digestion can dissolve in the lipid of the brush-border membrane. The concentration gradient between the lipids in the brush border and those in the intracellular compartment of the enterocytes favors initial diffusion of these products into the cell. The rapid reesterification of the intracellular lipids by enzymes of the endoplasmic reticulum (ER) to form triacylglycerols, phospholipids, and cholesteryl esters helps maintain low intracellular concentrations of these lipids, thus favoring the continued uptake or diffusion of these lipids into the intracellular compartment of the enterocytes. The postprandial luminal content of fatty acids and 2-monoacylglycerol achieves a combined concentration of as much as 50 mmol/L (Hernell et al., 1990), and the movement of fatty acids from the intestinal lumen into the enterocyte has generally been considered to be driven by the high concentration of fatty acids in the lumen after a meal containing fat. The more water-soluble products of lipid digestion, such as glycerol and short-chain fatty acids, if present, are efficiently taken up by diffusion.

The involvement of a transporter in the uptake of digestion products of triacylglycerols has also been considered. Stahl and colleagues (1999) identified an intestinal protein (FATP4) of the class of fatty acid transport proteins (FATPs) that increased the rate of uptake in transfected cells. These studies were performed with a total fatty acid concentration of 100 μmol/L, which is considerably less than that present in the intestinal lumen following a meal. It is possible that the transporter does facilitate fatty acid absorption when fat concentrations are extremely low, and perhaps it evolved as a protective means to ensure efficient uptake of essential fatty acids in times of fat deprivation. Mice with targeted disruption of the *FATP4* gene exhibited a neonatal lethal restrictive dermopathy, suggesting a role of FATP4 in skin development (Hermann et al., 2003). FATP4 may also function as a very long chain acyl-CoA synthetase (Hermann et al., 2001).

The intestinal absorption of lipid-soluble vitamins is discussed in Chapters 28 through 31.

Fat-soluble vitamins generally behave like the lipid digestion products and are solubilized in mixed bile salt micelles to ensure their efficient passage through the unstirred water layer. Whether they are taken up by the enterocytes by simple diffusion or by specific transporters located at the brush-border membrane or by both mechanisms is unclear.

INTRACELLULAR METABOLISM OF ABSORBED LIPIDS

Once in the cytosol of the enterocyte, lipid compounds are again in an aqueous environment. Thus, various lipids must be transported intracellularly from the apical region, where they are absorbed, to the ER, where the enzymes involved in their metabolism are located. These lipid digestion products are largely reesterified in the enterocyte in preparation for export in chylomicrons.

INTRACELLULAR TRANSPORT OF ABSORBED LIPIDS

As yet, it is not fully understood how the various absorbed lipids migrate from the site of absorption to the ER where biosynthesis of complex lipids takes place. A fatty acid–binding protein (FABP) present in the small intestine was first isolated and characterized by Ockner and Manning (1974), who proposed that this FABP plays an important role in the intracellular transport of fatty acids. This hypothesis is partly supported by the finding that the concentration of FABP is greater in villi than in crypt cells, greater in jejunum than in ileum, and greater in intestinal mucosa of animals fed a high-fat diet than in mucosa of animals fed a low fat diet (Ockner and Manning, 1974).

There are at least two cytosolic FABPs in enterocytes. These are the I-FABP (intestinal FABP) and L-FABP (liver FABP). These two FABPs differ in their binding specificity (Besnard et al., 1996). I-FABP strongly binds only with fatty acids, but L-FABP will bind not only long-chain fatty acids but also lysophosphatidylcholine, retinoids, bilirubin, carcinogens, and even selenium (Bansal et al., 1989; Bass, 1988; Glatz and Veerkamp, 1985). Based on nuclear magnetic resonance (NMR) binding studies, Cistola and colleagues (1990) speculated that the I-FABP facilitates the intracellular transport of fatty acids, whereas L-FABP probably facilitates the intracellular transport of monoacylglycerol and lysophosphatidylcholine. Future studies in mice with various FABP genes "knocked out" may shed some light on the function of these proteins in the intracellular transport of lipids.

Two cytosolic carrier proteins for sterols have been isolated and characterized: sterol carrier protein-1 (SCP-1) and sterol carrier protein-2 (SCP-2). Experimental evidence thus far seems to indicate that SCP-2 may play a role in the intracellular transport of cholesterol.

REESTERIFICATION OF LIPID DIGESTION PRODUCTS

2-Monoacylglycerols and fatty acids are reconstituted to form triacylglycerol, mainly via the monoacylglycerol pathway. As shown in Figure 10-3, 2-monoacylglycerol is reacylated into triacylglycerol by the consecutive action of monoacylglycerol acyltransferase and diacylglycerol acyltransferase. The enzymes involved in this monoacylglycerol pathway are present in a complex called triacylglycerol synthetase, and this has been purified (Lehner and Kuksis, 1995). This enzyme complex is located on the cytosolic surface of the ER, and this finding has important bearing on our understanding of the intracellular formation of chylomicrons. It appears that triacylglycerols are formed at the cytosolic surface of the ER, and they then gain access to the inside, or lumen, of the ER.

Wetterau and Zilversmit (1984) demonstrated the presence of a protein in the liver, the small intestine, and a number of other organs that promotes the transfer of triacylglycerol and cholesteryl ester between membranes; they proposed that this transfer activity may play a role in the movement of lipids into the ER. Wetterau and colleagues (1992) provided convincing evidence that this may indeed be the case. In studies of patients with abetalipoproteinemia, who lack the ability to make chylomicrons, they found that apolipoprotein B (apo B) was synthesized, but the triacylglycerol and apo B failed to associate with each other because of a lack of the microsomal (ER) triacylglycerol transfer protein.

The other pathway present in intestinal mucosa for the formation of triacylglycerol is called the glycerol 3-phosphate pathway.

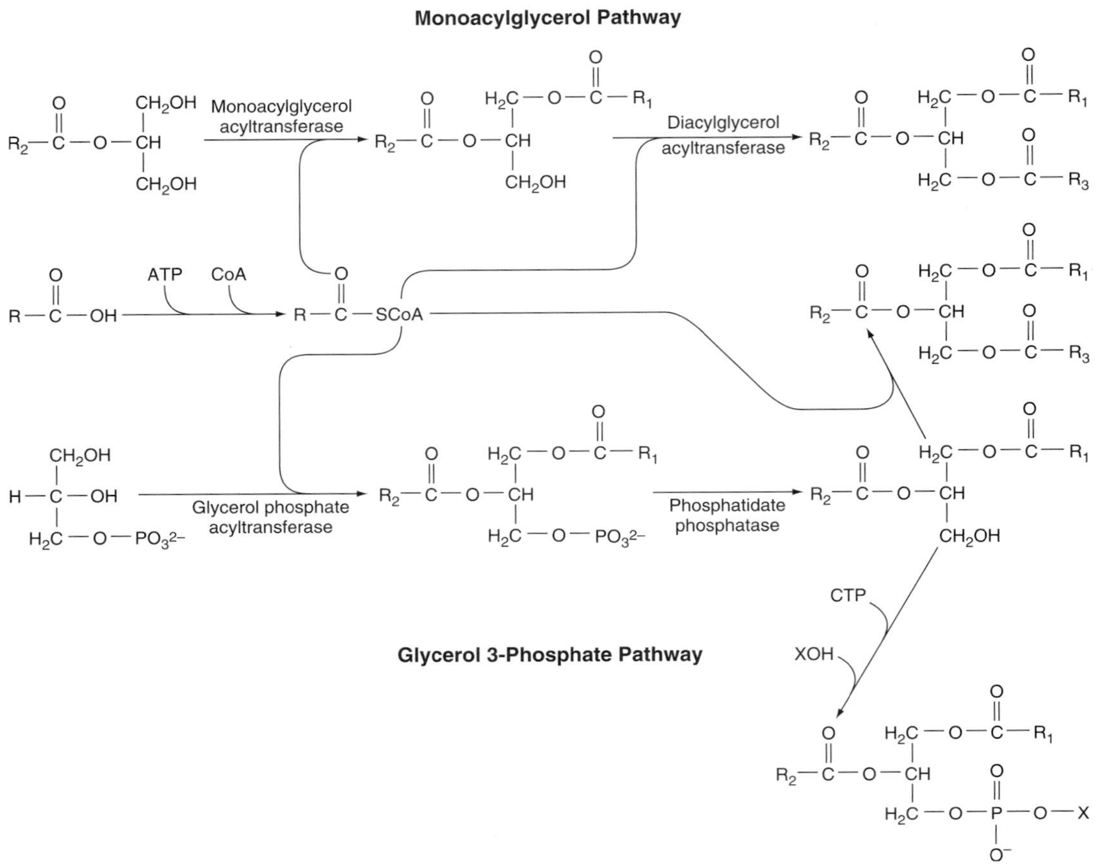

Figure 10-3 Pathways of triacylglycerol biosynthesis in the intestinal mucosal cells (enterocytes). *RCOOH,* Fatty acid; *XOH,* alcohol (e.g., choline or serine).

As shown in Figure 10-3, this pathway involves the stepwise acylation of glycerol 3-phosphate to form phosphatidic acid. In the presence of phosphatidate phosphatase, phosphatidic acid is hydrolyzed to release inorganic phosphate and to form diacylglycerol, which is then further esterified to form triacylglycerol.

The relative importance of the monoacylglycerol pathway and the glycerol phosphate pathway depends on the supply of 2-monoacylglycerol and fatty acid. During normal lipid absorption, the monoacylglycerol pathway is much more important than the glycerol phosphate pathway in enterocytes because of the abundant supply of 2-monoacylglycerol and fatty acid and their efficient conversion to triacylglycerol, and also because 2-monoacylglycerol inhibits the glycerol phosphate pathway. However, when the supply of 2-monoacylglycerol is lacking or insufficient, the glycerol phosphate pathway becomes the major pathway for the formation of triacylglycerol.

PHOSPHOLIPIDS

Lysophosphatidylcholine and other lysophospholipids inside the enterocytes can be reacylated to form phosphatidylcholine and other phospholipids, or these lysophospholipids can be hydrolyzed to form glycerol 3-phosphorylcholine. The liberated fatty acids can be used for triacylglycerol synthesis, whereas the glycerol 3-phosphorylcholine can be readily transported via the portal blood for use in the liver. Another reaction that occurs in intestinal mucosal cells is the combination of two molecules of lysophosphatidylcholine to yield one molecule of phosphatidylcholine and one molecule of glycerol 3-phosphorylcholine.

Nutrition Insight

Use of Structured Triacylglycerols to Enhance Absorption of Fatty Acids Into the Lymphatics

Structured triacylglycerols are mixtures of long- and medium-chain fatty acids incorporated on the same glycerol backbone by hydrolysis and random reesterification of the constituent oils. Structured triacylglycerols may have different actions than do identical physical mixtures of oils that have not been reesterified. Because triacylglycerols are hydrolyzed to 2-monoacylglycerols and fatty acids in the gastrointestinal tract and because the 2-monoacylglycerols may be taken up and converted to triacylglycerol without further hydrolysis, fatty acids esterified to the 2-position of glycerol may be more likely to be absorbed into the lymphatics. For example, fatty acids with less than 12 carbons are generally transported via the portal route as free fatty acids bound to plasma albumin, but medium-chain fatty acids esterified to the 2-position may be readily absorbed as 2-monoacylglycerols, which are further acylated with long-chain fatty acids in the 1- and 3-positions for lymphatic transport.

Jensen and colleagues (1994) studied the lymphatic absorption of a structured triacylglycerol versus an equivalent physical mixture of the constituent medium-chain triacylglycerol and fish oils. Enhanced lymphatic absorption of medium-chain fatty acids in rats was observed when they were delivered as a structured triacylglycerol containing medium-chain fatty acid in the 2-position and long-chain fatty acids in the 1- and 3-positions, compared with the physical mixture. Fish-oil fatty acids (long- and very-long-chain polyunsaturated fatty acids) are generally not well absorbed unless they are in the 2-position of the dietary triacylglycerol. However, because most of the long-chain polyunsaturated fatty acids in fish oils are in the 2-position naturally, there was little difference in lymphatic absorption of fish-oil fatty acids when structured triacylglycerols and physical mixes were compared.

CHOLESTEROL

Dietary or exogenous cholesterol absorbed by the enterocytes enters a free cholesterol pool. This free cholesterol pool in the enterocyte also derives cholesterol from endogenous sources, including nondietary cholesterol (biliary cholesterol and cholesterol from cells shed from the intestinal mucosa) absorbed from the lumen of the small intestine, cholesterol derived from circulating plasma lipoproteins, and cholesterol synthesized de novo. However, enterocytes handle cholesterol from various sources quite differently. For instance, the cholesterol derived from the intestinal lumen does not mix freely with the free cholesterol pool in the enterocyte and is preferentially esterified in the enterocyte for incorporation into chylomicrons and export into the lymph. Stange and Dietschy (1985) found that very little newly synthesized cholesterol is transported into lymph during fasting; however, during active lipid absorption and chylomicron synthesis, some of the newly synthesized cholesterol is incorporated into chylomicrons and transported in lymph.

Cholesterol is transported almost exclusively by the lymphatic system, mainly as esterified cholesterol. Therefore, the rate of esterification of cholesterol probably regulates the rate of its lymphatic transport. Two enzymes have been proposed to play a role in cholesterol esterification; these are cholesterol esterase and acyl CoA:cholesterol acyltransferase (ACAT). The distribution and regulation of ACAT in the small intestinal epithelium has been studied in considerable detail. Both the jejunum and ileum have high activities of this enzyme, with the jejunum having significantly higher levels than the ileum. The activity of this enzyme can be increased by feeding a high-cholesterol diet. By using immunocytochemistry, Gallo and colleagues (1980) demonstrated that intracellular cholesterol esterase is derived from the uptake of pancreatic cholesterol esterase. It is hypothesized that this cholesterol esterase could catalyze esterification instead of hydrolysis, given the relatively high intracellular concentrations of free cholesterol and fatty acids. As yet we do not understand the process of how pancreatic cholesterol esterase is taken up by the enterocyte, but elucidation of this process may enhance our general understanding of how intact proteins are taken up by the enterocytes. (See Chapter 9 for a description of the uptake of intact proteins from the intestine.)

There is still lack of a general agreement about whether cholesterol esterase or ACAT plays a more important role in the esterification of cholesterol by enterocytes. However, prevailing evidence supports a more important role of ACAT. For instance, a higher activity of ACAT is found in the segment of the small intestine most actively involved in cholesterol absorption. Furthermore, the activity present in the intestinal epithelium can adequately account for all the cholesteryl ester transported by the small intestine. Lastly, in studies employing a number of specific ACAT inhibitors, it has been demonstrated that these inhibitors significantly reduce the transport of cholesterol by the small intestine.

There is recent evidence that another protein in the intestinal mucosa may play a significant role in cholesterol uptake. The protein that has been identified is Niemann-Pick C1 Like 1 protein (NPC1L1) (Altmann et al., 2004). It is expressed primarily in the small intestine of the rat and mouse, and in the small intestine and liver in humans. NPC1L1 knockout mice were found to absorb less than 20% of dietary cholesterol, compared with a value of approximately 50% for wild type mice (Altmann et al., 2004). In addition, the addition of oral ezetimibe, a potent inhibitor of cholesterol absorption (Rosenblum et al., 1998), caused a decrease in cholesterol absorption in the wild-type mice but not in the knockout mice. The NPC1L1 null mice also had substantially reduced uptake of sitosterol and dramatically reduced plasma phytosterol levels (Davis et al., 2004). The cholesterol- and phytosterol-uptake protein NPC1L1 will undoubtedly be the subject of much study in the future.

PLANT STEROLS

It has been well documented that plant sterols are handled differently from cholesterol by the mammalian gut. A typical Western diet contains 150 to 350 mg of cholesterol and approximately 100 to 400 mg of noncholesterol sterols (mostly plant sterols such as β-sitosterol and campesterol, and some shellfish sterols). Plant sterols differ from cholesterol only by a methyl or ethyl group in the side chain. Although structurally quite similar to cholesterol, only a small percentage (<1%) of ingested noncholesterol sterols are absorbed and retained in the body, compared with approximately 50% to 60% of dietary cholesterol being absorbed and retained. This tremendous ability of the small intestine to discriminate against the plant sterols seems to be lost in patients with β-sitosterolemia, a rare autosomal recessive disorder characterized by hyperabsorption of all sterols (Salen et al., 1997). Bhattacharyya and Connor (1974) first described this disorder in two sisters who had plasma cholesterol concentrations of 200 to 210 mg/dL (5.1 to 5.4 mmol/L) and plasma plant sterol concentrations of 26 to 37 mg/100 mL (0.7 to 0.9 mmol/L, two thirds as β-sitosterol and the rest as campesterol). In most humans, the level of total plant sterols in plasma is less than 0.9 mg/100 mL. High levels of plant sterols are also present in erythrocytes, adipose tissue, and skin of patients with β-sitosterolemia, and patients develop xanthomatosis—a condition characterized by the presence of xanthomas, which are nodules composed of lipid-laden foam cells. Recently, mutations in the ABCG5 or ABCG8 genes, which code for an ATP-binding cassette transporter family heterodimer expressed in intestine and liver, were identified as the causes of β-sitosterolemia (Lu et al., 2001). Many of these mutations seem to prevent formation of stable heterodimers and to impair transport of the sterol transporter to the apical surface of the cells (Graf et al., 2004). The ABCG5-ABCG8 heterodimer is believed to mediate the export of absorbed plant sterols and cholesterol into the gut lumen, thereby reducing intestinal absorption of sterols. This transporter may also play an important role in promoting biliary excretion of cholesterol and other sterols. These two genes are regulated by the nuclear hormone receptor LXR (liver X receptor).

As mentioned previously, noncholesterol sterol uptake, as well as cholesterol uptake, into the enterocyte may occur via NPC1L1 (Davis et al., 2004). Ezetimibe effectively reduced plasma cholesterol and plant sterol concentrations in patients with sitosterolemia (Salen et al., 2004). However, despite their apparent uptake by the same transport system, the presence of plant sterols in the intestinal lumen has been shown to inhibit the intestinal absorption of cholesterol. One mechanism for this inhibition is the displacement of cholesterol from the bile salt–mixed micelles by plant sterols (Nissinen et al., 2002). Another possible mechanism is the inhibition of the rate of cholesterol esterification in the intestinal mucosa (Field and Mathur, 1983). Some evidence suggests that efflux of cholesterol via transporter ABCA1 may also be involved in the regulation of cholesterol uptake (Knight, 2004).

Margarines and vegetable oil spreads and salad dressings containing esters of plant sterols or plant stanols (hydrogenated sterols, no double bond) have been promoted as functional foods for lowering cholesterol levels. Fatty acid esters of plant sterols are used in these products because the fatty acid esters are more soluble in triacylglycerol than are the unesterified plant sterols. These esters are hydrolyzed in the small intestine to produce the free sterols that can hinder cholesterol solubility in micelles. Intake of 2 to 3 g of phytostanol ester or phytosterol ester per day has been associated with a decrease of approximately 10% in serum LDL-cholesterol level; this reduction is less than that predicted from estimates of decreased cholesterol absorption, but compensatory mechanisms may increase the rate of endogenous cholesterol synthesis (Lichtenstein and Deckelbaum, 2001).

ASSEMBLY OF INTESTINAL LIPOPROTEINS

Lipoproteins are lipid–protein complexes formed by the small intestine and the liver for the export of lipids from these organs. The cannulation of the lymphatic vessel of rats and a number of other animal species has been used extensively for the study of chylomicron secretion by the small intestine. This method allows the direct sampling and analysis of lipoproteins secreted by the small intestine before they enter the general circulation.

LIPOPROTEINS SECRETED BY THE SMALL INTESTINE

The small intestine secretes the following three lipoproteins: (1) chylomicrons; (2) intestinal very low density lipoproteins (VLDLs, small chylomicrons); and (3) high density lipoproteins (HDLs). Both chylomicrons and intestinal VLDLs are triacylglycerol-rich lipoproteins. In this chapter, only chylomicrons and intestinal VLDLs are discussed because the small intestine secretes only a small amount of HDLs. HDLs are discussed in Chapters 16 and 17. During fasting, the major lipoproteins secreted by the small intestine are the intestinal (apo B-48–containing) VLDLs. Chylomicrons are the major lipoproteins secreted by the small intestine following a lipid-rich meal.

ASSEMBLY AND SECRETION OF CHYLOMICRONS

Only the small intestine secretes chylomicrons. The composition of the chylomicron is described in Table 10-1. The major apolipoproteins associated with chylomicrons are apo A-I, apo A-IV, and apo B-48. Traces of apo E and apo C are added to the chylomicrons after their entry into the circulation. Data from both animals and humans indicate that the fatty acid composition of the triacylglycerol of chylomicrons closely resembles that of the dietary lipid consumed. In the example shown in Table 10-2, Kayden and colleagues (1963) studied the changes in human lymph triacylglycerol composition after a subject ingested 100 g of corn oil. The fatty acid composition of chylomicron triacylglycerol collected 8 hours after the lipid dose was virtually identical to that of the corn oil ingested.

The fatty acid composition of the phospholipids of lymph chylomicrons is less influenced by the dietary fatty acids than is the fatty acid composition of triacylglycerols in the chylomicron. This is because phosphatidylcholine from bile represents the major source of phospholipids in the intestinal lumen and, thus, is the major source of phospholipids for coating the chylomicrons. The fatty acid composition of biliary phosphatidylcholine is rather unique.

The intestinal triacylglycerol-rich lipoproteins are transported from the ER to the Golgi apparatus. The Golgi apparatus serves as the final site of assembly for many proteins and also lipoproteins. Consequently, a block in the trafficking between ER and the Golgi apparatus results in impairment in the formation of chylomicrons. Apo B is involved in this process. *N*-glycosylation of apo B begins in the ER and

Table 10-1
Composition and Characteristics of Nascent Intestinal Chylomicrons and Intestinal VLDLs*

	Chylomicron	Intestinal VLDL
Density	<0.95 g/mL	0.95 to 1.006 g/mL
Size	80 to 500 nm	30 to 80 nm
Total lipid	~98% of particle mass	~90% of particle mass
Triacylglycerol	~86%	~60%
Cholesterol (mostly as cholesteryl ester)	~4%	~15%
Phospholipids	~8%	~15%
Total protein	~2% of particle weight	~10% of particle weight
Major	B-48, A-1, A-IV, and A-II	Probably similar to chylomicron
Minor	C and E (both acquired through interaction with other plasma lipoproteins)	Same as chylomicron

VLDLs, Very low density lipoproteins.
*Nascent intestinal chylomicrons and VLDLs harvested from intestinal lymph.

Table 10-2
Alteration of Fatty Acid Composition (% by Weight) of Human Lymph Chylomicron Triacylglycerol After Feeding Corn Oil (100 g)

		Lymph	
Fatty Acid	Corn Oil (%)	Fasting (%)	8 to 10 hr* (%)
C 12:0		4	0
C 14:0		13	0
C 16:0	11	28	10
C 18:0		10	2
C 18:1	27	32	22
C 18:2	61	10	64

Data from Kayden HJ, Karmen A, Dumont A (1963) Alterations in the fatty acid composition of human lymph and serum lipoproteins by single feeding. J Clin Invest 42:1373-1381.
*Time after corn-oil feeding.

terminal glycosylation occurs at the Golgi apparatus. Golgi-derived vesicles containing the prechylomicrons have been clearly demonstrated by Sabesin and Frase (1977) in enterocytes actively absorbing lipid. This is illustrated in Figure 10-4. The Golgi vesicles containing the prechylomicrons migrate toward the basolateral membrane of the enterocytes, and prechylomicrons are discharged into the intercellular space through exocytosis.

ASSEMBLY AND SECRETION OF VERY LOW DENSITY LIPOPROTEINS

As shown in Table 10-1, intestinal VLDLs are smaller than chylomicrons, and they have a different lipid composition than chylomicrons. In contrast, the apolipoprotein composition is not different between lymph chylomicrons and intestinal VLDLs.

FACTORS AFFECTING FORMATION AND SECRETION OF CHYLOMICRONS

The formation and the secretion of chylomicrons are tightly regulated by the synthesis of apolipoproteins and lipids in the enterocytes. Although considerable information regarding these factors has been gathered, the mechanisms of how these factors regulate the formation and secretion of chylomicrons remain largely unknown. A major reason for our limited knowledge of this is the lack of good cell models for studying these processes: it is extremely difficult to maintain intestinal epithelial cells in culture.

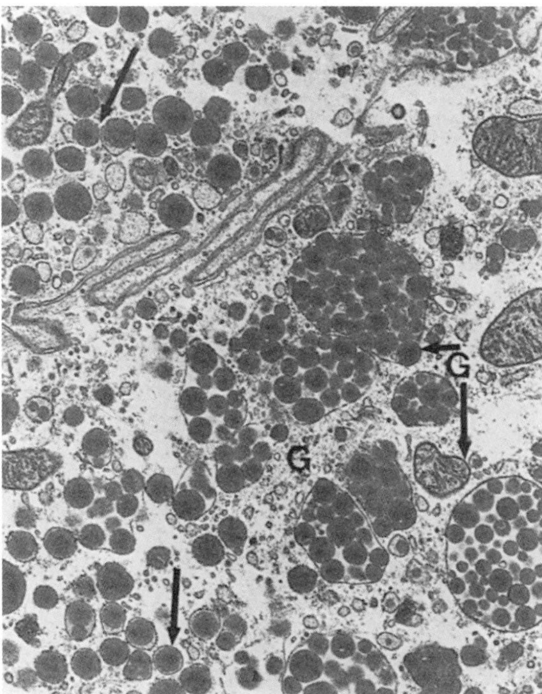

Figure 10-4 After fat digestion, the cell is filled with numerous fat droplets located within vesiculated channels of the smooth endoplasmic reticulum (ER) *(long arrows)*. A Golgi zone (*arrows denoted by G*) contains many vesicles filled with prechylomicrons measuring 600 to 3500 Å (× 11,420). *(From Sabesin SM, Frase S [1977] Electron microscopic studies of the assembly, intracellular transport, and secretion of chylomicrons by rat intestine. J Lipid Res 18:496-511.)*

Nutrition Insight

Absorption of Lipophilic Drugs and Toxins

Many lipophilic compounds, including drugs, fat-soluble vitamins, and other compounds present in food or present on food as contaminants, are incorporated into chylomicrons in the intestinal mucosal cells and transported via the lymph. Hence, absorption of these compounds depends upon normal fat digestion and absorption and upon chylomicron formation and secretion. The role of dietary fat in the absorption of fat-soluble vitamins is well known. Uptake of lipophilic drugs and toxins also may be promoted when ingested along with dietary fat. Factors that limit lipid digestion, such as blockage of biliary flow or chylomicron formation, may interfere with or protect from absorption of these compounds.

Patients are often advised to take lipophilic medications together with their meals to enhance the absorption of the drug by the gastrointestinal tract. Delivery of lipophilic drugs in forms that enhance their absorption and thus require smaller doses is of interest to pharmaceutical manufacturers. Enhancement of absorption of lipophilic compounds by the presence of dietary fat also may affect absorption of environmental contaminants or toxins. For example, absorption of DDT (1,1-*bis*-(p-chlorophenyl)-2,2,2-trichloroethane), a toxic chlorinated hydrocarbon pesticide now banned in the United States, is enhanced by concomitant fat feeding. Enhancement of absorption of lipophilic compounds by dietary fat also may account for the observation that tetrachloroethylene, a drug used for treating hookworm infections that is not ordinarily absorbed from the gastrointestinal tract, causes toxic effects when fed with a high-fat meal.

SYNTHESIS OF APOLIPOPROTEIN B

Two major forms of apolipoprotein B are made by humans, apo B-100 and apo B-48. Apo B-100 and apo B-48 refer to the relative apparent molecular masses obtained by sodium dodecyl sulfate (SDS) gel electrophoresis. According to this nomenclature, the large apo B-100 was assigned an arbitrary value of 100, whereas apo B-48 was assigned the number 48 because its apparent molecular mass is 48% that of apo B-100. In humans, the liver secretes only apo B-100, and the small intestine secretes only apo B-48. Both apo B-100 and apo B-48 are encoded by the same gene. The biogenesis of apo B-48 involves a unique mechanism of mRNA editing by which a CAA (cytosine-adenine-adenine) codon encoding glutamine is changed to a UAA (uracil-adenine-adenine) stop codon in the apo B mRNA, and thus translation is terminated earlier to form apo B-48 (Chen et al., 1987; Powell et al., 1987). This mRNA editing is done by a cytidine deaminase called apobec-1.

Although apo B is required for the formation of chylomicrons, the supply of apo B is probably not the rate-limiting step for lipid output in chylomicrons. Hayashi and colleagues (1990) demonstrated that apo B output by the small intestine did not change after intraduodenal infusion of lipid, despite the fact that lymphatic triacylglycerol output increased several fold. It appears that the number of chylomicron particles made by the small intestine remains relatively constant during fasting and active lipid absorption. Instead of making more chylomicrons during active lipid absorption, the enterocyte simply fills each chylomicron particle with more triacylglycerol molecules, making them larger and less dense.

Apo-B48 is clearly not obligatory for chylomicron assembly, because mice without the gene for editing apo B-100 to apo B-48 (apobec-1 knockout mice), which produce only apo-B100, absorb dietary fat. Nevertheless, studies of chylomicron secretion by apobec-1 knockout and wild-type mice suggest that apo-B48 is superior over apo-B100 in chylomicron assembly and fat absorption. Kendrick and colleagues (2001) found markedly reduced chylomicron secretion in fasted apobec-1 knockout mice relative to wild-type. However, after a fat-containing meal, secretion of preexisting chylomicrons was stimulated in the apobec-1 knockout animals. These observations are consistent with the proposed model for chylomicron assembly in which apo-B-rich, lipid-poor particles and triacylglycerol-rich particles are transferred separately into the lumen of the smooth ER, followed by fusion of the two types of particles to form chylomicrons. When dietary fat is low, the formation of apo-B–containing particles or an early stage of chylomicron assembly appears to be rate-limiting. Microsomal triglyceride transfer protein (MTP) appears to be involved in the lipidation of nascent apo B. When dietary fat is high, the rate-limiting step in chylomicron assembly and secretion appears to be the addition of the lipid droplet to the apo-B–containing particle. The size of these lipid droplets is thought to determine the size of the chylomicrons produced.

SYNTHESIS OF APOLIPOPROTEINS A-I AND A-IV

The human small intestine synthesizes both apo A-I and A-IV. These apoproteins are secreted in association with chylomicrons. Despite the marked increase in the amount of lipid secreted in chylomicrons following the ingestion of a lipid-rich meal, the synthesis and secretion of apo A-I is only marginally stimulated (20% to 30% compared with the fasting condition). In contrast, the synthesis and secretion of apo A-IV is markedly stimulated by the ingestion of fat. The roles of apo A-I and apo A-IV in the formation and secretion of chylomicrons are not clear.

When chylomicrons are metabolized in the body by lipoprotein lipase, apo A-IV detaches from these particles and circulates in the plasma either bound to HDLs or as a free protein. Although the amino acid sequence and the gene locus of apo A-IV have been known since 1984, the physiological role of apo A-IV remained unclear until recently. A number of recent reports indicate that apoA-IV has a unique physiological role: apo A-IV appears to be a circulating signal released in response to fat feeding that may mediate the anorectic (inhibition of food intake) effect of a lipid meal; this function of apo A-IV is discussed further in subsequent text of this chapter.

ROLE OF LUMINAL PHOSPHATIDYLCHOLINE

An adequate supply of luminal phosphatidylcholine is important for the formation and secretion of intestinal chylomicrons and intestinal VLDLs. This intestinal phosphatidyl choline may be important because it is a major component of the surface coat of chylomicrons. The observation that bile phosphatidylcholine has a unique fatty acid composition that closely resembles the fatty acid composition of the phosphatidylcholine in the surface coat of chylomicrons suggests that bile or luminal phosphatidylcholine is preferentially used for the coating of chylomicrons. In a model system, the lipolysis of triacylglycerol emulsions and the rates of clearance of particles from the plasma by hepatocytes versus reticuloendothelial cells depended on the cholesterol content and the phosphatidylcholine species of the lipid emulsion particles (Clark et al., 1991). Consequently, the specific fatty acid composition of the phosphatidylcholine in the chylomicron surface coat may play an important role in the metabolism of chylomicrons by the body.

Luminal phosphatidylcholine also may be important in maintaining the normal composition, turnover, and integrity of the membranes of the subcellular organelles of the enterocytes. Normal membrane composition and integrity are important not only for membrane function but also for the function of the enzymes associated with the membrane.

HORMONES

Relatively little is known of how intestinal lipid absorption is regulated by hormones. It has been reported that the intestinal peptide called neurotensin enhances lymphatic lipid transport in the rat by enhancing the processing of absorbed dietary fat. However, neurotensin also induces hemodynamic changes in the gastrointestinal tract (e.g., increased lymph flow). Further experiments are needed to ascertain whether this effect of neurotensin on intestinal lipid transport is an intracellular effect or simply a hemodynamic effect. The role of gastrointestinal hormones on intestinal lipid transport is largely unknown.

DISORDERS OF INTESTINAL LIPID ABSORPTION

The determination of the amount of fat in the stool is a common test for assessment of intestinal malabsorption. Normal humans excrete in their stool less than 6 g of fat per 24-hour period, which is less than 5% of their fat intake. Therefore, they absorb more than 95% of the fat consumed in their diet. Moreover, the capacity of the enzymatic and transport processes involved in dietary fat absorption greatly exceeds that required during normal fat absorption. Complete absorption of dietary fat at intakes of more than 300 g/day and toleration of intakes of more than 600 g/day for a period of 20 days have been reported (Kasper, 1970). The efficiency of fat absorption can be calculated as fat intake (in g/day) minus fecal fat (g/day) divided by fat intake in g/day, with the dividend multiplied by 100 to express the fraction as a percentage. Intestinal lipid malabsorption can be caused by a number of clinical conditions.

DISORDERS OF THE SMALL INTESTINE

A common disorder of the small intestine that results in malabsorption of nutrients, including lipids, is celiac sprue. Celiac sprue is characterized by lesions of the small intestinal mucosa. It is caused by gluten (a protein rich in proline and glutamine that is found in wheat, barley, oats, and some other cereals). This malabsorptive state can be corrected by feeding a gluten-free diet. The mechanism of gluten toxicity is still unclear.

DEFECTIVE DIGESTION CAUSED BY PANCREATIC DEFICIENCY

A major feature of pancreatic deficiency is severe abdominal pain and steatorrhea (the passage of large, pale, frothy stools), caused by the presence of a large amount of undigested fat owing to a disease of the pancreas, which results in lack of pancreatic digestive enzymes. Pancreatic deficiency is treated by prescribing a low-fat diet or by supplementation of enterically coated pancreatic enzymes with meals; severe deficiency may require diets containing partial hydrolysates of protein and starch as well. Medium-chain triacylglycerols (MCT oil, comprising principally octanoic and decanoic acid triacylglycerols) have also been used in the diet of patients with pancreatic insufficiency. MCT oil is more readily hydrolyzed than are long-chain fatty acid triacylglycerols, but it does not provide the essential fatty acids, linoleic and α-linolenic acid.

DEFECTIVE UPTAKE OF LIPIDS CAUSED BY BILE-SALT DEFICIENCY

Bile-salt deficiency results in poor micellar solubilization of lipid digestion products. Unlike pancreatic deficiency, bile-salt deficiency does not affect the digestion of triacylglycerol by pancreatic lipase, and, therefore, the fats present in the stool are mainly lipid digestion products in the form of fatty acid salts (soaps). As described in the preceding text, the solubilization of lipid digestion products in micelles formed by the bile salts is an important method for delivery of lipid molecules to the small intestinal epithelial cells. However, because vesicles may also play a role in the delivery of lipid digestion products to the small intestine, patients with bile salt deficiency caused by liver disease or gallstone disease often can absorb a significant amount of lipids.

ABETALIPOPROTEINEMIA

Patients with abetalipoproteinemia have a near-complete lack of apo B–containing lipoproteins in the circulation. For a long time it was believed that these patients lacked the ability to synthesize apo B. However, studies clearly showed that apo B is being synthesized by the enterocytes of abetalipoproteinemic patients and that the apo B gene is normal in patients with abetalipoproteinemia (Talmud et al., 1988). The genetic basis of abetalipoproteinemia is now known to be mutations in the gene for the large subunit of MTP (Berriot-Varoqueaux et al., 2000; Wetterau et al., 1992). MTP is thought to transfer lipids to the apo-B protein as it is translated, allowing it to attain the proper conformation for lipoprotein assembly. Consequently, triacylglycerol droplets accumulate in the intestinal mucosa of these subjects as lipid absorption progresses (Dobbins, 1970; Fig. 10-5). Abetalipoproteinemia also causes a defect in VLDL formation by the liver. Patients have neurologic disorders and exhibit acanthocytosis.

CHYLOMICRON RETENTION DISORDER

Chylomicron retention disorder appears to be an intestinal defect in the final assembly of chylomicrons or in the mechanism of their exocytosis. Chylomicrons are absent from the postprandial plasma. There is a failure in the discharge of prechylomicrons from the Golgi-derived vesicles into the intercellular space through exocytosis. Prechylomicrons refer to the chylomicrons that are still inside the intestinal epithelial cells. Consequently, despite the presence of numerous Golgi-derived vesicles in the cytoplasm, there is an absence of chylomicrons in the intercellular space (Roy et al., 1987). Compared with abetalipoproteinemia, chylomicron retention disorder involves a defect that is further along the chylomicron packaging pathway, probably in the trafficking of Golgi vesicles containing prechylomicrons to the plasma membrane. Patients with chylomicron retention disorder have an apparently normal capacity to secrete lipoproteins from the liver. This disorder is associated with chronic diarrhea and steatorrhea, abdominal distention, and failure to thrive in infants and needs to be recognized and treated early.

INTESTINAL LIPID ABSORPTION AND MUCOSAL INJURY

A number of investigators have shown that long-chain fatty acids can be injurious to the intestine, especially the developing intestine. Velasquez and colleagues (1994) reported that the magnitude of injury caused by the presence of fatty acids in the intestinal lumen was significantly higher in piglets less than 2 weeks of age than in 1-month-old animals, suggesting that a developmental process that renders the intestinal mucosa more resistant to lipid-induced injury occurred in the piglets. The lipid-induced injury was reversible. This interesting observation is of potential clinical relevance. Immaturity or disruption of the

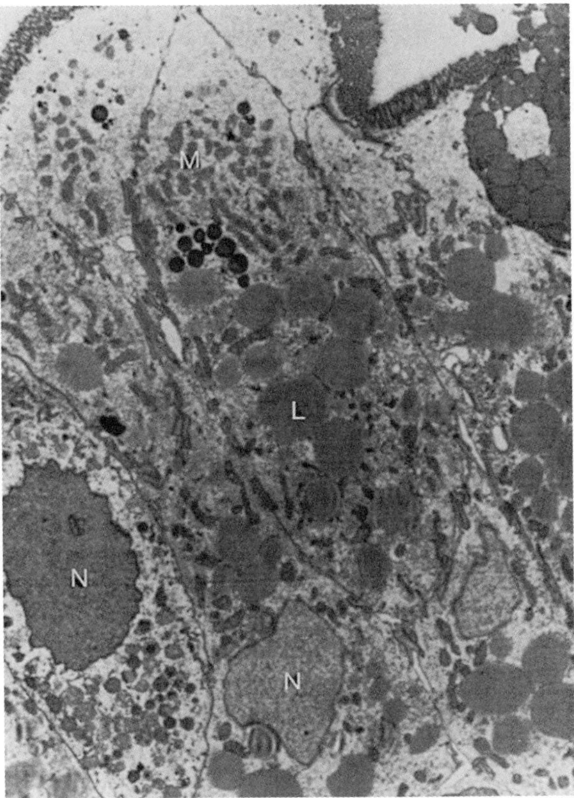

Figure 10-5 Electron micrograph of intestinal absorptive cells from a biopsy specimen of an abetalipoproteinemic patient. The enterocytes contain massive amounts of lipid *(L)*. Otherwise, the cells appear normal. The cell nucleus is labeled *N*, and a mitochondrion is labeled *M*. *(From Dobbins WO [1970] An ultrastructural study of the intestinal mucosa in congenital β-lipoprotein deficiency, with particular emphasis on intestinal absorptive cells. Gastroenterology 50:195-210.)*

intestinal mucosal barrier by fatty acids may result in clinical disease states to which the newborn infant is susceptible, such as necrotizing enterocolitis or toxigenic diarrhea. Velasquez and colleagues (1994) also showed that esterification of the injurious long-chain fatty acids with ethanol abolished their cytotoxic effects on the intestinal mucosa. Furthermore, they showed that the ethyl esters of the long-chain fatty acids are absorbed and utilized by the developing intestine.

REGIONAL DIFFERENCES IN INTESTINAL LIPID ABSORPTION

A difference in the abilities of the proximal and distal small intestine to absorb fat has been described in rats (Wu et al., 1980; Sabesin et al., 1975). Not only was the distal intestine much less efficient than the proximal intestine in chylomicron production (Sabesin et al., 1975), but also the chylomicrons produced by the distal intestine were larger (Wu et al., 1980). The investigators suggested that this difference between intestinal segments could be due to the availability of phospholipids for the coating of prechylomicrons or to altered intracellular membrane lipid composition. Most phospholipids are absorbed before the digesta reaches the distal small intestine. Therefore, the proximal intestine is supplied with biliary phospholipids, whereas the distal small intestine has to meet most of its phospholipid requirements by either de novo synthesis or uptake of lipoproteins from the plasma.

PORTAL TRANSPORT OF LONG-CHAIN FATTY ACIDS

The majority of absorbed fatty acids are transported by intestinal lymph as chylomicrons and intestinal VLDLs. However, there is evidence for portal transport of long-chain fatty acids, and this transport is increased when there is a defect in the intracellular esterification of fatty acids to form triacylglycerol or an impairment in chylomicron formation. In patients with abetalipoproteinemia, some dietary fat (fatty acids) may be absorbed in the virtual absence of chylomicron formation (Ways et al., 1967).

McDonald and colleagues (1980) demonstrated that a substantial amount of the absorbed fatty acid (e.g., 58% for linoleic acid) was transported in the portal blood of normal rats when the rates of lipid absorption were low. Mansbach and colleagues (1991) reported that considerable amounts of endogenous and exogenous fatty acids are transported by the portal blood. The amount of exogenous fatty acid transported via the portal route can be as much as 39% of the fatty acid infused into the small intestinal lumen. The portal transport of absorbed fatty acids by the small intestine, therefore, may be more important than previously recognized.

The absorption of fatty acids or fatty acid derivatives that do not produce 2-monoacylglycerol may in part be absorbed into the portal vein rather than the lymph. Because the majority of synthesis of triacylglycerol in the enterocyte follows a pathway that utilizes 2-monoacylglycerol (Mattson and Volpenheim, 1964), it has been suggested that a deficit of 2-monoacylglycerol can limit the resynthesis of triacylglycerol in the enterocyte, and fatty acids will leave the cell into the portal vein rather than the lymph. It should be noted, however, that endogenous glycerol and glycerol resulting from the hydrolysis of 1-monoacylglycerol are converted to 1-glycerol phosphate, which is a precursor to newly synthesized triacylglycerol (Mattson and Volpenheim, 1964). Therefore an alternative pathway for triacylglcyerol synthesis exists when 2-monoacylglycerol is absent.

Long-chain fatty acids in the form of 1,3-diacylglycerol do not provide 2-monoacylglycerol during the processes of ingestion and digestion. Murase and colleagues (2002) proposed that a dietary oil enriched in 1,3-diacylglycerol may result in a larger portion of the fatty acids being absorbed portally than would occur when triacylglycerol with the same fatty acid composition is fed.

SATIETY EFFECTS OF FAT FEEDING

There is compelling evidence in the literature showing that the ingestion of fat results in satiation and the inhibition of food intake. A number of characteristics of this lipid-induced satiety provide important clues about the mechanism involved. First, long-chain fatty acids are significantly more potent in inducing satiety than are short- or medium-chain fatty acids. Long-chain fatty acids are transported by the small intestine mainly as chylomicrons, whereas medium-chain fatty acids are transported mainly in the portal blood. This observation would imply that chylomicrons are somehow involved in this lipid-induced satiety. Second, fatty acids introduced into the small intestinal lumen are more potent in inducing satiety than are fatty acids delivered by direct peripheral venous, portal, or caval routes. Again, this would imply that the gastrointestinal tract, and probably the production of chylomicrons, is somehow involved in this lipid-induced satiety. Third, the lipid-induced satiety is abolished by the presence of orlistat (an inhibitor of pancreatic lipase) in the intestinal lumen, indicating that it is the digestion products and not triacylglycerols per se that elicit the satiety response. Therefore, most of the observations concerning lipid-induced satiety seem to imply that intestinal lipid absorption, in particular the formation and secretion of chylomicrons, is involved in this physiological response to the ingestion of lipid.

There is evidence that satiety results from the lipolytic products of ingested fat rather than from the undigested triacylglycerol. Meyer and colleagues (1998) suggested that satiety is attained by the interaction of these products with sensors in the regions of the mid and distal small intestine.

Fujimoto and colleagues (1992) reported that apo A-IV, an apolipoprotein made and secreted as part of the chylomicrons by the small intestinal epithelial cells, may be involved in this lipid-induced satiety. The synthesis and secretion of apolipoprotein A-IV is markedly stimulated by the ingestion of fat. It apparently acts on the central nervous system to elicit the satiety response, but the mechanism by which apo A-IV inhibits food intake is not understood. Okumura and colleagues (1994, 1996) suggested that apo A-IV may act as a modulator of upper gastrointestinal tract function by inhibiting gastric emptying as well as gastric acid secretion. Therefore, apo A-IV appears to play an important role in the integrated control of digestive function and ingestive behavior.

REFERENCES

Altmann SW, Davis HR, Zhu L, Yao X, Hoos LM, Tetzloff G, Iyer SPN, Maguire M, Golovko A, Zeng M, Wang L, Murgolo N, Graziano MP (2004) Niemann-Pick C1 Like 1 protein is critical for intestinal cholesterol absorption. Science 303:1201-1204.

Bansal MP, Cook RG, Danielson KG, Medina D (1989) A 14-kilodalton selenium-binding protein in mouse liver is fatty acid–binding protein. J Biol Chem 264:13780-13784.

Bass NM (1988) The cellular fatty acid–binding proteins: aspects of structure, regulation, and function. Int Rev Cytol 111:143-184.

Berriot-Varoqueaux N, Aggerbeck LP, Samson-Bouma M, Wetterau JR (2000) The role of the microsomal triglyceride transfer protein in abetalipoproteinemia. Annu Rev Nutr 20:663-697.

Besnard P, Niot I, Bernard A, Carlier H (1996) Cellular and molecular aspects of fat metabolism in the small intestine. Proc Nutr Soc 55:19-37.

Bhattacharyya AK, Connor WE (1974) β-Sitosterolemia and xanthomatosis. A newly described lipid storage disease in two sisters. J Clin Invest 53:1033-1043.

Borgstrom B (1976) Phospholipid absorption. In: Rommel K, Boohmer R (eds) Lipid Absorption: Biochemical and Clinical Aspects. MTP Press Ltd, London, pp 65-72.

Borgstrom B (1986) Luminal digestion of fats. In: Go VL (ed) The Exocrine Pancreas. Raven Press, New York, pp 361-373.9/**Cardell RR, Badenhausen S, Porter KR (1967) Intestinal triglyceride absorption in the rat. An electron microscopical study. J Cell Biol 54:123-155.

Carey MC, Small DM, Bliss CM (1983) Lipid digestion and absorption. Annu Rev Physiol 45:651-677.

Chen SH, Habib G, Yang CY, Gu ZW, Lee BR, Weng SA, Silberman SR, Cai SJ, Deslypere JP, Rosseneu M, Gotto AM, Jr, Li WH, Chan L (1987) Apolipoprotein B-48 is the product of a messenger RNA with an organ-specific in-frame stop codon. Science 238:363-366.

Cistola DP, Sacchettini JC, Gordon JI. (1990) ^{13}C NMR studies of fatty acid–protein interactions: comparison of homologous fatty acid–binding proteins produced in the intestinal epithelium. Mol Cell Biochem 98:101-110.

Clark SB, Derksen A, Small DM (1991) Plasma clearance of emulsified triolein in conscious rats: Effects of phosphatidylcholine species, cholesterol content, and emulsion surface physical state. Exp Physiol 76:39-52.

Davis HR Jr, Zhu LJ, Hoos LM, Tetzloff G, Maguire M, Liu J, Yao X, Iyer SP, Lam MH, Lund EG, Detmers PA, Graziano MP, Altmass SW (2004) Niemann-Pick C1 Like 1 (NPC1L1) is the intestinal phytosterol and cholesterol transporter and a key modulator of whole-body cholesterol homeostasis. J Biol Chem 279:333586-333592.

Dobbins WO (1970) An ultrastructural study of the intestinal mucosa in congenital β-lipoprotein deficiency with particular emphasis on intestinal absorptive cells. Gastroenterology 50:195-210.

Field FJ, Mathur S (1983) β-Sitosterol: esterification by intestinal acyl coenzyme A: cholesterol acyltransferase (ACAT) and its effect on cholesterol esterification. J Lipid Res 24:409-417.

Fujimoto K, Cardelli JA, Tso P (1992) Increased apolipoprotein A-IV in rat mesenteric lymph after lipid meal as a physiological signal for satiation. Am J Physiol 262:G1002-G1006.

Gallo LL, Chiang Y, Vahouny GV, Treadwell CR (1980) Localization and origin at rat intestinal cholesterol esterase determined by immunocytochemistry. J Lipid Res 21:537-545.

Genzel-Baroviczeny O, Wahle J, Koletzko B (1997). Fatty acid composition of human milk during the 1st month after term and preterm delivery. Eur J Pediatr 156:142-147.

Glatz JFC, Veerkamp JH (1985) Intracellular fatty acid–binding proteins. Int J Biochem 17:13-22.

Graf GA, Cohen JC, Hobbs HH (2004) Missense mutations in ABCG5 and ABCG8 disrupt heterodimerization and trafficking. J Biol Chem 279:24881-24888.

Hadvary P, Sidler W, Meister W, Vetter W, Wolfer, H (1991). The lipase inhibitor tetrahydrolipstatin binds covalently to the putative active site serine of pancreatic lipase. J Biol Chem 266:2021-2027.

Hamosh M (1996). Digestion in the newborn. Clin Perinatol 23:191-209.

Hartmann D, Hussain Y, Guzelhan C, Odink J (1993) Effect on dietary fat absorption of orlistat, administered at different times relative to food intake. Br J Clin Pharmacol 36:266-270.

Hayashi H, Fujimoto K, Cardelli JA, Nutting DF, Bergstedt S, Tso P (1990) Fat feeding increases size, but not number, of chylomicrons produced by small intestine. Am J Physiol 259:G709-G719.

Hermann T, Buchkremer F, Gosch I, Hall AM, Berhnlohr DA, Stremmel W (2001) Mouse fatty acid transport protein 4 (FATP4): characterization of the gene and functional assessment as a very long chain acyl-CoA synthesize. Gene 2001:31-40.

Hermann T, van der Hoeven F, Grone HJ, Stewart AF, Langbein L, Kaiser I, Liebisch G, Gosch I, Buchkremer F, Drobnik W, Schmitz G, Stremmel W (2003) Mice with targeted disruption of the fatty acid transport protein 4 (Fatp 4, Slc27a4)gene show features of lethal restrictive dermopathy. J Cell Biol 161:1105-1115.

Hernell O, Staggers JE, Carey MC (1990) Physical-chemical behavior of dietary and biliary lipids during intestinal digestion and absorption. 2. Phase analysis and aggregations states of luminal lipids during duodenal fat digestion in healthy adult human beings. Biochemistry 29:2041-2056.

Hofmann AF (1966). A physicochemical approach to the intraluminal phase of fat absorption. Gastroenterology 50:56-64.

Hofmann AF, Borgstrom B (1962) Physico-chemical state of lipids in intestinal content during their digestion and absorption. Federation Proc 21:43-50.

Jensen GL, McGarvey N, Taraszewski R, Wixson SK, Seidner DL, Pai T, Yeh YY, Lee TW, DeMichele SJ (1994) Lymphatic absorption of enterally fed structured triacylglycerol vs. physical mix in a canine model. Am J Clin Nutr 60:518-524.

Kasper H (1970) Faecal fat excretion, diarrhea, and subjective complaints with highly dosed oral fat intake. Digestion 3:321-330.

Kayden HJ, Karmen A, Dumont A (1963) Alterations in the fatty acid composition of human lymph and serum lipoproteins by single feeding. J Clin Invest 42:1373-1381.

Kendrick JS, Chan L, Higgins JA (2001) Superior role of apolipoprotein B48 over apolipoprotein B100 in chylomicron assembly and fat absorption: an investigation of apobec-1 knockout and wild-type mice. Biochem J 356:821-827.

Knight BL (2004) ATP-binding cassette transporter A1: regulation of cholesterol efflux. Biochem Soc Trans 32:124-127.

Lehner R, Kuksis A (1995) Triacylglycerol synthesis by purified triacylglycerol synthetase of rat intestinal mucosa: role of acyl-CoA acyltransferase. J Biol Chem 270:13630-13636.

Lichtenstein AH, Deckelbaum RJ (2001) Stanol/sterol ester-containing foods and blood cholesterol levels. Circulation 103:1177-1179.

Lu K, Lee MH, Hazard S, Brooks-Wilson A, Hidaka H, Kojima H, Ose L, Stalenhoef AF, Mietinnen T, Bjorkhem I, Bruckert E, Pandya A, Brewer HB Jr, Salen G, Dean M, Srivastava A, Patel SB (2001) Two genes that map to the STSL locus cause sitosterolemia: genomic structure and specturm of mutations involving sterolin-1 and sterolin-2, encoded by ABCG5 and ABCG8, respectively. Am J Hum Genet 69:278–290.

Mansbach CM II, Dowell RF, Pritchett D (1991) Portal transport of absorbed lipids in rats. Am J Physiol 261:G530-G538.

Mansbach CM II, Newton D, Stevens RD (1980) Fat digestion in patients with bile acid malabsorption but minimal steatorrhea. Dig Dis Sci 25:353-362.

Mattson FH, Volpenhein RA (1964) The digestion and absorption of triglycerides. J Biol Chem 239:2772-2777.

Mattson FH, Volpenhein RA (1972a) Hydrolysis of fully esterified alcohols containing from one to eight hydroxyl groups by the lipolytic enzymes of rat pancreatic juice. J Lipid Res 13:325-328.

Mattson FH, Volpenhein RA (1972b) Rate and extent of absorption of the fatty acids of fully esterified glycerol, erythritol, xylitol, and sucrose as measured in thoracic duct cannulated rats, J Nutr 102:1177-1180.

McDonald GB, Saunders DR, Weidman M, Fisher L (1980) Portal venous transport of long-chain fatty acids absorbed from rat intestine. Am J Physiol 239:G141-G150.

Meyer JH, Hlinka M, Khatibi A, Raybold HE, Tso P (1998) Role of small intestine in caloric compensation to oil premeals in rats. Am J Physiol 275:R1320-R1333.

Murase T, Aoki M, Wakisaka T, Hase T, Tokimitsu I (2002) Anti-obesity effect of dietary diacylglycerol in C57BL/6J mice: dietary diacylglycerol stimulates intestinal lipid metabolism. J Lipid Res 43:1312-1319.

Nissinen M, Gylling H, Miettenen TA (2002) Micellar distribution of cholesterol and phytosterols after duodenal sitosterol infusion. Am J Physiol Gastrointest Liver Physiol 282:G1009-G1015.

Northfield TC, Hofmann AF (1975) Biliary lipid output during three meals and an overnight fast. 1. Relationship to bile acid pool size and cholesterol saturation of bile in gallstone and control subjects. Gut 16:1-11.

Ockner R K, Manning JA (1974) Fatty acid–binding protein in small intestine. Identification, isolation and evidence for its role in cellular fatty acid transport. J Clin Invest 54:326-338.

Okumura T, Fukagawa K, Tso P, Taylor IL, Pappas TN (1996) Apolipoprotein A-IV acts in the brain to inhibit gastric emptying in the rat. Am J Physiol 270:G49-G53.

Okumura T, Fukagawa K, Tso P, Taylor IL, Pappas TN (1994) Intracisternal injection of apolipoprotein A-IV inhibits gastric secretion in pylorusligated conscious rats. Gastroenterology 107:1861-1864.

Palay SL, Karlin LJ (1959) An electron microscopic study of the intestinal villus. II. The pathway of fat absorption. J Biophys Biochem Cytol 5:373-383.

Porter HP, Saunders DR (1971) Isolation of the aqueous phase of human intestinal contents during the digestion of a fatty meal. Gastroenterology 60:997-1007.

Porter HP, Saunders DR, Tytgat G, Brunster O, Rubin CE (1971) Fat absorption in bile fistula man. A morphological and biochemical study. Gastroenterology 60:1008-1019.

Powell LM, Wallis SC, Pease RJ, Edwards YH, Knott TJ, Scott J (1987) A novel form of tissue-specific RNA processing produces apolipoprotein B-48 in intestine. Cell 50:831-840.

Rosenblum SB, Huynh T, Afonso A, Davis HR Jr, Yumibe N, Clader JW, Burnett DA (1998) Discovery of 1-(4-fluorophenyl)-(3R)-[3-(4-fluorophenyl)-(3S)-hydroxypropyl]-(4S)-(4-hydroxyphenyl)-2-azedidinone (SCH58235): a designed, potent, orally active inhibitor of cholesterol absorption. J Med Chem 41:973-980.

Roy CC, Levy E, Green PHR, Sniderman A, Letarte J, Buts JP, Orquin J, Brochu P, Weber AM, Morin CL, Marcel Y, Deckelbaum RJ (1987) Malabsorption, hypocholesterolemia, and fat-filled enterocytes with increased intestinal apoprotein B. Gastroenterology 92:390-399.

Sabesin SM, Bennett-Clark S, Holt PR (1975) Intestinal lipid absorption: Evidence for an intrinsic defect in chylomicron secretion in normal rat distal intestine. Lipids 10:840-846.

Sabesin SM, Frase S (1977) Electron microscopic studies of the assembly, intracellular transport, and secretion of chylomicrons by rat intestine. J Lipid Res 18:496-511.

Salen G, von Bergmann K, Lutjohann D, Kwiterovich P, Kane J, Patel SB, Musliner T, Stein P, Musser B (2004) Ezetimibe effectively reduces plasma plant sterols in patients with sitosterolemia. Circulation 109:966-971.

Salen G, Shefer S, Nguyen, L, Ness GC, Tint GS, Batta AK (1997) Sitosterolemia. Subcell Biochem 28:453-476.

Stahl A, Hirsch DJ, Gimeno RE, Punreddy S, Ge P, Watson N, Patel S, Kotler M, Alejandra A, Tartaglia LA, Lodish HF (1999) Identification of the major intestinal fatty acid transport protein. Mol Cell 4:299-308.

Stange EF, Dietschy JM (1985) The origin of cholesterol in the mesenteric lymph of the rat. J Lipid Res 26:175-184.

Talmud PJ, Lloyd JK, Muller DPR, Collins DR, Scott J, Humphries S (1988) Genetic evidence from two families that the apolipoprotein B gene is not involved in abetalipoproteinemia. J Clin Invest 82:1803-1806.

Velasquez OR, Place AR, Tso P, Crissinger KD (1994) Developing intestine is injured during absorption of oleic acid but not its ethyl ester. J Clin Invest 93:479-485.

Ways PO, Paramentier CM, Kayden HD, Jones JW, Saunders DR, Rubin CE (1967) Studies on the absorptive defect for triglyceride in abetalipoproteinemia. J Clin Invest 46:35-46.

Wetterau JR, Aggerbeck LP, Bouma ME, Eisenberg C, Munck A, Hermier M, Schmitz J, Gay G, Rader DJ, Gregg RE (1992) Absence of microsomal triglyceride transfer protein in individuals with abetalipoproteinemia. Science 258:999-1001.

Wetterau JR, Zilversmit DB (1984) A triglyceride and cholesteryl ester transfer protein associated with liver microsomes. J Biol Chem 259: 10863-10866.

Wu AL, Bennett-Clark S, Holt PR (1980) Composition of lymph chylomicrons from proximal or distal rat small intestine. Am J Clin Nutr 33:582-589.

RECOMMENDED READINGS

Thomson ABR, Keelan M, Garg ML, Clandinin MT (1989) Intestinal aspects of lipid absorption: In review. Can J Physiol Pharmacol 67:179-191.

Tso P (1994) Intestinal lipid absorption. In: Johnson LR (ed) Physiology of the Gastrointestinal Tract, 3rd ed. Raven Press, New York, pp 1867-1907.

Chapter 11

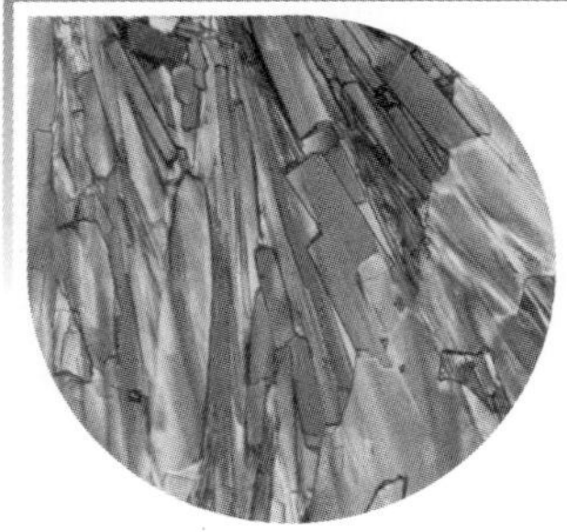

Dietary Fiber

Joanne R. Lupton, PhD, and Nancy D. Turner, PhD

OUTLINE

DEFINITION OF FIBER

Although fiber is recognized as an important dietary component, it is not a truly essential nutrient, as evidenced by the survival of Eskimos in Arctic regions and the Masai tribes of East Africa, both of whom consume no foods of vegetable origin in their traditional diets. In fact, the benefits of fiber stem not from its assimilation by the body, but from its almost completely indigestible nature. This results in fiber being retained within the gastrointestinal tract. The presence of fiber in the gastrointestinal tract as well as the fermentation of fiber by large intestinal microflora results in effects on gastrointestinal function that are important in health and in the prevention and management of a variety of disease states.

Currently the United States relies on an "analytical approach" to determine what is or is not considered fiber for purposes of noting the amount of fiber on food labels. This is in contrast to what is done in Canada, where a formal definition of fiber is used to determine the appropriate analytical techniques to measure fiber content of foods (Health and Welfare

Canada, 1985). In 2001 the Institute of Medicine (IOM) developed the following set of working definitions for fiber in the food supply:

> *Dietary Fiber* consists of nondigestible carbohydrates and lignin that are intrinsic and intact in plants.
> *Functional Fiber* consists of isolated, nondigestible carbohydrates that have beneficial physiological effects in humans.
> *Total Fiber* is the sum of *Dietary Fiber* and *Functional Fiber* (IOM, 2001, p. 2)

These new working definitions recognize the diversity of nondigestible carbohydrates in the food supply. Although this definition has yet to be formally adopted by the U.S. Food and Drug Administration (FDA), it would allow consideration of plant, animal, and manufactured fiber sources that exhibit beneficial physiological effects in humans.

There is still considerable debate concerning whether this new definition is appropriate. Most would accept that fiber is plant material not digested by mammalian enzymes. But some consider limiting fiber to "plant material" to be too restrictive. Some would include chitosan, which forms the exoskeleton of crustaceans, or certain heat-treated animal proteins that are not readily digestible by mammalian enzymes and thus reach the large intestine relatively intact. Others include "resistant starch" in their definition of fiber, which is not truly undigested by mammalian enzymes but may not be digested and absorbed in the small intestine and thus have characteristics similar to those of fiber, under certain circumstances. Resistant starches occur in some foods normally, but resistant starch may also develop as a result of manufacturing or processing of foods. Another question arises concerning the inclusion of oligosaccharides present in beans (raffinose, stachyose, and verbacose) and of the fructans (storage poly- and oligosaccharides) in vegetables and fruits such as onions and artichokes. The alcohol precipitation steps used in analytical techniques would exclude these two classes of substances, yet they have biological effects similar to those of other nondigested polysaccharides.

Another point of discussion concerning the new definition is whether dietary fiber has to be intact in the food to be characterized as fiber, or whether it can be extracted from food, or even manufactured, and still be called dietary fiber. The basis for this argument is that most of the data describing physiological effects and thus the potential health benefits from fiber were generated using high fiber foods. It is not completely clear whether the same benefits would accrue from consuming isolated or manufactured fibers. The converse could be true; isolated sources may in fact be more effective, but the extensive data that would be necessary to draw this conclusion do not currently exist.

Finally, many carbohydrate chemists prefer to have a chemical, rather than a physiological, definition of fiber. They argue that there needs to be a simple, universally accepted assay for dietary fiber in order to simplify compliance with and enforcement of labeling laws. The procedure should be suitable for the analysis of any food or food component to determine how much fiber it contains.

CHEMICAL CHARACTERIZATION

The major botanical categories of fiber are cellulose, hemicellulose, pectic substances, gums, mucilage, algal polysaccharides, and lignin. With the exception of lignin (a polyphenol), all fibers are complex, nonstarch polysaccharides. They differ from each other in the sugar residues making up the polysaccharide and in the arrangement of the residues. The principal residues in fibers are glucose, galactose, mannose, and certain pentoses. A description of the structure and bonds found in various fiber types is presented in Chapter 4 (see Table 4-2 and Fig. 4-13).

Cellulose is the most widely distributed fiber in the plant kingdom. It is found in plant cell walls and is a polymer of glucose with a β-1,4 linkage between glucose molecules. It is the only truly "fibrous" fiber. Hemicelluloses include a wide variety of polysaccharides, which contain both pentoses and hexoses. Although these compounds are called hemicellulose, they are chemically unrelated to cellulose. Pectic substances are water-soluble polysaccharides rich in galacturonic acid. Gums are secreted by plants in response to injury, and as such are not part of the plant cell wall. However, gums are classified as dietary fiber because of the way in which mammalian systems use and respond to them. Mucilages are similar to gums in that they are polysaccharides that form viscous solutions. Because of the water-retaining ability of mucilages, they protect seeds from desiccation. Algal polysaccharides are extracted from algae and represent a diverse group of fibers. Lignin, a polyphenolic compound, is found in the woody parts of plants, such as the stem.

Arrangement of the sugar residues in the polysaccharide is often more important to the physiological effect of the fiber than are the residues themselves. Branching and substitutions on the primary carbohydrate chain can have major consequences with respect to physical properties. The degree of methoxylation or sulfation of certain fibers also affects the physiological properties of the fiber. For example, if the galacturonic acid residues in pectin are methoxylated, there is no ionic group available for calcium binding or to trap water. This will not affect the gel-forming properties of pectin as long as there are sufficient nonmethoxylated portions of the molecule to form the gel. However, if methoxylation is randomly distributed throughout the molecule, a significant impact on gel-forming ability can occur.

In addition to the primary structure of fiber, which is determined by the bonds between residues, the molecule's secondary structure also can affect digestibility. For example, the α-1,4 glucose linkage in starch is readily cleaved by mammalian enzymes. However, modification of the same starch molecule to produce a different three-dimensional organization may render it resistant to human digestive enzymes. In other words, the packing or arrangement of the molecule can restrict access of enzymes to the bonds they normally hydrolyze. This is why starch can become "resistant" to enzymatic hydrolysis and act like dietary fiber. Raw starches, such as raw potato and banana starch, are almost completely resistant to pancreatic amylase and thus reach the colon relatively intact. This characteristic is the basis behind some arguments that resistant starch should be included in the definition of fiber.

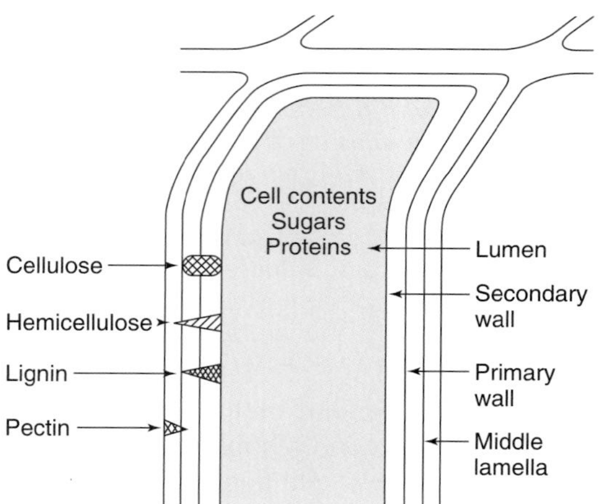

Figure 11-1 A diagram of a plant cell showing the location of fibrous components. The more digestible cell contents are contained within the lumen of the cell. Various fiber components are found primarily within the cell wall. The cell wall must be broken up by chewing, processing, or cooking in order for the cell contents to be made available for digestion and absorption. This also increases the surface area of the particle, increasing the ability of microbes to attach and begin fermentation of the fibrous components (cellulose, hemicellulose, lignin, and pectin). The location of greatest concentration for the various fibrous components is indicated by the hatched structures. *(Modified from Maynard LA, Loosli JK, Hintz HF, Warner RG [1979] Animal Nutrition, 7th ed. McGraw-Hill, New York, p 88.)*

The location of fiber components within the plant, and whether or not fiber is extracted from the plant or eaten intact, may have significant physiological consequences. If the fiber is contained within an intact plant cell, the cell wall must first be disrupted for the physiological effects of the particular fibers to be exerted (Fig. 11-1). Resistance to breakage of the cell wall depends on the structure of the cell wall and its degree of lignification. The number of plant cells per particle ingested (particle size) also may determine the accessibility of the cell wall to digestive enzymes (Slavin, 2003), as may cooking, processing, and mastication of the food (Bjorck et al., 1994).

PHYSIOLOGICAL CHARACTERIZATION

Fibers are also routinely categorized by their physiological effects. The primary physiological categories have been soluble versus insoluble. However, more recently fibers have been characterized as being viscous versus nonviscous, or fermentable versus nonfermentable. In general, the structural fibers (cellulose, lignin, and some hemicelluloses) are insoluble, nonviscous, and poorly fermentable. In contrast, the gel-forming fibers (pectins, gums, mucilages, and the remaining hemicelluloses) are soluble, viscous, and fermentable, and these fibers exert effects on digestion and absorption in the upper gastrointestinal tract. Although these generalizations are useful, there are exceptions to these generalizations. Gum arabic, for example, is a soluble fiber that does not form a viscous solution. Therefore current trends are to no longer characterize fibers based on solubility, but to characterize them based on their functionality, which is more dependent on viscosity and fermentability. The most important characteristic of fibers with respect to upper gastrointestinal physiology is viscosity, and that with respect to colon physiology is fermentability.

MAJOR PHYSIOLOGICAL EFFECTS OF FIBER AND STRUCTURE/FUNCTION RELATIONSHIPS

The role that fiber plays within the upper and lower gastrointestinal tract depends on the fiber's physical and chemical attributes. Therefore, the following sections describe the various effects fibers may have within the gastrointestinal tract segments, as well as how the chemical nature of the fiber generates these results.

EFFECTS OF FIBER ON THE UPPER GASTROINTESTINAL TRACT

Gastric Emptying and Satiety

One of the neurological pathways involved in the feeling of satiety is that of distention or physical fullness. Because fibers are resistant to digestion in the stomach, the bulk they add to the diet produces a feeling of fullness. Therefore, even though caloric intake may be similar, distention resulting from an increased fiber intake leads to a feeling of satiety (French and Read, 1994).

The viscosity of polysaccharides and their ability to form gels in the stomach appear to slow gastric emptying (Marlett et al., 2002). This, in turn, results in a more uniform presentation of the meal to the small intestine for absorption. Therefore gel-forming fibers further contribute toward a feeling of satiety by maintaining a feeling of fullness for a longer period after a meal (IOM, 2002). In contrast, fibers that do not form gels (such as wheat bran and cellulose) have little effect on the rate at which the meal exits from the stomach.

Effects on Absorption From the Small Intestine

Polysaccharides that produce a viscous solution can delay and even interfere with the absorption of nutrients such as carbohydrates, lipids, and proteins from the small intestine. The reasons for this effect on absorption include delayed gastric emptying (mentioned earlier), entrapment of nutrients in the gel-like structure, interference with micelle formation, and decreased access of enzymes to the nutrients. Fiber-rich foods may also contain lipase inhibitors. In addition, the mixing of intestinal contents appears to be impeded by the presence of viscous polysaccharides. This delayed or diminished nutrient absorption has both positive and negative health benefits.

Positive Effects of Delayed Nutrient Absorption

Positive benefits of delayed nutrient absorption include an improvement of glucose tolerance and a lowering of serum cholesterol levels. Delayed absorption of carbohydrate results in a lower postprandial glucose level. In general, the more viscous the fiber, the greater the effect on blood glucose. This is similar to the effect seen with eating several small meals rather than one large meal (nibbling versus gorging). When glucose is absorbed in small amounts over an extended period, such as seen with viscous fibers, the insulin response is attenuated (Pick et al., 1996). Because high amounts of glucose appear to trigger sustained insulin secretion and insulin secretion stimulates 3-hydroxy-3-methylglutaryl coenzyme A (HMG-CoA) reductase activity, high blood glucose concentrations promote cholesterol biosynthesis. Therefore fiber may also reduce plasma cholesterol levels via its effect on glucose tolerance. Because of the flattened glucose curves seen with ingestion of viscous fibers, these fibers are often recommended for diabetics, who typically have lipid profiles that indicate an elevated risk of cardiovascular disease.

Effects on Properties of Lipoproteins and Serum Cholesterol

Not much is known about the effect of different fibers on the formation of lipoproteins. However, it now appears that some fibers may affect very low density lipoproteins formed in the liver, whereas others exert their primary effect on chylomicrons formed in the intestine. This means that fiber may have a different effect on lipoproteins (and thus cholesterol and triacylglycerols) depending on whether the person has eaten or is fasting. It is also clear that the effect of fiber depends on the amount of fat in the diet and the energy status of the host. Certain viscous fibers have been shown to lower serum cholesterol both in laboratory animals (Fernandez et al., 1997) and in humans (Jensen et al., 1997). These fibers include guar gum, pectin, psyllium, and oat bran. Bean products also produce this effect. In contrast, wheat bran and cellulose do not lower plasma cholesterol.

Nutrition Insight

Cholesterol Manipulation

Elevated serum cholesterol can be the result of both genetic and dietary problems. Inclusion of soluble fiber in the diet can reduce serum cholesterol as well as alter the lipoprotein profile.

Thinking Critically

1. What is the expected effect on serum cholesterol of including cellulose-containing foods in the diet?
2. What are some potential mechanisms by which a water-soluble, viscous, gel-forming fiber could reduce serum cholesterol?

Possible Mechanisms by Which Fibers Lower Serum Cholesterol

The mechanism by which fibers lower serum cholesterol is still a subject of debate and is likely multifactorial. Alternatively, different fibers may work by different mechanisms. The major hypotheses are summarized in Table 11-1. These hypotheses include the binding of bile acids to fiber, which then interferes with their enterohepatic recirculation. By this hypothesis, more bile acids are excreted in the feces, requiring additional synthesis of bile acids from cholesterol, thus lowering the body's cholesterol pool. An additional consequence of binding bile acids is that they would be less available for micelle formation, which in turn could interfere with the absorption of cholesterol and triacylglycerols. A different mechanism, which remains controversial, is the production of the short-chain fatty acid propionate from fermentation of fiber in the colon. Propionate is absorbed from the colon, through the portal vein, and has been shown by some investigators to inhibit HMG-CoA reductase, the rate-limiting enzyme for cholesterol biosynthesis.

Potential Interference With Mineral Absorption

Large amounts of dietary fiber also have the potential to interfere with mineral bioavailability. Because the charged groups on polysaccharides are usually negatively charged, the tendency of dietary fiber is to bind cations such as calcium, magnesium, sodium, and potassium. This may limit the absorption of these minerals from the small intestine. This is not generally considered a public health concern, but it may be pertinent in certain cases when individuals have very high-fiber diets and low intakes of minerals such as calcium and magnesium.

EFFECTS OF FIBER ON THE LOWER GASTROINTESTINAL TRACT

Fermentation

The primary way in which fiber affects the colonic luminal environment is through its fermentation, as illustrated in Figure 11-2.

Table 11-1
Possible Mechanisms by Which Fibers Lower Serum Cholesterol

Mechanism	Effect
Delayed gastric emptying	Fiber affects the entrance of chyme into the small intestine. This in turn may affect the rate of carbohydrate and lipid absorption, which influences insulin secretion and lipoprotein formation.
Interference with digestive enzymes	Viscous fibers may sequester lipids, proteins, and carbohydrates from digestive enzymes, thereby impairing their absorption.
Interference with micelle formation	Fibers may bind to the bile acids or interfere with micelle formation, impairing the absorption of cholesterol, bile acids, and lipids.
Interference with mixing of intestinal contents	Fibers may interfere with micelle formation and with the ability of digestive enzymes to hydrolyze lipids, proteins, and starch.
Inhibition of cholesterol biosynthesis	Fermentation of fiber in the colon results in the production of propionate, a short-chain fatty acid. Once absorbed through the portal vein, this short-chain fatty acid is thought to inhibit HMG-CoA reductase activity, the rate-limiting enzyme for cholesterol biosynthesis.

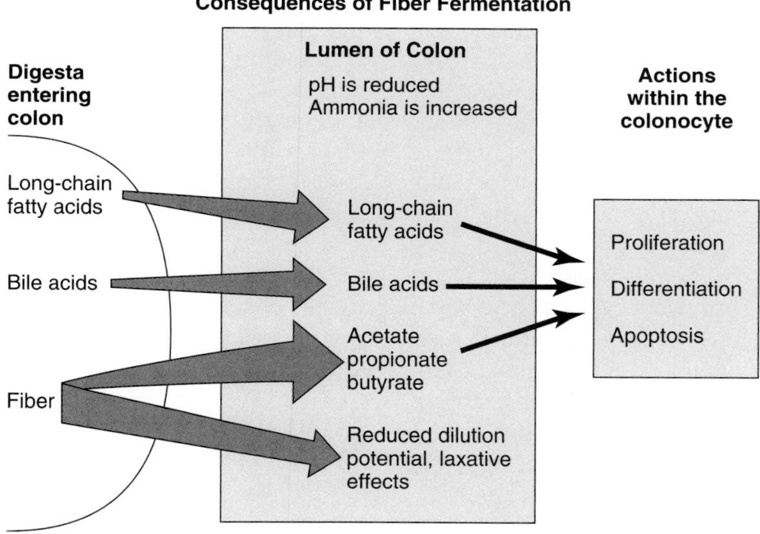

Figure 11-2 Intestinal contents entering the colon are fermented by bacteria, resulting in an increase in the amount of short-chain fatty acids and a reduction in pH. As fiber is fermented, its mass is reduced as the fecal stream passes through the colon. Therefore, because the mass of fiber decreases while the mass of short-chain fatty acids increases, and the mass of bile acids and long-chain fatty acids remains the same but has less fiber with which to associate, the concentrations of short-chain fatty acids, as well as long-chain fatty acids and bile acids, increase in the fecal stream. Luminal pH and these molecules affect colonocyte proliferation, differentiation, and apoptosis. Absorption of these molecules can be concentration-dependent, making their concentration within the fecal milieu a key determinant of cell cycle activity.

Clinical Correlation

Ulcerative Colitis

Ulcerative colitis occurs predominantly in the distal colon (Chapman et al., 1994), a segment of the colon that is more dependent on butyrate oxidation as its metabolic fuel supply than is the proximal colon. In fact, Mortensen and Clausen (1996) proposed that ulcerative colitis is an energy-deficiency disease. The results of Scheppach and colleagues (1992) indicate that supplying butyrate by enemas of short-chain fatty acids induces remission of colitis.

Thinking Critically

Patients receiving parenteral feeding for extended periods often develop ulcerative colitis. What would you recommend in order to alleviate this condition?

Fermentable fiber is metabolized by the colonic microflora in an anaerobic process with the production of short-chain fatty acids, hydrogen, carbon dioxide, and biomass. Fiber may be fermented to different amounts and types of short-chain fatty acids (such as acetate, propionate, and butyrate), each of which has specific properties. Foods containing dietary fiber composed of hemicellulose, pectin, or resistant starch provide highly fermentable substrates, whereas those containing high cellulose content provide less fermentable substrates. Currently, there is no evidence that a relationship exists between the quantity of fiber consumed and its fermentability, until very high levels of a fiber are consumed (IOM, 2002).

Roles of Acetate, Propionate, and Butyrate

The short-chain fatty acids are the major carbon products of fermentation. Acetate is rapidly absorbed from the colonic lumen into the portal blood and then goes to the liver before entering the general circulation. Acetate is used as an energy source by most nonhepatic tissues in the body. Propionate, like acetate, is also rapidly absorbed and enters the portal vein, by which it is transported to the liver. In contrast to acetate, however, propionate is used by the liver. Some studies show that propionate inhibits HMG-CoA reductase activity. Butyrate is unique in that it is the preferred energy source for colonocytes (epithelial cells lining the colon). Colonocytes metabolize butyrate to CO_2, which in part spares the use of glucose. Butyrate may also be incorporated into membrane lipids.

Dilution Potential of Fiber and Its Consequences

Different fibers have different bulking properties, depending on their degree of fermentation. Naturally, as a fiber is fermented, it is no longer available to contribute to fecal bulk; therefore, the poorly fermentable fibers are the best in vivo dilutors (Fig. 11-3). This is significant because colon cancer develops and progresses in response to certain factors in the fecal stream. For example, ingested carcinogens (cancer-causing agents) have less access to the cells lining the colon if they are dispersed in a larger, rather than smaller, volume. Other factors that affect the colonocytes and are subject to dilution by dietary fibers include bile acids, diacylglycerols, long-chain fatty acids, and ammonia. There are important health consequences to keeping these factors diluted in the feces, which are explained later. The responses to increased fiber intake may explain the reduction in colon cancer incidence observed in the European Prospective Investigation into Cancer and Nutrition (EPIC) study (Bingham et al., 2003).

Fermentability and Its Relationship to Colonic Luminal pH

As a fiber is fermented to short-chain fatty acids, the pH of luminal contents decreases. This is significant because many bacterial reactions are pH-sensitive. For example, the bacterial enzyme responsible for forming secondary bile acids from primary bile acids (7α-dehydroxylase) is inactivated below a pH of 6.5. Colon contents often can reach this pH when fiber is fermented. The significance of luminal pH in the colon and its relation to colon cancer is discussed in detail elsewhere (Newmark and Lupton, 1990).

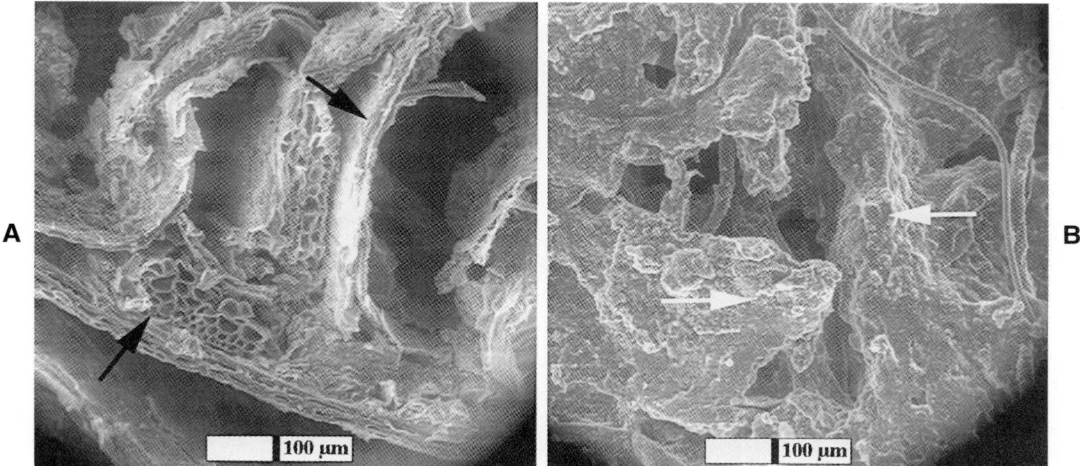

Figure 11-3 Effect of fiber in diluting fecal constituents by increasing fecal mass. Environmental scanning electron micrographs of fecal pellets from rats consuming diets containing either wheat bran **(A)** or oat bran **(B)**. More fiber *(black arrows)* remained in the feces of rats that consumed wheat bran than in those consuming oat bran. The extensive amount of wheat bran fiber remaining increases the porosity (empty spaces in picture) of the feces and is able to sequester undesirable constituents in the fecal stream, thereby reducing their absorption by colonocytes. In contrast, oat bran was extensively fermented, leaving a less porous fecal pellet that was composed primarily of undigested food, endogenous secretions, and bacteria *(white arrows)*. This increases availability of the more undesirable components and thus the potential for their absorption by colonocytes. *(Assistance in image acquisition was provided by C.M. McDonough, Texas A&M University, College Station, TX.)*

Colonic Epithelial Cell Proliferation, Differentiation, and Apoptosis

The cells lining the colon are only one epithelial cell deep. Unlike the case with the small intestine, no villi are found in the large intestine. Instead, the colonic mucosa consists of crypts that are depressions in an otherwise smooth surface epithelium (Fig. 11-4). Cells are formed toward the base of the crypt and migrate upward, making several divisions in transit. A cell differentiates as it reaches the upper part of the crypt and eventually is exfoliated and excreted by way of the feces. This process takes from 3 to 30 days, depending on the location within the colon.

During the progression of normal healthy cells to colonic tumors, the normal controls on cell division are lost. Through a series of genetic changes, cells continue to divide higher up the crypt, instead of differentiating. They may accumulate at the top of the crypt and form polyps, which then may become tumors. Tumors may invade down through the crypt and into the underlying muscle area. Because changes in colonic crypt cell proliferation have been shown both to precede and to accompany neoplasia, an upregulation of cell proliferation in the colon is considered an important marker for colon tumorigenesis. More recently other surrogate markers for colon cancer include a downregulation of cell differentiation and/or colon cell death (apoptosis) (Chang et al., 1997). Agents or diet ingredients that stimulate cells to divide are considered to promote cancer, because dividing cells are much more vulnerable to attack by carcinogens. In contrast, dietary factors that result in a more quiescent proliferative pattern or enhance differentiation or apoptosis are considered to protect against colon cancer.

How Fiber Affects Turnover of Colonic Epithelial Cells

Fibers can affect cell division by either increasing or decreasing the luminal concentration of certain mitogenic factors. As a fiber ferments, short-chain fatty acids are formed.

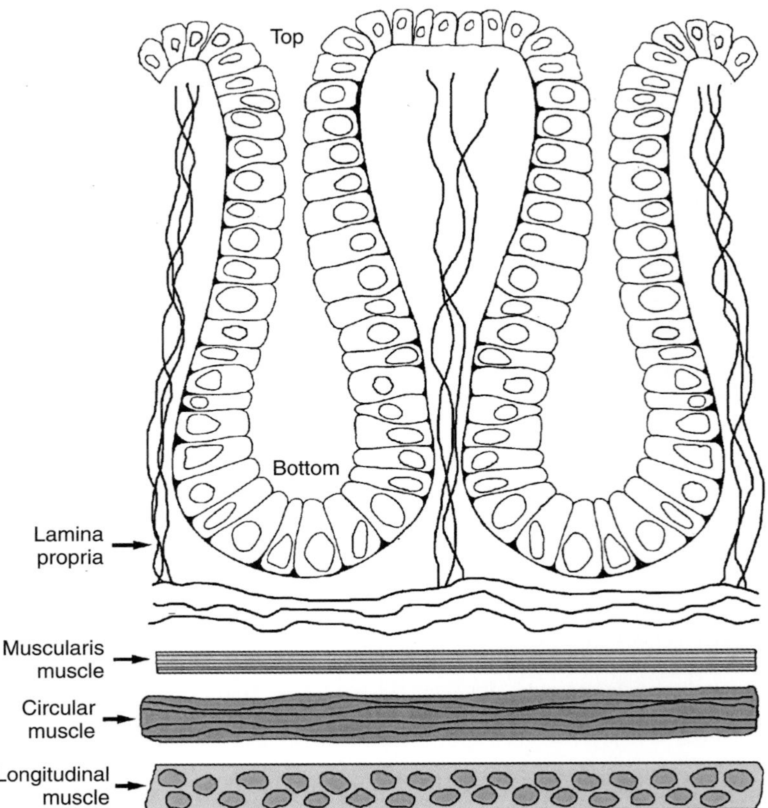

Figure 11-4 An illustration of a histological section of colon crypts, showing the arrangement of epithelial cells. The colon lumen is at the top of the picture, whereas the muscle layers surrounding the colon are represented at the bottom. Cells at the top of the crypt form the surface lining of the colon lumen. Crypts are invaginations within the colon, as opposed to the villi of the small intestine that protrude out into the lumen.

These short-chain fatty acids increase cell proliferation in the colon. Under normal circumstances, this may be a healthy role for dietary fiber. However, in the presence of a carcinogen, this may actually enhance the tumorigenic process. Also, as a fiber is fermented, it is no longer able to dilute constituents in the fecal stream. Fecal constituents, such as bile acids, long-chain fatty acids, diacyglycerols, and ammonia may also be mitogenic to colonocytes. With respect to the healthy colon, the poorly fermented fibers would protect against colon cancer by diluting mitogenic compounds, whereas, the fermentable fibers would provide the substrates necessary for normal colonocyte metabolism.

Transit Time and Constipation

Colonic motility is the largest determinant of overall gastrointestinal transit times, because gastric emptying time averages between 2 to 5 hours, and small intestinal emptying time averages between 3 to 6 hours, compared to 40 to 70 hours for residue from a particular meal to make its way through the lower portion of the gastrointestinal tract (Hillemeier, 1995). Adding fiber to the diet affects transit times in all three segments of the gastrointestinal tract. Within the stomach, food is processed to reduce particle size before it is released into the intestine. Extending the amount of time required for processing in the stomach through the addition of fiber slows the passage of nutrients into the small intestine. This has benefits for individuals who need to reduce the glycemic response to certain foods (Pick et al., 1996). The presence of fiber in the diet also delays absorption of some nutrients in the small intestine because of the dilution potential that fibers have, which reduces exposure to and absorption of nutrients by epithelial cells.

Within the colon, the ability of fiber to reduce transit time depends on whether or not it is soluble. Soluble fibers are more readily fermented by colonic bacteria than are insoluble fibers. Therefore, more of the insoluble fiber remains in the fecal stream, creating much more bulk than do the soluble fibers. The increase in bulk also increases the amount of water-holding capacity within the feces (Hillemeier, 1995). The combination of greater mass and greater moisture content contributes to a decrease in transit time within the colon. Hillemeier (1995) reported that including bran in the diets of control and constipated patients reduced transit time for both groups. Including bran in the diets of constipated individuals successfully decreased the time that digesta was present in the intestinal tract by almost half.

Constipation refers to a persistent condition in which defecation is difficult or infrequent (Camilleri et al., 1994). Whether the prevalence of constipation is related to age is currently being debated, with levels of reported constipation ranging from 3% to 20%, depending on the definitions used by the study investigators. Yet Camilleri and colleagues (1994) noted that, regardless of the study evaluated, as individual age increased to older than 65 years, those individuals reporting constipation increased to 10% to 30% of the population studied. Most cases of constipation are attributed to unknown causes, and most of these individuals can be treated by increasing hydration, exercise, and fiber intake (Dukas et al., 2003; Camilleri et al., 1994). Approximately 1% of individuals may have intractable constipation, meaning it is not easily managed or cured. Further study to determine the cause of this condition is warranted, because many physiological conditions could predispose a person to intractable constipation. Even in individuals with intractable constipation, the treatment regimen may include fiber as a means of decreasing constipation (Camilleri et al., 1994).

EFFECTS OF FIBER ON WHOLE-BODY ENERGY STATUS

Because fibers may be fermented to short-chain fatty acids, which can be absorbed from the colon and utilized for metabolism, the concept that dietary fiber contributes no energy to the host is clearly inaccurate. However, an attempt to assign a caloric value to dietary fiber is very difficult. First, one has to measure the amount of fiber in the diet, which, as discussed previously in this chapter, is a complex problem. Second, one needs to know how that particular fiber is processed within the gastrointestinal tract. Even if we were to consider only a single fiber source, there would be much variation between persons in how that fiber is handled in the gastrointestinal tract. In particular, differences in the other components of the diet, the colonic microflora, or the presence or absence of antibiotics could affect the degree of fermentation that occurs. Third, one would need to know how much of each fermentation product is absorbed and metabolized. Not all of the fermentation products are absorbed. Some energy is used to support bacterial growth, and bacteria, fiber, short-chain fatty acids, and other organic acids may be eliminated in the feces. The best estimate of energy yield generated by fiber fermentation in humans is between 6.2 to 10.4 kJ/g (1.5 to 2.5 kcal/g) of fiber (IOM, 2002), compared with 16.7 kJ/g (4.0 kcal/g) for starch.

RECOMMENDATIONS FOR FIBER INTAKE AND TYPICAL INTAKES

In establishing the dietary recommended intakes, the IOM (2002) recommended an adequate intake (AI) level of 14 g of fiber for each 1,000 kcal of energy consumed for all individuals from 1 year of age throughout the remainder of their lives. On the basis of median energy intakes, this equates to 25 g/day for women and 38 g/day for men ages 19 to 50. The AI was set at 21 g/day and 30 g/day, respectively, for women and men age 51 and older based on lower median energy intakes

Clinical Correlation

Short-Bowel Patients

Some diseases require the removal of segments of the small intestine, leaving patients with only a short segment of the bowel remaining, with or without a preserved colon. In many of these patients, only half the calories consumed are absorbed, making dietary manipulation critical if they are to consume enough food so as not to require parenteral nutritional support. In those patients with a functional colon, energy recovery through microbial fermentation can contribute significantly to total energy availability. Mortensen and Clausen (1996) noted that an increase in carbohydrate consumption from 20% to 60% of total caloric intake provided patients with an additional 465 kcal/day, which was about 30% of the total energy absorbed. Unfortunately, there was no additional energy availability with similar diet modifications in patients without functional colons.

Thinking Critically

1. Which type of fiber would you suggest that short-bowel patients with a functional colon include in their diet? Why?
2. How would the particle size of the fiber affect its ability to serve as a source of available energy in these patients?

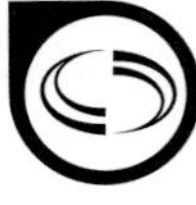

RECOMMENDED INTAKES (ADEQUATE INTAKES) FOR FIBER ACROSS THE LIFE CYCLE

	g Fiber per Day
Infants	
0 to 1 yr	(none set)
Children	
1 to 3 yr	19
4 to 8 yr	25
Males	
9 to 13 yr	31
14 to 18 yr	38
19 to 50 yr	38
>50 yr	30
Females	
9 to 18 yr	26
19 to 50 yr	25
>50 yr	21
Pregnant	28
Lactating	29

Data from Institute of Medicine (2002) Dietary, functional, and total fiber. In: Dietary Reference Intakes for Energy, Carbohydrate, Fiber, Fat, Fatty Acids, Cholesterol, Protein, and Amino Acids. National Academy Press, Washington, DC, pp 7-1–7-69.
AIs for dietary fiber were calculated by multiplying mean energy intake by 14 g fiber per 1,000 kcal.

for older adults. There are no data suggesting that pregnant or lactating women would benefit from increased fiber intake, yet because energy intakes increase for these two groups, the recommended AIs are 28 g/day and 29 g/day, for pregnant and lactating women, respectively.

Recommendations are not provided for infants younger than 1 year of age. An AI was not developed for this age-group because milk, which contains no fiber, is the primary recommended food source through 6 months of age, and there are no data on fiber intake in infants until after 1 year of age. On the basis of median energy intakes, the AI for children from 1 to 3 years was set at 19 g/day and for children from 4 to 8 years at 25 g/day.

Once children reach 9 years of age, the difference in energy intake between boys and girls differs sufficiently that the AI for them is also different. Therefore, the AI for boys aged 9 to 13 years is 31 g/day, and the AI for boys aged 14 to 18 years is 38 g/day. The AIs for girls aged 9 to 18 is 26 g/day.

Unfortunately, American women and men consume an average of only 13 to 17 g of fiber per day, respectively, which is far short of the suggested AI levels. However, it is possible to meet the recommended AI levels without drastically altering food choices (IOM, 2002). Many times, the limitation that prevents people from meeting these goals is that they do not know which foods provide desirable levels of dietary fiber. Food sources of fiber include whole grain products, legumes, vegetables, and fruits. There is also confusion about what foods would meet the criteria used to define whole grain foods, making it hard for consumers to increase the consumption of

Table 11-2
Examples of Food Sources of Total Dietary Fiber

Item	Quantity	Content (g)
Breads and Grains		
Cornbread	1 piece	1.4
Pumpernickel bread	1 slice	2.1
White bread	1 slice	0.6
Whole wheat bread	1 slice	1.9
Rice, brown	½ cup	1.7
Rice, white	½ cup	0.3
Cereals		
Kellogg's All Bran Original	1/2 cup	8.8
Kellogg's Product 19	1 cup	1.0
Kellogg's Raisin Bran	1 cup	7.3
Wheat Chex, General Mills	1 cup	3.3
Rice Chex, General Mills	1 1/4 cups	0.3
Shredded wheat	2 biscuits	5.5
Oatmeal	1 cup	4.0
Fruits		
Apple, with skin	each	3.3
Figs, dried, uncooked	2	3.7
Orange	each	3.1
Prunes, dried, uncooked	5	3.0
Raspberries	½ cup	4.0
Vegetables and Legumes		
Broccoli, raw	½ cup	1.1
Cauliflower, raw	½ cup	1.2
Corn, sweet, yellow	½ cup	2.1
Cowpeas, common, cooked	½ cup	5.6
Lettuce, iceberg, raw	½ cup	0.35
Kidney beans	½ cup	6.6
Peas, green, young	½ cup	4.4
Pinto beans	½ cup	7.7
Potato, baked, flesh	each	2.3
Squash, yellow, cooked	½ cup	1.25

Data from U.S. Department of Agriculture, Agricultural Research Service (2005) USDA Nutrient Database for Standard Reference, Release 18. U.S. Department of Agriculture, Washington, DC. Retrieved December 13, 2005, from www.ars.usda.gov/ba/bhnrc/ndl.

these foods. However, recognition of the importance of whole grain foods has led to compilation of product lists that can be used by consumers to increase incorporation of these foods into their diets (Marquart et al., 2003). Table 11-2 provides a short list of foods to demonstrate differences in fiber contents of similar types of foods. To acquire more information, readers should refer to the U.S. Department of Agriculture's (USDA's) Nutrient Data Laboratory website (USDA, 2004), which provides the dietary fiber content of most foods commonly consumed in the United States.

Although the presentation in this chapter has indicated why it may be advantageous to discuss dietary fiber in terms of its ability to be fermented or to form a viscous solution, the USDA database does not include any information about dietary fiber other than total fiber content. The levels of fiber contained within a class of foods are quite variable, so some knowledge of the fiber content of specific foods is necessary if one wants to increase fiber intake. For example, the fiber content of legumes ranges from 19 g per cup of cooked navy beans to 2.6 g per cup of canned green beans. Ready-to-eat cereals can be a good source of fiber, but the fiber content ranges from 5 to 8 g per serving of wheat bran cereals to 0.1 to 0.3 g per serving of rice cereals.

The incidences of heart disease, colon cancer, and obesity in populations consuming a Western-type diet are typically much higher, partly because of lower intake of fiber-rich foods, than are observed in most developing countries. As described previously, the presence of fiber in the diet can have a considerable impact on many diseases and appears to promote a healthier gastrointestinal tract. Therefore, all people should strive to include a variety of fiber-rich foods in their diets to prevent disease onset and at least to minimize the severity of disease once it has developed.

Many difficulties are associated with the study of fiber intake and health, and with interpretation of the results of published studies. The major problem is that of defining what type of fiber is being consumed and then adequately describing how much is being consumed and how much is utilized within the intestinal tract. In addition, it is difficult to separate the effect of a change in dietary fiber from the accompanying changes in nutrient density and nutrient intake that accompany the addition of fiber sources to a diet. A comparison of a high-fiber versus low-fiber diet usually indicates an alteration in the caloric density of the diet and often results in a lower intake of energy sources and other nutrients, unless the bulk quantity of diet consumed is increased. In addition, a high-fiber diet may imply the intake of additional biologically active compounds such as phytochemicals that are not present in the low-fiber diet. Experimental diets should be designed to contain the same amount of all nutrients and nonnutrient compounds other than the fiber sources chosen for comparison. The simplest design involves use of purified fiber sources, but purified fiber sources may not have the same effect as intact food sources. Therefore, much more research must be performed under tightly controlled protocols before the real value of dietary fiber can be fully evaluated.

REFERENCES

Bingham SA, Day NE, Luben R, Ferrari P, Slimani N, Norat T, Clavel-Chapelon F, Kesse E, Nieters A, Boeing H, Tjønneland A, Overvad K, Martinez C, Dorronsoro M, Gonzalez CA, Key TJ, Trichopoulou A, Naska A, Vineis P, Tumino R, Krogh V, Bueno-de-Mesquita HB, Peeters PHM, Berglund F, Hallmans G, et al. (2003) Dietary fibre in food and protection against colorectal cancer in the European Prospective Investigation into cancer and nutrition (EPIC): an observational study. Lancet 361:1496-1501.

Bjorck I, Granfeldt Y, Liljeberg H, Tovar J, Asp NG (1994) Food properties affecting the digestion and absorption of carbohydrates. Am J Clin Nutr 59(Suppl 3):699S-705S.

Camilleri M, Thompson WG, Fleshman JW, Pemberton JH (1994) Clinical management of intractable constipation. Ann Intern Med 121:520-528.

Chang W-CL, Chapkin RS, Lupton JR (1997) Predictive value of proliferation, differentiation and apoptosis as intermediate markers for colon tumorigenesis. Carcinogenesis 18:721-730.

Chapman MA, Grahn MF, Boyle MA, Hutton M, Rogers J, Williams NS (1994) Butyrate oxidation is impaired in the colonic mucosa of sufferers of quiescent ulcerative colitis. Gut 35:73-76.

Dukas L, Willett WC, Giovannucci EL (2003) Association between physical activity, fiber intake, and other lifestyle variables and constipation in a study of women. Am J Gastroenterology 98:1790-1796.

Fernandez ML, Vergara-Jimenez M, Conde K, Behr T, Abdel-Fattah G (1997) Regulation of apolipoprotein B-containing lipoproteins by dietary soluble fiber in guinea pigs. Am J Clin Nutr 65:814-822.

French SJ, Read NW (1994) Effect of guar gum on hunger and satiety after meals of differing fat content: relationship with gastric emptying. Am J Clin Nutr 59:87-91.

Health and Welfare Canada (1985) Report of the Expert Advisory Committee on Dietary Fibre. Supply and Services Canada, Ottawa.

Hillemeier C (1995) An overview of the effects of dietary fiber on gastrointestinal transit. Pediatrics 96:997-999.

Institute of Medicine (2001) Dietary Reference Intakes: Proposed Definition of Dietary Fiber. National Academy Press, Washington, DC.

Institute of Medicine (2002) Dietary, functional, and total fiber. In: Dietary Reference Intakes for Energy, Carbohydrate, Fiber, Fat, Fatty Acids,

Cholesterol, Protein, and Amino Acids. National Academy Press, Washington, DC, pp 7-1–7-69.

Jensen CD, Haskell W, Whittam JH (1997) Long-term effects of water-soluble dietary fiber in the management of hypercholesterolemia in healthy men and women. Am J Cardiol 79:34-37.

Marlett JA, McBurney MI, Slavin JL (2002) Position of the American Dietetic Association: Health implications of dietary fiber. J Am Diet Assoc 102:993-1000.

Marquart L, Wiemer KL, Jones JM, Jacob B (2003) Whole grain health claims in the USA and other efforts to increase whole-grain consumption. Proc Nutr Soc 62:151-160.

Mortensen PB, Clausen MR (1996) Short-chain fatty acids in the human colon: relation to gastrointestinal health and disease. Scand J Gastroenterol 31(Suppl 216):132-148.

Newmark HL, Lupton JR (1990) Determinants and consequences of colonic luminal pH: implications for colon cancer. Nutr Cancer 14:161-173.

Pick ME, Hawrysh ZJ, Gee MI, Toth E, Garg ML, Hardin RT (1996) Oat bran concentrate bread products improve long-term control of diabetes: a pilot study. J Am Diet Assoc 96:1254-1261.

Scheppach W, Sommer H, Kirchner T, Paganelli GM, Bartram P, Christl S, Richter F, Dusel G, Kasper H (1992) Effect of butyrate enemas on the colonic mucosa in distal ulcerative colitis. Gastroenterology 70:211-215.

Slavin J (2003) Why whole grains are protective: biological mechanisms. Proc Nutr Soc 62:129-134.

U.S. Department of Agriculture, Agricultural Research Service (2005) USDA Nutrient Database for Standard Reference, Release 18. U.S. Department of Agriculture, Washington, DC. Retrieved December 13, 2005, from www.ars.usda.gov/ba/bhnrc/ndl.

RECOMMENDED READINGS

Cho SC, Dreher ML (eds) (2001) Handbook of Dietary Fiber. Marcel Dekker, New York.

Institute of Medicine (2001) Dietary Reference Intakes: Proposed Definition of Dietary Fiber. National Academy Press, Washington, DC.

Institute of Medicine (2002) Dietary, functional, and total fiber. In: Dietary Reference Intakes for Energy, Carbohydrate, Fiber, Fat, Fatty Acids, Cholesterol, Protein, and Amino Acids. National Academy Press, Washington, DC, pp 7-1–7-69.

Kritchevsky D, Bonfield C (eds) (1995) Dietary Fiber in Health and Disease. Eagan Press, St. Paul, MN.

Marlett JA, McBurney MI, Slavin JL (2002) Position of the American Dietetic Association: Health implications of dietary fiber. J Am Diet Assoc 102:993-1000.

McNeil NI (1984) The contribution of the large intestine to energy supplies in man. Am J Clin Nutr 39:338-342.

Pilch SM (ed) (1987) Physiological Effects and Health Consequences of Dietary Fiber. Federation of American Societies for Experimental Biology, Bethesda, MD.

Ripsin CM, Keenan JM, Jacobs DR, Elmer PJ, Welch RR, Van Horn L, Liu K, Turnbull WH, Thye FW, Kestin M, Hegsted M, Davidson DM, Davidson MH, Dugan LD, Demark-Wahnefried W, Beling S (1992) Oat products and lipid lowering: A meta-analysis. JAMA 267: 3317-3325.

Unit IV

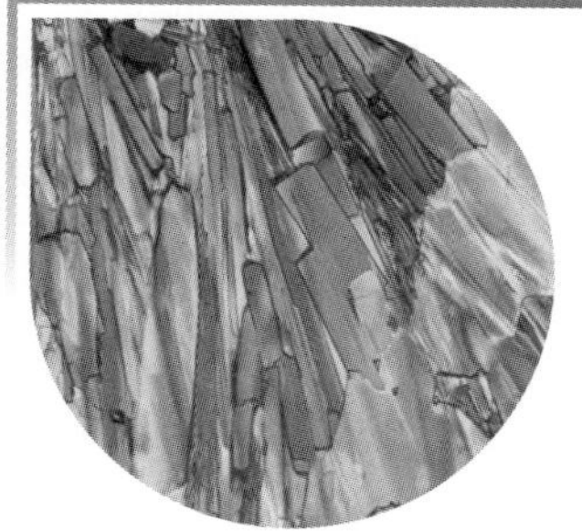

Metabolism of the Macronutrients

After the products of digestion are absorbed across the intestinal epithelium and enter the circulation, they are delivered to various tissues for use. The metabolism of the macronutrients by different tissues of the body is the subject of this unit. Metabolism is a term used to describe the sum of the processes by which a particular substance is handled by the living body; this includes the chemical changes occurring in cells by which energy is provided for vital processes and activities and the processes by which the body assimilates new tissue. The metabolic processes involved in the synthesis of macromolecules such as proteins, glycogen, various lipids, and nucleic acids are called anabolic pathways or anabolism. The metabolic processes involved in the breakdown of organic compounds to CO_2 and H_2O with release of energy (which may be captured as reducing equivalents or as nucleotide triphosphate bonds) are described as catabolic pathways or catabolism. Other pathways that connect anabolism and catabolism are described as amphibolic pathways; these include pathways that serve both catabolic and anabolic purposes, such as the citric acid cycle and oxidative phosphorylation.

Nutrients are needed for the formation of the structural and functional components of tissues. Proteins, phospholipids, cholesterol, glycosaminoglycans, and nucleic acids are important structural components of cell membranes, cellular organelles, and connective tissues. In addition to these obviously structural components of the body, numerous proteins and small, nonprotein organic molecules are distributed in the body fluids, including the intracellular fluid, extracellular fluid, and plasma; these tissue components play important functions and also are essential. All these body components must increase during growth, reproduction, and repair of injured tissues. In addition, the body must have nutrients for maintenance—for replacement of constituents lost during the normal processes of metabolism. The chemical components of the human body are not static but are all in a state of constant turnover (breakdown or catabolism followed by resynthesis or anabolism). For example, as proteins are broken down and resynthesized, some of the amino acids are oxidized and must be replaced via the dietary supply. Small amounts of nutrients, as well as degradation products from nutrient utilization in the body, are lost from the body via the urine or via secretion in the bile and excretion in the feces. Thus, the body requires nutrients for the formation of new tissues and for the replacement or maintenance of existing ones. The processes involved in the synthesis of glycogen, glycosaminoglycans, lipids, proteins, and nonprotein, nitrogen-containing compounds such as nucleotides are discussed in this unit.

The body, of course, must have a source of energy, and dietary macronutrients serve this purpose. Cells within the body are able to use glucose, fatty acids, ketone bodies (derived from fatty acids, especially during starvation), amino acids, and other gluconeogenic (and ketogenic) precursors, such as glycerol, lactate, and propionate, as cellular fuels. Energy substrates that are taken in beyond the amount the body is able to consume immediately are converted to glycogen or fat for storage. The body's capacity for storage of glycogen is very limited. Triacylglycerol storage in adipose tissue is the major way in which animals and humans store energy, and the body's capacity for this is very large, perhaps unlimited. Therefore, the body uses macronutrients in the diet as fuels and converts excess substrates to stored fuels, mainly triacylglycerol, which can be broken down when exogenous fuels are not available. These stored fuels serve an important function in providing fuels between meals and during strenuous exercise, in protecting lean body mass from immediate catabolism in the absence of food, and in extending the length of time an individual can survive with an inadequate caloric intake. The processes involved in the storage and utilization of fuels are described in this unit.

The intake of energy from carbohydrates, proteins, and fats from the diet should balance the overall needs of the body for energy and growth. Although carbohydrates, proteins, and lipids are all important components of the diet, specific compounds within these classes may be classified as essential or nonessential components, depending upon whether the body is able to synthesize them in sufficient amounts. This classification relates to metabolism; the body tissues have the enzymatic capacity to synthesize certain compounds but not others. For example, although carbohydrates make up a large proportion of healthy diets, the actual minimum requirement for carbohydrate per se is probably quite low. Certain cells or tissues of the body do have an absolute requirement for glucose as a fuel, but the liver is able to synthesize glucose from other sugars and from gluconeogenic substrates such as the carbon chains of amino acids or the glycerol backbone of triacylglycerols. Likewise, the body is able to synthesize the other various sugar units required for glycoprotein, glycosaminoglycan, and nucleic acid synthesis. We could say that the diet must provide either a source of glucose or a source of gluconeogenic substrate.

Protein is required in ample amounts because it serves as the source of essential amino acids and as a source of available nitrogen for synthesis of proteins and numerous other essential compounds, including purine and pyrimidine bases of nucleic acids, neurotransmitters, hormones such as thyroid hormone and epinephrine, creatine phosphate, carnitine, porphyrins, 1-carbon fragments of the folate coenzyme system, and small peptides such as glutathione and carnosine. Eleven of the 20 amino acids commonly found in proteins are considered essential or semi-essential for humans. Although the nine so-called nonessential or dispensable amino acids are not strictly essential, because the body can synthesize their carbon chains from intermediates in glucose metabolism or from other amino acids, the diet still must contain a sufficient total amount of amino acids to supply amino groups for synthesis of all the nonessential amino acids.

Dietary fat is not essential as a fuel because the body can convert carbon chains of amino acids or sugars into fatty acids and glycerol phosphate and, hence, triacylglycerol and other lipids. However, certain fatty acids cannot be synthesized completely in the body. The body requires an exogenous source of the so-called essential fatty acids; a fatty acid in both the ω6 (e.g., linoleate) and the ω3 (e.g., linolenate) classes must be provided by the diet. Essential fatty acids play important structural roles in membrane phospholipids and skin ceramides and serve as precursors for synthesis of eicosanoids.

Martha H. Stipanuk

Chapter 12

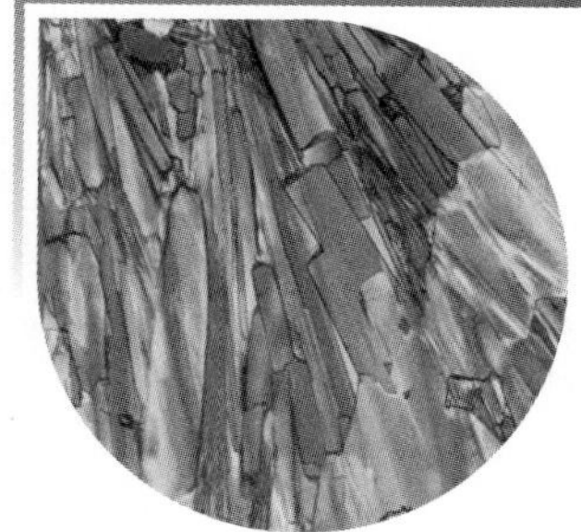

Carbohydrate Metabolism: Synthesis and Oxidation

Mary M. McGrane, PhD

OUTLINE

COMMON ABBREVIATIONS

GLUT *glucose transporter*

SGLT *sodium glucose transporter*

OVERVIEW OF CARBOHYDRATE METABOLISM

Carbohydrates present in food provide from 32% to 70% of the energy in diets of the American and Canadian populations. Carbohydrates, consumed as disaccharides, oligosaccharides, and polysaccharides, are digested, absorbed, and transported through the body primarily as glucose, although fructose and galactose are present as well. Glucose is the primary metabolic fuel in humans. All tissues in the human body are able to utilize glucose for energy production, and some specialized cell types such as red blood cells are completely dependent on glucose for their energy needs. Glucose is derived from dietary carbohydrate, body glycogen stores, or endogenous biosynthesis from nonhexose precursors; these sources provide for the constant availability of glucose in the blood, which is maintained within a strictly regulated concentration range. The balance among glucose oxidation, glucose biosynthesis, and glucose storage is dependent upon the hormonal and nutritional status of the cell, the tissue, and the whole organism.

The predominant pathways of glucose metabolism vary in different cell types, depending upon physiological demand (Fig. 12-1). The liver, for example, plays the central role in glucose homeostasis in the body. In liver parenchymal cells (hepatocytes), glucose can be completely oxidized for energy, can be stored as glycogen, or can provide carbons for the biosynthesis of fatty acids or amino acids. It is important to note that the liver also can release glucose from glycogen degradation or synthesize glucose de novo under conditions of low blood glucose. The hepatocyte, like other cell types, also has the ability to utilize glucose for NADPH and ribose 5-phosphate production via the pentose phosphate pathway. Other tissues, such as adipose tissue, skeletal and cardiac muscle, and brain, respond to blood glucose changes by altering their internal usage, but they do not contribute to whole-body glucose homeostasis by releasing glucose to the blood.

In skeletal muscle and heart, glucose can be completely oxidized or it can be stored in the form of glycogen. Although glycogen is degraded in muscle and cardiac cells, the glucose 6-phosphate so produced is oxidized endogenously. Glucose is not released to the circulating blood from either skeletal or cardiac muscle. The metabolic needs of cardiac tissue, however, differ from those of skeletal tissue; the heart has a continuous need for energy to conduct regular contractions, whereas skeletal muscle has periods of high and low energy demand. In the heart, metabolism is aerobic at all times. This is in contrast to skeletal muscle, which can function metabolically with insufficient oxygen for limited periods.

Adipose tissue presents another metabolic paradigm. In adipose cells, glucose can be partially degraded by glycolysis to provide glycerol

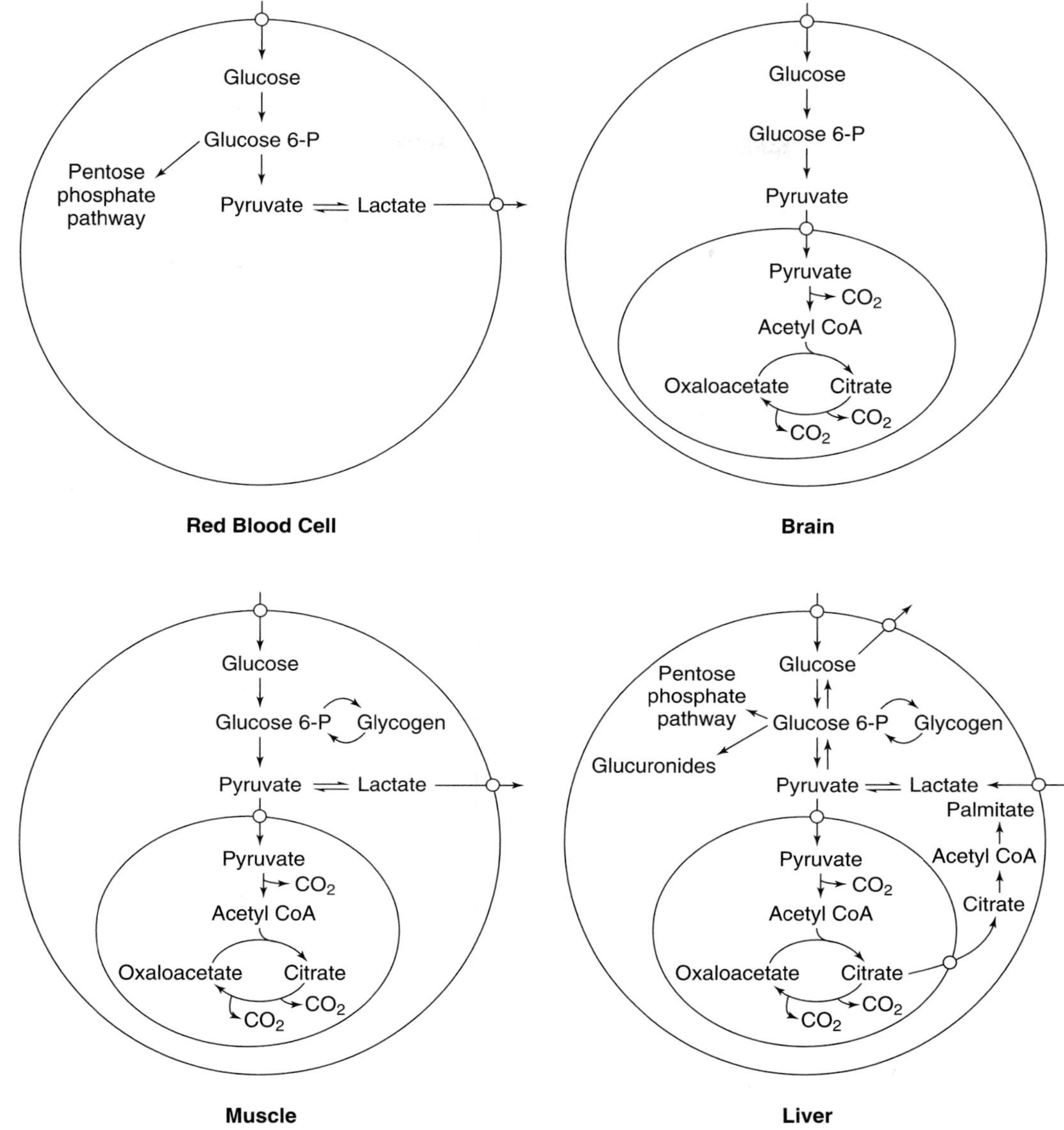

Figure 12-1 Overview of glucose metabolism in selected cell types.

for triacylglycerol synthesis, glucose can be completely oxidized, or, under conditions of high carbohydrate intake, glucose can be metabolized to acetyl CoA and the acetyl moiety channeled to de novo fatty acid synthesis for storage. Under conditions of energy need, adipose cells release metabolic fuel in the form of fatty acids to the circulating blood supply.

The brain, which is completely dependent upon glucose for its energy needs (under normal dietary conditions), is capable of the complete oxidation of glucose to CO_2 and H_2O via glycolysis and the citric acid cycle. The brain requires a continuous supply of glucose from the blood, as there is little storage of glucose in the form of glycogen in the brain. Red blood cells, on the other hand, have a limited ability to metabolize glucose because they lack mitochondria. In red blood cells, glucose is metabolized to lactate, and lactate is released to the circulation. Other specialized cells are also primarily glycolytic because of a relative lack of mitochondria or limited blood or oxygen supply relative to their rates of metabolism; these include some cells of the cornea, lens, and retina, as well as leukocytes, white muscle fibers, cells of the testis, and the renal medulla. Intestinal cells have the capacity to oxidize glucose, but they also utilize the amino acid glutamine for their energy needs.

Overall, there are significant tissue-specific differences in the pathways of glucose oxidation, glucose storage, glucose biosynthesis, and the utilization of glucose for the synthesis of other biomolecules. It is important to keep in mind the physiological context of the metabolic pathways as they occur in specific tissues.

TRANSPORT OF GLUCOSE ACROSS CELL MEMBRANES

The liver is the metabolic center of the human body and is anatomically located so that it is the first tissue exposed to elevated glucose after a carbohydrate-containing meal. After digestion, glucose and other monosaccharides are absorbed by the small intestine and transported via the portal vein to the liver. The liver has two sources of glucose: that derived from the portal vein and that derived from the hepatic artery. Dietary glucose presented via the portal route significantly increases the net uptake of glucose by the liver. A high glucose concentration in the portal vein creates a negative arterial-portal venous difference and activates hepatic glucose uptake. Hepatic glucose uptake is favored both by the sympathetic inhibition of glucose uptake and also by the direct stimulation of hepatic glucose uptake by the parasympathetic innervation to the liver (Moore and Cherrington, 1996). Overall, the liver disposes of approximately 30% to 35% of the ingested glucose.

Glucose is taken up by cells in an insulin-independent manner in liver and certain nonhepatic tissues such as brain and red blood cells and in an insulin-dependent manner by cells in muscle and adipose tissue. Cellular uptake of blood glucose occurs by a facilitated transport process. Facilitated glucose uptake is mediated by a family of structurally related glucose transport proteins that have a specific tissue distribution. Five different isoforms of the glucose transporter have been identified: GLUT1 in red blood cells and brain, GLUT2 in liver and pancreas, GLUT3 in brain, GLUT4 (insulin-responsive) in skeletal and cardiac muscle and adipose tissue, and GLUT5 in the small intestine. Although different glucose transporters predominate in specific tissues, a given tissue may contain more than one isoform. These glucose transporters are encoded by genes in the *SLC2A* family of solute carriers.

Exceptions to facilitated glucose uptake occur in the brush-border membrane of the small intestinal mucosal cells and the renal proximal tubules, where glucose is taken up into the epithelial cells by an active symport process mediated by the sodium ion (Na^+)–dependent glucose transporter (SGLT1). In active symport, glucose is moved into the cell by a transport protein, which first binds Na^+. The energy for this process is provided by a Na^+, K^+-ATPase, which maintains the low intracellular Na^+ concentration. Glucose, after entry into the epithelial cell, dissociates from the transport protein and exits from the distal side by facilitated transport. (See Chapters 7 and 8 for more discussion of glucose transport in the intestine.) The SGLT1 protein is encoded by the human gene *SLC5A1*.

The demands of glucose uptake vary depending on the tissue involved and the physiologic environment of the cell. The glucose transporter isoforms serve different functions to meet these variable demands. GLUT1 is a high-affinity glucose transporter found at high levels in the brain, placenta, and fetal tissues; these are tissues in which GLUT1 mediates glucose uptake across a blood–tissue barrier (e.g., the blood–brain barrier). GLUT1, however, is also found at low levels in erythrocytes and most tissues and may be involved in the underlying constitutive glucose uptake of the whole organism. GLUT2 is restricted primarily to the liver and the β cells of the pancreas, but it is also found in the small intestine and kidney. In liver, GLUT2 is involved in the uptake or release of glucose by hepatocytes, depending on the blood glucose concentration and the metabolic state of the tissue. In the pancreatic β cell, glucose uptake via GLUT2 results in glucose catabolism, which serves as a sensor of blood glucose levels and results in stimulation of insulin secretion by the β cell. In the small intestine and kidney tubules, GLUT2 is involved in glucose absorption and reabsorption, respectively, across the basolateral membranes of the epithelial cell barriers of these two tissues. GLUT2 is a low-affinity transporter for glucose.

GLUT3 is present at high levels in brain and placenta. Like GLUT1, GLUT3 mRNA is also found at low levels in most adult tissues, but the GLUT3 protein distribution is restricted to brain, sperm, and skeletal muscle (mainly slow-twitch fibers). GLUT3 has a high affinity for glucose. GLUT4, present primarily in skeletal and cardiac muscle and in white and brown adipose tissue, differs from the other isoforms in that it is stimulated by the hormone insulin. GLUT4 is responsible for insulin-stimulated glucose uptake in the aforementioned tissues in the postprandial (absorptive) state. Lastly, GLUT5 is found primarily in the jejunum of the small intestine but also in some other tissues including kidney and sperm. GLUT5 has the capacity to transport fructose but does not seem to contribute to glucose transport in humans.

Both GLUT1 and GLUT3 have a low K_m for glucose and transport glucose even when circulating levels are low. GLUT1 and GLUT3 appear to be responsible for basal glucose transport in most tissues of the body. This can be contrasted with glucose transport by GLUT2; GLUT2 has a high K_m for glucose and is a key transport protein involved in responding to elevated blood glucose in humans. In liver, because of the expression of GLUT2, maximal glucose uptake occurs when blood glucose levels are high, such as after a carbohydrate-containing meal. In the pancreatic β cell, glucose uptake via GLUT2 signals the cell that the blood glucose concentration has increased and begins the process by which the β cell responds to elevated blood glucose with secretion of insulin into the bloodstream. Glucose is transported into the β cell where it is rapidly phosphorylated to glucose 6-phosphate by the coupled action of a high K_m glucokinase (see subsequent text). The increase in glycolysis and oxidative metabolism of glucose increases the ATP/ADP ratio leading to a series of intracellular changes that result in the fusion of insulin-containing storage vesicles with the cell membrane and the release of insulin to the bloodstream (Fig. 12-2). The combined action of GLUT2 and glucokinase allow the pancreatic β cell to "sense" the blood glucose concentration and respond by increased secretion of insulin (Postic et al., 2001).

The insulin-responsive glucose transporter, GLUT4, has a unique physiological role in whole-body glucose homeostasis. In effect, GLUT4 mediates the second-tier response to elevated

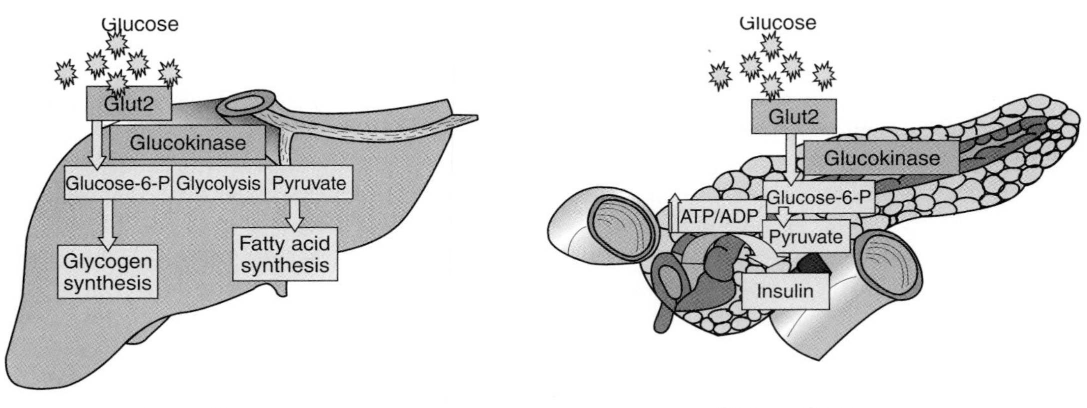

Figure 12-2 The combined action of high K_m GLUT2 and glucokinase produce "glucose sensing" in (1) the liver for energy storage and (2) the pancreatic β cell for insulin secretion. The GLUT2/glucokinase system is very active in both tissues when blood glucose levels are high.

blood glucose. In skeletal and cardiac muscle, as well as in adipose tissue, insulin stimulates a rapid translocation of preformed GLUT4 from intracellular vesicles in the cytosol to the surface of the plasma membrane of the cell (Czech, 1995). This translocation increases the concentration of glucose transporters at the cell surface, and, hence, the capacity for glucose uptake. Exercise can also stimulate GLUT4 translocation to the plasma membrane, but this involves a different signaling pathway than that initiated by insulin (Uldry and Thorens, 2004). GLUT1 is also present in these tissues at a lower level. GLUT1 is present on the plasma membrane at a relative abundance that is higher than GLUT4 under basal conditions, but GLUT1 cell surface abundance is not affected by insulin. There is, therefore, a specific insulin-responsive mechanism for the stimulation of GLUT4-mediated glucose uptake in muscle and adipose tissue. In addition, fasting and refeeding, as well as insulin, can affect the expression of the GLUT4 gene itself (as is discussed in subsequent text of this chapter). Overall, the different glucose transporter isoforms, with variability in their kinetics and mechanisms of action, respond to the physiological demands of the body and maintain blood glucose levels within the range of 4 to 5 mmol/L.

GLYCOLYSIS

At the cellular level, the breakdown of glucose for energy can be divided into two major pathways based on the intracellular location of the enzymatic machinery involved, and on the ability of different cell types to perform the enzymatic reactions. The first of these pathways is glycolysis, the anaerobic breakdown of glucose to pyruvate. The enzymes involved in glycolysis are present in the cytosol of all cell types. The second pathway is the citric acid cycle, in which acetyl CoA is completely oxidized to CO_2 and H_2O. The citric acid cycle occurs in mitochondria and is dependent on the presence of molecular oxygen. This pathway is restricted to cells that possess mitochondria. Glycolysis and the citric acid cycle are linked by the pyruvate dehydrogenase reaction, which also takes place in the mitochondria of the cell. As a result of glycolysis, the pyruvate dehydrogenase reaction, and the citric acid cycle, energy is conserved in the chemical form of ATP, with ATP synthesis occurring both by substrate-level phosphorylation and by electron transport linked to oxidative phosphorylation.

The series of enzymatic reactions that together constitute the glycolytic pathway convert one molecule of glucose to two molecules of pyruvate. All cells of the human body contain the full complement of glycolytic enzymes and can break down glucose to this extent. The metabolic fate of pyruvate, however, is variable and depends on the cell type and the availability of oxygen. Under anaerobic conditions, when tissues such as skeletal muscle are not supplied with enough oxygen to meet the metabolic need, pyruvate is reduced to lactate in the cytosol of the cells. Other tissues, such as red blood cells, produce lactate from glucose under aerobic conditions because of their lack or low abundance of mitochondria. Most tissues, under aerobic conditions, can oxidize pyruvate to acetyl CoA and CO_2 via the pyruvate dehydrogenase reaction in the mitochondria, followed by either complete oxidation of acetyl CoA to CO_2 and H_2O via the citric acid cycle or the synthesis of fatty acids from the acetyl moiety of acetyl CoA. The overall energy transfer of the glycolytic series of enzymatic reactions is exergonic, and a portion of this energy is stored as the high-energy phosphate bond of ATP. Glycolysis, however, provides a minor percentage of the ATP produced when compared with the complete oxidation of glucose to CO_2 and H_2O.

The series of enzymatic reactions that make up the glycolytic pathway are subdivided into two stages, as shown in Figure 12-3: (1) the priming of glucose, which requires ATP expenditure to generate phosphorylated intermediates, and (2) the production of reducing equivalents and the synthesis of ATP for energy provision. The enzymes that catalyze the reactions of glycolysis are present in the cytosol of the cell, organized into multienzyme complexes that function together to channel the intermediates from one enzyme to another so that they do not become diluted in the cytosol. The glycolytic enzymes are associated with cellular structures such as actin filaments, microtubules, or the outer membranes of mitochondria (Lehninger et al., 1993).

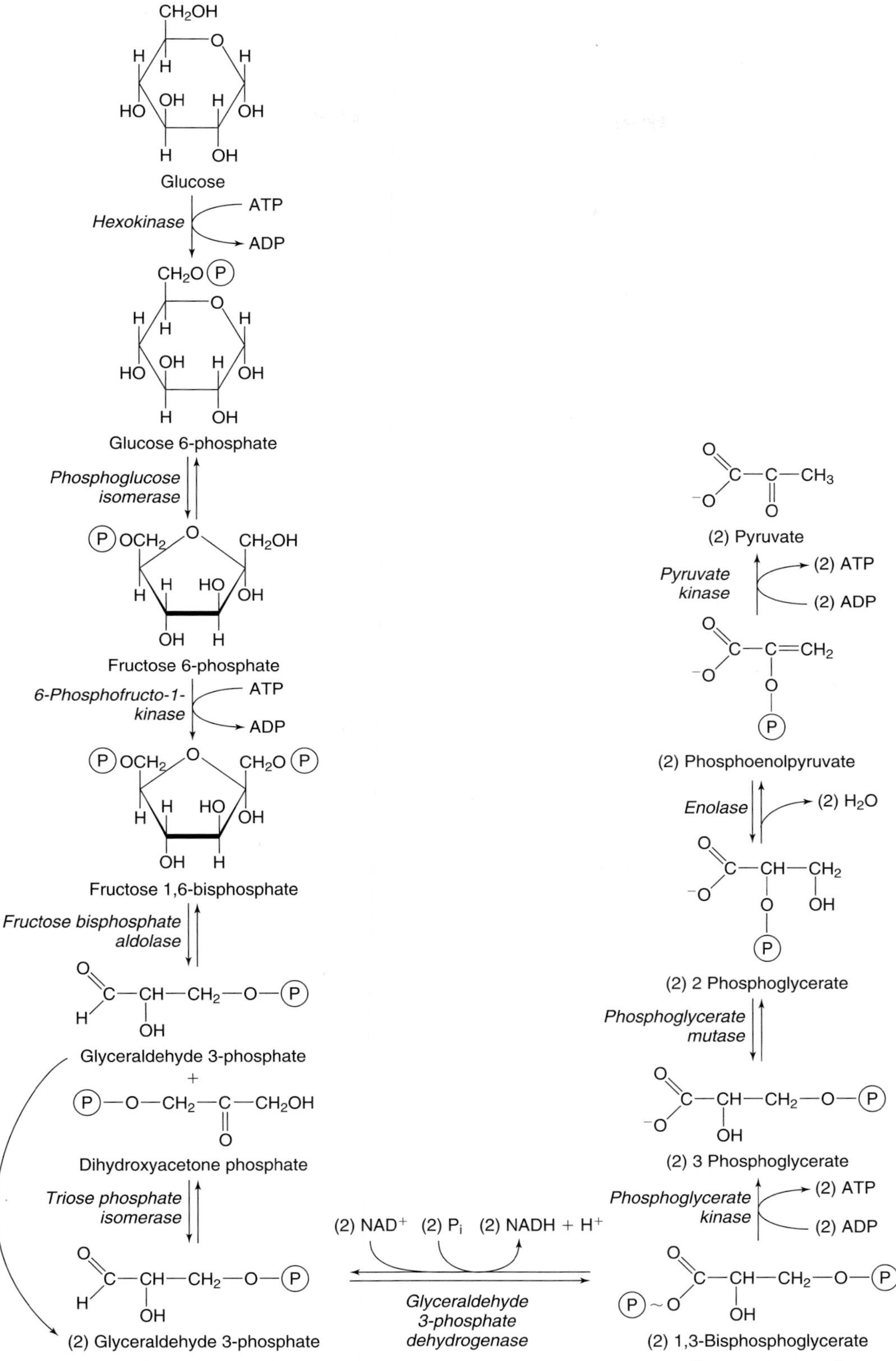

Figure 12-3 The glycolytic pathway for conversion of glucose to pyruvate. Ⓟ represents PO_3^{2-}.

THE GLYCOLYTIC PATHWAY

The series of enzymatic reactions that make up glycolysis utilize glucose, which enters the cell by carrier-mediated transport or glucose 6-phosphate, which is generated from glycogen degradation. Glucose, once transported inside the cell, is rapidly phosphorylated to glucose 6-phosphate in the following reaction:

$$\text{Glucose} + \text{ATP} \xrightarrow{Mg^{2+}} \text{Glucose 6-Phosphate} + \text{ADP}$$

The mechanism of glucose phosphorylation involves the transfer of the γ phosphate from ATP to the C-6 of glucose. This essentially irreversible reaction sequesters glucose within the cell, because the phosphorylated form of glucose does not readily cross the plasma membrane. This phosphorylation reaction is catalyzed by hexokinase in most cell types and by glucokinase (hexokinase IV) in liver cells and pancreatic β cells. In all cells, the product of this reaction, glucose 6-phosphate, can be broken down in the subsequent enzymatic steps of the glycolytic pathway. However, under anabolic conditions the production of glucose 6-phosphate is also the first step in the addition of glucose to the glucose polymer, glycogen, which is synthesized and stored mainly in liver and muscle tissue. In addition to glycolysis and glycogen synthesis, glucose-6-phosphate is also metabolized by the pentose phosphate pathway. This pathway serves to provide cells with reducing equivalents in the form of NADPH and with ribose-5-phosphate for nucleotide synthesis. The hexokinases of most cell types have a high affinity for glucose; the K_m for glucose is less than 0.1 mM (the concentration of glucose at which the enzymatic reaction is at half-maximal velocity). Glucokinase, on the other hand, has a low affinity for glucose; the K_m for glucose is approximately 10 mM. Therefore, glucokinase in liver and the pancreatic β cell has the ability to rapidly convert glucose to glucose 6-phosphate when blood glucose concentrations are elevated (e.g., after a carbohydrate-containing meal). This allows the liver to maintain blood glucose levels in the normal physiological range and the pancreas to sense elevations in blood glucose concentrations and respond with insulin secretion.

The second enzymatic reaction in glycolysis is the isomerization of glucose 6-phosphate (an aldose) to fructose 6-phosphate (a ketose), catalyzed by phosphoglucose isomerase.

$$\text{Glucose 6-Phosphate} \xleftrightarrow{Mg^{2+}} \text{Fructose-6-Phosphate}$$

In this reaction, there is an intramolecular shift of a hydrogen atom, changing the location of the double bond. Phosphoglucose isomerase functions close to equilibrium and, therefore, the reaction is reversible under intracellular conditions.

6-Phosphofructo-1-kinase catalyzes the next irreversible step in the glycolytic pathway, the phosphorylation of fructose 6-phosphate to fructose 1,6-bisphosphate:

$$\text{Fructose 6-Phosphate} + \text{ATP} \xrightarrow{Mg^{2+}} \text{Fructose 1,6-Bisphosphate} + \text{ADP}$$

The 6-phosphofructo-1-kinase reaction utilizes a second molecule of ATP and is the first committed step in glycolysis. Unlike glucose 6-phosphate, fructose 1,6-bisphosphate cannot be used directly as substrate for alternative pathways such as glycogen synthesis. It should be noted that in skeletal muscle, glucose 6-phosphate from glycogen breakdown is a major substrate for glycolysis and this does not require the hexokinase reaction. The 6-phosphofructo-1-kinase reaction is highly regulated by allosteric modifiers and is one of the major determinants of the rate of glycolytic conversion of glucose to pyruvate.

The next reaction involves the division of the 6-carbon sugar diphosphate, fructose 1,6-bisphosphate, to two 3-carbon phosphorylated intermediates. The aldol cleavage reaction is catalyzed by aldolase as follows:

$$\text{Fructose 1,6-Bisphosphate} \longleftrightarrow \text{Dihydroxyacetone Phosphate} + \text{Glyceraldehyde 3-Phosphate}$$

Glyceraldehyde 3-phosphate is in the direct path of glycolysis, but dihydroxyacetone phosphate is not. Dihydroxyacetone phosphate is isomerized to glyceraldehyde 3-phosphate via the action of triose phosphate isomerase.

The net result of the aldolase and triose phosphate isomerase reactions is the production of two molecules of glyceraldehyde 3-phosphate. The series of reactions that convert one molecule of glucose to two molecules of glyceraldehyde 3-phosphate constitute the first phase of glycolysis in which the chemical energy of ATP is utilized in the generation of phosphorylated intermediates. The dihydroxyacetone phosphate generated by the aldolase reaction may also be reduced to glycerol 3-phosphate and used for synthesis of glycerolipids such as triacylglycerols; this is a particularly important source of glycerol 3-phosphate in small intestine and adipose tissue.

The second stage of glycolysis results in the generation of reducing equivalents and the synthesis of ATP. Reducing equivalents in the form NADH are produced by the reaction catalyzed by glyceraldehyde 3-phosphate dehydrogenase:

$$\text{Glyceraldehyde 3-Phosphate} + \text{NAD}^+ + \text{P}_i \leftrightarrow \text{1,3-Bisphosphoglycerate} + \text{NADH} + \text{H}^+$$

This reaction incorporates inorganic phosphate (P_i) to produce a high-energy phosphate bond in 1,3-bisphosphoglycerate. The second product of the reaction, NADH, provides reducing equivalents for the energy conversion of electron transport and production of ATP by oxidative phosphorylation. This is the only glycolytic reaction that generates reducing equivalents for electron transport. It is important to note that the coenzyme NAD^+ is present in limited amounts in the cytosol of the cell. For this reason, the NAD^+ utilized in the glyceraldehyde-3-phosphate reaction needs to be replaced in the cytosolic compartment so that NAD^+ availability does not limit glycolysis.

The acyl-phosphate bond of 1,3-bisphosphoglycerate has a high-energy phosphoryl transfer potential that is used to generate ATP in the next reaction of glycolysis. This is the conversion of 1,3-bisphosphoglycerate to 3-phosphoglycerate:

$$\text{1,3-Bisphosphoglycerate} + \text{ADP} \longleftrightarrow \text{3-Phosphoglycerate} + \text{ATP}$$

The enzyme that catalyzes this reaction is phosphoglycerate kinase. This is the first reaction in glycolysis that generates ATP. The formation of ATP by transfer of the phosphate group from 1,3-bisphosphoglycerate to ADP is a substrate-level phosphorylation.

The next step in the glycolytic pathway is the conversion of 3-phosphoglycerate to 2-phosphoglycerate, catalyzed by phosphoglycerate mutase. The mechanism of this enzymatic reaction is complex and involves a phosphoenzyme intermediate. The end products of this reaction are 2-phosphoglycerate and the regenerated phosphoenzyme. The overall series of reactions can be summarized as follows:

$$\text{Enzyme-Phosphate} + \text{3-Phosphoglycerate} \leftrightarrow \text{Enzyme} + \text{2,3-Bisphosphoglycerate}$$

$$\text{Enzyme} + \text{2,3-Bisphosphoglycerate} \leftrightarrow \text{Enzyme-Phosphate} + \text{2-Phosphoglycerate}$$

A second glycolytic intermediate with a high-energy phosphate bond is generated when 2-phosphoglycerate is converted to phosphoenolpyruvate via a dehydration reaction catalyzed by enolase.

$$\text{2-Phosphoglycerate} \longleftrightarrow \text{Phosphoenolpyruvate} + H_2O$$

The phosphoenolpyruvate generated by the enolase reaction is substrate for the last reaction of glycolysis, the conversion of phosphoenolpyruvate to pyruvate with the generation of ATP.

$$\text{Phosphoenolpyruvate} + \text{ADP} \xrightarrow{Mg^{2+},\,K^+} \text{Pyruvate} + \text{ATP}$$

This reaction is catalyzed by pyruvate kinase and is the second substrate-level phosphorylation that occurs in glycolysis. The pyruvate kinase reaction is essentially irreversible under intracellular conditions. This enzyme is highly regulated by allosteric and covalent modification, much like 6-phosphofructose-1-kinase, as is discussed in subsequent text of this chapter.

The total ATP produced from the reactions of glycolysis can be calculated. In this pathway, one molecule of glucose is converted to two molecules of pyruvate. Two molecules of ATP are utilized in the priming of glucose; however, four molecules of ATP are produced by substrate-level phosphorylation in the second phase, yielding a net increase of two molecules of ATP. In addition, two molecules of NADH are produced in the glyceraldehyde 3-phosphate dehydrogenase reaction in the cytosol of the cell. The energy gain can be summarized as follows:

$$\text{Glucose} + 2\ \text{ATP} + 2\ \text{NAD}^+ + 4\ \text{ADP} + 2\ \text{P}_i \rightarrow 2\ \text{Pyruvate} + 2\ \text{ADP} + 2\ \text{NADH} + 2\ \text{H}^+ + 4\ \text{ATP} + 2\ \text{H}_2\text{O}$$

or a net of

$$\text{Glucose} + 2\ \text{NAD}^+ + 2\ \text{ADP} + 2\ \text{P}_i \rightarrow 2\ \text{Pyruvate} + 2\ \text{NADH} + 2\ \text{H}^+ + 2\ \text{ATP} + 2\ \text{H}_2\text{O}$$

In electron transport, NADH transfers electrons to carrier molecules in the mitochondria of the cell, and these reactions release sufficient energy for the production of two to three molecules of ATP per pair of electrons by oxidative phosphorylation. The total amount of ATP generated from NADH depends upon the mechanism by which the reducing equivalents from NADH enter the mitochondria. The net production of ATP from glycolysis is six to eight molecules of ATP from the oxidation of one molecule of glucose to two molecules of pyruvate.

Pyruvate produced by glycolysis can be metabolized in different ways, depending upon the availability of oxygen and the metabolic state of the cell. Pyruvate may enter the mitochondrion where it is converted to acetyl CoA in a complex series of reactions catalyzed by the multienzyme pyruvate dehydrogenase complex. Acetyl CoA so produced can enter the citric acid cycle for complete oxidation to CO_2 and H_2O, or it can be utilized for de novo fatty acid synthesis in certain cell types. In the absence of sufficient oxygen or in cells lacking mitochondria, pyruvate has a different fate; it is reduced to lactate by the cytosolic enzyme lactate dehydrogenase.

$$\text{Pyruvate} + \text{NADH} + \text{H}^+ \longleftrightarrow \text{Lactate} + \text{NAD}^+$$

Metabolism of glucose by this anaerobic pathway may occur in active skeletal muscle, and lactate can build up when molecular oxygen becomes insufficient to meet the metabolic need for aerobic metabolism. Pyruvate is also reduced to lactate in red blood cells, which do not have mitochondria. The reduction of two molecules of pyruvate to lactate generates two molecules of NAD^+ from two molecules of NADH. This replaces the two NAD^+ molecules that were reduced in the glyceraldehyde 3-phosphate dehydrogenase reaction of glycolysis. Therefore, these two reactions balance the utilization and regeneration of NAD^+ so that glycolysis can continue with no net loss of NAD^+. The lactate formed in this process can be recycled to the liver to regenerate glucose via gluconeogenesis. Heart muscle, on the other hand, is able to take up lactate and use it as a fuel for ATP production. Under conditions of heavy exercise, the heart may take up lactate released by exercising skeletal muscle and use it as a fuel.

In the presence of sufficient molecular oxygen and in cells with mitochondria, reducing equivalents ($NADH + H^+$) produced by the glyceraldehyde 3-phosphate dehydrogenase reaction can be shuttled to the mitochondria by the reduction of metabolic intermediates in the cytosol, regenerating NAD^+ in this compartment. The reduced intermediate is shuttled across the inner mitochondrial membrane with subsequent oxidation, thereby regenerating $NADH + H^+$ from NAD^+ in the mitochondria. NADH in the mitochondria is an electron donor, transferring reducing equivalents to Complex I (NADH dehydrogenase complex) in the series of oxidation/reduction reactions of electron transport (see Fig. 24-2). Under these conditions, the reduction of pyruvate to lactate is not required for the regeneration of NAD^+ in the cytosol.

METABOLISM OF MONOSACCHARIDES OTHER THAN GLUCOSE

In addition to glucose, monosaccharides obtained from the ingestion and digestion of common foods include fructose, galactose, and, in lesser amounts, mannose. Fructose, galactose, and mannose are converted to intermediates in glycolysis, as shown in Figure 12-4. There are two major pathways for the metabolism of fructose; one pathway is prominent in liver and the other in skeletal muscle. In skeletal muscle, the catabolism of fructose closely resembles that of glucose; fructose is phosphorylated to fructose 6-phosphate by

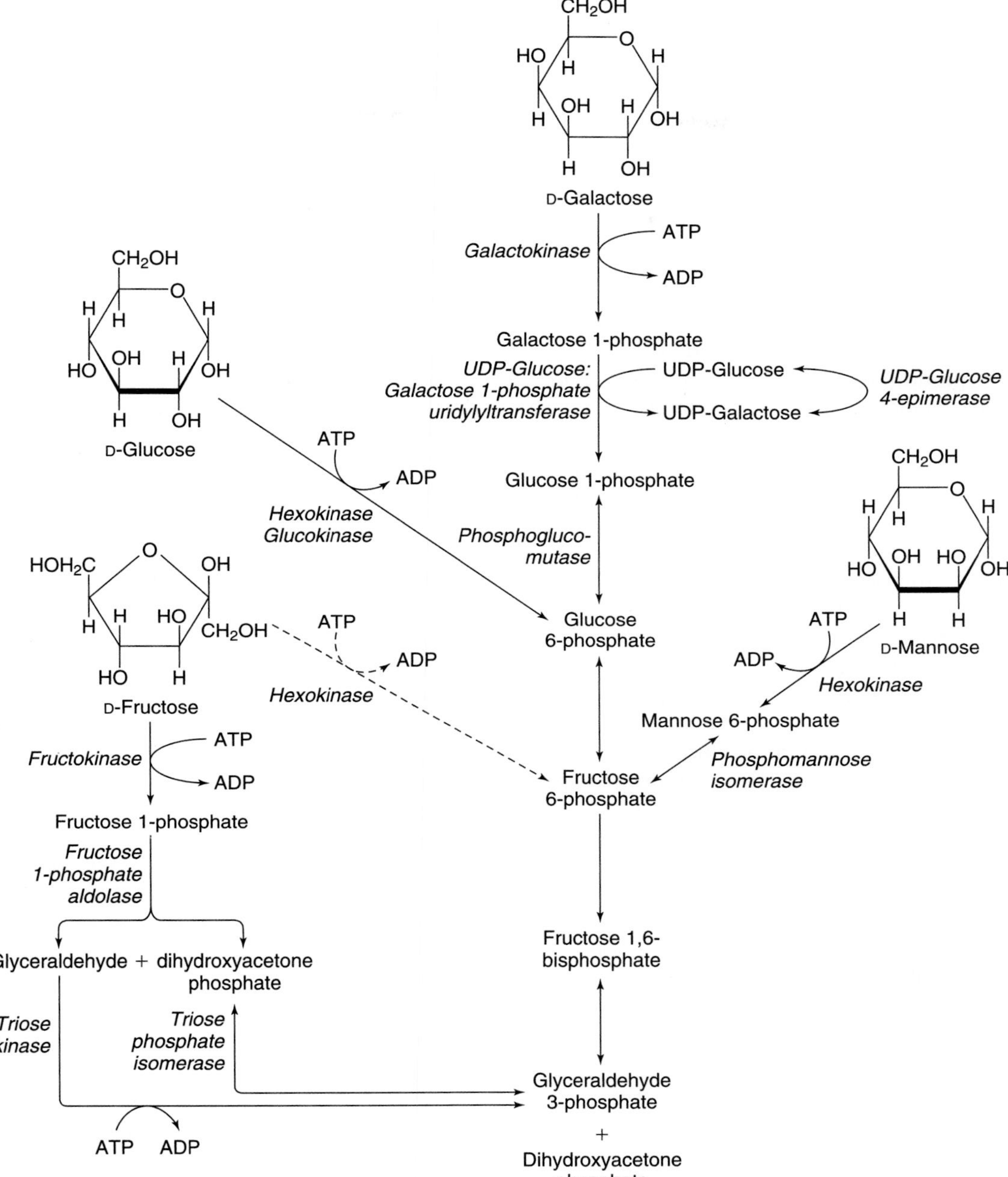

Figure 12-4 Conversion of absorbed monosaccharides to glycolytic intermediates in the liver.

the action of hexokinase, similar to the conversion of glucose to glucose 6-phosphate by the same enzyme. The fructose 6-phosphate is further metabolized via glycolysis in the muscle, being converted to fructose 1,6-bisphosphate, which is the hydrolyzed by aldolase A (the predominant form of aldolase in skeletal muscle) to glyceraldehyde 3-phosphate + dihydroxyacetone phosphate. In the liver, on the other hand, glucose and fructose are handled differently.

The liver has a high level of glucokinase and a relatively low level of hexokinase. Glucokinase is specific for glucose and does not phosphorylate fructose. Unlike skeletal muscle, liver has a relatively high concentration of fructokinase, an enzyme that catalyzes the phosphorylation of fructose at C-1 to generate fructose 1-phosphate. Therefore, the initial product is fructose 6-phosphate in muscle but fructose 1-phosphate in liver. Similar to glycolysis, the next step in what is referred to as fructolysis, is the aldolase reaction that hydrolyses the six-carbon fructose to two three-carbon intermediates. The liver has predominantly aldolase B, which hydrolyzes fructose 1,6-diphosphate and fructose 1-phosphate. Therefore, aldolase B continues the catabolism of fructose by hydrolyzing fructose 1-phosphate to dihydroxyacetone phosphate and glyceraldehyde. (The muscle isozyme of aldolase hydrolyzes only fructose 1,6-diphosphate and not fructose 1-phosphate.) The remaining reactions of fructolysis in liver are detailed in subsequent text. Although the catabolic end products of the metabolism of fructose are similar to those of glucose, fructose does not elicit the same glucose-induced hormonal response after absorption (i.e., a large increase in insulin secretion from the pancreas). Overall, fructose is metabolized mainly by the liver, whereas glucose is metabolized by all tissues of the body, with only 30% to 40% of glucose intake being metabolized by the liver. A brief description of the entry of fructose and the other monosaccharides into the glycolytic sequence of enzymatic reactions in the liver is presented here.

Fructose is a major sweetening agent in the human diet and is especially high in the American diet due to a high intake of sucrose and high fructose corn syrup in sweetened products. It is present in the monosaccharide form in honey, fruit, commercially produced high fructose corn syrup, and many vegetables, and in the disaccharide sucrose (a disaccharide of fructose and glucose) in common table (cane or beet) sugar. Sorbitol, present in many fruits and vegetables, is also converted to fructose in the liver via the sorbitol dehydrogenase reaction. As mentioned in the preceding text, the process of fructose degradation is referred to as fructolysis. In the liver, fructose is converted to fructose 1-phosphate by the action of fructokinase, as follows:

$$\text{Fructose} + \text{ATP} \xrightarrow{Mg^{2+}} \text{Fructose 1-Phosphate} + \text{ADP}$$

Fructose 1-phosphate is then hydrolyzed to glyceraldehyde and dihydroxyacetone phosphate by aldolase B (fructose 1-phosphate aldolase):

$$\text{Fructose 1-Phosphate} \longleftrightarrow \text{Dihydroxyacetone Phosphate} + \text{Glyceraldehyde}$$

Glyceraldehyde is then phosphorylated to glyceraldehyde 3-phosphate by glyceraldehyde kinase.

$$\text{Glyceraldehyde} + \text{ATP} \xrightarrow{Mg^{2+}} \text{Glyceraldehyde 3-Phosphate} + \text{ATP}$$

Dihydroxyacetone phosphate produced from the hydrolysis of fructose 1-phosphate is converted to glyceraldehyde 3-phosphate by triose phosphate isomerase, the enzyme that catalyzes the same conversion of triose phosphates in the glycolytic breakdown of glucose. Overall, one molecule of fructose is converted to two molecules of glyceraldehyde 3-phosphate. Glyceraldehyde 3-phosphate is then substrate for further glycolytic conversion.

The majority of the triose phosphates generated from fructose are catabolized to pyruvate, which is then converted to lactate or further degraded via the pyruvate dehydrogenase complex and the citric acid cycle. This is due, in part, to the fact that fructolysis bypasses the phosphofructo-1-kinase step, which is highly regulated and plays a major role in regulating glycolytic flux. Alternatively, to a small extent, the triose phosphates from fructose can be metabolized via gluconeogenic reactions to glucose or glycogen. Overall, because fructolysis provides the liver with an abundance of pyruvate and lactate, metabolites of the citric acid cycle, such as citrate and malate, also build up. Citrate can be transported from the mitochondria and converted to acetyl CoA via the action of citrate lyase in the cytosol; acetyl CoA then serves as a precursor for fatty acid synthesis or cholesterol synthesis (as discussed in Chapters 16 and 17). Overall, a long-term increase in fructose or sucrose consumption can lead to increased hepatic lipogenesis (Shafrir, 1991). These lipids are then secreted from the liver as components of lipoprotein particles, causing hyperlipidemia and increased lipid storage in adipose tissue, or retained in the liver if lipogenesis is in excess of lipoprotein export.

In men, fructose is the major fuel utilized by a specialized cell type, spermatozoa. Cells in the seminal vesicles have the ability to synthesize fructose from glucose. Fructose synthesis involves an NADPH-dependent reduction of glucose to sorbitol, followed by an NAD^+-dependent oxidation of sorbitol to fructose. Fructose is taken up by sperm cells and oxidized completely to CO_2 and H_2O by fructolysis and the citric acid cycle.

Another dietary monosaccharide, galactose, is derived from the digestion of lactose, a disaccharide of galactose and glucose. Lactose is the major carbohydrate in milk. In liver, galactose is phosphorylated by galactokinase as follows:

$$\text{Galactose} + \text{ATP} \xrightarrow{Mg^{2+}} \text{Galactose 1-Phosphate} + \text{ADP}$$

Galactose 1-phosphate then undergoes a conversion to its epimer glucose 1-phosphate through the action of UDP glucose:galactose 1-phosphate uridylyltransferase. In this reaction, uridine diphosphate (UDP) serves as a hexose carrier, and the two substrates for this reaction are galactose-1-phosphate and UDP-glucose. UDP glucose:galactose 1-phosphate uridylyltransferase catalyzes the transfer of the uridyl group from UDP-glucose to galactose 1-phosphate, generating a molecule of free glucose 1-phosphate and UDP-galactose as the end products. UDP-galactose is then converted back to UDP-glucose by UDP-galactose 4-epimerase. Glucose 1-phosphate is an

Clinical Correlation

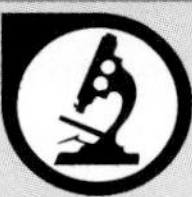

Fructose Intolerance and Essential Fructosuria

Two genetic defects in fructose metabolism are known: fructose intolerance and essential fructosuria (Van den Berghe, 1995). Fructose intolerance is caused by an autosomal recessive defect in the liver fructose 1-phosphate aldolase (aldolase B) gene. The symptoms of hereditary fructose intolerance are absent in infancy if the infant is breast-fed. However, the introduction of sweetened milk formulas or the later introduction of fruits and vegetables provokes the symptoms of this disorder due to exposure to fructose. The deficiency in aldolase B leads to the buildup of fructose 1-phosphate and the depletion of P_i for ATP production in liver. The accumulation of fructose 1-phosphate blocks both glycogenolysis, owing to inhibition of glycogen phosphorylase by fructose 1-phosphate, and gluconeogenesis, owing to inhibition of the aldolase and phosphoglucose isomerase reactions in the reversal of glycolysis (Van den Berghe, 1995). Furthermore, the depletion of P_i and ATP leads to a series of imbalances, including the inhibition of protein synthesis, that cause liver cell damage and a decline in liver function.

In contrast to fructose intolerance, the symptoms of essential fructosuria are essentially those of a "nondisease" (Van den Berghe, 1995). Essential fructosuria is caused by a defect in fructokinase, which is normally found in liver, kidney, and intestinal mucosa. This relatively harmless disorder results in the excretion of fructose in the urine, as well as some metabolism of fructose to fructose 6-phosphate by hexokinase in adipose and muscle tissue.

Thinking Critically

In normal individuals, the capacity of the liver to phosphorylate fructose (fructokinase activity) greatly exceeds the liver's capacity to split fructose 1-phosphate (aldolase B activity). Why is a deficiency of fructokinase a less serious genetic defect than a deficiency of fructose 1-phosphate aldolase? Consider what happens to fructose in each case and what effect this has on hepatic metabolism.

intermediate that can be channeled to glycogen synthesis under conditions that favor glucose storage. Under conditions that favor glucose utilization for energy, however, glucose 1-phosphate is converted to glucose 6-phosphate in the reversible phosphoglucomutase reaction:

$$\text{Glucose 1-Phosphate} \longleftrightarrow \text{Glucose 6-Phosphate}$$

Glucose 6-phosphate can then be utilized by the liver cell for glycolysis or dephosphorylated to glucose by the enzyme glucose 6-phosphatase for release to the circulating blood.

Mannose is the end product of the digestion of various polysaccharides and glycoproteins present in the diet. In the liver, mannose is phosphorylated by hexokinase at the C-6 position, generating mannose 6-phosphate:

$$\text{Mannose} + \text{ATP} \xrightarrow{Mg^{2+}} \text{Mannose 6-Phosphate} + \text{ADP}$$

The mannose 6-phosphate so produced is converted to fructose 6-phosphate by the action of phosphomannose isomerase. Therefore mannose can be converted to the glycolytic intermediate fructose 6-phosphate.

GLUCONEOGENESIS

The series of enzymatic reactions that make up the gluconeogenic pathway produce glucose from pyruvate, lactate, and other nonhexose precursors. The biosynthesis of glucose involves an essential reversal of glycolysis; however, the enzymatic reactions are not all a direct reversal of those of glycolysis (Fig. 12-5). Enzyme reactions specific to gluconeogenesis bypass the irreversible steps of glycolysis. Furthermore, unlike glycolysis, gluconeogenesis does not occur in all cell types—it occurs primarily in liver and to a lesser extent in kidney. In addition to having the enzymes that catalyze the reversible steps of glycolysis, liver and kidney have glycerol kinase activity, which allows glycerol to serve as a gluconeogenic substrate, entering the gluconeogenic pathway at the level of dihydroxyacetone phosphate.

The de novo synthesis of glucose by the body is critical for the maintenance of blood glucose for those tissues that are dependent upon glucose for their energy needs. In humans, in the absence of dietary carbohydrate intake, liver glycogen is depleted within 18 hours. After this time, the liver must synthesize glucose from

Clinical Correlation

Hereditary Defects in Galactose Metabolism

Three inborn errors in galactose metabolism have been characterized. These are due to rare autosomal recessive defects in either galactokinase, UDP-glucose:galactose 1-phosphate uridylyltransferase, or UDP-glucose 4-epimerase. Because galactose consumption is high during infancy, the clinical symptoms of these metabolic defects are exhibited early.

Galactokinase deficiency leads to the excretion of most of the ingested galactose or its conversion to the reduced metabolite galactitol because galactose is not phosphorylated to galactose 1-phosphate due to the defect. In newborn infants, galactitol concentrates in the lens, and the accumulation of galactitol results in the development of cataracts (Gitzelmann, 1995).

With UDP-glucose:galactose 1-phosphate uridylyltransferase deficiency, galactose 1-phosphate and galactose build up and galactitol is produced. This deficiency occurs in two forms: near-complete lack of the enzyme (classic galactosemia) and partial lack of the enzyme. Classic galactosemia affects the liver, kidney, and brain, as well as the eye, and can be life-threatening.

The third inborn error of galactose metabolism, caused by UDP-glucose 4-epimerase deficiency, also occurs in both a mild and a severe form. Severe epimerase deficiency is very rare, and the symptoms are similar to those of classical galactosemia.

nonhexose precursors to maintain blood glucose levels. The liver is the central gluconeogenic tissue of the human body and responds to low blood glucose by secreting newly synthesized glucose into the blood for transport to other tissues.

Although gluconeogenesis also occurs in the kidney, the kidney is smaller than the liver and is less productive in de novo glucose synthesis. Overall, the liver contributes approximately 90% of gluconeogenically derived glucose, whereas the kidney contributes approximately 10%. The contribution of glucose synthesis by the kidney becomes more important, however, during prolonged starvation.

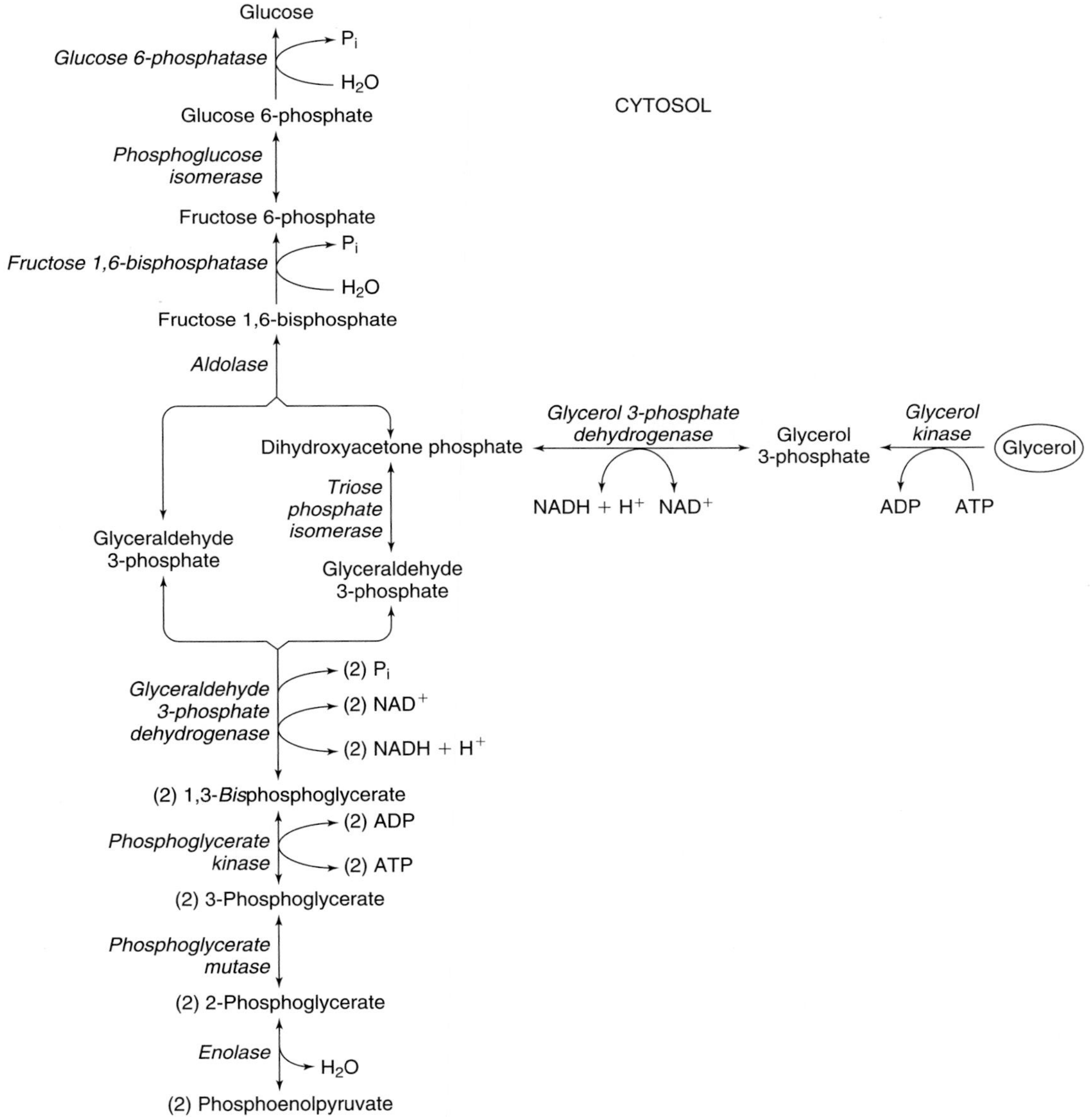

Figure 12-5 Gluconeogenesis from pyruvate, other precursors of phosphoenolpyruvate, and glycerol.

Continued

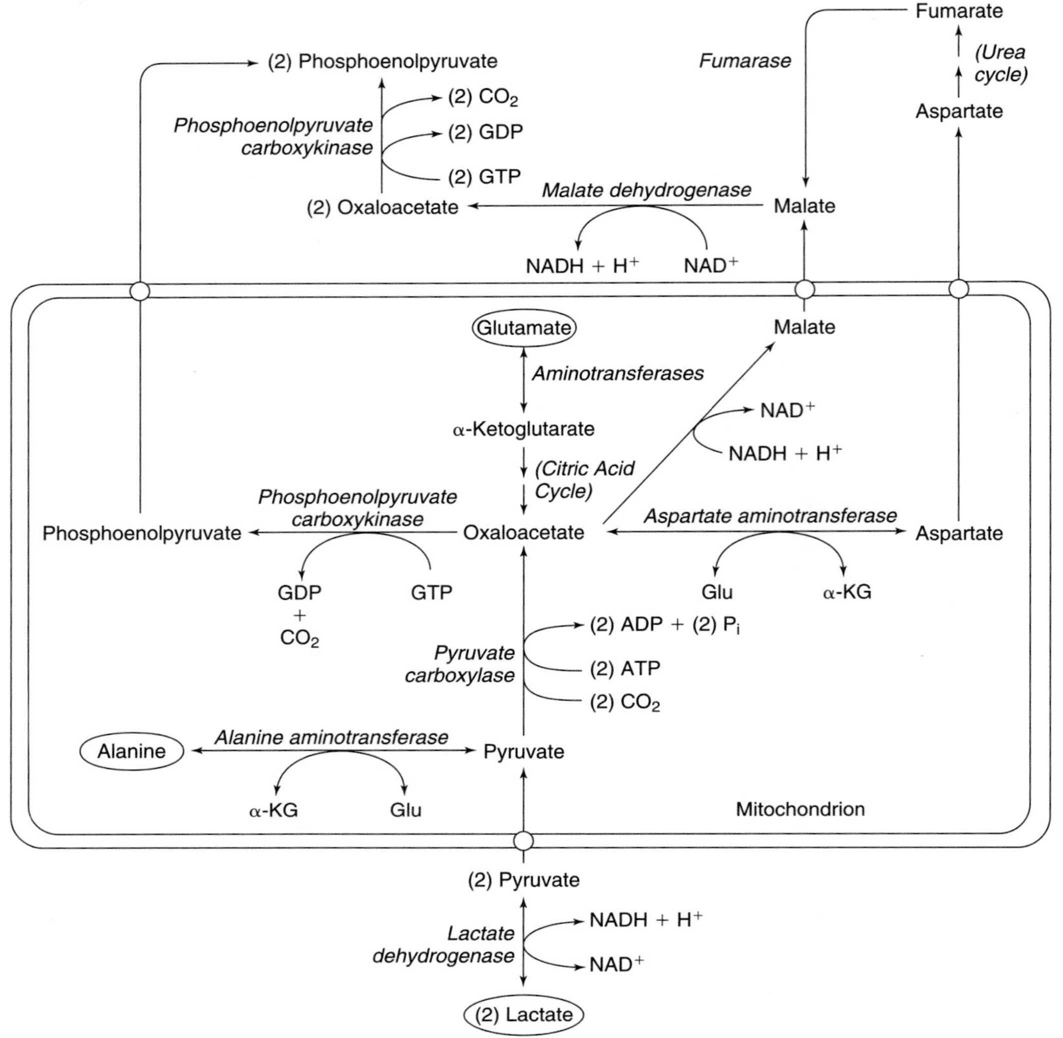

Figure 12-5—Cont'd

THE GLUCONEOGENIC PATHWAY

The first step in gluconeogenesis that bypasses an irreversible glycolytic reaction is the conversion of pyruvate to phosphoenolpyruvate. This involves the activity of two enzymes, pyruvate carboxylase and phosphoenolpyruvate carboxykinase. Pyruvate is transferred from the cytosol to the mitochondrial compartment where it is substrate for mitochondrial pyruvate carboxylase. (Pyruvate also can be generated by transamination of alanine in the mitochondrion itself.) In the mitochondrion, pyruvate is carboxylated to produce oxaloacetate. One molecule of ATP is hydrolyzed to ADP + P_i in this reaction. Pyruvate carboxylase is a biotin-dependent enzyme in which the covalently bound coenzyme functions as the carboxyl group carrier. The reaction can be described in two stages as follows:

$$\text{Enzyme-Biotin} + \text{ATP} + \text{HCO}_3^- \rightarrow \text{Enzyme-Biotin-CO}_2 + \text{ADP} + \text{P}_i$$

$$\text{Enzyme-Biotin-CO}_2 + \text{Pyruvate} \rightarrow \text{Enzyme-Biotin} + \text{Oxaloacetate}$$

In addition to the requirement for biotin as a coenzyme, this reaction also requires acetyl CoA as a positive allosteric activator.

When acetyl CoA is in excess, it becomes available for activation of pyruvate carboxylase. This promotes the anabolic utilization of pyruvate, stimulating the conversion of pyruvate to oxaloacetate for gluconeogenesis. However, during metabolic conditions when there is inadequate oxaloacetate for condensation with acetyl CoA in the citric acid cycle, oxaloacetate produced by the pyruvate carboxylase reaction is used for the continuation of the citric acid cycle rather than for gluconeogenic conversion to phosphoenolpyruvate. This is referred to as an anaplerotic reaction because citric acid cycle intermediates are replenished.

In the second enzymatic step in glucose biosynthesis from pyruvate, oxaloacetate is converted to phosphoenolpyruvate. This reaction is catalyzed by phosphoenolpyruvate carboxykinase. One molecule of the high energy compound, guanosine triphosphate (GTP), is hydrolyzed in this reaction, as follows:

$$\text{Oxaloacetate} + \text{GTP} \xrightarrow{Mg^{2+}} \text{Phosphoenolpyruvate} + CO_2 + \text{GDP}$$

Although this is a reversible reaction, it is essentially irreversible in the cell because phosphoenolpyruvate is rapidly utilized.

In human liver, phosphoenolpyruvate carboxykinase is present in approximately equal concentrations in the mitochondria and the cytosol of the hepatocyte. Oxaloacetate is metabolized differently depending upon whether it is the substrate for the mitochondrial or cytosolic enzyme and whether it is derived from pyruvate or lactate. When the gluconeogenic precursor is lactate, lactate must first be converted to pyruvate by lactate dehydrogenase, a reaction that generates NADH in the cytosol. Pyruvate then enters the mitochondrion and is converted to oxaloacetate by pyruvate carboxylase. Oxaloacetate is converted to phosphoenolpyruvate by mitochondrial phosphoenolpyruvate carboxykinase, and phosphoenolpyruvate can be transported across the mitochondrial membrane to the cytosol, where the remaining enzymes for gluconeogenesis are located. The lactate dehydrogenase reaction provides the required cytosolic NADH for a distal gluconeogenic step, the reversal of the glyceraldehyde 3-phosphate dehydrogenase reaction. Without this provision of cytosolic NADH, gluconeogenesis cannot continue.

A more complex process occurs when pyruvate is the gluconeogenic precursor because mitochondrial reducing equivalents must be shuttled to the cytosol to support gluconeogenesis. Pyruvate enters the mitochondrion and is converted to oxaloacetate by pyruvate carboxylase, but oxaloacetate leaves the mitochondrion as malate or aspartate. In the cytosol, malate, either directly from the mitochondria or generated by cytosolic fumarase from the fumarate released from aspartate during ureagenesis (see Chapter 14, Fig. 14-10), is converted back to oxaloacetate by cytosolic malate dehydrogenase, with the concomitant reduction of NAD^+ to NADH. Oxaloacetate is then available as substrate for cytosolic phosphoenolpyruvate carboxykinase.

In effect, these shuttles move potential NADH from the mitochondrion to the cytosol, providing the required reduced coenzyme for the glyceraldehyde 3-phosphate dehydrogenase reaction as well as carbon substrate for gluconeogenesis. The successive actions of pyruvate carboxylase and phosphoenolpyruvate carboxykinase effectively bypass the pyruvate kinase reaction. Overall, these two reactions result in the net hydrolysis of one molecule each of ATP and GTP as the energy cost.

The second bypass reaction that is unique to gluconeogenesis is that catalyzed by fructose 1,6-bisphosphatase, as follows:

$$\text{Fructose 1,6-Bisphosphate} + H_2O \rightarrow \text{Fructose 6-Phosphate} + P_i$$

This reaction reverses the 6-phosphofructo-1-kinase reaction and is essentially irreversible under intracellular conditions. It should be noted that inorganic phosphate, not ATP, is generated from the bisphosphatase reaction.

The terminal catalytic step in gluconeogenesis is the conversion of glucose 6-phosphate to glucose. This reaction provides free glucose for transport from the liver. The reaction is catalyzed by glucose 6-phosphatase and is essentially irreversible, as follows:

$$\text{Glucose 6-Phosphate} + H_2O \rightarrow \text{Glucose} + P_i$$

The glucose 6-phosphatase reaction reverses the glucokinase or hexokinase reaction. Glucose 6-phosphatase is important in both gluconeogenesis and glycogenolysis (glycogen breakdown) because glucose 6-phosphate is produced in both of these pathways. Tissues that do not synthesize this enzyme do not have the ability to release glucose to the circulation, with the exception of glucose residues at branch points in glycogen, which can be released from glycogen as free glucose by the debranching enzyme as discussed later in this chapter.

Glucose 6-phosphatase has a unique intracellular location. It is a membrane-bound enzyme in the endoplasmic reticulum (ER). Glucose 6-phosphatase activity is the result of the combined action of a glucose 6-phosphate translocase that moves glucose 6-phosphate into the lumen of the ER, the catalytic subunit that is responsible for the phosphohydrolase activity, and lastly, the glucose and P_i transporters that move the end products of the reaction back to the cytosol (Nordlie et al., 1993).

It should be noted that the gluconeogenic pathway is not active until after birth because the levels of phosphoenolpyruvate carboxykinase are very low until the neonatal period. Within a few hours after birth, phosphoenolpyruvate carboxykinase activity increases several-fold and the gluconeogenic pathway becomes viable. In the human neonate, the brain is dependent on glucose for its energy needs and, therefore, is dependent on gluconeogenically derived glucose during times of carbohydrate deprivation. The premature infant is prone to hypoglycemia due to small glycogen stores and the delay in induction of phosphoenolpyruvate carboxykinase activity after birth.

Overall, the de novo synthesis of glucose requires energy in the form of ATP. Six molecules of ATP are utilized for the synthesis of one molecule of glucose from two molecules of pyruvate. In the liver, ATP is usually generated for this process by the oxidation of fatty acids or by the partial oxidation of amino acid carbon chains, depending on fuel availability.

THE CORI AND ALANINE CYCLES

There is a metabolic connection between the liver and other tissues that depend upon glucose for their energy needs. Both lactate and alanine generated in peripheral tissues can be carried in the circulation to the liver, where they serve as substrates for hepatic gluconeogenesis. The glucose produced from these precursors can be transported from the liver and carried back to peripheral tissues for glycolytic catabolism and energy generation. This occurs in two well-defined cycles: the Cori cycle (Fig. 12-6) and the alanine cycle.

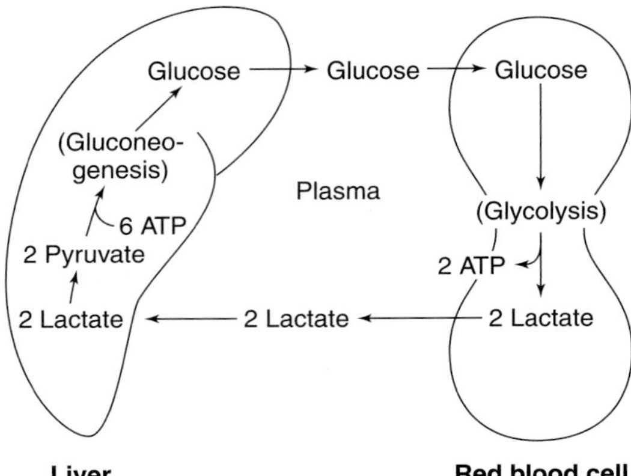

Figure 12-6 The Cori cycle, or lactate–glucose cycle. Tissues that either lack mitochondria or have a limited blood supply depend upon glycolysis to lactate a source of ATP. Obligate glycolytic tissues include mature red blood cells; regions of the eye including the cornea, lens, and parts of the retina; and the renal medulla.

In the Cori cycle, lactate generated from pyruvate, the end product of glycolysis, is released from tissues such as muscle or red blood cells and is transported to the liver. In the liver, lactate is converted back to pyruvate by lactate dehydrogenase, and pyruvate can be used to synthesize glucose by gluconeogenesis. Gluconeogenically derived glucose is then transported from liver cells and recirculated to muscle or red blood cells for glycolysis.

A second cycle, the alanine cycle (see Chapter 14, Fig. 14-12), involves the circulation of alanine from skeletal muscle to the liver. In muscle, alanine is generated from the transamination of glycolytically derived pyruvate and released. Liver cells take up the alanine and deaminate it to pyruvate, which serves as substrate for hepatic gluconeogenesis. Gluconeogenically derived glucose is then

Clinical Correlation

Inherited Deficiencies in Gluconeogenic Enzymes

In humans, defects in both the cytosolic and mitochondrial forms of phosphoenolpyruvate carboxykinase occur as rare, inherited autosomal recessive disorders. Defects in mitochondrial phosphoenolpyruvate carboxykinase are more common. A deficiency in either isoenzyme leads to hypoglycemia and lactic acidosis because sufficient glucose is not produced from pyruvate, lactate, or amino acid precursors. Therefore, individuals with this disorder are dependent upon glycogenolysis for glucose during a fast and become hypoglycemic when glycogen is depleted. The symptoms of this disorder usually present early in life. The hypoglycemia can cause seizures, coma, or lethargy. Typically, this disorder is associated with progressive neurological damage (Buist, 1995). Other symptoms include hepatomegaly, kidney dysfunction, and cardiomyopathy. This disorder can be fatal.

Inherited fructose 1,6-bisphosphatase deficiency results in impaired gluconeogenesis from any gluconeogenic precursor, including glycerol, lactate, and alanine. This disorder usually presents within the first few days of life, although in milder cases, presentation can be in early childhood. Symptoms of this disorder are similar to those described for phosphoenolpyruvate carboxykinase deficiency, that is, hypoglycemia and lactic acidosis. Fructose 1,6-bisphosphatase deficiency, however, does not result in neurodegenerative disorders as does phosphoenolpyruvate carboxykinase deficiency.

One of the most common genetic diseases to affect carbohydrate metabolism in humans is Von Gierke's disease, which is caused by an autosomal recessive genetic defect in glucose 6-phosphatase. This defect results in a block in release of glucose 6-phosphate from liver as glucose. Individuals with this disease have impaired gluconeogenesis because glucose 6-phosphate cannot be converted to glucose. This defect also affects hepatic glucose export from the breakdown of glycogen. Because the glucose 6-phosphate is "trapped" in the liver, excessive accumulation of glycogen is observed.

recycled from the liver back to muscle tissue. In the alanine cycle, unlike the Cori cycle, the NADH generated in skeletal muscle during glycolysis is not used for the reduction of pyruvate to lactate; therefore, the NADH is available for mitochondrial electron transport and ATP production assuming oxygen is sufficient.

REGULATION OF GLYCOLYSIS AND GLUCONEOGENESIS

In liver, the interconnected series of enzymatic reactions that constitute the glycolytic and gluconeogenic pathways are regulated in concert to ensure that cellular energy needs are met and that blood glucose levels are maintained. The mechanisms by which these pathways are regulated are complex and involve short-term regulation by allosteric or covalent modification of enzymes and long-term regulation by changes in expression of the genes that encode these enzymes.

THE SUBSTRATE CYCLE

The fine-tuned regulation of glycolysis and gluconeogenesis in liver can be understood by examining the functional concept of the substrate cycle. A substrate cycle consists of two opposing enzymatic reactions, with the potential to continuously cycle substrate and product (Fig. 12-7). If this occurs, energy is lost, with no net movement of product in either the glycolytic or gluconeogenic direction. In liver, three substrate cycles involve the essentially irreversible reactions of glycolysis (catalyzed by glucokinase, 6-phosphofructo-1-kinase, and pyruvate kinase) and gluconeogenesis (catalyzed by pyruvate carboxylase and phosphoenolpyruvate carboxykinase, fructose 1,6-bisphosphatase, and glucose 6-phosphatase).

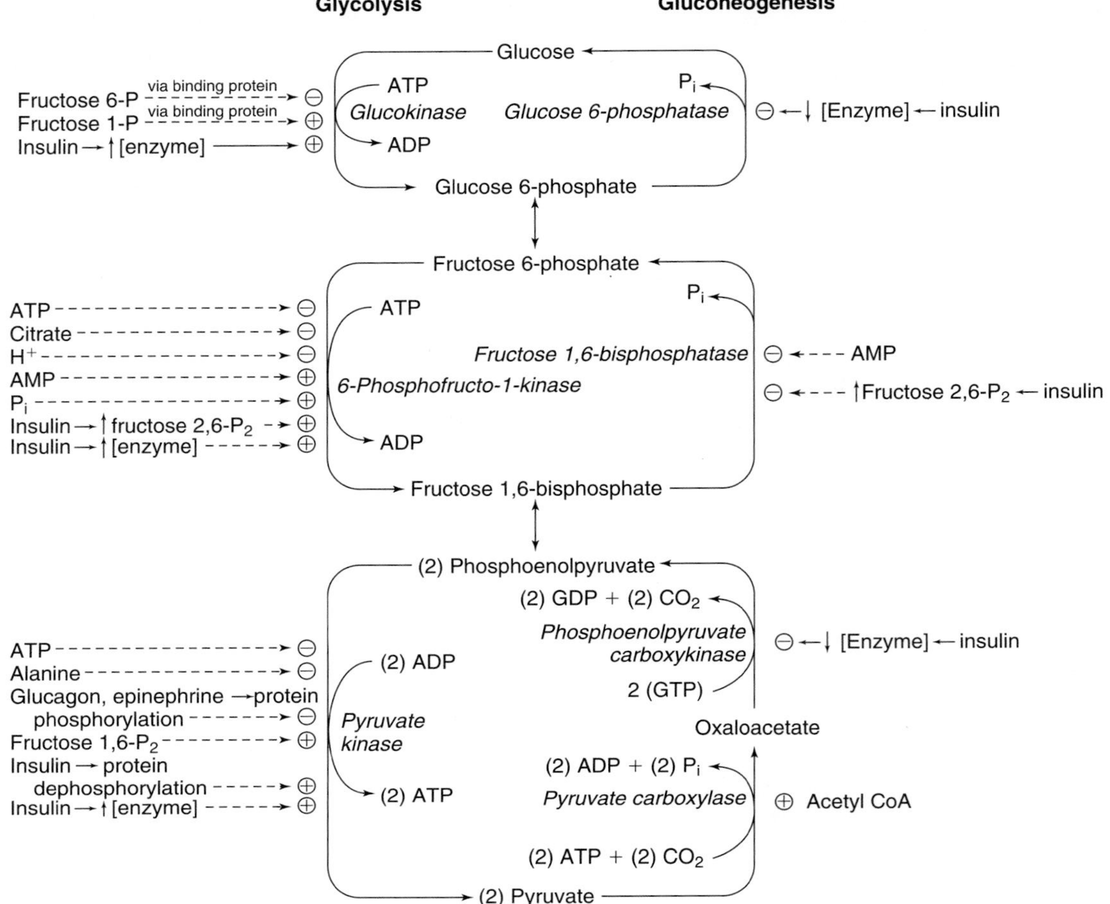

Figure 12-7 Substrate cycles and regulation of glycolysis and gluconeogenesis in liver.

The paired enzymes of each specific substrate cycle are regulated in a coordinated fashion so that the stimulation of one is accompanied by the inhibition of the other, although both enzymes function simultaneously with one functioning at a higher and the other at a lower percentage of its maximum activity. This coordinated regulation allows for a magnification of the regulatory effect and decreases the potential for futile cycling of substrate and product (Pilkis and Claus, 1991). The rate of these enzyme reactions can be affected by allosteric modification, covalent modification, or changes in enzyme concentration. The former two mechanisms are rapid, occurring within seconds, whereas the latter mechanism is described as long-term and may require minutes to hours.

HORMONAL REGULATION OF GLYCOLYSIS AND GLUCONEOGENESIS

In response to nutrient and physiological stimuli, hormones mediate both short- and long-term regulation of substrate cycle enzymes. Insulin, glucagon, epinephrine, and glucocorticoids are the predominant hormones that regulate enzymatic activity in carbohydrate metabolism.

Regulation of Hormone Levels

When blood glucose levels are elevated, such as occurs after a carbohydrate-containing meal, the anabolic hormone insulin is secreted from the β cells of the pancreas. The portal vein carries blood draining the digestive tract and pancreas to the liver, thereby ensuring the transport of pancreatic hormones like insulin directly to the liver sinusoids along with the absorbed monosaccharides. In the postabsorptive state, the insulin concentration is approximately threefold greater in the portal vein than in the peripheral blood. At these levels, approximately 180 pmol/L, insulin effectively decreases hepatic glucose production as well as increases hepatic glycogen storage (see subsequent text). Although insulin does not stimulate glucose uptake by liver, insulin does signal increased glycogen storage and glycolysis at the same time that it decreases glycogenolysis and gluconeogenesis. The net result is that glucose secretion from the liver is decreased. In peripheral tissues, particularly skeletal muscle and adipose tissue, insulin stimulates glucose uptake via increased translocation of the glucose transporter GLUT4 to the cell surface. In the long term, insulin regulates the expression of genes that encode key enzymes in carbohydrate metabolism; insulin activates expression of the glucokinase gene and inhibits expression of the phosphoenolpyruvate carboxykinase and glucose 6-phosphatase genes. Overall, insulin acts to decrease blood glucose levels by increasing the uptake of glucose from the blood by peripheral tissues and by decreasing glucose production/secretion by the liver.

When blood glucose levels are low, as in fasting or starvation, the α cells of the pancreas respond by releasing the polypeptide hormone glucagon to the bloodstream. In humans, liver is the main target tissue for glucagon action. Glucagon promotes increased blood glucose levels by increasing hepatic glucose production via enhanced glycogenolysis and gluconeogenesis. Glucagon, acting via 3′,5′cyclic AMP (cAMP), regulates the expression of numerous genes encoding rate-determining enzymes, such as phosphoenolpyruvate carboxykinase. In general, glucagon stimulates increased hepatic glucose output and is a counterregulatory hormone to insulin, as are the glucocorticoids and epinephrine.

Glucocorticoids and epinephrine, from the adrenal cortex and adrenal medulla, respectively, are also released in response to decreased blood glucose. Glucocorticoids are steroid hormones that are permissive for the action of other hormones such as glucagon. Epinephrine is a catecholamine that acts on many different tissues in the human body; the response of a given tissue to epinephrine (adrenaline) depends on the predominance of specific adrenergic receptor types on the cell surface. The adrenergic receptors are grouped into α (α1, α2) and β (β1, β2, β3) subtypes. Epinephrine stimulation of β-receptors increases glycogenolysis and gluconeogenesis, as well as lipolysis. Epinephrine stimulation of α1-receptors results in increased glycogenolysis, whereas stimulation of α2-receptors results in decreased lipolysis. Epinephrine increases hepatic glucose output as well as lipolysis in response to fasting or starvation.

Insulin: Signal Transduction

The insulin signal transduction pathway has been difficult to elucidate, but recently significant progress has been made in our understanding of the insulin receptor and the mechanism of insulin action, as described further in Chapter 19 (see Fig. 19-11). The insulin receptor is a member of the receptor tyrosine kinase family, a diverse family of glycoprotein transmembrane receptors with a cytoplasmic domain that has tyrosine kinase activity. The insulin receptor is a dimer made up of two α and two β subunits. The α subunits are on the extracellular face of the plasma membrane and contain the hormone-binding domains of the receptor. The two β subunits are transmembrane proteins with the carboxyl termini on the cytosolic side of the plasma membrane. The β subunits have tyrosine kinase activity, that is, they catalyze the phosphorylation of substrate at tyrosyl residues. Insulin binding to the α subunits initiates a conformational change in the β subunits, which stimulates the tyrosine kinase domains. The initiation of tyrosine kinase activity results in autophosphorylation of tyrosyl residues in the β subunits of the receptor itself at three specific tyrosine residues: Tyr 1158, Tyr1162, and Tyr1163. Autophosphorylation activates the tyrosine kinase domain to phosphorylate other target proteins in the cytosol and the membrane. Studies indicate that the tyrosine kinase activity of the insulin receptor increases with the degree of phosphorylation of these tyrosyl resides.

Insulin signal transduction is highly complex, and activation of the insulin receptor stimulates several signaling pathways within the cell. Insulin signaling has pleiotropic effects on different metabolic pathways, as well as effects on gene expression, cell growth, and cell differentiation. Relative to carbohydrate metabolism, the signaling pathway that involves insulin receptor phosphorylation of the insulin receptor substrate (IRS) effects both activation/inhibition of enzyme activities as well as activation/inhibition of the expression of metabolic genes. Currently, a family of four IRS proteins has been identified (IRS1, IRS2, IRS3, and IRS4) that are immediate targets of insulin receptor tyrosine kinase activity. The phosphorylation of the IRS proteins converts them to docking molecules that form platforms to bind other downstream signaling proteins that have SH2 (Src homology domain 2) domains. The SH2 domain is a conserved approximately 100-amino-acid residue region that binds phosphotyrosine residues, such as those on IRS proteins, with a high affinity. Amplification of the insulin response can occur at the level of IRS docking action, independent of insulin binding to the insulin receptor or of receptor tyrosine kinase activity (White, 1998).

One outcome of the phosphorylation of IRS proteins is the recruitment of phosphatidylinositol 3-kinase (PI 3-kinase) to the inner face of the plasma membrane via binding of its SH2 domain to the IRS phosphotyrosine residues. PI 3-kinase phosphorylates PI-(4,5)-bisphosphate [PI(4,5)P_2] and generates PI(3,4,5)P_3, an important second messenger that is involved in many of the metabolic effects of insulin (Cohen et al., 1997). Certain of these insulin effects occur in the nucleus of the cell where gene expression is activated or inhibited (e.g., the suppression of phosphoenolpyruvate carboxykinase and glucose 6-phosphatase gene expression by insulin). Other intracellular events initiated by insulin binding to the insulin receptor include increased glucose transport via GLUT4. In addition, insulin stimulates cyclic nucleotide phosphodiesterase, the enzyme that degrades cAMP, and stimulates a phosphoprotein phosphatase that dephosphorylates the bifunctional enzyme 6-phosphofructo-2-kinase/fructose 2,6-bisphosphatase, thereby activating the kinase function and favoring glycolysis over gluconeogenesis. Insulin also relieves inhibition of the phosphoprotein phosphatase that dephosphorylates and activates glycogen synthase and that also dephosphorylates and inhibits glycogen phosphorylase, thereby activating the glycogen synthesis pathway overall.

Glucagon and Epinephrine: Signal Transduction

The signal transduction mechanisms for glucagon and epinephrine are similar, albeit predominant in different tissues; both involve the activation of cognate receptors that are members of the heterotrimeric G protein–coupled receptor superfamily. Glucagon and epinephrine bind to glucagon receptors and adrenergic receptors, respectively, on the plasma membrane of target cells, as described further in Chapter 19 (see Fig. 19-10). These receptors are integral membrane proteins that span the lipid bilayer of the plasma membrane. The signal initiated by both glucagon binding to its receptor and epinephrine binding to β-adrenergic receptors involves a heterotrimeric G protein (e.g., the stimulatory GTP-binding protein G_s). Binding of hormone to the cognate receptor causes a conformational change in the receptor that alters the cytoplasmic face of the receptor. This conformational change brings the hormone-receptor complex in contact with the multisubunit cytosolic protein G_s. This association causes a molecule of GDP to be exchanged for a molecule of GTP at an allosteric site of the α subunit of G_s. The binding of GTP stimulates G_s, causing the G_s α subunit to disassociate from the β and γ subunits that remain anchored to the receptor; the released G_s α subunit then activates the adjoining adenylate cyclase. Adenylate cyclase, in turn, catalyzes the formation of cAMP, the intracellular second messenger of glucagon and epinephrine. Liver cells respond to both glucagon and epinephrine, indeed the cAMP signal is the accumulated total of cAMP produced by the stimulation of both the glucagon and β-adrenergic receptors.

The production of cAMP stimulates the cAMP-dependent protein kinase, referred to as protein kinase A. cAMP activates protein kinase A by binding to the two regulatory subunits of the tetrameric enzyme and releasing the two catalytic subunits. The catalytic subunit of protein kinase A has numerous intracellular substrates. Relevant to the regulation of glycolysis and gluconeogenesis, protein kinase A phosphorylates both pyruvate kinase and the bifunctional enzyme, 6-phosphofructo-2-kinase/fructose 2,6-bisphosphatase (described in subsequent text), both of which stimulate glycolysis. Protein kinase A also enters the nucleus of the cell and phosphorylates nuclear proteins, which can activate or inhibit the transcription of genes that encode certain glycolytic and gluconeogenic enzymes.

It should be noted that epinephrine also binds to α2-adrenergic receptors. The activated α2-receptor stimulates a series of intracellular events similar to those initiated by the β-adrenergic receptors, except that an inhibitory GTP-binding protein (G_i) is released and becomes associated with adenylate cyclase. G_i binding inhibits adenylate cyclase and leads to an overall decrease in intracellular cAMP levels. Another regulatory mechanism is contributed by epinephrine binding to α1-adrenergic receptors. Activation of the α1-adrenergic receptor stimulates phospholipase C on the cytoplasmic face of the plasma membrane by a GTP-binding protein mechanism similar to that for activation of adenylate cyclase. Phospholipase C hydrolyzes phosphatidylinositol 4,5-bisphosphate (PIP_2), present in the plasma membrane, to inositol 1,4,5-triphosphate (IP_3) and diacylglycerol. Diacylglycerol, in turn, stimulates protein kinase C. Protein kinase C has numerous substrates in the cell, some of which are key enzymes in hepatic glycogen metabolism, as described later in this chapter. IP_3 stimulates the release of Ca^{2+} from the ER, and calcium efflux activates the calcium/calmodulin-dependent protein kinase, as well as other enzymes. The calcium/calmodulin-dependent protein kinase catalyzes the phosphorylation and inactivation of pyruvate kinase, contributing to the diminution of the glycolytic rate (Pilkis and Claus, 1991).

Glucocorticoids

Glucocorticoids differ from the polypeptide hormones, such as insulin and glucagon, and the catecholamines in that the steroid hormones do not bind to plasma membrane receptors and initiate a series of intracellular events. Glucocorticoids, because they are lipid soluble, can traverse the lipid bilayer of the plasma membrane and enter the cell. Within the cytoplasm of the cell, glucocorticoids bind to their cognate receptors and subsequently enter the nucleus as an activated ligand–receptor complex. In the nucleus, the activated receptors take on the role of transcription factors and bind to regulatory regions of target genes, thereby increasing or decreasing expression of these responsive genes, many of which encode metabolic enzymes.

Coordinated Regulation in Response to Glucose Levels

In the liver, the rate of an enzymatic reaction in one substrate cycle is usually coordinated with the rates of other substrate cycle enzymes in the same pathway. For example, when blood glucose levels are low, glucagon levels increase and insulin levels decrease, resulting in an overall decrease in the insulin-glucagon ratio in the blood. This activates (by different mechanisms) phosphoenolpyruvate carboxykinase, fructose 1,6-bisphosphatase, and glucose 6-phosphatase and also inhibits pyruvate kinase, 6-phosphofructo-1-kinase, and glucokinase. These changes favor gluconeogenesis, which contributes to reestablishing normal blood glucose levels. Conversely, a high-carbohydrate diet, particularly following a fast, stimulates the release of insulin and decreases the release of glucagon from the pancreas. The rise in the insulin-glucagon ratio causes an increase in the activity of the glycolytic enzymes of the respective substrate cycles, with a concomitant decrease in the specific enzymes of gluconeogenesis. This response favors glucose utilization for energy or the synthesis of other biomolecules such as fatty acids. Clearly, this coordinated regulation allows the liver to respond to changes in the diet by determining the predominant enzymatic reaction at each substrate cycle, which in turn, determines the overall glycolytic or gluconeogenic rate of the tissue.

REGULATION OF THE ACTIVITY OF HEXOKINASE/GLUCOKINASE AND GLUCOSE 6-PHOSPHATASE

Differential Location, Insulin Responsiveness, and Kinetic Properties of Hexokinase Isozymes

Hexokinase, which catalyzes the initial phosphorylation of glucose when it enters the cell, has different tissue-specific isoenzyme forms. Isoenzymes are different molecular forms of an enzyme that catalyze the same reaction but differ in kinetics, regulatory mechanisms, and/or tissue localization. In humans, hexokinase I predominates in skeletal muscle and other peripheral tissues. Hexokinase I has a low K_m for glucose (less than 0.1 mmol/L) relative to blood glucose concentrations (4 to 5 mmol/L). The activity of hexokinase I is coordinated with that of the low K_m glucose carrier GLUT4, which specifically transports glucose in response to insulin stimulation. The combined action of hexokinase I and GLUT4 maintains a balance between glucose uptake and glucose phosphorylation. Hexokinase I is allosterically inhibited by its product, glucose 6-phosphate. This negative feedback ensures that glucose 6-phosphate does not build up in the cell.

In liver, the predominant hexokinase is glucokinase (hexokinase IV). This isoenzyme has a high K_m for glucose (10 mmol/L) and is not inhibited by glucose 6-phosphate. The activity of glucokinase is linked to that of the high K_m glucose transporter GLUT2, which is the major glucose carrier in liver parenchymal cells. The glucokinase/GLUT2 system is very active when blood glucose levels are high. Under these conditions, the rates of glucose uptake and phosphorylation are determined by the blood glucose concentration itself. A similar coupling of GLUT2 and the high K_m glucokinase occurs in the β cells of the pancreas. In the pancreatic β cell, GLUT2 and glucokinase allow the intracellular glucose 6-phosphate concentration to equilibrate with the blood glucose concentration, thereby allowing the β cells to detect elevated blood glucose levels and respond by the secretion of insulin.

Glucokinase Regulatory Protein

Although glucokinase in liver is not modified by its end-product, glucose 6-phosphate, it is subject to allosteric control by other intermediary metabolites. Glucokinase is indirectly inhibited by fructose 6-phosphate and activated by fructose 1-phosphate. This regulatory mechanism involves an inhibitory protein that binds to glucokinase; this inhibitory protein is referred to as glucokinase regulatory protein (GKRP) (Fig. 12-8). The affinity of GKRP for glucokinase is increased by fructose 6-phosphate; conversely, fructose 1-phosphate decreases the affinity of this inhibitory protein for glucokinase. Fructose 6-phosphate is present in the cell in equilibrium with glucose 6-phosphate because of the reversibility of the phosphoglucose isomerase reaction; therefore fructose 6-phosphate is a negative feedback metabolite that signals the cell that glucokinase activity should decrease to prevent the buildup of this intermediate. Fructose 1-phosphate, on the other hand, is present in the liver parenchymal cell only when fructose is being metabolized; therefore, when fructose is available, the negative feedback inhibition of glucokinase is released. Overall, the availability of fructose, most often via dietary sucrose, is coordinated indirectly with increased uptake of glucose via this relief of inhibition of glucokinase activity. Regulation of glucokinase by GKRP is further complicated by the intracellular localization of glucokinase. Glucokinase is unique among glycolytic enzymes in that it can translocate between the cytoplasm and the nucleus of the cell. Interestingly, the GKRP is localized in the nucleus where it can sequester glucokinase. In the presence of fructose or high glucose concentrations, glucokinase is released from GKRP and translocates to the cytoplasm where it is active in glucose phosphorylation (de la Iglesia et al., 1999; Nordlie et al., 1999). Conversely, under conditions of low glucose, glucokinase remains bound to GKRP in the nucleus of the cell and, therefore, unavailable for the conversion of glucose to glucose 6-phosphate, thereby limiting glucose/glucose 6-phosphate futile cycling (see Fig. 12-8).

Glucose 6-Phosphatase

In the liver, reversal of the glucokinase reaction is catalyzed by glucose 6-phosphatase.

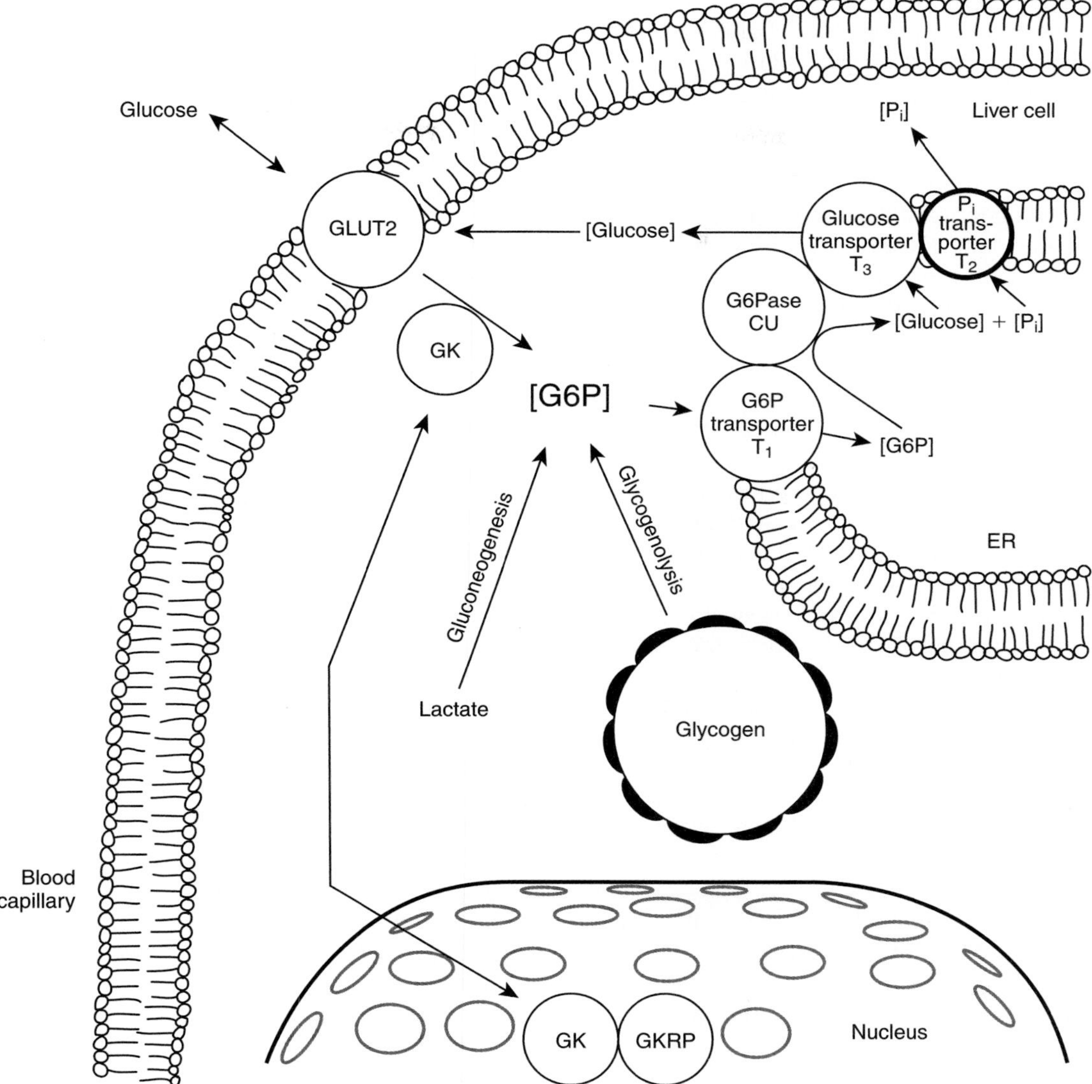

Figure 12-8 Diagram of the initial steps in glucose uptake and the terminal steps in glucose secretion from the liver parenchymal cell. Highlighted are GLUT2, the glucose transporter that conducts glucose import or export depending on the blood and cellular glucose concentrations; glucokinase (GK), the enzyme that is sequestered in the nucleus by the inhibitory protein, glucokinase regulatory protein (GKRP), under conditions of low glucose and high fructose 6-phosphate but is released from GKRP to the cytoplasm in the presence of fructose-1-phosphate or high glucose concentrations; and the multi-subunit glucose 6-phosphatase, which is associated with the endoplasmic reticulum (ER) and is made up of a catalytic subunit (CU) and at least three translocase (T) subunits that are involved in the import of glucose 6-phosphate into the ER and the export of glucose and P_i from the ER. Also shown are sources of glucose 6-phosphate (G6P), from either gluconeogenesis or glycogenolysis. *(Modified from Nordlie RC, Foster JD, Lange AJ [1999] Regulation of glucose production by the liver. Annu Rev Nutr 19:379-406.)*

Glucose 6-phosphatase is responsible for the last step in the production of glucose by either gluconeogenesis or glycogen breakdown and is required for the terminal transport of glucose from the liver cell. As indicated in the preceding text, glucose 6-phosphatase activity occurs in the ER and is the result of the combined action of a glucose 6-phosphate translocase (T_1) in the ER membrane, the catalytic subunit on the luminal side of the ER that is responsible for the phosphatase activity, and the glucose and P_i transporters (T_3 and T_2) that move the end products of the reaction back to the cytosol (see Fig. 12-8). Without glucose 6-phosphatase activity, glucose cannot be released to the circulation in response to low blood glucose. Glucose 6-phosphatase has a relatively high K_m for its substrate, glucose 6-phosphate (3 mmol/L). Because the intracellular glucose 6-phosphate concentration is 0.2 mmol/L, the rate of this enzymatic reaction primarily depends upon the substrate concentration.

In liver, a substrate cycle is established between the actions of glucokinase and glucose 6-phosphatase. In the long term, the glucokinase concentration is increased in response to insulin-induced changes in expression of the glucokinase gene itself. For example, the increased insulin–glucagon ratio that occurs in response to a high carbohydrate diet stimulates expression of the glucokinase gene. Expression of the gene for the glucose 6-phosphatase catalytic subunit, on the other hand, is inhibited by insulin. Therefore the ingestion of dietary carbohydrate results in an increase in glucokinase activity and a decrease in glucose 6-phosphatase activity, thereby favoring the net production of glucose 6-phosphate.

REGULATION OF 6-PHOSPHOFRUCTO-1-KINASE AND FRUCTOSE 1,6-BISPHOSPHATASE

In liver, the central regulatory site in glycolysis and gluconeogenesis is the substrate cycle established by the 6-phosphofructo-1-kinase and fructose 1,6-bisphosphatase reactions. Short-term regulation of this substrate cycle is critically important. Unlike the product of the glucokinase reaction, glucose 6-phosphate, which can enter glycolysis, glycogen synthesis, or the pentose phosphate pathway, the product of the 6-phosphofructo-1-kinase reaction provides a glycolytic intermediate or a substrate cycle intermediate. This reaction is the first committed step in glycolysis and, therefore, is subject to allosteric regulation by numerous metabolites that signal the energy level, pH, and hormonal status of the cell. Positive regulators of 6-phosphofructo-1-kinase include AMP, P_i, and fructose 2,6-bisphosphate (described in subsequent text); negative regulators include ATP, hydrogen ions, and citrate. ATP, AMP, and P_i signal the energy state of the cell; hydrogen ions signal the pH of the cell; citrate, the first metabolite of the citric acid cycle, signals the availability of sources of fuel; and fructose 2,6-bisphosphate signals the insulin–glucagon ratio.

The gluconeogenic enzyme fructose 1, 6-bisphosphatase is also allosterically regulated. AMP is a strong allosteric inhibitor of this enzyme, as are fructose 2,6-bisphosphate and possibly fructose 1,6-bisphosphate. There is a synergistic inhibition of fructose 1,6-bisphosphatase by the combined action of fructose 2,6-bisphosphate and AMP (Pilkis and Claus, 1991). When fuel for the citric acid cycle and oxygen are sufficient for oxidative phosphorylation, ATP levels in the cell are high, 6-phosphofructo-1-kinase is inhibited, and the rate of glycolysis is slow. Under the same conditions, AMP and P_i levels are low. The low concentrations of AMP and P_i contribute to the overall low 6-phosphofructo-1-kinase activity and high fructose 1-6-bisphosphatase activity.

Conversely, when oxygen pressure is low (e.g., hypoxia) or when ATP expenditure exceeds the mitochondrial capacity for oxidative metabolism and oxidative phosphorylation (e.g., when work is near or above VO_{2max}, when there are defects in mitochondrial metabolism, or in tissues with a relative or complete lack of mitochondria), lactate and hydrogen ions are increased as the end products of limited glucose catabolism. The cell releases lactate and hydrogen ions into the blood which, when in excess, can cause lactic acidosis. However, because hydrogen ions inhibit 6-phosphofructo-1-kinase activity, the glycolytic rate can be controlled to protect against lactate buildup.

A third inhibitory metabolite, citrate, signals the cell that fuel for the citric acid cycle, both oxaloacetate and acetyl CoA, is plentiful. Under these conditions, citrate is transported from the mitochondria to the cytosol, where it allosterically inhibits 6-phosphofructo-1-kinase, thereby decreasing the rate of glycolysis and sparing glucose.

The allosteric regulator fructose 2,6-bisphosphate is a potent activator of 6-phosphofructo-1-kinase and an inhibitor of fructose 1,6-bisphosphatase. The level of hepatic fructose 2,6-bisphosphate is increased by carbohydrate feeding or insulin administration. Overall, when insulin levels increase, fructose 2,6-bisphosphate levels rise and the rate of the 6-phosphofructo-1-kinase reaction is increased, thereby stimulating glycolysis. In contrast, when glucagon or epinephrine levels are elevated, fructose 2,6-bisphosphate levels are low and fructose 1,6-bisphosphatase activity is increased, resulting in an increase in gluconeogenesis. Regulation of this substrate cycle by fructose 2,6-bisphosphate is central in determining the overall flux of carbon to either glycolysis or gluconeogenesis in the liver. The end products, fructose 1,6-bisphosphate or fructose 6-phosphate, have positive feedforward effects on subsequent substrate cycles.

REGULATION OF 6-PHOSPHOFRUCTO-2-KINASE/ FRUCTOSE 2,6-BISPHOSPHATASE

Discovery of fructose 2,6-bisphosphate as an allosteric molecule in 1980 significantly advanced our understanding of the regulation of key enzymes involved in glucose metabolism. In liver, fructose 2,6-bisphosphate is a major regulatory molecule, controlling the overall direction of carbon flux toward either glycolysis or gluconeogenesis (Pilkis et al., 1990). When 6-phosphofructo-1-kinase activity is increased by fructose 2,6-bisphosphate, the increase in product, fructose 1,6-bisphosphate, allosterically activates pyruvate kinase by a feedforward mechanism. Conversely, when fructose 1,6-bisphosphatase activity is increased by a decrease in fructose 2,6-bisphosphate, more fructose 6-phosphate is produced. Fructose 6-phosphate is rapidly converted to glucose 6-phosphate, thereby providing increased substrate for glucose 6-phosphatase.

The carbohydrate content of the diet controls insulin and glucagon concentrations in the blood, which in turn regulate the production of fructose 2,6-bisphosphate. The levels of fructose 2,6-bisphosphate are controlled by a bifunctional enzyme that has both 6-phosphofructo-2-kinase and fructose 2,6-bisphosphatase activity. Regulation of the bifunctional enzyme by glucagon and insulin occurs by changes in the phosphorylation state of the enzyme. After a carbohydrate-containing meal, circulating blood glucose levels increase and stimulate insulin secretion from the β cells of the pancreas. Insulin activates phosphoprotein phosphatase 2A, which dephosphorylates the bifunctional enzyme, thereby stimulating 6-phosphofructo-2-kinase activity and favoring fructose 2,6-bisphosphate synthesis from fructose 6-phosphate and ATP. Overall, when insulin levels increase, fructose 2,6-bisphosphate levels rise and the rate of the 6-phosphofructo-1-kinase reaction is increased, thereby stimulating glycolysis (Fig. 12-9, *A*).

Conversely, as an individual begins to fast, circulating insulin levels decrease and the α cells of the pancreas respond to low blood glucose by secreting glucagon. Glucagon initiates an increase in intracellular cAMP and, therefore, activates protein kinase A. Protein kinase A phosphorylates the bifunctional enzyme at a specific serine residue. This alters the conformation of the bifunctional enzyme, decreasing the 6-phosphofructo-2-kinase activity and increasing the fructose 2,6-bisphosphatase activity. This rapidly decreases fructose 2,6-bisphosphate levels in liver, which releases the inhibition of fructose 1,6-bisphosphatase and favors gluconeogenesis (see Fig. 12-9, *B*). Both the 6-phosphofructo-2-kinase and the fructose 2,6-bisphosphatase reactions are also inhibited by the end products of their respective reactions, fructose 2,6-bisphosphate and fructose 6-phosphate. Overall, the predominant factors that determine fructose 2,6-bisphosphate levels in liver are the concentration of fructose 6-phosphate and the phosphorylation state of the bifunctional enzyme.

Studies done in rat liver indicate that in the fed state, fructose 6-phosphate levels are in

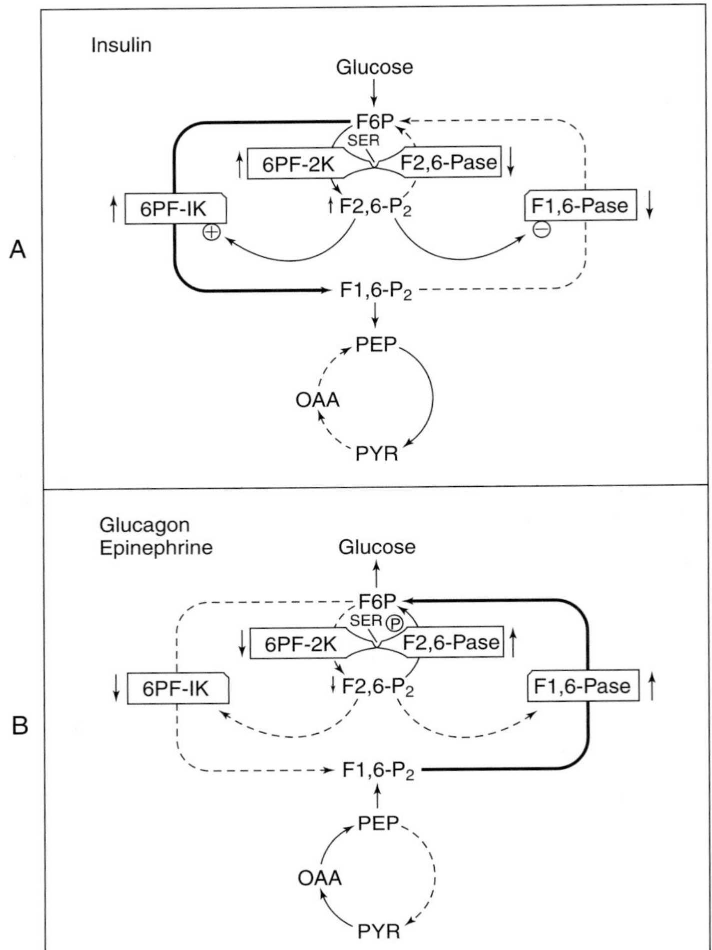

Figure 12-9 Regulation of the bifunctional enzyme 6-phosphofructo-2-kinase (6PF-2K)/fructose 2,6-bisphosphatase (F2,6-Pase) by phosphorylation (**B,** glucagon, or catecholamines) and dephosphorylation (**A,** insulin), and the allosteric regulation of 6-phosphofructo-1-kinase (6PF-1K) and fructose 1,6-bisphosphatase (F1,6-Pase) by fructose 2,6-bisphosphate (F2,6-P_2). *F6P,* Fructose 6-phosphate; *SER,* serine residue; *PEP,* phosphoenolpyruvate; *OAA,* oxaloacetate; *PYR,* pyruvate; *P,* $-PO_3^{2-}$.

the 0.1 to 0.2 μmol/g range, and the bifunctional enzyme is in the dephosphorylated state. In this conformation, the 6-phosphofructo-2-kinase reaction is favored by a decrease in the K_m for substrate, fructose 6-phosphate. Therefore, the intracellular substrate concentration is significantly higher than the K_m, maximizing the rate of fructose 2,6-bisphosphate production. During fasting (or diabetes) the bifunctional enzyme becomes phosphorylated at an amino-terminal serine residue, which activates the fructose 2,6-bisphosphatase and inhibits the 6-phosphofructo-2-kinase. The conformational change induced at the active site of 6-phosphofructo-2-kinase increases the K_m for substrate, fructose 6-phosphate. At the same time, during fasting, intracellular levels of fructose 6-phosphate decrease to below the K_m, and the rate of fructose 2,6-bisphosphate production is concomitantly slowed (Pilkis et al., 1995). Fructose 6-phosphate is also a substrate for 6-phosphofructo-1-kinase;

however, the rate of this reaction is two to three orders of magnitude greater than that of the 6-phosphofructo-2-kinase reaction. Therefore, the shunting of fructose 6-phosphate to fructose 2,6-bisphosphate production occurs at a much slower rate; the amount of glycolytic fuel used for the synthesis of this regulatory molecule is thus small.

REGULATION OF PYRUVATE KINASE AND PHOSPHOENOLPYRUVATE CARBOXYKINASE

The final substrate cycle in liver involves pyruvate kinase activity in the glycolytic direction and the combined action of pyruvate carboxylase and phosphoenolpyruvate carboxykinase in the gluconeogenic direction. The pyruvate kinase reaction is an important site of hormonal and nutritional regulation in glycolysis. In the liver, the momentum of glycolysis is maintained by pyruvate kinase under conditions that increase 6-phosphofructo-1-kinase activity. This is because the end product of the 6-phosphofructo-1-kinase reaction, fructose 1,6-bisphosphate, is a positive allosteric regulator of pyruvate kinase. Pyruvate kinase is also allosterically inhibited by ATP and alanine. At physiologic concentrations of substrate (phosphoenolpyruvate) and inhibitors (ATP and alanine), pyruvate kinase would be completely inhibited without the stimulatory effect of fructose 1,6-bisphosphate.

In the liver, pyruvate kinase is also regulated by phosphorylation. It is a substrate for both protein kinase A, induced by interaction of glucagon with glucagon receptors or of epinephrine with β-adrenergic receptors, and the calcium/calmodulin-dependent protein kinase, induced by epinephrine interaction with α1-adrenergic receptors. Phosphorylation of pyruvate kinase decreases the activity of the enzyme by increasing the K_m for its substrate, thereby slowing the rate of glycolysis. The reversal of this response is initiated by an increase in the insulin–glucagon ratio, which decreases cAMP and thus decreases protein kinase A activity, resulting in the dephosphorylation of pyruvate kinase and activation of the enzyme. It should be noted that the phosphorylated form of pyruvate kinase is less readily stimulated by fructose 1,6-bisphosphate and more readily inhibited by ATP and alanine. Conversely, in the dephosphorylated state, pyruvate kinase is more sensitive to allosteric activators and less sensitive to allosteric inhibitors. In the presence of fructose 1,6-bisphosphate, the protein kinase A–dependent phosphorylation of the enzyme is inhibited.

The gluconeogenic enzymes that oppose pyruvate kinase are pyruvate carboxylase and phosphoenolpyruvate carboxykinase. Pyruvate carboxylase is positively regulated by a buildup of acetyl CoA in the mitochondria, which signals the need for more oxaloacetate. However, it is the phosphoenolpyruvate carboxykinase reaction that is rate-determining for gluconeogenesis. Changes in the rate of the phosphoenolpyruvate carboxykinase reaction are not in response to allosteric or covalent modifiers; instead, enzyme concentration is highly regulated. The enzyme concentration is determined by regulation of the gene that encodes phosphoenolpyruvate carboxykinase.

REGULATION OF THE EXPRESSION OF GENES ENCODING GLYCOLYTIC AND GLUCONEOGENETIC ENZYMES

The pathways of glycolysis and gluconeogenesis function differently in the various tissues of the body. In liver, the rate of glycolysis is slow; the liver is more dependent on amino acids for metabolic fuel in the fed state and on fatty acids for metabolic fuel during food deprivation. Red blood cells, on the other hand, are completely dependent on glycolysis for their energy needs. Gluconeogenesis has a more restricted tissue distribution than does glycolysis; it is limited primarily to the liver and kidney. During starvation, gluconeogenesis in liver and kidney provides glucose for the body. It is clear, therefore, that different regulatory mechanisms are involved in the metabolic roles these pathways play in different tissues. Long-term regulation of the expression of specific genes dictates the concentrations of certain glycolytic and gluconeogenic enzymes as well as of transport proteins in the different cell types. Selective expression of specific genes plays a major role in determining the tissue distribution of these metabolic pathways.

A new era of metabolic investigation has been made possible by the identification and characterization of genes encoding glycolytic and gluconeogenic enzymes. Our knowledge of long-term regulation of glycolysis and gluconeogenesis is based upon studies of individual genes that have been cloned. Genes for the key regulatory enzymes of glycolysis and gluconeogenesis: glucokinase, glucose 6-phosphatase, 6-phosphofructo-1-kinase, fructose 1,6-bisphosphatase, pyruvate kinase, phosphoenolpyruvate carboxykinase, and 6-phosphofructo-2-kinase/fructose 2,6-bisphosphatase have been isolated and sequenced. DNA elements that are responsive to hormonal and nutrient stimuli have been characterized in several of the promoter/regulatory domains of these genes. Collectively, there are a number of similarities in hormonal regulation of genes encoding the key glycolytic and gluconeogenic enzymes. Insulin increases messenger RNA (mRNA) levels and transcription rates of the glycolytic genes and decreases mRNA levels and transcription rates of the gluconeogenic genes; glucagon, acting via cAMP, has the opposite effect (Pilkis and Granner, 1992). The genes encoding the different glucose transporters and other glycolytic enzymes also have been characterized.

EXPRESSION OF GLUCOSE TRANSPORTER GENES

The various tissue-specific glucose transporter proteins are encoded by separate genes. Expression of some of these genes is regulated by fluctuations in diet and hormones. In adipose tissue, for example, the gene for GLUT4 *(SLC2A4)* is regulated by fasting and carbohydrate refeeding (Charron et al., 1999). Fasting or type 2 diabetes leads to a significant decrease in *SLC2A4* mRNA and GLUT4 protein in adipocytes. This decrease can be reversed by carbohydrate refeeding or insulin treatment. A depletion in *SLC2A4* mRNA and protein results in a decrease in the vesicular GLUT4 pool that is available for translocation to the plasma membrane. The decrease in *SLC2A4* gene expression and the decrease in insulin-stimulated GLUT4 translocation both contribute to the decrease in glucose uptake in adipocytes with insulin deprivation (Fig. 12-10). Although the gene for GLUT1 *(SLC2A1)* is also expressed in adipose tissue, *SLC2A1* mRNA levels are not significantly changed by dietary carbohydrate or insulin status.

Expression of the *SLC2A4* gene has also been investigated in skeletal muscle. Because the red and white muscle fiber types have different insulin sensitivities and GLUT4 concentrations, it has been difficult to determine the hormonal responsiveness of the *SLC2A4* gene in this tissue. Most studies indicate that *SLC2A4* expression is not decreased with the insulin resistance characteristic of type 2 diabetes. This is surprising as skeletal muscle is responsible for at least 50% of glucose uptake from the blood after a carbohydrate-containing meal, whereas adipose tissue is responsible for much less. Studies in *SLC2A4* "knockout" mice, where the gene is selectively ablated in specific tissues such as skeletal muscle and adipose tissue indicate that there is "cross-talk" between these two tissues such that a decrease in adipose GLUT4 (and, therefore, glucose uptake) effects decreased glucose uptake in skeletal muscle as well (Minokoshi et al., 2003).

The major glucose transporter isoform in liver is GLUT2. The hepatic gene for GLUT2 *(SCL2A2)* does not appear to be regulated by dietary carbohydrate or insulin in different experimental models. Overall, *SCL2A2* mRNA and protein levels in liver have not been found to change consistently in response to altered metabolic states. However, it has been shown that *SCL2A2* gene expression in pancreatic β cells is decreased when blood glucose levels are low. Conversely, a rise in blood glucose levels results in an increase in *SCL2A2* mRNA and protein levels. *SCL2A2* "knockout" mice exhibit a loss of ability to sense glucose concentrations in the blood as well as impaired insulin secretion. This can be rescued by reexpression of the *SCL2A2* gene in pancreatic cells, which restores the insulin-secretory function of the pancreas (Thorens, 2002). The differential responsiveness of the *SCL2A2* gene in liver and pancreas provides a good example of tissue specificity in the regulation of gene expression.

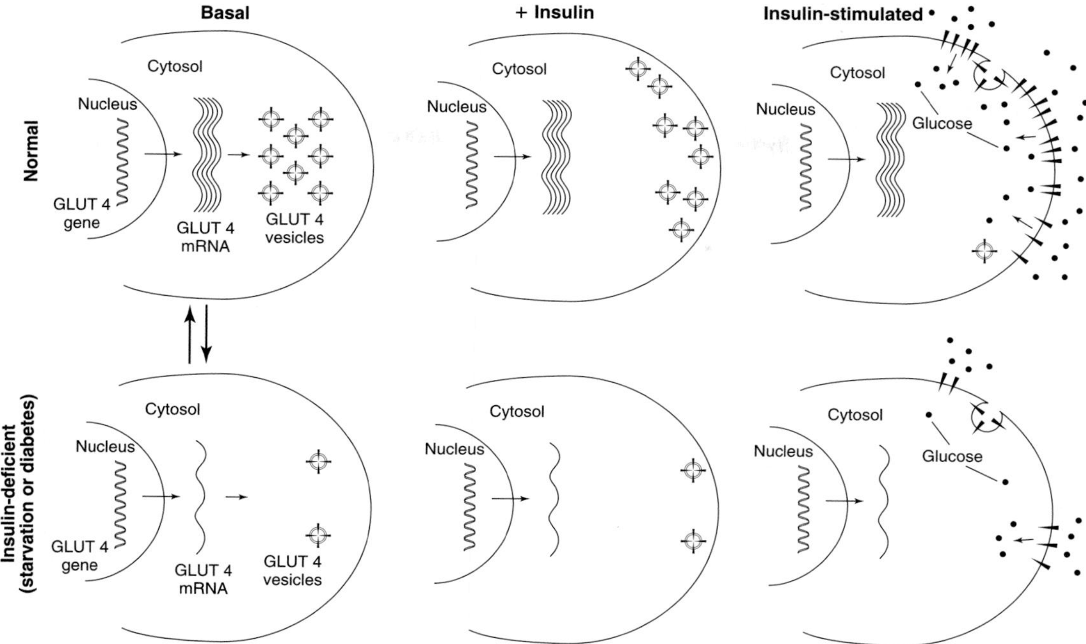

Figure 12-10 Effect of insulin on expression and translocation of the GLUT4 glucose transporter in adipocytes.

EXPRESSION OF THE GLUCOKINASE *(GCK)* GENE

Glucokinase (hexokinase IV), which converts glucose to glucose 6-phosphate, is the predominant hexokinase isoform in both the liver and pancreatic β cell. However, glucokinase plays a different metabolic role in these two tissues. In liver, glucose uptake is responsible for removal of approximately 35% to 40% of portal vein glucose after a carbohydrate-containing meal. The high K_m glucokinase maintains a glucose concentration deficit across the liver cell membrane, as glucose that enters the cell is rapidly converted to glucose 6-phosphate. In pancreatic β cells, glucokinase is part of the cells' machinery for detecting the levels of glucose in the blood. The high K_m for glucose allows β cell glucose utilization to vary with alterations in the blood glucose concentration. Because glucokinase activity is optimal at elevated blood glucose concentrations, the rate of glycolytic flux increases with elevated blood glucose, thereby increasing the ATP–ADP ratio. It is postulated that this ratio is involved in the complex signal that controls the rate of insulin secretion from the pancreatic β cell. Both the hepatic and pancreatic glucokinase catalyze the same reaction, but the metabolic function that is served is different in liver and pancreas. Underlying this functional difference is a divergence in expression and regulation of the *GCK* gene.

In humans, the *GCK* gene has two transcription start sites and two alternative splicing patterns that are used differentially in the liver and the pancreatic β cells (Postic et al., 2001. Magnuson and Jetton, 1993). Transcription of the *GCK* gene and processing of the primary transcript proceed differently in these two tissues. These are common regulatory mechanisms that increase the flexibility of gene expression in eukaryotic cells. In this case, two different promoter–regulatory domains are used to determine the transcription rate of the *GCK* gene from the different transcription start sites; these promoters are located at different positions in the 5′ noncoding region of the gene, upstream of their respective transcription start sites. On the basis of liver- and pancreas-specific usage of each promoter, there can be two different start sites for transcription initiation and two different first exons (or expressed sequences) in the primary transcript for *GCK*. Each first exon is linked by alternative splicing to a common second exon during processing in the nucleus of the cell. The remaining exons (2-10) are the same for both the liver and pancreatic forms of *GCK* mRNA. Therefore, different *GCK* mRNAs are produced in the liver and the pancreatic β cell. The translation of these mRNAs results in two glucokinase isoforms that differ in the first 15 amino acids of the protein structure. Altogether, the liver- and pancreas-specific differences in expression of the *GCK* gene involve two different promoter domains, two different start sites of transcription, alternative splicing of the primary transcript, and ultimately two different protein products.

What is the functional significance of this type of tissue-specific variation in expression of the *GCK* gene? This divergence allows for specific tissue responses to hormones and/or nutrients. In liver, but not in the pancreatic β cell, insulin stimulates transcription of the *GCK* gene and glucagon inhibits it. In the pancreatic β cell, but not in liver, expression of the *GCK* gene is responsive to glucose. Therefore there are distinct differences in the regulation of expression of the *GCK* gene in these two tissues. It is the insulin–glucagon ratio that regulates liver glucokinase expression, whereas it is the blood glucose concentration that regulates pancreatic β cell *GCK* expression. Differences between the glucokinase isoforms themselves (e.g., kinetic parameters) remain to be determined (Magnuson and Jetton, 1993). Of clinical significance is the fact that mutations in the *GCK* gene in humans are associated with maturity onset diabetes of the young, type 2 (MODY-2).

EXPRESSION OF THE 6-PHOSPHOFRUCTO-1-KINASE *(PFK)* GENE

6-Phosphofructo-1-kinase catalyzes the first committed step of glycolysis and is involved in the fructose 6-phosphate/fructose 1,6-bisphosphate substrate cycle. In humans, there are three isoenzymes of 6-phosphofructo-1-kinase, each of which is encoded by a separate gene. The expression of the liver form has been examined under conditions of fasting and carbohydrate refeeding. Hepatic *PFK* mRNA levels are increased in response to carbohydrate refeeding after a fast, and this response can be partially blocked by the administration of cAMP. Hepatic *PFK* mRNA levels are also increased in response to insulin treatment of diabetic animals. Therefore, *PFK* mRNA levels in liver appear to be determined by the counterregulatory signals of insulin and glucagon (Granner and Pilkis, 1990). 6-Phosphofructo-1-kinase also is subject to short-term regulation by insulin and glucagon, as discussed previously. In skeletal muscle there are no changes in expression of the *PFK* gene with either diabetes, insulin treatment, or exercise (Vestergaard, 1999).

EXPRESSION OF THE ALDOLASE *(ALDO)* GENES

Aldolase converts fructose 1,6-bisphosphate to glyceraldehyde 3-phosphate in glycolysis. Under intracellular conditions, the aldolase reaction is reversible; therefore, it is active in both glycolysis and gluconeogenesis. Notably, aldolase is also active in fructose catabolism. The aldolase enzyme is made up of four subunits, consisting of different combinations of three subunit types (A, B, and C). Each of the subunits is encoded by a separate gene. The aldolase A subunit is found in most tissues but is most abundant in muscle. The distribution of the aldolase B subunit is more restricted; it is found in liver, kidney proximal tubules, and enterocytes of the small intestine. Aldolase C is present in brain, fetal tissues, and cancer cells.

Of the genes for the three subunits, the aldolase B *(ALDOB)* gene has been the best-characterized (Lemaigre and Rousseau, 1994). The structure of the *ALDOB* gene has been determined for humans and other species. This gene has a single promoter directing aldolase expression in liver, kidney, and the small intestine. The effects of dietary changes, as tested in experimental rats, show that during starvation there is a significant decrease in *ALDOB* mRNA abundance in liver and small intestine, but not in kidney. Refeeding a high-carbohydrate diet returns *ALDOB* mRNA levels to normal. The effect of refeeding on *ALDOB* mRNA can be blocked in liver by glucagon or cAMP. Neither glucagon nor cAMP, however, has this effect in the small intestine. It is interesting that refeeding rats a high-fructose diet increases *ALDOB* mRNA in kidney as well as in liver in diabetic rats. Hereditary fructose intolerance in humans is caused by a deficiency in *ALDOB* that is due to mutations in the *ALDOB* gene. The increased consumption of sucrose and fructose in Western diets probably accounts for the increased recognition of hereditary fructose intolerance as a nutritional disease, as well as increased recognition of the prevalence of the *ALDOB* mutation in the population (Ali et al., 1998). Current evidence shows that mutations in the *ALDOB* gene are relatively common, particularly in Western Europe where more than 1% of the population is heterozygous for one of the 20 known mutations in the *ALDOB* gene (Kullberg-Lindh et al., 2002).

EXPRESSION OF THE GLYCERALDEHYDE 3-PHOSPHATE DEHYDROGENASE *(GAPDH)* GENE

Glyceraldehyde 3-phosphate dehydrogenase catalyzes the conversion of glyceraldehyde 3-phosphate to 1,3-bisphosphoglycerate, with the generation of NADH. The enzyme is a tetramer of four identical subunits encoded by one gene. The tissue distribution of glyceraldehyde 3-phosphate dehydrogenase is ubiquitous; however, the *GAPDH* gene is regulated by nutrients and hormones in a tissue-specific manner (Sirover, 1997). *GAPDH* mRNA levels increase in liver when fasting is followed by carbohydrate refeeding and in adipose tissue in response to insulin treatment. Regulation of the *GAPDH* gene is localized to these lipogenic tissues where *GAPDH* mRNA levels increase in response to elevated blood glucose and insulin.

It should be noted that glyceraldehyde 3-phosphate dehydrogenase also has nonglycolytic functions. Recently it has been shown that glyceraldehyde 3-phosphate dehydrogenase is also present in the nuclei of certain cell types such as neurons in the brain. Glyceraldehyde 3-phosphate dehydrogenase, in this location, has been shown to mediate apoptosis (programmed cell death). Overexpression of the *GAPDH* gene in rats has been shown to initiate apoptotic cascades that may be involved in certain neurodegenerative diseases such as Parkinson's, Huntington's or Alzheimer's disease (Ishitani et al., 2003).

EXPRESSION OF THE PYRUVATE KINASE *(PK)* GENE

Pyruvate kinase catalyzes the conversion of phosphoenolpyruvate to pyruvate in the last enzymatic step of glycolysis. Four pyruvate kinase isoenzymes have been characterized: the M_1 form is the predominant form in muscle, heart, and brain; the M_2 form is found in fetal tissue and in most adult tissues; the L′ (or R) form is the major form in red blood cells; and the L form is the major liver form but is also present in kidney and the small intestine. Two *PK* genes have been isolated that code for the four isoenzymes identified. The *PKLR* and *PKM2* genes encode the L and L′ isoenzymes and the M_1 and M_2 isoenzymes, respectively. The *PKLR* gene has two promoters, which regulate two distinct transcription start sites, generating two unique first exons in the pyruvate kinase transcript. The *PKM2* gene, on the other hand, is alternatively spliced so that the mRNAs contain either the 9th (M_1) or the 10th (M_2) exon, each expressed in the aforementioned tissue-specific manner (Noguchi and Tanaka, 1993).

In liver, regulation of the *PKLR* gene involves both direct nutrient and indirect hormonal effects. Keep in mind that pyruvate kinase is also considered a lipogenic enzyme because in the presence of excess carbohydrate intake, glucose (or fructose) can be converted to fatty acids. As such, the *PK* genes are regulated in a manner similar to other lipogenic genes. Refeeding fasted rats a high-carbohydrate diet increases PK-L mRNA levels in liver, and this stimulation is dependent on the presence of insulin. Dietary fructose also increases PK-L mRNA levels, and it does so more rapidly than does glucose and without the insulin requirement. Glucose stimulation of PK-L mRNA abundance appears to require the catabolism of glucose to glucose 6-phosphate or another downstream metabolite. Therefore in liver, insulin may be required for glucose stimulation of the expression of the *PKLR* gene because it stimulates glucose 6-phosphate production by increasing transcription of the glucokinase gene. Dietary glycerol is also a potent stimulant of the *PKLR* gene in liver. It is possible that a downstream metabolite, common to glucose, fructose, and glycerol, is the regulatory intermediate involved in regulating *PKLR* gene expression.

The first glucose response element to be identified in the promoter region of a gene was in the *PKLR* gene. Two repeated DNA sequences of six nucleotides in length, referred to as "E box motifs," are required for glucose responsiveness of the *PKLR* gene when tested in cell culture or whole animal experimental models (Vaulont and Kahn, 1993). Recently, the transcription factor that binds the E box domains of the *PKLR* gene to signal the presence of increased glucose, or a metabolic intermediate, has been identified. It is referred to as the carbohydrate response element–binding protein (ChREBP). ChREBP is regulated at two different levels: its entry into the nucleus of the cell and its binding to the DNA of the *PKLR* gene. These processes, in turn, are regulated by both glucose and cAMP. There are two functional cAMP-dependent protein kinase phosphorylation sites in ChREBP; phosphorylation of serine residue 196 causes impaired nuclear localization of ChREBP and phosphorylation of threonine residue 666 causes loss of ChREBP DNA binding and activation of *PKLR* gene transcription (Kawaguchi et al., 2001).

PK-L is the predominant mRNA isoform in liver; however, it is also found in kidney and small intestine. All three of these tissues are major sites of fructose metabolism, and liver and kidney are major sites of glycerol metabolism. It stands to reason that PK-L mRNA levels would be regulated by dietary fructose and glycerol in those tissues involved in their metabolism. Consistent with this assumption, refeeding a high-fructose diet to fasted rats increased PK-L mRNA in kidney and in the small intestine, whereas refeeding a high-glycerol diet increased PK-L mRNA in kidney alone. A high-glucose diet did not increase PK-L mRNA in kidney or the small intestine (Noguchi and Tanaka, 1993).

EXPRESSION OF THE PHOSPHOENOLPYRUVATE CARBOXYKINASE *(PCK)* GENE

Countering the activity of pyruvate kinase in liver cytosol is the activity of phosphoenolpyruvate carboxykinase, which determines gluconeogenic flux by catalyzing the conversion of oxaloacetate to phosphoenolpyruvate. A single gene (*PCK1*) encodes the cytosolic enzyme, with one promoter–regulatory domain directing transcription of the gene. This single promoter, however, is composed of a complex network of interrelated DNA response elements that are affected by nutrients, hormones, and tissue-specific transcription factors (Gurney et al., 1994). These direct the expression of the *PCK1* gene at high levels in liver, kidney, and adipose tissue and at lower levels in the intestinal epithelium and mammary gland. In addition to this tissue specificity, there is a cell-specific pattern of *PC1K* mRNA localization in liver. In liver, *PCK1* mRNA is present in highest concentration in the hepatocytes surrounding the portal vein. *PCK1* mRNA is localized to the same periportal cells as phosphoenolpyruvate carboxykinase enzyme activity; therefore, this zonation of enzyme activity appears to be determined at the mRNA level. Other gluconeogenic enzymes and urea cycle enzymes share this periportal distribution.

Expression of the *PC1K* gene is highly regulated by diet and hormones. It is well known that fasting increases *PCK1* mRNA levels, and that refeeding a high-carbohydrate diet decreases *PCK1* mRNA abundance (Hanson and Reshef, 1997). In the fasted state, both the transcription rate of the *PCK1* gene and the stability of the *PCK1* mRNA are increased by cAMP. PPARγ coactivator (PGC-1) is a critical activator of *PCK1* gene expression and of gluconeogenesis overall (Rhee et al., 2003; Yoon et al., 2001) PGC-1 is induced synergistically by the combined action of cAMP and glucocorticoids. PGC-1 interacts with, and coactivates, both the glucocorticoid receptor and the liver-specific transcription factor HNF-4α (hepatic nuclear factor-4α) to mediate increased *PCK1* gene expression (Yoon et al., 2001). Carbohydrate refeeding, which increases the insulin level in the blood, decreases the transcription rate of the *PCK1* gene, probably mediated by active PI 3-kinase (Sutherland et al., 1996). Insulin is the dominant negative regulator of *PCK1* gene expression and will inhibit cAMP- or glucocorticoid-stimulated increases in the rate of transcription of this gene. However, glucose alone decreases *PCK1* mRNA levels by decreasing the transcription rate and the stability of the mRNA in hepatocytes cultured in the absence of insulin (Kahn et al., 1989). Therefore the inhibition of *PCK1* gene expression imposed by refeeding a high-carbohydrate diet may be due, in part, to a direct effect of glucose or a metabolite of glucose on the *PCK1* promoter.

Both the *PCK1* and glucose 6-phosphatase *(G6PC)* genes are negatively regulated by insulin. Recently, it has been shown that both of the genes encoding these enzymes have a DNA response element in common in their respective promoter–regulatory regions referred to as an insulin response element (IRE). Sutherland and colleagues have shown that glycogen synthase kinase 3 is an essential component in the signaling pathway between the insulin signal and the IREs of both genes (Finlay et al., 2004, Lochhead et al., 2001). Another important potential mediator of insulin regulation of the *PCK1* gene is the liver X receptor that is involved in carbohydrate and lipid metabolism in liver and other tissues. LXR (liver X receptor) has been shown to mediate the inhibition of all three gluconeogenic genes: those encoding phosphoenolpyruvate carboxykinase *(PCK1)*, fructose 1,6-bisphosphatase, and glucose 6-phosphatase *(G6PC)*. Furthermore, LXR agonists have been shown to decrease plasma glucose in diabetic rats (Steffensen and Gustafsson, 2004).

EXPRESSION OF THE GLUCOSE 6-PHOSPHATASE *(G6PC)* GENE

Glucose 6-phosphatase catalyzes the terminal reaction in both the gluconeogenic and the glycogenolytic pathways—the conversion of glucose 6-phosphate to free glucose. As indicated previously, the enzyme activity is conferred by the action of three separate enzymes. The gene for the catalytic subunit *(G6PC)* has been isolated and partially characterized. The rate of transcription of the gene for the catalytic subunit of glucose 6-phosphatase is increased by glucocorticoids, and both basal and glucocorticoid-stimulated transcription are inhibited by insulin. The promoter for the *G6PC* gene contains an insulin response element, similar to the *PCK1* promoter. It is likely that the two genes are coordinately regulated either to increase or decrease hepatic glucose output (Streeper et al., 1997). In addition to the aforementioned role of glycogen synthase kinase 3 in mediating the coordinated insulin response of the *G6PC* and *PCK1* genes, there is evidence that insulin controls the expression of the *G6PC* gene via the transcription factor FOXO1a that is regulated by protein kinase B (Orth et al., 2004). The counterregulatory mechanism that is induced by the glucagon/cAMP signal involves transcription factors activated by cAMP-dependent protein kinase A phosphorylation as well as recruitment of the coactivator CBP (cAMP-response element binding protein [CREB] binding protein) to cAMP response elements in the promoter/regulatory domain of the *G6PC* gene (Gautier-Stein et al., 2005).

EXPRESSION OF THE 6-PHOSPHOFRUCTO-2-KINASE/ FRUCTOSE 2,6-BIPHOSPHATASE *(PFKFB)* GENE

The bifunctional enzyme 6-phosphofructo-2-kinase/fructose 2,6-bisphosphatase catalyzes both the synthesis and breakdown of the allosteric regulator fructose 2,6-bisphosphate. There are different 6-phosphofructo-2-kinase/fructose 2,6-bisphosphatase isoenzymes, which have specific catalytic properties, tissue distributions, and responses to regulatory molecules. Four genes have been identified in mammals encoding the different isoenzymes; they are called *PFKFB1* (liver/muscle isoenzyme), *PFKFB2* (heart isoenzyme), *PFKFB3* (brain/placenta isoenzyme), and *PFKFB4* (testis isoenzyme) (Rider et al., 2004). Each of the *PFKFB* genes are located on different chromosomes. The *PFKFB1* gene contains three promoters (L, M, and F) in its 5′ regulatory sequence. The L promoter is active in liver, adipose tissue, and skeletal muscle; the M promoter is active in a number of tissues and is predominant in muscle; and the F-type promoter is active primarily in fetal tissues, fibroblasts, and proliferating cells. In the fasted state, glucagon inhibits transcription from the L promoter of the *PFKFB1* gene and decreases the stability of the L-type mRNA. Refeeding (or insulin treatment of a diabetic) increases *PFKFB1* mRNA levels in liver within 24 to 48 hours (Lemaigre and Rousseau, 1994). Insulin and glucocorticoids control the *PFKFB1* gene via a glucocorticoid response unit (GRU) located in the first intron of the coding sequence of the gene (rather than the upstream promoter–regulatory domain). Glucocorticoids stimulate the nuclear glucocorticoid receptor, whereas insulin inhibits this stimulation. Glucose also has a positive stimulatory effect on the L promoter of the *PFKFB1* gene although the transcription factors involved in the glucose effect have not been identified (Rider et al., 2004). Nutrient and hormonal conditions that increase the amount of *PFKFB1* mRNA, also increase the amount of enzyme and increase the hepatic levels of fructose 2,6-bisphosphate, whereas those conditions that decrease *PFKFB1* mRNA and protein levels decrease hepatic fructose 2,6-bisphosphate levels.

GLUCOSE REGULATION OF TARGET GENES

In the liver, under physiological conditions, insulin and glucose together are involved in regulating the expression of metabolic genes when nutritional conditions change, such as in the fasted-to-fed transition. Genes encoding enzymes of carbohydrate metabolism that are upregulated in the fasted-to-fed transition are *GCK* and *PK-L* and those that are downregulated are *PCK1* and *G6PC*. Lipogenic and ketogenic genes are regulated as well. Experimentally, when the insulin signal is separated from increased glucose concentrations, certain genes were directly regulated by insulin, others by insulin and glucose, and others by glucose alone. In glycolysis, *GCK* is regulated by insulin, whereas *PK-L* is regulated by glucose. In gluconeogenesis, *PCK1* is regulated by insulin and glucose, whereas *G6PC* is regulated by insulin alone. However, the effect of glucose alone on gene expression requires insulin-stimulated glucokinase activity and, therefore, the production of glucose-6-P, making insulin permissive for the effects of glucose on the previously mentioned metabolic genes.

LIVER COMPARTMENTALIZATION OF GLUCONEOGENIC ENZYMES

In liver, the catabolism of glucose via glycolysis occurs at a low rate under aerobic conditions when glucose levels in the blood are not high. Gluconeogenesis, on the other hand, is carried out at a higher rate. It is interesting that there is a gradient of gluconeogenic enzyme activity, compartmentalized to different zones in the liver. These zones arise in functional subdivisions of the liver that are defined by the microcirculation of the tissue. The smallest functional unit of the liver is the acinus, and each acinus is circumscribed by terminal hepatic veins at the periphery and a terminal portal vein and terminal hepatic artery at the center (Fig. 12-11). The portal vein supplies approximately 70% of the blood that comes to the liver, and the hepatic artery supplies the rest.

The hepatocytes that surround the incoming portal venule are referred to as periportal cells, and those that surround the outgoing central venule are referred to as perivenous cells. Distinct metabolic zones occur between these regions of afferent and efferent blood flow (Jungermann, 1992). At the proximal side of the circulatory supply to the liver acinus, the cells are receiving oxygen and nutrient-rich blood from the portal vein and hepatic artery. As the blood traverses the cell population, it becomes relatively depleted of oxygen and dietary nutrients as it moves toward the hepatic central vein. It is generally accepted that the activity of gluconeogenic and urea cycle enzymes is higher in hepatocytes at the periportal side of the liver acinus. There is some debate as to whether the limited glycolysis that occurs in liver is more predominant in perivenous cells or is less compartmentalized overall than is gluconeogenesis. Because perivenous cells receive blood with a somewhat lower oxygen tension than do periportal hepatocytes, perivenous cells are thought to be more dependent upon glycolysis. It is documented that the low K_m glucose transporter GLUT1 is localized to a layer of cells surrounding the hepatic venule. The high affinity of GLUT1 for glucose assures that perivenous cells take up glucose to provide for increased glycolysis. GLUT2, on the other hand, is distributed evenly across the liver acinus.

The compartmentalization of specific enzymes and transporters of glucose metabolism appears to be due to localized gene expression. The pattern of gene expression and compartmentalization changes with alterations in dietary state. For example, the periportal to perivenous ratios of the activities of phosphoenolpyruvate carboxykinase, fructose

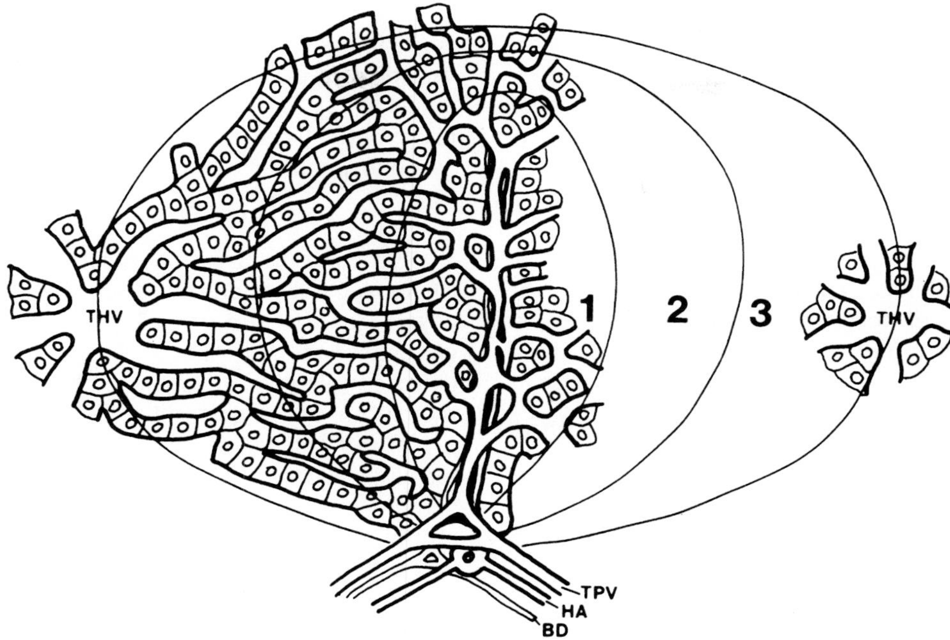

Figure 12-11 Hepatic acinus. This three-dimensional structure is the microvascular unit of hepatic parenchyma. The acinar axis is formed by the terminal portal venule (TPV), the hepatic arteriole (HA), and the bile ductule (BD). The perfusion of this unit is unidirectional from the acinar axis to the acinar periphery where two or more terminal hepatic venules (THV) empty the acinus. The arbitrary division of the acinus into functional zones is represented by 1 (periportal), 2, and 3 (perivenous). *(From Gumucio, JJ, Chianale J [1988] Liver cell heterogeneity and liver function. In: Arias IM, Jakoby WB, Popper H, Schachter D, Shafritz DA [eds] The Liver: Biology and Pathobiology, 2nd ed. Raven Press, New York, pp 931-947.)*

1,6-bisphosphatase, and glucose 6-phosphatase decrease with fasting. These decreases in the periportal to perivenous ratios are due to increases in gluconeogenic enzyme activity in the perivenous cells during a fast, when total hepatic glucose output increases. Under these conditions, gluconeogenesis is activated in the larger hepatocyte population, and compartmentalization is decreased.

GLYCOGEN METABOLISM

Glucose is stored in liver and muscle tissue as glycogen, a branched-chain polymer of glucose. In humans, liver has the capacity to store glycogen up to approximately 10% of its weight. Skeletal muscle, on the other hand, has a more limited capacity to store glycogen, to approximately 1% of its weight. In humans, the overall mass of skeletal muscle is greater than that of liver, so total muscle glycogen is approximately double the amount of liver glycogen. Glycogen is stored in the postprandial state for future use when glucose levels decrease in the blood. When blood glucose levels decline, the body's first line of defense is to degrade hepatic glycogen to its individual glucose units via glycogenolysis. Glucose 6-phosphate derived from glycogenolysis has different fates in liver and skeletal muscle. The liver secretes glucose to the blood to maintain circulating blood levels for those tissues that are dependent upon glucose for energy. Skeletal muscle, on the other hand, utilizes glucose 6-phosphate produced by glycogenolysis for glycolysis and ATP production within the same cell.

GLYCOGEN SYNTHESIS

The glycogen polymer is a linear array of glucose residues linked by $\alpha 1 \rightarrow 4$-glycosidic bonds, with branch points in $\alpha 1 \rightarrow 6$-glycosidic linkage. The branching structure of the molecule is not random; branch points occur approximately every fourth glucose residue along the linear chains of the polymer. The series of enzymes that catalyze the steps of glycogen synthesis are responsible for the specificity of this structure.

The first enzymatic reaction in glycogen synthesis from glucose is the same as that in glycolysis, the glucokinase reaction in liver, or the hexokinase reaction in skeletal muscle. The product of these reactions, glucose 6-phosphate, is further metabolized to glucose 1-phosphate by the action of phosphoglucomutase.

$$\text{Glucose 6-Phosphate} \longleftrightarrow \text{Glucose 1-Phosphate}$$

The third reaction in this series prepares glucose for storage as glycogen. This reaction is catalyzed by glucose 1-phosphate uridylyltransferase.

$$\text{Glucose 1-Phosphate} + \text{UTP} \rightarrow \text{UDP-Glucose} + PP_i$$

This is an energy-requiring step, but it is made essentially irreversible by the hydrolysis of one of the end products, pyrophosphate (PP_i), to two molecules of inorganic phosphate. This reaction is catalyzed by pyrophosphatase:

$$PP_i + H_2O \rightarrow 2\ P_i$$

Glycogen synthase catalyzes the addition of single glucosyl residues to a growing polymer of glycogen. The substrates for this reaction are glycogen and UDP-glucose (Fig. 12-12). The glucose moiety is added to the glycogen polymer in an $\alpha1\rightarrow4$-glycosidic linkage between C-1 of the "activated" glucose and C-4 of the terminal glucose of a linear chain of the glycogen polymer. For each new glycogen molecule, a primer is required for the attachment of the first molecule of glucose. The protein glycogenin serves this function; the first glucose moiety in a nascent chain is attached to a specific tyrosine residue in glycogenin. Glycogen

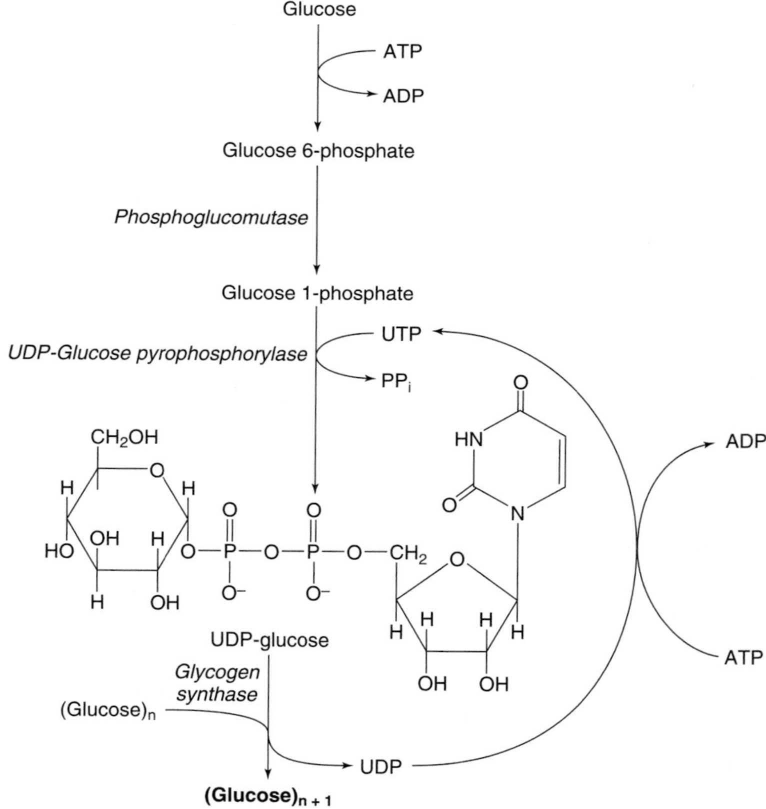

Figure 12-12 Addition of glucosyl residues to the linear $\alpha1\rightarrow4$-linked chains of glycogen.

synthase then forms a complex with glucose-bound glycogenin, and extension of the polysaccharide chain is autocatalyzed by the glucosyltransferase activity of glycogenin until the linear glycogen chain reaches 8 units in length (Smythe and Cohen, 1991). The nascent glycogen chain then becomes the substrate for glycogen synthase. The glycogen synthase reaction can be represented as follows:

$$(\text{Glucose})_n + \text{UDP-Glucose} \rightarrow (\text{Glucose})_{n+1} + \text{UDP}$$

Because of the UTP requirement for glycogen synthesis, an "ATP" equivalent is required for the glycogen synthase reaction. When added to the ATP used in the glucokinase reaction, this generates an overall energy expenditure of two molecules of ATP for the addition of one glucose unit to the glycogen polymer.

Glycogen synthase specifically catalyzes the addition of the glucose moiety in the $\alpha 1 \rightarrow 4$ orientation; it is not involved in branching, which is the formation of an $\alpha 1 \rightarrow 6$-glycosidic bond. A second enzyme, 1,4-α-glucan branching enzyme, is involved in the formation of branch points in the growing glycogen polymer. This branching enzyme catalyzes the transfer of an oligosaccharide chain of approximately seven glucose residues from the nonreducing end (the outer terminal glucosyl residue) of a linear glycogen segment to an interior C-6 of a glucose residue at least 4 units away from the last branch site, thereby creating a new branch (Fig. 12-13).

ROLE OF GLUCONEOGENESIS IN GLYCOGEN FORMATION

There is an interesting paradox in the synthesis of glycogen in liver. A significant amount of glycogen synthesis in liver is dependent on gluconeogenically derived substrate rather than on glucose entering the hepatocyte directly by facilitated transport. Gluconeogenically derived glucose 6-phosphate in liver is utilized for glycogen synthesis even in the fed state when blood glucose is elevated. In contrast, muscle cells directly utilize glucose for synthesis of glycogen.

In humans, approximately one third of the glucose 6-phosphate utilized for glycogen synthesis in liver is gluconeogenically derived. It is postulated that the indirect route of glycogen synthesis in liver utilizes lactate from extrahepatic tissues such as skeletal muscle and red blood cells. In the absorptive phase, it appears that a certain amount of dietary glucose may be metabolized to lactate in peripheral tissues, with the lactate being recirculated to the liver where it becomes a substrate for gluconeogenesis. In the absorptive state, other substrates present in the portal blood, such as amino acids and glycerol, are also potential sources of gluconeogenic carbon for glycogen synthesis.

GLYCOGENOLYSIS

The glycogen polymer may contain as many as 100,000 glucose units in its branched-chain structure. In humans, the liver is completely depleted of glycogen by 24 hours of fasting. The degradation of this complex molecule begins at the nonreducing ends of the multiple branches and involves the phosphorolysis of single glucose units by glycogen phosphorylase.

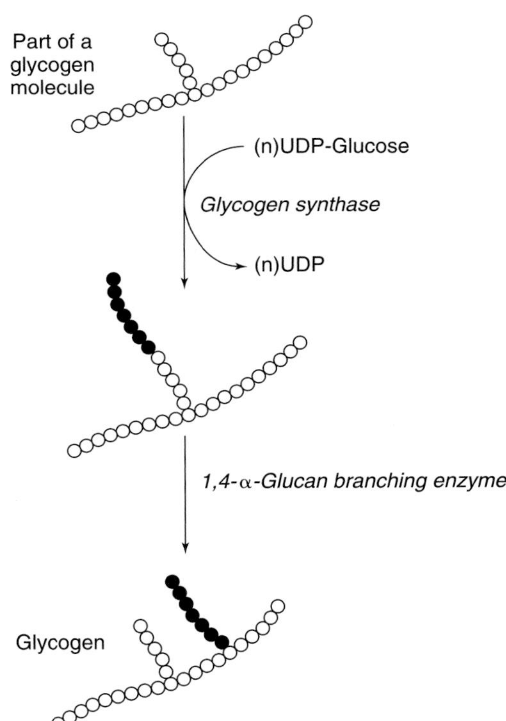

Figure 12-13 Pictorial illustration of the growth of glycogen chains and the role of the branching enzyme in the translocation of linear segments of growing chains to create $\alpha 1 \rightarrow 6$-linkages and, hence, new branch points.

Clinical Correlation

Glycogen Storage Diseases

A lack of glucose 6-phosphatase in liver, kidney, and intestinal mucosa causes Von Gierke's disease (Type I glycogen storage disease). This is caused by a genetic defect in the glucose 6-phosphatase gene that occurs as an autosomal recessive trait in 1 of 200,000 people. This deficiency usually presents in early infancy, and the symptoms include fasting hypoglycemia, hepatomegaly, and recurrent acidosis (Dunger and Holton, 1994). A genetic defect in either the glucose 6-phosphatase enzyme (Type Ia), the glucose 6-phosphatase translocase (Type Ib), or the pyrophosphate transporter (Type Ic) can occur. Individuals with this disease lack the ability to respond to low blood glucose by releasing glucose from either glycogenolysis or gluconeogenesis. This particularly affects the liver's ability to maintain glucose balance in the body by releasing glucose from either of the latter two metabolic sources. The symptoms of this disease can be modified by providing dietary carbohydrate throughout the day so that low blood glucose does not occur.

Tissue-specific mutations in both the liver and muscle glycogen phosphorylase genes occur as rare autosomal recessive disorders. In liver, the metabolic disorder is called Hers' disease (Type VI) and presents in childhood. In this condition, liver glycogen accumulates because the first step in the degradation of glycogen is impaired. Clinical symptoms of this disorder include hypoglycemia, hepatomegaly (which develops slowly), and some growth delay (Fernandes and Chen, 1995). In muscle, the metabolic disorder is referred to as McArdle's disease (Type V), which usually presents in adult life. In early adult life, progressive muscle weakness occurs; however, hepatomegaly and fasting hypoglycemia do not. Individuals with this disease accumulate glycogen in muscle tissue and are exercise intolerant because glucose cannot be released from glycogen to meet the energy demand. There are also genetic disorders in the phosphorylase kinase gene that lead to phosphorylase kinase deficiency in liver and muscle. Phosphorylase kinase deficiency is more common than phosphorylase deficiency and is inherited as an X chromosome–linked recessive trait. Symptoms associated with this disorder are similar to those for phosphorylase deficiency.

A mutation in the gene that encodes "debranching enzyme" can occur in the liver or as a mixed liver–muscle defect. The disorder is referred to as Cori's disease (Type III). Cori's disease leads to the accumulation of glycogen in liver and muscle in the form of branched short chains. Cori's disease usually presents in infancy with symptoms of fasting hypoglycemic convulsions, hepatomegaly, and myopathy (Dunger and Holton, 1994). However, the hypoglycemia and hepatomegaly usually abate by puberty.

Thinking Critically

1. Explain the underlying metabolic basis for development of (a) hypoglycemia, (b) lactic acidosis, and (c) hypertriglyceridemia in patients with glycogen storage disease Type I.
2. What effect does treatment of patients with glycogen storage disease Type I by providing carbohydrate throughout the day (and during the night via infusion of carbohydrate into the gut through a nasogastric tube) have on the overproduction of lactate and triacylglycerol? Explain.

In the glycogen phosphorylase reaction, an $\alpha1\rightarrow4$-glycosidic bond is attacked by inorganic phosphate (P_i), generating glucose 1-phosphate and a shortened glycogen polymer (Fig. 12-14).

$$(\text{Glucose})_n + P_i \rightarrow (\text{Glucose})_{n-1} + \text{Glucose 1-Phosphate}$$

The phosphorylase reaction is repeated successively until the fourth glucose unit from a branch point is reached. Then the bifunctional debranching enzyme (4-α-D-glucano-transferase/amylo-α ($1\rightarrow6$)glucosidase) comes into play. It catalyzes the transfer of three of the four glucose units to the closest nonreducing

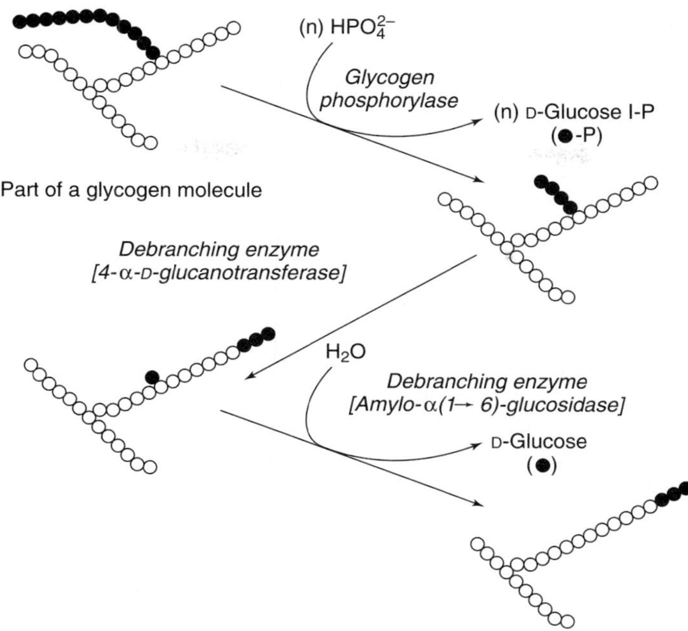

Figure 12-14 Pictorial illustration of the breakdown of glycogen by glycogen phosphorylase and the activities of the debranching enzyme.

end to which they are attached in a new α1→4-glycosidic linkage. The debranching enzyme also has α1→6-glucosidase activity and removes the remaining glucose by hydrolysis of the α1→6 linkage at the branch point; this glucosyl residue is released as free glucose (see Fig. 12-14). The remaining linear array is now the substrate for continued glycogen phosphorylase activity.

The product of the glycogen phosphorylase reaction, glucose 1-phosphate, is converted to glucose 6-phosphate by phosphoglucomutase. In muscle tissue, the glucose 6-phosphate produced in this reaction is broken down via the glycolytic pathway. In liver, where there is significant glucose 6-phosphatase activity, and glycolysis is inhibited under the hormonal conditions that favor hepatic glycogenolysis, most glucose 6-phosphate is converted to free glucose, which is transported from the cell.

REGULATION OF GLYCOGENESIS AND GLYCOGENOLYSIS

The regulatory mechanisms affecting glycogen synthesis and degradation have been well characterized. Glycogen synthase and glycogen phosphorylase are the hormonally regulated enzymes in glycogen synthesis and degradation, respectively. The anabolic hormone insulin stimulates glycogen synthesis in liver and muscle in the absorptive state. Glucagon, on the other hand, stimulates glycogen degradation in liver when blood glucose levels decline. Epinephrine promotes glycogen degradation in both the liver and skeletal muscle. In the liver, both β-adrenergic and α-adrenergic receptors mediate the response to epinephrine via different signal-transduction mechanisms. In skeletal muscle there are no glucagon receptors, but β-adrenergic receptors are stimulated by epinephrine, inducing the cAMP cascade of signaling events. Neural control of glycogen degradation is also important in skeletal muscle.

REGULATION OF GLYCOGEN SYNTHASE

Glycogen synthase is present in the cell in two different forms; the active form (*a*) is active in the absence of the allosteric modifier, glucose 6-phosphate, and the inactive form (*b*) is dependent on glucose 6-phosphate for activity. Covalent modification of glycogen synthase by phosphorylation converts the enzyme from the *a* to the *b* form. Glycogen synthase is a substrate for numerous protein kinases, including the cAMP-dependent protein kinase A. The various protein kinases are activated as the result of different intracellular signal transduction pathways responding to different hormonal and nutrient signals. In addition to protein kinase A, the following protein kinases phosphorylate glycogen synthase: phosphorylase kinase, which itself is phosphorylated by protein kinase A; the calmodulin-dependent protein kinase, which is regulated by calcium binding to calmodulin (see subsequent text in this section); protein kinase C, which is activated by diacylglycerol; and glycogen synthase kinase-3 and casein kinases I and II, which are signal transduction enzymes with unidentified stimuli as related to glycogen synthase inhibition. Interestingly, glycogen synthase kinase-3 has been shown to have numerous effects on cellular function, independent of its role in the phosphorylation of glycogen synthase. Glycogen synthase kinase-3 has a role in cell structure and function, as well as cell survival. Furthermore, glycogen synthase kinase-3 has been implicated in the metabolic dysregulation that occurs in type 2 diabetes and Alzheimer's disease (Jope and Johnson, 2004).

Each of these protein kinases can convert glycogen synthase *a* to glycogen synthase *b* (Fig. 12-15). The reciprocal regulation of both

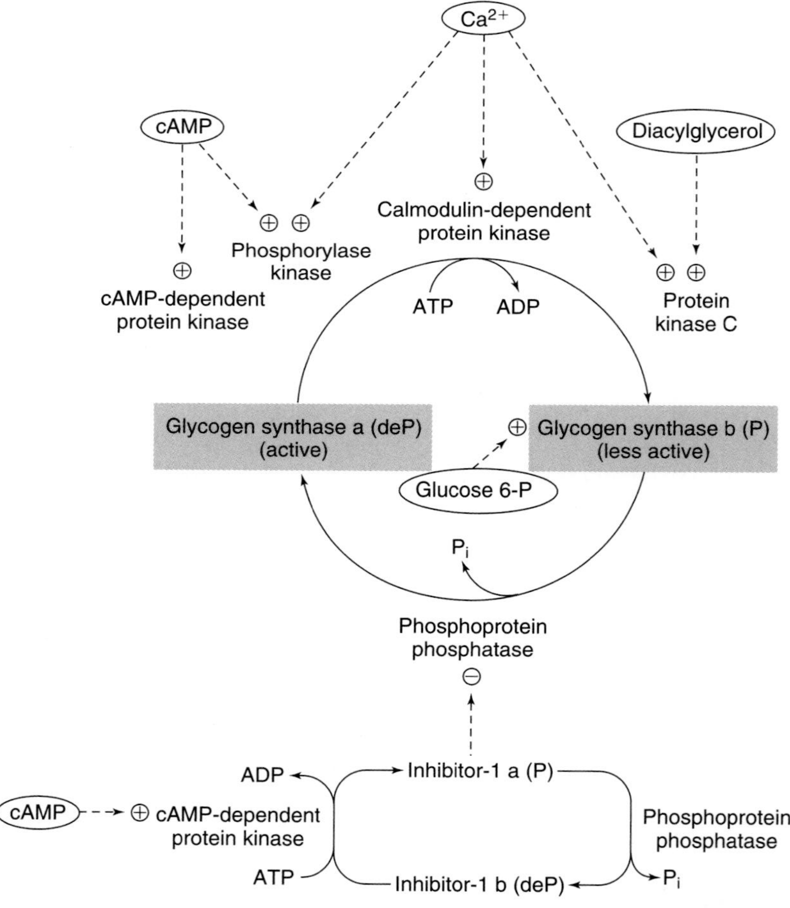

Figure 12-15 Regulation of glycogen synthase by hormone-induced second messenger and intracellular Ca^{2+} concentrations. Phosphorylated and dephosphorylated proteins are indicated by (P) and (deP), respectively.

glycogen synthase and glycogen phosphorylase, however, is modulated primarily in response to changes in the intracellular concentration of cAMP and the activation of protein kinase A. In liver, both glucagon receptors and β-adrenergic receptors activate adenylate cyclase and induce the cAMP response; in skeletal muscle, β-adrenergic receptors are responsible for adenylate cyclase activation and increased cAMP production.

Glycogen synthase is dephosphorylated and converted back to the *a* form by the enzyme phosphoprotein phosphatase. This enzyme, in turn, is regulated by inhibitor-1, present in certain tissues and well-characterized in skeletal muscle. The inhibitor decreases phosphoprotein phosphatase activity, thereby maintaining glycogen synthase in the inactive phosphorylated state. Inhibitor-1, itself, is also a substrate for protein kinase A and phosphoprotein phosphatase; it is active in the phosphorylated state and inactive in the dephosphorylated state (see Fig. 12-15). Therefore cAMP is involved in another activation-inhibition cycle in muscle tissue. When glucagon levels rise, cAMP levels increase, protein kinase A is activated, and glycogen synthase is phosphorylated and converted to the inactive *b* form. At the same time, inhibitor-1 is activated by phosphorylation and inhibits phosphoprotein phosphatase. The inhibition of phosphoprotein phosphatase activity maintains glycogen synthase in the *b* form. Therefore, both phosphorylation of glycogen synthase and of inhibitor-1 contribute to the "turning off" of glycogen synthase.

REGULATION OF GLYCOGEN PHOSPHORYLASE

Glycogen phosphorylase is subject to covalent modification by phosphorylation and allosteric activation by AMP and inhibition by ATP (Fig. 12-16). In skeletal muscle, glycogen phosphorylase has an active form, phosphorylase *a*, and an inactive form, phosphorylase *b*. Phosphorylation at a single serine residue causes a conformational change to the phosphorylase *a* form. AMP can stimulate glycogen phosphorylase *b*, but not the active glycogen phosphorylase *a*. Overall, in skeletal muscle, the rate of glycogen breakdown depends on the ratio of phosphorylase *a* to phosphorylase *b*. In this tissue, the glucose 1-phosphate produced by the action of glycogen phosphorylase is converted to glucose 6-phosphate and metabolized by the glycolytic pathway to produce ATP for muscle contraction.

The phosphorylation of glycogen phosphorylase is catalyzed by phosphorylase kinase. This protein kinase, itself, is phosphorylated by protein kinase A in response to increased intracellular cAMP. The intracellular cAMP level is increased in skeletal muscle cells in response to epinephrine. The overall effect is that of a protein kinase cascade that leads to the activation of glycogen phosphorylase. In the presence of cAMP, inhibitor-1 is phosphorylated and active; it inhibits phosphoprotein phosphatase, thereby preventing dephosphorylation of glycogen phosphorylase to its less active form.

Phosphorylase kinase is also regulated by a Ca^{2+}-calmodulin regulatory mechanism. Phosphorylase kinase has a complex molecular structure and consists of four subunits. The γ subunit is catalytic, and the α, β, and δ subunits are regulatory. The α and β subunits are phosphorylated by protein kinase A in the activation process. The δ subunit is a Ca^{2+}-binding protein, calmodulin. Calmodulin is an intracellular Ca^{2+} receptor, and it is found in different locations in the cell, either unbound or in association with different enzymes. The calmodulin subunit of phosphorylase kinase binds Ca^{2+} when there is Ca^{2+} influx into the cytosol of the cell. This induces a conformational change that activates phosphorylase kinase. Phosphorylation of the α and β subunits by protein kinase A makes phosphorylase kinase more sensitive to further stimulation by calcium. Maximal activation of phosphorylase kinase is achieved by phosphorylation of the α and β subunits, plus calcium binding to the calmodulin subunit.

The importance of this regulation can be seen in skeletal muscle cells, where nerve impulses in muscle contraction depolarize the cell membrane and stimulate calcium efflux from the sarcoplasmic reticulum to the cytosol. The efflux of calcium stimulates phosphorylase kinase by calcium binding to the calmodulin subunit. At the same time, epinephrine

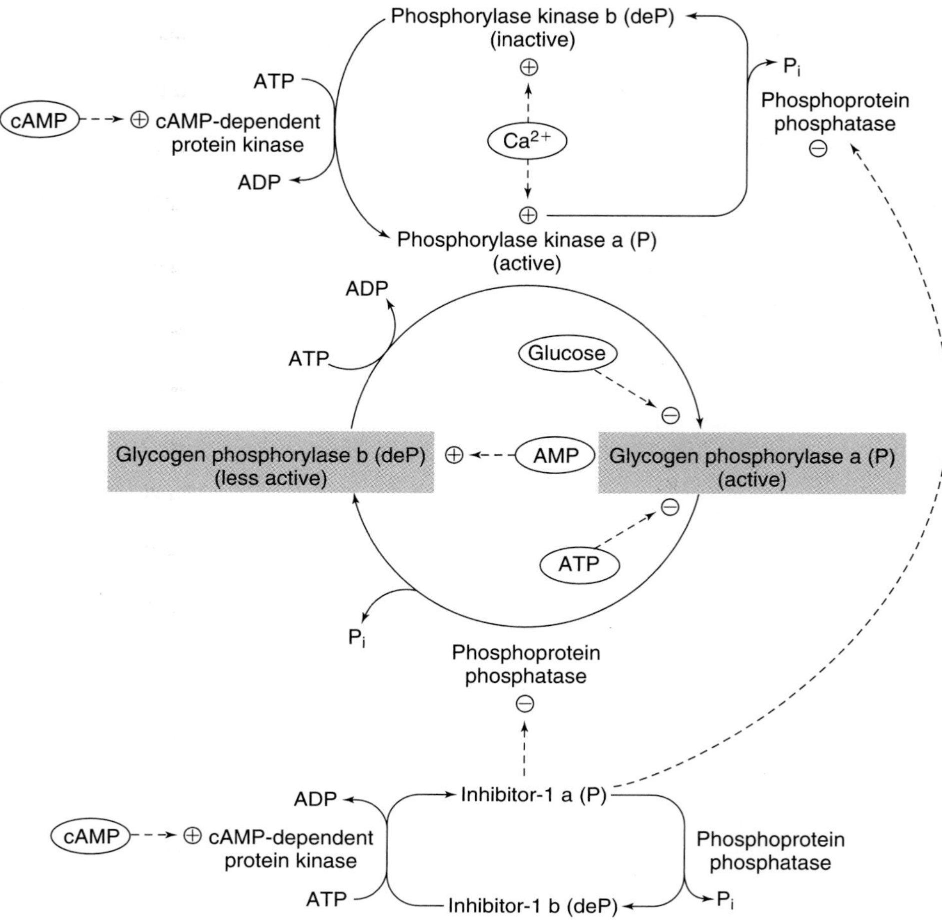

Figure 12-16 Regulation of glycogen phosphorylase in muscle in response to cAMP and intracellular Ca^{2+} concentrations. Phosphorylated and dephosphorylated proteins are indicated by (P) and (deP), respectively.

released from the adrenal medulla stimulates the intracellular cAMP cascade, which leads to phosphorylation of the α and β subunits of phosphorylase kinase. The synergistic effects of Ca^{2+} and cAMP maximally stimulate phosphorylase kinase. Phosphorylase kinase, in turn, activates glycogen phosphorylase and thereby increases the rate of glycogen breakdown. This assures that glucose is available to meet the increased fuel demands of muscle contraction. Concurrently, Ca^{2+} stimulates the calmodulin-dependent protein kinase, which phosphorylates and inhibits the anabolic enzyme glycogen synthase.

Allosteric modification of glycogen phosphorylase by ATP and AMP is a faster mechanism (milliseconds) of regulation than is hormone-induced covalent modification (seconds to minutes). In general, these two mechanisms function in an ordered sequence. For example, in muscle contraction, glycogen phosphorylase *b*, but not glycogen phosphorylase *a*, is allosterically stimulated by AMP. When resting muscle begins to contract and AMP levels increase, this rapidly stimulates phosphorylase *b*. As muscle contraction continues, however, epinephrine stimulation of the cAMP-induced protein kinase cascade increases the concentration of phosphorylase *a*, thereby continuing the breakdown of glycogen regardless of the AMP concentration. Conversely, in the resting state, the phosphorylase *b* form predominates and ATP levels are high. Under these conditions, ATP inhibits any AMP stimulation of phosphorylase *b*, and there is no stimulation of phosphorylase *a* formation by epinephrine. Therefore, when muscle is at rest, glycogenolysis is inactive.

In the liver, glycogen breakdown serves a different metabolic function than it does in muscle tissue. Glycogenolysis provides glucose for release into the circulation to maintain normal blood glucose levels (4 to 5 mmol/L). Glycogenolysis, therefore, is regulated somewhat differently in liver than in muscle tissue. Although there is an *a* and a *b* form of glycogen phosphorylase in liver, as in muscle, the hormonal stimulus for this conversion is primarily glucagon. Furthermore, in liver, glycogen phosphorylase is allosterically regulated by glucose and not by the AMP/ATP ratio. In hepatocytes, glucose can bind to an allosteric site on phosphorylase *a* and change the conformation of the enzyme so that it becomes a good substrate for phosphoprotein phosphatase. Glucose, therefore, stimulates the dephosphorylation of phosphorylase *a* to phosphorylase *b* in liver. This regulatory mechanism ensures that glycogenolysis will be slowed under conditions of elevated blood glucose.

Although glucagon is the major hormonal stimuli for hepatic glycogenolysis, epinephrine can also stimulate the mobilization of glycogen in liver. In humans, this response involves either epinephrine stimulation of the pancreatic α cells to secrete glucagon, or the binding of epinephrine to β-adrenergic receptors on liver cells to stimulate adenylate cyclase and increase intracellular cAMP. A third mechanism of epinephrine action involves epinephrine binding to α1-adrenergic receptors on liver cells. Activation of the α1-adrenergic receptor stimulates phospholipase C on the cytoplasmic face of the plasma membrane by a GTP-binding protein mechanism. Phospholipase C cleaves phosphatidylinositol bisphosphate (PIP_2), present in the membrane, to inositol triphosphate (IP_3) and diacylglycerol. Diacylglycerol, in turn, stimulates protein kinase C. Protein kinase C has numerous substrates in the cell; among these is glycogen synthase a, which is inactivated by phosphorylation. At the same time, IP_3 stimulates the release of Ca^{2+} from the ER, and calcium efflux activates phosphorylase kinase, which activates glycogen phosphorylase. The combined effect of the second messengers derived from PIP_2 is the enhancement of glycogenolysis in response to epinephrine in liver. It is not known, however, which of the preceding mechanisms of epinephrine stimulation of hepatic glycogenolysis is physiologically predominant in humans.

REGULATION OF GENE EXPRESSION

There is less information on the genes that encode the enzymes of glycogen synthesis and degradation than there is on certain of the glycolytic and gluconeogenic genes. The genes for glycogen synthase *(GYS)*, glycogen phosphorylase *(PYG)*, glycogen synthase kinase 3 *(GSK3)*, and the phosphorylase kinase *(PHK)* catalytic subunit have been isolated. Regulation of these genes has been studied to a limited extent. Starvation significantly decreases hepatic glycogen synthase concentration in an experimental rat model, whereas refeeding returns the glycogen synthase concentration to control values. This is thought to be due to changes in *GYS2* mRNA translation; *GYS2* mRNA levels do not change significantly with starvation and refeeding. There are three isoforms of glycogen phosphorylase and each is encoded by a separate gene for liver, muscle, and brain: *PYGL*, *PYGM*, and *PYGB*, respectively (Lockyer and McCracken, 1991). Of these, the *PYGM* gene has been the best characterized, and transcription factors that regulate the *PYGM* promoter have been identified (Ferrer-Martinez et al., 2004). The *PYGL* gene has been shown to be regulated by chronic diabetes and insulin treatment. *PYGL* mRNA stability and abundance are decreased by the diabetic state and can be normalized by insulin treatment (Rao et al., 1995). The gene that encodes the catalytic subunit (gamma) of phosphorylase kinase, *PHKG*, is highly regulated in a tissue-specific manner. In muscle, the expression of the *PHKG* determines the rate of expression of the genes encoding the regulatory subunits of *PHK* (O'Mahony and Walsh, 2002). This ensures that all of the subunits are expressed in a coordinated way such that production of excess free catalytic subunit, which would cause excess glycogen breakdown, is prevented.

Currently, there is a focus on the role of *GSK3* in a number of disease states, including insulin resistance and type 2 diabetes. Although *GS* expression is not changed in skeletal muscle of persons with type 2 diabetes, *GSK3* expression is increased, thereby altering the glycogen synthase–glycogen synthase kinase 3 ratio in type 2 diabetic muscle. Higher levels of glycogen synthase kinase 3 would favor greater inhibition of glycogen synthase and, therefore, decreased glycogen storage in skeletal muscle of persons with type 2 diabetes (Nikoulina et al., 2002).

PYRUVATE DEHYDROGENASE COMPLEX AND CITRIC ACID CYCLE

The aerobic phase of macronutrient catabolism is referred to as cellular respiration. The metabolic stages involved in cellular respiration are the production of acetyl CoA from pyruvate (or fatty acids or specific amino acids), the complete oxidation of the acetyl moiety of acetyl CoA via the citric acid cycle, the utilization of reducing equivalents from the citric acid cycle for electron transport, and the production of ATP by oxidative phosphorylation (Fig. 12-17).

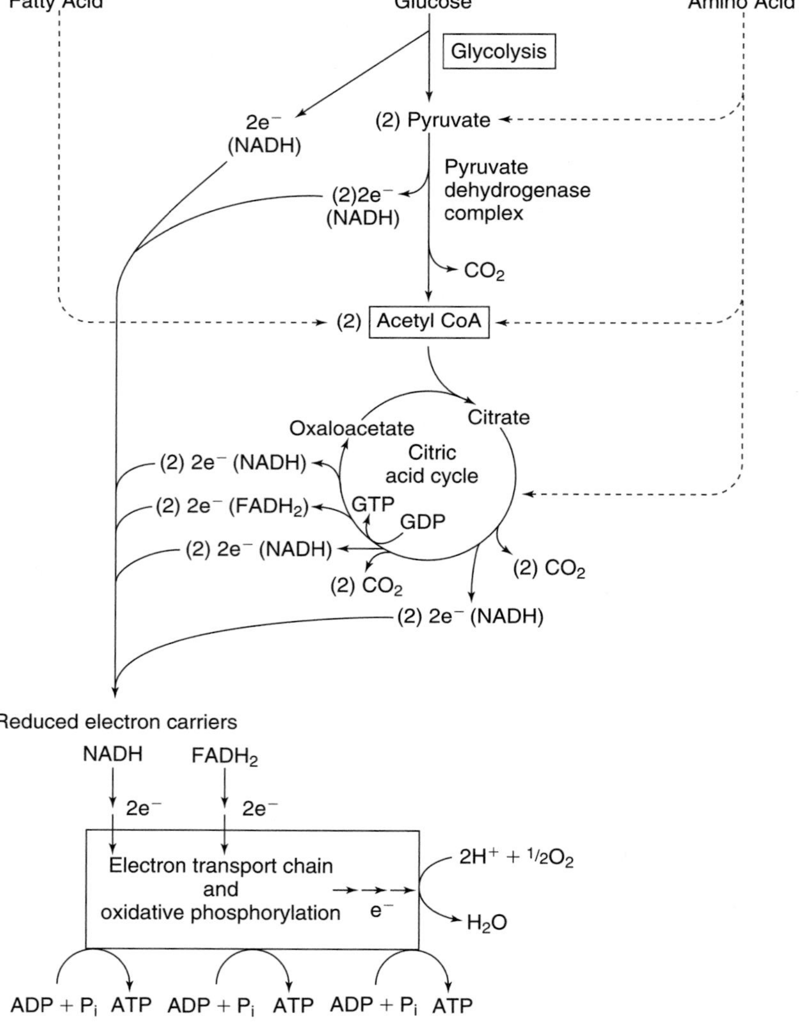

Figure 12-17 Complete oxidation of pyruvate in the mitochondria via the pyruvate dehydrogenase complex (oxidative decarboxylation), the citric acid cycle, and the electron (e^-) transport chain.

Together with the pyruvate dehydrogenase complex, the enzymes of the citric acid cycle are present in the mitochondrial compartment of the cell. The reactions of glycolysis take place in the cytosol of the cell; therefore pyruvate produced as the end product of glycolysis needs to be translocated to the mitochondria. Pyruvate is transported across the inner mitochondrial membrane by a monocarboxylate carrier and is then converted to acetyl CoA by the pyruvate dehydrogenase complex. The acetyl CoA so produced then enters the citric acid cycle. The citric acid cycle is usually referred to as a cycle because one of the "substrates" (oxaloacetate) is regenerated in the process of oxidation of the other substrate, acetyl CoA. Although the complete citric acid cycle functions only in the mitochondria, it should be noted that some enzymes of the citric acid cycle also have cytosolic forms (i.e., cytosolic aconitase, isocitrate dehydrogenase, fumarase, and malate dehydrogenase) and that particular citric acid cycle enzymes in the mitochondria also may play other roles in metabolism.

PYRUVATE DEHYDROGENASE COMPLEX

The pyruvate dehydrogenase complex, associated with the mitochondrial inner membrane of mammalian cells, catalyzes the conversion of pyruvate to acetyl CoA. The overall reaction involves the activity of three individual enzymes, the activities of which are coordinated by association in a multienzyme complex. There are multiple copies of the three enzymes in this complex; the complex includes pyruvate dehydrogenase (E_1), dihydrolipoyl transacetylase (E_2), and dihydrolipoyl dehydrogenase (E_3) (Fig. 12-18). The overall reaction is essentially irreversible and converts the 3-carbon intermediate, pyruvate, to acetyl CoA. Acetyl CoA, in turn, can be either oxidized via the citric acid cycle or utilized for fatty acid synthesis, isoprenoid/cholesterol/steroid synthesis, or ketone body synthesis, as discussed in Chapters 16 and 17.

The pyruvate dehydrogenase complex in mammals contains numerous coenzymes derived primarily from the B vitamin family. These coenzymes include thiamin pyrophosphate (TPP), derived from thiamin; flavin adenine dinucleotide (FAD), derived from riboflavin; coenzyme A (CoA), derived from pantothenic acid; nicotinamide adenine dinucleotide (NAD), derived from niacin; and lipoate. These coenzymes perform specific functions in the activity of the three individual enzymes of the pyruvate dehydrogenase complex.

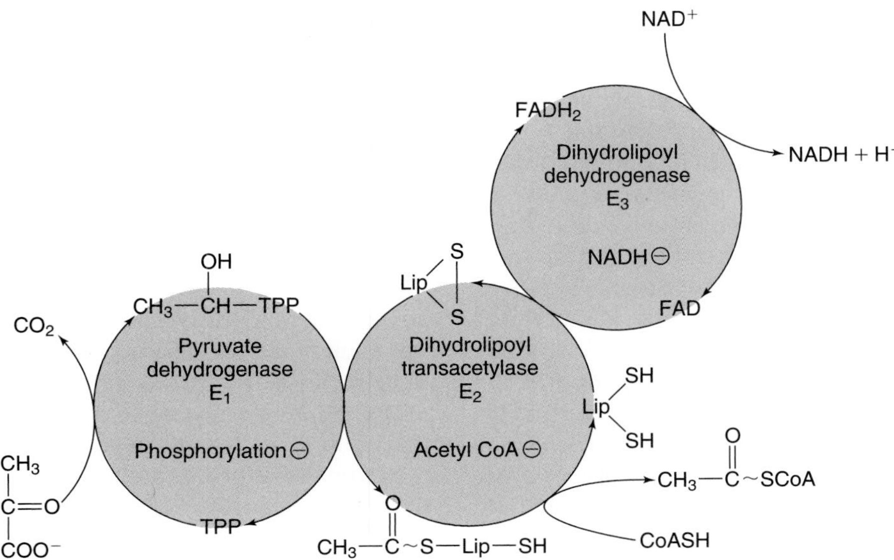

Figure 12-18 Oxidative decarboxylation of pyruvate by the pyruvate dehydrogenase complex. *FAD*, Flavin adenine dinucleotide; *Lip*, enzyme-bound lipoate; *NAD*, nicotinamide adenine dinucleotide; *TPP*, thiamin pyrophosphate. Negative effectors of E_1, E_2, and E_3 enzymes are shown.

These coenzymes are discussed in Chapters 24 and 26.

The first reaction of the multienzyme series is the decarboxylation of pyruvate, catalyzed by pyruvate dehydrogenase (E_1), requiring the coenzyme TPP (see Fig. 12-18). The two electrons removed in this reaction and the acetyl group are transferred by E_1 to lipoate, which is attached to the second enzyme, dihydrolipoyl transacetylase (E_2). In the next reaction, the acetyl group is transferred by a transesterification reaction to CoA, generating acetyl CoA; concomitantly, lipoate is fully reduced. The third enzyme, dihydrolipoyl dehydrogenase (E_3) transfers two hydrogen atoms from reduced lipoate to the coenzyme FAD bound to E_3, generating $FADH_2$ and regenerating the oxidized form of lipoate on E_2. A subsequent oxidation–reduction reaction transfers the hydrogen atoms of $FADH_2$ to NAD^+, forming $NADH + H^+$. The completion of these reactions produces CO_2, acetyl CoA, reducing equivalents in the form of NADH, and the regenerated enzyme complex prepared for another catalytic cycle.

Because the reaction catalyzed by the pyruvate dehydrogenase complex commits carbon intermediates from glucose and amino acid catabolism to either the citric acid cycle or lipid synthesis, the enzymes of the complex are tightly regulated. The pyruvate dehydrogenase complex is regulated primarily by end product inhibition and covalent modification (Behal et al., 1993). The products of the individual enzyme reactions, acetyl CoA and NADH, act as negative feedback inhibitors of their respective reactions; acetyl CoA inhibits E_2 and NADH inhibits E_3. The multienzyme complex is also inactivated by phosphorylation of E_1 by a specific protein kinase that is bound to the enzyme.

The end product inhibitors acetyl CoA and NADH also stimulate phosphorylation of E_1, whereas pyruvate, free CoA, and NAD^+ inhibit this phosphorylation. Therefore, when the mitochondrial [NADH]/[NAD] or [acetyl CoA]/[CoA] ratio is maintained relatively high by the oxidation of fatty acids for energy, the production of acetyl CoA from pyruvate is restrained via inhibition of the activity of the pyruvate dehydrogenase complex. This allows tissues, such as the heart, to "spare" glucose and utilize fatty acids or ketone bodies for energy needs.

Fasting decreases pyruvate dehydrogenase complex activity significantly in tissues such as heart, kidney, and skeletal muscle, and this can be reversed by refeeding. Conversely, in the brain, the pyruvate dehydrogenase complex is necessary for ATP production, and activity of the pyruvate dehydrogenase complex is not reduced with fasting or starvation.

CITRIC ACID CYCLE

The metabolic fate of acetyl CoA varies, depending upon dietary carbohydrate intake, the energy level of the cell, and the cell type. To meet the energy needs of the cell, acetyl CoA can be completely oxidized by the enzymes of the citric acid cycle (Fig. 12-19). If the energy needs of the cell have been met, an alternative route for acetyl CoA utilization is for the biosynthesis of fatty acids in liver and other lipogenic tissues. Only the oxidation of acetyl CoA via the citric acid cycle is considered in this chapter; other fates of acetyl CoA are discussed in Chapters 16, 17, and 26. This cycle is also referred to as the tricarboxylic acid (TCA) cycle or as the Krebs cycle, after Sir Hans Krebs, who proposed this pathway in 1937.

The condensation of acetyl CoA and oxaloacetate to form citrate marks the beginning of one round of the citric acid cycle, and the regeneration of oxaloacetate marks the completion of one round of the citric acid cycle. The energy transferred in the catabolism of acetyl CoA via the citric acid cycle is carried in the reduced coenzymes and in GTP produced by substrate level phosphorylation (see Fig. 12-19). For each molecule of acetyl CoA that enters the cycle, two molecules of CO_2 are formed from the acetate moiety, and reducing equivalents are produced in the form of three molecules of NADH and one molecule of $FADH_2$. From one molecule of NADH entering the electron transport chain, a maximum of three molecules of ATP are produced by oxidative phosphorylation. $FADH_2$ generates a maximum of two molecules of ATP by oxidative phosphorylation. Therefore the reducing equivalents produced in one round of the citric acid cycle generate a maximum of 11 molecules

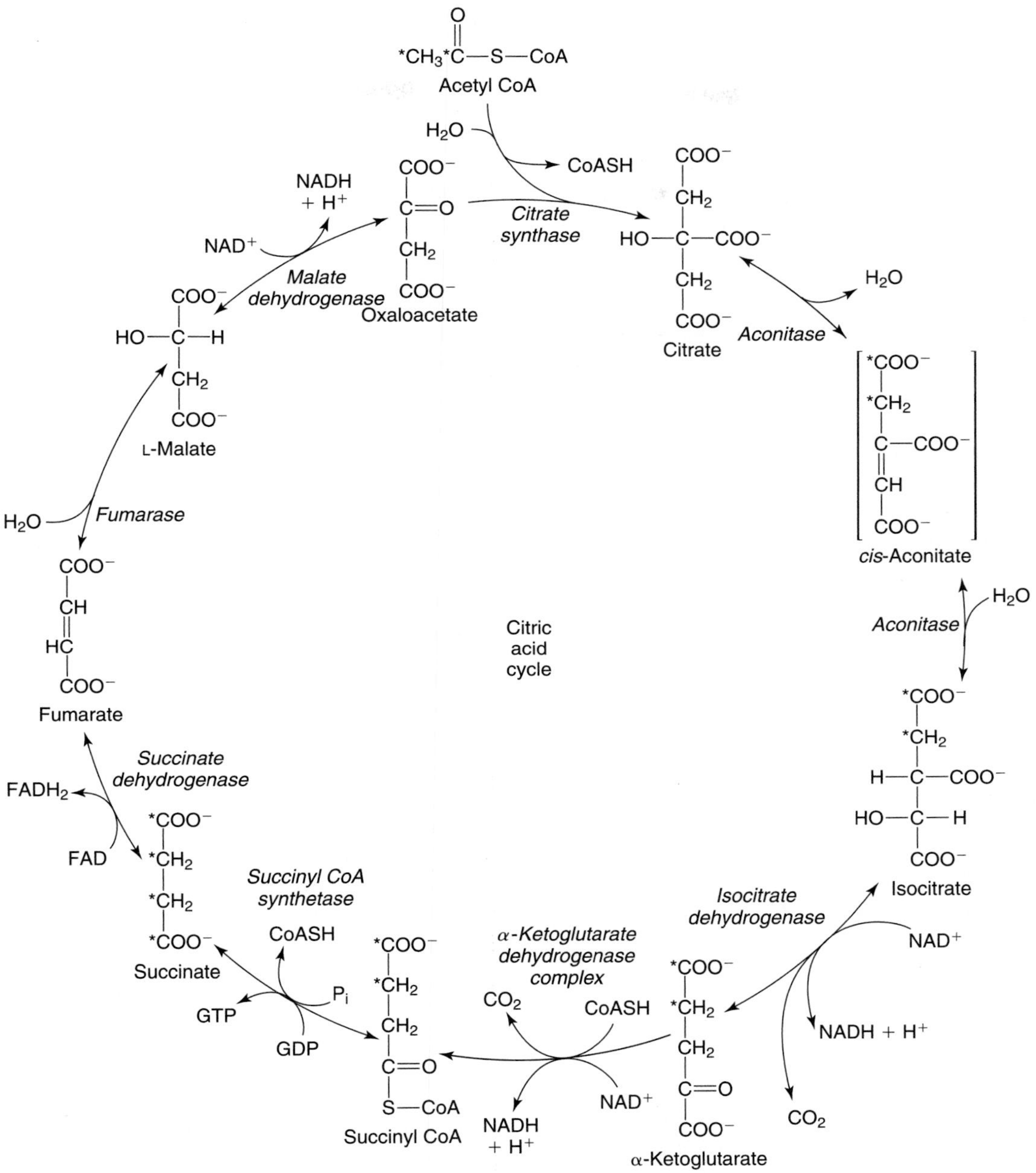

Figure 12-19 The oxidation of acetyl CoA and generation of reducing equivalents and ATP equivalents by the citric acid cycle. Although these reactions result in the net oxidation of the acetyl group to two CO_2, the actual carbons lost as CO_2 in a single round of the cycle are derived from oxaloacetate. The carbons denoted by the asterisks are those from the acetate moiety of acetyl CoA. Because succinate and fumarate are symmetrical molecules, C-1 and C-2 cannot be distinguished from C-3 and C-4 once these intermediates are formed.

of ATP. To this can be added the molecule of ATP (from GTP) produced by substrate-level phosphorylation at the succinyl CoA synthetase step. Taken together, a maximum of 12 molecules of ATP are produced as a result of the complete oxidation of acetate from acetyl CoA through the citric acid cycle.

The total amount of ATP produced from the complete oxidation of glucose to CO_2 and H_2O can be summarized at this point. In glycolysis, the conversion of one molecule of glucose to two molecules of pyruvate produces a net gain of two molecules of ATP from substrate-level phosphorylation. Reducing equivalents (two molecules of NADH) are also generated in the glyceraldehyde 3-phosphate dehydrogenase reaction. These reducing equivalents generate a maximum of four to six molecules of ATP after translocation of electrons to the mitochondrion (depending on the mode of transport across the inner membrane of the mitochondrion). Therefore, under aerobic conditions in those cells with mitochondria, six to eight molecules of ATP are produced as a result of the breakdown of one molecule of glucose to two molecules of pyruvate. The pyruvate dehydrogenase reaction in the mitochondrion generates reducing equivalents as well; two molecules of NADH are produced from the conversion of two molecules of pyruvate to two molecules of acetyl CoA. Therefore, this step generates up to six molecules of ATP from electron transport and oxidative phosphorylation.

As detailed, 24 molecules of ATP are generated in the mitochondria from oxidation of two acetate moieties by the citric acid cycle coupled with the electron transport chain and oxidative phosphorylation. These ATPs are derived from one substrate-level ATP, three NADH, and one $FADH_2$ formed per acetyl CoA that is completely oxidized by the citric acid cycle. Overall, the total energy generated from the complete oxidation of one molecule of glucose to six molecules of CO_2 and H_2O is as much as 36 to 38 molecules of ATP.

ELECTRON TRANSPORT AND OXIDATIVE PHOSPHORYLATION

The ability of a cell to generate energy from macronutrients under aerobic conditions is dependent on the number of mitochondria contained by that cell. Cardiac muscle cells are highly dependent on aerobic metabolism; these cells contain a high concentration of mitochondria, more so than skeletal muscle cells. The mitochondrial space takes up approximately 50% of the total cytoplasmic volume in cardiac muscle cells. Liver cells contain a similarly high concentration of mitochondria. The amount of oxygen consumed by various tissues in the human adult varies depending upon the mitochondrial respiratory capacity of the tissue and upon physiological activity. Skeletal muscle utilizes approximately 30% of consumed oxygen at rest, but with heavy exercise, skeletal muscle may use more than 86% of consumed oxygen. The brain and abdominal tissues also consume large percentages of oxygen at rest.

To understand the enzymatic reactions that occur during electron transport with subsequent oxidative phosphorylation and ATP production, it is important to understand the cellular physiology that makes it possible. This requires a description of the structure of the mitochondrion as it occupies space within the cytoplasm of the cell. The mitochondrion is a membranous organelle. The membrane structures effectively divide the mitochondrion into functional subcompartments. There is an outer membrane and an inner membrane, with numerous invaginations referred to as cristae; between these two membranes is the intermembrane space. Notably, in cells with a high rate of cellular respiration such as cardiac muscle cells, the cristae are more numerous. The space inside the inner membrane is the matrix that contains the enzymes of the pyruvate dehydrogenase complex and the citric acid cycle. Associated with the inner membrane are most of the enzymes involved in electron transport and oxidative phosphorylation, as well as carrier proteins for metabolic intermediates that are transported between the cytosol and the mitochondrial matrix. The inner membrane is much less permeable than the outer membrane to the metabolic intermediates and nucleotides that are important in energy metabolism. The outer membrane is permeable because it contains large, channel-forming proteins called porins. In effect, the intermembrane space is similar in composition to the cytosolic space because the outer membrane is so permeable. Consequently, it is the inner membrane that effectively separates the mitochondrial and cytosolic domains of the cell. This inner membrane is not permeable to oxaloacetate, NADH, or NAD^+, but it does have transporters for malate/α-ketoglutarate, aspartate/glutamate, and phosphoenolpyruvate, as well as pyruvate, citrate/malate, ATP, ADP, and phosphate. The movement of H^+ across the inner mitochondrial membrane normally is coupled with ATP synthesis by the F_1F_0 ATPase, but can also occur via uncoupling proteins.

SHUTTLE OF REDUCING EQUIVALENTS ACROSS THE INNER MITOCHONDRIAL MEMBRANE

The oxidation–reduction pairs that are involved in electron transport (e.g., NAD^+/NADH, $NADP^+$/NADPH, and FAD/$FADH_2$) cannot diffuse across the inner mitochondrial membrane. Specific transport mechanisms compensate for the impermeability of this membrane to these cofactors. The transport of reducing equivalents (protons and electrons) from the cytosol to the mitochondrial matrix is accomplished via substrate shuttles. The most active of these shuttle systems is the malate–aspartate shuttle. Malate carries reducing equivalents, which were generated as NADH and then used to reduce oxaloacetate to malate in the cytosol, to the mitochondrial matrix. In the mitochondria, NADH is regenerated by conversion of malate back to oxaloacetate, which can then be transaminated to aspartate and exit from the mitochondria. Cytosolic and mitochondrial isozymes of malate dehydrogenase catalyze the interconversion of malate and oxaloacetate. The malate–aspartate shuttle functions primarily in liver, heart muscle, and kidney. NADH, whether regenerated in the mitochondrial matrix from cytosolic reducing equivalents or generated within the mitochondrial matrix by the citric acid cycle and other reactions, can be oxidized by the mitochondrial respiratory chain.

In skeletal muscle and brain, another NADH shuttle mechanism occurs. This is the glycerol 3-phosphate shuttle, which does not involve transport of organic compounds but of electrons by the inner membrane flavoprotein, glycerol 3-phosphate dehydrogenase. Dihydroxyacetone phosphate, substrate for the cytosolic glycerol 3-phosphate dehydrogenase, accepts two reducing equivalents from NADH, producing glycerol 3-phosphate and NAD^+ in the cytosol. Another isozyme of glycerol 3-phosphate dehydrogenase, located on the outer face of the inner mitochondrial membrane, transfers two reducing equivalents from glycerol 3-phosphate in the intermembrane space, via an FAD coenzyme, to ubiquinone within the inner mitochondrial membrane. The glycerol 3-phosphate shuttle is different from the malate–aspartate shuttle in that the reducing equivalents are transferred from ubiquinone to complex III (the cytochrome bc_1 complex), thereby bypassing the NADH dehydrogenase complex of the electron transport chain and leading to the synthesis of a maximum of only two molecules of ATP rather than the three molecules of ATP possible when electrons enter the chain at the level of NADH (see Chapters 21 and 24, Figs. 21-2 and 24-7).

Another critical transport step that occurs at the inner mitochondrial membrane is the transfer of adenine nucleotides by the adenine nucleotide translocator. In this case, cytosolic ADP produced in the hydrolysis of ATP is exchanged across the inner membrane for ATP produced by oxidative phosphorylation. This exchanger provides ADP as substrate for oxidative phosphorylation at the same time as it removes the product from the mitochondrial compartment.

Although the focus of the preceding discussion has been on the flow of reducing equivalents into the mitochondria, shuttles also exist that carry potential reducing equivalents from the mitochondrial compartment into the cytosol for use in reductive synthetic processes. The transfer of substrate as well as reducing equivalents from the mitochondria to the cytosol is discussed in Chapter 14 for gluconeogenesis from amino acids and in Chapters 16 and 17 for lipogenesis from acetyl CoA.

ELECTRON TRANSPORT

The electron transport chain is another example of a pathway channeling metabolic intermediates in a series of linked enzymatic reactions. These are oxidation–reduction reactions, in which electrons are passed through protein complexes that have numerous redox centers with increasingly greater affinity for electrons (or increased standard reduction potential). The protein complexes involved in electron transport are integral membrane proteins, with cofactors or fat-soluble molecules that can freely diffuse across the inner membrane. At three distinct steps (at complexes I, III, and IV), the free energy generated from electron transport is utilized to pump protons from the mitochondrial matrix to the intermembrane space between the inner and outer membranes; this establishes an electrochemical gradient across the inner mitochondrial membrane. The amount of energy trapped in the proton gradient at each step is sufficient to drive the synthesis of the gamma phosphate bond in one molecule of ATP (7.3 kcal, or 30.5 kJ). The three electron transfer steps where this occurs are the reduction of FMN by NADH in complex I, the reduction of cytochrome c_1 by cytochrome b in complex III, and the reduction of molecular oxygen by cytochrome a_3 in complex IV (cytochrome c oxidase). These oxidation–reduction reactions produce sufficient energy to effectively pump protons from the mitochondrial matrix to the intermembrane space. A proton concentration gradient is established, which changes the pH (rendering the matrix more alkaline) and electrical charge (rendering the matrix more negative) across the inner mitochondrial membrane.

The movement of electrons via a series of oxidation–reduction reactions that make up the electron transport chain in the inner membrane of the mitochondrion is a specific example of energy transfer in linked, exergonic reactions. The large free energy generated from this process is capable of producing ATP. The question remains: What is the mechanism by which energy generated by electron transport is coupled to the production of ATP? The accepted theory is the chemiosmotic theory, which postulates that the proton-motive force generated from the proton concentration difference across the inner mitochondrial membrane conserves energy for ATP production. ATP is produced when the movement of protons according to their downhill concentration gradient releases this energy. Protons return to the matrix via specific proton pores in the membrane. The pore or channel through which protons move is provided by a subunit structure of the mitochondrial ATP synthase that spans the inner membrane.

This mitochondrial ATP synthase is an F-type ATPase, which is characterized as an ATP-dependent proton pump. Generally, F-type ATPases utilize the energy of ATP hydrolysis to move protons against a concentration gradient. The reverse, however, occurs in oxidative phosphorylation. The spontaneous flow of protons through the channel, provided by the ATP synthase subunit (F_0) in the inner membrane, releases energy for the synthesis of ATP from enzyme-bound ADP and P_i. The latter enzymatic reaction is catalyzed by the second ATP synthase subunit (F_1), which is on the interior side of the inner mitochondrial membrane.

Therefore the three sites in electron transport that pump protons to the intermembrane space generate the electrochemical energy for ATP synthesis. The electrochemical energy

Clinical Correlation

Mutations in Mitochondrial DNA

Autosomal recessive defects occur in the proteins of the respiratory chain. Two genomes are involved in the coding of respiratory chain proteins: the nuclear genome and the mitochondrial genome. Mitochondrial DNA (mtDNA) is circular and encodes 13 proteins, which are synthesized in this compartment of the cell. These proteins include seven subunits of complex I, one subunit of complex III, three subunits of cytochrome C oxidase, and two subunits of the ATP synthase (Bindoff and Turnbull, 1994).

Current evidence shows that mutations in the mtDNA are responsible for numerous degenerative disorders of skeletal muscle, heart, central nervous system, and the eye (Shoffner and Wallace, 1994). Biochemical analyses indicate that many of the clinical syndromes caused by mtDNA mutations involve multiple respiratory chain defects, although single deficiencies have also been reported.

difference generated across the inner mitochondrial membrane is referred to as the proton-motive force. This force is the amount of free energy available to do work when protons flow passively back into the mitochondrial matrix. The electrochemical energy generated by complexes I, III, and IV is each sufficient for, and coupled to, ATP synthesis. Therefore, three molecules of ATP are generated from the oxidation-reduction reactions initiated by NADH entry into the electron transport chain. Only two molecules of ATP are generated from $FADH_2$, which donates electrons to oxidized ubiquinone, bypassing the oxidation–reduction reactions of complex I and the energy derived therefrom. Approximately 40% of the energy from electron transport is conserved in the form of ATP; the remaining energy is dissipated as heat. (See Chapter 21 for more about electron transport and oxidative phosphorylation.)

OTHER PATHWAYS OF CARBOHYDRATE METABOLISM

PENTOSE PHOSPHATE PATHWAY

The pentose phosphate pathway serves as a secondary pathway of glucose oxidation, a source of reducing equivalents in the form of NADPH, and as a means of generation of 5-carbon sugar phosphates, particularly ribose 5-phosphate. The pentose phosphate pathway is also called the hexose monophosphate shunt or the phosphogluconate pathway. The first three steps of the pathway shown in Figure 12-20 are involved in the oxidation of glucose 6-phosphate to ribulose 5-phosphate, which can be transformed to ribose 5-phosphate or xylulose 5-phosphate.

NADPH is formed in the first and third steps, which are catalyzed by glucose 6-phosphate dehydrogenase and phosphogluconate dehydrogenase, respectively. Glucose 6-phosphate dehydrogenase is regulated by the $NADP^+$ concentration (substrate availability), and the need for NADPH regeneration determines flux through this pathway. Glucose 6-phosphate dehydrogenase is considered a lipogenic enzyme because the NADPH generated by the pentose phosphate pathway is required for synthesis of fatty acids, cholesterol, and other sterols. The tissues most heavily involved in fatty acid and cholesterol biosynthesis (mammary gland, adipose tissue, liver, adrenal cortex, and testis) are rich in pentose phosphate pathway enzymes. The gene that encodes glucose 6-phosphate dehydrogenase is regulated by fasting and refeeding and by dietary fatty acids in the liver, consistent with the important role of the encoded enzyme in lipogenesis in liver (Stabile et al., 1996). The pentose phosphate pathway is also active in red blood cells, which require NADPH for reduction of glutathione. Reduced glutathione is required by red blood cells for maintenance of their redox state and thus of the integrity of the red blood cell membrane. Without adequate NADPH, the red blood cell membrane lyses and hemolytic anemia results. Oxidation of glucose by the pentose phosphate pathway occurs in the cytosol and is not dependent upon the presence of mitochondria.

The ribulose 5-phosphate produced from glucose 6-phosphate by the first three steps of the pentose phosphate pathway serves as a source of ribose 5-phosphate, which can be formed by isomerization of ribulose 5-phosphate. Ribose 5-phosphate is essential for the biosynthesis of nucleotides and nucleic acids, including ATP, coenzyme A, NAD, NADP, FAD, RNA, and DNA. If the cell needs the pentose phosphates produced from glucose 6-phosphate, the pathway may stop at the level of the pentose phosphates. Alternatively, a series of reversible reactions can convert excess ribose 5-phosphate and xylulose 5-phosphate to the glycolytic intermediates fructose 6-phosphate and glyceraldehyde 3-phosphate, as shown in part 2 of Fig. 12-20. Fructose 6-phosphate and glyceraldehyde 3-phosphate can reenter glycolysis or be converted to glucose 6-phosphate and enter other pathways of glucose metabolism. These sugar rearrangements also allow for degradation of ribose 5-phosphate from nucleotide degradation. Because the reactions involved in these sugar rearrangements are freely reversible, cells that need pentose phosphates also can form them by conversion of glycolytic intermediates to pentoses without net oxidation of glucose to CO_2 and without NADPH production.

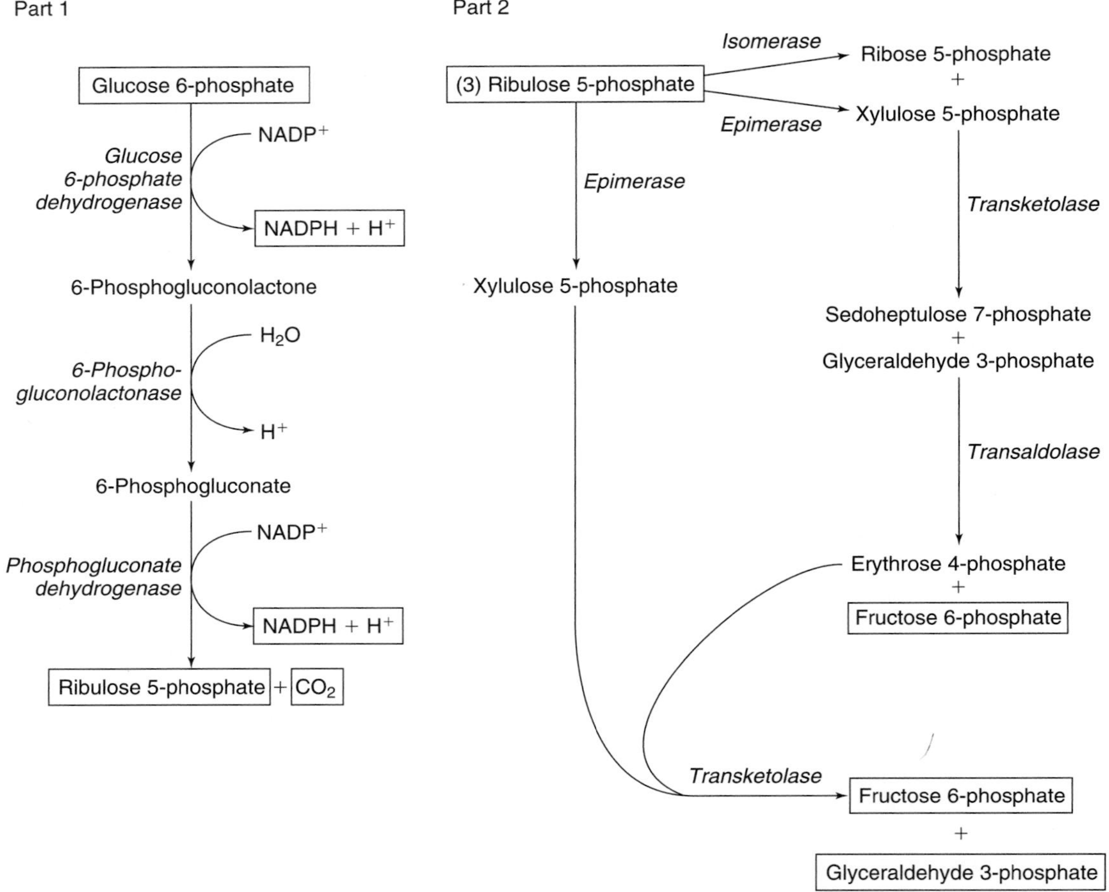

Figure 12-20 The pentose phosphate pathway. Oxidation of glucose occurs in part I of the pathway. Part II of the pathway shows the rearrangement of three molecules of ribulose 5-P to re-form glycolytic intermediates, fructose 6-phosphate and glyceraldehyde 3-phosphate.

Although only the 1-carbon of glucose 6-phosphate is lost as CO_2 in the pentose phosphate pathway, net oxidation of glucose can occur if both parts 1 and 2 of the pathway, as shown in Figure 12-20, are operative. This occurs when the need for NADPH is greater than the need for ribose 5-phosphate. If six molecules of glucose 6-phosphate are oxidized to six molecules of pentose 5-phosphate, and these pentoses are further rearranged to form four molecules of fructose 6-phosphate and two molecules of glyceraldehyde 3-phosphate (the equivalent of five molecules of hexose), net conversion of one molecule of glucose to 6 molecules of CO_2 will have occurred with net production of 12 molecules of NADPH.

FORMATION OF SUGAR DERIVATIVES FOR SYNTHESIS OF GLUCURONIDES, LACTOSE, AND OTHER CARBOHYDRATES

Various sugars and sugar derivatives are formed from glucose phosphate. These have a variety of functions in the body, including serving as substrate for glucuronidation pathways; for synthesis of glycosaminoglycans, glycoproteins, and glycolipids; and as substrate for lactose synthesis by the mammary gland. The amount of glucose that is consumed by these pathways is generally small relative to the amount that is catabolized via glycolysis and the citric acid cycle.

Glucuronide formation is an important pathway of glucose consumption in the liver.

UDP-glucose, formed by reaction of glucose 1-phosphate with UTP, is oxidized to UDP-glucuronate. UDP-glucuronate serves as the glucuronosyl donor in various detoxification and elimination reactions in which conjugates of glucuronate and nonpolar acceptor molecules are formed.

UDP-Glucuronate + R-OH →
R-O-Glucuronate + UDP

Many drugs, such as the anti-AIDS drug 3′-azido-2′-3′-dideoxythymidine (AZT) or the over-the-counter drug acetaminophen, and endogenous compounds, such as bilirubin, are conjugated with glucuronate to form more polar compounds that are more readily excreted in the urine and bile. UDP-glucuronate can be converted to glucuronate, which can be converted to xylulose 5-phosphate, a pentose phosphate pathway intermediate. In most species other than primates, glucuronate serves as a substrate for ascorbic acid synthesis (see Chapter 27, Fig. 27-1). Because humans and other primates lack one of the enzymes in this pathway, gulonolactone oxidase, ascorbic acid must be supplied in the diet.

Pathways for interconversion of galactose, glucose, fructose, and mannose were shown in Figure 12-4. Additional pathways exist to form a number of other sugar derivatives, many in the form of nucleotide diphosphate sugars. These include GDP-L-fucose from GDP-mannose; UDP-*N*-acetylglucosamine, UDP-*N*-acetylgalactosamine, and CMP-*N*-acetylneuraminic acid (one of the sialic acids) from glucose phosphate or fructose phosphate; dTDP-rhamnose from glucose phosphate; and UDP-galactose from galactose phosphate or UDP-glucose.

The disaccharide lactose is synthesized by the lactating mammary gland. The mammary enzyme lactose synthase is induced in response to release of the hormone prolactin. UDP-galactose and glucose are substrates; a glycosidic bond is formed between galactose and glucose to form β-galactosyl(1→4)glucose, commonly known as lactose.

SYNTHESIS OF GLYCOSAMINOGLYCANS AND PROTEOGLYCANS

Glycosaminoglycan chains are long, unbranched, heteropolysaccharide chains made up largely of disaccharide repeating units, with a hexosamine and a uronic acid commonly found in the repeating structure. In many glycosaminoglycans, the sugars are sulfated. Both the carboxylate groups of the uronic acid units and the sulfate groups that are linked either to hydroxyl groups of the sugar residues or to amino groups of the hexosamine residues are responsible for the large number of negative charges associated with these compounds. Six classes of glycosaminoglycans are recognized: hyaluronate, chondroitin sulfate, dermatan sulfate, heparin, heparan sulfate, and keratan sulfate. Most of these are found covalently attached to protein in proteoglycan and are present mainly in the extracellular matrix of tissues. Exceptions include hyaluronate, which is not known to exist covalently attached to protein, and heparin, which is found as an intracellular component of mast cells.

The oligosaccharide chains of glycosaminoglycans contain sugars linked to other sugars by glycosidic bonds. Chondroitin sulfate, dermatan sulfate, heparin, heparan sulfate, and keratan sulfate chains are synthesized in the lumen of the ER by transfer of glycosyl units from nucleotide diphosphate (NDP) derivatives to the nonreducing end of an acceptor sugar or oligosaccharide chain.

NDP-Sugar (Donor) +
Sugar or Oligosaccharide (Acceptor) →
Glycosyl-*O*-Glycose (Glycoside) + NDP

Conversely, hyaluronic acid is synthesized in association with the plasma membrane using UDP-glucuronate and UDP-*N*-acetylglucosamine as precursors; sugar units are added to the reducing end of the chain by hyaluronan synthase.

Proteoglycans are high-molecular-weight polyanionic substances that consist of many different glycosaminoglycan chains linked covalently to a protein core. Because proteoglycans may contain as much as 95% carbohydrate, their properties tend to resemble those of polysaccharides more than those of proteins. The polysaccharide chains (glycosaminoglycan chains) of proteoglycans are assembled by the sequential action of a series of glycosyltransferases in the lumen of the ER. These glycosyltransferases catalyze the transfer of a monosaccharide from an NDP—sugar to the appropriate acceptor, either the nonreducing end of another sugar or an amino acid side chain on a polypeptide. In chondroitin sulfate proteoglycan formation, for example, sugar units are added to the core protein to form a tetrasaccharide linkage region followed by alternate addition of the characteristic repeating *N*-acetylgalactosamine and glucuronate units of chondroitin sulfate and by sulfation of the *N*-acetylgalactosamine residues on either C-4 or C-6.

Proteoglycans are found in tissues such as cartilage, tendons, ligaments, aorta, skin, blood vessels, and heart valves. Proteoglycans are usually found together with fibrous proteins, such as collagen and elastin, in the extracellular matrix. The network of proteoglycans and the cross-linked fibers of collagen or elastin provide the extracellular matrix with tensile strength, as is found in tendons, or elasticity, as is found in ligaments. In addition, an intricate attachment is formed between cells and the proteoglycans of extracellular matrix. Integrins, integral membrane proteins of the cell, have an extracellular domain that binds members of a family of adhesion proteins, and these adhesion proteins also bind to proteoglycans. Therefore integrins and the extracellular adhesion proteins form an attachment between cells and the surrounding proteoglycans of the extracellular matrix. Common adhesion proteins are fibrin and laminin.

Chondroitin sulfate is the most abundant class of glycosaminoglycans in the body. Most chondroitin sulfate chains consist of between 60 and 100 sugar residues made up mainly of alternating *N*-acetylgalactosamine and glucuronate units. A typical chondroitin sulfate proteoglycan has about 100 chondroitin sulfate chains attached to the protein core. These chondroitin sulfate proteoglycans are abundant in cartilage, tendons, ligaments, and aorta.

Although hyaluronate chains are not covalently attached to proteins, hyaluronate can serve as a central strand around which proteoglycan molecules are organized. Hyaluronate chains can be very long (approximately 10^6 sugar residues). Because of its large molecular weight and anionic character, hyaluronate holds large volumes of water and serves as an effective lubricant and shock absorbent. It is found predominantly in the synovial fluid of the joints and the vitreous humor of the eye.

SYNTHESIS OF GLYCOPROTEINS

Glycoproteins are defined as proteins that contain one or more saccharide chains (usually less than 12 to 15 sugar residues per chain) that lack serial repeat units and that are bound covalently to the polypeptide chain. This definition distinguishes them from the carbohydrate-rich proteoglycans. Glycoproteins are found in cell membranes with the oligosaccharide portion of the glycoprotein on the external face of the plasma membrane. The carbohydrate portion of glycoproteins can range from 1% to 70% of the glycoprotein by weight. The carbohydrate chains are covalently linked to glycoproteins by *N*- or *O*-glycosyl bonds. A variety of monosaccharide units linked by either α- or β-glycosidic bonds result in the diversity of oligosaccharide moieties that are found in glycoproteins.

Glycosylation of proteins occurs in the ER and Golgi apparatus. Glycosylation serves to alter the properties of proteins, and the oligosaccharide structures also act as recognition signals for various aspects of protein targeting and for cellular recognition of proteins and of other cells. The *O*-linked oligosaccharides are synthesized in the Golgi apparatus by serial addition of monosaccharide units to a completed polypeptide chain. The sugar residues are added by the sequential action of a series of glycosyltransferases. This process begins with transfer of a sugar such as *N*-acetylgalactosamine from UDP-*N*-acetylgalactosamine to a serine or threonine residue on the polypeptide. This is then followed by stepwise addition of other sugars.

The *N*-linked oligosaccharides are synthesized somewhat differently and usually contain a core structure made up of mannose and *N*-acetylglucosamine residues. This common core is preassembled as a dolichol-linked oligosaccharide prior to incorporation into the polypeptide. First *N*-acetylglucosamine from UDP-*N*-acetylglucosamine is attached to dolichol phosphate to form *N*-acetylglucosaminylpyrophosphoryldolichol, with release of UMP from the nucleotide sugar. The addition of other core sugars occurs and, in the final step, the core oligosaccharide is transferred from the dolichol pyrophosphate to an asparagine residue in the polypeptide chain. After synthesis and transfer of the specific core region, extensive processing of the oligosaccharide chain occurs in the Golgi apparatus. Processing involves removal of some of the core oligosaccharide's sugar units followed by addition of other sugar residues to the remaining core oligosaccharide; these reactions are catalyzed by glycosyltransferases and do not require the participation of dolichol intermediates.

Glycoproteins are important components of cell membranes where the oligosaccharide portion of the glycoprotein is on the external face of the plasma membrane. Glycoproteins make up a major part of the mucus secreted by epithelial cells. Many secreted proteins such as follicle-stimulating hormone, chorionic gonadotropin, and luteinizing hormone are glycoproteins, and many plasma proteins such as immunoglobulins, prothrombin, plasminogen, and ceruloplasmin are also glycoproteins. A well-characterized erythrocyte glycoprotein called glycophorin is widely studied as a model of plasma membrane glycoproteins. The glycophorin C complex in human erythrocyte membranes regulates the stability and mechanical properties of the plasma membrane. Components of the glycophorin C complex are implicated in ion channel clustering, cytoskeletal organization, cell signaling, and cell proliferation (Chishti, 1998). The oligosaccharide component of glycoproteins also marks soluble glycoproteins in the plasma for continued circulation or degradation by the liver. A specific unit of the oligosaccharide, a sialic acid residue at the terminus of the oligosaccharide chain, marks glycoproteins for continued circulation; the loss of this sialic acid residue results in the uptake of the asialoglycoprotein and its degradation by the liver. Liver contains asialoglycoprotein receptors that recognize, bind, and internalize glycoproteins that lack terminal sialic acid residues.

SYNTHESIS OF GLYCOLIPIDS

Sphingoglycolipids are glycosyl derivatives of sphingolipids. Structure and synthesis of the glycosphingolipids, including glucocerebrosides, galactocerebrosides, globosides, and gangliosides, are discussed in Chapters 4, 6, and 17. The more complex globosides and gangliosides contain glucose and/or galactose as well as additional sugars such as L-fucose, *N*-acetylgalactosamine, and sialic acids (e.g., *N*-acetylneuraminic acid).

Another important glycolipid is glycosyl phosphatidylinositol (GPI), which functions to anchor a variety of proteins to the exterior surface of the plasma membrane. The core GPI is synthesized on the luminal side of the ER from phosphatidylinositol, UDP-*N*-acetylglucosamine, dolicholphosphomannose, and phosphatidylethanolamine. The core GPI structure is modified by the addition of a variety of additional sugar residues, which vary with the protein to which the GPI attaches. Target proteins in the ER become attached to preformed GPI when the amino group of the GPI phosphoethanolamine moiety nucleophilically attacks a specific residue of the protein near its C-terminus, resulting in a transamidation reaction that releases a 20- to 30-amino acid residue C-terminal peptide and attaches GPI to the new C-terminal amino acid residue of the target protein. These GPI-anchored proteins are found on the exterior surface of the plasma membrane of cells; the fatty acids of GPI are inserted into the lipid membrane to provide the anchor.

DIETARY REFERENCE INTAKES AND TYPICAL INTAKES OF CARBOHYDRATES

The Institute of Medicine (IOM) set a recommended dietary allowance (RDA) for carbohydrate for the first time in 2002 (IOM, 2002). The estimated average requirement (EAR) was based on the minimum amount of glucose utilized by the brain under circumstances of adequate energy intake. The amount of glucose required by the central nervous system when there is no increase in plasma concentrations of acetoacetate and β-hydroxybutyrate was estimated to be approximately 100 g/day. The estimated utilization of glucose by brain of children from 1 year onward is similar to that of adults, so the EAR is set as 100 g/day of carbohydrate for all groups

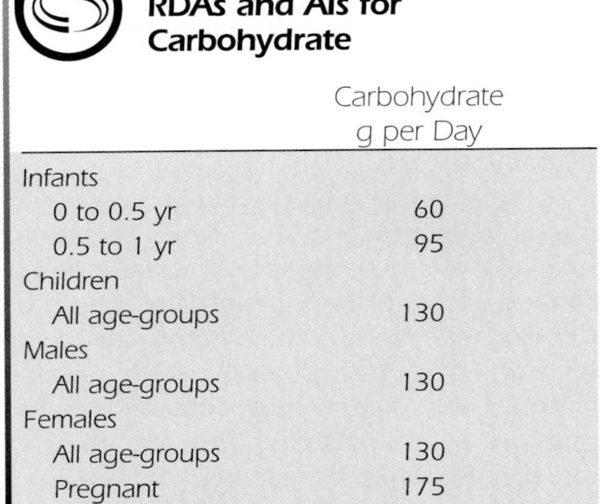

RDAs and AIs for Carbohydrate

	Carbohydrate g per Day
Infants	
0 to 0.5 yr	60
0.5 to 1 yr	95
Children	
All age-groups	130
Males	
All age-groups	130
Females	
All age-groups	130
Pregnant	175
Lactating	210

Data from Institute of Medicine (2002) Dietary Reference Intakes for Energy, Carbohydrate, Fiber, Fat, Fatty Acids, Cholesterol, Protein, and Amino Acids. National Academy Press, Washington, DC.
AI, Adequate intake.

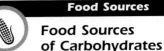

except infants, for whom AIs are based on dietary intake. The RDA was set using a coefficient of variation of 15% [100 g/day + 2(15)] to yield an RDA of 130 g/day.

Although it is recognized that humans can adapt to diet that contains essentially no carbohydrate by using amino acids and glycerol (from fat) for gluconeogenesis, this adaptation involves increased production of β-hydroxybutyric and acetoacetic acids. The plasma concentration of these keto acids is normally very low, even after an overnight fast. The ability of the body to adapt to extended starvation involves a rise in circulating nonesterified fatty acid and keto acid concentrations. Similar increases in keto acid concentrations have been observed in children with epilepsy being treated with "ketogenic diets" for extended periods (Vining, 1999; Swink et al., 1997). It is not known if these adaptations have negative consequences for the health of individuals consuming adequate energy but no carbohydrate, but they may have adverse effects on bone mineral, cholesterol levels, development and function of the central nervous system, one's general sense of well being, or glycogen stores.

According to the Continuing Survey of Food Intakes by Individuals (CSFII, 1994-1996, 1998) food intake data for the United States population, median total carbohydrate intake was 294 g/day for men (19 to 70 years) and 210 g/day for women. The range (1st and 99th percentiles) for carbohydrate intake of adults (19 to 70 years) was 112 to 589 g/day for men and 91 to 384 g/day for women. Median intakes clearly exceed the RDA. Carbohydrate intake as a percentage of total calories ranged from 34% to 65% (1st to 99th percentiles) with a median of 49% for adult men (19 to 70 years). For adult women, the range was 36% to 68% with a median of 52%. For all age and sex groups, the range was 36% to 68% with a median of 52%.

An increment of 35 g/day was added to the adult EAR to establish the EAR for pregnant women. This increment was based on the newborn infant brain weight (~380 g) and the daily glucose consumption rate of adults (8.64 g/100 g brain) to yield a glucose requirement of the fetal brain at the end of pregnancy of 32.5 g/day.

Food Sources

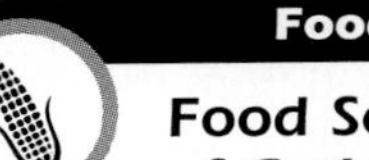

Food Sources of Carbohydrates

Fruits
25 to 38 g per ½ cup canned or frozen sweetened fruit
13 to 20 g per ½ cup canned or frozen unsweetened fruit
17 to 22 g per ¾ cup fruit juice

Soda
38 to 40 g per 12 oz carbonated sweetened soda

Grain Products
17 to 23 g per ½ cup rice, barley, couscous, bulgar, or buckwheat
20 g per ½ cup pasta or noodles
22 to 46 g per cup ready-to-eat cereal
21 to 30 g per 2-oz roll, bun, or croissant

Vegetables
17 to 29 g per ½ cup white, navy, kidney, or garbanzo beans
11 to 16 g per ½ cup potatoes, sweet corn, mixed vegetables, or green peas

Data from U.S. Department of Agriculture, Agricultural Research Service (2005) USDA Nutrient Database for Standard Reference, Release 18. U.S. Department of Agriculture, Washington, DC. Retrieved March 1, 2005, from www.ars.usda.gov/ba/bhnrc/ndl.

For lactating women, the EAR was set as the adult EAR plus an increment of 60 g calculated as the lactose content of human milk (74 g/L) times the volume of milk secreted (0.78 L/day). Therefore, the EARs of carbohydrate for pregnant and lactating women are 135 and 160 g/day, respectively. The RDAs (EARs + 30%) are 175 g/day and 210 g/day.

The IOM (2002) set AIs for infants based on the average intake of carbohydrate consumed from human milk and complementary foods. These AIs were calculated as the carbohydrate (lactose) content of human milk (74 g/L) times the intake of milk (0.78 L/day) for infants from 0 to 6 months of age; and as the carbohydrate intake from human milk (0.78 L/day times 0.6 L/day) plus the intake from complementary foods (51 g/day) for older infants. Therefore the AIs are 60 and 95 g/day of carbohydrate for 0 to 6-month-old and 7- to 12-month-old infants, respectively.

The IOM (2002) considered the possibilities of setting tolerable upper intake levels (ULs) for high glycemic index carbohydrates and for sugars but did not do so because of the lack of a critical mass of evidence. However, they highlighted a need for more research to elucidate the health effects resulting from ingestion of high versus low glycemic index carbohydrates and the possible effects of sugars and energy density on energy expenditure, food intake, and weight reduction. Although a UL was not set, a maximal intake level of 25% or less of energy from added sugars was suggested based on the decreased intake of some micronutrients by American subpopulations who exceed this level of sugar intake. The National Health and Nutrition Examination Survey (NHANES III) data indicated that added sugar intakes are particularly high in young adults, especially in males, being as high as 57 teaspoons (228 g or 912 kcal) per day for male adolescents.

REFERENCES

Ali M, Rellos R, Cox TM (1998) Hereditary fructose intolerance. J Med Genet 35:353-365.

Behal RH, Buxton DB, Robertson JG, Olson MS (1993) Regulation of the pyruvate dehydrogenase multienzyme complex. Annu Rev Nutr 13:497-520.

Bindoff LA, Turnbull DM (1994) Defects of the mitochondrial respiratory chain. In: Holton JB (ed) The Inherited Metabolic Diseases, 2nd ed. Churchill Livingstone, London, pp 265-295.

Buist NRM (1995) Disorders of gluconeogenesis. In: Fernandes J, Saudubray J-M, van den Berghe G. (eds) Inborn Metabolic Diseases: Diagnosis and Treatment. Springer-Verlag, Berlin, pp 101-106.

Charron MJ, Katz EB, Olson AL (1999) GLUT4 gene regulation and manipulation. J Biol Chem 274:3253-3256.

Chishti AH (1998) Function of p55 and its nonerythroid homologues. Curr Opin Hematol 5:116-121.

Cohen PT, Alessi DR, Cross DA (1997) PDK1, one of the missing links in insulin signal transduction? FEBS Lett 410:3-10.

Czech MP (1995) Molecular actions of insulin on glucose transport. Annu Rev Nutr 15:441-471.

Dunger DB, Holton JB (1994) Disorders of carbohydrate metabolism. In: Holton JB (ed) The Inherited Metabolic Diseases, 2nd ed. Churchill Livingstone, London, pp 21-65.

Ferrer-Martinez A, Marotta M, Baldan A, Haro D, Gomez-Foix A (2004) Chicken ovalbumin upstream promoter-transcription factor I represses the transcriptional activity of the human muscle glycogen phosphorylase promoter in C2C12 cells. Biochim Biophys Acta 1678:157-162.

Fernandes J, Chen Y-T (1995) Carbohydrate metabolism: Glycogen storage diseases. In: Fernandes J, Saudubray J-M, van den Berghe G. (eds) Inborn Metabolic Diseases: Diagnosis and Treatment. Springer-Verlag, Berlin, pp 71-131.

Finlay D, Patel S, Kidkson MM, Phipiro N, Marquez R, Rhodes CJ, Sutherland C (2004) Glycogen synthase kinase-3 regulated IGFBP-1 gene transcription through the thymine-rich insulin response element. BMC Mol Biol 5:15.

Gautier-Stein A, Mithieux G, Rajas F (2005) A distal region involving hepatocyte nuclear factor 4alpha and CAAT/enhancer binding protein markedly potentiates the protein kinase a stimulation of the glucose-6-phosphatase promoter. Mol Endocrinol 19:163-174.

Gitzelmann R (1995) Disorders of galactose metabolism. In: Fernandes J, Saudubray J-M, van den Berghe G. (eds) Inborn Metabolic Diseases: Diagnosis and Treatment. Springer-Verlag, Berlin, pp 87-92.

Granner DK, Pilkis SJ (1990) The genes of hepatic glucose metabolism. J Biol Chem 265:10173-10176.

Gurney AL, Park EA, Liu J, Giralt M, McGrane MM, Patel YM, Crawford DR, Nizielski SE, Savon S, Hanson RW (1994) Metabolic regulation of gene transcription. J Nutr 124:1533S-1539S.

Hanson RW, Reshef L (1997) Regulation of phosphoenolpyruvate carboxykinase (GTP) gene expression. Annu Rev Biochem 66:581-611.

de la Iglesia N, Veiga-daCunha M, Van Schaftingen E, Guinovart JJ, Ferrer JC (1999) Glucokinase regulatory protein is essential for the proper subcellular localization of liver glucokinase FEBS Lett 456:332-338.

Institute of Medicine (2002) Dietary Reference Intakes for Energy, Carbohydrate, Fiber, Fat, Fatty Acids, Cholesterol, Protein and Amino Acids. National Academy Press, Washington, DC.

Ishitani R, Tajima H, Takata H, Tsuchiya K, Kuwae T, Yamada M, Takahashi H, Tatton N, Katsube N (2003) Proapoptotic protein glyceraldehydes-3-phosphate dehydrogenase: a possible site of action of antiapoptotic drugs. Prog Neuropsychopharmacol Biol Psychiatry 27:291-301.

Jope RS, Johnson GV (2004) The glamour and gloom of glycogen synthase kinase-3. Trends Biochem Sci 29:95-102.

Jungermann K (1992) Zonal liver cell heterogeneity. Enzyme 46:5-7.

Kahn CR, Lauris W, Koch S, Crettaz M, Granner DK (1989) Acute and chronic regulation of phosphoenolpyruvate carboxykinase mRNA by insulin and glucose. Mol Endocrinol 3:840-845.

Kawaguchi T, Takenoshita M, Kabashima T, Uyeda K (2001) Glucose and cAMP regulate the L-type pyruvate kinase gene by phosphorylation/dephosphorylation of the carbohydrate response element binding protein. Proc Natl Acad Sci 98:13710-13715.

Kullberg-Lindh C, Hannoun C, Lindh M (2002) Simple method for detection of mutations causing hereditary fructose intolerance. J Inherit Metab Dis 25:571-575.

Lehninger AL, Nelson DL, Cox MM (1993) Glycolysis and the catabolism of hexoses. In: Principles of Biochemistry, 2nd ed. Worth Publishers, New York, pp 400-439.

Lemaigre FP, Rousseau GG (1994) Transcriptional control of genes that regulate glycolysis and gluconeogenesis in adult liver. Biochem J 303:1-14.

Lochhead PA, Coghlan M, Rice SQJ, Sutherland C (2001) Inhibition of GSK-3 selectively reduces glucose-6-phosphatase and phosphoenolpyruvate carboxykinase gene expression. Diabetes 50:937-946.

Lockyer JM, McCracken JB (1991) Identification of a tissue-specific regulatory element within the human muscle glycogen phosphorylase gene. J Biol Chem 266:20262-20269.

Magnuson MA, Jetton TL (1993) Tissue-specific regulation of glucokinase. In: Berdanier CD, Hargrove JL (eds) Nutrition and Gene Expression. CRC Press, Boca Raton, FL, pp 143-167.

Minokoski Y, Kahn CR, Kahn BB (2003) Tissue-specific ablation of the GLUT4 glucose transporter or the insulin receptor challenges assumptions about insulin action and glucose homeostasis. J Biol Chem 278: 33609-33612.

Moore MC, Cherrington AD (1996) Regulation of net hepatic glucose uptake: interaction of neural and pancreatic mechanisms. Reprod Nutr Dev 36:399-406.

Nikoulina SE, Ciaraldi TP, Mudaliar N, Carter L, Johnson K, Henry RR (2002) Inhibition of glycogen synthase kinase 3 improves insulin action and glucose metabolism in human skeletal muscle. Diabetes 51:2190-2198.

Noguchi T, Tanaka T (1993) Dietary and hormonal regulation of L-type pyruvate kinase gene expression. In: Berdanier CD, Hargrove JL (eds) Nutrition and Gene Expression. CRC Press, Boca Raton, FL, pp 143-167.

Nordlie RC, Bode AM, Foster JD (1993) Recent advances in hepatic glucose 6-phosphatase regulation and function. Proc Soc Exp Biol Med 203:274-285.

Nordlie RC, Foster JD, Lange AJ (1999) Regulation of glucose production by the liver. Annu Rev Nutr 19:379-406.

O'Mahony AM, Walsh DA (2002) Differentiation-dependent mechanisms of transcriptional regulation of the catalytic subunit of phosphorylase kinase. Biochem J 362:199-211.

Orth HM, Kruger DK, Schmoll D, Grempler R, Scherbaum WA, Joost HG, Bornstein SR, Barthel A (2004) Cellular models for the analysis of signaling by protein kinase B and the forkhead transcription factor FKHR (Foxo1a). Regul Pept 121:19-24.

Pilkis SJ, El-Maghrabi MR, Claus TH (1990) Fructose-2,6-bisphosphate in control of hepatic gluconeogenesis. From metabolites to molecular genetics. Diabetes Care 13:582-599.

Pilkis SJ, Claus TH (1991) Hepatic gluconeogenesis/glycolysis: regulation and structure/function relationships of substrate cycles. Annu Rev Nutr 11:465-515.

Pilkis SJ, Claus TH, Kurland IJ, Lange AJ (1995) 6-Phosphofructo-2-kinase/fructose-2,6-bisphosphatase: A metabolic signaling enzyme. Annu Rev Biochem 64:799-835.

Pilkis SJ, Granner DK (1992) Molecular physiology of the regulation of hepatic gluconeogenesis and glycolysis. Annu Rev Physiol 54:885-909.

Postic C, Shiota M, Magnuson MA (2001) Cell-specific roles of glucokinase in glucose homeostasis. Recent Prog Horm Res 56:195-217.

Rao PV, Pugazhenthi S, Khandelwal RL (1995) The effects of streptozotocin-induced diabetes and insulin supplementation on expression of the glycogen phosphorylase gene in rat liver. J Biol Chem 270:24955-24960.

Rhee J, InooueY, Yoon JC, Puigserver P, Fan M, Gonzales FJ, Spiegelman BM (2003) Regulation of hepatic fasting response by PPAR gamma coactivator-1alpha (PGC-1): requirement for hepatocyte nuclear factor 4 alpha in gluconeogenesis. Proc Natl Acad Sci USA 100:4012-4017.

Rider MH, Bertrand L, Vertommen D, Michels PA, Rousseau GG, Hue L (2004) 6-Phosphofructo-2-kinase/fructose-2,6-bisphosphatase: head-to-head with a bifunctional enzyme that controls glycolysis. Biochem J 381:561-579

Shafrir E (1991) Metabolism of disaccharides and monosaccharides with emphasis on sucrose and fructose and their lipogenic potential. In: Gracey M, Kretchmer N, Rossi E (eds) Sugars in Nutrition. Nestle Nutrition Workshop Series, Vol. 25. Raven Press, New York, pp 131-152.

Shoffner JM, Wallace DC (1994) Oxidative phosphorylation diseases and mitochondrial DNA mutations: diagnosis and treatment. Annu Rev Nutr 14:535-568.

Sirover MA (1997) Role of the glycolytic protein, glyceraldehyde-3-phosphate dehydrogenase, in normal cell function and in cell pathology. J Cell Biochem 66:133-140.

Smythe C, Cohen P (1991) The discovery of glycogenin and the priming mechanism for glycogen biogenesis. Eur J Biochem 200:625-631.

Stabile LP, Hodge DL, Klautky SA, Salati LM (1996) Posttranscriptional regulation of glucose-6-phosphate dehydrogenase by dietary polyunsaturated fat. Arch Biochem Biophys 332:269-279.

Steffensen KR, Gustafsson JA (2004) Putative metabolic effects of the liver X receptor. Diabetes, 53:S36-S42.

Streeper RS, Svitek CA, Chapman S, Greenbaum LE, Taub R, O'Brien RM (1997) A multicomponent insulin response sequence mediates a strong repression of mouse glucose-6-phosphatase gene transcription by insulin. J Biol Chem 272:11698-11701.

Sutherland C, O'Brien RM, Granner DK (1996) New connections in the regulation of PEPCK gene expression by insulin. Philos Trans R Soc Lond B Biol Sci 351:191-199.

Swink TD, Vining EP, Freeman JM (1997) The ketogenic diet. Adv Pediatr 44:297-329.

Thorens B (2002) A gene knockout approach in mice to identify glucose sensors controlling glucose homeostasis. Pflugers Arch—Eur J Physiol 445:482-490.

Uldry M, Thorens B (2004) The SLC2 family of facilitated hexose and polyol transporters. Pflugers Archiv—Eur J Physiol 447:480-489.

Van den Berghe G (1995) Disorders of fructose metabolism. In: Fernandes J, Saudubray J-M, van den Berghe G (eds) Inborn Metabolic Diseases: Diagnosis and Treatment. Springer-Verlag, Berlin, pp 95-99.

Vaulont S, Kahn A (1993) Transcriptional control of metabolic regulation genes by carbohydrates. FASEB J 8:28-36.

Vestergaard H (1999) Studies of gene expression and activity of hexokinase, phosphofructokinase and glycogen synthase in human skeletal muscle in states of altered insulin-stimulated glucose metabolism. Dan Med Bull 46:13-34.

Vining EP (1999) Clinical efficacy of the ketogenic diet. Epilepsy Res 37:181-190.

White M (1998) The IRS-signalling system: a network of docking proteins that mediate insulin action. Mol Cell Biochem 182:3-11.

Yoon JC, Puigserver P, Chen G, Donovan J, Wu Z, Rhee J, Adelmant G, Stafford J, Kahn CR, Granner DK, Newgard CB, Speigelman BM (2001) Control of hepatic gluconeogenesis through the transcriptional coactivator PGC-1. Nature 413:131-138.

RECOMMENDED READINGS

Berdanier CD (1995) Advanced Nutrition: Macronutrients. CRC Press, Boca Raton, FL, pp 160-207.

Devlin TM, ed. (2002) Textbook of Biochemistry with Clinical Correlations, 5th ed. Wiley-Liss, New York, pp 537-692.

Guyton AC, Hall JE (2000) Textbook of Medical Physiology, 10th ed. W.B. Saunders, Philadelphia, pp 772-780.

Lehninger AL, Nelson DL, Cox MM (2000) Principles of Biochemistry, 3rd ed. Worth Publishers, New York, pp 293-324, 527-597, 722-779.
Magnuson MA, She P, Shiota M (2003) Gene altered mice and metabolic flux control. J Biol Chem 278, 32485-32488.
Nordlie RC, Foster JD, Lange AJ (1999) Regulation of glucose production by the liver. Annu Rev Nutr 19: 379-406.
Rider MH, Bertrand L, Vertommen D, Michels PA, Rousseau GG (2004) 6-Phosphofructo-2-kinase/fructose-2,6-bisphosphatase: head-to head with a bifunctional enzyme that controls glycolysis. Biochem J 381:561-579.
Voet D, Voet JG (2004) Biochemistry: Biomolecules, Mechanisms of Enzyme Action and Metabolism, 3rd ed. John Wiley & Sons, Inc., New York, pp 549-682.

Chapter 13

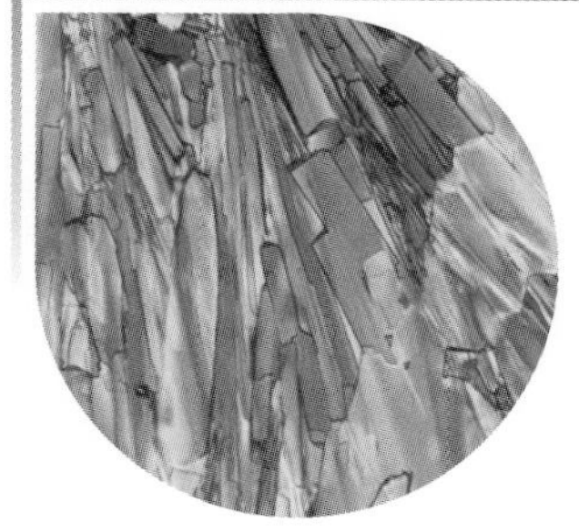

Protein Synthesis and Degradation

Margaret A. McNurlan, PhD, and Tracy G. Anthony, PhD

OUTLINE

This chapter is a revision of the chapter contributed by Margaret A. McNurlan, PhD, and Peter Garlick, PhD, for the first edition.

COMMON ABBREVIATIONS

DNA	deoxyribonucleic acid
eEF	eukaryotic elongation factor
eIF	eukaryotic initiation factor
eRF	eukaryotic release factor
ER	endoplasmic reticulum
ERAD	endoplasmic reticulum–associated degradation
hnRNA	heterogeneous nuclear RNA
IGF	insulin like growth factor
IL	interleukin
mRNA	messenger ribonucleic acid
rRNA	ribosomal ribonucleic acid
tRNA	transfer ribonucleic acid
TNF	tumor necrosis factor
UPR	unfolded protein response

ESSENTIALITY OF PROTEIN

The importance of dietary protein to life was demonstrated in the early 1800s by the nutritional experiments of François Magendie. He found that adult dogs fed on diets containing only flour (carbohydrate) or oil (fat) died, whereas dogs lived indefinitely on diets of eggs or cheese; that is, on diets containing protein (Munro, 1964).

In the young, the provision of dietary protein is not only necessary for maintaining body protein but for the increase in protein mass associated with growth. If either dietary protein or energy is limited, growth is retarded. In the adult, an adequate intake of protein maintains the body protein mass and the capacity to adapt to changing conditions. Loss of body protein is not compatible with health and accompanies many disease states. Renal, gastrointestinal, and liver disease, as well as cancer and infections such as human immunodeficiency virus (HIV), are associated with the loss of body protein, which in turn is associated with increased mortality. In HIV-infected individuals, for example, the loss of less than 30% of body protein mass is associated with about 80% survival. When the loss of body protein exceeds 30%, the survival rate drops to about 20% (Suttmann et al., 1995). It is imperative, therefore, to understand what functions proteins serve, why body protein is lost, and how these losses can be prevented.

FUNCTIONS AND DISTRIBUTION OF BODY PROTEIN

Proteins consist of linear polymers of amino acids and make up approximately 17% of the body mass. Protein molecules function to maintain body structure (e.g., collagen), to facilitate mobility (e.g., actin and myosin for muscle contraction), in transport (e.g., oxygen transport by hemoglobin, membrane transport systems), in metabolism (e.g., enzymes), in regulation (e.g., growth factors, transcription factors), and in immune function (e.g., immunoglobulins). Although the diversity in function of body proteins is reflected in the large number of different protein species, almost one half of body protein is contained in just four: the structural proteins collagen, actin, and myosin, and the oxygen-transporting protein hemoglobin.

Body protein is distributed throughout the various organs, with the majority (approximately 40%) in muscle tissue. In addition to providing for locomotion and work, muscle protein also provides amino acids that can be mobilized in times of stress. However, muscle protein is not a storage form, like glycogen or fat, and loss of muscle protein represents a loss of functional protein. The functions of muscle tissue are given a lower priority than the functions of the visceral tissues such as liver and intestine, which contain approximately 10% of body protein. The protein of these tissues is not mobilized rapidly in times of stress, thereby preserving the more vital functions of these tissues (Kinney, 1978). Another 30% of body protein is contained in skin and blood, and both skin lesions and anemia accompany deficits of dietary protein. Some proteins such as collagen are preserved during malnutrition, not because of their essential function but because their structure is such that they are not readily degraded.

NITROGEN BALANCE

Protein and amino acids are unique among the compounds of the body in the amount of nitrogen they contain. Although other compounds such as amino sugars and nucleic acids contain nitrogen, they do not contain the substantial amounts that are contained in body protein. On average, protein contains 16% nitrogen, leading to the familiar factor of 6.25 (i.e., 100/16) for converting measured values of nitrogen into corresponding amounts of protein. Because nitrogen is relatively easy to measure, changes in the protein mass of the body can be assessed by the difference between nitrogen intake and nitrogen excretion. Historically and clinically, one of the most common ways of assessing changes in body protein mass is through the assessment of the difference between the intake of nitrogen and the loss of nitrogen from the body, the nitrogen balance:

Nitrogen balance = Nitrogen intake − Nitrogen excretion

Using 6.25 as the average conversion factor for converting grams of nitrogen to grams of protein, protein balance can then be derived from nitrogen balance:

Nitrogen balance × 6.25 = Protein (gained or lost)

When the body is in nitrogen equilibrium, nitrogen excretion is equal to nitrogen intake. Thus, for a typical American adult consuming approximately 100 g of protein per day, both nitrogen intake and nitrogen excretion will be approximately 16 g per day. Whenever nitrogen intake exceeds excretion, protein is being retained by the body, which results in growth. When nitrogen excretion exceeds nitrogen intake, body protein is being lost, such as during starvation and disease.

Although the concept of nitrogen balance is useful in that it can provide information about the overall balance of body protein, this concept is a static one. For example, it cannot answer questions about whether negative balance arises from depressed protein synthesis or accelerated protein degradation. The nitrogen balance technique is neither able to determine which organs within the body are retaining protein and which are losing it nor able to assess details of the adaptive changes that occur in body protein metabolism in order to preserve balance. Questions such as these require a more dynamic assessment of protein metabolism.

DYNAMIC PROTEIN METABOLISM

During any day an adult human makes, and degrades, about 300 g of protein. In contrast, the normal intake of protein from the diet for an affluent, well-fed individual is approximately one third of that amount, or 100 g. This means that the body not only processes the protein that is taken in but also degrades about three times as much body protein. Therefore, approximately 400 g of protein is broken down to amino acids by digestion plus protein degradation. Amino acids are used to resynthesize about 300 g of body protein; most of the remaining amino acids are catabolized.

INTERCHANGE OF PROTEIN AND AMINO ACIDS

The interchange between body protein and the pool of free amino acids is depicted schematically in Figure 13-1. The process by which body protein is continually degraded and resynthesized is called protein turnover, a term that has been used collectively to include both protein synthesis and degradation. In addition to the exchange of amino acids into and out of protein, amino acids also are irreversibly lost through degradative pathways. For most adults who are in protein balance, the amount of amino acids degraded is equivalent to the amount in the diet. The degradative pathways are also shown schematically in Figure 13-1. Degradation involves the removal of nitrogen, primarily as urea and ammonia, and the degradation of the carbon skeleton. The end result of the degradation of the carbon skeleton of amino acids is the provision of energy either directly or through the formation of compounds such as glucose and fatty acids, which can then be stored or metabolized to provide energy. The pathways for the oxidative metabolism of amino acids and nitrogen excretion are discussed in detail in Chapter 14, but it is important to understand the integrated nature of protein metabolism that is represented by Figure 13-1. The needs of the body regulate the flux of amino acids through these possible pathways; that is, when amino acids are used for the synthesis of protein, when they are oxidized for energy, and when they are used to form glucose.

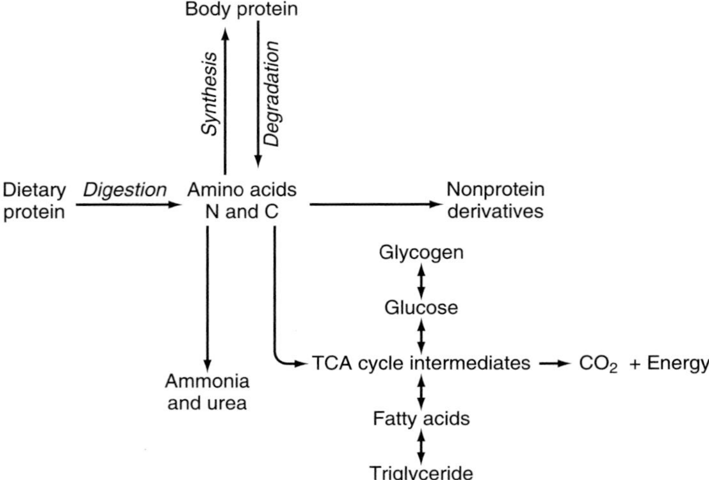

Figure 13-1 Overview of protein and amino acid metabolism. Amino acids are incorporated primarily into protein or degraded to provide energy. In general, the synthesis of nonprotein compounds does not consume quantitatively important amounts of amino acids. Degradation of amino acids involves removal of the nitrogen and catabolism of the carbon skeleton.

There are also pathways within the body for conversion of amino acids to end products other than protein. These reactions are depicted in Figure 13-1 as nonprotein derivatives. Nonprotein derivatives include compounds such as purine and pyrimidine bases, neurotransmitters (serotonin, tyramine), and nonpeptide hormones (catecholamines, thyroid hormones). The quantities of amino acids involved in these nonprotein pathways are, in general, much smaller than the amounts of amino acids involved in protein synthesis and degradation. Because the amounts of amino acids irreversibly consumed in the synthesis of nonprotein compounds are normally much smaller than those consumed either by protein synthesis or by amino acid oxidation, these pathways often are ignored in the assessment of protein turnover and nitrogen balance. However, the amounts of some of these compounds that are synthesized can be substantial (e.g., creatine, heme, and nucleic acids), and, for some amino acids, these pathways can become quantitatively significant during periods of protein deprivation. The synthesis of the peptide glutathione (γ-glutamylcysteinylglycine) accounts for a large amount of the body's cysteine flux, but most of the amino acids in glutathione are returned to the amino acid pool upon glutathione turnover.

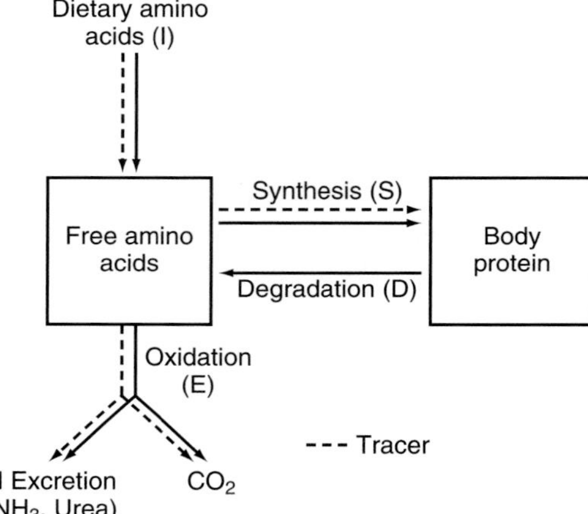

Figure 13-2 Protein turnover. The complexity of body protein and free amino acid pools is simplified in this two-compartment model, which can be used to assess kinetic data from labeled tracers (shown as *dashed lines*). In this model, amino acids enter a free amino acid pool via the diet *(I, for intake)* or from the degradation of body protein *(D)*. Amino acids leave the free amino acid pool through protein synthesis *(S)* and oxidation *(E, for excretion)*.

PROTEIN TURNOVER

The pathways shown in Figure 13-1 can be simplified to focus specifically on the interactions of amino acids with body protein through protein synthesis and protein degradation (Fig. 13-2).

In this simplified scheme, all the tissue and circulating proteins are considered together and, likewise, the free amino acid pool is simplified to a single, homogeneous pool, rather than the complex arrangements of pools in blood, individual tissues, and subcellular compartments that are known to exist. This simplification has proved helpful in conceptualizing and developing methods for measuring the exchange of amino acids between the free amino acid pool and the protein pool.

This simple model in Figure 13-2 highlights the exchange of free amino acids with body protein through the processes of protein synthesis and protein degradation, and also the entry and exit of amino acids by dietary intake and oxidation. Essential amino acids enter the body free pool from the digestion and absorption of dietary protein (I) and from the degradation of body protein (D). Removal of amino acids from the free pool occurs either by the synthesis of protein (S) or through excretion (E) via oxidation to CO_2 with the concurrent excretion of nitrogen, mainly as ammonia and urea.

If the amount of free amino acid in the pool is constant, then the sum of the processes that remove amino acids (protein synthesis + oxidation) is equal to the sum of the processes by which amino acids enter the free pool (protein degradation + dietary amino acid intake).

$$S + E = D + I = Q$$

Q, the sum of the rates of either entry or exit from the free amino acid pool, has been termed the flux rate. This is sometimes also known as the rate of appearance, R_a, or rate of disappearance, R_d. In an adult in nitrogen equilibrium or protein balance, nitrogen intake (I) is equal to nitrogen excretion (E), and protein synthesis (S) is equal to protein degradation (D). For an individual to be in positive nitrogen balance, there must be net protein synthesis or accretion (S>D), whereas there must be net protein degradation or loss for an individual to be in negative nitrogen balance (S<D).

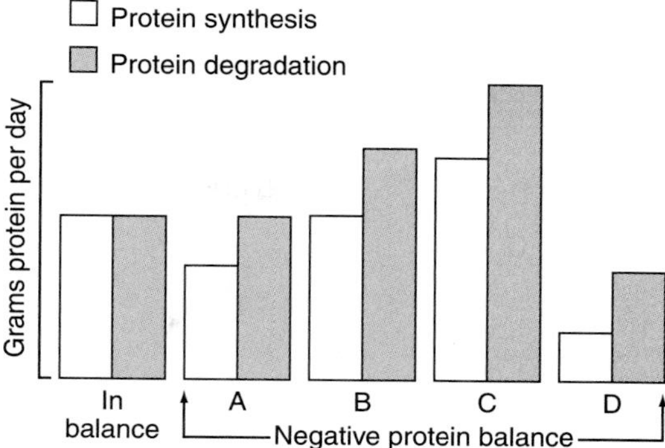

Figure 13-3 Four ways of achieving negative nitrogen balance. Negative nitrogen balance (degradation > synthesis) arises from changes in either protein synthesis *(A)* or protein degradation *(B)*, or from changes in both *(C, D)*. Similarly, positive balance (synthesis > degradation) arises whenever synthesis exceeds degradation. This can occur with changes in the rates of synthesis or degradation or with changes in both.

PROTEIN BALANCE = PROTEIN SYNTHESIS − PROTEIN DEGRADATION

From the aforementioned relationships, it is clear that protein is retained in the body when synthesis exceeds degradation and that protein is lost from the body when degradation exceeds synthesis. Unlike the technique of nitrogen balance, which measures only net changes in body protein, estimates of protein synthesis and degradation indicate that changes in balance arise in a number of different ways.

For example, as shown in Figure 13-3, loss of body protein can occur from a decrease in the synthesis of protein with no change in protein degradation (Fig. 13-3, *A*), an increase in the degradation with no change in protein synthesis (Fig. 13-3, *B*), or from either an increase (Fig. 13-3, *C*) or a decrease (Fig. 13-3, *D*) in both synthesis and degradation, with protein degradation exceeding protein synthesis. In a number of pathological conditions, body protein degradation exceeds synthesis, with both protein synthesis and degradation rates elevated over the rates in healthy individuals. In the case of infection in malnourished children, body protein is lost, but both synthesis and degradation rates are depressed.

Likewise, positive protein balance can be achieved by increases in protein synthesis, by decreases in protein degradation, or with changes in both protein synthesis and degradation, such that synthesis exceeds degradation. For example, in children recovering from malnutrition, both the rates of protein synthesis and degradation were increased, but the increase in synthesis was larger than the increase in protein degradation (Golden et al., 1977; also see Fig. 13-12 later in this chapter). Unlike the information from nitrogen balance studies, measurements of protein synthesis and degradation provide information about how the changes in balance are brought about.

Although the illustration of protein turnover in Figure 13-2 is presented in terms of whole-body protein, the balance between the processes of synthesis and degradation also determines the net protein balance at the level of individual tissues or organs and for individual proteins. Examples of this type of regulation are discussed later in this chapter.

MEASUREMENT OF PROTEIN SYNTHESIS AND DEGRADATION

The methods used for measuring protein synthesis, protein degradation, and amino acid oxidation, in general, require isotopic tracer techniques (Waterlow et al., 1978). Amino acids labeled with either radioactive (^{14}C, ^{3}H) or stable (^{15}N, ^{13}C, ^{2}H) isotopes have been used, although the trend is toward the exclusive use of stable isotopes for humans (Table 13-1). Like their radioactive counterparts, stable isotopes differ in atomic mass from the abundant natural form of the element, but they are not radioactive and occur as a small proportion of all naturally occurring materials. Because of this, they are totally harmless and can be used for multiple studies in the same subject. No radioactive isotope of nitrogen is suitable for use in laboratory studies; therefore, the stable isotope ^{15}N is the only commonly available tracer for this element. Measurement of stable isotopes is by mass spectrometry, which requires more expensive and elaborate equipment than radioactivity counting but has the advantage of greater selectivity and sensitivity.

The earliest work on protein turnover, performed by German scientist Rudolf Schoenheimer and his colleagues at Columbia University in the 1930s, used ^{15}N-labeled amino acids. Schoenheimer and colleagues (1939) first demonstrated the concept of turnover of protein by observing that a labeled amino acid was incorporated into body protein even when the animals were not growing. They reasoned that the body protein pool was turning over, so that some of the label was incorporated into protein, replacing some of the unlabeled body protein that was degraded and excreted.

Table 13-1
Stable Isotopes of Elements Commonly Used in Metabolic Research

Element	Normal*	Radioactive	Stable*
Hydrogen	^{1}H	^{3}H	^{2}H (0.015%)
Carbon	^{12}C	^{14}C	^{13}C (1.1%)
Nitrogen	^{14}N	—	^{15}N (0.37%)
Oxygen	^{16}O	—	^{17}O (0.037%)
			^{18}O (0.2%)

*The "normal" isotope is the most abundant naturally occurring form. The average natural abundance of the less abundant "stable" isotopes is shown in parentheses.

METHODS BASED ON THE DISAPPEARANCE OF LABEL FROM THE FREE POOL

Protein Turnover in the Whole Body

Since the time of Schoenheimer, various techniques for assessing protein turnover have been developed. The isotopic labeling procedure usually is performed by giving the tracer amino acid as an intravenous injection or infusion, although sometimes the less-invasive intragastric route is used. Two alternative methods of measurement have been developed. One method measures the disappearance of the label from the free amino acid pool, and the other method assesses the rate of appearance of label in protein. The former approach has been used extensively to measure rates of protein turnover in the whole body, because the free pool is easier to sample than the body protein pool. When a ^{13}C-labeled amino acid is given (e.g., L-[1-^{13}C]leucine), rates of whole-body protein synthesis and degradation, as well as amino acid oxidation, can be determined by monitoring the labeling of the amino acid in the blood and the labeling of expired CO_2 in the breath. The rates of whole-body synthesis in humans of different ages shown in Figure 13-4 were measured with this technique.

If the tracer is an amino acid labeled with ^{15}N (e.g., [^{15}N]glycine), the excretion of the label in urinary end products (urea or ammonia) can be used to calculate whole-body protein synthesis and degradation. This approach also assumes a single pool of free amino acid, which is sampled via urinary urea or ammonia. (The rates of protein synthesis and degradation in malnourished and recovering children shown in Figure 13-12 in this chapter were measured with [^{15}N]glycine.)

Measurements of Protein Turnover From Arterial–Venous Differences

Measurement of the disappearance of label from the free amino acid pool has also been used to determine rates of protein synthesis in individual organs or limbs by monitoring the extraction of the label as the blood passes through the tissue. Sampling of both arterial and venous blood allows for the estimation of extraction of label by the organ or limb. This measurement is referred to as the arterial–venous, or A–V, difference. A similar approach, the dilution of label in the free amino acid pool by release of unlabeled amino acids from tissue proteins as the blood passes through the organ or limb, has been used to determine rates of protein degradation.

METHODS BASED ON THE INCORPORATION OF A LABELED AMINO ACID INTO PROTEIN

Measurement of Protein Synthesis in Tissues

The determination of rates of protein synthesis in individual organs or tissues is based on the amount of a labeled amino acid that is incorporated into protein in a given amount of time.

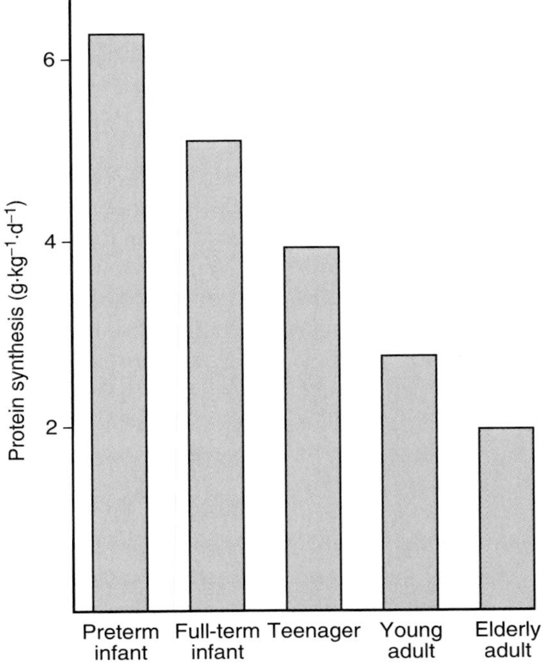

Figure 13-4 The decline in whole-body protein synthesis with advancing age. Rates of whole-body protein synthesis were measured with L-[1-^{13}C]leucine infusion in subjects of various ages. *(Data from Mitton SG, Calder AG, Garlick PJ [1991] Protein turnover rates in sick, premature neonates during the first few days of life. Pediatr Res 30:418-422; Denne SC, Kalhan SC [1987] Leucine metabolism in human newborns. Am J Physiol 253:E608-E615; Mauras N [1995] Estrogens do not affect whole-body protein metabolism in the prepubertal female. J Clin Endocrinol Metab 80:2842-2845; Mauras N, Haymond MW, Darmaun D, Vieira NE, Abrams SA, Yergey AL [1994] Calcium and protein kinetics in prepubertal boys. Positive effects of testosterone. J Clin Invest 93:1014-1019; and Welle S, Thornton C, Statt M, McHenry B [1994] Postprandial myofibrillar and whole body protein synthesis in young and old human subjects. Am J Physiol 267:E599-E604.)*

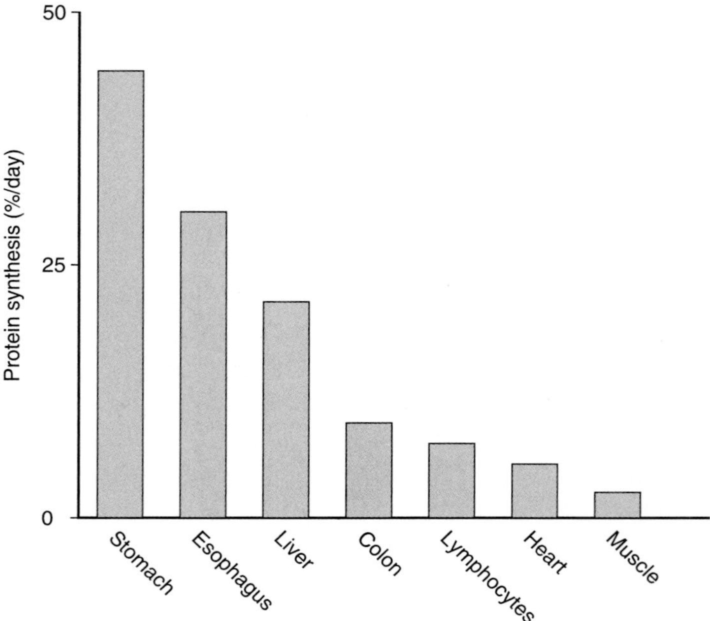

Figure 13-5 Fractional rates of protein synthesis in a range of human tissues. Rates of protein synthesis, assessed from the incorporation of L-[1-^{13}C]leucine or L-[$^{2}H_5$]phenylalanine into tissue protein, are expressed as a fractional rate; that is, as the fraction of the protein pool that is synthesized each day. *(Data from Garlick PJ, McNurlan MA, Essén P, Wernerman J [1994] Measurement of tissue protein synthesis rates in vivo: a critical analysis of contrasting methods. Am J Physiol 266:E287-E297.)*

A range of tissue protein synthetic rates measured from the incorporation of a labeled amino acid is shown in Figure 13-5. The technique does not yield estimates of protein degradation, but it has the advantage that individual tissue responses can be monitored, which is valuable in conditions in which there are different responses in different tissues. In cancer, for example, the responses in the tumor can be differentiated from the responses in the host tissues. The disadvantage of the technique based on the incorporation of label is that tissue samples must be obtained and, therefore, the technique is more invasive than the methods based on the disappearance of label from the free pool.

Turnover Rates of Individual Proteins

These are measured by basically the same technique as that used for individual tissues except that proteins from the tissue sample must be separated by electrophoresis, chromatography, or other methods. The range of turnover rates for individual proteins is extremely wide as illustrated by the examples listed in Table 13-2. Some proteins, such as hemoglobin, do not turn over unless their environment changes. Within the red blood cell, hemoglobin is stable and is degraded only when the cell is broken down. Other proteins turn over extremely rapidly. Rapid turnover facilitates a rapid change in the amount of protein present and is commonly found for regulatory proteins.

Isotopic Measurement of Protein Degradation in Tissues

Rates of protein degradation in tissues are more difficult to determine than are synthesis rates. The direct method involves isotopic labeling of protein and the determination of the rate at which label is lost. This technique, however, is complicated by the fact that label from degraded protein can be reincorporated into protein and, consequently, not be included in the measurement of the rate of degradation. A more indirect method, which is not affected by recycling, involves the measurement of synthesis rate together with the rate of change of

Table 13-2
Turnover Rates of Enzymes in Rat Liver

Enzyme	Cellular Compartment	$t_{1/2}$	k_d
Ornithine decarboxylase	Cytosol	11 minutes	91
5-Aminolevulinate synthetase	Cytosol	20 minutes	50
5-Aminolevulinate synthetase	Mitochondria	72 minutes	14
Hydroxymethylglutaryl CoA reductase	Endoplasmic reticulum	4.0 hours	4.2
Phosphoenolpyruvate carboxykinase	Cytosol	5.0 hours	3.3
Alanine-glyoxylate aminotransferase	Cytosol	3.5 days	0.20
Arginase	Cytosol	4.0 days	0.17
NAD+ nucleosidase	Endoplasmic reticulum	16 days	0.04

Data from Waterlow JC, Garlick PJ, Milward DJ (1978) Protein Turnover in Mammalian Tissues and in the Whole Body. North-Holland Publishing, Amsterdam, pp 490-492.
NOTE: Turnover rates are expressed as half-lives ($t_{1/2}$, the time to replace half the molecules originally present) and fractional turnover rates (k_d, fraction turned over per day).

protein mass. Protein degradation is determined from the difference between the rate of growth (or loss) of tissue and the rate of protein synthesis (i.e., growth = synthesis − degradation). Neither of these techniques is entirely satisfactory, however, because they cannot be used in humans and because they require measurements in a large number of animals over an extended period of time. This method also cannot be used for the many proteins that turn over very rapidly.

MYOFIBRILLAR DEGRADATION FROM 3-METHYLHISTIDINE

For muscle, a nonisotopic method can be used to measure protein degradation. The amino acid 3-methylhistidine (N^3-methylhistidine) is produced by posttranslational methylation of histidyl residues of actin and myosin. After release by protein degradation, the 3-methylhistidine cannot be reincorporated into protein, is not metabolized further in most species such as rats and humans, and is, therefore, excreted quantitatively in the urine. Consequently, the rate of 3-methylhistidine excretion is used as a measure of the rate of muscle or, more specifically, myofibrillar protein degradation. Although there are myofibrillar proteins in tissues other than muscle (e.g., the smooth muscle of the intestinal tract), studies on the release of 3-methylhistidine determined by arterial–venous difference across the leg, have shown good agreement with urinary 3-methylhistidine excretion (Sjolin et al., 1989), and urinary 3-methylhistidine excretion is used widely to estimate human muscle protein degradation. The excretion of 3-methylhistidine also depends on the total muscle mass, so that data are most often expressed as the ratio of 3-methylhistidine to creatinine, because urinary creatinine is an indicator of total muscle mass. The ratio of 3-methylhistidine to creatinine is, therefore, an indication of how actively protein is being degraded. However, because meat contains 3-methylhistidine as well as creatinine, which would complicate the interpretation of 3-methylhistidine excretion, the measurement of excretion must be made when subjects are on a meat-free diet. (See Figure 13-13 later in this chapter for an example of the assessment of muscle protein degradation from 3-methylhistidine excretion in patients with acquired immunodeficiency syndrome [AIDS].)

PROTEIN TURNOVER AND ADAPTATION

What are the advantages and disadvantages of this highly inefficient protein turnover system that uses energy to cycle proteins and amino acids? Obviously, the system is inefficient with respect to energy because energy is needed both for the degradation of protein and for the synthesis of new protein. Estimates of the energy cost of protein turnover suggest that 15% of basal energy expenditure is associated with the turnover of protein (Reeds and Garlick, 1984). However, substantial advantages also are conferred by the dynamism. Protein turnover allows the body to degrade and replace proteins that are oxidized, damaged, misfolded, or otherwise nonfunctional. It also allows the body to change the relative amounts of different proteins to respond to changes in nutritional and physiological conditions. One example of the value of this capacity to adapt is seen in the response of malnourished children to infection with measles. Whereas well-nourished children with measles increase both protein synthesis and degradation with a net loss of body protein, malnourished children respond to the infection with both a blunted increase in protein turnover and a blunted loss of body protein. Although the loss of body protein is smaller in the malnourished children, the impact of the disease is greater, and these children often die from measles infection (Tomkins et al., 1983). Protein turnover provides benefit in the capacity to adapt to infection, at the expense of the loss of some body protein and the expenditure of energy.

Individual proteins vary in their rate of turnover (see Table 13-2), and the higher rates of turnover are found in regulatory proteins. The higher rates of turnover of regulatory proteins allow for more rapid adaptation in the levels of these proteins in response to changing conditions. Levels of proteins with very slow turnover rates, such as collagen with a half-life of approximately 300 days, remain relatively constant.

At the level of individual tissues, higher turnover rates are associated with a capacity of the tissue to respond more rapidly to changes in the environment. The turnover rates for a selection of human tissues are shown in Figure 13-5. The high rates of protein synthesis in tissues like stomach and esophagus reflect both the secretory function and the rapid replacement of cells of the gastric and esophageal mucosa. The liver also has a relatively high rate of turnover, which facilitates adaptation to changes such as alterations in nutrient intake. By contrast, the rate of protein synthesis is relatively slower in muscle tissue, and the response of this tissue to altered conditions (e.g., work-induced hypertrophy) occurs more slowly.

In response to altered demands or alterations in the environment, tissues can respond both by altering the overall rates of protein synthesis and degradation and by changing the spectrum of individual proteins being made. This adaptation allows the body to meet continuously changing demands such as those associated with growth and development, health and illness, and pregnancy and lactation. Protein turnover is, therefore, a substrate cycle (or futile cycle; see Chapters 12 and 21 for related discussions relative to energy metabolism); that is, there is continual synthesis and degradation, which requires energy but accomplishes no net change in amount of protein. The benefit is that protein turnover provides the capacity for rapid adaptation when needed.

MOLECULAR MECHANISMS OF PROTEIN SYNTHESIS

In its most global sense, the term protein synthesis describes the processes required for a gene to be transcribed, processed, translated, folded, and packaged into a functional protein. Each process comprises multiple steps, and regulation can occur at one or more of the steps within each process, as outlined in Figure 13-6. Major advances in understanding the regulation of protein synthesis at the molecular level have been made in the last 25 years. From elucidating the molecules that make up the transcriptional and translational machinery to identifying the factors that influence regulation of each step, enough information has been gained to encompass many volumes of text. Furthermore, with whole-genome sequences now available for a growing number of different organisms, including rodents and humans, new information clarifying and extending our current understanding of the regulation of protein synthesis is accumulating at a faster rate than ever before. Therefore, although the following general overview is meant to be a solid foundation for the nutrition professional, it is but merely a starting point for those interested in the finer details of the cellular and molecular events that influence the making of protein.

The recent revelation that the human genome contains approximately 30,000 genes, only about twice as many as found in invertebrates, has caused the scientific community

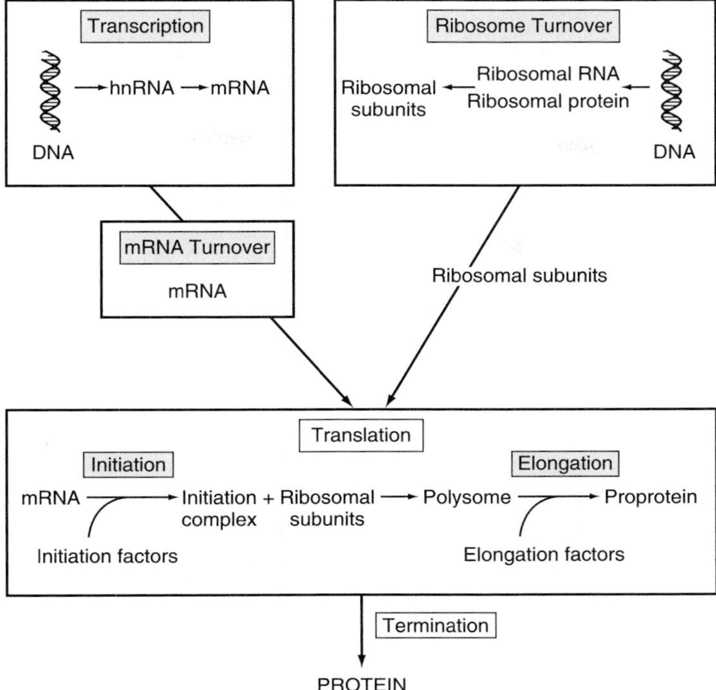

Figure 13-6 Protein synthesis. The scheme shows the processes involved in the synthesis of protein. The boxes all denote points of regulation. Transcription of DNA produces heterogeneous nuclear RNA (hnRNA), much of which is processed into messenger RNA (mRNA). mRNA undergoes continuous synthesis and degradation, shown as mRNA turnover. Ribosomal subunits cycle between subunits and polyribosomes. Both ribosomal RNA (rRNA) and ribosomal proteins also undergo synthesis and degradation. Translation of mRNA into protein involves the processes of initiation and elongation, which are regulated by initiation and elongation factors. The final step in protein formation is termination, the separation of the protein from the polyribosome.

to re-evaluate the influence of the genome in determining animal variety and organismal complexity. It is now believed that the regulation of protein synthesis is the driver in determining cellular diversity. In eukaryotic cells, the ability to express biologically active or functional proteins comes under major regulation at several points: deoxyribonucleic acid (DNA) transcription, ribonucleic acid (RNA) processing, messenger RNA (mRNA) stability, mRNA translation, and posttranslational protein modifications and folding.

TRANSCRIPTION OF DNA

DNA transcription comprises the first level at which the "reading of the DNA cookbook" can be regulated. Transcription is the mechanism by which a template strand of DNA is accessed and utilized to generate different classes of RNA:

1. *Messenger RNAs (mRNAs),* which are the genetic coding templates used by the translational machinery to determine the order of amino acids incorporated into an elongating polypeptide during the process of mRNA translation.
2. *Transfer RNAs (tRNAs),* which carry individual amino acids to the mRNA template, thereby allowing correct insertion of amino acids into the growing polypeptide chain.
3. *Ribosomal RNAs (rRNAs),* which are assembled with numerous ribosomal proteins to form the ribosomes, and which, in eukaryotic cells, include (designated by centrifugal sedimentation size) the 28S, 5S, and 5.8S RNAs that are associated with the large

(60S) ribosomal subunit and the 18S rRNA that is associated with the small (40S) ribosomal subunit.

4. *Small nuclear RNAs (snRNAs),* which are involved in processing RNA within the nucleus.
5. Other types of RNAs, including small nucleolar RNA and microRNA.

DNA transcription (i.e., RNA synthesis) is catalyzed by a family of enzymes called RNA polymerases. All RNA polymerases are dependent upon a DNA template in order to synthesize RNA. Transcription of the three different classes of RNAs in eukaryotes is carried out by three different polymerases. RNA polymerase I synthesizes the rRNAs, excluding the 5S species. RNA polymerase II synthesizes the mRNAs and some snRNAs involved in RNA splicing. RNA polymerase III synthesizes the tRNAs, 5S rRNA, and some other snRNAs. All RNA polymerases contain a core group of proteins, defined as the basic enzymatic unit required for transcription to proceed. In addition, multisubunit protein cofactors have been identified that associate with the various RNA polymerases to increase enzyme stability and regulate the rate of elongation.

RNA synthesis by RNA polymerase occurs in three stages: initiation, elongation, and termination. The most important mode for control of eukaryotic gene expression lies at the level of transcription initiation. Transcription initiation involves the binding of the RNA polymerase to the transcription start site. Following this is the elongation step, in which the incorporation of ribonucleotides to the elongating RNA is the hallmark event. Finally, termination is defined as the dissociation of RNA polymerase from the DNA template, with concomitant release of the nascent transcript.

The most complex controls observed in eukaryotic genes are those that regulate the expression of the genes encoding mRNAs. These eukaryotic genes contain a basic structure consisting of coding exons and noncoding introns and any number of different domains, both transcribed and nontranscribed, that serve to regulate transcription. Signals present within the DNA template that act to modulate the rate of transcription are called *cis*-acting elements. *Cis*-elements that serve to stimulate the initiation of transcription are termed promoters and enhancers, whereas *cis*-elements that serve to inhibit or downregulate transcription are called repressor domains. Promoters are sequences that increase the ability of RNA polymerases to recognize the site at which initiation begins. Almost all eukaryotic genes contain basal promoters of two types that are termed CCAAT-boxes and TATA-boxes based on their conserved nucleotide sequences. In addition to promoters, other *cis*-elements may enhance polymerase activity even further. These sequence elements are termed enhancers or activating sequences. Regulatory sequences in DNA are predominantly located upstream (5′) of the transcription initiation site, although some *cis*-elements occur downstream (3′) or even within the genes themselves. The number and type of *cis*-elements vary with each gene.

Proteins that bind *cis*-elements are termed *trans*-acting factors, or, more commonly, transcription factors. Transcription factors are DNA binding proteins that can act to enhance or repress mRNA gene expression. For example, numerous proteins identified as TFII (for transcription factors regulating RNA polymerase II) have been observed to interact with the TATA-box, and the protein identified as C/EBP (for CCAAT-box/enhancer binding protein) binds to the CCAAT-box element. Recent estimates report that there may be as many as 3,000 transcription factors in humans (Levine and Tjian, 2003). Transcription factors afford a means of coordinately regulating a number of genes. For example, the pathway for the synthesis of cholesterol (see Chapter 17), involves at least 23 enzymes, and many of the genes for enzymes in this pathway are regulated by a family of transcription factors called sterol regulatory element binding proteins (SREBPs). Confirmation of the genes regulated by SREBP has been provided by microarray analysis of mRNAs in strains of mice that either over or under express SREBP (Horton et al., 2003). Another family of transcription factors responsible for coordinate regulation of genes are vitamin A derivatives involved in regulation of differentiation (see Chapter 30). Transcription factors often pair up with a second DNA binding protein that is either identical to itself (forming a homodimer) or different (forming a heterodimer).

Each cell type expresses characteristic combinations of activator proteins and repressor proteins, and many signaling pathways converge at the level of transcription factors to alter their activity or interaction. The absolute number, ratio, and interaction of transcription factors all confer detailed control of mRNA synthesis. In addition, the presence of multiple *cis*-acting elements within each template strand of DNA results in a diverse array of binding sites for different regulatory proteins, revealing an even greater level of combinatorial complexity. All of the above factors permit exquisite control of mRNA gene expression.

Eukaryotic DNA is organized in a complex structure called chromatin. Although a primary function of chromatin is compaction of DNA, chromatin is much more dynamic than was previously thought. The changes in chromatin structure that accompany transcriptional activation or repression are collectively called chromatin remodeling. Chromatin is remodeled before and during transcription initiation (by ATP-dependent remodelers) and during transcript elongation. Much evidence now suggests that the physical structure of the DNA, compacted into chromatin, affects the ability of the various transcription factors and RNA polymerases to gain access to specific genes and to activate transcription from them (Studitsky et al., 2004).

PRE-mRNA PROCESSING AND SPLICING

Newly transcribed pre-mRNA undergoes significant post transcriptional processing as illustrated in Figure 13-7. First, the 5′ end of eukaryotic mRNAs is "capped" with a 7-methylguanosine residue (m^7GTP). The covalently

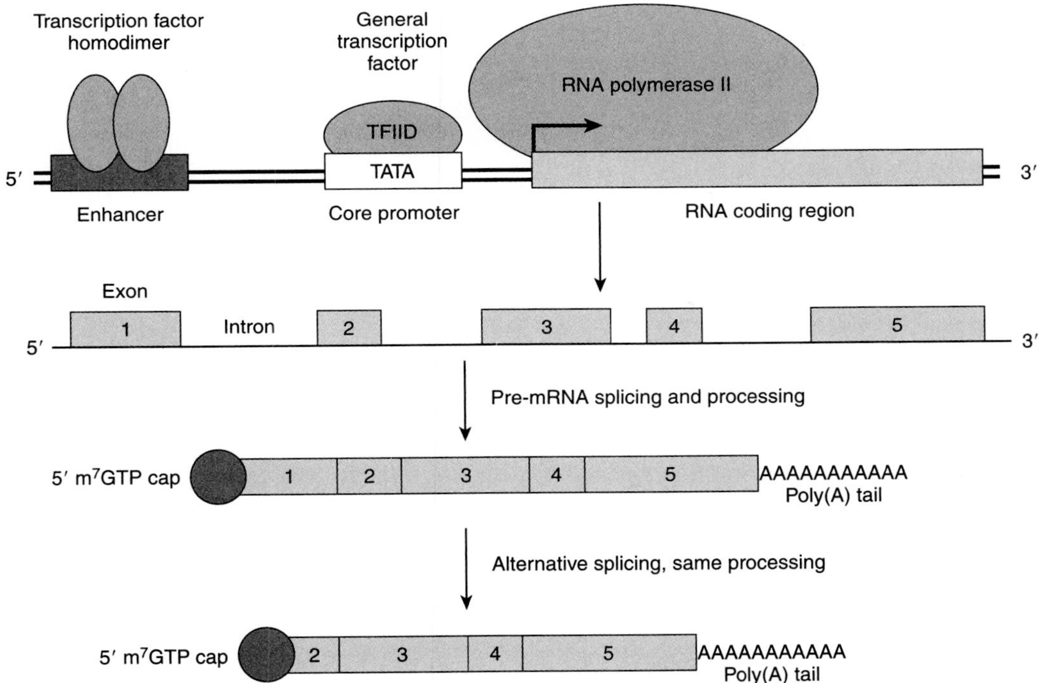

Figure 13-7 The basic eukaryotic transcription apparatus and assembly of an mRNA transcript. *Top,* A simple core promoter (TATA) and enhancer element found upstream of the transcription start site (noted as an *arrow*) is bound by DNA binding proteins called transcription factors to activate or repress the synthesis of RNA. *Middle,* After transcription, the RNA species is edited by the spliceosome to form an mRNA species that contains only coding exons. After RNA splicing, the transcript is processed for mRNA translation via capping and polyadenylation. *Bottom,* The process of alternative splicing can produce multiple transcripts from a single RNA species, thereby enhancing genetic diversity from a limited number of genes.

attached m^7GTP molecule serves to protect the mRNA from exonucleases and more importantly is recognized by specific proteins of the translational machinery (Wilkie et al., 2003). Next, capped mRNA is polyadenylated at the 3′ end. A stretch of 20 to 250 adenosine residues added by polyadenylate polymerase serves among other things as a binding region for the protein, poly(A)-binding protein, which functions in the circularization of mRNA during translation and increases mRNA stability (Wilkie et al., 2003). Following polyadenylation, the pre-mRNA undergoes a process which separates the noncoding regions of the primary transcript (introns) from the biologically active coding regions (exons). Exons are then joined together to generate a mature mRNA product. This process of intron removal and exon ligation is called RNA splicing. Introns are either self-splicing or require a specialized RNA-protein complex called a spliceosome. Spliceosomes are multicomponent ribonucleoprotein complexes containing small nuclear ribonucleoprotein particles (snRNPs) and more than 100 other proteins.

Alternative pre-mRNA splicing is responsible for the production of multiple mature mRNAs from a single gene. By altering the pattern of exons from a single primary transcript that are spliced together, biologically different proteins can arise from a single gene, increasing genetic diversity. Nearly three-quarters of human multi-exon genes undergo tissue-specific patterns of alternative splicing. Alternative splicing can occur either at specific developmental stages or in different cell types. Many human diseases, such as cancer, are linked to alternative splicing. For example, the tumor suppressor genes BRCA1 and BRCA2 are involved in 90% of familial breast cancers and are also known to be involved in ovarian and prostate cancers (Orban and Olah, 2003). Splice variants of the BRCA1 and BRCA2 transcripts encode altered or truncated proteins that malfunction in controlling processes such as transcriptional regulation and DNA repair. Following transcription, capping, polyadenylation and splicing, the final mRNA product is then exported out of the nucleus and made available for translation into protein.

TURNOVER OF mRNA

Increases in the cellular abundance of a particular mRNA species can occur as a result of increased formation by transcription or by increased stability (i.e., decreased rate of degradation or turnover) of the mRNA. When the decay of a particular mRNA is reduced, that mRNA accumulates and hence the total amount of protein translated from that mRNA increases. The stability of a given mRNA transcript is determined by the presence of specific sequence elements, which can be bound by RNA-binding proteins to inhibit or enhance mRNA degradation. These interactions are controlled by a wide variety of factors including hypoxia, hormones, and cytokines. For example, the stability of the mRNA for phosphoenolpyruvate carboxykinase (PEPCK), a key regulatory enzyme in gluconeogenesis (see Chapter 12), is enhanced by cyclic adenosine monophosphate (cAMP), which functions as a second messenger between hormonal signals and regulation of PEPCK mRNA (Nachaliel et al., 1993). Stabilizing the mRNA for PEPCK increases the amount of enzyme protein within the cell. Dysregulation of mRNA stability has been associated with human diseases including α-thalassemia, Alzheimer's disease, inflammatory disease, and cancer.

TRANSLATION OF mRNA

The levels of a number of specific proteins are regulated at the level of translation of their mRNAs. If cellular abundance of all proteins was determined at the level of transcription, the relationship between molar protein and mRNA levels would be linear. In fact, the correlation between mRNA levels and protein abundance in a single cell is poor, emphasizing the fact that posttranscriptional processes dominate the regulation of cellular protein abundance. In the past decades, the control of gene expression at the translational level has emerged as a means of regulation of cell growth, proliferation, malignant transformation, and apoptosis (programmed cell death) (Thornton et al., 2003).

Regulation of mRNA translation may involve changes that alter the overall translational or ribosomal capacity of the cell (i.e., change in the number of ribosomes) or changes that alter the translational or ribosomal efficiency (i.e., amount of protein synthesized per ribosome). Furthermore, changes in translational efficiency may be restricted to regulation of expression of specific proteins (e.g., ferritin mRNA) or affect the translational rate of specific proteins that are subsequently involved in mRNA translation and, thus, have global effects on the capacity and efficiency of mRNA translation (e.g., the TOP mRNAs, which are discussed in the following text).

A change in translational capacity implies alteration in the cellular abundance of the ribosomal proteins and rRNA. Each ribosome is composed of 80 different proteins and four RNA species (5S, 5.8S, 18S, and 28S). The time needed to modify these populations dictates that only chronic or sustained conditions, such as prolonged starvation or tumor growth, can alter overall protein synthesis at the level of ribosomal capacity. Three of the RNA species (5S, 8S, 18S, and 28S) are transcribed from one gene (the 45S rDNA gene) by RNA polymerase I. Transcription of RNA polymerase I is enhanced by the transcription factor UBF (upstream binding factor). Conditions promoting anabolic growth may be accompanied by increased expression and/or activity of the UBF protein, resulting in increased 45S rDNA transcription (Hannan et al., 1996).

Translational capacity can also be influenced by ribosomal protein synthesis. Regulation of ribosomal protein synthesis occurs via the presence of a stretch of pyrimidines in the 5′-untranslated region of the gene. This terminal oligopyrimidine (TOP) motif is predominantly found in mRNAs that encode proteins that are involved in ribosome biogenesis. These TOP mRNAs include those that encode the ribosomal proteins, mRNA translation factors such as eukaryotic elongation factors eEF1A and eEF2, and poly(A)-binding protein. Reduction in translation of TOP mRNAs reduces the overall translational, or protein-synthetic, capacity of the cell because TOP mRNAs encode for proteins involved in translation. A number of studies have implicated the phosphoinositide 3-kinase (PI3K) and mammalian target of rapamycin (mTOR) signaling pathways in the translational activation of TOP mRNAs, but the precise role of each pathway in this process has not been defined at present. Feeding a protein-containing meal enhances TOP mRNA translation, whereas feeding an amino acid–deficient meal reduces translation of TOP mRNAs (Anthony et al., 2001). Although deprivation of amino acids can cause a decrease in the synthesis of essentially any protein, the synthesis of those proteins encoded by TOP mRNAs are repressed to a much greater extent than most proteins. The exaggerated inhibition of TOP mRNAs by protein undernutrition is due to an 'all or none' binary control mechanism that shifts the association of TOP mRNAs with polysomes (the translating population of ribosomes) into the sub-polysomes (the nontranslating ribosome population).

The regulation of translational capacity provides the organism with an ability to adapt to chronic or sustained conditions of change. In contrast, changes in translational efficiency can be accomplished as needed without delay because all the protein synthetic machinery is already present. Conditions that alter translational efficiency include nutrient intake, hypoxia, and fluctuations in levels of hormones such as insulin. A change in translational efficiency implies regulation at the level of mRNA translation.

The translation of mRNA is a highly organized and multicomponent pathway that, like DNA transcription, can be divided into three stages or steps: (1) initiation, (2) elongation, and (3) termination. During the initiation step, the small (40S) ribosomal subunit is recruited to a selected mRNA and joined with the large (60S) ribosomal subunit to form an 80S ribosome competent to identify the translation start codon and begin the process of elongation. The process of elongation involves the energy-expensive process of adding amino acids one after the other to the growing peptide chain. The termination step consists of recognition of the stop or termination codon and dissociation of the ribosomal subunits from the mRNA. Each of these steps is regulated by separate categories of protein factors called eukaryotic initiation factors (eIF), eukaryotic elongation factors (eEF), and eukaryotic release factors (eRF), respectively. Most of the protein factors regulating translation have multiple subunits and contain binding sites for interaction with other translation factors as well as for association with the ribosome. In addition, several are capable of catalytic activity that can be exploited to stimulate or inhibit translation.

The majority of translational control lies at the initiation step, which is summarized in Figure 13-8. This step can be further subdivided into three events that determine overall initiation activity. The first event involves the binding of the initiating tRNA (specifically, a methionyl-tRNA, or Met-tRNA$_i$) to the small ribosomal subunit. The Met-tRNA$_i$ is brought to the 40S ribosomal subunit by the protein factor eIF-2. The ability of eIF-2 and GTP (guanosine 5′-triphosphate) to associate with the initiating Met-tRNA$_i$ is regulated in a major way by the phosphorylation state of eIF-2. Increases in phosphorylated eIF-2 prevent association of Met-tRNA$_i$ with the small ribosomal subunit and stall the process of initiation, resulting in global downregulation of mRNA translation. Under conditions of cellular stress, phosphorylation of eIF-2 also signals the need for increased expression of specific mRNAs that function to manage or alleviate cell stress. This paradoxical concept will be covered in greater detail in subsequent text.

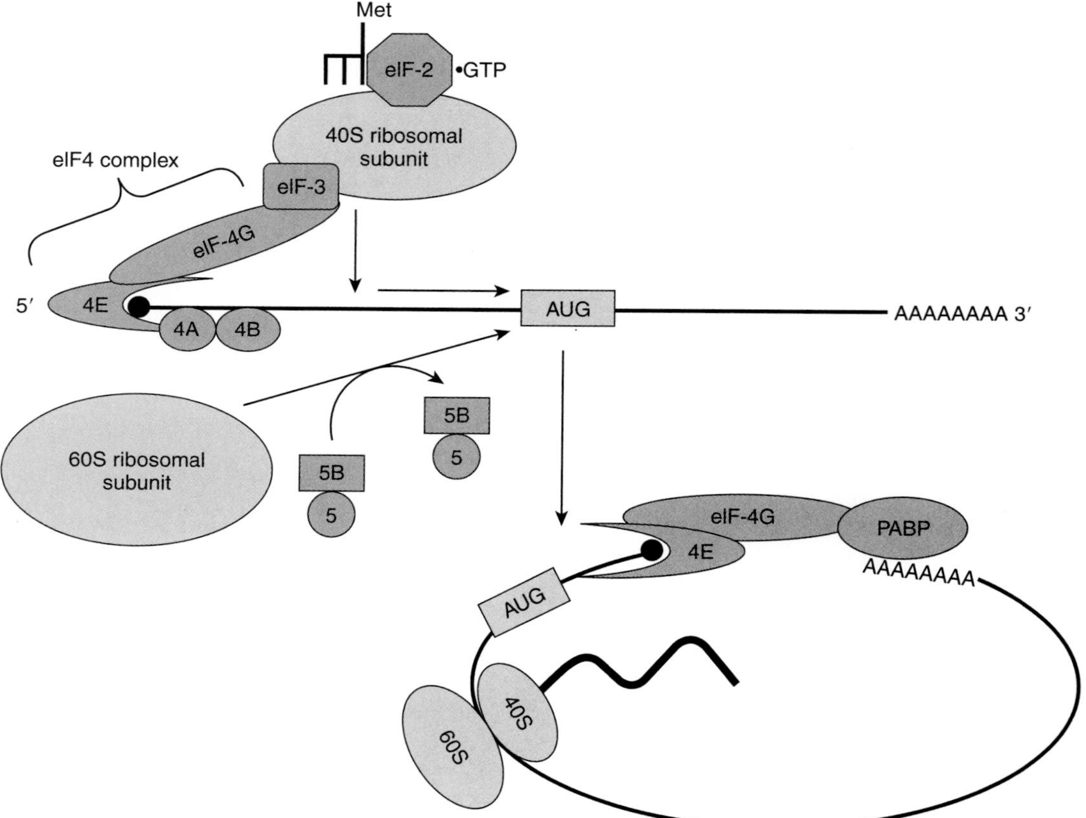

Figure 13-8 The pathway of initiation of eukaryotic mRNA translation. Eukaryotic initiation factor 2 (eIF-2) binding to GTP is a necessary event that allows the binding of itself and the initiating tRNA (Met-tRNA$_i$) to the 40S ribosomal subunit. The AUG codon (i.e., the methionine start codon) signals the start of translation. After this preinitiation complex formation, the mRNA targeted for translation is selected by the eIF-4 group of translation factors, which includes the mRNA cap binding protein eIF-4E and the scaffold protein eIF-4G. eIF-4G is important for bringing the small ribosomal subunit into proximity with the mRNA and has a role in mRNA circularization by binding the poly(A)-binding protein. After selection of mRNA, the 60S ribosomal subunit joins the 40S to form a competent 80S ribosome in a reaction catalyzed by eIF-5 and eIF-5B, along with the help of eIF-2 and eIF-3.

The second event in translation initiation subject to regulation involves the binding of the small ribosomal subunit to the selected mRNA. This event requires several initiation factors, collectively called eIF-4 (or eIF-4F). One of the proteins in this group, named eIF-4E, selects the mRNA to be translated by binding its 5′-m^{7}GTP cap structure. A second member of the eIF4 group, called eIF-4G, functions to bring the small ribosomal subunit and the mRNA into proximity to each other. It accomplishes this task by binding both eIF-4E and a protein factor (eIF-3) associated with the 40S ribosome. A family of repressor proteins (named 4E-BPs) can prevent eIF-4G from interacting with eIF-4E and thereby inhibit the 40S ribosome from binding mRNA. A second function of eIF-4G is to associate with poly(A)-binding protein, permitting 5′→3′circularization of mRNA. Circularization of mRNA is believed to be important for stabilizing recruited 40S ribosomal subunits and for efficient recycling of terminating ribosomes for another round of translation of the same mRNA (Wilkie et al., 2003). The final event involves the joining of the small ribosomal subunit (bound to mRNA) to the large ribosomal subunit. This event is catalyzed by several eIFs, including eIF-2, eIF-3, and eIF-5B. Although the factors involved and their interactions have been explored, details surrounding potential regulation at this step are poorly understood.

After initiation, the polypeptide is assembled with the amino acid sequence being specified by the mRNA sequence, as illustrated in Figure 13-9. This process requires a substantial amount of metabolic energy, cleaving two molecules of GTP for every added amino acid. The elongation step of mRNA translation involves fewer protein factors than the initiation step (just three eEFs versus more than a dozen eIFs), but the eEFs required are considered the workhorses of protein synthesis on the ribosome. At the start of elongation, the Met-tRNA$_i$ is base-paired with the mRNA start codon in a location named the peptidyl or "P" site within the ribosome. The protein factor eEF-1A (bound to GTP) then delivers the next correct aminoacyl-tRNA to the ribosome at the aminoacyl or "A" site. Upon correct codon–anticodon interaction, energy is released from eEF-1A in the form of GTP hydrolysis. A second factor, named eEF-1B, assists in regenerating active eEF-1A, ensuring continued deliverance of aminoacyl-tRNAs to the ribosome.

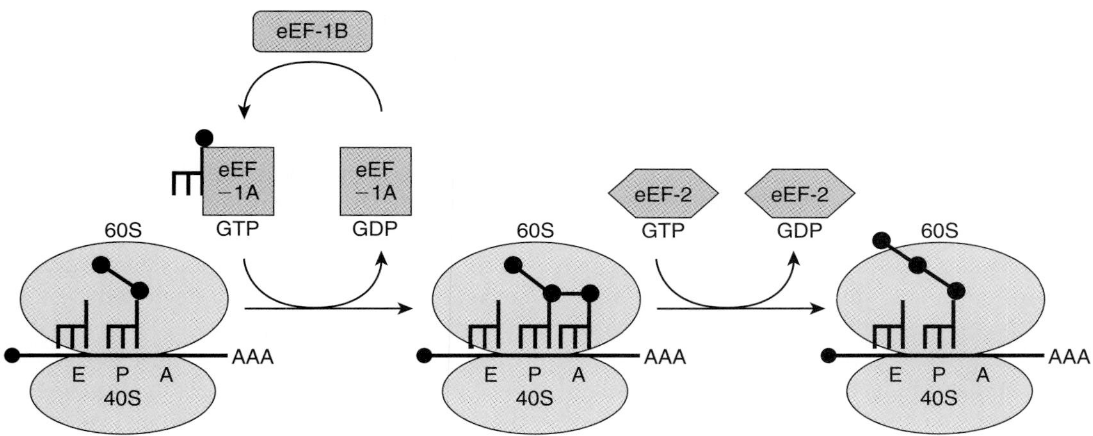

Figure 13-9 The pathway of elongation of eukaryotic mRNA translation. Eukaryotic elongation factor 1A (eEF-1A) bound to GTP delivers an aminoacylated tRNA to the A-site of the ribosome. When the appropriate codon–anticodon interaction occurs, GTP is hydrolyzed and eEF-1A is released from the ribosome bound to GDP. eEF-1B functions to regenerate the GTP-bound form of eEF-1A. The protein factor eEF-2 serves to catalyze the linking of the new amino acid to the growing peptide chain as well as the movement of the ribosome along the mRNA.

A third and final factor, named eEF-2, mediates translocation of the peptidyl-tRNA from the P site to the A site, and facilitates movement of the ribosome along the mRNA. This ribosomal translocation also requires energy in the form of GTP hydrolysis.

All three eEFs are subject to phosphorylation in mammalian cells. Phosphorylation of eEF-1A stimulates elongation activity whereas phosphorylation of eEF-1B has no reported influence on elongation rates. On the other hand, eEF-2 is inactivated by phosphorylation in response to stimuli that increase energy demand or reduce its supply. This likely serves to slow down protein synthesis and thus conserve energy under such circumstances (Andersen et al., 2003).

The final step in translation, that of termination, occurs when the stop codon is positioned in the A site of the ribosome. This event is recognized by the protein eRF-1, which binds to the ribosome and, in a GTP-dependent fashion, catalyzes the cleavage of the bond between the nascent peptide and the tRNA, thereby releasing the protein. A second release factor called eRF-3 serves to stimulate eRF-1 activity in the presence of GTP.

POSTTRANSLATIONAL MODIFICATIONS AND FOLDING OF PROTEINS

Co-translational and posttranslational modifications are essential steps for the translocation, activation, regulation, and, ultimately, the degradation of proteins. In fact, there are probably only a small number of proteins that do not undergo some type of chemical change during or following their synthesis. The N-terminal methionine residue is removed from many proteins, and other unnecessary regions of some proteins undergo cleavage. Other common modifications include, but are not limited to, glycosylation, acetylation, fatty acylation, and disulfide bond formation. Despite the omnipresence of protein modification in nature, much remains unknown about how these alterations affect the activity of each individual protein. This is mostly because a singular type of modification imparts different functions, depending on the target protein. For example, asparagine-linked glycosylation may stabilize the folding process of one polypeptide, whereas in a different protein, it may play an important role in cellular recognition or function. The mechanism for these and other protein modifications during and following translation is varied and complex. Nevertheless, it is important to point out that mutations in genes encoding proteins involved in protein modifications, such as glycosylation, have been identified in various neuromuscular disorders such as muscular dystrophy, muscle-eye-brain disease, Walker-Warburg syndrome, and congenital disorders of glycosylation (Paschen, 2003). These human diseases emphasize the fact that co-translational and posttranslational modifications are germane events in regulating protein synthesis and also protein degradation, as will be detailed later in this chapter.

The majority of mRNA translation is initiated on cytosolic ribosomes. For distinct classes of proteins, the nascent polypeptide is targeted (via the signal recognition particle) to the endoplasmic reticulum (ER) for completion and for certain co-translational and posttranslational modifications to occur. These classes of proteins include ER and Golgi-resident proteins, membrane-associated proteins, proteins of the endosomal–lysosomal system, and proteins destined for secretion. Following translation and modification, nascent peptides located in the ER must be correctly folded and assembled prior to transit to intracellular organelles or the cell surface. A family of proteins referred to as molecular chaperones accomplishes this task, functioning as a quality control system in nascent peptide synthesis. Unfolded or misfolded proteins linger in the ER lumen for a time, awaiting proper assembly. Proteins unable to be correctly assembled are eventually translocated from the ER and targeted for degradation in the cytosol by the proteasome.

ER homeostasis requires that the capacity of the protein-folding apparatus remains in balance with the demand. This balance can be disrupted by environmental stress (e.g., glucose starvation or disturbance of Ca^{2+} homeostasis during hypoxia), genetic mutations in proteins requiring ER assembly (e.g., cystic fibrosis transmembrane conductance regulator), or malfunctions in the folding machinery itself. When the balance becomes disrupted, unfolded or misfolded proteins accumulate in the lumen of the ER. This buildup of "cellular trash" initiates an adaptive mechanism, termed the unfolded protein response (UPR, or ER stress response), which is summarized in Figure 13-10 (Kaufman, 2004). The UPR encompasses three separate processes. First, the global rate of protein synthesis is slowed down to reduce the ER protein-folding load. Second, ER resident chaperones are transcriptionally induced to increase the folding capacity in these organelles. Third, a protein degrading system named endoplasmic reticulum–associated degradation (ERAD) is initiated to help clear the accumulating cellular waste. Activation of ERAD is important for the degradation of unfolded proteins through the ubiquitin–proteasomal pathway (McCracken and Brodsky, 2003). If the ER stress cannot be alleviated by these three processes, then cellular pathways will be activated to induce programmed cell death.

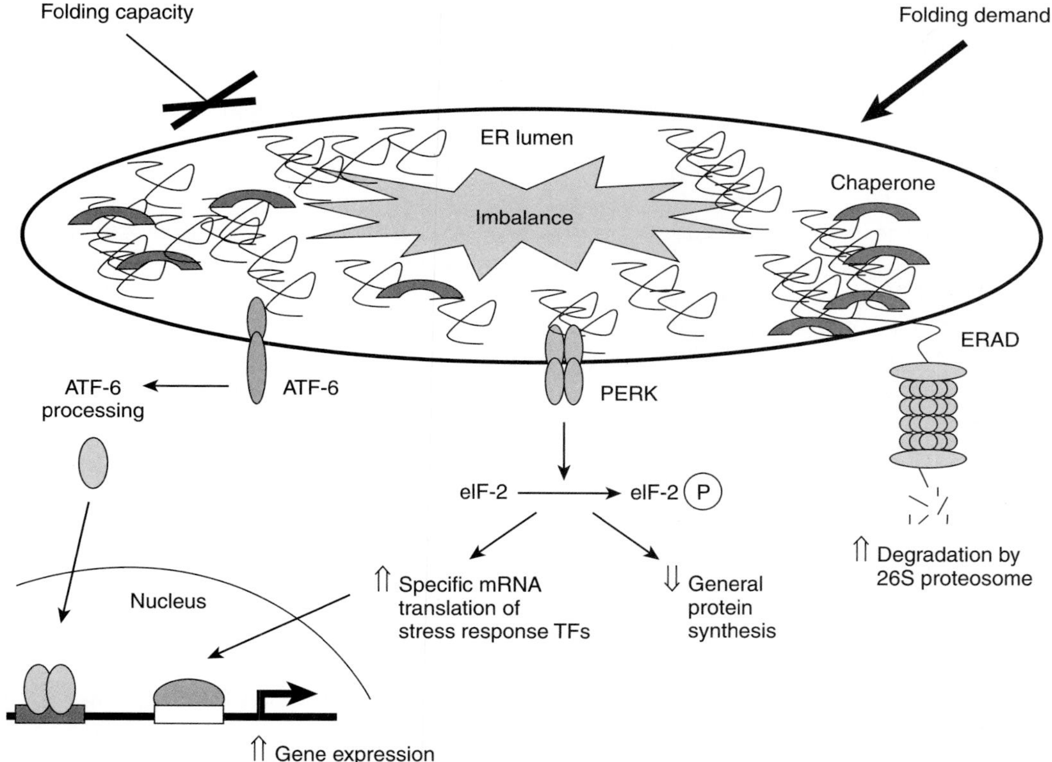

Figure 13-10 The functional components of the mammalian unfolded protein response (endoplasmic reticulum [ER] stress response). An imbalance between protein folding demand and protein folding capacity imposes stress on the ER resulting in a tripartite response. First, the transcription and translation of genes necessary for stress remediation are increased by increasing specific mRNA translation and promoting DNA binding of transcription factors originating from proteins associated with the ER membrane. Second, general protein synthesis is inhibited to reduce the load on the folding apparatus. Third, ER-associated degradation (ERAD) is increased via molecular chaperones guiding unfolded or misfolded proteins from the ER to the 26S proteasome. Both the general reduction in protein synthesis and the upregulation of gene-specific translation occur in association with the phosphorylation of eIF-2 by the protein kinase, PERK.

Clinical Correlation

Protein Misfolding: The Basis of Cystic Fibrosis and Alzheimer's Disease

All the information for protein folding is contained in the polypeptide sequence. Because the rate of the folding process is significantly faster than the rate of translation, the folding process must be regulated to hold back the polypeptide from folding until all of the relevant sequence is available and to prevent hydrophobic regions in the newly synthesized polypeptide from intermolecular aggregation. Folding mediators or chaperones are proteins responsible for sequestering nascent polypeptides and mediating folding. Some of these chaperones (holdases) are involved in sequestering nascent polypeptides on the ribosomes. They bind to short, linear sequences with hydrophobic character as they emerge from the ribosomes, maintaining them in an extended state until productive folding can occur. This prevents premature folding that may lead to incorrectly folded aggregates. Other chaperones (foldases) are multimeric complexes that act as "cages" to isolate a molecule of folding polypeptide to prevent any intermolecular encounters so that it folds on itself.

Researchers now understand that proteins must pass through partially folded states in which they are delicately poised between folding all the way to the correct state and becoming seriously stuck as a result of premature entanglement with other molecules. Misfolding of a protein can lead to its degradation (too little of the protein) or to its aggregation (formation of toxic deposits, of excessive quantities of wrongly folded proteins). This insight has opened the way to understanding some aspects of a range of human diseases.

Cystic fibrosis is the most common fatal genetic disease in humans, affecting approximately 1 in 2,000 live births among populations of Caucasians of Northern European descent. The autosomal recessive disorder is due to lack of a protein that regulates the transport of the chloride ion across cell membranes. The most common mutation underlying cystic fibrosis (~70% of the disease alleles; >90% of CF patients) is a deletion of Phe508 in the N-terminal region of this approximately 160-kDa protein. The deletion of this single amino acid acts to hinder the dissociation of the chloride ion transport regulator protein (cystic fibrosis transmembrane conductance regulator, CFTR) from one of its chaperones. This prevents the final steps for normal folding of CFTR, and, therefore, normal amounts of active CFTR are not produced. Interestingly, the ΔPhe508 mutant protein, if folded into a native state, is functional under physiological conditions. The problem is that nearly all of the newly synthesized protein is shunted to the degradation pathway before it has an opportunity to form functional chloride channels in the ER membrane. The trapped, partially folded protein is subsequently degraded.

Misfolding or folding too slowly can also lead to inappropriate association of partially folded chains, giving rise to cellular pathologies due to the formation of insoluble aggregates rather than from a lack of native protein. Some diseases known as amyloidoses, of which Alzheimer's disease is the best-known example, are characterized by the accumulation of plaques of insoluble protein in the extracellular tissue. Different proteins, each associated with a different disease, act as the building blocks of these plaques. Alzheimer's disease is characterized by the accumulation of plaques of insoluble β-amyloid in the brain. Normally, the body processes amyloid precursor protein by hydrolysis into soluble amyloid-β peptide fragments that are 40 to 42 amino acids in length. Under certain circumstances, these peptides aggregate into long filaments that then form the insoluble β-amyloid that makes up the neuritic plaque in patients with Alzheimer's. The implication of misfolding of the amyloid α-peptides as a basis of Alzheimer's disease is strongly supported by the finding that premature or early onset Alzheimer's disease is due to mutations in the amyloid precursor protein.

Several ER-resident molecules detect the accumulation of unfolded proteins. One of these is named protein kinase R-like ER-resident kinase (PERK, also named pancreatic eIF2 kinase, or PEK). PERK/PEK induces phosphorylation of the translation factor eIF-2, resulting in a shutdown of translation at the initiation step. This response blocks new synthesis of proteins and prevents further accumulation of unfolded proteins that form toxic aggregates. At the same time, increases in the phosphorylation of eIF-2 allow the translation of a specific mRNA that encodes activating transcription factor-4 (ATF-4). ATF-4 promotes the transcription of stress-remediation genes as well as genes that are linked to programmed cell death. The upregulation of specific mRNA translation in the face of global repression is a coordinated process that highlights the capacity of the cell to sequester and channel multiple biological processes in an organized fashion. In addition, other ER-resident proteins, such as IRE-1 (a transmembrane protein with both kinase and endoribonuclease functions) and ATF-6 (a transmembrane transcription factor), respond to the accumulation of unfolded proteins by activating the transcription of other stress-response genes, all serving to increase folding capacity in the ER (Kaufman, 2004).

Although cellular stress is certainly a major activator of the UPR, it should be mentioned that not only harmful events trigger the UPR. To the contrary, recent studies show that cell differentiation associated with increased secretory-protein production is coupled with activation of these same signaling pathways. For example, terminal differentiation of a B lymphocyte into a mature antibody-secreting plasma cell requires the ER to assemble and ship out large quantities of antibodies with remarkable efficiency. This task requires enormous expansion of the ER protein-folding capacity during B cell differentiation. The UPR mediates ER homeostasis as B cells transition into high-rate antibody secretion and serves to regulate events required for humoral immunity (Gass et al., 2004).

It is also clear that the UPR is required for normal cellular function. Patients with the rare autosomal-recessive disorder Wolcott-Rallison syndrome experience a severe form of neonatal or early infancy insulin-dependent diabetes along with multiple defects in bone formation and growth retardation (Delepine et al., 2000). The genetic mutation in these patients lies in the *EIF2AK3* gene, which encodes the human form of the eIF-2 kinase PERK. Mice with a functionally disrupted *EIF2AK3/PERK* gene demonstrate massive apoptosis of the exocrine pancreas a few weeks after birth, destroying the insulin-producing β cells (Zhang et al., 2002). It is interesting to note that apoptosis of the endocrine pancreas occurs as the animal begins to establish a pattern of meal feeding. Meal feeding requires the coordinated task of matching insulin production with large swings in glucose availability. The early steps of insulin biosynthesis occur in the ER, and the pancreatic β cell has a highly developed and active ER. The inability to phosphorylate eIF-2 in the β cell leads to an inability to properly regulate folding capacity during times of high glucose intake, sending the cell into apoptotic pathways.

Finally, several studies indicate that signaling pathways related to the UPR have evolved to couple nutritional needs with some metabolic processes. A cellular stress response that is related to but distinct from the UPR involves the cellular response to amino acid deprivation. In response to limitation of essential amino acids, another eIF-2 kinase named GCN2 (for general control nondepressible-2 kinase) phosphorylates the translation factor to reduce protein synthesis and initiate a cascade of events, not linked to protein folding, which results in the upregulation of genes involved in amino acid metabolism and transport. Animals lacking GCN2 are not able to cope with dietary essential amino acid deprivation and become moribund within days of feeding on a leucine-devoid diet (Anthony et al., 2004).

REGULATION OF PROTEIN SYNTHESIS AT THE TISSUE LEVEL

In addition to regulation that alters the synthesis of individual proteins or, coordinately, of multiple enzymes in a biochemical pathway, regulation of protein synthesis and degradation also occurs at the level of the tissue by changes that affect all the proteins of that tissue or organ.

Protein synthesis at the tissue level is regulated by the number of ribosomes in the cell and also by the amount of work done by each ribosome.

An example of the regulation of protein synthesis at the tissue level is seen in the responses to starvation during which there is a substantial loss of protein from skeletal muscle. Within hours of food withdrawal, there is a fall in the rate of synthesis per ribosome, followed by a slower decline in the total number of ribosomes that becomes the dominant factor as starvation progresses. There are also changes in protein degradation with starvation that are discussed later in this chapter.

The exact manner in which protein synthesis is controlled in response to any particular stimulus depends on the particular tissue or cell type. Each tissue responds in a way determined by the needs of the body as a whole. This is observed in tumor-bearing mice, in which protein synthesis in muscle declines while the synthesis of liver proteins is enhanced, presumably because liver function is more important to survival than preservation of function in skeletal muscle. In rats with malaria, there is also evidence of priority among tissues. In response to the anemia that accompanies infection with malaria, heart and spleen protein synthesis is maintained, whereas that in skeletal muscle declines.

MOLECULAR MECHANISMS OF PROTEIN DEGRADATION

Once a protein is made, it is immediately a target for degradation. Some proteins, such as collagen and hemoglobin, are relatively resistant to degradation and therefore turn over slowly. Other proteins are readily degraded, especially those that have an important regulatory function or those that are damaged in some way or that have errors in amino acid sequence due to errors in transcription. The details of the molecular basis of protein degradation, or proteolysis, have not been as fully described as for the system of protein synthesis. However, like synthesis, the regulation of protein degradation includes both a component that targets specific proteins and a component that regulates the overall rate of protein degradation in a tissue and facilitates changes in protein content. An example of the alterations in the degradation of a single protein is the stabilization of the enzyme tryptophan dioxygenase by the substrate, tryptophan (Cihak et al., 1973). When animals are fed high levels of tryptophan, there is an increased need to catabolize this amino acid. Tryptophan dioxygenase catalyzes the initial step of tryptophan catabolism, and a reduction in the degradation or turnover of tryptophan dioxygenase in response to tryptophan ensures that the capacity for tryptophan catabolism will increase whenever levels of tryptophan are high. An example of coordinated increases in the rate of degradation of all the proteins of a tissue, allowing the whole tissue to adapt to alterations in its environment, is the increased proteolysis of muscle tissue proteins that occurs in response to a number of stresses including fasting, acidosis, denervation, cancer, and thermal injury (Mitch and Goldberg, 1996).

Protein degradation, or proteolysis, in eukaryotic cells is accomplished by a large number of specific and nonspecific proteases. Most of these degradative enzymes can be associated with one of three major systems of cellular protein breakdown: the ubiquitin–proteasome pathway, the autophagy–lysosomal system, and the calcium- or calpain-dependent system. In general, the ubiquitin–proteasome system degrades most intracellular proteins, whereas the autophagy-lysosomal system degrades membrane and endocytosed proteins. The calcium-dependent thiol proteases, known as calpains, are widely expressed and have been implicated in a number of basic cellular processes, although their physiological function in vivo is not well understood. Investigations of the pathways directing protein degradation have proved that these processes are as complicated and as exquisitely controlled as are the processes for protein synthesis.

UBIQUITIN–PROTEASOME PATHWAY

The majority (up to 80% to 90%) of intracellular protein degradation is accomplished by the ubiquitin–proteasome pathway (Herrmann et al., 2004; Kee et al., 2003). The ubiquitin–proteasome pathway is present in both the nucleus and cytoplasm of eukaryotic cells and plays a role in the degradation of both normal and abnormal proteins. This pathway is responsible for the regulated degradation of many critical proteins, including those required for the control of cell growth and proliferation, cell differentiation, immune and inflammatory responses, apoptosis, and metabolic adaptation. The ubiquitin–proteasome pathway also carries out housekeeping functions in basal protein turnover and the elimination of abnormal proteins that are miscoded, misfolded, mislocalized, damaged, or otherwise rendered inoperative. The ubiquitin–proteasome pathway plays a critical role in the control of muscle mass, and its activity is increased during muscle wasting (e.g., during denervation atrophy, atrophy due to immobilization, or starvation). It also plays an important role in muscle recovery and remodeling (Taillandier et al., 2004). There is some evidence that the activity of the ubiquitin–proteasome pathway is decreased with regular endurance exercise, which is known to have hypertrophic effects in skeletal muscle.

As illustrated in Figure 13-11, the ubiquitin–proteasome pathway can be considered as made up of three sequential processes: (1) recognition of a protein substrate for degradation; (2) covalent addition of a polyubiquitin chain to mark the protein for degradation; and (3) proteolysis of the protein by a 2,500 kDa complex called the 26S proteasome. The recognition of a protein for degradation typically takes advantage of certain structural changes in the protein, including the exposure of specific amino acid sequences that are normally buried, posttranslational modifications such as phosphorylation or hydroxylation, binding

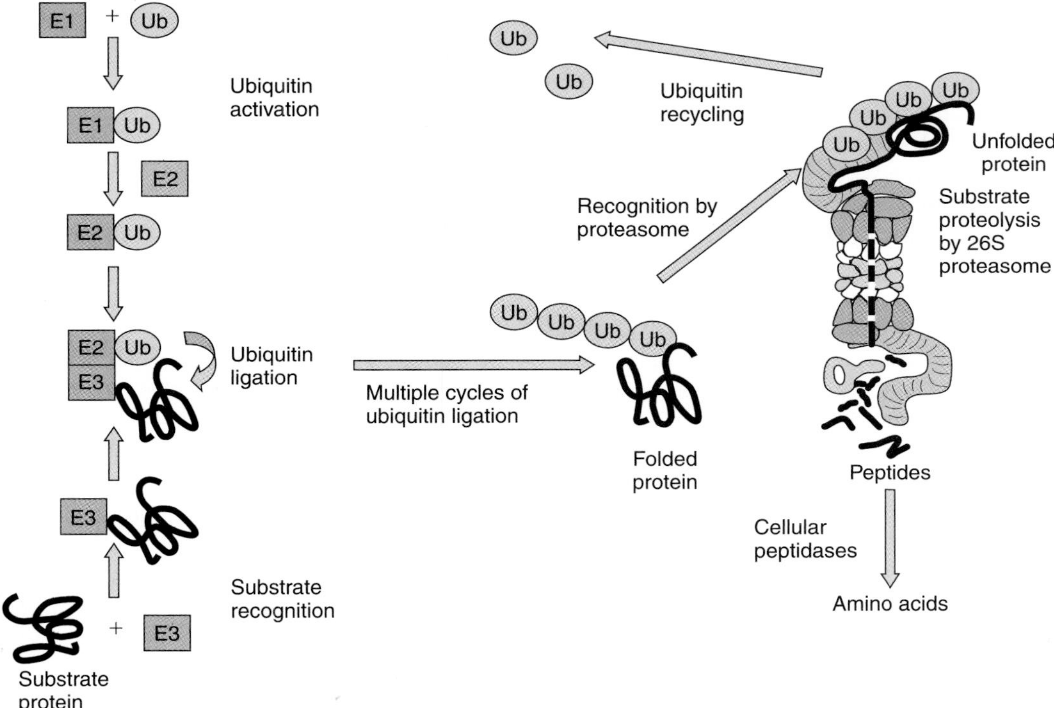

Figure 13-11 Major steps in the degradation of a protein by the ubiquitin–proteasome pathway. The protein substrate for degradation is recognized by a ubiquitin ligase E3, and ubiquitin (Ub) is activated by a ubiquitin activating E1 and then transferred to a ubiquitin conjugating E2. An E3-E2-substrate complex forms and Ub is transferred from the E2 (in some cases, via transfer to E3) to the substrate to form a polyubiquitin chain attached to the protein substrate. The polyubiquitin-tagged protein is recognized by the 26S proteasome and is degraded in an ATP-dependent manner to small peptides, which are released and further hydrolyzed by intracellular peptidases.

to or release from its ligand, interaction with an adaptor protein or chaperone (e.g., the export of misfolded proteins via chaperones from the ER into the cytosol), or specific damage incurred to the protein such as oxidation or nitrosylation.

Once a protein has been identified as a substrate for degradation, it is covalently tagged with ubiquitin. Ubiquitin, a protein so-named because of its omnipresence in all cell types, is made up of 76 amino acid residues including a C-terminal glycine and a lysine residue at position 48. Ubiquitin is covalently attached to the protein destined for degradation in a series of three reactions or steps catalyzed by enzymes known as E1 (ubiquitin-activating enzyme), E2 (ubiquitin-conjugating enzyme), and E3 (ubiquitin-ligating enzyme), (Doherty et al., 2002). There are a few isoforms of E1, multiple isoforms of E2, and a very large number of E3 enzymes, allowing for much tissue and substrate-specific regulation of this process. In the first step, a molecule of ubiquitin is activated by binding to E1 in an ATP-dependent reaction, and the ubiquitin moiety is then transferred to an E2. Both E1s and E2s have active site cysteine residues that form thioesters with the C-terminal glycine of ubiquitin. Finally, the ubiquitin attached to E2 is transferred, directly or via E3, to a lysine residue on the substrate protein; E3 plays a critical function in recognition of a substrate protein for degradation and in mediating the formation of an E2-E3–substrate complex. Additional ubiquitins are similarly added to the monoubiquitinated substrate by forming isopeptide bonds between the C-terminal glycine of the ubiquitin molecule being added and lysine 48 of the ubiquitin molecule previously added. A chain of at least four ubiquitin molecules is required for polyubiquitinated proteins to be readily recognized and targeted to the 26S proteasome for destruction.

The actual degradation of ubiquitinated proteins takes place within an inner chamber of the proteasome, but the ubiquitin molecules are first released so they can be reused. The 26S proteasome is a large, multisubunit complex that consists of a core 20S proteolytic complex with a regulatory 19S complex attached to one or both ends. The regulatory units are involved in recognition of tagged proteins, removal of the ubiquitin tag, and in the ATP-dependent unfolding and guiding of the client protein into the tunnel-shaped proteolytic core. The 20S core complex is composed of four stacked ring-like structures (αββα) of seven subunits each, which together form a barrel-like structure. The central catalytic cavity of the structure contains a total of six proteolytic sites, contributed by the three separate catalytic subunits of each β ring. These catalytic subunits are classified as N-terminal threonine hydrolases because the N-terminal threonine acts as the nucleophile catalyst. However, the three different subunits in each of the two rings differ in their preference for cleaving peptide bonds immediately after basic, hydrophobic, or acidic residues. The 20S core hydrolyzes incoming substrate into peptide fragments of approximately 3 to 30 amino acid residues. These peptide products are released from the proteasome and are further hydrolyzed by other proteases and aminopeptidases in the cell.

Regulation of proteolysis by the proteasome occurs on three levels. First, substrate recognition is regulated by features that uniquely specify the targeted protein for polyubiquitination. These are largely unidentified for most proteins and include phosphorylation, hydroxylation of a proline residue, or unmasking of a degradation signal contained in the primary sequence. Ubiquitination signals on target proteins may be acquired posttranslationally, or the signal may be constitutively active. Second, regulated degradation of specific classes of substrates may be achieved by association of E2-E3 complexes with different ancillary factors. For example, in some cases it is the E3 that must be modified or switched "on" by undergoing posttranslational modification to yield an active form that recognizes the substrate. In other cases, the stability of the protein substrate depends on its association with ancillary proteins such as molecular chaperones that act as recognition elements in *trans* and serve as a link to the appropriate ligase. Others, such as certain transcription factors, have to dissociate from the specific DNA sequence to which they bind in order to be recognized by the system. Finally, the ubiquitin–proteasome pathway can be regulated overall at the level of ubiquitination or at the level of proteasome activity, such as by increased expression of ubiquitin or proteasome subunits. An example of an overall increase in capacity of the ubiquitin–proteasome pathway is the acceleration of muscle degradation in cancer cachexia, which has been associated with increased expression of ubiquitin and proteasome subunits or with increased proteasomal proteolytic activity (Costelli and Baccino, 2003; Sakamoto, 2002).

A special example of change in proteasome activity that results from changes in the expression level of particular proteasomal subunits is the change in proteasomal catalytic specificity induced by interferon γ. Special proteasome subunits are expressed upon induction by interferon γ, resulting in formation of immunoproteasomes that generate different patterns of cleavage products. It is thought that these proteasomes are involved in regulating the production of antigenic peptides (8 to 9 amino acids in length) or in presentation of antigens by major histocompatibility complex (MHC) class I molecules (Kloetzel, 2004).

ER-ASSOCIATED DEGRADATION

The ER-associated degradation (ERAD) pathway functions in ER quality control, directing ubiquitin-mediated degradation of a variety of ER-associated misfolded and normal proteins. Proteins located in the ER that are targeted for destruction are retrotranslocated (or dislocated) from the ER into the cytosol where the ubiquitin-conjugating enzymes and 26S proteosome are located. ERAD comprises three events: substrate selection, transport to the cytosol, and ubiquitin-mediated degradation. Substrate selection is mediated by the various molecular chaperones located in the ER, which facilitate gating and movement to the cytosol through a specific translocation. Dysfunctions in ERAD result in the buildup of cellular protein waste, and are linked to human disease states such as cystic fibrosis, Tay-Sachs disease, hypercholesterolemia, type A insulin resistance, and several neuromuscular disorders (McCracken and Brodsky, 2003).

AUTOPHAGY-LYSOSOMAL SYSTEM

Separate from the proteasome, cellular proteins are degraded within an intracellular compartment called the lysosome. Lysosomes are budded off from the membrane of the Golgi apparatus and dispersed throughout the cytosol, and they also form more gradually from later endosomes. Lysosomes contain a variety of hydrolytic enzymes that degrade proteins and other substances. The lysosomal system is less selective in targeting specific proteins for breakdown than is the ubiquitin–proteasome system.

Extracellular components, including plasma membrane components, enter the lysosomal system via endocytosis, whereas intracellular components (portions of the cytoplasm, including certain organelles) are sequestered by autophagy. In the process of autophagy, cytosolic components, including old organelles, destined for degradation by the lysosome are surrounded by a membrane donated by the ER to form an autophagic vacuole. This autophagic vacuole then fuses with a lysosome (Klionsky and Emr, 2000). On the other hand, in the process of endocytosis, vesicles are formed at the plasma membrane by pinching off and enclosing a portion of the extracellular matrix to bring it into the cell. The early endosome matures to a late endosome as lysosomal hydrolases and an acidic luminal environment are acquired. Then, the late endosome fuses with a lysosome. In both cases, within the lysosomes, the vesicular contents are broken down by degradative enzymes such as the cathepsins, and the degraded cellular components are then either recycled back into the cytosol or exported out of the cell via exocytosis.

Much of the information about the regulation of the lysosomal system is derived from studies in rats. Under conditions of nutrient starvation, autophagic proteolysis is induced to high levels and is referred to as macroautophagy. Although the lysosomal system is believed to be present in all tissues, macroautophagy is most actively expressed in the liver. Macroautophagy is believed to be a major source of amino acids during starvation. The rate of autophagy is physiologically controlled by amino acid concentrations, with activation of the system when amino acid supply is reduced and inhibition of the system when amino acid supply is increased (Lee and Marzella, 1994). Another example of regulation of lysosomal degradation is the increased degradation of certain membrane receptor proteins that is invoked in response to specific hormones. For example, some plasma membrane-bound receptors (e.g., the insulin receptor, the growth hormone receptor, and the epidermal growth factor receptor) are routed to the lysosomes for degradation in response to binding to their hormone ligands. Similarly, GLUT4 glucose transporters are internalized and degraded in response to binding to glucose.

CALPAINS

A third mechanism of cellular degradation that is emerging as important to human health and disease is the calcium and/or calpain-dependent system. The calpain system consists of a widely expressed family of at least 14 Ca^{2+}-activated proteolytic enzymes. The precise physiological functions of the calpains remain to be determined, but so far they have been implicated in basic cellular processes including cell proliferation, cell motility, and apoptosis. Experimental evidence suggests that overactivation of calpain following loss of Ca^{2+} homeostasis is associated with a variety of degenerative conditions and processes such as Alzheimer's disease, cataract formation, myocardial infarctions, multiple sclerosis, various muscular dystrophies, and stroke (Goll et al., 2003). Interestingly, mammalian calpains have a ubiquitous endogenous inhibitor protein, calpastatin, which is actually a group of at least eight polypeptide isoforms that are produced from a single gene by alternative splicing or use of alternate promoters. How calpastatin regulates calpain activity in living cells is not well understood.

REGULATION OF PROTEIN METABOLISM

Each step in the synthesis or degradation of protein is a potential site of regulation. Some steps of protein synthesis and degradation are controlled through the action of mediators such as hormones and cytokines. Although these mediators do not act in isolation, an understanding of the individual actions of hormones and cytokines is necessary for understanding the coordinated regulation involved in the responses of protein turnover to feeding, growth, and injury. These aspects of regulation are under study, but some examples of the ways in which protein metabolism is controlled are given in the following section.

HORMONES AND CYTOKINES

Anabolic Hormones

Growth hormone and insulin are both considered to be anabolic in that reduced circulating levels of these hormones are associated with loss of body protein or decreased growth. Normally, the blood insulin concentration increases with feeding and decreases with fasting, and is associated with cyclic responses of carbohydrate, fat, and protein metabolism between anabolism and catabolism. An inability to mount an anabolic response to the influx of nutrients is accompanied by a loss of body protein, and individuals who lack insulin because of diabetes lose body protein. Measurements in animal models show that insulin stimulates the synthesis of protein, although some human studies suggest that provision of amino acids is also required for this response. The most consistent finding in human studies is that protein degradation is inhibited by insulin in both the whole body and in skeletal muscle (Long and Lowry, 1990).

The mechanism for the acute action of insulin to stimulate protein synthesis occurs at the level of the initiation of translation of mRNA via phosphorylation of initiation factors (e.g., eIF-2) already present in the cell. The precise way in which insulin inhibits protein degradation is not known, but some depression in protein degradation, particularly in the liver, may be brought about through increased amino acid concentrations that inhibit lysosomal degradation (Lee and Marzella, 1994).

Growth hormone is associated with longer-term regulation of growth. Growth hormone levels are higher in children, especially during growth spurts, and children are dwarfed when growth hormone is absent. The effect of growth hormone is, in part, mediated by insulin-like growth factors IGF-1 and IGF-II, which are peptides produced by the liver in response to circulating growth hormone. The activity and availability of IGFs are also regulated by a number of binding proteins. IGFs in the blood are bound to these binding proteins, which tend to reduce the bioactivity of the hormone (Lang and Frost, 2002). Local production of IGFs at their sites of action in tissues might also be important in regulating protein metabolism. Muscle protein synthesis in adults is stimulated by provision of growth hormone or IGF-I, whereas there is no observable stimulation of whole-body protein synthesis. Muscle degradation is also enhanced by growth hormone, as evidenced by an increase in the excretion of 3-methylhistidine. This response may be a necessary consequence of the remodeling needed for the growth of muscle, but the precise details of how these hormones regulate protein metabolism are not yet fully understood.

In addition to growth hormone and insulin, the male sex hormone testosterone also promotes protein synthesis, particularly in muscle. Testosterone can also reduce protein degradation (Ferrando et al., 2002). Low levels of testosterone are associated not only with a lack of lean body mass, but also with an increase in adipose tissue. Replacement of testosterone is associated with increased muscle tissue, and this increase is associated with an increase in the number of satellite cells (myogenic stem cells that can fuse with muscle fibers), which suggests that androgens may affect differentiation (Sinha-Hikim et al., 2003). Synthetic testosterone-like compounds, classed as anabolic steroids, are also capable of promoting the retention of body protein, and have been used in animal production.

Catabolic Hormones

The three hormones cortisol, glucagon, and epinephrine are often collectively termed the stress hormones because their plasma concentrations are elevated after injury or during infection. Infusion of these hormones together mimics stress, causing loss of body protein and an inhibition of muscle protein synthesis. Glucagon promotes gluconeogenesis from amino acids and from lactate. The ratio of glucagon to insulin levels is an important factor in both acute regulation (such as after a meal) and in long-term regulation (such as with prolonged dietary deprivation). At physiological levels, glucagon is not known to have a direct effect on tissue or whole-body protein synthesis, but elevated glucagon does interfere with the ability of insulin to inhibit protein degradation (Long and Lowry, 1990).

Cortisol, from the adrenal cortex, is a glucocorticoid hormone that has a catabolic effect similar to that of glucagon. In addition, cortisol decreases protein synthesis and increases protein degradation in muscle. The mechanism for enhanced protein degradation in response to elevated glucocorticoids involves activation of the ubiquitin–proteasome pathway in muscle (Combaret et al., 2004). The synthesis of several liver proteins is increased, including the synthesis of enzymes involved in amino acid oxidation, which facilitates the conversion of amino acids into energy-yielding compounds or gluconeogenic precursors.

Few studies have been performed with epinephrine, but it appears that protein metabolism is not affected at moderate levels of the hormone, whereas protein degradation in the whole body and in muscle may be reduced at higher levels of epinephrine (Matthews et al., 1990). This anabolic action of epinephrine may act to limit the loss of body protein brought about by elevated cortisol and glucagon levels.

Cytokines

Cytokines are peptides produced by cells of the immune system (macrophages) in response to injury or inflammation. High circulating levels of cytokines, particularly interleukin-1β (IL-1β), interleukin-6 (IL-6), and tumor necrosis factor-α (TNF-α), are associated with catabolism of body protein. Direct action of these cytokines on muscle has not been demonstrated in vitro. However, when given to growing rats, both IL-1β and TNF-α stimulate protein synthesis in liver and depress protein synthesis in muscle. Protein degradation is inhibited in liver and stimulated in muscle by TNF-α, and these effects are potentiated by treatment with IL-1β. These effects on muscle protein synthesis and degradation mimic those observed in injury or inflammation. Further evidence for cytokine involvement in the catabolic response to infection is provided by studies that show a diminished catabolic state in septic animals treated with TNF-α antibody and IL-1β receptor antagonist (Garlick and Wernerman, 1997).

In addition to effects on muscle protein synthesis and degradation, cytokines such as TNF-α may also induce muscle loss by affecting the ability of precursor cells to differentiate into mature muscle cells. Muscle differentiation in response to injury is under the control of a family of transcription factors including MyoD. Elevated levels of TNF-α and interferon-γ are accompanied by reduced expression of MyoD and by reduced muscle cell differentiation (Black and Olson, 1998).

RESPONSES OF PROTEIN METABOLISM TO NUTRIENT SUPPLY

Anabolic Responses to Eating

One of the most fundamental anabolic responses is that observed after the ingestion of a meal. Substrates in the form of amino acids and energy-yielding substances are provided by the influx of nutrients. The hormonal responses include an increase in the circulating levels of insulin and a decrease in the levels of catabolic hormones such as glucagon. Rates of protein degradation are decreased in the whole body, and rates of synthesis might, in addition, be stimulated. Although the oxidation of amino acids is increased in the immediate postprandial period due to their elevated concentrations, there is a net positive balance of protein.

Nutrient intake affects protein synthesis at the level of ribosomal efficiency, that is, at the level of initiation of mRNA translation. In this regard, both the hormone insulin and dietary amino acids are necessary to drive postprandial changes in protein synthesis, particularly in liver and skeletal muscle. This is accomplished in two ways. First, balanced nutrient intake relieves phosphorylation of eIF-2, allowing the 40S ribosome to bind the initiating tRNA. Second, balanced nutrition promotes formation of the mRNA cap-binding complex, eIF-4. In the skeletal muscle of young animals, both insulin and oral intake of the essential amino acid leucine can independently stimulate eIF-4 complex formation and general protein synthesis rates (Prod'homme et al., 2004; Anthony et al., 2000). However, feeding a protein-free meal to humans or animals does not stimulate protein synthesis despite a significant increase in plasma insulin, suggesting that actual stimulation of protein synthesis is largely an amino acid- (perhaps leucine-) dependent process. Nevertheless, both insulin and leucine appear to function separately as a means to "jump-start" the translational machinery by relieving the chemical inhibition of the assembly of the 80S ribosome on the mRNA, and the effect of amino acid plus insulin is greater than the effect of either amino acid or insulin alone (Anthony et al., 2002).

In addition to stimulating protein synthesis, food intake also decreases overall protein degradation, but the mechanisms by which this is accomplished within the whole animal are not well understood. Amino acid intake is known to reduce lysosomal proteolysis. This effect is best studied in liver, where macroautophagy is inhibited by a group of amino acids that include leucine (Kanazawa et al., 2004). Available evidence suggests that an extracellular leucine sensor is involved, but its identity remains unknown. The ubiquitin–proteasome pathway is the major proteolytic system responsible for starvation- and refeeding-induced changes in proteolysis. However, this system is slow to respond to changes in nutritional status. Although four hours of refeeding was sufficient to normalize muscle protein synthesis rates in starved rats, ten hours of refeeding was required to normalize the starvation-induced elevation in ubiquitin–proteasome-dependent proteolysis in skeletal muscle of these rats (Kee et al., 2003). Thus protein degradation in response to feeding does not appear to be acutely linked to changes in protein synthesis.

Catabolism Associated With Brief Fasting

As the body moves from the absorptive period following a meal (also known as postprandial) to the postabsorptive period before the consumption of the next meal, protein balance changes from net accumulation to net loss. At the level of the whole body, the change is predominantly due to an increase in protein degradation. Amino acids are mobilized from tissues such as muscle and redirected to maintain protein synthesis in tissues such as the liver, as well as to provide substrates for gluconeogenesis and maintenance of the blood glucose level. The hormonal changes associated with fasting include a reduction in the circulating level of insulin and an increase in the level of glucagon.

Starvation

If fasting is prolonged and the body's stores of liver glycogen are exhausted, the body adapts to use muscle protein to meet most of the needs for glucose production. Although body fat is mobilized to meet most of the energy needs, this results in only limited usable energy for the brain and obligate glycolytic tissues such as red blood cells and the renal medulla. These tissues cannot use fatty acids as an energy source, and only a small amount of glucose can be formed from the small glycerol backbone component of fat. During starvation, the major portion of the brain's glucose requirement is met by mobilization of amino acids from body protein with subsequent gluconeogenesis by the liver. Increased mobilization of body protein for glucose production is evidenced by a relatively high excretion of urinary nitrogen during early starvation.

If gluconeogenesis were to continue at the accelerated rate observed during early starvation, skeletal muscle would soon be exhausted. An adaptation in lipid metabolism occurs in longer-term starvation, so that ketone bodies (acetoacetate, β-hydroxybutyrate) are formed. Ketone bodies can cross the blood-brain barrier to provide energy for the brain and thereby reduce the need for gluconeogenesis and spare body protein. Production and utilization of ketone bodies are associated with other adaptations that result in reductions in protein synthesis and degradation and in oxidation of amino acids. These adaptations help conserve both energy and amino acids and are reflected in the output of nitrogen, which is decreased from approximately 12 g in early starvation to approximately 3 g nitrogen per day by several weeks of starvation (Cahill, 1976). When body fat stores are exhausted, body protein is again mobilized for energy by means of an increase in muscle protein degradation. This final increase in the degradation of body protein cannot be sustained for long; if feeding does not occur, death ensues.

The hormonal changes that bring about alterations in protein metabolism in starvation are, for the most part, an amplification of the response to an overnight fast, with a further reduction in insulin and a further elevation in glucagon. In addition, the level of thyroid hormone decreases. Reduced levels of thyroid hormones result in a reduction in proteolysis by both lysosomal and ubiquitin–proteasome pathways (Mitch and Goldberg, 1996). In addition, reduced levels of thyroid hormones reduce basal energy expenditure and this helps to spare body protein stores.

Malnutrition

Prolonged undernutrition of energy and protein (see Chapters 15, 19, and 23) shares many of the same characteristics as starvation, but these develop over a longer time-frame. In protein-energy malnutrition, circulating levels of insulin decrease and those of glucagon increase. Growth hormone is elevated, but the level of IGF-I is depressed. Thyroid hormone level is reduced, with a similar conservation of energy and amino acids as is seen in starvation. The oxidation of amino acids is reduced, as is protein turnover (both synthesis and degradation).

In children, a reduction in food intake is accompanied by a cessation of growth. Chronic malnutrition results in both stunting (reduction in height for age) and wasting (reduction in weight for height). Nutrient deprivation also results in reductions of particular proteins. Albumin concentration often is reduced, as scarce amino acids are directed to more essential proteins. This selective reduction in albumin is mediated through a reduction in the amount of mRNA for albumin in the liver. Because circulating levels of albumin respond to nutritional intake, albumin concentration has been used to assess nutritional status, but the relation of albumin levels to nutritional status often is confused by the fall in albumin associated with injury or disease. Immunity and the resistance to infection are also impaired by chronic undernutrition;in the undernourished, infections both are more frequent than normal and are accompanied by increases in mortality and morbidity.

The data in Figure 13-12 demonstrate the reduction in protein synthesis and degradation in malnourished children in Jamaica. These children were studied at sequential time points as they recovered from their malnutrition. During recovery from malnutrition, both synthesis and degradation were accelerated compared with measurements made either when the children were malnourished or after they had recovered from malnutrition.

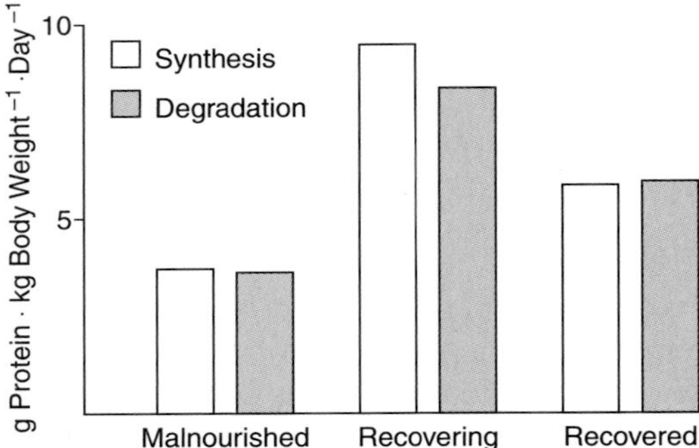

Figure 13-12 Rates of protein synthesis and degradation in children with malnutrition, during the recovery process (recovering), and when recovery is complete (recovered). The rates of protein synthesis and degradation, expressed in grams of protein per kilogram of body weight per day, were assessed with [^{15}N]glycine. *(Data from Golden MHN, Waterlow JC, Picou D [1977] Protein turnover, synthesis and breakdown before and after recovery from protein-energy malnutrition. Clin Sci Mol Med 53:473-477.)*

This increased synthesis and degradation was associated with catch-up growth (i.e., growth rates that are more rapid than normal). When children recovering from protein-energy malnutrition reached more appropriate weights and heights for age, their growth slowed to more age-appropriate rates.

PROTEIN METABOLISM IN GROWTH AND DEVELOPMENT

Normal Growth

Growth is an anabolic process that occurs over a much longer period than do the acute responses to the intake of nutrients. Although the overall process of growth includes a net increase in the amount of body protein, this is often accompanied by significant remodeling so that protein degradation is also elevated. The capacity for growth can be seen in the difference in turnover rates between growing children and adults. In newborn infants, fractional rates of protein synthesis are about twice those in adults.

Growth rates for children recovering from malnutrition are greater than those observed in healthy children, and the rate of growth is positively correlated with the rate of protein synthesis, even though protein degradation also is increased to some extent. A similar phenomenon with increases in both synthesis and degradation associated with protein accumulation can occur in specific tissues under certain conditions, an example being hypertrophy of muscle in response to increased work. In this latter case, net protein is retained within the tissue, and this is accomplished by an increase in protein synthesis that exceeds the increase in degradation.

Increased protein synthesis sustained during growth is accomplished with increased levels of RNA in the tissue, including both mRNA and rRNA, so that the capacity of the body to make protein is increased. Growth is under the influence of hormones, primarily growth hormone and IGF-I. The capacity for growth may also include responses to other anabolic agents that do not occur in the adult. For example, insulin has the capacity to stimulate protein synthesis in the young, growing rat, but this anabolic response to insulin is diminished in the nongrowing adult rat.

In addition to an acceleration of the overall process of turnover and the positive balance between protein synthesis and degradation, growth and development also involve the selective accumulation of specific proteins at the appropriate period of development. At puberty and during pregnancy and lactation, for example, appropriate hormone concentrations are increased by the selective transcription of the appropriate genes. These hormones, in turn, provide for further alterations in protein metabolism. Androgens, for example, are anabolic, providing for an increase in protein mass. This androgen effect may be mediated, in part, through a potentiation of the effect of growth hormone or by a reduction in the catabolic action of corticosteroids.

Hypertrophy and Atrophy

Certain organs are capable of growth even in the adult; most notably, an increase in muscle tissue can be brought about by increased use of the muscle. This phenomenon, known as work-induced hypertrophy, is associated with increased levels of protein synthesis and smaller increases in protein degradation. One of the most common forms of muscle hypertrophy is that which accompanies resistance exercise. Following weight-bearing exercise, rates of protein synthesis in human muscle increase relative to rates of protein degradation, resulting in net positive protein balance (Wolfe, 2001). Although this response is well documented, little is known about the mechanism by which resistance exercise regulates protein synthesis. Most of the molecular events revealed thus far have been discovered with the use of animal models, particularly rats. Resistance exercise in rats resulted in immediate, but transient, increases in the phosphorylation of 4E-BP1 and association of the active eIF-4 complex in skeletal muscle (Bolster et al., 2003). Later, but more substantial, increases in the amount (both protein and mRNA) and activity of eIF-2 GDP–GTP exchange factor (eIF-2B) were observed (Kubica et al., 2004). Studies of the response to acute resistance exercise indicated that regulation of peptide chain initiation after exercise is more dependent on eIF-2B than on the eIF-4 complex (Farrell et al., 2000). Whereas resistance exercise is associated with muscle hypertrophy, endurance exercise is not. After a bout of treadmill running, skeletal muscle protein synthesis and eIF-4 complex formation in rats were decreased rather than increased. This decrease was minimized by ingestion of a protein-containing meal immediately after exercise (Gautsch et al., 1998).

Protein can be lost from individual tissues during disuse. In humans, the loss of muscle tissue is apparent during immobilization, such as that which accompanies bone fracture. This disuse atrophy is associated with decreased synthesis of muscle protein with little change in protein degradation (Gibson et al., 1987).

PROTEIN LOSS IN INJURY AND DISEASE

Loss of body protein accompanies many disease states, such as trauma, cancer, and infection. These disease states contrast with malnutrition and overt starvation in that adaptation to preserve lean body mass does not occur. In response to starvation, energy is conserved with a lowering of metabolic rate, whereas disease states are hypermetabolic; that is, the basal metabolic rate is higher than in healthy individuals. In addition to the increased demands for energy, there is an accompanying metabolic abnormality that prevents adaptation to the use of ketone bodies for energy. The lack of this adaptive response means that body protein is not preserved but rather continues to be the supply of substrate for energy through the formation of glucose. The mobilization of amino acids from muscle involves an acceleration in the rate of protein degradation. Although some amino acids, particularly leucine, valine, and isoleucine, are oxidized in muscle tissue, other amino acids pass into the bloodstream for transport to the liver. Within the liver, the amino acids are available for gluconeogenesis and for the synthesis of liver proteins, especially acute-phase proteins, including C-reactive protein and fibrinogen, which increase in concentration after injury or during illness.

Burns, Surgery, and Sepsis

Conditions such as burn injury, surgery, and systemic infection or sepsis are all accompanied by a set of metabolic responses that are often collectively referred to as stress responses. Stress responses include increased energy expenditure, loss of body protein, and the synthesis of acute-phase proteins. The magnitude of the response varies with the condition and the severity of the injury. In patients with burn injury, for example, there is loss of body heat to the environment, and energy expenditure is increased to compensate for this loss. Raising the ambient temperature and humidity can reduce the loss of body heat. With major surgery, the degree of surgical trauma has an impact on the magnitude of the response. At the level of the whole body, there is an observable increase in both protein synthesis and degradation following surgery, with degradation increased more than synthesis, so that there is net loss of body protein. However, this whole-body response is a composite of different responses in different tissues. For example, the rate of protein synthesis in skeletal muscle is depressed after surgery or in sepsis, whereas sepsis and a variety of inflammatory conditions cause an increase in protein synthesis in the liver.

In general, the response to stress involves the mobilization of muscle amino acids through decreased protein synthesis along with accelerated degradation in skeletal muscle and the production of acute-phase proteins by the liver. These effects are primarily mediated by the concerted actions of stress hormones—glucagon, cortisol, and epinephrine. However, production of cytokines, a decreased efficacy of anabolic hormones such as insulin, growth hormone, and IGF-I, and reduced levels of other anabolic hormones such as testosterone also contribute to the complete response to stress.

At the molecular level, depression of protein synthesis in skeletal muscle in sepsis is associated with decreased activity of eIF-2B for catalyzing GTP–GDP exchange on eIF-2. This reduces the formation of 40S-Met-tRNA pre-initiation complexes. Alterations in the eIF-4 system in sepsis are minor (Vary and Kimball, 2000). In the liver, sepsis-stimulated protein synthesis is associated with an increase in the total RNA content, the content of eIF-2, and the phosphorylation of the kinase responsible for the phosphorylation of ribosomal protein S6 (Cooney et al., 2000). Accelerated muscle protein degradation during sepsis is associated with increased levels of mRNAs for ubiquitin and the 20S proteosome subunit, HC3 (Tiao et al., 1997). Head trauma is also associated with an increased rate of muscle protein breakdown. Muscle biopsies from patients with severe head trauma showed increased levels of mRNAs for cathepsin D, m-calpain, and critical components of the ubiquitin–proteasome pathway (Mansoor et al., 1996). Activation of proteolysis in these patients may be promoted by their elevated circulating levels of cortisol and the cytokines, IL-1β and IL-6. Although multiple proteolytic processes may play a role in muscle proteolysis, proteosome-mediated proteolysis is believed to be the most active in the degradation of myofibrillar proteins.

In addition to direct effects of stress hormones in stimulating catabolic processes such as muscle protein degradation, higher levels of stress hormones are also associated with a failure of normal anabolic responses such as the ability of insulin to reduce the rate of protein degradation. Resistance to another anabolic hormone, growth hormone, also occurs in trauma and sepsis. Growth hormone secretion is normally associated with elevated levels of IGF-I. In sepsis, however, levels of IGF-I are reduced despite normal or elevated levels of growth hormone. In animal models of sepsis, reduction in IGF-I is associated with a reduction in the rate of protein synthesis and a reduction in the formation of the eIF-4E–eIF-4G complex (Lang et al., 2000). The inability of growth hormone to increase IGF-I may be mediated through the STAT (signal transducers and activators of transcription) family of transcription factors. In mice, the deletion of STAT 5 is associated with an inability of growth hormone to increase IGF-I synthesis (Davey et al., 2001). In addition to reduced levels of IGF-I, trauma and sepsis are associated with alterations in the IGF-I regulatory or binding proteins, the IGFBPs. In sepsis and burn injury, levels of IGFBP-I are increased, leading to reduced bioavailability of IGF-I as a result of increased cytokine activity.

A multitude of cytokines are produced by leukocytes in response to stress; those particularly associated with protein catabolism include TNF-α, IL-1, and IL-6. In burn injury, the strongest correlations of increased whole-body protein degradation are observed with IL-6 (Long and Lowry, 1990). The interaction of these multiple hormones and cytokines exacerbates the catabolic stimuli and the loss of muscle protein during stress.

Immobilization also contributes to muscle loss in critical illness, and the loss of protein is greater than with immobilization alone because of the hormonal changes that accompany critical illness. The inactivity associated with 14 days of bed rest, in a healthy individual, results in a 50% suppression of the rate of muscle protein synthesis with no alteration in the rate of muscle degradation. When elevated levels of cortisol are also present, the loss of muscle is exacerbated by acceleration of protein degradation associated with a reduction in circulating levels of anabolic hormones, such as testosterone (Ferrando et al., 1999).

For some types of surgery, an attenuation of the increase in plasma cortisol can be achieved by epidural anesthesia, with a reduction in the negative nitrogen balance that normally accompanies surgical stress. This suggests that neural regulation also is an important factor in the catabolic response to trauma. Burn patients have elevated levels of cortisol and reduced levels of testosterone. When testosterone is administered to burn patients, they show improved protein balance, which is due to reduced protein degradation, not to a stimulation of protein synthesis as would be expected from testosterone replacement therapy in healthy subjects. This response may be mediated by an effect of testosterone on the cortisol receptor that diminishes the activity of cortisol (Danhaive and Rousseau, 1986). Giving growth hormone to patients with critical illness to overcome growth hormone resistance and stimulate an anabolic response has been less successful. Although growth hormone treatment is beneficial in reducing the catabolic response, use of growth hormone in treatment of critically ill adults (both burn patients and non-burned critically ill patients) is associated with increased morbidity and mortality (Herndon and Tompkins, 2004; Takala et al., 1999).

Muscle wasting is part of the response to stress and may be viewed as beneficial in that amino acids are mobilized from expendable to essential tissues to provide substrate for more vital functions such as the synthesis of acute-phase proteins. As with starvation, such short-term adaptation may be beneficial to the organism; however, the longer this state continues, the more detrimental it becomes. Nutritional support therefore becomes obligatory in long-term critical illness, and there is much active research on strategies for optimizing nutrition by altering the composition of nutrients given in particular illnesses and also by combining nutrition with anabolic agents such as growth hormone.

Cancer

In catabolic conditions such as cancer, the loss of body protein can be due in part to the anorexia that accompanies the disease. However, some forms of cancer, such as small cell cancer of the lung, are associated with loss of body protein even when nutrients are supplied. This wasting condition is called cachexia. The mechanism by which this loss is mediated is not fully delineated, but both reduction in dietary intake and diversion of nutrients to the tumor contribute to the loss of lean body mass.

Rapid proliferation of the tumor contributes to loss of muscle protein in the cancer patient by sequestering available substrate (amino acids) away from healthy tissues to support malignant growth. Dysregulated growth of the cell can occur at the level of mRNA translation, contributing to both cancer formation and progression. Increased expression of several translation factors, including eIF-2, eIF-4E (the protein in the eIF-4 complex that specifically binds the mRNA cap), and eIF-5B has been observed in benign and malignant tumors of the breast, head and neck, colon, prostate, bladder, cervix, and lung (De Benedetti and Graff, 2004; Guan et al., 2004; Hii et al., 2004; Ruggero et al., 2004; Rosenwald et al., 2003). In addition, overexpression of certain eIFs, such as eIF-4E, enhances cellular proliferation of human cell lines and is related to tumor progression (Ruggero et al., 2004).

Studies in human cancer cell lines have shown that blocking eIF function by antisense RNA or overexpression of an inhibitory protein (such as one of the eIF-2 kinases or the eIF-4 repressor proteins) can suppress cellular transformation and tumor growth (De Benedetti and Graff, 2004; Shir et al., 2003). Translation factor function can also be blocked nutritionally by amino acid depleting enzymes such as asparaginase, which depletes blood levels of asparagine (and, to a lesser extent, glutamine). Leukemic cells do not synthesize asparagine in amounts adequate to support their enhanced rate of growth and so depend on an exogenous source. As it turns out, asparaginase is a very effective inhibitor of protein synthesis via downregulation of signaling pathways controlling eIF-4 complex formation (Liboshi et al., 1999). Side effects of asparaginase include liver dysfunction and immunosuppression, both related to a decrease in protein synthesis. The challenge of retarding loss of body protein by nutritional means in cancer patients must, therefore, be considered in terms of the effects on both body tissue and the tumor. The challenge is to devise feeding regimens or cancer treatments that block translation factor function (and thus, protein synthesis) in the tumor but not in healthy tissues.

Loss of body protein in cancer is also associated with upregulation of protein degradation (Bossola et al., 2003). Although extensive involvement of the lysosomal system has not been demonstrated, increased activity of calpains is observed in tumor-bearing animals. Cancer cachexia is associated with activation of the ATP-dependent ubiquitin–proteasome proteolytic system. Patients with gastric cancer, for example, have increased expression of mRNA for ubiquitin in skeletal muscle, with the highest levels of expression in patients with the most advanced disease. Increased ubiquitin expression is accompanied by increased proteasomal activity in skeletal muscle biopsies of these patients. Interestingly, increased ubiquitin expression in skeletal muscle is evident even before patients begin to lose weight. This elevation in ubiquitin mRNA may be cytokine-mediated. Proinflammatory cytokines (e.g., TNF-α) are elevated in patients with cancer, but antibodies to TNF-α reduce both ubiquitin mRNA levels and body protein loss in animal models. Inhibitors of the proteosome system are being explored as potential cancer therapies (Adams et al., 1999).

Researchers have also hypothesized that there may be a factor that induces the loss of protein in cancer patients. Patients with a variety of cancers (pancreatic, breast, ovary, lung, colon, and rectal) excrete a tumor-derived proteolysis-inducing factor (PIF), which can induce cachexia in mice (Cariuk et al., 1997). PIF-induced cachexia is associated with increased expression of both ubiquitin and proteasome subunits (Gomes-Marcondes et al., 2002). In animal models, PIF action can be inhibited by eicosapentaenoic acid (EPA) via downregulation of genes for proteasome subunits and ubiquitin-conjugating enzymes (Whitehouse et al., 2001).

It has been suggested that energy expenditure might be elevated in cancer, thereby contributing to body weight loss, but this has not been a consistent finding. Studies on whole-body protein metabolism in cancer have, in general, demonstrated elevations in both synthesis and degradation. In animal studies in which it is possible to study the responses at the tissue level, differential responses among different tissues have been reported. For example, in tumor-bearing mice, the rate of muscle protein synthesis was depressed, whereas the synthesis of liver protein was enhanced. This is similar to the response pattern observed with other forms of stress.

Clinical Correlation

Is AIDS Wasting Simply Starvation?

Infection with HIV is associated with a profound and selective loss of body protein that gives rise to the condition known as AIDS wasting. Although AIDS wasting superficially appears to be like simple starvation in that there is a loss of body protein, there are a number of differences between this state of stress and uncomplicated starvation.

Thinking Critically

1. What are the similarities/differences between starvation and AIDS wasting?
2. Which hormones might potentially be involved in AIDS wasting? What other possible mediators might be different in the adaptation to starvation compared with adaptation to the stress of HIV infection?

Human Immunodeficiency Virus

Infection with human immunodeficiency virus (HIV) results in substantial loss of body weight, known as acquired immunodeficiency syndrome (AIDS) wasting. This condition is somewhat different from starvation and other wasting conditions in that body fat is preserved but lean tissue is lost. Poor nutrient intake may contribute to AIDS wasting through anorexia, diarrhea, and malabsorption. However, the wasting associated with AIDS is not simply due to poor nutrient intake but has many features of other catabolic states such as those associated with burns, surgery, and sepsis. The loss of body protein arises from the use of amino acids for the formation of glucose, similar to the mobilization of amino acids during the early stages of starvation. Unlike in starvation, however, in AIDS the adaptive responses to spare body protein are blunted. HIV disease is associated with increased rates of whole-body protein synthesis and degradation.

At the level of muscle tissue, the catabolic condition of AIDS wasting can be seen in the measurements of protein synthesis and protein degradation shown in Figure 13-13. The rates of muscle protein synthesis are similar in healthy controls and AIDS patients, but the rates of muscle protein degradation, based on the excretion of 3-methylhistidine, are higher. Moreover, increased rates of protein degradation in muscle are apparent in AIDS patients who have not lost weight, indicating that changes in muscle metabolism precede the onset of significant weight loss.

Resting energy expenditure is also increased in patients with AIDS, particularly during the periods of secondary infection that frequently accompany the disease. This increase may be due in part to the increased energy requirement imposed by increased protein turnover. Adaptive mechanisms to reduce voluntary energy expenditure (i.e., by reduced physical activity) may balance some of the increase in resting energy expenditure, so that total energy expenditure is not elevated.

Circulating levels of several anabolic hormones are reduced in AIDS patients, including growth hormone, IGF-I, and insulin. Glucagon and cortisol levels are elevated, as they are in other conditions of stress and trauma. Levels of thyroid hormone (T_3) and of gonadal hormones such as testosterone are also reduced. Testosterone replacement in HIV-infected men with low testosterone levels results in improvement in both muscle mass and function (Bhasin et al., 2000). The hormonal changes are, in general, similar to the changes seen in starvation (Sellmeyer and Grunfeld, 1996), but the failure of the adaptive responses suggests resistance to hormonal effects at the level of the tissue. Furthermore, the levels of catabolic cytokines, TNF-α, interferon α and γ, and IL-1 and IL-6, are increased in the later stages of HIV disease, particularly during episodes of secondary infections (Grunfeld and Feingold, 1992). These cytokines may contribute directly to wasting and may also mediate hormonal resistance, exacerbating the loss of body protein that is characteristic of this disease.

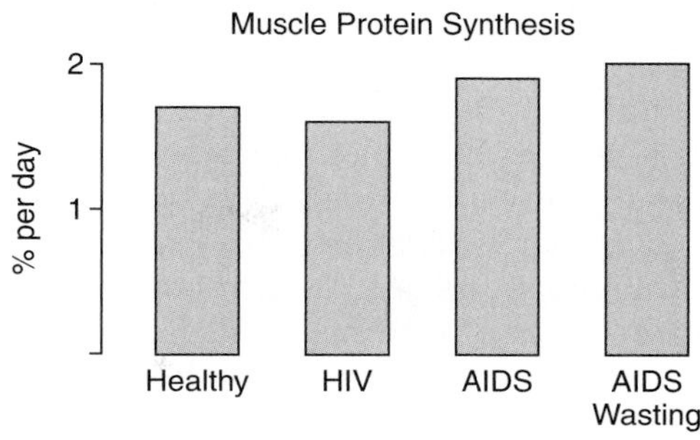

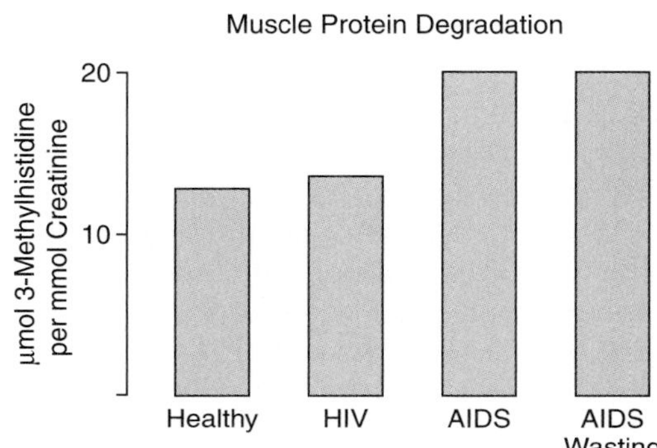

Figure 13-13 Muscle protein metabolism in healthy subjects and in patients in infected with human immunodeficiency virus (HIV), in patients with acquired immunodeficiency syndrome (AIDS) but no weight loss, and in patients with AIDS wasting. The rate of synthesis of vastus lateralis muscle was determined from the incorporation of L-[$^2H_5$]phenylalanine. Muscle protein degradation was measured from the ratio of urinary 3-methylhistidine to urinary creatinine. HIV subjects were asymptomatic. AIDS patients previously had an AIDS-defining illness but no significant weight loss. Patients with AIDS wasting had lost more than 10% of their pre-illness weight. *(Data from McNurlan MA, Garlick PJ, Steigbigel RT, DeCristofaro KA, Frost RA, Lang CH, Johnson RW, Santasier AM, Cabahug CJ, Fuhrer J, Gelato MC [1997] Responsiveness of muscle protein synthesis to growth hormone administration in HIV-infected individuals declines with severity of disease. J Clin Invest 100:2125-2132.)*

CURRENT CHALLENGES IN PROTEIN METABOLISM

The preservation of body protein in diseases such as HIV and other long-term illnesses is one of the current challenges in the field of protein metabolism. The approach to solving this problem has been both to understand the underlying mechanisms and to reverse the loss of body protein, either by nutritional means or by combining specific nutritional regimens with anabolic agents. For example, investigations into stress responses have delineated both hormonal mechanisms and those involving cytokines such as TNF-α. The link to cytokines has led to treatment modalities that include antibodies to either a cytokine or its receptor. But greater understanding of underlying mechanisms has also illuminated the vast complexity of the systems that regulate levels of body proteins. Researchers are only beginning to understand the interplay of hormones with each other and with cytokines.

An understanding of the molecular mechanisms involved in protein processing may lead to new therapies. Many degenerative neuromuscular diseases, including Parkinson's, Alzheimer's, various muscular dystrophies, and even prion-associated diseases, appear to be associated with defects in the ability of the ER to regulate the tasks of protein synthesis, protein folding, and protein breakdown. An important challenge for both basic scientists and clinicians is to identify the defects leading to disease and then to treat or prevent the onset of symptoms related to these defects. Inhibition of proteasome-associated proteolysis is also providing new lines of investigation for retarding loss of body protein and for novel forms of cancer therapy.

Feeding regimens can also alter the course of disease progression, and more beneficial regimens would be helpful. Although early parenteral nutrition does not completely prevent the loss of body protein associated with stresses such as surgery, it clearly does attenuate the loss of body protein compared to that observed when nutrition is not provided. The amino acids that are supplied help preserve body tissue and also may facilitate responses by the body such as the synthesis of acute-phase proteins, activation of the immune system, or synthesis of specific proteins involved in wound healing. Provision of anabolic agents (such as insulin; oxandrolone, a weak analog of testosterone; or propranolol, a beta blocker drug that attenuates the release of catecholamines) in conjunction with adequate nutrition has been demonstrated to be more effective than nutrition alone in preventing the loss of body protein (Herndon and Tompkins, 2004).

Increasingly, the focus in catabolic illness is not only on the provision of adequate nutrition but also on altering nutrition to address the particular problems associated with different diseases. For example, patients with severe liver disease may benefit from the provision of nutrition enriched with branched-chain amino acids. As the capacity of the liver to degrade amino acids such as methionine, phenylalanine, and tyrosine is diminished, plasma levels of these amino acids rise, whereas concentrations of branched-chain amino acids, which are degraded in the periphery, fall. Enhancing the supply of branched-chain amino acids may help correct the amino acid imbalance caused by the liver disease.

The provision of extra amounts of single amino acids sometimes has been demonstrated to have therapeutic benefit. For example, glutamine-enriched nutrition has been used clinically in both critically ill patients and in patients after surgery. Glutamine is released from muscle tissue in response to stress, and provision of glutamine-containing nutritional regimens to surgical patients reduces negative nitrogen balance and may reduce infections and complications (Novak et al., 2002). Both glutamine and arginine have been used in conjunction with adequate nutrition to stimulate the immune system and to promote healing. Ongoing research seeks to understand how protein metabolism is altered by disease states and how nutrition may be employed for benefit.

Lastly, increased understanding of the genes that regulate muscle cell differentiation also has the potential to lead to better therapies for the loss of protein. The protein, myostatin, has been shown to have an inhibitory role on muscle mass (Lee and McPherron, 2001). Mutations in the gene that encodes myostatin are associated with increased body weight and muscle mass (Schuelke et al., 2004). Myostatin is a transforming growth factor beta (TGF-β) family member that functions to inhibit the differentiation and proliferation of myoblasts. Muscle contains satellite cells, quiescent muscle stem cells that can be activated to promote postnatal muscle growth and repair. Myostatin is a potent negative regulator of satellite cell activation and, thus, acts to maintain muscle satellite cells in a quiescent state. When myostatin activity is blocked, satellite cells are activated and fuse with muscle fibers, leading to muscle hypertrophy (Thomas et al., 2000). In a mouse model of muscular dystrophy, blocking myostatin was associated with improved muscle mass and function (Bogdanovich et al., 2002).

Recent studies have also identified two genes that encode E3 ubiquitin ligases [muscle ring finger 1 (MuRF1) and muscle atrophy F-box (MAFbx)] whose expressions are upregulated during loss of muscle due to conditions such as immobilization or glucocorticoid treatment (Bodine et al., 2001; Gomes et al., 2001). Animals with disruptions of these genes do not lose as much muscle as normal mice during muscle atrophy. These genes also represent potential targets for gene-based therapy to prevent muscle loss. The expansion of research tools including transgenic animals, genomics, and proteomics are all contributing to enhanced understanding of the way body protein is regulated, and each addition to our understanding has the potential to provide clinical benefit for conditions in which body protein is lost.

REFERENCES

Adams J, Palombella VJ, Sausville EA, Johnson J, Destree A, Lazarus DD, Maas J, Pien CS, Prakash S, Elliott PJ (1999) Proteasome inhibitors: a novel class of potent and effective antitumor agents. Cancer Res 59:2615-2622.

Andersen GR, Nissen P, Nyborg J (2003) Elongation factors in protein biosynthesis. Trends Biochem Sci 28:434-441.

Anthony JC, Lang CH, Crozier SJ, Anthony TG, MacLean DA, Kimball SR, Jefferson LS (2002) Contribution of insulin to the translational control of protein synthesis in skeletal muscle by leucine. Am J Physiol Endocrinol Metab 282:E1092-E1101.

Anthony JC, Yoshizawa F, Anthony TG, Vary TC, Jefferson LS, Kimball SR (2000) Leucine stimulates translation initiation in skeletal muscle of postabsorptive rats via a rapamycin-sensitive pathway. J Nutr 130:2413-2419.

Anthony TG, McDaniel BJ, Byerley RL, McGrath BC, Cavener DR, McNurlan MA, Wek RC (2004) Preservation of liver protein synthesis during dietary leucine deprivation occurs at the expense of skeletal muscle mass in mice deleted for eIF-2 kinase GCN2. J Biol Chem 279:36553-36561.

Anthony TG, Reiter AK, Anthony JC, Kimball SR, Jefferson LS (2001) Deficiency of dietary EAA preferentially inhibits mRNA translation of ribosomal proteins in liver of meal-fed rats. Am J Physiol Endocrinol Metab 281:E430-E439.

Bhasin S, Storer TW, Javanbakht M, Berman N, Yarasheski KE, Phillips J, Dike M, Sinha-Hikim I, Shen R, Hays RD, Beall G (2000) Testosterone replacement and resistance exercise in HIV-infected men with weight loss and low testosterone levels. JAMA 283:763-770.

Black BL, Olson EN (1998) Transcriptional control of muscle development by myocyte enhancer factor-2 (MEF2) proteins. Annu Rev Cell Dev Biol 14:167-196.

Bodine SC, Latres E, Baumhueter S, Lai VK, Nunez L, Clarke BA, Poueymirou WT, Panaro FJ, Na E, Dharmarajan K, Pan ZQ, Valenzuela DM, DeChiara TM, Stitt TN, Yancopoulos GD, Glass DJ (2001) Identification of ubiquitin ligases required for skeletal muscle atrophy. Science 294:1704-1708.

Bogdanovich S, Krag TO, Barton ER, Morris LD, Whittemore LA, Ahima RS, Khurana TS (2002) Functional improvement of dystrophic muscle by myostatin blockade. Nature 420:418-421.

Bolster DR, Kubica N, Crozier SJ, Williamson DL, Farrell PA, Kimball SR, Jefferson LS (2003) Immediate response of mammalian target of rapamycin (mTOR)-mediated signalling following acute resistance exercise in rat skeletal muscle. J Physiol 553:213-220.

Bossola M, Muscaritoli M, Costelli P, Grieco G, Bonelli G, Pacelli F, Fanelli FR, Doglietto GB, Baccino FM (2003) Increased muscle proteasome activity correlates with disease severity in gastric cancer patients. Ann Surg 237:384-389.

Cahill GF, Jr. (1976) Starvation in man. Clin Endocrinol Metab 5:397-415.

Cariuk P, Lorite MJ, Todorov PT, Field WN, Wigmore SJ, Tisdale MJ (1997) Induction of cachexia in mice by a product isolated from the urine of cachectic cancer patients. Br J Cancer 76:606-613.

Cihak A, Lamar C, Jr., Pitot HC (1973) L-Tryptophan inhibition of tyrosine aminotransferase degradation in rat liver in vivo. Arch Biochem Biophys 156:188-194.

Combaret L, Taillandier D, Dardevet D, Bechet D, Ralliere C, Claustre A, Grizard J, Attaix D (2004) Glucocorticoids regulate mRNA levels for subunits of the 19S regulatory complex of the 26S proteasome in fast-twitch skeletal muscles. Biochem J 378:239-246.

Cooney RN, Kimball SR, Maish G, 3rd, Shumate M, Vary TC (2000) Effects of tumor necrosis factor-binding protein on hepatic protein synthesis during chronic sepsis. J Surg Res 93:257-264.

Costelli P, Baccino FM (2003) Mechanisms of skeletal muscle depletion in wasting syndromes: role of ATP-ubiquitin-dependent proteolysis. Curr Opin Clin Nutr Metab Care 6:407-412.

Danhaive PA, Rousseau GG (1986) Binding of glucocorticoid antagonists to androgen and glucocorticoid hormone receptors in rat skeletal muscle. J Steroid Biochem 24: 481-487.

Davey HW, Xie T, McLachlan MJ, Wilkins RJ, Waxman DJ, Grattan DR (2001) STAT5b is required for GH-induced liver IGF-I gene expression. Endocrinology 142:3836-3841.

De Benedetti A, Graff JR (2004) eIF-4E Expression and its role in malignancies and metastases. Oncogene 23:3189-3199.

Delepine M, Nicolino M, Barrett T, Golamaully M, Lathrop GM, Julier C (2000) EIF2AK3, encoding translation initiation factor 2-alpha kinase 3, is mutated in patients with Wolcott-Rallison syndrome. Nat Genet 25:406-409.

Doherty FJ, Dawson S, Mayer RJ (2002) The ubiquitin-proteasome pathway of intracellular proteolysis. Essays Biochem 38:51-63.

Farrell PA, Hernandex JM, Fedele MJ, Vary TC, Kimball SR, Jefferson LS (2000) Eukaryotic initiation factors and protein synthesis after resistance exercise in rats. J Appl Physiol 88:1046-1052.

Ferrando AA, Sheffield-Moore M, Yeckel CW, Gilkison C, Jiang J, Achacosa A, Lieberman SA, Tipton K, Wolfe RR, Urban RJ (2002) Testosterone administration to older men improves muscle function: molecular and physiological mechanisms. Am J Physiol Endocrinol Metab 282:E601-E607.

Ferrando AA, Stuart CA, Sheffield-Moore M, Wolfe RR (1999) Inactivity amplifies the catabolic response of skeletal muscle to cortisol. J Clin Endocrinol Metab 84:3515-3521.

Garlick PJ, Wernerman J (1997) Protein Metabolism in Injury. In: Cooper GJ, Dudley HAF, Gann DS, Little RA, Maynard RL (eds) Scientific Foundations of Trauma. Butterworth-Heinemann, Oxford, pp 690-728.

Gass JN, Gunn KE, Sriburi R, Brewer JW (2004) Stressed-out B cells? Plasma-cell differentiation and the unfolded protein response. Trends Immunol 25:17-24.

Gautsch TA, Anthony JC, Kimball SR, Paul GL, Layman DK, Jefferson LS (1998) Availability of eIF4E regulates skeletal muscle protein synthesis during recovery from exercise. Am J Physiol 274:C406-C414.

Gibson JN, Halliday D, Morrison WL, Stoward PJ, Hornsby GA, Watt PW, Murdoch G, Rennie AJ (1987) Decrease in human quadriceps muscle protein turnover consequent upon leg immobilization. Clin Sci (Lond) 72:503-509.

Golden MHN, Waterlow JC, Picou D (1977) Protein turnover, synthesis and breakdown before and after recovery from protein-energy malnutrition. Clin Sci Mol Med 53:473-477.

Goll DE, Thompson VF, Li H, Wei W, Cong J (2003) The calpain system. Physiol Rev 83:731-801.

Gomes MD, Lecker SH, Jagoe RT, Navon A, Goldberg AL (2001) Atrogin-1, a muscle-specific F-box protein highly expressed during muscle atrophy. Proc Natl Acad Sci U S A 98:14440-14445.

Gomes-Marcondes MC, Smith HJ, Cooper JC, Tisdale MJ (2002) Development of an in-vitro model system to investigate the mechanism of muscle protein catabolism induced by proteolysis-inducing factor. Br J Cancer 86:1628-1633.

Grunfeld C, Feingold KR (1992) Metabolic disturbances and wasting in the acquired immunodeficiency syndrome. N Engl J Med 327:329-337.

Guan XY, Fung JM, Ma NF, Lau SH, Tai LS, Xie D, Zhang Y, Hu L, Wu QL, Fang Y, Sham JS (2004) Oncogenic role of eIF-5A2 in the development of ovarian cancer. Cancer Res 64:4197-4200.

Hannan RD, Luyken J, Rothblum LI (1996) Regulation of ribosomal DNA transcription during contraction-induced hypertrophy of neonatal cardiomyocytes. J Biol Chem 271:3213-3220.

Herndon DN, Tompkins RG (2004) Support of the metabolic response to burn injury. Lancet 363:1895-1902.

Herrmann J, Ciechanover A, Lerman LO, Lerman A (2004) The ubiquitin-proteasome system in cardiovascular diseases—a hypothesis extended. Cardiovasc Res 61:11-21.

Hii SI, Hardy L, Crough T, Payne EJ, Grimmett K, Gill D, McMillan NA (2004) Loss of PKR activity in chronic lymphocytic leukemia. Int J Cancer 109:329-335.

Horton JD, Shah NA, Warrington JA, Anderson NN, Park SW, Brown MS, Goldstein JL (2003) Combined analysis of oligonucleotide microarray data from transgenic and knockout mice identifies direct SREBP target genes. Proc Natl Acad Sci U S A 100:12027-12032.

Kanazawa T, Taneike I, Akaishi R, Yoshizawa F, Furuya N, Fujimura S, Kadowaki M (2004) Amino acids and insulin control autophagic proteolysis through different signaling pathways in relation to mTOR in isolated rat hepatocytes. J Biol Chem 279:8452-8459.

Kaufman RJ (2004) Regulation of mRNA translation by protein folding in the endoplasmic reticulum. Trends Biochem Sci 29:152-158.

Kee AJ, Combaret L, Tilignac T, Souweine B, Aurousseau E, Dalle M, Taillandier D, Attaix D (2003) Ubiquitin-proteasome-dependent muscle proteolysis responds slowly to insulin release and refeeding in starved rats. J Physiol 546:765-776.

Kinney JM (1978) The tissue composition of surgical weight loss. In: Johnson JA (ed) Advances in Parenteral Nutrition. Medical and Technical Press, Lancaster, England, pp 511-520.

Klionsky DJ, Emr SD (2000) Autophagy as a regulated pathway of cellular degradation. Science 290:1717-1721.

Kloetzel PM (2004) Generation of major histocompatibility complex class I antigens: functional interplay between proteasomes and TPPII. Nat Immunol 5:661-669.

Kubica N, Kimball SR, Jefferson LS, Farrell PA (2004) Alterations in the expression of mRNAs and proteins that code for species relevant to eIF2B activity after an acute bout of resistance exercise. J Appl Physiol 96:679-687.

Lang CH, Frost RA (2002) Role of growth hormone, insulin-like growth factor-I, and insulin-like growth factor binding proteins in the catabolic response to injury and infection. Curr Opin Clin Nutr Metab Care 5:271-279.

Lang CH, Frost RA, Jefferson LS, Kimball SR, Vary TC (2000) Endotoxin-induced decrease in muscle protein synthesis is associated with changes in eIF2B, eIF4E, and IGF-I. Am J Physiol Endocrinol Metab 278:E1133-E1143.

Lee HK, Marzella L (1994) Regulation of intracellular protein degradation with special reference to lysosomes: role in cell physiology and pathology. Int Rev Exp Pathol 35:39-147.

Lee SJ, McPherron AC (2001) Regulation of myostatin activity and muscle growth. Proc Natl Acad Sci U S A 98:9306-9311.

Levine M, Tjian R (2003) Transcription regulation and animal diversity. Nature 424:147-151.

Liboshi Y, Papst PJ, Hunger SP, Terada N (1999) L-Asparaginase inhibits the rapamycin-targeted signaling pathway. Biochem Biophys Res Commun 260:534-539.

Long CL, Lowry SF (1990) Hormonal regulation of protein metabolism. JPEN J Parenter Enteral Nutr 14:555-562.

Mansoor O, Beaufrere B, Boirie Y, Ralliere C, Taillandier D, Aurousseau E, Schoeffler P, Arnal M, Attaix D (1996) Increased mRNA levels for components of the lysosomal, Ca2+-activated, and ATP-ubiquitin-dependent proteolytic pathways in skeletal muscle from head trauma patients. Proc Natl Acad Sci U S A 93:2714-2718.

Matthews DE, Pesola G, Campbell RG (1990) Effect of epinephrine on amino acid and energy metabolism in humans. Am J Physiol 258:E948-E956.

McCracken AA, Brodsky JL (2003) Evolving questions and paradigm shifts in endoplasmic-reticulum-associated degradation (ERAD). Bioessays 25:868-877.

Mitch WE, Goldberg AL (1996) Mechanisms of muscle wasting. The role of the ubiquitin-proteasome pathway. N Engl J Med 335: 1897-1905.

Munro HN (1964) Historical introduction: The origin and growth of our present concepts of protein metabolism. In: Munro HN, Allison JB (eds) Mammalian Protein Metabolism. Vol 1. Academic Press, New York, pp 1-29.

Nachaliel N, Jain D, Hod Y (1993) A cAMP-regulated RNA-binding protein that interacts with phosphoenolpyruvate carboxykinase (GTP) mRNA. J Biol Chem 268:24203-24209.

Novak F, Heyland DK, Avenell A, Drover JW, Su X (2002) Glutamine supplementation in serious illness: a systematic review of the evidence. Crit Care Med 30:2022-2029.

Orban TI, Olah E (2003) Emerging roles of BRCA1 alternative splicing. Mol Pathol 56:191-197.

Paschen W (2003) Endoplasmic reticulum: a primary target in various acute disorders and degenerative diseases of the brain. Cell Calcium 34:365-383.

Prod'homme M, Rieu I, Balage M, Dardevet D, Grizard J (2004) Insulin and amino acids both strongly participate to the regulation of protein metabolism. Curr Opin Clin Nutr Metab Care 7:71-77.

Reeds PJ, Garlick PJ (1984) Nutrition and protein turnover in man. In: Draper HH (ed) Advances in Nutritional Research. Vol 6. Plenum Press, New York, pp 93-138.

Rosenwald IB, Wang S, Savas L, Woda B, Pullman J (2003) Expression of translation initiation factor eIF-2alpha is increased in benign and malignant melanocytic and colonic epithelial neoplasms. Cancer 98:1080-1088.

Ruggero D, Montanaro L, Ma L, Xu W, Londei P, Cordon-Cardo C, Pandolfi PP (2004) The translation factor eIF-4E promotes tumor formation and cooperates with c-Myc in lymphomagenesis. Nat Med 10:484-486.

Sakamoto KM (2002) Ubiquitin-dependent proteolysis: its role in human diseases and the design of therapeutic strategies. Mol Genet Metab 77:44-56.

Schoenheimer R, Ratner S, Rittenberg D (1939) Studies in protein metabolism. VII. The metabolism of tyrosine. J Biol Chem 127:333-344.

Schuelke M, Wagner KR, Stolz LE, Hubner C, Riebel T, Komen W, Braun T, Tobin JF, Lee SJ (2004) Myostatin mutation associated with gross muscle hypertrophy in a child. N Engl J Med 350:2682-2688.

Sellmeyer DE, Grunfeld C (1996) Endocrine and metabolic disturbances in human immunodeficiency virus infection and the acquired immune deficiency syndrome. Endocr Rev 17:518-532.

Shir A, Friedrich I, Levitzki A (2003) Tumor specific activation of PKR as a non-toxic modality of cancer treatment. Semin Cancer Biol 13:309-314.

Sinha-Hikim I, Roth SM, Lee MI, Bhasin S (2003) Testosterone-induced muscle hypertrophy is associated with an increase in satellite cell number in healthy, young men. Am J Physiol Endocrinol Metab 285:E197-E205.

Sjolin J, Stjernstrom H, Henneberg S, Andersson E, Martensson J, Friman G, Larsson J (1989) Splanchnic and peripheral release of 3-methylhistidine in relation to its urinary excretion in human infection. Metabolism 38:23-29.

Studitsky VM, Walter W, Kireeva M, Kashlev M, Felsenfeld G (2004) Chromatin remodeling by RNA polymerases. Trends Biochem Sci 29:127-135.

Suttmann U, Ockenga J, Selberg O, Hoogestraat L, Deicher H, Muller MJ (1995) Incidence and prognostic value of malnutrition and wasting in human immunodeficiency virus-infected outpatients. J Acquir Immune Defic Syndr Hum Retrovirol 8:239-246.

Takala J, Ruokonen E, Webster NR, Nielsen MS, Zandstra DF, Vundelinckx G, Hinds CJ (1999) Increased mortality associated with growth hormone treatment in critically ill adults. N Engl J Med 341:785-792.

Tailliandier D, Combaret L, Pouch M-N, Samuels SE, Bechet D, Attaix D (2004) The role of ubiquitin-proteasome-dependent proteolysis in the remodeling of skeletal muscle. Proc Nutr Soc 63:357-361.

Thomas M, Langley B, Berry C, Sharma M, Kirk S, Bass J, Kambadur R (2000) Myostatin, a negative regulator of muscle growth, functions by inhibiting myoblast proliferation. J Biol Chem 275:40235-40243.

Thornton S, Anand N, Purcell D, Lee J (2003) Not just for housekeeping: protein initiation and elongation factors in cell growth and tumorigenesis. J Mol Med 81:536-548.

Tiao G, Hobler S, Wang JJ, Meyer TA, Luchette FA, Fischer JE, Hasselgren PO (1997) Sepsis is associated with increased mRNAs of the ubiquitin-proteasome proteolytic pathway in human skeletal muscle. J Clin Invest 99:163-168.

Tomkins AM, Garlick PJ, Schofield WN, Waterlow JC (1983) The combined effects of infection and malnutrition on protein metabolism in children. Clin Sci (Lond) 65:313-324.

Vary TC, Kimball SR (2000) Effect of sepsis on eIE4E availability in skeletal muscle. Am J Physiol Endocrinol Metab 279: E1178-E1184.

Waterlow JC, Garlick PJ, Millward DJ (1978) Protein Turnover in Mammalian Tissues and in the Whole Body. North-Holland Publishing, Amsterdam.

Whitehouse AS, Smith HJ, Drake JL, Tisdale MJ (2001) Mechanism of attenuation of skeletal muscle protein catabolism in cancer cachexia by eicosapentaenoic acid. Cancer Res 61:3604-3609.

Wilkie GS, Dickson KS, Gray NK (2003) Regulation of mRNA translation by 5'- and 3'-UTR-binding factors. Trends Biochem Sci 28:182-188.

Wolfe RR (2001) Control of muscle protein breakdown: effects of activity and nutritional states.

Int J Sport Nutr Exerc Metab 11 Suppl: S164-S169.

Zhang P, McGrath B, Li S, Frank A, Zambito F, Reinert J, Gannon M, Ma K, McNaughton K, Cavener DR (2002) The PERK eukaryotic initiation factor 2 alpha kinase is required for the development of the skeletal system, postnatal growth, and the function and viability of the pancreas. Mol Cell Biol 22:3864-3874.

RECOMMENDED READINGS

Frayn KN (1996) Metabolic Regulation and Human Perspective. Portland Press, London.

Garlick PJ, Wernerman J (1997) Protein metabolism in injury. In: Cooper GJ, Dudley HAF, Gann DS, Little RA, Maynard RL (eds) Scientific Foundations of Trauma. Butterworth-Heinemann Reed, Oxford, England, pp 690-728.

Chapter 14

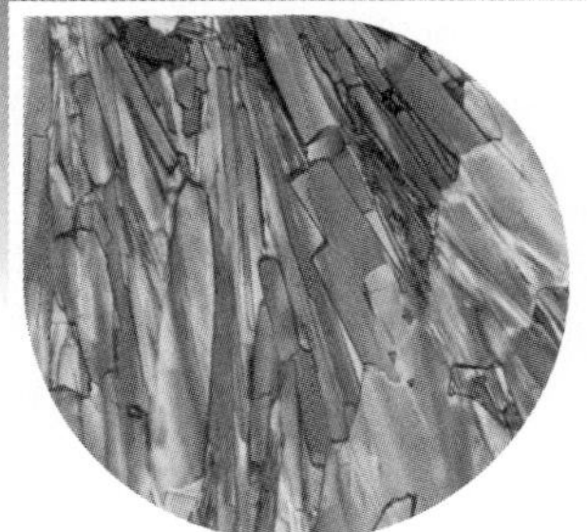

Amino Acid Metabolism

Martha H. Stipanuk, PhD, and Malcolm Watford, DPhil

OUTLINE

OVERVIEW OF AMINO ACID METABOLISM

This discussion of amino acid metabolism focuses on the 20 α-amino (or -imino, in the case of proline) α-carboxylic acids that are the precursors for protein synthesis. Many other compounds in the body, perhaps as many as 300, also could be considered amino acids, because this term can be used more broadly to describe any compound with an amine group and an acidic group. For example, other amino acids are formed when some of the 20 amino acids used for protein synthesis undergo limited posttranslational modification to form derivatized residues that are released as free amino acids during proteolysis; these include *N*-methylhistidine, γ-carboxyglutamate, hydroxyproline, and hydroxylysine. In addition, some serine is specifically converted to selenocysteine cotranslationally. A number of other amino acids (including citrulline, ornithine, γ-aminobutyrate, homocysteine, and taurine) are formed during metabolism of specific amino acids. In addition, these and other amino acid derivatives, including some that are not synthesized by mammalian tissues, are consumed in the diet.

The 20 amino acids required for protein synthesis include some for which the carbon chains cannot be synthesized in the body (essential, or indispensable, amino acids) and others for which the carbon skeletons can be made from common intermediates in metabolism (nonessential, or dispensable, amino acids). The nutritional requirement for protein is actually a requirement for the indispensable (essential) amino acids and a source of nitrogen for synthesis of dispensable (nonessential) amino acids, as is discussed in more detail in Chapter 15. Most of the nitrogen for synthesis of dispensable amino acids must be provided by α-amino groups of amino acids because the body has a limited ability to incorporate inorganic nitrogen (i.e., NH_3 and NH_4^+) into amino acids. The indispensable amino acids for humans include leucine, isoleucine, valine, lysine, threonine, tryptophan, phenylalanine, methionine, and histidine. Tyrosine and cysteine are termed semi-essential because they can be synthesized only if their indispensable amino acid precursors (phenylalanine and methionine, respectively) are provided. Many, but not all, of these indispensable amino acids actually can be made from their keto acid or hydroxy acid analogs if these are fed instead of the amino acids; this is possible because of widespread transamination reactions in mammalian tissues that convert keto acids to the respective amino acids. In practice, food proteins provide all 20 amino acids, but the body can adjust the proportions by transferring nitrogen to nonessential carbon skeletons and by catabolizing excess amino acids. An overview of amino acid metabolism is shown in Figure 14-1. The free amino acid pool is shown in the center of this figure; free amino acid pool is the term used to describe the amino acids that exist in the body in free form at any moment and to distinguish these free amino acids from those that exist in peptide or polypeptide/protein form. The size of this free amino acid pool in humans is approximately 150 g, and the flux of amino acids through this pool typically amounts to 400 to 500 g per day (Jungas et al., 1992; Bergstrom et al., 1974).

As can be seen by arrows leading toward the free amino acid pool, there are three major sources of amino acids, as follows:

1. Digestion of endogenous proteins and peptides secreted or sloughed off into the gastrointestinal tract and absorption of the resulting amino acids into the circulation (~70 g/day)
2. Dietary protein after digestion and absorption of the resulting amino acids into the circulation (~100 g/day depending on diet)
3. Intracellular protein turnover or degradation (~230 g/day)

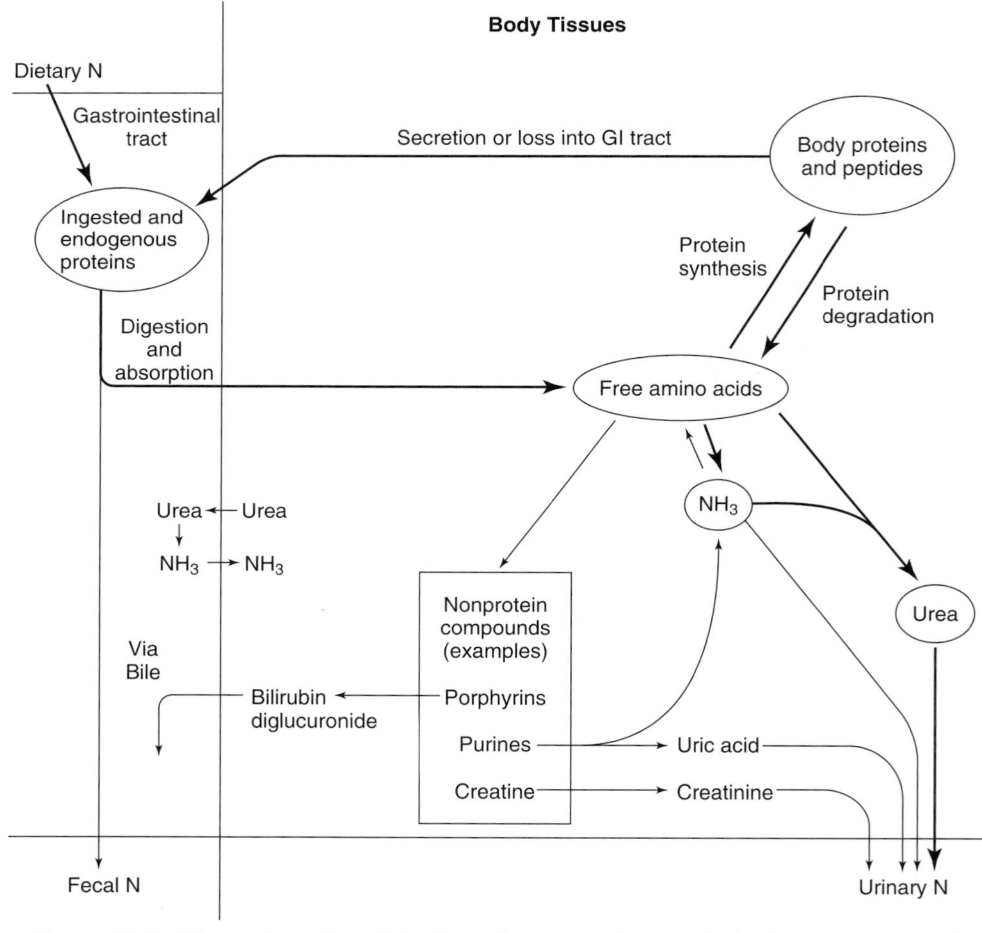

Figure 14-1 Schematic outline of the flow of nitrogen through the body. Major routes of nitrogen movement are indicated by the *heavy lines*.

These processes are discussed in Chapters 9 and 13. As shown by the arrows leading away from the free amino acid pool, the major metabolic fates of amino acids include (1) their use for protein synthesis, (2) their use as precursors for the synthesis of numerous nonprotein nitrogenous molecules, and (3) their catabolism with excretion of nitrogen and use of carbon chains as energy substrates. Note that the amino acids incorporated into proteins may eventually reenter the amino acid pool as a result of protein degradation and become available for reutilization, but those amino acids that were irreversibly modified or used for synthesis of nonpeptide metabolites, or that underwent oxidative catabolism, will, for the most part, no longer exist as amino acids.

The utilization of amino acids for protein synthesis was discussed in Chapter 13. Catabolism of amino acids with the use of their carbon chains as fuels is described in the present chapter. These two fates of amino acids account for most of the amino acids that move through the amino acid pool. Although only small quantities of amino acids are involved, the very important role of amino acids in synthesis of a large range of nonprotein compounds with specialized functions also is described in this chapter under the sections for metabolism of individual amino acids. Synthesis of dispensable amino acids, a process which is often simply the reverse of their catabolism and which involves catabolism of another amino acid to provide the α-amino group, is also discussed.

In discussing the metabolism of amino acids in the body, it is important to recognize that amino groups can be transferred from one carbon skeleton to another by a number of reactions. Hence, the fate of amino groups and carbon skeletons must be considered somewhat separately, and the amino acid via which nitrogen enters a particular cell or tissue may be the same as or different from the amino acid that carries the nitrogen out of the cell or tissue. For example, glutamine or glutamate catabolism by the small intestine can result in release of the carbon chain as CO_2 and pyruvate, lactate, or alanine, and release of the nitrogens as alanine, ammonia, or both. The small intestine also converts glutamine to citrulline and proline, which contain both carbon and the α-amino nitrogen from glutamine or glutamate.

TRANSPORT OF AMINO ACIDS

As discussed in Chapter 9, amino acids taken up from the gastrointestinal tract are released by intestinal mucosal cells into the portal circulation. Specific transport proteins with overlapping specificities are responsible for the uptake and release of amino acids from cells. A number of transport systems for amino acids have been categorized in mammalian cells (Hyde et al., 2003; Christensen, 1990) as summarized in Table 14-1. The Human Genome Project has classified 298 known solute carrier (SLC) systems into 43 families of proteins, and amino acid carriers fall into a number of these different families (see Table 14-1) (Hediger et al., 2004). Major systems for the transport of small aliphatic amino acids include Na^+-dependent systems A *(SLC38A1, A2,* and *A3)* and ASC *(SLC7A10)* and the Na^+-independent system L *(SLC7A5* and *A8)*. Other, more restricted systems are probably responsible for the transport of glutamine, acidic amino acids, basic amino acids, and imino acids. In general, the amino acid transport systems serve to carry several amino acids across the cell membrane, and the transport of a particular amino acid is subject to competitive inhibition by other amino acids that share the same transport system.

Amino acid transport is subject to short- and long-term regulation. Although most of the amino acid transporters have now been identified (Hyde et al., 2003), relatively little is known about their regulation. System A has been studied most extensively, particularly in hepatocytes and hepatoma cells, in which it is subject to a variety of regulatory signals. System A activity is rapidly increased in response to glucagon or epidermal growth factor (EGF) by mechanisms that involve hyperpolarization of the cell membrane by changes in Na^+/H^+ exchange. In addition, system A is sensitive to pH changes. In response to acidosis, there is evidence that amino acid transport in the liver may be decreased, with a resultant decrease in urea synthesis.

System A is also subject to long-term regulation brought about by changes in the amount

Table 14-1
The Human Genome Organization Nomenclature for Solute Carrier Gene Families That Code for Amino Acid Transporters

HUGO Solute Carrier Family Series	General Description	Transport System/ Functional Names
SLC1	The high-affinity glutamate and neutral amino acid transporter family	ASC, B^0, X_{AG}^-
SLC3	The heavy subunits of the heteromeric amino acid transporters	4f2hc/CD98
SLC7	The cationic amino acid transporter/glycoprotein-associated amino acid transporter family; the light subunits of the heteromeric amino acid transporters	asc, L, x_c^-, y^+L, $b^{0,+}$, y^+
SLC6	The sodium- and chloride-dependent neurotransmitter transporter family (for GABA, taurine, betaine transporters)	Beta, GLY, PROT, $B^{0,+}$
SLC16	The monocarboxylate transporter family (including aromatic amino acids)	T
SLC36	The proton-coupled amino acid transporter family (for small neutral amino acids)	imino
SLC38	The system A and N, sodium-coupled neutral amino acid transporter family	A, N
SLC43	The sodium-independent, system L–like amino acid transporter family	L-like
SLC17	The vesicular glutamate transporter family	
SLC18	The vesicular amine transporter family	
SLC32	The vesicular inhibitory amino acid transporter family	

Data from Hediger MA, Romero MF, Peng J-B, Rolfs A, Takanaga H, Bruford EA (2004) The ABCs of solute carriers: physiological, pathological and therapeutic implications of human membrane transport proteins. Pflugers Arch Eur J Physiol 447:465-468; and Hyde R, Taylor PM, Hundal HS (2003) Amino acid transporters: roles in amino acid sensing and signaling in animal cells. Biochem J 373:1-18.
A complete list is available at www.gene.ucl.ac.uk/nomenclature/activities.shtml.
HUGO, Human Genome Organization; *SLC,* solute carrier.

of transporter protein. System A can be induced by insulin in most cell types and by either insulin or glucagon in liver cells. This apparent paradox of induction of system A in liver by two opposing hormones probably is explained by the increased hepatic uptake of amino acids required in response to food intake (when protein synthesis and catabolism of excess exogenous amino acids predominate in the liver) and in response to starvation or diabetes (when amino acids from muscle protein degradation are taken up and catabolized by the liver as gluconeogenic precursors).

Dipeptides and tripeptides are transported into cells by two proton-linked carriers (SLC15 family): PepT1, found in intestine and possibly kidney, and PepT2, expressed in kidney, brain, mammary gland, and lung (Pinsonneault et al., 2004; Adibi, 2003). In addition, urea is transported by two distinct transporters, UTA and UTB (SLC14 family), which are found in many tissues and highly expressed in the kidney, where they play an important role in concentrating urine.

Several genes coding for amino acid transporters have been shown to contain amino acid response elements (AAREs), which are responsible for transcriptional upregulation of the expression of these genes under conditions of amino acid starvation (Palii et al., 2004; Sato et al., 2004; Fernandez et al., 2003). These include the sodium-coupled neutral amino acid transporter system A gene (*SNAT2* or *SLC38A2*), the arginine/lysine transporter (y^+) gene (*CAT-1* or *SLC7A1*), and the cystine/glutamate transporter (X_c^-) gene (*xCT* or *SLC7A11*). Transcription factors that belong to the ATF (activating transcription factor) and C/EBP

$$\underset{\text{Amino acid}}{H_3\overset{+}{N}-\underset{R_1}{\overset{COO^-}{C}}-H} + \underset{\text{Keto acid}}{O=\underset{R_2}{\overset{COO^-}{C}}} \xrightleftharpoons[\text{Aminotransferase}]{\text{(PLP)}} \underset{\text{Keto acid}}{O=\underset{R_1}{\overset{COO^-}{C}}} + \underset{\text{Amino acid}}{H_3\overset{+}{N}-\underset{R_2}{\overset{COO^-}{C}}-H}$$

Figure 14-2 Example of a transamination reaction. The amino acid substrate is converted to a keto acid product, whereas the keto acid cosubstrate is converted to an amino acid product. *PLP*, Pyridoxal 5′-phosphate.

(CCAAT/enhancer binding protein) families appear to be involved in binding to the AARE or AARE-like sequences in these genes.

REACTIONS INVOLVED IN THE TRANSFER, RELEASE, AND INCORPORATION OF NITROGEN

Because each amino acid has one or more individual pathways for metabolism, it is difficult to present a simplified scheme for amino acid metabolism. Some general types of reactions that are involved in the movement of amino groups and fixation of inorganic nitrogen (NH_3 or NH_4^+) are described first, followed by a summary of the fate of the carbon skeletons released by amino acid catabolism. This is followed by a summary of specific metabolic pathways for each amino acid or related group of amino acids. Finally, the pathways for excretion of nitrogen from the body are summarized. The reader should also refer to Chapter 25 for a discussion of the roles vitamin B_6, vitamin B_{12}, and folate coenzymes play in many of the reactions of amino acid metabolism.

TRANSAMINATION

The α-amino group may be moved from one carbon chain to another by transamination reactions to form the respective amino and keto acids. Transamination is the most general route for removing nitrogen from an amino acid and transferring it to another carbon skeleton. The transfer of the amino group from an amino acid to a keto acid to form another amino acid is catalyzed by aminotransferases, which are pyridoxal 5′-phosphate–dependent enzymes. The general reaction catalyzed by an aminotransferase is shown in Figure 14-2. Most physiologically important aminotransferases have a preferred amino acid–keto acid substrate and utilize α-ketoglutarate/glutamate as the counter keto acid/amino acid; an example is aspartate aminotransferase, which accepts aspartate or oxaloacetate as substrate and uses glutamate or α-ketoglutarate as cosubstrate. Alanine, aspartate, glutamate, tyrosine, serine, valine, isoleucine, and leucine are actively transaminated in human tissues. Histidine, phenylalanine, methionine, cysteine, glutamine, asparagine, and glycine also may undergo transamination in human tissues, but these amino acids are metabolized primarily by other types of reactions under normal physiological conditions. In contrast, threonine, lysine, proline, tryptophan, and arginine do not participate directly in transamination reactions in mammalian tissues; intermediates in the degradation pathways of lysine, proline, tryptophan, and arginine may, however, undergo transamination for transfer of the amino group. Because α-ketoglutarate is used widely as the acceptor of amino groups in transamination reactions, the α-amino groups of numerous amino acids are funneled through glutamate in the process of amino acid catabolism. Aspartate and alanine aminotransferases are widespread in tissues, which allows the movement of amino groups between glutamate/α-ketoglutarate and aspartate/oxaloacetate and alanine/pyruvate.

DEAMINATION

A limited number of reactions in the body is capable of direct deamination of amino acids to release ammonia and form a keto acid. The major reaction in the body in which α-amino groups are released as ammonia is catalyzed by glutamate dehydrogenase. As shown in Figure 14-3, glutamate dehydrogenase brings about the interconversion of glutamate with α-ketoglutarate and ammonia. Glutamate dehydrogenase is mitochondrial and is present at high activity in liver, kidney cortex, and brain. The fates of the products released by glutamate dehydrogenase are tissue specific. In liver, the ammonia is mainly incorporated into urea; in the kidney, it can be excreted as urinary ammonium; in the brain, the reaction functions toward glutamate formation in some cells and in other cells toward production of ammonia, which is then incorporated into glutamine.

Specific reactions in the metabolism of individual amino acids also give rise to free ammonia from the α-amino nitrogen. In particular, ammonia is released from histidine by histidine ammonia lyase (commonly called histidase), from methionine in the process of transsulfuration (in the reaction catalyzed by cystathionine γ-lyase, commonly called cystathionase), from glycine by the glycine cleavage system, and from serine or threonine by serine-threonine dehydratase. In some tissues that lack significant glutamate dehydrogenase activity, such as skeletal muscle, the purine nucleotide cycle can function to release ammonia from adenosine via adenosine deaminase, with the subsequent resynthesis of adenosine using nitrogen obtained from aspartate (Lowenstein, 1972). The net effect of this purine nucleotide cycle is the release of the amino group from aspartate (or indirectly from glutamate following transamination of glutamate with oxaloacetate to form aspartate) as ammonia and with salvage of the aspartate (or glutamate) carbon chain. L-Amino acid oxidase activity is very low in mammals and is likely of little importance in amino acid catabolism in humans. However, some foodstuffs contain small amounts of D-amino acids, and these appear to be degraded mainly by D-amino acid oxidase, which is expressed at high levels in the kidney (D'Aniello et al., 1993). The overall reaction catalyzed by amino acid oxidase is shown in Figure 14-4.

$$\underset{\text{Glutamate}}{^{-}OOC{-}CH_2{-}CH_2{-}CH(\overset{+}{N}H_3){-}COO^{-}} + NAD^{+}\ (\text{or } NADP^{+}) + H_2O \xrightleftharpoons[\text{dehydrogenase}]{\text{Glutamate}} \underset{\alpha\text{-Ketoglutarate}}{^{-}OOC{-}CH_2{-}CH_2{-}C({=}O){-}COO^{-}} + NH_4^{+} + NADH\ (\text{or } NADPH) + H^{+}$$

Figure 14-3 Interconversion of glutamate and α-ketoglutarate plus ammonia by glutamate dehydrogenase.

$$\underset{\text{D-Amino acid}}{H{-}C(R)(COO^{-}){-}\overset{+}{N}H_3} + O_2 \xrightarrow[\text{D-Amino acid oxidase}]{(FAD)} \underset{\text{Unstable amino acid}}{\left[R{-}C(COO^{-}){=}NH_2^{+} \right]} + H_2O_2$$

$$\left[R{-}C(COO^{-}){=}NH_2^{+} \right] + H_2O \xrightarrow{\text{Spontaneous}} \underset{\alpha\text{-Keto acid}}{R{-}C(COO^{-}){=}O} + NH_4^{+}$$

Figure 14-4 Oxidative deamination of a D-amino acid by D-amino acid oxidase.

Once a keto acid is formed from a D-amino acid, the keto acid can be transaminated by an L-amino acid aminotransferase to form an L-amino acid, allowing some utilization of D-amino acid carbon chains. In addition to D-amino acids arising from the diet, recent evidence suggests that some D-serine is formed in the brain through the action of serine racemase, and that D-serine is a ligand (co-activator) for the *N*-methyl-D-aspartate (NMDA) subtype of glutamate receptor (Boehning and Snyder, 2003).

DEAMIDATION AND TRANSAMIDATION

Glutamine and asparagine contain carboxamide groups, from which the amide nitrogen can be released by glutaminase or asparaginase. The reaction catalyzed by glutaminase is shown in Figure 14-5. The hydrolysis of glutamine to glutamate and ammonia occurs in many tissues and is catalyzed by phosphate-activated glutaminase, which is located in the mitochondria. In most cells, the liberated ammonia is released from the cell without further modification. The glutaminase of liver is a different isozyme from that found in most other tissues; in the liver, the ammonia generated by this reaction may be used by the carbamoyl phosphate synthetase I reaction and incorporated into urea. In a similar reaction catalyzed by asparaginase, asparagine is deamidated to yield aspartate plus ammonia. Transfer of the amide group from glutamine also plays an important role in synthetic reactions, including the synthesis of purine and pyrimidine nucleotides, NAD^+, and amino sugars, as is discussed further in a subsequent section of this chapter.

INCORPORATION OF AMMONIA INTO THE α-AMINO POOL

Although most of the interconversions and metabolism of amino acids and other nitrogenous compounds within the body occur with organic nitrogen, primarily amino and amide groups, some reactions can utilize ammonia. Glutamate dehydrogenase (see Fig. 14-3), which was discussed as the mitochondrial enzyme responsible for release of α-amino nitrogen as ammonia, can also function in the reverse direction to allow incorporation of ammonia into glutamate and, hence, into the α-amino nitrogen pool. This enzyme catalyzes a near-equilibrium reaction in tissues with high activity (liver, kidney, and brain) and can operate to either incorporate ammonia into or release ammonia from the α-amino acid pool. The direction of flux depends on the provision and removal of reactants. Because glutamate and α-ketoglutarate are key intermediates in many transamination reactions, the glutamate dehydrogenase reaction plays a central role in the movement of nitrogen between the inorganic and organic pools, as illustrated in Figure 14-6. The equilibrium nature of the glutamate dehydrogenase and transamination reactions in these tissues also acts to maintain intracellular ammonia levels in a narrow range.

INCORPORATION OF AMMONIA INTO GLUTAMINE AS AN AMIDE GROUP

A second major ammonia-fixing reaction in the body is the synthesis of glutamine from glutamate and ammonia; this reaction is catalyzed by glutamine synthetase and involves the addition of ammonia to form a carboxamide

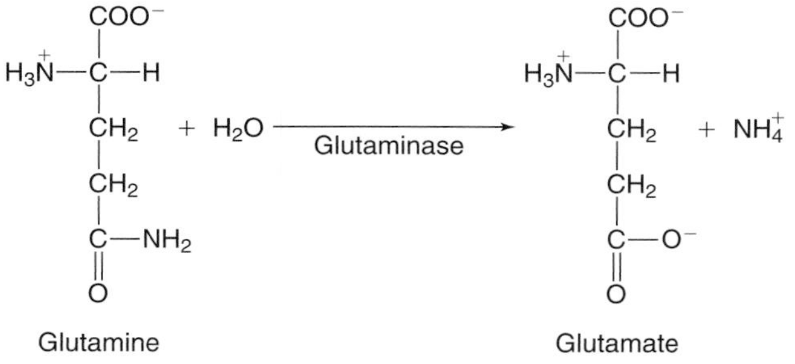

$$\mathrm{H_3\overset{+}{N}{-}CH(COO^-){-}CH_2{-}CH_2{-}C({=}O){-}NH_2} + H_2O \xrightarrow{\text{Glutaminase}} \mathrm{H_3\overset{+}{N}{-}CH(COO^-){-}CH_2{-}CH_2{-}C({=}O){-}O^-} + NH_4^+$$

Glutamine Glutamate

Figure 14-5 Hydrolysis of amide nitrogen from glutamine by glutaminase.

group from the γ-carboxyl group of glutamate (Fig. 14-7). Glutamine, which has two nitrogenous groups, plays an important role in the transfer of nitrogen between cells and tissues, and glutamine synthetase activity is particularly high in muscle, adipose tissue, lung, brain, and the perivenous parenchymal cells of the liver (the cells located closest to the terminal hepatic venules or central veins by which blood exits the liver; see Chapter 12, Fig. 12-11).

Asparagine synthetase catalyzes a similar reaction by which asparagine is synthesized from aspartate, but this enzyme can use either ammonia or glutamine as the substrate for the amidation reaction. This reaction plays a small role in overall nitrogen transfer in the body compared with that of glutamine synthetase.

INCORPORATION OF AMMONIA INTO CARBAMOYL PHOSPHATE FOR FORMATION OF UREA CYCLE INTERMEDIATES AND UREA

Although it does not result in incorporation of inorganic nitrogen into the amino acid pool (except into the guanidinium group of arginine), carbamoyl phosphate synthetase I, which is found in the mitochondria of liver and small intestinal cells, produces carbamoyl phosphate for citrulline production (Fig. 14-8). Within the liver, this citrulline is an integral part of the urea cycle, but in the intestine the citrulline may be released into the circulation as citrulline for further metabolism to arginine in the kidney.

METABOLISM OF THE CARBON CHAINS OF AMINO ACIDS

The use of an amino acid as a fuel requires the removal of the amino group and the conversion of the carbon chain to an intermediate that can enter the central pathways of fuel metabolism. The processes of amino acid catabolism, excretion of nitrogen as urea or ammonia, conversion of amino acid carbon chains to glucose or other fuels, and the eventual complete oxidation of the amino acid carbon skeleton are all metabolically interrelated.

CATABOLISM OF AMINO ACID CARBON CHAINS

The rate of amino acid catabolism varies with amino acid supply. When amino acids are abundant, after a meal or during conditions of net proteolysis (e.g., uncontrolled diabetes, hypercatabolic states, or starvation), the extent of amino acid catabolism increases markedly.

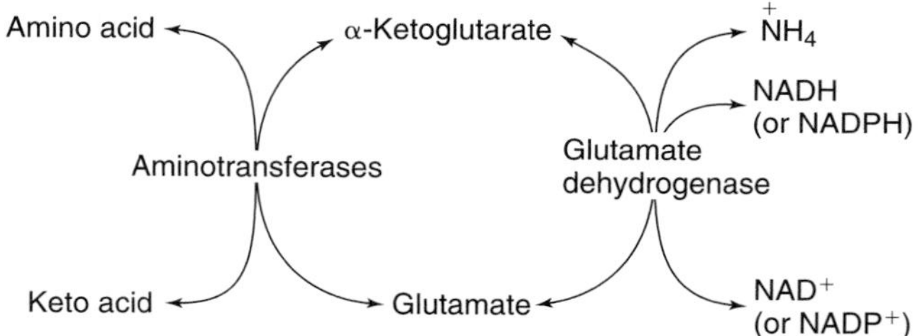

Figure 14-6 The equilibrium nature of aminotransferases and glutamate dehydrogenase activities in brain, liver, and kidney maintain ammonia, amino acid, and keto acid levels.

$$\underset{\text{Glutamate}}{{}^{-}OOC{-}CH_2{-}CH_2{-}CH(\overset{+}{N}H_3){-}COO^{-}} + NH_3 + ATP \xrightarrow[\text{synthetase}]{\text{Glutamine}} \underset{\text{Glutamine}}{H_2NOC{-}CH_2{-}CH_2{-}CH(\overset{+}{N}H_3){-}COO^{-}} + ADP + P_i$$

Figure 14-7 Synthesis of glutamine from glutamate and NH_3 by glutamine synthetase.

Conversely, when the diet is adequate in energy but deficient in amino acids, the catabolism of amino acids is reduced significantly.

The points at which the carbon skeletons of various amino acids enter central pathways of metabolism during their catabolism are shown in Figure 14-9. The carbon skeletons of most amino acids are metabolized to glycolytic or citric acid cycle intermediates and hence have the potential to be used for gluconeogenesis. Isoleucine, phenylalanine, tryptophan, and tyrosine also give rise to acetyl coenzyme A (CoA) in addition to a potentially glucogenic intermediate, whereas catabolism of leucine and lysine results only in the formation of acetyl units (as acetyl CoA or as acetoacetate). Amino acids often are classified as glucogenic, ketogenic, or both glucogenic and ketogenic based on their metabolic fates, but any amino acid that is potentially glucogenic is also potentially ketogenic. Once the carbon skeleton of an amino acid enters central pathways of fuel metabolism, it may be further oxidized for energy or used for synthesis of other compounds such as dispensable amino acids, glucose and glycogen, cholesterol, or triacylglycerols.

It is often stated that amino acids are oxidized in the liver, which is the major site of amino acid catabolism and urea production. In addition, similar statements are made about

$$NH_3 + CO_2 + 2\,ATP \xrightarrow[\text{Carbamoyl phosphate synthetase I}]{N\text{-Acetylglutamate}} H_2N{-}\overset{\overset{\displaystyle O}{\|}}{C}{-}O{-}\overset{\overset{\displaystyle O}{\|}}{\underset{\underset{\displaystyle O^-}{|}}{P}}{-}O^- + 2\,ADP + P_i$$

Carbamoyl phosphate

Figure 14-8 Synthesis of carbamoyl phosphate from NH_3 and CO_2 in mitochondria of hepatocytes and enterocytes.

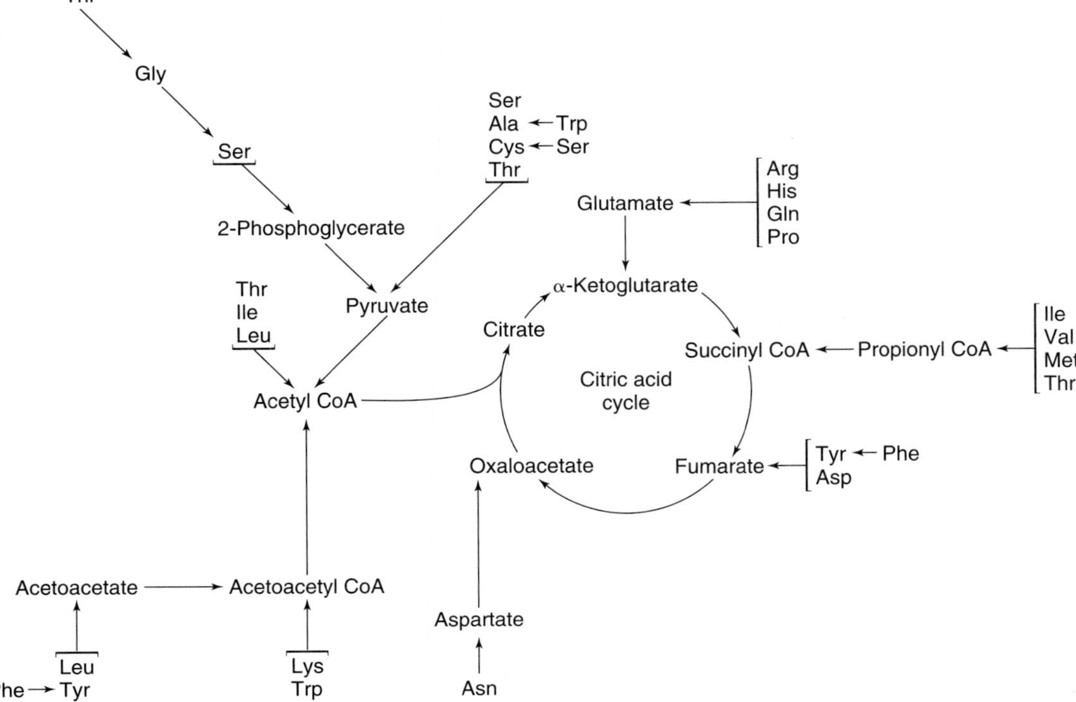

Figure 14-9 Formation of amphibolic intermediates from the carbon skeletons of amino acids.

amino acid catabolism in other tissues, such as glutamine oxidation in the small intestine or branched-chain amino acid oxidation in the muscle. Such statements seem to imply that the amino acids are completely oxidized to CO_2 and H_2O. However, apart from some evidence for leucine oxidation in skeletal muscle, the complete oxidation of amino acids does not occur in any single tissue. Jungas and colleagues (1992) calculated that the amount of energy that would be produced by complete catabolism of amino acids at a rate equivalent to their net uptake by the liver would exceed the total energy used by the liver. Therefore amino acids not used for protein or peptide synthesis in the liver are only partially oxidized within the liver, and the carbon skeletons are converted to glucose, glycogen, carbon chains of dispensable amino acids, lipids, and small amounts of ketone bodies for utilization or storage by various tissues. Like the liver, other tissues that utilize amino acids for energy do not completely catabolize amino acids.

Amino acids are quantitatively important as a fuel for the liver, small intestine, and other specialized cells such as reticulocytes and cells of the immune system. It has been estimated that liver derives at least half of its ATP need from the partial oxidation of amino acids, and that the small intestinal jejunum may derive up to 80% of its fuel needs from amino acids. The intestinal jejunum uses glutamine, glutamate, and aspartate taken up from the luminal contents (digesta), as well as arterial glutamine (Reeds and Burrin, 2001). Although branched-chain amino acid oxidation at least partially occurs in muscle, nonprotein fuels are quantitatively much more important for muscle; muscle releases nitrogen primarily as glutamine and alanine (Darmaun and Dechelotte, 1991; Elia and Livesey, 1983). The kidneys consume large amounts of glutamine and significant, but lesser, amounts of glycine (Tizianello et al., 1982). The kidneys also release serine. The net uptake of amino acids by the liver (from the arterial and portal circulation) differs substantially from the dietary input. In particular, the uptakes of alanine and serine are high, whereas net uptakes of aspartate, glutamate, and the branched-chain amino acids are very low, and the liver may actually exhibit net glutamate release. Although the gastrointestinal tract extracts large amounts of glutamine from the circulation and also metabolizes dietary glutamine (and glutamate), there is evidence that human liver also takes up considerable amounts of glutamine (Watford, 2000; Elia, 1993; Felig et al., 1973).

GLUCONEOGENESIS

In the liver, amino acid catabolism is accompanied by both ureagenesis and gluconeogenesis, which is the synthesis of glucose from nonglucose precursors. Amino acids are an important source of carbon skeletons for gluconeogenesis, and gluconeogenesis plays an important role in the process of amino acid catabolism in the liver. Although gluconeogenesis in the liver traditionally has been considered to operate predominantly during fasting or starvation in response to hypoglycemia and breakdown of muscle protein, it is now apparent that gluconeogenesis also functions postprandially while amino acids are being absorbed and processed. Estimates of glucose synthesis from amino acid carbon in the fed human are 50 to 60 g of glucose per 100 g of protein partially oxidized (Jungas et al., 1992). Therefore ureagenesis can be viewed as operating together to produce glucose (or glycogen), urea, and CO_2 from amino acids whenever the liver is processing amino acids.

A general overview of the processes by which the liver converts amino acid carbon chains to the "universal fuel" glucose and at the same time incorporates the nitrogen groups into urea for excretion is shown in Figure 14-10. This scheme demonstrates that, when a balanced mixture of amino acids is being oxidized, most of the glucogenic carbon will be carried out of the mitochondria as aspartate, which also serves as the immediate donor of one of the two nitrogens for urea synthesis. Within the mitochondria, pyruvate is carboxylated to oxaloacetate by pyruvate carboxylase, whereas α-ketoglutarate and other glucogenic carbon chains of amino acids are converted to oxaloacetate by citric acid cycle enzymes. Gluconeogenesis and ureagenesis can be considered as sharing the common steps (catalyzed by argininosuccinate synthetase and lyase) by which aspartate is converted to fumarate and citrulline is converted to arginine (Jungas et al., 1992). Because metabolism of

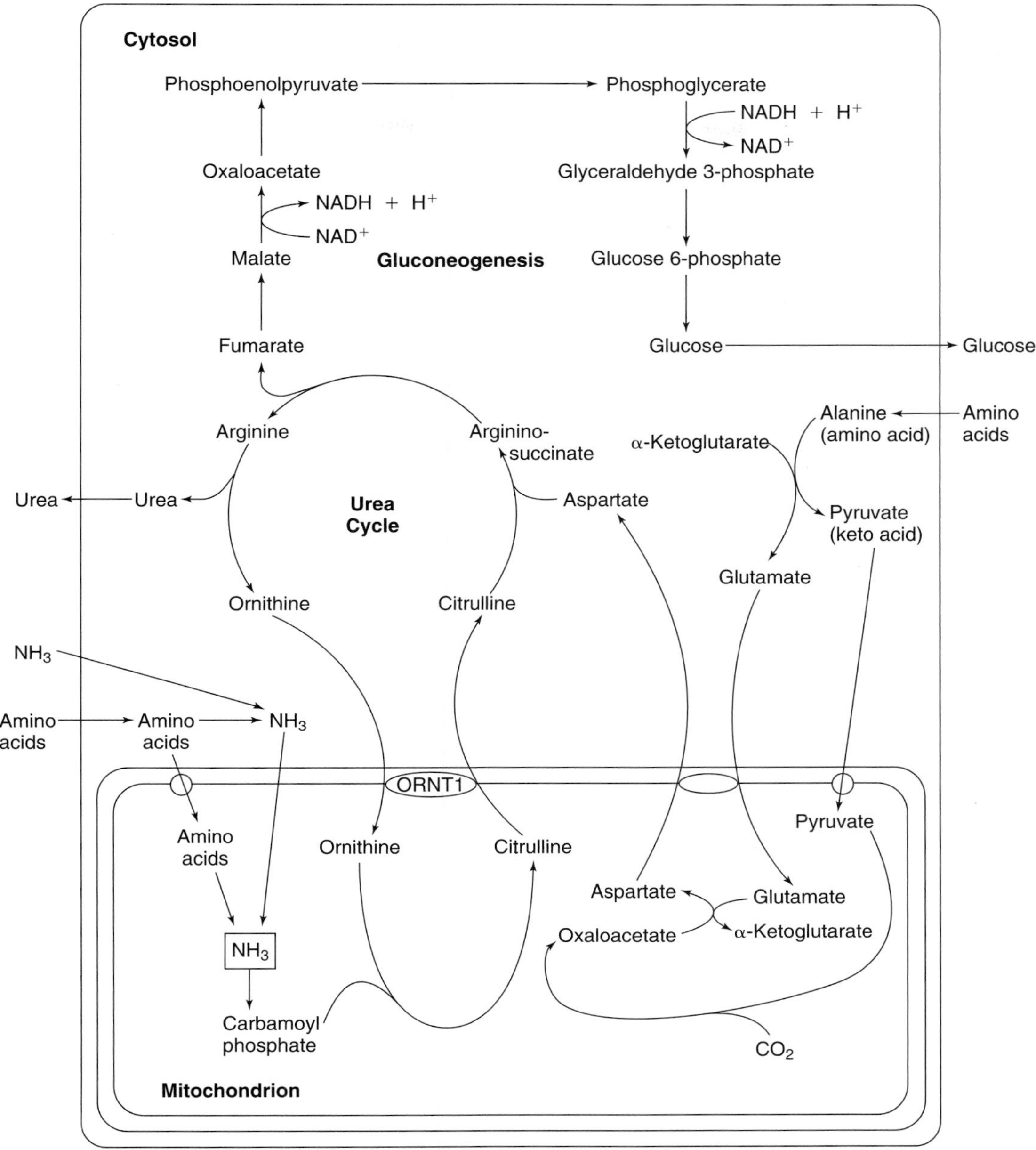

Figure 14-10 Metabolism of amino acids by the liver, including the partial oxidation of amino acids, gluconeogenesis, and ureagenesis. Although not shown in the figure, α-ketoglutarate generated in the mitochondria can be transported from the mitochondria to replenish the cytosolic α-ketoglutarate pool.

aspartate by argininosuccinate synthetase and lyase releases the carbon as fumarate (a precursor of malate, which in turn is oxidized to oxaloacetate in a reaction that generates cytosolic NADH + H^+), aspartate also carries reducing equivalents out of the mitochondria to the cytosol, where they are needed for gluconeogenesis. Gluconeogenesis is discussed in detail in Chapter 12. Urea synthesis is discussed in more detail in the last section of this chapter.

ENERGETICS OF AMINO ACID OXIDATION

Jungas and colleagues (1992) detailed the processes involved in amino acid oxidation in liver and calculated that the partial oxidation of dietary amino acids provides sufficient energy to support the ATP requirements for synthesis of both glucose and urea; hence, the liver is not dependent on oxidation of another fuel besides amino acids to provide ATP to support these processes. On the basis of the detailed calculations of Jungas and colleagues (1992), complete oxidation of 1 g of meat protein by the body yields a net gain of approximately 195 mmoles of ATP (an average of 21.5 moles of ATP per mole of amino acids). They also estimated that, on a whole-body basis, approximately 35% of this net ATP production results from amino acid oxidation in muscle and small intestine, 60% from oxidation of the glucose generated by hepatic gluconeogenesis, and 5% from oxidation of acetoacetate generated from amino acid carbon chains.

REGULATION OF AMINO ACID OXIDATION AND GLUCONEOGENESIS

Clearly, amino acid oxidation, gluconeogenesis, and ureagenesis are processes that are metabolically interrelated in the liver. These metabolic pathways are predominantly expressed in the periportal parenchymal cells (cells that surround the terminal portal venule and hepatic arteriole by which blood enters the liver) rather than in the perivenous cells. These processes are active in both the fed (protein-containing meal) and in the starved states. Glucagon, glucocorticoids, and thyroid hormones play a role in increasing the rates of amino acid catabolism as well as ureagenesis and gluconeogenesis in the liver, whereas insulin may decrease these metabolic processes. Many amino acid catabolic enzyme activities are increased under conditions that result in higher rates of amino acid catabolism, and some of these changes involve responses to hormonal signals, whereas others seem to be specific responses to high concentrations of amino acid substrates. Glucocorticoids, catecholamines, and cytokines—which are elevated during stress, infection, and trauma—play a role in increasing net muscle protein breakdown and, thus, the availability of amino acids to the liver for gluconeogenesis.

In the fed state, dietary glutamine, glutamate, and aspartate (~20% of dietary protein) are metabolized within the enterocyte with the resultant production of alanine. Therefore, the portal blood contains higher amounts of alanine but lower amounts of glutamine, glutamate, and aspartate when compared with the amino acid pattern of dietary protein. In addition, the portal-drained viscera also extract glutamine from the arterial circulation, even during protein feeding. Because the intestine catabolizes glutamine, glutamate, and aspartate to alanine, which is subsequently released and taken up by the liver, the gluconeogenic potential of amino acid carbon chains largely is conserved despite the intestine's use of these amino acids as fuels (Watford, 1994). Uptake of alanine by the liver exceeds gut release (with additional alanine originating from the peripheral tissues), whereas hepatic uptake of branched-chain amino acids is substantially less than gut output such that the systemic blood levels of valine, leucine, and isoleucine rise in response to protein ingestion. There is a net uptake of these branched-chain amino acids by peripheral tissues (muscle, brain) during the absorptive period.

In the starved state, large amounts of glutamine and large amounts of alanine are released from muscle, and these can be utilized as fuels or substrate for gluconeogenesis. The increases in hepatic removal of alanine and in hepatic gluconeogenesis in early starvation or uncontrolled diabetes probably are related to a rise in glucagon and a fall in insulin. A rise in the concentrations of plasma branched-chain amino acids is noted in early starvation and probably is due to the hypoinsulinemia of starvation and decreased net uptake of amino acids by the muscle. Although the initial response to starvation is directed at maintenance of hepatic glucose output by increasing gluconeogenesis, the later response is directed at maintenance of body protein reserves by minimizing protein catabolism. The replacement of glucose by ketone bodies as the major oxidative fuel utilized by the brain is accompanied by a decrease in hepatic gluconeogenesis and urinary nitrogen excretion (particularly as urea, such that the ratio of ammonium to urea in the urine markedly increases). A general decline in plasma amino acid levels is observed, but the fall in plasma alanine is most obvious.

Decreased output of alanine from muscle contributes to the decreased alanine uptake and decreased gluconeogenesis by liver. The availability of ketone bodies as a fuel for muscle and other tissues seems to contribute to protein conservation by limiting amino acid (alanine) availability for gluconeogenesis.

ACID–BASE CONSIDERATIONS OF AMINO ACID OXIDATION

Amino acid oxidation generates nonvolatile or fixed acids, primarily SO_4^{2-} (+2 H^+) from catabolism of the sulfur-containing amino acids methionine and cysteine. The body can compensate for some of this excess fixed anion by increasing its excretion of dietary HPO_4^{2-} as $H_2PO_4^-$ (titratable acidity) or by consumption of HCO_3^- (bicarbonate) generated from the metabolism of dietary carboxylate anions (e.g., malate or citrate). The kidney excretes additional acid by generating NH_3 from glutamine (and to a lesser extent glycine) catabolism and then excreting it as NH_4^+ (net acid) while simultaneously producing and retaining HCO_3^- (net base) from the amino acid carbon skeleton. Note that ureagenesis in the liver is not capable of adjusting acid–base balance because both HCO_3^- and NH_4^+ are consumed in ureagenesis.

Metabolic acidosis results in an increased release of glutamine from skeletal muscle. Within the kidney, a stimulation of α-ketoglutarate dehydrogenase by the lower pH results in increased glutamine utilization and ammonia production. The glutamine carbon skeleton is then further metabolized to bicarbonate and, in some species, glucose. Long-term regulation during metabolic acidosis involves increased synthesis of the key kidney enzymes glutaminase and phosphoenolpyruvate carboxykinase (Curthoys and Watford, 1995).

SYNTHESIS OF DISPENSABLE AMINO ACIDS

For the synthesis of the carbon chains of dispensable amino acids, glucose or glucogenic substrates (such as the carbon skeletons of most amino acids) are required. Pyruvate or other 3-carbon glycolytic intermediates serve as substrates for synthesis of alanine, serine, and glycine. Oxaloacetate, a 4-carbon keto acid, is the carbon skeleton of aspartate and asparagine. The 5-carbon keto acid α-ketoglutarate, or its metabolites, provides the carbon skeleton for glutamate, glutamine, proline, and arginine (Fig. 14-11). Nitrogenous groups

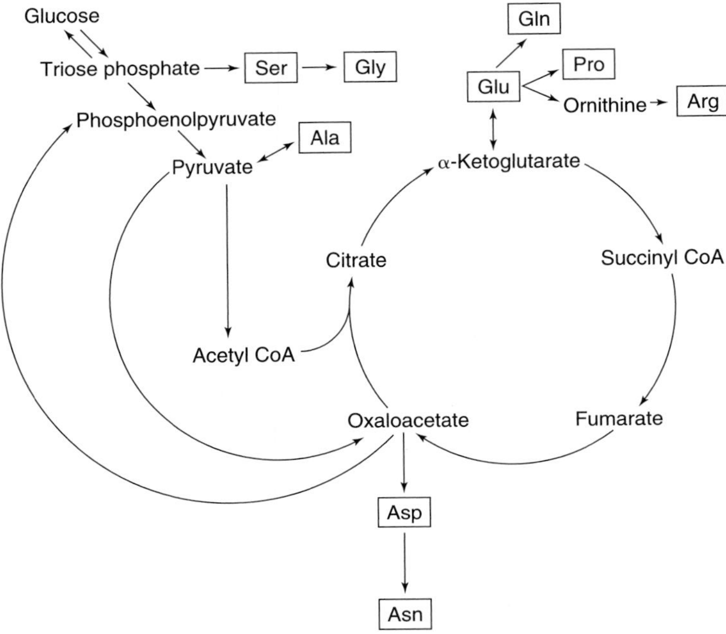

Figure 14-11 Synthesis of dispensable amino acids from the carbon skeletons of amphibolic intermediates.

are added to these carbon chains by direct transamination of pyruvate, 3-phosphohydroxypyruvate, oxaloacetate, and α-ketoglutarate with other amino acids; by amidation of glutamate and aspartate; and by the formation of metabolites of pyrroline 5-carboxylate as is discussed in more detail in the section on proline and arginine.

Synthesis of nonessential amino acids is regulated. Synthesis of asparagine from aspartate and glutamine is transcriptionally regulated in response to amino acid or glucose starvation; the asparagine synthetase gene contains a nutrient-sensing response unit that is responsible for regulation of this gene by nutrient starvation (Chen et al., 2004). Synthesis of arginine from proline in enterally fed neonatal piglets was upregulated when the diet was deficient in arginine, apparently by increased extraction of proline from the plasma (Wilkinson et al., 2004).

METABOLISM OF SPECIFIC AMINO ACIDS

For the reader who is interested in the metabolism of individual amino acids, details of the pathways by which amino acid carbon chains are used as fuels, by which amino acids are used for synthesis of numerous nonprotein compounds, and by which dispensable amino acids are synthesized are discussed in this section. To the extent possible, an effort has been made to describe the pathways and interorgan fluxes that are most significant in humans. The dispensable amino acids are discussed first, followed by discussion of the indispensable amino acids.

ALANINE

The only reactions that use alanine in mammalian tissues are those involving its incorporation into proteins and its participation in transamination. In skeletal muscle, liver, and small intestine, alanine aminotransferase catalyzes a reaction close to equilibrium, and alanine flux increases when a high carbohydrate diet is ingested and tissues are using glucose as a major fuel (Yang et al., 1986). (A minor source of alanine is its formation from the aliphatic portion of tryptophan during tryptophan catabolism.)

As already mentioned, alanine is a major amino acid that is released from muscle and small intestine. The muscle normally releases large quantities of alanine in the postabsorptive, or basal, state, and this release of alanine from muscle is increased during early starvation. However, the release of alanine by muscle is reduced when branched-chain amino acids from a protein-containing meal are abundantly available as a fuel for muscle, in which case glutamine is the major amino acid released by muscle. The carbon skeleton of alanine is derived primarily from glucose in muscle; the nitrogen (as well as a small amount of the carbon of alanine) is derived from catabolism of branched-chain and other amino acids in muscle. The catabolism of dietary glutamate, aspartate, and glutamine, together with arterial glutamine, in the enterocytes of the small intestine results in the synthesis and release of lactate, pyruvate, and alanine. Hence, these cells only partially oxidize these amino acids, and the gluconeogenic potential is conserved within the body (Watford, 1994).

Alanine is removed from the circulation primarily by the liver, which uses the alanine for ureagenesis and gluconeogenesis (Jungas et al., 1992; Felig, 1975). Alanine alone accounts for more than 25% of the total amino acids removed from the blood by the liver. It should be noted, however, that most of the production of alanine in muscle, especially during exercise when glycolytic activity is high, does not represent a net contribution of alanine to body glucose because most of the pyruvate for alanine synthesis in muscle is derived from glycolysis of glucose. The role of the glucose–alanine cycle in transporting nitrogen to the liver for ureagenesis is shown in Figure 14-12. This cycle serves to transport nitrogen out of the muscle but does not generate any new glucogenic substrates. In contrast, the synthesis and release of glutamine by skeletal muscle does represent the provision of new gluconeogenic substrate (Nurjhan et al., 1995). Although not definitively known, because of problems in sampling the portal vein in humans, there is evidence that approximately 30% to 40% of the glutamine used by the splanchnic bed (portal-drained viscera) is taken up directly by the liver (Elia, 1993; Felig et al., 1973).

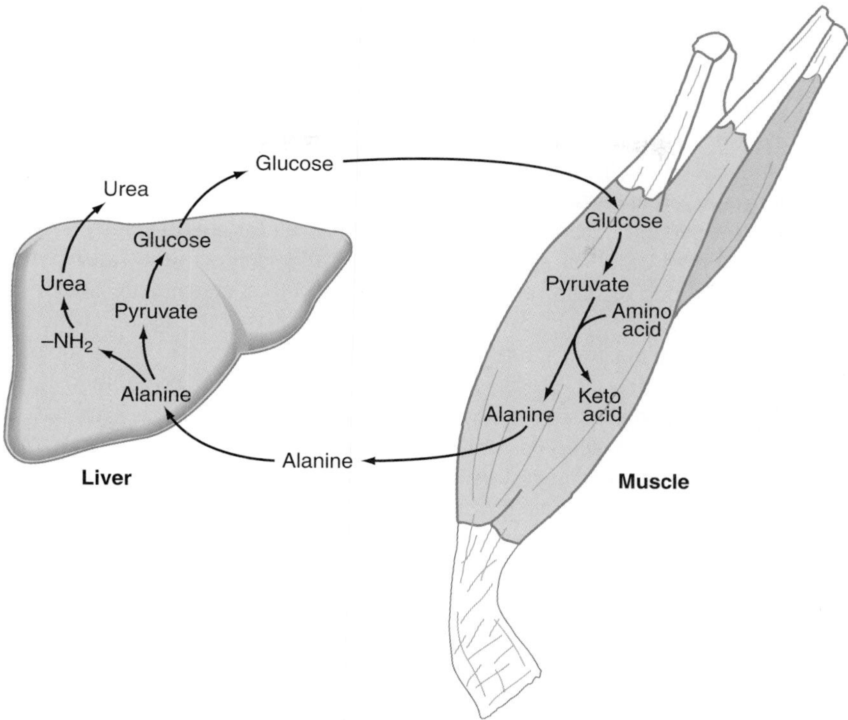

Figure 14-12 The glucose–alanine cycle for amino group transport. The carbon chain is cycled between glucose and pyruvate.

As indicated previously, intestinal glutamine catabolism also results in the synthesis of alanine, which is then taken up by the liver for gluconeogenesis.

GLUTAMATE, GLUTAMINE, ASPARTATE, AND ASPARAGINE

Roles of Glutamate, Glutamine, and Aspartate in the Movement of Amino Acid Nitrogen and Carbon in the Body

Glutamate, glutamine, and aspartate play central roles in nitrogen metabolism within the body. Glutamate and aspartate are involved in numerous reactions, such as the transfer of α-amino acid nitrogen in the synthesis of dispensable amino acids, purines, and pyrimidines. Most glutamate and aspartate metabolism is intracellular, and the turnover of the plasma pools is relatively low (Battezzati et al., 1995). Glutamine, in contrast, not only plays a major role in intracellular metabolism (e.g., pyrimidine and purine synthesis), but also is the major transport form of nitrogen among tissues in the circulation.

Glutamate and aspartate are interconvertible with two citric acid cycle intermediates, α-ketoglutarate and oxaloacetate, respectively. Hence, like alanine, they have carbon skeletons that play central roles as amphibolic intermediates (serving both anabolic and catabolic purposes) in metabolism. Aspartate aminotransferase catalyzes the interconversion of aspartate and oxaloacetate, and two isozymes of aspartate aminotransferase, cytosolic and mitochondrial, play important roles in the movement of carbon and reducing equivalents across mitochondrial membranes by the malate–aspartate shuttle. In addition, during ureagenesis and gluconeogenesis in the liver, as shown in Figure 14-10, aspartate carries carbon and reducing equivalents for hepatic gluconeogenesis as well as nitrogen for ureagenesis from the mitochondria to the cytosol. Glutamate and α-ketoglutarate are interconverted by a number of other aminotransferases, especially alanine aminotransferase and branched-chain aminotransferase, in addition to aspartate aminotransferase. In some tissues, glutamate is also interconverted with its keto acid via the mitochondrial glutamate dehydrogenase reaction (see Fig. 14-6).

In addition to the α-carboxylic acid group, aspartate and glutamate (or aspartic acid and glutamic acid) possess a second carboxylic acid group. The β-carboxylic acid group of aspartate and the γ-carboxylic acid group of glutamate can be amidated to form amino acids with carboxamide groups; these amino acids are asparagine and glutamine, respectively. Their synthesis was described previously in the discussion of the assimilation of inorganic nitrogen (see Fig. 14-7).

Glutamine catabolism occurs predominantly by the hydrolysis of the amide group from the carboxamide, a process called deamidation. A mitochondrial enzyme, glutaminase, catalyzes the reaction, which results in the production of glutamate and ammonia (see Fig. 14-5). Asparagine catabolism occurs in the same manner in a reaction catalyzed by asparaginase; aspartate and ammonia are released. Glutamine also serves as a donor of its carboxamide nitrogen via transamidation reactions. Although of minor physiological importance, both asparagine and glutamine can also undergo transamination with keto acids, especially in the mitochondria of some cells, to produce α-ketosuccinamate or α-ketoglutaramate. These keto acids can be deamidated to form ammonia plus oxaloacetate or α-ketoglutarate.

Tissue-Specific Metabolism of Glutamine

Glutamine is the most abundant free α-amino acid in the body; the body contains approximately 80 g of free glutamine, with more than 95% of this located intracellularly. The branched-chain amino acids are a major source of carbon and nitrogen for glutamine synthesis (as well as of the nitrogen for alanine synthesis) by muscle. In addition to branched-chain amino acids, there is evidence that muscle also takes up some glutamate from the circulation. During the fed state, large amounts of dietary branched-chain amino acids are taken up and catabolized in the muscle. During times of net proteolysis, the branched-chain amino acids from muscle proteins are catabolized within the muscle. In both cases, the release of glutamine serves to transport carbon and nitrogen that originated from the branched-chain amino acids to other tissues such as small intestine, immune cells, kidney, and liver.

The source of the carbon skeleton for net glutamine synthesis in muscle is not firmly established, but the propionyl CoA derived from valine and isoleucine metabolism may be carboxylated to succinyl CoA. Succinyl CoA is then converted to oxaloacetate, which in turn may condense with acetyl CoA to form citrate, which may then be converted to α-ketoglutarate as shown in Figure 14-13. This can be transaminated to glutamate (probably in concert with the transamination of a branched-chain amino acid to form a branched-chain keto acid) and amidated to glutamine by glutamine synthetase (using ammonia released from glutamate or other amino acids). Thus glutamine seems to transport branched-chain amino acid carbons as well as nitrogen out of the muscle. Net synthesis of glutamine also occurs in the lungs, adipose tissue, brain, and, under certain conditions, in liver.

In the healthy individual, the major site of glutamine catabolism is the small intestine,

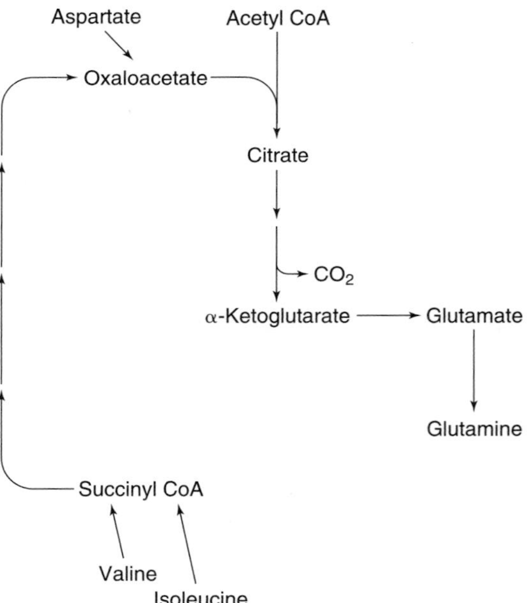

Figure 14-13 Proposed pathway for de novo synthesis of glutamine in skeletal muscle. The carbon-chain precursors are aspartate and branched-chain amino acids.

where glutamine is the principal respiratory fuel of enterocytes during the postabsorptive state (Reeds and Burrin, 2001). The catabolism of glutamine in the intestine results in the production of CO_2, alanine, pyruvate, and lactate from the carbon skeleton, and of ammonia and alanine from the amide and amino groups. Proline and citrulline are additional products of intestinal glutamine/glutamate catabolism. Thymocytes, lymphocytes, and macrophages all use glutamine as the principal respiratory fuel, and these cells show increased rates of glutamine utilization when they are activated. In these immune system cells, the major carbon end product is aspartate, with little or no production of alanine, proline, or citrulline. Glutamine plays an important role in acid–base balance and is taken up by the kidney during metabolic acidosis. The kidney uses the glutamine to produce ammonia, bicarbonate, and glucose, which allows the excretion of acid and conservation of important cations. In the liver, glutamine is taken up and catabolized in periportal cells with the resultant production of urea and glucose, whereas perivenous cells synthesize glutamine for release into the circulation.

Roles of Aspartate and *N*-Acetylglutamate in Urea Synthesis

In the urea cycle (see Fig. 14-10), aspartate serves as the donor of an α-amino group to citrulline to form argininosuccinate. This nitrogen, along with the nitrogen (from ammonia) plus carbon and oxygen (from HCO_3^-) contributed via carbamoyl phosphate, ultimately is released as urea. Hence, aspartate serves as a direct donor of α-amino nitrogen to the urea cycle, with release of the aspartate carbon chain as fumarate, whereas carbamoyl phosphate serves as a direct donor of inorganic nitrogen to the urea cycle. Both nitrogen donors serve to funnel nitrogen that originated in various dietary and endogenous amino acids into the urea cycle for ultimate excretion from the body. As discussed in the preceding text (see Fig. 14-10), the fumarate derived from aspartate metabolism in the urea cycle serves as a carrier of both carbon and reducing equivalents that can be used for the process of gluconeogenesis from amino acid carbon skeletons.

N-Acetylglutamate, an allosteric activator of carbamoyl phosphate synthetase I, is synthesized from acetyl CoA and glutamate in the liver and in the small intestine (the two tissues that have carbamoyl phosphate synthetase I activity). *N*-Acetylglutamate can be hydrolyzed by a specific deacylase.

Roles of Aspartate and Glutamine in Purine and Pyrimidine Nucleotide Synthesis

Purine nucleotides (adenine and guanine nucleotides) are synthesized by a sequence of reactions that involve glutamine and aspartate, as well as glycine, as direct participants (Fig. 14-14). Both of the carbons and the nitrogen of glycine are incorporated into purines; the amide nitrogen of two glutamine molecules and the α-amino nitrogen of one aspartate molecule (with the aspartate carbons being released as fumarate) are contributed to each purine molecule that is synthesized. Two one-carbon units from the folate coenzyme system are also required; these likely originate from serine or other amino acids. This process results in the formation of inosine monophosphate, from which the other purine nucleotides can be formed. Formation of adenosine monophosphate (AMP) requires transfer of one more amine group from aspartate, with subsequent release of the aspartate carbon chain as fumarate. Formation of guanosine monophosphate (GMP) requires transfer of an additional amide nitrogen from glutamine.

Pyrimidine nucleotides (uridine, thymidine, and cytidine nucleotides) are synthesized by a sequence of reactions that involve glutamine and aspartate (Fig. 14-15). Glutamine donates only a nitrogen, whereas aspartate donates carbons and nitrogen. The synthetic sequence begins with formation of carbamoyl phosphate by the carbamoyl phosphate synthetase II cytosolic reaction, which uses glutamine (amide group) as the nitrogen donor. Carbamoyl phosphate is condensed with aspartate to form *N*-carbamoyl aspartate. Three of the four carbons of aspartate become part of the newly synthesized pyrimidine, whereas the α-carboxyl carbon of aspartate is lost as CO_2 in the conversion of orotidine 5′-phosphate to uridine 5′-phosphate. Conversion of uridine triphosphate (UTP)

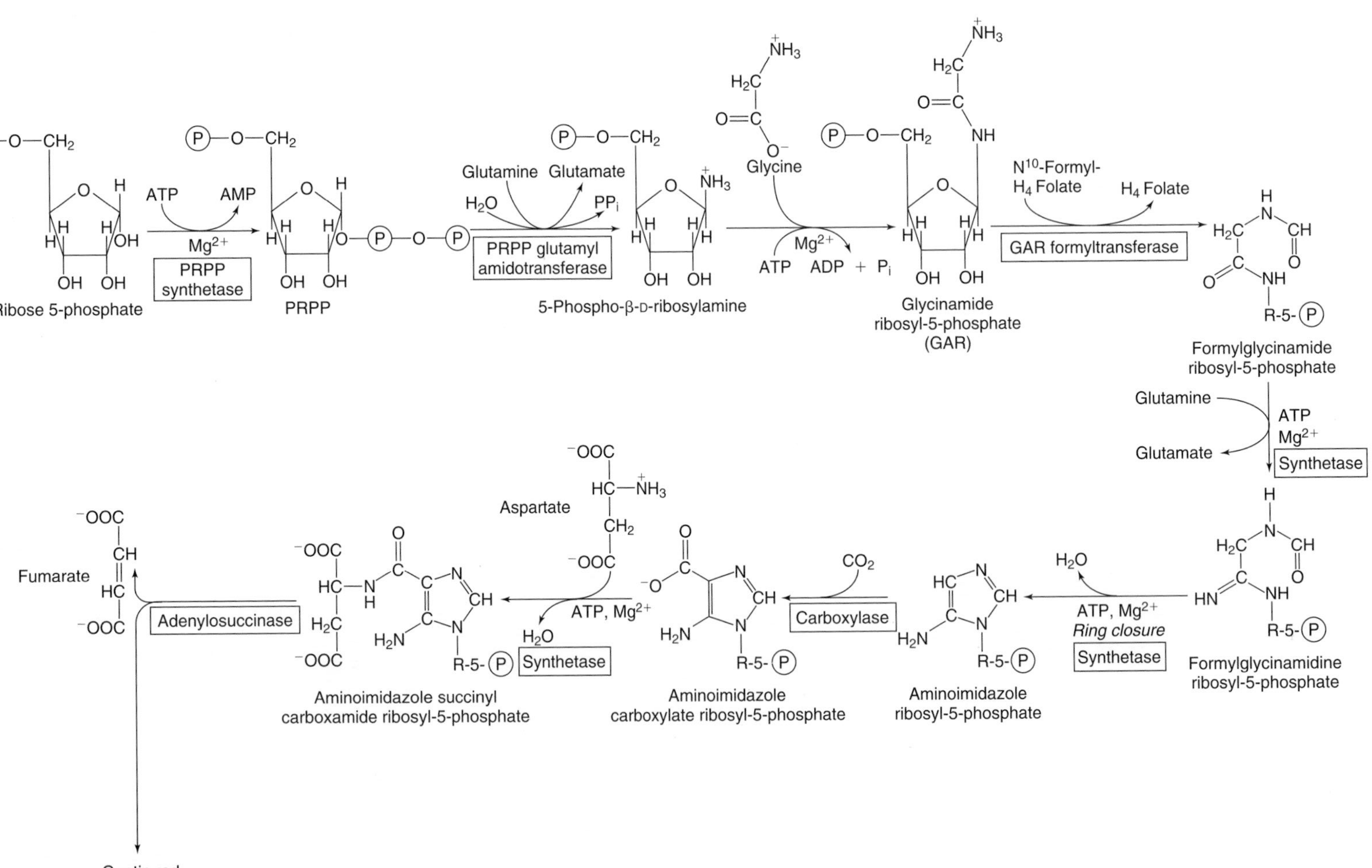
α-D-Ribose 5-phosphate
ATP
AMP
Mg^{2+}
PRPP synthetase
PRPP
Glutamine Glutamate
H_2O
PP_i
PRPP glutamyl amidotransferase
5-Phospho-β-D-ribosylamine
Glycine
Mg^{2+}
ATP ADP + P_i
Glycinamide ribosyl-5-phosphate (GAR)
N^{10}-Formyl-H_4 Folate
H_4 Folate
GAR formyltransferase
Formylglycinamide ribosyl-5-phosphate
Glutamine
Glutamate
ATP
Mg^{2+}
Synthetase
Formylglycinamidine ribosyl-5-phosphate
H_2O
ATP, Mg^{2+}
Ring closure
Synthetase
Aminoimidazole ribosyl-5-phosphate
CO_2
Carboxylase
Aminoimidazole carboxylate ribosyl-5-phosphate
Aspartate
ATP, Mg^{2+}
H_2O
Synthetase
Aminoimidazole succinyl carboxamide ribosyl-5-phosphate
Adenylosuccinase
Fumarate
Continued

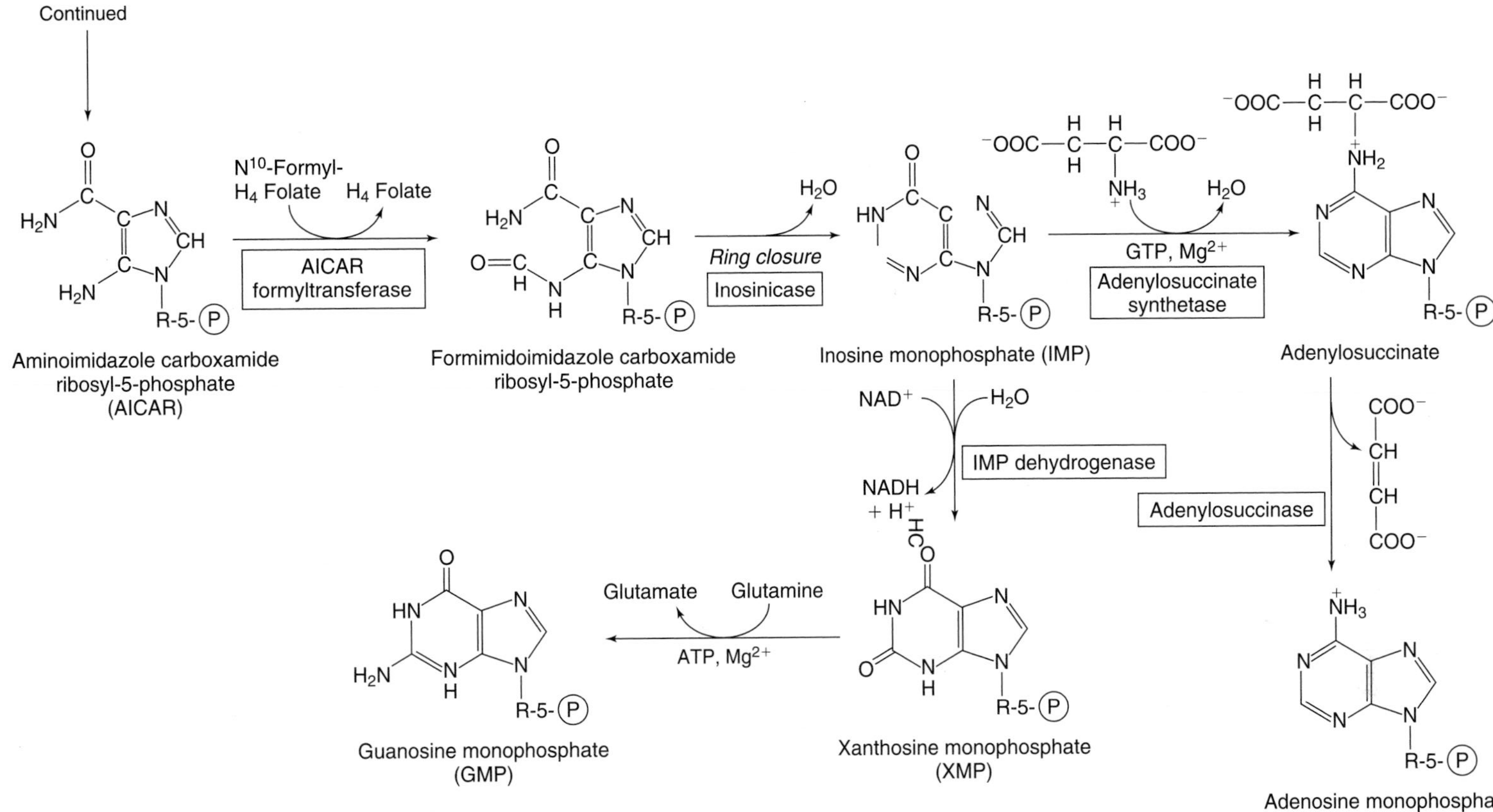

Figure 14-14 Pathway of de novo purine nucleotide biosynthesis from ribose 5-phosphate, ATP, glycine, glutamine amide groups, aspartate amino group, and one-carbon units from the folate coenzyme system. *R-5-Ⓟ*, Ribosyl-5-phosphate; *PRPP*, 5-phosphoribosyl-1-pyrophosphate; P_i, inorganic phosphate; PP_i, inorganic pyrophosphate.

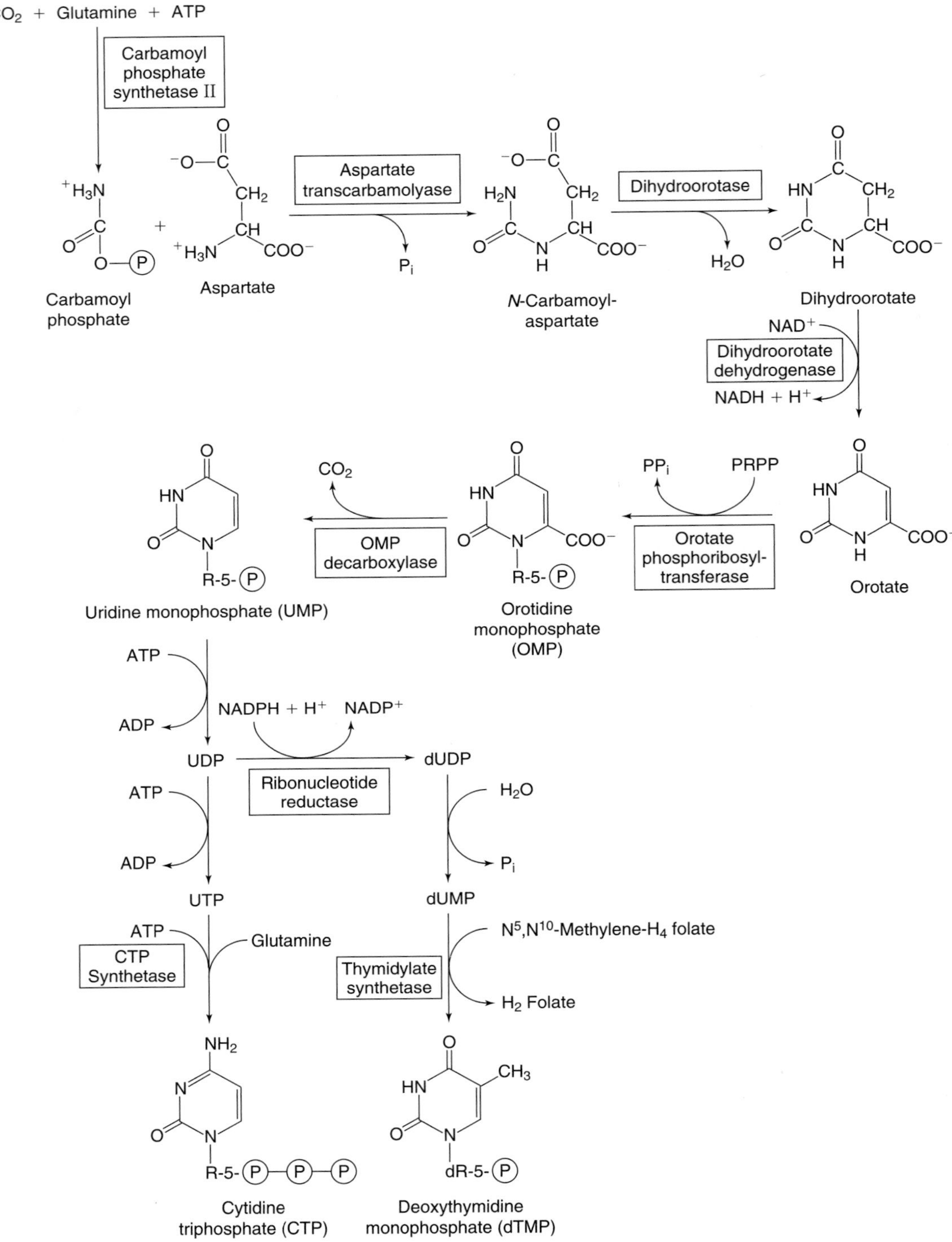

Figure 14-15 Pathway of de novo synthesis of pyrimidine nucleotides from CO_2, ATP, glutamine amide groups, aspartate, ribose phosphate, and one-carbon units from the folate coenzyme system. *R-5-(P)*, Ribosyl-5-phosphate; *dRP*, deoxyribosyl-5-phosphate; *PRPP*, 5-phosphoribosyl-1-pyrophosphate; P_i, inorganic phosphate; PP_i, inorganic pyrophosphate.

to cytidine triphosphate (CTP) requires donation of an additional amide nitrogen from glutamine. Conversion of deoxyuridine monophosphate (dUMP) to deoxythymidine monophosphate (dTMP) requires donation of a methyl group from the folate coenzyme system; again, this 1-carbon fragment likely originates from serine or another amino acid.

Other Processes That Require Glutamate or Glutamine

In the central nervous system, glutamate is an important excitatory neurotransmitter, and it also serves as the precursor for γ-aminobutyric acid (GABA), an important inhibitory neurotransmitter. The conversion of glutamate to γ-aminobutyrate is catalyzed by glutamate decarboxylase, which releases the α-carboxyl group as CO_2, as shown in Figure 14-16. GABA is removed by transamination with α-ketoglutarate to yield glutamate and succinate semialdehyde; this is then oxidized to succinate, which can be used to regenerate α-ketoglutarate via citric acid cycle enzymes. The cycling of α-ketoglutarate to glutamate to GABA to

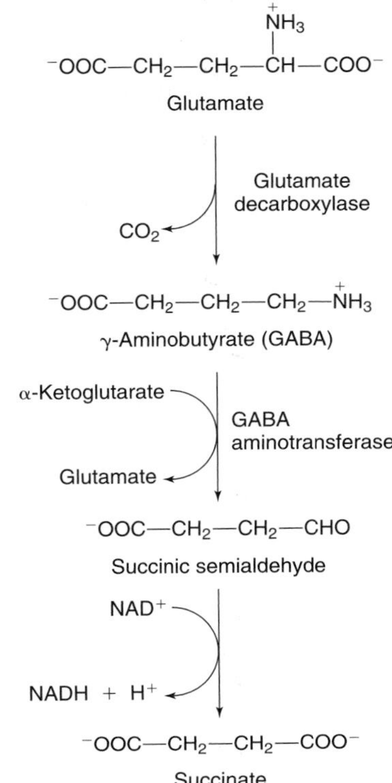

Figure 14-16 Synthesis and degradation of γ-aminobutyric acid (GABA).

Nutrition Insight

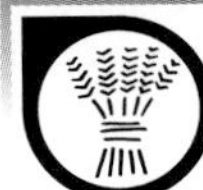

Neurotransmitters

The nervous system uses many biogenic amines and neuropeptides as neurotransmitters. The biogenic amines include the amino acids glutamate and glycine, as well as many decarboxylation products or derivatives of amino acids such as GABA (γ-aminobutyric acid), serotonin, catecholamines, and histamine.

Glycine and GABA are the major neuroinhibitory peptides in the central nervous system. Glycine acts predominantly in the spinal cord and brainstem, and GABA acts predominantly in all other parts of the brain. The receptors for glycine and GABA are ligand-gated channels that are selectively permeable to Cl^-. When these channels are open, the membrane potential becomes more negative (hyperpolarized) rather than depolarized (as occurs when excitatory cation channels are opened). A neuron inhibited by hyperpolarization requires a more intense depolarization than is otherwise required to trigger an action potential. In the brain cortex, glycine acts as an excitatory agonist of the *N*-methyl-D-aspartate (NMDA)–type of glutamate receptor–channel complex.

Nonketotic hyperglycinemia is an inborn error caused by a biochemical defect in one of the components of the glycine cleavage system complex that results in the accumulation of large quantities of glycine in all body tissues. Most individuals born with nonketotic hyperglycinemia show severe neurological abnormalities, including lethargy, hypotonia and myoclonic jerks, and apnea, often progressing to coma and death. Those who regain spontaneous respiration develop intractable seizures and profound mental retardation. It is thought that the apnea and hiccupping seen early in the course of the disease is the result of the neuroinhibitory effects of glycine in the spinal cord and brainstem. The intractable seizures and brain damage observed in individuals with nonketotic hyperglycinemia may be related to excessive stimulation of excitatory NMDA-glutamate receptors.

succinate and back to α-ketoglutarate is called the GABA shunt. Nerve terminals and neurons also may use glutamine for synthesis of glutamate (and hence GABA) because neurons have high glutaminase activity. Some of the glutamate and GABA released by neurons is taken up by glial cells, which have high glutamine synthetase activity, and is used in the resynthesis of glutamine.

Glutamate is part of the tripeptide glutathione, in which its γ-carboxyl group is in peptide linkage to the α-amino group of cysteine. (Glutathione synthesis is covered in the discussion of sulfur amino acids in this chapter.) Glutamate forms a similar linkage with other glutamate residues to form the polyglutamate chain that is added to folate coenzymes in cells (see Chapter 25).

Glutamine is the donor of nitrogen for synthesis of amino sugars such as glucosamine 6-phosphate (formed from fructose 6-phosphate and glutamine). Glucosamine is further metabolized to synthesize *N*-acetylglucosamine and sialic acids. Other amino sugars include galactosamine and *N*-acetylgalactosamine. Amino sugars are found in both glycoproteins and proteoglycans. The transfer of glutamine amido nitrogen is catalyzed by a family of eight amidotransferases, all of which possess a conserved active site sequence.

Asparagine

In contrast to the major role played by glutamine, asparagine does not widely participate in the transfer of nitrogen among compounds. As with many other amino acid residues, asparagine residues in proteins may undergo posttranslational modifications. Asparagine residues undergo deamidation and intra-chain bond rearrangements to form isoaspartate residues, which may play a useful function in some proteins. Asparagine residues also undergo hydroxylation, and hydroxyasparagine formation is involved in oxidative modification of hypoxia-inducible factor-α and the posttranslational modification of vitamin K–dependent protein S. In some glycoproteins, the oligosaccharide unit is attached to the side chain of an asparagine residue in the protein by an *N*-glycosidic linkage with the carboxamide group. This linkage is formed by transfer of the oligosaccharide chain from dolichol pyrophosphate. (See Chapter 5 for a discussion of posttranslational modification of amino acid residues and Chapters 4 and 12 for a discussion of glycoproteins.)

PROLINE AND ARGININE

Proline and Arginine Synthesis and Degradation: Interconversion of Proline and Arginine With Glutamate, Ornithine, and Citrulline

Glutamate and ornithine are key intermediates in the metabolism of proline and arginine, because all these amino acids share the same 5-carbon skeleton. The dispensability of proline and arginine (Carey et al., 1987) is related to the body's ability to synthesize these two amino acids from glutamate or α-ketoglutarate and amino groups (Cynober et al., 1995; Rabier and Kamoun, 1995). These interrelationships are illustrated in Figure 14-17. The reactions shown are intended to illustrate whole body metabolism of these amino acids and not metabolism within any single tissue. Of particular importance for arginine and proline synthesis are ornithine carbamoyltransferase, carbamoyl phosphate synthetase I, and *N*-acetylglutamate synthetase, which are expressed in both liver and small intestine, and pyrroline 5-carboxylate synthase, which is abundant only in small intestine. The synthesis of both arginine and proline from glutamate depends on the presence of an adequate level of pyrroline 5-carboxylate synthase (the enzyme that catalyzes the step that allows the glutamate carbon and nitrogen to enter the proline/ornithine/citrulline/arginine pool) in the small intestine. Two siblings with pyrroline 5-carboxylate synthase deficiency have recently been described. These children had low levels of plasma ornithine, citrulline, arginine, and proline and mild hyperammonemia; clinical symptoms included neurodegeneration with peripheral neuropathy, cataracts, and connective tissue manifestations (Baumgartner et al., 2005). Hence, the small intestine plays a critical role in the synthesis of both arginine and proline (or their precursors, citrulline and ornithine) from glutamate or glutamine.

In adults, metabolism of glutamate and glutamine within small intestinal cells (enterocytes)

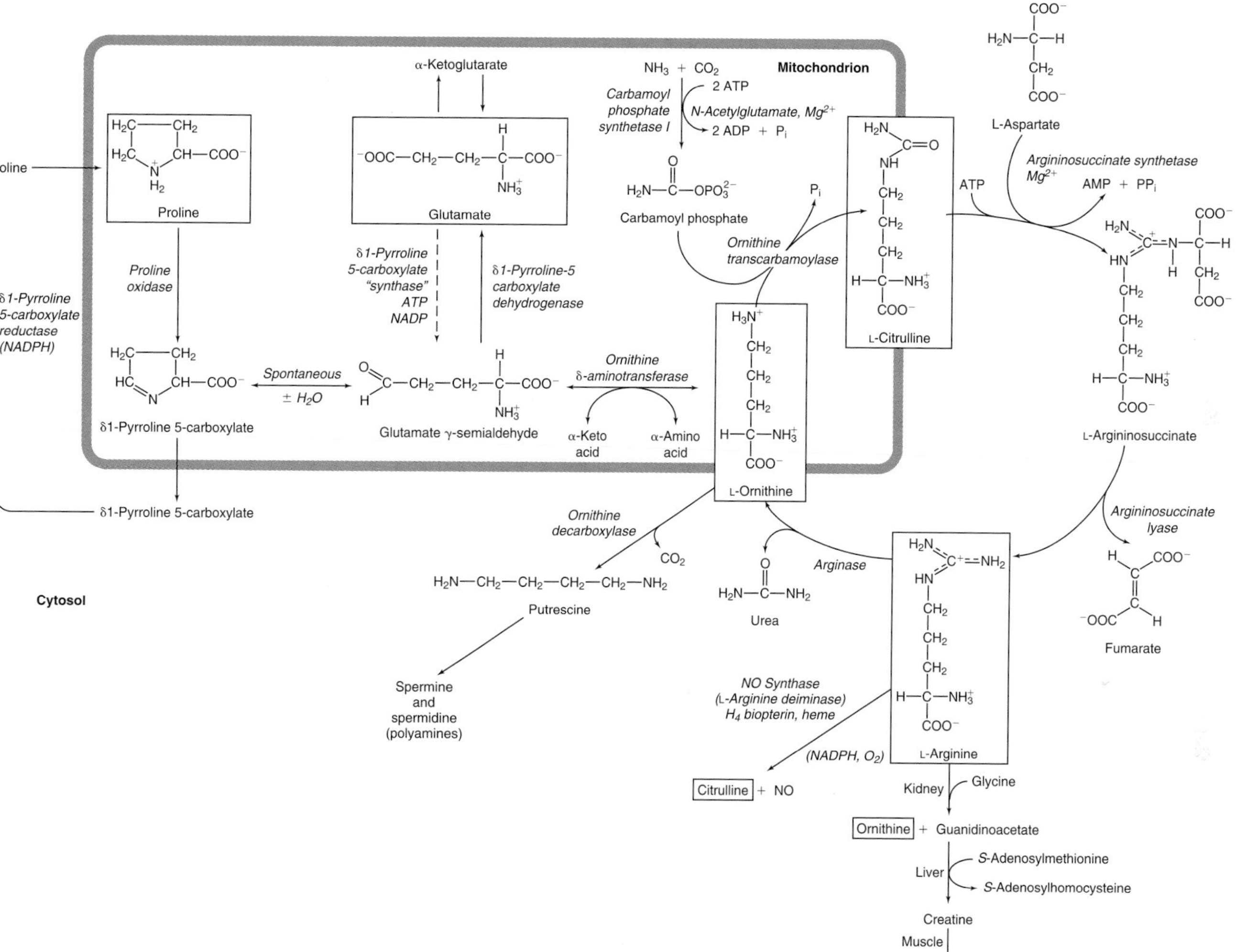

Figure 14-17 Reactions involved in the metabolism of arginine and proline, illustrating the interconversion of the 5-carbon skeletons and α-amino group of glutamate, ornithine, citrulline, arginine, and proline.

results in the formation and release of proline and citrulline and lesser amounts of arginine and ornithine. These amino acids are released into the portal circulation and provide arginine and proline or their precursors to various tissues. Ornithine is readily used for proline synthesis through ornithine aminotransferase and pyrroline 5-carboxylate reductase activities; the liver and intestine probably are important sites of proline synthesis. Plasma citrulline is not actively taken up from the circulation by the liver, but rather passes through to be removed by other tissues, especially by the kidney. The kidney has relatively high levels of argininosuccinate synthetase and argininosuccinate lyase, which allows the kidney to convert citrulline to arginine for use by peripheral tissues. Although the liver has an active urea cycle, it cannot use glutamate to produce ornithine/citrulline/arginine or proline. Extensive hydrolysis of arginine to ornithine occurs in liver, but the ornithine is recycled back to citrulline and arginine via the urea cycle.

The rate of arginine synthesis in the adult has been estimated to be about 25 mmoles/day (Castillo et al., 1994), and arginine synthesis seemed adequate to meet arginine requirements of adults who consumed an arginine-devoid diet for several days (Carey et al., 1987). In adult subjects, the rate of de novo synthesis of arginine did not change in response to changes in arginine intake or need, but the rate of arginine catabolism (formation and oxidation of ornithine) was diminished in subjects with low arginine intakes; arginine catabolism rather than arginine synthesis seems to be regulated to conserve arginine when arginine availability is low (Beaumier et al., 1995).

The pre-weanling pig, which is often used as a model for human infants, has a low rate of intestinal proline and arginine synthesis due to low intestinal pyrroline 5-carboxylate synthase activity, which limits the formation of citrulline/arginine/ornithine or proline from glutamate carbons in enterocytes (Wu et al., 2004). An arginine requirement (despite an adequate supply of dietary proline) can be demonstrated when intestinal synthesis of citrulline is limited or blocked, but it has been difficult in practice to demonstrate a requirement for proline (when arginine supply is adequate) even in pigs that have undergone massive resection of the small intestine. Apparently, the rate of arginine catabolism in the body is sufficiently high to allow ornithine to be used for proline synthesis, whereas use of proline for arginine synthesis does not occur at an adequate rate.

Conditions that result in a decreased capacity for synthesis (premature birth of an infant or intravenous feeding) or increased demand (tissue injury and repair) for arginine and proline may result in a need for dietary arginine. Because of the role of urea cycle enzymes in arginine synthesis, individuals with inborn errors of the urea cycle (other than a lack of arginase) require arginine in the diet.

Use of the Guanidinium Group of Arginine in the Synthesis of Creatine, Nitric Oxide, and Urea

The guanidinium group of arginine is crucial for synthesis of urea, nitric oxide, and creatine (Grillo and Colombatto, 2004; Morris, 2004; Cynober et al., 1995; Rabier and Kamoun, 1995). In the liver, which has a complete urea cycle, arginine is formed from ornithine, carbamoyl phosphate, and the amino group of aspartate. The terminal guanidinium group of arginine is cleaved in the final step of the urea cycle to release the amidino portion of the guanidinium group as urea and to replenish the ornithine used as the starting substrate. This cyclic process consumes nitrogen and bicarbonate but does not result in any net synthesis of arginine. In the urea cycle, urea essentially is synthesized by forming and cleaving the amidino portion of the guanidinium group of arginine.

Some of the arginine made in the kidney is used for synthesis of guanidinoacetate, which then goes to the liver to be used for creatine synthesis. The amidino group of arginine is transferred to glycine to form guanidinoacetate, and the 5-carbon skeleton of arginine is released as ornithine; this reaction is catalyzed by a transamidinase. Arginine is also the substrate for nitric oxide synthase, which forms nitric oxide (NO) and citrulline. Nitric oxide is an effector molecule that is produced by cells of the immune system, including macrophages, which use it for cytotoxicity, and endothelial

Clinical Correlation

Role of Extrahepatic Tissues in Arginine Synthesis

The urea cycle enzymes are required to prevent the accumulation of toxic nitrogenous compounds and for the de novo synthesis of arginine. Genetic defects that result in abnormal synthesis of carbamoyl phosphate synthetase I, ornithine transcarbamoylase, argininosuccinate synthetase, and argininosuccinate lyase are characterized by the accumulation of ammonia and glutamine.

Rabier and colleagues (1991) reported their experience with two patients with urea cycle defects. One patient was a girl who presented at 18 months of age with hyperammonemic coma. She had high urinary orotate levels, and a diagnosis of ornithine transcarbamoylase deficiency was made following liver biopsy. The second patient was a boy who developed hyperammonemia on the third day after birth. He had a high plasma concentration of citrulline, and a diagnosis of argininosuccinate synthetase deficiency was confirmed by enzyme assay on liver biopsy. Both patients were placed on a protein-restricted diet supplemented with arginine and sodium benzoate.

Both patients subsequently underwent orthotopic liver transplantation because of recurrent ammonia intoxication; liver transplantation was done at 6 years of age for the girl and 3 years of age for the boy. Following liver transplantation, both patients were placed on diets with 50 g of protein per day through normal meals. Liver transplantation was effective in normalizing plasma ammonia concentration in both patients, and it reduced the urinary excretion of orotate in the female patient. However, plasma citrulline and arginine concentrations did not return to normal values. In the patient with ornithine transcarbamoylase deficiency, citrulline remained significantly lower than control values. In the patient with argininosuccinate synthetase deficiency, plasma citrulline was decreased compared with values observed before transplantation but was still higher than control values. Both patients had low plasma arginine concentrations before the liver transplantation despite arginine supplementation, and their plasma arginine concentrations remained low, compared with control levels, after transplantation.

Thinking Critically

1. Why did citrulline and arginine levels remain low after liver transplantation? What is the role of extrahepatic tissues in arginine synthesis?
2. What was the purpose of the conventional diet/supplement therapies used prior to liver transplantation? What specific dietary recommendations would you have made for these patients who had undergone successful liver transplantation?
3. In total parenteral (intravenous) nutrition, the gut is bypassed in supplying nutrients. What effect might this have on the synthesis of arginine and proline from precursor glutamate?

cells, which produce it as a vasodilator of smooth muscle in blood vessels. Two general types of NO synthase have been identified: a calcium-dependent form found in most tissues including endothelial cells and neurons, and a calcium-independent inducible form found in cells that are stimulated by inflammatory cytokines (e.g., macrophages). Analogs of arginine such as *N*-monomethyl arginine are effective inhibitors of nitric acid synthase and can be used to lower NO production.

Although the amidino portion of arginine's guanidinium group is used for urea synthesis, creatine synthesis, and NO synthesis, none of these processes consumes the 5-carbon skeleton of arginine. The citrulline or ornithine released by arginine guanidinium group metabolism can be recycled back to arginine or, alternatively, used for proline synthesis or catabolized to α-ketoglutarate.

Other Requirements for Arginine and Proline

In mammalian brain, arginine decarboxylase brings about decarboxylation of arginine to agmatine, which may, like other bioactive amines, serve as a neurotransmitter or neuromodulator (Satriano, 2003, 2004).

The 5-carbon skeleton of arginine or proline (as ornithine) is substrate for polyamine synthesis (Pegg et al., 1995; Cynober et al., 1995). Arginase is present in many extrahepatic tissues, where it can function to produce the ornithine needed for polyamine synthesis. The major polyamines include putrescine and derivatives of putrescine, spermine, and spermidine, which are formed by transfer of one or two aminopropyl groups from decarboxylated *S*-adenosylmethionine to the 5-carbon skeleton of putrescine. These compounds are found in all tissues and appear to play important roles in cell growth and division.

Additional dietary arginine may be beneficial in times of tissue injury and repair because arginine is required for synthesis of NO (an effector molecule produced in response to cytokines/inflammation), polyamines (as mediators of cell growth/tissue repair), and proline (needed for collagen synthesis/fibrogenesis). In this context, dietary arginine might be considered as a conditionally indispensable amino acid in states of tissue injury and repair.

Catabolism of Proline and Arginine via Conversion to α-Ketoglutarate

As shown in Figure 14-17, the 5-carbon skeletons of proline and ornithine and the 5-carbon portions of arginine and citrulline are degraded mainly via glutamate and α-ketoglutarate. Thus, the ultimate fate of the α-amino nitrogen of these amino acids depends largely on the fate of glutamate. The 5-carbon portion of arginine is released as citrulline or ornithine in the synthesis of urea, NO, and creatine, allowing salvage of the carbon skeleton and some of the nitrogen atoms. Some loss of 5-carbon skeleton and α-amino nitrogen occurs via the conversion of ornithine to putrescine and other polyamines.

GLYCINE AND SERINE

Glycine Degradation by the Glycine Cleavage System

Glycine and serine play very important roles in nitrogen homeostasis and in 1-carbon metabolism, as illustrated in Figure 14-18. Glycine is degraded by a complex enzyme system, the glycine cleavage system. In mammals, the expression of this enzyme system is restricted to liver, kidney, and brain astrocytes; it is located on the inner mitochondrial membrane of these cells. Primarily it operates to degrade glycine and not to synthesize it. The overall reaction mechanism consists of a pyridoxal 5′-phosphate–dependent glycine decarboxylation, followed by transfer of the aminomethyl group to a lipoyl-aminomethyltransferase and finally to an N^5,N^{10}-methylenetetrahydrofolate–synthesizing protein. The overall products are CO_2, ammonia, and N^5,N^{10}-methylenetetrahydrofolate. (NAD^+ is reduced to NADH + H^+ in order to oxidize the dihydrolipoyl-dehydrogenase component of the system; this enzyme is the same as the lipoyl-dehydrogenase that is present in the α-keto acid dehydrogenase complexes discussed in Chapters 12 and 24.) The importance of the glycine cleavage system in humans is well established due to inborn errors of metabolism that result in absent or very low glycine cleavage system activity in the tissues that normally express this activity. These defects give rise to nonketotic hyperglycinemia, a condition in which glycine accumulates in body fluids. In rats, the activity of the glycine cleavage system in liver is stimulated rapidly by high protein intakes, by glucagon administration, or by Ca^{2+} (dependent on presence of inorganic phosphate); the activity of the system is increased in the kidneys of rats with metabolic acidosis, which is associated with net ammonia production from glycine (Ewart et al., 1992; Lowry et al., 1985).

Other minor pathways of glycine catabolism have been described, including the deamination and transamination pathways that lead to glyoxylate production. These enzymes seem to be of little physiological importance in glycine catabolism in mammals. In vitamin B_6–deficient animals, increased excretion of oxalate in the urine is thought to be caused by decreased serine hydroxymethyltransferase (see next section) or decreased glycine cleavage system activity that results in increased metabolism of glycine by deamination to oxalate.

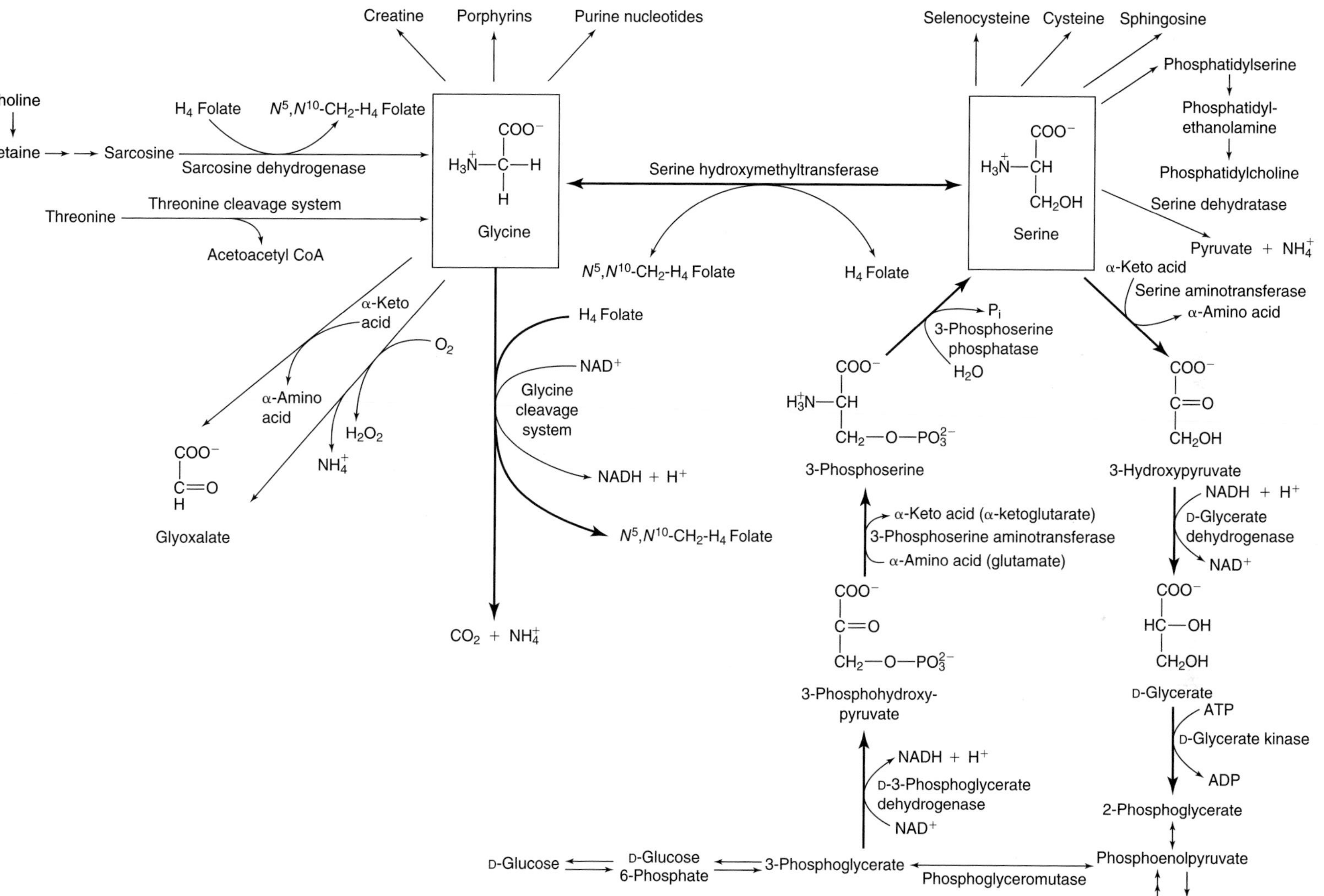

Figure 14-18 Reactions of glycine and serine metabolism. Major pathways of glycine and serine metabolism are indicated by the *heavy lines.*

Interconversion of Glycine and Serine via Serine Hydroxymethyltransferase

Serine and glycine are freely interconvertible via the enzyme serine hydroxymethyltransferase. Serine hydroxymethyltransferase is a pyridoxal 5′-phosphate–dependent enzyme; it uses tetrahydrofolate as a substrate and transfers the C-3 of serine, which is at the oxidation level of formaldehyde, to the tetrahydrofolate acceptor, where it bridges the nitrogen atoms at positions 5 and 10. From this reaction, serine serves as the major donor of 1-carbon units to the folate coenzyme system. The product, N^5,N^{10}-methylenetetrahydrofolate, can transfer the 1-carbon element back to glycine. Hence, this enzyme allows synthesis of either serine or glycine, provided that the other amino acid is available, or this reaction can permit serine catabolism via conversion to glycine with further catabolism of glycine. Although glycine contains only two carbon atoms, it can be considered glucogenic because of its ability to be converted to serine and hence to glucose.

Both mitochondrial and cytosolic forms of serine hydroxymethyltransferase are found in tissues. The mitochondrial serine hydroxymethyltransferase is distributed widely in tissues and seems to be involved mainly in serine catabolism to glycine plus formate (via N^5,N^{10}-methylenetetrahydrofolate). Serine degradation is the major route of glycine synthesis. A cytosolic form of serine hydroxymethyltransferase is abundant only in liver and kidney of humans, with some activity also being found in skeletal muscle (Girgis et al., 1998). The cytosolic serine hydroxymethyltransferase seems to be involved in net synthesis of serine from glycine in these tissues.

The combined action of the glycine cleavage system and serine hydroxymethyltransferase allows conversion of two molecules of glycine to one molecule each of serine, ammonia, and CO_2 (Cowan et al., 1996). This allows the kidney to use glycine as a contributor to net ammoniagenesis (by taking up glycine, releasing serine, and excreting ammonium). Glycine contributes approximately 5% of the urinary ammonium, much less than is contributed by glutamine. In addition, the combined action of glycine cleavage and serine hydroxymethyltransferase allows glycine to potentially supply all three carbons (via serine and hydroxypyruvate) for gluconeogenesis in liver. Glycine seems to play an important role in nitrogen–carbon transfer among organs and in renal ammoniagenesis. Glycine, in addition to alanine and glutamine, is released by muscle during starvation, and the renal uptake of glycine is increased in prolonged starvation.

Serine Synthesis From Glycolytic Intermediates

In addition to being synthesized from glycine via serine hydroxymethyltransferase, serine can be synthesized from the glycolytic intermediate 3-phosphoglycerate via an NAD^+-linked dehydrogenase that converts this intermediate to 3-phosphohydroxypyruvate. The latter then undergoes transamination with glutamate to 3-phosphoserine, followed by the irreversible removal of the phosphate by a phosphatase. This cytosolic pathway from 3-phosphoglycerate is distributed widely and is considered the major pathway of serine synthesis de novo in mammals. Once serine is formed from glycolytic intermediates, it can be converted to glycine via serine hydroxymethyltransferase, permitting de novo synthesis of glycine as well.

Other Routes of Glycine Synthesis

A limited amount of glycine can be synthesized from catabolism of threonine by the threonine cleavage complex (Darling et al., 1997). Glycine also can be produced from metabolism of betaine (or its precursor, choline) by successive removal of the methyl groups from the amine group of betaine. This leads to sequential formation of dimethylglycine, monomethylglycine (sarcosine), and, ultimately, glycine, via transfer of the first methyl group to homocysteine to form methionine and donation of the second and third methyl groups to the folate coenzyme system to form N^5,N^{10}-methylenetetrahydrofolate. Direct methylation of glycine also occurs; this is catalyzed by glycine methyltransferase, which transfers the methyl group from *S*-adenosylmethionine to glycine to form sarcosine. Sarcosine formation by methylation of glycine seems to be an important route for removal of excess methyl groups via the folate system, and, ultimately, for their release as CO_2; this glycine methyltransferase reaction plays an important role in the regulation of *S*-adenosylmethionine/*S*-adenosylhomocysteine ratios (see Fig. 14-21 and Chapter 25). The significance of the betaine/sarcosine pathway in glycine production/turnover depends on the dietary intake of choline or betaine and on the turnover of choline-containing phospholipids. Nevertheless, the major route of glycine synthesis is clearly the serine hydroxymethyltransferase reaction.

Other Pathways of Serine Degradation

As discussed previously, serine degradation can be accomplished by conversion of serine to glycine by serine hydroxymethyltransferase, followed by catabolism of glycine by the glycine cleavage system. Serine also can be degraded by other routes. Transamination of serine to yield 3-hydroxypyruvate is a major route of serine degradation in human liver; the serine:pyruvate/alanine aminotransferase is located in peroxisomes of human liver (Xue et al., 1999). The 3-hydroxypyruvate can be further converted to glycerate and phosphorylated to 2-phosphoglycerate, an intermediate in glycolysis and gluconeogenesis. In some species, serine (as well as threonine) is degraded by a cytosolic enzyme called serine (threonine) dehydratase, which increases markedly in liver of rats fed high-protein diets. Serine dehydratase catalyzes the deamination of serine to pyruvate plus ammonia. The activity of serine dehydratase is reported to be low in human liver (Ogawa et al., 1989), and serine deamination to pyruvate seems unlikely to be quantitatively significant in human liver. The relative roles of various pathways of serine synthesis and degradation, however, remain to be clarified for human tissues.

Essential Roles of Glycine in the Synthesis of Nonprotein Compounds

Glycine is a substrate for synthesis of purine nucleotides, porphyrins, creatine, 1-carbon fragments for the folate coenzyme system, glutathione, and glycine-conjugated bile acids. The glycine cleavage system is involved in the donation of 1-carbon units to the folate coenzyme system, as shown in Figure 14-17. Glycine is incorporated (as an intact molecule) into purine nucleotides, as shown in Figure 14-13. Delta-aminolevulinate, a precursor of porphyrins, is synthesized from glycine and succinyl CoA with the α-carbon and the α-amino group of glycine retained in the porphobilinogen, but with the carboxyl carbon lost as CO_2. Some of the glycine nitrogen is lost when porphobilinogen is converted to porphyrinogen in the process of porphyrin/heme synthesis. Glycine is used by the kidney in the synthesis of guanidinoacetate, a precursor of creatine phosphate. Both the glycine carbons and nitrogen remain in creatine phosphate or its elimination product, creatinine.

Glycine is a major inhibitory neurotransmitter in the central nervous system. Glycine, along with glutamate and cysteine, is a component of the tripeptide glutathione, and glycine is released during glutathione turnover by γ-glutamyltranspeptidase and dipeptidases. Glycine is used to conjugate bile acids in the liver, and glycine-conjugated bile acids are secreted in the bile. Other compounds also can form glycine conjugates; the best-known example is the conjugation of glycine with benzoic acid to form hippuric acid, which is excreted in the urine. The conjugation of benzoic acid with glycine facilitates the excretion of nitrogen from the body (as glycine), and this is presumed to be the basis of its therapeutic effect in patients with hyperammonemia.

Essential Roles of Serine in the Synthesis of Nonprotein Compounds

Large amounts of D-serine have been found in mammalian brain, where it is formed by a pyridoxal-5′-phosphate–dependent serine racemase and acts as an endogenous coagonist of NMDA receptors (De Miranda et al., 2000). Serine is a precursor for synthesis of 1-carbon fragments for the folate coenzyme system, for synthesis of phospholipids and sphingosine, and for synthesis of cysteine and selenocysteine. The 3-carbon of serine is the major source of 1-carbon fragments for the folate coenzyme system via the reaction catalyzed by serine hydroxymethyltransferase (see Fig. 14-18 and Chapter 25). This same reaction allows serine to be converted to glycine.

Serine is used in the production of phosphatidylserine, phosphatidylethanolamine, and phosphatidylcholine (see Chapter 16, Fig. 16-20). Thus serine serves as the precursor of choline. The details of the conversion are not well established, but phosphatidylserine undergoes decarboxylation to phosphatidylethanolamine, followed by transfer of three methyl groups from *S*-adenosylmethionine to form phosphatidylcholine. Because choline can be degraded to betaine, sarcosine, and glycine, this synthetic route provides another possible route of glycine synthesis from serine or from dietary choline or betaine. Serine, along with palmitoyl CoA, is used for the synthesis of the amino alcohol sphingosine, which is a component of ceramide and other sphingolipids (see Chapter 16, Fig. 16-22).

Serine is the precursor of the carbon chain of both cysteine and selenocysteine. The incorporation of the 3-carbon chain of serine into cysteine is accomplished enzymatically in the methionine transsulfuration pathway, by which the sulfur of methionine is transferred to serine to form cysteine (see Fig. 14-21). The utilization of the carbon chain of serine for synthesis of selenocysteine is accomplished in a very different manner. A limited number of proteins contains the modified amino acid selenocysteine in specific location(s). This amino acid is named selenocysteine because it has the structure of cysteine except that the sulfur is replaced by selenium. Unlike other modified amino acid residues found in proteins, selenocysteine is formed by cotranslational, rather than by posttranslational, modification of an amino acid residue. Serine esterified to a specific transfer RNA (tRNA) that contains an anticodon complementary to the stop codon UGA (uracil-guanine-adenine) is the substrate for selenocysteine synthesis. In certain messenger RNAs (mRNAs), this codon acts as a codon for selenocysteine rather than as a termination sequence. (See Chapter 39 for details of selenocysteine synthesis.) Proteins also may contain selenomethionine residues at random locations owing to incorporation of selenomethionine in place of methionine; this incorporation reflects dietary intake of selenomethionine and not its specific synthesis and incorporation.

THREONINE

Threonine Catabolism

Threonine is an indispensable amino acid for humans; its carbon skeleton cannot be synthesized in the body. The major pathway of threonine degradation in humans is uncertain. Threonine is catabolized in mammals by cytosolic threonine (serine) dehydratase or by a mitochondrial threonine cleavage complex, as shown in Figure 14-19.

Although threonine (serine) dehydratase does not seem to play a major role in serine catabolism in human liver, this cytosolic enzyme may play a significant role in threonine catabolism. Darling and colleagues (1997) conducted kinetic studies in humans that suggested threonine was metabolized predominantly to CO_2. They attributed threonine oxidation to the conversion of threonine to α-ketobutyrate plus ammonia (catalyzed by threonine dehydratase), with only a small proportion of threonine being converted to glycine (via the mitochondrial threonine cleavage complex). The α-ketobutyrate, which is formed from both threonine and methionine catabolism, is oxidatively decarboxylated to propionyl CoA by the action of the branched-chain keto acid dehydrogenase or pyruvate dehydrogenase complex (Paxton et al., 1986). Propionyl CoA can be converted to succinyl CoA, a glucogenic precursor, and further metabolized.

Studies in pigs have suggested that this species, which has low serine (threonine) dehydratase activity, converts threonine to glycine through the threonine cleavage complex in both liver and extrahepatic tissues (Ballevre et al., 1991). Studies involving liver mitochondria suggest that the coupled activities of threonine dehydrogenase and 2-amino-3-ketobutyrate CoA ligase act as a threonine cleavage complex, which converts threonine to glycine plus acetyl CoA in the presence of coenzyme A and NAD^+. However, when coenzyme A is limiting, threonine carbon may be released from the enzyme complex as

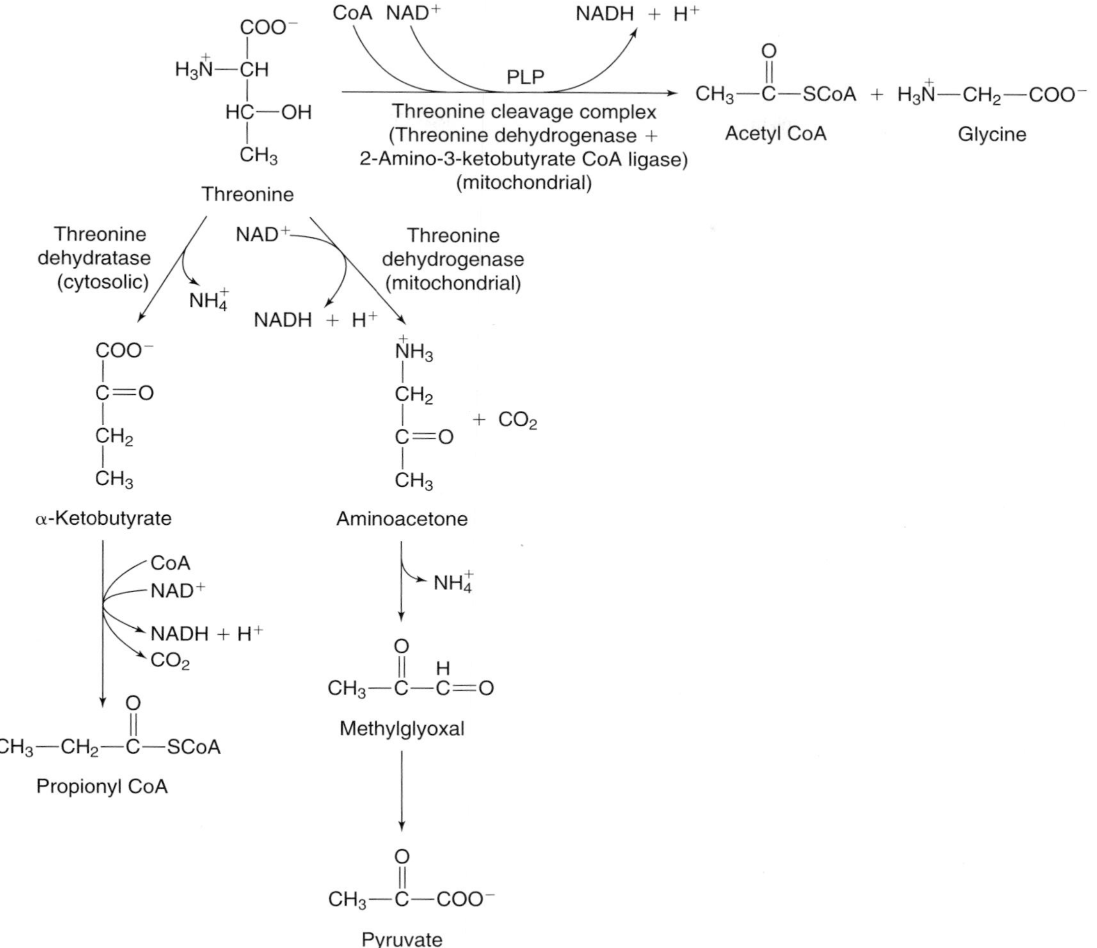

Figure 14-19 Catabolism of threonine in mammalian cells.

aminoacetone + CO_2 as a result of the threonine dehydrogenase activity. Bird and colleagues (1984) calculated that, at physiological concentrations of threonine and coenzyme A, at least 65% of threonine in intact rat liver mitochondria was metabolized to glycine and acetyl CoA. At higher threonine concentrations, more aminoacetone was formed (and excretion of aminoacetone in the urine increased); at lower threonine levels, more glycine was formed. Hence, mitochondrial threonine catabolism can give rise to either a glucogenic metabolite (aminoacetone) or to both a glucogenic (glycine) and a ketogenic metabolite (acetyl CoA) upon its degradation.

Aminoacetone can be converted to pyruvate by the reactions shown in Figure 14-19, and glycine can be converted to pyruvate via serine, as shown in Figure 14-18.

HISTIDINE

Essentiality of Histidine

Histidine is essential in infants, but it has been difficult to establish adult requirements. In long-term studies, histidine is essential for maintenance of nitrogen balance of adults (Cho et al., 1984). There is very little evidence of de novo histidine synthesis in humans, and no pathway for histidine synthesis in mammalian tissues has been described. The presence of histidine in dipeptides (carnosine and anserine), which are found in very high concentrations in human skeletal muscle and which can be degraded to release histidine, and the ability of the body to selectively degrade hemoglobin, a histidine-rich protein, may allow the body to maintain a supply of histidine in the face of a deficiency. Adults fed a histidine-free diet for 48 days experienced a decline in whole-body protein turnover and diminished levels of plasma albumin, transferrin, and hemoglobin (Kriengsinyos et al., 2002).

Histidine Catabolism

The first step in histidine degradation involves the conversion of histidine to urocanate with release of the α-amino group as ammonia; this step is catalyzed by histidine ammonia lyase, more commonly called histidase. Histidase activity is located only in the liver and in the surface layer (stratum corneum) of the skin. In the skin, the breakdown of histidine stops with the production of urocanic acid, which is an ultraviolet-absorbing compound that plays an important protective role. Urocanate is found in the sweat. The inborn error of metabolism called histidinemia, which is relatively benign, is due to a lack of histidase activity.

In the liver, the urocanate formed from histidine is further metabolized to ammonia (2 moles ammonia per mole of histidine), glutamate, and a 1-carbon fragment for the folate coenzyme system (Fig. 14-20). Additional steps convert the urocanate to *N*-formiminoglutamate (Figlu), which participates in the transfer of the formimino group, a 1-carbon fragment bearing a nitrogen atom, to the N^5 of tetrahydrofolate, with release of glutamate. Hence, the α-amino group of histidine is lost, as ammonia, the 2-carbon of the imidazole ring, is donated to the folate coenzyme system, and the adjacent imidazole nitrogen is lost as ammonia in conversion of N^5-formiminotetrahydrofolate to N^{10}-formyltetrahydrofolate; the other carbons and the second ring nitrogen are converted to glutamate. The histidine catabolic pathway in liver is regulated at the level of histidase; transcription of the hepatic histidase gene is induced by glucagon, glucocorticoids, and estrogens. Hepatic histidase activity also increases in the livers of animals fed high levels of high-quality protein, but not histidine alone; the type and amount of protein consumed alter

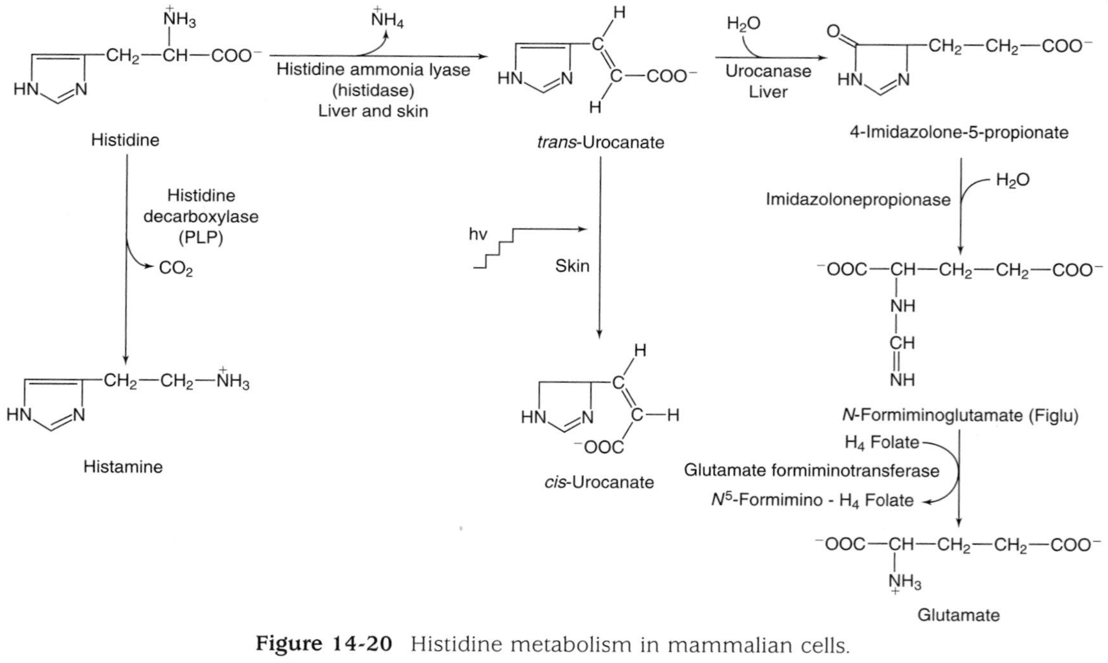

Figure 14-20 Histidine metabolism in mammalian cells.

histidase gene expression through changes in the plasma glucagon level (Tovar et al., 2002; Torres et al., 1998).

Although the liver possesses high histidine aminotransferase activity, this does not appear to be of much physiological importance under normal conditions. However, individuals with a histidase deficiency, who have decreased or blocked urocanate formation, do transaminate histidine to imidazolepyruvate, and this keto acid and its metabolites (imidazoleacetate and imidazolelactate) are excreted in their urine (Lam et al., 1996).

Synthesis of Nonprotein Compounds From Histidine

The decarboxylation of histidine to the corresponding amine, histamine, occurs in various organs. Histamine synthesis is catalyzed by a specific histidine decarboxylase, as shown in Figure 14-20. In most tissues, histamine is located predominantly in mast cells. Most tissues contain type H_1-histamine receptors, and histamine acts as a paracrine agent in the physiological control of various functions. In the stomach, histamine acts on type H_2-receptors to stimulate the secretion of gastric acid by the parietal cells. H_2-receptor antagonists are used to treat gastric and duodenal ulcers. Histamine-containing neurons are present in the hypothalamus, and histamine acts as a neurotransmitter in histaminergic pathways. In addition, histamine release is part of immune cell function. Binding of antigen to immunoglobulin E (IgE) molecules bound to mast cells stimulates the release of granules that contain histamine. Excess reaction to histamine causes the symptoms of asthma and various allergic reactions. Antihistamine medications are H_1-receptor blockers; they minimize the symptoms caused by histamine release. Histamine is inactivated by deamination to imidazoleacetate or by methylation followed by oxidation by monoamine oxidase.

Two unusual peptides that contain histidine, carnosine and homocarnosine, are synthesized in human tissues and may be present at concentrations near 1 mmol/g in skeletal and cardiac muscle and in central nervous tissues (MacFarlane et al., 1991). Carnosine (β-alanyl-L-histidine) is synthesized in muscle from histidine and β-alanine (a catabolite of cytosine as well as of β-alanylpeptides). Homocarnosine (γ-aminobutyryl-L-histidine) is synthesized in brain from histidine and GABA or putrescine (an ornithine catabolite that serves as the donor of the GABA moiety). Both are synthesized by carnosine synthetase and degraded by plasma or brain carnosinase. The roles of these peptides are not well established, although a number of protective roles have been proposed. Carnosine may play a functional role in the skeletal muscle and heart, and homocarnosine could be an alternate route of GABA synthesis in brain. Two other histidine-containing peptides are present in foods and are concentrated by some tissues; these are ergothioneine (2′-thiolhistidine betaine), which accumulates in red blood cells, and anserine (β-alanyl-L-l-methylhistidine), which accumulates in skeletal muscle.

METHIONINE AND CYSTEINE

Methionine Metabolism: Transmethylation and Transsulfuration

Methionine is metabolized almost entirely via the transmethylation/transsulfuration pathway, as shown in Figure 14-21 (Stipanuk, 2004, 1986). Liver is the most active site of methionine metabolism. Methionine is activated by synthesis of *S*-adenosylmethionine, which converts the sulfur of methionine (a thioether) to a positively charged sulfonium atom. *S*-Adenosylmethionine serves as the methyl donor for numerous methyltransferases, which transfer the methyl group from *S*-adenosylmethionine to acceptor substrates. *S*-Adenosylmethionine is the direct donor of methyl groups for almost all transmethylation reactions in the body. The *S*-adenosylhomocysteine that is generated by transfer of the methyl group subsequently is hydrolyzed to release homocysteine and adenosine. These reactions are collectively referred to as the methionine transmethylation pathway.

Homocysteine may be remethylated to methionine by a widespread N^5-methyltetrahydrofolate:homocysteine methyltransferase (methionine synthase) or by a liver-specific betaine:homocysteine methyltransferase. The remethylation of homocysteine allows the body

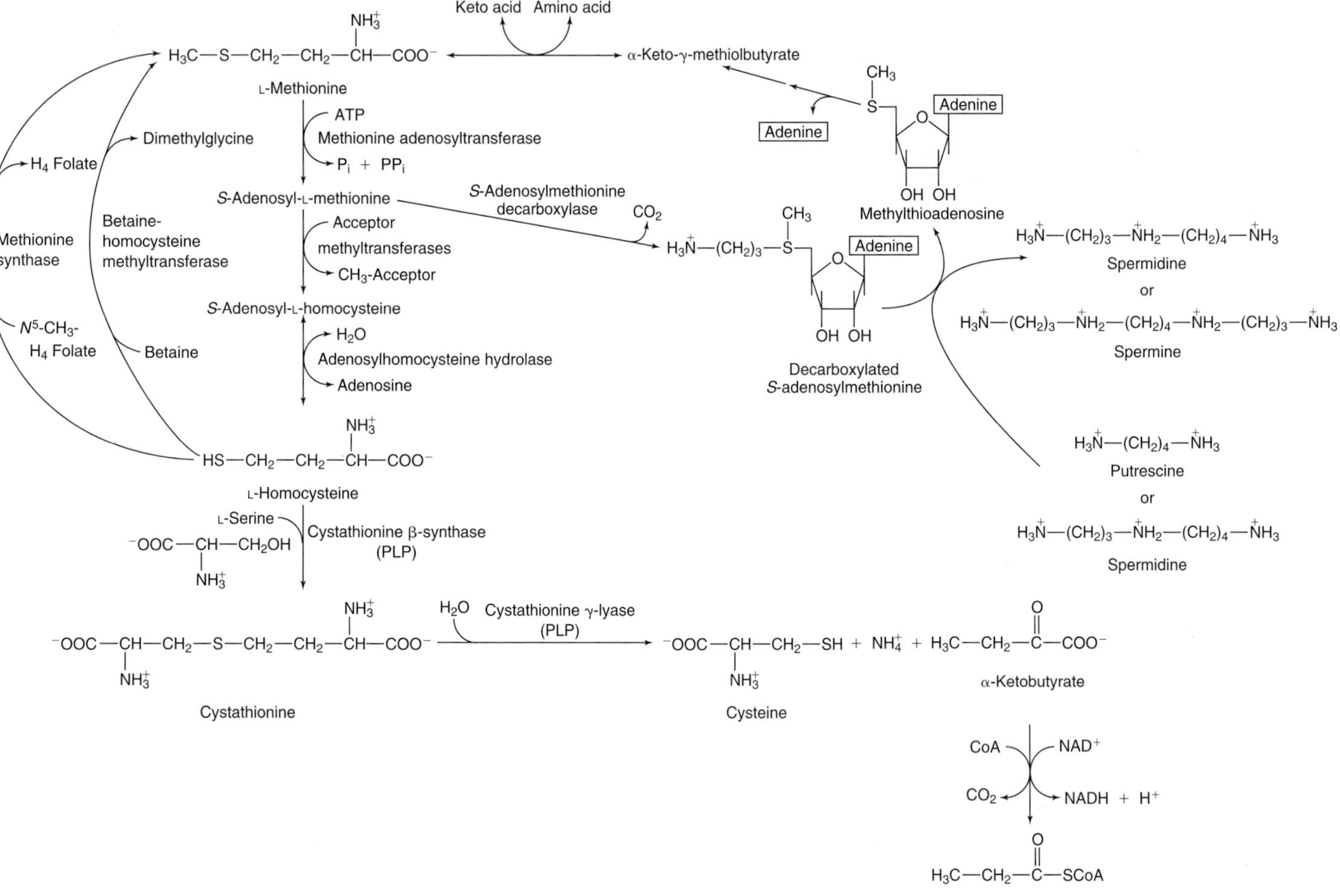

Figure 14-21 Pathways of methionine transmethylation, transsulfuration, and polyamine synthesis. Note that the remethylation allows the body to use methyl groups from de novo synthesis in the folate coenzyme system or from choline/betaine for *S*-adenosylmethionine–dependent transmethylation reactions. The transsulfuration pathway is required for cysteine synthesis and for methionine catabolism. Polyamine synthesis transfers aminopropyl groups from decarboxylated *S*-adenosylmethionine to putrescine (formed from ornithine) with salvage of the methylthioribose moiety of *S*-adenosylmethionine for resynthesis of methionine.

to use methyl groups from choline (betaine) or from de novo synthesis from 1-carbon fragments via the folate coenzyme system for the numerous methylation reactions for which *S*-adenosylmethionine serves as the immediate methyl donor. In male subjects fed methionine-adequate diets, approximately 40% of the homocysteine formed per transmethylation cycle underwent remethylation to methionine (Storch et al., 1990). The extent of remethylation increased in subjects fed methionine-deficient diets.

Homocysteine that is not remethylated condenses with serine to form the thioether cystathionine, as shown in Figure 14-21. This step commits the methionine molecule to degradation via the transsulfuration pathway. Cystathionine is cleaved on the other side of the sulfur atom to release α-ketobutyrate and ammonia as products of the homocysteine moiety, and cysteine, which contains the sulfur from homocysteine and the carbon chain and nitrogen donated by serine. Therefore, transsulfuration allows cysteine to be synthesized from serine and the methionine sulfur atom and also accomplishes the process of methionine degradation. The carbon skeleton of methionine, α-ketobutyrate, is oxidatively decarboxylated to propionyl CoA, which enters the citric acid cycle at the level of succinyl CoA. Because transsulfuration permits methionine to serve as the precursor of cysteine sulfur, the sulfur amino acid requirement can be met either by methionine alone or by a mixture of methionine and cysteine. Studies in young men have indicated that approximately 50% of the total sulfur amino acid requirement can be supplied as cysteine (Storch et al., 1990).

A number of inborn errors of sulfur amino acid metabolism have served to verify the steps in the methionine metabolic pathway in humans. Inborn errors or vitamin deficiencies that limit the removal of homocysteine, either by remethylation to methionine or by transsulfuration, result in elevated levels of homocysteine in the blood and urine. A mildly elevated level of plasma homocysteine is considered a risk factor for vascular disease and neural tube defects (Guba et al., 1996; Robinson et al., 1994). In patients with inborn errors associated with homocystinuria, numerous abnormalities are observed, including premature thromboembolic and atherosclerotic disease and mental deficiencies. Treatment by restriction of methionine intake and supplementation with betaine has been found to lower the homocysteine level in these homocystinuric patients.

Methionine also can be degraded by transamination to its keto acid and further catabolism of that keto acid, but this does not appear to be a substantial route of methionine degradation in humans under normal conditions. Therefore, methionine degradation depends almost entirely on the transmethylation and transsulfuration pathways, with transfer of the methionine sulfur to cysteine.

Role of Methionine as the Donor of Aminopropyl Groups for Polyamine Synthesis

An alternative route of *S*-adenosylmethionine metabolism is polyamine synthesis (Pegg et al., 1995). This pathway involves the decarboxylation of *S*-adenosylmethionine and the transfer of the aminopropyl group from the decarboxylated *S*-adenosylmethionine (*S*-adenosylmethylthiopropylamine) to putrescine to form spermidine or to spermidine to form spermine (see Fig. 14-21). Polyamines are essential molecules that seem to be involved in cell division and cell growth. The byproduct of polyamine synthesis, methylthioadenosine, is efficiently salvaged with little loss of sulfur. The sulfur atom, methyl carbon, and ribose chain of methylthioadenosine all are reincorporated into methionine by a series of reactions in which α-keto-γ-methiolbutyrate (methionine keto acid) is formed and then transaminated to methionine in the final step.

Cysteine Catabolism to Pyruvate and Inorganic Sulfur to Taurine

Cysteine catabolism results in production of several essential compounds, including taurine, reduced inorganic sulfur, and sulfate or 3′-phosphoadenosine-5′-phosphosulfate (Stipanuk, 2004). Formation of these metabolites is accomplished by the cysteine catabolic pathways, as shown in Figure 14-22. Cysteine catabolism may occur by desulfuration of cysteine to yield pyruvate and reduced sulfur (often in the form of a persulfide such as thiocysteine or thiosulfate). Cysteine desulfuration can be catalyzed by the β-cleavage of cysteine (or cystine) by cystathionine γ-lyase or by transamination of cysteine to β-mercaptopyruvate followed by de- or transsulfuration by mercaptopyruvate sulfurtransferase (Stipanuk and Beck, 1982). Desulfuration is also catalyzed by cystathionine β-synthase, which can use cysteine in place of serine. Individuals with a rare inborn error of metabolism in which β-mercaptopyruvate sulfurtransferase is deficient excrete the mixed disulfide of cysteine and β-mercaptolactate, suggesting that transamination of cysteine to mercaptopyruvate occurs to some extent in humans. These patients excrete normal levels of urinary sulfate, indicating that overall cysteine catabolism is not impaired. The reduced sulfur may be used for synthesis of iron-sulfur proteins or other molecules that require a source of reduced sulfur or sulfide, or the reduced inorganic sulfur is further oxidized to thiosulfate (inner sulfur), sulfite, and, finally, sulfate. H_2S appears to act as a smooth muscle relaxant, and it is produced in the brain in response to neuronal excitation (Dominy and Stipanuk, 2004).

In the liver of animals that are fed high-protein or high-sulfur amino acid–containing diets, the major pathway of cysteine catabolism involves the oxidation of cysteine to cysteinesulfinate by cysteine dioxygenase. Cysteine dioxygenase is robustly regulated in response to dietary protein or sulfur amino acid intake via a cysteine-mediated inhibition of its polyubiquitination and, hence, degradation by the 26S proteasome (Stipanuk, 2004). Cysteinesulfinate may be decarboxylated to hypotaurine, which is subsequently oxidized to taurine, or cysteinesulfinate may be transaminated (with α-ketoglutarate) to the putative intermediate β-sulfinylpyruvate, which spontaneously decomposes to pyruvate and sulfite. Sulfite is further oxidized to sulfate by sulfite oxidase. In all pathways except that which results in taurine formation, the carbon chain of cysteine is released as pyruvate, the sulfur is released as inorganic sulfur (reduced or oxidized), and the amino group is released as ammonia or transferred to a keto acid acceptor. When taurine is the end product, only the carboxyl carbon of the cysteine is released, and the other three carbons as well as the nitrogen and sulfur atoms remain in the end product. Both sulfate and taurine are excreted in the urine, but sulfate normally accounts for more than 80% of the total sulfur excreted. The inorganic sulfate produced from methionine and cysteine sulfur largely accounts for the acidogenic potential of protein-containing diets (Bella and Stipanuk, 1995).

Inorganic sulfur and taurine are not necessarily essential dietary nutrients because they are provided via sulfur amino acid degradation. Nevertheless, both taurine and inorganic sulfur are essential nutrients for many nonhepatic cells that cannot synthesize these nutrients at adequate rates. Reduced sulfur is required for synthesis of iron–sulfur proteins and other compounds. The activated form of sulfate, 3′-phosphoadenosine-5′-phosphosulfate (PAPS), serves as the substrate for sulfation of a number of molecules. Many structural compounds are sulfated. In particular, proteoglycans contain oligosaccharide chains with many sulfated sugar residues. In addition, many compounds of both endogenous and exogenous origin are excreted as sulfo-esters; sulfo-esters of steroid hormones and of the drug acetaminophen are examples.

Taurine, like glycine, is used for conjugation of bile acids in the liver. (See Chapters 7 and 10 for the role of bile acids in digestion and absorption.) In addition, taurine seems to be essential for other physiological functions; studies with animal models, including primates, indicate that abnormalities in retinal and neurological development and function may occur when taurine is deficient (Huxtable, 1992). Taurine is present in high concentrations in human milk and is added to infant formulas in the United States.

Role of Cysteine in the Synthesis of Glutathione and Coenzyme A

A large amount of available cysteine is used for synthesis of the tripeptide γ-glutamylcysteinylglycine, as illustrated in Figure 14-22; this tripeptide is better known as glutathione. At sulfur amino acid intakes near the requirement, a large proportion of available cysteine is used

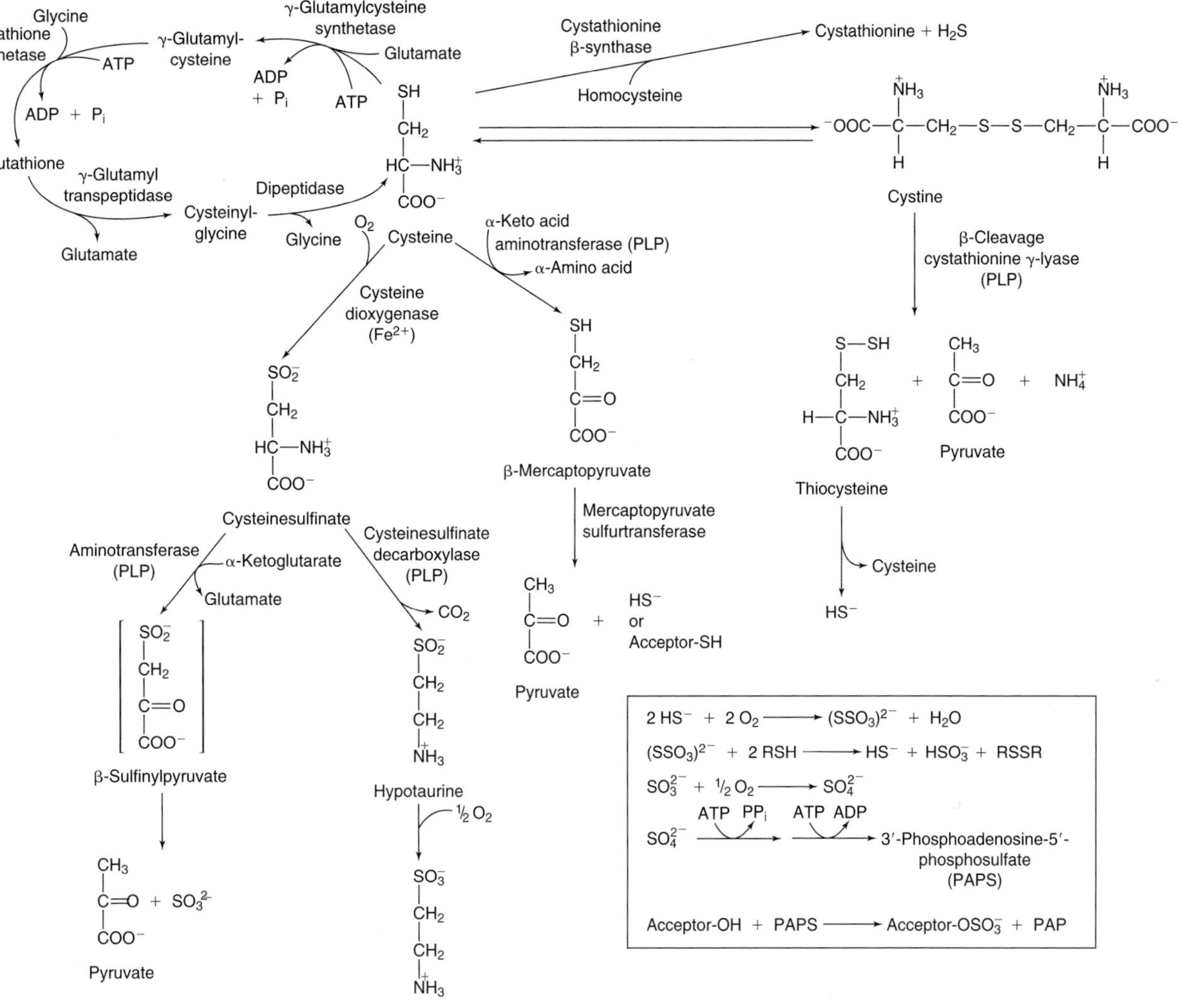

Figure 14-22 Pathways of cysteine and inorganic sulfur metabolism, including glutathione synthesis and degradation.

for synthesis of glutathione; the normal turnover of glutathione in adults has been estimated to be 40 mmol/day, which is slightly greater than the estimated normal turnover of cysteine in protein (Fukagawa et al., 1996). A large part of the normal glutathione turnover is related to glutathione's role as a reservoir of cysteine and as a means for transporting cysteine. The enzyme γ-glutamyltranspeptidase is located on the outer surface of the plasma membrane of cells in extrahepatic tissues such as kidney and lung, and it can hydrolyze the γ-glutamyl linkage of glutathione to yield cysteinylglycine (with or without transpeptidation of glutamate to another amino acid). The cysteinylglycine dipeptide can be hydrolyzed to cysteine and glycine, either extracellularly or intracellularly by dipeptidases. Therefore, cysteine may be released into the plasma or provided to peripheral tissues by hepatic glutathione synthesis and extrahepatic glutathione hydrolysis. (If a γ-glutamyl amino acid is formed, this dipeptide is transported into cells and then hydrolyzed; the glutamate spontaneously undergoes cyclization to form 5-oxoproline, which can be used to regenerate glutamate.)

Glutathione (GSH) has a reactive sulfhydryl group and can readily form disulfides with itself (oxidized glutathione or GSSG) or with other thiol compounds (GSSR). The ratio of GSH to GSSG in most cells is greater than 500, and GSH serves as a supply of reducing equivalents or electrons. Glutathione is involved in protection of cells from oxidative damage because of its role in the reduction of hydrogen peroxide and organic peroxides via glutathione peroxidases and because of its ability to inactivate free radicals by donating hydrogen to the radical; these processes result in oxidation of GSH to GSSG (White et al., 1994; DeLeve and Kaplowitz, 1991). Oxidized glutathione and GSH can be interconverted via the glutathione reductase reaction, which uses $NADP^+$/NADPH as the oxidant–reductant; hence, glutathione plays a role in maintenance of the cellular redox state.

Glutathione also serves as cosubstrate for several reactions, including certain steps in leukotriene synthesis and melanin polymer synthesis. Glutathione is the substrate for a group of enzymes, the glutathione *S*-transferases, which form glutathione conjugates from a variety of acceptor compounds, including various xenobiotics (foreign compounds such as drugs and carcinogens). These conjugates are normally degraded by γ-glutamyl transpeptidase and cysteinylglycine dipeptidase to yield the cysteinyl derivatives, which may be acetylated using acetyl CoA to become mercapturic acids, which are excreted in the urine. This process usually is a detoxification and excretion process.

Cysteine is necessary for the synthesis of the cysteamine (decarboxylated cysteine) portion of the CoA molecule (see Chapter 26). It contributes the reactive sulfhydryl group that forms thioesters with fatty acids and related metabolites.

Formation of Cystine and Cysteine

Cysteine readily reacts with itself or other thiols to form disulfides. The disulfide formed from two molecules of cysteine is cystine. Most of the cyst(e)ine present in the plasma is present as cystine. Also, some cysteinyl residues in proteins react to form disulfide bridges; when the protein is hydrolyzed, these residues are released as cystine. Hence, there is a need to reduce cystine and other disulfides in order to release cysteine for use in metabolic reactions that require cysteine as substrate. Glutathione is an important source of reducing equivalents for this reduction, which can occur by thiol-disulfide exchange or enzymatically by thioltransferase, with glutathione providing the reducing equivalents.

High concentrations of cystine are found in the urine of patients with cystinuria, an inborn error of cystine and dibasic amino acid transport by the brush-border membranes of the small intestinal mucosa and the renal tubules. Because cystine is insoluble, it causes cystine stones to form in the renal tubules if it is present at levels higher than its aqueous solubility limit (250 mg/L, or 1 mmol/L). In another genetic disease, cystinosis, there is a defect in the transport of cystine out of lysosomes, and high concentrations of cystine accumulate in lysosomes of various tissues.

Nutrition Insight

Detoxification of Acetaminophen

Role of Sulfur Amino Acids in Providing Sulfate and Glutathione for Phase II Enzymes

Metabolism of xenobiotic compounds or drugs is normally accomplished by two groups of enzymes. The phase I activating enzymes convert hydrophobic compounds to more hydrophilic, but often more reactive, forms. The phase II detoxification enzymes convert compounds, including the products of the phase I enzymes, to water-soluble conjugates that can readily be eliminated from the body. The phase I activating enzymes include the cytochrome P450 family of enzymes, aldehyde oxidase, xanthine oxidases, and peroxidases. The phase II enzymes include the multigene family of glutathione S-transferases, UDP-glucuronosyltransferases, and sulfotransferases. Because, the products of the phase I enzymes are often very reactive, they must be removed rapidly to avoid cellular toxicity, cell injury, or carcinogenesis.

As an example of the detoxification of a drug, we will consider acetaminophen. Acetaminophen is widely used as an analgesic and antipyretic drug and has been marketed in the United States as an over-the-counter preparation since 1960. Acetaminophen is largely metabolized by phase II enzyme systems, and undergoes conjugation with glucuronate and sulfate in the liver. These nontoxic conjugates are excreted by the kidney. Most of an acetaminophen dose can be recovered in the urine within 24 hours as glucuronide conjugates (~50% to 65%) and sulfate conjugates (~30% to 45%). Only approximately 1% of the dose is excreted in the urine as free acetaminophen. The extent of metabolism to glucuronide versus sulfate conjugates, but not total conjugation, has been shown to be influenced by diet, with a high-carbohydrate, low-protein diet favoring glucuronidation and a high-protein, low-carbohydrate diet favoring sulfation (Pantuck et al., 1991).

A smaller fraction of an acetaminophen dose is metabolized by a phase I enzyme system to a hepatotoxic reactive intermediate. If this reactive intermediate is not detoxified by conjugation with glutathione, it can covalently bind to cellular macromolecules or cause other injurious effects that lead to hepatocellular necrosis. Glutathione conjugates are further metabolized to form cysteine conjugates and *N*-acetylcysteine conjugates (mercapturic acids), which together account for 2% to 3% of the acetaminophen excreted in the urine. A small amount of glutathione-derived conjugates may also be excreted in the bile. A study of acetaminophen disposition in subjects with Gilbert's syndrome, which is an inherited deficiency of UDP-glucuronosyltransferase, demonstrated an inverse relationship between glucuronidation and bioactivation (De Morais et al., 1992). This observation suggests that a decrease in a major pathway of elimination (phase II system) can shunt more drug through the toxifying route (phase I system).

Although acetaminophen is generally considered to be safe at doses of less than 6 g/day, it is a potential hepatotoxin. The upper recommended dose is 4 g/day. Overdoses (usually single doses of more than 15 g) can be fatal. The toxicity of acetaminophen is enhanced by alcohol intake, which decreases phase II and increases phase I metabolism. There have been a number of reports of liver damage related to therapeutic use of acetaminophen (in some cases, at reported acetaminophen doses of less than 4 g/day) by alcoholics or regular alcohol consumers. The effect of ethanol on acetaminophen hepatotoxicity is thought to result primarily from the induction of cytochrome P450(2E1) by ethanol, which allows greater conversion of acetaminophen to its active metabolite. Depletion of hepatic glutathione and malnutrition may also play a role. Based on analysis of 161 cases of hepatic injury in alcohol consumers who took acetaminophen with therapeutic intent, Zimmerman and Maddrey (1995) recommended that individuals who ingest more than 60 g/day of ethanol should take no more than 2 g/day of acetaminophen. (Approximately 60 g of ethanol is contained in 5 fluid ounces of 80-proof liquor, such as whiskey, gin, or vodka, 15 to 20 fluid ounces of wine, or 50 fluid ounces of beer.)

Clinical Correlation

Cystinosis

Cystinosis is a rare, autosomal recessively inherited disorder caused by a defect in the lysosomal transport system for the amino acid cystine. In cystinosis, free cystine accumulates to 15 to 1,000 times normal concentrations in the lysosomes. The cystine forms crystals within the lysosomes of most tissues, which are damaged at different rates.

Children born with cystinosis are normal at birth, but signs of the renal tubular Fanconi syndrome (failure of the kidney to reabsorb small molecules properly) develop, usually when the child is between 6 and 12 months of age. Symptoms of renal tubular Fanconi syndrome include dehydration, acidosis, vomiting, electrolyte imbalances, hypophosphatemic rickets, and failure to grow. The renal glomerular damage progresses, and children typically require dialysis or transplantation by 6 to 12 years of age. In individuals who receive a kidney transplant, cystine accumulation does not occur in the transplanted kidney but continues in other tissues, resulting in retinal blindness, corneal erosions, diabetes mellitus, distal myopathy, swallowing difficulties, pancreatic insufficiency, and primary hypogonadism in patients between 13 and 35 years of age. Plasma cystine concentrations and the intestinal absorption of cystine are normal in individuals with cystinosis, unlike in the disorder known as cystinuria (described in Chapter 9). Urinary cystine levels are slightly elevated due to renal damage, but the cystine levels are no more elevated than those of other amino acids.

The reasons for the variable rates of cystine accumulation among different tissues are unknown, but they may be related to different rates of protein turnover and lysosomal protein degradation. Lysosomes are involved in protein degradation, and cysteinyl residues in protein that have formed disulfide linkages give rise to free cystine upon hydrolysis of the peptide linkages. Oral cysteamine (β-mercaptoethylamine) has been used successfully to lower the cystine content of cystinotic fibroblasts. The cysteine–cysteamine mixed disulfide resembles lysine structurally and is transported across cystinotic lysosomal membranes in a carrier-mediated fashion by the intact lysine transporter, whereas cystine remains trapped inside the lysosomes. Long-term oral cysteamine therapy lowers the cystine content of tissues, preserves renal function, and improves growth. Cysteamine also is used in eyedrops to dissolve corneal crystals in children and to remove the haziness from the corneas of older patients.

PHENYLALANINE AND TYROSINE

Conversion of Phenylalanine to Tyrosine

The major catabolism of phenylalanine and tyrosine occurs in the liver, but tyrosine is an important precursor for synthesis of several essential compounds in other tissues. As shown in Figure 14-23, phenylalanine is converted to tyrosine by phenylalanine hydroxylase, which is a tetrahydrobiopterin-dependent, mixed-function oxidase that hydroxylates phenylalanine at the C-4 of the aromatic ring. This reaction is the first step in phenylalanine degradation and also is the step that allows phenylalanine to serve as a dietary precursor of tyrosine (Clarke and Bier, 1982). The reverse reaction does not occur, so tyrosine cannot totally replace phenylalanine in the diet; only approximately 50% of the total phenylalanine and tyrosine requirement can be provided as tyrosine.

Conversion of phenylalanine to tyrosine and, hence, phenylalanine catabolism, is regulated by changes in the activity of phenylalanine hydroxylase, which is regulated by its phosphorylation state (Doskeland et al., 1996; Kaufman, 1993) and by effects of phenylalanine on its conformation (McKinney et al., 2001; Knappskog et al., 1996). Phosphorylation of a serine residue in a regulatory domain of the enzyme activates phenylalanine hydroxylase by increasing its specific activity. The potency of phenylalanine as an

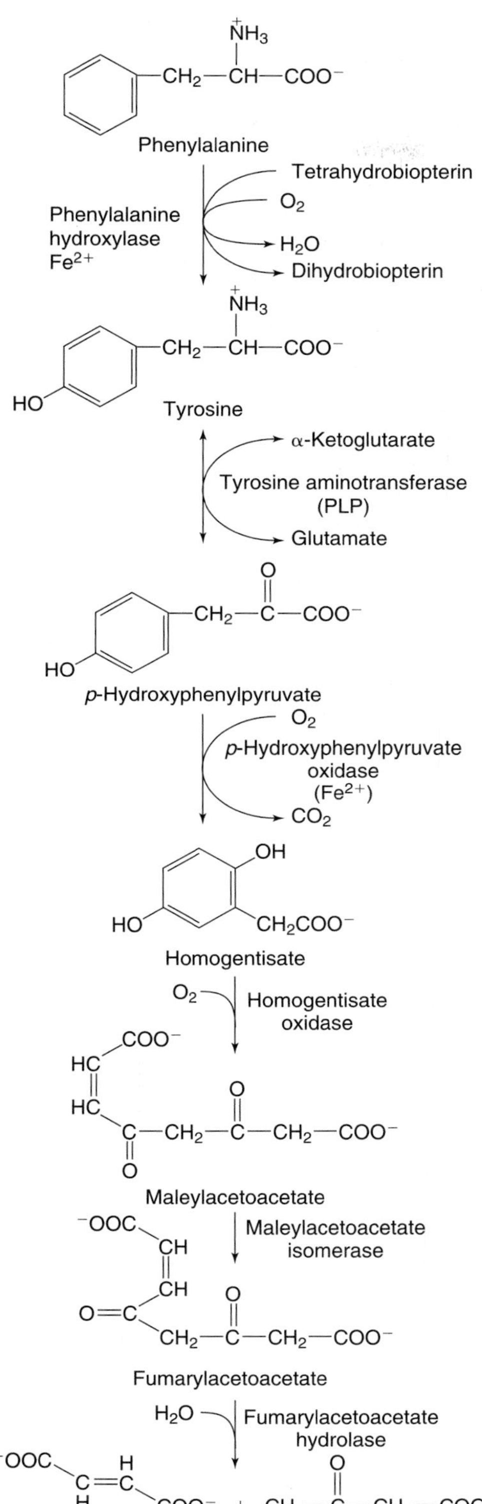

Figure 14-23 Metabolism of phenylalanine and tyrosine.

activator of phenylalanine hydroxylase is greater for the phosphorylated form of the enzyme. An increase in phenylalanine concentration induces conformational changes that favor tetramer formation and high-affinity phenylalanine binding. The tetrameric form of phenylalanine hydroxylase exhibits cooperative binding of phenylalanine. Therefore, either an increase in phenylalanine concentration (high-protein diet) or an increase in the circulating glucagon level acts to increase phenylalanine hydroxylase activity. In the rat, phosphorylation of the enzyme is catalyzed by both cAMP-dependent protein kinase and calcium/calmodulin-dependent protein kinase. (See Chapter 19 for a discussion of these signal transduction pathways.)

The absence of phenylalanine hydroxylase activity is the basis of the inborn error of metabolism, phenylketonuria (PKU); PKU is the most common disease caused by a deficiency of an enzyme of amino acid metabolism, and infants routinely are screened at birth for this defect (Erlandsen et al., 2003). Children with an absence of phenylalanine hydroxylase accumulate high levels of phenylalanine in their tissues and also metabolize some phenylalanine via abnormal routes such as transamination. The keto acid of phenylalanine, phenylpyruvate, along with its products phenyllactate and phenylacetate, accumulates in body fluids and is excreted in the urine of individuals with phenylketonuria who are not treated with a low-phenylalanine (adequate tyrosine) diet. In normal individuals, transamination of phenylalanine plays a very small role because the K_m for phenylalanine transamination is much higher than normal hepatic phenylalanine concentrations.

Tyrosine Catabolism

Tyrosine is primarily catabolized via transamination to *p*-hydroxyphenylpyruvate (see Fig. 14-23). Tyrosine aminotransferase is expressed only in the liver, has a short half-life, and is subject to regulation by a number of hormones, including insulin, glucagon, and glucocorticoids. The keto acid *p*-hydroxyphenylpyruvate is further metabolized to homogentisate and ultimately to fumarate plus acetoacetate.

The role of the tyrosine transamination pathway in phenylalanine and tyrosine catabolism is demonstrated by the inborn error of metabolism called alcaptonuria. Alcaptonuria results from a deficiency of homogentisate oxidase. Individuals with alcaptonuria excrete almost all ingested tyrosine (and phenylalanine) as homogentisate in their urine. If urine that contains homogentisate is allowed to stand or if alkali is added, it gradually turns dark as the homogentisate is oxidized to a melanin-like product. This darkening of the urine led to early recognition of this disease, and alcaptonuria was the first condition to be identified as an inborn error of metabolism. Alcaptonuria and other inborn errors of metabolism have provided much information about metabolism of amino acids in humans.

Role of Tyrosine in the Synthesis of Neuroactive Amines, Hormones, and Pigments

In catecholamine-producing neurons and chromaffin granules, tyrosine is hydroxylated to 3,4-dihydroxyphenylalanine (DOPA) by tyrosine hydroxylase, which is a tetrahydrobiopterin-dependent enzyme similar to phenylalanine hydroxylase (Eisenhofer et al., 2003; Dix et al., 1987). DOPA is further metabolized to various products, depending on the tissue (Fig. 14-24). In specific regions of the brain, DOPA is decarboxylated to dopamine, which functions as a neurotransmitter. Decreased production of dopamine is the cause of Parkinson's disease. In noradrenergic neurons, DOPA is converted to dopamine and further hydroxylated to norepinephrine. Norepinephrine is the chemical transmitter at most sympathetic postganglionic nerve endings. Norepinephrine is synthesized by the noradrenergic neurons and stored in vesicles in the termini of the axons; these cells also have an active mechanism for reuptake of norepinephrine.

In chromaffin granules in the adrenal medulla, dopamine and norepinephrine also are produced, but most of the norepinephrine is methylated (by a transmethylase that uses *S*-adenosylmethionine) to epinephrine, the major hormone secreted by the adrenal medulla of humans. Epinephrine, norepinephrine, and dopamine, collectively called catecholamines, are stored in these chromaffin granules and are subsequently released from these granules into the blood. Inactivation of catecholamines is accomplished by the reactions catalyzed by monoamine oxidase and catechol-*O*-methyltransferase and by conjugation of catecholamines with sulfate or glucuronate.

In melanin-producing cells (melanocytes), DOPA formed by tyrosine hydroxylase is oxidized by tyrosinase to form dopaquinone and various derivatives of dopaquinone. These compounds condense to form melanins or dark pigments, which are contained in cellular organelles called melanosomes. Melanins are a family of high-molecular-weight polymers that contain various metabolites of dopaquinone and, in the case of reddish pigments, cysteine. Melanins are concentrated in the skin, hair, and parts of the eye and brain. Genetic defects in melanin synthesis are responsible for albinism.

Tyrosine residues in the protein thyroglobulin serve as precursors of thyroid hormones. Thyroglobulin in the thyroid gland contains iodinated aromatic amino acids derived from tyrosine. Posttranslational iodination and coupling of tyrosine residues in thyroglobulin is followed by release of triiodothyronine (T_3) and thyroxin (T_4) from the thyroid gland after proteolysis of thyroglobulin (see Chapter 38).

TRYPTOPHAN

Tryptophan Catabolism and NAD Synthesis

Tryptophan is degraded primarily in the liver. The first step in the catabolic pathway is an oxygenation that opens the 5-member ring of the indole nucleus of tryptophan to yield *N*-formylkynurenine. This reaction is catalyzed by tryptophan dioxygenase (also called tryptophan pyrrolase) in the liver, but it can also be catalyzed by indoleamine 2,3-dioxygenase in other tissues (Fig. 14-25). Hepatic tryptophan 2,3-dioxygenase has a short half-life and is highly regulated. Glucagon and other hormones such as glucocorticoids increase the amount of the enzyme; high levels of nicotinamide nucleotide coenzymes can inhibit the enzyme; and tryptophan can stabilize the enzyme against proteolysis, resulting in higher steady-state levels of enzyme.

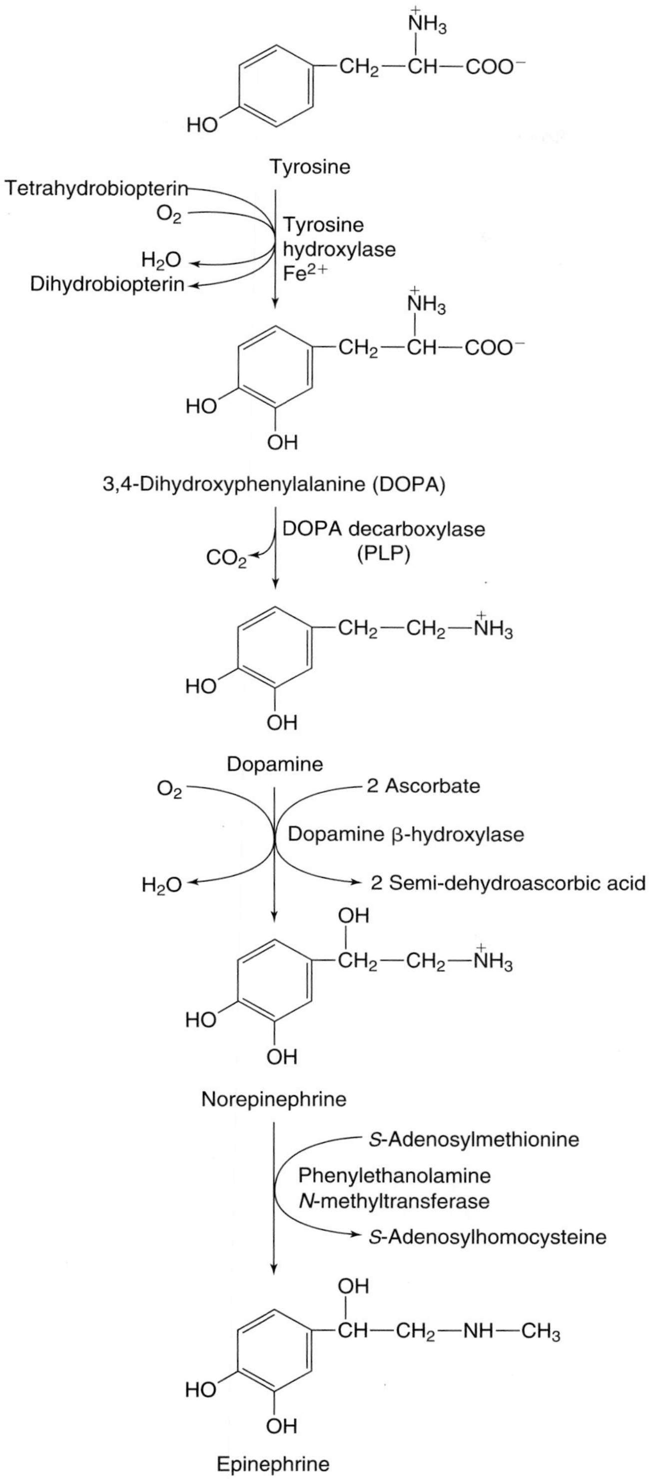

Tyrosine

Tetrahydrobiopterin, O_2 → H_2O, Dihydrobiopterin
Tyrosine hydroxylase Fe^{2+}

3,4-Dihydroxyphenylalanine (DOPA)

DOPA decarboxylase (PLP) → CO_2

Dopamine

O_2, 2 Ascorbate → H_2O, 2 Semi-dehydroascorbic acid
Dopamine β-hydroxylase

Norepinephrine

S-Adenosylmethionine → S-Adenosylhomocysteine
Phenylethanolamine N-methyltransferase

Epinephrine

Figure 14-24 Synthesis of catecholamines from tyrosine.

The hydrolytic removal of formate (which can be used by the folate coenzyme system) from *N*-formylkynurenine yields kynurenine, a compound that lies at the first branch point of the tryptophan catabolic pathway (Peters, 1991). As shown in Figure 14-25, kynurenine can be converted to kynurenate, anthranilate, or 3-hydroxykynurenine. Another branch-point occurs at 3-hydroxykynurenine: 3-hydroxykynurenine can be metabolized to 2-amino-3-carboxymuconate semialdehyde or to xanthurenate. The major metabolite produced as a result of the second branch of normal tryptophan catabolism, 2-amino-3-carboxymuconate semialdehyde, lies at a third important branch-point in tryptophan metabolism, leading to the production of NAD^+ (nicotinamide adenine dinucleotide) by one route and aminomuconate by the other route. Hence, tryptophan catabolism by the various branches of the catabolic pathway results in formation of kynurenate, anthranilate, xanthurenate, NAD^+, or aminomuconate semialdehyde from the ring structure of tryptophan.

Both kynurenine and 3-hydroxykynurenine are converted to anthranilate or 3-hydroxyanthranilate by kynureninase, which is a pyridoxal 5′-phosphate–dependent enzyme. The kynureninase-catalyzed steps result in production of anthranilate or 3-hydroxyanthranilate from the benzene ring of tryptophan and of alanine from the 3-carbon aliphatic portion of the amino acid, including its α-amino and carboxyl groups. In contrast, in the branches of the pathway that lead to formation of kynurenate and xanthurenate, kynurenine or 3-hydroxykynurenine undergoes transamination with α-ketoglutarate, such that the amino group of tryptophan is incorporated into glutamate, and the remainder of the aliphatic side chain condenses to form a second 6-member ring.

Loss of kynurenine, kynurenate, 3-hydroxykynurenine, or xanthurenate in the urine represents a loss of both gluconeogenic and ketogenic precursors; the basal excretion of these tryptophan catabolites normally accounts for approximately 3% to 6% of the ingested tryptophan (Leklem, 1971). A deficiency of vitamin B_6 results in decreased kynurenase activity and increased excretion of kynurenine, 3-hydroxykynurenine, kynurenate, and xanthurenate in the urine. During pregnancy, increased urinary excretion of these same tryptophan metabolites is observed; this seems to result from a pregnancy-specific decrease in kynureninase activity that is not related to a vitamin B_6 deficiency (Van De Kamp and Smolen, 1995).

At the 2-amino-3-carboxymuconate semialdehyde branch-point, the 2-amino-3-carboxymuconate semialdehyde can undergo nonenzymatic cyclization to quinolinate, which can be converted to NAD^+ or $NADP^+$ by a pathway similar to that used for conversion of nicotinic acid to NAD^+ or $NADP^+$, or it can be decarboxylated by picolinate carboxylase to form 2-aminomuconate semialdehyde (Ikeda et al., 1965). (The 2-aminomuconate semialdehyde also can spontaneously undergo cyclization to form picolinate, which is the basis for the name of the enzyme that forms 2-aminomuconate semialdehyde.) Hence, the synthesis of quinolinate and subsequently $NAD(P)^+$ depends on a nonenzymatic step that competes with an enzymatic route of tryptophan catabolism. Species with high picolinate carboxylase activity rapidly metabolize 2-amino-3-carboxymuconate semialdehyde by the enzymatic reaction and, hence, convert little tryptophan to NAD^+. Humans have moderate levels of picolinate carboxylase, and the synthesis of NAD^+ and $NADP^+$ (the niacin-containing coenzymes) from tryptophan is sufficient to provide a major portion of the body's need for the vitamin niacin, provided that dietary tryptophan intake is sufficient, even though this pathway is a minor route of tryptophan catabolism. (See Chapter 24 for more discussion of $NAD(P)^+$ synthesis from tryptophan.)

In humans, most of the 2-aminomuconate semialdehyde formed in the picolinate carboxylase–catalyzed reaction, at the last major branch-point of tryptophan metabolism, is dehydrogenated, deaminated, and further oxidized. The pathway for further oxidation of 2-aminomuconate semialdehyde involves its conversion via poorly understood reactions to α-ketoadipate, which is oxidatively decarboxylated to glutaryl CoA. Glutaryl CoA ultimately is converted to acetoacetyl CoA by a sequence of reactions that are similar to those involved in the metabolism of the α-aminoadipate that is formed in lysine catabolism (see Fig. 14-27).

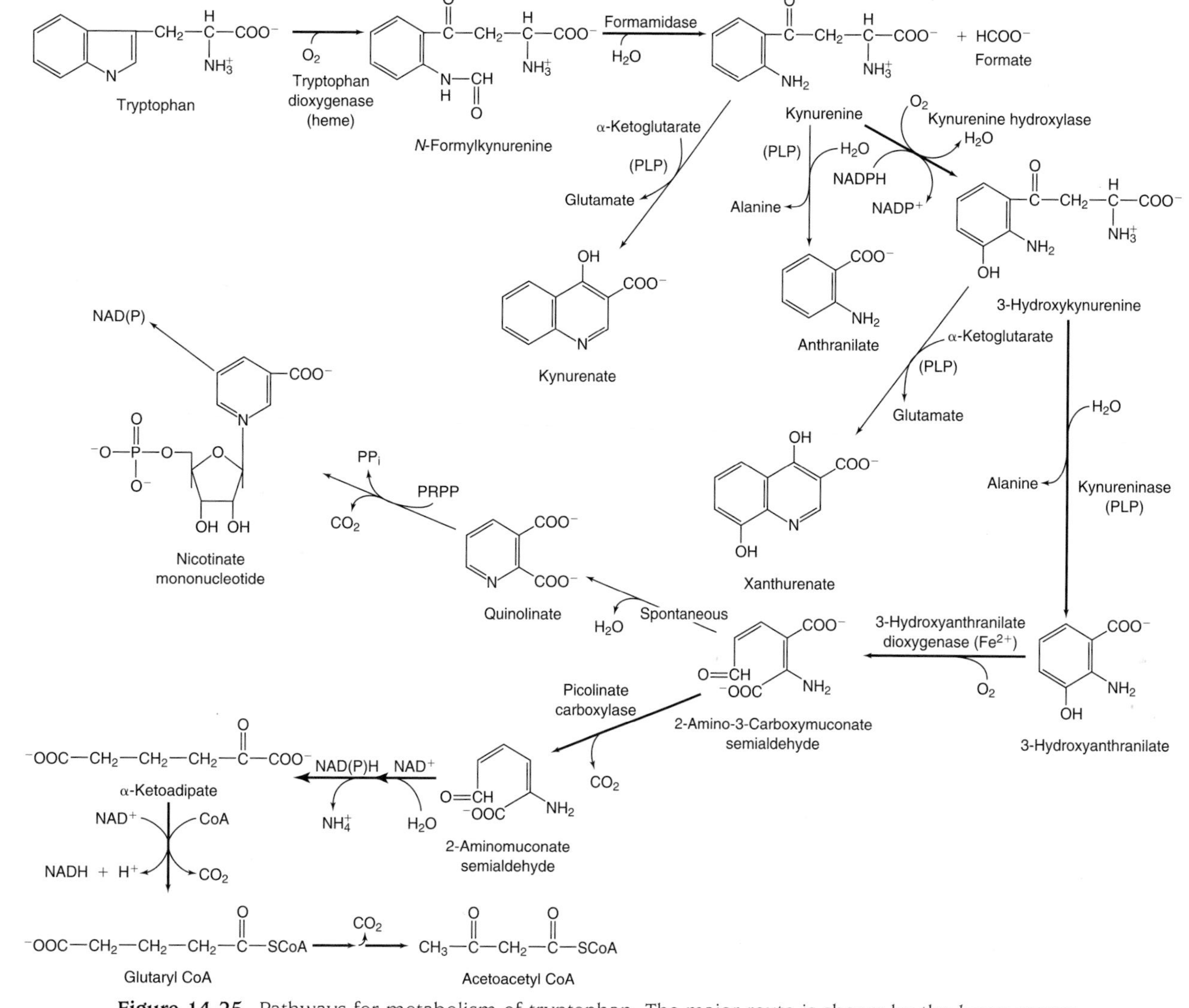

Figure 14-25 Pathways for metabolism of tryptophan. The major route is shown by the *heavy arrows.*

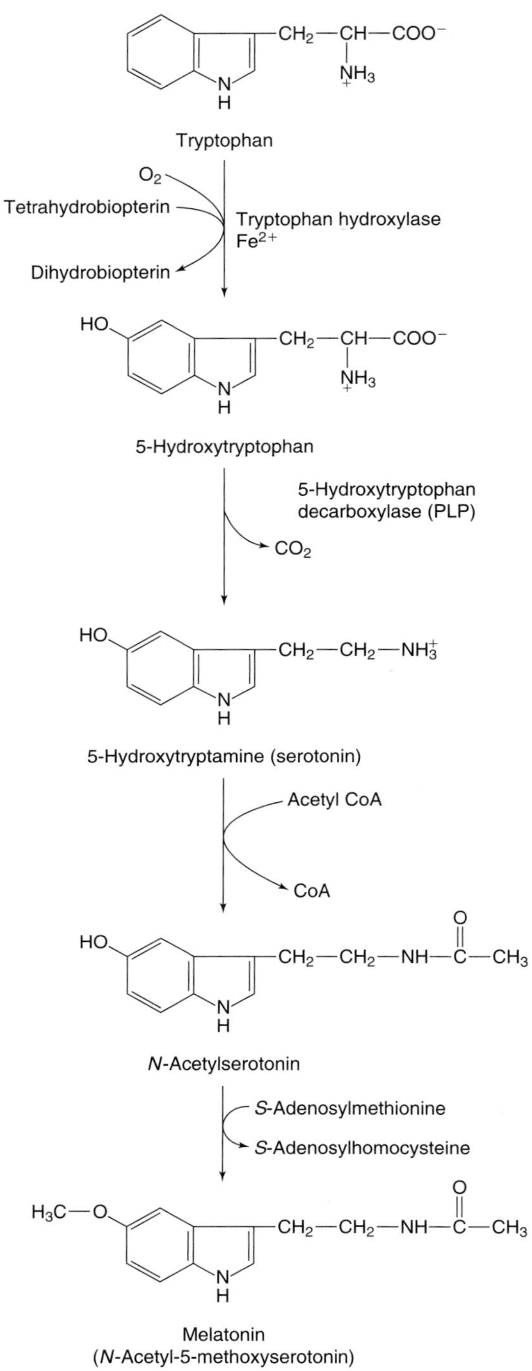

Tryptophan

O_2, Tetrahydrobiopterin → Dihydrobiopterin; Tryptophan hydroxylase Fe^{2+}

5-Hydroxytryptophan

5-Hydroxytryptophan decarboxylase (PLP) → CO_2

5-Hydroxytryptamine (serotonin)

Acetyl CoA → CoA

N-Acetylserotonin

S-Adenosylmethionine → *S*-Adenosylhomocysteine

Melatonin (*N*-Acetyl-5-methoxyserotonin)

Figure 14-26 Synthesis of serotonin and melatonin from tryptophan.

Glutaric aciduria type I results from a deficiency of glutaryl CoA dehydrogenase; when patients with this inborn error of metabolism are treated with dietary restrictions of both tryptophan and lysine, the urinary excretion of glutarate is decreased (Yannicelli et al., 1994). (Compare with glutaric aciduria type II discussed in Chapter 24.) This, along with the observed patterns of metabolite excretion, suggests that metabolism of tryptophan via kynurenine, 3-hydroxykynurenine, 2-amino-3-carboxymuconate semialdehyde, 2-aminomuconate semialdehyde, and glutaryl CoA is the major route of tryptophan catabolism under normal conditions.

Most of the tryptophan carbon skeleton is ultimately funneled into central pathways of energy metabolism. The formation of alanine in the two reactions catalyzed by kynureninase (conversion of kynurenine to anthranilate or conversion of 3-hydroxykynurenine to 3-hydroxyanthranilate) would be considered glucogenic, and the formation of acetoacetyl CoA from 2-aminomuconate semialdehyde in the major branch of the catabolic pathway would be considered ketogenic.

Conversion of Tryptophan to Serotonin and Melatonin

Tryptophan is also converted to serotonin, an important neurotransmitter that also may have functions outside the central nervous system (Peters, 1991). Serotonin synthesis involves the hydroxylation of tryptophan at C-5 by a mixed-function oxygenase that uses tetrahydrobiopterin as a cosubstrate, followed by decarboxylation of the resulting 5-hydroxytryptophan by a pyridoxal 5′-phosphate–dependent enzyme to give 5-hydroxytryptamine (serotonin), as shown in Figure 14-26. Tryptophan hydroxylase normally is not saturated with substrate, and increased uptake of tryptophan by a tissue can result in increased serotonin synthesis. Serotonergic neurons have an active reuptake mechanism, and they can inactivate the serotonin by oxidation to 5-hydroxyindoleacetic acid and by methylation. The inactive metabolites and their conjugates are excreted in the urine. Serotonin is methylated and acetylated to form melatonin

(*N*-acetyl-5-methoxytryptamine) in the pineal gland and, perhaps, other tissues. Melatonin production in the pineal gland is elevated during the dark phase of the daily cycle and is believed to play a role in maintenance of daily and seasonal rhythms.

Metabolism of Tryptophan by the Kynurenine Pathway in Nonhepatic Tissues

Whereas tryptophan dioxygenase is present in liver and is involved in the major pathway of tryptophan catabolism, the enzyme indoleamine 2,3-dioxygenase is present in other tissues (placenta, lung, and intestine) and also catalyzes the conversion of tryptophan to *N*-formylkynurenine and, hence, kynurenine. Indoleamine 2,3-dioxygenase is inducible by the proinflammatory cytokine interferon-γ, and accelerated tryptophan degradation is observed concomitant to cellular immune activation (Wirleitner et al., 2003; Maes et al., 2002). Low plasma tryptophan levels occur when there is persistent immune activation as during infectious, autoimmune, and malignant diseases and during pregnancy. Depletion of circulating tryptophan may lead to reduced serotonin production, which may contribute to the development of anxiety and depression in individuals with chronic disease and in women in the early puerperium. Indolamine 2,3-dioxygenase is present in the lens of the eye where the tryptophan catabolites, kynurenine and 3-hydroxykynurenine glucoside, bind to lens proteins to form yellow and fluorescent adducts (Takikawa et al., 2001). These adducts are responsible for the yellowing of the lens with age.

LYSINE

Lysine Catabolism

Most degradation of lysine occurs by the saccharopine pathway, shown in Figure 14-27, which is present in liver mitochondria of mammals (Vianey-Liaud et al., 1991). This pathway involves the reaction of the ε-amino group of lysine with the carbonyl group of α-ketoglutarate to form saccharopine, which is further metabolized to α-aminoadipic semialdehyde plus glutamate. These two reactions result in transfer of the ε-amino group of lysine to the α-ketoglutarate that was used to form saccharopine; the net effect of these two reactions is to incorporate the ε-amino group of lysine into the α-amino nitrogen pool via glutamate. The α-aminoadipate semialdehyde is oxidized to α-aminoadipate, which undergoes a conventional transamination with α-ketoglutarate to transfer the α-amino group of lysine to glutamate with formation of α-ketoadipate from the lysine carbon chain. The α-ketoadipate, which is a higher homologue of α-ketoglutarate, is oxidized to glutaryl CoA and ultimately to acetoacetyl CoA (Yannicelli et al., 1994); these final steps of lysine catabolism are analogous to those involved in the final steps of tryptophan catabolism (see Fig. 14-25).

The formation and dehydrogenation of saccharopine are catalyzed by a bifunctional protein (α-aminoadipic semialdehyde synthase). A rare inborn error of metabolism in which both lysine-α-ketoglutarate reductase and saccharopine dehydrogenase activities are deficient results in hyperlysinemia and excretion of lysine and smaller amounts of saccharopine in the urine (Sacksteder et al., 2000; Divry et al., 1991). The saccharopine pathway is regulated by changes in the activity of α-aminoadipic semialdehyde synthase, which is increased in animals fed diets high in lysine or protein (increased amount of enzyme protein) and in rats treated with glucagon (increased activity state) (Scislowski et al., 1994).

Although not sufficient to compensate for deficiency in the saccharopine pathway, other pathways of lysine degradation may play a role, especially in nonhepatic tissues (Broquist, 1990). The α-amino group of lysine can be released as ammonia by a lysine α-oxidase reaction with formation of a cyclic derivative, piperideine-2-carboxylate, which is reduced to form pipecolate, a cyclic imino acid. The pipecolate is oxidized by pipecolate peroxidase, which is found in peroxisomes in human liver, brain, and kidney (and perhaps in brain mitochondria). Pipecolate accumulates in individuals with peroxisomal disorders. The oxidation of pipecolate by pipecolate peroxidase yields hydrogen peroxide and piperideine-6-carboxylate, which is

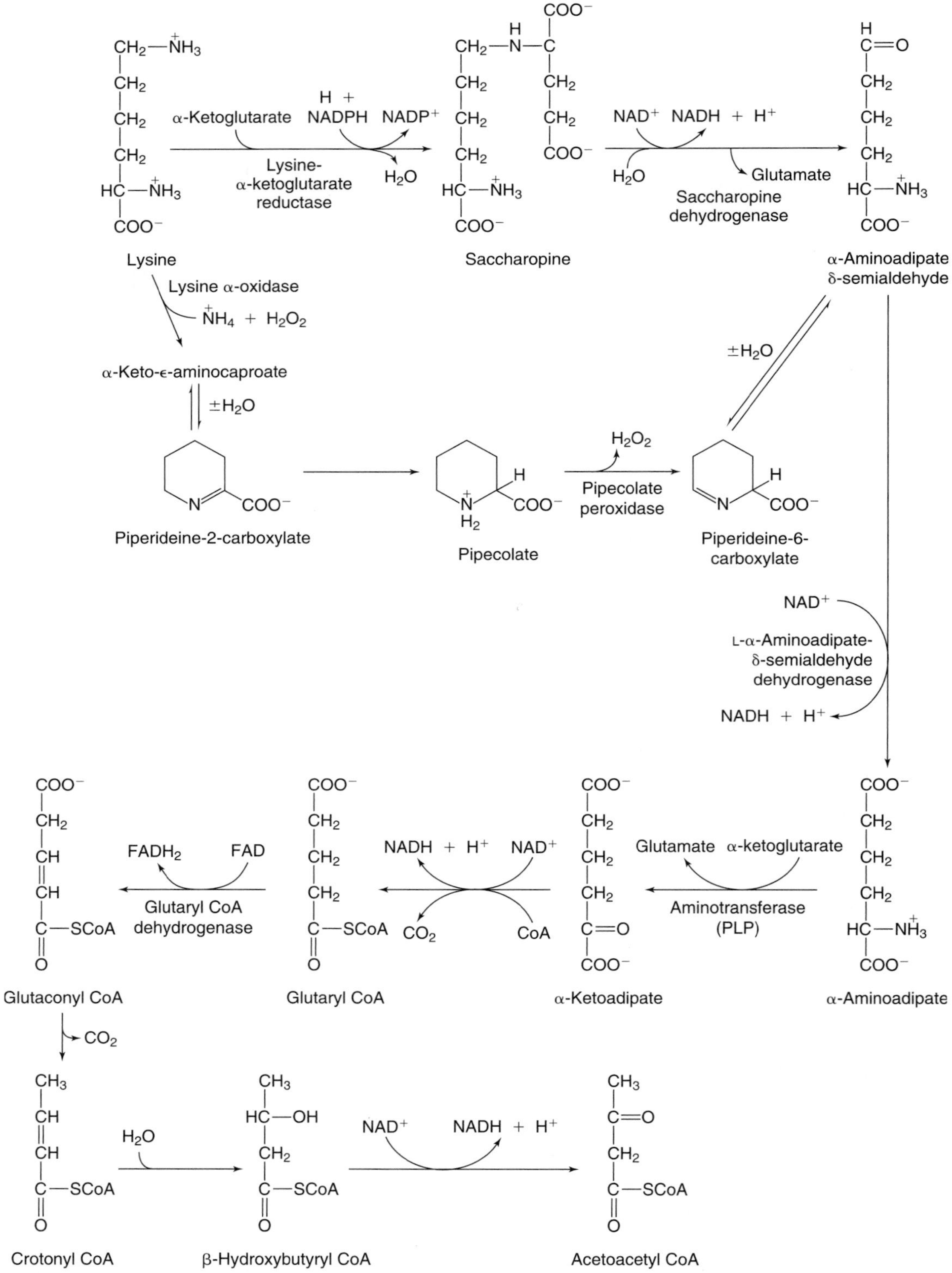

Lysine

α-Ketoglutarate, H^+ + NADPH, $NADP^+$, H_2O

Lysine-α-ketoglutarate reductase

Saccharopine

NAD^+, NADH + H^+, H_2O, Glutamate

Saccharopine dehydrogenase

α-Aminoadipate δ-semialdehyde

Lysine α-oxidase

NH_4^+ + H_2O_2

α-Keto-ϵ-aminocaproate

±H_2O

Piperideine-2-carboxylate

Pipecolate

H_2O_2

Pipecolate peroxidase

Piperideine-6-carboxylate

±H_2O

NAD^+

L-α-Aminoadipate-δ-semialdehyde dehydrogenase

NADH + H^+

α-Aminoadipate

Glutamate, α-ketoglutarate

Aminotransferase (PLP)

α-Ketoadipate

NADH + H^+, NAD^+, CO_2, CoA

Glutaryl CoA

$FADH_2$, FAD

Glutaryl CoA dehydrogenase

Glutaconyl CoA

CO_2

Crotonyl CoA

H_2O

β-Hydroxybutyryl CoA

NAD^+, NADH + H^+

Acetoacetyl CoA

Figure 14-27 The saccharopine and the pipecolate pathways of lysine catabolism. The two pathways merge at the intermediate, α-aminoadipate semialdehyde.

hydrolyzed spontaneously to α-aminoadipate δ-semialdehyde, an early intermediate in the saccharopine pathway of lysine catabolism. Hence, the two pathways converge, and the process of lysine catabolism is completed by the same series of reactions.

Carnitine Formation From Lysine

The ε-amino groups of lysyl residues in many proteins are methylated to monomethyllsyl, dimethyllsyl, or trimethyllysyl residues by an *N*-methyltransferase that uses *S*-adenosylmethionine as the methyl donor. Trimethyllysine is released when these proteins undergo proteolysis, and this trimethyllysine serves as the precursor of carnitine (Rebouche, 1988). Carnitine synthesis is discussed in Chapter 27 (see Fig. 27-8). The synthesis of carnitine and the role of carnitine in the transport of long-chain fatty acids into the mitochondria are discussed in Chapters 16, 26, and 27.

LEUCINE, ISOLEUCINE, AND VALINE

Branched-Chain Amino Acid Catabolism

The branched-chain amino acids (leucine, isoleucine, and valine) make up a considerable part of the diet (20% to 30% of all amino acids). In contrast to other amino acids, these amino acids are not metabolized substantially by the human intestine or by liver, both of which have low levels of branched-chain amino acid transaminase activity and very low levels of the branched-chain keto acid dehydrogenase complex (Suryawan et al., 1998; Taniguchi et al., 1996). Although some transamination of branched-chain amino acids may occur in the splanchnic organs, the transamination is probably reversible due to the slow removal of branched-chain keto acids. Hence, the concentration of branched-chain amino acids in peripheral plasma rises considerably after a meal. Branched-chain amino acids in excess of amounts needed for protein synthesis are catabolized in peripheral tissues such as skeletal muscle, heart, pancreas, kidney, and brain. Catabolism begins by transamination of the amino acids with α-ketoglutarate to form the corresponding branched-chain α-keto acids, as shown in Figure 14-28. Both mitochondrial and cytosolic forms of branched-chain aminotransferase exist, and the mitochondrial form is widespread in human tissues (Suryawan et al., 1998). Both isoenzymes are capable of using all three branched-chain amino or keto acids as substrate.

The branched-chain keto acids formed as a result of transamination are oxidized via a mitochondrial branched-chain keto acid dehydrogenase complex to CO_2, NADH, and the branched-chain acyl CoAs. The branched-chain keto acid dehydrogenase complex is similar to the pyruvate and α-ketoglutarate dehydrogenase complexes and is composed of three enzymes known as E1, E2 and E3 (see Chapter 12, Fig. 12-18). This is the most important regulatory enzyme in the catabolic pathways of the branched-chain amino acids. In the rat, much of the branched-chain keto acid formed in muscle is released into the circulation to be further metabolized in the liver, but the oxidative decarboxylation of branched-chain keto acids in humans occurs predominantly in muscle and also in kidney, liver, and brain (Suryawan et al., 1998).

The branched-chain keto acid dehydrogenase complex is subject to feedback regulation by high ratios of NADH/NAD^+ and acyl CoA/CoA and also is regulated by phosphorylation/dephosphorylation. The activity state of the branched-chain keto acid dehydrogenase complex is regulated by the phosphorylation state of specific serine residues of the E1 component of the complex, which in turn is regulated by the relative activities of a specific mitochondrial kinase and phosphatase (Harris et al., 2004). The complex is inactive in its phosphorylated state. In animals, adaptation to higher protein diets results in the association of less kinase with the branched-chain keto acid dehydrogenase complex, which favors the dephosphorylated, active state. Short-term regulation of the complex is achieved by inhibition of the branched-chain keto acid dehydrogenase kinase by branched-chain keto acids (especially by α-ketoisocaproate), which are the substrates for the branched-chain dehydrogenase complex. This mechanism allows leucine to regulate its own catabolism or tissue concentrations and, thus, to self-limit its positive effects on protein

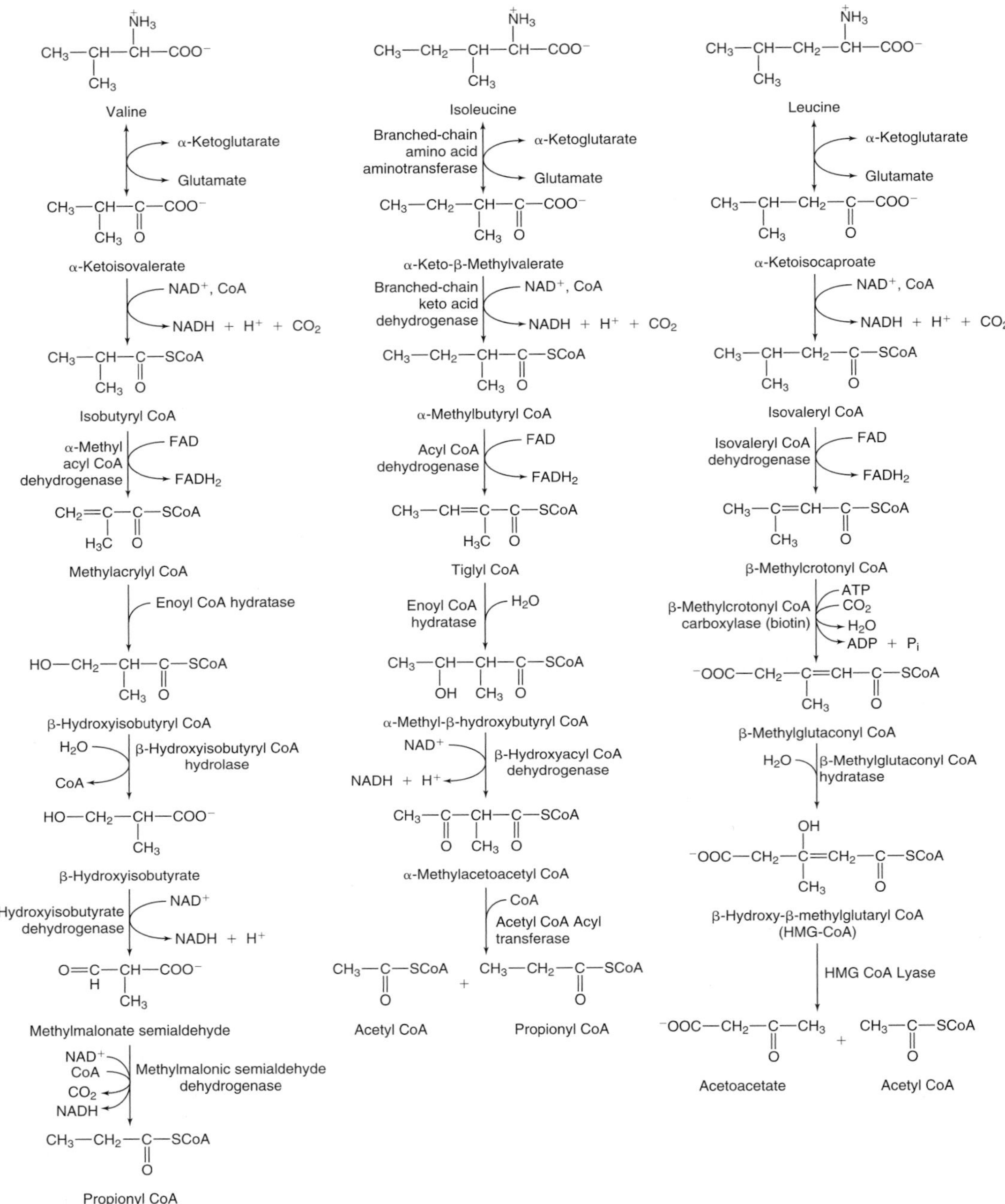

Figure 14-28 Catabolism of the branched-chain amino acids.

accretion (increased synthesis, decreased degradation, and increased insulin as discussed in Chapter 13). Medium-chain fatty acids such as octanoate also inhibit the kinase, probably because they are structurally related to α-ketoisocaproate. (See Chapters 24 and 26 for the roles of coenzymes in the catabolism of the branched-chain keto acids.)

Long-term control mechanisms include the transcriptional regulation of the expression of the branched-chain keto acid dehydrogenase subunits and of branched-chain keto acid dehydrogenase kinase. The expression of the branched-chain keto acid dehydrogenase subunits is markedly reduced in rats fed a low-protein diet. In contrast, expression of the kinase is upregulated by low protein feeding and by thyroid hormone and downregulated by high protein feeding, starvation, and glucocorticoids. Activation of the transcription factor PPARα (peroxisome proliferator-activated receptor-α) appears to be involved in both the transcriptional upregulation of the expression of the branched-chain keto acid dehydrogenase subunits and the downregulation of the branched-chain keto acid dehydrogenase kinase. Promotion of fatty acid oxidation, such as during starvation or exercise, may increase branched-chain amino acid oxidation via long-chain fatty acids acting as ligands for PPARα.

An inborn error of branched-chain amino acid metabolism, called maple syrup urine disease because of the odor of the urine, results from mutations affecting different subunits of the mitochondrial branched-chain keto acid dehydrogenase complex. A thiamine-responsive form of maple syrup urine disease has been characterized due to mutations in the gene for the E2 subunit (Chuang et al., 2004). Plasma and urinary levels of branched-chain amino acids and their α-keto acids are elevated. Small amounts of branched-chain α-hydroxy acids (formed by reduction of α-keto acids) also are found in the urine of patients with this inborn error (Parsons et al., 1990). This rare inborn error is associated with severe neurological symptoms if not diagnosed early and treated with a protein-modified diet.

The branched-chain acyl CoAs are further oxidized by specific branched-chain acyl CoA dehydrogenases to form the corresponding α,β-unsaturated compounds (Taniguchi et al., 1996). Catabolism of valine and isoleucine then continues through several steps to produce propionyl CoA from valine and both propionyl CoA and acetyl CoA from isoleucine. Release of β-hydroxyisobutyrate from muscle and heart has been observed in animals; this valine catabolite can be converted to glucose in the liver or kidney. The branched-chain acyl CoA formed from leucine, isovaleryl CoA, is catabolized to yield β-hydroxy-β-methylglutaryl CoA (HMG CoA). A biotin-dependent carboxylation step is required for conversion of β-methylcrotonyl CoA to β-methylglutaconyl CoA prior to HMG CoA formation in the leucine catabolic pathway. The HMG CoA can be further catabolized to yield acetoacetate and acetyl CoA. As discussed previously, much of the branched-chain amino acid nitrogen is carried out of muscle as alanine and glutamine (Darmaun and Dechelotte, 1991). Defects in branched-chain amino acid metabolism that affect a number of these intermediary steps have been identified in human patients (Gibson et al., 1994).

NITROGEN EXCRETION

The major end products of amino acid catabolism in humans are CO_2, H_2O, and urea, with a small amount of ammonia. Because energy is required for urea synthesis and urea has a heat of combustion of 151.6 kcal per mole, the net physiological fuel value mammals can gain from dietary protein is less than would be predicted based on complete oxidation of protein. In adults in nitrogen balance, nitrogen excretion as urea approximates the daily intake of nitrogen from protein. Urine also contains smaller amounts of other nitrogenous end products formed from catabolism of amino acids or of nonprotein compounds formed from amino acids (Table 14-2). Although most of the body's loss of nitrogen occurs via the

Table 14-2
Major Nitrogen-Containing Components of Normal Human Urine

End Product	Excreted Nitrogen (g N/24 hours)
Urea	10-15*
Creatinine	0.3-0.8
NH_3^+, NH_4^+	0.4-1.0
Uric acid	0.1-0.2
Amino acids	0.1-0.2
Other nitrogen	0.2-0.8†
TOTAL NITROGEN	12-18

*Urea N depends heavily on the amount of dietary protein and may vary from less than 2 to more than 20 g per day.
†Other N includes trace amount of proteins, δ-aminolevulinic acid, porphobilinogen, 5-hydroxyindole acetic acid, catecholamine metabolites, and tryptophan metabolites.

urine, nitrogen is also lost via the feces (including loss of remnants from digestion of dietary and endogenous proteins in the gastrointestinal tract and endogenous nitrogenous compounds excreted by the liver in the bile) and via loss of proteins and other nitrogenous compounds in the hair, nails, sloughed-off skin, various bodily secretions, and blood losses.

INCORPORATION OF NITROGEN INTO UREA BY THE UREA CYCLE IN THE LIVER

The urea cycle was first described by Hans Krebs and Kurt Henseleit in 1932, based on experiments in which they found that ornithine stimulated urea synthesis by rat liver without itself being utilized in the process. In mammals, a complete urea cycle functions only in liver, the major site of urea synthesis. (Some urea cycle enzymes are expressed in the intestine, kidney, and other tissues, where they play a role in the synthesis of citrulline, arginine, and ornithine, as discussed in the preceding text of this chapter.) The urea cycle is shown in Figures 14-10 and 14-17. The pathway begins with the incorporation of ammonia and carbon dioxide into carbamoyl phosphate by the mitochondrial enzyme carbamoyl phosphate synthetase I. The carbamoyl phosphate then combines with ornithine to form citrulline, which exits from the mitochondria in exchange for ornithine (Indiveri et al., 1992) on the ORNT 1 carrier. In the cytosol, argininosuccinate synthetase and argininosuccinate lyase effectively add a nitrogen (from aspartate) to the citrulline to produce arginine. The arginine is then hydrolyzed by arginase, thereby liberating urea and ornithine; ornithine reenters the mitochondria to begin a new cycle.

The urea cycle is subject to both short- and long-term regulation. The first step, catalyzed by carbamoyl phosphate synthetase I, is subject to activation by *N*-acetylglutamate (Watford, 2003); although *N*-acetylglutamate levels always change in parallel with changes in the rate of urea synthesis, *N*-acetylglutamate does not control flux through the cycle. Rather, changes in *N*-acetylglutamate levels allow changes in flux through the cycle to occur at relatively constant ammonia levels. Therefore, increased rates of amino acid catabolism result in increased levels of both ammonia and *N*-acetylglutamate, and the *N*-acetylglutamate stimulates carbamoyl phosphate synthetase I activity to effectively buffer the ammonia levels. With an increase in carbamoyl phosphate synthesis, flux through the rest of the urea cycle also increases because all the subsequent enzymes have K_m values that are below or near the physiological concentrations of their substrates.

Long-term regulation is brought about by adaptive changes in the amounts of urea cycle enzymes. Conditions that result in high rates of urea synthesis (high-protein diets and hypercatabolic states) are accompanied by increases in the activities of all the urea cycle enzymes, whereas conditions that result in low rates of urea synthesis (low-protein diets) result in decreased activities of the urea cycle enzymes. Although the enzymes of the urea cycle appear to be coordinately regulated, the mechanisms involved in regulation of different enzymes vary. Regulation occurs both by changes in the rate of protein degradation and by changes in the rate of enzyme synthesis, with changes in protein synthesis being primarily due to changes in the rate of gene transcription (Takiguchi and Mori, 1995).

In the postabsorptive state, the principal extrahepatic sources of nitrogen used for ureagenesis are glutamine and alanine, which are released by muscle and ammonia from the portal blood. Glutamine is largely taken up by the intestine, and glutamine nitrogen is released back into the portal blood as citrulline, alanine, proline, and ammonia. The ammonia delivered to the liver via the portal blood originates predominately from glutamine catabolism in the small intestinal cells (enterocytes) and from bacterial metabolism of urea in the lumen of the large intestine. It is estimated that nearly 25% of the urea that is synthesized by the liver over the course of a day is broken down to ammonia in the large intestine and returned to the liver as ammonia for reincorporation into urea. Alanine and ammonia are readily removed by the liver. In the fed state, most amino acids that reach the liver can serve as precursors for ureagenesis. For each molecule of urea, one nitrogen is derived from ammonia via the carbamoyl phosphate synthetase I reaction; the second nitrogen is donated to the urea cycle from the α-amino nitrogen of aspartate, with the carbon chain of aspartate being released as fumarate. The immediate sources of hepatic ammonia funneling into the urea cycle have been estimated to include ammonia from the portal blood (33%), glutamine deamidation (6% to 13%), release of α-amino nitrogen from glutamate by the glutamate dehydrogenase–catalyzed reaction, with the amino groups of various amino acids being transferred to glutamate via transamination (20%), and direct catabolism of certain amino acids such as glycine to release ammonia (33% to 40%) (Meijer et al., 1990). A variety of amino acids, especially alanine, contribute amino groups to aspartate (via the coupled activities of alanine or another aminotransferase and aspartate aminotransferase), with glutamate being the direct donor of the amino group to oxaloacetate to form aspartate. These α-amino groups are funneled into the urea cycle to provide the second nitrogen atom for urea synthesis.

EXCRETION OF AMMONIUM BY THE KIDNEY

Ammonia excretion usually is low, because most ammonia is incorporated into urea. However, in metabolic acidosis (resulting from diabetic ketosis, lactic acidosis, or excess protein catabolism), the urinary output of ammonium is increased. The production and excretion of strong acids (such as acetoacetic, β-hydroxybutyric, lactic, and sulfuric acids) requires the co-excretion of a cation. Excretion of ammonia as the cation ammonium (NH_4^+) allows the body to conserve cations such as Na^+, K^+, and Ca^{2+}; facilitates the excretion of excess H^+; and has the net effect of conserving bicarbonate ion (HCO_3^-), which serves as an important buffer. The ammonia that is excreted by the kidney is generated predominantly in the kidney by deamidation of glutamine by glutaminase, followed by deamination of glutamate by glutamate dehydrogenase. The process of acidosis-increased ammonia excretion also is facilitated by net glutamine production by the liver and increased release of glutamine from skeletal muscle during acidosis. A small proportion of ammoniagenesis in the kidney is accomplished by the metabolism of glycine.

NITROGENOUS END PRODUCTS OF PURINE AND PYRIMIDINE CATABOLISM

Purines are present in relatively large amounts in the body because they are present both in nucleic acids and in the form of free adenine and guanine nucleotides (including ATP, ADP, AMP, GTP, NAD, and FAD). Purine degradation results in formation of uric acid rather than urea; uric acid is excreted in the urine. Purine degradation involves the deamination of AMP or adenosine to release ammonia and form inosine. Inosine and guanosine undergo phosphorolysis by purine nucleoside phosphorylase to yield hypoxanthine (from inosine) and guanine (from guanosine). The guanine is deaminated to yield xanthine, and the hypoxanthine is oxidized to xanthine. Finally, xanthine is converted to uric acid by xanthine oxidase. Hence, both ammonia and uric acid result from catabolism of purine bases. Uric acid is not very soluble in water, and deposition of urate in the joints causes gout. Gout usually is treated with the drug allopurinol, which inhibits oxidation of xanthine to uric acid and results in excretion of soluble purine metabolites (hypoxanthine, xanthine, and guanine).

Degradation of pyrimidines results in the release of β-amino acids and ammonia. Cytidine monophosphate (CMP) loses ammonia in its degradation to uridine monophosphate (UMP) or uridine. Degradation of the pyrimidine base, uracil, results in release of ammonia and formation of β-alanine. Degradation of the base of dTMP, thymine, results in the release of ammonia and the formation of β-aminoisobutyrate. The β-amino acids may be excreted in the urine, but further metabolism of these amino acids does occur and the nitrogen from pyrimidine degradation is thought to be excreted largely as urea. β-Aminoisobutyrate is a specific product of thymine catabolism, and the level of β-aminoisobutyrate in urine increases in cancer patients undergoing chemotherapy or radiation therapy due to the increased death of cells and degradation of DNA.

β-Alanine is found in the urine, but it is not a specific product of pyrimidine metabolism because it is also formed from pantothenic acid, carnosine, and other peptides. In comparison with purine degradation, pyrimidine degradation makes a smaller contribution to urinary nitrogen because of the more limited occurrence of pyrimidines in the body (mainly in the nucleic acids) compared with purines.

EXCRETION OF CREATININE

Creatine phosphate is present in muscle cells at a high concentration of approximately 25 mmoles per kg. Both creatine and creatine phosphate undergo spontaneous loss of water and cyclization to creatinine, and this creatinine is excreted from the body in the urine. Approximately 1.7% (~12 mmoles) of the total body creatine is replaced each day by synthesis from glycine, arginine, and *S*-adenosylmethionine. The rate of creatinine formation reflects the amount of creatine/creatine phosphate present in the muscle mass and is relatively constant from day to day in adults who are not losing or gaining muscle mass. Because of this relation, creatinine excretion has been used to estimate the completeness of 24-hour urine collections, as a basis for normalizing urinary concentrations of various metabolites, and to estimate the lean body mass of individuals; the contribution of meat intake to creatinine excretion can limit the usefulness of urinary creatinine for these purposes, however. Because the renal tubules do not reabsorb creatinine, creatinine excretion also can be used to calculate the volume of plasma filtered by the kidneys, which is used as a measure of renal clearance or renal function.

REABSORPTION OF AMINO ACIDS FROM THE RENAL FILTRATE

Amino acids are efficiently reabsorbed from the renal filtrate, and only small amounts are lost in the urine. A few milligrams of nitrogen per day are accounted for by excretion of derivatives of amino acids such as N^3-methylhistidine and hydroxyproline. Trace amounts of a large variety of other compounds also are normal constituents of urine. These include trace amounts of albumin and other proteins, δ-aminolevulinate, porphobilinogen, tryptophan metabolites, and catecholamine catabolites. Together, amino acids, proteins, and miscellaneous nitrogenous metabolites account for approximately 0.3 to 1.0 g of urinary nitrogen per day.

REFERENCES

Adibi SA (2003) Regulation of expression of the intestinal oligopeptide transporter (Pept-1) in health and disease. Am J Physiol 285: G779-G788.

Ballevre O, Houlier M-L, Prugnaud J, Bayle G, Bercovici D, Seve B, Arnal M (1991) Altered partition of threonine metabolism in pigs by protein-free feeding or starvation. Am J Physiol 261:E748-E757.

Battezzati A, Brillon DJ, Matthews DE (1995) Oxidation of glutamic acid by the splanchnic bed in humans. Am J Physiol 269:E269-E276.

Baumgartner MR, Rabier D, Nassogne MC, Dufier JL, Padovani JP, Kamoun P, Valle D, Saudubray JM (2005) Δ^1-pyrrolide-5-carboxylate synthase deficiency neurodegeneration, cataracts and connective tissue manifestations combined with hyperammonaemia and reduced ornithine, citrulline, arginine and proline. Eur J Pediatr 164:31-36.

Beaumier L, Castillo L, Ajamik AM, Young VR (1995) Urea cycle intermediate kinetics and nitrate excretion at normal and "therapeutic" intakes of arginine in humans. Am J Physiol 269:E884-E896.

Bella DL, Stipanuk MH (1995) Effects of protein, methionine, or chloride on acid-base balance and on cysteine catabolism. Am J Physiol 269:E910-E917.

Bergstrom J, Furst P, Noree L-O, Vinnars E (1974) Intracellular free amino acid concentration in human muscle tissue. J Appl Physiol 36:693-697.

Bird MI, Nunn PB, Lord LAJ (1984) Formation of glycine and aminoacetone from L-threonine by rat liver mitochondria. Biochim Biophys Acta 802:229-236.

Boehning D, Snyder SH (2003) Novel neural modulators. Annu Rev Neurosci 26:105-131.

Broquist HP (1990) Lysine-pipecolic acid metabolic relationships in microbes and mammals. Annu Rev Nutr 11:435-448.

Carey GP, Kime Z, Rogers QR, Morris JG, Hargrove D, Buffington CA, Brusilow SW (1987) An arginine-deficient diet in humans does not evoke hyperammonemia or orotic aciduria. J Nutr 117:1734-1739.

Castillo L, Sanchez M, Chapman TE, Ajami A, Burke JF, Young VR (1994) The plasma flux and oxidation rate of ornithine adaptively decline with restricted arginine intake. Proc Natl Acad Sci USA 91:6393-6397.

Chen H, Pan YX, Dudenhausen EE, Kilberg MS (2004) Amino acid deprivation induces the transcription rate of the human asparagine synthetase gene through a timed program of expression and promoter binding of nutrient-responsive basic region/leucine zipper transcription factors as well as localized histone acetylation. J Biol Chem 279:50829-50839.

Cho ES, Anderson HL, Wixom RL, Hanson KC, Krause GF (1984) Long-term effects of low histidine intake on men. J Nutr 114:369-384.

Christensen H (1990) Role of amino acid transport and countertransport in nutrition and metabolism. Physiol Rev 70:43-77.

Chuang JL, Wynn RM, Moss CC, Song J, Li J, Awad N, Mandel H, Chuang DT (2004) Structural and biochemical basis for novel mutations in homozygous Israeli maple syrup urine disease patients. J Biol Chem 279:17792-17800.

Clarke JTR, Bier DM (1982) The conversion of phenylalanine to tyrosine in man. Direct measurement by continuous intravenous tracer infusions of L-[ring-$^2H_5$]phenylalanine and L-[1-^{13}C]tyrosine in the postabsorptive state. Metabolism 31:999-1005.

Cowan GJ, Willgoss DA, Bartley J, Endre ZH (1996) Serine isotopomer analysis by ^{13}C-NMR defines glycine-serine interconversion in situ in the renal proximal tubule. Biochim Biophys Acta 1310:32-40.

Curthoys NP, Watford M (1995) Regulation of glutaminase activity and glutamine metabolism. Annu Rev Nutr 15:133-159.

Cynober L, Le Boucher J, Vasdson M-P (1995) Arginine metabolism in mammals. J Nutr Biochem 6:402-413.

D'Aniello A, Vetere A, Petrucelli L (1993) Further study on the specificity of D-amino acid oxidase and of D-aspartate oxidase and time course for complete oxidation of D-amino acids. Comp Biochem Physiol 105B:731-734.

Darling P, Rafii M, Grunow J, Ball RO, Brookes S, Pencharz PB (1997) Threonine dehydrogenase is not the major pathway of threonine catabolism in adult humans. FASEB J 11:A149.

Darmaun D, Dechelotte P (1991) Role of leucine as a precursor of glutamine α-amino nitrogen in vivo in humans. Am J Physiol 260:E326-329.

DeLeve LD, Kaplowitz N (1991) Glutathione metabolism and its role in hepatotoxicity. Pharmacol Ther 52:287-305.

De Miranda J, Santoro A, Gngelender S, Wolosker H (2000) Human serine racemase: molecular cloning, genomic organization and functional analysis. Gene 256:183-188.

De Morais SMF, Uetrecht JP, Wells PG (1992) Decreased glucuronidation and increased bioactivation of acetaminophen in Gilbert's syndrome. Gastroenterology 102:577-586.

Divry P, Vianey-Liaud C, Mathieu M (1991) Inborn errors of lysine metabolism. Ann Biol Clin 49:27-35.

Dix TA, Kuhn DM, Benkovic SJ (1987) Mechanism of oxygen activation by tyrosine hydroxylase. Biochemistry 26:3354-3361.

Dominy JE, Stipanuk MH (2004) New roles for cysteine and transsulfuration enzymes: production of H2S, a neuromodulator and smooth muscle relaxant. Nutr Rev 62:348-353.

Doskeland AP, Martinez A, Knappskog PM, Flatmark T (1996) Phosphorylation of recombinant human phenylalanine hydroxylase: effect on catalytic activity, substrate activation and protection against non-specific cleavage of the fusion protein by restriction protease. Biochem J 313:409-414.

Eisenhofer G, Tian H, Holmes C, Matsunaga J, Roffler-Tarlov S, Hearing VJ (2003) Tyrosinase: a developmentally specific major determinant of peripheral dopamine. FASEB J 17:1248-1255.

Elia M (1993) Glutamine metabolism in human adipose tissue in vivo. Clin Nutr 12:51-53.

Elia M, Livesey G (1983) Effects of ingested steak and infused leucine on forelimb metabolism in man and the fate of the carbon skeletons and amino groups of branched-chain amino acids. Sci Lond 64:517-526.

Erlandsen H, Patch MG, Gamez A, Straub M, Stevens RC (2003) Structural studies on phenylalanine hydroxylase and implications toward understanding and treating phenylketonuria. Pediatrics 112:1557-1565.

Ewart HS, Jois M, Brosnan JT (1992) Rapid stimulation of the hepatic glycine-cleavage system in rats fed on a single high-protein meal. Biochem J 283:441-447.

Felig P (1975) Amino acid metabolism in man. Annu Rev Nutr 44:933-955.

Felig P, Wahren J, Raf L (1973) Evidence of interorgan amino acid transport by blood cells in man. Proc Natl Acad Sci USA 70:1775-1779.

Fernandez J, Lopez AB, Wang C, Mishra R, Zhou L, Yaman I, Snider MD, Hatzolgou M (2003) Transcriptional control of the arginine/lysine transporter, Cat-1, by physiological stress. J Biol Chem 278:50000-50009.

Fukagawa NK, Ajami AM, Young VR (1996) Plasma methionine and cysteine kinetics in response to an intravenous glutathione infusion in adult humans. Am J Physiol 270:E209-E214.

Gibson KM, Lee CF, Hoffmann GF (1994) Screening for defects of branched-chain amino acid metabolism. Eur J Pediatr 153:S62-S67.

Girgis S, Nasrallah IM, Suh JR, Oppenheim E, Zanetti KA, Mastri MG, Stover PJ (1998) Molecular cloning, characterization and alternative splicing of the human cytoplasmic serine hydroxymethyltransferase gene. Gene 210:315-324.

Grillo MA, Colombatto S (2004) Arginine revisited: mini review article. Amino Acids 26:345-351.

Guba SC, Fink LM, Fonseca V (1996) Hyperhomocysteinemia: an emerging and important risk factor for thromboembolic and cardiovascular disease. Am J Clin Pathol 105:709-722.

Harris RA, Joshi M, Jeoung NH (2004) Mechanisms responsible for regulation of branched-chain amino acid catabolism. Biochem Biophys Res Comm 313:391-396.

Hediger MA, Romero MF, Peng J-B, Rolfs A, Takanaga H, Bruford EA (2004) The ABCs of solute carriers: physiological, pathological and therapeutic implications of human membrane transport proteins. Pflugers Arch Eur J Physiol 447:465-468.

Hyde R, Taylor PM, Hundal HS (2003) Amino acid transporters: roles in amino acid sensing and signaling in animal cells. Biochem J 373:1-18.

Huxtable RJ (1992) Physiological actions of taurine. Physiol Rev 72:101-163.

Ikeda M, Tsuji H, Nakamura S, Ichiyama A, Nishizuka Y, Hayaishi O (1965) Studies on the biosynthesis of nicotinamide adenine dinucleotide. J Biol Chem 240:1395-1401.

Indiveri C, Tonazzi A, Palmieri F (1992) Identification and purification of the ornithine/citrulline carrier from rat liver mitochondria. Eur J Biochem 207:449-454.

Jungas RL, Halperin ML, Brosnan JT (1992) Quantitative analysis of amino acid oxidation and related gluconeogenesis in humans. Physiol Rev 72:419-448.

Kaufman S (1993) The phenylalanine hydroxylating system. Adv Enzymol Relat Areas Mol Biol 67:77-264.

Knappskog PM, Flatmark T, Aarden JM, Haavik J, Martinez A (1996) Structure-function relationships in human phenylalanine hydroxylase. Effect of terminal deletions on the oligomerization, activation and cooperativity of substrate binding to the enzyme. Eur J Biochem 242:813-821.

Kriengsinyos W, Rafii M, Wykes LJ, Ball RO, Pencharz PB (2002) Long-term effects of histidine depletion on whole-body protein metabolism in healthy adults. J Nutr 132:3340-3348.

Lam WK, Cleary MA, Wraith JE, Walter JH (1996) Histidinaemia: a benign metabolic disorder. Arch Dis Child 74:343-346.

Leklem JE (1971) Quantitative aspects of tryptophan metabolism in humans and other species: a review. Am J Clin Nutr 24:659-672.

Lowenstein JM (1972) Ammonia production in muscle and other tissues: the purine nucleotide cycle. Physiol Rev 52:383-414.

Lowry M, Hall DE, Brosnan JT (1985) Increased activity of renal glycine-cleavage-enzyme complex in metabolic acidosis. Biochem J 231:477-480.

MacFarlane N, McMurray J, O'Dowd JJ, Dargie HJ, Miller DJ (1991) Synergism of histidyl dipeptides as antioxidants. J Mol Cell Cardiol 23:1205-1208.

Maes M, Verkerk R, Bonaccorso S, Ombelet W, Bosmans E, Sharpe S (2002) Depressive and anxiety symptoms in the early puerperium are related to increased degradation of tryptophan into kynurenine, a phenomenon which is related to immune activation. Life Sci 71:1837-1848.

McKinney J, Teigen K, Froystein NA, Salaun C, Knappskog PM, Haavik J, Martinez A (2001) Conformation of the substrate and pterin cofactor bound to human tryptophan hydroxylase Biochemistry 40:15591-15601.

Meijer AJ, Lamers WH, Chamuleau RAFM (1990) Nitrogen metabolism and ornithine cycle function. Physiol Rev 70:701-749.

Morris SM Jr (2004) Enzymes of arginine metabolism. J Nutr 134:2743S-2747S.

Nurjhan N, Bucci A, Stumvoll M, Bailey G, Bier DM, Toft I, Jenssen TG, Gerich JE (1995) Glutamine: a major gluconeogenic precursor and vehicle for interorgan carbon transport in man. J Clin Invest 95:272-277.

Ogawa H, Gomi T, Konishi K, Date T, Nakashima H, Nose K, Matsuda Y, Peraino C, Pitot HC, Fujioka M (1989) Human liver serine dehydratase: cDNA cloning and sequence homology with hydroxyamino acid dehydratases from other sources. J Biol Chem 264:15818-15823.

Palii SS, Chen H, Kilberg MS (2004) Transcriptional control of the human sodium-coupled neutral amino acid transporter system A gene by amino acid availability is mediated by an intronic element. J Biol Chem 279:3463-3471.

Pantuck EJ, Pantuck CB, Kappas A, Conney A, Anderson KE (1991) Effects of protein and carbohydrate content of diet on drug conjugation. Clin Pharmacol Ther 50:254-258.

Parsons HG, Carter RJ, Unrath M, Snyder FF (1990) Evaluation of branched-chain amino acid intake in children with maple syrup urine disease and methylmalonic aciduria. J Inherit Metab Dis 13:125-136.

Paxton R, Scislowski PWD, Davis EJ, Harris RA (1986) Role of branched-chain 2-oxo acid dehydrogenase and pyruvate dehydrogenase in 2-oxobutyrate metabolism. Biochem J 234:295-303.

Pegg AE, Poulin R, Coward JK (1995) Use of aminopropyltransferase inhibitors and of non-metabolizable analogs to study polyamine regulation and function. Int J Biochem Cell Biol 27:425-442.

Peters JC (1991) Tryptophan nutrition and metabolism: an overview. In: Schwarcz R., Young SN, Brown RR (eds) Kynurenine and Serotonin Pathways. Plenum Press, New York, pp 345-358.

Pinsonneault JK, Nielsen CU, Sadee W (2004) Genetic variants of the humans H^+/dipeptide transporter PEPT2: analysis of haplotype functions. J Pharmacol Exp Ther 311:1088-1096.

Rabier D, Kamoun P (1995) Metabolism of citrulline in man. Amino Acids 9:209-316.

Rabier D, Narcy C, Bardet J, Parvy P, Saudubray JM, Kamoun P (1991) Arginine remains an essential amino acid after liver transplantation in urea cycle enzyme deficiencies. J Inherit Metab Dis 14:277-280.

Rebouche CJ (1988) Carnitine metabolism and human nutrition. J Appl Nutr 40:99-111.

Reeds PJ, Burrin DG (2001) Glutamine and the bowel. J Nutr 131:2505S-2508S.

Robinson K, Mayer E, Jacobsen DW (1994) Homocysteine and coronary artery disease. Cleve Clin J Med 61:438-450.

Sacksteder KA, Biery BJ, Morrell JC, Goodman BK, Geisbrecht BV, Cox RP, Gould SJ, Geraghty MT (2000) Identification of the alpha-aminoadipic semialdehyde synthase gene, which is defective in familial hyperlysinemia. Am J Hum Genet 66:1736-1743.

Sato H, Nomura S, Maebara K, Sato K, Tamba M, Bannai S (2004) Transcriptional control of cystine/glutamate transporter gene by amino acid deprivation. Biochem Biophys Res Commun 325:109-116.

Satriano J (2004) Arginine pathways and the inflammatory response: interregulation of nitric oxide and polyamines. Amino Acids 4:321-329.

Satriano J (2003) Agmatine: at the crossroads of the arginine pathways. Ann N Y Acad Sci 1009:34-43.

Scislowski PWD, Foster AR, Fuller MF (1994) Regulation of oxidative degradation of L-lysine in rat liver mitochondria. Biochem J 300:887-891.

Stipanuk MH (1986) Metabolism of sulfur-containing amino acids. Annu Rev Nutr 6:179-209.

Stipanuk MH (2004) Sulfur Amino Acid metabolism: pathways for production and removal of homocysteine and cysteine. Annu Rev Nutr 24:539-577.

Stipanuk MH, Beck PW (1982) Characterization of the enzymic capacity for cysteine desulphydration in liver and kidney of the rat. Biochem J 206:267-277.

Storch KJ, Wagner DA, Burke JF, Young VR (1990) [$1\text{-}^{13}C$;*methyl*-$^2H_3$]methionine kinetics in humans: methionine conservation and cystine sparing. Am J Physiol 258:E790-E798.

Suryawan A, Hawes JW, Harris RA, Shimomura Y, Jenkins AE, Hutson SM (1998) A molecular model of human branched-chain amino acid metabolism. Am J Clin Nutr 68:72-81.

Takiguchi M, Mori M (1995) Transcriptional regulation of genes for ornithine cycle enzymes. Biochem J 312:649-659.

Takikawa O, Littlejohn TK, Truscott RJW (2001) Indoleamine 2,3-dioxygenase in the human lens, the first enzyme in the synthesis of UV filters. Exp Eye Res 72:271-277.

Taniguchi K, Nonami T, Nakao A, Harada A, Kurokawa T, Sugiyama S, Fujitsuka N, Shimomura Y, Hutson SM, Harris RA, Takagi H (1996) The valine catabolic pathway in human liver: effect of cirrhosis on enzyme activities. Hepatology 24:1395-1398.

Tizianello A, Deferrari G, Garibotto G, Robaudod C, Acquarone N, Ghiggeri GM (1982) Renal ammoniagenesis in an early stage of metabolic acidosis in man. J Clin Invest 69:240-250.

Torres N, Martinez L, Aleman G, Bourges H, Tovar AR (1998) Histidase expression is regulated by dietary protein at the pretranslational level in rat liver. J Nutr 128:818-824.

Tovar AR, Ascencio C, Torres N (2002) Soy protein, casein, and zein regulate histidase gene expression by modulating serum glucagons. Am J Physiol Endocrinol Metab 283:E1016-E1022.

Van De Kamp JL, Smolen A (1995) Response of kynurenine pathway enzymes to pregnancy and dietary level of vitamin B-6. Pharmacol Biochem Behav 51:753-758.

Vianey-Liaud C, Divry P, Poinas C, Mathieu M (1991) Lysine metabolism in man. Ann Biol Clin 49:18-26.

Watford M (1994) Glutamine metabolism in rat small intestine: Synthesis of three-carbon products in isolated enterocytes. Biochim Biophys Acta 1200:73-78.

Watford M (2000) Glutamine and glutamate metabolism across the liver sinusoid. J Nutr 130:983S-987S.

Watford M (2003) The urea cycle. Biochem Mol Biol Ed 31:289-297.

White AC, Thannickal VJ, Fanburg BL (1994) Glutathione deficiency in human disease. J Nutr Biochem 5:218-226.

Wilkinson DL, Bertolo RF, Brunton JA, Shoveller AK, Pencharz PB, Ball RO (2004) Arginine synthesis is regulated by dietary arginine intake in the enterally fed neonatal piglet. Am J Physiol Endocrinol Metab 287:E454-E462.

Wirleitner B, Neurauter G, Schrocksnadel K, Frick B, Fuchs D (2003) Interferon-gamma-induced conversion of tryptophan: immunologic and neuropsychiatric aspects. Curr Med Chem 10:1581-1591.

Wu G, Jaeger LA, Bazer FW, Rhoads JM (2004) Arginine deficiency in preterm infants: biochemical mechanisms and nutritional implications. J Nutr Biochem 15:442-451.

Xue HH, Sakaguchi T, Fujie M, Ogawa H, Ichiyama A (1999) Flux of the L-serine metabolism in rabbit, human, and dog livers. J Biol Chem 274:16028-16033.

Yang RD, Matthews DE, Bier DM, Wen ZM, Young VR (1986) Response of alanine metabolism in humans to manipulation of dietary protein and energy intakes. Am J Physiol 250:E39-E46.

Yannicelli S, Rohr F, Warman ML (1994) Nutrition support for glutaric acidemia type I. J Am Diet Assoc 94:183-191.

Zimmerman HJ, Maddrey WC (1955) Acetaminophen (paracetamol) hepatotoxicity with regular intake of alcohol: Analysis of instances of therapeutic misadventure. Hepatology 22:767-773.

RECOMMENDED READINGS

Jungas RL, Halperin ML, Brosnan JT (1992) Quantitative analysis of amino acid oxidation and related gluconeogenesis in humans. Physiol Rev 72:419-448.

Morris SM Jr (2002) Regulation of enzymes of the urea cycle and arginine metabolism. Annu Rev Nutr 22:87-105.

Stipanuk MH (2004) Sulfur amino acid metabolism: pathways for production and removal of homocysteine and cysteine. Annu Rev Nutr 24:539-577.

Watford M (2003) The urea cycle. Biochem Mol Biol Ed 31:289-297.

Chapter 15

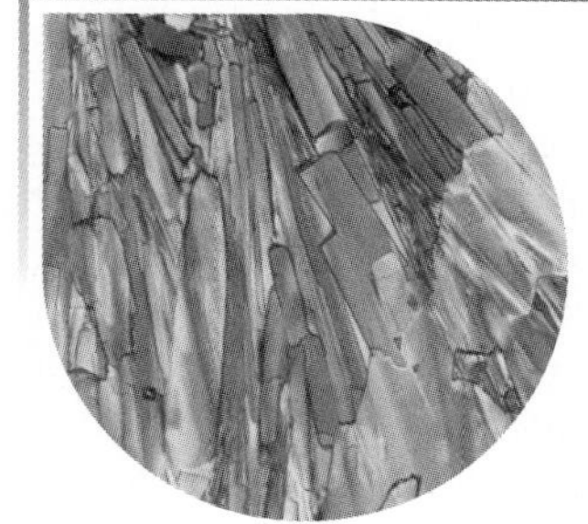

Protein and Amino Acid Requirements

Martha H. Stipanuk, PhD

OUTLINE

COMMON ABBREVIATIONS

BV	biological value
NPU	net protein utilization
PER	protein efficiency ratio
PDCAAS	protein digestibility corrected amino acid score
PEM	protein energy malnutrition
P/E ratio	energy from protein/total energy in diet, expressed as fraction or percentage

This chapter is a revision of the chapter contributed by Macolm F. Fuller, PhD, for the first edition.

PHYSIOLOGICAL BASIS OF PROTEIN AND AMINO ACID REQUIREMENTS

In the early part of the nineteenth century, it was discovered that protein (or a substance containing nitrogen) was required in the diet, but it was more than a century later (the 1930s) before all the constituent amino acids were identified and work could begin on assessing human requirements for these nutrients. Because adults are such a large proportion of the total human population, it is appropriate that most efforts have been directed toward establishing the requirements of this population, although the special needs of infants and children have also received attention.

DISPENSABLE AND INDISPENSABLE AMINO ACIDS

It is normally considered that the dietary requirement for protein represents only the need for the amino acids that constitute it. By convention, the 20 amino acids required for protein synthesis have been divided into two categories: (1) indispensable (or essential) and (2) dispensable (or nonessential). The term dispensable is preferred by some nutritionists instead of the term nonessential because all the amino acids found in protein are metabolically essential, even though some are dispensable in the diet. Borman and colleagues (1946) defined an indispensable amino acid as, "one which cannot be synthesized by the animal organism, out of materials ordinarily available to the cells, at a speed commensurate with the demands for normal growth" (p. 593). Nine amino acids are clearly indispensable for humans, who do not possess the pathways for their synthesis from compounds ordinarily available to cells. These indispensable amino acids are histidine, isoleucine, leucine, lysine, methionine, phenylalanine, threonine, tryptophan, and valine.

The other eleven amino acids (alanine, arginine, asparagine, aspartate, cysteine, glutamate, glutamine, glycine, proline, serine, and tyrosine) can be synthesized by cells from materials ordinarily available to the cells. It should be noted, however, that, although the carbon skeletons of these dispensable amino acids can be synthesized de novo, the amino groups for their synthesis are derived from other amino acids via transamination reactions. Thus, the total supply of amino acids also is an important dietary consideration. The extent of synthesis of some of these amino acids may depend upon the dietary supply of particular precursors or the biosynthetic capacity of the organism. In addition, the metabolic demand for an amino acid may be increased or the capacity to synthesize an amino acid may be decreased in instances of injury, disease, or parenteral nutrition, thereby affecting an individual's dietary need for that amino acid. These factors have led to subclassifications of the dispensable amino acids and the use of the terms semi-essential, conditionally indispensable, and truly dispensable (Reeds, 2000; Institute of Medicine [IOM], 2002). Only alanine, aspartate, asparagine, glutamate, and serine are classified as truly dispensable.

Cysteine, or its disulfide cystine, and tyrosine are considered semi-essential (or semi-indispensable) because their synthesis depends upon an adequate dietary supply of an indispensable amino acid precursor. Cysteine can be synthesized in the body from serine and the sulfur group of methionine. Tyrosine can be formed in the body by the hydroxylation of phenylalanine. Both of these syntheses are irreversible. This means that, whereas a lack of tyrosine in the diet can be compensated by an excess of phenylalanine, the reverse is not true: no matter how much tyrosine is provided by the diet, tyrosine cannot compensate for a deficiency of phenylalanine. Likewise, methionine cannot be synthesized from cyst(e)ine. Each of these semiessential amino acids must be considered along with its indispensable amino acid precursor when evaluating indispensable amino acid intake for adequacy; both the sum and the proportion of methionine and cyst(e)ine or of phenylalanine and tyrosine must be taken into account.

Other dispensable amino acids are considered to be conditionally indispensable from a dietary viewpoint because the rate at which they are provided by endogenous synthesis may fall below the rate at which they are utilized. Arginine, proline, glutamine, and glycine are classified as conditionally indispensable; their synthesis is dependent upon the provision of dispensable amino acid precursors. Arginine, proline, and glutamine synthesis requires the glutamate skeleton as a precursor, and synthesis of arginine requires additional nitrogen donated via carbamoyl phosphate and aspartate. Glycine synthesis is dependent upon serine or choline as a precursor. The synthesis of both arginine and proline appears to be dependent upon intestinal metabolism of dietary glutamate, such that alterations in either intestinal metabolism or the route of nutrition can significantly affect dietary requirements (Brunton et al., 1999). In some circumstances, when the requirement is particularly high, the rate of endogenous production may be less than the rate of utilization; this appears to particularly be the case for glycine during recovery (catch-up growth) from severe childhood malnutrition (Badaloo et al., 1999). There are suggestions that glycine may similarly behave as an indispensable amino acid in infants (especially premature infants), who have a limited capacity for glycine synthesis and who are usually fed milk, which is low in glycine (Jackson et al., 1981). Therefore, an amino acid cannot be classified as dispensable solely because a pathway for its synthesis exists; whether it behaves as a dispensable or an indispensable amino acid depends on the functional state of that pathway relative to the rate of metabolic utilization of the product.

NEEDS FOR DIETARY AMINO ACIDS TO REPLACE LOSSES AND TO ALLOW FOR GROWTH

Amino acids are used for a great variety of functions in the body, as discussed in Chapters 13 and 14. Both dispensable and indispensable amino acids are required for the synthesis of protein; as intermediates in various pathways of metabolism, including the transport of nitrogen between organs; and for synthesis of numerous nonprotein compounds that require amino acids as precursors. The requirements for indispensable amino acids and total amino acid nitrogen are basically a requirement for net tissue accretion (during growth, pregnancy, and lactation) and for maintenance or replacement of obligatory losses. The major routes of obligatory amino acid or protein loss are by irreversible modification (see Chapters 5 and 13), loss of proteins through the epithelia, loss of amino acids in the urine, use of amino acids for synthesis of nonprotein substances (see Chapter 14), and oxidation of amino acids as fuels (see Chapter 14).

As discussed in Chapter 13, the rate of utilization of amino acids for protein synthesis usually accounts for several-fold the daily intake, with a significant rate of amino acid reutilization. During growth and in pregnancy, when protein synthesis is greater than protein degradation, the use of amino acids for body protein accretion is a major component of requirements. Likewise, in lactation, the needs of the mammary gland for milk protein synthesis become a large component of requirements. However, when there is no change in body protein mass, protein synthesis does not in and of itself result in much net disposal of amino acids because the concomitant process of protein degradation returns amino acids almost entirely to the free pool. Nevertheless, protein turnover in the adult does result in some irreversible loss of amino acids. Some amino acids, after they are incorporated into proteins, are irreversibly modified by processes such as methylation (methylhistidine, methyllysine) or hydroxylation (hydroxylysine, hydroxyproline); these modified amino acids cannot be reutilized for protein synthesis and are excreted in the urine.

Protein and amino acid losses also occur via integumental losses and miscellaneous secretions and via the gastrointestinal tract. Integumental and miscellaneous losses together account for a protein loss of approximately 0.03 g/kg/day (or ~2 g/day for an adult). Dermal losses of protein include the keratins of skin, hair, and nails. Because keratins are very rich in cystine, these losses may account for approximately 5% of the methionine and cyst(e)ine requirements for maintenance. Additional and highly variable quantities of nitrogen are lost in sweat; loss of nitrogen in sweat is particularly significant for individuals living in tropical climates. Although the loss of nitrogen in sweat is mainly urea and represents little loss of amino acids per se, it does represent a loss of nitrogen from amino acid catabolism that must be accounted for in nitrogen balance studies. Miscellaneous losses of protein include minor routes of nitrogen loss such as sputum, nasal fluids, menstrual fluids, seminal fluids, and ammonia in the breath. Loss of protein via the gastrointestinal tract is substantially greater than that lost via integumental and miscellaneous routes. Proteins, including mucins and digestive enzymes, are continuously secreted into the gastrointestinal tract via salivary, gastric, pancreatic, hepatic (bile), and intestinal secretions. Furthermore, the enterocytes, which form the gastrointestinal epithelium, are themselves continuously shed from the villi. Although much of the protein passing into the gastrointestinal tract from these sources is itself digested, with the resulting amino acids and small peptides being reabsorbed, a substantial amount, especially of mucins and other proteins that are inherently resistant to proteolysis, escapes digestion, and the nitrogen is excreted in the feces.

Those incompletely digested proteins that pass into the large intestine may be utilized by the gastrointestinal microflora, and a large proportion of this nitrogen is voided in the microbial biomass of the feces. There is experimental evidence, mainly from animal studies, that little absorption of amino acids occurs in the large intestine. There is, however, substantial absorption of nitrogen from the large intestine, most of it as ammonia and much of it originating from hydrolysis of urea secreted into the gastrointestinal tract. Measurement of amino acid losses in ileostomy fluid when subjects were given protein-free diets suggested that losses of nitrogen via the gastrointestinal tract may account for approximately 10% to 15% of maintenance requirements for most indispensable amino acids and an even greater percentage (~25%) of the requirement for threonine (Fuller et al., 1994).

Small amounts of amino acids and an even smaller amount of protein is lost in the urine. The highly efficient reabsorption of nutrients by the kidneys means that losses of amino acids through urine are small: for most amino acids, urinary excretion accounts for less than 5% of total requirements, although some derivatized amino acids such as *N*-methylhistidine and hydroxyproline are essentially quantitatively excreted.

Amino acids, both dispensable and indispensable, are precursors or donors of essential groups for the synthesis of many essential substances such as hormones, neurotransmitters, pyrimidines, and purines. Although the amounts of amino acids that are used over the course of a day for synthesis of nonprotein compounds are generally much less than the amounts used for protein synthesis, the irreversible disposal of amino acids into the various nonprotein synthetic pathways accounts for a small but significant proportion of the requirements for indispensable amino acids and amino acid nitrogen. The rates at which amino acids are consumed for these nonprotein purposes depend, to some extent, on the turnover rate of the pools of the individual compounds and on net tissue accretion. For example, the amount of glycine required for synthesis of creatine and other nonprotein compounds or the amount of lysine used for synthesis of carnitine may impact nutritional requirements under some circumstances.

Whether nitrogen intake is large or small, the major loss of amino acids is due to oxidation or catabolism. Amino acid catabolism is usually assessed by measuring the amount of nitrogen (mainly urea) excreted in the urine. Replacement of obligatory losses due to oxidation or catabolism of amino acids is the largest single component of maintenance requirements. The rate of amino acid oxidation is modulated so as to dispose of amino acids in excess of needs for maintenance and growth—not only preventing their potentially toxic accumulation, but also converting them into energy-yielding substrates (see Chapter 14, Fig. 14-9). This control is exercised partly as a direct response to alterations in plasma or intracellular amino acid concentrations and partly by activation or induction (or both) of the relevant oxidative enzymes. When the dietary intake is less than the requirement, oxidation is suppressed to conserve the limited supply. However, oxidation is not shut down completely and the residual rate of oxidation, although small compared with the rate in normal diets, is nevertheless the major route of obligatory loss. Minimum rates of oxidation have been measured directly for only a few amino acids, but the overall obligatory loss of amino acids due to oxidation can be estimated from the urinary excretion of the nitrogenous byproducts of amino acid catabolism (urea and ammonium) by subjects adapted to protein-free diets. The collective needs for replacement of nitrogen losses are normally estimated for protein rather than for individual amino acids because nitrogen losses (mainly as urea) cannot be related directly to the catabolism or loss of specific amino acids.

MAINTENANCE REQUIREMENTS

All individuals require amino acids for maintenance, simply to replace inevitable losses due to irreversible modification, loss of proteins through the epithelia, loss of amino acids in the urine, use of amino acids for synthesis of nonprotein substances, and oxidation of amino acids as fuels. The obligatory loss of an amino acid is the sum of the losses by all routes, and the maintenance requirement is the dietary intake needed to replace this obligatory loss. The association between obligatory nitrogen losses of individuals adapted to protein-free diets and the magnitude of the negative nitrogen balance experienced by these subjects is illustrated in Table 15-1.

In the context of protein metabolism, maintenance is the condition in which there is no change in the amino acid content of the body; this is usually considered to occur at nitrogen equilibrium. In this condition, the dietary intake of every amino acid is exactly balanced by losses in digestion, secretion, and metabolism. Because dietary intake can vary enormously, it is obvious that the body has mechanisms to adjust the rate of amino acid disposal according to the supply, the major mechanism being the modulation of amino acid oxidation. This adaptive component changes only slowly with a sustained change in intake, as illustrated by the pattern of urinary nitrogen excretion by subjects switched from a diet containing adequate protein to one providing only a minimal level of protein; an example is shown in Figure 15-1. Because the body can maintain nitrogen equilibrium over a wide range of intakes, the protein or amino acid "requirement" is usually defined as the minimum intake consistent with nitrogen equilibrium. Furthermore, a period of adaptation to the test diet is essential for studies of minimal protein requirements.

The following equations apply to an individual in nitrogen (N) equilibrium or zero N balance:

- Supply of amino acid N to free amino acid pool = Removal of amino acid N from free amino acid pool
- Amino acid N intake + Amino acid N from endogenous protein degradation = Amino acid N used for protein synthesis + Amino acid N liberated by endogenous protein degradation
- N balance = Amino acid N intake − Nitrogen loss or excretion = Amino acid N used for protein synthesis − Amino acid N liberated by endogenous protein degradation = 0

The efficiency with which absorbed amino acids are used for either body protein accretion

Table 15-1
Obligatory Nitrogen Losses in Healthy Adults on Protein-Free Diets

	Nitrogen (mg/kg/day)	Protein (g/kg/day)	Protein (g/day for 70-kg adult man)
Urinary N	32	0.2	14
Fecal N	11	0.07	4.9
Integumental and miscellaneous losses of N	5	0.03	2.1
Sum of obligatory losses	**48**	**0.3**	**21**
N balance of adults consuming ≤5 mg/kg/day/	−48	−0.3	−21

Based on data summarized by Rand WM, Pellett PL, Young VR (2003) Meta-analysis of nitrogen balance studies for estimating protein requirements in healthy adults. Am J Clin Nutr 77:109-127.

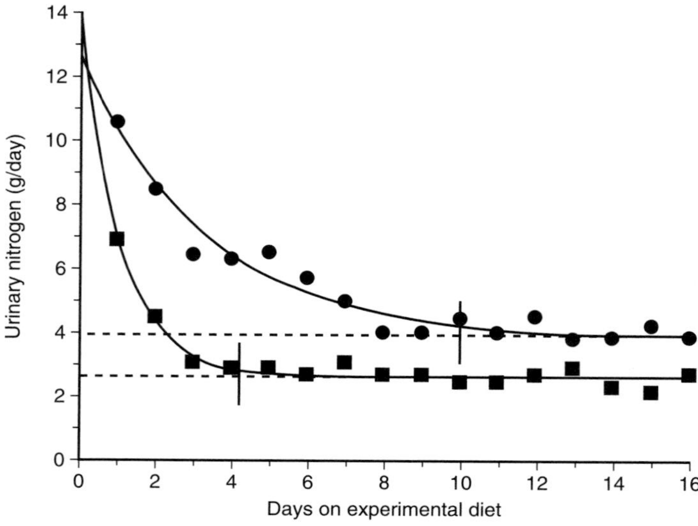

Figure 15-1 Time course of changes in the urinary nitrogen (N) excretion of two subjects (■;●) on changing, at day 0, from a high to a minimal level of protein intake. The vertical lines at 4.2 and 10.0 days represent the time to reach a new plateau or stable rate of urinary N excretion. *Data from Rand WM, Young VR, Scrimshaw NS (1976) Change of urinary nitrogen excretion in response to low-protein diets in adults. Am J Clin Nutr 29:639-644.*

or maintenance is not complete. The overall efficiencies of protein utilization that were estimated from nitrogen balance experiments summarized by Rand and colleagues (2003), and used by the Institute of Medicine (IOM) in establishing the current dietary reference intakes (DRIs) for protein and amino acids, were 58% for children up to age 13 years and 47% for adults (IOM, 2002). Therefore, a dietary intake of 1.7 g (1/0.58) or 2.13 g (1/0.47) of protein or amino acid is needed to retain 1 g of protein or amino acid in children or adults, respectively. Likewise, the obligatory loss of protein on a protein-free diet (0.3 g/kg/day), as shown in Table 15-1, is less than the amount of protein required to maintain zero balance in adults (estimated average requirement [EAR] = 0.66 g/kg/day).

Rand and colleagues (2003) used a linear model to interpret nitrogen balance data or graphs of N intake (x) versus N balance (y), such that the y-intercept represents the obligatory nitrogen loss on a protein-free diet (N intake = 0), with the overall slope representing the efficiency of dietary protein utilization (units N balance/units N intake). In reality, nitrogen balance curves tend to be nonlinear, with steeper slopes (i.e., higher efficiency of dietary N utilization) at submaintenance intakes and shallower slopes (i.e., lower efficiency of dietary N utilization) at intakes near the maintenance level or at supramaintenance levels, as illustrated in Figure 15-2. The slope or efficiency derived by linear regression will actually be an average of several slopes or efficiencies. The rate of free amino acid oxidation will be lowest in subjects fed submaintenance amounts and highest in subjects fed supramaintenance amounts of protein.

REQUIREMENTS FOR BODY PROTEIN ACCRETION AND FOR MILK PROTEIN SECRETION

In addition to their maintenance needs, children require additional quantities of amino acids for the growth of their body protein mass. During the first months of life, an infant's requirement for growth exceeds the infant's requirement for maintenance, and protein accretion still represents a relatively large proportion (~37%) of the total protein need of infants at 7 to 12 months. The proportion of the total requirement due to growth decreases with age to approximately 20% at

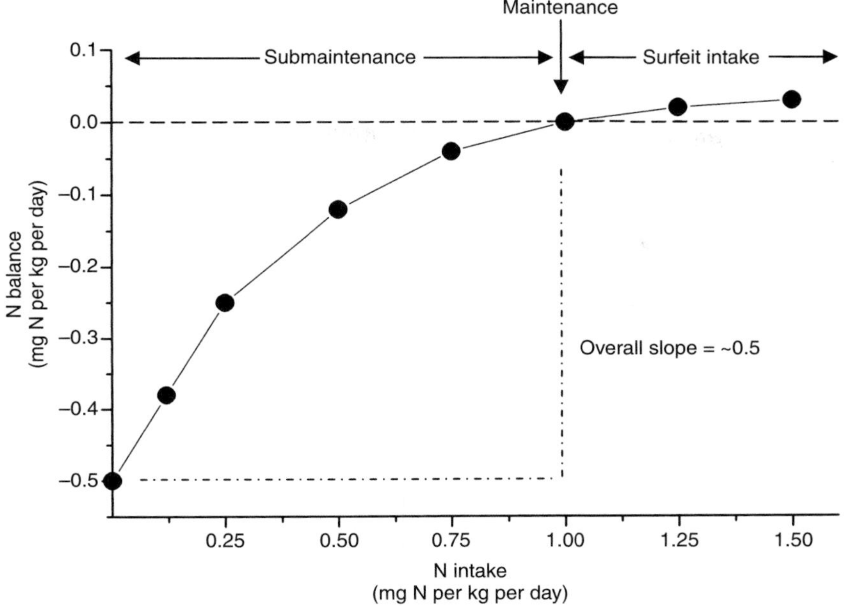

Figure 15-2 Schematic representation of the change in efficiency of dietary nitrogen (N) retention with changes in the submaintenance and surfeit ranges of N (protein) intake. The slope of the N balance curve ($\Delta y/\Delta x$) gives the efficiency of dietary protein utilization. The y-axis intercept can be taken to represent the obligatory N loss on a protein-free diet. The N intake (x-axis value) that gives an N balance of zero ($y = 0$) is taken as the maintenance requirement.

Nutrition Insight

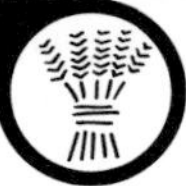

Does Muscular Work Require the Breakdown of Muscle Protein for Fuel?

Justus Liebig, in his influential *Animal Chemistry* published in 1840, stated that protein broke down during the release of energy, with the nitrogenous fraction being converted to urea and excreted by the kidney, so that the total amount of work performed (both internally and externally) was proportional to the nitrogen excreted. These points were tested by two Swiss physiologists, Adolf Fick and Johannes Wislicenus, in 1866 (Carpenter, 1994). Using themselves as subjects, Fick and Wislicenus spent a day walking up a steep mountain path carrying urine collection equipment. From noon the day before the climb and until 6 hours after the climb, Fick and Wislicenus ate only cakes from starch paste fried in fat. Both men excreted approximately 5.6 g of N during a 14-hour period including the 8-hour climb plus the 6-hour period after the climb. Relying on the concurrent studies of Sir Edward Frankland on the heat of oxidation of organic materials and of James Prescott Joule in establishing the mechanical equivalent of heat, they calculated that the urinary N was equivalent to the breakdown of approximately 35 g of protein, and that 35 g of protein would be equivalent to approximately 154 kcal or a work equivalent of 65×10^3 kg-m. The net external work required to ascend the 1,956-m path was calculated to be approximately 139×10^3 kg-m. Even without considering the energy required for basal or internal work or a correction for incomplete efficiency of the muscle in converting chemical energy to work, the quantity of protein metabolized was clearly insufficient to have provided the energy needed for their climb. Therefore, Fick and Wislicenus (1866) concluded that the burning of protein could not be the only source of muscular power, and, although their conclusion was not immediately accepted, we now know this to be true.

age 1 to 3 years, approximately 10% at age 4 to 13 years, and less than 2% by age 18 years. Therefore, except for the first months of life, maintenance requirements account for the major proportion of the dietary protein needs of children and adolescents.

In establishing the current DRIs for protein and amino acids for children, an estimated efficiency of utilization of amino acids of 58% for children up to age 13 years was used (IOM, 2002). Although the number of nitrogen balance studies used to obtain the estimate for children was fewer than that used for adults, the slightly higher estimate of efficiency for children suggests that the overall efficiency of utilization of amino acids may possibly be greater for growth than for maintenance. Thus, an estimated dietary intake of 1.7 g (1/0.58) of protein or amino acid is needed to retain 1 g of protein or amino acid in children.

Based on an average deposition of 5.4 g/day of additional protein during the second and third trimesters of pregnancy, and using a conservative estimate of efficiency for protein utilization (43%), the IOM calculated a need of an average of 12.6 g of additional protein per day during the second and third trimesters of pregnancy for growth of the fetus and maternal tissues. The additional need for protein for pregnant women was calculated as the protein requirement for deposition (12.6 g/day) plus an increase in the maintenance requirement to allow for maintenance of this new tissue (+8.4 g/day), a total of 21 g/day.

As with growth, the additional amino acid requirements for lactation derive primarily from the quantity and composition of the protein and amino acids secreted in the milk. The average milk output over the first 6 months of lactation contains approximately 10 g of protein per day. Assuming an efficiency of protein utilization of 47% for lactating women, an increase in protein intake of 21.2 g/day is required (IOM, 2002). The increased requirement for protein during lactation, therefore, is similar to that during pregnancy (+21 g/day). In both pregnancy and lactation, the increase in protein requirement of 21 g/day is roughly equivalent to one third of the prepregnancy requirement or one fourth of the total requirement during pregnancy or lactation.

CONCEPT OF LABILE PROTEIN RESERVES

A feature of the response to a change in protein intake is the short-term loss and gain of body nitrogen. The apparent rapid short-term change in body nitrogen content that occurs in response to a change in protein intake, as opposed to a slower losses that occur with continued inadequate intake or fasting, has given rise to the concept of labile protein reserves. This does not imply, however, that the protein lost or gained (i.e., the labile protein) is different from the main mass of body protein. The more rapid changes in body nitrogen content may be due to changes in the body urea and free amino acid pools and in the size and protein content of splanchnic organs such as the liver. A slow adaptation of amino acid oxidative capacity could be a contributing factor in the apparent depletion/repletion of body nitrogen that occurs with a decrease/increase in dietary protein intake or in response to the fasting/feeding transition.

FOOD PROTEINS AND PROTEIN QUALITY

Although the physiological requirement is for a mixture of indispensable amino acids plus other amino acids to provide the total amount of required amino acid nitrogen, these requirements normally are met by a mixture of food proteins. Consequently, requirements and recommended dietary intakes are usually expressed in terms of dietary protein rather than amounts of individual amino acids. Different individual proteins (e.g., casein, gelatin) or different food proteins, which are actually mixtures of proteins (e.g., milk proteins, soy proteins), are not identical in terms of their amino acid composition, and, hence, are not identical in their ability to replace losses or support net protein accretion. Consequently, we need a way to describe the ability of particular proteins or mixtures of proteins to meet requirements. The term *protein quality* has been developed for this purpose. Therefore, the protein or mixture of proteins in the food or diet can be described both in terms of quantity and quality.

Dietary protein is usually measured not as protein but as nitrogen, and then nitrogen is converted to protein by use of a factor. Factors have been developed for the conversion of weight of nitrogen to weight of protein. Most frequently this is done using an average factor of 6.25 g protein per g of N (or equivalently, an average of 0.16 g of N per g protein). The term *crude protein* implies the use of the factor 6.25. For mixed diets, the factor 6.25 is used to calculate protein content as a matter of convenience. Most studies of protein requirements and of food protein content have been based on measurements of nitrogen and application of the 6.25 factor to convert g of N to g of protein. Therefore, this general factor is usually appropriate when considering nitrogen balance or protein requirements.

Nevertheless, it must be borne in mind that this average factor may be substantially in error for particular foods. For example, the actual factor for milk is 6.38 g protein per g N and that for wheat is 5.7 g protein per g N. The amino acid composition of individual proteins varies, resulting in different percentages of nitrogen in different proteins. That this would occur is obvious if one simply considers that the nitrogen content of tyrosine is 77 mg/g, whereas that of arginine is 322 mg/g. It must be noted, too, that not all the nitrogen in food is in the form of amino acids. Substances such as nitrates, amides, urea, amino sugars, and nucleic acids may account for a significant proportion of the total nitrogen in some foods, and these components affect the relationship between nitrogen and protein contents. Again, however, most studies of protein requirements and most calculations of dietary protein content have been based on measurements of total N and application of the 6.25 factor.

DEFINITION OF PROTEIN QUALITY

Protein quality, or the ability of a given amount of a particular protein or mixture of proteins to meet the body's amino acid requirements, depends on three attributes of the protein: its digestibility, the availability of its amino acids, and the pattern of amino acids making up the protein.

Digestibility

It is obvious that only that part of the protein that is digested can contribute amino acids to meet requirements. Apparent protein digestibility (d) is conventionally described as

$$d = (I - F)/I$$

where I is the protein or nitrogen intake, and F is fecal nitrogen or protein excretion, with both measured in the same units (e.g., g/day, usually as nitrogen). This is called *apparent digestibility* in recognition of the fact that the fecal nitrogen output does not consist entirely of undigested dietary matter, but includes nitrogen from endogenous sources (i.e., secretions and sloughed intestinal cells). By deducting this endogenous component, which can be estimated by measuring fecal nitrogen in individuals consuming protein-free diets, a value for the *true digestibility* of the dietary protein can be derived. True digestibility is higher than apparent digestibility because of this correction. In practice, these measurements are not routinely made in human subjects but commonly are made when protein quality is evaluated in experimental animals. As illustrated in Table 15-2, the true digestibility of most animal proteins such as milk, meat, and eggs is high: between 90% and 99%.

Table 15-2
Protein Digestibility Values

Protein Source	True Digestibility (5%)
Egg	97
Milk, cheese	95
Meat, fish	94
Peanut butter	95
Soy protein isolate	95
Soy flour	86
Wheat, refined	96
Wheat, whole	86
Rice, polished	88
Corn, whole	87
Millet	79
Maize	85
Oatmeal	86
Peas, nature	88
Beans	78
Indian rice and bean diet	78
American mixed diet	96

Data from Food and Agriculture Organization of the United Nations (1991) Protein Quality Evaluation: Report of Joint FAO/WHO Expert Consultation. FAO Food and Nutrition Paper #51. FAO, Rome.

Many plant proteins, conversely, especially when eaten raw, are less digestible (70 % to 90 % digestibility), partly because they are contained within cell walls, which are resistant to mammalian digestive enzymes and are broken down only by the gastrointestinal microflora. Some dietary proteins, such as legumes, contain antinutritional factors such as trypsin inhibitors that affect digestibility.

Availability

There is some confusion about the use of the terms *digestibility* and *availability,* and these terms are sometimes used interchangeably. The original use of availability was to describe the chemical integrity of an amino acid, which is an attribute separate from its digestibility, and it seems preferable to preserve the distinction. Loss of availability is principally associated with Maillard reactions, which modify lysine residues through conjugation of lysine's ε-amino group with sugar residues. These reactions occur readily during drying of milk, meat, fish, and other animal proteins. Severe heat damage can also reduce the availability of methionine and tryptophan and of protein as a whole.

Amino Acid Pattern

The major factor determining the quality of a protein is usually its amino acid composition: essentially, how closely the pattern of its amino acids conforms to the needs of the subject. It is, therefore, not a fixed attribute of the protein, but a measure of its suitability for a particular use. In practice, the protein's quality is determined by the amino acid that is most deficient in the protein relative to the requirements. This is the limiting amino acid. A protein that supplies indispensable amino acids in exactly the same pattern as the requirements, along with a sufficient supply of dispensable amino acids, can be considered an "ideal" or "complete" protein. In order to establish which amino acid is limiting and how closely a given protein conforms to the ideal, both a reference pattern and a method for comparing the dietary protein with the reference pattern are needed. This pattern must include a value for each of the indispensable amino acids, together with the sum of the dispensable amino acids. The pattern of the dispensable amino acids is of little consequence in terms of protein quality, although a mixture of dispensable amino acids such as occurs in proteins is preferable to one or a few of the dispensable amino acids (e.g., glutamate). The rate of dispensable amino acid synthesis may become limiting when all of the dispensable amino acids must be synthesized from a single nitrogen source. Excess indispensable amino acids also can be used to provide amino acid nitrogen for synthesis of dispensable amino acids that are needed by the body.

METHODS OF EVALUATING PROTEIN QUALITY

Methods of assessing protein quality are basically of two kinds. Those in the first category, which can be considered integrative assays, simply describe the utilization of the dietary protein without regard for its amino acid composition. Those in the second category are based on comparing the amino acid composition of the protein with an "ideal" or reference pattern.

Integrative Bioassays

In the earliest of the integrative assays, proteins were compared in terms of their growth-promoting values, most commonly using rats or chicks as the test species. Protein efficiency ratio (PER) is defined as the weight gain per gram of protein consumed. However, weight gain reflects aspects of the diet other than the quality of the protein, and PER gives no information on the value of a protein for meeting maintenance requirements. These two factors limit the usefulness of PER as a measure of the quality of protein for use in human diets. Other methods such as biological value (BV) and net protein utilization (NPU) are based on the nitrogen gained. BV describes the efficiency with which absorbed dietary nitrogen is utilized for both maintenance and body nitrogen gain. It is calculated as

$$BV = (N_{int} - [N_u - N_{eu}] - [N_f - N_{mf}]) \div (N_{int} - [N_f - N_{mf}])$$

where N_{int} is nitrogen intake, N_u is urinary nitrogen excretion, N_{eu} is endogenous urinary nitrogen excretion, N_f is fecal nitrogen excretion, and N_{mf} is metabolic fecal nitrogen. N_{eu} and N_{mf} are measured as the urinary and fecal nitrogen excretion of comparable animals given a protein-free diet or, alternatively, as their total body nitrogen loss. NPU is similar to BV in being a measure of nitrogen utilization for both maintenance and body protein accretion, but is expressed in relation to nitrogen intake rather than nitrogen actually absorbed; NPU is numerically equal to BV multiplied by true digestibility and is likewise determined using two groups of animals, one fed the test protein and the other fed a protein-free diet.

The values obtained with integrative assays are meaningful when determined for whole diets, but are of limited usefulness when applied to individual foods that are components of mixed diets. Values for the protein quality of individual foods are additive only when the limiting amino acid in all the foods happens to be the same. If not, the deficiency of a particular amino acid in one of the foods can be compensated by a relative excess of that amino acid in another; this effect is called complementation. The complementation of cereals, which typically are limiting in lysine, and legumes, which typically are limiting in sulfur amino acids but higher in lysine, is an important example.

Amino Acid Scoring

The protein quality of proteins in individual foods or in mixtures of foods may be evaluated on the basis of amino acid composition. In order to evaluate proteins on the basis of their amino acid composition, a reference pattern is needed against which to compare them. Block and Mitchell (1946) devised the system of chemical score, in which the concentration of each amino acid in the test protein is expressed as a proportion of the corresponding concentration in the reference pattern. The lowest of these proportions identifies the limiting amino acid and defines the score of the protein, which is usually expressed as a percentage.

When this method of protein evaluation was first devised, Block and Mitchell (1946) used egg protein as the standard, because in assays with rapidly growing rats, chicks, or other animals, egg protein was found to be unsurpassable in quality (i.e., a minimum amount of protein was required to support maximal weight gain). The high quality of egg protein, however, does not mean that this protein's amino acid pattern closely matches the "ideal" pattern; it could contain excesses of some of the essential amino acids relative to the total amino acid requirement. In addition, because young, rapidly growing animals utilize most of their amino acid intake for growth whereas the amino acid requirements of humans (at least after the first 2 months of postnatal life) are dominated by maintenance needs, egg protein is not necessarily an appropriate reference pattern for humans. As a consequence of one or both of these factors, the egg protein reference pattern is not appropriate for application to human diets and undervalues some proteins used in human nutrition. However, the same scoring principle can be used with reference patterns more appropriate to the needs of the human population.

Several amino acid patterns are shown in Table 15-3, including the reference pattern recommended by the IOM (2002). Because there were relatively small differences between the amino acid requirement patterns for 1- to 3-year-old children and for adults, the 1- to 3-year-old requirement pattern is recommended as the reference pattern for the purposes of assessing and planning the protein component of diets. The IOM pattern has uniformly higher proportions of all the indispensable amino acids than does the widely used Food and Agriculture Organization (FAO)/World Health Organization (WHO)/United Nations University (UNU) pattern, which was based on earlier nitrogen balance studies of amino acid requirements that may have underestimated amino acid needs (WHO,1985). The marked increases in the amounts of lysine and threonine in the new IOM reference pattern compared to patterns used earlier (e.g., FAO/WHO/UNU 1985 pattern) has significant implications for protein scoring based on the first limiting amino acid.

Compared with the IOM recommended pattern, the pattern of indispensable amino acids found in whole-body protein of animals (Smith, 1980) has higher proportions of indispensable amino acids relative to total protein (12% to 50% higher) but a fairly similar dispensable amino acid pattern on a relative basis (i.e., the pattern × 0.76). Although there have been no studies in humans to confirm the point, we can extrapolate the animal data to suggest

Table 15-3
Amino Acid Patterns Based on Estimates of Amino Acid and Protein Requirements or the Composition of Human Milk or Whole Body Protein

	Preschool Child (1-3 yr of age) Requirement Pattern and IOM Recommended Scoring Pattern (IOM, 2002)	Adult Maintenance Requirement Pattern (IOM, 2002)	Human Milk and Pattern for Infants (IOM, 2002)	FAO/WHO/ UNU Pattern (WHO, 1985)	Whole Body Protein (Smith, 1980)
	mg amino acid/g protein				
Histidine	18	17	23	—	24
Isoleucine	25	23	57	13	37
Leucine	55	52	101	19	66
Lysine	51	47	69	16	68
Methionine + cysteine	25	23	38	17	33
Phenylalanine + tyrosine	47	41	87	19	63
Threonine	27	24	47	9	39
Tryptophan	8	6	18	5	9
Valine	32	29	56	13	49

Based on data reported by Institute of Medicine (2002) Dietary Reference Intakes: Energy, Carbohydrate, Fiber, Fat, Fatty Acids, Cholesterol, Protein, and Amino Acids. Part 2. National Academy Press, Washington, DC; World Health Organization (1985) Energy and Protein Requirements. Report of a Joint FAO/WHO/UNU Expert Consultation. WHO Technical Report Series 724. World Health Organization, Geneva; and Smith RH (1980) Comparative amino acid requirements. Proc Nutr Soc 39:71-78. The whole-body protein values are based on average values for whole-body protein of rat, pig, calf, and chicken, plus a calculated value based on the amino acid content of various types of cellular protein.

that the pattern of amino acids required for growth is fairly close to the composition of whole-body protein. (One outcome of the similarity of the amino acid requirement patterns and the relative pattern of amino acids in body protein is a basis for the assumption that all of the indispensable amino acids are used with much the same efficiency such that application of general values for efficiency of protein utilization is appropriate.) Conversely, the pattern of amino acids in human milk is quite different from that of the recommended scoring pattern, both in relative pattern and amount of each indispensable amino acid per gram of protein: the lysine level is 35% greater and the aromatic amino acid level is 85% greater in human milk than in the IOM-recommended pattern. Because very little direct work on amino acid requirements of infants has been done, we do not know how closely the milk pattern matches the actual requirement pattern for infants. The human milk pattern is generally viewed as a "safe and adequate" pattern for infants.

As for animal bioassay values, chemical score values for various food proteins are not additive (unless the limiting amino acid is the same for all proteins). However, amino acid contents of individual proteins can be added, and the overall chemical score for the diet can be calculated. Thus, the only general approach for using information about individual proteins to evaluate a mixture of these proteins requires addition of the amounts of amino acids in the components of the mixture followed by calculation of a single chemical score for the mixture. This method is illustrated in Tables 15-4 and 15-5.

Chemical score methods yield values that closely correlate with BV determinations. The chemical score method provides no information about protein digestibility or amino acid availability. Digestibility can be determined separately and applied to correct the chemical score value, but possible differences in the availability of different amino acids within the protein would not be detected. Another assumption of the chemical score method that is not made in the animal bioassay methods is that excesses of nonlimiting amino acids do not affect the utilization of the protein. This is not entirely true: relative excesses of some amino acids can affect the

Table 15-4

Sample Calculation of Amino Acid Score and PDCAAS for Peanut and Wheat Proteins and a Mixture of the Two Proteins (Peanut Butter Sandwich)

	Peanut Butter			White Bread (Wheat)			Peanut Butter Sandwich			IOM Reference Pattern
	mg/g Protein	mg/2 Tbsp or mg/8 g Protein	Amino Acid Score %	mg/g Protein	mg/2 Slices or mg/3.8 g Protein	Amino Acid Score %	mg/Sandwich or mg/11.8 g Protein	mg/g Protein	Amino Acid Score %	mg/g Protein
Histidine	30	240		18	68		308	26		18
Isoleucine	40	320		34	129		449	38		25
Leucine	77	616		62	236		852	72		55
Lysine	39	312	76	17	65	33	377	32	63	51
Methionine + Cysteine	24	192	(96)	36	137		336	28		25
Phenylalanine + Tyrosine	108	864		64	243		1107	94		47
Threonine	30	240		24	91	(89)	331	28		27
Tryptophan	12	96		10	38		134	11		8
Valine	46	368		38	144		512	43		32

Amino acid scores were calculated only for amino acids present below the requirement pattern; all others would be 100%. The correct method for calculating the amino acid score for a mixture of protein is shown above: the amino acids in each component of the mixture must be added and the sum is then divided by the total grams of protein in the mixture to get the pattern (mg amino acid per g protein). In the unique case, where the same amino acid is the first limiting amino acid of each protein in a mixture, the chemical score for each component multiplied by its fractional contribution to the total mixture can be added: in this example where lysine is first limiting in both bread and peanut butter, and peanut butter contributes 8/11.8 g or 68% of the total protein in the sandwich whereas bread contributes 3.8/11.8 g or 32% of the total protein in the sandwich, the amino acid score for the sandwich = (76 × 0.68) + (33 × 0.32) = 52 + 11 = 63.

Table 15-5

Illustration of the Concept of Amino Acid Complementation and Calculation of Amino Acid Scores for Mixtures of Proteins

				Mixture (% of protein)			
	Rice	Red Beans	Milk	1/2 Rice + 1/2 Beans	2/3 Rice + 1/3 Milk	1/3 Rice + 1/3 Beans + 1/3 Milk	IOM 2002 Reference Pattern
	mg amino acid/g protein						
Lysine	39	75	80	57	51	65	51
Sulfur amino acids	44	20	30	32	36	31	25
Threonine	44	34	37	39	41	38	25
Tryptophan	11	10	12	10.5	11	11	7
Amino acid score (%)	76 (Lys)	80 (SAA)	100 (124- SAA)	100 (112-Lys)	100 (100-Lys)	100 (124-SAA)	

For this table, only lysine, sulfur amino acids (methionine + cysteine), threonine, and tryptophan were considered because they are the only amino acids that are limiting in common foods. Lysine is first limiting for rice, and sulfur amino acids are first limiting for red beans. Milk provides a complete protein compared to the pattern. Fractional composition of the mixtures refers to the food protein, not to the entire food.

utilization of others with which they interact in metabolism. In practice, significant effects are likely to be confined to situations in which there are gross imbalances among the branched-chain amino acids or between lysine and arginine. Despite these limitations, amino acid pattern is the major factor determining protein quality, and chemical scores and protein utilization have been shown to be closely correlated in animal studies. Although all indispensable amino acids are considered in determination of chemical score, only lysine, methionine + cyst(e)ine, tryptophan, or threonine are normally limiting in the mixed proteins of human diets (see Table 15-5).

Because most population groups consume a mixture of dietary proteins, the quality of individual proteins is of less concern than the quality of the mixture of proteins present in the total diet. When mixtures of proteins are consumed, complementation occurs such that the amino acid score for the mixture of proteins may be higher than that of any of the individual proteins (see Table 15-5). Protein quality is most likely to be a concern when a very limited variety of protein sources is consumed, particularly when the major dietary staple contains a small amount of total protein and that protein has a low amino acid score. In these cases, complementation of proteins (e.g., corn and beans) or supplementation of the diet with a small amount of high-quality protein can be of significant benefit.

An amino acid score (AAS) can be calculated as follows:

$$\text{AAS}(\%) = \frac{\text{mg of limiting amino acid in 1 g of test protein or test protein mixture}}{\text{mg of same amino acid in 1 g of IOM recommended reference pattern}} \times 100\%$$

A protein digestibility corrected amino acid score (PDCAAS) can be calculated as follows:

$$\text{PDCAAS}(\%) = \frac{\text{mg of limiting amino acid in 1 g of test protein or test protein mixture}}{\text{mg of same amino acid in 1 g of IOM recommended reference pattern}} \times \text{true digestibility}(\%)$$

ASSESSMENT OF REQUIREMENTS FOR DIETARY PROTEIN OR AMINO ACIDS

Essentially three approaches have been used to assess protein and amino acid requirements. The first and simplest approach is to examine the protein and amino acid contents of diets that are found to be satisfactory in practice. An example is the derivation of infant requirements from the volume and composition of milk consumed by normally growing breast-fed infants.

The second approach is an empirical analysis of dose responses. In experiments of this kind, the response of growth rate or nitrogen balance, or a related parameter, is measured at various intakes of protein or amino acid. Nitrogen balance studies have been used widely for determination of protein requirements for maintenance. The criterion of nitrogen balance provided the basis of the first quantitative estimates of the amino acid needs of human adults, but breakpoint approaches for direct amino acid oxidation or indicator amino acid oxidation have been used more recently to assess the intakes of individual indispensable amino acids that are required for optimal rates of protein synthesis or amino acid retention.

The third approach is the factorial method, in which the relevant components of the requirement (maintenance, growth, accretion of tissues and growth of the fetus during pregnancy, and milk secretion during lactation) are estimated separately and then added. Although this approach ostensibly provides a logical system for determination of requirements, the direct estimation of the component requirements is difficult.

CONTENT IN SATISFACTORY DIETS

Requirements for infants are based on intake data because of the difficulty in accurately determining requirements for growth and development. Infant formula or human milk will meet an infant's needs for protein up to 4 to 6 months of age if energy needs are met. Healthy full-term infants who are exclusively breast-fed do not manifest any signs of protein deficiency. The average protein intake of

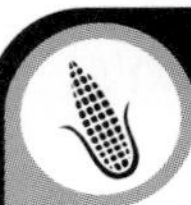

Food Sources

Food Sources of Protein

Meats
- 15 to 23 g per 3 oz fish
- 16 to 26 g per 3 oz beef
- 22 to 26 g per 3 oz chicken

Dairy Products
- 8 g per cup milk
- 2.5 g per ½ cup ice cream
- 7 g per ounce cheddar cheese

Cereals and Legumes
- 2 g per ½ cup cooked white rice
- 6 g per cup cooked oatmeal
- 2 g per cup cornflakes
- 8 g per ounce peanuts
- 8 g per ½ cup black beans
- 9 g per ½ cup tofu

Eggs
- 6 g per egg

Data from U.S. Department of Agriculture/Agricultural Research Service (2005) National Nutrient Database for Standard Reference, Release 18. USDA/ARS, Washington, DC. Retrieved March 7, 2005, from www.ars.usda.gov/ba/bhnrc/ndl/.

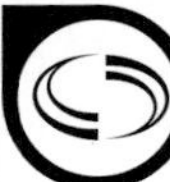

RDAs Across the Life Cycle

	g Protein per day
Infants	
0 to 0.5 yr	9 (AI)
0.5 to 1.0 yr	13 (AI)
Children	
1 to 3 yr	13
4 to 8 yr	19
9 to 13 yr	34
Males	
14 to 18 yr	52
≥19 yr	56
Females	
14 to 18 yr	46
≥19 yr	46
Pregnant	71
Lactating	71

All values are recommended dietary allowances (RDAs) except those indicated as adequate intakes (AIs).
Data from Institute of Medicine (2002) Dietary Reference Intakes for Energy, Carbohydrate, Fiber, Fat, Fatty Acids, Cholesterol, Protein, and Amino Acids. National Academy Press, Washington, DC.

breast-fed infants in the United States is about 1.68 g/kg/day. The IOM (2002) established an adequate intake (AI) of 9.1 g of protein per day for infants up to 6 months of age, based upon the average volume of milk intake (0.78 L/day) and the average protein content of human milk during the first 6 months of lactation (11.7 g/L). The AI can be stated as 1.52 g/kg/day, based on a reference weight of 6 kg for 2- to 6-month-old infants. Although this approach results in safe allowances, it does not yield a close estimate of the protein requirement or indicate that the established AI will be adequate if a different source of protein is used in infant diets. Adequate intakes of individual indispensable amino acids can be calculated in the same way from the amino acid content of human milk proteins. This approach has been used to derive a scoring pattern for adequacy of the quality of protein mixtures in infant diets.

DOSE-RESPONSE STUDIES FOR PROTEIN–NITROGEN BALANCE

Nitrogen balance data was used for estimation of the maintenance requirements of adults and children in establishing the DRIs for protein (IOM, 2002). In nitrogen balance experiments (Fig. 15-3), the rate of body nitrogen retention is estimated as the difference between the dietary nitrogen intake and the sum of the losses in urine and feces and by other routes (integumental and miscellaneous).

Nitrogen balance = Nitrogen intake − Nitrogen losses

In adults, it is generally presumed that the protein requirement is achieved when an individual is in zero nitrogen balance. Infants, children, and pregnant women, as well as individuals recovering from disease states in which lean body mass was lost, should be in positive nitrogen balance.

The IOM based the adult EAR for protein on a recent meta-analysis of published nitrogen balance studies (Rand et al., 2003). For each study, the lowest continuing intake of dietary

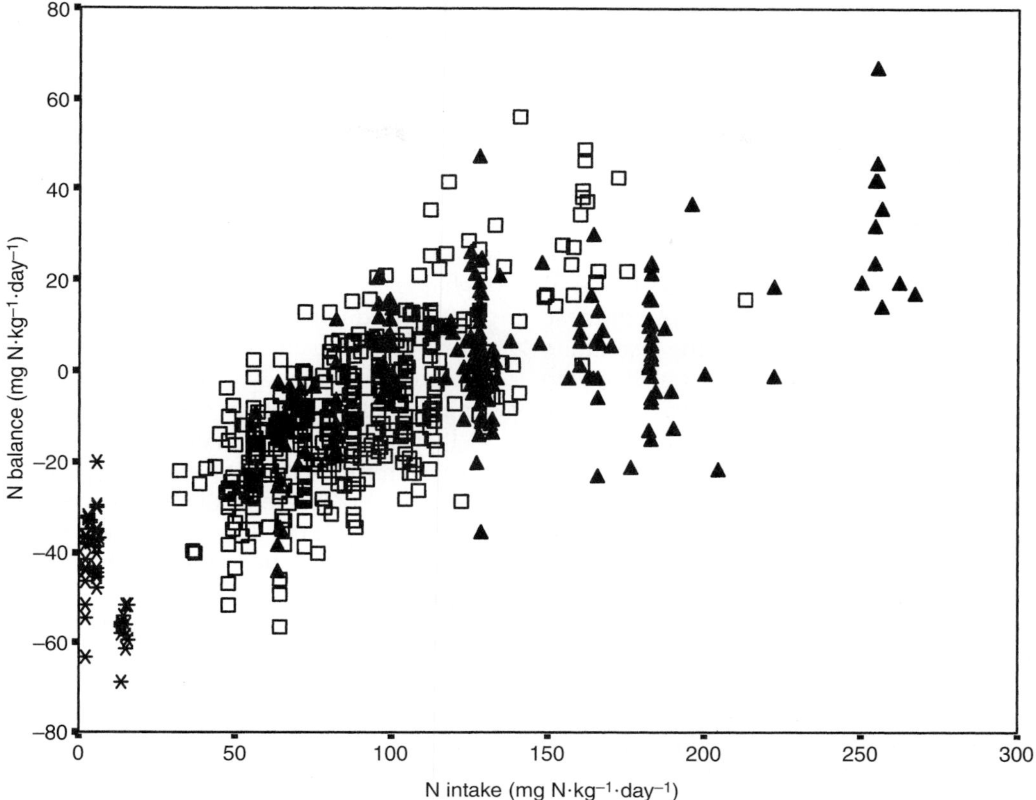

Figure 15-3 Relation between individual nitrogen balances, corrected for dermal and miscellaneous losses, and nitrogen intake in healthy adults. Each point represents an individual's observed response to a specific intake. The median nitrogen requirement is the intake needed for zero balance; this was determined to be approximately 105 mg/kg/day. *(From Rand WM, Pellett PL, Young VR [2003] Meta-analysis of nitrogen balance studies for estimating protein requirements in healthy adults. Am J Clin Nutr 77:109-127, with permission from the American Society for Clinical Nutrition.)*

protein that was sufficient to achieve body nitrogen equilibrium (zero balance) was considered as the individual requirement. The median nitrogen requirement derived from the meta-analysis was 105 mg nitrogen/kg/day, and this value was used as the best estimate of the nitrogen EAR in the healthy adult population (IOM, 2002). Using the conversion factor of 6.25 g protein per g of nitrogen, the EAR for protein was set as 0.66 g/kg/day for men and women (19 to 50 years of age). On the basis of reference body weights of 57 and 70 kg for women and men, respectively, the EAR for protein is 38 g/day for women and 47 g/day for men. To obtain a recommended dietary allowance (RDA) for protein, the EAR was increased by 25.7%, based on an estimate of the between-individual variance, to cover the needs of 97.5% of the healthy adult population. The RDA for protein is 0.80 g/kg/day for adults, or 46 g/day for the 57-kg reference woman and 56 g/day for the 70-kg reference man.

When evaluated in terms of amount needed per kilogram of body weight, no significant effect of age on the protein requirement of older adults was detected by the analyses of Rand and colleagues (2003). Therefore, for older adults, no additional protein allowance based on body weight beyond that of younger adults is warranted, and the EAR and RDA for older adults are the same as those for younger adults. However, the protein allowance as a percentage of energy need will increase for older adults because lean body mass, as a percentage of body weight, decreases with age and, hence, lowers basal energy expenditure.

Nitrogen balance studies have also been used to determine the maintenance needs of children. Many of these were summarized by the IOM (2002).

DOSE-RESPONSE STUDIES FOR AMINO ACIDS: AMINO ACID OXIDATION STUDIES AND NITROGEN BALANCE STUDIES

Several approaches have been used in determining amino acid requirements. All of these involve feeding graded levels of the test amino acid to the subject and looking for a change in amino acid utilization. Ideally, a range of amino acids levels greater than and less than the requirement (six or more levels) should be tested in each individual subject. The basal diet must be adequate in all other amino acids and energy, as well as all other essential nutrients, such that the amount of the amino acid being tested is the only factor that limits the extent of protein synthesis. Three patterns of response are possible for various biologic parameters that have been used to assess the adequacy of amino acid levels; these are illustrated in Figure 15-4.

One pattern is that seen when either nitrogen balance or growth is plotted against amino acid intake. Nitrogen balance or growth (in a child or growing animal) will increase as the intake of the limiting indispensable amino acid (i.e., the test amino acid) increases up until the requirement amount is reached. After the requirement is reached, nitrogen balance or growth will plateau despite the addition of higher levels of protein or limiting amino acid.

A second pattern occurs when oxidation of a test amino acid is observed directly. This approach usually involves labeling the test amino acid with ^{13}C in the α-carboxyl group (C-1 position) and measuring the loss of this carbon from the body bicarbonate pool by the appearance of labeled $^{13}CO_2$ in the breath. This method is called the direct amino acid oxidation (DAAO) method. The DAAO method is useful only for amino acids in which the labeled carbon is readily lost as CO_2 in an early irreversible step of its catabolic pathway. In this case, oxidation of the test amino acid remains low with little change until the requirement is approached or met, after which its oxidation increases progressively as intake is further increased. A similar

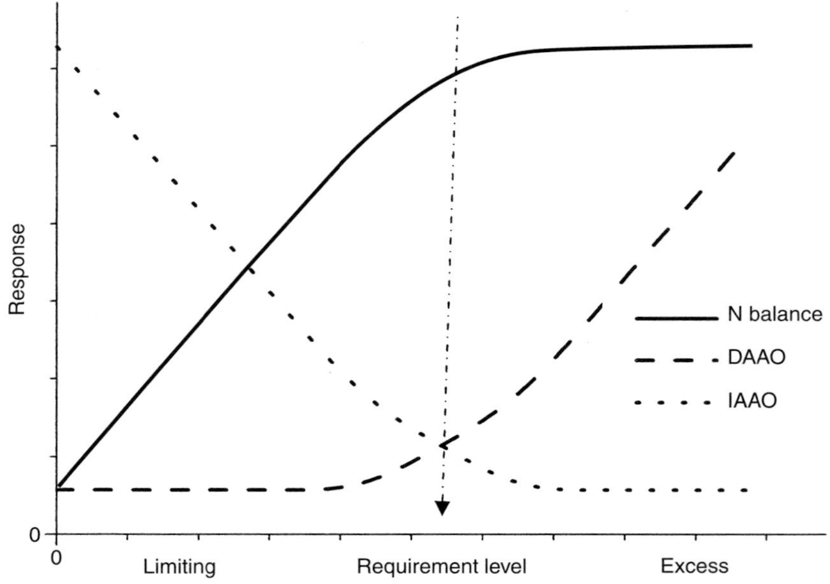

Figure 15-4 General patterns of metabolic responses to graded intakes of an indispensable amino acid. *DAAO*, Direct amino acid oxidation; IAAO, indicator amino acid oxidation. *(Modified from Pencharz PB, Ball RO [2003] Different approaches to define individual amino acid requirements. Annu Rev Nutr 23:101-116.)*

pattern may be observed by following the plasma amino acid level, which increases when intake exceeds the requirement.

A third response pattern is seen when an indicator amino acid is used in what is called the indicator amino acid oxidation (IAAO) method. In this case, an amino acid present in adequate amount is labeled. When intake of the test amino acid is low and protein synthesis is limited by a lack of the test amino acid, the excess non-test (and indicator) amino acids not used for protein synthesis will be oxidized. As the intake of the test amino acid is increased, incorporation of the non-test amino acids (including the indicator amino acid) into protein will increase, such that oxidation of the indicator amino acid to $^{13}CO_2$ will decrease. Once the requirement level is reached for the test amino acid, oxidation of the indicator amino acid will plateau at a low level. Plasma urea concentration may follow the same trend in this case, being high when amino acids are not being used maximally for protein synthesis and decreasing to a plateau when the requirement of limiting amino acid for protein synthesis is met. In some indicator amino acid oxidation studies, the 24-hour balance of the indicator amino acid, the intake of which is constant, is calculated:

$$\text{Balance} = \text{Indicator amino acid intake} - \text{Indicator amino acid oxidation}$$

In this case, indicator amino acid balance will be negative when test amino acid intakes are inadequate and will increase as test amino acid intake increases until zero balance is reached, after which indicator amino acid oxidation will plateau.

Although the data may appear to be curvilinear, bilinear models fit amino acid oxidation data well, yielding one line that has minimal or no slope and a second line with a slope. The crossover point of the two lines, or the breakpoint, is used to determine the requirement level as illustrated in Figure 15-4.

Nitrogen balance studies were used to obtain the first estimates of the amino acid requirements of human adults. Rose and colleagues, in a series of nitrogen balance studies in the 1940s, determined the amino acid requirements of young men (see Rose, 1957). First, men were given diets devoid of a single amino acid so as to establish which amino acids were dispensable and which were indispensable or dietary essentials. Eight amino acids were determined to be indispensable. (In these studies, removal of histidine from the diet did not lead to a negative nitrogen balance; this was interpreted to mean that histidine was dispensable, and this conclusion was only reversed much later by longer-term experiments.) Rose and colleagues then conducted a series of quantitative studies in which they gave each subject a succession of diets with different concentrations of the amino acid under investigation. From the changes in nitrogen balance that ensued, they attempted to identify the intake of each amino acid that was required for nitrogen equilibrium to be achieved. Similar experiments were conducted on young women, but using more subjects and with several improvements in experimental procedures (Leverton et al., 1959). The results of these early experiments in determining the amino acid requirements of men and women formed the basis of the widely used international estimates of adult amino acid requirements (WHO, 1985). These international estimates of amino acid requirements for various age-groups are low compared to the estimates published more recently by the IOM in the United States (IOM, 2002). FAO/WHO/UNU is currently reexamining the international recommendations.

The main problem with estimates based on nitrogen balance experiments is the well-known tendency for the balance technique to overestimate nitrogen retention. The size of the error depends on the procedures used. Commonly, nitrogen losses other than those in urine and feces were ignored in nitrogen balance studies, and this was true in both the experiments of Rose and of Leverton and associates described in the preceding text. In addition, failure to account for small amounts of unconsumed food (overestimation of intake) and small losses of urine or feces (underestimation of excretion) both tend to exaggerate retention in balance studies. This means that a subject apparently receiving sufficient amino acid (or protein) to maintain nitrogen equilibrium is actually in negative nitrogen balance and needs more of the amino acid (or protein) to maintain true nitrogen equilibrium. The overestimation of nitrogen retention in the experiments of Rose and co-workers (see Rose, 1957) and of Leverton and colleagues (1959) was probably about 300 mg/day; recalculating the estimates to correct for this overestimation gives substantially higher estimates for the amino acid requirements (IOM, 2002).

A further problem with the nitrogen balance approach, especially in short-term studies, may arise through the implicit assumption that a subject in nitrogen equilibrium must also be in amino acid equilibrium. This is not necessarily so. Histidine, for example, is stored in the form of the peptide carnosine (β-alanylhistidine). Carnosine, in experimental animals at least, is depleted during dietary histidine deficiency. This allows obligatory losses of histidine to be met for a time without loss of body protein, despite an inadequate histidine intake. There may also be a potential to adapt to an indispensable amino acid deficiency through modification of the amino acid composition of the body protein pool as a whole. Of course, it is not possible to modify the amino acid composition of any of the body's proteins, but it is possible to vary the relative amounts of the various proteins. Because proteins have different amino acid compositions, there is the potential to adapt, at least temporarily, to a deficiency of one amino acid by depleting the body of proteins rich in that amino acid. This also happens in histidine deficiency, in which hemoglobin, which is very rich in histidine, can be gradually depleted. The mechanism of this adaptation is not known. However, this ability of the body to use endogenous sources of histidine explains why histidine was not identified as an indispensable amino acid in the early balance studies.

It is also important to note that most estimates of amino acid requirements have been made using free amino acids. The use of diets based on natural foods may lead to higher estimates of requirements because the dietary proteins may be incompletely digested to amino acids.

More recently, indispensable amino acid requirements have been studied using DAAO or IAAO. To date, most of these studies have been done in adults. The DAAO method has been used to assess oxidation of amino acids whose carboxyl groups are released to the body bicarbonate pool in an early step of the amino acid's committed degradation pathway. The IAAO method is not dependent upon release of the carboxyl carbon of the test amino acid and, thus, can be used to assess the requirement of any indispensable amino acid. In the IAAO method, a different amino acid such as phenylalanine (in the presence of an excess of tyrosine) or lysine is used as an indicator amino acid. In setting up the current DRIs for indispensable amino acids in adults, the IOM (2002) used results from IAAO studies for leucine, lysine, methionine + cysteine, phenylalanine + tyrosine, threonine, and tryptophan; results from DAAO studies for leucine, valine, lysine, phenylalanine, and threonine; and results from nitrogen balance studies for lysine and methionine + cysteine to determine the EARs for amino acids (IOM, 2002). Only studies in which several levels of intake of the test amino acid were studied were included, and results of some studies were reanalyzed. Their conclusion was that, when the method was based on measuring a change in a particular end-point in response to graded levels of a test amino acid, results for N balance and DAAO and IAAO approaches were similar. Furthermore, for the DAAO and IAAO methods, results of 24-hour studies were similar to those done over only a few hours. Because no suitable studies had been done to determine the isoleucine and histidine requirements of adults, the isoleucine and histidine requirements were calculated from the EAR for protein and the amino acid composition of body protein with adjustments for the relationship between these values and the EARs for other amino acids. Amino acid EARs for pregnant and lactating women were set as 1.33 × the EAR for adult women based on the ratio of protein requirements for pregnant and nonpregnant women (0.88/0.66). As shown in Table 15-6, RDAs were calculated based on an approximate coefficient of variation (CV) of 12% such that the RDA is the EAR multiplied by 1.24. The amino acid reference or scoring pattern for adults was calculated by dividing the EARs for amino acids by the EAR for protein (i.e., by 0.66 g/kg/day).

Table 15-6
DRIs for Indispensable Amino Acids and Comparison to Median Intakes in the United States

	EAR (mg/kg/day)	RDA (mg/kg/day)	IOM (2002) Reference Pattern (mg amino acid/ g protein)	EAR (mg/day for 70-kg man)	RDA (mg/day for 70-kg man)	Median Intake of U.S. Men (mg/day)
Histidine	11	14	17	0.8	1.0	2.8
Isoleucine	15	19	23	1.1	1.3	4.4
Leucine	34	42	52	2.4	2.9	7.6
Lysine	31	38	47	2.2	2.7	6.7
Methionine + cysteine	15	19	23	1.1	1.3	1.3 + 2.2 = 3.5
Phenylalanine + tyrosine	27	33	41	1.9	2.3	4.2 + 3.5 = 7.7
Threonine	16	20	24	1.1	1.4	3.8
Tryptophan	4	5	6	0.28	0.35	1.1
Valine	19	24	29	1.3	1.7	5.0

DRIs from Institute of Medicine (2002) Dietary Reference Intakes for Energy, Carbohydrate, Fiber, Fat, Fatty Acids, Cholesterol, Protein, and Amino Acids. Part 2. National Academy Press, Washington, DC. Food intake data from U.S. Department of Health and Human Services and National Center for Health Statistics, as published by Institute of Medicine (2002). *EAR*, Estimated average requirement; *RDA*, recommended dietary allowance.

Table 15-7
DRIs for Children and Adults

	Protein EAR (g/kg/day)	Protein RDA (g/kg/day)	Protein RDA (g/day)
1-3 yr (12 kg)	0.88	1.10	13
4-8 yr (20 kg)	0.76	0.95	19
9-13 yr (36 kg)	0.76	0.95	34
14-18 yr			
Boys (61 kg)	0.73	0.85	52
Girls (54 kg)	0.71	0.85	46
19->70 yr			
Men (70 kg)	0.66	0.80	56
Women (57 kg)	0.66	0.80	46
Pregnant women	0.88	1.1	71
Lactating women	1.05	1.3	71

From Institute of Medicine (2002) Dietary Reference Intakes for Energy, Carbohydrate, Fiber, Fat, Fatty Acids, Cholesterol, Protein, and Amino Acids. Part 2. National Academy Press, Washington, DC.
DRI, Dietary reference intake; *EAR*, estimated average requirement; *RDA*, recommended dietary allowance.

FACTORIAL METHOD

In the factorial approach, the protein needs for each function (maintenance, body protein accretion, and milk protein secretion) are summed. In establishing the 2002 DRIs, the protein requirements of children were determined by the factorial method in that the requirements were estimated from maintenance needs plus requirements for growth (Table 15-7). Similarly, protein needs of pregnant or lactating women were determined by adding an allowance for protein accretion or secretion in the milk to their maintenance requirements.

In setting the 2002 DRIs for protein, the IOM relied on results of nitrogen balance studies for determination of maintenance requirements of children as well as of adults. The maintenance requirement for protein was calculated to be 0.688 g/kg/day for children from 7 months to age 13 and 0.656 g/kg/day for 14- to 18- year-olds and adults. For children, the additional protein needs for growth were calculated from average rates of body protein deposition for each age–gender group multiplied by a factor to correct for the inefficiency of protein utilization (IOM, 2002). The efficiency of protein utilization was estimated from results of nitrogen balance studies: an estimate of 58% was used for children from 7 months to 13 years, and the adult estimate of 47% was used for 14 to 18 year olds. These data were sufficient to set EARs for older infants and children: the EAR was 1.1 g/kg/day of protein for 7- to 12-month-old infants (i.e., 0.688 g/kg/day for maintenance + 0.412 g/kg/day for growth) and decreased to 0.88 g/kg/day for 1- to 3-year-old children, to 0.76 g/kg/day for 4- to 13-year-old children, and to 0.73 or 0.71 g/kg/day for 14- to 18-year-old boys and girls, respectively. RDAs for protein were set by adding two times the estimated CV of the protein requirement among individuals in each age–gender group to the EAR in order to establish a level of intake that should meet the needs of 97.5% of the population.

Similarly, protein requirements for pregnant women were established by adding their maintenance requirements to protein needs for deposition of new tissue accreted during pregnancy (IOM, 2002). Little protein is deposited during the first trimester, so a recommendation for additional dietary protein is made only for pregnant women during the second and third trimesters. Average protein deposition is 5.4 g/day during the second and third trimesters, which with correction for a conservative estimate of efficiency of protein utilization during pregnancy (43%) results in an additional protein need of 12.6 g/day for tissue accretion. This increased need for tissue accretion is equivalent to +0.22 g/kg/day for the 57-kg reference woman. Thus, this amount was added to the protein maintenance requirement of nonpregnant women (0.66 g/kg/day) to yield an EAR for pregnant women of 0.88 g/kg/day. It should be noted that the increased tissue mass also results in an increase in the normal maintenance requirement (e.g., 8.4 g protein for maintenance of an additional 12.7 kg of body weight), so that the total protein requirement of a pregnant woman is about 21 g more than her pre-pregnant requirement. The factorial approach was also utilized to set the EAR for lactating women (IOM, 2002). The additional protein requirement for lactation is based on the output of total nitrogen (protein and nonprotein nitrogen) in the milk, which was 10 g/day, corrected for the adult efficiency of protein utilization (47%). Therefore, the incremental protein required by lactating women is 21 g/day (10 g/day ÷ 0.47), or 0.39 g/kg/day for a 57-kg woman. Consequently, the protein EAR for lactating women is 0.66 g/kg/day + 0.39 g/kg/day = 1.05 g/kg/day. The RDAs for pregnant and lactating women were set as the respective EAR + 24%, or as the woman's non-pregnant RDA plus 25 g protein/day.

Indispensable amino acid requirements for children and lactating women were set using similar approaches. The amino acid EARs for adults were used as an estimate of maintenance requirements of amino acids, and the additional requirements for accretion of protein or milk production were based on the amino acid composition of body proteins or human milk, respectively.

FACTORS THAT AFFECT AMINO ACID REQUIREMENTS

Protein and amino acid requirements of healthy individuals are affected by several important factors—some intrinsic (mainly genetic) and others extrinsic (mainly dietary).

DIETARY ENERGY

Perhaps the most important dietary factor affecting protein utilization is dietary nonprotein energy (carbohydrate and fat). If energy is insufficient, amino acids will be used as a fuel rather than for protein synthesis. When amino acids are oxidized as a fuel, most of their carbon enters the citric acid cycle and other central pathways of fuel metabolism via pyruvate, oxaloacetate, α-ketoglutarate, or acetyl CoA (see Chapter 14, Fig. 14-9). The ability of amino acids to substitute for other energy sources is important, for example, in starvation, when body protein is depleted to provide amino acids both as precursors for important synthetic pathways and as a source of glucose and other energy-yielding substrates. However, when energy is available in other forms, either from body glycogen and fat or from dietary carbohydrate and fat, the need for net breakdown of body protein with oxidation of amino acids is diminished.

Dietary energy, in the form of carbohydrate or fat, has a profound effect on protein utilization in both the growing and adult states. With generous intakes of nonprotein energy, in excess of immediate energy needs, amino acid oxidation is minimized and amino acids are utilized with maximum efficiency. This is called the protein-sparing effect of dietary carbohydrate and fat. In adults, the effect is typically to spare 2 mg of nitrogen for each kcal added to a nutritionally adequate basal diet, which is associated with an increase in lean body mass that accompanies the deposition of body fat. In growing animals, the magnitude of the effect is similar, or even greater, and diminishes as the highest levels of energy intake are approached. Thus, excess energy has the effect of lowering apparent amino acid requirements for maintenance in adults and for normal growth in the immature. Conversely, when carbohydrate and fat intakes are limited, amino acid oxidation rises and apparent amino acid requirements are increased. This means that amino acid requirements cannot be stated without reference to the provision of other nutrients, particularly carbohydrate and fat. Deficiencies of many other nutrients, such as vitamins and minerals, also can limit the utilization of dietary protein. In published estimates of requirements, it is assumed that other nutrients are also provided at the appropriate levels and that adult subjects are not gaining weight.

POSSIBLE CONTRIBUTION OF MICROBIAL SYNTHESIS OF AMINO ACIDS

It is normally assumed that the indispensable amino acids can be derived only from the diet. However, this may not be entirely true. Evidence from both human and animal studies indicates that some amino acids synthesized by gastrointestinal microorganisms may be absorbed, augmenting the dietary supply. It has not been established whether this route makes a significant net contribution to meeting human requirements, but the available evidence suggests that it may (Metges et al., 1999).

CRITERION OF ADEQUACY

As we have seen, amino acid requirements may be derived in a number of different ways. It is perhaps not surprising that these should yield rather different estimates. However, most have been based on some measure of body protein status. In considering maintenance requirements, for example, it has been assumed that the requirement is that amount needed to preserve the total protein or amino acid content of the body. This may be too limited a definition on which to base dietary recommendations. We need to ask if there are aspects of health and well-being that would benefit from amounts of protein or individual amino acids that are greater than those that are needed simply to maintain protein homeostasis. Is the diet optimal for protein-related health such as immune function, bone health, or growth in height?

Higher tryptophan intakes are associated with greater synthesis of nicotinamide-adenine dinucleotide (NAD), and higher sulfur amino acid intakes are associated with greater synthesis of glutathione and taurine. However, the relation of dietary supply to optimal production or tissue concentrations of these nonprotein metabolites is not considered by current methods used for establishing amino acid and protein requirements and allowances. In addition, it is possible that intakes of specific dispensable amino acids affect metabolic state and health. For example, arginine supplements have been shown to enhance aspects of immune function and to have beneficial effects on wound healing, possibly due to the function of arginine in the formation of nitric oxide and polyamines. Likewise, glutamine, another amino acid normally considered dispensable, may improve recovery from injury or disease. This may relate to the fact that glutamine is a major fuel for rapidly proliferating cells, including lymphocytes. There is, however, little reliable evidence for any beneficial effect of higher habitual protein intakes on mortality, morbidity, and longevity.

Although the question of whether protein intakes somewhat greater than those needed for maintenance would be beneficial to health of adults has not been studied to any extent, it does seem clear that the optimum level of protein is not likely to be lower than the current EAR. In a study designed to evaluate the safe level of protein that had been set by FAO/WHO in 1973, young men were fed egg protein at a level of 0.59 g/kg/day for 12 weeks (Garza et al., 1977). Four of the six subjects were in negative nitrogen balance and experienced loss of lean body mass (based on total body potassium measurements and creatinine excretion). Two of the six subjects exhibited an excessive rise in serum aspartate aminotransferase and alanine aminotransferase, which rapidly fell to normal levels when the subjects were switched to a diet higher in protein. These findings suggest that 0.59 g of high quality protein per kg per day is not adequate for long-term maintenance of most healthy young men, and that the current estimate of the adult EAR for protein (0.66 g/kg/day) is close to the actual requirement, despite the limitations of nitrogen balance studies.

BENEFITS OF INTACT DIETARY PROTEINS AND PEPTIDES

Although dietary requirements for protein are correctly viewed as requirements for the amino acids contained in the proteins, there are some examples of intact peptides and proteins that are of nutritional significance, such as the immunoglobulins and lactoferrin passed to the infant in mother's milk. Other bioactive proteins, such as retinol-binding protein, transforming growth factor, and epidermal growth factor, may also be derived from maternal milk. It is also possible that certain peptides resulting from the incomplete hydrolysis of dietary proteins may sufficiently resemble bioactive peptides as to mimic their function in the body. Proteins in the diet also include antigens, toxins, and proteins with antinutritional effects such as the trypsin inhibitors in a number of legumes. Some of these exert their effects in the gut lumen; others are absorbed. All of these could be important in determining the extent to which protein nutriture may amount to more than simply the provision of amino acids and nitrogen.

TYPICAL INTAKES OF PROTEIN AND AMINO ACIDS AND SIGNIFICANCE OF PROTEIN-ENERGY RATIOS

Median intake of protein by adults in the United States was 97 and 64 g/day for 31 to 50-year-old men and women, respectively (Continuing Survey of Food Intake by Individuals [CSFII] 1994-96, 1998). For all adult age–gender groups, median intake ranged from 55 to 101 g/day. Overall, intake of adults ranged from approximately 27 g/day for some elderly women to 190 g/day for some young men. Median protein intakes for young individuals ranged from 15 g/day for 0 to 6-month-old infants and 50 g/day for 1- to 3-year-old children to 97 g and 65 g/day for 14- to 18-year-old males and females, respectively. In a recent nutrition survey of adults in the United Kingdom, protein intake of adults was found to be similar to that reported for the United States: 88 ± 32 g/day for men and 64 ± 17 g/day for women (mean ± SD) (Henderson et al., 2003).

The protein to energy (P/E) ratio, expressed as the percentage or fraction of total energy that is derived from protein, is a useful calculation. According to the Continuing Survey of Food Intakes by Individuals (CSFII, 1994-96, 1998, data for all individuals), the median percentage of total energy from protein consumed in the United States from 1994 to 1998 was 15.1% (IOM, 2002). This, however, ranged from a median of 8.8% for 0 to 6-month-old infants to 16% for adults, with intermediate values of 10.4% for 7- to 12-month-old infants and 14% for children 1 to 18 years of age. Although the median percentage of total energy from protein was 16% for adults, protein intake as a percentage of energy ranged from low values of approximately 9% to high values of approximately 24%. Food intake data for the United Kingdom gave P/E values, expressed as a percentage, of 14.2% for omnivores and 12.7% for vegetarians (Millward and Jackson, 2003).

Because protein EARs and RDAs are defined as a constant function of body weight (kg), variation in basal metabolic rate and variation in the level of energy expenditure will affect the percentage of energy that needs to be supplied as protein. If calculations are made based on the DRIs for protein and the estimated energy requirements (EERs), the percentage of total energy needed in the form of protein increases with age, is higher for females than males, is higher for small compared with large adults at any age, and decreases with physical activity. Therefore, the breast-fed infant is able to satisfy a high demand for protein by consuming large quantities of a very-low-protein food. Because the energy requirement per kilogram is very high during infancy and decreases with age at a greater rate than does the protein requirement per kilogram, the P/E ratio of the requirements for infants is relatively low and increases with age.

This concept is illustrated in Figure 15-5. By using adult weights representative of those in developed countries, Millward and Jackson (2003) calculated desirable P/E ratios for population groups of various ages and at three levels of physical activity. They then compared these with the protein-quality adjusted P/E ratios of four diets: the diet of adult omnivores in the United Kingdom; the diet of adult vegetarians (meat-free) in the United Kingdom; the average diet of India; and the average diet of West Bengal (a state in eastern India). Assuming that approaches to determining protein requirements and protein quality are correct and that the energy density or bulk of the diet does not limit consumption to a quantity that fails to satisfy energy requirements, this figure indicates that protein deficiency would most likely occur in elderly sedentary women and would least likely occur in moderately active young children, the opposite of what has usually been assumed. Adolescent females would also be a vulnerable group.

Unadjusted P/E ratios for various foods are given in Table 15-8, along with P/E ratios adjusted for the food's protein digestibility corrected amino acid score (PDCAAS) (Millward and Jackson, 2003). The majority of the world's population live in developing countries where plant proteins constitute the major source of proteins, with wheat, rice, and maize accounting for the bulk of the cereal intake. Digestibility and availability of plant proteins ranges from 50% to 90% due to resistant plant cell walls, antinutritional factors, and effects of processing and heat treatment. Lysine is the most important limiting amino acid in cereal-based diets, and estimates of BV depend heavily on the level of lysine in the scoring pattern that is applied. Note that the P/E ratios drop markedly for many staple cereals and root vegetables when they are corrected for protein quality. Millward and Jackson (2003) calculated an average P/E ratio of 0.111 for India, but the P/E ratio was lower for certain states within India (e.g., 0.088 in West Bengal). Food balance data sheets from the FAO for the period 1961-1992 show P/E ratios of 0.080 for Sierra Leone and 0.084 for Bangladesh. If adjusted for protein quality (digestibility and biologic value), the ratios for West Bengal, Sierra Leone, and Bangladesh fall to less than 0.070. Therefore, both the quantity and quality of protein are limiting features of many cereal-based diets.

Although the exact interpretation of the type of calculation illustrated in Figure 15-5

Table 15-8

Protein/Energy Ratios of Foods

	P/E Ratio	PDCAAS-Adjusted P/E Ratio
Beef	0.660	0.660
Egg	0.340	0.340
Cow's milk	0.194	0.194
Breast milk	0.060	0.060
Soy	0.388	0.349
Wheat	0.166	0.089
Maize	0.135	0.071
Improved variety of maize (variety o2 or o2s2)	0.140	0.102
Potatoes	0.097	0.079
Rice	0.072	0.047
Yam	0.061	0.045
Cassava	0.034	0.019
Cassava–soy mix (90% kcal from cassava/10% kcal from soy)	0.069	0.059

Data from Millward DJ, Jackson AA (2003) Protein/energy ratios of current diets in developed and developing countries compared with a safe protein/energy ratio: implications for recommended protein and amino acid intakes. Public Health Nutr 7:387-405.

PDCAAS, Protein digestibility corrected amino acid score.

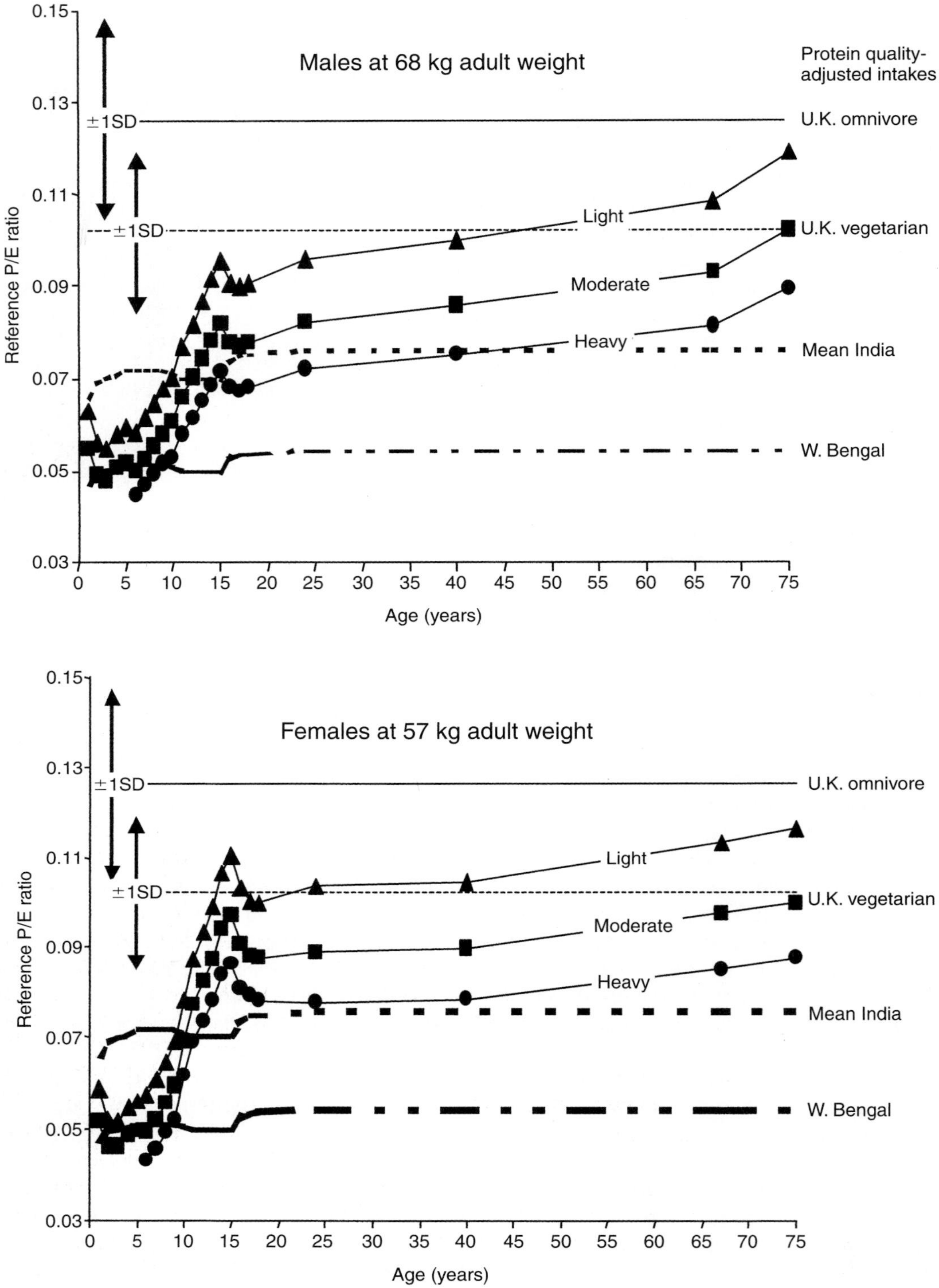

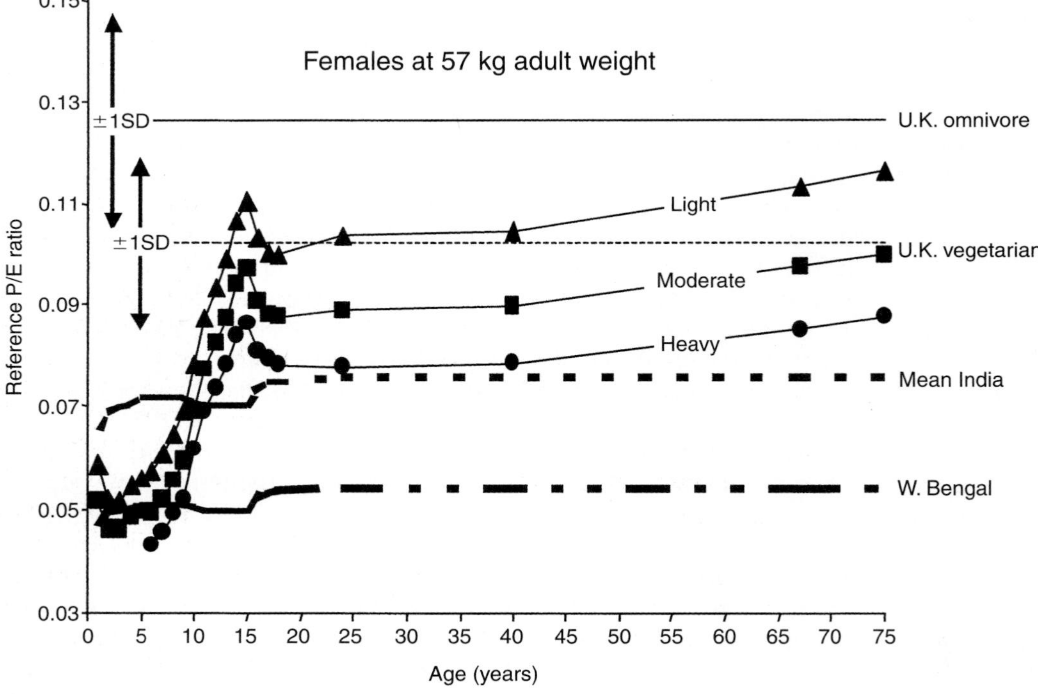

Figure 15-5 Reference P/E ratios (energy from protein/total energy in diet, expressed as a fraction) for men and women compared with the adjusted P/E ratios of diets. *(From Millward DJ, Jackson AA [2003] Protein/energy ratios of current diets in developed and developing countries compared with a safe protein/energy ratio: implications for recommended protein and amino acid intakes. Public Health Nutr 7:387-405.)*

can be debated, two conclusions are clear. First, food supplies or diets with adjusted P/E ratios of less than 0.07 are likely to be suboptimal for a substantial fraction of any population, and this will be especially true for individuals with low energy expenditures who need higher P/E ratios. Second, any population with a low energy intake is at greater risk of protein deficiency because protein will be used as a fuel when energy from fat and carbohydrate are insufficient.

In addressing needs of populations of protein-energy malnourished individuals, it is often the bulk and low energy density of the habitual diet or the lack of an adequate quantity of food that results in low intakes of both protein and energy. In some cases, such as when starchy roots, tubers, or fruits (especially cassava, plantain, or Ethiopian banana) or purified forms of starch or sugar are a major component of the diet, protein density of the diet is a constraint. Children recovering from severe protein-energy malnutrition and/or infection are particularly vulnerable to these constraints, and improvement in the quality, not just the quantity, of the diet is required. When children whose growth has been retarded by malnutrition are switched to a nutritious diet, their fractional growth rate may then reach 2% to 3% per day, and the amino acid needs for this rapid rate of body protein gain may increase requirements to two or three times the normal levels. Although catch-up growth requires an increased intake of both protein and energy, the fold-increase for protein is greater than that for energy. For children recovering from protein-energy malnutrition, infection, or other stress, diets with up to 12% of calories from protein may be appropriate (Badaloo et al., 1999).

EFFECTS OF INADEQUATE PROTEIN INTAKE AND ASSESSMENT OF PROTEIN STATUS

Protein-energy malnutrition (PEM) is common in both children and adults throughout the world. WHO estimates that PEM affects one in four children younger than 5 years of age on a worldwide basis (WHO, 2000). Of these, 150 million children (27%) are underweight and 182 million (32%) have stunted growth. PEM is associated with the deaths of approximately 5 million children each year. More than 70% of children affected by PEM live in Asia, especially southern Asia, and 26% live in Africa. In developed countries, PEM occurs primarily as a secondary complication of illnesses that impair the body's ability to absorb or use nutrients or to compensate for nutrient losses.

The most commonly used method to clinically evaluate protein status is the measurement of plasma proteins. Serum or plasma albumin and transferrin are the best measures of protein malnutrition, but the levels of these two proteins may also be affected by disease, infection, injury, or iron-deficiency. Because the skin and hair are rapidly growing tissues, physical examination of these tissues is useful. In protein malnutrition, the skin becomes thinner and appears dull, whereas the hair first does not grow and then may fall out or show color changes. Over a longer period, a loss of lean body mass occurs. In infants and children, borderline inadequate protein intake is reflected in failure to grow in length or height and in increased vulnerability to infections. Mid-upper-arm muscle circumference (or diameter) has been used as a measure of protein nutritional status in children.

The more severe expressions of PEM are typically seen in young children. Kwashiorkor, also called wet protein-energy malnutrition, is a form of PEM that results from a deficiency of primarily protein rather than energy. This condition usually appears at the age of about 12 months when breastfeeding is discontinued. In kwashiorkor, adequate energy consumption and decreased protein intake lead to decreased synthesis of visceral proteins. The resulting hypoalbuminemia contributes to extravascular fluid accumulation. Impaired synthesis of hepatic proteins results in fatty liver. The liver enlargement and fluid accumulation can distend the abdomen and disguise weight loss. Dry or peeling skin, hair discoloration, anemia, diarrhea, and fluid and electrolyte disorders are also commonly observed in children with kwashiorkor. In developed countries, kwashiorkor-like secondary PEM is observed primarily in patients who have been severely burned or who have had trauma or sepsis.

Clinical Correlation

Protein-Energy Malnutrition

Protein-energy malnutrition (PEM) is currently the most common deficiency disease in the world. As its name implies, PEM is a macronutrient deficiency disease resulting from an inadequate intake and/or utilization of protein and calories. Often the energy deficiency is more important than that the protein deficiency because proper protein utilization by the body depends on adequate energy intake. PEM ranges from mild to moderate forms, where the only obvious symptoms are inadequate growth in children, to the severe forms, kwashiorkor and marasmus, which can lead to death. PEM is often associated with micronutrient deficiencies; a diet that is lacking in calories and protein is also likely to be lacking in micronutrients. PEM is also associated with infections, which can increase nutrient requirements and/or decrease absorption and utilization of nutrients in the diet. Although adults can have PEM, it is most commonly seen in early childhood. This is partially because of a young child's relatively higher needs for protein and calories per kilogram body weight compared to older children or adults. Young children also have more parasitic and infectious diseases that can reduce appetite and food intake, decrease absorption and utilization of nutrients, and increase nutrient losses and requirements.

The classic theory of PEM is illustrated in the following diagram, along with some examples of diets that might result in kwashiorkor or marasmus.

All forms of PEM can be treated with a diet high in protein and calories. The more severe forms are life-threatening and usually require hospitalization to deal with the dehydration, electrolyte disturbance, and infections that often accompany severe PEM. Micronutrient deficiencies also need to be identified and treated. Although the immediate cause of PEM is an inadequate diet, it is important to remember that the underlying causes are poverty, inequity in food distribution, unsanitary conditions, and lack of knowledge. These underlying causes must be corrected if PEM is to be prevented. Even in developed countries, PEM is sometimes observed due to neglect or inadequate feeding of young children or substitution of low-protein products (e.g., rice milk) for milk or infant formula.

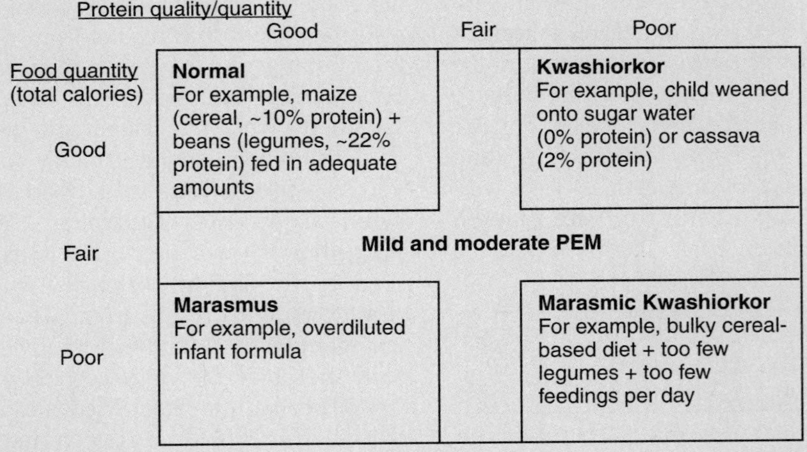

HOW MUCH PROTEIN IS TOO MUCH?

The major problem with intake of protein has to do with the allergenic sensitivity of some individuals to certain proteins. Relatively few food proteins cause most allergic reactions. Milk, eggs, peanuts, and soy are the most problematic for children, whereas fish, shellfish, peanuts, and nuts tend to be most allergenic for adults.

Although a tolerable upper intake level (UL) for protein has not been set by the IOM (2002), caution should be exercised in terms of very high levels of protein intake. An all-meat diet that provided 20% and 35% of energy as protein was consumed by explorers, trappers, and hunters during winters in northern America. These men survived exclusively on "pemmican," a concentrated food made by mixing lean dried meat (powdered jerked bison or caribou meat) with melted fat (Stefansson, 1944). A 1930 report described a study of two men, who had been arctic explorers, which involved their eating a meat-only diet for an entire year while living in a temperate climate (New York City) and under medical supervision. The diet was made up of muscle, liver, kidney, brain, bone marrow, bacon, and fat from beef, lamb, veal, pork, and chicken, and provided ~21% of energy as protein, 78% of energy as fat, and less than 2% of energy as carbohydrate (McClellan and Du Bois, 1930). These men lost weight during the first week, due to a shift in the water content of the body while it adjusted itself to the low-carbohydrate diet, but their weights remained constant thereafter. No ill effects of the all-meat diet were evident, but total acidity of the urine and calcium loss in the urine were both increased above control levels (mixed diet) and ketoaciduria was present throughout the study period. No evidence of renal hypertrophy or damage was observed.

Protein intakes exceeding 30% of calories (diets made up of essentially all meat or all animal products) have been described for the Masai of southern Kenya and northern Tanzania (~30% to 35% of calories as protein), the Ache hunters in the forests of eastern Paraguay (~39% of calories as protein), and Eskimos on the east coast of Greenland studied in the mid-1930s (45% of calories as protein), as summarized by Speth (1989). Ill effects of consumption of large portions of lean meat (>45% of calories as protein) have been reported, including a condition known as "rabbit starvation" that resulted in death of early American explorers who ate rabbit meat, which contains very little fat (Speth and Spielmann, 1983). Animal studies have clearly demonstrated that renal hypertrophy and damage occurs with very high protein intakes, and high protein intakes have adverse effects on patients with renal failure. In general, it seems wise to avoid protein intakes of greater than 250 g/day or more than 40% of energy.

No ULs have been set for intakes of individual amino acids, but available information about hazards of high intakes of amino acids was summarized by the IOM (2002). There is no reason to believe that levels of amino acids consumed as part of food proteins, even at high protein intakes near ~40% of energy, are of concern. However, caution should be used with either amino acid or protein supplements and with additives that contain amino acids (e.g., aspartame).

REFERENCES

Badaloo A, Boyne M, Reid M, Persaud C, Forrester T, Millward DJ, Jackson AA (1999) Dietary protein, growth and urea kinetics in severely malnourished children and during recovery. J Nutr 129:969-979.

Block RJ, Mitchell HH (1946) The correlation of the amino-acid composition of proteins with their nutritive value. Nutr Abstr Rev 16:249-278.

Borman A, Wood TR, Black HC, Anderson EG, Oesterling MJ, Wormack M, Rose WC (1946) The role of arginine in growth with some observations on the effects of argininic acid. J Biol Chem 166:585-594.

Brunton JA, Bertolo RF, Pencharz PB, Ball RO (1999) Proline ameliorates arginine deficiency during enteral but not parenteral feeding in neonatal piglets. Am J Physiol 277:E223-E231.

Carpenter KJ (1994) Protein and Energy: A Study of Changing Ideas in Nutrition. Cambridge University Press, New York.

Fick A, Wislicenus J (1866) On the origin of muscular power. Phil Mag Lond (4th ser.) 31: 485-503.

Food and Agriculture Organization of the United Nations (FAO) (1991) Protein Quality Evaluation: Report of Joint FAO/WHO Expert Consultation. FAO Food and Nutrition Paper #51. FAO, Rome.

Fuller MF, Milne A, Harris CI, Reid TMS, Keenan R (1994) Amino acid losses in ileostomy fluid on a protein-free diet. Am J Clin Nutr 59:70-73.

Garza C, Scrimshaw NS, Young VR (1977) Human protein requirements: a long-term metabolic nitrogen balance study in young men to evaluate the 1973 FAO-WHO safe level of egg protein intake. J Nutr 107:335-352.

Henderson L, Gregory J, Irving K, Swan G (2003) The National Diet and Nutrition Survey: Adults aged 19 to 64 years. Vol. 2. Energy, Protein, Carbohydrate, Fat and Alcohol Intake. Office for National Statistics and Food Standards Agency, London.

Institute of Medicine (IOM) (2002) Dietary Reference Intakes: Energy, Carbohydrate, Fiber, Fat, Fatty Acids, Cholesterol, Protein, and Amino Acids. Part 2. National Academy Press, Washington, DC.

Jackson AA, Shaw JCL, Barber A, Golden MHN (1981) Nitrogen metabolism in preterm infants fed human donor breast milk: the possible essentiality of glycine. Pediatr Res 15: 1454-1461.

Leverton RM, Waddill FS, Skellenger M (1959) The urinary excretion of five essential amino acids by young women. J Nutr 67:19-28.

McClellan WS, Du Bois EF (1930) Clinical calorimetry: XLV. Prolonged meat diets with a study of kidney function and ketosis. J Biol Chem 87:651-668.

Metges CC, Petzke KJ, El-Khoury AE, Henneman L, Grant I, Bedri S, Regan MM, Fuller MF, Young VR (1999) Incorporation of urea and ammonia nitrogen into ileal and fecal microbial proteins and plasma free amino acids in normal men and ileostomates. Am J Clin Nutr 70:1046-1158.

Millward DJ (2003) An adaptive metabolic demand model for protein and amino acid requirements. Br J Nutr 90:249-260.

Millward DJ, Jackson AA (2003) Protein/energy ratios of current diets in developed and developing countries compared with a safe protein/energy ratio: implications for recommended protein and amino acid intakes. Public Health Nutr 7:387-405.

Rand WM, Pellett PL, Young VR (2003) Meta-analysis of nitrogen balance studies for estimating protein requirements in healthy adults. Am J Clin Nutr 77:109-127.

Reeds PJ (2000) Dispensable and indispensable amino acids for humans. J Nutr 130: 1835S-1840S.

Rose WC (1957) The amino acid requirements of adult man. Nutr Abstr Rev 27:631-647.

Smith RH (1980) Comparative amino acid requirements. Proc Nutr Soc 39:71-78.

Speth JD (1989) Early hominid hunting and scavenging: the role of meat as an energy source. J Hum Evol 18:329-343.

Speth JD, Spielmann KA (1983) Energy source, protein metabolism, and hunter-gatherer subsistence strategies. J Anthropol Archaeol 2:1-31.

Stefansson V (1944) Pemmican. Military Surgeon 95:89-98.

World Health Organization (WHO) (1985) Energy and Protein Requirements. Report of a Joint FAO/WHO/UNU Expert Consultation. WHO Technical Report Series 724. World Health Organization, Geneva.

World Health Organization (WHO) (2000) Nutrition for Health and Development: A global agenda for combating malnutrition. Progress Report. World Health Organization, Geneva.

RECOMMENDED READINGS

Millward DJ (2003) An adaptive metabolic demand model for protein and amino acid requirements. Br J Nutr 90:249-260.

Millward DJ, Jackson AA (2003) Protein/energy ratios of current diets in developed and developing countries compared with a safe protein/energy ratio: implications for recommended protein and amino acid intakes. Public Health Nutr 7:387-405.

Pencharz PB, Ball RO (2003) Different approaches to define individual amino acid requirements. Annu Rev Nutr 23:101-116.

Rand WM, Pellett PL, Young VR (2003) Meta-analysis of nitrogen balance studies for estimating protein requirements in healthy adults. Am J Clin Nutr 77:109-127.

Chapter 16

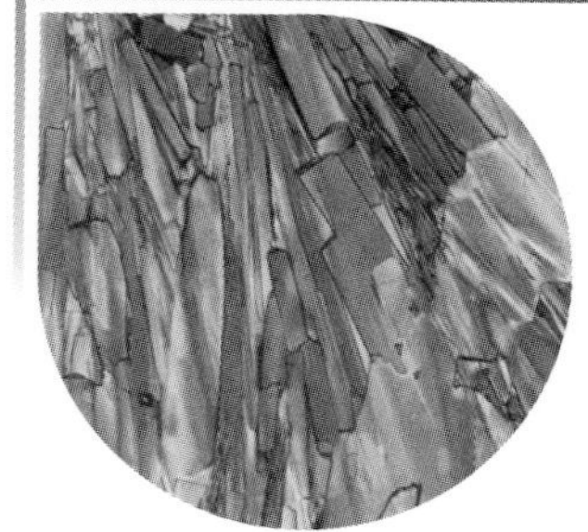

Metabolism of Fatty Acids, Acylglycerols, and Sphingolipids

Hei Sook Sul, PhD

OUTLINE

This chapter is a revision of a chapter written by Alan G. Goodridge, PhD, and Hei Sook Sul, PhD, for the first edition.

COMMON ABBREVIATIONS

ACP	acyl carrier protein
CPT	carnitine palmitoyltransferase
HSL	hormone sensitive lipase
PPAR	peroxisome proliferator-activated receptor
SREBP	sterol regulatory element binding protein

BIOLOGICAL ROLES FOR LIPIDS

There are four major and a multitude of minor roles for lipids in living organisms. Major roles include serving as an energy source or fuel, as structural components of membranes, as lubricants (especially of the body surfaces), and as signaling molecules. These four major functions require specific classes of lipids that differ in general structure. Each class contains numerous members with small but substantial structural differences. These lipid structures and their characteristics are discussed in Chapter 6.

Acylglycerols are the major lipids in the body. Lipids in the form of triacylglycerol play a critical role in metabolism as the primary form of stored energy in the mammalian body. Approximately 85% of the energy stored in the body of a 70-kg normal-weight man is in the form of triacylglycerol, primarily stored in adipose tissue. Triacylglycerol in the diet provides a concentrated source of energy. Triacylglycerol in milk is important for supplying calories to the newborn infant. When the caloric content of the diet exceeds the immediate energetic requirements of the individual, carbohydrates (and to some extent amino acids) may be converted to fatty acids and esterified to glycerol to form triacylglycerol. Triacylglycerol is a very efficient chemical form for storing energy because it contains approximately 9 kcal/g as opposed to approximately 4 kcal/g for carbohydrate and protein. In addition, triacylglycerol is advantageous because it can be stored in a relatively anhydrous form requiring about 1 g of water per gram of fat, whereas carbohydrate and protein require about 4 g of water per gram of glycogen or protein. Conversion of carbohydrate and protein to triacylglycerol is regulated by diet; the conversion is high in the fed state, especially if the diet is rich in carbohydrate, and is low in the fasting state. Storage of triacylglycerol also is high in the fed state and low in the fasting state, regardless of the composition of the diet.

The principal structural role of lipids is in the membranes—both the plasma membrane and subcellular membranes. A lipid bilayer constitutes the external boundary of every mammalian cell. Similarly, lipid membranes form the boundaries of numerous subcellular organelles. The principal components of the lipid bilayer are acylglycerols, phospholipids, sphingolipids, and cholesterol, the proportions of which vary with the membrane type.

Lipids also play an important role in lubrication and conditioning of body surfaces. Most sebaceous glands, which are microscopic, are found in skin and the mucous membranes of external orifices of the mammalian body. These glands secrete a lipid product composed of triacylglycerol, squalene, and wax esters. This secretion lubricates mucous membranes and conditions skin and hair. Some larger glands are modified sebaceous glands with specific functions. The meibomian glands in the eyelids, for example, provide lubricant and protection for the surface of the eye.

Lipids are important signaling molecules, both outside and inside cells. Sex hormones, adrenocortical hormones, and vitamin D are derived from cholesterol and play important extracellular signaling roles. Eicosanoids derived from arachidonic acid, and platelet-activating factor, which is a phospholipid-like compound, are also important in extracellular signaling. Inside cells, diacylglycerol and molecules derived from phospholipids and sphingolipids are involved in the transmission of signals from the plasma membrane to enzymes in the cytosol or other subcellular compartments and to proteins that regulate the expression of specific genes in the nucleus. In this chapter, synthesis and oxidation of fatty acids and acylglycerols as well as sphingolipids are discussed. Cholesterol and lipoprotein metabolism and transport are discussed in Chapter 17.

SYNTHESIS OF LONG-CHAIN FATTY ACIDS FROM ACETYL CoA

The primary anatomical sites for synthesis of fatty acids are the liver and adipose tissue. In humans, the extent and the contribution of each of these tissues to de novo lipogenesis are still debated (Hellerstein 1999). The lipogenic pathway may be suppressed by the high fat content of the modern diet (~40% of total energy). Therefore, in most individuals consuming typical Western diets, de novo lipogenesis may not contribute significantly to triacylglycerol biosynthesis. However, low but regulated rates of lipogenesis still may be critical for overall control of fatty acid metabolism in humans. The substrates and intermediates in pathways of lipid synthesis and oxidation are mainly esters of fatty acids and coenzyme A (CoA). As discussed in subsequent text, malonyl coenzyme A (CoA), the product of the acetyl CoA carboxylase reaction, inhibits fatty acid oxidation. In addition, in some physiological and pathophysiological conditions, de novo lipogenesis may play a quantitatively significant role. For example, developmental needs for lipid in the fetus may be met by de novo lipogenesis, the rate of which is extremely high in premature infants. De novo lipogenesis also contributes significantly to the hypertriglyceridemia of alcoholic liver diseases. Some of the metabolic abnormalities in untreated type 1 diabetes mellitus arise from the impaired fatty acid synthesis caused by low insulin levels. Another calorically important site of fat synthesis is the lactating mammary gland, in which medium-chain fatty acids are synthesized and esterified to glycerol for milk fat. Branched-chain fatty acids for conditioning body surfaces are synthesized in sebaceous and other more specialized glands.

TRANSFER OF ACETYL CoA FROM INSIDE THE MITOCHONDRIA TO THE CYTOSOL

The enzymes that catalyze the reactions for fatty acid synthesis are cytosolic. This localization is important because it separates processes of fatty acid synthesis from mitochondrial fatty acid oxidation (mitochondrial). Although the enzymes that catalyze the reactions in these two pathways are different, the substrate of one pathway is the product of the other and vice versa. Because the reactions occur in different compartments, the strategy for regulating these competing processes is different from that used in gluconeogenesis and glycolysis, in which most of the competing reactions are in the same compartment. Therefore, fatty acid synthesis is regulated by both phosphorylation and allosteric control of the key regulatory enzyme of fatty acid synthesis, acetyl CoA carboxylase, whereas fatty acid oxidation is regulated primarily by the rate of uptake of substrate by the mitochondria.

The substrate for fatty acid synthesis, acetyl CoA, is formed from pyruvate in the mitochondria. The inner mitochondrial membrane is impermeable to acetyl CoA and does not contain a carrier to transport the acetyl CoA into the cytosol. When production of acetyl CoA from pyruvate is high, the rate of formation of citrate catalyzed by citrate synthase in the citric acid cycle also is elevated, resulting in the accumulation of intramitochondrial citrate. Under these conditions, citrate can be translocated to the cytosol in exchange for a dicarboxylate anion, probably malate, by the tricarboxylate anion carrier in the inner mitochondrial membrane (Fig. 16-1). Citrate, therefore, serves as the intermediary for the transfer of acetyl CoA from mitochondria to cytosol. As described in subsequent text of this chapter, citrate as a feed-forward activator of acetyl CoA carboxylase plays a key role in regulating fatty acid synthesis. In the cytosol, therefore, fatty acid synthesis actually starts by cleavage of citrate back to acetyl CoA.

Cytosolic citrate is cleaved to acetyl CoA and oxaloacetate in a reaction that is catalyzed by adenosine triphosphate (ATP)–citrate lyase:

$$\text{Citrate} + \text{CoA} + \text{ATP} + H_2O \rightarrow \text{Acetyl CoA} + \text{Oxaloacetate} + \text{ADP} + P_i$$

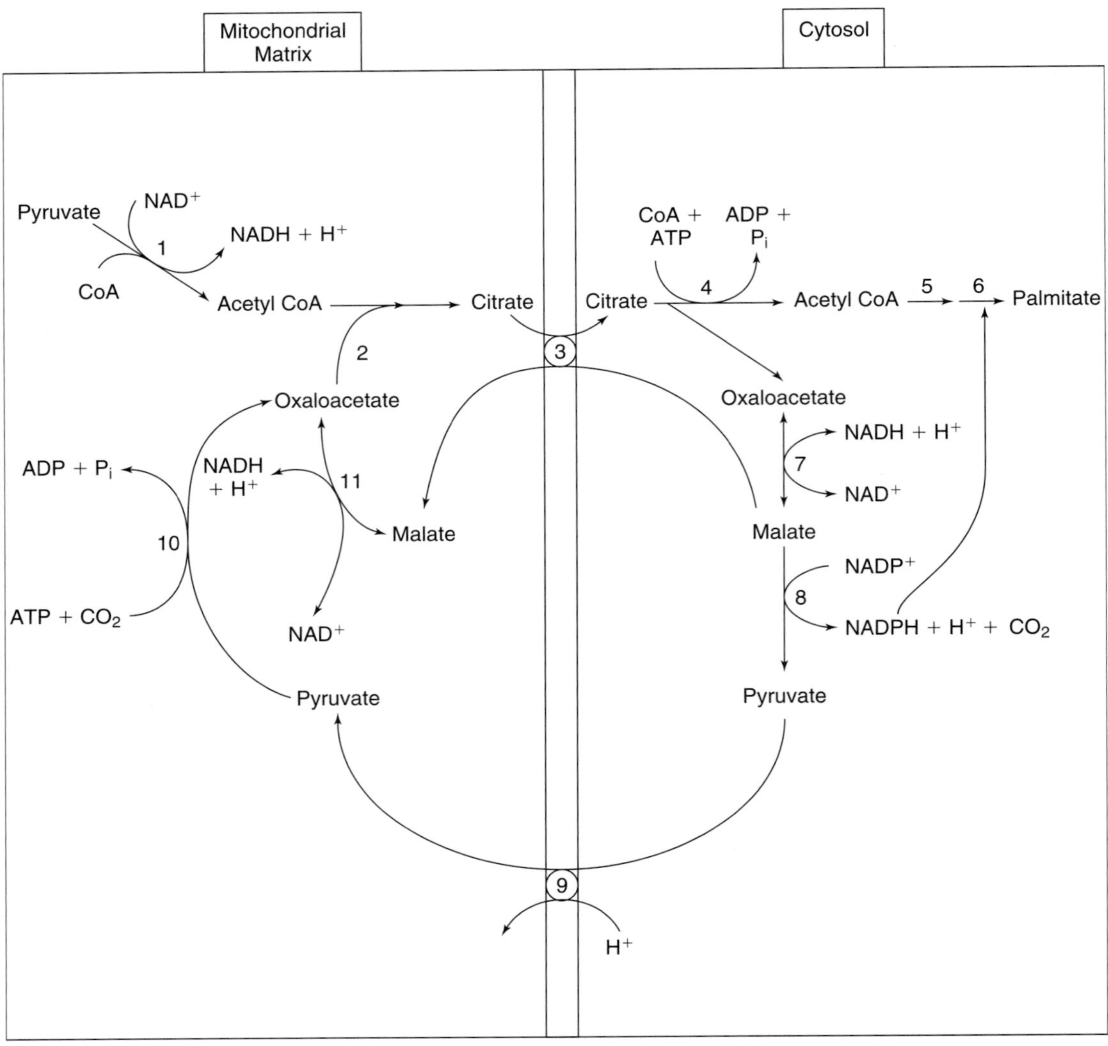

Figure 16-1 A schematic diagram of the pathways involved in the synthesis of fatty acids. *1*, Pyruvate dehydrogenase; *2*, citrate synthase; *3*, tricarboxylate transporter; *4*, ATP-citrate lyase; *5*, acetyl CoA carboxylase; *6*, fatty acid synthase; *7*, malate dehydrogenase; *8*, malic enzyme; *9*, pyruvate transporter; *10*, pyruvate carboxylase; *11*, malate dehydrogenase.

Oxaloacetate formed in the cytosol cannot be returned to the mitochondria because the mitochondrial membrane lacks the necessary transporter. Oxaloacetate can be reduced to malate by cytosolic malate dehydrogenase:

$$\text{Oxaloacetate} + \text{NADH} + \text{H}^+ \leftrightarrow \text{Malate} + \text{NAD}^+$$

Malate can be returned to mitochondria on a tricarboxylate anion carrier in exchange for another molecule of citrate. Malate can then be converted back to oxaloacetate by mitochondrial malate dehydrogenase. This cycle results in the net transport of acetyl CoA at an energetic cost of 1 mole of ATP per mole of acetyl CoA translocated. In addition, it results in transfer of NADH formed in the cytosol to the mitochondria, where it can contribute to the generation of ATP via oxidative phosphorylation.

Alternatively, or perhaps in addition, malate generated by reduction of oxaloacetate in the cytosol can, in turn, be oxidized to pyruvate and carbon dioxide by malic enzyme in the cytosol. The pyruvate can then be returned to the mitochondria. Oxidation of malate to pyruvate by the malic enzyme requires NADP as the hydrogen acceptor and generates NADPH. As discussed in subsequent text, NADPH is the required donor for the reductive step in fatty acid biosynthesis. This longer cycle is then completed in the mitochondria by the ATP-dependent carboxylation of pyruvate to oxaloacetate that is catalyzed by pyruvate carboxylase. The malic enzyme cycle thus translocates 1 mole of acetyl CoA and generates 1 mole of NADPH per 2 moles of ATP expended. By this pathway, reducing equivalents from cytosolic NADH are transferred to NADP so that the resulting NADPH is used for fatty acid synthesis along with NADPH produced by the pentose phosphate pathway.

CONVERSION OF ACETYL CoA TO MALONYL CoA

The next reaction in the synthesis of fatty acids is catalyzed by acetyl CoA carboxylase and involves an ATP-dependent carboxylation of acetyl CoA to malonyl CoA (see Chapter 26, Fig. 26-8). This is the first committed step in fatty acid synthesis and is highly regulated. Like pyruvate carboxylase, acetyl CoA carboxylase utilizes bicarbonate as a source of carbon dioxide, has a two-step reaction mechanism, and requires a covalently bound biotin:

$$HCO_3^- + \text{ATP} + \text{Biotin-Enzyme} \rightarrow \text{Carboxybiotin-Enzyme} + \text{ADP} + P_i$$

$$\text{Carboxybiotin-Enzyme} + \text{Acetyl CoA} \rightarrow \text{Malonyl CoA} + \text{Biotin-Enzyme}$$

$$\text{NET: Acetyl CoA} + HCO_3^- + \text{ATP} \rightarrow \text{Malonyl CoA} + \text{ADP} + P_i$$

In the first step, the biotin, which is bound to a specific lysyl residue of the enzyme, is carboxylated with the energy furnished by the hydrolysis of ATP (biotin carboxylation). In the second step (transcarboxylation), the activated, biotin-bound carboxyl group is transferred to acetyl CoA, regenerating enzyme-bound biotin and synthesizing malonyl CoA. Both of these reactions are catalyzed by a single polypeptide chain that also contains a domain for the covalently linked biotin. In biotin deficiency, the acetyl CoA carboxylase reaction is impaired, and thus fatty acid synthesis from acetyl CoA is decreased. (See Chapter 26 for further discussion of biotin dependent carboxylation.)

Acetyl CoA carboxylase is regulated by an array of control mechanisms, thereby permitting the rate of fatty acid synthesis to fluctuate in response to physiological and developmental conditions (Hillgartner et al., 1995; Munday, 2002). At the same time, because malonyl CoA, the product of acetyl CoA carboxylase, is a potent inhibitor of carnitine palmitoyltransferase-I (CPT-I), the rate of fatty acid oxidation in mitochondria is reciprocally regulated (as discussed in subsequent text). There are two isoforms of acetyl CoA carboxylase: ACC1 is for acetyl CoA synthesis in lipogenic tissues (i.e., liver and adipose tissue), whereas ACC2 present in muscle is for formation of malonyl CoA for regulating fatty acid oxidation. The activity of acetyl CoA carboxylase is stimulated by citrate, an allosteric activator, and inhibited by long-chain acyl CoA, an allosteric inhibitor. Production of cytosolic citrate is increased under conditions favoring fatty acid synthesis. The level of long-chain acyl CoAs increases during starvation when fatty acid synthesis is inhibited and, conversely, the long-chain acyl CoA level decreases in the fed state when fatty acid synthesis is stimulated. These allosteric mechanisms thus represent examples of feed-forward and feedback regulation.

Acetyl CoA carboxylase also is regulated by covalent modification. Each molecule of enzyme contains up to seven serine residues that can be phosphorylated. The phosphorylated enzyme is less active, less sensitive to the stimulatory effects of citrate, and more sensitive to the inhibitory action of long-chain acyl CoA. A number of different protein kinases catalyze phosphorylation of acetyl CoA carboxylase and do so at different specific serine residues on the enzyme. AMP activated protein kinase is the important physiological kinase that phosphorylates acetyl CoA carboxylase. Therefore, when cellular energy state is low, with increased intracellular AMP levels, AMP-activated protein kinase is allosterically activated by AMP and in turn phosphorylates acetyl CoA carboxylase resulting in a decrease in its activity. AMP-activated protein kinase is phosphorylated and activated by an upstream protein kinase. The identity of the upstream kinase is not clear; LKB1 is a possible candidate (Woods et al., 2004). In liver, glucagon is an important

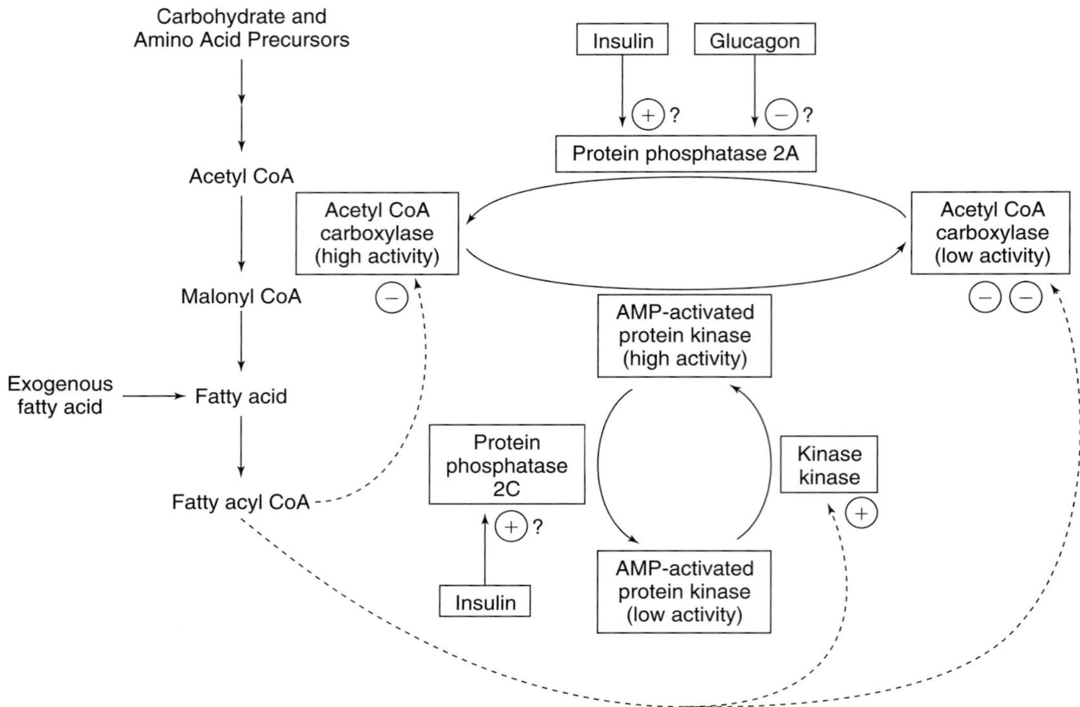

Figure 16-2 Model for the regulation of acetyl CoA carboxylase. Acetyl CoA carboxylase is phosphorylated and converted to a less active form by AMP-activated protein kinase. The latter enzyme is phosphorylated and activated by a kinase. Arrows with dotted lines indicate either positive (+) or negative (–) allosteric effects of fatty acyl CoA on the specified enzyme. Extent of allosteric inhibition is indicated by the number of (–) symbols. The phosphatases that inactivate AMP-activated protein kinase or activate glucagon inhibition of this step have not been demonstrated definitively.

effector increasing production of cAMP, which, in turn, activates protein kinase A (Fig. 16-2). There is a potential physiological role for protein kinase A in the hormonally mediated inactivation of acetyl CoA carboxylase. However, unlike glucagon regulation of other enzymes via direct phosphorylation of the enzyme by protein kinase A, regulation of acetyl CoA carboxylase via protein kinase A may not be by direct phosphorylation of acetyl CoA carboxylase by protein kinase A.

In addition to regulation by allosteric and phosphorylation–dephosphorylation mechanisms, acetyl CoA carboxylase also is regulated by changes in the number of molecules present in the cell. The concentration of the enzyme is low in the liver of starved animals and high in the liver of fed animals, especially if the diet is high in carbohydrate. The acetyl CoA carboxylase protein concentration in cells is controlled primarily by changes in the rate of transcription of the acetyl CoA carboxylase gene. Changes in circulating insulin and glucagon, as well as glucose levels during the fasting and fed states, participate in regulating acetyl CoA carboxylase gene transcription; insulin and glucose increase and cAMP decreases the rate of transcription.

SYNTHESIS OF PALMITATE FROM MALONYL CoA, ACETYL CoA, AND NADPH BY FATTY ACID SYNTHASE

The second and final committed step in fatty acid synthesis is catalyzed by a multifunctional polypeptide, fatty acid synthase that contains an acyl carrier protein (ACP) domain with a 4′-phosphopantetheine prosthetic group. The substrates for this reaction are 7 molecules of malonyl CoA, 1 of acetyl CoA, 14 of NADPH,

1. Acyl transferase

$$CH_3\overset{O}{\overset{\|}{C}}-S-\text{CoA} + \text{HS}-\text{pan}-\text{E} \longleftrightarrow CH_3\overset{O}{\overset{\|}{C}}-S-\text{pan}-\text{E} + \text{CoA}$$

2. β-Ketoacyl synthase

$$CH_3\overset{O}{\overset{\|}{C}}-S-\text{pan}-\text{E} + \text{HS}-\text{cys}-\text{E} \longleftrightarrow CH_3\overset{O}{\overset{\|}{C}}-S-\text{cys}-\text{E} + \text{HS}-\text{pan}-\text{E}$$

3. Acyl transferase

$$^{-}O\overset{O}{\overset{\|}{C}}CH_2\overset{O}{\overset{\|}{C}}-S-\text{CoA} + \text{HS}-\text{pan}-\text{E} \longleftrightarrow {}^{-}O\overset{O}{\overset{\|}{C}}CH_2\overset{O}{\overset{\|}{C}}-S-\text{pan}-\text{E} + \text{CoA}$$

4. β-Ketoacyl synthase

$$CH_3\overset{O}{\overset{\|}{C}}-S-\text{cys}-\text{E} + {}^{-}O\overset{O}{\overset{\|}{C}}CH_2\overset{O}{\overset{\|}{C}}-S-\text{pan}-\text{E} \longrightarrow CH_3\overset{O}{\overset{\|}{C}}CH_2\overset{O}{\overset{\|}{C}}-S-\text{pan}-\text{E} + \text{HS}-\text{cys}-\text{E} + CO_2$$

5. β-Ketoacyl reductase

$$CH_3\overset{O}{\overset{\|}{C}}CH_2\overset{O}{\overset{\|}{C}}-S-\text{pan}-\text{E} + \text{NADPH} + H^+ \longrightarrow CH_3\underset{OH}{\underset{|}{\overset{H}{\overset{|}{C}}}}CH_2\overset{O}{\overset{\|}{C}}-S-\text{pan}-\text{E} + \text{NADP}^+$$

6. β-Hydroxyacyl dehydratase

$$CH_3\underset{OH}{\underset{|}{\overset{H}{\overset{|}{C}}}}CH_2\overset{O}{\overset{\|}{C}}-S-\text{pan}-\text{E} \longleftrightarrow CH_3\overset{H}{\overset{|}{C}}=\underset{H}{\underset{|}{C}}\overset{O}{\overset{\|}{C}}-S-\text{pan}-\text{E} + H_2O$$

Figure 16-3 The component reactions of fatty acid synthase. The abbreviations HS–cys–E and HS–pan–E indicate an enzyme-bound cysteine residue and an enzyme-bound 4′-phosphopantetheine group, respectively.

Continued

and 14 of H^+. The products are 1 molecule of palmitate (C16), 8 of CoA, 7 of CO_2, 14 of $NADP^+$, and 6 of H_2O. The reaction is complex in two ways. First, the fatty acid is built up by the serial addition of two-carbon fragments to a growing chain. Second, after each addition, the added carbons are reduced, dehydrated, and reduced again. The process then repeats itself—condensation, reduction, dehydration, and reduction—until a 16-carbon fatty acid has been formed and is released from the enzyme (Fig. 16-3).

The first step in this complicated process involves an acyl transferase activity that transfers the acetyl moiety of acetyl CoA to a serine residue in the acyltransferase domain of the enzyme. The acetyl group is then transferred from the serine residue in the acyltransferase domain to the 4′-phosphopantetheine if the sulfhydryl of the covalently linked 4′-phosphopantetheine group in the acyl carrier protein domain of the enzyme is free. The 4′-phosphopantetheine group of the ACP domain of fatty acid synthase is described in Chapter 26. The β-ketoacyl synthase (the "condensing enzyme") activity of fatty acid synthase then catalyzes transfer of the acetyl group to a cysteine residue at the active site of the condensation reaction. The serine residue in the acyl transferase domain is now free to accept a malonyl group. The malonyl group is then transferred to the sulfhydryl group of the

7. Enoyl reductase

$$CH_3C(H){=}C(H)C({=}O){-}S{-}pan{-}E + NADPH + H^+ \longrightarrow CH_3CH_2CH_2C({=}O){-}S{-}pan{-}E + NADP^+$$

8. β-Ketoacyl synthase (#2)

$$CH_3CH_2CH_2C({=}O){-}S{-}pan{-}E + HS{-}cys{-}E \longleftrightarrow CH_3CH_2CH_2C({=}O){-}S{-}cys{-}E + HS{-}pan{-}E$$

9. Acyl transferase (#3)

$$^{-}OC({=}O)CH_2C({=}O){-}S{-}CoA + HS{-}pan{-}E \longleftrightarrow {}^{-}OC({=}O)CH_2C({=}O){-}S{-}pan{-}E + CoA$$

10. β-Ketoacyl synthase (#4)

$$CH_3CH_2CH_2C({=}O){-}S{-}cys{-}E + {}^{-}OC({=}O)CH_2C({=}O){-}S{-}pan{-}E \longrightarrow CH_3CH_2CH_2C({=}O){-}CH_2C({=}O){-}S{-}pan{-}E + HS{-}cys{-}E + CO_2$$

11-13. Repeat 5-7; Forming Hexanoyl—pan—E

14-38. Five Repeats of Reactions 3-7; Forming Palmitoyl—pan—E

39. Thioesterase

$$Palmitoyl{-}pan{-}E + H_2O \longrightarrow Palmitate + HS{-}pan{-}E$$

Figure 16-3—Cont'd

phosphopantetheine side arm (see Fig. 16-3), which has been freed of its acetyl group, and the enzyme is poised to carry out the first condensation reaction.

During the condensation reaction, the methylene carbon of the malonyl-phosphopantetheine form of the enzyme attacks the carbonyl group of the acetyl moiety in the active site of the β-ketoacyl transferase, forming the acetoacetyl-phosphopantetheine form of the enzyme and releasing the carboxyl group at C-2 of the malonyl moiety as CO_2. The energy for this reaction is provided by coupling condensation of the acetyl and malonyl groups with decarboxylation. A condensation that started with two acetyl CoAs would be energetically unfavorable. As a result, the energy for this reaction really comes from the hydrolysis of ATP during the carboxylation of acetyl CoA to form malonyl CoA; malonyl CoA is thus an activated form of acetyl CoA. The carboxyl group added by acetyl CoA carboxylase is the same one that is removed during the condensation reaction. Thus, even though bicarbonate is a required substrate for the fatty acid synthesis pathway, net incorporation of bicarbonate into the fatty acid does not occur.

The phosphopantetheine side arm in the acyl carrier protein (ACP) domain of fatty acid synthase is long and flexible, so that its attached acetoacetyl group can interact sequentially with the active sites of the β-ketoacyl reductase, β-hydroxyacyl dehydratase, and enoyl reductase domains to form a 4-carbon saturated fatty acyl group. At the end of this reaction sequence, the butyryl moiety remains attached to the phosphopantetheinyl moiety, but it is then transferred to the cysteine residue in the active site of the β-ketoacyl synthase domain. This leaves the sulfhydryl of the phosphopantetheinyl moiety free to receive a new malonyl CoA moiety from the serine residue in the

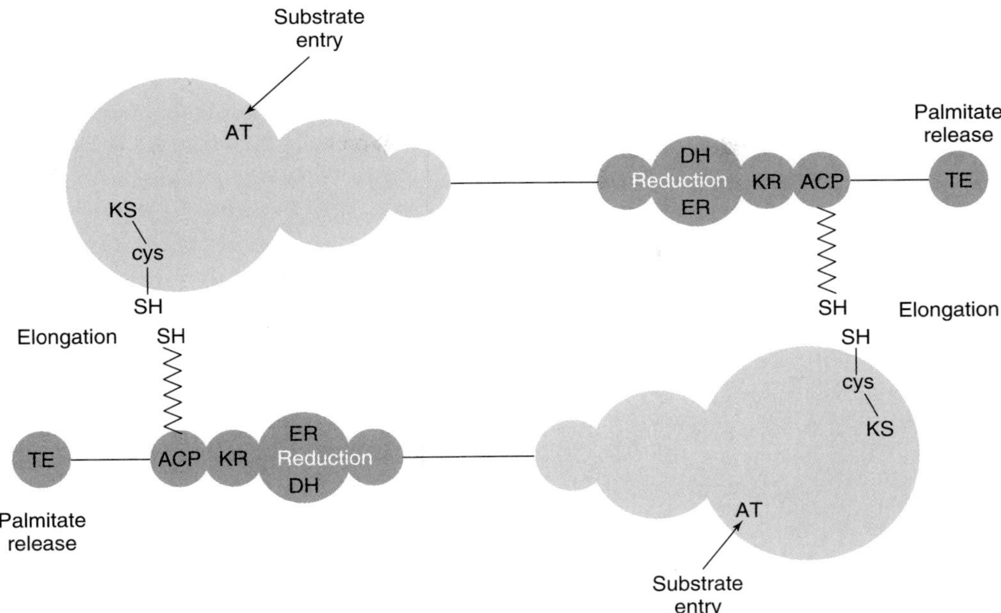

Figure 16-4 The fatty acid synthase model. Two identical subunits of fatty acid synthase are juxtaposed head-to-tail. Two centers for acyl chain assembly and release are shown. *ACP,* Acyl carrier protein; *AT,* acyl transferase; *DH,* β-hydroxyacyl dehydratase; *ER,* enoyl reductase; *KR,* β-ketoacyl reductase; *KS,* β-ketoacyl synthase; *SH,* the free sulfhydryl group of the 4′-phosphopantetheine moiety of ACP or of a cysteine residue of KS; *TE,* thioesterase.

acyltransferase domain. The next cycle of condensation, reduction, dehydration, and reduction then forms a 6-carbon saturated fatty-acyl group (hexanoyl) attached to the phosphopantetheine side arm. The hexanoyl group is transferred to the active site cysteine residue of the β-ketoacyl synthase domain, and another malonyl group is condensed, reduced, dehydrated, and reduced. After seven cycles, the growing acyl chain reaches 16 carbons, and a thioesterase activity in the thioesterase domain of fatty acid synthase cleaves the free fatty acid from the enzyme (see Fig. 16-3).

All the reactions required for fatty acid synthesis from acetyl CoA and malonyl CoA are catalyzed by a single polypeptide that contains all the activities in separate domains. The multifunctional fatty acid synthase can provide a greater efficiency by channeling intermediates from one active site to the next rather than relying on diffusion of intermediates between separate enzymes. In addition, the amounts of each enzyme can be regulated simultaneously by controlling expression of a single gene. Mammalian fatty acid synthase is synthesized as an inactive monomer of about 270 kDa. The active enzyme is a homodimer. The dimer is assembled with the head of one monomer bound to the tail of the other, resulting in the formation of two catalytic centers in each homodimer. Each catalytic center has components from each monomer (Fig. 16-4).

The activity of fatty acid synthase, similar to that of acetyl CoA carboxylase and other enzymes involved in fatty acid synthesis, such as ATP-citrate lyase, malic enzyme, and some of the enzymes in the pentose phosphate pathway, is high in the fed state (especially if the diet is high in carbohydrate) and low in the fasting state. Fat, especially polyunsaturated fatty acids in the diet, decreases fatty acid synthase activity. Neither allosteric nor phosphorylation–dephosphorylation mechanisms appear to contribute to these changes in fatty acid synthase activity. Regulation is at the level of protein concentration, and both transcriptional and posttranscriptional mechanisms are involved. Sterol regulatory element binding protein-1c (SREBP-1c), which is expressed predominantly in the lipogenic tissues, is itself suppressed in the fasted state but induced by high carbohydrate feeding. SREBP-1c is the major transcription factor involved in the coordinated transcriptional regulation of lipogenic enzymes including fatty acid synthase (Latasa et al., 2003). The function of SREBP is discussed in more detail in Chapter 17.

SYNTHESIS OF FATTY ACIDS OTHER THAN PALMITATE

The product of the reaction catalyzed by fatty acid synthase is exclusively palmitate, a 16-carbon saturated fatty acid. However, fatty acids with chain lengths of 18 or more carbons, in both saturated and unsaturated forms, are abundant in animal tissues. For example, more than 50% of the human adipose tissue triacylglycerol contains fatty acids of 18 carbons in length. Acyl chain length and the degree of saturation can influence membrane function, and polyunsaturated long-chain fatty acids serve as precursors for biologically active signaling molecules such as eicosanoids. Therefore, although a variety of fatty acids are provided by the diet, the capacity to modify and elongate fatty acid chains prior to esterification is required to maintain specific fatty acid composition in cells. Many specialized organs, such as mammary and sebaceous glands, synthesize fatty acids with shorter acyl chains and branched acyl chains. The de novo synthesis of these fatty acids requires separate enzymes and enzyme systems.

ELONGATION OF FATTY ACIDS

Fatty acids can be elongated in two-carbon steps. There are two systems for elongating fatty acids, one in the endoplasmic reticulum (ER) and the other in mitochondria. Although neither system is well characterized, the ER system is more active and better understood; it uses both saturated and unsaturated fatty acyl CoAs as substrates. The individual reactions are analogous to those catalyzed by fatty acid synthase, except that only long-chain acyl CoAs are used as primers, and different gene products catalyze the individual reactions. The sequence of reactions is condensation, reduction, dehydration, and reduction. Malonyl CoA is the elongating group, and NADPH is the electron donor. The mitochondrial system appears to utilize acetyl CoA as the elongating unit and NADH or NADH plus NADPH as electron donors. The mitochondrial elongation system is not a simple reversal of fatty acid oxidation involving two-carbon units (β-oxidation) because flavoenzymes are not involved in catalysis for either the first or second reduction in each cycle.

DESATURATION OF FATTY ACIDS

Monounsaturated fatty acids are formed by direct oxidative desaturation of preformed long-chain saturated fatty acids in reactions catalyzed by a complex of enzymes located in the ER. The first double bond introduced into a saturated acyl chain is generally in the $\Delta9$ position. The $\Delta9$ desaturase complex (also called stearoyl CoA desaturase, SCD) uses saturated fatty acids with 14 to 18 carbons; stearate is the most active. This complex, sometimes called a mixed function oxidase, utilizes two electrons and two protons donated by NADH ($+H^+$) and two electrons and two protons from the fatty acid, plus oxygen as an electron acceptor, to generate the oxidized fatty acid and two water molecules. The substrates and products are the acyl CoA derivatives of the fatty acid. Electrons donated by NADH are passed via $FADH_2$ to the heme iron of cytochrome b_5, reducing it to the ferrous form, in a reaction catalyzed by NADH:cytochrome b_5 reductase. Cytochrome b_5 then donates two electrons to the nonheme iron of the desaturase component, reducing it to the ferrous form. This form then interacts with molecular oxygen and the fatty acyl CoA to form water and the unsaturated fatty acyl CoA (Fig. 16-5). The desaturase activity regulates the overall reaction. Multiple forms of desaturases are present with differing tissue distribution and regulation. The activity of SCD1, the isozyme present mostly in liver and adipose tissue, is controlled by diet and hormones in much the same manner as are the activities of the lipogenic enzymes, mainly by regulation of enzyme concentration.

Polyunsaturated fatty acids, usually containing double bonds interrupted by methylene groups, are produced in mammalian tissues. By using the enzymatic mechanism just described for the first desaturation at the $\Delta9$ position,

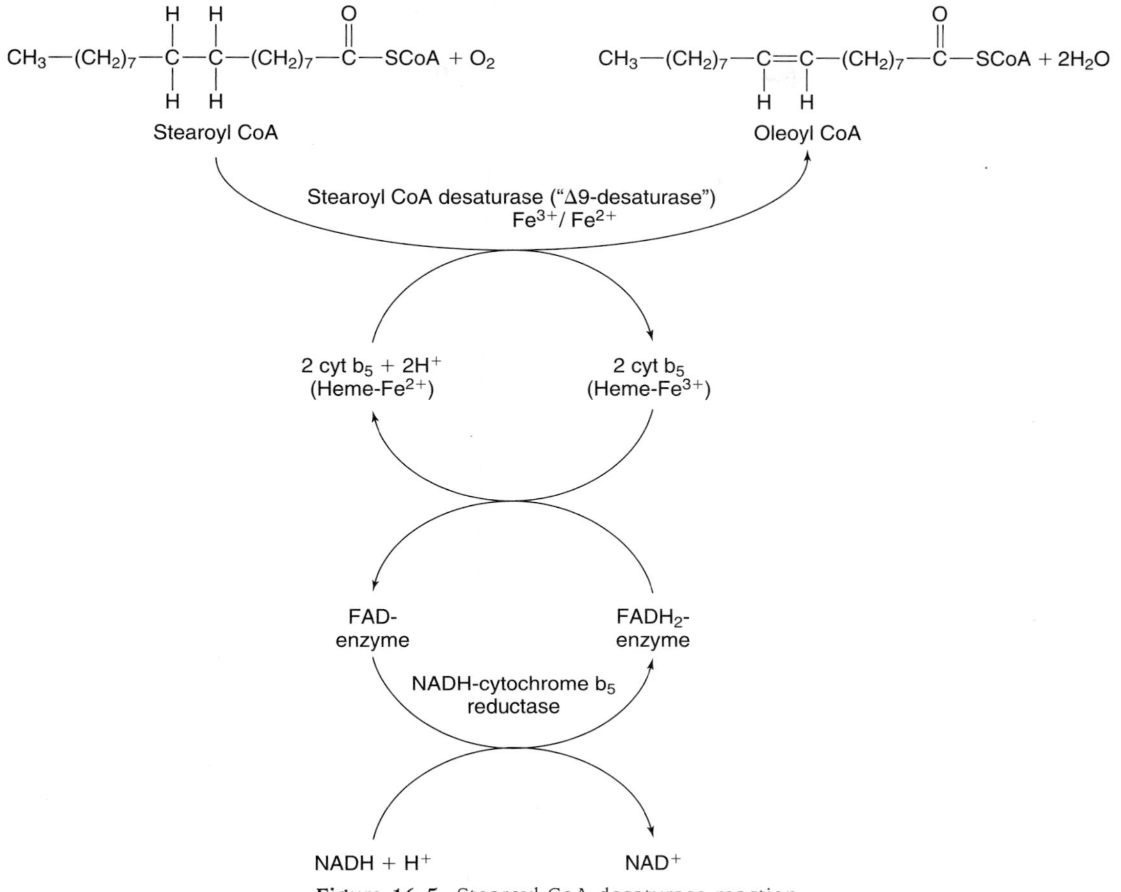

Figure 16-5 Stearoyl CoA desaturase reaction.

mammalian cells can further introduce double bonds into long-chain fatty acids at the Δ5 and Δ6 positions. However, due to the lack of Δ12 and Δ15 desaturases, double bonds cannot be introduced beyond the Δ9 position. As a consequence, linoleate (18:2, Δ9, Δ12) or linolenate (18:3, Δ9, Δ12, Δ15) cannot be synthesized in humans, and they or longer chain members of the ω3 or ω6 classes must be provided in the diet. These fatty acids are essential for the synthesis of polyunsaturated fatty acids such as arachidonate (20:4, Δ5, Δ8, Δ11, Δ14) or docosahexaenoate (22:6, Δ4, Δ7, Δ10, Δ13, Δ16, Δ19). An alternating pattern of desaturation and elongation produces arachidonate from the essential fatty acid linoleate; these reactions, plus a retroconversion step, are involved in synthesis of docosahexaenoate from α-linolenate. (See Chapters 6 and 18, including Fig. 18-2, for further discussion of essential fatty acids and fatty acid nomenclature.)

SYNTHESIS OF MEDIUM-CHAIN FATTY ACIDS

Medium-chain fatty acids are synthesized in mammary gland and are present as triacylglycerol in milk. Mammary gland has the same fatty acid synthase as does liver. Therefore, fatty acid synthase purified from either tissue can synthesize palmitate because the thioesterase activity of fatty acid synthase is specific for 16-carbon acyl groups. However, secretory cells of the mammary gland contain a second thioesterase that is specific for medium-chain fatty acids. This enzyme interacts with growing acyl chains on the fatty acid synthase and cleaves them from fatty acid synthase when they are 8 to 12 carbons in length.

PRODUCTION OF SIMPLE BRANCHED-CHAIN FATTY ACIDS

Sebaceous glands and certain derivatives of sebaceous glands, such as the meibomian glands in the eyelids, synthesize fatty acids with 1-carbon side chains. The "normal" fatty acid synthase carries out these reactions using unusual substrates. Therefore, propionyl CoA can be used as a primer for fatty acid synthase rather than acetyl CoA, and the resulting fatty acid will have a methyl branch at the 2(α) position. Methyl groups also can be inserted at other positions along the fatty acid chain. Although it has a lower affinity for the condensing enzyme than does malonyl CoA, methylmalonyl CoA is used as an elongating group if the concentration of malonyl CoA is lower than that of methylmalonyl CoA. In sebaceous glands and their derivatives, propionyl CoA is converted to methylmalonyl CoA in a reaction catalyzed by acetyl CoA carboxylase. The enzyme uses both acetyl CoA and propionyl CoA equally efficiently so that the group actually incorporated depends on the relative concentrations of the two substrates. In sebaceous glands, a soluble malonyl CoA carboxylase keeps malonyl CoA levels low. The mechanism for generating high levels of propionyl CoA is not known.

SYNTHESIS AND STORAGE OF TRIACYLGLYCEROL

ESTERIFICATION OF FATTY ACIDS

Triacylglycerols are esters of glycerol and three molecules of fatty acids. The substrates for this pathway are glycerol 3-phosphate and fatty acyl CoA. Two reactions catalyze formation of glycerol 3-phosphate. First, dihydroxyacetone phosphate, a glycolytic (and gluconeogenic) intermediate, can be reduced to glycerol 3-phosphate. NADH is the electron donor in the reaction catalyzed by glycerol 3-phosphate dehydrogenase:

$$\text{Dihydroxyacetone Phosphate} + \text{NADH} + \text{H}^+ \leftrightarrow \text{Glycerol 3-Phosphate} + \text{NAD}^+$$

This reaction is freely reversible, allowing glycerol 3-phosphate to enter the glycolytic or gluconeogenic pathways under certain conditions. Second, in some tissues such as liver, but not appreciably in adipose or muscle tissues, glycerol can be phosphorylated to glycerol 3-phosphate in a reaction catalyzed by glycerol kinase:

$$\text{Glycerol} + \text{ATP} \rightarrow \text{Glycerol 3-Phosphate} + \text{ADP}$$

Fatty acids to be used for synthesis of triacylglycerol comprise fatty acids from de novo synthesis or those from hydrolysis of triacylglycerols in the cell, as well as fatty acids taken up from the circulation. Free fatty acids or fatty acids from lipoproteins generated by the action of lipases are taken up by the cell either by passive diffusion or by plasma membrane fatty acid transporters such as fatty acid translocase (FAT/CD36), fatty acid transport protein (FATP), or plasma membrane fatty acid binding protein (FABPpm) (Kalant and Cianflone, 2004). Because of their hydrophobic properties, long-chain fatty acids are bound to fatty acid binding proteins (FABPs) to be transferred from membrane to membrane within the cell (Haunerland and Spener, 2004). Prior to esterification or oxidation in the cell, these fatty acids must be activated to their CoA derivatives. This reaction is catalyzed by fatty acyl CoA synthetase (also called fatty acyl CoA ligase or fatty acid thiokinase). Fatty acyl CoA synthetase is present in the membranes of mitochondria, ER, and peroxisomes, where fatty acids are utilized for either esterification or oxidation. One of the proposed fatty acid transporters FATP, in fact, has intrinsic fatty acyl CoA synthetase activity and may function to trap fatty acids in the cell and thereby facilitate fatty acid transport (Hall et al., 2003).

The ATP-dependent fatty acyl CoA synthetase reaction has three steps. In the first step, fatty acid reacts with ATP to form a fatty acyl-AMP intermediate plus pyrophosphate. In the second step, the acyl moiety is transferred to CoA, and AMP is generated:

(1) $\text{Fatty Acid} + \text{ATP} \leftrightarrow \text{Fatty Acyl-AMP} + \text{PP}_i$

(2) $\text{Fatty Acyl-AMP} + \text{CoASH} \leftrightarrow \text{Fatty Acyl CoA} + \text{AMP}$

As written, the reactions are freely reversible: one high-energy bond is cleaved between PP_i and AMP, and one is formed between the fatty acid and CoA. In the third step, the reaction is driven in the direction of formation of fatty acyl CoA by a ubiquitous pyrophosphatase that rapidly cleaves pyrophosphate to inorganic phosphate:

(3) $PP_i + H_2O \rightarrow 2\ P_i$

NET: Fatty Acid + ATP + CoASH →
Fatty Acyl CoA + AMP + $2P_i$

As will be shown in other pathways in this chapter, the hydrolysis of pyrophosphate is a relatively common mechanism for driving reactions to completion.

The glycerol 3-phosphate reaction pathway for the synthesis of triacylglycerols starts with fatty acyl CoA and glycerol 3-phosphate (Fig. 16-6). The acyl group of a fatty acyl CoA is transferred to the *sn*-1 position of glycerol 3-phosphate in the reaction catalyzed by glycerol 3-phosphate acyltransferase. This is the first committed step in glycerolipid biosynthesis. The 1-acylglycerol 3-phosphate (lysophosphatidic acid) is esterified by a second molecule of fatty acyl CoA to form 1,2-diacylglycerol 3-phosphate (phosphatidic acid). The enzyme that catalyzes this reaction is 1-acylglycerol 3-phosphate acyltransferase. Although their distinctive roles are not known, several isoforms for each of these acyltransferases have been found (Cases et al., 2001). Usually, the *sn*-1 position of the glycerol backbone is esterified with a saturated fatty acid, whereas the *sn*-2 position is esterified with an unsaturated fatty acid. However, the fatty acid composition of lipids in the diet influences the fatty acid composition of triacylglycerol in adipose tissue:

(1) Glycerol 3-Phosphate + Fatty Acyl CoA →
1-Acylglycerol 3-Phosphate + CoA

(2) 1-Acylglycerol 3-Phosphate + Fatty Acyl CoA →
1,2-Diacylglycerol 3-Phosphate + CoA

In the third reaction of this pathway, 1,2-diacylglycerol 3-phosphate is dephosphorylated to 1,2-diacylglycerol and inorganic phosphate. The enzyme that catalyzes this reaction is 1,2-diacylglycerol 3-phosphate phosphatase (also called phosphatidic acid phosphohydrolase):

(3) 1,2-Diacylglycerol 3-Phosphate →
1,2-Diacylglycerol + P_i

Up to this point the reactions of triacylglycerol synthesis are the same as those leading to synthesis of phospholipids, some of which utilize 1,2-diacylglycerol 3-phosphate as substrate and some of which utilize diacylglycerol. The final reaction for triacylglycerol synthesis involves acylation of diacylglycerol to form triacylglycerol. This reaction is catalyzed by 1,2-diacylglycerol acyltransferase, which is particularly active in liver and adipose tissue:

(4) 1,2-Diacylglycerol + Fatty Acyl CoA →
Triacylglycerol + CoA

Dihydroxyacetone phosphate also can be used in the first acylation of fatty acyl CoA. The first reaction, catalyzed by a dihydroxyacetone acyltransferase, which is present in ER and also in peroxisomes, forms 1-acyl dihydroxyacetone as the product. This compound is then reduced by 1-acyl dihydroxyacetone reductase with NADPH as the electron donor and 1-acylglycerol 3-phosphate and $NADP^+$ as products. The remaining steps are the same as outlined for the glycerol 3-phosphate pathway. The role of this second pathway in phosphatidic acid biosynthesis is not clear. It is generally accepted that 1-acyl dihydroxyacetone phosphate is an intermediate in the synthesis of alkyl and alkenyl lipids, a process that occurs exclusively in peroxisomes.

Glycerolipid biosynthesis occurs mostly in ER. The enzymes reside on the ER membrane, but the catalytic activities face the cytosol where substrates reside. Because these enzymes are membrane-bound, their characterization has been difficult, and their regulation is largely unknown. It is presumed that 1,2-diacylglycerol 3-phosphate phosphatase may be a rate-controlling step in triacylglycerol synthesis, and that the enzyme activity is regulated via translocation of the enzyme from the cytosol to the ER where it becomes active. However, 1,2-diacylglycerol acyltransferase also may be involved in regulating triacylglycerol synthesis, because this is the only unique step not involved in phospholipid synthesis. Glycerol 3-phosphate acyltransferase also may be a regulatory step. An isoform of glycerol 3-phosphate acyltransferase, with characteristics different from those of the form present in ER, is present in mitochondrial membrane. The mitochondrial enzyme is expressed mostly in lipogenic tissues (the liver and adipose tissue) and is regulated by nutritional changes as described earlier for the enzymes involved in fatty acid synthesis (Coleman and

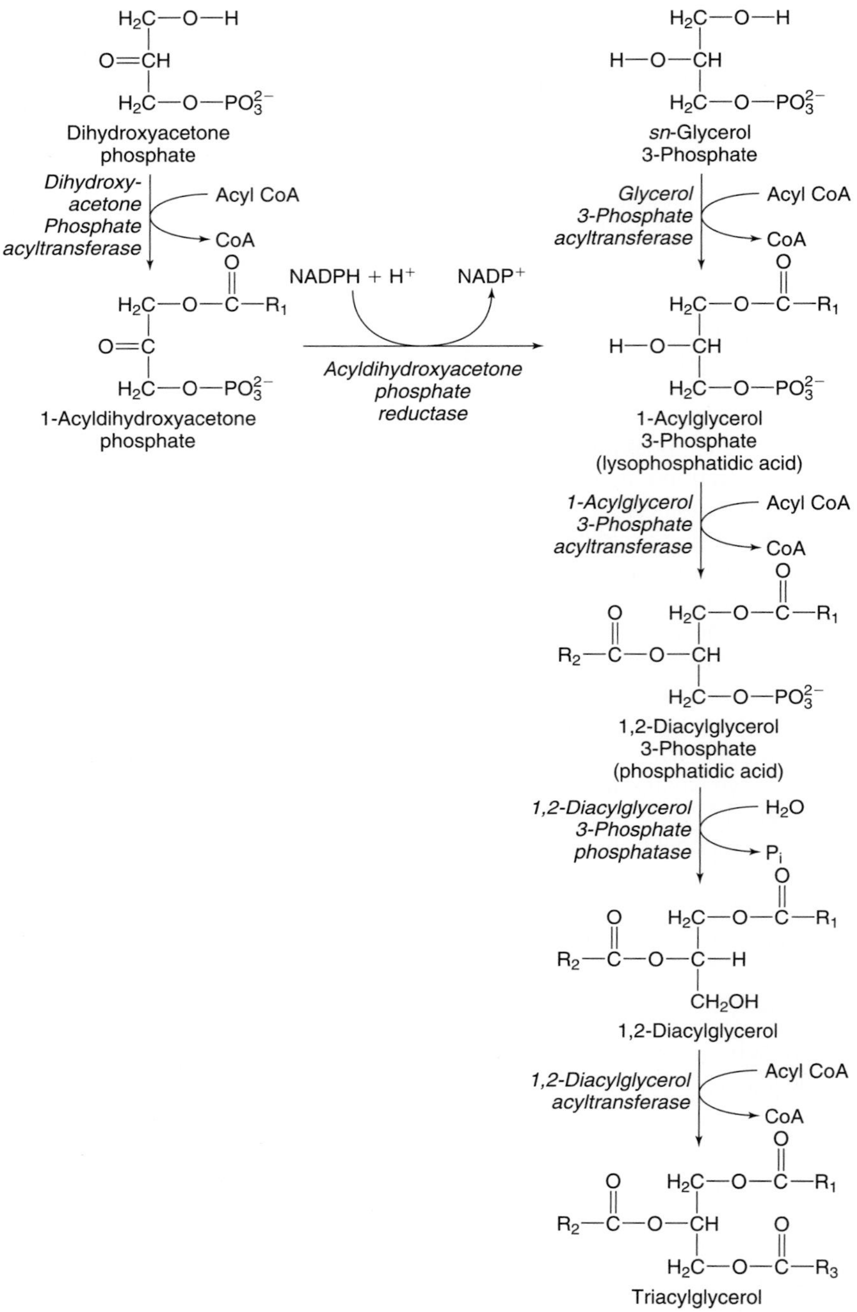

Dihydroxyacetone phosphate

Dihydroxyacetone Phosphate acyltransferase

Acyl CoA → CoA

1-Acyldihydroxyacetone phosphate

NADPH + H^+ → $NADP^+$

Acyldihydroxyacetone phosphate reductase

sn-Glycerol 3-Phosphate

Glycerol 3-Phosphate acyltransferase

Acyl CoA → CoA

1-Acylglycerol 3-Phosphate (lysophosphatidic acid)

1-Acylglycerol 3-Phosphate acyltransferase

Acyl CoA → CoA

1,2-Diacylglycerol 3-Phosphate (phosphatidic acid)

1,2-Diacylglycerol 3-Phosphate phosphatase

H_2O → P_i

1,2-Diacylglycerol

1,2-Diacylglycerol acyltransferase

Acyl CoA → CoA

Triacylglycerol

Figure 16-6 Triacylglycerol biosynthesis.

Lee, 2004; Dircks and Sul, 1999). During the fasting state, the activity of glycerol 3-phosphate acyltransferase is very low; in the fed state, especially on a high carbohydrate diet, enzyme activity increases. Regulation is at the transcriptional level.

Much of the triacylglycerol synthesized in the liver is destined for export to peripheral tissues, especially to adipose tissue where it is stored. Triacylglycerol is not soluble in water, so special arrangements must be made to permit its transport in the blood. Lipoproteins

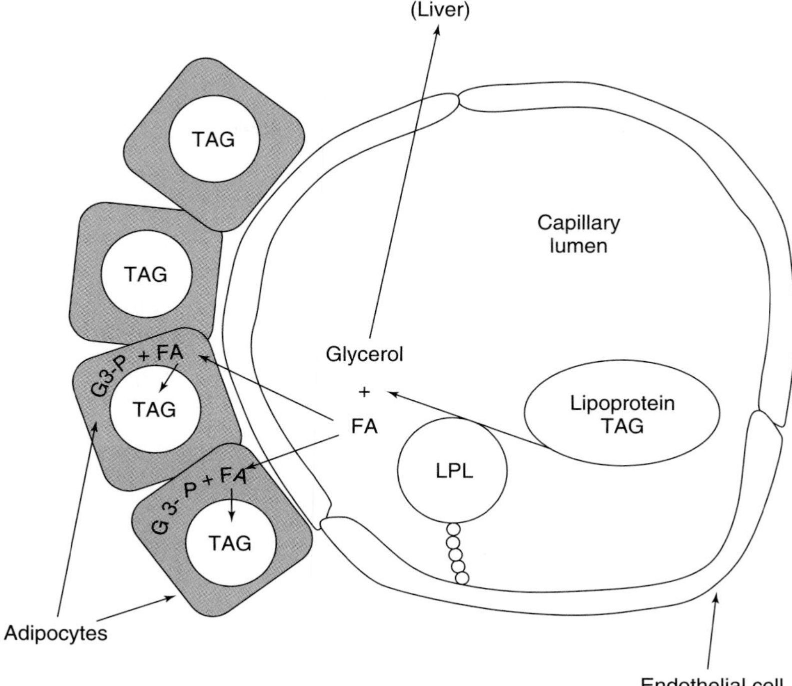

Figure 16-7 Model for hydrolysis of lipoprotein-bound triacylglycerol *(TAG)* and uptake of fatty acid *(FA)* into adipocytes resulting in assimilation of TAG for storage. Hydrolysis of FA from TAG-rich lipoproteins by lipoprotein lipase *(LPL)* bound to the capillary endothelial surface via sulfated proteoglycans is shown. Released FA are then taken up by adipocytes and reesterified to TAG for storage.

perform this function, as described in detail in Chapter 17. Triacylglycerols synthesized in liver from fatty acids derived from dietary fat or from de novo synthesis are packaged into lipoproteins in liver and secreted into the blood as VLDL.

Synthesis of triacylglycerol in enterocytes (intestinal cells) follows a somewhat different pathway than that just described for liver and adipose tissue and is described in Chapter 10. The products of the hydrolysis of triacylglycerol in the lumen of the intestine are unesterified fatty acids and 2-monoacylglycerol. These compounds are taken up by enterocytes and recombined to form triacylglycerol. The triacylglycerol is then packaged into lipoproteins and secreted into the lymph; ultimately it passes into the bloodstream as chylomicrons. In the first reaction of triacylglycerol resynthesis in enterocytes, 2-monoacylglycerol reacts with fatty acyl CoA to form diacylglycerol (2-monoacylglycerol acyltransferase). The next step is the same as that in other tissues and is catalyzed by the same enzyme, diacylglycerol acyltransferase. The 2-monoacylglycerol pathway is dominant in enterocytes, but because some triacylglycerol is hydrolyzed to glycerol and fatty acids in the intestinal lumen, the glycerol 3-phosphate pathway also is essential.

UPTAKE AND STORAGE OF TRIACYLGLYCEROL IN LIPOPROTEINS

Fatty acids derived from triacylglycerol in lipoproteins are taken up by extrahepatic tissues such as muscle, where they provide a source of oxidizable fatty acids, and adipose tissue, where they are reconverted to triacylglycerol and stored in the "signet ring–like" adipocytes until needed. Lipoprotein lipase facilitates uptake of fatty acids by extrahepatic tissues from blood by hydrolyzing plasma triacylglycerol in the circulating lipoproteins. Lipoprotein lipase is localized on the luminal face of the endothelial cells that form the "walls" of capillaries (Fig. 16-7). The enzyme is synthesized by myocytes (muscle cells) or adipocytes (adipose cells) and secreted into the interstitial space (Preiss-Landl et al., 2002). It then is taken up at the interstitial (basal) side of the endothelial cells, transported across those cells, secreted, and bound to the plasma side of the luminal surface. As discussed in more detail in Chapter 17, triacylglycerol in lipoproteins is hydrolyzed by lipoprotein lipase, producing unesterified fatty acids. The unesterified fatty acids cross the endothelial cells by an unknown mechanism (by diffusion or by a protein-mediated transport) and are taken up by adipocytes or myocytes. Synthesis and secretion of lipoprotein lipase in muscle and adipose tissue are regulated differentially. In the fed state, synthesis and secretion of adipose tissue lipoprotein lipase are increased. During a shortage of energy (such as overnight fasting or exercise), muscle lipoprotein lipase is increased. Inside adipocytes, the fatty acids are activated to their CoA derivatives, esterified to triacylglycerol via the glycerol 3-phosphate pathway, and stored as a lipid droplet in those cells. Inside myocytes the fatty acids are used primarily for oxidation.

MOBILIZATION OF STORED TRIACYLGLYCEROL

Another lipase, hormone-sensitive lipase (HSL), catalyzes release of fatty acids from the lipid droplet stored in the adipocytes. It acts at the surface of the triacylglycerol droplet and hydrolyzes fatty acids at the *sn*-1 and *sn*-3 positions preferentially. However, it appears that HSL hydrolyzes diacylglycerol more efficiently than triacylglycerol. A triacylglycerol hydrolase, which prefers triacylglycerol, has recently been found to be present specifically in adipose tissue (Villena et al., 2004). Subsequently, monoacylglycerol lipase present at high activity hydrolyzes the fatty acids at the *sn*-2 position. HSL is regulated by a phosphorylation–dephosphorylation mechanism. In the fed state, the insulin level in the blood rises and brings about dephosphorylation and inactivation of HSL in adipocytes (Fig. 16-8). Fat mobilization from adipose tissue is, therefore, decreased. In addition, insulin promotes uptake of glucose into the adipocyte. Because the rate of glycolysis is limited by the rate of uptake of glucose, the enhancement of glucose uptake ensures a steady production of triose phosphate and glycerol 3-phosphate under these conditions. As a consequence, in fed animals, any fatty acid produced by the adipose tissue is reesterified.

On the other hand, in the fasting state, stored triacylglycerol in adipose tissue is the major source of energy. HSL is phosphorylated by protein kinase A, which is activated by increased intracellular cAMP. In isolated rat adipocytes, glucagon, which rises during starvation, is a potent stimulator of fat mobilization. In humans, however, epinephrine and norepinephrine probably play the major role in increasing intracellular cAMP levels and thus phosphorylation and activation of HSL. This leads to the accelerated hydrolysis of triacylglycerol (Fig. 16-8). HSL is present in the cytosol of adipocytes and translocates to the surface of lipid droplets upon phosphorylation by hormonal stimulation (Yeaman, 2004; Holm, 2003). Lipid droplets are normally coated with proteins such as perilipin. Phosphorylation of both HSL and perilipin is necessary for HSL translocation and for HSL activation. The antilipolytic action of insulin mentioned earlier is due, to a large extent, to insulin-mediated activation of phosphodiesterase, which lowers the cAMP levels and, hence, reduces activation of HSL.

During starvation, the decrease in insulin levels inhibits glucose uptake and, therefore, production of triose phosphate. Because adipose tissue lacks or has extremely low levels of glycerol kinase, the glycerol 3-phosphate required for esterification of fatty acids is mainly derived from glycolysis (Reshef et al., 2003). As a consequence, during starvation, there is little reesterification to restrain the increased production of fatty acids by the activated HSL, and release of fatty acids to the blood proceeds at a high rate. Once in the blood, unesterified fatty acids are bound noncovalently to albumin and transported in that form to other tissues, primarily destined for oxidation. Glycerol produced in adipose tissue during triacylglycerol hydrolysis also is released to the blood and is transported to the liver for reutilization.

Blood

Cytosol of Adipocyte

Epinephrine

Glucagon

Adenylate Cyclase

ATP

cAMP + PP_i → $R_2(cAMP)_4$ + 2 C [cAMP-Dependent protein kinase A (active)]

R_2C_2 [cAMP-Dependent protein kinase A (inactive)]

Hormone-sensitive lipase Ⓟ (active) → *Hormone-sensitive lipase* (deP) (inactive)

(+ Monoacylglycerol lipase)

Glycerol ← Glycerol

Triacylglycerol

Albumin-bound fatty acids ← 3 Fatty acids

Glucose → Glucose → Glucose 6-phosphate → → → Glycerol 3-phosphate

Insulin

Figure 16-8 Hydrolysis of stored triacylglycerol in adipose tissue by hormone-sensitive lipase. *R* and *C* represent the regulatory and catalytic subunits of cAMP-dependent protein kinase A.

Nutrition Insight

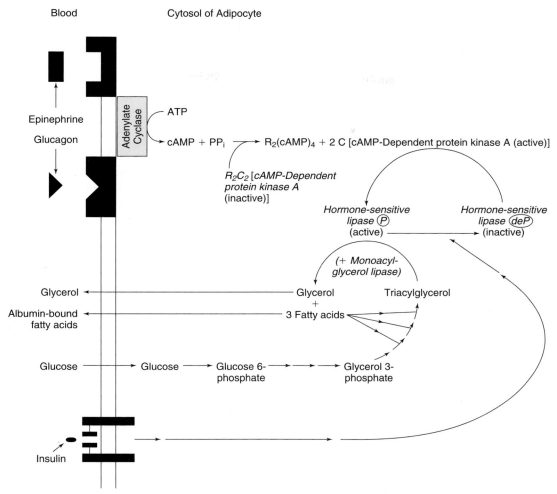

Malonyl CoA, AMPK, and Regulation of Food Intake

Obesity, a major health issue in modern society, is a disorder of energy imbalance in which energy intake exceeds energy expenditure. As discussed in Chapter 22, many neuromodulators as well as peripheral signals, including leptin, are involved in the control of food intake. Malonyl CoA is a critical metabolite in fatty acid metabolism in peripheral tissues. It is an intermediate of fatty acid synthesis by providing acetyl groups. It also regulates fatty acid oxidation by inhibiting CPT-I. There may be separate pools of malonyl CoA for fatty acid synthesis and CPT-I inhibition. Malonyl CoA generated by cytoplasmic acetyl CoA carboxylase-I is used for fatty acid synthesis, whereas malonyl CoA produced by the mitochondrial isoform acetyl CoA carboxylase-II inhibits CPT-I. Recently, malonyl CoA has been implicated in the regulation of food intake. Pharmacological inhibition of fatty acid synthase activity, which causes

Continued

Nutrition Insight

Malonyl CoA, AMPK, and Regulation of Food Intake—cont'd

accumulation of malonyl CoA, causes a reduction in food intake in rodents (Shimokawa et al., 2002). Conversely, genetic knockout of acetyl CoA carboxylase in mice, and, therefore, a block in production of malonyl CoA, increased food intake (Abu-Elheiga et al., 2003). The lipogenic enzymes are present at a high level in neurons in many brain regions, including hypothalamic neurons that regulate feeding behavior. Malonyl CoA may act as a signal of energy status for the brain, causing changes in neuropeptide levels and thereby decreasing food intake.

The enzyme 5′-AMP-activated protein kinase (AMPK), which is known to be an energy sensor of the cell, may be involved in the control of food intake (Unger, 2004). Direct injection of an AMPK activator AICAR (5-aminoimidazole 4-carboxamide riboside) into the hypothalamus or expression of an activated mutant form of AMPK in the hypothalamus increases food intake in mice. Conversely, expression of a dominant-negative inhibitory mutant of AMPK decreases food intake (Minokoshi et al., 2004). Interestingly, the adipose tissue hormone leptin has been suggested to stimulate dephosphorylation and inactivation of AMPK in hypothalamus, and the decrease in AMPK activity can, in turn, change neuropeptide levels to regulate food intake. These effects of AMPK on food intake are also consistent with the fact that AMPK can phosphorylate and inhibit acetyl CoA carboxylase, causing a decrease in malonyl CoA levels. Further studies will clarify the circumstantial evidence linking malonyl CoA and/or AMPK to hypothalamic control of energy metabolism and food intake.

OXIDATION OF FATTY ACIDS

Long-chain fatty acids are supplied to most tissues via circulation in which fatty acids, due to their insolubility in water, are largely bound to albumin and are present at 0.3 to 2.0 mmol/L. The rate of oxidation of fatty acids is proportional to their concentration in the plasma. Fatty acid oxidation is high in muscle and liver during starvation because rapid mobilization of fatty acids in adipose tissue causes an increase in the level of plasma unesterified fatty acids. The converse is true in the fed state. The positive correlation between plasma fatty acid concentration and the rate of fatty acid oxidation is due to the fact that uptake of fatty acids from the plasma and the rate of activation of intracellular fatty acid to the acyl CoA derivative are proportional to the concentration of unesterified fatty acids in the plasma. During exercise, fatty acid oxidation in muscle also increases, although the plasma fatty acid level may remain the same. This is mainly due to the increase in delivery of fatty acids that accompanies higher blood flow during exercise.

ROLE OF CARNITINE IN TRANSPORT OF ACYL GROUPS FROM CYTOSOL TO MITOCHONDRIA

Synthesis of fatty acyl CoA is catalyzed by fatty acyl CoA synthetase, as outlined earlier in this chapter. Oxidation of fatty acids is mostly localized in the mitochondrial compartment. Neither unesterified long-chain fatty acids nor their fatty acyl CoA derivatives can diffuse across the inner mitochondrial membrane. Entry of the acyl groups is catalyzed by a "carnitine" cycle (Fig. 16-9) (Foster, 2004). On the outer mitochondrial membrane, an enzyme called carnitine palmitoyltransferase-I (CPT-I) catalyzes the transfer of long-chain acyl groups from CoA to carnitine:

$$\text{Fatty Acyl CoA} + \text{Carnitine} \leftrightarrow \text{Fatty Acylcarnitine} + \text{CoA}$$

Carnitine–palmitoylcarnitine translocase catalyzes transport of the acylcarnitine across the impermeable inner mitochondrial membrane in exchange for free carnitine. On the inner surface of the inner mitochondrial membrane, carnitine palmitoyltransferase-II (CPT-II)

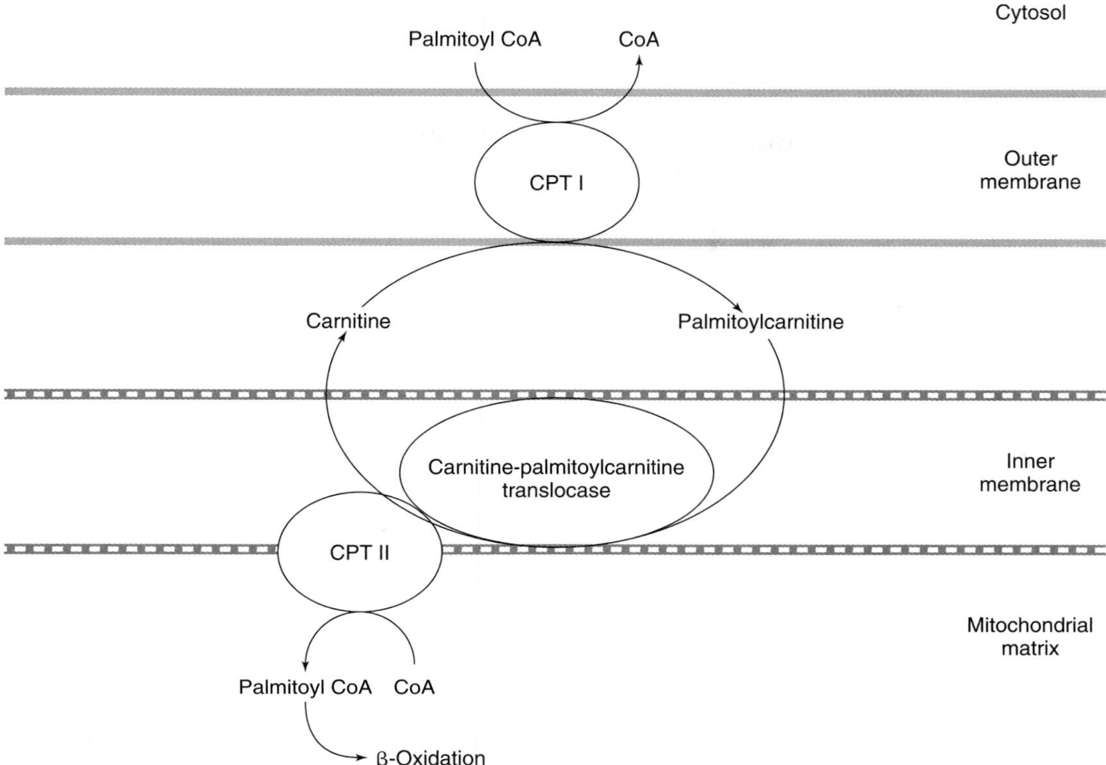

Figure 16-9 Transport of long-chain fatty acyl CoA into mitochondria. *CPT,* Carnitine palmitoyl transferase.

catalyzes the reesterification of acylcarnitines to form acyl CoA esters:

Fatty Acylcarnitine + CoA ↔
Fatty Acyl CoA + Carnitine

The free carnitine is exchanged for acylcarnitine, allowing the process to continue. Rapid oxidation of the fatty acyl CoA in the β-oxidation pathway likely provides the driving force to keep everything moving in the same direction through these largely freely reversible reactions. Both saturated and unsaturated long-chain fatty acids are metabolized via this pathway.

In the fed state, the rate of lipolysis in adipose tissue is slow, and the concentration of plasma free fatty acids and hence their availability for β-oxidation in other tissues are decreased. In liver, the rate of production of malonyl CoA and its intracellular concentration are elevated in the fed state, because acetyl CoA carboxylase, the key regulatory enzyme in de novo lipogenesis, is activated by insulin. Malonyl CoA is a potent allosteric inhibitor of CPT-I. Malonyl CoA limits entry of fatty acyl CoA into the mitochondrial compartment and consequently depresses β-oxidation. This reciprocal regulatory mechanism minimizes futile cycling by ensuring that the opposing processes of β-oxidation and fatty acid biosynthesis are not activated simultaneously.

MITOCHONDRIAL β-OXIDATION

Fatty acids are oxidized by a series of reactions that overall are the reverse of those catalyzed by fatty acid synthase. The two processes, however, are catalyzed by different enzymes, have different subcellular localizations, and have a number of chemical differences (Eaton, 2002). Instead of the condensation, reduction, dehydration, and reduction involved in fatty acid

Clinical Correlation

Defects in Fatty Acid Transport Into Mitochondria for Oxidation

Genetic disorders in any of the enzymes in the carnitine cycle, including carnitine palmitoyltransferases-I and -II (CPT-I and CPT-II) and carnitine-acylcarnitine translocase (see Fig. 16-9), block oxidation of long-chain fatty acids due to impaired transport of long-chain fatty acids into the mitochondrial matrix (Scriver et al., 2001). There are two tissue-specific isoforms of CPT-I encoded by separate genes: the liver form is expressed mainly in liver and kidney, and the muscle form is expressed in muscle and heart. Conversely, there appears to be only one form of CPT-II.

Reported cases of CPT-I deficiency involve defects of liver metabolism: enlarged fatty livers, hypoketotic hypoglycemia, and possibly coma during fasting. Neither muscle weakness nor cardiomyopathy was associated with CPT-I deficiency. Although the molecular basis of CPT-I deficiency has not been elucidated, the finding that patients diagnosed with this genetic defect mainly have liver defects suggests that only the liver isoform of CPT-I is defective.

CPT-II deficiency can take two distinct clinical forms. Classical CPT-II deficiency in adults affects primarily fatty acid metabolism in skeletal and/or cardiac muscle. In these patients, long-chain acylcarnitine translocated across the inner mitochondrial membrane is not reconverted to acyl CoAs. The accumulated long-chain acylcarnitine species are then transported from the mitochondria and into plasma. Under normal conditions, fuel metabolism is still adequate. During sustained exercise or starvation, however, fatty acid oxidation is important quantitatively, and patients experience cramps and fatigue. Although the CPT-II deficiency primarily affects muscle, defects in CPT-II also occur in other tissues. The manifestation of a severe infantile form of CPT-II deficiency is hypoketotic hypoglycemia with cardiomyopathy; it is usually fatal. In the adult-onset form, there is a partial deficiency of CPT-II activity. In the more severe infantile form, CPT-II activity is less than 10% of normal. CPT-II in a patient with an infantile form of the disease was shown to have an arginine-to-cysteine substitution at amino acid residue 631; this variant CPT-II has decreased CPT-II activity.

Carnitine deficiency causes a similar impairment of fatty acid oxidation, but fatty acid oxidation in this case can be restored by administering carnitine. Carnitine in the diet is absorbed in the intestine. In addition, human tissues can synthesize carnitine de novo, mostly in liver and kidney. Endogenous synthesis normally meets the metabolic need, provided the diet contains sufficient lysine and methionine (precursors) and ascorbic acid, vitamin B_6, niacin, and iron (cofactors) for the biosynthesis. (Synthesis of carnitine is outlined in Fig. 27-9 and is discussed in Chapters 14 and 27.) Carnitine deficiency is rare in adults. However, patients undergoing kidney dialysis or those with organic aciduria may lose large amounts of carnitine; they and patients receiving long-term parenteral nutrition may exhibit carnitine deficiency. Carnitine deficiency also may occur in neonates, particularly in premature infants.

Thinking Critically

1. Why does hypoketotic hypoglycemia occur in CPT-I deficiency?
2. What dietary recommendations would you make for patients with CPT-I or CPT-II deficiency?
3. Why are the symptoms of CPT-I and CPT-II deficiencies in patients more severe during starvation?
4. What changes in plasma carnitine and acylcarnitine levels could be used to distinguish between CPT-I and CPT-II deficiencies?

synthesis, the β-oxidation cycle involves oxidation, hydration, oxidation, and cleavage, catalyzed by four enzymes (Fig. 16-10). The intermediates of β-oxidation, however, have not been detected. It is probable that the product of one reaction is transferred directly to the next enzyme. In fact, some of the steps in β-oxidation are catalyzed by a multifunctional enzyme. β-Oxidation occurs in two-carbon steps, as with fatty acid synthesis.

The first step in β-oxidation is catalyzed by acyl CoA dehydrogenase. In contrast to fatty acid synthesis in which NADPH is the electron donor, a tightly but noncovalently linked flavin

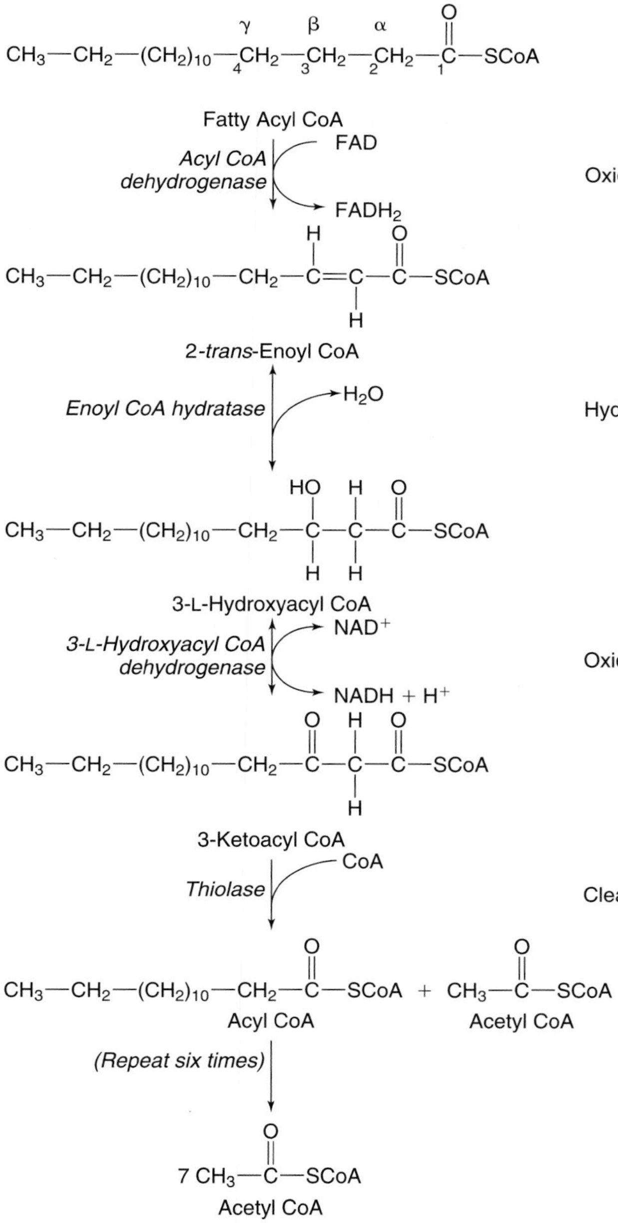

$CH_3—CH_2—(CH_2)_{10}—\overset{\gamma}{C}H_2—\overset{\beta}{C}H_2—\overset{\alpha}{C}H_2—C(=O)—SCoA$ (carbons numbered 4, 3, 2, 1)

Fatty Acyl CoA

Acyl CoA dehydrogenase — FAD → $FADH_2$ — Oxidize

$CH_3—CH_2—(CH_2)_{10}—CH_2—CH=CH—C(=O)—SCoA$

2-*trans*-Enoyl CoA

Enoyl CoA hydratase — H_2O — Hydrate

$CH_3—CH_2—(CH_2)_{10}—CH_2—CH(OH)—CH_2—C(=O)—SCoA$

3-L-Hydroxyacyl CoA

3-L-Hydroxyacyl CoA dehydrogenase — NAD^+ → $NADH + H^+$ — Oxidize

$CH_3—CH_2—(CH_2)_{10}—CH_2—C(=O)—CH_2—C(=O)—SCoA$

3-Ketoacyl CoA

Thiolase — CoA — Cleave

$CH_3—CH_2—(CH_2)_{10}—CH_2—C(=O)—SCoA + CH_3—C(=O)—SCoA$

Acyl CoA + Acetyl CoA

(Repeat six times)

$7\ CH_3—C(=O)—SCoA$

Acetyl CoA

Figure 16-10 β-Oxidation of fatty acids. Example is for oxidation of palmitoyl CoA.

adenine dinucleotide (FAD) is the electron acceptor in the first reaction of β-oxidation:

Acyl CoA + Enzyme-FAD → 2-*trans*-Enoyl CoA + Enzyme-$FADH_2$

FAD is used as the electron acceptor because the ΔG of this reaction is not sufficient to drive production of NADH. The $FADH_2$ generated in this first reaction of β-oxidation donates its electrons to the FAD prosthetic group of electron-transferring flavoprotein, which, in turn, transfers its electrons to ubiquinone in the electron transfer chain (see Chapter 24, Fig. 24-7). Oxidation of each mole of $FADH_2$ generates a maximum of 2 moles of ATP. Separate acyl CoA dehydrogenases encoded by different genes catalyze the oxidation of long-, medium-, and short-chain fatty acids.

The second step in β-oxidation is catalyzed by enoyl CoA hydratase and involves hydration of the *trans* double bond created by the first oxidation:

2-*trans*-Enoyl CoA + H_2O ↔ L-3-Hydroxyacyl CoA

Hydration of the double bond is stereospecific; L-3-hydroxyacyl CoA is the product when a *trans* double bond is hydrated. Enoyl CoA hydratase also hydrates *cis* double bonds; this produces the D-isomer of 3-hydroxyacyl CoA. Two enoyl CoA hydratases, one specific for long-chain fatty acids and the other for short- and medium-chain fatty acids, are present in the mitochondria and cooperate in the hydration of fatty acyl chains of different lengths.

In the third step, a dehydrogenase that is specific for the L-isomer of hydroxyacyl CoA catalyzes a second oxidation step. NAD^+ is the electron acceptor. (See Chapter 24, Fig. 24-7, for reactions involved in transfer of electrons through the electron transport chain.)

L-3-Hydroxyacyl CoA + NAD^+ ↔ 3-Ketoacyl CoA + NADH + H^+

Two dehydrogenases, one specific for long-chain fatty acids and the other for short- and medium-chain fatty acids, cooperate in the oxidation of 3-hydroxyacyl CoA chains of different lengths.

In the final step of each 2-carbon cycle of β-oxidation, 3-ketothiolase catalyzes the thiolytic cleavage of the 3-ketoacyl CoA to acetyl CoA plus an acyl CoA that is two carbons shorter:

3-Ketoacyl CoA + CoASH → Acetyl CoA + Acyl CoA (n−2)

Several types of thiolases have been described. Mitochondria contain two: acetoacetyl CoA thiolase, which cleaves acetoacetyl CoA and functions during ketone metabolism, and 3-ketothiolase, which catalyzes the thiolytic cleavages that occur during β-oxidation of fatty acids. A single 3-ketothiolase appears to catalyze the cleavage of acyl groups of all chain lengths.

Deficiencies in each of the enzymes in the β-oxidation pathway, including specific short-, medium-, and long-chain fatty acyl CoA dehydrogenase deficiencies, cause disorders in metabolic adaptation during starvation owing to an impairment of fatty acid oxidation. The most common deficiency is that of medium-chain fatty acyl CoA dehydrogenase, an inherited disease with an incidence similar to that of phenylketonuria (Scriver et al., 2001). Intermediates of fatty acid oxidation accumulate and result in increased levels of related plasma and urinary metabolites, especially during conditions such as fasting and infection when the rate of lipolysis is increased. Accumulation of some intermediates, such as dicarboxylic acids, is due to the metabolic block of fatty acid oxidation in general. Accumulation of some others, such as *cis*-4-decanoic acid, phenylpropionylglycine, and octanoyl- and *cis*-4-decenoylcarnitine, is unique to the deficiency of medium-chain fatty acyl CoA dehydrogenase.

Carnitine supplementation has been used to treat patients with medium-chain acyl CoA dehydrogenase deficiency. Although the supplementation does not correct the underlying defect, it may help remove these potentially toxic intermediates as acylcarnitines. In patients with this deficiency, nonketotic hypoglycemia can be provoked by fasting during the first 2 years of life. Avoidance of fasting and administration of glucose in acute episodes of hypoglycemia are recommended. Deficiencies in long-chain fatty acyl CoA dehydrogenase, long-chain 3-hydroxyacyl CoA dehydrogenase, and short-chain acyl CoA dehydrogenase cause muscle weakness similar to that caused by a deficiency of CPT-II. A deficiency in mitochondrial acetoacetyl CoA thiolase does not impair fatty acid oxidation but affects isoleucine and ketone body metabolism.

The function of mitochondrial fatty acid oxidation is primarily to supply energy. Peroxisomes also carry out β-oxidation, and some fatty acids, including very-long-chain fatty acids, are preferentially oxidized in peroxisomes. Peroxisomes do not contain an energy-coupled electron transport system to generate ATP but use flavin oxidases and release energy as heat. Fatty acid oxidation can be increased upon treatment with synthetic ligands of lipid-activated peroxisomal proliferator-activated receptors (PPARs), which belong to the nuclear hormone receptor family. PPAR ligands not only induce the expression of some of the enzymes in β-oxidation including acyl CoA oxidase that catalyzes the first step in peroxisomal fatty acid oxidation, but also cause the proliferation of peroxisomes in the liver of rodents. One function of peroxisomal β-oxidation may be to supply acetyl CoA for anabolic reactions. As discussed in subsequent text of this chapter, diagnosis of peroxisome defects such as Zellweger's syndrome can be based on measurement of the concentrations of very-long-chain fatty acids (Wanders, 2004).

ENERGY YIELD FROM β-OXIDATION OF PALMITATE

For each cycle of β-oxidation—oxidation, hydration, oxidation, and cleavage—an acyl CoA is shortened by 2 carbons, and 1 molecule each of $FADH_2$, NADH, hydrogen ion, and acetyl CoA are produced. For the oxidation of palmitate, therefore, the balanced equation is:

$$\text{Palmitoyl CoA} + 7\ \text{CoASH} + 7\ \text{FAD} + 7\ \text{NAD} + 7\ H_2O \rightarrow 8\ \text{Acetyl CoA} + 7\ FADH_2 + 7\ \text{NADH} + 7\ H^+$$

Each $FADH_2$ yields a maximum of 2 ATPs as it passes its electrons down the electron transport chain; each NADH yields a maximum of 3 ATPs. Therefore, oxidation of palmitoyl CoA as shown in the preceding equation yields a maximum of 35 ATPs. As noted in Chapter 12, the complete oxidation of acetyl CoA to CO_2, H_2O, and CoASH yields a maximum of 12 ATPs. In sum, the complete oxidation of palmitoyl CoA yields 131 ATPs. Two high-energy bonds are used up in the activation of palmitate to palmitoyl CoA because ATP is split into AMP and PP_i (which is further hydrolyzed to $2P_i$). The complete oxidation of palmitate to CO_2 and H_2O thus yields a net of a maximum of 129 moles of ATP per mole of palmitate.

The standard free energy for the complete oxidation of palmitate is about 9,800 kJ/mol (2,344 kcal/mol). The standard free energy for the hydrolysis of ATP is 30.5 kJ/mol (7.3 kcal/mol). Therefore, palmitate oxidation in the living cell, if it were under standard conditions (1 atm pressure, 1 mol/L concentration of substrates), would conserve a maximum of 129×30.5, or 3,935 kJ/mol (940 kcal/mol) in ATP. This represents a very respectable efficiency of approximately 40%. However, if the free energy changes are calculated under the conditions that exist in vivo, the energy conservation is closer to 80%. Living cells are remarkably efficient at capturing the energy available in lipid foodstuffs.

ADDITIONAL REACTIONS REQUIRED FOR β-OXIDATION OF UNSATURATED FATTY ACIDS

Unsaturated fatty acids are abundant in nature and are also degraded via β-oxidation. Most of the double bonds in natural mono- and polyunsaturated fatty acids are in the *cis* configuration. For the purpose of this discussion, it is convenient to place these fatty acids into two classes: ones that extend from odd- (e.g., Δ9 of oleic acid or Δ9 of linoleic acid) or from even-numbered (e.g., Δ12 of linoleic acid) carbons in the fatty acid chain. Neither of these double bonds is a natural intermediate in β-oxidation, so auxiliary enzymes must rearrange the double bonds to permit complete oxidation. The simplest of these rearrangements involves double bonds extending from odd-numbered carbons (Fig. 16-11). Oleoyl CoA (9-*cis*-octadecenoyl CoA) undergoes three rounds of β-oxidation to form 3-*cis*-dodecenoyl CoA. This intermediate is not a substrate for either of the dehydrogenases or enoyl CoA hydratase. This problem is circumvented by isomerization of the double bond to yield 2-*trans*-dodecenoyl CoA. The auxiliary enzyme that catalyzes this reaction is 3-*cis*, 2-*trans*-enoyl CoA isomerase

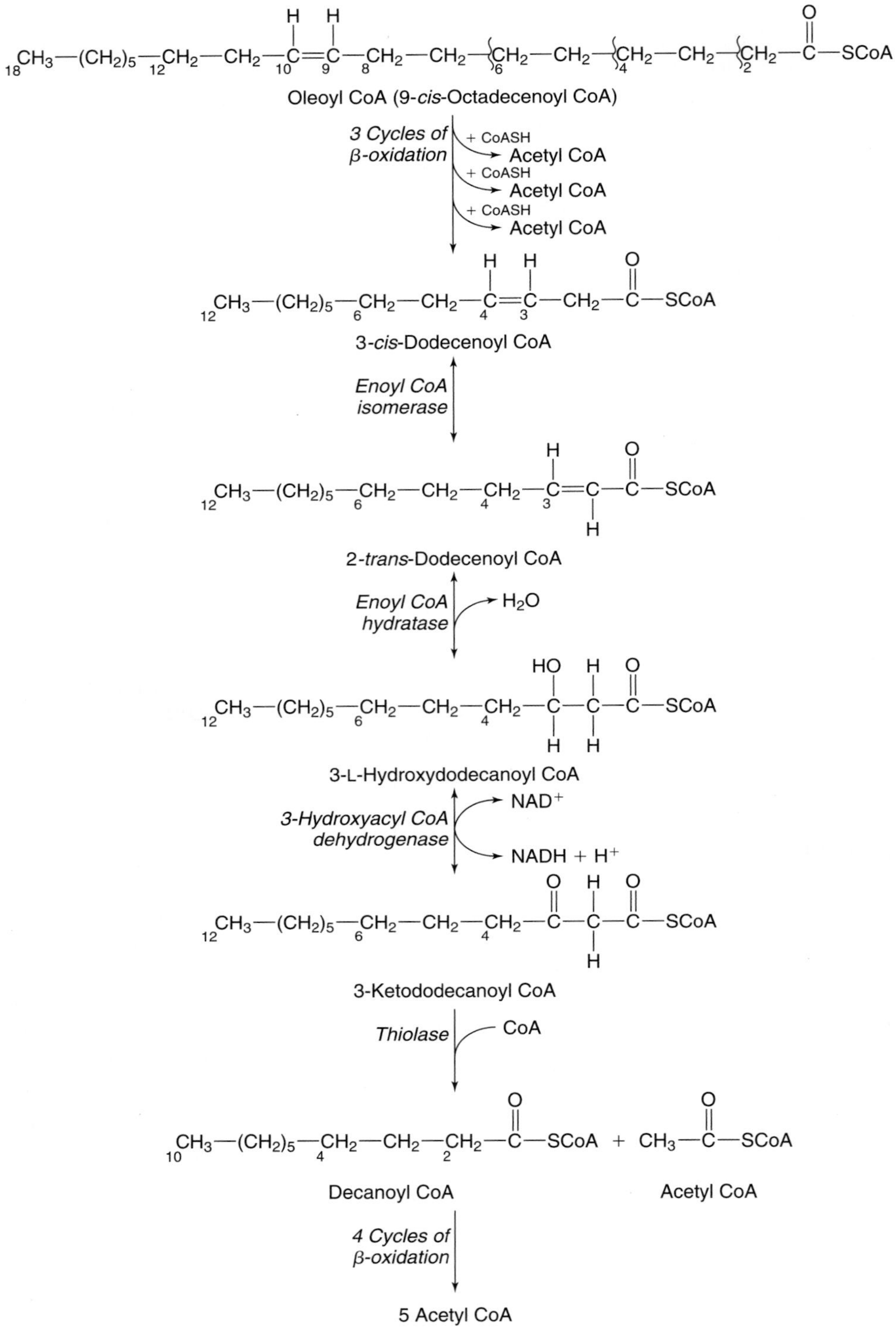

$_{18}CH_3{-}(CH_2)_5{-}\underset{12}{C}H_2{-}CH_2{-}\underset{10}{\overset{H}{C}}{=}\underset{9}{\overset{H}{C}}{-}\underset{8}{C}H_2{-}CH_2{-}\underset{6}{C}H_2{-}CH_2{-}\underset{4}{C}H_2{-}CH_2{-}\underset{2}{C}H_2{-}\overset{O}{\overset{\|}{C}}{-}SCoA$

Oleoyl CoA (9-*cis*-Octadecenoyl CoA)

3 Cycles of β-oxidation

+ CoASH → Acetyl CoA

+ CoASH → Acetyl CoA

+ CoASH → Acetyl CoA

$_{12}CH_3{-}(CH_2)_5{-}\underset{6}{C}H_2{-}CH_2{-}\underset{4}{\overset{H}{C}}{=}\underset{3}{\overset{H}{C}}{-}CH_2{-}\overset{O}{\overset{\|}{C}}{-}SCoA$

3-*cis*-Dodecenoyl CoA

Enoyl CoA isomerase

$_{12}CH_3{-}(CH_2)_5{-}\underset{6}{C}H_2{-}CH_2{-}\underset{4}{C}H_2{-}\underset{3}{\overset{H}{C}}{=}\underset{H}{C}{-}\overset{O}{\overset{\|}{C}}{-}SCoA$

2-*trans*-Dodecenoyl CoA

Enoyl CoA hydratase → H_2O

$_{12}CH_3{-}(CH_2)_5{-}\underset{6}{C}H_2{-}CH_2{-}\underset{4}{C}H_2{-}\overset{HO}{\underset{H}{C}}{-}\overset{H}{\underset{H}{C}}{-}\overset{O}{\overset{\|}{C}}{-}SCoA$

3-L-Hydroxydodecanoyl CoA

3-Hydroxyacyl CoA dehydrogenase

→ NAD^+

→ $NADH + H^+$

$_{12}CH_3{-}(CH_2)_5{-}\underset{6}{C}H_2{-}CH_2{-}\underset{4}{C}H_2{-}\overset{O}{\overset{\|}{C}}{-}\overset{H}{\underset{H}{C}}{-}\overset{O}{\overset{\|}{C}}{-}SCoA$

3-Ketododecanoyl CoA

Thiolase CoA

$_{10}CH_3{-}(CH_2)_5{-}\underset{4}{C}H_2{-}CH_2{-}\underset{2}{C}H_2{-}\overset{O}{\overset{\|}{C}}{-}SCoA + CH_3{-}\overset{O}{\overset{\|}{C}}{-}SCoA$

Decanoyl CoA Acetyl CoA

4 Cycles of β-oxidation

5 Acetyl CoA

Figure 16-11 Oxidation of oleoyl CoA.

(enoyl CoA isomerase). This enzyme also isomerizes 3-*trans*-enoyl CoA to its 2-*trans*-enoyl CoA isomer. The product of the enoyl CoA isomerase–catalyzed reaction is 2-*trans*-dodecenoyl CoA, a substrate for enoyl CoA reductase. This reaction allows β-oxidation to continue, but, in the fourth cycle of β-oxidation, the first dehydrogenase step catalyzed by acyl CoA dehydrogenase is omitted. Therefore, complete oxidation of oleate (18:1) yields one less $FADH_2$—or 2 less ATPs—than complete oxidation of stearate (18:0).

The oxidation of linoleate (Fig. 16-12) proceeds like that of oleate, including the isomerase step just described, for four cycles plus the first dehydrogenase reaction of the fifth cycle. At this point the product is 2-*trans*, 4-*cis*-decadienoyl CoA, an intermediate that is not a substrate for the enoyl CoA hydratase or the β-hydroxyacyl CoA dehydrogenase. This potential block to β-oxidation is circumvented by two reactions catalyzed by auxiliary enzymes. First, 2-*trans*, 4-*cis*-decadienoyl CoA is reduced to 3-*trans*-decenoyl CoA. This reaction utilizes NADPH as the electron donor and is catalyzed by 2,4-dienoyl CoA reductase. The product of this reaction, 3-*trans*-decenoyl CoA, is not a substrate for the enzymes of β-oxidation and must be isomerized to 2-*trans*-decenoyl CoA, a substrate for the enoyl CoA hydratase. β-Oxidation then continues to complete the fifth cycle and three more complete cycles as shown in Figure 16-12. In the oxidation of linoleate, one $FADH_2$ (2 ATPs) is lost in the third cycle, as with oleate. The fifth cycle utilizes both dehydrogenases, generating both $FADH_2$ and NADH. However, the utilization of 1 NADPH balances the production of 1 NADH, meaning that 3 ATPs are lost. Overall then, the complete oxidation of linoleate (18:2) generates 5 less ATPs than that of stearate (18:0).

Although most naturally occurring unsaturated fatty acids contain *cis* double bonds, small amounts of *trans* fatty acids are found in cow's milk fat. During hydrogenation of polyunsaturated fatty acids by rumen microorganisms, the double bonds are isomerized from the *cis* to the *trans* configuration. A similar process occurs during hydrogenation in manufacturing margarine and other hydrogenated vegetable fats, and considerable amounts of *trans* fatty acids are found in margarine products. Although they have a lower affinity for isomerases, *trans* fatty acids are oxidized by the isomerases. Dietary *trans* fatty acids seem to have effects similar to, or potentially worse than, saturated fatty acids in promoting atherosclerosis. (See Chapter 17 for a discussion of dietary fat and cardiovascular disease.)

β-OXIDATION OF FATTY ACIDS WITH AN ODD NUMBER OF CARBONS OR WITH METHYL SIDE CHAINS TO GENERATE PROPIONYL CoA

Fatty acids of odd-chain length are not synthesized in animals and, therefore, are not commonly found in meat. However, small amounts of odd-chain fatty acids are found in vegetables. The β-oxidation of straight-chain fatty acids containing an odd number of carbons requires three auxiliary enzymes (Fig. 16-13). Oxidation proceeds as described in the preceding text for other saturated fatty acids until the last step of the last cycle, producing $FADH_2$, NADH, and acetyl CoA in each cycle. However, the product of the final cleavage reaction is 1 acetyl CoA and 1 propionyl CoA instead of 2 acetyl CoA molecules. Propionyl CoA is more abundantly generated by metabolism of certain amino acids (valine, isoleucine, threonine, and methionine), as described in Chapter 14, than by fatty acid oxidation. Propionyl CoA is carboxylated to D-methylmalonyl CoA in an ATP-dependent reaction catalyzed by propionyl CoA carboxylase. The reaction mechanism is similar to that for acetyl CoA carboxylase. The enzyme methylmalonyl CoA racemase catalyzes the isomerization of the D-isomer to the L-isomer, and L-methylmalonyl CoA is isomerized to succinyl CoA in a reaction catalyzed by methylmalonyl CoA mutase. Succinyl CoA is an intermediate in the citric acid cycle. Unlike acetyl CoA, which is the final product of β-oxidation of fatty acids containing an even number of carbons, succinyl CoA can be converted to phosphoenolpyruvate and hence to glucose. Therefore, fatty acids with an odd number of carbons, especially propionic acid, can be considered gluconeogenic. Methylmalonyl CoA mutase requires deoxyadenosylcobalamin, a derivative of vitamin B_{12}, as a cofactor. Individuals develop pernicious anemia when they

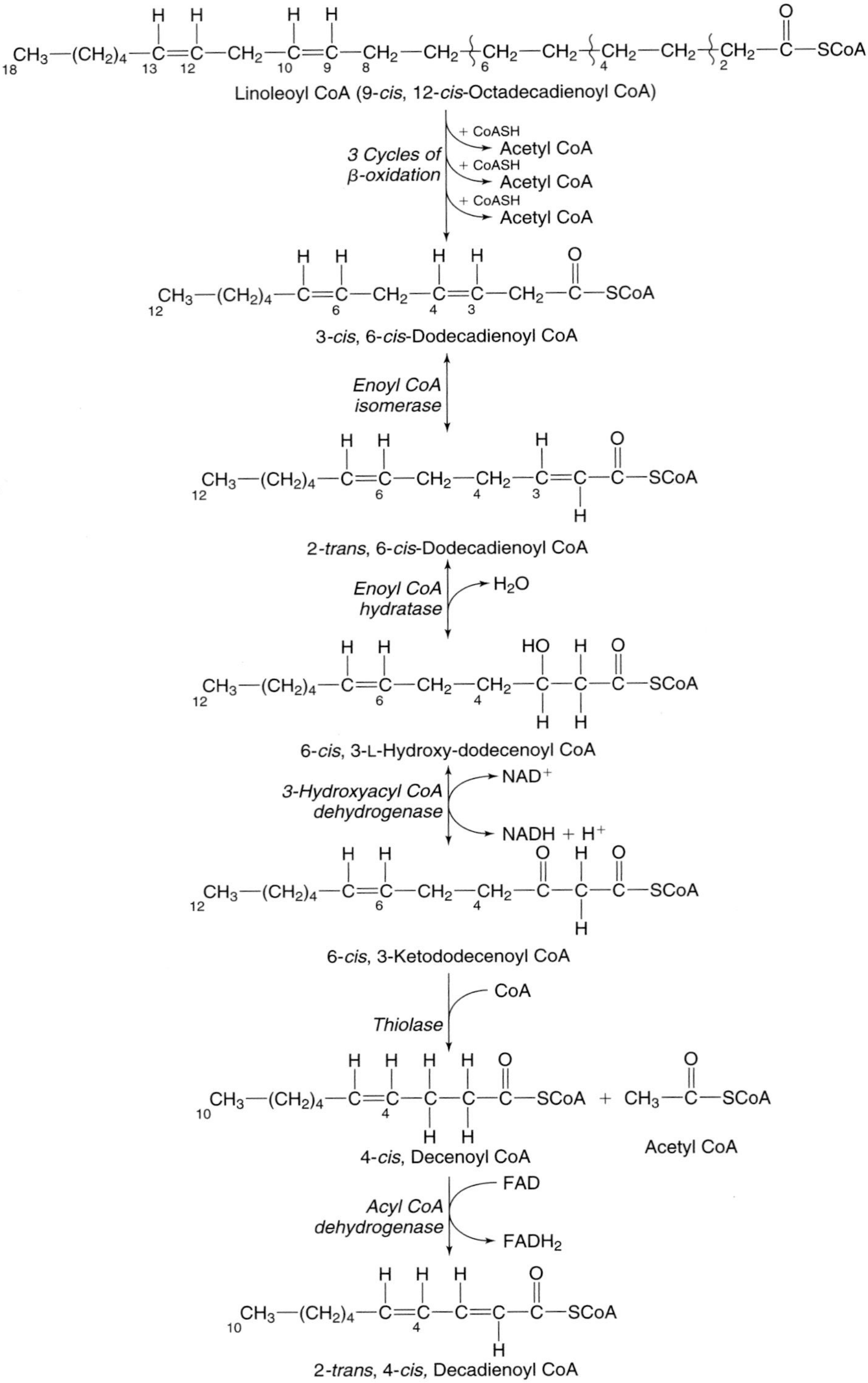

$CH_3-(CH_2)_4-CH=CH-CH_2-CH=CH-CH_2-CH_2-CH_2-CH_2-CH_2-CH_2-CH_2-C(=O)-SCoA$ (carbons numbered 18, 13, 12, 10, 9, 8, 6, 4, 2)

Linoleoyl CoA (9-*cis*, 12-*cis*-Octadecadienoyl CoA)

3 Cycles of β-oxidation: + CoASH → Acetyl CoA; + CoASH → Acetyl CoA; + CoASH → Acetyl CoA

$CH_3-(CH_2)_4-CH=CH-CH_2-CH=CH-CH_2-C(=O)-SCoA$ (carbons numbered 12, 6, 4, 3)

3-*cis*, 6-*cis*-Dodecadienoyl CoA

Enoyl CoA isomerase

$CH_3-(CH_2)_4-CH=CH-CH_2-CH_2-CH=CH-C(=O)-SCoA$ (carbons numbered 12, 6, 4, 3)

2-*trans*, 6-*cis*-Dodecadienoyl CoA

Enoyl CoA hydratase: → H_2O

$CH_3-(CH_2)_4-CH=CH-CH_2-CH_2-CH(OH)-CH_2-C(=O)-SCoA$ (carbons numbered 12, 6, 4)

6-*cis*, 3-L-Hydroxy-dodecenoyl CoA

3-Hydroxyacyl CoA dehydrogenase: → NAD^+; → $NADH + H^+$

$CH_3-(CH_2)_4-CH=CH-CH_2-CH_2-C(=O)-CH_2-C(=O)-SCoA$ (carbons numbered 12, 6, 4)

6-*cis*, 3-Ketododecenoyl CoA

Thiolase: CoA

$CH_3-(CH_2)_4-CH=CH-CH_2-CH_2-C(=O)-SCoA$ (carbons numbered 10, 4) + $CH_3-C(=O)-SCoA$

4-*cis*, Decenoyl CoA   Acetyl CoA

Acyl CoA dehydrogenase: FAD → $FADH_2$

$CH_3-(CH_2)_4-CH=CH-CH=CH-C(=O)-SCoA$ (carbons numbered 10, 4)

2-*trans*, 4-*cis*, Decadienoyl CoA

Figure 16-12 Oxidation of linoleoyl CoA.

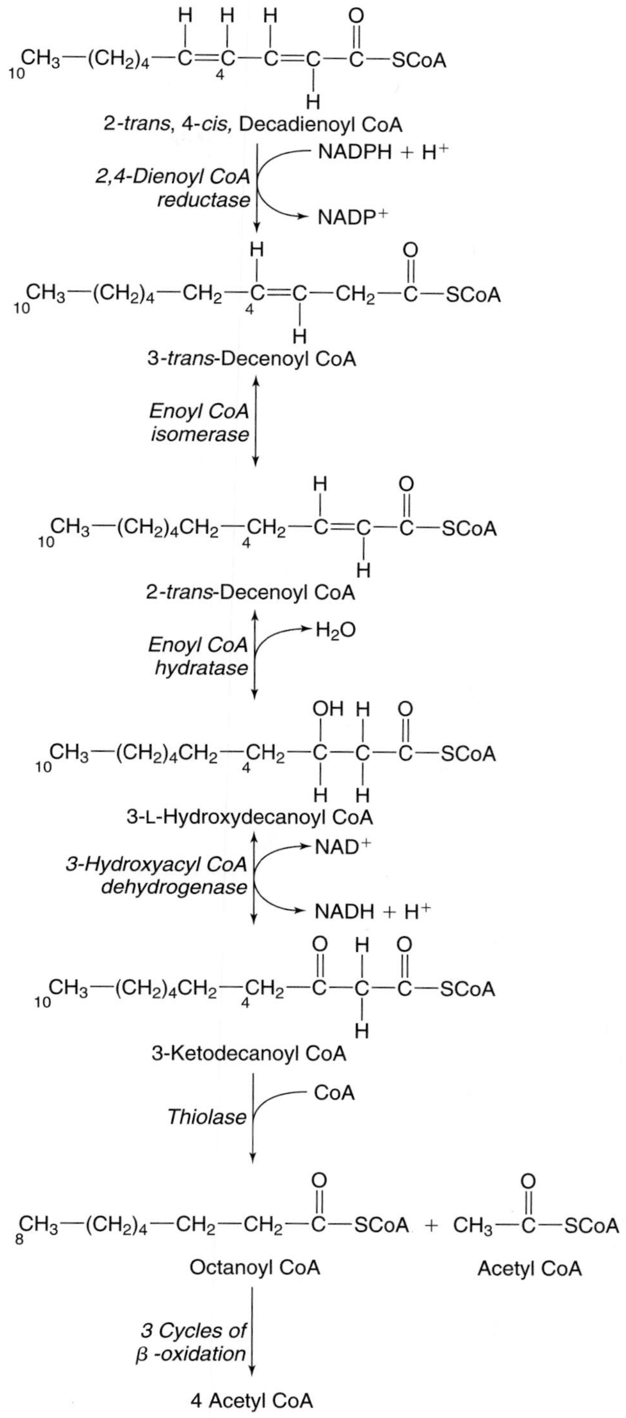

$_{10}CH_3-(CH_2)_4-CH=\underset{4}{C}H-CH=CH-C(=O)-SCoA$

2-*trans*, 4-*cis*, Decadienoyl CoA

↓ *2,4-Dienoyl CoA reductase* ($NADPH + H^+ \rightarrow NADP^+$)

$_{10}CH_3-(CH_2)_4-CH_2-\underset{4}{C}H=CH-CH_2-C(=O)-SCoA$

3-*trans*-Decenoyl CoA

↕ *Enoyl CoA isomerase*

$_{10}CH_3-(CH_2)_4CH_2-\underset{4}{C}H_2-CH=CH-C(=O)-SCoA$

2-*trans*-Decenoyl CoA

↕ *Enoyl CoA hydratase* (H_2O)

$_{10}CH_3-(CH_2)_4CH_2-\underset{4}{C}H_2-CH(OH)-CH_2-C(=O)-SCoA$

3-L-Hydroxydecanoyl CoA

↕ *3-Hydroxyacyl CoA dehydrogenase* ($NAD^+ \rightarrow NADH + H^+$)

$_{10}CH_3-(CH_2)_4CH_2-\underset{4}{C}H_2-C(=O)-CH_2-C(=O)-SCoA$

3-Ketodecanoyl CoA

↓ *Thiolase* (CoA)

$_{8}CH_3-(CH_2)_4-CH_2-CH_2-C(=O)-SCoA + CH_3-C(=O)-SCoA$

Octanoyl CoA Acetyl CoA

↓ *3 Cycles of β-oxidation*

4 Acetyl CoA

Figure 16-12—Cont'd

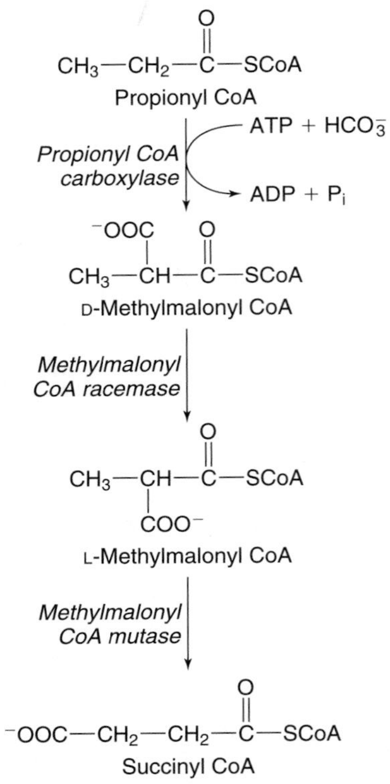

$CH_3—CH_2—C(=O)—SCoA$
Propionyl CoA

Propionyl CoA carboxylase
ATP + HCO_3^- → ADP + P_i

$^-OOC—CH(CH_3)—C(=O)—SCoA$
D-Methylmalonyl CoA

Methylmalonyl CoA racemase

$CH_3—CH(COO^-)—C(=O)—SCoA$
L-Methylmalonyl CoA

Methylmalonyl CoA mutase

$^-OOC—CH_2—CH_2—C(=O)—SCoA$
Succinyl CoA

Figure 16-13 Propionate metabolism.

lack intrinsic factor, a specific vitamin B_{12}-binding glycoprotein required for vitamin B_{12} absorption. These patients have impaired conversion of methylmalonyl CoA to succinyl CoA and excrete methylmalonate in their urine.

Odd- or even-numbered fatty acids that contain methyl side chains are oxidized by the usual β-oxidation scheme. A methyl side chain on the carbon does not interfere with β-oxidation. The products of the thiolytic cleavage are propionyl CoA and chain-shortened acyl CoA. The latter continues through additional cycles of β-oxidation. Propionyl CoA is metabolized to succinyl CoA as described previously.

FORMATION OF KETONE BODIES FROM ACETYL COA IN THE LIVER AS A FUEL FOR EXTRAHEPATIC TISSUES

In muscle and other nonhepatic tissues in any nutritional state, and in the liver in the well-fed state, acetyl CoA formed during the β-oxidation of fatty acids is oxidized to CO_2 and H_2O in the citric acid cycle. When the rate of mobilization of fatty acids from adipose depots is accelerated, as, for example, during starvation, the liver converts acetyl CoA generated from fatty acid oxidation into ketone bodies—acetoacetate and 3-hydroxybutyrate. The rate of formation of ketone bodies is directly proportional to the rate of fatty acid oxidation. Therefore, when the rate of mobilization of fatty acids from adipose tissue is high, hepatic oxidation of fatty acids with production of acetoacetate and 3-hydroxybutyrate is high. Ketone bodies are "water-soluble" metabolites of fatty acids that are readily transported to other organs for oxidation to CO_2 and H_2O.

SYNTHESIS OF ACETOACETATE AND 3-HYDROXYBUTYRATE IN LIVER MITOCHONDRIA

Ketone bodies are synthesized in mitochondria. This is important because production of acetyl CoA, the substrate for synthesis of ketone bodies, occurs in the mitochondria via β-oxidation of fatty acids. Furthermore, initial steps for the de novo synthesis of cholesterol utilize some of the same reactions, but the enzymes for synthesis of cholesterol precursors are present in the cytosol of the liver as discussed in Chapter 17. Differential localization permits independent regulation of ketone body production and cholesterol synthesis.

The first step in ketone body synthesis is condensation of two molecules of acetyl CoA to form acetoacetyl CoA (Fig. 16-14). This reaction is catalyzed by β-ketothiolase:

Acetyl CoA + Acetyl CoA →
Acetoacetyl CoA + CoA

The second step involves condensation of a third molecule of acetyl CoA with acetoacetyl CoA to form 3-hydroxy-3-methylglutaryl CoA (HMG CoA). This reaction is catalyzed by HMG CoA synthase:

Acetyl CoA + Acetoacetyl CoA →
3-Hydroxy-3-Methylglutaryl CoA + CoA

In the third step of ketone body synthesis, HMG CoA is cleaved to acetoacetate and acetyl CoA in a reaction catalyzed by HMG CoA lyase:

3-Hydroxy-3-Methylglutaryl CoA →
Acetoacetate + Acetyl CoA

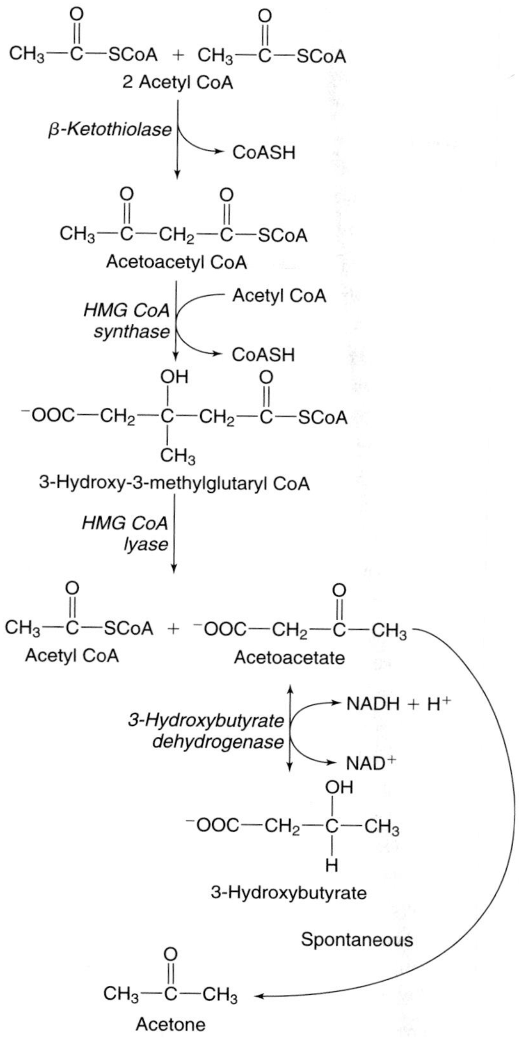

$CH_3-CO-SCoA + CH_3-CO-SCoA$
2 Acetyl CoA
β-Ketothiolase → CoASH
$CH_3-CO-CH_2-CO-SCoA$
Acetoacetyl CoA
HMG CoA synthase (Acetyl CoA → CoASH)
$^-OOC-CH_2-C(OH)(CH_3)-CH_2-CO-SCoA$
3-Hydroxy-3-methylglutaryl CoA
HMG CoA lyase
$CH_3-CO-SCoA + {}^-OOC-CH_2-CO-CH_3$
Acetyl CoA Acetoacetate
3-Hydroxybutyrate dehydrogenase (NADH + H^+ → NAD^+)
$^-OOC-CH_2-CH(OH)-CH_3$
3-Hydroxybutyrate
Spontaneous
$CH_3-CO-CH_3$
Acetone

Figure 16-14 Ketone body formation.

Both acetoacetate and 3-hydroxybutyrate are considered ketone bodies because they are rapidly interconverted via a reaction catalyzed by 3-hydroxybutyrate dehydrogenase. This NAD^+-requiring enzyme catalyzes a reversible reaction in which the concentrations of the products are nearly in thermodynamic equilibrium with NAD^+ and NADH in the mitochondria. Both acetoacetate and 3-hydroxybutyrate circulate in the blood. The ratio of their concentrations reflects the molar ratio of NAD^+ to NADH in liver mitochondria:

$$\text{Acetoacetate} + \text{NADH} + H^+ \leftrightarrow \text{3-Hydroxybutyrate} + NAD^+$$

Of the two "ketone bodies," only one is a keto compound. So, how did these compounds become known as ketone bodies? Acetoacetate decarboxylates slowly and spontaneously to acetone in the blood. When the plasma concentration of ketone bodies is very high—as in untreated diabetics—sufficient acetone accumulates in the blood to be detectable by breath odor. This led early investigators to give the name "ketone bodies" to the chemically uncharacterized material that accumulated in the blood of diabetics. The name has been retained even though we now know that acetone is only a minor component, and 3-hydroxybutyrate, a non-keto compound, is the major component.

OXIDATION OF KETONE BODIES IN PERIPHERAL TISSUES

The liver produces ketone bodies, but it cannot utilize them because it lacks the mitochondrial enzyme succinyl CoA:3-keto acid CoA transferase required for activation of acetoacetate to acetoacetyl CoA. This results in the net flow of ketone bodies from the liver to extrahepatic tissues for use as a fuel. The plasma concentration of albumin-bound fatty acids can increase from approximately 0.5 mmol/L in the fed state to 2 mmol/L in the fasting state. During prolonged starvation, glucose concentration can decrease from 5.5 mmol/L to 3.5 mmol/L. The concentration of ketone bodies is approximately 0.01 mmol/L in the fed state and 0.1 mmol/L after an overnight fast, but the concentration of ketone bodies can reach 2 mmol/L after 3 days of starvation or more than 5 mmol/L after a week of starvation. At these increased concentrations, ketone bodies become significant fuels. In peripheral tissues such as muscle, ketone bodies are an important source of energy, especially when fatty acid mobilization has been activated. The brain also requires a large and constant source of energy. In the fed state, the brain depends exclusively on glucose for energy, because the blood-brain barrier limits uptake of long-chain fatty acids and the circulating level of ketone bodies is low in the fed individual. During starvation, however, ketone body concentration is elevated in the plasma and acetoacetate and 3-hydroxybutyrate become important energy sources for the brain, sparing the limited sources of glucose. In untreated type I diabetes mellitus, ketosis (i.e., ketonemia and ketonuria) can occur. Because acetoacetic and 3-hydroxybutyric acids are moderately strong acids, ketonuria causes loss of sodium ions and metabolic acidosis, causing coma and death.

Both 3-hydroxybutyrate and acetoacetate diffuse into peripheral tissues along their concentration gradients. The rates of their metabolism are related directly to their concentrations in the blood, which, in turn, are proportional to the rate of release of fatty acids from adipose tissue. The reaction pathway is shown in Figure 16-15. 3-Hydroxybutyrate must be converted to acetoacetate before it can be used. The same enzyme, 3-hydroxybutyrate dehydrogenase, that catalyzes interconversion of 3-hydroxybutyrate and acetoacetate in liver also does so in peripheral tissues. In peripheral tissues, acetoacetate is then activated to acetoacetyl CoA in a reaction catalyzed by acetoacetate:succinyl CoA transferase:

Acetoacetate + Succinyl CoA → Acetoacetyl CoA + Succinate

Acetoacetyl CoA is then cleaved to two molecules of acetyl CoA by the action of β–ketothiolase.

Acetoacetyl CoA → 2 Acetyl CoA

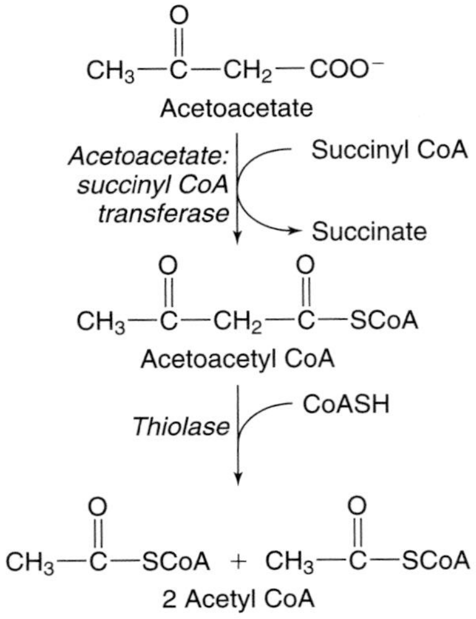

$CH_3—CO—CH_2—COO^-$
Acetoacetate
Acetoacetate: succinyl CoA transferase (Succinyl CoA → Succinate)
$CH_3—CO—CH_2—CO—SCoA$
Acetoacetyl CoA
Thiolase (CoASH)
$CH_3—CO—SCoA + CH_3—CO—SCoA$
2 Acetyl CoA

Figure 16-15 Ketone body metabolism.

The reactions of ketone body metabolism are localized in mitochondria, so that the acetyl CoA that is formed enters the citric acid cycle and is oxidized to CO_2 and water.

ENERGY YIELD FROM OXIDATION OF PALMITATE VIA THE KETONE BODY PATHWAY

Oxidation of palmitoyl CoA to acetyl CoA in the liver will yield 8 acetyl CoA, 7 $FADH_2$, and 7 NADH and, therefore, a maximum of 35 moles of ATP per mole of palmitoyl CoA—as described previously in this chapter. An additional 96 moles of ATP can be generated from the oxidation of the 8 moles of acetyl CoA in the mitochondria of peripheral tissues. However, ketone body utilization in extrahepatic tissues requires energy expenditure. Conversion of acetoacetate to 2 acetyl CoAs utilizes the equivalent of 1 ATP (succinate + CoA+ GTP→succinyl CoA + GDP + P_i). The β-ketothiolase–catalyzed synthesis of 2 acetyl CoAs from 1 acetoacetyl CoA utilizes the energy released in the cleavage of the 4-carbon ketone body to drive synthesis of the second molecule of CoA derivative. The NADH used to reduce acetoacetate to 3-hydroxybutyrate in the liver is recovered in the peripheral organs when the 3-hydroxybutyrate is converted back to acetoacetate via the same reaction. The net result is utilization of 1 mole of ATP per mole of ketone body. Because there are 4 molecules of acetoacetyl group per molecule of palmitoyl CoA, oxidation of palmitoyl CoA via ketone body formation costs 4 moles of ATP per mole of palmitoyl CoA, resulting in the net production of a maximum of 127 moles of ATP instead of 131 moles of ATP per mole of palmitoyl CoA oxidized (or 125 instead of 129 moles per mole of palmitate oxidized).

Why has this apparently wasteful pathway of ketone body formation been preserved during evolution? A simple explanation is that the brain cannot metabolize fatty acids and, therefore, needs ketone bodies as a fuel during prolonged starvation. Moreover, by generating ketone bodies, the liver does not completely use the energy derived from fatty acids but distributes it as ketone bodies for other tissues to use during metabolic adaptation to starvation (or other dietary conditions that cause production and utilization of ketone bodies).

PHOSPHATIDATE AND DIACYLGLYCEROL AS PRECURSORS OF PHOSPHOLIPIDS

Phospholipids are amphipathic lipids that contain acyl groups esterified to the *sn*-1 and *sn*-2 positions of the glycerol moiety. The amphipathic nature of phospholipids makes them suitable for their roles as components of membranes and as surfactants. They contain an alcohol in the *sn*-3 position that is linked to the diacylglycerol by a phosphodiester bond. In eukaryotic phospholipids, the most common alcohols are choline, ethanolamine, serine, glycerol, and inositol. The number of different molecular species of phospholipids is enormous because the long-chain fatty acyl groups in the *sn*-1 or *sn*-2 positions vary in length and degree of unsaturation. Synthesis of triacylglycerols and phospholipids follows a common pathway up to the diacylglycerol stage. In this section, the reactions that occur in higher animals are described (Vance and Vance, 2004). Most of the reactions occur in the ER, as do those of triacylglycerol biosynthesis.

SYNTHESIS OF PHOSPHATIDYLCHOLINE FROM ACTIVATED CHOLINE AND DIACYLGLYCEROL

Phosphatidylcholine (lecithin) is the most abundant phospholipid in eukaryotic cells. Choline from the diet is phosphorylated to phosphocholine by choline kinase (Fig. 16-16).

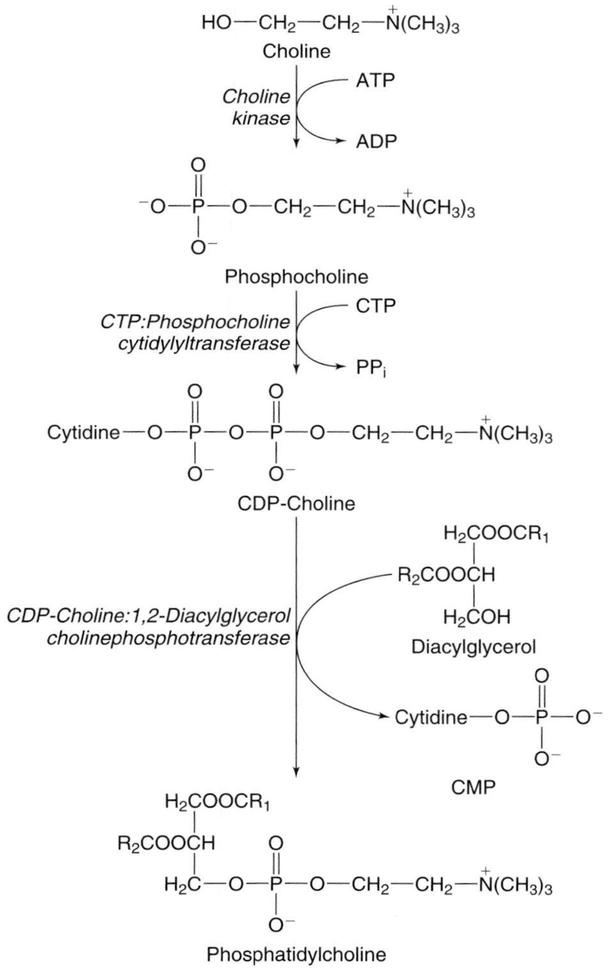

$HO-CH_2-CH_2-\overset{+}{N}(CH_3)_3$

Choline

Choline kinase (ATP → ADP)

$^-O-P(=O)(O^-)-O-CH_2-CH_2-\overset{+}{N}(CH_3)_3$

Phosphocholine

CTP:Phosphocholine cytidylyltransferase (CTP → PP_i)

$Cytidine-O-P(=O)(O^-)-O-P(=O)(O^-)-O-CH_2-CH_2-\overset{+}{N}(CH_3)_3$

CDP-Choline

CDP-Choline:1,2-Diacylglycerol cholinephosphotransferase (Diacylglycerol: H_2COOCR_1 / R_2COOCH / H_2COH → CMP: $Cytidine-O-P(=O)(O^-)-O^-$)

H_2COOCR_1 / R_2COOCH / $H_2C-O-P(=O)(O^-)-O-CH_2-CH_2-\overset{+}{N}(CH_3)_3$

Phosphatidylcholine

Figure 16-16 Phosphatidylcholine synthesis from choline and diacylglycerol. R_1COOH and R_2COOH represent fatty acids.

Choline kinase also uses ethanolamine as a substrate. This lack of substrate specificity suggests that it is not a regulatory step but may serve as a means of trapping choline inside the cell:

$$\text{Choline} + \text{ATP} \rightarrow \text{Phosphocholine} + \text{ADP}$$

Phosphocholine then reacts with cytidine triphosphate (CTP) to yield the activated form of choline, cytidine diphosphate (CDP)–choline. The other product, pyrophosphate, is rapidly degraded to two inorganic phosphates by the ubiquitous pyrophosphatase. As noted previously, this ensures that the reaction will proceed in the direction of CDP-choline synthesis. The enzyme CTP:phosphocholine cytidylyltransferase catalyzes this reaction:

$$\text{Phosphocholine} + \text{CTP} \rightarrow \text{CDP-Choline} + PP_i$$
$$PP_i + H_2O \rightarrow 2\ P_i$$

Cytidylyltransferase catalyzes the main regulatory step in this pathway and is found in both soluble and membrane fractions. The enzyme requires phospholipid for activity so translocation between the ER membrane (with phospholipid, active enzyme) and the cytosol (no phospholipid, inactive enzyme) is a regulatory mechanism. Diacylglycerol and phosphatidylcholine are potential feed-forward (positive) and feedback (negative) regulators of cytidylyltransferase activity, respectively.

In the final reaction in this pathway, CDP-choline reacts with diacylglycerol to form phosphatidylcholine (CDP-choline:1,2-diacylglycerol cholinephosphotransferase):

$$\text{CDP-choline} + \text{Diacylglycerol} \rightarrow \text{Phosphatidylcholine} + \text{CMP}$$

The enzyme catalyzing this reaction is localized in the ER and does not appear to be limiting for phosphatidylcholine synthesis.

Phosphatidylcholine also is formed from phosphatidylethanolamine (Fig. 16-17). The three methyl groups are donated by S-adenosylmethionine in a series of three reactions catalyzed by phosphatidylethanolamine *N*-methyltransferase:

$$3\ \text{S-Adenosylmethionine} + \text{Phosphatidylethanolamine} \rightarrow 3\ \text{S-Adenosylhomocysteine} + \text{Phosphatidylcholine}$$

Normal diets provide sufficient choline. In humans, choline cannot be synthesized directly but is produced indirectly via the foregoing phosphatidylethanolamine *N*-methyltransferase reaction. The metabolism of choline, methionine, and folate is closely interrelated. The three methyl groups of choline can be made available for one-carbon metabolism upon conversion of choline to betaine. One-carbon metabolism is discussed in detail in Chapter 25. In malnutrition, when stores of choline, methionine, and folate are depleted, or in total parenteral nutrition, choline may become deficient. Carbohydrate loading, due to enhanced hepatic triacylglycerol synthesis, also increases the amount of choline required. Phosphatidylcholine is required for lipoprotein synthesis and secretion. In choline deficiency, biosynthesis of phosphatidylcholine is inhibited, causing development of fatty liver.

PATHWAYS FOR THE SYNTHESIS OF PHOSPHATIDYLETHANOLAMINE AND PHOSPHATIDYLSERINE

The first and most prevalent pathway for synthesis of phosphatidylethanolamine is de novo synthesis. This pathway involves phosphorylation of ethanolamine, which is catalyzed by choline kinase, the same enzyme that is involved in the synthesis of phosphatidylcholine. The remainder of the pathway is also similar to that for the de novo pathway for synthesis of phosphatidylcholine (see Fig. 16-16). Ethanolamine reacts with CTP to produce its activated form, CDP-ethanolamine, in a reaction catalyzed by CTP:ethanolaminephosphate cytidylyltransferase. CDP-ethanolamine:1,2-diacylglycerol ethanolaminephosphotransferase then catalyzes the reaction of CDP-ethanolamine with diacylglycerol to form phosphatidylethanolamine.

In addition, there are two pathways for synthesis of phosphatidylethanolamine via modification of preexisting phospholipids. First, phosphatidylserine decarboxylase catalyzes the decarboxylation of phosphatidylserine to form phosphatidylethanolamine (see Fig. 16-17):

$$\text{Phosphatidylserine}^- + H^+ \rightarrow \text{Phosphatidylethanolamine} + CO_2$$

The second route involves an exchange reaction with phosphatidylserine in which

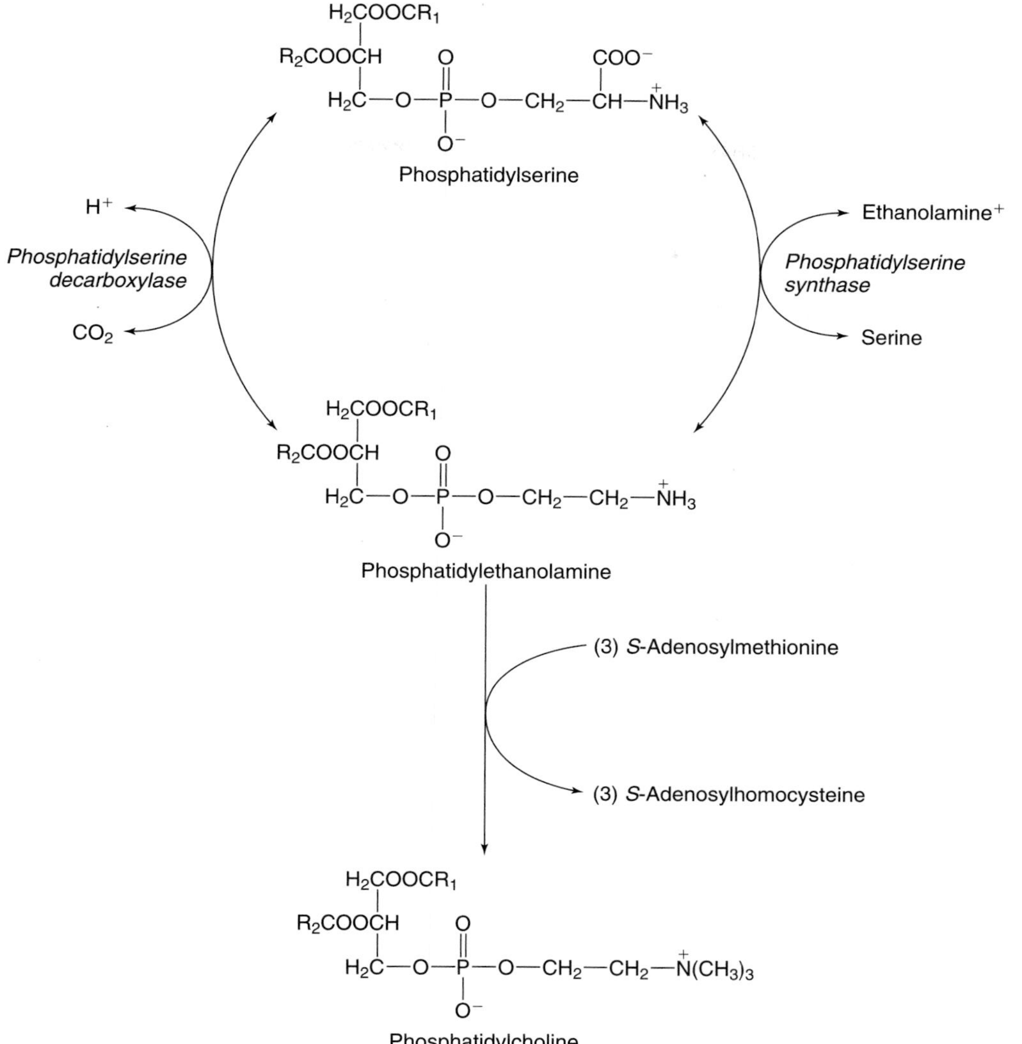

Figure 16-17 Synthesis of phosphatidylcholine from phosphatidylethanolamine and interconversion of phosphatidylserine and phosphatidylethanolamine. R_1 and R_2 represent fatty acid chains.

phosphatidylserine reacts with ethanolamine to form phosphatidylethanolamine and serine. The reaction is catalyzed by phosphatidylserine synthase (see Fig. 16-17):

$$\text{Phosphatidylserine}^- + \text{Ethanolamine}^+ \rightarrow \text{Phosphatidylethanolamine} + \text{Serine}$$

Phosphatidylserine constitutes only 5% to 15% of phospholipids in cells. Although the CDP-diacylglycerol pathway, similar to that described in the next section for phosphatidylglycerol, is used in the de novo synthesis of phosphatidylserine in bacteria, the enzyme catalyzing the reaction of CDP-diacylglycerol and serine does not appear to be present in mammalian tissue. Instead, phosphatidylethanolamine or phosphatidylcholine reacts with serine to undergo base exchange to form phosphatidylserine and ethanolamine or choline (phosphatidylserine synthase).

CDP-DIACYLGLYCEROL AS AN INTERMEDIATE IN THE SYNTHESIS OF PHOSPHATIDYLGLYCEROL AND DIPHOSPHATIDYLGLYCEROL

In this pathway, CTP is used to activate diacylglycerol to CDP-diacylglycerol. Pyrophosphate is the other product in this reaction catalyzed by phosphatidate cytidylyltransferase. Cleavage of the resulting pyrophosphate drives the reaction toward completion:

Diacylglycerol + CTP →
CDP-Diacylglycerol + PP_i

$$PP_i + H_2O \rightarrow 2\ P_i$$

In the next reaction, CDP-diacylglycerol reacts with *sn*-glycerol 3-phosphate to form phosphatidylglycerol phosphate and CMP. The reaction is catalyzed by glycerophosphate phosphatidyltransferase (Fig. 16-18):

CDP-Diacylglycerol + *sn*-Glycerol 3-Phosphate →
Phosphatidylglycerol Phosphate + CMP

In the second step, phosphatidylglycerol phosphate phosphatase catalyzes hydrolysis of phosphate from phosphatidylglycerol phosphate to form phosphatidylglycerol:

Phosphatidylglycerol Phosphate →
Phosphatidylglycerol + P_i

Another molecule of CDP-diacylglycerol may react with phosphatidylglycerol to form diphosphatidylglycerol and CMP (see Fig. 16-18, reaction catalyzed by phosphatidate phosphatidyltransferase). Diphosphati-dylglycerol (cardiolipin) is synthesized exclusively in the mitochondria and is found only in these organelles. Cardiolipin is rich in unsaturated 18-carbon fatty acids such as oleate and linoleate:

Phosphatidylglycerol + CDP-Diacylglycerol →
Diphosphatidylglycerol + CMP

CDP-DIACYLGLYCEROL AS AN INTERMEDIATE IN INOSITOL PHOSPHOLIPID SYNTHESIS

Inositol reacts with CDP-diacylglycerol to form phosphatidylinositol in a reaction localized in the ER and catalyzed by phosphatidylinositol synthase:

Inositol + CDP-Diacylglycerol →
Phosphatidylinositol + CMP

The inositol phospholipids (Fig. 16-19) are constituents of membranes. A small portion of the phosphatidylinositols that are phosphorylated serves as precursors to the important intracellular second messengers diacylglycerol and inositol polyphosphates as described in subsequent text of this chapter. Phosphatidylinositol phosphate and phosphatidylinositol bisphosphate are formed by the sequential addition of phosphate using ATP; the reactions are catalyzed by phosphatidylinositol kinase and phosphatidylinositol phosphate kinase, respectively. Several inositol polyphosphates with more than three phosphates can be derived from the inositol triphosphate released by the hydrolysis of phosphatidylinositol bisphosphate catalyzed by phospholipase C. The additional phosphorylations of inositol triphosphate to form polyphosphates are catalyzed by kinases that use free inositol polyphosphates as substrates.

ETHER-LINKED LIPIDS

There are two major classes of ether-linked lipids in the cells. Glycerol ethers have *O*-alkyl groups; plasmalogens have *O*-alk-1-enyl groups. In each case, the ether linkage is to the *sn*-1 position. Some ether-linked lipids have potent biological activity. Platelet activating factor, 1-alkyl-2-acetyl-*sn*-glycerol 3-phosphocholine, for example, causes aggregation of blood platelets at concentrations as low as 10^{-11} mol/L. Plasmalogens, the other class of ether-linked lipids, constitute approximately 5% to 20% of the phospholipids of cell membranes. Although the exact biological function(s) of these compounds is not known, their importance is suggested by the symptoms of plasmalogen deficiency (Zellweger's syndrome) described in subsequent text. Plasmalogen is especially abundant in nervous tissue and in the membranes of the myelin sheath; for example, ethanolamine plasmalogen may represent as much as 80% of phospholipids in the myelin sheath membranes. High levels of choline plasmalogens are found in heart tissue.

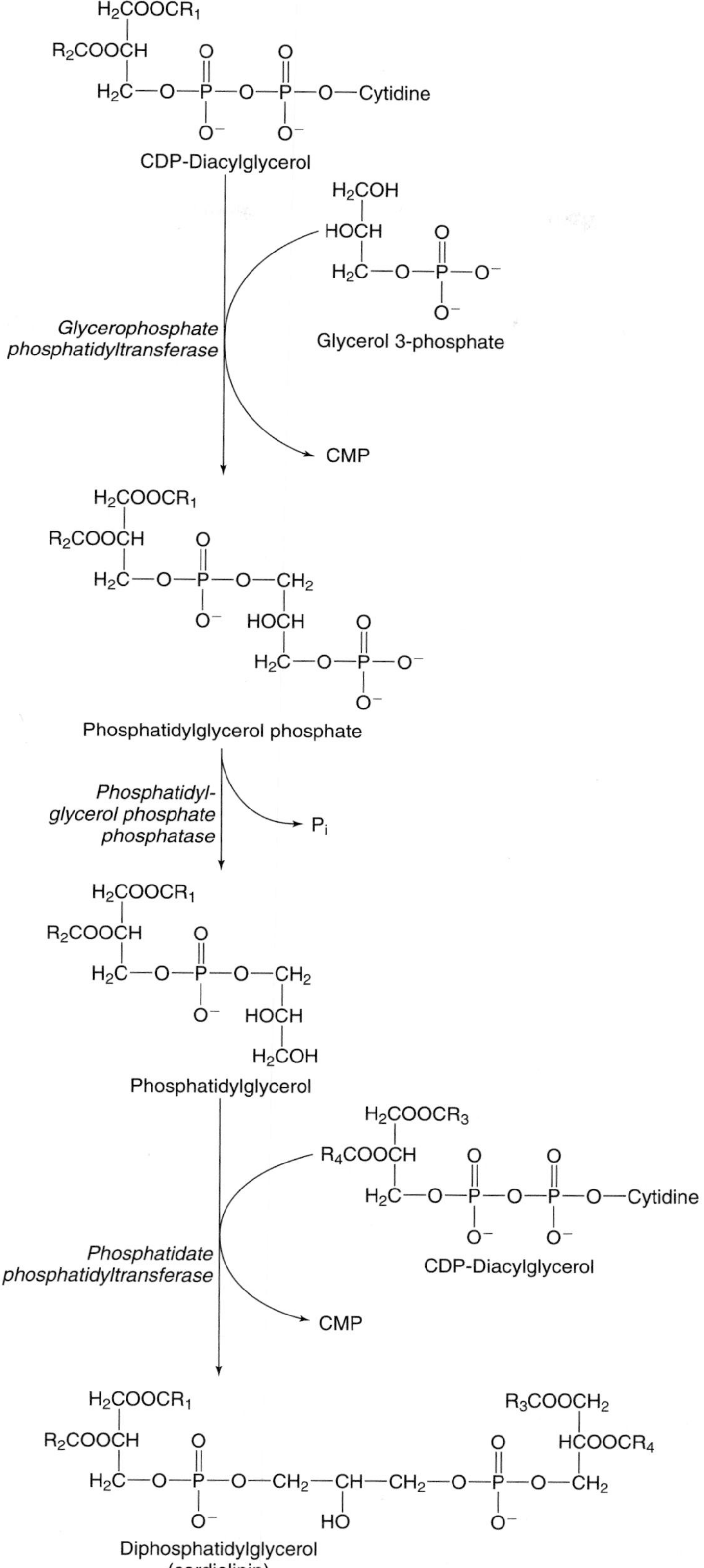

Figure 16-18 Synthesis of phosphatidylglycerol and cardiolipin. Fatty acids are represented as *R_1COOH, R_2COOH, R_3COOH,* and *R_4COOH.*

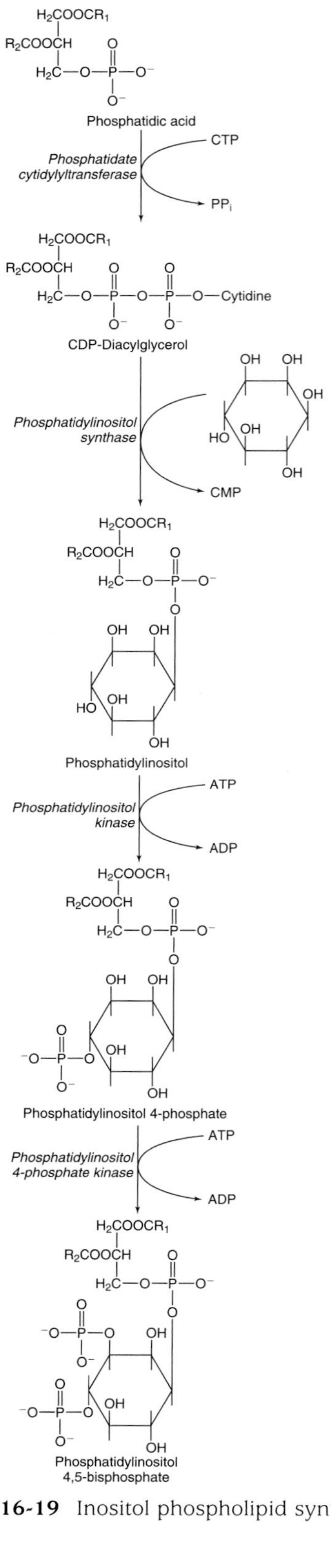

Figure 16-19 Inositol phospholipid synthesis.

One of the substrates for the synthesis of ether-linked lipids is a fatty alcohol. This compound is produced from acyl CoA in a reaction that requires NADPH. This reaction involves an aldehyde intermediate and is catalyzed by a membrane-associated acyl CoA reductase:

(1) Acyl CoA + NADPH + H^+ → Fatty Aldehyde + $NADP^+$ + CoA

(2) Fatty Aldehyde + NADPH + H^+ → Fatty Alcohol + $NADP^+$

The other substrate for synthesis of ether-linked lipids is 1-acyldihydroxyacetone phosphate. This is produced by the dihydroxyacetone phosphate acyltransferase that was described in the section on synthesis of triacylglycerol:

Dihydroxyacetone Phosphate + Fatty Acyl CoA → 1-Acyldihydroxyacetone Phosphate + CoA

In triacylglycerol synthesis, the next step is reduction of the keto group to a hydroxyl group to form lysophosphatidic acid. In ether–lipid synthesis, the next step is an exchange reaction with a fatty alcohol to produce 1-alkyldihydroxyacetone phosphate in a reaction catalyzed by 1-alkyldihydroxyacetone phosphate synthase (Fig. 16-20):

1-Acyldihydroxyacetone Phosphate + Fatty Alcohol → 1-Alkyldihydroxyacetone Phosphate + Fatty Acid

This reaction is specific for a substrate with a ketone function. Synthesis of ether lipids thus utilizes only the dihydroxyacetone phosphate pathway. The next reaction is a reduction of the keto group of alkyldihydroxyacetone phosphate to yield alkylglycerol 3-phosphate. This reaction is catalyzed by NADPH-dependent alkyldihydroxyacetone phosphate reductase. This reductase is capable of reducing both acyl and alkyl analogs of dihydroxyacetone phosphate:

1-Alkyldihydroxyacetone Phosphate + NADPH + H^+ → 1-Alkylglycerol 3-Phosphate + $NADP^+$

In the next reaction, the alkyl analog of phosphatidic acid is synthesized by adding an acyl group to the *sn*-2 position. This reaction is catalyzed by 1-alkylglycerol phosphate acyltransferase:

1-Alkylglycerol 3-Phosphate + Acyl CoA $\rightarrow$
1-Alkyl-2-Acylglycerol 3-Phosphate + CoA

The next step in this pathway creates an alkylacylglycerol by dephosphorylation. This compound represents a branch point in ether–lipid synthesis in much the same way as diacylglycerol is at a branch point for synthesis of triacylglycerol and glycerophospholipids:

1-Alkyl-2-Acylglycerol 3-Phosphate + H_2O $\rightarrow$
1-Alkyl-2-Acylglycerol + P_i

Next, analogous to the reactions that form phosphatidylethanolamine or phosphatidylcholine, an alcohol base is transferred to 1-alkyl-2-acylglycerol from CDP-ethanolamine or CDP-choline:

1-Alkyl-2-Acylglycerol + CDP-Ethanolamine $\rightarrow$
1-Alkyl-2-Acylglycerol 3-Phosphoethanolamine
+ CMP

Plasmalogens are formed by desaturation of the alkyl moiety of the ethanolamine or choline derivative to form an *O*-alk-1-enyl substituent. Platelet activating factor is synthesized from 1-alkyl-2-acetylglycerol and is 1-alkyl-2-acetylglycerol 3-phosphocholine.

The enzymatic reaction that creates the double bond in 1-alkyl-2-acylglycerol 3-phosphoethanolamine is unusual in that the intact phospholipid is the substrate for the desaturase. Fatty acyl groups are usually desaturated prior to making them part of more complex lipids. Δ1-Alkyl desaturase behaves like a typical acyl CoA desaturase; it is a mixed function oxidase that requires O_2, NADH, cytochrome b_5 reductase, and a terminal desaturase protein (see Fig. 16-5, which illustrates a similar reaction mechanism for stearoyl CoA desaturase).

Dihydroxyacetone phosphate acyltransferase and 1-alkyldihydroxyacetone phosphate synthase catalyze the first two reactions in ether–lipid biosynthesis and are localized in peroxisomes. One of the manifestations of Zellweger's syndrome, a block in peroxisome biogenesis, is decreased tissue plasmalogen levels, and these deficiencies may contribute to pathological features of this disease, including profound neurological deficits and death within

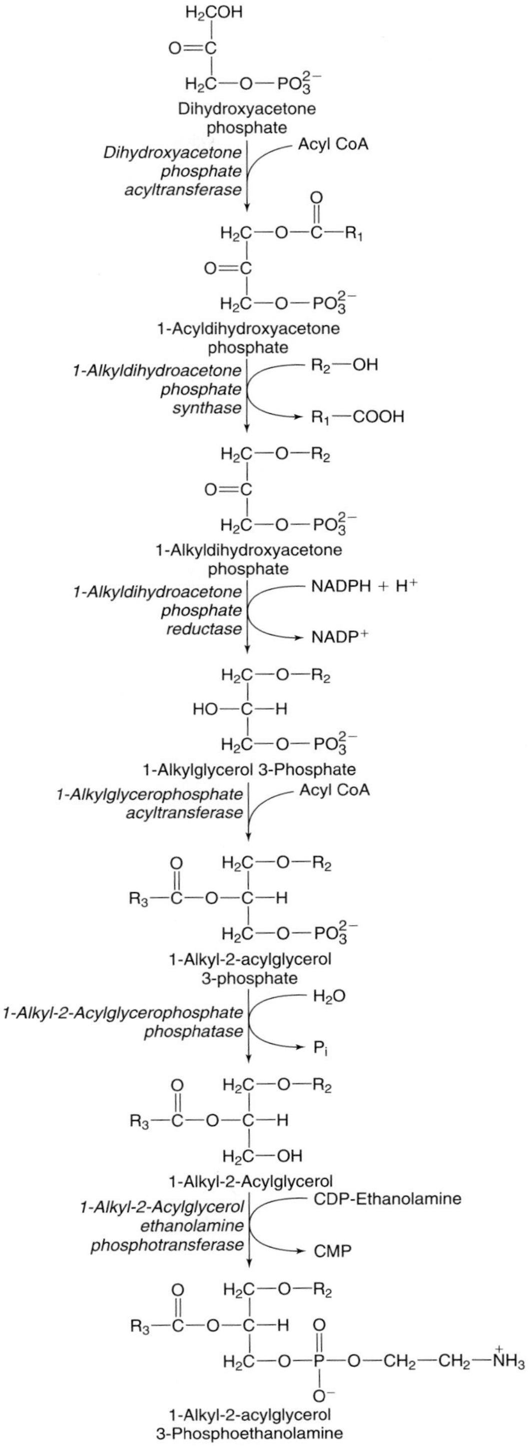

Figure 16-20 Ether-lipid synthesis. R_1COOH represents a fatty acid, and R_2OH represents a fatty alcohol.

the first year of life. Some types of β-oxidation of fatty acids, including oxidation of very-long-chain fatty acids, polyunsaturated fatty acids, and dicarboxylic fatty acids, occur in peroxisomes. Patients with Zellweger's syndrome, therefore, show both accumulation of very-long-chain fatty acids and decreased plasmalogen levels.

REMODELING OF PHOSPHOLIPIDS IN SITU

The phospholipid composition of different cellular membranes is usually specific for each organelle. Differences involve both the fatty acyl groups in the *sn*-1 and *sn*-2 positions and the alcohol base in the *sn*-3 position. In general, the *sn*-1 position of phospholipids contains saturated fatty acids, whereas the *sn*-2 position contains unsaturated fatty acids. However, dietary content of fatty acids influences fatty acid composition of phospholipids. The specificity of insertion of fatty acids at the *sn*-1 and *sn*-2 positions is usually determined by the specificities of glycerol 3-phosphate acyltransferase and 1-acylglycerol 3-phosphate acyltransferase. An additional mechanism for generating and/or maintaining these specific compositions is to remove acyl groups from phospholipids through the action of phospholipases and to reesterify with a specific acyl group. The abundance of polyunsaturated fatty acids at the *sn*-2 position is due to phospholipid remodeling. The alcohol bases also can be rearranged when a specific phospholipase generates diacylglycerol or phosphatidic acid.

The phospholipases that cleave acyl groups or alcohol bases can be put into five groups, based on the specific phospholipid bond that they attack (Fig. 16-21). Phospholipases A and B are acyl hydrolases. Phospholipase A_1 cleaves the ester bond between the *sn*-1 position and its acyl group, generating 2-acylglycerol 3-phospholipid. Phospholipase A_2 attacks the ester bond between the *sn*-2 position and its acyl group, generating 1-acylglycerol 3-phospholipid. Phospholipase B cleaves the ester bonds at either the *sn*-1 or *sn*-2 position but is relatively rare. Phospholipases C and D are phosphodiesterases. Phospholipase C cleaves the bond between the *sn*-3 position and the phosphate (glycerophosphate bond) and encompasses a family of enzymes that generate diacylglycerol and the free phosphorylated alcohol as products. Phospholipase D attacks the bond between the alcohol base and the glycerol phosphate.

GENERATION OF SIGNALING MOLECULES BY REGULATED PHOSPHOLIPASES

In addition to the remodeling of molecular species of membrane lipids, some of the phospholipases play important roles in cell signaling. When certain hormones or growth factors occupy their cell surface receptors, phosphoinositide-specific plasma membrane phospholipase Cs are activated. The reaction catalyzed by phospholipase C generates the second messengers inositol 1,4,5-triphosphate and diacylglycerol, which cause Ca^{2+} release and activation of protein kinase C, respectively. This mechanism is discussed in more detail in Chapters 18 and 19. Inositol polyphosphates and diacylglycerol are recycled, and recycling accomplishes

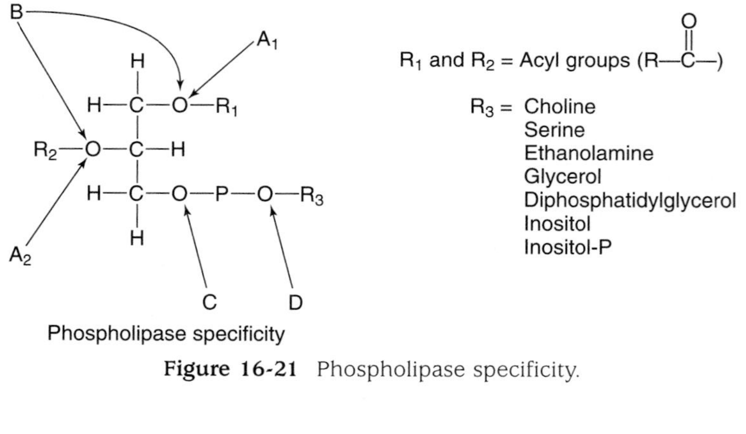

Figure 16-21 Phospholipase specificity.

two purposes. First, it ends the action of the second messenger, and, second, it regenerates the substrates upon which phospholipases can act. Specific phosphatases act on inositol polyphosphates to remove the phosphates, ultimately yielding free inositol. The diacylglycerol can be converted to phosphatidic acid via the action of diacylglycerol kinase, or it can react with CDP-inositol to form phosphatidylinositol or with other compounds activated with CDP to yield other phospholipids. Lithium, a drug that is used to treat bipolar disorders, exerts its therapeutic effects by inhibiting hydrolysis of inositol monophosphate to inositol. This depletes the intracellular supply of inositol and, therefore, interrupts the phosphatidylinositol signaling pathway, which is presumably hyperactive in bipolar disorders.

Phospholipase A_2 also can be activated by extracellular stimuli, including local mediators, by a receptor-mediated process. Arachidonic acid released by phospholipase A_2 can be used for synthesis of prostaglandins and thromboxanes via the cyclooxygenase pathway and for synthesis of leukotrienes via the lipoxygenase pathway (see Chapter 18 for further discussion of these eicosanoids). Antiinflammatory corticosteroids induce an inhibitory protein for phospholipase A_2, lipocortin, and thereby decrease arachidonic acid release and, hence, decrease the synthesis of eicosanoids.

SPHINGOLIPIDS AS STRUCTURAL AND SIGNALING MOLECULES

More than 300 structurally distinct sphingolipids occur in nature. The hydrophobic portion of sphingolipids is ceramide; ceramide contains a fatty acid that is amide-linked to sphingosine or a related sphingoid base. Sphingolipids also contain a hydrophilic moiety, usually phosphocholine (as in sphingomyelin) or one or more sugar residues (as in cerebrosides and gangliosides). Sphingolipids are particularly abundant in the central nervous system. Sphingolipids play both structural and regulatory roles. After glycerophospholipids, the most abundant lipids in membranes are sphingolipids. Ceramide and sphingosine likely play important physiological roles in intracellular signaling (Payne et al., 2004; Pettus et al., 2004). Numerous gangliosides are displayed on the external face of mammalian cells and probably play roles in recognition of other cells and basement membranes. Many bacteria have developed specific adhesion mechanisms that recognize and result in their binding to specific gangliosides. Further evidence for the importance of these compounds is that inherited mutations in the pathway for degradation of sphingolipids result in the accumulation of specific gangliosides, cerebrosides, and ceramides. These lipid accumulations account for the pathologies of several lipid storage diseases.

CERAMIDE, THE PRECURSOR OF MOST MAMMALIAN SPHINGOLIPIDS

Enzymes involved in the synthesis of ceramide are localized in the ER. In the first reaction, palmitoyl CoA reacts with serine to form 3-ketosphinganine. This reaction requires pyridoxal 5′-phosphate (vitamin B_6 coenzyme) for decarboxylation and is catalyzed by serine palmitoyltransferase (Fig. 16-22):

$$\text{Palmitoyl CoA} + \text{Serine} \rightarrow \text{3-Ketosphinganine} + \text{CoA} + CO_2$$

The next reaction is a reductase that requires NADPH and converts the keto group at C-3 of the long-chain base to a hydroxyl, forming sphinganine (dihydrosphingosine):

$$\text{3-Ketosphinganine} + \text{NADPH} + H^+ \rightarrow \text{Sphinganine} + \text{NADP}^+$$

Addition of a long-chain acyl group to sphinganine to produce dihydroceramide is catalyzed by ceramide synthase:

$$\text{Sphinganine} + \text{Fatty Acyl CoA} \rightarrow \text{Dihydroceramide} + \text{CoA}$$

Finally, dihydroceramide is converted to ceramide by the introduction of a 4,5-*trans*-double bond. Ceramide is the precursor of all complex sphingolipids.

SPHINGOMYELIN

Sphingomyelin is the only major sphingolipid that contains phosphate. Sphingomyelin is synthesized when ceramide reacts with

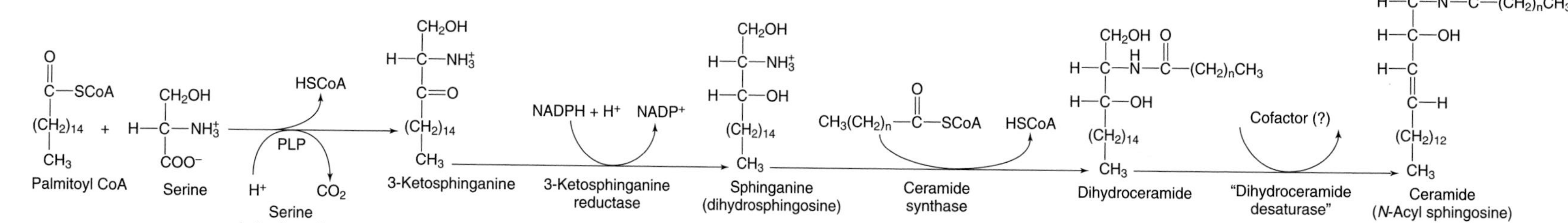

Figure 16-22 Ceramide synthesis.

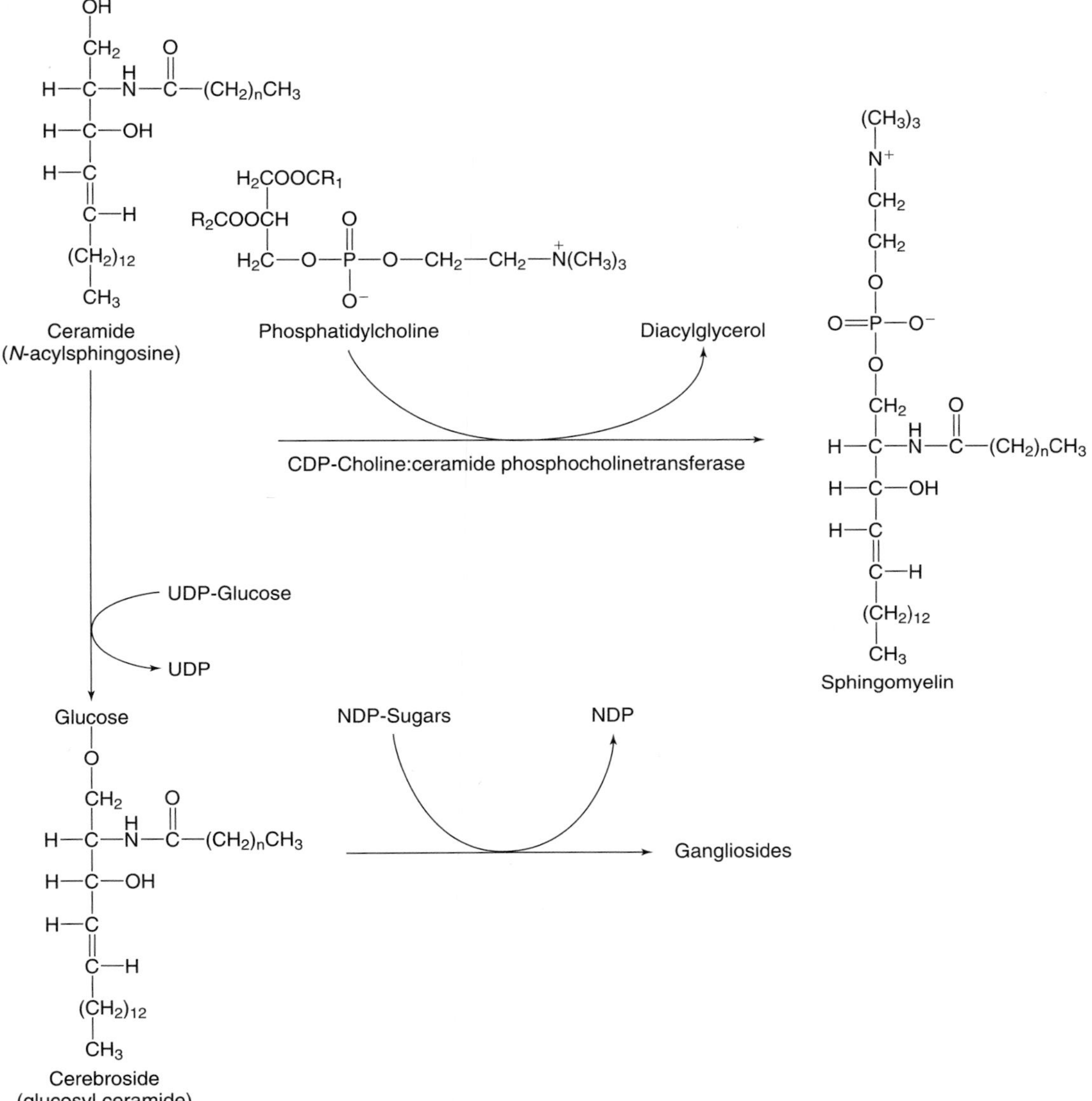

Figure 16-23 Sphingolipid synthesis from ceramide.

phosphatidylcholine to form sphingomyelin and diacylglycerol (Fig. 16-23):

Ceramide + Phosphatidylcholine →
Sphingomyelin + Diacylglycerol

Sphingomyelin is hydrolyzed by sphingomyelinase to produce ceramide and phosphocholine. Ceramide is hydrolyzed by ceramidase to produce the sphingoid base sphingosine. Activations of sphingomyelinase and ceramidase are linked to activation of cell surface receptors that initiate multiple cellular responses. Ceramide acts as a second messenger in a signaling cascade regulating cell growth and differentiation, cellular functions, and programmed cell death. Sphingosine also activates or inhibits a number of cellular events.

GANGLIOSIDES AND SULFATOGLYCOSPHINGOLIPIDS

Gangliosides are built up from cerebroside by the addition of sugars. The neutral glycosphingolipids, galactosylceramide and glucosylceramide, are intermediates in the synthesis of more complex gangliosides and sulfatoglycosphingolipids. They are formed by the reaction of ceramide with uridine diphosphate (UDP)-galactose or UDP-glucose to form the corresponding cerebroside and UDP (Fig. 16-23):

$$\text{Ceramide} + \text{UDP-Glucose} \rightarrow \text{Cerebroside} + \text{UDP}$$

Gangliosides are created by adding one or more sugars to the nonreducing end of the carbohydrate moiety of cerebroside or of the growing carbohydrate chain. Specific glycosyl transferases catalyze these reactions. The sugar donors are nucleotide diphosphate sugars. The "terminal" sugar of all gangliosides is *N*-acetyl neuraminic acid.

Galactocerebroside 3-sulfate is a major sulfolipid. It is synthesized by the reaction of galactosyl ceramide with 3′-phosphoadenosine-5′-phosphosulfate (PAPS). PAPS is a common donor of sulfate groups in the synthesis of sulfated compounds.

DEGRADATION OF GANGLIOSIDES BY SPECIFIC LYSOSOMAL EXOGLYCOSIDASES

Specific acid hydrolases localized in lysosomes degrade plasma membrane–bound and extracellular gangliosides. The pathway for this sequential removal of sugars has been worked out based on the metabolic consequences of known genetic defects in humans that are often manifested in childhood. In Tay-Sachs, Fabry's, Sandhoff's, and Gaucher's diseases, specific gangliosides accumulate because degradation of a specific ganglioside is blocked while synthesis and the initial steps of degradation occur at normal rates. Abnormal accumulations of these lipids, particularly in nervous tissues, cause the pathologies of these diseases, including mental retardation.

Lysosomal defects in acid ceramidase (Farber's lipogranulomatosis) and acid sphingomyelinase (Niemann-Pick disease) result in tissue accumulation of ceramide and sphingomyelin, respectively, and metabolic disturbances. Acid ceramidase catalyzes the hydrolysis of ceramide to release sphingosine and long-chain fatty acid. Acid sphingomyelinase catalyzes the degradation of sphingomyelin to form ceramide plus phosphocholine. All of these defects are lysosomal disorders of sphingolipid catabolism. Nonlysosomal ceramidases and sphingomyelinases, which have optimal activity at neutral or slightly alkaline pH, probably are involved in turnover of ceramide and sphingomyelin, respectively, for cell signaling.

REFERENCES

Abu-Elheiga L, Oh W, Kordari P, Wakil SJ (2003) Acetyl-CoA carboxylase 2 mutant mice are protected against obesity and diabetes induced by high-fat/high-carbohydrate diets. Proc Natl Acad Sci U S A 100:10207-10212.

Cases S, Stone SJ, Zhou P, Yen E, Tow B, Lardizabal KD, Voelker T, Farese RV Jr (2001) Cloning of DGAT2, a second mammalian diacylglycerol acyltransferase, and related family members. J Biol Chem 276:38870-38876.

Coleman RA, Lee DP (2004) Enzymes of triacylglycerol synthesis and their regulation. Prog Lipid Res 43:134-176.

Dircks LK, Sul HS (1999) Acyltransferases of the de novo glycerophospholipid biosynthesis. Prog Lipid Res 38:461-479

Eaton S (2002) Control of mitochondrial beta-oxidation flux. Prog Lipid Res 41:197-239.

Foster DW (2004) The role of the carnitine system in human metabolism. Ann N Y Acad Sci 1033:1-16.

Hall AM, Smith AJ, Bernlohr DA (2003) Characterization of the acyl-CoA synthetase activity of purified murine fatty acid transport protein 1. J Biol Chem 278:43008-43013.

Haunerland NH, Spener F (2004) Fatty acid-binding proteins—insights from genetic manipulations. Prog Lipid Res 43:328-349.

Hellerstein MK (1999) De novo lipogenesis in humans: metabolic and regulatory aspects. Eur J Clin Nutr 53:553-565.

Hillgartner FB, Salati LM, Goodridge AG (1995) Physiological and molecular mechanisms involved in nutritional regulation of fatty acid synthesis. Physiol Rev 75:47-76.

Holm C (2003) Molecular mechanisms regulating hormone-sensitive lipase and lipolysis. Biochem Soc Trans 31:1120-1124.

Kalant D, Cianflone K (2004) Regulation of fatty acid transport. Curr Opin Lipidol 15:309-314.

Latasa MJ, Griffin MJ, Moon YS, Kang C, Sul HS (2003) Occupancy and function of the -150 sterol regulatory element and -65 E-box in nutritional regulation of the fatty acid synthase gene in living animals. Mol Cell Biol 23:5896-5907.

Minokoshi Y, Alquier T, Furukawa N, Kim Y-B, Lee A, Xue B, Mu J, Foufelle F, Ferre P, Birnbaum MJ, Stuck BJ, Kahn BB (2004) AMP-kinase regulates food intake by responding to hormonal and nutrient signals in the hypothalamus. Nature 428:569-574.

Munday MR (2002) Regulation of mammalian acetyl-CoA carboxylase. Biochem Soc Trans 30:1059-1064.

Payne SG, Milstien S, Barbour SE, Spiegel S (2004) Modulation of adaptive immune responses by sphingosine-1-phosphate. Semin Cell Dev Biol 15:521-527.

Pettus BJ, Chalfant CE, Hannun YA (2004) Sphingolipids in inflammation: roles and implications. Curr Mol Med 4:405-418.

Preiss-Landl K, Zimmermann R, Hammerle G, Zechner R (2002) Lipoprotein lipase: the regulation of tissue specific expression and its role in lipid and energy metabolism. Curr Opin Lipidol 13:471-481.

Reshef L, Olswang Y, Cassuto H, Blum B, Croniger CM, Kalhan SC, Tilghman SM, Hanson RW (2003) Glyceroneogenesis and the triglyceride/fatty acid cycle. J Biol Chem 278:30413-30416.

Scriver CR, Beaudet AL, Valle D, Sly WS, Childs B, Kinzler KW, Bert Vogelstein B (eds) (2001) The Metabolic and Molecular Bases of Inherited Disease, 8th edition. McGraw-Hill, New York.

Shimokawa T, Kumar MV, Lane MD (2002) Effect of a fatty acid synthase inhibitor on food intake and expression of hypothalamic neuropeptides. Proc Natl Acad Sci U S A 99:66-71.

Unger RH (2004) The hyperleptinemia of obesity-regulation of caloric surpluses. Cell 116:145-151.

Vance JE, Vance DE (2004) Phospholipid biosynthesis in mammalian cells. Biochem Cell Biol 82:113-128.

Villena JA, Roy S, Sarkadi-Nagy E, Kim KH, Sul HS (2004) Desnutrin, an adipocyte gene encoding a novel patatin domain-containing protein, is induced by fasting and glucocorticoids: ectopic expression of desnutrin increases triglyceride hydrolysis. J Biol Chem 279:47066-47075.

Wanders RJA (2004) Metabolic and molecular basis of peroxisomal disorders: a review. Am J Med Genet 126A:355-375.

Woods A, Johnstone SR, Dickerson K, Leiper FC, Fryer LGD, Neumann D, Schlattner U, Wallimann T, Calson M, Carling D (2004) LKB1 is the upstream kinase in the AMP-activated protein kinase cascade. Curr Biol 13:2004-2008.

Yeaman SJ (2004) Hormone-sensitive lipase—new roles for an old enzyme. Biochem J 379:11-22.

RECOMMENDED READINGS

Anderson RG (2003) Joe Goldstein and Mike Brown: from cholesterol homeostasis to new paradigms in membrane biology. Trends Cell Biol 13:534-539.

Scriver CR, Beaudet AL, Valle D, Sly WS, Childs B, Kinzler KW, Bert Vogelstein B (eds) (2001) The Metabolic and Molecular Bases of Inherited Disease, 8th edition. McGraw-Hill, New York.

Vance DE, Vance JE (2002) Biochemistry of Lipids, Lipoproteins and Membranes, 4th edition. New Comprehensive Biochemistry Vol 36. Elsevier Science, BV, New York.

Chapter 17

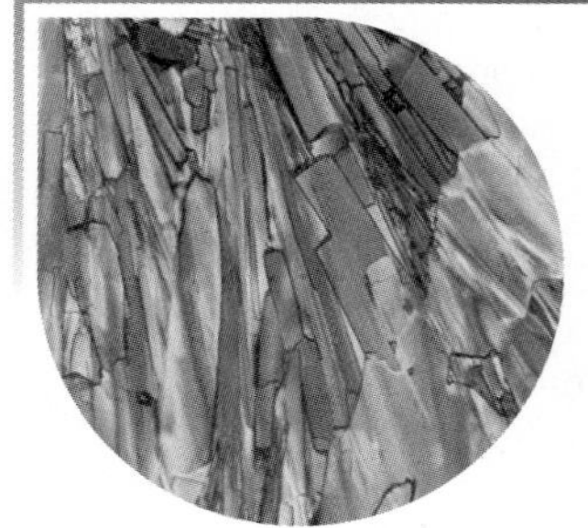

Cholesterol and Lipoproteins: Synthesis, Transport, and Metabolism

Hei Sook Sul, PhD, and Judith Storch, PhD

OUTLINE

COMMON ABBREVIATIONS

ABCA1	ATP-binding cassette transporter A1
ACAT	acyl-CoA cholesterol acyltransferase
apo A-I	apolipoprotein A-I
apo B	apolipoprotein B
apo C-II	apolipoprotein C-II
apo E	apolipoprotein E
CAD	coronary artery disease
CETP	cholesteryl ester transfer protein
FXR	farnesoid X receptor
HDL	high density lipoprotein
HMG CoA	3-hydroxy-3-methylglutaryl coenzyme A
HSL	hormone-sensitive lipase
IDL	intermediate density lipoprotein
LCAT	lecithin:cholesterol acyltransferase
LDL	low density lipoprotein

LPL	lipoprotein lipase
LXR	liver X receptor
MTP	microsomal triacylglycerol transfer protein
PLTP	phospholipid transfer protein
SCAP	SREBP cleavage-activating protein
SRE	sterol regulatory element
SREBP	sterol regulatory element binding protein
VLDL	very low density lipoprotein

BIOLOGICAL ROLES FOR CHOLESTEROL AND ISOPRENOIDS

Cholesterol is a sterol molecule with critical biological importance. It is an essential structural component of cell membranes. It is also a precursor of the sex and adrenal steroid hormones, and of bile acids. Oxysterol metabolites of cholesterol are also important regulators of lipid metabolic pathways. Moreover, isoprenoids, intermediates in the cholesterol biosynthetic pathway, are used for production of small amounts of molecules that have important biological functions. These include dolichol, which is required for glycoprotein synthesis, and ubiquinone (coenzyme Q), which is involved in electron transport in mitochondria. Isoprenoids also are used for posttranslational farnesylation or geranylgeranylation (called prenylation) of a variety of proteins including heterotrimeric G-proteins and small GTP binding proteins. Cholesterol itself is also used for modification of specific proteins. These covalently attached lipids, isoprenoid groups or cholesterol, serve in most cases as anchors for targeting proteins to certain membrane compartments or submembrane domains.

Synthesis and disposal of cholesterol must be tightly regulated both to meet cellular cholesterol needs and to prevent cholesterol accumulation. However, abnormal deposition of cholesterol and cholesterol-rich lipoproteins in the coronary arteries eventually leads to atherosclerosis, a major contributory factor of cardiovascular diseases.

SYNTHESIS OF CHOLESTEROL FROM ACETYL CoA UNITS

Cholesterol is provided by foods of animal origin. Although the exact mechanism of intestinal cholesterol absorption remains under active investigation, its marked inhibition by the drug ezetimibe provides strong evidence for a regulatable protein-mediated process. Indeed, a protein known as NPC1-L1, for Niemann-Pick C1-like protein 1, was recently shown to be involved in the actions of ezetimibe in blocking the intestinal absorption of dietary cholesterol (Altmann et al., 2004; Davis et al., 2004). In addition to dietary sources, de novo synthesis of cholesterol occurs in all nucleated cells, and is regulated by the availability of cholesterol in the blood. Quantitatively, the liver and intestine are the major sites of cholesterol synthesis. On average, cholesterol intake from the diet is approximately 0.6 g/day, whereas cholesterol from synthesis is approximately 1 g/day. The enzymes of cholesterol synthesis are extramitochondrial. Mevalonate and squalene are intermediates in the synthesis of cholesterol.

CONVERSION OF ACETYL COA TO MEVALONATE IN THE CYTOSOL

Synthesis of 3-hydroxy-3-methylglutaryl coenzyme A (HMG CoA) (Fig. 17-1) follows the same pathway described in Chapter 16 for the synthesis of ketone bodies, except that it occurs in the cytosol instead of the mitochondria. Two molecules of acetyl CoA condense to form acetoacetyl CoA (acetyl CoA:acetoacetyl CoA acetyltransferase). Another molecule of acetyl CoA then condenses with a molecule of acetoacetyl CoA to form HMG CoA, a reaction catalyzed by HMG CoA synthase. HMG CoA is converted to mevalonate (see Fig. 17-1) by HMG CoA reductase in the ER:

$$\text{HMG CoA} + 2\ \text{NADPH} + 2\ \text{H}^+ \rightarrow \text{Mevalonate} + 2\ \text{NADP}^+ + \text{CoA}$$

This NADPH-requiring enzyme catalyzes the committed step in isoprenoid synthesis. It is the regulatory step in cholesterol biosynthesis and is regulated by several mechanisms, as described in the material that follows.

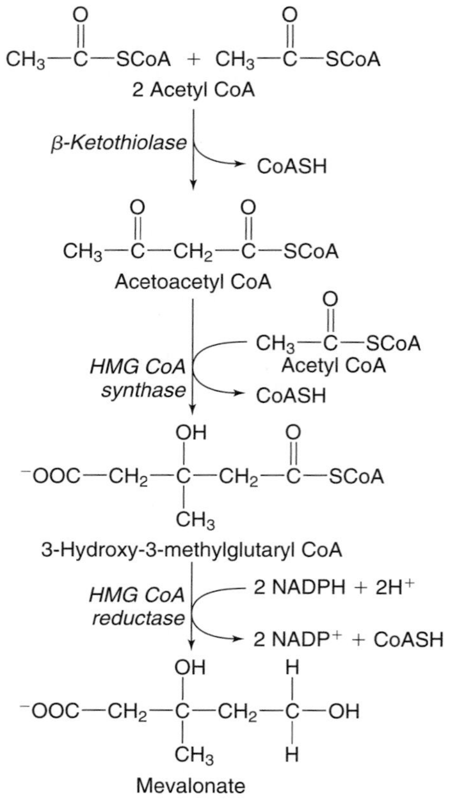

Figure 17-1 Mevalonate biosynthesis.

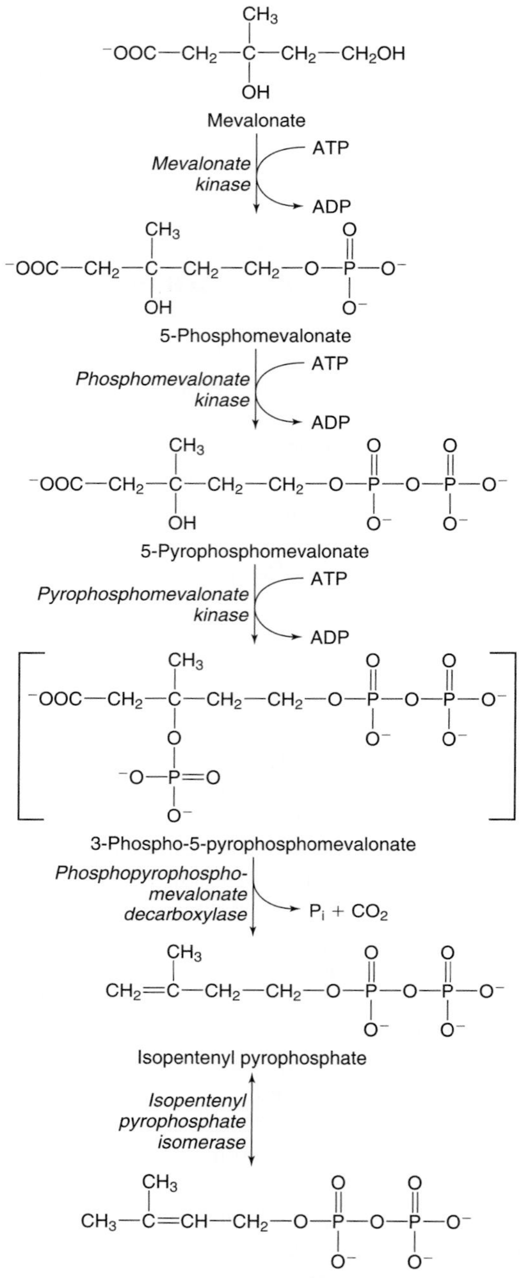

Figure 17-2 Synthesis of isoprenoid units.

SYNTHESIS OF SQUALENE FROM MEVALONATE

Mevalonate is converted to 3-phospho-5-pyrophosphomevalonate by three sequential phosphorylations (Fig. 17-2):

(1) Mevalonate + ATP $\rightarrow$
5-Phosphomevalonate + ADP

(2) 5-Phosphomevalonate + ATP $\rightarrow$
5-Pyrophosphomevalonate + ADP

Synthesis of isopentenyl pyrophosphate from 5-pyrophosphomevalonate involves transient formation of a phosphorylated intermediate, 3-phospho-5-pyrophosphomevalonate and decarboxylation of the 5-pyrophosphomevalonate to form isopentenyl pyrophosphate:

(3) 5-Pyrophosphomevalonate + ATP $\rightarrow$
Isopentenyl Pyrophosphate + CO_2 + ADP + P_i

Squalene, and thus the sterol molecule, is built from multiple isopentenyl groups. The reaction sequence involves condensation of two 5-carbon molecules to form one of 10 carbons. A third 5-carbon molecule is added to form a 15-carbon intermediate. Two 15-carbon intermediates are linked to form the 30-carbon squalene (Fig. 17-3):

$$C5 \rightarrow C10 \rightarrow C15 \rightarrow C30$$

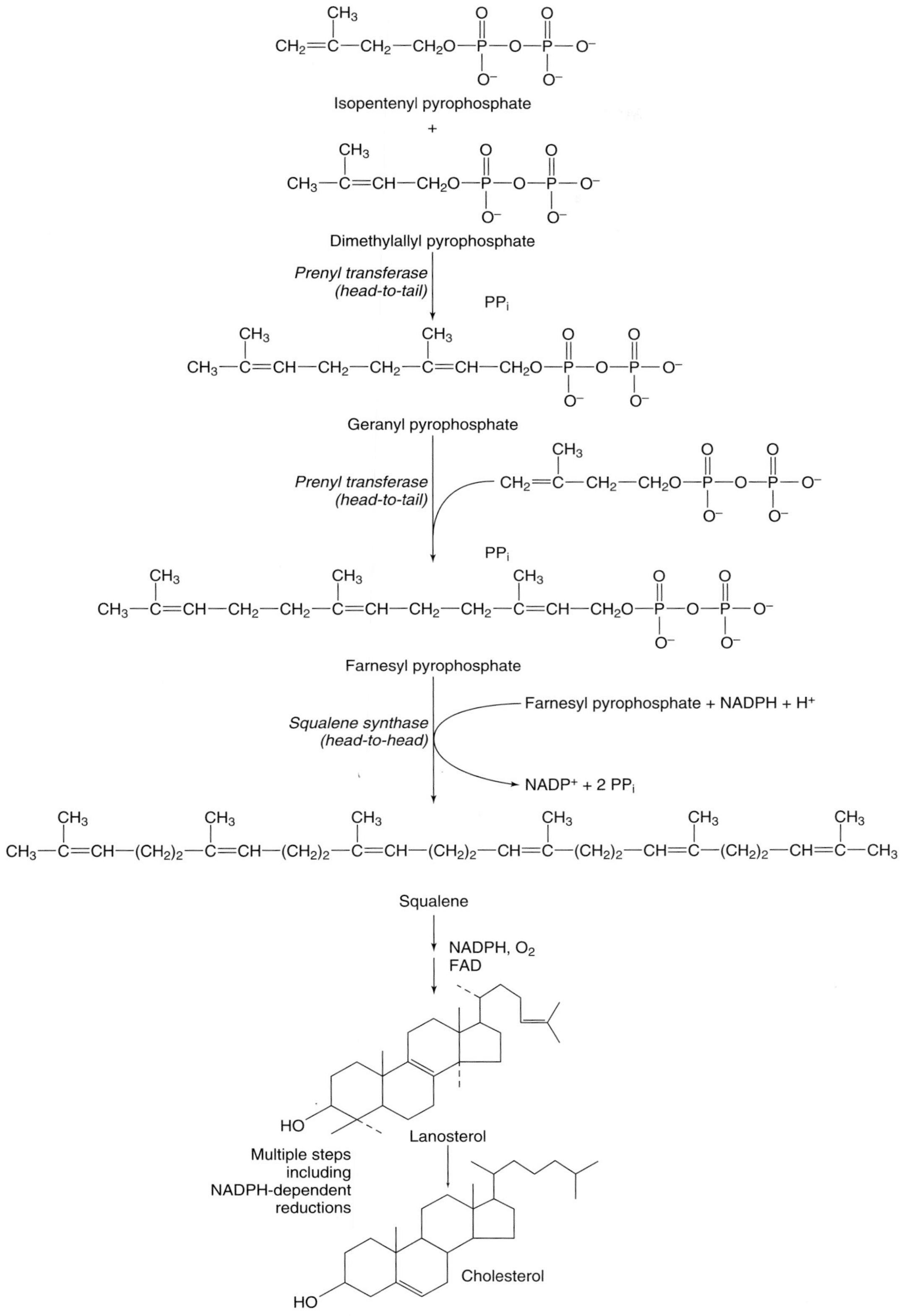

$CH_2{=}C(CH_3){-}CH_2{-}CH_2O{-}P(=O)(O^-){-}O{-}P(=O)(O^-){-}O^-$

Isopentenyl pyrophosphate

+

$CH_3{-}C(CH_3){=}CH{-}CH_2O{-}P(=O)(O^-){-}O{-}P(=O)(O^-){-}O^-$

Dimethylallyl pyrophosphate

Prenyl transferase (head-to-tail)

PP_i

$CH_3{-}C(CH_3){=}CH{-}CH_2{-}CH_2{-}C(CH_3){=}CH{-}CH_2O{-}P(=O)(O^-){-}O{-}P(=O)(O^-){-}O^-$

Geranyl pyrophosphate

Prenyl transferase (head-to-tail)

$CH_2{=}C(CH_3){-}CH_2{-}CH_2O{-}P(=O)(O^-){-}O{-}P(=O)(O^-){-}O^-$

PP_i

$CH_3{-}C(CH_3){=}CH{-}CH_2{-}CH_2{-}C(CH_3){=}CH{-}CH_2{-}CH_2{-}C(CH_3){=}CH{-}CH_2O{-}P(=O)(O^-){-}O{-}P(=O)(O^-){-}O^-$

Farnesyl pyrophosphate

Squalene synthase (head-to-head)

Farnesyl pyrophosphate + NADPH + H^+

$NADP^+$ + 2 PP_i

$CH_3{-}C(CH_3){=}CH{-}(CH_2)_2{-}C(CH_3){=}CH{-}(CH_2)_2{-}C(CH_3){=}CH{-}(CH_2)_2{-}CH{=}C(CH_3){-}(CH_2)_2{-}CH{=}C(CH_3){-}(CH_2)_2{-}CH{=}C(CH_3){-}CH_3$

Squalene

NADPH, O_2
FAD

HO

Lanosterol

Multiple steps including NADPH-dependent reductions

Cholesterol

HO

Figure 17-3 Synthesis of squalene and cholesterol.

Formation of the 10-carbon geranyl pyrophosphate involves two enzymatic reactions. First, isopentenyl pyrophosphate isomerase catalyzes the isomerization of isopentenyl pyrophosphate to dimethylallyl pyrophosphate (as shown in Fig. 17-2). Then one molecule of each of these two activated isoprenes condenses. As shown in Figure 17-3, C-1 of one isoprene bonds with C-5 of the other (head-to-tail) to form geranyl pyrophosphate:

Isopentenyl Pyrophosphate + Dimethylallyl Pyrophosphate → Geranyl Pyrophosphate + PP_i

In a mechanistically similar reaction, a third 5-carbon isopentenyl pyrophosphate condenses with geranyl pyrophosphate—in a head-to-tail manner—to form farnesyl pyrophosphate. Farnesyl pyrophosphate is a precursor of cholesterol, dolichol, ubiquinone, and the isoprenoid groups on a number of proteins and thus represents a branch-point in the synthesis of steroid and isoprenoid compounds.

Squalene synthase, the next step in cholesterol biosynthesis, is the committed step in sterol biosynthesis. This enzyme catalyzes the head-to-head condensation of two farnesyl pyrophosphates to form an intermediate, presqualene pyrophosphate. Presqualene pyrophosphate then undergoes NADPH-dependent reduction and pyrophosphate elimination to form squalene. Several further rearrangements, with lanosterol as one of the intermediates, convert the 30-carbon squalene to the 27-carbon cholesterol.

In Chapter 16, we noted that activation of fatty acids to their acyl CoA derivatives involves hydrolysis of ATP to AMP and PP_i. Ubiquitous pyrophosphatases in cells then rapidly degrade PP_i to two inorganic phosphates. This biochemical mechanism is used to drive to completion several of the intermediate reactions in cholesterol biosynthesis.

REGULATION OF CHOLESTEROL SYNTHESIS

Cholesterol synthesis is tightly regulated in cells. Along with the low density lipoprotein (LDL) receptor, the enzymes in the cholesterol biosynthetic pathway—HMG CoA synthase, HMG CoA reductase, farnesyl diphosphate synthase, and squalene synthase—are regulated coordinately at the transcriptional level. Therefore, cholesterol synthesis in the cell, as well as cholesterol uptake via the LDL receptor as described later, is under negative feedback control. The primary target for regulation in the cholesterol biosynthetic pathway is HMG CoA reductase, which catalyzes the main regulatory step in the overall cholesterol biosynthetic pathway. This enzyme is inhibited by a class of drugs called statins, which are potent competitive inhibitors with K_i values in the nanomolar range that are used therapeutically for lowering plasma cholesterol levels. HMG CoA reductase is under negative feedback control by mevalonate, its immediate product, and by the eventual main product, cholesterol. The principal mechanism of regulation involves changes in the number of enzyme molecules per cell, which results from several levels of regulation from transcription of the gene to stability of the protein.

Cholesterol itself regulates transcription of HMG CoA reductase, as well as various genes mentioned in the preceding text, by a mechanism that senses cellular cholesterol levels (Radhakrishnan et al., 2004; Gibbons, 2003; Horton et al., 2002). Transcriptional control by cholesterol requires the presence of a sterol regulatory element (SRE) in the promoter regions of those genes where the transcription factor termed SRE binding protein (SREBP) binds. There are three SREBPs: SREBP-1a and SREBP-1c, which are both encoded by the *SREBP-1* gene by alternative exon usage, and SREBP-2. Although not directly involved in cholesterol metabolism, SREBP-1c expression is increased by insulin and/or feeding and mediates the induction of enzymes in fatty acid and fat synthesis as described in Chapter 16. All SREBPs contain two transmembrane helices that anchor these proteins in the endoplasmic reticulum (ER). The N-terminal domain faces the cytosol and contains a basic-helix-loop-helix-leucine-zipper transcription factor motif. When the cholesterol level in the cell is low, SREBP cleavage–activating protein (SCAP), which has a cholesterol sensing domain, functions as an escort protein to transport SREBP to the Golgi apparatus, where two proteases cleave SREBP to release the N-terminal domain. The N-terminal domain can then enter the nucleus, where it binds to SREs to activate transcription of the

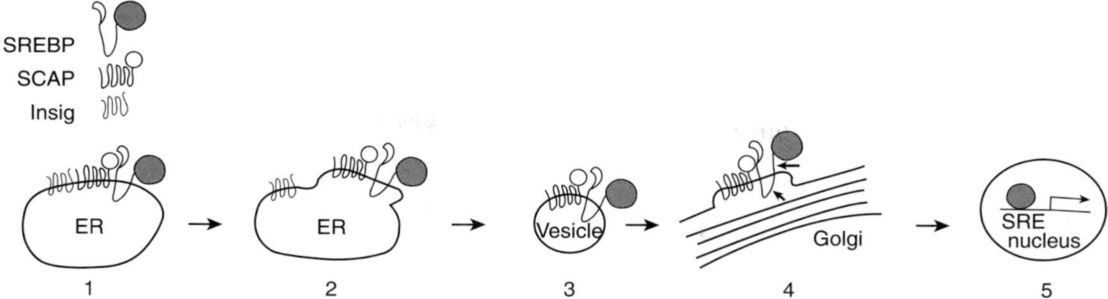

Figure 17-4 Cholesterol-dependent SREBP processing. When cellular cholesterol is high, the sterol regulatory element binding protein (SREBP)/SREBP cleavage-activating protein (SCAP) complex is associated with Insig in the endoplasmic reticulum (ER) *(1)*. A low cellular cholesterol level in the ER membrane causes release of Insig *(2)*, which allows SCAP to escort SREBP to COP II-coated buds *(3)*. COP II vesicles form and deliver SCAP/SREBP to the Golgi apparatus *(4)*, where SREBP is cleaved at two sites (marked with *arrows*). Mature SREBP can then move to nucleus where it can bind to sterol regulatory elements (SREs) in the promoters of various genes and, thus, function as a transcriptional activator *(5)*.

genes for HMG CoA reductase, LDL receptor, and other enzymes of cholesterol and fatty acid metabolism. When cholesterol builds up in the ER membrane, SCAP undergoes a conformational change that allows it to bind to another ER resident protein called Insig. Insig serves as an anchor, preventing the SCAP/SREBP complex from moving to the Golgi and thereby decreasing cholesterol synthesis and uptake (Fig. 17-4) (Rawson, 2003).

The level of HMG CoA reductase protein also is regulated at the step of degradation of the enzyme. HMG CoA reductase, an ER membrane protein, also contains a cholesterol sensing domain similar to that in SCAP. When the cellular cholesterol level is high, HMG CoA reductase protein is ubiquitinated and consequently recognized by the proteasome for degradation.

In addition to regulation of enzyme protein levels, the activity of HMG CoA reductase is regulated by a phosphorylation–dephosphorylation mechanism. HMG CoA reductase is less active in the phosphorylated state. The enzyme is phosphorylated by AMP-activated protein kinase (AMPK), a kinase that is activated by cellular AMP as well as by phosphorylation by another upstream kinase. This phosphorylation–dephosphorylation mechanism explains why HMG CoA reductase activity can respond rapidly to nutritional or hormonal perturbations, even when there has been little change in the concentration of HMG CoA reductase protein.

BILE ACID SYNTHESIS FROM CHOLESTEROL

As mentioned in Chapter 7, conversion of cholesterol to bile acids occurs exclusively in the liver. Bile acids, as well as free cholesterol, are incorporated into bile, which is destined for secretion into the proximal small intestine. The ultimate excretion of bile acids and free cholesterol in bile is the major route for removing excess cholesterol from the body. Synthesis of bile acids involves a cascade of reactions catalyzed by enzymes located in the ER, mitochondria, cytosol, and peroxisomes. The steroid nucleus is modified in the ER and mitochondria, and the cholesterol side chain is removed in peroxisomes. The major steps for the two pathways for bile acid synthesis are shown in Figure 17-5 (Russell, 2003). In the major or "classic" pathway, the steroid nucleus modification includes 7α-hydroxylation catalyzed by cholesterol 7α-hydroxyase (CYP7A1), epimerization of the 3β-hydroxyl group (to 3α-), and saturation of the steroid nucleus. There is also a 12α-hydroxylation in the case of cholic acid synthesis, but not in chenodeoxycholic acid synthesis. These reactions precede the removal of the terminal three carbons of the cholesterol side chain by oxidative cleavage. In an alternative pathway, hydroxylation of the side chain, catalyzed by cholesterol 27-hydroxyase (CYP27A1), precedes the modification

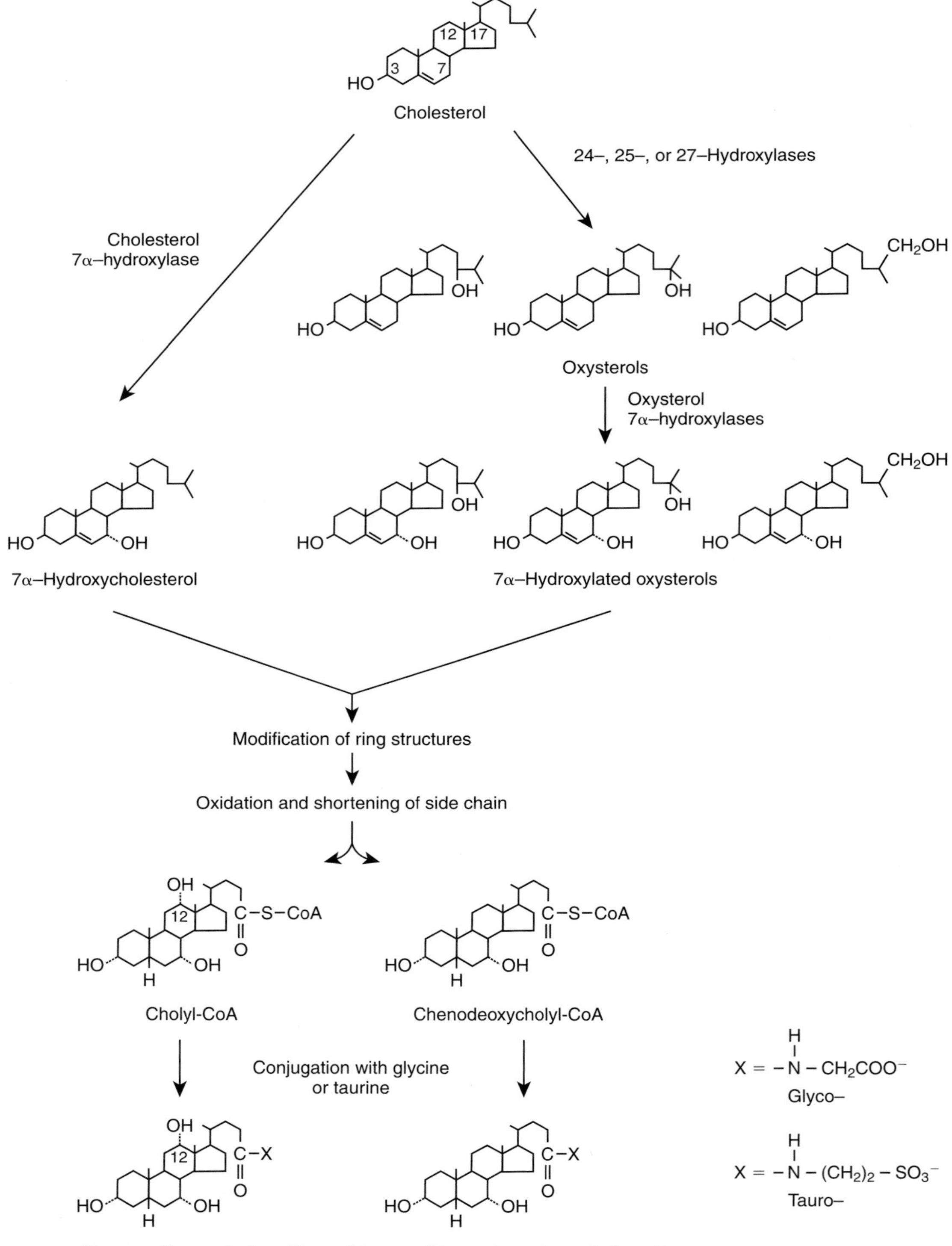

Figure 17-5 Synthesis of bile acids from cholesterol.

of the steroid nucleus. Cholic acid and chenodeoxycholic acid are the two primary bile acids in human bile. Further modification of the primary bile acids by gut bacteria form secondary bile acids, which may be reabsorbed and are thus found in the liver and bile along with the primary bile acids.

The rate of bile acid synthesis parallels the activity of CYP7A, the rate-limiting step in the bile acid synthetic pathway. This step is under feedback regulation. Bile acids excreted from the liver are reabsorbed in the distal small intestine and transported back to the liver by the enterohepatic recirculation as mentioned in Chapter 7. Therefore, bile acid reabsorption is the means to control the overall rate of bile acid synthesis in the liver. Identification of farnesoid X receptor (FXR), which belongs to the nuclear receptor family, as a bile acid receptor provides a mechanism for the feedback regulation. The genes coding for several enzymes in the two bile acid synthetic pathways, including *CYP7A1* and *CYP27A1*, contain a bile acid response element where FXR can bind to prevent a transactivating factor from binding to the site.

Oxysterols, potent regulators of cholesterol synthesis and lipid metabolism, can be formed from cholesterol by enzymatic as well as nonenzymatic reactions (Bjorkhem, 2002; Schroepfer, 2000). An intermediate in bile acid biosynthesis, 27-hydroxycholesterol, is the most abundant oxysterol in human plasma. Oxysterols are ligands for liver X receptor (LXR), another member of the nuclear receptor family (Chiang, 2002; Edwards et al., 2002; Repa and Mangelsdorf, 2002). The LXR response element is present in the promoter region of the *CYP7A1* gene, and LXR binding activates *CYP7A1* gene transcription. Therefore, regulation of *CYP7A1* transcription and bile acid synthesis depends on the balance between the positive LXR control and negative FXR control. LXR also activates a variety of other genes involved in cholesterol and fat metabolism. LXR activates transcription of genes encoding ATP-binding cassette transporters and other proteins involved in reverse cholesterol transport, mentioned later in this chapter. In addition, activation of the *SREBP-1c* gene by LXR stimulates transcription of enzymes in fatty acid and fat synthesis.

INTRACELLULAR TRAFFICKING OF CHOLESTEROL

Cellular cholesterol trafficking comprises numerous individual steps, since cholesterol is synthesized endogenously and obtained exogenously, and acts at many sites, including incorporation into membranes and conversion to a number of different products in the ER and mitochondria. Because cholesterol is a hydrophobic molecule, almost all of it is found in membranes or lipid droplets, and little is found in the soluble fraction. Most of the cellular free cholesterol (60% to 80%) is found in the plasma membrane. Because cholesterol originates either in the ER where it is synthesized, or in the endosomal–lysosomal system where it is brought in via LDL-receptor–mediated endocytosis, the high levels of cholesterol in the plasma membrane indicate the movement of cholesterol within the cell to maintain this distribution.

There are two main mechanisms for intracellular cholesterol trafficking (Soccio and Breslow, 2004). One mechanism is through vesicular transport, in which cholesterol incorporated into membranes moves as part of the membrane vesicle. The second way in which cholesterol can move from one subcellular location to another is by the monomolecular diffusion of protein-bound or, perhaps, unbound cholesterol, within the aqueous cytosol.

Distinct trafficking pathways exist for cholesterol synthesized de novo and for cholesterol obtained via receptor-mediated endocytosis of LDLs. Newly synthesized cholesterol moves from the ER primarily to the plasma membrane. A small fraction of this occurs by vesicular trafficking through the Golgi apparatus. The remainder of cholesterol movement from the ER to the plasma membrane likely occurs by nonvesicular, protein-mediated pathways, but the proteins involved are not known. Excess ER cholesterol can be esterified to form cholesteryl esters, which are stored in lipid droplets that are often found in proximity to the ER. The cholesteryl ester in these droplets can be hydrolyzed to liberate free cholesterol, which is then thought to be trafficked to the ER by protein-mediated diffusional transfer.

The enrichment of cholesterol in the plasma membrane is important for the structural properties of this important barrier. Excess cholesterol can be trafficked to the ER for esterification and storage in lipid droplets. As with transport from the ER to the plasma membrane, transport of cholesterol from the plasma membrane to the ER also involves both vesicular and diffusional processes, although they do not appear to be the same steps in reverse.

As is detailed in subsequent text of this chapter, cholesteryl ester–rich LDLs are taken up by receptor-mediated endocytosis, thereby delivering exogenous cholesterol into the endosomal–lysosomal system. Acid lipases liberate free cholesterol, some of which recycles back to the plasma membrane in the so-called endocytic recycling compartment, which also delivers the LDL-receptor back to the plasma membrane. The rest of the cholesterol remains in vesicles, which are processed into the late endosome–lysosome compartment.

In order for exogenously derived LDL cholesterol to activate cholesterol-mediated homeostatic responses, the cholesterol must exit the endosome–lysosome compartment. Specific proteins in this compartment are thought to be involved in this egress of cholesterol. Evidence for a role of NPC1 and NPC2 in cholesterol trafficking or transport comes from abnormalities observed in patients with the inherited lysosomal storage disease Niemann-Pick type C (NPC). NPC disease is caused by defects in either NPC1 or NPC2, suggesting that these two proteins function in a coordinated manner. In patients with NPC disease, unesterified cholesterol, as well as glycolipids, is trapped in the endosomal–lysosomal compartment, resulting in an ultimately fatal progression of neurological deterioration and premature death. NPC1 has multiple membrane-spanning domains and localizes in late endosomes. NPCI contains a sterol-sensing domain similar to that found in several proteins involved in cholesterol homeostasis, including the LDL receptor and HMG CoA reductase as described later in the chapter. NPC2 is a soluble intralysosomal protein that binds cholesterol. Cholesterol from the endosomal–lysosomal compartment trafficks primarily to the plasma membrane, with some of this cholesterol going through the Golgi apparatus before reaching the plasma membrane. Only a small portion of exogenously derived cholesterol moves from the endosome–lysosome compartment directly to the ER.

Although mitochondria have very low cholesterol levels, they nevertheless perform several important steps in sterol metabolism, including cholesterol conversion to steroid hormones in steroidogenic cells and the production of the oxysterol 27-hydrocholesterol. Both of these reactions occur on the inner leaflet of the inner mitochondrial membrane. Mitochondrial cholesterol may be trafficked from the plasma membrane, from the endosomal–lysosomal compartment, or perhaps from lipid droplets. The movement of cholesterol into the mitochondria is accomplished by steroidogenic acute regulatory protein (StAR) or StAR-related lipid transport proteins (START proteins) that are present at the outer mitochondrial membrane. The movement across the inner mitochondrial membrane is thought to involve a peripheral-type benzodiazepine receptor (PBR), which is also located at the outer mitochondrial membrane but concentrated at contact sites with the inner mitochondrial membrane.

MAJOR GROUPS OF PLASMA LIPOPROTEINS

For transport in aqueous blood plasma, the small intestine and liver package the nonpolar lipids (triacylglycerol and cholesteryl esters) in the core of large lipoprotein particles with amphipathic cholesterol and phospholipids, along with certain apolipoproteins, on the surface, as mentioned in Chapters 10 and 16. The particles from the intestine are nascent chylomicrons and those from the liver are nascent very low density lipoproteins (VLDLs). These lipoprotein particles consist of a neutral lipid core of many molecules of triacylglycerol, and cholesteryl ester surrounded by a surface monolayer of phospholipids and cholesterol and a smaller number of various apolipoproteins. Chylomicrons secreted by the intestine after a fat-containing meal can have average molecular weights greater than 100 times those of the VLDLs secreted by the liver. Once the nascent lipoproteins enter the plasma, they pick up additional apolipoproteins (such as apo C and apo E apoproteins) from circulating HDLs to become mature chylomicrons and VLDLs. Largely due to the loss of triacylglycerol from the core of the lipoprotein complexes, chylomicrons and VLDLs become smaller and denser in the plasma (they become chylomicron remnants; intermediate density lipoproteins [IDLs], also known as VLDL remnants; and LDLs). Nascent high density lipoproteins (HDLs) are involved in chylomicron and VLDL metabolism as well as in cholesterol transport back to liver. In contrast to chylomicrons and VLDLs, which are secreted as lipid-rich particles, HDLs are thought of as being generated in the plasma. In the plasma, HDLs are generated by the association of apo A-I, which is secreted by the liver and to a lesser extent intestine, with cell-derived phospholipids to form lipid-poor HDLs that can accumulate cell-derived cholesterol as they circulate.

The plasma lipoproteins can be separated by ultracentrifugation or electrophoresis. Their names are based on their density or electrophoretic migration. Density is inversely proportional to the lipid content (%) of the lipoproteins, with HDLs being denser than VLDLs, for example. In agarose gel electrophoresis, lipoprotein complexes are mainly separated on the basis of their charge-to-mass ratio, with α-lipoproteins (HDLs) migrating farther than β-(LDL) or pre-β-(VLDL) particles. The lipoproteins found in normal plasma are listed in Table 17-1. The most abundant of the circulating lipoproteins in fasting plasma are HDLs and LDLs.

Plasma lipoproteins may also be grouped into two classes of particles according to the presence of an essential apolipoprotein: the apolipoprotein A-I (apo A-I)–containing lipoproteins and the apolipoprotein B (apo B)–containing lipoproteins. Apo A-I is found only in HDLs. HDLs are small particles with a "core" of cholesteryl esters and a small amount of triacylglycerol and a surface composed of free cholesterol, phospholipids (particularly phosphatidylcholine, commonly called lecithin), and apoproteins. The amino acid sequence of apo A-I contains a series of amphipathic helical repeats of 22 amino acids in length. Lipid-binding, hydrophobic amino acids are preferentially localized to one face of the helix and turned toward the lipid core, whereas charged and other hydrophilic residues are turned out to face the aqueous medium. Apo A-I is flexible, and is weakly associated with the surface of HDLs. As a result, the shape of apo A-I on the surface of HDLs can adapt as the lipid core of the particle expands. If the diameter of the HDL particles is reduced by loss of core lipids (cholesteryl ester and triacylglycerol), lipid-poor apo A-I easily dissociates from the surface of HDLs. Many HDL particles contain smaller amounts of other apolipoproteins in addition to apo A-I (i.e., apo A-II, apo A-IV, apo C-I, apo C-III, and apo E). The functions of several of these proteins are clearly established, and their mechanisms of lipid binding are similar to that described for apo A-I. In addition to being an essential structural component of HDL, apo A-I promotes desorption of free cholesterol from cell membranes and activates cholesterol esterification by the lecithin:cholesterol acyltransferase (LCAT).

The apo B–containing lipoproteins are chylomicrons, VLDLs, and their circulating lipoprotein lipolysis products (so-called remnants).

Table 17-1
Classification of Plasma Lipoproteins

Major Lipoproteins		Other Major Apolipoproteins	Density (g/mL)
Apo B-48 lipoproteins:	Chylomicrons	Apo C-II, apo C-III, apo E	<1.00
Apo B-100 lipoproteins:	VLDLs	Apo C-II, apo C-III, apo E	<1.006
	IDLs	Apo E	1.006-1.019
	LDLs	None	1.019-1.063
Apo A-I lipoproteins:	Pre-β-HDLs	None	>1.21
	α-HDLs	Apo A-II	1.063-1.21

HDLs, High-density lipoproteins; *IDL,* intermediate-density lipoprotein; *LDL,* low-density lipoprotein; *VLDL,* very-low-density lipoprotein.

Each VLDL particle contains a single molecule of apo B-100, a large protein comprising 4,536 amino acid residues. As mentioned in Chapter 10, chylomicrons contain one molecule of a shorter form of apo B (2,152 amino acids in length, 48% of apoB-100), apo B-48. Apo B-48 is encoded by the same gene as apo B-100, but is made only in intestine where an intestine-specific cytosine deaminase converts a cytosine to a uracil creating a premature stop codon in the apo B mRNA. IDLs and LDLs are formed in the circulation as lipolysis products of VLDL, and, therefore, these particles also contain one copy of apo B-100. Apo B-100 is synthesized only in liver and makes a single turn around the circumference of an LDL particle. Other apolipoproteins adsorbed to the VLDL surface include the lipoprotein lipase cofactor apo C-II and the receptor ligand apo E. These increase the stability of the large particles, regulate the catabolism of VLDL lipids, and control the removal of partially lipolyzed VLDL particles (IDLs) from the circulation by receptor-mediated uptake into cells.

The large apo B-48 and B-100 polypeptides, like apo A-I, contain stretches of amphipathic helix, but these helical regions form a smaller proportion of the whole sequence in apo B than in apo A-I. Apo B-100 contains at least 11 cystine bridges, most of them in the N-terminal region. Apo B does not dissociate during the metabolism of VLDL to IDL and LDL. Apo B plays an essential role in VLDL and chylomicron secretion, in the binding of triacylglycerol-rich lipoproteins to the capillary endothelium prior to lipolysis, and in the removal of apo B-100–containing lipoprotein particles from the circulation. The amino acid sequence that binds to the high-affinity apo B (LDL) receptor of liver cells is in the C-terminal half of apo B-100 and is absent from apo B-48. Whereas the removal of VLDL remnants by the LDL receptor in the liver is mediated by apo B, the removal of chylomicron remnants is mediated mainly by apo E. A small proportion of chylomicron remnants may be internalized via an LDL receptor-like protein (LRP)-mediated endocytosis (Twinckler et al., 2004; Yu et al., 2001).

Plasma normally contains a relatively large amount of apo B-100 and only a very small amount of apo B-48 because chylomicrons are very rapidly cleared from the circulation by lipase catabolism and hepatic receptors. Most of the circulating apo B-100 is in LDLs, with only small amounts in IDLs and VLDLs, because VLDL particles are relatively rapidly catabolized by lipases. Some VLDL particles are removed as IDLs (i.e., VLDL remnants), but most are converted to LDL particles, which have a much longer circulation time (~2 days) than the lighter apo B–containing lipoproteins.

The contributions of the major lipoprotein fractions to the triacylglycerol and total cholesterol content of normal plasma are shown in Table 17-2.

Table 17-2
Distribution of Triacylglycerol and Cholesterol Among Fasting Plasma Lipoproteins

	Cholesterol	Triacylglycerol
	mg/100 mL Plasma	
Total	176.4±20 (100%)	84.9±19.1 (100%)
VLDL	9.1±3.7 (5.1%)	46.5±12.8 (54.8%)
IDL	3.5±4.3 (1.9%)	5.8±6.2 (6.6%)
LDL	114.8±28 (65.1%)	15.9±8.8 (18.7%)
HDL	45.3±11.8 (25.7%)	12.2±1.6 (14.3%)

Recalculated from Fielding, PE, Fielding CJ (1996) Dynamics of lipoprotein transport in the circulatory system. In: Vance DE, Vance J (eds) Biochemistry of Lipids. Amsterdam, Elsevier Science-NL, pp 495-516.
HDL, High-density lipoprotein; *IDL,* intermediate-density lipoprotein; *LDL,* low-density lipoprotein; *VLDL,* very-low-density lipoprotein.

SYNTHESIS AND SECRETION OF TRIACYLGLYCEROL-RICH LIPOPROTEINS: CHYLOMICRONS AND VLDLs

As mentioned in Chapter 10, intestinal cells make apo B-48, the structural protein of chylomicrons. Initially, the intracellular precursor chylomicron particle is a lipid-poor phospholipid monolayer encapsulating most of the cholesteryl ester found in mature chylomicrons and a much smaller proportion of their triacylglycerol. The first addition of triacylglycerol to chylomicron precursor particles requires the microsomal triacylglycerol transfer protein (MTP). A second step of triacylglycerol addition, which leads to the formation of mature, triacylglycerol-rich chylomicrons, is considered to be independent of MTP, but a second, as yet unidentified, transfer protein may be involved. The importance of MTP is evident from the human disorder called abetalipoproteinemia. In this hereditary disease, mutations in the gene encoding MTP result in an inability of patients with this disease to produce chylomicrons and VLDLs in the intestine and liver, respectively.

Nascent chylomicrons, thus assembled within the ER and Golgi apparatus, are released from the enterocyte within mature Golgi vesicles that fuse with the basolateral region of the plasma membrane. These newly secreted particles are too large to penetrate the capillary membrane. Therefore, they are secreted into the lymphatic system via the lacteals of the intestinal villi and subsequently enter the venous plasma compartment via the left thoracic lymph duct. Chylomicron secretion into the lymphatics rather than directly into the portal vein is thought to be important for delivery of dietary lipid to peripheral tissue without prior hepatic catabolism as well as for the removal of associated toxins by lymphatic leukocytes.

The assembly of VLDL within the hepatocyte follows a similar two-step assembly process, with the initial formation of precursor particles of a phospholipid shell with apo B-100 and a hydrophobic core of cholesteryl ester, and some triacylglycerol that is added via MTP. The second step of VLDL assembly involves the addition of triacylglycerol to precursor particles in the ER, probably by molecular transfer. Whereas triacylglycerol in chylomicrons originates mainly from the dietary fat, some of the fatty acids in the VLDL triacylglycerol are synthesized de novo from dietary carbohydrate. VLDL triacylglycerol secretion and circulating concentrations both increase after a carbohydrate-rich meal. Other fatty acids in the triacylglycerol of VLDLs originate from long-chain free fatty acids that are internalized by the liver from plasma lipoprotein remnants or unesterified circulating fatty acids. Regardless of the origin of the fatty acids in the triacylglycerol, triacylglycerol in VLDL is thought to be produced by esterification and not from existing triacylglycerol.

CLEARANCE OF TRIACYLGLYCEROL IN CHYLOMICRONS AND VLDLs BY LIPOPROTEIN LIPASE

Due to their hydrophobicity, most of the triacylglycerol and cholesteryl ester is concentrated in the core of plasma lipoprotein particles, but this core is in rapid equilibrium with small amounts of the same lipids dissolved within the surface monolayer, which is made up mainly of phospholipids and free cholesterol. The hydrolysis or transfer of triacylglycerol of apo B–containing lipoproteins by plasma lipases or transfer proteins, respectively, depletes only the surface pool of lipids. The surface lipids are replenished by equilibration from the core of the particle. Lipoprotein lipase (LPL) is a triacylglycerol hydrolase present on the capillary endothelium of various tissues, with highest concentrations present in muscle and adipose tissues (Merkel et al., 2002). LPL is synthesized by the parenchymal cells of these tissues and is then secreted. The secreted LPL migrates to the vascular face of the endothelial cells within the tissue, where it is anchored by glycosaminoglycans, with its active site facing the circulation. Only LPLs found in the endothelial fraction of adipose or muscle tissue can hydrolyze triacylglycerol present in lipoprotein particles.

Chylomicrons and VLDLs are the substrates for LPLs that are bound to the endothelial surface of adipose and muscle tissues. Much of the free fatty acid produced by lipolysis is taken up locally, although some escapes into the general circulation. During fasting, the VLDL (hepatic) triacylglycerol concentration in plasma is relatively low and chylomicron (intestinal) triacylglycerol is almost absent. Also during fasting, the expression of LPL in adipose tissue is downregulated due to the lack of insulin, whereas LPL levels in heart and other muscle tissues are maintained. LPL on the capillary endothelial surface of the heart has a higher affinity (lower K_m) for lipoprotein substrate than does LPL in the adipose tissue. This difference in affinity of LPL for lipoprotein substrate may provide a mechanism for regulating the partitioning of lipoprotein triacylglycerol–derived fatty acids between storage in adipose tissue and oxidation in muscle tissues.

According to this model, triacylglycerol hydrolysis by the vascular bed of the heart would be determined mainly by the endothelial LPL levels, because heart LPL has a low K_m, and, as a result, is saturated at low circulating VLDL concentrations. In contrast, in adipose tissue, where the apparent K_m exceeds normal circulating triacylglycerol concentrations, triacylglycerol hydrolysis would be influenced by VLDL and chylomicron concentrations. In this way, the energy needs of muscle cells (such as those of the heart) that use fatty acids from lipoprotein triacylglcerol hydrolysis as a fuel would receive priority, particularly during fasting. Adipose tissue, on the other hand, would reesterify and store most of the fatty acids released from hydrolysis of excess lipoprotein triacylglycerol by adipose endothelial LPL after a fatty meal, due both to the higher K_m of adipose tissue LPL and the increased level of adipose LPL in adipose tissue in the fed state. The stored triacylglcerol in adipose tissue can be hydrolyzed to generate fatty acids during extended periods of exercise or fasting, by activation of adipose tissue hormone-sensitive lipase (HSL), as described in Chapter 16.

The hydrolysis of triacylglycerol by LPL depends on the presence of its activator (apo C-II) on the surface of chylomicron and VLDL particles. Apo C-II preferentially transfers from other lipoproteins (e.g., HDLs) to the newly secreted nascent VLDLs and chylomicrons as these particles are released into the plasma.

As the triacylglycerol of a chylomicron is hydrolyzed by LPL, the chylomicron decreases in size within an hour after a meal, and apo C-II dissociates from its surface. After approximately 80% of the initial triacylglycerol has been lost, insufficient apo C-II remains to support LPL activity. The chylomicron remnants contain residual triacylglycerol together with most of the cholesteryl ester in the initial chylomicron.

VLDLs, IDLs, and LDLs make up a lipolysis cascade, as illustrated in Figure 17-6. All LDLs in the plasma are formed from the catabolism of VLDLs and IDLs, but not all VLDLs become LDLs. As VLDL triacylglcyerol is catabolized, apo C-II dissociates, as it does from chylomicrons, leaving VLDL remnants (usually called

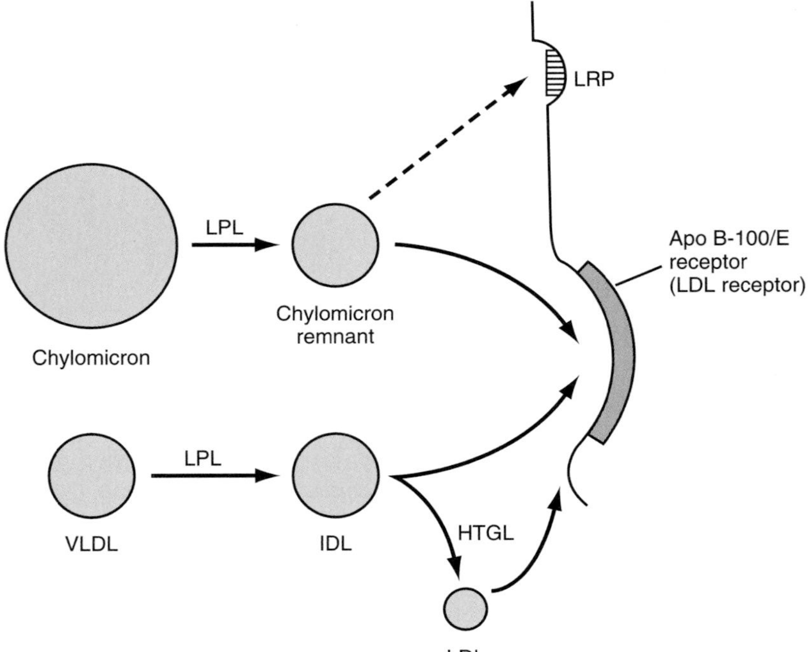

Figure 17-6 Catabolism of apolipoprotein B–containing lipoproteins in human plasma. *HTGL*, Hepatic triacylglycerol lipase; *LDL*, low density lipoprotein; *LPL*, lipoprotein lipase; *LRP*, low density lipoprotein related protein.

IDLs) that still contain both apo B-100 and apo E. Some of the IDL particles become LDLs by losing additional triacylglcyerol at the hepatocyte surface. Another lipase, hepatic triacylglycerol lipase (HTGL) at the endothelial surface of the liver, hydrolyzes IDL triacylglcerol. HTGL is structurally related to the LPL found in muscle and adipose tissue. Apo E also is transferred from IDL to HDL during the transition of IDL to LDL. HTGL also plays an important role in hydrolyzing HDL triacylglycerol and probably HDL phospholipids.

CHOLESTEROL UPTAKE BY LDL RECEPTOR–MEDIATED ENDOCYTOSIS

Cholesterol-rich LDLs as well as VLDL remnants (IDLs) and chylomicron remnants, which have lost triacylglycerols but are rich in cholesteryl esters, are all taken up into cells via the high-affinity LDL receptor (also called the apo B-100/apo E receptor), which recognizes both apo B-100 and apo E (Fig. 17-7). The LDL receptor spans the plasma membrane. An extracellular domain contains the apo B-100/apo E binding site. The intracellular domain directs clustering of LDL receptors into regions of the plasma membrane called clathrin-coated pits. Once LDL binds to the LDL receptor, the complex is rapidly internalized by the process of endocytosis. The receptor/LDL complex undergoes invagination within the coated pit, which is internalized, uncoated (i.e., clathrin coat is removed from the internalized endosome), and then acidified due to the action of an ATP-dependent proton pump. In this acidified endosome, LDL and the LDL receptor dissociate. The endosomal membranes harboring the receptor are then recycled to the plasma membrane, while the LDL-containing endosomes fuse with lysosomes. Acid hydrolases in the lysosomes degrade the apoprotein to free amino acids, and cholesteryl esters to fatty acids and cholesterol.

The greatest number of functional LDL receptors is expressed in the liver. Lesser amounts are present in adrenal and gonadal cells. Familial hypercholesterolemia (FH) is caused by a mutation in the LDL receptor gene and is a prevalent disorder of lipoprotein metabolism. Because the circulating concentration of apo B lipoproteins exceeds that required for saturation of the high-affinity LDL receptors, the rate of internalization of LDL by the liver is determined by the number of LDL receptors rather than by the concentration of LDL. Although receptor-mediated endocytosis is the predominant mechanism for uptake of lipopoteins, there are other minor processes of nonspecific (receptor-independent) uptake of intact LDL particles by the liver, especially when circulating LDL levels are high.

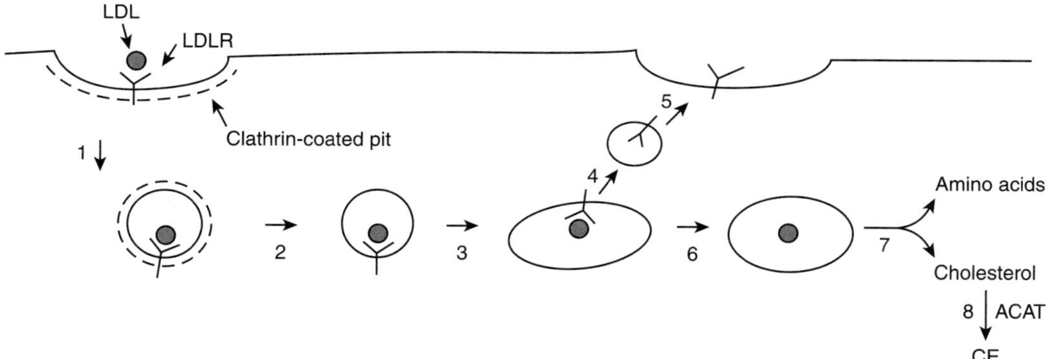

Figure 17-7 Receptor-mediated endocytosis of lipoproteins. When a low density lipoprotein (LDL) particle binds to an LDL receptor at a clathrin-coated pit, a coated vesicle is invaginated and internalized *(1)*. The vesicle is uncoated *(2)* and fuses with an endosome *(3)*. In the early endosome, LDL/LDL receptor (LDLR) dissociates *(4)* and budding of a transport vesicle makes the LDL receptor recycle back to the membrane *(5)*. The LDL-containing endosome fuses with a lysosome *(6)*, and hydrolytic enzymes in the lysosome produce amino acids as well as free cholesterol *(7)*. Cholesterol can be esterified to cholesteryl ester (CE) by acyl CoA cholesterol acyltransferase (ACAT) in the endoplasmic reticulum ER *(8)*.

Clinical Correlation

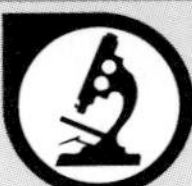

Familial Hypercholesterolemia

Familial hypercholesterolemia (FH) is characterized by a genetic defect in low density lipoprotein (LDL) receptors. A variety of mutations in the LDL receptor gene have been identified that affect synthesis, processing, binding, or clustering of the receptor on the cell surface. The homozygous phenotype may result from a compound heterozygote with two different genetic defects that affect the same gene. Homozygotes for FH have high levels of LDL in their plasma, resulting in plasma cholesterol levels that are typically six or more times normal levels.

Patients with FH often deposit cholesterol in their skin and tendons, forming nodules known as xanthomas. When cultured in lipoprotein-containing media, fibroblasts taken from either normal subjects or FH homozygotes do not express LDL receptors at their cell surfaces. However, when these cells are equilibrated in vitro in lipoprotein-deficient plasma to reduce their cellular free cholesterol content, normal cells express LDL receptors but cells from FH homozygotes do not. Cells from heterozygotes remove LDL at about half the normal rate. These results with fibroblasts are considered to model in vivo hepatic clearance of LDL.

Coronary artery disease typically occurs during childhood in homozygotes, and it occurs early in adulthood, with a prevalence of approximately 25 times that of the general population in heterozygotes. The occurrence of heterozygotes for FH in the population is about 1 in 500 individuals. The prevalence of homozygotes is rare and is estimated at 1 in 1 million people.

Thinking Critically

What effects [direction of change (increase/decrease) and degree of change (little/moderate/major)] would you anticipate a genetic defect in the LDL receptor to have on the following features of plasma lipid concentration and metabolism in vivo? Why?

- Plasma cholesterol in very low density lipoprotein (VLDL) and high density lipoprotein (HDL)
- Extrahepatic cholesterol synthesis
- Nonspecific uptake of LDL by the liver
- Lecithin:cholesterol acyltransferase (LCAT) activity

In the cell, free cholesterol is esterified by acyl-CoA cholesterol acyltransferase (ACAT) and stored as cholesteryl ester:

$$\text{Cholesterol} + \text{Fatty Acyl CoA} \xrightarrow{\text{ACAT}} \text{Cholesteryl Ester}$$

This esterification is catalyzed by ACAT present in the ER. Esterification of cholesterol is a means to remove excess free cholesterol (Chang et al., 2001). The cholesteryl esters are deposited in cytosolic lipid droplets. ACAT plays an important role in establishing the cellular free cholesterol pool that provides substrates for synthesis of bile acids or steroid hormones in liver and adrenal cortex, respectively. ACAT is also critical for supplying cholesteryl esters as a core lipid for chylomicron and VLDL synthesis in intestine and liver, respectively, as well as in the formation of cholesteryl-ester–laden foam cells from macrophages, as will be described later in this chapter. The stored cholesteryl esters are hydrolyzed to generate free cholesterol when it is needed. Although there may be additional cholesteryl ester hydrolases, HSL is known to function as a cholesteryl ester hydrolase in addition to its major action as a triacylglycerol–diacylglycerol hydrolase. In this regard, HSL and perilipin, a lipid droplet surface protein that regulates HSL translocation and activation, are found on the surface of cholesteryl ester droplets in steroidogenic cells, such as adrenal cortical cells (Tansey et al., 2004).

REVERSE CHOLESTEROL TRANSPORT AND HDLs

The apo B–containing lipoproteins, particularly LDLs, are thought to deliver several hundred milligrams of cholesterol to peripheral tissues daily. Consequently, there must be some mechanism to balance that delivery system to maintain homeostasis. HDL plays an important role in cholesterol homeostasis by transporting cholesterol from peripheral tissues back to liver for conversion to bile acids and excretion into the bile, a process called reverse cholesterol transport (Barter, 2002; Fielding and Fielding, 1995).

Approximately 95% of HDL in plasma consists of spherical particles with a hydrophobic lipid core; these are called α-HDL because they migrate fast (so-called α-migration) in agarose gel electrophoresis. The hallmark of all HDL is the presence of apo A-I. In addition to a few molecules of apo A-I, these particles also contain apo A-II, a small protein implicated in HDL turnover. A small proportion of spherical HDL also contains other lipoproteins (including apo C-II and apo E) that can be transferred to apo B–containing lipoproteins and the main functions of which are involved in the metabolism of plasma VLDL and chylomicron triacylglycerol. The remaining HDLs are very small particles (6 to 7 nm in diameter), unlike α-HDL, composed of apo A-I and phospholipids, without a significant lipid core. These HDLs migrate slowly (so-called pre-β migration) in gel electrophoresis and are called pre-β–HDL or lipid-poor HDL.

The majority of pre-β–HDLs are formed from spherical α-HDL by several reactions, all of which reduce the surface-to-volume ratio of the particle. Reduction of HDL core volume leads to dissociation of some of the apo A-I, probably as a complex with a small amount of phospholipid. The hydrolysis of HDL triacylglycerol by hepatic triacylglycerol lipase, the activity of plasma phospholipid transfer protein (PLTP), and a hepatic cell-surface receptor SR-BI (scavenger receptor class B type I) that selectively internalizes cholesteryl esters from HDL all probably contribute to pre-β–HDL formation (Connelly and Williams, 2004). As shown in Figure 17-8, pre-β–HDLs (molecular mass: 65 to 70 kDa) cross the endothelium freely.

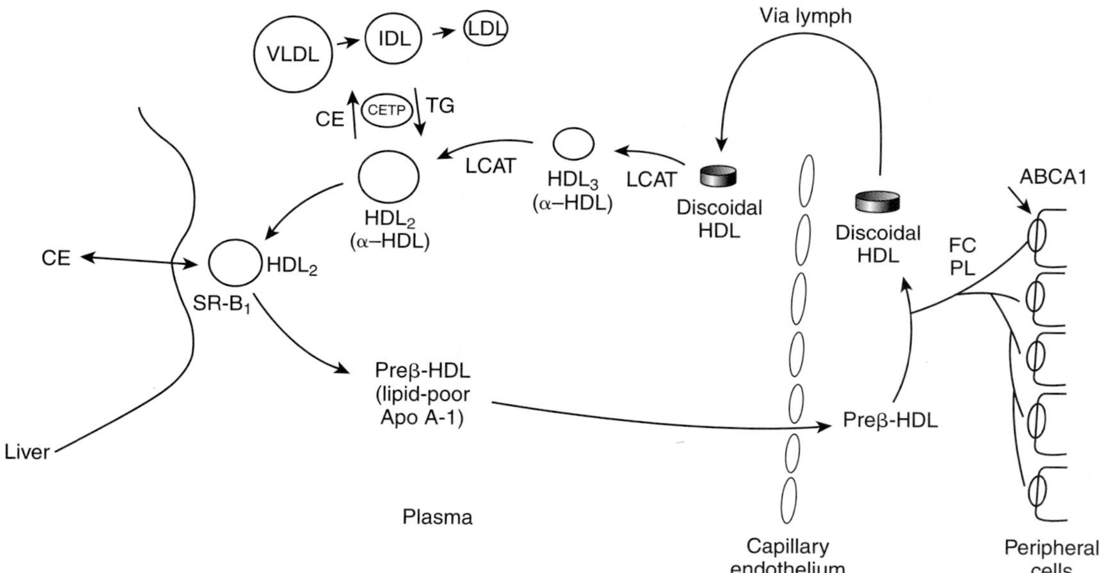

Figure 17-8 The high density lipoprotein (HDL) cycle. Lipid-poor apo A-I (pre-β–HDL) passes through the vascular bed to the extravascular space and accumulates free cholesterol (FC) and phospholipid (PL) from the parenchymal cells of peripheral tissues via ABC-cassette transporter A1 (ABCA1). The discoidal HDLs that form reenter the plasma compartment via the lymph. Free cholesterol in HDL is esterified by LCAT (lecithin: cholesterol acyltransferase) as HDL discs become spheres and then larger spheres (α-HDLs from HDL_3 to HDL_2). After hepatic triacylglycerol lipase (HTGL) and/or cholesteryl ester transfer protein (CETP) activity, cholesterol is selectively taken up by the liver via scavenger receptor- B1(SR-B1) and pre-β–HDL or lipid-poor apo A-I is released for recycling.

Pre-β–HDLs are enriched in the extracellular fluid of peripheral tissues, compared with the larger spherical α-HDLs, most of which have a molecular mass of 180 to 250 kDa. Pre-β–HDLs are exceptionally active as acceptors of free cholesterol and phospholipids from the parenchymal cells of extrahepatic tissues. Many peripheral tissues are rich in caveolae. Caveolae are microdomains of the plasma membrane that are rich in cholesterol and represent a major location from which free cholesterol in these tissues is transferred to pre-β–HDLs.

Free cholesterol efflux to pre-β–HDL is directly, or indirectly via phospholipid efflux, dependent on the cell membrane transporter ABCA1 (ATP-binding cassette transporter A1) (Ory, 2004; Attie et al., 2001). Normally, within the extracellular space, the small pre-β–HDLs become enlarged into disc-shaped particles by the continuing transfer of phosphatidylcholine and free cholesterol from cell membranes via ABCA1. Discoidal HDLs formed in this way reenter the plasma via the main lymph trunks. Within the plasma, LCAT esterifies the free cholesterol with a fatty acid (e.g., linoleate) from phosphatidylcholine (lecithin). This reaction preferentially uses the *sn*-2 acyl chain of phosphatidylcholine as the fatty acid (Jonas, 2000). The LCAT reaction is as follows:

$$\text{Cholesterol} + \text{Phosphatidylcholine} \xrightarrow{\text{LCAT}} \text{Lysophosphatidylcholine} + \text{Cholesteryl Ester}$$

Apo A-I present in the HDL particles activates plasma LCAT, probably by directly interacting with the enzyme. The hydrophobic cholesteryl ester formed then moves from the surface of the HDL into the core, a process that allows more free cholesterol to adsorb onto the surface. As the cholesteryl ester core builds up, the nascent discoidal HDL particle becomes spherical, grows in size, and becomes less dense. The transfer of phospholipids from tissues is much slower than that of free cholesterol. As a result, much of the phosphatidylcholine needed for the LCAT reaction may come from transfer of the phospholipids from apo B-100–containing lipoproteins (VLDLs, IDLs, and LDLs) by the reaction catalyzed in the plasma by PLTP.

Approximately one third of the cholesteryl ester made by the LCAT reaction is transferred from HDL to apo B-100–containing lipoproteins through the action of the plasma cholesteryl ester transfer protein (CETP) (De Grooth et al., 2004). The optimal substrate of CETP (i.e., the recipient of the HDL cholesteryl ester) appears to be an apo B-100–containing particle, with a density near that of IDL or LDL, that can be taken up by the LDL receptor. However, some HDL-derived cholesteryl ester is also transferred to VLDL. In fact, most of the cholesterol in lipoproteins circulates as cholesteryl ester that has been produced by the LCAT-catalyzed reaction. Triacylglycerol is moved from the apo B-100–containing particles to HDL in exchange for the cholesteryl ester. This CETP-mediated exchange would not modify the core volume of HDL appreciably, unless this was followed by hepatic lipase–mediated hydrolysis of HDL triacylglycerol. The rest of the cholesteryl ester generated by the LCAT reaction is selectively taken up from HDL by hepatocytes, and to a lesser extent by adrenal and gonadal cells, via the scavenger receptor SR-BI without the concomitant uptake of the entire HDL particle. These cells use the cholesteryl ester for bile acid and steroid hormone synthesis, respectively. Pre-β–HDL (lipid-poor apo A-I) is rapidly removed from the circulation when there is insufficient cholesterol efflux, and apo A-I is excreted in the urine.

Tangier disease, caused by mutations of the *ABCA1* gene, is a rare recessive genetic disorder characterized by an almost complete absence of HDL in plasma, accumulation of cholesteryl esters in macrophages and, as a result, increased susceptibility to atherosclerosis. As discussed previously, *ABCA1* appears to be necessary for the efflux of tissue cholesterol and phospholipids from peripheral cells into the reverse cholesterol transport pathway. In patients affected by Tangier disease, because cells are unable to efflux cholesterol onto nascent HDL particles, rapid degradation of the nascent HDL and loss of apo A in the urine occur. Infiltration of cholesteryl ester in hematopoietic organs occurs also.

POSTPRANDIAL LIPOPROTEIN METABOLISM

The concentration and proportions of plasma lipoproteins following an overnight (16-hour) fast are often used as a baseline state from which the effects of postprandial lipemia can be evaluated. The proportions and types of dietary fat and carbohydrate consumed have major effects upon postprandial plasma lipid levels. The effects of a moderate meal (one third of daily caloric requirements) can be observed over a 9- to 12-hour period postprandially as changes (from the fasting baseline) in plasma lipid concentrations and in activities of lipoprotein-metabolizing enzymes. This means that humans who consume regular meals are in a nonfasting or absorptive state for most of each day or 24-hour period.

CHANGES IN PLASMA TRIACYLGLYCEROL AND CHOLESTEROL CONCENTRATIONS IN RESPONSE TO A MEAL

In humans, the size, frequency, and composition of meals are often unpredictable. Lipid metabolic rates must respond rapidly to continually changing inputs of cholesterol and fatty acids. Lipid and carbohydrate in excess of immediate needs must be selectively transferred to appropriate storage sites and released later upon demand.

Plasma triacylglycerol levels peak about 3 hours after a moderate meal, although the magnitude and duration of the postprandial response depend on the fat content of the meal. After ingestion of a normal meal containing one third of the daily caloric intake, plasma triacylglycerol levels typically double by 3 hours, then decrease toward or even below fasting levels by 9 hours, and finally rebound to fasting levels again by 12 hours.

The concentrations of circulating apo B-48 and apo B-100 in triacylglycerol-rich lipoproteins increase postprandially, but, even at peak triacylglycerol levels, apo B-48 makes up only a small part of the total apo B lipoproteins circulating within the triacylglycerol-rich lipoproteins. The greater abundance of apo B-100 than of apo B-48 in plasma is due to several factors. The triacylglycerol content of a newly secreted chylomicron is 10-fold to 100-fold greater than that of a nascent hepatic VLDL particle, yet both lipoprotein particles contain a single apo B polypeptide. As a result, the apo B-48 to apo B-100 ratio greatly underrepresents the proportion of triacylglycerol of intestinal origin that is present in postprandial plasma. In addition, chylomicron triacylglycerol is hydrolyzed more rapidly by LPL ($t_{1/2}$ = 5 to 15 minutes) than is triacylglycerol in VLDL ($t_{1/2}$ = 1 to 5 hours). Chylomicron or apo B-48–containing remnants also are cleared rapidly, whereas the plasma concentration of apo B-100–containing LDL remains relatively high at all times.

Dietary cholesterol appears as cholesteryl ester in chylomicrons. It is retained within the chylomicron remnant and taken up rapidly by the liver. Because of their relatively rapid clearance, chylomicrons contain an insignificant part of total plasma cholesterol, even after a meal rich in free cholesterol. Loss of free cholesterol from LDL and a comparable increase within the triacylglycerol-rich lipoprotein fractions have been observed during the postprandial response. This probably reflects mainly a passive transfer of free cholesterol, driven by the low free cholesterol content of newly secreted VLDL. There is little change postprandially in the cholesterol or triacylglycerol content of HDL.

POSTPRANDIAL CHANGES IN PLASMA LIPID METABOLISM

Adipose tissue LPL regulates fatty acid storage after a meal. After a meal, the level of LPL activity at the endothelial surface of adipose tissue is increased. The principal factor mediating this effect is a rise in the circulating level of insulin. Insulin increases the transcription of LPL in the adipocyte and stimulates the processing of polysaccharide chains in newly synthesized LPL to the trimmed state found in the secreted lipase.

Lipemia in postprandial plasma also stimulates the activity of CETP in exchanging VLDL triacylglycerol for HDL cholesteryl ester. Because the proportion of plasma triacylglycerol in acceptor lipoproteins (VLDLs, IDLs, and LDLs) increases after a meal, there is a greater likelihood, on average, that a cholesteryl ester molecule transferred from HDL to VLDL or

LDL will be replaced by transfer of a triacylglycerol molecule—rather than by a cholesteryl ester molecule—from VLDL or LDL back to HDL. As a result, the net exchange of HDL cholesteryl ester mass (e.g., from HDL to VLDL) for triacylglycerol mass (e.g., from VLDL to HDL) increases. There is no increase in the plasma concentration of CETP protein postprandially. By 9 hours after a meal, the flux of cholesteryl ester through CETP has usually decreased again to baseline fasting levels.

Postprandial lipemia also stimulates free cholesterol mass transfer from cells into plasma. Increased transfer of triacylglycerol to HDL in exchange for cholesteryl ester, followed by hydrolysis of the triacylglycerol by hepatic triacylglycerol lipase, leads to a significant decrease in the size of HDL particles. If sequential plasma samples obtained during the course of postprandial lipemia are incubated in vitro with monolayers of peripheral cells, an increase in the mass transfer of free cholesterol from the cells to plasma lipoproteins is seen for plasma samples obtained 6 to 9 hours postprandially. The model shown in Figure 17-8 suggests that small, lipid-poor pre-β–HDL (generated from HDL) first cross the endothelium into the interstitial space of the peripheral tissues. "Discoidal" HDLs are then formed extravascularly from small pre-β–HDLs by accumulation of phospholipids and free cholesterol from peripheral cells; they accumulate in the lymph and they are returned to the plasma via the lymphatic ducts. Finally, LCAT activity (but not the plasma concentration of LCAT protein) also increases postprandially. This increase normally peaks after about 9 hours and favors esterification of the free cholesterol picked up by the pre-β–HDLs. Therefore, postprandial lipemia is associated with stimulation of the reverse transport of cholesterol from peripheral tissues to the liver.

The extravascular phase of postprandial lipid metabolism is likely to explain the 3-hour lag between the increase in net exchange of HDL cholesteryl ester for triacylglycerol (catalyzed by CETP) and the subsequent rise of LCAT activity (esterification of free cholesterol to form HDL cholesteryl ester). This lag is characteristic of postprandial lipemia (Fig. 17-9). The difference in the shape of the response curves of LCAT and CETP activities means that the ratio of LCAT to

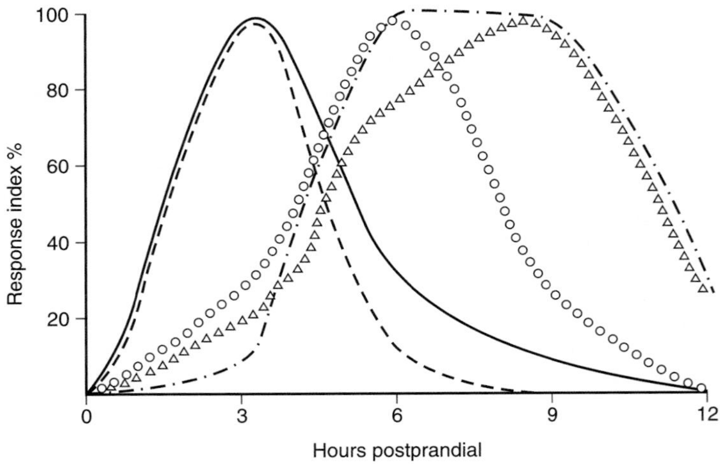

Figure 17-9 The postprandial response of triacylglycerol and plasma metabolic activities following a moderate meal (approximately one third of daily calories) of whole foods. Shown on the figure are plasma triacylglycerol concentration (*solid line*); net exchange of cholesteryl ester in HDL for triacylglycerol, catalyzed by CETP (*dashed line*); transfer of cellular free cholesterol to plasma (*open circles*); cholesterol esterification by LCAT (*dashed-and-dotted line*); and phospholipid transfer catalyzed by PLTP (*triangles*). Values have been scaled between 0% (fasting) and 100% (peak postprandial response) to facilitate comparison among different factors. *(Data from Castro GR, Fielding CJ [1985] Effects of postprandial lipemia on plasma cholesterol metabolism. J Clin Invest 75:874-882.)*

CETP activity is increased at 6 hours postprandially compared to fasting levels. As a result, the mean diameter of HDL, which decreases early in postprandial metabolism (3 hours), increases back to its fasting value later in the postprandial period (6 hours) as LCAT-derived cholesteryl ester accumulates in the spherical, α-migrating particles.

The sequential changes that characterize postprandial lipid metabolism in plasma (see Fig. 17-9) have several effects. Fatty acids in triacylglycerols are directed for storage to adipose tissue through the properties and regulation of adipose tissue LPLs. The accumulation of unstable, cholesterol-enriched remnant lipoproteins is prevented by the efficient removal of these particles by the liver. Fat-soluble vitamins are delivered efficiently to the liver as part of the chylomicron remnants. Finally, postprandial lipemia promotes reverse cholesterol transport from peripheral tissues to the liver by accelerating the recycling of apo A-I through pre-β–HDL.

ATHEROSCLEROTIC CARDIOVASCULAR DISEASE

Epidemiological studies have generated an enormous database linking diets high in saturated fat and cholesterol to human diseases. These observational studies were paralleled by the rapid development of the field of lipid and lipoprotein metabolism, with studies stretching from human dietary investigations to studies of diet and atherosclerosis in transgenic and "knockout" mouse models of human dyslipidemia.

PATHOPHYSIOLOGY OF ATHEROSCLEROSIS

Atherosclerosis is a vascular disease characterized by fatty plaques in the intima of arteries. These plaques not only block blood flow but can undergo rupture and precipitate blood clots within arteries, thereby leading to heart attack, stroke, or peripheral vascular disease. The key event in atherogenesis is retention of apo B–containing lipoproteins in the intima of arterial walls (Tulenko and Sumner, 2002). To carry out their role as transporters for cholesterol, the smaller apo B–containing lipoproteins move across the endothelial cells lining the blood vessels to reach the extracellular space and then normally return to the circulation. LDL is the predominant lipoprotein passing through the endothelial layer, but there is evidence that chylomicron remnants and VLDL remnants (IDLs) can do so as well. In certain focal areas of arteries, usually at branching points with disturbed flow, lipoproteins may be retained by the extracellular proteoglycans, which make lipoproteins susceptible to being "modified." Modification may include oxidation of phospholipids with accumulation of lipid hydroperoxides as well as oxidation of apo B-100. Alternatively, modified apo B–containing lipoproteins may be prone to aggregate or stick to extracellular matrix molecules in the subendothelial space. In either case, greater numbers of circulating lipoproteins will infiltrate the endothelium and be retained.

As illustrated in Figure 17-10, modification and retention of apo B–containing lipoproteins, particularly LDLs, signal endothelial cells to produce cell adhesion molecules, monocyte chemotactic proteins, and monocyte colony-stimulating factor. Together, these molecules stimulate formation, migration, and sequestation of monocytes at sites where lipoproteins are retained in the subendothelial space. These monocytes are then activated and perpetuate a local inflammatory response, take up modified LDLs, and transform into macrophages. The inflammatory response includes T-cell recruitment, cytokine secretion, and monocyte chemotaxis. The accumulated macrophages further oxidize and internalize the retained lipoproteins to become lipid-laden foam cells. They also secrete growth factors that stimulate smooth muscle cell proliferation and migration. Both the monocytes and macrophages and the activated smooth muscle cells begin to secrete extracellular matrix molecules as well. At this point, all the components of the advanced lesion are in place and atherogenesis is well under way.

Because atherosclerosis is an inflammatory disease, markers of inflammation such as C-reactive protein (CRP) are suggested to be risk factors for coronary artery disease (CAD) (Willerson and Ridker, 2004). Statins, mentioned in the preceding text as inhibitors of

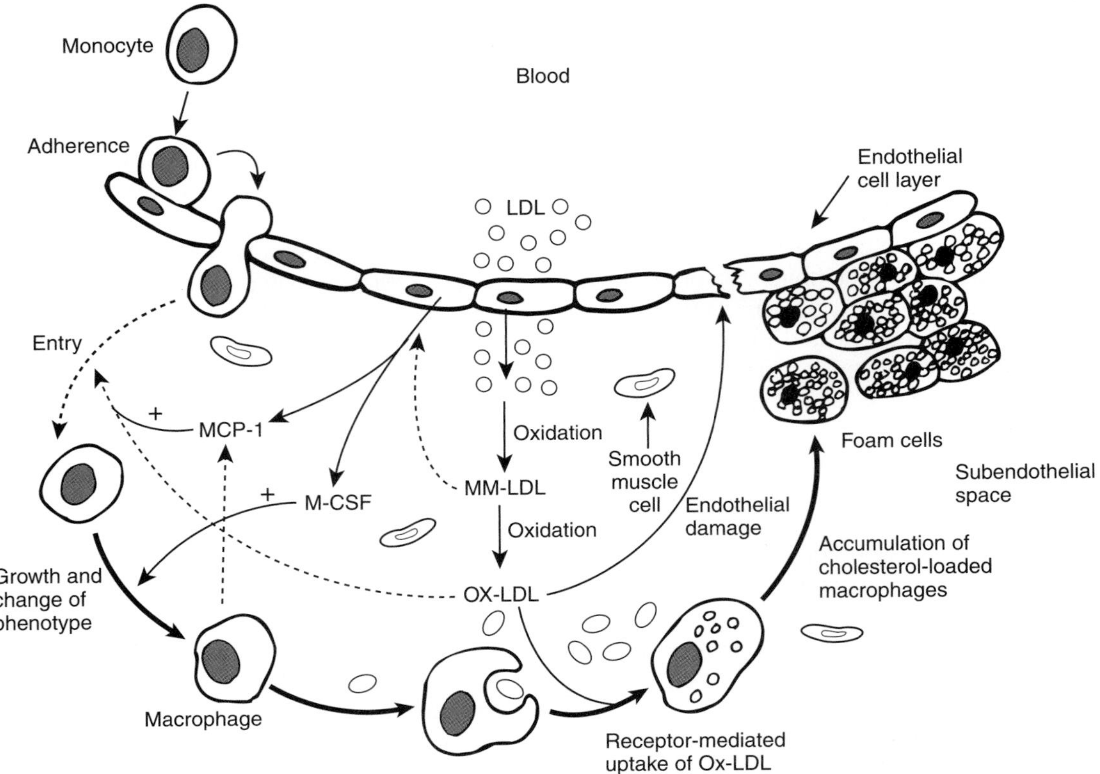

Figure 17-10 Depiction of the early stages of atheroma formation, including low density lipoprotein (LDL) entry into the vessel wall, endothelial damage or dysfunction, LDL modification and oxidation, recruitment of monocytes into the vessel wall, and uptake of modified/oxidized LDL by monocyte-derived macrophages. *MM-LDL,* Lightly oxidized LDL; *OX-LDL,* oxidized LDL; *M-CSF,* macrophage colony-stimulating factor; *MCP-1,* monocyte chemotactic protein. *(From Steinberg D [1991] Antioxidants and atherosclerosis: A current assessment. Circulation 84:1420-1425.)*

HMG CoA reductase activity, are potent cholesterol-lowering drugs that reduce the risk of heart attack and stroke. Increasing evidence suggests that the beneficial effects of statins are due not only to their cholesterol-lowering effects but also to their direct effects on endothelial cell function, including antiinflammatory and antithrombotic effects. This may be due to inhibition of protein prenylation (geranylgeranylation) (Endres and Laufs, 2004; Liao, 2002). Recent evidence also links the statins to decreased levels of CRP, independent of the cholesterol-lowering actions of the drug.

LIPID AND LIPOPROTEINS AS RISK FACTORS FOR ATHEROSCLEROTIC CARDIOVASCULAR DISEASE

Lipids and lipoproteins as risk factors for CAD have been well established. Disorders of lipoprotein metabolism can lead to alterations in plasma cholesterol and triacylglycerol levels, and these disorders are usually associated with increased risk of cardiovascular disease. Plasma total cholesterol is strongly associated with CAD, but this association is confounded by the distribution of cholesterol among the lipoprotein classes. High total cholesterol level in blood is usually paralleled by high plasma concentration of LDL cholesterol, and LDL-cholesterol level is a significant indicator of risk for atherosclerosis. Nevertheless, LDL is not a homogeneous class. Small, dense LDLs, which are commonly found in individuals with higher triacylglycerol and lower HDL cholesterol levels, have been proposed to be more atherogenic (Austin et al., 1990). Small, dense LDLs may be more atherogenic because they may penetrate into the artery wall more easily or be more readily oxidized. However, patients with FH have large, cholesteryl ester–enriched LDLs that are quite atherogenic. Because oxidized LDLs affect endothelial cells, convert macrophages into foam cells, and cause inflammation, oxidized LDL levels in plasma are implicated as a risk factor for CAD. However, it is not known whether the level of oxidized LDL in plasma reflects that in subendothelial space. Lipoprotein (a) [Lp(a)] is composed of LDL with a second protein, apo(a), covalently linked to apo B. Apo(a) is a large protein with a highly variable size (200 to 700 kDa), which is synthesized in the liver and present only in humans. It is believed that apo(a) interacts with LDL apo B in plasma. A high plasma level of Lp(a) has been linked to increased risk for atherosclerotic cardiovascular disease, although the mechanism remains unclear (Berglund and Ramakrishnan, 2004).

In contrast to LDL cholesterol, the HDL cholesterol level is inversely related to risk for CAD (Barter, 2002). As described previously, HDL is critical for the reverse transport of cholesterol from tissues throughout the body back to the liver. HDL, or the apo A-I–containing lipoproteins, appears to have protective effects against atherosclerosis. Some studies have indicated that only the larger, more cholesteryl ester–rich HDL_2 (density of 1.063 to 1.12 g/mL) is protective against CAD in comparison with HDL_3 (density of 1.12 to 1.21 g/mL), but other investigators have failed to see a difference between the two types of HDLs. HDLs are also antiatherogenic due to their potential role as an antioxidant that counteracts LDL oxidation. Inhibition of LDL oxidation by HDL is usually attributed to HDL's high content of lipid-soluble antioxidants (e.g., vitamin E), the antioxidative properties of apo A-I, and the presence of several enzymes in HDL that prevent LDL oxidation or degrade active products. HDLs also may exert an antiatherogenic effect by protecting endothelial cells from dysfunction (Gotto and Brinton, 2004).

The role of plasma triacylglycerol level as an independent risk factor has been controversial. The controversy stems from several observations, including triacylglycerols accounting for only a minor component of lipids in vessel-wall lesions, the inverse relationship between triacylglycerols and HDL cholesterol, and the lack of strong evidence that triacylglycerols are independent predictors of disease. However, triacylglycerols may play a role in atherogenesis as a source of free fatty acids that can be converted into lipids that are bioactive in the formation of lesions. Postprandial hypertriglyceridemia is a risk factor for CAD, and fibrate drugs that decrease plasma triacylglycerol levels can prevent CAD. So-called remnant-like particles (RLPs) are considered equivalent to remnants of triacylglycerol-rich lipoproteins. Plasma RLP–cholesterol level may also be a risk factor, and RLP–cholesterol and plasma triacylglycerol levels are correlated. Cholesterol transported in VLDLs with triacylglycerols can accumulate in arterial wall macrophages. This suggests that an elevated triacylglycerol level may be a marker of increased delivery of non-LDL cholesterol to lesion sites.

CHRONIC EFFECTS OF DIETARY LIPIDS ON PLASMA LIPOPROTEINS AND LIPID METABOLISM

The major differences among diets that affect plasma lipids are the percentage of total calories consumed as fat, the proportions of saturated and polyunsaturated fats (monounsaturated fats being considered neutral), and the amount of dietary cholesterol. The major effects of dietary lipids are on circulating levels of triacylglycerol and of LDL cholesterol.

EFFECTS OF TOTAL DIETARY FAT ON FASTING PLASMA LIPID LEVELS

Switching from a typical American diet to a low-fat diet, in which fat has been replaced isocalorically by carbohydrate, typically increases the fasting triacylglycerol levels and decreases, probably by a CETP-mediated process, both fasting LDL and HDL cholesterol levels. This increase in serum triacylglycerol has been attributed to the influence of carbohydrate in stimulating fatty acid synthesis and the secretion of triacylglycerol-rich VLDL from the liver. An increase in dietary fat is associated with modest increases (10% to 20%) in the levels of LPL and hepatic triacylglycerol lipase. It is not clear whether corresponding decreases in lipase activities occur when individuals switch to low-fat diets, but such reductions would be consistent with the modest hypertriglyceridemia that is observed.

EFFECTS OF DIETARY FAT SATURATION ON FASTING PLASMA LIPID LEVELS

The degree of dietary fat saturation is often expressed as a P/S (polyunsaturated/saturated) ratio. The effects of dietary fat saturation depend upon the dietary cholesterol level. For example, Hayes and Khosla (1992) showed that when cholesterol intake was low (~200 mg/day), there was no significant effect of P/S ratios (0.8 to 0.2 at constant total fat and constant monounsaturated fat) on the plasma cholesterol level. In contrast, when the cholesterol intake was approximately 600 mg/day, a decrease in the P/S ratio from 0.8 to 0.2 resulted in a doubling of the fasting plasma cholesterol levels. In contrast to the effects of saturated fat on plasma cholesterol, plasma triacylglycerol level was minimally affected by an increase in saturated fat (with constant dietary cholesterol and total fat calories) when there was no change in body weight. Polyunsaturated fatty acids may be of the n-6 family or the n-3 family, as described in Chapter 18. The n-3 or so-called fish oil fatty acids have been shown to decrease the risk of cardiovascular disease by lowering plasma triacylglycerol and cholesterol levels and by virtue of their metabolic conversion to antithrombotic and antiinflammatory eicosanoids (Connor and Connor, 1997). The incorporation of *trans*-unsaturated fatty acids (arising during hydrogenation of vegetable oil) in dietary fat has been shown to be atherogenic, with increases in LDL cholesterol levels and decreases in HDL cholesterol levels found in several clinical trials (Zock and Katan, 1997). When considering effects of dietary fat saturation on plasma lipid levels, *trans*-unsaturated fatty acids are typically thought of as akin to saturated fatty acids rather than as unsaturated fatty acids. Monounsaturated fatty acids, found in high amounts in Mediterranean diets, are often considered "neutral" for serum lipid levels. However, some studies suggest that monounsaturated fatty acids act similarly, although not as potently, as polyunsaturated fatty acids, lowering LDL-cholesterol and increasing HDL-cholesterol levels (Lada and Rudel, 2003; Perez-Jimenez et al., 2002).

Nutrition Insight

Effect of Degree of Fat Saturation on Plasma Lipids

A typical American diet might provide a total of 15% of calories as protein and 36% of calories as fat. If this fat is made up of equal parts of saturated, monounsaturated, and polyunsaturated fats, the polyunsaturated/saturated (P/S) ratio of this diet would be about 1.0. If 80% of the polyunsaturated fat is replaced isocalorically with saturated fat, the P/S ratio would be markedly reduced to 0.11.

Thinking Critically

Assuming that no other changes are made in the diet and that no changes in body weight result from this dietary change, what effect would you predict on the following parameters? Give the direction of change (increase/decrease) and the magnitude of the change (little/moderate/major).

- Plasma fasting triacylglycerol concentration
- Plasma high density lipoprotein (HDL) cholesterol concentration
- Plasma postprandial triacylglycerol concentration
- Plasma low density lipoprotein (LDL) cholesterol concentration

EFFECTS OF DIETARY CHOLESTEROL ON FASTING PLASMA LIPID LEVELS

In responsive individuals, increased dietary cholesterol is generally associated with increased LDL cholesterol without significant changes in the cholesterol content of other lipoprotein fractions. This effect is mediated, at least in part, by downregulation of hepatic LDL receptor expression. Increases in dietary cholesterol (+400 to 600 mg/day), at different levels of total fat and fat saturation, are usually associated with approximately 20% increases in the flux of lipids through both LCAT and CETP. Because of the long circulation time of LDL ($t_{1/2}$ = ~2 days), even modest changes in CETP activity alone could lead to significant redistribution of cholesteryl esters among plasma lipoproteins. CETP activity could affect the circulating level of LDL cholesterol in human plasma, but more information is needed to determine the importance of CETP activity relative to that of hepatic LDL receptor levels.

RECOMMENDATIONS AND TYPICAL INTAKES FOR DIETARY FAT

Fat is important in the diet because it is a major source of fuel for the body, it aids in the absorption of fat-soluble vitamins and carotenoids, and it provides the essential n-3 and n-6 fatty acids. The Institute of Medicine (IOM, 2002) did not establish a recommended dietary allowance (RDA) or adequate intake (AI) for total fat intake, except for infants, because of insufficient data for determination of the level of fat intake at which risk of inadequacy or lack of promotion of chronic disease occurs. Any increase in incremental intake of saturated fatty acids, as well as of *trans* fatty acids, appears to be associated with increased risk of coronary artery disease, but it is not feasible or advisable to eliminate saturated or *trans* fat from a typical whole-food diet because fat and oil sources contain mixtures of fatty acids. The acceptable macronutrient distribution range (AMDR) for total fat is set at 20% to 35% of energy. Diets low in saturated fatty acids and as low as possible in *trans* fatty acids are advised.

The IOM (2002) summarized surveys of fat intake in the United States and Canada. Median total fat intake ranged from 65 to 100 g/day for men and 48 to 63 g/day for women in the United States, as determined in the Continuing Survey of Food Intakes of Individuals (USDA, 1998). These intake ranges represented about 32% to 34% of total energy intake. Median saturated fatty acid intake ranged from 21 to 34 g/day for men and 15 to 21 g/day for women, providing about 11% to 12% of total energy in adult diets. Monounsaturated fatty acid intake ranged from 25 to 39 g/day for men and 18 to 24 g/day for women, providing about 14% of total energy. Median n-6 polyunsaturated fatty acid intake ranged from about 12 to 17 g/day for men and 9 to 11 g/day for women, contributing about 5% to 7% of total energy intake in the diets of adults. Approximately 85% to 90% of the n-6 polyunsaturated fatty acid intake was in the form of linoleic acid. Total n-3 polyunsaturated fatty acid intake was 1.3 to 1.8 g/day for men and 1.0 to 1.2 g/day for women, contributing about 0.7% of total energy intake. Approximately 90% of the n-3 polyunsaturated fatty acid intake was from α-linolenic acid, with approximately 5% from docosahexaenoic acid (DHA). Rough estimates of *trans* fatty acid intake suggest that these accounted for about 2.6% of total energy intake. Estimates of the typical intake of conjugated linoleic acid (a possible bioactive compound discussed in Chapter 2) in the United States and Canada fall in the range of 0.15 to 0.33 g/day.

Food Sources

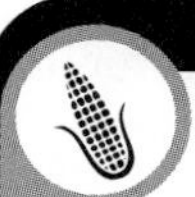

Typical Food Sources of Dietary Fats and Cholesterol

Saturated Fatty Acids

Dairy fat: whole milk, cream, butter, cheese
Meat fats: pork, beef
Certain plant oils: coconut, palm, palm kernel

Monounsaturated Fatty Acids

Meat fats: pork, lamb
Nuts: macadamia, hazelnuts, pecans
Plant oils: canola, olive

Polyunsaturated Fatty Acids

n-6 (linoleic acid)

Nuts and seeds: walnuts, sunflower seeds, pinenuts, pecans
Plant oils: soybean, safflower, corn

n-3

Fish: sardines, salmon (eicosapentaenoic acid and docosahexaenoic acid)
Plant oils: soybean, flax seed (α-linolenic acid)

***Trans* Fatty Acids**

Hydrogenated oils: margarines and vegetable shortenings
Dairy fats: whole milk, butter, cheese
Ruminant meat fats: beef, lamb

Conjugated Linoleic Acids

Dairy fats: milk, cheese
Ruminant meat fats: beef, lamb

Cholesterol

Meat, poultry, and fish fats: chicken, salmon, lamb, pork, crab
Eggs
Dairy fats: whole milk, butter, cheese

AIs for total fat intake of infants were based on the intake of fat from human milk and from complementary foods during the second half of the first year of life. The AIs are 31 g/day for infants from 0 to 6 months of age and 30 g/day for infants from 7 to 12 months of age. Therefore, fat provides 55% and 40% of total energy intake for infants during the first and second 6 months of life, respectively. Human milk contains 20% to 25% of energy as saturated fatty acids, 6% of energy as n-6 fatty acids, 1% to 5% of total energy as *trans* fatty acids, 1% as n-3 fatty acids, and the remainder (~23%) as monounsaturated fatty acids.

The IOM (2002) did establish AIs for the essential polyunsaturated fatty acid classes for all age and gender groups. These are described in more detail in Chapter 18. The AIs for n-6 polyunsaturated fatty acids (linoleic acid) are 17 g/day for young men and 12 g/day for young women. AIs for n-3 polyunsaturated fatty acids (e.g., α-linolenic acid) are 1.6 and 1.1 g/day for men and women, respectively.

REFERENCES

Altmann SW, Davis HR Jr, Zhu L-j, Yao X, Hoos LM, Tetzloff G, Lyer SPN, Maguire M, Golovko A, Zeng M, Wang L, Murgolo N, Graziano MP (2004) Niemann-Pick C1 like 1 protein is critical for intestinal cholesterol absorption. Science 303:1201-1204.

Attie AD, Kastelein JP, Hayden MR (2001) Pivotal role of ABCA1 in reverse cholesterol transport influencing HDL levels and susceptibility to atherosclerosis. J Lipid Res 42:1717-1726.

Austin MA, King MC, Vranizan KM, Krauss RM (1990) Atherogenic lipoprotein phenotype. A proposed genetic marker for coronary heart disease risk. Circulation 82:495-506.

Barter PJ (2002) Hugh Sinclair lecture: the regulation and remodeling of HDL by plasma factors. Atherosclerosis S3:39-47.

Berglund L, Ramakrishnan R (2004) Lipoprotein(a): an elusive cardiovascular risk factor. Arteriscler Thromb Vasc Biol 24:1-8.

Bjorkhem I (2002) Do oxysterols control cholesterol homeostasis? J Clin Invest 110:725-730.

Chang TY, Chang CCY, Lin S, Yu C, Li B-L, Miyazaki A (2001) Roles of acyl-coenzyme A: cholesterol acyltransferase-1 and -2. Curr Opin Lipidol 12:289-296.

Chiang JYL (2002) Bile acid regulation of gene expression: roles of nuclear hormone receptors. Endoc Rev 23:443-463.

Connelly MA, Williams DL (2004) Scavenger receptor B1: a scavenger receptor with a mission to transport high density lipoprotein lipids. Curr Opin Lipidol 15:287-295.

Connor SL, Connor WE (1997) Are fish oils beneficial in the prevention and treatment of coronary artery disease? Am J Clin Nutr 66:1020S-1031S.

Davis HR Jr, Zhu LJ, Hoos LM, Tetzloff G, Maguire M, Liu J, Yao X, Iyer SP, Lam MH, Lund EG, Detmers PA, Graziano MP, Altmann SW (2004) Niemann-Pick C1 Like 1 (NPC1L1) is the intestinal phytosterol and cholesterol transporter and a key modulator of whole-body cholesterol homeostasis. J Biol Chem 279:33586-33592.

De Grooth GJ, Klerkx AHEM, Stroes ESG, Stalenhoef AFH, Kastelein JJP, Kuivenhoven JA (2004) A review of CETP and its relation to atherosclerosis. J Lipid Res 45:1967-1974.

Edwards PA, Kast HR, Anisfeld AM (2002) BAREing it all: the adoption of LXR and FXR and their roles in lipid homeostasis. J Lipid Res 43:2-12.

Endres M, Laufs U (2004) Effects of statins on endothelium and signaling mechanisms. Stroke 35 I:2708-2711.

Fielding CJ, Fielding PE (1995) Molecular physiology of reverse cholesterol transport. J Lipid Res 36:211-228.

Gibbons GF (2003) Regulation of fatty acid and cholesterol synthesis: co-operation or competition? Prog Lipid Res 42:479-497.

Gotto AM Jr, Brinton EA (2004) Assessing low levels of high-density lipoprotein cholesterol as a risk factor in coronary heart disease. J Am Coll Cardiol 43:717-724.

Hayes KC, Khosla (1992) Dietary fatty acid thresholds and cholesterolemia. FASEB J 6:2600-2607.

Horton JD, Goldstein JL, Brown MS (2002) SREBPs: activators of the complete program of cholesterol and fatty acid synthesis in the liver. J Clin Invest 109:1125-1131.

Institute of Medicine (2002) Dietary Reference Intakes for Energy, Carbohydrate, Fiber, Fat, Fatty Acids, Cholesterol, Protein, and Amino Acids (Macronutrients). National Academy Press, Washington, DC.

Jonas A (2000) Lecithin cholesterol acyltransferase. Biochim Biophys Acta 1529:245-256.

Lada AT, Rudel LL (2003) Dietary monounsaturated versus polyunsaturated fatty acids: which is really better for protection from coronary heart Disease? Curr Opin Lipidol 14:41-6.

Liao JK (2002) Isoprenoids as mediators of the biological effects of statins. J Clin Invest 110:285-288.

Merkel M, Eckel RH, Goldberg IJ (2002) Lipoprotein lipase: genetics, lipid uptake, and regulation. J Lipid Res 43:1997-2006.

Ory DS (2004) The Niemann-Pick disease genes regulators of cellular cholesterol homeostasis. Trends Cardiovasc Med 14:66-72.

Perez-Jimenez F, Lopez-Miranda J, Mata P (2002) Protective effect of dietary monounsaturated fat on arteriosclerosis. Atherosclerosis 163: 385-398.

Radhakrishnan A, Sun L-P, Dwon HJ, Brown MS, Goldstein JL (2004) Direct binding of cholesterol to the purified membrane region of SCAP: mechanism for a sterol-sensing domain. Mol Cell 15:259-268.

Rawson RB (2003) The SREBP pathway—insights from insigs and insects. Nature Rev 4:631-640.

Repa JJ, Mangelsdorf DJ (2002) The liver X receptor gene team: potential new players in atherosclerosis. Nature 8:1245.

Russell DW (2003) The enzymes, regulation, and genetics of bile acid synthesis. Annu Rev Biochem 72:137-174.

Schroepfer GJ Jr (2000) Oxysterols: modulators of cholesterol metabolism and other processes. Physiol Rev 80:361-554.

Soccio RE, Breslow JL (2004) Intracellular cholesterol transport. Arterioscler Thromb Vasc Biol 24:1-12.

Tansey JT, Sztalryd C, Hlavin EM, Kimmel AR, Londos C (2004) The central role of perilipin A in lipid metabolism and adipocyte lipolysis. IUBMB Life 56:379-385.

Tulenko TN, Sumner AE (2002) The physiology of lipoproteins. J Nucl Cardiol 9:638-649.

Twinckler TB, Dallinga-Thie GM, Cohn JS, Chapman MJ (2004) Elevated remnant-like particle cholesterol concentration. A characteristic feature of the atherogenic lipoprotein phenotype. Circulation 109:1918-1925.

U.S. Department of Agriculture (1998) Continuing Survey of Food Intakes of Individuals (1994-1996, 1998). Diet and Health Knowledge Survey CD-ROM. National Technical Information Service, Springfield, VA.

Willerson JT, Ridker PM (2004) Inflammation as a cardiovascular risk factor. Circulation 109:II-2-10.

Yu KC-W, Chen W, Cooper AD (2001) LDL receptor-related protein mediates cell-surface clustering and hepatic sequestration of chylomicron remnants in LDLR-deficient mice. J Clin Invest 107:1387-1394.

Zock PL, Katan MB (1997) Butter, margarine and serum lipoproteins. Atherosclerosis 131:7-16.

RECOMMENDED READINGS

Ginsberg HN, Stalenhoef AF (2003) The metabolic syndrome: targeting dyslipidaemia to reduce coronary risk. J Cardiovasc Risk 10:121-128.

Vance DE, Vance J (2002) Biochemistry of Lipids, Lipoproteins and Membranes, 4th edition. New Comprehensive Biochemistry, Vol 36. New York, Elsevier Science, BV.

Chapter 18

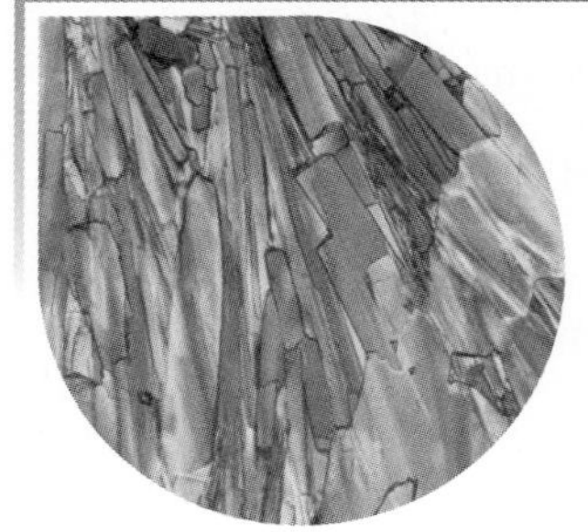

Essential Fatty Acids

Arthur A. Spector, MD

OUTLINE

COMMON ABBREVIATIONS

COX	cyclooxygenase
DHA	docosahexaenoic acid
ER	endoplasmic reticulum
EPA	eicosapentaenoic acid
G-protein	GTP-binding protein
LDL	low density lipoprotein
PG	prostaglandin
PPAR	peroxisome proliferator-activated receptor
RXR	retinoid X receptor
SREBP	sterol regulatory element binding protein

Essential fatty acids are polyunsaturated fatty acids that are necessary for growth and normal physiological function but cannot be completely synthesized in the body. There are two classes of essential fatty acids, omega (ω)6 and ω3. They cannot be interconverted. Therefore, the dietary fat intake must contain both of these classes in order to maintain good health and prevent an eventual deficiency. Plants have the ability to synthesize the first 18-carbon member of each class, linoleic acid (ω6) and α-linolenic acid (ω3), and plant products are the ultimate sources of essential fatty acids in the human food chain.

HISTORICAL PERSPECTIVE

Early work demonstrated that a small amount of dietary fat was necessary for laboratory rats to grow normally, remain healthy, and reproduce. Two opposing views were put forward to explain this observation. Some thought that the protective action was due entirely to the vitamin E present in the dietary fat. Others thought that, in addition to vitamin E, some component of the fat itself was an essential nutrient. This controversy was resolved in 1929 when George O. Burr and Mildred M. Burr demonstrated that linoleic acid, the 18-carbon ω6 fatty acid that contains two double bonds, was an essential nutrient for the rat. The syndrome produced in rats by a lack of ω6 fatty acids, called essential fatty acid deficiency, was characterized by a cessation of growth, dermatitis, loss of water through the skin, loss of blood in the urine, fatty liver, and loss of reproductive capacity. Subsequent work showed that linoleic acid also is an essential nutrient for other mammals, including humans.

No well-defined disease occurred when experimental animals were fed a diet deficient in α-linolenic acid, the corresponding 18-carbon member of the ω3 class. Therefore, it initially appeared that ω3 fatty acids were not essential nutrients and were present in the body simply because small amounts ordinarily are contained in the diet. This view gradually changed during the last 35 years because of increasing evidence that ω3 fatty acids are required for optimum vision and nervous system development (Lauritzen et al., 2001). A consensus now exists that, like the ω6 class, the ω3 fatty acids are essential nutrients for humans.

STRUCTURE OF POLYUNSATURATED FATTY ACIDS

Fatty acids contain a hydrocarbon chain and a carboxyl group. All fatty acids that have two or more double bonds in the hydrocarbon chain are classified as polyunsaturated. In humans and other mammals almost all of the polyunsaturated fatty acids present in the blood and tissues contain between 18 and 22 carbons and from two to six double bonds. The double bonds normally are three carbons apart; a carbon atom that is fully saturated (called a methylene carbon) separates them:

$$-CH=CH-CH_2-CH=CH-$$

The presence of the methylene carbon between each pair of double bonds reduces the tendency of polyunsaturated fatty acids to undergo spontaneous oxidation in air, a process called lipid peroxidation.

The double bonds in all unsaturated fatty acids synthesized by plants and animals are in the *cis* configuration. This introduces a rigid 45-degree bend at each double bond in the fatty acid chain. The bent conformation reduces the tightness with which adjacent fatty acid chains can pack, producing a more mobile physical state and thereby decreasing the melting point.

The carbon atoms of fatty acids are numbered in two different ways. In the delta (Δ) numbering system, the carboxyl carbon is designated as carbon 1. The reverse occurs in the ω numbering system; the carbon at the methyl end of the hydrocarbon chain is designated as carbon 1. Another designation for the ω notation is n, and both ω and n notations are used interchangeably for numbering double bonds from the methyl end of a fatty acid (see below).

When the methyl end notations are used, a minus sign and number often are placed after them to indicate the location of the first double bond with respect to the methyl carbon; for

	CH_3-	CH_2-	CH_2-	CH_2-	CH_2-	$COOH$
Δ Numbering system	6	5	4	3	2	1
ω or n Numbering system	1	2	3	4	5	6

example, n-3 indicates that the first double bond is located 3-carbons from the methyl group. The location of double bonds in the Δ numbering system can be determined from the ω or n notation if the number of carbons that the fatty acid contains is known. For example, a double bond located in the n-3 position of an 18-carbon fatty acid is at C-15 in the Δ nomenclature, and an n-6 double bond in an 18-carbon fatty acid is at C-12 in the Δ nomenclature.

Fatty acids are abbreviated as the number of carbons and a colon followed by the number of double bonds (e.g., 18:2 represents a fatty acid with 18 carbons and two double bonds). If the fatty acid is unsaturated, the location of the double bonds is placed before the number of carbons. Therefore, the notation for a polyunsaturated fatty acid that contains 18 carbons and two double bonds that are present at C-9 and C-12 is 9,12-18:2. However, the position of the double bonds often is omitted, and the commonly used notation for this fatty acid is 18:2. Although this shortened notation is more convenient, it is best to include the position of the double bonds to avoid confusion in situations where ambiguity might occur.

In every member of the ω3 class, the double bond closest to the methyl end is located 3 carbons from the methyl end:

$$\omega 3\quad \underset{1}{CH_3} - \underset{2}{CH_2} - \underset{3}{CH} = CH -$$

The double bond closest to the methyl end is located 6 carbons from the methyl end in every member of the ω6 class:

$$\omega 6\quad \underset{1}{CH_3} - \underset{2}{CH_2} - \underset{3}{CH_2} - \underset{4}{CH_2} - \underset{5}{CH_2} - \underset{6}{CH} = CH -$$

Humans and other mammals do not have the enzymes necessary to form either the ω3 or ω6 double bonds that are present in essential fatty acids. However, plants have the capacity to synthesize 18-carbon polyunsaturated fatty acids containing these double bonds and are the ultimate sources of essential fatty acids in the human food chain.

Figure 18-1 illustrates the chemical structures of the major ω6 and ω3 fatty acids present in humans and animals. The ω6 fatty acids are shown on the left and the ω3 fatty acids on the right. Although each class contains eight fatty acids, the six fatty acids shown in this figure account for more than 90% of the polyunsaturated fatty acids present in the plasma and tissues under normal physiological conditions.

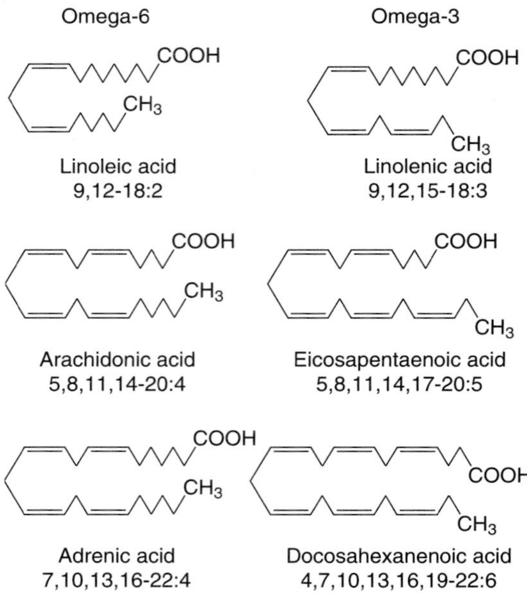

Figure 18-1 Structures of the most prominent ω6 and ω3 essential fatty acids.

ω6 POLYUNSATURATED FATTY ACIDS

Linoleic acid (18:2), the first member of the ω6 series, is the main polyunsaturated fatty acid synthesized by terrestrial plants. It is the most abundant fatty acid contained in the triacylglycerols of corn oil, sunflower seed oil, and safflower oil, and linoleic acid accounts for most of the ω6 fatty acid obtained from the diet. Moreover, because there is much more ω6 than ω3 fatty acid in most foods that we eat, linoleic acid usually is the most abundant polyunsaturated fatty acid in the diet.

The most prominent member of the ω6 series from a functional standpoint is arachidonic acid (20:4). It is the main substrate utilized for the synthesis of the eicosanoid biomediators, such as the prostaglandins and leukotrienes, and it is also a major fatty acid component of the inositol phosphoglycerides.

Although a small amount of arachidonic acid is present in meat and other animal products in the diet, most of the arachidonic acid contained in the body is synthesized from dietary linoleic acid. Adrenic acid (22:4), the elongation product of arachidonic acid, accumulates in tissues that have a high content of arachidonic acid. When necessary, adrenic acid can be converted back to arachidonic acid by removal of two carbons from its carboxyl end.

ω3 POLYUNSATURATED FATTY ACIDS

The ω3 fatty acids are present in large amounts in the retina and certain areas of the brain. Like their ω6 counterparts, ω3 fatty acids can be structurally modified but cannot be synthesized completely in the body and ultimately must be obtained from the diet. The structures of the most important ω3 fatty acids are shown on the right side of Figure 18-1. α-Linolenic acid (18:3), the 18-carbon member, is structurally similar to linoleic acid except for the presence of an additional double bond at C-15. Some terrestrial plants synthesize small amounts of this fatty acid, and α-linolenic is present in soybean oil and canola oil. Larger amounts of α-linolenic acid are produced by vegetation that grows in cold water, and it is a prominent component in the food chain of fish and other marine animals. Although the intestinal mucosa can desaturate α-linolenic acid, most of the dietary intake is incorporated into the intestinal lipoproteins and absorbed by humans without structural modification. α-Linolenic acid (18:3ω3) is commonly called linolenic acid, but α-linolenic is used here to avoid confusion with γ-linolenic acid (18:3ω6).

Members of the ω3 fatty acid class that have five and six double bonds are present in fish, other marine animals, and foods that contain fish oils. The most abundant are eicosapentaenoic acid (20:5; EPA) and docosahexaenoic acid (22:6; DHA), which are often referred to as the fish oil fatty acids. Fish and other marine animals feed on cold-water vegetation and convert the α-linolenic acid to EPA and DHA. Therefore, humans typically ingest a mixture of ω3 fatty acids, with the proportion of α-linolenic acid compared to EPA and DHA depending on the relative intake of plant products as compared with intake of seafood and products containing fish oil. This differs from the ω6 fatty acid dietary intake, which is mostly in the form of linoleic acid.

HIGHLY UNSATURATED FATTY ACIDS

The term "highly unsaturated fatty acids" is used for polyunsaturated fatty acids that contain four or more double bonds. It generally is applied to arachidonic acid (20:4) and adrenic acid (22:4) of the ω6 series and to EPA (20:5) and DHA (22:6) of the ω3 class (see Fig. 18-1). The term was introduced recently to distinguish between the 20- and 22-carbon polyunsaturated fatty acids, which produce most of the functional effects of essential fatty acids, and their 18-carbon precursors, which serve primarily as substrates for the synthesis of these more highly unsaturated derivatives.

ESSENTIAL FATTY ACID METABOLISM

Humans cannot completely synthesize either ω3 or ω6 fatty acids. However, all humans, even infants, can convert the 18-carbon members of each class to the corresponding 20- and 22-carbon products (Salem et al., 1996). It is generally agreed that the human requirement for ω6 fatty acid can be fully satisfied by synthesis from dietary linoleic acid. However, there is ongoing debate as to whether humans, especially infants, can synthesize enough 20- and 22-carbon ω3 fatty acids from α-linolenic acid for optimum growth and development of the neural and visual systems.

The synthesis of the longer, more highly unsaturated derivatives from the 18-carbon members of the ω3 and ω6 classes occurs through the pathway illustrated in Figure 18-2. Three types of reactions are involved; fatty acid chain elongation, desaturation, and retroconversion (Sprecher, 2000). These reactions occur with both ω6 and ω3 fatty acids, but the two classes cannot be interconverted. Therefore, an ω6 fatty acid can be converted only to another ω6 fatty acid, and likewise, an ω3 fatty acid can be converted only to another ω3 fatty acid. Therefore, both classes of essential fatty acids are necessary in the diet.

All the reactions in the polyunsaturated fatty acid metabolic pathway utilize fatty acids in

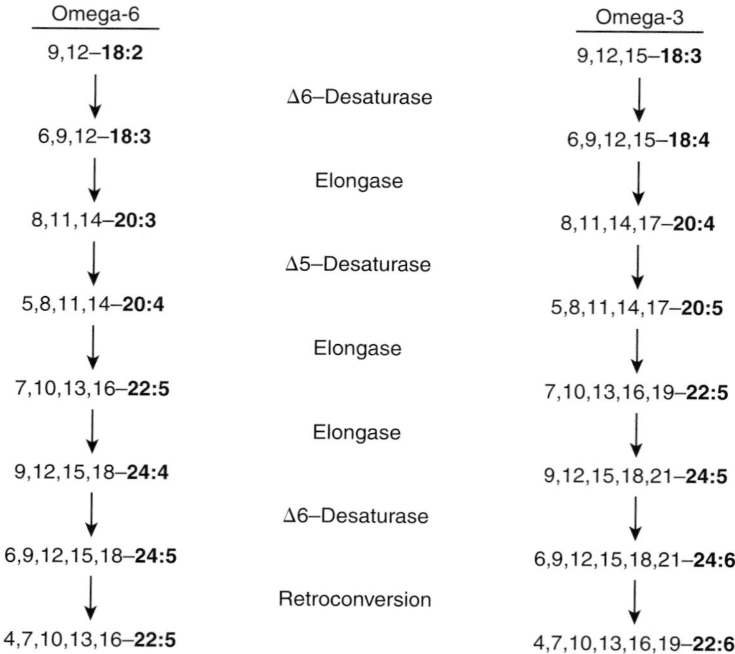

Figure 18-2 Pathway for the conversion of the 18-carbon ω6 and ω3 essential fatty acids to their elongated and more highly unsaturated products in mammalian tissues. The fatty acids are abbreviated as number of carbons and the number of double bonds, separated by a colon. This is preceded by the locations of the double bonds counting from the carboxyl end. Although not evident from the figure, this enzymatic pathway only utilizes fatty acids in the form of fatty acyl CoA.

the form of their esters with coenzyme A (acyl CoAs). The complete pathway involves three elongation reactions, three desaturation reactions, and one retroconversion reaction. Fatty acids containing similar numbers of carbons and double bonds occur in the ω3 and ω6 classes (e.g., 18:3, 20:4, and 22:5). They are positional isomers, not identical compounds. Therefore, the 18:3 in the ω3 pathway is α-linolenic acid (9,12,15-18:3), whereas the 18:3 in the ω6 pathway is γ-linolenic acid (6,9,12-18:3). Likewise, the 20:4 and 22:5 fatty acids that occur in both pathways are isomeric pairs. The 24-carbon fatty acids present in each class are metabolic intermediates that normally do not accumulate in either the plasma or tissues.

Although each of the seven reactions in polyunsaturated fatty acid metabolism can utilize either ω3 or ω6 fatty acids, the pathway functions differently with the two classes of essential fatty acids under normal physiological conditions. The ω3 fatty acids ordinarily pass through the entire pathway, and the most abundant product is DHA. By contrast, the main ω6 fatty acid product normally is arachidonic acid, and the last product normally formed is 22:4. The final three reactions in the ω6 fatty acid metabolic pathway—(1) elongation to a 24-carbon intermediate, (2) Δ6-desaturation of this intermediate, and (3) retroconversion to the 22-carbon end-product—only become prominent when there is an ω3 fatty acid deficiency.

Figure 18-3 shows the fatty acid composition of normal human erythrocytes as determined by gas-liquid chromatography. Much more ω6 than ω3 fatty acids are contained in the erythrocyte lipids. The ω6 fatty acids present are 18:2, 20:3, 20:4, and 22:4, with linoleic acid (18:2) and arachidonic acid (20:4) accounting for about 80% of the total. The small amount of ω3 fatty acid is distributed almost equally between 22:5 and DHA (22:6). A similar distribution normally is present in human plasma and many other human tissues. This distribution reflects the large excess

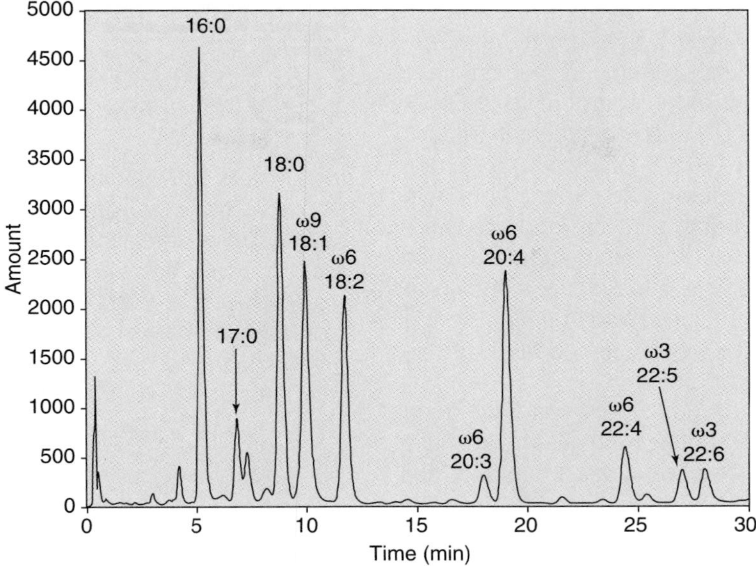

Figure 18-3 Fatty acid composition of the human erythrocyte as determined by gas chromatography. The fatty acids are indicated as the number of carbons followed by a colon and then the number of double bonds. Margaric acid, 17:0, was added as an internal standard for the analysis and is not ordinarily present in erythrocyte lipids. The classes of the unsaturated fatty acids detected in the erythrocyte lipids are ω9, 18:1; ω6, 18:2, 20:3, 20:4, 22:4; ω3, 22:5, 22:6.

of ω6 fatty acids typically present in the diet and the differences in the products that ordinarily accumulate in ω3 as compared with ω6 fatty acid metabolism. The most notable exceptions to this typical fatty acid distribution are the lipids of the retina and brain, which have a very high DHA content.

FATTY ACID ELONGATION

Fatty acids are elongated in the endoplasmic reticulum (ER) through the mechanism illustrated in Figure 18-4. The fatty acid must be in the form of an acyl CoA, and malonyl CoA is the elongating agent. In the condensation reaction, which is the rate-limiting step, the free carboxyl group of malonyl CoA is released as CO_2 and the remaining 2-carbon fragment is attached to the fatty acid carbonyl group by displacement of CoA. Finally, the carbonyl group, which is C-3 in the elongated product, is reduced in a three-step process that utilizes two NADPH molecules.

The position of the double bonds does not shift relative to the methyl end when a polyunsaturated fatty acid is elongated, and their

R—C(=O)—CoA + $^-$OOC—CH$_2$—C(=O)—CoA → R—C(=O)—CH$_2$—C(=O)—CoA + CO_2 + CoA

R—C(=O)—CH$_2$—C(=O)—CoA + NADPH + H^+ → R—CH(OH)—CH$_2$—C(=O)—CoA + $NADP^+$

R—CH(OH)—CH$_2$—C(=O)—CoA → R—CH=CH—C(=O)—CoA + H_2O

R—CH=CH—C(=O)—CoA + NADPH + H^+ → R—CH$_2$—CH$_2$—C(=O)—CoA + $NADP^+$

Figure 18-4 Mechanism of fatty acid chain elongation.

numbering remains the same in the ω or n nomenclature. However, the numbering of the double bonds changes in the Δ nomenclature because the 2-carbon fragment that adds becomes C-1 and C-2 of the lengthened product. Therefore, when 6,9,12-18:3 undergoes one elongation, the resulting 20-carbon fatty acid is 8,11,14-20:3. A fatty acid can undergo more than one elongation. Each elongation sequence consists of the enzymatic reactions shown in Figure 18-4 and utilizes two NADPH, and the fatty acid is lengthened by the addition of two carbons to the carboxyl end.

All the elongation enzymes that have been studied effectively utilize both ω3 and ω6 fatty acids. However, there are at least five different human long-chain fatty acid elongase genes, denoted *ELOVL1-5* (Leonard et al., 2004). The expression of these genes is tissue dependent. Furthermore, each ELOVL enzyme has different substrate specificity, although there is some overlap. For example, ELOVL5 acts on 18- and 20-carbon fatty acids, whereas ELOVL2 and ELOVL4 act on 20- and 22-carbon fatty acids. Consequently, at least two different fatty acid elongation enzymes operating in sequence are needed to convert an 18-carbon polyunsaturated fatty acid to the 24-carbon intermediate, and the enzymes that act in one tissue may be different from those that act in another tissue. These factors make elongation a complicated process that still is not fully understood.

Clinical Correlation

Fatty Acid Δ6-Desaturase Deficiency

A 4-year-old girl who had persistent health problems since birth was referred to a pediatric genetic disease specialist for evaluation because of poor growth, ulcerated cornea, severe photophobia, scaly skin lesions over her arms and legs, and cracking of the skin at the corners of her mouth. Analysis of her plasma revealed abnormally low levels of arachidonic acid and DHA. Supplements of fish oil and of black currant seed oil, which contains γ-linolenic acid (18:3ω6), was prescribed. This treatment corrected the deficiencies of arachidonic acid and DHA in the plasma, and many of her symptoms gradually improved. A skin biopsy subsequently was obtained and fibroblasts were grown in culture. Biochemical studies revealed that the fatty acid Δ6-desaturase activity of the fibroblasts was very low as compared with normal human skin fibroblasts (Williard et al., 2001).

Thinking Critically

1. Why was black current seed oil prescribed instead of corn oil as a source of ω6 fatty acids for this patient?
2. Could capsules containing purified EPA ethyl ester be used instead of fish oil to effectively treat the DHA deficiency in this patient?
3. Would you expect to find an elevation in 20:3ω9 in the patient's plasma?

FATTY ACID DESATURATION

Double bonds are inserted into fatty acids by desaturation, a process that also occurs in the ER. The double bonds that are formed are always in the *cis* configuration. There are two classes of desaturase enzymes: (1) the stearoyl CoA (Δ9) desaturases (SCDs) that act on saturated fatty acids and (2) the fatty acyl CoA desaturases (FADS) that act on polyunsaturated fatty acids.

The FADS enzymes are encoded by two genes: (1) *FADS1* and (2) *FADS2*. *FADS1* encodes the fatty acid Δ5-desaturase, and *FADS2* encodes the fatty acid Δ6-desaturase. The *FADS1* and *FADS2* are located on human chromosome 11q12-q13.1 in reverse orientation, separated by about 10,000 bp (Marquardt et al., 2000). The expression of these two genes is coordinately regulated (Cho et al., 1999). In addition, a third desaturase gene, *FADS3*, is located in the 11q12-q13.1 region, but its function is unknown. Figure 18-2 illustrates where the fatty acid Δ5- and Δ6-desaturases act in essential fatty acid metabolism.

Both fatty acid desaturases can utilize either ω3 or ω6 polyunsaturated acyl CoA substrates, and they both require O_2, NADH, cytochrome b_5, and cytochrome b_5 reductase. Figure 18-5 illustrates the two reactions. The desaturases act on the segment of the acyl CoA chain between the carboxyl group and the first existing double bond. The Δ5-desaturase acts on polyunsaturated acyl CoAs that have

$$R-CH_2-\underset{9}{CH}=\underset{8}{CH}-CH_2-CH_2-CH_2-CH_2-CH_2-CH_2-CO-CoA$$

$$\xrightarrow[\Delta 5\text{-Desaturase}]{O_2,\ NADH + H^+,\ \text{Cytochrome } b_5}$$

$$R-CH_2-\underset{9}{CH}=\underset{8}{CH}-CH_2-\underset{6}{CH}=\underset{5}{CH}-CH_2-CH_2-CH_2-CO-CoA$$

$$R-\underset{10}{CH}=\underset{9}{CH}-CH_2-CH_2-CH_2-CH_2-CH_2-CH_2-CH_2-CO-CoA$$

$$\xrightarrow[\Delta 6\text{-Desaturase}]{O_2,\ NADH + H^+,\ \text{Cytochrome } b_5}$$

$$R-\underset{10}{CH}=\underset{9}{CH}-CH_2-\underset{7}{CH}=\underset{6}{CH}-CH_2-CH_2-CH_2-CH_2-CO-CoA$$

Figure 18-5 Positional differences in the double bonds inserted by the fatty acid Δ5- and Δ6-desaturases.

the first double bond at C-8, inserting the new double bond at C-5. This enzyme acts at only one point in the metabolic pathway, converting 20:3ω6 to arachidonic acid in ω6 fatty acid metabolism and 20:4ω3 to EPA in ω3 fatty acid metabolism. The Δ6-desaturase acts on polyunsaturated fatty acyl CoA substrates that have the first double bond at C-9, and inserts the new double bond at C-6. There is only one fatty acid Δ6-desaturase, and this enzyme functions twice in ω3 fatty acid metabolism, converting α-linolenic acid to 18:4ω3 and 24:5ω3 to 24:6ω3 (Sprecher, 2000). The Δ6-desaturase ordinarily functions only once in ω6 fatty acid metabolism, converting linoleic acid to 18:3ω6. It also is capable of converting 24:4ω6 to 24:5ω6, but this occurs to an appreciable extent only if there is a deficiency of ω3 fatty acids.

RETROCONVERSION

Conversion of the 24-carbon acyl CoA intermediates to the 22-carbon end products occurs through peroxisomal fatty acid oxidation, a β-oxidation system that functions to shorten very long-chain fatty acids. This process requires transport of the 24-carbon intermediate from the ER to the peroxisomes and, subsequently, transport of the 22-carbon product back to the ER where it is incorporated into tissue lipids. Recent evidence suggests that these transport processes may be mediated by cytosolic fatty acid binding proteins (Norris and Spector, 2002).

As shown in Figure 18-6, the retroconversion reaction requires O_2, FAD, NAD^+, and CoA, and it removes two carbons in the form of acetyl CoA from the carboxyl end of the fatty acyl CoA. The peroxisomal enzymes that catalyze this β-oxidation process are straight-chain acyl CoA oxidase, D-bifunctional protein (D-3-hydroxyacyl CoA dehydrogenase) and either 3-ketoacyl CoA thiolase or sterol carrier protein X (Ferdinandusse et al., 2001). In ω3 fatty acid metabolism, this process converts 24:6ω3 to DHA (22:6ω3). The numbering of the carbons in the Δ nomenclature changes when retroconversion occurs because the carbons that were numbered 1 and 2 in the original fatty acid are removed. Therefore, the C-6 double bond in the 24-carbon intermediate becomes the C-4 double bond of DHA, the 22-carbon product.

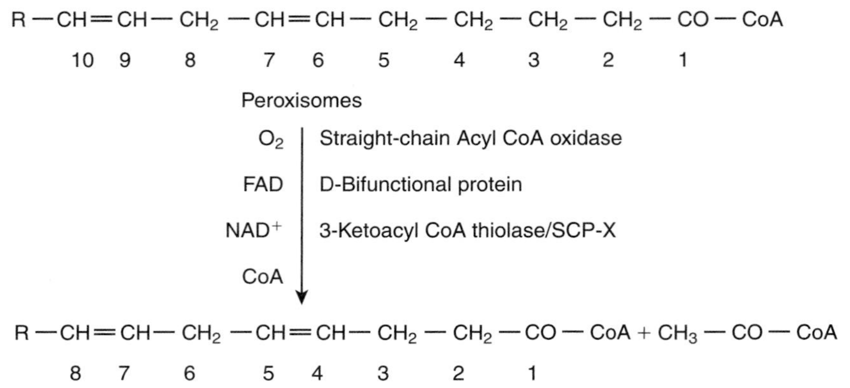

$R-CH=CH-CH_2-CH=CH-CH_2-CH_2-CH_2-CH_2-CO-CoA$

10 9 8 7 6 5 4 3 2 1

Peroxisomes

O_2 | Straight-chain Acyl CoA oxidase

FAD | D-Bifunctional protein

NAD^+ | 3-Ketoacyl CoA thiolase/SCP-X

CoA ↓

$R-CH=CH-CH_2-CH=CH-CH_2-CH_2-CO-CoA + CH_3-CO-CoA$

8 7 6 5 4 3 2 1

Figure 18-6 Retroconversion reaction that occurs in essential fatty acid metabolism. *SCP-X* is the abbreviation for sterol carrier protein-X.

Although a similar process can occur with ω6 fatty acids to produce 22:5ω6, the main function of retroconversion in ω6 fatty acid metabolism is to produce arachidonic acid from 22:4ω6. Likewise, in the ω3 pathway, DHA can be retroconverted to EPA. Therefore, just as linoleic and α-linolenic acids can be converted to their longer, more highly unsaturated derivatives, the 22-carbon members of the ω3 and ω6 classes can serve as a source of the corresponding shorter 20-carbon fatty acids. This enables the body to utilize whichever ω3 and ω6 fatty acids are available in the diet to produce all of the necessary members of these essential fatty acid classes.

Peroxisomal fatty acid β-oxidation is deficient in cells of patients with Zellweger's syndrome, a genetic defect in the biogenesis of peroxisomes. Patients who inherit this severe neurological disease have low levels of DHA because they cannot carry out the peroxisomal retroconversion step needed to produce DHA from ω3 fatty acid precursors. Dietary supplements containing DHA appear to improve the clinical condition in some of these patients (Martinez, 2001).

TISSUE DIFFERENCES

Differences in dietary intake and metabolism lead to the accumulation of different types of essential fatty acids in the body. Linoleic acid is the most abundant polyunsaturated fatty acid in the diet and, therefore, the ω6 fatty acids predominate in the plasma and most tissues. Many tissues are able to convert linoleic to arachidonic acid through the pathway illustrated in Figure 18-2, and linoleic and arachidonic acids are the main ω6 fatty acids that accumulate in the body.

Very little α-linolenic acid ordinarily is present in the plasma or tissues, and unless the diet is supplemented with fish oil or ω3 fatty acid ethyl esters, there also is little EPA. Tissues like the retina and brain that have a high content of ω3 fatty acids contain mostly DHA. Some DHA is obtained directly from the diet, and dietary DHA is an important source of DHA for the brain (Su et al., 1999). The remainder is obtained by synthesis from α-linolenic acid and other ω3 fatty acids that may be present in the diet. Hepatocytes express the complete metabolic pathway shown in Figure 18-2, but many other cells normally do not convert α-linolenic acid to DHA and depend on the circulation for a supply of DHA synthesized elsewhere in the body. For example, the retina utilizes DHA that is formed in the liver from ω3 fatty acid precursors (Scott and Bazan, 1989). Similarly, neurons utilize DHA that is synthesized from α-linolenic acid by the combined actions of the astrocytes (neuroglial cells) and the microvascular endothelial cells that form the blood-brain barrier (Edmond, 2001; Moore, 2001).

ESSENTIAL FATTY ACID COMPOSITION OF PLASMA AND TISSUE LIPIDS

Human plasma contains a wide variety of essential fatty acids. The data in Table 18-1 were

Table 18-1

Essential Fatty Acid Composition of Normal Human Serum Lipids

		Lipoprotein Lipids		
Fatty Acid*	**Free Fatty Acids**	**Phospholipids†**	**Triacylglycerols**	**Cholesteryl Esters‡**
	(Fraction of Total Fatty Acids [% by Weight])			
ω3				
18:3	0.71 ± 0.11	0.21 ± 0.03	1.18 ± 0.08	0.50 ± 0.06
22:6	0.34 ± 0.06	2.23 ± 0.14	0.35 ± 0.04	0.49 ± 0.08
ω6§				
18:2	15.60 ± 0.63	22.94 ± 0.57	19.54 ± 0.84	49.82 ± 1.79
20:3	0.14 ± 0.04	3.11 ± 0.12	0.36 ± 0.05	0.91 ± 0.06
20:4	1.25 ± 0.17	10.95 ± 0.45	1.64 ± 0.14	8.08 ± 0.39

Modified from data compiled by Edelstein C (1986) General properties of plasma lipoproteins and apoproteins. In: Scanu AM, Spector AA (eds) Biochemistry and Biology of the Plasma Lipoproteins. Marcel Dekker, New York, pp 495-505.
*Abbreviated as the number of carbons and number of double bonds.
†Phospholipids contain 0.65 ± 0.08% 20:5ω3 and 0.77 ± 0.03% 22:5ω3. The other lipid fractions contain only trace amounts (<0.3%) of these ω3 fatty acids.
‡Cholesteryl esters contain 1.07 ± 0.07% 18:3ω6, but the other lipid fractions contain only trace amounts.
§The lipids contain only trace amounts (<0.5%) of 22:4ω6 and 22:5ω6.

obtained from human subjects who consumed Western diets, which ordinarily contain about 10 times more ω6 than ω3 fatty acids. These data show that ω3 fatty acids comprise only 1% to 3% of the total fatty acids in any of the serum lipid fractions. By contrast, ω6 fatty acids account for 17% of the fatty acids in the plasma free fatty acid fraction, 37% in phospholipids, 22% in triacylglycerols, and 60% in cholesteryl esters. Linoleic and arachidonic acids comprise most of the ω6 fatty acids contained in these serum lipids.

After an individual eats, the fatty acid composition of the triacylglycerols contained in chylomicrons, the lipoproteins produced by the small intestine, reflects that of the dietary fat. Therefore, in the immediate postprandial state, chylomicrons are a major source of essential fatty acids for the tissues. The other plasma lipoproteins and albumin continue to provide essential fatty acids to the tissues after the chylomicrons are removed from the circulation. Even though the concentrations of arachidonic acid and DHA are very low in the plasma free fatty acid pool, studies in the rat indicate that the rates of utilization of these unesterified fatty acids are sufficiently rapid to supply the needs of the brain (Rapoport et al., 2001).

Essential fatty acids in tissues are contained primarily in phospholipids. They are located almost entirely in the phospholipid *sn*-2 position, the middle carbon of the glycerol moiety. Although each phospholipid class contains a mixture of essential fatty acids, one or two fatty acids usually predominate in each phospholipid class. Arachidonic acid is highly enriched in the inositol phosphoglycerides, whereas linoleic and arachidonic acids are contained in large amounts in the choline phosphoglycerides. The 22-carbon members, DHA and adrenic acid (22:4ω6), tend to accumulate in the ethanolamine and serine phosphoglycerides, and DHA is highly enriched in the ethanolamine plasmalogens. These differences in fatty acid distribution are due primarily to the substrate specificities of the acyltransferases that incorporate the acyl CoAs into the *sn*-2 position of the phospholipids.

ESSENTIAL FATTY ACID FUNCTION

The ω3 and ω6 classes of fatty acids are essential primarily because they are required for two important physiological processes, the synthesis of lipid biomediators and the production of membrane phospholipids that have optimal structural and signal transduction properties. Because these are fundamental processes, it is surprising that some animal cell lines can grow in culture for many passages in the absence of

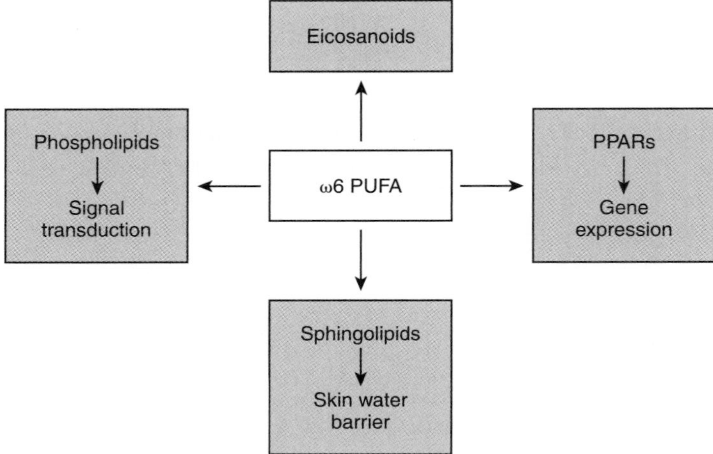

Figure 18-7 Physiological functions of the ω6 essential fatty acids. *PUFA,* Polyunsaturated fatty acid; *PPARs,* peroxisome proliferator-activated receptors.

Nutrition Insight

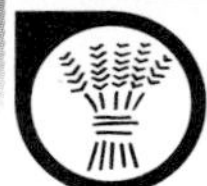

Dietary Effects on Membrane Fatty Acid Composition

Modifying the dietary fat intake can alter the fatty acid composition of membrane phospholipids. Even the fatty acid composition of the heart, which one might think of as a very stable tissue, can be modified rapidly in experimental animals. The brain is the only organ that is resistant to such diet-induced changes. Except for those in the brain, the fatty acid composition of most membranes adapts to some extent to the type of fat available in the diet. This flexibility is surprising, considering the vital role that membranes play in so many cellular functions. Diet-induced changes in membrane lipid composition support the old saying that "you are what you eat." However, there are limits to the extent of change that can take place in mammalian cells. Most of the variation occurs in the relative proportions of unsaturated fatty acids. For example, if the diet is enriched in sunflower seed oil, which contains 70% linoleic acid, the ω6 fatty acid content of the membrane phospholipids increases and is counterbalanced by a decrease in oleic acid. This reduction in monounsaturated fatty acid content is a compensation that protects against an excessive increase in membrane fluidity due to overabundance of unsaturated fatty acid in the membrane phospholipids. The relative amounts of ω3 and ω6 fatty acids in membrane phospholipids also is dependent on the dietary intake of these essential fatty acids.

any detectable essential fatty acids. Many of these cell lines were derived from rodent malignant tumors that do not express the fatty acid Δ6-desaturase. Although a few biochemical functions are slightly compromised in these cells, they are viable and grow well. Therefore, essential fatty acids apparently are not required for the maintenance of basic life processes in a mammalian cell. The functions of essential fatty acids appear to become necessary when cells differentiate and form multicellular organisms, where intercellular communication, highly specialized membrane functions, and coordination of gene expression become vital.

ω6 POLYUNSATURATED FATTY ACIDS

Figure 18-7 illustrates the main functions of the ω6 fatty acids. These processes must operate properly for the body to function normally. Linoleic and arachidonic acid have membrane structural effects, and linoleic acid is especially required as a component of sphingolipids that prevent water loss from the skin. Arachidonic acid is the primary substrate for eicosanoid synthesis, and it is a major component of the inositol phosphoglycerides that are involved in membrane signal transduction. In addition, ω6 fatty acids and some of the eicosanoids are ligands for the peroxisome proliferator-activated receptors (PPARs), and thereby affect the expression of many genes involved in lipid metabolism.

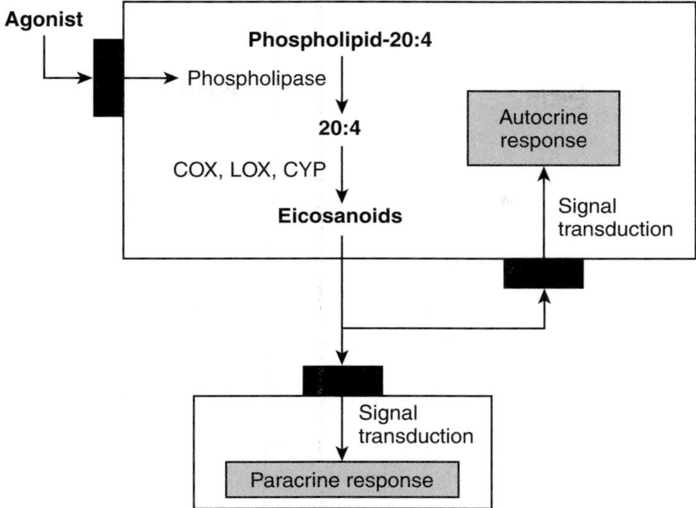

Figure 18-8 Synthesis and mechanism of action of eicosanoids. *COX,* Cyclooxygenase; *CYP,* cytochrome P450; *LOX,* lipoxygenase.

Arachidonic Acid and Eicosanoids

Eicosanoids synthesized from arachidonic acid are lipid biomediators that regulate many cellular functions. Figure 18-8 illustrates the production and action of these compounds. The binding of a cytokine or hormone to a plasma membrane receptor triggers eicosanoid production by the target cell via activation of a calcium-dependent cytoplasmic phospholipase A_2. This phospholipase hydrolyzes arachidonic acid from the *sn*-2 position of intracellular membrane phospholipids, primarily choline phosphoglycerides. The cyclooxygenase (COX), lipoxygenase, and/or cytochrome P450 pathways contained in the cell convert the arachidonic acid to one or more eicosanoid products. A major function of eicosanoids is cell-to-cell communication. These compounds are released into the extracellular fluid and function as autocrine and paracrine mediators by binding to plasma membrane GTP-binding protein (G-protein)–coupled receptors that either activate or modulate the activity of intracellular signaling pathways. Some of the responses occur very rapidly, whereas others that involve transcriptional mechanisms occur more slowly.

Figure 18-9 lists the types of eicosanoids formed by the COX, lipoxygenase, and cytochrome P450 pathways and illustrates the structures of several representative products. The cyclooxygenase pathway produces prostaglandins and thromboxanes. There are two cyclooxygenase isozymes, a constitutive form (COX-1) and an inducible form (COX-2). The structure of prostaglandin E_2 (PGE_2), one of the major prostaglandins, is shown. The subscript 2 denotes that the eicosanoid has two double bonds outside the ring structure, a characteristic of all COX products synthesized from arachidonic acid. Eicosanoids formed by the COX pathway have many physiological actions, including modulation of cardiovascular and renal function, blood coagulation, and inflammation.

Lipoxygenases convert arachidonic acid to a hydroperoxyeicosatetraenoic acid (HPETE). There are three isozymes, 5-, 12-, and 15-lipoxygenase, which differ in their positional specificity for the arachidonic acid double bonds. The HPETE then is converted to a hydroxyeicosatetraenoic acid (HETE), leukotriene, or lipoxin. The structure of leukotriene B_4 (LTB_4), one of the main leukotrienes, is shown. Lipoxygenase products function primarily in the tissue response to inflammatory stimuli.

Cytochrome P450 epoxygenases convert arachidonic acid to epoxyeicosatrienoic acids (EETs). The structure of 5,6-EET, one of the four EET positional isomers, is shown. Another class of cytochrome P450 enzymes, the ω-oxidases, insert a hydroxyl group at or

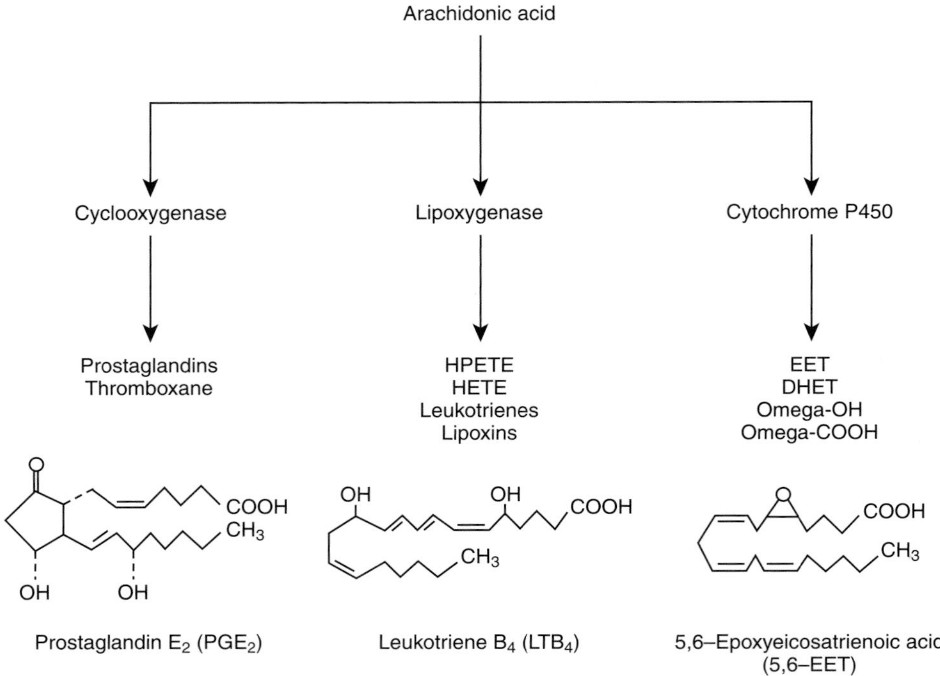

Figure 18-9 Pathways of eicosanoid synthesis and structures of some representative products. *HPETE,* Hydroperoxyeicosatetraenoic acid; *HETE,* hydroxyeicosatetraenoic acid; *EET,* epoxyeicosatrienoic acid; *DHET,* dihydroxyeicosatrienoic acid; *omega-OH* and *omega-COOH* refer to 20-hydroxy or 20-carboxy eicosatetraenoic products.

near the methyl terminus of arachidonic acid; 20-HETE is the main product. Eicosanoids formed by the cytochrome P450 pathway act on small arteries and in the kidney. They modulate vascular resistance and blood pressure.

Table 18-2 lists the prostaglandin receptors, the main prostanoids that they bind, the biochemical mechanism of action, and the physiological responses that are produced. Eight different types of prostaglandin receptors have been cloned; they are all G protein–coupled receptors. Although there is some overlap in substrate specificity, each type is designated according to the main product that it binds. For example, IP is the PGI receptor, and EP is a PGE receptor. The four subtypes of EP receptors have different tissue distributions, are linked to different G-proteins, and produce different functional responses.

Prostaglandin-mediated signaling is a very complicated process that can occur in different ways, depending on the type of prostaglandin and the receptor to which it binds. One mechanism is activation of adenylate cyclase. PGI_2 functions in this way. It binds to the IP receptor, which is coupled to a G_s protein. This activates adenylate cyclase, causing a large increase in cyclic adenosine monophosphate (cAMP) within the target cell. PGE_2 produces a similar response when it binds to the EP_2 receptor. However, when PGE_2 binds to the EP_3 receptor, it activates a G_i protein that reduces adenylate cyclase activity, thereby decreasing cAMP production. To further complicate matters, PGE_2 also can bind to EP_1 receptors, which are coupled to G-proteins that activate phospholipase C. This stimulates hydrolysis of phosphatidylinositol 4,5-bisphosphate, producing an increase in the cytosolic calcium concentration.

Inositol Phosphoglycerides

Another important function of arachidonic acid is phospholipid-mediated signal transduction. In particular, the inositol phosphoglycerides that activate the intracellular protein kinase C signaling pathway contain a relatively high percentage of arachidonic acid. When phospholipase C is activated and hydrolyzes

Table 18-2
Prostaglandin Receptors

Receptor	Main Ligand	Signal Transduction Mechanism	Major Physiological Functions
DP	PGD_2	Inositol phospholipids Increases intracellular Ca^{2+}	Platelet aggregation Smooth muscle contraction
EP_1	PGE_2	Inositol phospholipids Increases intracellular Ca^{2+}	Smooth muscle contraction
EP_2	PGE_2	Adenylate cyclase Increases cAMP	Smooth muscle relaxation
EP_3	PGE_2	Adenylate cyclase Decreases cAMP	Decreases water reabsorption Inhibits gastric acid secretion Uterine contraction
EP_4	PGE_2	Adenylate cyclase Increases cAMP	Smooth muscle relaxation
FP	$PGF_{2\alpha}$	Inositol phospholipids Increases intracellular Ca^{2+}	Smooth muscle contraction
IP	PGI_2	Adenylate cyclase Increases cAMP	Arterial smooth muscle relaxation Inhibits platelet aggregation
TP	TXA_2	Inositol phospholipids Increases intracellular Ca^{2+}	Platelet aggregation Vasoconstriction Bronchoconstriction

PG, Prostaglandin; *TX,* thromboxane.

phosphatidylinositol 4,5-bisphosphate, the resulting 1,2-diacylglycerol that is involved in activating protein kinase C contains the arachidonic acid. The function of the high arachidonic acid content is not known. The possibilities include targeting to specific membrane domains or imparting special binding properties to the diacylglycerol. Alternatively, the diacylglycerol may be hydrolyzed by a diacylglycerol lipase, releasing the arachidonic acid for eicosanoid production.

Linoleic Acid

The average intake of ω6 fatty acids in healthy adults, 11 to 17 g/day, greatly exceeds the amount of arachidonic acid needed for the synthesis of the eicosanoid biomediators. This suggests either that there are other actions of arachidonic acid or that other ω6 fatty acids have essential functions. Emphasis has focused on the skin because essential fatty acid deficiency leads to a breakdown of the epidermal barrier to water loss. Linoleic acid is strongly preferred for the synthesis of two sphingolipids, acylceramide, and acylglucosylceramide, which maintain the structure of the stratum corneum, the outer layer of the skin. This suggests that linoleic acid is required to impart an optimal barrier property to the skin surface sphingolipids, thereby preventing excessive water loss.

Lipoxygenase enzymes can oxygenate linoleic acid, adding oxygen at one of its double bonds. 15-Lipoxygenase is the main lipoxygenase that acts on linoleic acid in human tissues, forming the 13-hydroperoxyoctadecadienoic acid. This product is reduced to the corresponding hydroxy-derivative, 13-hydroxyoctadecadienoic acid (13-HODE). No physiological requirement for this or other oxygenated linoleic acid derivatives has been established, and it is uncertain as to whether the lipoxygenase pathway of linoleic acid metabolism has any essential function.

A decrease in the level of plasma low density lipoproteins (LDLs) occurs when fats enriched in linoleic acid, such as corn oil or safflower oil, are substituted for dietary saturated fats. LDLs contain the highest percentage of cholesterol in the plasma, and a decrease in

LDL level reduces the risk of developing coronary heart disease. The mechanism producing the decrease in LDL level is complex and may depend more on the reduction in saturated fat intake rather than a direct biochemical effect produced by linoleic acid or one of its ω6 fatty acid products. Although it is unlikely that reduction of the LDL level is an essential function of linoleic acid, it certainly is one that has health benefits.

ω3 POLYUNSATURATED FATTY ACIDS

Two approaches have been used to investigate the functions of ω3 fatty acids. One is to determine the effects of ω3 fatty acid–deficient diets in experimental animals. The other is to study humans who consume a diet high in ω3 fatty acids or who are treated with dietary supplements containing either fish oil or ω3 fatty acid ethyl esters. Table 18-3 lists the biochemical and biophysical functions of ω3 fatty acids. EPA produces some of these effects, and DHA produces the others. No unique functional effects have been reported for α-linolenic acid in humans or animals, except to serve the substrate for EPA and DHA synthesis.

Table 18-3
Biochemical and Biophysical Functions of ω3 Fatty Acids

Fatty Acid	Function
EPA	Production of ω3 eicosanoids
EPA	Inhibition of ω6 eicosanoid production
EPA	Inhibition of hepatic triglyceride synthesis
DHA	Enhanced coupling of rhodopsin to the retinal G protein
DHA	Increased plasmalogen synthesis
DHA	Ligand for brain RXR nuclear receptor
DHA	Docosanoid synthesis
DHA	Nonbilayer phospholipid configuration
Not specified	Modulation of sodium ion channel conductance
Not specified	Ligand for PPAR nuclear receptors

DHA, Docosahexaenoic acid; *EPA,* eicosapentaenoic acid; *PPAR,* peroxisome proliferator-activated receptor; *RXR,* retinoid X receptor.

Eicosapentaenoic Acid

EPA is primarily responsible for the antithrombotic and antiinflammatory actions produced by ω3 fatty acid dietary supplements. This occurs through an effect on eicosanoid production. The suggested mechanism is illustrated schematically in Figure 18-10.

The COX and lipoxygenase pathways can convert EPA to eicosanoids. Although these EPA products have bioactivity, no unique or vital function has been demonstrated for them. Furthermore, EPA is a poor substrate for COX as compared with arachidonic acid, but it effectively inhibits the conversion of arachidonic acid to COX products, especially thromboxane A_2, which triggers platelet aggregation and thrombosis. EPA may produce its inhibitory effects by competing with arachidonic acid for incorporation into the tissue phospholipids that supply

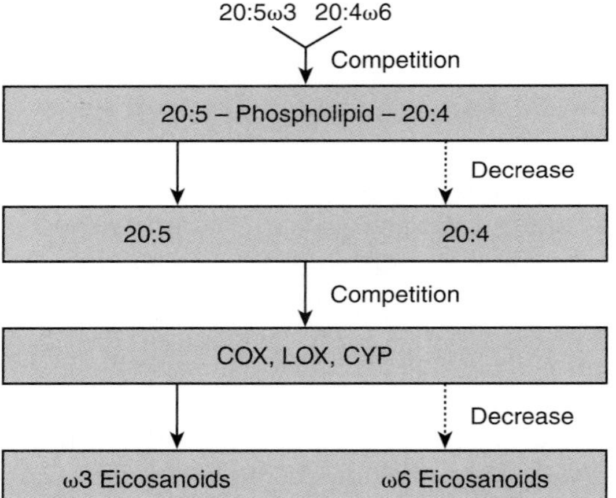

Figure 18-10 Competition between EPA (20:5ω3) and arachidonic acid (20:4ω6) for eicosanoid synthesis. These essential fatty acids compete for incorporation into the membrane phospholipids that provide the fatty acid substrate for eicosanoid synthesis. Both fatty acids are released when phospholipase A_2 hydrolyzes the phospholipids. Although they compete effectively for access to the eicosanoid-producing enzymes, EPA is a less effective substrate. As a result there is a reduction in the quantity of eicosanoids synthesized from arachidonic acid without a compensatory replacement by products formed from EPA. In some cases, the products formed from EPA also have less bioactivity. The overall effect is a reduction in the eicosanoid response to cellular activation. The abbreviations are the same as in Figure 18-8.

substrate for eicosanoid synthesis. When cells are exposed to supplemental EPA, the arachidonic acid content of the phospholipids decreases and is replaced by EPA and its elongation product 22:5ω3. As a result, less arachidonic acid is released when phospholipases are activated, so that less is available for eicosanoid synthesis. The amount of COX products synthesized from EPA is either too small to compensate for the decrease in arachidonic acid products, or the eicosanoids produced from EPA have less bioactivity. This, combined with reduction in arachidonic acid availability, makes EPA an effective modulator of arachidonic acid function.

EPA also produces the hypotriglyceridemic effect of fish oil, primarily by increasing mitochondrial β-oxidation (Frøyland et al., 1997). In addition, it probably contributes the antihypertensive effects of fish oil. These actions, together with its antiinflammatory and antithrombotic effects, can prevent or reduce the severity of life-threatening illnesses. However, none of these effects is likely to be essential for the maintenance of normal bodily function. Therefore, EPA probably is not the essential component of the ω3 fatty acids.

Clinical Correlation

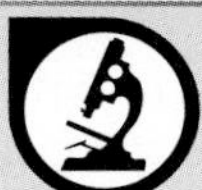

Fish Oil for the Prevention of Coronary Thrombosis

Daily fish oil supplements are being recommended by some physicians to reduce the risk of coronary thrombosis. Patients usually take between 1 and 3 g/day, administered either in the form of fish oil capsules or capsules containing purified EPA and DHA ethyl esters.

Thinking Critically

1. How might ω3 fatty acids act to reduce the risk of coronary thrombosis?
2. Would the administration of canola oil, which contains α-linolenic acid as the only source of ω3 fatty acid, be as effective as fish oil for this purpose?

Docosahexaenoic Acid

DHA, which is highly enriched in retinal and brain phospholipids, is responsible for the visual and cognitive actions of the ω3 fatty acids. It is present in the phospholipids of cell membranes, primarily in the ethanolamine and serine phosphoglycerides and ethanolamine plasmalogens. These phospholipids are contained primarily in the inner (cytoplasmic) leaflet of the membrane lipid bilayer, so the functional effects produced by DHA most likely occur in this region of the membrane. The DHA chains contained in phospholipids are highly flexible and transition very rapidly between a large number of conformations, providing an optimum microenvironment for the function of certain proteins that are embedded in the membrane (Gawrisch et al., 2003).

Phospholipids enriched in DHA augment the response of the retina to light and enhance the transmission of the visual signal. The retinal light receptor, rhodopsin, is a G protein–coupled receptor. When rhodopsin is activated by light, the structure of the surrounding phospholipid DHA fatty acyl chains facilitates the conformational change of rhodopsin to the metarhodopsin II state, increasing the rate of coupling to the retinal G-protein. This enhances the amplification in the first stage of the visual pathway. The high DHA content of the retinal phospholipids also increases the activity of the phosphodiesterase, which is a measure of the integrated visual signal response (Mitchell et al., 2003). The need for DHA to produce optimum membrane lipid bilayer properties in the retina for the visual response is one reason why ω3 fatty acids are essential nutrients. If a similar DHA-mediated mechanism applies to G protein–coupled receptor signaling in the brain, it also may explain the cognitive benefits produced by ω3 fatty acids (Moriguchi et al., 2000).

Biophysical studies indicate that some phospholipids have a tendency not to form a bilayer structure. One of the alternate arrangements is a hexagonal structure, an inverted configuration in which the polar head groups of the phospholipids cluster together on the inside and the hydrocarbon chains point outward. Phosphatidylethanolamine has an increased tendency to form this type of hexagonal arrangement when it contains a high percentage of DHA. The tendency to form such a structure may affect the packing of the phospholipid head groups at the surface of the lipid bilayer and thereby change the surface properties of the membrane. This is likely to facilitate vesicle formation and membrane–vesicle fusion. Furthermore, the transient formation of a hexagonal structure in a membrane domain might allow the passage of a polar solute through the lipid bilayer by creating a temporary aqueous channel in the center of the clustered phospholipid head groups. The unique properties of phospholipids enriched in DHA might be necessary for the optimum function of membranes such as neural synapses that must rapidly respond to excitation, and this probably is another reason why ω3 fatty acids are essential.

A relationship exists between DHA and plasmalogens, a class of membrane phospholipids that contains a vinyl ether group (Nagan and Zoeller, 2001). Low tissue levels of DHA occur in genetic diseases associated with plasmalogen deficiency, and mutant cell lines that are deficient in plasmalogens incorporate less than the usual amount of DHA. The functions of plasmalogens include membrane–vesicle fusion, intracellular signal transduction, and protection against oxidant stress. However, it is uncertain whether supplying DHA for plasmalogen synthesis is an essential function of ω3 fatty acids.

DHA also can be oxygenated stereospecifically, producing bioactive hydroxylated derivatives called docosanoids. These compounds are antiinflammatory and protect against brain injury due to ischemia-reperfusion (Marcheselli et al., 2003). One pathway that is initiated by 15-lipoxygenase produces a group of DHA derivatives that contain a 17(S)-hydroxyl group. Two of the products formed are 10,17(S)-docosatriene and 4,17(S)-dihydroxy-DHA. A second pathway that converts DHA to resolvins is initiated when COX-2 is inhibited by aspirin. Resolvins are DHA derivatives that contain a 17(R)-hydroxyl group, such as 7,8,17(R)-trihydroxy-DHA. Additional studies are needed to determine whether docosanoids have an essential function and, hence, whether another reason for the essentiality of ω3 fatty acids is to supply DHA for the synthesis of this recently discovered class of bioactive compounds.

The ω3 fatty acids also decrease fatal heart arrhythmias in experimental models by modulating the conductance of ion channels in cardiac myocyte membranes (Leaf et al., 2003). The interaction of the ion channel with ω3 fatty acyl chains causes a conformational change that alters the conductance of the channel. Although this effect can be life-saving, the modulation of ion channel conductance probably is a pharmacological action rather than an essential function of ω3 fatty acids.

REGULATION OF GENE EXPRESSION BY ESSENTIAL FATTY ACIDS

Essential fatty acids regulate the expression of many genes involved in fatty acid and glucose metabolism (Jump, 2002; Ntambi and Bené, 2001). Dietary studies with corn oil and fish oil indicate that Δ6-desaturation must occur before either ω3 or ω6 fatty acids become transcriptionally active; in other words, linoleic acid (9,12-18:2) is inactive, but its derivatives such as arachidonic acid (5,8,11,14-20:4) that have undergone Δ6-desaturation are effective. Table 18-4 lists some of the genes that are regulated by the highly unsaturated forms of essential fatty acids. These genes control fatty acid synthesis, mitochondrial and peroxisomal fatty acid oxidation, saturated fatty acid desaturation, the synthesis of fatty acid binding proteins, and insulin-mediated glucose utilization.

Essential fatty acids exert their transcriptional effects by regulating the activity of three major classes of transcription factors; PPAR, liver X receptor (LXR), and sterol regulatory element binding protein (SREBP). PPARs become activated when they bind either polyunsaturated fatty acids or their eicosanoid derivatives. Lipid binding also activates LXR, but SREBP activation occurs through an entirely different mechanism. Increases in polyunsaturated fatty acids inhibit the proteolytic process that releases the transcription factor domain from intact SREBP. This decreases the amount of active SREBP available for transport to the nucleus. SREBP-1c, the form that regulates fatty acid metabolism, is especially responsive to polyunsaturated fatty acids. Dietary fish oil

Table 18-4
Representative Genes Regulated by Essential Fatty Acids or their Products

Gene	Function
Acyl CoA oxidase	Peroxisomal fatty acid β-oxidation
Acyl CoA synthase	Conversion of fatty acids to fatty acyl CoA
Adipocyte-fatty acid binding protein	Intracellular fatty acid transport
CYP4A6	Fatty acid ω-oxidation
D-Bifunctional protein	Peroxisomal fatty acid β-oxidation
Fatty acid synthase	Synthesis of saturated fatty acids from acetyl CoA
Glucose 6-phosphate dehydrogenase	NADPH production
Liver–fatty acid binding protein	Intracellular fatty acid transport
Malic enzyme	NADPH production
Medium-chain acyl CoA dehydrogenase	Mitochondrial fatty acid β-oxidation
Stearoyl CoA desaturase	Desaturation of saturated fatty acids

is more effective than safflower oil in suppressing SREBP-1c processing, indicating that this is primarily an effect of ω3 fatty acids. These fatty acids also regulate the transcription of the *SREBP-1c* gene and the stability of the SREBP-1c mRNA.

In addition, DHA can modulate gene expression through a different mechanism. It binds to and activates the retinoid X receptor (RXR) in the brain (Mata de Urquiza et al., 2000). The activated RXR forms heterodimers with PPAR and LXR, as well as with the thyroid hormone receptor, vitamin D receptor, and retinoic acid receptor. Each of these transcription factors must form a heterodimer with RXR in order to bind to the response elements in the promoter of their target genes (see Chapter 30). Therefore, DHA has the potential to exert widespread and very complex effects on gene expression in the central nervous system.

RECOMMENDATIONS FOR ESSENTIAL FATTY ACID INTAKE

Recommended dietary allowances have not been established for either ω6 or ω3 fatty acids because available information is not adequate to estimate average requirements. However, the Institute of Medicine ([IOM] 2002), in setting the dietary reference intakes, did establish adequate intakes (AIs) for essential fatty acids. The AIs for infants in the first 6 months of life were calculated from the ω3 and ω6 contents of human milk (5.6 g ω6/L and 0.63 g ω3/L) and the average intake of milk (0.78 L/day). Those for infants in the second 6 months of life were calculated based on intake of milk plus complementary foods. The AIs for children and adults, as well as for pregnant and lactating women, were set as the median intakes of linoleic acid (18:2ω6) and of α-linolenic acid (18:3ω3) for each age/sex group in the United States. It was assumed that median intakes in the United States are adequate because essential fatty acid deficiency is essentially nonexistent in healthy individuals in this population. Linoleic acid is the primary ω6 fatty acid in the diet, and the body readily converts linoleic to arachidonic acid. However, both EPA and DHA, in addition to α-linolenic acid, may be important sources of ω3 fatty acid intake, particularly if fish products are part of the diet. The IOM (2002) also established acceptable macronutrient distribution ranges (AMDRs) for the essential fatty acids. The AMDR for linoleic acid is 5% to 10% of energy and that for α-linolenic acid is 0.6% to 1.2 % of energy.

Upper tolerable limits were not set for essential fatty acids because of the lack of a defined level at which adverse effects can occur. Although there is some evidence suggesting that high intakes of ω3 fatty acids, particularly EPA and DHA, may impair immune response and result in prolonged bleeding times, the highest intakes of EPA and DHA reported in the Continuing Survey of Food Intakes by Individuals (CSFII, 1994-1996, 1998) were 0.66 and 0.65 g/day, respectively, which are only about one fifth of the intake of Greenland Eskimos.

ESSENTIAL FATTY ACID DEFICIENCY

An illness develops if the diet is deficient in essential fatty acids over a prolonged period. Although the dietary deficiency usually involves both classes of essential fatty acids, the ω6 fatty acids are depleted from the tissues much more rapidly than DHA. Therefore, the symptoms observed when the disease manifests itself are due to a deficiency in ω6 fatty acids. In practical terms, essential fatty acid deficiency is caused by a dietary deficiency of linoleic acid. The diagnostic signs are dermatitis, poor wound healing, and in infants and children, failure to grow. A relatively small linoleic acid intake, between 3 and 5 g/day for the average adult, is sufficient to prevent this disease. Because most diets contain far more linoleic acid, often 20 g/day or more, essential fatty acid deficiency is extremely rare. It occurs primarily in patients who are not able to eat because of serious injury or major surgery and who receive total parenteral nutrition without an adequate source of essential fatty acids for an extended period.

A biomarker that is diagnostic for essential fatty acid deficiency is a large increase in the plasma concentration of the ω9 eicosatrienoic acid (5,8,11-20:3), associated with a decrease in arachidonic acid. The pathway for the synthesis of the ω9 eicosatrienoic acid and its elongation product, 7,10,13-22:3ω9, is shown in Figure 18-11. Oleic acid, the most abundant monounsaturated fatty acid, is an intermediate in this pathway. The ω9 class of polyunsaturated fatty acids can be completely synthesized from acetyl CoA or from dietary fatty acids. The desaturation and elongation enzymes are the same as those that normally act on ω3 and ω6 fatty acids, but the fatty acid Δ6-desaturase does not utilize appreciable quantities of oleic acid as a substrate unless there is a deficiency of linoleic acid. Therefore, only very small amounts of ω9 polyunsaturated fatty acids ordinarily are present in the

RDAs across the Life Cycle

	ω6 or Linoleic acid (g/day)	ω3 or α-Linolenic acid (g/day)
Infants		
0 to 0.5 yr	4.4	0.5
0.5 to 1 yr	4.6	0.5
Children		
1 to 3 yr	7	0.7
4 to 8 yr	10	0.9
Males		
9 to 13 yr	12	1.2
14 to 18 yr	16	1.6
19 to 50 yr	17	1.6
51 to >70 yr	14	1.6
Females		
9 to 13 yr	10	1.0
14 to 18 yr	11	1.1
19 to 50 yr	12	1.1
51 to 70 yr	11	1.1
Pregnant	13	1.1
Lactating	13	1.1

Data from Institute of Medicine (2002) Dietary Reference Intakes for Energy, Carbohydrate, Fiber, Fat, Fatty Acids, Cholesterol, Protein, and Amino Acids. National Academy Press, Washington, DC.

Food Sources

Food Sources of Essential Fatty Acids

	18:2ω6	18:3ω3
Oils		
Canola oil, 1 Tbsp	3 g	1.5 g
Soybean oil, 1 Tbsp	7 g	1 g
Olive oil, 1 Tbsp	1 g	0.1 g
Corn oil, 1 Tbsp	8 g	tr
Margarine, soybean oil, 1 Tbsp	2 g	0.2 g
Nuts, Seeds, and Grains		
Flax seeds, 2 Tbsp, ground	1 g	3 g
English walnuts, 2 Tbsp	5 g	1 g
Wheat germ	1 g	0.1 g
Legumes		
Soybeans, ½ cup	4 g	0.5 g
Tofu, ½ cup	4 g	0.5 g

Rich Sources of Highly Unsaturated ω3 Fatty Acids (20:5 and 22:6)

Cod liver oil (~21% 20:5 + 22:6)

Salmon oil (~20% 20:5 + 22:6)

plasma and tissues. The 5,8,11-20:3 and 7,10,13-22:3 that are synthesized compensate for some of the abnormalities by substituting for essential fatty acids in structural lipids. However, 5,8,11-20:3 cannot be converted to prostaglandins, so it does not prevent the abnormalities caused by insufficient eicosanoid production. The fact that 5,8,11-20:3 ω9 and 7,10,13-22:3 ω9 are produced by the body as an attempt to compensate for the essential fatty acid deficiency emphasizes the importance of essential fatty acids for normal physiological function.

Clinical Correlation

Triene–Tetraene Ratio in Essential Fatty Acid Deficiency

Clinicians often use the term triene/tetraene ratio in evaluating the essential fatty acid status of a patient. Triene and tetraene refer to the number of double bonds in polyunsaturated fatty acids. A trienoic fatty acid has three double bonds; a tetraenoic fatty acid has four. Arachidonate is the main tetraenoic fatty acid in plasma, and it normally comprises 8% to 10% of the plasma fatty acids. Because little trienoic fatty acid ordinarily is present, the triene to tetraene ratio normally is very low, about 0.1. This ratio becomes abnormally high in essential fatty acid deficiency. Due to a lack of ω6 fatty acid, the arachidonate content of the plasma decreases and is replaced by the ω9 eicosatrienoic acid (5,8,11-20:3) that is synthesized from oleic acid. This produces an increase in the triene to tetraene ratio of the plasma. Thus, the triene/tetraene ratio is used as a biomarker to confirm the clinical diagnosis of essential fatty acid deficiency.

Decreased visual acuity and peripheral neuropathy are the signs of an ω3 fatty acid deficiency in humans. This is consistent with findings in experimental animals indicating that ω3 fatty acid deficiency affects the development and function of the visual and central nervous system (Salem et al., 2001). Although it is possible that large segments of the population may be consuming less than the amount of ω3 fatty acid needed for optimum health, the frequency of an obvious ω3 fatty acid deficiency disease is extremely rare for several reasons. If the diet is deficient in all essential fatty acids, the symptoms of ω6 fatty acid deficiency appear first and predominate because of the longer retention of DHA in the brain and retina. In the rare case in which the dietary deficiency involves only ω3 fatty acids, some of the functional deficits are compensated by replacement with ω6 fatty acids. For example, when DHA becomes deficient, ω6 fatty acids are taken through the entire polyunsaturated fatty acid metabolic pathway shown in Figure 18-2. The ω6 analog of DHA, 22:5ω6, is produced and is incorporated into the tissue phospholipids that normally contain DHA. Although the structural

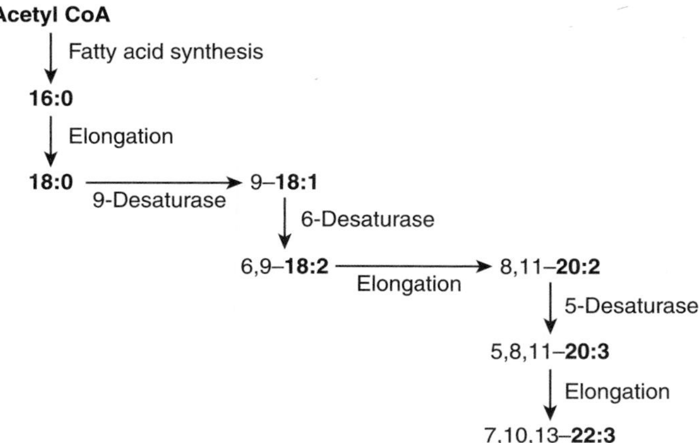

Figure 18-11 Pathway for the synthesis of the ω9 polyunsaturated fatty acids. This enzymatic pathway can utilize fatty acids in the form of fatty acyl CoA only. The fatty acids are designated by abbreviated nomenclature as indicated in Figure 18-2.

properties of 22:5ω6 are different from those of DHA (Eldho et al., 2003), there is enough similarity to allow the system to operate. The resulting function is not optimal, but it is sufficient to prevent a readily apparent disease phenotype.

PEROXIDATION OF POLYUNSATURATED FATTY ACIDS

Although essential fatty acids are required for normal physiological function and optimum health, they are susceptible to lipid peroxidation. This can cause tissue damage. Lipid peroxidation is a nonenzymatic process initiated when a free radical attacks the methylene carbon present between a pair of double bonds. The process is autocatalytic and is propagated by the presence of oxygen and transition metal ions such as Fe^{2+}. When a polyunsaturated fatty acid is converted to a free radical, it reacts with oxygen and attacks an adjacent polyunsaturated fatty acid. As a result, the second fatty acid also is converted to a free radical and attacks a third polyunsaturated fatty acid, and so on, continually spreading the process. Peroxidation perturbs the structural integrity of the membrane lipid bilayer. In addition, some of the radicals that are generated can attack proteins and DNA, injuring or even killing the cell. (Lipid peroxidation is discussed further in Chapter 29.)

Isoprostanes are arachidonic acid products formed by lipid peroxidation that have a prostaglandin-like structure. They are produced while the arachidonic acid is still attached to phospholipids. The isoprostane is then hydrolyzed by a phospholipase, released into the plasma, and excreted in the urine. Isoprostanes can be measured either by gas chromatography combined with mass spectrometry or by immunoassay, and they are considered to be the best biomarker of oxidant stress (Morrow and Roberts, 1997). Similar products called neuroprostanes are formed by lipid peroxidation of DHA. This process occurs in the brain, and an increase in neuroprostanes in the cerebrospinal fluid is considered to be a biomarker of oxidative injury in the brain (Roberts et al., 1998).

Tissues are protected against lipid peroxidation by antioxidants such as vitamin E (see Chapter 29) and by antioxidant enzymes such as superoxide dismutase, catalase, and glutathione peroxidase. Because many tissues contain substantial quantities of essential fatty acids, it is important that they also

Clinical Correlation

Oxidized Low Density Lipoproteins and Atherosclerosis

Lipid peroxidation appears to be a key event in atherosclerosis, the disease caused by cholesterol accumulation in the arterial wall. When plasma low density lipoproteins (LDLs) penetrate into the arterial wall, the LDLs are exposed to reactive oxygen species and undergo lipid peroxidation, forming oxidized LDL. Oxidation converts LDL into a form that can be taken up by macrophages that are attracted into the arterial wall. The cholesterol contained in the LDL cannot be degraded and is converted to cholesteryl esters that accumulate in the macrophages as cytoplasmic lipid droplets. The lipid-filled macrophages, called foam cells, form fatty streak lesions in the arterial intima. In the process, the macrophages become activated and induce a locally damaging inflammatory reaction that eventually progresses into an atherosclerotic plaque. The plaques can increase in size and gradually obstruct the artery, or they can rupture and cause thrombosis. The recognition that lipid peroxidation probably is involved in the pathogenesis of atherosclerosis suggests that antioxidants might be beneficial in preventing this disease and its most serious complications, coronary thrombosis and stroke. However, the clinical trials that have been done so far with vitamin E have been disappointing and have not demonstrated any protective effect.

Nutrition Insight

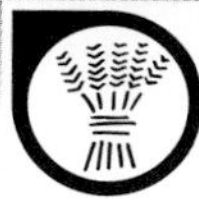

Olive Oil in the Treatment of Hypercholesterolemia

It has been known for 50 years that replacement of dietary saturated fat with plant oils rich in linoleic acid, such as corn, sunflower seed, or safflower oil, reduces the plasma LDL-cholesterol concentration. This is considered to be a beneficial effect because LDL-cholesterol is a major risk factor for atherosclerotic cardiovascular disease. Recent studies indicate that substitution of olive oil for saturated fat produces a similar effect. Olive oil contains large amounts of oleic acid, the most abundant monounsaturated fatty acid in the plasma and tissues. Therefore, it appears that the cholesterol-lowering effect of dietary fat modification results primarily from a reduction in saturated fatty acid intake rather than from any specific effect of the type of unsaturated fat that replaces it. Because of concerns about the susceptibility of LDL to lipid peroxidation and the role of oxidized LDL in atherosclerosis, there is an increasing tendency to recommend diets rich in olive oil rather than linoleic acid when dietary therapy is utilized in patients with hypercholesterolemia.

contain an adequate supply of antioxidants as well as properly functioning antioxidant enzyme systems to protect against lipid peroxidation.

REFERENCES

Cho HP, Nakamura MT, Clarke SD (1999) Cloning, expression, and nutritional regulation of the human Δ-5 desaturase. J Biol Chem 274:37335-37339.

Edmond J (2001) Essential polyunsaturated fatty acids and the barrier to the brain: the components of a model for transport. J Mol Neurosci 16:181-193.

Eldho NV, Feller SE, Tristram-Nagle S, Polozov IV, Gawrisch K (2003). Polyunsaturated docosahexaenoic vs docosapentaenoic acid—differences in lipid matrix properties from the loss of one double bond. J Am Chem Soc 125:6409-6421.

Ferdinandusse S, Denis S, Mooijer PAW, Zhang Z, Reddy JK, Spector AA, Wanders RJA (2001) Identification of the peroxisomal β-oxidation enzymes involved in the biosynthesis of docosahexaenoic acid. J Lipid Res 42:1987-1995.

Frøyland L, Madsen L, Vaagenes H, Totland GK, Auwerx, J, Kryvi H, Staels B, Berge RK (1997). Mitochondrion is the principal target for nutritional and pharmacological control of triglyceride metabolism. J Lipid Res 38:1851-1858.

Gawrisch K, Eldho NV, Holte LL (2003) The structure of DHA in phospholipid membranes. Lipids 38:445-452.

Institute of Medicine. (2002) Dietary Reference Intakes for Energy, Carbohydrate, Fiber, Fat, Fatty Acids, Cholesterol, Protein, and Amino Acids. Part 2. The National Academy Press, Washington, DC.

Jump DB (2002) Dietary polyunsaturated fatty acids and regulation of gene transcription. Curr Opin Lipidol 13:155-164.

Lauritzen L, Hansen HS, Jørgensen MH, Michaelsen KF (2001) The essentiality of long chain *n-3* fatty acids in relation to development and function of the brain and retina. Prog Lipid Res 40:1-94.

Leaf A, Kang JX, Xiao Y-F, Billman GE (2003) Clinical Prevention of sudden cardiac death by n-3 polyunsaturated fatty acids and mechanism of prevention of arrhythmias by n-3 fish oils. Circulation 107:2646-2652.

Leonard AE, Pereria SL, Sprecher H, Huang Y-S (2004) Elongation of long-chain fatty acids. Prog Lipid Res 43:36-54.

Marcheselli VL, Hong S, Lukiw WJ, Tian XH, Gronert K, Musto A, Hardy M, Gimenez JM, Chiang N, Serhan CN, Bazan NG (2003) Novel docosanoids inhibit brain ischemia-reperfusion-mediated leukocyte infiltration and pro-inflammatory gene expression. J Biol Chem 278: 43807-43817.

Marquardt A, Stor H, White K, Weber BHF (2000) cDNA cloning, genomic structure, and chromosomal localization of three members of the human fatty acid desaturase family. Genomics 66:175-183.

Martinez M (2001) Restoring the DHA levels in the brains of Zellweger patients. J Mol Neurosci 16:309-316.

Mata de Urquiza M, Liu S, Sjoberg M, Zetterstrom RH, Griffiths W, Sjovall J, Perlmann T (2000) Docosahexaenoic acid, a ligand for the retinoid X receptor in mouse brain. Science 290:2140-2144.

Mitchell DC, Niu SL, Litman BJ (2003) Enhancement of G protein-coupled signaling by DHA phospholipids. Lipids 38:437-443.

Moore SA (2001) Polyunsaturated fatty acid synthesis and release by brain-derived cells in vitro. J Mol Neurosci 16:195-200.

Moriguchi T, Greiner RS, Salem N Jr (2000) Behavioral deficits associated with dietary induction of decreased brain docosahexaenoic acid concentration. J Neurochem 75:2563-2573.

Morrow JD, Roberts LJ II (1997) The isoprostanes: unique bioactive products of lipid peroxidation. Prog Lipid Res 36:1-21.

Nagan N, Zoeller RA (2001) Plasmalogens: biosynthesis and functions. Prog Lipid Res 40:199-229.

Norris AW, Spector AA (2002) Very long chain n-3 and n-6 polyunsaturated fatty acids bind strongly to liver fatty acid-binding protein. J Lipid Res 43:646-653.

Ntambi JM, Bené H (2001) Polyunsaturated fatty acid regulation of gene expression. J Mol Neurosci 16:273-278.

Rapoport SI, Chang MCJ, Spector AA (2001) Delivery and turnover of plasma-derived essential PUFAs in mammalian brain. J Lipid Res 42:678-685.

Roberts LJ II, Montine TJ, Marksberry WR, Tapper AR, Hardy P, Chemtob S, Dettbarn WD, Morrow JD (1998) Formation of isoprostane-like compounds (neuroprostanes) in vivo from docosahexaenoic acid. J Biol Chem 273:13605-13612.

Salem N Jr, Moriguchi T, Greiner RS, McBride K, Ahmad A, Catalan JN, Slotnick B (2001) Alterations in brain function after loss of docosahexaenoate due to dietary restriction of n-3 fatty acids. J Mol Neurosci 16:299-307.

Salem N Jr, Wegher B, Mena P, Uauy R (1996) Arachidonic and docosahexaenoic acids are biosynthesized from their 18-carbon precursors in human infants. Proc Natl Acad Sci USA 93:49-54.

Scott BL, Bazan NJ (1989) Membrane docosahexaenoate is supplied to the developing brain and retina by the liver. Proc Natl Acad Sci USA 86:2903-2907.

Sprecher H (2000) Metabolism of highly unsaturated n-3 and n-6 fatty acids. Biochim Biophys Acta 1486:219-231.

Su HM, Bernardo L, Mirmiran M, Ma XH, Corso TN, Nathanielsz PW, Brenna JT (1999) Bioequivalence of dietary α-linolenic and docosahexaenoic acid as sources of docosahexaenoate accretion in brain and associated organs of neonatal baboons. Pediatr Res 45:87-93.

Williard DE, Nwankwo JO, Kaduce TL, Harmon SD, Irons M, Moser HW, Raymond GV, Spector AA (2001). Identification of a fatty acid Δ^6-desaturase deficiency in human skin fibroblasts. J Lipid Res 42:501-508.

RECOMMENDED READINGS

Brenna JT (2002) Efficiency of conversion of α-linolenic acid to long chain n-3 fatty acids in man. Curr Opin Clin Nutr Metab Care 5:127-32.

Clarke SD (2001) Polyunsaturated fatty acid regulation of gene transcription: a molecular mechanism to improve the metabolic syndrome. J Nutr 131:1129-1132.

Cunnane SC (2003) Problems with essential fatty acids: time for a new paradigm? Prog Lipid Res 42:544-568.

Salem N Jr, Litman B, Kim HY, Gawrisch K (2001). Mechanisms of action of docosahexaenoic acid in the nervous system. Lipids 36: 945-959.

Spector AA (1999) Essentiality of fatty acids. Lipids 34:S1-S3.

Spector AA (2001) Plasma free fatty acid and lipoproteins as sources of polyunsaturated fatty acid for the brain. J Mol Neurosci 16:159-165.

Chapter 19

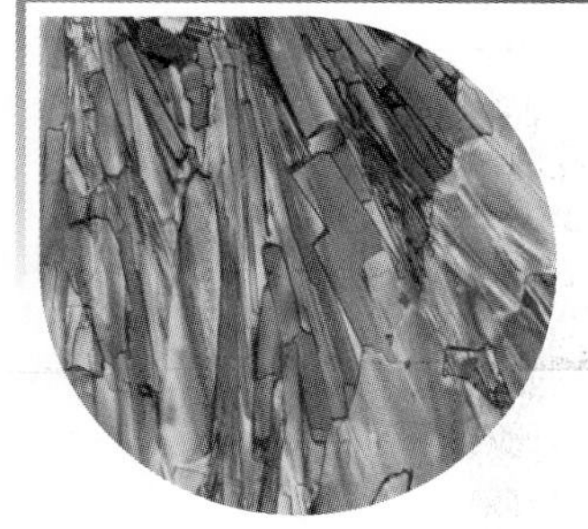

Regulation of Fuel Utilization in Response to Food Intake

Malcolm Watford, DPhil

OUTLINE

FUELS

The macronutrients—carbohydrates, lipids, and proteins—are the sources of energy in the diet. Although the protein requirement is based on the need to maintain protein synthesis, and all macronutrients are involved in numerous biosynthetic functions, the bulk of macronutrients consumed each day are catabolized for energy production. A metabolic fuel may be defined as a circulating compound that is taken up by tissues for energy production. The major fuels are glucose, free fatty acids, triacylglycerols in lipoprotein complexes, ketone bodies, and amino acids. Lactate, glycerol, and alcohol also serve as fuels. Not all fuels are available at the same time, and their replenishment from exogenous (dietary) or endogenous (body) sources must be balanced and regulated in order to maintain homeostasis.

CONSTRAINTS ON FUEL UTILIZATION

Organisms may be confronted with a supply of macronutrients that is inadequate to meet current needs with respect to total calories or specific nutrients. One solution potentially available to any mobile organism is to move to another location that has an adequate supply of nutrients. In many cases this is not feasible, and nature has provided a number of alternative strategies. Regulation of the uptake and metabolism of nutrients provides the basis for adjustments. Prokaryotes and unicellular eukaryotes, such as yeast, can induce a new set of enzymes that takes advantage of other nutrients in the existing environment. Alternatively, many prokaryotes can sporulate; growth and metabolic rates in bacterial spores are reduced to very low levels, and nutrient requirements are minimal. Such spores then await the development of conditions more propitious to growth.

This chapter is a revision of the chapter contributed by Malcolm Watford and Alan G. Goodridge, PhD, for the first edition.

Both cold-blooded (poikilothermic) and warm-blooded (homeothermic) vertebrates that hibernate have a solution that, in principle, is analogous to sporulation; they lower their energy requirements by lowering their body temperatures. Hibernation does not provide as long-term a potential for survival as does sporulation, but it does allow the organism to survive extended periods of unfavorable conditions. Most homeothermic vertebrates, however, cannot hibernate. Furthermore, lowering body temperature is not always a feasible strategy by which poikilothermic animals can survive periods of food deprivation. Vertebrates deal with the inevitable periods of food deprivation by storing fuel when food is available and using the stored fuel during times of deprivation.

Birds and mammals are homeothermic animals, which means that they maintain a constant body temperature irrespective of the ambient temperature (within limits). Homeotherms have minimal (resting) metabolic rates that are related to their respective rates of heat loss. From the mouse to the elephant, minimal heat loss and basal metabolic rate are proportional to surface area. Small animals have much higher surface area to body weight ratios than do large animals, and they have higher rates of heat loss and hence higher energy utilization per unit of volume than do larger animals. It is this energy turnover, plus that resulting from physical activity and a small component for the thermic effect of food, that must be balanced with an adequate source of energy, as discussed in more detail in Chapters 21 through 23. Energy consumed must equal energy utilized, as follows, or changes in body energy stores will result:

$$\text{Changes in body energy stores} = \text{Energy intake} - \text{Energy expenditure}$$

When food is abundant, calories in excess of current energy needs are stored, first as glycogen and then as triacylglycerol. When food is unavailable, the stored energy is used for current needs. Because the nature and amounts of fuels provided by the diet are not identical to those of fuels consumed or stored by the body, the synthesis, oxidation, and storage of each of the individual macronutrients must be regulated.

TISSUE-SPECIFIC METABOLISM OF FUELS

Perhaps the most important concept for understanding metabolism is tissue specificity; different tissues show different and characteristic patterns of fuel utilization, storage, and release (Table 19-1). In this respect, the brain and other structures of the central nervous system are important tissues to consider. The brain must receive a constant supply of fuel, but it is only capable of using glucose and ketone bodies. In key regions of the brain the blood-brain barrier limits the rate of transfer of long-chain fatty acids. Therefore, the rate of oxidation of long-chain fatty acids is limited so that even when their level in the circulation rises they do not contribute significantly as a fuel for the brain (Vannucci and Hawkins, 1983). Similarly, although many amino acids undergo a variety of interconversions within the brain, they do not play a major role in overall energy supply.

Under most conditions the brain utilizes glucose, which it oxidizes completely. There is some evidence that in extreme pathological conditions the brain can take up lactate, but normally lactate levels are not sufficiently high for this to occur. Similarly, the use of ketone bodies is usually minimal because the level of circulating ketones is low in the healthy, fed individual. However, after a few days of starvation, and in some pathological conditions, the levels of ketone bodies rise, and the brain oxidizes them in preference to glucose. Even when ketone bodies are available, parts of the brain still require glucose. Although some glucose is still completely oxidized when ketone bodies are being used, the metabolism of most glucose under this condition is restricted to glycolysis with a resultant release of lactate. This regulation of brain energy metabolism is very important, because the brain is unable to obtain sufficient glucose to maintain function at glucose levels of less than 3 mmol/L (54 mg/100 mL of plasma). To maintain blood glucose levels higher than this minimum, particularly during starvation when the only sources of glucose are endogenous (hepatic glycogen breakdown and gluconeogenesis), it is important to provide alternative fuels such as fatty acids and ketone bodies in order to decrease the body's need for glucose.

Table 19-1
Tissue-Specific Metabolism

Tissue	Fuel Used	Fuel Released
Brain	Glucose Ketone bodies	Lactate (only in prolonged starvation; brain is able to utilize lactate in some pathological conditions)
Skeletal muscle	Glucose Free fatty acids Triacylglycerols Branched-chain amino acids	Lactate Alanine Glutamine
Heart	Free fatty acids Triacylglycerols Ketone bodies Glucose Lactate	
Liver*	Amino acids (partial oxidation) Free fatty acids Lactate Glycerol Glucose Alcohol	Glucose Ketone bodies Lactate (during absorptive phase) Triacylglycerols
Intestine†	Glucose Glutamine	Lactate Alanine
Red blood cells	Glucose	Lactate
Kidney	Glucose Free fatty acids Ketone bodies Lactate Glutamine	Glucose (renal gluconeogenesis is important only in prolonged starvation)
Adipose tissue	Glucose Triacylglycerols	Lactate Glycerol Free fatty acids

*The liver is also the site of galactose and fructose metabolism.
†The small intestine also releases dietary glucose, galactose, fructose, amino acids, and lipids.

Skeletal muscle makes up most of the lean body mass and accounts for much of the daily energy metabolism, although this varies greatly depending on the amount of physical work performed. Different types of muscle can, and do, use different fuels, but in general, skeletal muscle is capable of using glucose, fatty acids (including those derived from both circulating and intramyocellular triacylglycerol), ketone bodies, and the branched-chain amino acids (leucine, isoleucine, and valine). In addition, skeletal muscle takes up and stores considerable amounts of glucose (stored as glycogen) and free fatty acids (stored as triacylglycerol) for later use during contraction. Not all of these fuels are completely oxidized in skeletal muscle; considerable amounts of lactate may be released from glucose metabolism. Furthermore, the breakdown of branched-chain amino acids and some other amino acids in the muscle results in the formation and release of alanine and glutamine. Muscle glycogen is used as a local fuel store and is not able to contribute directly to the circulating glucose supply because muscle lacks glucose 6-phosphatase. Heart muscle represents a special case because it is constantly working. It is highly aerobic and largely dependent on fatty acid oxidation for its energy requirements; the heart will oxidize glucose during times of glucose excess, and it may even take up and oxidize lactate when circulating lactate levels rise. Further discussion of fuel utilization by muscle during rest and exercise can be found in Chapter 20.

The liver plays a major regulatory role because, in effect, it monitors the intake of nutrients. It takes up glucose and other monosaccharides and stores them as glycogen to be released later as glucose. It takes up lactate, amino acids, and glycerol and converts them to glucose 6-phosphate, either to be stored as glycogen or released directly as glucose (gluconeogenesis); and it takes up fatty acids either for reesterification or for β-oxidation and ketone body production. In addition, alcohol is metabolized exclusively in the liver. Although the liver has the capacity to oxidize completely each of the macronutrients, this is probably not a major fate of most macronutrients. Indeed, partial oxidation of dietary amino acids (protein) alone would provide more than enough energy for the liver. Thus, hepatic amino acid metabolism conserves most of the carbon skeletons as glucose; hepatic fatty acid oxidation is limited mainly to the production of ketone bodies; and hepatic glucose metabolism results in net lactate release across the liver in the absorptive period. In theory, the liver could utilize excess carbohydrate and amino acids for de novo fatty acid synthesis. Based on measurements, however, net synthesis of fat is not of quantitative importance for energy storage in humans consuming typical Western diets (>30% of calories as fat). Indeed, excess dietary carbohydrate and protein are normally oxidized before dietary fat is catabolized (Horton et al., 1995; see Chapter 22).

In addition to the liver, the kidneys are the only organs capable of gluconeogenesis. Renal gluconeogenesis is probably of quantitative importance only during prolonged starvation or metabolic acidosis. This issue is uncertain because certain cells in the kidney utilize glucose at high rates at the same time that other cells are producing glucose. Although the kidneys account for less than 0.5% of body mass, they account for about 10% of total oxygen consumption at rest, indicating their quantitative importance in energy metabolism. The kidneys are very heterogeneous, and different cells show marked differences in metabolism of specific fuels; different types of renal cells have differing capacities to use glucose, lactate, fatty acids, ketone bodies, and certain amino acids, especially glutamine.

Another metabolically active tissue, accounting for 20% of resting oxygen consumption, is the intestinal tract, where dietary glutamine and glutamate and circulating glutamine are major respiratory fuels for the absorptive epithelial cells (Reeds and Burrin, 2001). Glucose is utilized and, if available, free fatty acids and ketone bodies are used. Within enterocytes, glucose is not oxidized completely; partially metabolized glucose carbons are released as lactate. Glutamine also undergoes partial oxidation; the carbon skeleton is probably partially conserved as the 3-carbon compounds lactate, pyruvate, and alanine. In addition, the metabolism of glutamine in these cells results in the production of ammonia, proline, and citrulline. The colonic mucosa demonstrates a specific and unique metabolism in that colonocytes derive most of their energy from the oxidation of butyrate, which is produced during the fermentation of dietary fiber and resistant starch by the microflora in the lumen of the colon (Roediger, 1982).

A few tissues contain obligatory glycolytic cells: these cells are able to obtain energy only from the metabolism of glucose to lactate (with a little via the pentose phosphate pathway). The best known example is the mammalian red blood cell, which, lacking mitochondria, is unable to extensively oxidize any fuels because the principal oxidative pathways are intramitochondrial and dependent upon oxygen as a terminal electron acceptor (via the electron transport chain). This group of tissues also includes the retina and the renal medulla. Although these cells always require some glucose as an obligatory fuel, they produce lactate as the end product. This lactate then returns to the liver to be converted back into glucose; this cycling of lactate and glucose between tissues and liver is known as the Cori cycle (see Chapter 12).

Although adipose tissue can be the largest tissue mass in the body, its role in energy metabolism is primarily to store and release fatty acids. In the fed state, circulating triacylglycerols are hydrolyzed by lipoprotein lipase in the adipose tissue capillary bed, and the fatty acids are taken up by the adipocytes to be stored as triacylglycerol. Because adipose tissue lacks glycerol kinase activity, the glycerol 3-phosphate required for reesterification is derived from glucose or glycolytic intermediates. During starvation, the stored triacylglycerols are hydrolyzed intracellularly by hormone-sensitive lipase, and the free fatty acids and glycerol are released into the circulation. One important aspect of adipose tissue metabolism is that anatomically different depots show different rates of metabolism and responsiveness to hormones and other signals. In general, intraabdominal adipose tissue is more active metabolically than subcutaneous adipose tissue (Leibel et al., 1989).

Other tissues have various specialized patterns of metabolism but are not generally considered to be of quantitative importance. However, the mammary gland during lactation, the fetus and placenta during gestation, various organs during certain pathological conditions such as hypercatabolic states, or large tumors can have major effects on whole-body energy metabolism.

METABOLIC FATE OF MACRONUTRIENTS

There are two sources of fuels for the body: (1) exogenous, those that are derived directly from the diet, and (2) endogenous, those that arise from tissues either directly from fuel stores (such as glycogen or triacylglycerol) or from the metabolism of other fuels (such as lactate or ketone bodies). Most individuals eat discrete meals, and the macronutrients are absorbed, processed, and stored during the absorptive phase after a meal. (The stores of fuel are listed in Table 21-1, Chapter 21.) The size of the carbohydrate store is limited (~350 g in an adult), and a purely storage form of protein does not exist. Conversely, triacylglycerol stores appear to be without limit. In the late 1960s, Cahill (1970) studied a group of obese men undergoing therapeutic starvation for 6 weeks. This work led to the concept that glucose homeostasis could be divided into different stages (Fig. 19-1). In this model of glucose homeostasis, the body maintains circulating glucose levels through five major phases, using different physiological mechanisms to regulate glucose production and utilization and providing alternative fuels (Ruderman et al., 1976; Cahill, 1970). The following section briefly outlines the fate of macronutrients in a typical meal and how the body adapts to maintain glucose homeostasis as starvation progresses in subsequent phases. Details of the pathways and specific regulatory mechanisms are provided in Chapters 12 through 17.

ABSORPTIVE OR POSTPRANDIAL PHASE

The macronutrients in a standard meal of 90 g of carbohydrate, 30 g of protein, and 20 g of fat (27% of the calories as fat) will be utilized by the body in a characteristic manner. Dietary glucose is taken up from the intestinal lumen into the enterocyte by the sodium-linked glucose transporter SGLT1. A small amount of glucose is utilized by these cells for glycolysis with resultant lactate production, but most passes out of the cell down a concentration gradient via the facilitative glucose (hexose) transporter GLUT2 and into the portal vein. Although dietary carbohydrate also may be absorbed into the portal system as galactose or fructose, these two sugars probably are normally metabolized exclusively by the liver (see Chapter 12) and hence are not considered part of peripheral carbohydrate metabolism.

The absorption of dietary carbohydrate causes a rise in circulating glucose level, which together with other signals triggers release of insulin. Although insulin does not stimulate hepatic glucose transporters directly, it is required for the uptake and utilization of glucose by the liver. During this phase, the level of glucose in the portal vein rises considerably (up to 15 mmol/L). The liver appears to be able to sense the glucose concentration difference between the portal vein and the hepatic artery (liver receives ~80% of its blood supply via the portal vein and only ~20% via the artery), and the liver shows only net glucose uptake when a large portal to arterial glucose gradient exists together with an elevated level of insulin (Stumpel and Jungerman, 1997). The liver is able to take up considerable amounts of glucose because it possesses a unique isozyme of hexokinase, hexokinase IV, or glucokinase. Glucokinase has a much lower affinity for glucose (and other hexoses) than the other hexokinases, being half saturated at approximately 5 mmol/L of glucose, such that it can respond to increases in glucose concentration. In addition, unlike the other hexokinases, glucokinase is not subject to inhibition by physiological levels of glucose 6-phosphate.

These differences in glucokinase kinetics enable the liver to take up glucose and store it as glycogen when glucose is abundant even as

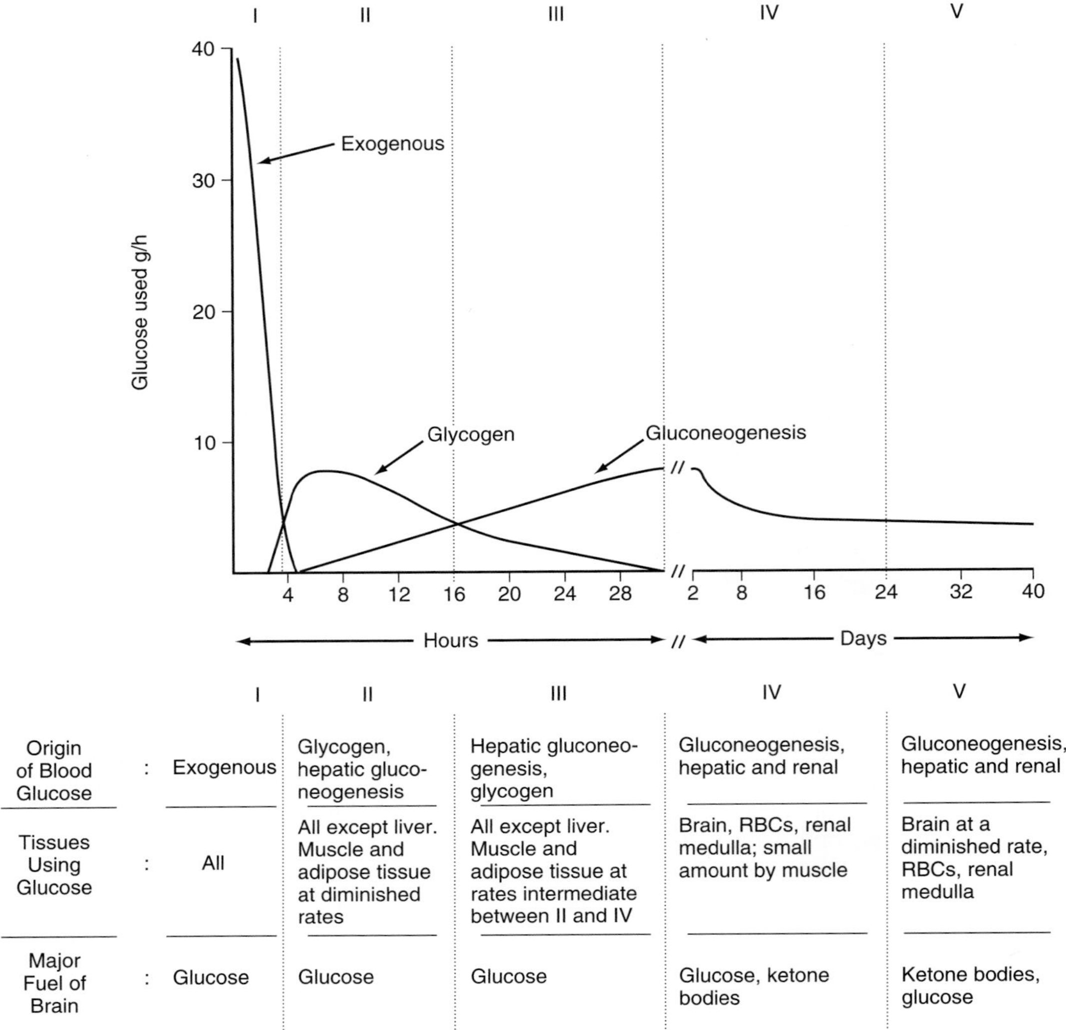

Figure 19-1 Glucose utilization versus time in the five phases of glucose homeostasis. Stage I refers to the absorptive or postprandial period; II, to the postabsorptive period; III, to early starvation; IV, to intermediate starvation; and V, to prolonged starvation. *(From Ruderman NB, Aoki TT, Cahill GF Jr [1976] Gluconeogenesis and its disorders in man. In: Hanson RW, Mehlman MA, [eds] Gluconeogenesis: Its Regulation in Mammalian Species. John Wiley & Sons, New York, Wiley Interscience.)*

the levels of intracellular glucose 6-phosphate increase. Therefore, the liver takes up glucose, and perhaps as much as 20 g of the glucose in a meal is deposited as glycogen. In addition, the liver may partially catabolize some glucose and may demonstrate net lactate release at this time. However, there also is evidence of lactate uptake by some liver cells, and some glycogen synthesis (perhaps as much as 30% to 40%) may occur via the gluconeogenic (indirect) pathway from the carbon skeletons of lactate and amino acids (Shulman and Landau, 1992).

The remainder of the glucose from the meal (70 g) passes through the liver, causing peripheral plasma glucose levels to rise to 6 to 7 mmol/L. Over the next 2 hours, the brain will take up approximately 15 to 20 g of glucose to be oxidized directly as fuel (Fig. 19-2). The obligatory glycolytic cells will use some glucose

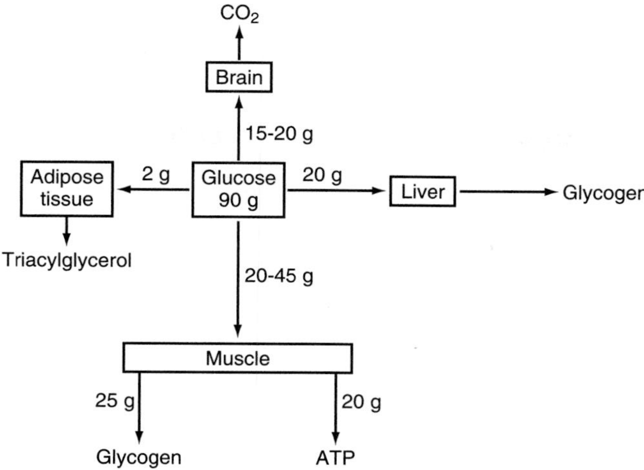

Figure 19-2 Fate of dietary carbohydrate (glucose) from one meal during the absorptive phase (~2 hours). Glucose provides the glycerol moiety for triacylglycerol synthesis. In addition to the fates shown, 2 to 3 g of glucose is required by the obligatory glycolytic cells.

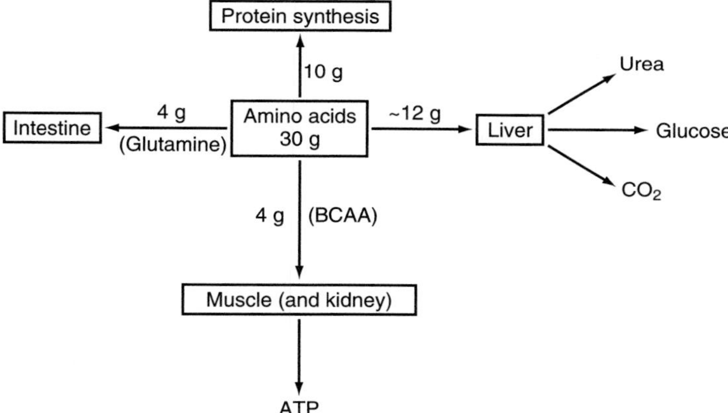

Figure 19-3 Fate of dietary protein (amino acids) from one meal during the absorptive phase (~2 hours).

(2 to 3 g/hour), and when circulating glucose levels are high and those of free fatty acids are low (e.g., as in the absorptive phase), all tissues capable of using glucose probably will be using it as fuel. Most of the glucose, however, will be taken up in an insulin-dependent manner (facilitative transporter GLUT4; see Chapter 12) by skeletal muscle (45 g) and adipose tissue (2 g). In skeletal muscle, approximately half will be oxidized and half stored as glycogen. In adipose tissue, most will be used for the synthesis of glycerol 3-phosphate for triacylglycerol synthesis, and a small quantity may be metabolized to lactate. During the absorptive phase, there is evidence that the net production of lactate by the liver and other tissues provides an important fuel for the kidneys, heart, and possibly colon.

The ingestion of 100 g of protein per day presents the body with a problem because amino acids must be used for protein synthesis or degraded. After a meal, a large surge of amino acids (i.e., ~30 g from the standard meal we are considering) enters the circulation, generating signals for increased protein synthesis. Approximately 10 g will be converted to protein, but this leaves 20 g to be catabolized because the body lacks a purely storage form of protein (Fig. 19-3). Much of the glutamine, glutamate, and aspartate in the meal (4 g) will be metabolized by the intestine, with resultant production of alanine, proline, citrulline, ammonia, and lactate. The remaining amino acids are mainly absorbed unmodified, which causes a rise in amino acid levels in portal blood that, in turn, stimulates their catabolism in the liver. The branched-chain amino acids, which comprise just more than 25% of dietary protein (8 g of those in the meal), are not catabolized by the liver; after about 4 g have been used for protein synthesis, the remaining 4 g will be catabolized in extrahepatic tissues such as skeletal muscle with lesser roles played by the kidneys and adipose tissue. Therefore, approximately 40% to 50% of the amino acid load is catabolized by the liver, with the resulting synthesis of approximately 7 to 9 g of glucose (stored as glycogen). Jungas and colleagues (1992) calculated that the complete oxidation of the amino acids from dietary protein could result in excessive ATP production in the liver, and they proposed that the synthesis of glucose (glycogen) and urea, and perhaps even protein, from dietary amino acids could be viewed as mechanisms to regenerate ADP and so allow continued degradation of amino acids by the liver. This analysis suggests that the liver does not oxidize amino acids completely in vivo, and that in the fed/absorptive state the major energy source for synthesis of ATP in the liver is the partial oxidation of amino acids.

Dietary fats are perhaps the simplest to describe in terms of their immediate fate after a meal. Although the digestion, processing, and storage of fats require repeated cycles of hydrolysis and resynthesis of triacylglycerols (see Chapters 10 and 16), most of the fat in a meal will be deposited, mainly in adipose tissue (with limited amounts in liver and skeletal muscle), and stored for utilization at a later time. During the postabsorptive period, the level of free fatty acids in the circulation is low because lipids are transported to tissues as triacylglycerols in lipoproteins. Although dietary fatty acids may undergo some modification, the profile of fatty acids laid down in adipose tissue triacylglycerol is essentially the same as that in the diet.

Synthesis of fatty acids de novo is a minor pathway of energy storage in humans consuming Western diets (>30% of calories as fat) (Hellerstein et al., 1996). In calorimetry studies of subjects eating hypercaloric, very low-fat (3% of calories as fat), high-carbohydrate diets, glycogen accumulated up to 1 kg, and net fatty acid synthesis in excess of fatty acid oxidation was detectable only after 5 days of such an extreme regimen (Minehira et al. 2004; Acheson et al., 1988). However, calorimetry is limited in that it cannot detect de novo fatty acid synthesis directly. Studies with stable isotopes did demonstrate de novo fatty acid synthesis in subjects consuming low-fat diets (10% of calories as fat), although there was no net synthesis (i.e., fatty acid synthesis was not in excess of fatty acid oxidation) (Hudgins et al., 1996). De novo fatty acid synthesis was not detectable in subjects consuming a higher fat diet (40% of energy as fat). Most people find it difficult to maintain a hypercaloric, low-fat, high-carbohydrate diet for more than a few days. Thus, experimental data indicate that the role of de novo fatty acid synthesis in energy storage and weight gain in the normal population is minimal. However, in a study of subjects consuming 10% of calories as fat, in whom de novo fatty acid synthesis was detected, the low-fat, high-carbohydrate diet did result in an increase in circulating triacylglycerols and, perhaps more significantly, in an increase in the degree of saturation of those triacylglycerols, because de novo fatty acid synthesis produces saturated fatty acids, predominantly palmitate (Hudgins et al., 1996).

During the absorptive phase, approximately 40 g of glucose is taken out of the circulation per hour. This occurs because insulin stimulates glucose uptake and metabolism in skeletal muscle and to a lesser extent in adipose tissue, insulin stimulates glycogen synthesis in liver, and most other tissues use glucose as a fuel. Consequently, 2 to 3 hours after a meal, about one third of the glucose has been stored and the rest has been oxidized. One third of the amino acids has been used for protein synthesis, and most other amino acids have undergone catabolism, providing the major source of energy for the liver together with some conversion of carbon chains to glucose with storage as hepatic glycogen. Lipids have been absorbed more slowly, and have been transported in the circulation as triacylglycerols in lipoproteins, thereby limiting their availability and oxidation. The majority of the fatty acids from dietary lipids will be stored in adipose tissue depots for future use.

POSTABSORPTIVE OR FASTING GLUCOSE HOMEOSTASIS

Once the nutrients in a meal have been absorbed, the body relies on endogenous sources for its energy. The brain requires about 120 g of glucose per day, and the glycolytic tissues will use another 50 to 60 g. Blood glucose levels must be maintained to allow brain function, so the body responds in a coordinated and tissue-specific manner to regulate provision and utilization of fuels. Falling blood glucose levels (Fig. 19-4) cause decreased insulin secretion and increased glucagon secretion (Fig. 19-5). At physiological levels in humans, glucagon is known only to act on the liver, where one of its prime actions is to stimulate the breakdown of glycogen. Because liver contains glucose 6-phosphatase, it releases glucose 6-phosphate derived from glycogenolysis into the circulation as free glucose and so maintains glucose levels. However, if all tissues continued to use glucose as the major fuel, the reserves of liver glycogen would not last very long. Therefore, as hepatic glycogen is mobilized, some tissues switch to alternative fuels, decreasing use of glucose and prolonging the availability of liver glycogen. Insulin is a very strong inhibitor of lipolysis in adipose tissue, and the fall in circulating insulin levels relieves such inhibition. A simultaneous rise in catecholamines stimulates lipolysis in adipose tissue. The combined effects of the fall in insulin and rise in catecholamine concentrations result in a rise in the level of free fatty acids in the circulation (see Fig. 19-4).

Tissues such as skeletal muscle have a defined hierarchy for the fuels that they oxidize. When free fatty acids are available, skeletal muscle oxidizes them in preference to glucose. Thus, the decrease in circulating glucose and insulin results in an increased availability of free fatty acids, which are then used as a fuel instead of glucose. This is known as the glucose–fatty acid cycle or the Randle cycle (Fig. 19-6) (Randle et al., 1963). Higher levels of fatty acids result in activation of malonyl CoA decarboxylase

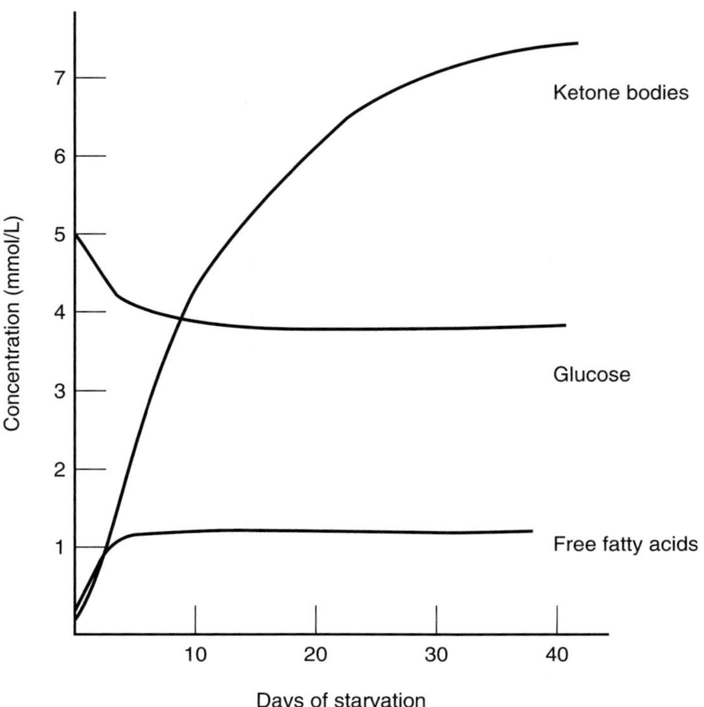

Figure 19-4 Plasma concentrations of fuels during prolonged starvation.

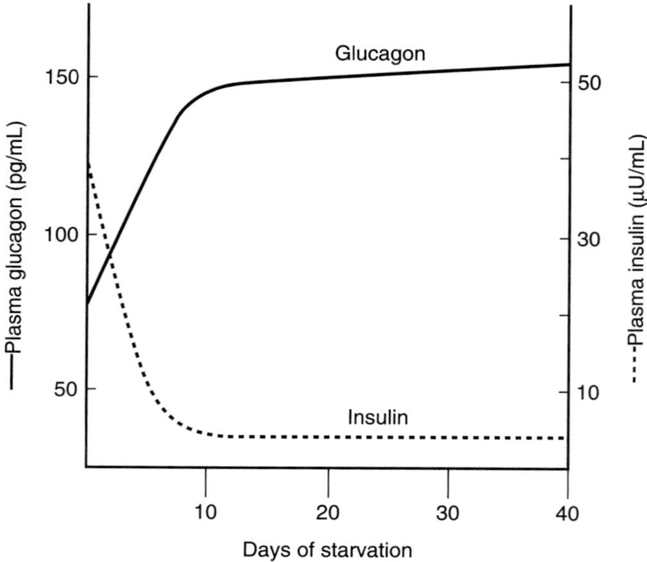

Figure 19-5 Plasma levels of insulin and glucagon during prolonged starvation.

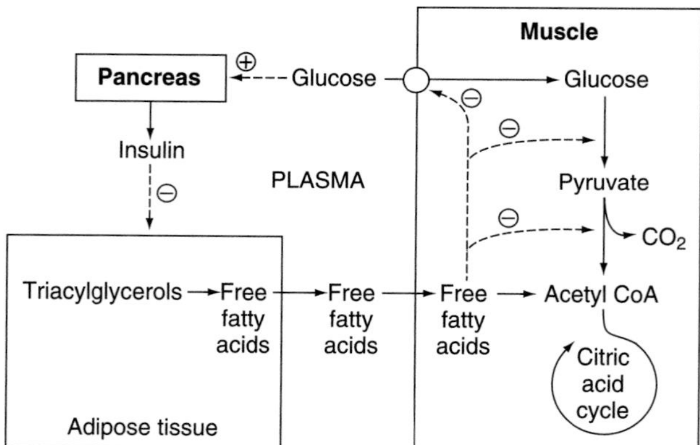

Figure 19-6 The glucose–fatty acid (Randle) cycle. A rise in plasma glucose stimulates insulin release by the pancreas. When plasma glucose levels decrease, insulin levels will also decrease. This results in increased mobilization of free fatty acids from adipose tissue; the fatty acids are then utilized in tissues such as muscle with a resultant inhibition of glucose utilization. (The production of ketone bodies by the liver and their resultant utilization in peripheral tissues spare glucose oxidation in a similar manner. Overall, this is known as the glucose-sparing effect of fat-derived fuels.)

and inhibition of acety CoA carboxylase, both via AMP kinase (Assifi et al., 2005; Gibson and Harris, 2002), which decreases malonyl CoA levels, removing inhibition of carnitine palmitoyltransferase I, and further increasing the oxidation of fatty acids within the mitochondrial matrix. The oxidation of fatty acids and ketone bodies generates large amounts of acetyl CoA, NADH, ATP, and citrate. Elevated levels of these compounds inhibit glucose metabolism through feedback inhibition of pyruvate dehydrogenase and allosteric inhibition of 6-phosphofructo-1-kinase (see Chapter 12). Together with inhibition of pyruvate dehydrogenase in response to phosphorylation of pyruvate dehydrogenase due to the lower insulin levels, this effectively spares glucose utilization in skeletal muscle.

During the postabsorptive phase, circulating glucose is maintained by the breakdown of liver glycogen. The brain accounts for 50% of glucose utilization at this stage. Although other tissues are still using glucose, it is at a reduced rate, and they are beginning to substitute other fuels. This glucose-sparing effect of fat-derived fuels means that as starvation develops, less glucose is used by the body.

Liver glycogen stores are not limitless, and after approximately 24 hours of starvation, they become depleted. Once this has occurred, the only source of glucose is gluconeogenesis (the synthesis of glucose from noncarbohydrate precursors). Therefore, as liver glycogen stores begin to decline, gluconeogenesis becomes increasingly more important, and gluconeogenesis is the only source of blood glucose after approximately 24 hours of starvation. Gluconeogenesis, however, is very costly in terms of substrate. The only substrates for gluconeogenesis during starvation are lactate (and pyruvate), glycerol, and amino acids. The body is not able to make glucose from the 2-carbon units released as acetyl CoA during fatty acid oxidation, and hence fatty acids are not gluconeogenic substrates. Also important is the fact that hepatic gluconeogenesis, in addition to providing "new" glucose for the brain to oxidize, is involved in the recycling of lactate and alanine carbons back to glucose.

Throughout starvation the obligatory glycolytic tissues continue to utilize glucose, but they conserve the carbon skeleton as lactate, which is recycled into glucose (Cori cycle). Therefore, these tissues do not represent a drain on the circulating glucose pool, but they do demand continuing gluconeogenesis from lactate in liver. The energy for the synthesis of glucose within the liver is provided from the partial oxidation of fatty acids. Similarly, although alanine is quantitatively the most important amino acid taken up by the liver for glucose synthesis, the carbon skeleton of this alanine is derived primarily from glucose metabolism in peripheral tissues and likewise simply recycles glucose carbon via the glucose-alanine cycle (see also Chapters 12 and 14). Thus, recycled glucose cannot contribute to the net amount of glucose required by the brain because net use of glucose from this pool would compromise the metabolism of a number of tissues and lead to hypoglycemia. Therefore, the brain relies on gluconeogenesis to provide "new" glucose synthesized from glycerol and amino acids. The amount of glucose synthesized from glycerol is relatively small (~18 g/day) and remains fairly constant throughout starvation. The major gluconeogenic substrates providing "new" glucose are amino acids that are derived from the net breakdown of body protein. Initially, the principal source may be hepatic proteins, but within a few hours the bulk of amino acids will be derived from increased net proteolysis in skeletal muscle. Not all amino acid carbon will yield glucose; on average, 1.6 g of amino acid is required to synthesize 1 g of glucose. Therefore, to keep the brain supplied with glucose at a rate of 110 to 120 g/day, the breakdown of 160 to 200 g of protein, or close to 1 kg of muscle tissue, per day would be required. This is clearly undesirable, and the body limits glucose utilization to reduce the need for gluconeogenesis and thereby spare body protein.

High levels of fatty acids in the circulation result in their partial oxidation in the liver and the resultant production of ketone bodies. The ketone bodies are released into the circulation during starvation, and their concentration rises (see Fig. 19-4). Many tissues, including the brain, use ketone bodies as fuels; this spares glucose metabolism via a mechanism similar to the sparing of glucose by oxidation of fatty acids as an alternative fuel. The use of ketone bodies, therefore, replaces some of the glucose required by the brain. In addition, it decreases glucose oxidation in the brain by limiting the extent of some glucose metabolism to glycolysis to lactate. Thus, after 4 to 6 days of starvation, utilization of blood glucose has decreased to 1 to 2 g/hour for oxidation in the brain and perhaps a similar amount for the Cori and glucose-alanine cycles in other tissues.

The high levels of ketone bodies in the circulation produce a metabolic acidosis and also result in excretion of considerable quantities of ketone bodies in the urine. The loss of some energy in the urine seems to be a price that is paid in order to provide the brain with an alternative substrate. In response to the ketoacidosis,

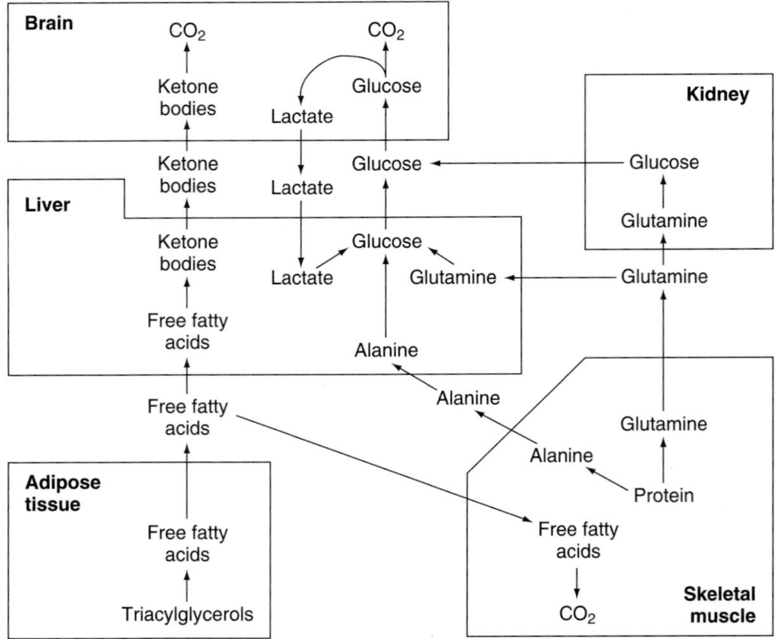

Figure 19-7 Fuel utilization during prolonged starvation. The only tissues utilizing glucose are the brain and the obligatory glycolytic tissues (omitted for clarity). Fatty acids have become the major fuel for tissues such as liver and muscle, and ketone bodies have replaced a considerable amount of the brain's glucose utilization. In addition, the brain has restricted some of its glucose utilization to glycolysis with the release of lactate, thereby reducing glucose oxidation to CO_2 to extremely low rates.

both to maintain pH and to limit excretion of inorganic cations, the kidneys produce large amounts of ammonia and bicarbonate and excrete ammonium ions (NH_4^+). The substrate for renal ammonia production is glutamine (derived from muscle proteolysis), and the carbon skeleton of glutamine is recovered as glucose through renal gluconeogenesis. Thus, during the ketoacidotic phase of starvation, the kidney becomes a major gluconeogenic organ; this occurs at a time when the liver has decreased its rate of gluconeogenesis considerably.

Consequently, in long-term starvation (Fig. 19-7), the brain is the only tissue that completely oxidizes glucose. However, the brain's consumption of glucose occurs at a reduced rate, with ketone bodies providing most of the fuel to the brain. Glucose use in other tissues is limited to glycolysis to lactate (or alanine), which conserves the gluconeogenic potential. The liver derives most of its energy from the partial oxidation of fatty acids, and most other tissues are using either fatty acids or ketone bodies as the major fuel.

HORMONAL SIGNALS FOR REGULATION OF FUEL UTILIZATION

The coordinated regulation of metabolism, as is illustrated by the maintenance of glucose homeostasis, requires key signals that can communicate the state of alimentation of the body to the tissues. Substrate supply (e.g., glucose uptake by the liver at high portal glucose levels or use of free fatty acids and ketone bodies only when they are available) can and does play a very important role. However, the main circulating signaling agents are hormones, especially insulin, glucagon, catecholamines, glucocorticoids, and thyroid hormones. A number of other hormones and circulating factors, together with paracrine and autocrine agents, also participate in the regulation of tissue metabolism.

Clinical Correlation

Diabetes Mellitus

Diabetes mellitus is a chronic disease that results from a lack of secretion of insulin in sufficient amounts or from a lack of insulin stimulation of its target cells. Diabetes mellitus is often diagnosed by an elevated fasting blood glucose level, by excretion of glucose in the urine, or by an abnormal glucose tolerance test. Diabetes mellitus is the third leading cause of death in the United States, following heart disease and cancer.

Diabetes mellitus occurs in two major forms: (1) type 1, insulin-dependent, juvenile-onset diabetes mellitus and (2) type 2, non–insulin-dependent, maturity-onset diabetes mellitus. In insulin-dependent diabetes mellitus (IDDM), the pancreas lacks or has defective β cells and secretes no, or essentially no, insulin. Onset is thought to occur when 80% or more of the pancreatic β cells have been destroyed by the immune system. Because the patients do not synthesize or secrete insulin, daily insulin injections are essential.

Non–insulin-dependent diabetes mellitus (NIDDM) is a more complex disease that may be present for many years prior to diagnosis and that has a strong genetic component. NIDDM accounts for the majority (>80%) of the diagnosed cases of diabetes. It usually occurs after age 40 years and is often (>80%) associated with obesity. Patients with NIDDM exhibit varying levels of plasma insulin, but their tissues are resistant to its actions. Prior to the onset of diabetes, the bodies of these patients probably maintained blood glucose homeostasis by increasing the release of insulin in response to a glucose load. Ultimately, as insulin resistance develops, the pancreas is not able to secrete sufficient insulin to maintain blood glucose levels. Insulin resistance means that insulin fails to control key functions in liver, skeletal muscle, and adipose tissue. Changes in diet, together with a loss of weight and increased physical activity, or the use of drugs that enhance insulin secretion and action often can control NIDDM without the need for exogenous insulin administration.

Thinking Critically

1. In untreated NIDDM, the plasma glucose level is high due to both reduced clearance of glucose from the plasma and increased release of glucose into the plasma. Explain how a reduced response to insulin might (a) decrease the removal of glucose from the circulation and (b) increase glucose release into the circulation.
2. In what ways are the fuel supply and hormonal signals similar in untreated diabetes mellitus and starvation? In what ways are they dissimilar?
3. Untreated IDDM is associated with high levels of ketone bodies in the circulation. Explain.

HORMONES AND THEIR ACTIONS IN THE REGULATION OF FUEL METABOLISM

Insulin is a polypeptide hormone synthesized and secreted by the β cells of the islets of Langerhans in the pancreas. It is secreted in response to changes in circulating glucose; a change of as little as 2 mg/100 mL of plasma can be detected by the pancreas. Insulin release also can be stimulated in response to certain amino acids in the circulation. Other important signals for insulin secretion include gut hormones and nervous stimulation.

Insulin has many effects in a variety of tissues. The insulin-stimulated uptake of glucose in skeletal muscle and adipose tissue involves the transporter GLUT4 and is well characterized (see Chapter 12). However, even in the liver where glucose transport is not directly stimulated by insulin, the hormone still signals glucose storage and utilization. Insulin is a major signal in decreasing hepatic glucose output after feeding and in increasing hepatic glucose use for glycogen synthesis and the flux of glucose through glycolysis, pyruvate dehydrogenase, and the citric acid cycle. In adipose tissue,

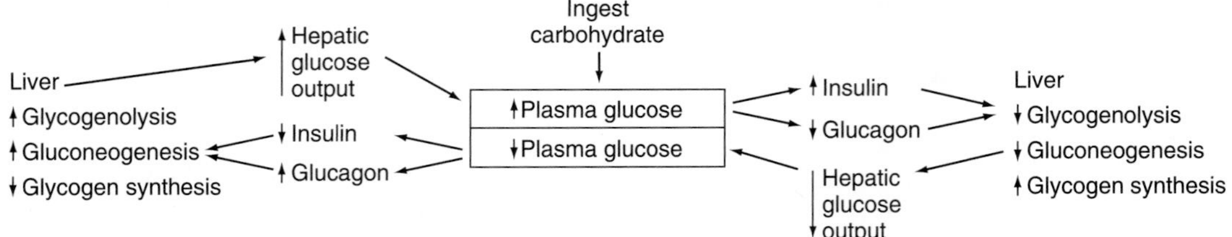

Figure 19-8 Insulin and glucagon regulate hepatic glucose output. Insulin also lowers plasma glucose levels by increasing uptake into skeletal muscle and adipose tissue.

insulin increases fatty acid uptake and triacylglycerol storage via increases in lipoprotein lipase activity and, at the same time, decreases lipolysis by decreasing hormone-sensitive lipase activity. The latter may be one of insulin's strongest actions because it occurs at very low insulin levels and effectively lowers the levels of free fatty acids in the circulation, thereby decreasing their utilization as a fuel.

In addition, insulin brings about other changes, including stimulation of amino acid transport and protein synthesis and a decrease in protein degradation in a variety of tissues. Insulin also regulates the expression of a number of genes; for example, expression of glucokinase (glucose utilization) in the liver is increased by insulin, whereas expression of phosphoenolpyruvate carboxykinase (glucose production) is decreased. Some actions of insulin, particularly those seen at very high concentrations, may be related to its structural similarity to growth factors; these actions include an increase in DNA synthesis and an overall increase in cell growth. Insulin is an anabolic hormone in that it increases storage of glycogen and triacylglycerols; decreases glycogenolysis, gluconeogenesis, and lipolysis; and generally stimulates net protein synthesis. As insulin stimulates the removal of blood glucose into the tissues, circulating levels of glucose drop and insulin secretion consequently slows; thus, insulin and glucose effectively form a negative feedback loop (Fig. 19-8).

Glucagon is a polypeptide hormone secreted by the α cells of the islets of Langerhans in the pancreas. Glucagon secretion is inhibited by high blood glucose, and, therefore, regulation of its concentration is usually opposite to that for insulin. However, glucagon secretion also is increased by some amino acids. Because these two hormones tend to have opposite effects on fuel metabolism, the ratio of insulin to glucagon is commonly used as a way to incorporate changes in both hormones into one value. Although the insulin to glucagon ratio is a useful concept, reference to this ratio should not be taken to mean that there is any direct competition of insulin and glucagon for the same receptors. In humans, glucagon acts only on the liver, where it works through a cyclic AMP (cAMP)–dependent mechanism to increase hepatic glucose output by stimulation of glycogen breakdown and gluconeogenesis. It also stimulates β-oxidation, proteolysis, amino acid transport and catabolism, and urea synthesis. Long-term effects of glucagon include increased expression of the phosphoenolpyruvate carboxykinase gene and of the genes encoding the urea cycle enzymes. By increasing hepatic glycogen breakdown and gluconeogenesis, glucagon causes an increase in blood glucose levels (see Fig. 19-8).

Adrenergic hormones are catecholamines secreted by the adrenal medulla (mainly epinephrine, which is also called adrenaline) and from the sympathetic nervous system (norepinephrine, which is also called noradrenaline). (Synthesis of catecholamines is discussed in Chapters 14 and 27; see Fig. 14-24.) Epinephrine is released into the circulation at times of stress, the fight or flight response, and during starvation. In contrast, the neurological release of norepinephrine occurs directly at nerve endings in the tissues to provide a localized signal. The actions of the catecholamines depend largely on the type of receptor(s) present on the cell surface, as detailed in Table 19-2.

Broadly, adrenergic receptors can be classified into two α (α_1, α_2) and three β (β_1, β_2, and β_3) types (Frayn, 2003; Lafontan and

Table 19-2
Adrenergic Receptors

	Receptor Type		
	β	α_1	α_2
Second Messenger	cAMP	Ca^{2+}	Decrease of cAMP
Effects	Glycogenolysis Lipolysis Vasodilation	Glycogenolysis Vasoconstriction	Inhibition of lipolysis Vasoconstriction

Modified from Frayn, KN (1996) Metabolic Regulation: A Human Perspective. Portland Press, London, p. 100.

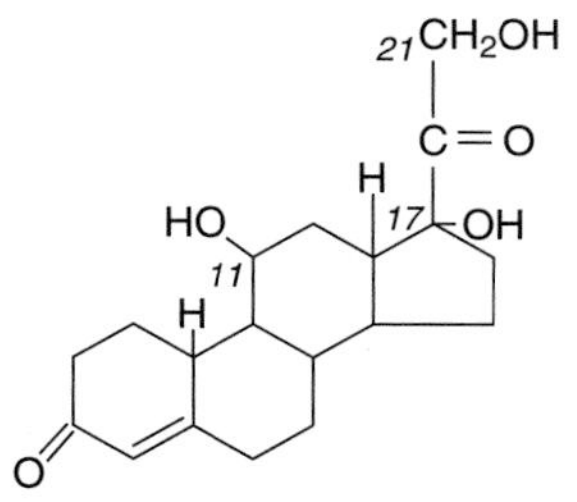

Figure 19-9 Structure of cortisol, a glucocorticoid hormone.

Berlan, 1993). All three β-receptors signal increased lipolysis, glycogenolysis, and gluconeogenesis, and α_1-receptors are involved in stimulating glycogenolysis. In contrast, α_2-receptors inhibit lipolysis. It is interesting that there are marked tissue differences in the expression of adrenergic receptors. Subcutaneous adipose tissue usually has relatively more α_2-receptors, whereas intraabdominal adipose tissue has relatively more β-receptors. This could account for the observation that intraabdominal lipid stores are more rapidly lost than subcutaneous stores during caloric restriction. Despite the somewhat contradictory actions of catecholamines, the elevated levels observed during starvation result in net increases in lipolysis and in hepatic glucose output. Adrenergic hormones also have marked effects on the circulation: β-adrenergic actions include increased heart rate and blood vessel dilation, whereas binding of catecholamines to both types of α-adrenergic receptors generally causes constriction of blood vessels.

Glucocorticoids, predominantly cortisol (Fig. 19-9), are steroid hormones synthesized by the adrenal cortex, and although their levels do not change markedly during starvation or after feeding, they do appear to be essential for the action of a number of other hormones, especially those involving changes in specific gene expression. The action of glucocorticoids is often described as permissive because the action of other hormones is compromised if cortisol levels are low. In general, cortisol stimulates hepatic glucose output and expression of hepatic genes encoding gluconeogenic enzymes. Glucocorticoids are also involved in maintaining elevated rates of proteolysis in skeletal muscle in conditions of net protein breakdown.

The thyroid hormones, triiodothyronine (T_3, active form) and thyroxine (T_4), are synthesized in the thyroid gland and by conversion of T_4 to T_3 in other tissues as described in Chapter 38 (see Fig. 38-1 for hormone structures). The level of T_3 falls in starvation, whereas the concentration of an inactive form, reverse T_3, rises. The thyroid hormones regulate metabolism in a long-term manner by changing gene expression and by modulating the effects of other hormones. For example, although the rise in circulating epinephrine during starvation would be expected to increase the rate of metabolism, this does not occur, perhaps because lower levels of thyroid hormones decrease the rate of metabolism.

MECHANISMS OF HORMONE ACTION

Hormones initiate their actions by binding to receptors. The presence, abundance, and specificity of certain receptors in a given tissue determine its responsiveness to these hormones. The actual physiological responses depend upon various signal transduction mechanisms or upon changes in gene expression or protein synthesis.

There are two general types of hormone receptors in mammalian cells: (1) those on the cell surface that bind the hormone and then transmit the signal to the inside of the cell via a second messenger, and (2) those that bind the hormone inside the cell such that the ligand–receptor complex is the intracellular signaling agent, often acting in the nucleus. Glucagon, insulin, and the catecholamines (adrenergic hormones) are examples of the first type; glucocorticoids and thyroid hormones are examples of the second type.

Glucagon, insulin, and catecholamines bind to specific receptors on the cell membrane. Such receptors contain an extracellular domain that binds the hormone and transmembrane and intracellular domains that anchor the receptor in the membrane and transmit the signal to the inside of the cell. The glucagon receptor and the β- and α-adrenergic receptors share some common mechanisms, including use of cAMP as the intracellular messenger. The initial intracellular event after hormone binding is interaction of the receptor with a specific guanosine triphosphate (GTP)–binding protein (called a G-protein) located on the inner surface of the plasma membrane (Fig. 19-10). There are a variety of G-proteins, but classes important in signal transduction via regulation of cAMP production are G_s, stimulatory proteins, and G_i, inhibitory proteins. G-proteins are composed of three subunits: G_α, G_β, and G_γ. The specificity resides mainly in the α subunit of these heterodimeric proteins.

Effects mediated by glucagon or β-adrenergic receptors involve G_s-proteins. As shown in Figure 19-10, when glucagon or β-adrenergic receptors are activated by hormone binding, $G_{s\alpha}$ binds GTP in exchange for guanosine diphosphate (GDP) with simultaneous dissociation of the α subunit from the β,γ complex. The dissociated $G_{s\alpha}$-GTP subunit then interacts with and activates adenylate cyclase, which is also located on the inner surface of the membrane. This results in synthesis of cAMP from ATP as long as the $G_{s\alpha}$-GTP/adenylate cyclase complex exists. $G_{s\alpha}$ also has a low level of GTPase activity that slowly hydrolyzes GTP to GDP. This renders $G_{s\alpha}$ inactive, and $G_{s\alpha}$-GDP recomplexes with the β,γ subunits to form the inactive heterodimer. The cycle can proceed only in the direction indicated because activation involves an exchange of GDP for GTP, whereas inactivation involves hydrolysis of GTP to GDP.

In contrast to the glucagon or β-adrenergic receptors, which interact with G_s-proteins, effects of catecholamines are mediated through α_2-adrenergic receptors that involve inhibitory G-proteins (G_i-proteins). The GTP–GDP exchange and association–disassociation of subunits proceeds as described for the stimulatory G-proteins. In this case, however, the GTP-bound, activated form of $G_{i\alpha}$ inhibits the activity of adenylate cyclase and results in a decrease in cAMP concentration.

Adenylate cyclase catalyzes the synthesis of cAMP, which is a second messenger within the cell. The level of cAMP regulates the activity of protein kinase A (cAMP-dependent protein kinase). When the level of cAMP is low, the kinase exists as an inactive heterotetrameric complex containing two regulatory subunits (R) and two catalytic subunits (C). When cAMP binds to the regulatory subunits, the catalytic subunits are released in an active form, as follows:

$$R_2C_2 + 4\ \text{cAMP} \rightarrow R_2(\text{cAMP})_4 + 2\ \text{C}$$

Protein kinase A is responsible for the phosphorylation and consequent activation or inactivation of a variety of proteins involved in glycogen, glucose, lipid, and amino acid metabolism. Other targets of protein kinase A include transcription factors that regulate expression of metabolically important enzymes. The levels of cAMP in the cell also are regulated by the rate of hydrolysis of cAMP to AMP by phosphodiesterase.

Catecholamines also may react with α_1-adrenoreceptors that act via association with a G-protein (e.g., G_q) to activate phospholipase C. This occurs via a mechanism similar to that for activation of adenylate cyclase by G_s-proteins. As shown in Figure 19-11, phospholipase C hydrolyzes phosphatidylinositol 4,5-bisphosphate (PIP_2), a minor component of the inner leaflet of the plasma membrane and mainly the species 1-stearoyl-2-arachidonoyl-*sn*-glycerol, to inositol 1,4,5-triphosphate (IP_3) and diacylglycerol. IP_3 acts as a water-soluble second messenger: it opens a Ca^{2+} transport channel and thereby stimulates the release of Ca^{2+} from the endoplasmic reticulum into

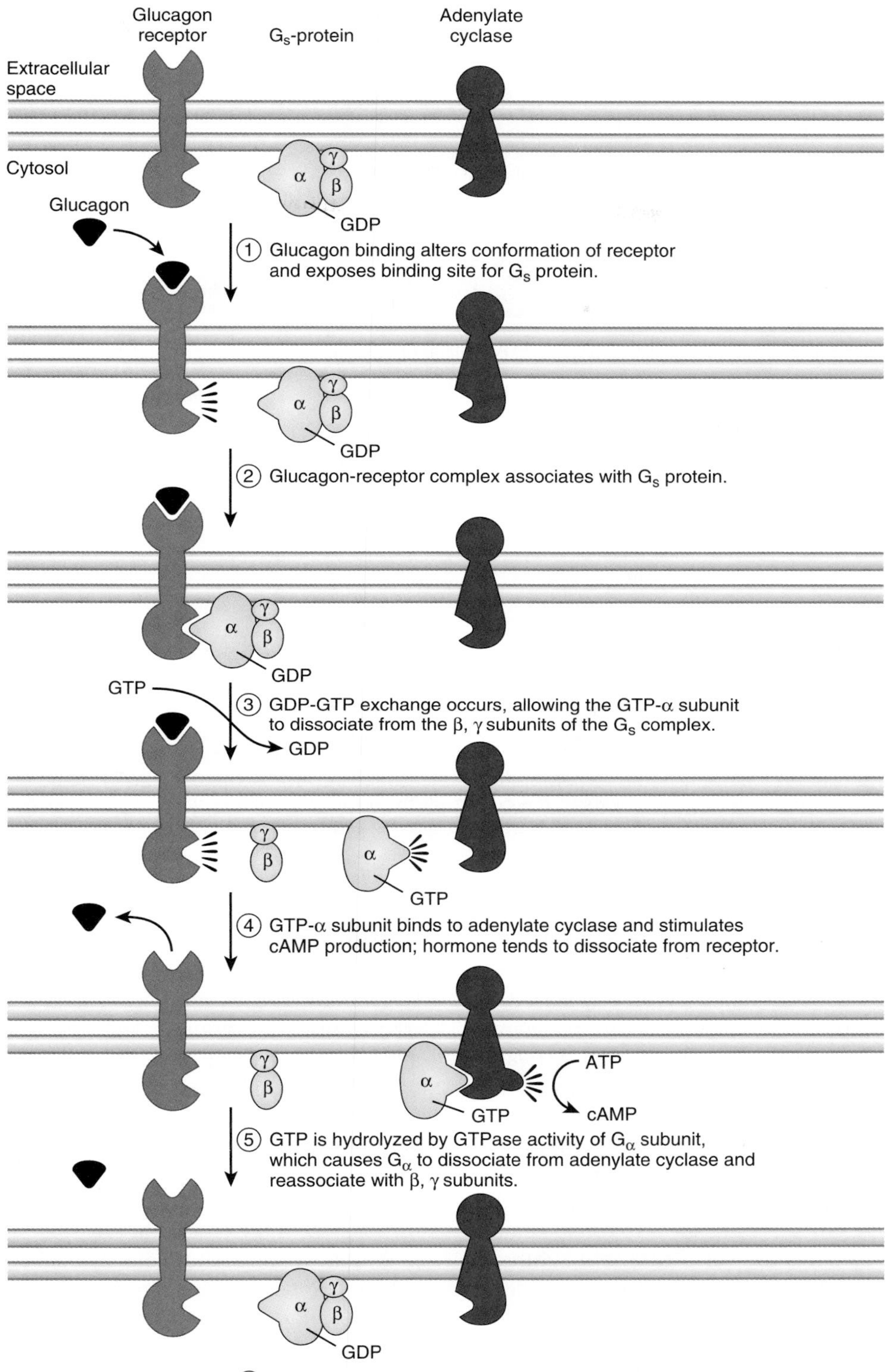
Glucagon receptor
Gs-protein
Adenylate cyclase
Extracellular space
Cytosol
Glucagon
α
γ
β
GDP
① Glucagon binding alters conformation of receptor and exposes binding site for Gs protein.
② Glucagon-receptor complex associates with Gs protein.
GTP
③ GDP-GTP exchange occurs, allowing the GTP-α subunit to dissociate from the β, γ subunits of the Gs complex.
④ GTP-α subunit binds to adenylate cyclase and stimulates cAMP production; hormone tends to dissociate from receptor.
ATP
cAMP
⑤ GTP is hydrolyzed by GTPase activity of Gα subunit, which causes Gα to dissociate from adenylate cyclase and reassociate with β, γ subunits.
⑥ Activation of Gs and of adenylate cyclase may be repeated by reassociation of glucagon with receptor.

Figure 19-10 Mechanism of glucagon action and of epinephrine action via β-adrenergic receptors. The role of a G_s-protein in stimulating adenylate cyclase activity (cAMP production) in response to glucagon is illustrated. Epinephrine acts in a similar mechanism via β-adrenergic receptors. Epinephrine also works via α_2-receptors, which are coupled to G_i-proteins and result in inhibition of adenylate cyclase activity and lower levels of cAMP.

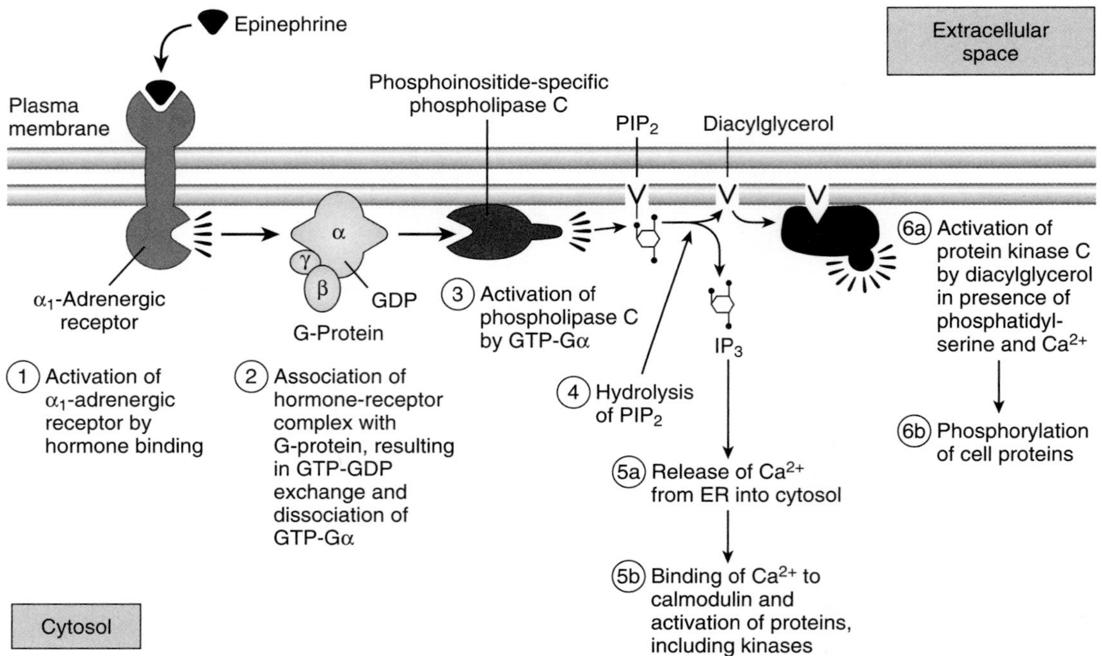

Figure 19-11 Mechanism of action of epinephrine via α_1-adrenergic receptors. Binding of epinephrine to an α_1-adrenergic receptor is coupled via a G-protein to activation of phospholipase C. Phospholipase C catalyzes the hydrolysis of phosphatidylinositol 4,5-bisphosphate (PIP_2) in the membrane to release inositol 1,4,5-triphosphate (IP_3) and diacylglycerol. Biological effects in the cell result from the stimulation by IP_3 of Ca^{2+} release from the endoplasmic reticulum (ER) into the cytosol and from the activation of protein kinase C by diacylglycerol.

the cytosol. The rise in intracytosolic Ca^{2+} stimulates various processes via binding to calmodulin. The diacylglycerol released by phospholipase C acts as a second messenger within the plasma membrane by activating protein kinase C in the presence of Ca^{2+} and phosphatidylserine. Protein kinase C phosphorylates and thereby modulates the activities of several proteins, including glycogen synthase. The diacylglycerol may be further degraded in some tissues to yield arachidonate as substrate for eicosanoid synthesis, as discussed in Chapter 18. Other agents or processes that regulate calcium levels include vasopressin and muscle contraction; the latter is very important in coordinating glycogen breakdown with ATP generation in muscle.

The insulin receptor is composed of two α and two β subunits linked by disulfide bonds (Fig. 19-12) (Kahn, 1994). The extracellular domain is composed of the α subunit, which binds insulin, and the N-terminus of the β subunit. The β subunit contains a single transmembrane domain that transmits the signal to the cytosol. The intracellular domain of the β subunit possesses tyrosine kinase activity. Insulin binding to the receptor activates this tyrosine kinase activity, which first autophosphorylates specific tyrosyl residues on the β subunit. This autophosphorylation in turn activates the β subunit tyrosine kinase so it is able to phosphorylate cytosolic protein substrates, such as insulin receptor substrate 1, which, in turn, bind to and activate other proteins. A variety of different signal transduction cascades is involved in mediating the actions of insulin in the cell.

Thyroid hormones and steroid hormones such as the glucocorticoids are highly lipophilic and circulate bound to specific carriers.

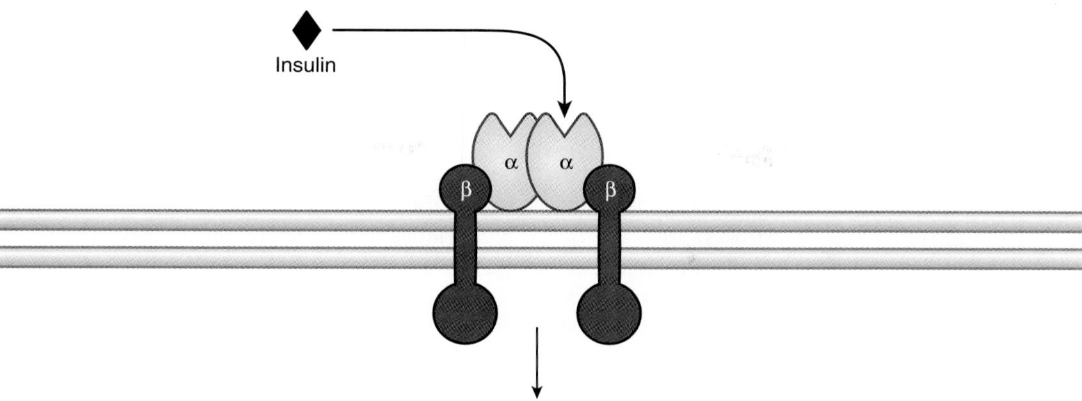

(1) Binding of insulin to the insulin receptor activates the tyrosine kinase activity of the cytosolic domains of the receptor's β subunits, which causes autophosphorylation of tyrosyl residues of the receptor's cytosolic domains.

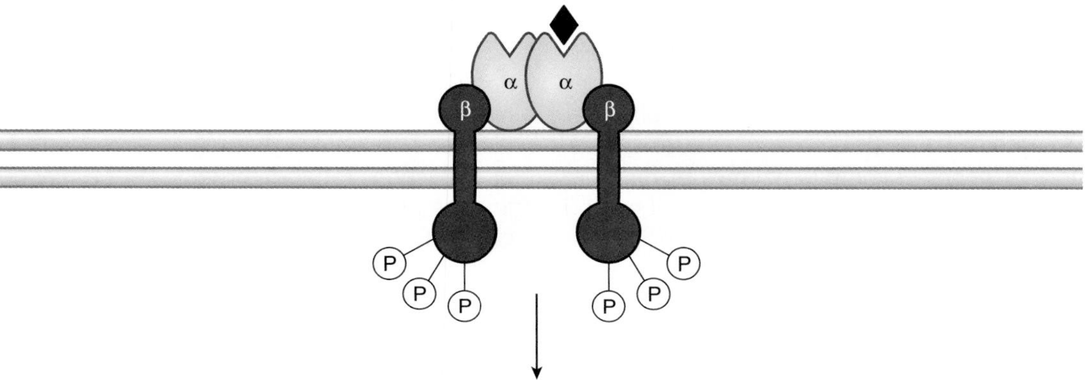

(2) Receptor tyrosine kinase phosphorylates cytosolic "relay" proteins (such as insulin receptor substrate 1, IRS-1), which then bind and activate other proteins. A number of different signal transduction cascades result in changes in cellular physiology and/or patterns of gene expression via serine/threonine phosphorylation/dephosphorylation.

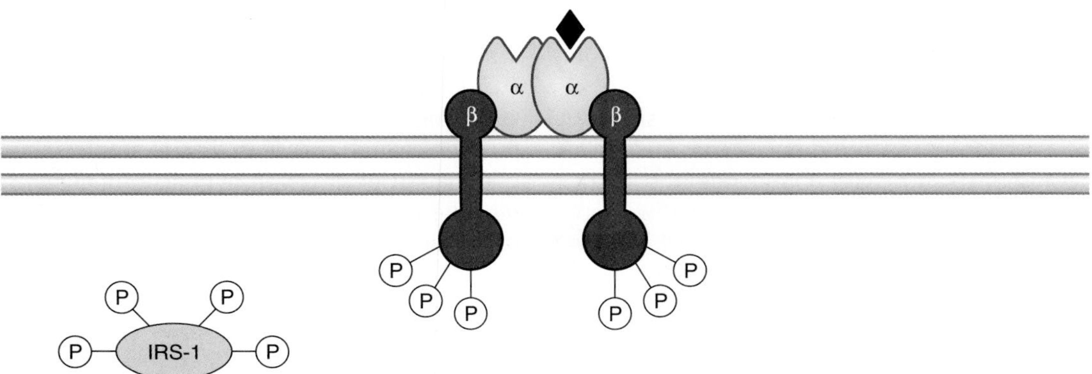

Figure 19-12 Mechanisms of insulin action. Insulin binding to the insulin receptor results in receptor tyrosine kinase activity of the β subunits of the insulin receptor, which first autophosphorylates specific tyrosyl residues on the β subunits. This autophosphorylation, in turn, activates the β subunit tyrosine kinase so it is able to phosphorylate cytosolic protein substrates, such as insulin receptor substrate 1 (IRS-1). IRS-1 then binds and activates other proteins, eventually bringing about its biological effects as a result of serine/threonine phosphorylation of target proteins.

They enter cells, probably by diffusion, and then bind to specific receptors that may be located in the nucleus (T_3) or the cytosol (glucocorticoid). The glucocorticoid–receptor complex is translocated from the cytosol to the nucleus. The activated ligand–receptor complexes then bind to specific sites on the chromosomes and regulate (enhance or repress) the rate of transcription of specific genes. (Further discussion of the action of hormones that are ligands for nuclear receptors can be found in Chapters 30, 31, and 38.)

REGULATION AND CONTROL OF FUEL UTILIZATION

The tissue-specific metabolism mentioned in the previous sections is clearly regulated. Not all pathways are operating in all tissues at all times. Tissue-specific metabolism is often due to the expression, or lack of expression, of genes encoding enzymes of different pathways, but this is a crude method of control that does not allow rapid regulation of flux. As explained in the previous sections, blood glucose levels are regulated, and regulation can be defined as a systemic property. Control, however, is a local property and is defined as the power to change the state of metabolism in response to an external signal. Thus, control is measurable as the degree of influence that an external factor has on the system. It can be said that insulin and glucagon regulate blood glucose levels by control of metabolism in various tissues.

When regulation and control are considered, it is important to remember that metabolic pathways do not exist independently in the body. A beginning and an end of a pathway are usually defined for convenience. In reality, even glycolysis in red blood cells, which appears to begin with glucose and end with lactate, actually requires the continued provision (from the intestine or liver) of glucose into the plasma and the continued removal of the lactate by the liver. Although this scheme is an oversimplification, it illustrates how a very simple pathway extends to other tissues and processes; the utilization of glucose by red blood cells is directly linked to the control of such processes as hepatic glycogen metabolism and gluconeogenesis.

CHARACTERISTICS OF REGULATORY ENZYMES

One of the major goals of the study of intermediary metabolism is to understand regulation and control. Although there has been a somewhat conventional paradigm in this area, it has become apparent that the traditional explanations have many limitations, and more quantitative methods are being developed. A number of terms have been introduced in an effort to aid in the identification and description of control; these include rate-limiting step, pacemaker, and flux-generating step. Although these concepts have been useful, they do not always accurately describe the physiological aspects of regulation and control and, unfortunately, often give the impression that control rests with a single enzyme. A brief consideration follows of qualities that are characteristic of regulation and control, and of some of the problems encountered with traditional explanations of regulation. A full description of the theories and problems of quantitative control analysis can be found in a monograph by Fell (1996).

The rate of flux through a metabolic pathway is controlled by regulatory enzymes and transporters. A regulatory enzyme is defined as one for which activity is controlled by external factors, not simply by substrate supply, and as one for which activity controls some pathway function. It is useful to define two types of regulatory enzymes: (1) those that stabilize (control) metabolite concentrations and maintain homeostasis and (2) those that change or control flux through the pathway. Both are regulatory, but not all regulatory enzymes are flux-controlling enzymes. For example, phosphorylation of glycogen synthase functions to regulate the concentrations of glucose 6-phosphate and other metabolites, rather than to control flux toward glycogen synthesis (Schafer et al., 2004). The two types of control often occur at different steps in a given pathway.

A number of properties have been described that are claimed to be characteristic of regulatory enzymes, but no property by itself can be taken as direct evidence that an enzyme is regulatory or controlling. Enzymes that catalyze reactions near the beginning of a pathway make teleologic sense as sites of control because regulation at this point would avoid the buildup of intermediates and prevent the waste of valuable cofactors. However, when flux in most pathways is changed, there is no major change in the levels of intermediates along the pathway. For example, when the rate of glycolysis in skeletal muscle changes by more than 1,000-fold, the levels of intermediates change by less than 10-fold, and most changes are trivial (Fell, 1996). Because such small changes in metabolite concentrations would result only in minor changes in flux through subsequent enzymes, the results indicate that the activity of more than one enzyme has been changed by external factors. Similarly, the argument has been made that the enzyme with the lowest maximal activity, as determined in vitro, would be easiest to control. At times this seems to have been interpreted as the enzyme with the lowest activity in vivo, but this is not valid because all enzymes in a pathway must be operating at the same rate in vivo, otherwise large excesses (and deficits) of intermediates would arise. In practice, all enzymes in most pathways show activities in vitro that are many times the maximal flux of the pathway in vivo. For example, the capacities (V_{max}, measured in vitro) of the enzymes of glycolysis in heart muscle are all at least ten times the maximal flux measured in the intact organ.

Another property used to identify regulatory enzymes is that they catalyze reactions that are far removed from equilibrium in the cell (i.e., enzymes that catalyze unidirectional reactions). The levels of metabolic intermediates in a cell are usually at a steady state, and there is no noticeable change with time. Even when there is a change in flux in the pathway, a new steady state is achieved relatively quickly. In part, this is due to the fact that most enzymes catalyze reactions in two directions, and the overall reaction will be close to equilibrium if the forward and back reactions are proceeding at nearly equal rates. In practice, this means that changing the activity in one direction will also change the activity in the other direction, with little net effect on overall flux; therefore, a change in activity of a reversible reaction is of little regulatory value.

However, some enzymatic reactions are effectively irreversible in the cell because the back reaction is very slow or nonexistent. These reactions exhibit very large negative changes in free energy (ΔG) (i.e., they are far removed from equilibrium). The position of the equilibrium is a thermodynamic property of the system; enzymes can speed up the rate at which equilibrium is achieved, but they cannot change the position of an equilibrium. Enzymes that catalyze nonequilibrium reactions in the cell are considered good candidates for regulation, because changes in activity in one direction are not immediately negated by changes in the rate of the back direction. However, it is not always easy to determine whether an enzyme catalyzes a nonequilibrium reaction in vivo; and, even when there is clear evidence that it does, this cannot be interpreted as definitive evidence that the enzyme controls flux in the pathway. Finally, even the existence of a well-defined regulatory mechanism cannot be taken as proof that the enzyme is regulatory.

Although all the foregoing criteria are useful in identifying potential regulatory enzymes, definitive conclusions can be drawn only from quantitative analysis of the entire pathway. Normally, hormones and other agents have effects on numerous enzymes in a pathway and in related pathways. For example, in the liver, glucagon will increase phosphorylation of pyruvate kinase and 6-phosphofructo-2-kinase, resulting in decreased flux in glycolysis, while at the same time increasing synthesis of the gluconeogenic enzyme phosphoenolpyruvate carboxykinase and consequently bringing about a net increase in gluconeogenesis. However, glucagon also regulates hepatic glycogen metabolism so that the glucose 6-phosphate produced via gluconeogenesis is not stored as glycogen. Thus, in order to change gluconeogenic flux, glucagon controls the activities of many enzymes, some of which are not directly linked to the pathway, and all of these play some role in the ultimate metabolic change. Therefore, modern quantitative methods are designed to address the question, how much does flux in the pathway change if the activity of a specific enzyme is changed? The experimental evidence points to multiple points of control in a pathway, with the degree of importance of different steps often changing with the physiological state.

MECHANISMS OF ENZYME CONTROL

Control of enzymatic activity can be conveniently split into two models: (1) short-term and (2) long-term. As their names imply, they are distinguished by the length of time required for bringing about changes, but this distinction does not apply absolutely. In reality, these two terms refer to two distinct mechanisms of regulation. *Short-term control* refers to changes in the specific activity of an enzyme, with no change in its concentration. *Long-term control* refers to changes in the amount of enzyme protein, with no change in kinetic properties. The two mechanisms are not exclusive, and some enzymes are subject to both short-term and long-term control in response to the same stimulus. In some cases, a short-term response can take as long as a long-term response; control of protein concentration is highly dependent on the half-life of the protein (see the following information and Chapter 13). All regulatory mechanisms must be reversible if they are to be of physiological importance.

Short-term control can be brought about by a variety of mechanisms. Many specific examples related to fuel metabolism are given in Chapters 12 through 18. Short-term regulation is often related to small changes in the levels of key intermediates such as ATP and NADH. Often this is due simply to changes in cosubstrate or coenzyme supply. For example, a change in NADH concentration will usually be mirrored by an opposite change in NAD^+, and a change in acyl CoA concentration will result in an opposite change in the free CoA concentration. Any change in these ratios will affect flux through reactions catalyzed by enzymes utilizing one of these couplets. Both allosteric activation and inhibition are important short-term mechanisms that involve the binding of a regulatory molecule to a distinct site on an enzyme. Several examples of short-term control can be seen in the pathway for glycolysis. For example, ATP is a strong inhibitor of 6-phosphofructo-1-kinase, and this inhibition can be relieved by a second allosteric factor, such as fructose 2, 6-bisphosphate in liver or AMP in muscle. Hexokinase is inhibited by glucose 6-phosphate. Hepatic pyruvate kinase is stimulated by fructose 1,6-bisphosphate and

Nutrition Insight

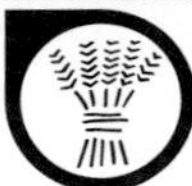

Alcohol Consumption and Hypoglycemia

Alcohol is metabolized in the liver by alcohol dehydrogenase, which catalyzes the oxidation of ethanol to acetaldehyde:

$$CH_3CH_2OH + NAD^+ \rightarrow CH_3CHO + NADH + H^+$$

Consumption of alcohol, especially by an undernourished individual, can cause hypoglycemia. Drinking alcohol after strenuous exercise can have the same effect. This hypoglycemia can be quite dangerous, especially because a person may be thought to be inebriated when, in fact, he or she has hypoglycemia that may lead to irreversible damage to the central nervous system.

Thinking Critically

1. What is the normal source of glucose for maintenance of normoglycemia between meals? How might this source of glucose be affected by fasting/starvation or by strenuous exercise? What role would this play in the development of hypoglycemia subsequent to alcohol consumption?
2. Metabolism of ethanol to acetaldehyde is accompanied by the conversion of NAD^+ to NADH and a potentially dramatic increase in the ratio of NADH to NAD^+ in the cytosol of liver cells. Considering the role of NAD^+ in ethanol and pyruvate/lactate metabolism, how would gluconeogenesis from pyruvate (alanine) or lactate be affected by alcohol consumption? What role might this play in development of hypoglycemia?

inhibited by alanine. In addition, hepatic pyruvate kinase is subject to covalent modification and is phosphorylated by cAMP-dependent protein kinase (e.g., in response to glucagon); this makes it more sensitive to allosteric inhibition.

Reversible covalent modification of enzymes is an important short-term regulatory mechanism. A number of covalent modifications have been described (Lehninger et al., 1993), and one of the most common types is phosphorylation–dephosphorylation. Since the first description of activation of an enzyme (glycogen phosphorylase) by phosphorylation, there have been numerous reports of protein phosphorylation. Such phosphorylations usually occur on serine, threonine, or tyrosine residues. Phosphorylation results in activation of some enzymes and in inhibition of others. Many cases of protein phosphorylation have been reported that do not change the kinetic properties of the enzyme and, therefore, are of unknown function.

Important examples of enzymes that are controlled by phosphorylation–dephosphorylation include hormone-sensitive lipase in adipose tissue (activated by phosphorylation in response to catecholamines and inactivated by dephosphorylation in response to insulin), glycogen synthase (inactivated by phosphorylation in response to glucagon in liver), and 6-phosphofructo-2-kinase (a bifunctional enzyme, which loses kinase activity while its fructose 2,6-bisphosphatase activity is enhanced in response to glucagon in liver). Another very important phosphorylation is that of pyruvate dehydrogenase, which is inactivated by phosphorylation catalyzed by a specific kinase bound to the enzyme complex. Phosphorylation (inactivation) of pyruvate dehydrogenase is stimulated by acetyl CoA and NADH and inhibited by high CoA, NAD^+, or pyruvate. Dephosphorylation (activation) of the enzyme is stimulated by insulin. The pyruvate dehydrogenase reaction is a crucial step in maintaining the body's glucose reserves, because inhibition of the oxidative decarboxylation of pyruvate (a 3-carbon compound) to acetyl CoA (a 2-carbon compound) conserves the gluconeogenic potential; the body lacks a mechanism to reverse this reaction. Pyruvate dehydrogenase can be phosphorylated on three distinct sites with phosphorylation on site 1 inactivating the complex. Phosphorylation on the other two sites appears to play a role in determining the rate at which the complex is reactivated by dephosphorylation after glucose again becomes abundant. The tissue-specific expression of different isoforms of pyruvate dehydrogenase kinase and phosphatase allows different tissues to respond differently in terms of pyruvate dehydrogenase inactivation during starvation. Therefore, the brain, in contrast to the liver, maintains its pyruvate dehydrogenase activity well into starvation (Sugden and Holness, 2003; Harris et al., 2002).

A somewhat different form of short-term control is the physical movement of proteins within a cell. A well-known example of this is the insulin-regulated movement of GLUT4 glucose transporters to the cell surface of skeletal muscle and adipocytes, which increases the glucose transport capacity of these cells. Another example is the movement and activation of certain enzymes within the liver in response to hormones or substrate availability, a process that results in the enzymes becoming physically close to or removed from their substrates (Watford, 2002). For example, in the postabsorptive state glucokinase is present within the nucleus where it is bound by a regulatory protein together with fructose 6-phosphate. During the absorptive period fructose 1-phosphate binds to the regulatory protein, and this releases the glucokinase that then translocates to the cytosol where it is active.

Changes in the amount of enzyme protein (long-term control) are brought about by changes in the synthesis and/or degradation of the protein and consequently can be rather slow, often taking days or hours to achieve a new steady state. However, some enzymes can show these long-term changes within relatively short time-periods (<1 hour), whereas some short-term covalent modifications can take almost as long. The steady-state concentrations of proteins (enzymes) are functions of the rates of their synthesis and degradation. Enzyme synthesis is a zero-order reaction: the rate is linear with time and can be described by a constant, k_s. However, enzyme degradation follows first-order reaction kinetics, meaning that the actual rate is dependent on the amount of enzyme present (e.g., when enzyme synthesis decreases, the absolute degradation rate will decrease exponentially with time). The rate of enzyme degradation can be described as the product of the enzyme concentration at time zero, E, and a degradation constant, k_d, so that the rate of enzyme degradation is $E \cdot k_d$. Therefore, it is generally not meaningful to describe degradation in absolute rates because the absolute rate changes depending on the amount of enzyme present. Instead, either the k_d or the apparent half-life is typically used to describe the rate of protein degradation. Half-life ($t_{1/2}$) can be defined as the time taken for 50% of the original enzyme to be degraded. Different proteins exhibit half-lives that range from a few minutes to many days. Proteins with very short half-lives not only will be degraded rapidly, but they also will respond rapidly to changes in the synthesis or degradation rate, and so are able to establish new steady-state concentrations much more quickly than proteins with long half-lives. Such proteins are ideal candidates for regulation (Walker, 1983; Schimke, 1973).

An example of a highly regulated key enzyme of glucose metabolism is phosphoenolpyruvate carboxykinase in liver. This enzyme has a half-life of about 6 hours and is regulated exclusively by long-term mechanisms. Most of this regulation is brought about by changes in the rate of transcription of the phosphoenolpyruvate carboxykinase gene. During starvation, one of the initial hormonal signals is increased glucagon, which increases glycogenolysis in liver via the second messenger cAMP. The increase in cAMP stimulates transcription of the phosphoenolpyruvate carboxykinase gene and results in higher rates of synthesis of the enzyme protein and hence higher enzyme activity. Thus, as starvation slowly develops and as liver glycogen stores are gradually depleted, the liver is synthesizing new phosphoenolpyruvate carboxykinase at an increased rate and thereby increasing its capacity to carry out gluconeogenesis. Such a mechanism is highly suited to a situation such as starvation in which changes in metabolism occur over several hours. On the other hand, this mechanism would not be suitable for rapid responses such as muscle contraction during which short-term mechanisms such as allosterism are used to allow responses in fractions of a second. Although changes in phosphoenolpyruvate carboxykinase level are largely the result of changes in transcription of the gene, changes in phosphoenolpyruvate carboxykinase protein level also can occur through changes in its mRNA turnover or changes in the rate of degradation of the enzyme protein itself.

As with all reports of regulation, evidence that an enzyme is itself regulated, even via long-term changes in the amount of enzyme protein, cannot be taken to indicate changes in flux in the pathway or to imply that such changes in the enzyme activity are in any way regulatory. They may be simply adaptive in nature; many such changes occur long after flux through the pathway has changed in response to more rapid control at various points in the pathway. In the final analysis, any theory of metabolic regulation and control must be consistent with the evidence for changes in flux in vivo.

REFERENCES

Acheson KJ, Schutz Y, Bessard T, Anantharaman K, Flatt JP, Jequier E (1988) Glycogen storage capacity and de novo lipogenesis during massive carbohydrate overfeeding in man. Am J Clin Nutr 48:240-247.

Assifi NM, Suchankova G, Constant S, Prentki M, Saha AK, Ruderman NB (2005) AMP-activated protein kinase and coordination of hepatic fatty acid metabolism of starved/carbohydrate-refed rats. Am J Physiol Endocrinol Metab 289: E794-E800.

Cahill GF Jr (1970) Starvation in man. N Engl J Med 282:668-675.

Fell D (1996) Understanding the Control of Metabolism. Portland Press, London.

Frayn K (2003) Metabolic Regulation: A Human Perspective. Blackwell Publishers, Oxford, pp 143-145.

Gibson DM, Harris RA (2002) Metabolic Regulation in Mammals. Taylor & Francis, London, pp 143-146,

Harris RA, Bowker-Kinley MM, Huang B, Wu P (2002) Regulation of the activity of the pyruvate dehydrogenase complex. Adv Enzymol Reg 43:249-259

Hellerstein M, Schwarz J-M, Neese RA (1996) Regulation of hepatic de novo lipogenesis in humans. Annu Rev Nutr 16:523-557.

Horton T J, Drougas H, Brachy A, Reed GW, Peters JC, Hill JO (1995) Fat and carbohydrate overfeeding in humans: different effects on energy storage. Am J Clin Nutr 62:19-29.

Hudgins LC, Hellerstein M. Seidman C, Neese R, Diakun J, Hirsch J (1996) Human fatty acid synthesis is stimulated by a eucaloric low fat, high carbohydrate diet. J Clin Invest 97: 2081-2091.

Jungas RL, Halperin ML, Brosnan J T (1992) Quantitative analysis of amino acid oxidation and related gluconeogenesis in humans. Physiol Rev 72:419-448.

Kahn CR (1994) Insulin action, diabetogenes, and the cause of type II diabetes. Diabetes 43:1066-1084.

Lafontan M, Berlan M (1993) Fat cell adrenergic receptors and their control of white and brown fat cell function. J Lipid Res 34:1057-1091.

Lehninger AL, Nelson DL, Cox MM (1993) Principles of Biochemistry. Worth Publishers, New York, pp 233-235.

Leibel RL, Edens NK, Fried SK (1989) Physiological basis for the control of body fat distribution in humans. Annu Rev Nutr 9:417-443.

Minehira K, Vega N, Vidal H, Acheson K, Tappy L (2004) Effect of carbohydrate overfeeding on whole body macronutrient metabolism and expression of lipogenic enzymes in adipose tissue of lean and overweight humans. Int J Obesity 28:1291-1298.

Randle PJ, Garland PB, Hales CN, Newsholme EA (1963) The glucose fatty acid cycle. Its role in insulin sensitivity and the metabolic disturbances of diabetes mellitus. Lancet i:785-794.

Reeds PJ, Burrin DG (2001) Glutamine and the bowel. J Nutr 131:2505S-2508S.

Roediger WE (1982) Utilization of nutrients by isolated epithelial cells of the rat colon. Gastroenterology 83:424-429.

Ruderman NB, Aoki TT, Cahill GF Jr (1976) Gluconeogenesis and its disorders in man. In: Hanson RW, Mehlman MA (eds) Gluconeogenesis: Its Regulation in Mammalian Species. Wiley Interscience, New York, pp 515-532.

Schafer JRA, Fell DA, Rothman D, Shulman RG (2004) Protein phosphorylation can regulate metabolite concentrations rather than control flux: the example of glycogen synthase. Proc Natl Acad Sci USA 101:1485-1490.

Schimke R (1973) Control of enzyme levels in mammalian tissues. Adv Enzymol 37: 135-187.

Shulman GI, Landau B R (1992) Pathways of glycogen repletion. Physiol Rev 72:1019-1035.

Stumpel F, Jungerman K (1997) Sensing by intrahepatic muscarinic nerves of a portal-arterial glucose concentration gradient as a signal for insulin-dependent glucose uptake in the perfused rat liver. FEBS Lett 406:119-122.

Sugden MC, Holness MJ (2003) Recent advances in mechanisms regulating glucose oxidation at the level of pyruvate dehydrogenase complex by PDKs. Am J Physiol Endocrinol Metab 284:E855-E862.

Vannucci S, Hawkins R (1983) Substrates for energy metabolism of the pituitary and pineal glands. J. Neurochem 41:1718-1725.

Walker R (1983) The Molecular Biology of Enzyme Synthesis: Regulatory Mechanisms of Enzyme Adaptation. Wiley Interscience, New York.

Watford M (2002) Small amounts of dietary fructose dramatically increase hepatic glucose uptake through a novel mechanism of glucokinase activation. Nutr Rev 60:252-257.

RECOMMENDED READINGS

DeFronzo RA (1997) Pathogenesis of type 2 diabetes: metabolic and molecular implications for identifying diabetes genes. Diabetes Rev 5:177-269.

Frayn KN (2003) Metabolic Regulation: A Human Perspective. Blackwell Publishing, Oxford.

Gibson DM, Harris RA (2002) Metabolic Regulation in Mammals. Taylor and Francis, London

Newsholme EA, Leech AR (1986) Biochemistry for the Medical Sciences. John Wiley and Sons, Chichester, UK.

Randle PJ (1986) Fuel selection in animals. Biochem Soc Trans 14:799-806.

Chapter 20

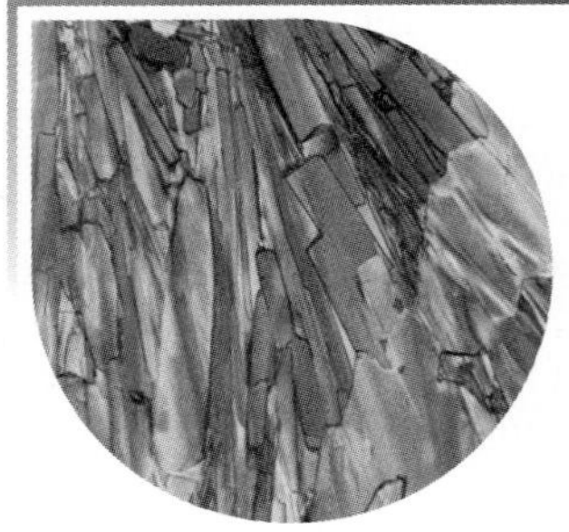

Regulation of Fuel Utilization in Response to Exercise

Martha H. Stipanuk, PhD

OUTLINE

COMMON ABBREVIATIONS

CPT I	carnitine palmitoyltransferase I
IMTG	intramyocellular triacylglycerol
RQ	respiratory quotient, defined as moles CO_2 produced/moles O_2 consumed; also known as respiratory exchange ratio (RER)
VO_{2max}	maximum aerobic capacity; measure of maximum volume of O_2 consumption

This chapter is a revision of the chapter contributed by Anton J. M. Wagenmakers, PhD, for the first edition.

OVERVIEW OF FUEL UTILIZATION IN MUSCLE

Carbohydrate and fat are the most important fuels for muscle. Under most conditions, the muscle uses a mixture of fat and carbohydrate as fuel. Although oxidation of branched-chain amino acids may serve as a fuel in muscle, the contribution of these amino acids is minimal and will not be considered in this chapter. The sources of the carbohydrate and lipid used by the muscle include those provided from the diet or from other tissues via the plasma and those stored within the muscle cells themselves.

Sources external to the muscle include glucose, which is obtained directly from the diet or released by the liver following glycogenolysis or gluconeogenesis, and fatty acids, which are released from adipose-tissue stores by action of hormone-sensitive lipase (mostly albumin-bound fatty acids, referred to as plasma free fatty acids) or released locally in the muscle capillaries from circulating lipoproteins (chylomicrons or very low density lipoproteins [VLDLs]) via the action of lipoprotein lipase. Liver typically has approximately 80 to 100 g of glycogen in the postabsorptive state. Adipose-tissue stores vary widely, but a 70-kg individual of normal body composition has approximately 16 kg of adipose tissue (composed of 12.5 kg of lipid, 3.1 kg of water, and 0.5 kg of protein). The composition of the diet will obviously affect the availability of dietary fuels. The availability of all of the external fuels is affected by cardiovascular mechanisms that affect blood flow to the muscle as well as by the actual plasma levels of the fuels.

Within the muscle fibers themselves there are glycogen stores (glycogen granules) and lipid droplets that contain intramyocellular triacylglycerol (IMTG). The content of intramuscular fuels depends on fiber type, training status, and diet. Muscle glycogen stores can vary from 50 g after strenuous exercise to 900 g in a well-fed, well-trained, muscular person. Typical muscle glycogen stores in an adult are approximately 350 g when intramuscular stores are full. IMTG is localized mostly adjacent to the mitochondria of the muscle fibers (Fig. 20-1). The intramuscular stores of triacylglycerol are relatively small compared to those of adipose tissue; the total IMTG amounts to approximately 300 g (Jeukendrup, 2003).

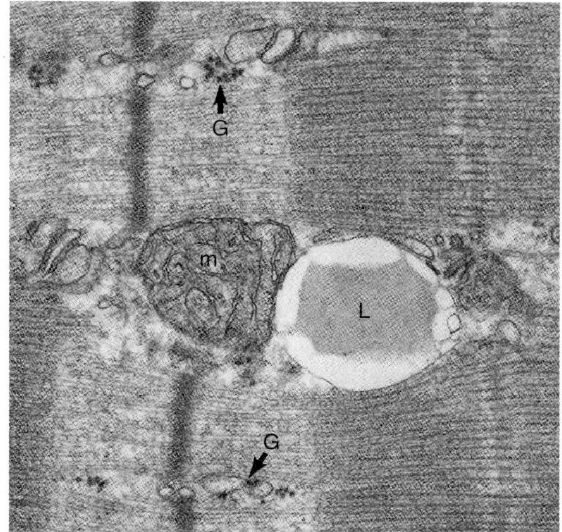

Figure 20-1 Electron micrograph of skeletal muscle showing mitochondria (*m*), lipid droplets (*L*), and glycogen granules (*G*). (Courtesy Dr. Hans Hoppeler, University of Berne, Berne, Switzerland.)

Because the muscle is dependent upon a mixture of fat and carbohydrate as fuel and because body stores of carbohydrate are much less than those of fat, depletion of muscle and liver glycogen reserves often coincides with exhaustion. This has led to efforts to enhance glycogen stores or provide glucose intake during exercise in order to enhance performance.

MUSCLE FIBER TYPES

Individual human muscles are a mixture of type 1 and type 2 muscle fibers. These muscle fibers are differentiated by their myosin heavy chain isoform contents and by their metabolic properties. Characteristics of type 1 and type 2 muscle fibers are given in Table 20-1. The myosin heavy-chain isoforms are an important determinant of the contractile characteristics of the muscle fiber. Type 1 fibers have relatively slow acting myosin ATPases and, hence, contract slowly, but they have a high capacity for oxidative metabolism (high activities of enzymes of the citric acid cycle, of fatty acid oxidation, and of the electron transport chain), a high content of triacylglycerols (IMTGs), high

Table 20-1
Characteristics of Major Skeletal Muscle Fiber Types

	Type 1 Red Fibers (Slow-Twitch, Slow-Oxidative, Fatigue-Resistant)	Type 2A Red Fibers (Fast-Twitch A, Fast-Oxidative, Fatigue-Resistant)	Type 2B White (Fast-Twitch B, Fast-Glycolytic, Fatigable)
Relative distribution (in average person)	~50 %	~40 %	~10 %
Fiber diameter	Intermediate	Small	Large
Myosin ATPase activity	Slow	Fast	Fast
Force production	Low	High	Very high
Contraction velocity	Slow	Fast	Very fast
Size of motor neuron	Small	Large	Very large
Resistance to fatigue	High	Intermediate	Low
Recruitment order	Early	Intermediate	Late
Activity used for	Aerobic (e.g., long-distance running)	Long-term aerobic plus anaerobic (e.g., middle distance running and swimming)	Short-term anaerobic (e.g., sprinting)
Myoglobin content	High	Intermediate	Low
Generate ATP by	Aerobic system	Aerobic system	Anaerobic system
Mitochondrial density	High	Intermediate	Low
Capillary density	High	Intermediate	Low
Oxidative capacity	High	High	Low
Glycolytic capacity (glycogen phosphorylase)	Low	High	High
Creatine phosphate content	Intermediate	High	High
Glycogen content	Intermediate	Intermediate	High
Triacylglycerol content	High	Intermediate	Low

hormone-sensitive lipase activity, and moderate glycolytic capacity. Type 2B fibers possess rapidly acting myosin ATPases and thus have fast contraction times. Type 2B fibers have a lower oxidative capacity and a very high glycolytic capacity and contain more glycogen and much less IMTG than do the type 1 fibers. Type 2A fibers also contain fast-acting myosin ATPases and have a high glycolytic capacity, like the type 2B fibers, but type 2A fibers also have a moderate oxidative capacity.

Although all three types of fibers are found within individual muscles, the proportions of fiber types vary depending on the action of that muscle. A mixture of fiber types is present within skeletal muscles; however, only one type of muscle fiber is contained within a particular motor unit. In fact, the muscle fiber type depends on the motor neuron (axon) supplying that particular fiber. Therefore, if a weak contraction is needed, only the type 1 motor units will be activated, whereas if a stronger contraction is needed, the type 2A fibers will also be activated to assist the type 1 fibers. Type 2B fibers are activated last and are needed for maximal contractions (e.g., ballistic activities), but these fibers tire easily.

It traditionally is assumed that type 2 fibers are specialized to perform sprinting exercise, whereas type 1 fibers are more suited to perform endurance exercise. In agreement with this, the better sprinters tend to have a high percentage of type 2 fibers, although some world-class sprinters have a 50 % type 1 and 50 % type 2 distribution. Conversely, a marathoner may have a much higher percentage of type 1 fibers. Certainly, genetic factors play a role in determining fiber type distribution. In addition, muscle fibers display a degree of plasticity that allows them to reversibly change their biochemical and morphological properties when exposed to different functional demands. For example, strength or resistance (low repetition, high load) training can lead to an increase in the myofibrillar volume (hypertrophy) of both type 1 and 2 fibers. High-intensity endurance (high repetition, low load) training can result in an increase in the proportion of type 1 fibers (increase in mitochondrial and capillary density), but it does not result in an increase in fiber size. It is thought that both metabolic and mechanical signals are involved in bringing about these changes (Putman et al., 2004; Hoppeler and Flück, 2002).

SKELETAL MUSCLE FUEL UTILIZATION DURING REST

Skeletal muscle is the largest body compartment in humans, accounting for 40% to 50% of body mass in an ordinary lean subject. As such, skeletal muscle can have major effects on human metabolism, whole-body energy expenditure, and nutritional requirements.

SKELETAL MUSCLE FUEL NEEDS DURING REST

During rest, energy expenditure is low, and resting skeletal muscle needs less energy on a per kilogram basis for maintenance than do intraabdominal tissues such as liver, gut, or kidney. The latter tissues not only have to take care of their own maintenance but also serve many essential functions in whole-body metabolism (e.g., digestion, absorption, fluid retention, urea synthesis, fatty acid synthesis, and lipoprotein synthesis), and are the sites of synthesis of many export proteins (e.g., albumin, fibrinogen, apolipoproteins, and digestive enzymes). Apart from a few muscles that are active continuously in the maintenance of posture, skeletal muscles in resting conditions have low energy expenditures. At rest, energy in the form of ATP, the universal energy donor, as in all other cells, is required only for the following functions:

- To maintain electrolyte and calcium gradients via ATP-dependent ion pumps
- To maintain amino acid gradients (much higher intracellular than extracellular concentrations)
- To replace fuel stores lost via oxidation (glycogen and intramuscular triacylglycerols)
- To keep substrate cycles going (e.g., the fructose 6-phosphate/fructose 1,6-bisphosphate cycle, and the triacylglycerol/free fatty acid cycle)
- To maintain the continuous synthesis and breakdown of proteins (protein turnover)

Even from the point of view of protein turnover, skeletal muscle needs less energy than intraabdominal tissues because the mean turnover rate of skeletal muscle protein (0.05% per hour) is lower than that of most other proteins of the human body and much lower than that of the intracellular and export proteins of liver and gut (e.g., apolipoprotein B-100, which is synthesized in the liver, with a turnover rate of 16% per hour). The need, therefore, for ATP synthesis during rest is easily met by aerobic metabolism (oxidation). For these reasons, skeletal muscle oxygen consumption constitutes only 25% of whole-body oxygen consumption during resting conditions, despite the fact that the skeletal muscle compartment constitutes 40% to 50% of body mass (see Chapter 21, Fig. 21-8).

Skeletal muscle oxidizes a mixture of carbohydrate and fat during rest. Although the impact of skeletal muscle gas exchange on the resting whole-body (systemic) respiratory quotient (RQ) is small, measurements of the arteriovenous difference for oxygen and carbon dioxide across skeletal muscle have demonstrated the relative importance of fat and carbohydrate as fuels for the resting muscle. The RQ is defined as moles CO_2 produced/moles O_2 consumed, and it is usually measured as volume of CO_2 produced/volume of O_2 consumed (see Chapter 21). Himwich and Rose (1927), using such techniques in dogs, observed that the RQ of skeletal muscle in fed dogs was about 0.92, whereas the RQ of skeletal muscle in starved dogs was 0.80 and lower. Because an RQ of 1.00 indicates 100% carbohydrate oxidation and a value of 0.70 indicates 100% fat oxidation, it is clear that skeletal muscle at rest always oxidizes a mixture of carbohydrate and fat. This finding has been confirmed in humans on many occasions, using the same techniques.

USE OF PLASMA GLUCOSE AND FATTY ACIDS OBTAINED FROM PLASMA FREE FATTY ACIDS AND LIPOPROTEINS DURING THE RESTING STATE

The next question is which carbohydrate sources and which fat sources are oxidized by skeletal muscle during the resting state. In both cases there is a choice between intramuscular and extracellular sources. For carbohydrates the sources are the glycogen stores in skeletal muscle and blood glucose. Blood glucose originates from the diet in the first hours after a meal (i.e., during the postprandial period) and originates from the liver in the postabsorptive and fasted state. The breakdown of liver glycogen to glucose is the major source of hepatic glucose output in the first 16 hours of fasting, whereas gluconeogenesis from glycerol and amino acids becomes the primary source of hepatic glucose output after 16 to 24 hours of fasting. Blood glucose is the major source of carbohydrate for oxidation in skeletal muscle at rest, and breakdown of muscle glycogen makes a minimal contribution to the energy needs of resting muscle.

Fatty acids for oxidation by muscle may be obtained from three potential sources. The first source consists of the free fatty acids circulating in the blood bound to albumin. Free fatty acids originate either from the diet or, in the postabsorptive state and during fasting, from mobilization from the large triacylglycerol stores in adipose tissue. The plasma concentration of fatty acids is about 0.3 mmol/L after ingestion of a mixed diet but are higher in the postabsorptive state, increasing to as much as 1.0 to 1.5 mmol/L after a few days of fasting. Plasma fatty acids are a major fuel for muscle during resting conditions.

The second potential source of fatty acids lies in the triacylglycerols circulating in the blood as lipoproteins. The endothelial wall of the capillary bed in skeletal muscle contains the enzyme called lipoprotein lipase, which liberates fatty acids from plasma lipoproteins. Skeletal muscle lipoprotein lipase activities are elevated during fasting, and this favors the hydrolysis of triacylglycerols in circulating VLDLs by muscle tissue, allowing the uptake and oxidation of the released fatty acids.

A third potential source of fatty acids lies in the IMTGs. These are present in the muscle fibers in small lipid droplets. In a study of IMTG turnover in leg muscle, a relatively high turnover rate of IMTG (~3.4% per hour) was observed in both the fed and postabsorptive states, but the rate of synthesis was balanced by the rate of breakdown such that the IMTG concentration did not change (Sacchetti et al., 2004). Skeletal muscle contains hormone-sensitive lipase, which can liberate fatty acids from the IMTG stores. Although a high constitutive level of hormone-sensitive lipase is found in human skeletal muscle, its activity in the resting and fed state is presumably minimized by the low levels of epinephrine and intracellular Ca^{+2} along with the resting levels of insulin.

TRANSITION FROM PREDOMINANT UTILIZATION OF CARBOHYDRATE IN THE POSTPRANDIAL STATE TO PREDOMINANT UTILIZATION OF FAT IN THE FASTED STATE

RQ measurements across the leg have shown that carbohydrates are the main fuel for skeletal muscle in the fed situation, whereas fat oxidation accounts for 80% to 90% or more of oxygen consumption in the postabsorptive and fasted situation. The transition from the fed to the fasted state is carefully controlled, as described in Chapters 12, 16, and 19.

In the postprandial situation, high plasma insulin concentrations lead to a rapid uptake of blood glucose by skeletal muscle. The insulin-stimulated translocation of glucose transporter-4 (GLUT4) from membranes of the sarcoplasmic reticulum into the sarcolemma plays an important role in the insulin-stimulated uptake of glucose into skeletal muscle (Brozinick et al., 1994). From a quantitative point of view, skeletal muscle is the most important tissue for the removal of glucose that enters the blood after oral ingestion of carbohydrates. Glucose uptake by skeletal muscle, therefore, is extremely important for glucose homeostasis and prevents large peaks in blood glucose concentration following meals. The glucose is used both for glycogen synthesis (especially in individuals who are regularly involved in exercise and who, therefore, regularly deplete their muscle glycogen stores) and for oxidation as a fuel.

Simultaneously, via inhibition of hormone-sensitive lipase, the high insulin concentration restricts lipolysis in adipose tissue and skeletal muscle so that no mobilization of fatty acid from these triacylglycerol stores occurs. The high glycolytic flux in muscle in the fed state results in high rates of pyruvate and acetyl CoA formation, which result in a relatively high malonyl CoA concentration. Malonyl CoA serves to keep the rate of fatty acid oxidation low by inhibiting carnitine palmitoyltransferase I (CPT-I) (Bezaire et al., 2004; Roepstorff et al., 2004; Sugden and Holness, 1994). The fatty acids present in the diet appear in the circulation mainly as triacylglycerols in chylomicrons. Lipids in circulating chylomicrons and VLDLs are primarily directed to the adipose tissue stores because the activity of lipoprotein lipase in adipose tissue is much higher than the activity of lipoprotein lipase in skeletal muscle in animals in the fed state (Sugden et al., 1993). Therefore, in the fed state, all of these mechanisms collectively act to limit fat utilization and make carbohydrate the main skeletal muscle fuel.

In the transition to the fasted state, the insulin concentration gradually falls, leading to a return of GLUT4 from the sarcolemma to the sarcoplasmic reticulum, and to a reduction of glucose uptake by the muscle. This is probably accompanied by a fall in pyruvate dehydrogenase and glycogen synthase activities. This is paralleled by a decrease of the malonyl CoA concentration in muscle and relief of inhibition of CPT-I, allowing fatty acids to enter the mitochondria for β-oxidation. Concurrently, free fatty acid mobilization from adipose tissue is accelerated owing to the removal of the inhibitory effect of insulin on hormone-sensitive lipase. As a result, the plasma concentrations of free fatty acids rise, making more free fatty acids available for oxidation in muscle.

During the latter decades of the twentieth century it was thought that increased oxidation of free fatty acids in skeletal muscle suppressed glucose oxidation and uptake via the glucose–fatty acid (Randle) cycle. The glucose–fatty acid cycle refers to the inhibition of glucose utilization when fatty acids are available as an alternative fuel, and vice versa. The glucose–fatty acid cycle may be involved in regulating glucose and fatty acid utilization by muscle under conditions of rest and low-intensity exercise. In the postabsorptive and fasted situation, the Randle cycle would operate to suppress glucose oxidation by muscle, thereby saving glucose for tissues that depend more heavily on glucose as a fuel (e.g., the brain). The basic mechanism proposed by the glucose–fatty acid cycle is that an increase in fatty acid availability will result in an increased uptake of fatty acids, which will undergo β-oxidation in the mitochondria to acetyl CoA. This will result in an accumulation of acetyl CoA that, in turn, results in inhibition of pyruvate dehydrogenase (which inhibits oxidative metabolism of pyruvate), the accumulation of citrate (which inhibits phosphofructokinase), and the accumulation of glucose 6-phosphate (which reduces hexokinase activity). Ultimately, these changes would inhibit glycolysis and mitochondrial pyruvate oxidation. The reduced glucose metabolism along with the increased availability of fatty acids would, consequently, favor fatty acid oxidation. However, in studies of the metabolic effects of increasing fatty acid availability by intravenous infusion of triacylglycerol during low-intensity exercise, changes in glucose uptake and acetyl CoA levels were not observed, although a decrease in pyruvate dehydrogenase activity and a small increase in citrate level were observed in leg muscle (Odland et al., 1998). Therefore, it is still not clear exactly what factors cause the reduction in glucose oxidation in skeletal muscle when fatty acids are present at elevated levels, although it appears that inhibition of pyruvate dehydrogenase activity via activation of pyruvate dehydrogenase kinase is involved (Jeukendrup, 2002).

Skeletal muscle lipoprotein lipase activities increased dramatically between 9 and 12 hours after fasting in rats, whereas adipose tissue lipoprotein lipase activities declined by 50% after 6 hours of fasting and continued to fall when fasting was continued for 24 hours (Sugden et al., 1993). During the first hours of refeeding, following 12 hours of fasting, skeletal muscle lipoprotein lipase remained high, not returning immediately to the level observed in rats fed ad libitum. A programmed shift in the expression of lipoprotein lipase in different tissues in response to the dietary intake, therefore, seems to direct fatty acids from chylomicrons and VLDLs into adipose tissue for storage in the fed state and to direct fatty acids from VLDLs into muscle for oxidation in the postabsorptive and fasted state.

The transition in fuel utilization by muscle as part of the fed to fasted transition illustrates the importance of substrate availability in determining the fuels that are used by muscle. The resting muscle uses mainly fatty acids derived from adipose tissue during fasting, but depends mainly on glucose when plasma glucose and insulin levels are elevated in the absorptive state. A number of studies have shown that fat oxidation by muscle is increased and carbohydrate disposal is decreased when the availability of fatty acids is increased by feeding high fat diets or by infusion of lipids. Likewise, other studies have shown that glucose infusion or loading can increase the muscle's utilization of glucose as fuel. An increase in glucose levels in response to a typical moderate carbohydrate diet causes an insulin-stimulated increase in GLUT4 translocation to the plasma membrane of muscle fibers, an increase in pyruvate dehydrogenase activity, and an increase in glycogen synthase activity in skeletal muscle. In contrast, a high fat/low carbohydrate diet does not promote the activation of glucose uptake, glucose oxidation, or glycogen storage in muscle.

This effect of substrate availability on fuel utilization was illustrated in a study of the short-term adaptation of aerobically trained men to a high fat/low carbohydrate diet (Pehleman et al., 2005). Adaptation to a high fat/low carbohydrate (73 % fat/5 % carbohydrate) diet increased pyruvate dehydrogenase kinase activity, which decreased pyruvate dehydrogenase activation to the "a" form, and decreased the oxidative disposal of glucose by skeletal muscle. The glycogen synthase activity in skeletal muscle was not affected by the high fat/low carbohydrate diet compared to the control diet (29 % fat, 51 % carbohydrate). Administration of an oral glucose load (glucose tolerance test) to these men, on either the control or high fat/low carbohydrate diet, resulted in both increases in glycogen synthase activity in muscle and in decreases in pyruvate kinase activity, which resulted in increases in pyruvate dehydrogenase activity. The extent of the changes in response to an oral glucose load was similar regardless of diet, but the absolute level of pyruvate dehydrogenase "a" remained lower in men fed the high fat/low carbohydrate diet.

THE ENERGY COST OF MOVEMENT

Muscle shortening and movement are brought about by repeated formation of cross-bridges between the thin (actin) and thick (myosin) filaments of the myofibrils. This process costs energy and requires hydrolysis of ATP by the myofibrillar ATPase. The contraction cycles are under nervous control. Whenever a sufficient number of nerve impulses during a limited time-period arrive at the muscle fiber, the following sequence is set into action: (1) the plasma membrane is depolarized by a short-term loss of potassium ions and uptake of sodium ions into the muscle fiber; (2) the formed action potential is propagated along the sarcolemma into the transverse (T) tubules, where (3) the signal is transmitted to the sarcoplasmic reticulum; this then leads to (4) a rapid release of calcium ions (Ca^{2+}) from the sarcoplasmic reticulum and a 1,000-fold increase in the cytosolic Ca^{2+} concentration. This increase in cytosolic Ca^{2+} leads to (5) cross-bridge formation between the actin and myosin filaments of the myofibrils and (6) activation of the myofibrillar ATPase and ATP hydrolysis to break the formed cross-bridges. The cytosolic Ca^{2+} concentration simultaneously is reduced again by the action of the calcium ATPase in the sarcoplasmic reticulum, and the muscle is ready for the next contraction.

The myofibrillar ATPase, the Na^+, K^+-ATPase (needed to restore the membrane potential following a depolarization), and the Ca^{2+}-ATPase are all much more active during exercise than at rest, and, therefore, greater amounts of ATP are needed during exercise. A muscle can in seconds increase its aerobic ATP turnover rate by more than 100-fold. The higher the exercise intensity, the more contraction cycles are needed per unit of time, the more the amount of ATP that needs to be synthesized per unit time, and the higher the amount of fuel that needs to be oxidized. Energy expenditure of skeletal muscle, therefore, is greatly influenced by the increased contractile activity needed to walk, work, or run.

At rest, whole-body energy expenditure of humans is about 80 watts or 68 kcal/hour (comparable to that of a light bulb), with approximately 25% (20 watts or 17 kcal/hour) being expended in the skeletal muscles. Energy expenditure during a marathon run covering 42 km in a little over 2 hours is about 20 times resting energy expenditure (1,600 watts or 1,377 kcal/hour). Because more than 90% of the increase in energy expenditure originates from fuel oxidation in the active muscle (part is needed for the cardiovascular response), and assuming that maximally about half of skeletal muscle mass is actively used in running a marathon, the energy expenditure of this active half of skeletal muscle can be estimated to increase by more than 130-fold (from 10 watts to 1,368 watts), as shown in Figure 20-2. Skeletal muscle, therefore, must have powerful mechanisms to increase the rates of ATP synthesis and fuel oxidation. In an individual running a marathon, most of the required ATP is produced by aerobic oxidation of carbohydrate and fat.

A top-class sprinter during a 100-m sprint can achieve a power output of around 3,600 watts—that is, approximately 45 times resting energy expenditure at whole-body level. Because more than 95% of the increase in energy expenditure originates from increased fuel metabolism in the active muscle during a sprint, the energy expenditure of the active muscle is estimated to increase by more than 300-fold. Most of the ATP for a 100-m sprint is produced anaerobically by net breakdown of muscle creatine phosphate and by conversion of glycogen to lactate.

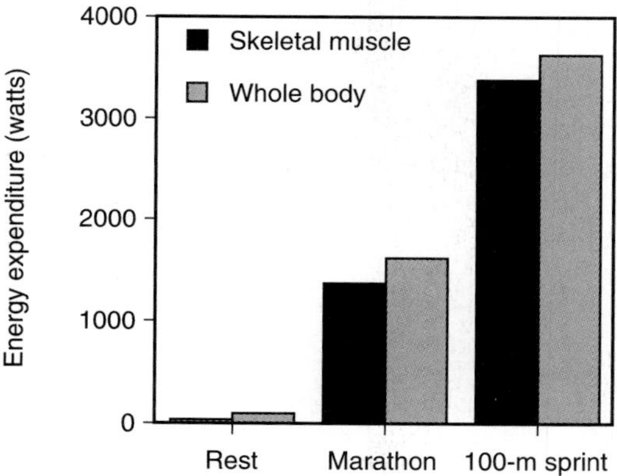

Figure 20-2 Whole-body and muscle energy expenditure at rest, during marathon running, and during a 100-m sprint. One watt is equivalent to 1 J/second or 2.39×10^{-4} kcal/second. One thousand watts, therefore, is equivalent to an energy expenditure of 0.239 kcal/second or 14 kcal/minute or 860 kcal/hour.

FUEL UTILIZATION BY WORKING MUSCLE

FUELS FOR MODERATE- INTENSITY TO HIGH-INTENSITY EXERCISE

The intensity of muscular work or exercise is often defined relative to a person's maximum aerobic capacity (VO_{2max}), with VO_{2max} being a measure of the maximum volume of O_2 consumption. For purposes of our discussion, we will define energy expenditure at approximately 25% VO_{2max} as low-intensity, approximately 60% of VO_{2max} as moderate-intensity, and approximately 80% of VO_{2max} as high-intensity exercise or work. The maximal aerobic work rate is defined as 100% VO_{2max}. As energy expenditure increases per unit time with exercise intensity, there are substantial changes in substrate utilization. As illustrated in Figure 20-3, utilization of both fat and carbohydrate increases as the intensity of exercise is increased from rest or low intensity to moderate intensity. Both plasma free fatty acids and triacylglycerol sources are used by muscle. Because it has been difficult to discriminate between utilization of fatty acids derived from the action of muscle lipoprotein lipase on circulating lipoprotein triacylglycerol and utilization of intramuscular lipid stores, these two sources are grouped together in the data used to generate Figure 20-3. Oxidation of fat increases with an increase in exercise intensity up to approximately 65% VO_{2max}, and then decreases, primarily due to decreased utilization of plasma free fatty acids, as intensity is further increased. Utilization of both plasma glucose and muscle glycogen stores increases progressively as exercise intensity increases from low to moderate to high. At the higher work intensities, muscle glycogen can provide more than half of the total energy used by the muscle.

The increase in fat oxidation with a shift from rest to moderate exercise intensity results mainly from increased fatty acid availability (Fig. 20-4). As a result of exercise initiation, the epinephrine concentration increases and the

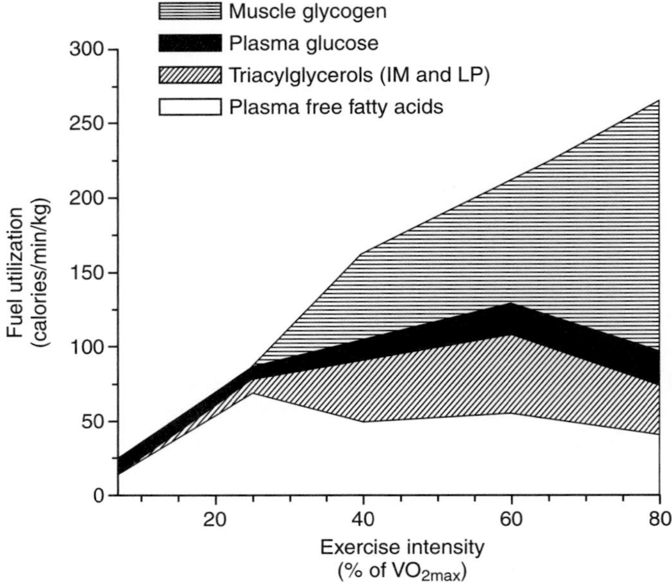

Figure 20-3 Utilization of fuel mixtures by the exercising muscle at different exercise intensities. Values are based on data for male cyclists who exercised while in the postabsorptive state following an overnight fast. *IM*, Intramuscular; *LP*, lipoprotein. *(Data from Romijn JA, Coyle EF, Sidossis LS, Gastaldelli A, Horowitz JF, Endert E, Wolfe RR [1993] Regulation of endogenous fat and carbohydrate metabolism in relation to exercise intensity and duration. Am J Physiol 265:E380–E391; and van Loon LJC, Greenhaff PL, Constantin-Teodosiu D, Saris WHM, Wagenmakers AJM [2001] The effects of increasing exercise intensity on muscle fuel utilization in humans. J Physiol 536:295.)*

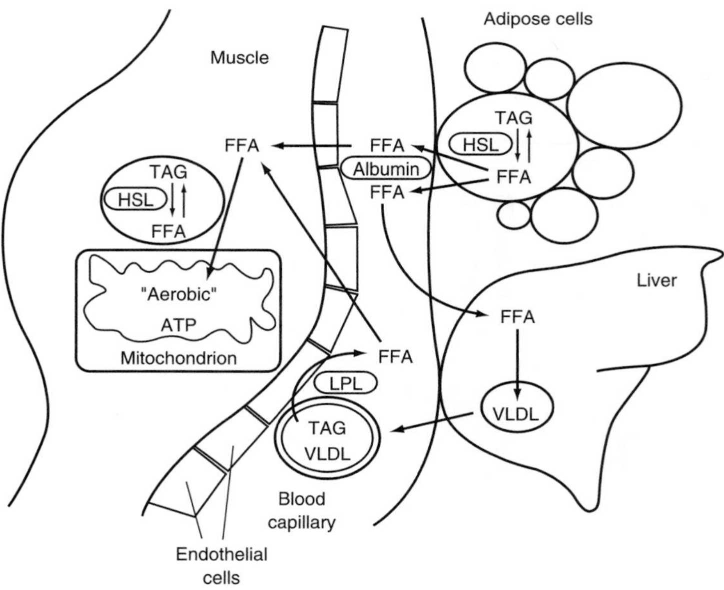

Figure 20-4 Sources of fatty acids for oxidation by skeletal muscle during prolonged exercise. *FFA*, Free fatty acid; *HSL*, hormone-sensitive lipase; *LPL*, lipoprotein lipase; *TAG*, triacylglycerol; *VLDL*, very low density lipoprotein.

insulin concentration decreases in response to the fall in the plasma glucose level. The rate of lipolysis in adipose tissues is increased to approximately three times the basal rate and re-esterification is decreased by more than 50%, such that up to six times as much fatty acid is released from adipose stores into the plasma (Achten and Jeukendrup, 2004). In addition, the blood flow to working skeletal muscle is increased dramatically during moderate- to high-intensity exercise, and this further increases the delivery of fatty acids to the muscle. When the plasma free fatty acid concentration is measured, a decrease in the plasma fatty acid concentration during the first 15 minutes of exercise (e.g., from ~0.3 mmol/L in the fed state to ~0.15 mmol/L) is frequently observed because the muscle is taking up fatty acids faster than fatty acids are appearing from lipolysis. However, the rate of appearance soon exceeds the rate of utilization by muscle, and the plasma fatty acid concentration rises to levels as high as 1.5 to 2.0 mmol/L. Therefore, an increase in plasma fatty acid concentration along with greater blood flow delivers more fatty acids to muscle to use as fuel during exercise.

In addition, fatty acids are mobilized from the IMTG within the muscle fibers by muscle hormone-sensitive lipase. In the initial minute of low and moderate aerobic exercise, muscle hormone-sensitive lipase is activated by contractions in the apparent absence of increases in circulating epinephrine (Watt and Spriet, 2004). This contraction-induced activation may be related to increased Ca^{2+} or other unknown intramuscular activators and probably involves phosphorylation (Langfort et al., 2003). As exercise continues beyond a few minutes, activation by epinephrine through the cAMP signaling cascade also may occur. IMTG content of muscle of male cyclists was measured before and after 120 minutes of moderate-intensity exercise (60% of VO_{2max}); the IMTG in type 1 fibers was decreased by 62% of the pre-exercise level, whereas the IMTG content of type 2 fibers was not significantly affected (van Loon et al., 2003).

In addition to an increase in fatty acid availability, fatty acid oxidation by muscle is upregulated in response to exercise. Biopsies of moderately trained men performing bicycle exercise (60 minutes, 65% VO_{2max}) demonstrated that the exercise period resulted in a decrease in the malonyl CoA concentration, which was associated with, and presumably secondary to, increased activity of AMP-activated protein kinase (AMPK) and inhibition of acetyl CoA carboxylase as a result of its phosphorylation by AMPK (Roepstorff et al., 2004). The decrease in malonyl CoA level relieves inhibition of CPT-I, facilitating entry of fatty acids into the mitochondria for β-oxidation.

Fat oxidation seems to peak at moderate exercise intensities (45% to 65% of VO_{2max}), but the exact intensity at which it peaks varies among individuals. The average maximal fat oxidation was 0.5 g per minute, or 8 mg /kg/minute in women and 7 mg/kg/minute in men (Venables et al., 2005).

As a result of exercise initiation, delivery of glucose to working muscle also increases (Fig. 20-5). Liver glycogen breakdown and the hepatic glucose output increase at the onset of exercise. Exercise mediates muscle glucose uptake via an insulin-like effect—via stimulation of GLUT4 translocation to the sarcolemma. Exercise-induced glucose transport does not require the action or signaling of insulin, however, and, although intracellular Ca^{+2} appears to contribute, the mechanism is not entirely clear.

The maximal contribution of plasma glucose is approximately 1 g/minute, and this seems to be limited by the rate of appearance of glucose into plasma. Exogenous carbohydrate oxidation was increased to as much as 1.7 g/minute in athletes who ingested a carbohydrate source that provided a mixture of glucose plus fructose instead of glucose only (Wallis et al., 2005; Jentjens et al., 2004). This latter observation is assumed to be due to the fact that glucose and fructose use different intestinal transporters for absorption such that the rate of total sugar absorption can be increased by providing both glucose and fructose (Jeukendrup, 2004).

Within muscle, glucose 1-phosphate generated from muscle glycogen breakdown is used along with plasma glucose. Glycogen phosphorylase in muscle is activated during exercise. Both the increase in intracellular Ca^{+2} and the elevation of the level of metabolites related to the energy status of the cell (ADP, AMP, and P_i)

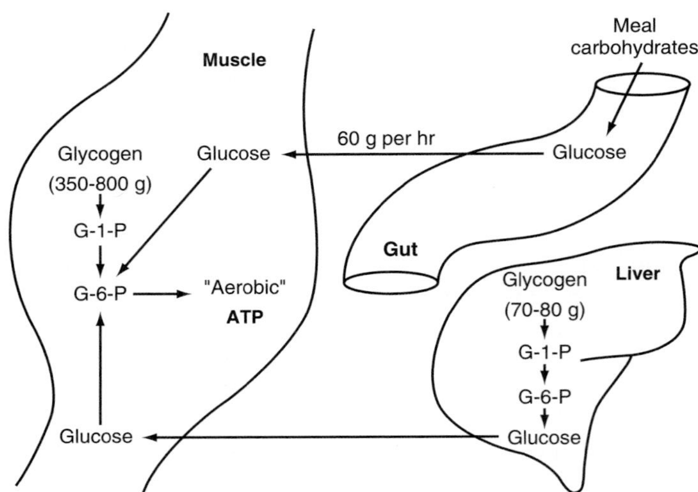

Figure 20-5 Sources of glucose available for oxidation by skeletal muscle during prolonged exercise.

upregulate glycogen phosphorylase as discussed in Chapter 12. Glycogen synthesis is minimal during exercise unless exercise intensity is very low. In fact, the muscle's capacity for glycogenolysis far exceeds that for glycogenesis, and glycogen breakdown under most conditions is independent of the activity of glycogen synthase. Therefore, most glucose disposal by muscle during periods of exercise or work is via its utilization as fuel.

Muscle glycogen stores are an important source of carbohydrate during moderate exercise, and the extent of muscle glycogen stores appears to influence the relative utilization of fat versus carbohydrate during moderate-intensity work. The muscle of glycogen-depleted subjects oxidized more fat and had lower pyruvate dehydrogenase activity, lower concentrations of acetyl CoA and acetylcarnitine, and a higher concentration of free carnitine (Roepstorff et al., 2005). Thus, muscle of glycogen-depleted subjects is poised to have lower levels of malonyl CoA and higher levels of carnitine, which favors transport of fatty acids into the mitochondria. Conversely, in subjects with high muscle glycogen, pyruvate dehydrogenation to acetyl CoA would be favored, and this would favor malonyl CoA synthesis. In addition, the formation of acetylcarnitine would limit the availability of free carnitine. Together, the higher malonyl CoA level and lower carnitine level would limit the transport of long-chain fatty acids into mitochondria and, thus, limit the use of fatty acids as fuel. To a more limited extent, similar effects could presumably be accomplished by increasing plasma glucose availability during exercise by glucose infusion or provision of glucose plus fructose–containing drinks.

As work intensity is increased from moderate to high, total fat utilization by muscle decreases slightly, whereas carbohydrate oxidation continues to increase markedly (see Fig. 20-3). Oxidation of plasma fatty acids decreases, whereas utilization of triacylglycerol remains fairly constant as exercise intensity is increased from moderate to high. Utilization of plasma glucose and muscle glycogen stores both continue to increase in magnitude as exercise intensity increases from moderate to high. When exercise intensity exceeds approximately 50% VO_{2max}, muscle glycogen becomes the substrate that provides the largest portion of the total fuel need.

The reduced utilization of fatty acids as fuel at high work intensities appears to be partially due to lowered fatty acid availability, as a result of a reduced rate of lipolysis. However, additional mechanisms are also involved. Regulation of fat metabolism inside skeletal muscle may involve fatty acid uptake from the vascular space across the sarcolemma into the sarcoplasm, the role of CPT-I and carnitine in

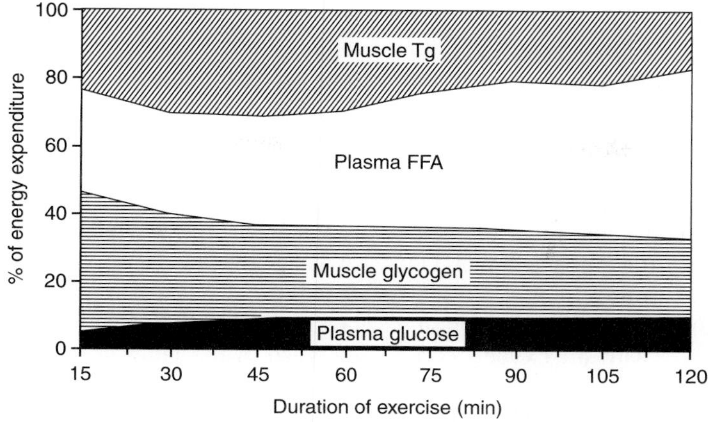

Figure 20-6 Relative contribution of carbohydrate and lipid fuels to energy production during 120 minutes of exercise at 65% VO_{2max} by endurance-trained cyclists who were in the postabsorptive state after a 10- to 12-hour fast. *(From Romijn JA, Coyle EF, Sidossis LS, Gastaldelli A., Horowitz JF, Endert E, Wolfe RR [1993] Regulation of endogenous fat and carbohydrate metabolism in relation to exercise intensity and duration. Am J Physiol 265:E380–E391, with permission from the American Physiological Society.)*

the transport of fatty acids across the mitochondrial membrane, or the release of fatty acids from IMTG under the influence of a hormone-sensitive lipase. The β-oxidation of fatty acids once they are in the mitochondria does not appear to be significantly regulated. Although malonyl CoA levels are decreased in rodent skeletal muscle with an increase from low- to moderate-intensity exercise (which relieves the inhibition of CPT-I that is exhibited under resting/fed conditions), malonyl CoA levels are increased in rodent muscle with an increase from moderate- to high-intensity exercise, perhaps as a result of an increase in acetyl CoA levels as substrate for malonyl CoA synthesis. However, the regulation of CPT-I and fatty acid transport into mitochondria is less clear for human muscle and may involve both malonyl CoA and other regulators such as hydrogen ion concentration. A decrease in pH from 7.1 to 6.8 reduced CPT-I activity by approximately 40% in mitochondria isolated from human skeletal muscle (Bezaire et al., 2004).

In individuals exercising at high intensities, it is possible to increase the use of fat as a fuel by increasing the plasma fatty acid concentration (via infusion). When this is done, the increased fatty acid availability results in decreased breakdown of muscle glycogen. In studies using ^{14}C-labeled medium-chain fatty acids (octanoate) and ^{13}C-labeled long-chain fatty acids (oleate), the percentage of oleate taken up and oxidized decreased at high exercise intensities, whereas there was no difference in oxidation of octanoate as exercise intensity increased (Sidossis et al., 1997). Because uptake of long-chain fatty acids is dependent on the CPT-I, whereas medium-chain fatty acids use a different system or cross the membrane by diffusion, this outcome suggested that transport across the sarcolemma or mitochondrial membrane may be involved.

Despite the increased reliance on carbohydrate fuels as exercise intensity increases, these carbohydrate fuels are limited. Prolonged exercise at moderate or high intensities will ultimately lead to depletion of muscle glycogen stores and a greater reliance on lipid fuels, as illustrated in Figure 20-6. A greater reliance on lipid fuels, however, will decrease the VO_{2max} at which one can work.

FUELS FOR PROLONGED ENDURANCE EXERCISE: THE MARATHON

The marathon distance is 42.195 km (26 miles, 385 yards) and is completed by elite runners in a little more than 2 hours. The total energy expenditure during a marathon is about 12 MJ (2,868 kcal), independent of running speed.

This is equivalent to burning about 750 g of carbohydrate or 330 g of fat. These numbers immediately illustrate that it is unlikely that a marathon is run solely on carbohydrate, because the human body in the fed state has only approximately 400 to 900 g of carbohydrate on board (~80 g in liver and the remainder in the combined skeletal muscles) and because only half of the muscle mass is involved in marathon running.

Recreational runners run a marathon at 70% to 80% of VO_{2max} with an oxygen consumption of 1,500 mL/minute up to 4,000 mL/minute, depending on how well trained they are. The slowest runners tend to slow down more than the better trained ones do during the latter part of the race. Both a reduction in running efficiency and a gradual reduction in exercise intensity (as a percentage of VO_{2max}) may contribute to the reduction in running speed. Whole-body RQ can be measured in the laboratory while simulating a marathon run using a treadmill, and the RQ can be used to estimate muscle fuel utilization. Such experiments reveal that the RQ in recreational runners falls from values of 0.90 to 1.00 in the first 30 minutes to approximately 0.80 to 0.85 after 2 hours of running. These observations indicate that carbohydrates are the most important fuel in the first hour of the marathon and that fat gradually increases in importance.

Elite runners are able to maintain a relatively constant pace during the marathon and run at a higher intensity (85% to 90% of VO_{2max} or 4,000 to 5,000 mL of O_2/minute). The gradual reduction in running efficiency is smaller in their case, and it also is assumed that these runners are able to maintain a more constant fuel mixture, with less pronounced switching from carbohydrate as the major fuel in the beginning to fat as the major fuel in the last part of the race. Studies in the laboratory investigating the effect of exercise intensity on RQ have shown that RQ becomes elevated with increasing work intensity in a given individual, indicating that the fractional contribution of fat to total energy expenditure is suppressed at high exercise intensities (see Fig. 20-3). Trained subjects, however, have a higher capacity to oxidize fat than do untrained subjects when comparisons are made at high absolute work rates. This increased capacity for fat oxidation leads to glycogen sparing and enables the trained subjects to use their glycogen stores more economically.

In recreational runners, high blood lactate concentrations are often observed during the first hour of exercise at 70% to 80% of maximal aerobic power, after which lactate falls to very low levels until the finish has been reached. Measurement of the arteriovenous lactate concentration difference during one-leg exercise in the laboratory also showed a substantial lactate release by the leg (Kiens et al., 1993). This indicates that part of the ATP production in the early period originates from lactate production via glycolysis. The oxygen tension in skeletal muscle is never decreased during submaximal exercise, so it is unlikely that this lactate production is driven by lack of oxygen. It also has been suggested that type 2 fibers are increasingly recruited in sedentary or moderately trained subjects during the first 30 minutes of exercise. These fibers start to produce lactate because of their low oxidative capacity. This release of lactate is reduced by training (Kiens et al., 1993). Elite marathon runners appear to metabolize muscle glycogen and blood glucose almost entirely aerobically from the first minute of a marathon until the last despite the fact that they run at a very high percentage (up to 90%) of aerobic power.

The body carbohydrate stores are too small to meet the energy cost of ultramarathons, triathlons, and cycling races. Distances covered in athletic events in recent years have tended to become greater, and the selected tracks have tended to become more difficult, often including many steep slopes in mountainous areas. Ultramarathons can be as long as 200 km. In the Tour de France, a professional cycling race, a distance of 3,000 km is covered in 3 weeks, and the daily energy expenditure ranges from 27 MJ (6,453 kcal) on a flat course to 38 MJ (9,082 kcal) when cycling over mountain passes. The latter represents more than three times the daily energy expenditure of a sedentary man. Extremely popular also is the triathlon. In Ironman triathlons, athletes first swim 3,800 m, then cycle 180 km, and finally run a full marathon (42 km, 195 m). Although the pace is slower than during a marathon run, elite athletes still are able to exercise at 70% to 80% of maximal aerobic power for continuous periods of 7 to 10 hours. At these high intensities, carbohydrates remain an important energy source, but the need for carbohydrates by far exceeds the size of the glycogen stores of the body. During these types of events, therefore, it is extremely important to ensure that the carbohydrate stores at the start of the race are as large as possible and that carbohydrates are ingested before and during the competition if possible.

FUEL UTILIZATION DURING THE POSTEXERCISE RECOVERY PERIOD

During the postexercise period, both fatty acids and glucose are taken up by muscle. The insulin sensitivity of muscle is greater when glycogen is depleted, so glucose uptake is upregulated. However, in studies of fuel utilization by endurance-trained male subjects over the 18-hour period after an exhaustive bout of exercise, plasma lipids appeared to be the major source of fuel even in subjects fed high-carbohydrate meals (66% of energy as carbohydrate, 21% as fat) at 1, 4, and 7 hours of recovery (Kimber et al., 2003). Despite the elevation of glucose and insulin following the high-carbohydrate meals, carbohydrate oxidation and pyruvate dehydrogenase activation were decreased, supporting the hypothesis that glycogen resynthesis is of high metabolic priority. Muscle glycogen increased significantly and progressively at 3, 6, and 18 hours of recovery. Consistent with less reliance on carbohydrate as fuel, the concentrations of acetyl CoA, acetylcarnitine, and pyruvate all declined during recovery. No net change in the content of IMTG was observed over the course of the recovery period. Therefore, plasma lipids (free fatty acids and/or lipoprotein triacylglycerol) were the major muscle fuels during recovery.

Repletion of IMTG stores in type 1 fibers requires a longer recovery period. In a study of trained male cyclists (van Loon et al., 2003), IMTG content was decreased by 21% by prolonged endurance cycling (3 hours at 55% VO_{2max}). During recovery, IMTG content at 24 and 48 hours postexercise was not increased in subjects consuming a carbohydrate-rich diet (24% energy from fat), but did increase in subjects consuming a higher fat diet (39% energy from fat), reaching pre-exercise levels within 48 hours. Other studies have indicated that replenishment occurs at a range of fat intakes if the carbohydrate intake is low. IMTG stores were nearly replenished by 5 hours in fasted subjects (Krssak et al., 2000). It appears that IMTG accumulates largely in response to elevations of plasma free fatty acids, and, in fact, the IMTG pool is dynamic during exercise, with both lipolysis and esterification occurring concurrently (Johnson et al., 2004).

FUELS FOR SHORT, SUPER-INTENSE EFFORTS: SPRINTING

Because the energy requirement of a 100-m sprint is extremely high and the sprint lasts only 10 seconds, only the fuels present in muscle can be used for ATP synthesis. Moreover, oxygen cannot be transported quickly enough to the active skeletal muscle mass. Even a top-class athlete does not consume more than 0.5 L of oxygen during the 100-m sprint. This implies that more than 95% of the phenomenal need for ATP synthesis (24 g/second, or 47 mmol/second) must be derived from anaerobic metabolism. This leaves only two energy sources as main contributors to the ATP production during the 100-m sprint: muscle creatine phosphate and muscle glycogen stores. The use of these fuels over the duration of a 10-second sprint is illustrated in Figure 20-7.

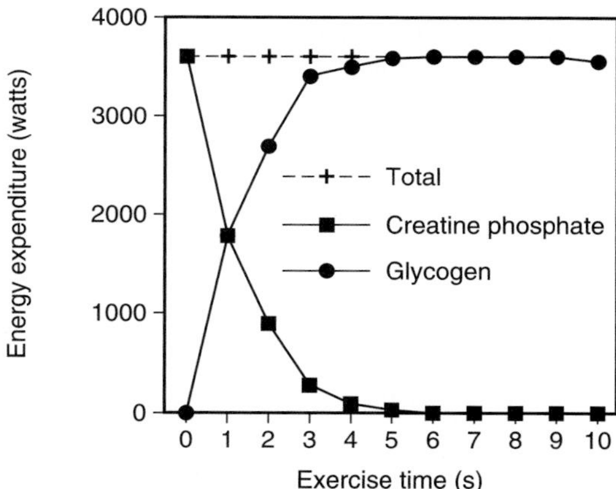

Figure 20-7 Utilization of creatine phosphate and muscle glycogen as fuels over the course of a 100-m sprint.

Use of Creatine Phosphate for Maintenance of ATP Levels During the First Few Seconds of Sprinting

In the first seconds after leaving the starting block, ATP is not yet synthesized by glycolysis at the required rate. At the same time, only approximately 20 % of the ATP content of the muscle is lost. Greater losses probably would lead locally to ATP concentrations that are too low to allow the myofibrillar ATPase and ion pumps to function at maximal velocity during exercise. Creatine phosphate plays a critical role in maintenance of ATP levels under these conditions. During the first seconds of the sprint, ATP lost during contraction is almost instantaneously regenerated from creatine phosphate. The concentration of creatine phosphate in human muscle is 80 to 85 μmol/g of dry muscle—that is, some four to five times higher than the ATP concentration. During the first 4 to 5 seconds of sprinting, approximately 80 % of the creatine phosphate pool is lost and used to regenerate ATP. The transfer of the phosphate group from creatine phosphate to ADP generated during contraction is catalyzed by the enzyme creatine kinase in the following reaction:

$$\text{Creatine phosphate} + \text{ADP} + \text{H}^{+} \leftrightarrow \text{Creatine} + \text{ATP}$$

Use of Glycogenolysis and Glycolysis (Lactate Production) to Provide Energy for Sprinting

The 20 % decrease in the ATP content during the first seconds of sprinting is also extremely important in muscle fuel utilization during anaerobic metabolism because it leads to a rapid increase in the concentration of free AMP and free ADP. (Note that most of the AMP and ADP in muscle is bound to myosin and actin; "free" refers to the portion of these nucleoside phosphates that is not bound to proteins and, hence, is available for metabolic regulation.) Free AMP and free ADP are important allosteric regulators of the key enzymes in the glycolytic pathway (glycogen phosphorylase and phosphofructokinase), and increases in their concentrations in combination with the contraction-induced rise in cytosolic Ca^{+2} (and changes in the concentrations of several other allosteric effectors) lead to a massive increase in the rate of glycogenolysis and glycolysis (lactate production) during the first seconds of sprinting.

The rise in free ADP in muscle fibers during the first meters of a sprint, coupled with the decrease in cytosolic pH (as a consequence of ATP hydrolysis and lactate production), also forces the creatine kinase equilibrium to rapid ATP production. The contribution of this reaction to ATP synthesis is greatest in the first second of sprinting and then gradually falls to zero in the next 4 seconds, during which glycolysis (lactate production) is coming up to full speed.

Breakdown of the glycogen stores and subsequent glycolysis with formation of lactate is quantitatively the most important process for ATP production during sprinting. In approximately 4 to 5 seconds from the start of a sprint, the rate of glycolysis increases to 1,000-fold or more. This increase in rate implies that the rate at which the muscle glycogen stores are broken down is very high during sprinting at top speed. Theoretically, there is enough glycogen in the muscle for about 800 to 1500 m of sprinting at maximal speed. However, even world-class athletes begin to slow down after 80 to 100 m and cannot maintain full speed. The reason for this is that fatigue processes come into operation and start to reduce the force-generating capacity of the muscle. The exact mechanism of fatigue during sprinting is not known, but the rapid increase in the concentration of inorganic phosphate, the decrease of the muscle pH (due to lactate accumulation), and the disturbed ion balances (K^+ and Ca^{2+}) have all been implicated in these mechanisms. (For a review of fatigue mechanisms, see Fitts [1994].) Most of the energy demand of the 100-m sprint is covered by anaerobic metabolism of muscle glycogen. During a 400-m sprint, athletes deliberately have to reduce maximal power output, so that fatigue develops less rapidly and a reasonable pace can be maintained. Part of the ATP production is covered, in that case, by aerobic oxidation of glycogen by glycolysis, pyruvate dehydrogenase, and the citric acid cycle, coupled with the electron transport chain and oxidative phosphorylation; the contribution of aerobic oxidation rapidly increases between the start and finish of a 400-m sprint.

FUELS FOR INTERMITTENT HIGH-INTENSITY EXERCISE

Sports like soccer, football, baseball, basketball, rugby, squash, tennis, and many others can be qualified as intermittent high-intensity exercise. Speed of running or intensity of work varies widely during a game in these sports. Soccer will be used here as an example of an intermittent, high-intensity sport, but similar considerations apply to all of these sports.

A game of soccer lasts 90 minutes in total with a 10-minute break after 45 minutes. The total distance covered by soccer players depends on the position of the player, but the mean distance covered is 10 km. The speed of running varies from zero to maximal, with a major part of the distance covered at a walking or dribbling pace. Soccer players, however, make many short sprints of 10 to 60 m at full speed throughout the game. The total distance run at full speed is between 800 and 1,500 m; this is the distance that theoretically could be covered while consuming muscle glycogen at the rate required to meet the energy demand of sprinting. Part of the energy demand for these sprints is met by creatine phosphate breakdown, with creatine phosphate resynthesis occurring between sprints. Muscle glycogen breakdown and subsequent lactate production is the other major supply of energy for these sprints. Each sprint empties part of the glycogen stores, until the glycogen stores are depleted and the sprints can no longer be run at full speed.

The mean heart rate during a game in the highest-class professional league is 85% of maximum; the average oxygen consumption is 80% of maximum; and the mean blood lactate is 8 to 10 mmol/L with peaks up to 12 mmol/L. The lactate produced during sprinting is used as a fuel by the heart and in the intervals at lower intensity also by skeletal muscle. Some lactate also may be converted to glucose by the liver (Cori cycle; see Chapters 12 and 19). Professional soccer players run about the same distance in the first and second halves and also run about the same distance at full speed in both halves of game. Recreational players tend to cover less distance in the second half, run less distance at full speed, and slow down during sprinting in the second half. Muscle biopsy studies have shown that recreational players who start with low muscle glycogen concentrations will have emptied most of their muscle glycogen by half-time.

It is as important for soccer players as for marathon runners to be endurance-trained. The better-trained players have a higher aerobic power and, therefore, depend on anaerobic glycolysis with lactate production less frequently during a game. During the intervals at lower intensity, they probably also can oxidize more fat, and in this way also save glycogen for a few more sprints (and scoring chances) at the end of the game. Soccer players also benefit from training at high intensity in order to increase speed and maximal anaerobic power, so that they can outrun their opponents during the short sprints.

SKELETAL MUSCLE ADAPTATIONS IN RESPONSE TO TRAINING AND THE CONSEQUENCES FOR FUEL UTILIZATION AND PERFORMANCE

Sedentary individuals can markedly increase their endurance by means of regularly performed exercise. After a few weeks of endurance training, individuals can exercise comfortably for prolonged periods at exercise intensities that they could maintain for only a few minutes prior to training. For a long time it was thought that the improved endurance was exclusively the result of the cardiovascular adaptations to endurance training (increased cardiac output, increased gas exchange in the lungs, and increased capillary density in skeletal muscle). However, we now know that training can affect the characteristics of the muscle fibers as well.

One of the most important training-induced adaptations is the increase in the number of mitochondria per unit mass of skeletal muscle. This results in increased activities of enzymes involved in the citric acid cycle, oxidative phosphorylation, and β-oxidation. Training can lead to a five-fold increase in the mitochondrial content of skeletal muscle of sedentary human subjects. In addition, in elite athletes the mitochondrial content may vary through the year as a function of training intensity. Cyclists in the Tour de France, which covers a distance of 3,000 km over 3 weeks, have only about half the mitochondrial content in the winter season (reduced frequency and intensity of training) that they have in the middle of summer when they are competing daily in cycling races covering 200 to 300 km and often including the ascent of several mountain passes. Their VO_{2max} is only 2% to 5% lower in winter than in summer because it takes much longer for the cardiovascular system to adapt. Their endurance performance, however, is much better in summer due to the higher mitochondrial content of skeletal muscle.

A major advantage of the increased number of mitochondria in muscle of trained subjects is that the disturbance of the energy status of the muscle is smaller at a given intensity of exercise. Decreases in the muscle ATP and creatine phosphate content, and increases in free ADP, free AMP, and inorganic phosphate, are smaller in trained muscles with a high mitochondrial content (Dudley et al., 1987). Because increases in free AMP, inorganic phosphate, and other allosteric regulators activate glycolysis (see Chapter 12, Fig. 12-7), the untrained muscle will produce more lactate than the trained muscle will. Therefore, elite runners with very high mitochondrial contents are able to run at very high exercise intensities without lactate production, whereas recreational runners and sedentary subjects start to produce lactate at much lower exercise intensities. Because aerobic oxidation of glycogen delivers much more energy than glycolysis alone (~38 versus 3 ATPs per glucose molecule), elite runners also are able to run a much greater distance using the same amount of muscle glycogen.

Increases in the muscle concentrations of inorganic phosphate, hydrogen ions (H^+), and lactate during exercise stimulate group III and group IV afferent nerve fibers in skeletal muscle, which signal to the brain that the muscle is approaching a critical energy deficit leading to contraction failure (Kaufman and Forster, 1996). This activates the muscle-heart reflex and leads to further increases of the heart rate, the ventilation rate, and the blood concentration of catecholamines, which are all experienced as an increase in exercise stress. In trained muscles with a high mitochondrial content, the increases in the muscle concentrations of inorganic phosphate, H^+, and lactate are lower at the same absolute exercise intensity, and, therefore, less exercise stress will be experienced. For these reasons, elite runners can run at a higher pace than untrained individuals yet experience only a similar or even lower amount of exercise stress.

Endurance training also reduces the reliance on carbohydrate as an energy source during submaximal exercise. Trained muscles extract a greater percentage of the plasma free fatty acids delivered to the muscle than do untrained muscles (Kiens et al., 1993). Endurance training results in increases in fatty acid transport proteins (FAT/CD36 and FABPm) in the sarcolemma. In addition, the IMTG content of muscle can be substantially greater in trained endurance athletes compared to sedentary subjects (van Loon et al., 2004). Endurance training also is associated with substantial increases in AMP kinase (AMPK) activity and increased phosphorylation of the AMPK target acetyl CoA carboxylase, which reduces acetyl CoA carboxylase activity and malonyl CoA formation, thereby favoring entrance of fatty acids into the mitochondria. The higher mitochondrial content also enhances the capacity for fatty acid oxidation. Therefore, training increases the ability to oxidize fat when working at 80% to 90% of maximal aerobic power. This results in a slower utilization of muscle glycogen and blood glucose, a greater reliance on fat oxidation, and less lactate production during exercise of moderate to high intensity. For all these reasons, elite marathoners can run at a speed of 20 km/hour for more than 2 hours, whereas most recreational runners are exhausted within minutes at such a speed.

INTERVENTIONS TO INCREASE MUSCLE GLYCOGEN: CARBOHYDRATE LOADING

Resting glycogen concentrations in human skeletal muscle range from about 10 to 23 g/kg of wet muscle. Between 350 and 800 g of glycogen are present in the combined skeletal muscles if one assumes that a lean, 70-kg subject has a skeletal muscle mass of about 35 kg. In highly trained athletes, the reported resting muscle glycogen concentrations tend to be higher than in sedentary subjects, suggesting that glucose deposition and glycogen resynthesis are increased by exercise training.

Muscle glycogen is the main fuel during marathon running, for both elite and recreational marathoners. Both types of athletes, therefore, have to ensure that they have enough carbohydrate on board to reach the finish while oxidizing aerobically a fuel mixture consisting of both carbohydrate and fat. If muscle glycogen is emptied a few kilometers before they reach the finish, then fatigue will occur (i.e., they "hit the wall"), and they have to reduce the pace. Several approaches are used by athletes to enhance their muscle glycogen stores prior to competition; this is called carbohydrate loading. Recreational runners cannot use their glycogen stores as efficiently as elite runners can, but carbohydrate loading leading to high glycogen content at the start still helps them maintain the pace chosen in the beginning of the race as long as possible. The traditional methods of increasing glycogen content prior to performance included a carbohydrate withdrawal or depletion stage followed by very high carbohydrate intakes. The current approach is usually 1 to 3 days of rest or reduced exercise training coupled with a high carbohydrate (>50 % of energy) intake.

Ingestion of a carbohydrate-rich meal 2 to 4 hours prior to competition also improves performance as it helps replenish the liver glycogen stores that have been emptied during overnight fasting. In competitions of less than 2 hours duration, these carbohydrates preferably should be taken as easily digestible food products or sports drinks. In more prolonged competitions, athletes often prefer solid products, such as bread, bananas, and energy bars. The percentage of protein and fat always should be low in the pre-exercise meal to prevent a reduction of the rate of gastric emptying and the occurrence of gastrointestinal disturbances during exercise. In very few subjects hypoglycemia may occur during the first minutes of exercise when the pre-exercise meal is taken less than 1 hour before exercise. Therefore, it is advised to build up experience with pre-exercise meals during training sessions.

Ingestion of carbohydrate drinks during cycling or running exercise of long duration (>2 hours) and moderate to high intensity (50 % to 90 % VO_{2max}) has been shown to improve performance in both elite and recreational athletes. Therefore, it is advised to refuel carbohydrates during competition. Carbohydrate ingestion maintains both blood glucose concentration and the glucose oxidation rate at higher values during prolonged exercise. The rate of muscle glycogen breakdown is not reduced by carbohydrate ingestion, but the supply of blood glucose to the exercising muscle is increased.

The ideal athletic drink also should supply water to compensate for the sweat losses during exercise. Dehydration due to excessive sweating is a well-known cause of a gradual reduction in performance during exercise in the heat. Large volumes of a low-carbohydrate drink should be ingested in the heat, whereas smaller volumes of a drink with higher carbohydrate content are advised in cold weather conditions. Sodium chloride should be added to increase intestinal glucose absorption and to replenish electrolytes. Again, it is advised that athletes build up personal experience with fluid losses (or needs) and fluid tolerance in training sessions under different weather conditions.

During ultra-endurance events, a high starting glycogen concentration also helps postpone the point in time when the muscle glycogen stores are empty and the pace has to be reduced. As these athletic events last for many hours, carbohydrates also should be ingested during exercise for the aforementioned reasons. During events like the Tour de France that requires a massively high energy expenditure continuously for 3 weeks, carbohydrates are ingested the whole day prior to, during, and after competition, as both carbohydrate-containing drinks and solid food. Easily digestible carbohydrates should be ingested at a high rate (100 g/hour or more) immediately after competition to start glycogen resynthesis as early as possible. Failure to have fully replenished glycogen stores by the

Nutrition Insight

Nutritional Ergogenic Aids

Athletes have long been searching for means that will give them an additional advantage over their competitors. Even small positive effects are considered to be important, as the time difference separating number one and two in competition in most cases is minimal. The battery of means in use to improve performance are generally known as ergogenic aids. The term ergogenic means "work-generating" and is derived from the Greek word *ergo,* meaning work. Ergogenic aids can be classified into different categories (Williams, 1992)—that is, mechanical aids (e.g., lighter sports equipment and improved aerodynamics); psychological aids (e.g., stress and anxiety control); pharmacological aids (e.g., caffeine, anabolic steroids, erythropoietin, and clenbuterol); physiological aids (e.g., sodium bicarbonate and blood infusion); and nutritional aids (e.g., carbohydrate loading and the use of dietary supplements like vitamins, carnitine, creatine, special amino acids, and special fatty acids).

Most pharmacological and physiological aids, when taken in abnormal quantities, meet the definition of doping and, therefore, are included in the list of substances banned by the International Olympic Committee. The reason for banning is that the use of many of these compounds also presents considerable health risks to the users, either in the acute period of usage or in the long term. For example, erythropoietin, a hormone that leads to an increase in the number of circulating red blood cells, may increase the viscosity of the blood so far that fatal circulatory problems could occur either during high-intensity exercise or during periods of low cardiac output (e.g., in the overnight resting state). The long-term use of clenbuterol, a drug with β-agonist action and a proven ability to reduce fat mass and increase muscle mass in meat-producing farm animals, could lead to a further increase in size of the already enlarged heart in a top athlete and increase the risk for development of cardiovascular complications.

In contrast to the use of pharmacological aids, the use of nutritional supplements that are expected to have performance-enhancing effects is generally accepted and has become very popular. Some of the most common nutritional supplements are creatine, carnitine, branched-chain amino acids, and medium-chain fatty acids. Despite their widespread use, there is little metabolic basis or evidence from controlled studies to support the beneficial claims made for most of these supplements (Wagenmakers, 1999).

start of exercise on the next day (e.g., due to insufficient carbohydrate intake or digestive problems) in most cases leads to the inability to follow the speed of the main group, and the cyclists will either give up voluntarily or be disqualified for finishing too late.

In intermittent high-intensity sports involving many repeated short distance sprints, the size of the glycogen stores in the muscle determines the total distance that can be covered at full speed. Carbohydrate loading, therefore, is very important. In those sports in which regular drinking is allowed (e.g., tennis) it is advisable to ingest carbohydrate-containing drinks so that orally ingested carbohydrates may contribute at least part of the carbohydrate oxidized during lower-intensity exercise, saving some of the muscle glycogen stores for a few more full-speed sprints at the end of the game. During sports with a break at half-time, the break can be used to refuel carbohydrate.

PROTEIN AND AMINO ACID METABOLISM IN SKELETAL MUSCLE DURING REST AND EXERCISE

In the middle of the nineteenth century, the renowned German physiologist Justus von Liebig assumed that the protein of skeletal muscle was consumed during muscular work as a fuel and that large quantities of meat and protein should be eaten by industrial workers to replenish the protein losses during physical exercise. This was shown to be incorrect in the late nineteenth century, when careful nitrogen balance studies failed to show increased nitrogen losses during periods of increased physical activity. Use of stable isotope studies to assess whole-body protein turnover have shown that net protein oxidation during periods of exercise do not differ from those observed in the resting state or during the postexercise period. Numerous studies have demonstrated that no increase in net breakdown or oxidation of muscle and whole-body protein occurs during exercise, especially when the exercise is performed in the fed state as athletes do in practice during competition (for references, see Rennie, 1996). Modest increases in plasma urea concentration and urinary urea excretion have been observed only during ultramarathons and during exercise in the laboratory after overnight or more prolonged fasting.

Therefore, the protein needs of athletes are at most only slightly higher than those of sedentary individuals, especially when the energy balance is adequate. A diet that provides 12% of total energy from protein should easily meet the protein requirement of athletes, especially when, due to the daily exercise and training sessions, they have an increased energy expenditure and, therefore, an increased energy and protein intake per kilogram of body weight.

Although athletes normally perform in the fed state, higher rates of net protein breakdown have been observed in subjects who exercised in the fasted state. Koopman and colleagues (2004) studied the effect of addition of protein to a carbohydrate-containing beverage on protein balance in trained male subjects who were studied after an overnight fast. Subjects were studied at rest prior to exercise, during a 6-hour period of cycling and treadmill at moderate intensity, and during a 4-hour recovery period. Combined ingestion of protein (0.25 g/kg every hour) and carbohydrate (0.7 g/kg every hour) improved net protein balance at rest as well as during exercise and postexercise recovery compared to intake of carbohydrate alone. In another study, untrained male subjects who had fasted overnight performed a resistance exercise protocol (Koopman et al., 2005). During a 6-hour post-exercise period, subjects were given solutions that contained carbohydrate (0.3 g/kg per hour) with or without protein (0.2 g/kg per hour) and leucine (0.1 g/kg per hour). The plasma insulin response and protein balance were greater for subjects given a beverage that contained protein plus leucine than in those given only carbohydrate or carbohydrate plus protein without leucine.

Supplementation of branched-chain amino acids have been shown to affect muscle protein synthesis in several studies. Whether long-term supplementation of branched-chain amino acids would have an effect on protein balance is uncertain. The effect of short-term supplements during or following exercise may be related to an enhanced oxidation of branched-chain amino acids by muscle during exercise as a result of activation of the branched-chain keto acid dehydrogenase complex, to effects of branched-chain amino acids on signal transduction pathways in the muscle, or to an amplification of insulin-induced protein synthesis by leucine (Koopman et al., 2005; Karlsson et al., 2004; Shimomura et al., 2004; Jefferson and Kimball, 2001).

SKELETAL MUSCLE ADAPTATIONS IN RESPONSE TO DISUSE AND DISEASE AND THE CONSEQUENCES FOR FUEL UTILIZATION AND WELL-BEING DURING NORMAL DAILY LIFE

Although the main part of this chapter focuses on fuel utilization in healthy people during sports events requiring high energy expenditures, a reduced use of skeletal muscle also has consequences for fuel utilization; exercise tolerance; and feelings of fitness, fatigue, and well-being in the daily life of inactive people. Not only training but also disuse (a reduction of muscular activity for a prolonged period) leads to a remarkable adaptation in skeletal muscle. Patients with very low energy outputs in habitual activities may have mitochondrial contents that are as little as 10% of those of sedentary individuals (Wagenmakers et al., 1988, 1987).

The ranges of the rates of palmitate oxidation and cytochrome *c* oxidase activity (both of which are mitochondrial oxidative processes and a reflection of mitochondrial content) in muscle homogenates of individuals with a wide range of habitual physical activities are shown in Figure 20-8. The lowest activities ever reported were observed in young children with Duchenne muscular dystrophy and with hypotonia due to spinal muscular atrophy type I. Their muscle contained as little as 3% to 4% of the mitochondrial activities observed in the muscle of elite marathoners. Low mitochondrial contents also are seen in the muscle of patients who have been bedridden for a long time due to an acquired disease; of subjects who are very inactive due to psychiatric problems; of those who prefer to avoid exercise-induced pains originating from metabolic defects or from unknown causes; of astronauts traveling through space in a weightless condition for several months; and of subjects deliberately subjected to hypokinesia for 90 days as part of a space research program (for references, see Wagenmakers et al. [1988]). An 80% to 90% decrease in the mitochondrial contents of skeletal muscle of patients entering intensive care units with severe trauma, sepsis, or septic shock is also seen within a period of days (Helliwell et al., 1990).

Subjects with such low mitochondrial contents have maximal aerobic powers of 60 to 120 watts or 50 to 100 kcal/hour (Wagenmakers et al., 1988), and during incremental cycle exercise they start to produce significant amounts of lactate at energy expenditure rates of 30 to 80 watts or 25 to 70 kcal/hour. This implies that they quite often experience the stress of severe exercise while performing normal daily activities and that they walk around in their home or at work with high heart and ventilation rates and high blood concentrations of catecholamines. They may empty their muscle glycogen stores while traveling to work or doing routine tasks. In such a condition it is not unusual for subjects who entered this situation without a clear causal disease to respond by trying to avoid exercise and then to spiral down in a vicious cycle of further inactivity leading to a further decrease of the mitochondrial contents of their muscle cells. Professional help and physiotherapy programs may be indicated to break this cycle.

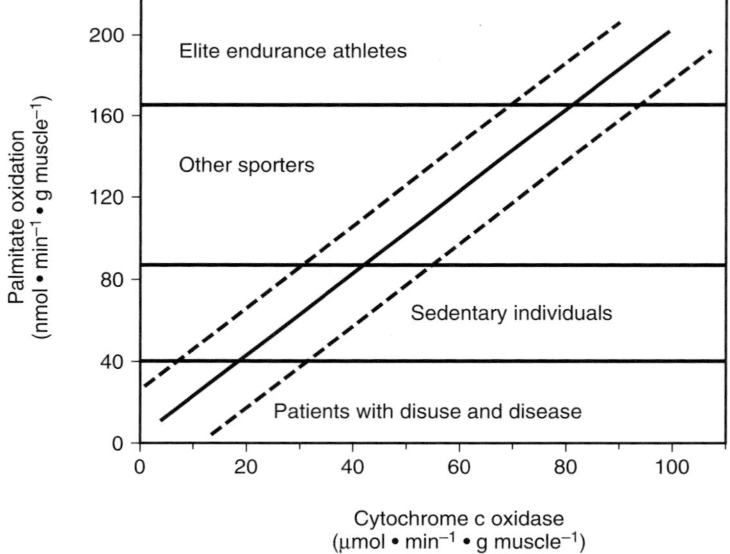

Figure 20-8 Ranges of the activities of two mitochondrial enzymes in populations with high, intermediate, and low habitual activities. *(Based on data from Wagenmakers AJM, Kaur N, Coakley JA, Griffiths RD, Edwards RHT [1987] Mitochondrial metabolism in myopathy and myalgia. In: Benzi G [ed] Advances in Myochemistry: 1. John Libbey [Eurotext Ltd.], London, pp. 219-230.)*

The adaptation to disuse is similar to adaptation to training, but in the reverse direction. Patients with low mitochondrial contents experience effort syndrome symptoms that may include palpitations, dizziness, disturbances of consciousness/vision, breathlessness, chest pain, epigastric pain, dysphagia, aerophagy, muscular pains especially in the neck and shoulder area, tremor, excessive sweating, fatigue, weakness, headache tension, and anxiety. These symptoms are experienced by all subjects with low mitochondrial contents independent of the reason leading to their physical inactivity. Therapeutic exercise programs may be useful to speed up recovery and improve fitness and the quality of life of patients recovering from prolonged acquired diseases or from an acute critical illness. Subjective muscle weakness and rapid fatigue often prevent these patients from taking up their professional life for periods of 6 to 12 months after discharge from the hospital. Therapeutic exercise programs also may slow down the gradual loss of muscle function and greatly improve the quality of life and well-being of patients who are disabled due to progressive inherited neuromuscular diseases.

REFERENCES

Achten J, Jeukendrup AE (2004) Optimizing fat oxidation through exercise and diet. Nutrition 20:716-727.

Bezaire V, Heigenhauser GJ, Spriet LL (2004) Regulation of CPT I activity in intermyofibrillar and subsarcolemmal mitochondria from human and rat skeletal muscle. Am J Physiol Endocrinol Metab 286:E85-E91.

Brozinick JT, Etgen GJ, Yaspelkis BB, Ivy JL (1994) The effects of muscle contraction and insulin on glucose-transporter translocation in rat skeletal muscle. Biochem J 297:539-545.

Dudley GA, Tullson PC, Terjung RL (1987) Influence of the mitochondrial content on the sensitivity of respiratory control. J Biol Chem 262:9109-9114.

Fitts RH (1994) Cellular mechanisms of muscle fatigue. Physiol Rev 74:49-94.

Helliwell TR, Griffiths RD, Coakley JH, Wagenmakers AJM, McClelland P, Campbell IT, Bone J M (1990) Muscle pathology and biochemistry in critically-ill patients. J Neurol Sci 98:329.

Himwich HE, Rose MI (1927) The respiratory quotient of exercising muscle. Am J Physiol 81:485-486.

Hoppeler H, Flück M (2002) Normal mammalian skeletal muscle and its phenotypic plasticity. J Exp Biol 205:2143-2152.

Jefferson LS, Kimball SR (2001) Translational control of protein synthesis: implications for understanding changes in skeletal muscle mass.Int J Sport Nutr Exerc Metab 11(Suppl):S143-S149.

Jentjens RL, Achten J, Jeukendrup AE (2004) High oxidation rates from combined carbohydrates ingested during exercise. Med Sci Sports Exerc 36:1551-1558.

Jeukendrup AE (2004) Carbohydrate intake during exercise and performance. Nutrition 20:669-677.

Jeukendrup AE (2003) Modulation of carbohydrate and fat utilization by diet, exercise and environment. Biochem Soc Trans 31: 1270-1273.

Jeukendrup AE (2002) Regulation of fat metabolism in skeletal muscle. Ann NY Acad Sci 967:217-235.

Johnson NA, Stannard SR, Thompson MW (2004) Muscle triglyceride and glycogen in endurance exercise: implications for performance. Sports Med 34:151-164.

Karlsson HK, Nilsson PA, Nilsson J, Chibalin AV, Zierath JR, Blomstrand E (2004) Branched-chain amino acids increase p70S6k phosphorylation in human skeletal muscle after resistance exercise. Am J Physiol Endocrinol Metab 287:E1-E7.

Kaufman MP, Forster HV (1996) Reflexes controlling circulatory, ventilatory and airway responses to exercise. In: Rowell LB, Shepherd JT (eds) Handbook of Physiology; Section 12, Exercise: Regulation and Integration of Multiple Systems. Oxford University Press, New York, pp 381-447.

Kiens B, Éssen-Gustavsson B, Christensen NJ, Saltin B (1993) Skeletal muscle substrate utilization during submaximal exercise in man: effect of endurance training. J Physiol 469:459-478.

Kimber NE, Heigenhauser GJ, Spriet LL, Dyck DJ (2003) Skeletal muscle fat and carbohydrate metabolism during recovery from glycogen-depleting exercise in humans. J Physiol 548:919-927.

Koopman R, Pannemans DL, Jeukendrup AE, Gijsen AP, Senden JM, Halliday D, Saris WH, van Loon LJ, Wagenmakers AJ (2004)

Combined ingestion of protein and carbohydrate improves protein balance during ultra-endurance exercise. Am J Physiol Endocrinol Metab 287:E712-E720.

Koopman R, Wagenmakers AJ, Manders RJ, Zorenc AH, Senden JM, Gorselink M, Keizer HA, van Loon LJ (2005) Combined ingestion of protein and free leucine with carbohydrate increases postexercise muscle protein synthesis in vivo in male subjects. Am J Physiol Endocrinol Metab 288:E645-E653.

Krssak M, Petersen KF, Bergeron R, Price T, Laurent D, Rothman DL, Roden M, Shulman GI (2000) Intramuscular glycogen and intramyocellular lipid utilization during prolonged exercise and recovery in man: a ^{13}C and ^{1}H nuclear magnetic resonance spectroscopy study. J Clin Endocrinol Metab 85:748-754.

Langfort J, Donsmark M, Ploug T, Holm C, Galbo H (2003) Hormone-sensitive lipase in skeletal muscle: regulatory mechanisms. Acta Physiol Scand 178:397-403.

Odland LM, Heigenhauser GJ, Wong D, Hollidge-Horvat MG, Spriet LL (1998) Effects of increased fat availability on fat-carbohydrate interaction during prolonged exercise in men. Am J Physiol 274:R894-R902.

Pehleman TL, Peters SJ, Heigenhauser GJ, Spriet LL (2005) Enzymatic regulation of glucose disposal in human skeletal muscle after a high-fat, low-carbohydrate diet. J Appl Physiol 98:100-107.

Putman CT, Xu X, Gillies E, MacLean IM, Bell GJ (2004) Effects of strength, endurance and combined training on myosin heavy chain content and fibre-type distribution in humans. Eur J Appl Physiol 92:376-384.

Rennie M J (1996) Influence of exercise on protein and amino acid metabolism. In: Rowell LB, Shepherd JT (eds) Handbook of Physiology; Section 12, Exercise: Regulation and Integration of Multiple Systems. Oxford University Press, New York, pp 995-1035.

Roepstorff C, Halberg N, Hillig T, Saha AK, Ruderman NB, Wojtaszewski JF, Richter EA, Kiens B (2005) Malonyl-CoA and carnitine in regulation of fat oxidation in human skeletal muscle during exercise. Am J Physiol Endocrinol Metab 288:E133-E142.

Roepstorff C, Vistisen B, Roepstorff K, Kiens B (2004) Regulation of plasma long-chain fatty acid oxidation in relation to uptake in human skeletal muscle during exercise. Am J Physiol Endocrinol Metab 287:E696-E705.

Sacchetti M, Saltin B, Olsen DB, van Hall G (2004) High triacylglycerol turnover rate in human skeletal muscle. J Physiol 561:883-891.

Shimomura Y, Murakami T, Nakai N, Nagasaki M, Harris RA (2004) Exercise promotes BCAA catabolism: effects of BCAA supplementation on skeletal muscle during exercise. J Nutr 134:1583S-1587S.

Sidossis LS, Gastaldelli A, Klein S, Wolfe RR (1997) Regulation of plasma fatty acid oxidation during low- and high-intensity exercise. Am J Physiol 272:E1065-E1070.

Sugden MC, Holness MJ (1994) Interactive regulation of the pyruvate dehydrogenase complex and the carnitine palmitoyltransferase system. FASEB J 8:54-61.

Sugden MC, Holness MJ, Howard RM (1993) Changes in lipoprotein lipase activities in adipose tissue, heart and skeletal muscle during continuous or interrupted feeding. Biochem J 292:113-119.

van Loon LJ, Koopman R, Manders R, van der Weegen W, van Kranenburg GP, Keizer HA (2004) Intramyocellular lipid content in type 2 diabetes patients compared with overweight sedentary men and highly trained endurance athletes. Am J Physiol Endocrinol Metab 287:E558-565.

van Loon LJ, Schrauwen-Hinderling VB, Koopman R, Wagenmakers AJ, Hesselink MK, Schaart G, Kooi ME, Saris WH (2003) Influence of prolonged endurance cycling and recovery diet on intramuscular triglyceride content in trained males. Am J Physiol Endocrinol Metab 285:E804-811.

Venables MC, Achten J, Jeukendrup AE (2005) Determinants of fat oxidation during exercise in healthy men and women: a cross-sectional study. J Appl Physiol 98:160-167.

Wagenmakers AJM (1999) Nutritional supplements: effects on exercise performance and metabolism. In: Lamb DR, Murray R (eds) Perspectives in Exercise Science and Sports Medicine; Vol. 12: The Metabolic Basis of Performance in Sport and Exercise. Cooper Publishing Group, Carmel, IN.

Wagenmakers AJM, Coakley JH, Edwards RHT (1988) The metabolic consequences of reduced habitual activities in patients with muscle pain and disease. Ergonomics 31:1519-1527.

Wagenmakers AJM, Kaur N, Coakley JH, Griffiths RD, Edwards RHT (1987) Mitochondrial metabolism in myopathy and myalgia. In: Benzi G (ed) Advances in Myochemistry: 1. John Libbey (Eurotext Ltd.), London, pp 219-230.

Wallis GA, Rowlands DS, Shaw C, Jentjens RL, Jeukendrup AE (2005) Oxidation of combined ingestion of maltodextrins and fructose during exercise. Med Sci Sports Exerc 37:426-432.

Watt MJ, Spriet LL (2004) Regulation and role of hormone-sensitive lipase activity in human skeletal muscle. Proc Nutr Soc 63:315-322.

Williams MH (1992) Ergogenic and ergolytic substances. Med Sci Sports Ex 24:S344-S348.

RECOMMENDED READINGS

Rowell LB, Shepherd JT (eds) (1996) Handbook of Physiology; Section 12, Exercise: Regulation and Integration of Multiple Systems. Oxford University Press, New York.

Jeukendrup AE (2002) Regulation of fat metabolism in skeletal muscle. Ann NY Acad Sci 967:217-235.

Unit V

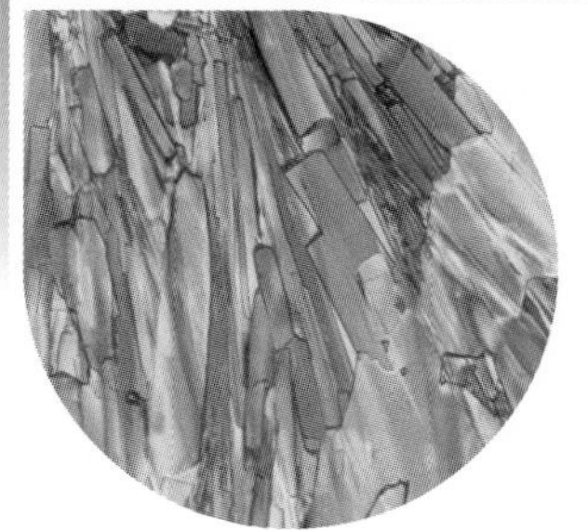

Energy

Energy is defined as the capacity for doing work. In the biological world, the various types of work that require energy include mechanical work, chemical work, and osmotic and electrical work. In animals and humans, the energy that sustains the various forms of biological work is derived from the carbohydrates, lipids, and proteins of the diet; this energy initially came from the sun and was stored by plants during photosynthesis at the beginning of the food chain. Some of the food energy is stored in the body as specific fuel reserves, mainly as glycogen and triacylglycerol, for use during the absence of food intake.

All forms of energy may be described as consisting of either potential or kinetic energy. For people, food is a source of potential energy. In the catabolism of carbohydrates, proteins, and lipids, some of this potential energy is stored or conserved in forms in which it can be used to support various energy-utilizing reactions. The first law of thermodynamics states that energy can neither be created nor destroyed. Some of the chemical energy available in glucose is converted in the process of catabolism to another form of chemical energy, adenosine 5′-triphosphate (ATP). The energy involved in the proton gradient produced across the inner mitochondrial membrane during electron transport is converted to chemical energy when the proton gradient is used to drive ATP synthesis. In skeletal and cardiac muscle, chemical energy involved in the energy-rich phosphate bonds of ATP is converted to mechanical energy during the process of muscle contraction. Ultimately, most of the potential energy taken in as food is converted to and lost from the body as heat.

The second law of thermodynamics states that all processes tend to progress toward a situation of maximum entropy (disorder or randomness). Entropy can be viewed as the energy in a system that is unavailable to perform useful work. The portion of the total energy in a system that is available for useful work is called the free energy and is usually denoted by G. Reactions with positive free-energy changes (endergonic reactions) may be coupled to and driven by reactions that have negative free-energy changes (exergonic reactions); the sum of the ΔG values for the individual reactions in a pathway must be negative in order for a metabolic sequence to be thermodynamically feasible.

Most biological work is mediated by hydrolysis of energy-rich bonds, particularly by hydrolysis of so-called high-energy phosphate bonds. These high-energy phosphate esters retain the energy in the structural, chemical, electrostatic, and resonant properties of the molecules. They release or transfer large amounts of free energy upon hydrolysis of the phosphate ester bonds because hydrolysis results in formation of products that are more stable (i.e., have more resonant forms or less electrostatic repulsion) than the high-energy phosphate substrate. The hydrolysis of simple phosphate esters, such as glucose 6-phosphate and glycerol 3-phosphate, has $\Delta G^{\circ\prime}$ values in the range of −1 to −3 kcal/mol. Hydrolysis of phosphoric acid anhydrides such as the β- and γ-phosphates of ATP, of enol phosphates such as phosphoenolpyruvate, and of thiol esters such as acetyl CoA is associated with $\Delta G^{\circ\prime}$ values of approximately −7.3, −14.8, and −7.7 kcal/mol, respectively.

ATP plays a central role in linking energy-producing and energy-utilizing pathways. Potential ATP "units" or "equivalents" are often counted as a means of expressing the amount of available energy, the rate at which energy can be produced and/or utilized, or the amount of energy that can be obtained from storage depots. In the cell, the hydrolysis of ATP must be balanced with the phosphorylation of adenosine diphosphate (ADP). During macronutrient catabolism, some ATP equivalents are formed as a result of substrate-level phosphorylation, but most ATP is formed in the final stages of fuel catabolism in the mitochondria, that is by the transfer of reducing equivalents to oxygen via the electron transport chain and oxidative phosphorylation driven by the proton gradient. Because of the central role of oxidative phosphorylation in conservation of chemical energy in ATP, the production of reducing equivalents, such as NADH + H^+ or $FADH_2$, by catabolic pathways and the transfer of these hydrogens (electrons and protons) to oxygen as the terminal acceptor are closely linked to overall energy expenditure by the body.

In this unit, energy nutrition is considered largely from a whole body perspective. Nutritionists have traditionally considered the energy requirement or expenditure as being constituted by three major categories: energy for support of the normal processes of growth and maintenance (called basal metabolism), energy for the assimilation or use of dietary fuels (called specific dynamic action or thermic effect of food), and energy for activity. For maintenance of body weight, energy intake must be balanced by energy expenditure. If energy intake is greater than energy expenditure, excess energy will be stored as triacylglycerol in adipose tissue and lead to obesity. If energy intake is less than energy expenditure, this will result in loss of body weight and, if severe, can lead to protein-energy malnutrition.

Martha H. Stipanuk

Chapter 21

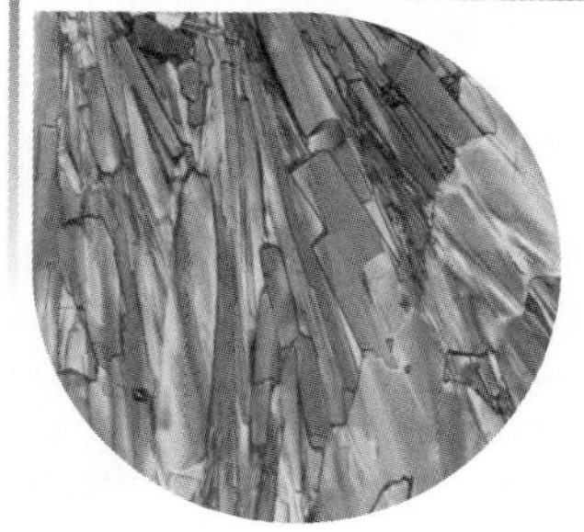

Cellular and Whole-Animal Energetics

James. A. Levine, MD, PhD, William T. Donahoo, MD, and Edward L. Melanson, PhD

OUTLINE

COMMON ABBREVIATIONS

ADP	adenosine diphosphate
ATP	adenosine triphosphate
BEE	basal energy expenditure, previously known as BEE, basal metabolic rate
EEPA	energy expenditure for physical activity
NEAT	nonexercise activity thermogenesis
PAL	physical activity level
RQ	respiratory quotient
TEE	total energy expenditure
TEF	thermic effect of food
RMR	resting metabolic rate

Total-body energy utilization is the sum of the myriad of energy-utilizing and energy-producing reactions occurring within individual cells and organ systems throughout the body. The various metabolic reactions that serve to sustain life are fueled by the energy released from the biological oxidation of energy-yielding nutrients in the food we consume. A fraction of the energy released from biological oxidation processes is captured in so-called high energy molecules, namely ATP (adenosine triphosphate), which is the main energy currency of the cell, and a few other specialized molecules such as creatine phosphate. These energy carriers fuel the various biochemical processes within cells that support basal metabolism, growth, and other essential functions. Chemical bond energy not captured in ATP synthesis is released as heat, which helps maintain body temperature.

This chapter is a revision of the chapter contributed by Adamandia D. Kriketos, PhD, John C. Peters, PhD, and James O. Hill, PhD, for the first edition.

METABOLIC SOURCES OF HEAT PRODUCTION

Current research suggests that heat production within cells has three components: (1) essential, (2) obligatory, and (3) regulatory (Fig. 21-1). Essential heat production is associated with the heat released during the reactions associated with the anabolic and catabolic cycles responsible for tissue turnover, primarily via the utilization and resynthesis of ATP molecules. Obligatory heat production originates from a variety of energy-utilizing molecular transport mechanisms. Examples of these obligatory processes include reactions involved in the absorption, digestion, and storage of nutrients, the Na^+,K^+-pump located in the cell membrane, and the proton pump located within the mitochondrial membrane. In homeothermic organisms (i.e., those that maintain a constant body temperature), regulatory heat production comprises a third component of cellular heat production.

Many neural and endocrine factors affect these various heat-producing reactions within cells (see Fig. 21-1). Thyroid hormone, for example, increases oxygen consumption and stimulates the metabolism of all warm-blooded animals. Thyroid hormone affects several components of the electron transport chain; the cell membrane Na^+,K^+-ATPase pump; and fat, carbohydrate, and protein metabolism. The effects of thyroid hormone on energy metabolism are discussed in more detail in Chapter 38.

Quantitatively, the energy expended in fueling various molecular transport mechanisms, many of which are responsible for maintaining essential electrochemical gradients across membranes, is responsible for a significant fraction of whole-body energy expenditure at rest. For example, it has been estimated that the Na^+,K^+-ATPase reaction, which is coupled to transport of K^+ into cells and movement of Na^+ out, accounts for 20% to 40% of whole-body resting energy expenditure (resting metabolic rate, or RMR) (McBride and Kelly, 1990). In highly metabolically active cell types, such as hepatocytes (liver cells), proton pumping across the mitochondrial membrane may represent up to 30% of the energy utilization of the cell (McBride and Kelly, 1990). Numerous other processes that transport amino acids, glucose, and nucleic acids, as well as reactions responsible for macromolecular synthesis and

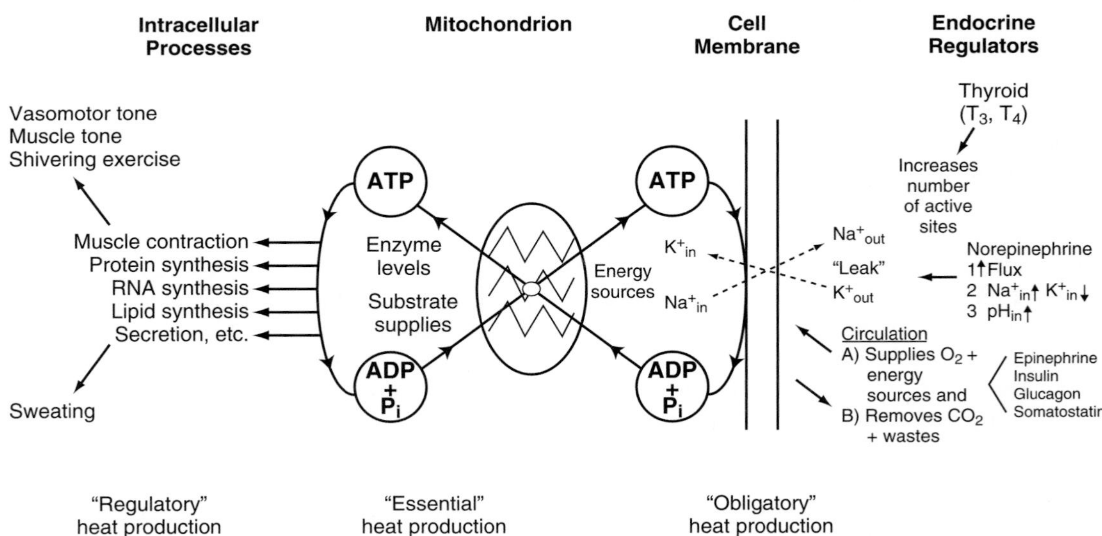

Figure 21-1 Nature of biochemical pathways for heat production. *(From Goldman RF [1980] Effect of environment on metabolism. In: Kinney JM [ed] Assessment of Energy Metabolism in Health and Disease. Report of the First Ross Conference on Medical Research. Ross Laboratories, Columbus, OH, pp 117-121.)*

degradation (e.g., membrane protein and phospholipid turnover), also contribute substantially to cellular and whole-body energy utilization.

Regulatory heat production, an essential function in homeotherms, is needed to maintain a constant body temperature in the face of fluctuating environmental temperature. Shivering, which is triggered in response to cold exposure, can involve a substantial increase in skeletal muscle contraction, which results in a significant increase in ATP turnover and subsequently increased heat production. Conversely, exposure of the individual to increased environmental temperature stimulates sweat production, which helps cool the body through the heat loss associated with evaporation. The processes of modulating heat production confer tremendous flexibility to many species so that they may survive in many different environmental conditions.

OXIDATIVE PHOSPHORYLATION

The coupling of fuel molecule oxidation to heat production and ATP synthesis is localized within the mitochondria of mammalian cells. The specialized proteins and enzymes required for the oxidative phosphorylation chain of reactions are specifically localized on the inner mitochondrial membrane. Oxidative phosphorylation is the process by which a molecule of inorganic phosphate is condensed with ADP (adenosine diphosphate) to form ATP, a process driven by the step-by-step transfer of electrons along a chain of electron carriers, as illustrated in Figure 21-2. The rate of ATP synthesis is governed or regulated by the availability of ADP. ADP is the "spent" end product of ATP-requiring reactions and is regenerated into ATP. Therefore, ATP production is directly coupled to ATP utilization through the generation and phosphorylation of the ADP intermediate.

The synthesis of ATP during oxidative phosphorylation is linked to the release of electrons carried by flavin and pyridine nucleotides to proteins of the electron transport chain. Hydrogen ions are pumped out of the mitochondrial matrix across the inner mitochondrial membrane at three sites along the electron transport chain to create an electrochemical gradient.

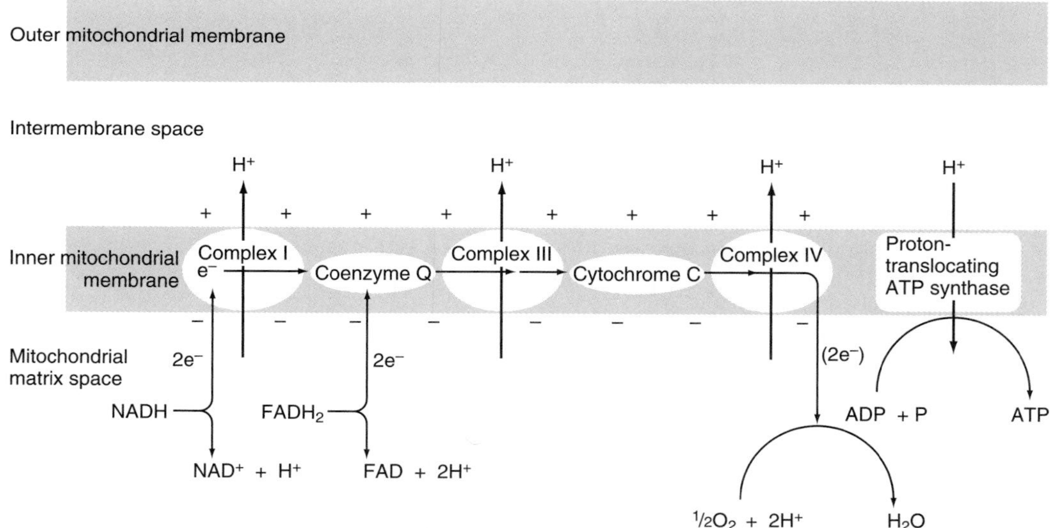

Figure 21-2 A general scheme for mitochondrial electron transport and oxidative phosphorylation. The transport of electrons from nicotinamide adenine dinucleotide, reduced form (NADH), and flavin adenine dinucleotide, reduced form ($FADH_2$), is accomplished by specific carrier molecules that constitute the electron transport chain. The terminal electron (and proton) acceptor is oxygen, and water is formed as a product of electron transport. The generation of the proton gradient by pumping protons out of the mitochondrial matrix is also shown. Dissipation of this proton gradient by the ATP synthase is coupled to ATP synthesis.

This proton gradient is subsequently dissipated as protons are allowed back through the membrane by the ATP synthase, which couples this process to ATP synthesis. Sufficient free energy may be collected at three sites along the electron transport chain (levels of complexes I, III, and IV, as shown in Fig. 21-2) to allow phosphorylation of ADP to ATP. A maximum of three molecules of ATP can be generated from each molecule of NADH that is oxidized via donation of its pair of electrons to the electron transport chain. The oxidation of $FADH_2$ occurs at a later step in the electron transport chain, and a maximum of only two molecules of ATP can be generated from each $FADH_2$ molecule. A thorough description of the electron transport chain can be found in most biochemistry textbooks (also see Chapter 24, Fig. 24-7).

The oxidation of fuel molecules utilizes molecular oxygen, especially as the terminal electron acceptor at the end of the electron transport chain, and the energy yield or heat production generated by these biochemical processes can be determined by measuring oxygen consumption. A frequently used index of the efficiency of oxidative phosphorylation is the P:O ratio. It is defined as the number of molecules of inorganic phosphate incorporated into organic form per atom of oxygen consumed (Murphy and Brand, 1987). At maximal biological efficiency, the complete oxidation of NADH yields 3 ATP molecules, and so the ratio observed for this process is 3. For the complete oxidation of $FADH_2$, the P:O ratio is 2. Few direct attempts to determine the P:O ratio in intact cells have been made because of difficulties encountered in trying to determine the rapid turnover of ATP molecules involved in the maintenance of a cell's metabolic activities without disturbing the cell's internal milieu. Nevertheless, the physiological P:O ratio is almost certainly somewhat less than the maximal values of 3 and 2 that are commonly used as a basis for calculating "ATP equivalents" of NADH and $FADH_2$, respectively.

OXIDATION OF FUEL MOLECULES

Free energy for the synthesis of ATP within cells comes from the oxidation of energy-yielding molecules in food, which include predominantly carbohydrate, fat, protein, and also alcohol if consumed (Flatt, 1985). The ATP yield per gram of glucose (from glycogen), fatty acid, or amino acid oxidized differs in proportion to the oxidation state of the different molecules. A molecule of glucose, for example, is more highly oxidized than a fatty acid molecule, and therefore less energy per gram is released in its complete oxidation to CO_2 than is released by complete oxidation of a fatty acid.

Net ATP yield depends on the amount of energy (ATP) the body must expend in the complete metabolism of the energy-yielding molecule as well as on that produced via substrate-level phosphorylation and oxidative phosphorylation. For example, the complete oxidation of 1 molecule of glucose via glycolysis, pyruvate dehydrogenase, and the citric acid cycle (as described in Chapter 12) results in synthesis of 40 ATPs, the expenditure of 2 ATPs, and a net yield of 38 ATPs. Furthermore, if the oxidation of fuels already stored in the body is considered—so that the inefficiencies or costs of digestion, absorption, and assimilation are not factors—the way in which net ATP yield may vary with the tissue and particular pathway (sequence of reactions) by which the fuel is catabolized may also be considered.

For example, if liver glycogen were released as glucose and the glucose were taken up and completely oxidized by muscle, the net ATP yield from the oxidation of this glucose derived from liver glycogen stores would be 38 moles of ATP per mole of glucose. However, if muscle glycogen were the source of the glucose, with breakdown of glycogen to glucose 1-phosphate, the complete metabolism of this glucose phosphate within the muscle could generate 39 moles of ATP per mole of glucose phosphate; one less ATP would be expended because ATP-dependent phosphorylation of glucose was not required. Alternatively, muscle might convert plasma glucose to lactate under anaerobic conditions (with a net yield of 2 moles of ATP per mole of glucose), but the conversion of lactate back to glucose by liver (with a net cost of 6 moles of ATP per 2 moles of lactate), followed by its complete oxidation to CO_2 + H_2O) (net release of 38 moles of ATP per mole of glucose) would result in the net generation of 34 moles of ATP per mole of glucose completely oxidized

Nutrition Insight

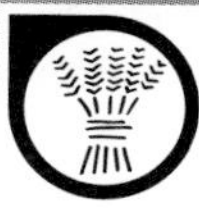

Physiological Fuel Values

Physiological fuel value is a term used to connote the energy from a food that is available to the body. Physiological fuel values of foods are obtained by subtracting energy lost in the excreta (feces and urine) from the total energy value of the food. Wilbour Olin Atwater and his associates at the Connecticut (Storrs) Agriculture Experiment Station determined the digestibility and fuel values of a number of food materials in the later 1800s and early 1900s and proposed the general physiological fuel equivalents of 4.0, 8.9, and 4.0 kcal/g dietary protein, fat, and carbohydrate, respectively, for application to the mixed American diet. In the years following the publication of Atwater's work, the 4, 9, and 4 (rounded) factors came into widespread usage in estimating the caloric value of foods.

It should be noted that factors for carbohydrate, fat, or protein in specific foods may vary considerably due to differences in digestibility or chemical composition. The general factors are intended for application to mixed diets. The carbohydrate factor is applied to total food carbohydrate, which includes nondigestible carbohydrate that is now referred to as dietary fiber. In addition, the derivation of the factors attributed all the energy lost in the urine to excretion of protein nitrogen as urea; this is not strictly correct, but the error associated with the calculation of energy value of foods by application of Atwater's protein factors to diets has been estimated to be small.

More recently, the data and values of Atwater were checked and confirmed by 108 digestion experiments conducted by Annabel L. Merrill and Bernice K. Watt at the U.S. Department of Agriculture (USDA) (Merrill and Watt, 1973). The available energy of the diets, determined from gross energy values of food, feces, and urine, showed close agreement with calculations based on the application of average energy factors to the protein, fat, and carbohydrate in the diet. Merrill and Watt also recalculated Atwater's general factors for protein, fat, and carbohydrate, based on a typical U.S. mixed diet in 1949. They obtained average values of 4.0, 8.9, and 3.9, which were essentially the same as the general factors Atwater reported in 1899.

The rounded 4, 9, and 4 factors for physiological fuel values derived by Atwater are still widely used today, more than a century later.

---

with intermediate cycling to lactate and back to glucose.

Not all the free energy of dietary fuel molecules is available to the body. Some energy is lost due to incomplete digestion and absorption of fuel molecules. In general, a small amount (usually no more than 5% to 10%) of the gross energy content of food is lost in feces due to incomplete digestion and absorption. The fate of absorbed fuel energy is shown in Figure 21-3. Once absorbed, an additional 5% to 10% of the energy in the food molecules is expended in the processes of transport, storage, and biochemical conversion of different fuels into appropriate storage forms (e.g., glucose is converted to glycogen, fatty acids are esterified to form triacylglycerol, and amino acids are utilized for tissue protein synthesis) (Acheson et al., 1984). In addition, some energy is lost within the body as heat during the oxidation of fuel molecules, whereas the rest of the energy is conserved in the high-energy phosphate bonds of ATP. Some absorbed energy is lost in the urine or in the feces (via the bile or other secretions) due to excretion of incompletely oxidized metabolites. In particular, the excretion of urea as a waste product of amino acid oxidation results in a loss of approximately 20% of the potential energy that could have been derived from amino acid oxidation. Therefore, the efficiency of energy capture from the processes of digestion, storage, and metabolism of fuel molecules determines the amount of ATP available for the body's use.

Roughly one half of the total energy released from oxidation of metabolic fuel is lost as heat to the environment without formation of ATP; this stems from the inherent inefficiency of converting the molecular bond energy in fuel molecules to ATP bond energy. The remaining

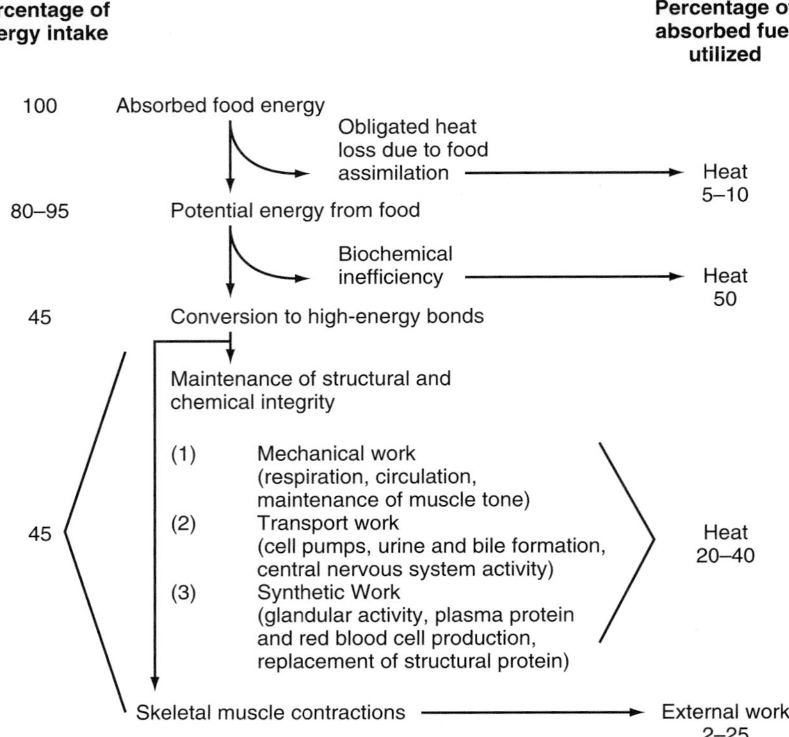

Figure 21-3 The conversion of absorbed fuel energy to heat and work.

energy that is captured in the form of ATP is used to fuel both internal (e.g., mechanical, transport, and synthetic) and external (skeletal muscle contraction) work. Some energy is also lost as heat when ATP is hydrolyzed for work.

EFFICIENCY OF ENERGY CONSERVATION FROM FUEL OXIDATION

The efficiency of energy conservation or the efficiency of the coupling of electron transfer to ATP synthesis can be affected by different pharmacological agents, such as dinitrophenol, caffeine, nicotine, and amphetamines. These agents dissipate the proton-motive force across the inner mitochondrial membrane, which is essential for driving ATP synthesis; so, while electron transport from NADH and $FADH_2$ to oxygen proceeds normally, ATP synthesis is disrupted. This loss of respiratory control leads to increased oxygen consumption and more rapid oxidation of NADH and $FADH_2$ that is not dependent on the regeneration of ATP from ADP (Argyropoulos et al., 1998).

In contrast to the uncoupling caused by pharmacological agents, the physiological uncoupling of oxidative phosphorylation can be useful in generating heat to maintain body temperature in hibernating animals, in some newborn animals (including humans), and in mammals adapted to cold climates (Kozak, 2000). Newborn infants have a significant amount of brown adipose tissue (BAT), but by adulthood only an insignificant amount (if any) of this specialized tissue is present in the body. The inner mitochondrial membrane of BAT contains thermogenin, also known as the uncoupling protein 1 (UCP1), which permits the reentry of protons into the mitochondrion independent of the synthesis of ATP, so that the potential energy represented by the proton gradient is lost as heat.

There are two other uncoupling proteins (UCP2 and UCP3) in many tissues of the human body. UCP2 and UCP3, unlike UCP1, are not solely affected by exposure to cold (Vidal-Puig et al., 1997). UCP2 expression increased when rats were fed a high-fat diet, suggesting it may be involved in regulating energy expenditure in response to excess caloric intake. The genetic expression of some uncoupling proteins has been linked to obesity, although there is no direct evidence to date that they play a significant role in the etiology of obesity. The UCP2 gene, for example, maps to regions of human chromosome 11 and mouse chromosome 7 that have been linked to hyperinsulinemia and obesity. It is possible that alterations in function or expression of the genes regulating these "energy-wasting" proteins may contribute to an underlying susceptibility to obesity stemming from increased energetic efficiency (Donahoo et al., 2004).

SUBSTRATE CYCLING

Substrate cycling denotes a situation in which a key enzyme in a metabolic pathway is opposed by another enzyme that catalyzes the reverse reaction and that may act simultaneously. Because ATP is consumed in these enzyme-catalyzed reactions but there is no net change in reactant or product concentrations, these reactions are often termed futile cycles. The ATP hydrolysis used to fuel these reactions contributes to heat production but is not coupled to net metabolic or external work. Changes in the rate of substrate cycling within cells may be one means by which the efficiency of energy utilization can be increased or decreased, leading to changes in the overall efficiency of metabolism and energy utilization by the whole body (Newsholme and Parry-Billings, 1992). One such enzyme–reaction couple is the interconversion of fructose 6-phosphate and fructose 1,6-bisphosphate by 6-phosphofructo-1-kinase and fructose 1,6-bisphosphatase. In this cycle, as in all futile cycles, ATP is expended but no net metabolism is accomplished. Other potentially important substrate cycles include conversions of glucose and glucose 6-phosphate, of protein and amino acids, and of fatty acids and triacylglycerols.

COMPONENTS OF ENERGY EXPENDITURE

There are three principal components of human energy expenditure: basal energy expenditure (BEE), thermic effect of food (TEF), and energy expenditure of physical activity (EEPA). There are also other small components of energy expenditure that may contribute to the whole such as the energetic costs of cold-adaptation, medications, and emotion. These components are sometimes referred to as adaptive thermogenesis, although this term is widely used but rarely specifically defined. Suffice it to point out that, although cold-adaptation is well documented in humans (van Marken Lichtenbelt and Daanen, 2003), the majority of humans are not exposed to extremes of cold temperature.

Most of the variance in daily energy expenditure is accounted for by BEE, TEF, and EEPA. BEE is the energy expended when an individual is supine at complete rest, in the morning, after sleep, and in the postabsorptive state. BEE accounts for approximately 60% of total daily energy expenditure in individuals with sedentary occupations. Because it is not always possible to measure BEE under rigidly defined conditions, resting metabolic rate (RMR) is often used as an approximation of BEE. RMR is slightly higher than BEE (or BMR), but BEE and RMR are sometimes used interchangeably. TEF is the increase in energy expenditure associated with the digestion, absorption, and storage of food and accounts for approximately 10% to 15% of total daily energy expenditure (Reed and Hill, 1996; Kinabo and Durnin, 1990; D'Alessio et al., 1988; Hill et al., 1985). EEPA is the sum of the daily energy expenditure for physical activities of all kinds.

The EEPA or activity thermogenesis can be separated into two components, as illustrated in Figure 21-4: (1) the energy expenditure related to planned exercise and (2) the remainder, which can be called nonexercise activity thermogenesis (NEAT). Exercise is most easily defined as the purposeful physical activity undertaken for health (e.g., sports; visiting the gym or club) and is defined in the *Merriam-Webster Dictionary* as "bodily exertion for the sake of developing and maintaining physical fitness." Information about the energy costs

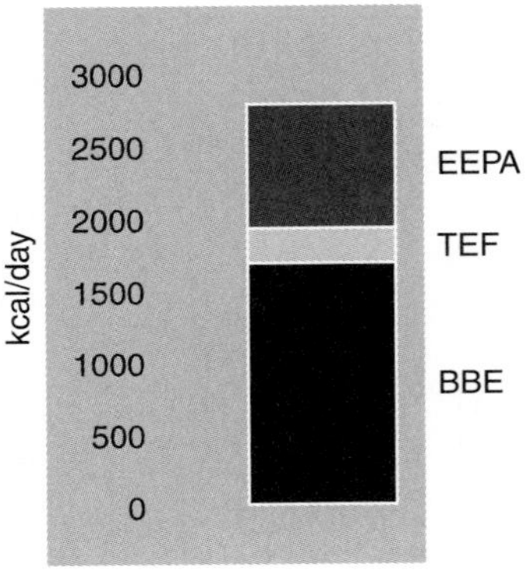

Figure 21-4 The components of energy expenditure in sedentary adults. *BEE*, Basal energy expenditure; *TEF*, thermic effect of food; *EEPA*, energy expenditure for physical activity.

of sporting-like exercise may be found in Pacy and colleagues (1986). However, most people do not participate in exercise, as so defined, and, hence, for them, exercise activity thermogenesis is zero. NEAT, even in most exercisers, is the predominant component of EEPA and is the energy expenditure associated with all the activities we undertake as vibrant, independent beings. NEAT includes the energy expenditure of occupational activities (e.g., construction work, office work, or housekeeping), leisure activities, sitting, standing, lifting, walking, talking, toe-tapping, playing guitar, dancing, and shopping.

MEASUREMENT OF ENERGY EXPENDITURE

Energy expenditure (heat production), whether in cells, tissues, or the whole body, is most often measured using the methods of direct and indirect calorimetry. Direct calorimetry measures the heat released from the cell, tissue, or body by directly measuring changes in the temperature of the environment surrounding the organism (usually a carefully controlled, closed environmental chamber) (Jequier and Schutz, 1983). In practice, direct calorimetry is not often used, in part because of the long delay between heat production and release of the heat to the surrounding environment. This delay occurs because the body has a large capacity for heat storage. A second reason for not using direct calorimetry is because of the cost and complexity of the equipment.

Indirect calorimetry measures oxygen consumption as a surrogate for heat production. This is valid, because in aerobic organisms most heat production originates from metabolic oxidation reactions, which utilize molecular oxygen in specific amounts depending on the substrate (or mixture of substrates) oxidized. For example, the oxidation of glucose yields the following stoichiometry:

$$C_6H_{12}O_6 + 6\ O_2 = 6\ H_2O + 6\ CO_2 + 673\ \text{kcal}$$

The energy yield per mole of O_2 utilized has been determined experimentally for the main oxidative substrates, and these factors can be used to calculate heat production from the quantity of oxygen consumed (Table 21-1).

Energy expenditure is measured increasingly by the combination of indirect calorimetry and tracer techniques in order to study details of substrate oxidation in tissues and in the whole body (Romijn et al., 2000). Because, in general, tracers are administered into and sampled from the blood compartment, they can trace the kinetics of blood-borne substrates, whereas calorimetry estimates whole-body (blood plus tissues) oxidation. Oxidation of tissue substrates that do not pass through the bloodstream in their pathways to oxidation is included when metabolic rate is measured by indirect calorimetry (precisely to the extent that their combustion consumes O_2 and releases CO_2), but it may not be detectable by changes in the concentration of a labeled tracer substrate in the blood. Therefore, in principle, the difference between calorimetric and tracer estimates of substrate oxidation should reflect phenomena that occur entirely at the tissue level (Wolfe and George, 1993).

The O_2 consumption of individual tissues in vivo can be estimated by making measurements of the arteriovenous concentration difference of oxygen across a tissue in conjunction with measurement of blood flow. Although muscle is the largest tissue in the adult whole body, accounting for approximately 40% of adult body weight, its estimated BEE is relatively low (~10 to 15 kcal/kg/day), so muscle's contribution to the total basal energy expenditure of the body is only approximately 20% to 25%.

Table 21-1

Energy and Respiratory Equivalent of Body Fuels

	Energy (kcal/g)			Respiratory Equivalent			Volume	
Food	Complete Oxidation of Food Component in Bomb Calorimeter	"Complete Oxidation" of Absorbed or Stored Fuel in Body*	Physiological Fuel Value of Consumed Foodstuff†	O_2 (kcal/L)	CO_2 (kcal/L)	RQ (V_{CO_2}/V_{O_2})	O_2 (L/g)	CO_2 (L/g)
Carbohydrate	4.1	4.1	4	5.05	5.05	1.00	0.81	0.81
Protein	5.4	4.2	4	4.46	5.57	0.80	0.94	0.75
Fat	9.3	9.3	9	4.74	6.67	0.71	1.96	1.39
Alcohol	7.1	7.1	7	4.86	7.25	0.67	1.46	0.98
Average				4.83	5.89	0.82		

*All energy in urine is attributed to N excretion in this calculation, and the calculated factor is 7.9 kcal/g N. N is excreted as urea, which has an energy content of 5.4 kcal/g N.
†Values are adjusted for digestibility (incomplete absorption) and incomplete oxidation.

In a resting subject consuming an average diet providing roughly 35% fat, 12% protein, and 53% carbohydrate (as percentages of total energy intake), who is studied in the postabsorptive state, approximately 4.83 kcal are expended for every liter of O_2 consumed. Although different amounts of oxygen are consumed during the biological oxidation of different energy-yielding foodstuffs, the multiplication of liters of O_2 consumed by 4.83 kcal per liter will provide an estimate of heat production to within approximately 8% of the actual value regardless of which nutrients are being oxidized.

Because the body's oxygen store is very small, measurement of oxygen consumption by indirect calorimetry can provide a rapid measure of heat production that is in close temporal association with metabolic energy utilization. An additional advantage of indirect calorimetry is the ability to measure substrate (fuel molecule) oxidation rates. The amount of heat released per liter of O_2 consumed depends on the type of nutrient being oxidized (i.e., protein, carbohydrate, or fat). By measuring CO_2 production and urinary nitrogen excretion in addition to O_2 consumption, it is possible to determine the proportion of the different nutrients that are oxidized and thus to calculate the heat released from each nutrient class (see Table 21-1).

Another indirect method was developed in the 1960s for measuring total energy expenditure in free-living individuals over periods of 10 to 14 days (Schoeller et al., 1986). This method uses water that has been doubly labeled with the isotopes ^2H (deuterium) and ^{18}O. The principle behind the doubly labeled water method is based on the fact that ^2H from the body's labeled water pool leaves as ^2H-labeled water, whereas the ^{18}O equilibrates with CO_2 (via $H_2CO_3 \rightleftharpoons CO_2 + H_2O$) and leaves the body as both ^{18}O-labeled water and ^{18}O-labeled CO_2. The difference in the disappearance rates of the two isotopes and a measure of the size of the body water pool provide an estimate of unlabeled CO_2 production from oxidation of fuels (Fig. 21-5). Oxygen consumption can then be calculated from an estimate of the respiratory quotient (RQ = CO_2 produced/O_2 consumed) of the diet; RQ can be measured or estimated from diet composition and tabled values.

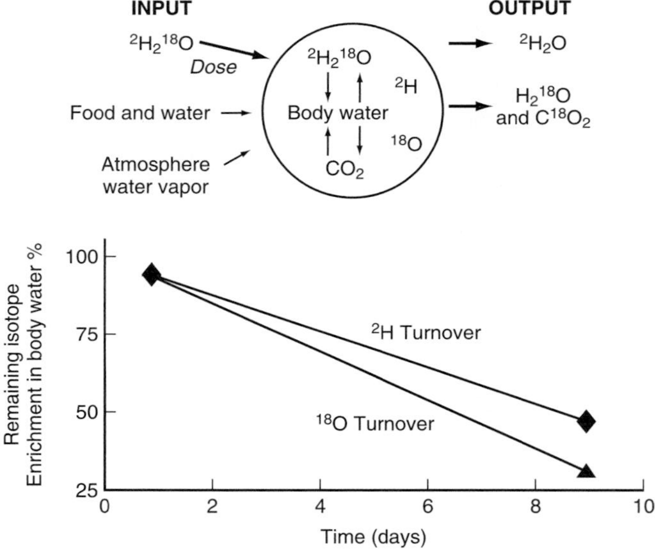

Figure 21-5 Model of doubly labeled water technique. Water labeled with ^2H and ^{18}O mixes with the total body water. ^2H is lost in H_2O, whereas ^{18}O equilibrates with CO_2 and is lost both with H_2O and CO_2. The difference in the rate of loss of ^2H and ^{18}O is related to the rate of CO_2 production from the fuel metabolized and O_2 utilized. From this analysis, energy expenditure can be determined in a free-living individual by sampling body fluids (H_2O) over time.

To understand the potential role of EEPA in human energy balance one must first appreciate the strengths and limitations of available techniques. Little information is available regarding the time-period of measurement needed to gain a representative assessment of EEPA. Approximately 7 days of measurement is likely to provide a representative assessment of activity thermogenesis for a given 3- or 4-month block of time (Marr and Heady, 1986). Such 7-day measurements can potentially be repeated to understand the importance of variables such as season or changing occupational roles. Broadly, EEPA can be measured by one of two approaches. The first approach is to measure or estimate total EEPA. Here, total daily energy expenditure is measured and from it, BEE-plus-TEF is subtracted. The second approach is the factoral approach whereby the components of EEPA are quantified using questionnaires or electronic devices and total EEPA is calculated by summing these components. The methodology for measuring EEPA will not be described herein but has been reviewed in detail (Levine, 2002). The most widely used statistic related to EEPA is the physical activity level (PAL), which is defined as the ratio of TEE:BEE. The calculation of PAL does not separate out TEF and, thus, does not require a determination of TEF. PAL values are optimally determined using doubly labeled water to measure TEE and indirect calorimetry to measure BEE.

VARIATION IN DAILY ENERGY EXPENDITURE

When trying to understand whether energy expenditure could play an important role in obesity and body weight modulation, one might first examine the variability in total daily energy expenditure. The question is: How variable is TEE?

Data suggest that TEE varies enormously even in industrialized countries, where use of machinery that promotes a sedentary lifestyle is commonplace. Data from Britain gathered using doubly labeled water demonstrate that TEE varies substantially among individuals (Fig. 21-6). The marked variance in TEE is even

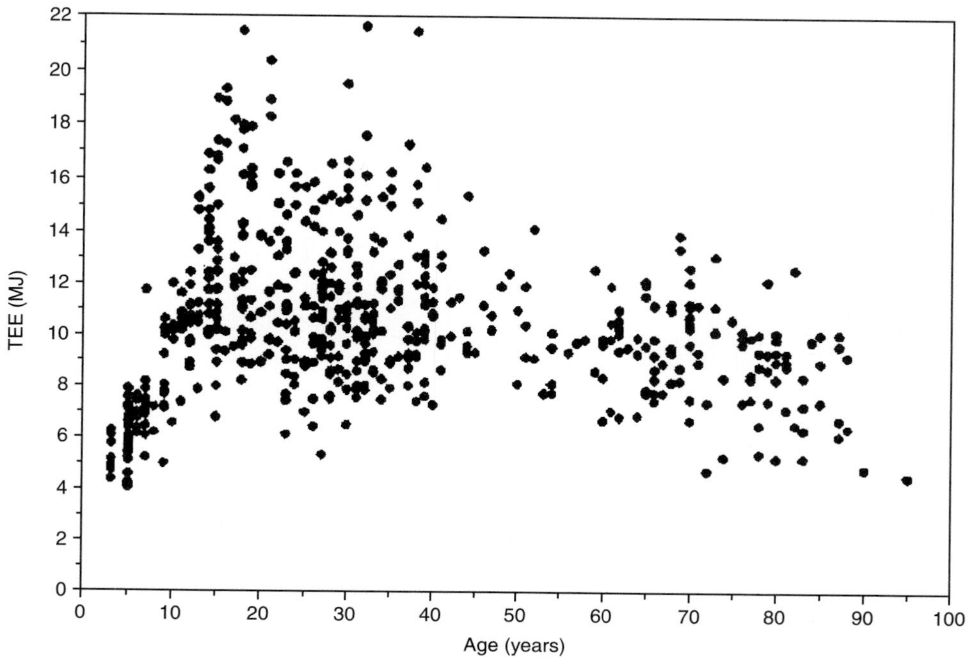

Figure 21-6 Total daily energy expenditure (TEE) for 574 persons aged 2 to 95 years. *(Redrawn from Black AE, Coward WA, Cole TJ, Prentice AM [1996] Human energy expenditure in affluent societies: an analysis of 574 doubly-labelled water measurements. Eur J Clin Nutr 50:72-92.)*

greater when data from nonindustrialized countries is considered (Levine et al., 2001; Coward, 1998).

For two adults of similar size, TEE can vary by as much as 1,500 kcal per day. Does this occur through BEE, TEF or EEPA?

BASAL ENERGY EXPENDITURE

The majority (83%) of variance in BEE and 24-hour energy expenditure is accounted for by fat-free mass (FFM); age and gender contribute modestly (Lucas et al., 1988). Figure 21-7 shows a strong tendency for 24-hour energy expenditure to aggregate closely within families compared with between families. This familial trait suggests, but does not prove, that metabolic rate is genetically determined (Bogardus et al., 1986). Bouchard and colleagues (1989) have studied the heritability of BEE in monozygotic and dizygotic twins and showed higher correlations in monozygotic twins than in dizygotic twins, whether BEE is expressed per kilogram of body weight or of FFM. These investigators suggest that the more genes are shared, the more similar the metabolic rate, independent of body size and composition. Under standard conditions the within-individual coefficient of variance (CV) in BEE of healthy adult humans is approximately 3% to 8% when measured on the same or different days (Adriaens et al., 2003; Gasic et al., 1997; Westrate, 1993; Zurlo et al., 1986).

The within-individual CV for BEE in prepubertal children (3%), prepubertal obese girls (6%), elderly men (4%), and elderly women (3%) is similar to that reported in healthy adult populations (Gibbons et al., 2004; Figueroa-Colon et al., 1996). BEE is elevated in certain disease states. Bell et al. (1999) reported that the within-individual CV for BEE measurements in patients with cystic fibrosis (4%) was significantly greater than that for measurements in age- and sex-matched controls (2%) but within the range of CVs reported in the

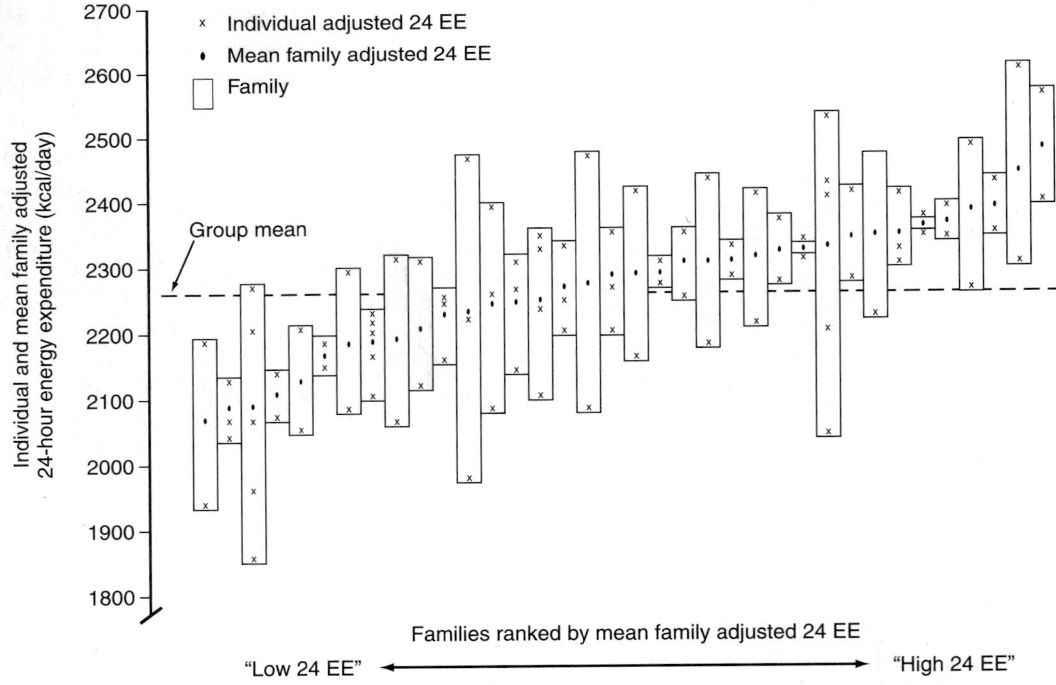

Figure 21-7 Individual and mean family total daily (24-hour) energy expenditure (24 EE) adjusted for fat-free body mass, fat mass, age, and sex. *(Based on the data of Bogardus C, Lillioja S, Ravussin E, Abbott W, Zawadzki JK, Young A, Knowler WC, Jacobowitz R, Moll PP [1986] Familial dependence of the resting metabolic rate. N Engl J Med 315:96-100.)*

aforementioned studies in healthy adults. Even in healthy adults, individual CVs vary from approximately 0% to 10% (Adriaens et al., 2003), suggesting that large errors in energy requirements are possible when based on a single measurement of BEE.

BEE exhibits a biphasic pattern during the menstrual cycle, with a greater BEE observed in the luteal compared to follicular phase, presumably due to elevated serum concentrations of estrogen and progesterone (Solomon et al., 1982). Nonetheless, a recent study by Henry and colleagues (2003) demonstrated that the within-individual CV for measurements of BEE across a single menstrual cycle ranged from 2% to 10%, which is similar to the range of CVs observed in the other populations described above.

One might expect that BEE measured in out-patient settings would be higher than that measured in an in-patient setting. However, studies in prepubertal girls (Figueroa-Colon et al., 1996) and adults (Turley et al., 1993) found no significant differences in BEE measured under inpatient and outpatient conditions. Unfortunately, neither of these studies reported within-subject CVs, so it is unclear to what extent within-individual BEE varied under inpatient and outpatient conditions. Individual differences in BEE measured under outpatient conditions would likely be influenced by physical activity in the period preceding the measurement. However, Adriaens and colleagues (2003) reported that differences in BEE (CV = 3.3 ± 2.1%) were not explained by differences in physical activity the day before the measurement. Furthermore, the CV in BEE fell from 5.2% to 3.3% when subjects who did not comply with the 12-hour fast were excluded, suggesting that prior food intake, rather than prior physical activity (exclusive of exercise), will have a much greater effect on BEE. Somewhat different results were obtained in another recent study. Haugen and colleagues (2003) found that BEE measured in the morning under standard testing conditions was 6% lower compared to an afternoon measurement obtained under less stringent conditions (4-hour fast, no exercise between measurements; RMR), but the change in BEE from morning to afternoon was not related to reported energy intake. Furthermore, despite the less stringent conditions for the afternoon measurements, the within-individual CV was lower for the afternoon measurements (2.8%) than for the morning measurements (4.5%). Nonetheless, these studies indicate that BEE measurements obtained in outpatient settings are highly reproducible, provided there is reasonable control for prior physical activity and food intake.

The partitioning of resting energy expenditure among the various body organ systems is shown in Figure 21-8. Brain, liver, kidney, and heart are the most metabolically active organs within the body at rest and comprise over half

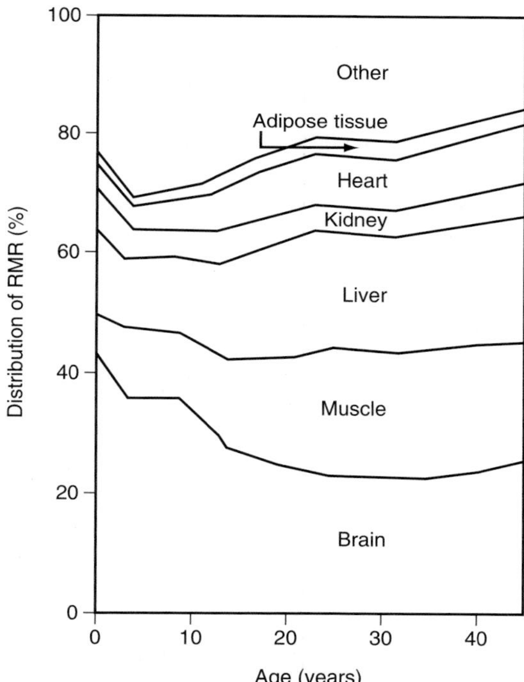

Figure 21-8 The contribution of energy expenditure by different organs to resting metabolic rate (*RMR*) or basal energy expenditure. Area is calculated from the product of the organ (tissue) weight and organ (tissue) metabolic rate. *(Modified from Elia M [1992] Organ and tissue contribution to metabolic rate. In: Kinney JM, Tucker HN [eds] Energy Metabolism: Tissue Determinants and Cellular Corollaries. Raven Press Ltd., New York, pp 61-79.)*

the resting energy expenditure, although they account for only 5% to 6% of body weight. In infants, the brain is the largest contributor to resting or basal energy expenditure, due to its exaggerated size per unit of body weight. The contribution to total metabolic rate of these organs is proportional to the blood flow to these tissues. These tissues have a metabolic rate that is 15 to 40 times greater than an equivalent mass of resting muscle and 50 to 100 times greater than adipose tissue. Skeletal muscle also represents a significant fraction of resting energy expenditure because of its large total mass, but on a per gram basis, skeletal muscle is much less active than these other organs. Of course, the contribution of muscle tissue to TEE increases markedly during physical activity (Elia, 1992).

As shown in Figure 21-9, the metabolic rate per unit of organ weight appears to change little throughout life for the main metabolic organs (brain, liver, heart, and kidney). However, the BEE for the whole body, expressed per unit of body weight, decreases with age. This decrease in BEE per unit of body weight with age is primarily caused by the much greater growth of the entire body (particularly skeletal muscle) compared to the metabolic organs (particularly the brain) over time. Throughout adulthood, however, the size and metabolic activity of these organs remain stable, and hence both the BEE per unit of body weight and the metabolic rate of the main metabolic organs per unit of organ weight remain relatively constant in the adult years.

Physiological stresses include injury, fever, surgery, renal failure, burns, infections, and even starvation or malnutrition (Elia, 2000). In these cases, characteristically catecholamine and hormone levels increase, BEE increases, and glucose and free fatty acid concentrations rise in the blood. Studies examining patients with severe illnesses accompanied by fever have shown up to a 13% increase in metabolic rate for each degree Celsius of increase in body temperature (Powanda and Beisel, 2003). During fever, there is an increase in the production and utilization of the metabolizable, energy-yielding substrates made available to cells; this is primarily an increased utilization of glucose as a result of accelerated rates of glycogenolysis and gluconeogenesis. In the

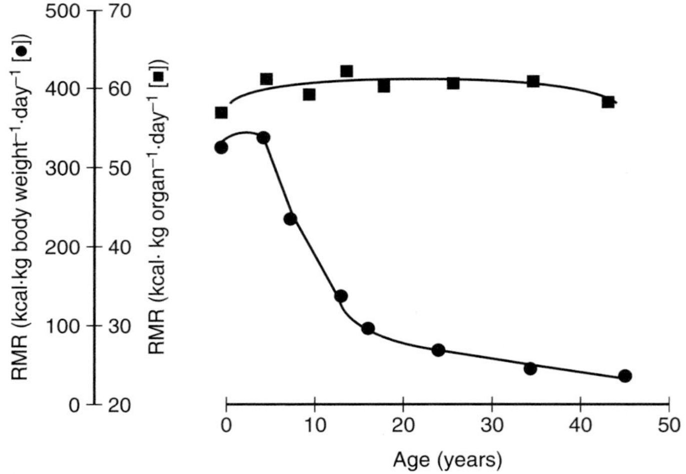

Figure 21-9 Changes in resting metabolic rate during growth and development. The whole body resting metabolic rate (RMR) per kg of body weight is shown along with the metabolic rate for liver, kidney, brain, and heart combined per kg of organ weight. (Organ weight refers to the sum of the weights of liver, kidney, brain, and heart.) *(Modified from Elia M [1992] Organ and tissue contribution to metabolic rate. In: Kinney JM, Tucker HN [eds] Energy Metabolism: Tissue Determinants and Cellular Corollaries. Raven Press Ltd., New York, pp 61-79.)*

situation of a patient with severe burns, the body requires an increased metabolic rate to ensure a stable body temperature when much of the body's insulation is lost by the injury to skin. In addition, in most illnesses increased energy is required as a result of the increased production of immune response agents such as cytokines and the subsequent energy-requiring processes associated with their actions.

Activation of the sympathetic nervous system causes the release of the catecholamines, epinephrine and norepinephrine, from the adrenal medulla. Activation of this system occurs predominantly in response to stress and is accompanied by the secretion of other hormones. These hormones act together to increase the metabolic rate of cells by altering the rate of numerous biochemical processes. The pancreatic hormones insulin and glucagon affect the rates of utilization of carbohydrate and fat metabolism predominantly via activation of transporters. Thyroid hormone affects the expression of specific proteins by altering nuclear transcription rates, thereby affecting metabolic rate and heat production. An accelerated cellular uptake of thyroid hormones, especially triiodothyronine (T_3), often occurs in response to infection. An increase in thyroid hormone promotes an increase in the metabolic rate of all cells, but, unlike for catecholamines, the effect of an increased level of thyroid hormone occurs over a period of days to weeks.

THERMIC EFFECT OF FOOD

The CV for TEF measured with indirect calorimetry is larger than the CV for BEE, typically approximately 20% (Miles et al., 1993; Piers et al., 1992). Although similar results are obtained with the use of a ventilated hood face mask or a mouthpiece (Segal et al., 1990), no study has evaluated the potential effect of sampling method on variation in TEF. The timing of measurements (intermittent versus continuous) has been shown to alter both the magnitude and variability of TEF, with intermittent measures giving a 50% lower, but a more replicable, value for TEF (Piers et al., 1992). TEF is increased when the ambient temperature is decreased from 22° to 16°C (Westerterp-Plantenga et al., 2002). The duration of measurements also contributes to the variation in TEF, with shorter measurements (<5 hours) yielding greater errors (Reed and Hill, 1996). The magnitude of TEF is proportional to the energy content (Reed and Hill, 1996) and the protein content (Karst et al., 1984) of the test meal. Both overfeeding and underfeeding on the days prior to measurement have been reported to alter TEF, although the reported effect varies dramatically among the studies (Granata and Brandon, 2002). Prior activity likely also affects TEF, as increased resting energy expenditure and increased macronutrient oxidation have been reported following an exercise session (Bielinski et al., 1985). Also activity (i.e., fidgeting) during the measurement period affects TEF measurement (Levine et al., 2000).

The degree to which interindividual characteristics contribute to variation in TEF is unclear. Lean body mass is a strong determinant of TEF (Reed and Hill, 1996). Weight gain increases and weight loss decreases TEF (Leibel et al., 1995), although some studies have not seen a decrease in TEF with weight loss (Miles et al., 1993). Interestingly, it has been reported that TEF falls up to the point where a 10% weight loss has been achieved, but does not change with further weight loss (Leibel et al., 1995). A reduced TEF has been reported in obese and insulin-resistant individuals (Segal et al., 1990), although the independent effect of obesity on TEF is controversial (Granata and Brandon, 2002). Likewise, age has been associated with a decline in TEF in some (Morgan and York, 1983) but not all studies (Melanson et al., 1998). A lower TEF has been reported in trained individuals (Poehlman et al., 1988), but another study reported a positive correlation between TEF and maximum oxygen consumption (Davis et al., 1983). It does not appear as though TEF varies over the menstrual cycle (Melanson et al., 1996). Most recently, genetic factors such as variations in the β3-adrenoceptor (Walston et al., 2003) have been shown to alter TEF. Variations in intestinal fatty acid binding proteins contribute to variations in fat absorption and oxidation and, therefore, might also contribute to variations in TEF (Dworatzek et al., 2004).

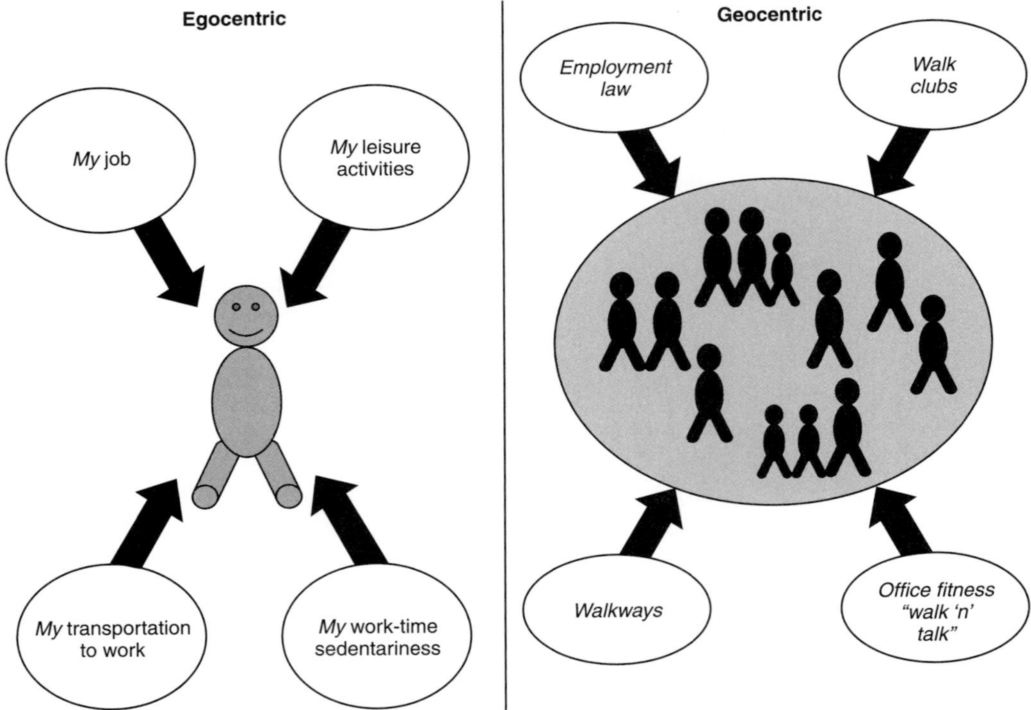

Figure 21-10 Illustration of egocentric and geocentric models of environmental influences on nonexercise activity thermogenesis (NEAT). Balloons contain examples of different factors.

NONEXERCISE ACTIVITY THERMOGENESIS

As noted in the preceding text, BEE is largely (80%) accounted for by body size, and TEF is a small component of TEE (6% to 12%), so the variance in TEE among people of similar size can be explained only by variance in EEPA. Because most people do not participate in volitional sporting-like exercise, variance in NEAT may be the critical component of energy expenditure that accounts for the interindividual variance in weight-independent energy expenditure. So, is it possible that NEAT could vary by 1,500 kcal day? The factors that account for the variability of NEAT can be categorized as environmental or biological.

Environmental Determinants of NEAT

It is self-evident that NEAT is affected by environment. Consider the effects on physical activity of holding meetings while seated, grasping the remote control at home, and of living or working in the "concrete jungle." Understanding how environment interacts with NEAT is important because of its potential impact on obesity and undernutrition. It is convenient to classify the environmental determinants of NEAT into two models: the egocentric model and the geocentric model. In the egocentric model we consider a single person as the focus. Hence the environmental factors that impact that person's NEAT (e.g., the activity associated with her occupation, her mode of transportation, and her leisure time) are considered. In the geocentric model we consider the environmental factors that affect NEAT (e.g., tax breaks to companies that include compulsory physical-activity breaks as part of the work day, or city planning to ensure walk-friendly or bike-accessible environments). These models are helpful as they provide a theoretical framework in which we can understand NEAT and how best to intervene to promote NEAT. The egocentric and geocentric models are illustrated in Figure 21-10 and Table 21-2.

A simple initial classification of egocentric factors is to divide a person's NEAT activities

Table 21-2
Examples of Egocentric and Geocentric Models to Examine the Interaction of NEAT and Environment

Question	Egocentric Model	Geocentric Model
Is walking important in NEAT?	Measure NEAT in subjects under intensive study (e.g., lean versus obese subjects) using high-level sensing technologies and doubly labeled water	Establish thermal surveillance system to detect differences in walk-through for walking paths that are well-lit compared to those that are poorly lit
Can a specified intervention decrease sitting time?	Measure sitting before, during, and after a specified anti-sitting intervention	Perform productivity analyses of companies that encourage "walk-'n'-talk" meetings and discourage interoffice e-mail
Does increasing NEAT improve diabetes control?	Clinical research center study comparing glucose values and insulin sensitivity before and after an experimental increase in NEAT	Evaluation of the use of statewide diabetes services before and after a statewide walking initiative targeted at patients with diabetes

NEAT, Nonexercise activity thermogenesis.

Table 21-3
Prediction of Physical Activity Level on the Basis of Occupation

Occupation Type	PAL
Chair-bound or bed-bound	1.2
Seated work with no option of moving around and little or no strenuous leisure activity	1.4-1.5
Seated work with discretion and requirement to move around but little or no strenuous leisure activity	1.6-1.7
Standing work (e.g., housewife, shop assistant)	1.8-1.9
Strenuous work or highly active leisure	2.0-2.4

PAL, Physical activity level.
From Black AE, Coward WA, Cole TJ, Prentice AM (1996) Human energy expenditure in affluent societies: an analysis of 574 doubly-labelled water measurements. Eur J Clin Nutr 50:72-92.

into those associated with occupation and those associated with leisure-time. Most of the variance in NEAT between people is associated with differences in occupation. Here, data are most commonly expressed as PAL values. PAL is TEE/BEE and essentially represents a correction of TEE for body size.

PAL values vary substantially among individuals engaged in different occupations as shown in Table 21-3. To illustrate this point, consider a sedentary office worker with a daily TEE of 2,400 kcal/day, a BEE of 1,500 kcal/day, and a PAL of 1.6. If he or she were to change occupations to achieve a PAL of 2.4, say by now working in agriculture or construction, NEAT could be increased by 1,200 kcal/day. Therefore, occupation has a major influence on NEAT and TEE.

The energy expended in a variety of activities is shown in Figure 21-11 (Levine et al., 2000). Consider again the same office worker. Argue that he or she returns home from work, by car, at 5 PM. From then until bedtime at 11 PM the primary activity is to operate the television remote control in a semirecumbent position. For these 6 hours, the average energy expenditure above resting would approximate 8% and NEAT would be approximately 30 kcal for the evening [0.08 × 1,500 kcal^{BEE} × (6/24) hours]. Now imagine that he or she instead uses the evening time to paint a bedroom and weed the garden and also chooses to cycle home from work. The increase in energy expenditure would be equivalent to walking approximately 1 to 2 mph for the same period of leisure-time (5 to 11 PM). NEAT then increases by 750 to 1,125 kcal for the evening [2 or 3 × $1{,}500^{\text{BEE}}$ × (6/24) hours]. Thus, for this hypothetical office worker, the variance in leisure-time NEAT has the potential of affecting TEE by approximately 1,000 kcal/day.

Thus, from an egocentric perspective, there are profound environmental influences on NEAT

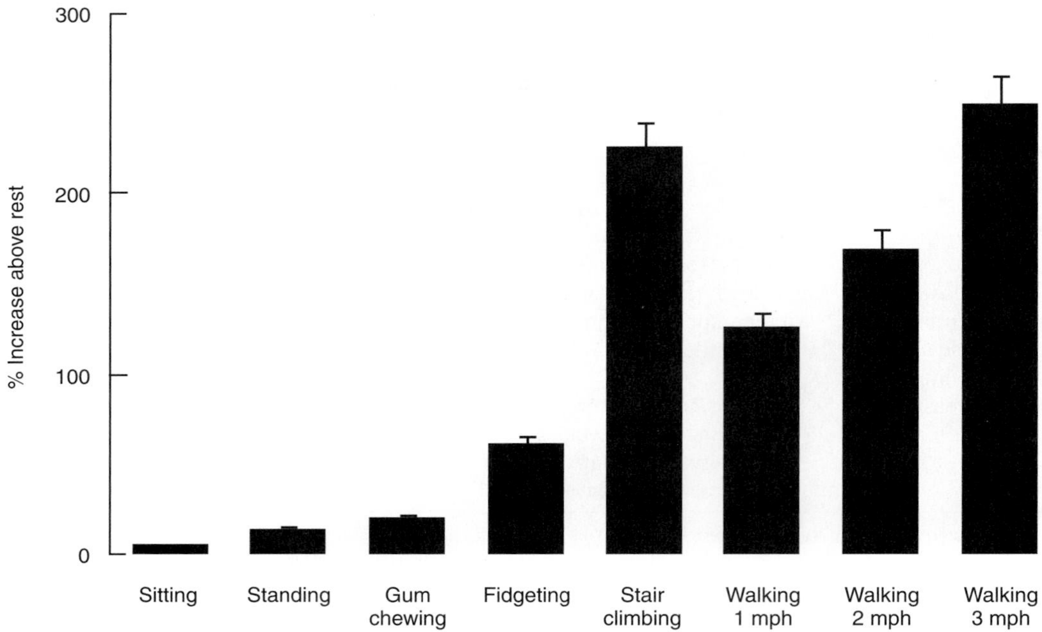

Figure 21-11 Energy expenditure above resting for a variety of activities.

that include occupational and leisure-time activities. The potential variance in NEAT is substantial and can vary for a given person by as much as 2,000 kcal/day. In fact several authors argue that a consistent energetic imbalance of only 100 kcal/day is sufficient to account for obesity (Hill et al., 2003; Lanningham-Foster et al., 2003; Garrow, 1986). Therefore, regulation of NEAT might be important in predisposition to fat gain and obesity.

A wide variety of geocentric environmental factors also impact NEAT (see Fig. 21-10). Sedentariness and a sedentary-promoting environment are pervasive features of the twenty-first century in high- and middle-income countries. The levels of physical activity have declined as individuals have moved from agricultural communities to urban environments and as industrialization has increased (Hill and Peters, 1998).

Sedentary cues are unmistakable in developed countries and often come through services designed to optimize convenience and throughput at the expense of locomotion. Examples include drive-through restaurants and banks, televisions, escalators, motorized walkways, and washing machines. Schools may be built beyond the walking-distance of the community served, suburbs may be built without sidewalks, city streets may be considered unsafe for leisure-time walking, and playgrounds may be considered unsafe spaces for children. A comparison between the energetic costs of mechanized tasks and the same tasks performed manually as would have occurred a century ago indicated that mechanization has decreased energy expenditure by approximately 110 kcal per day (Lanningham-Foster et al., 2003). This agrees well with Hill's estimate of 100 kcal per day as the cost of mechanization (Hill et al., 2003). It is worth noting also that sales of labor-saving devices track with obesity rates in the United States, whereas food intake data do not, as illustrated in Figure 21-12 (Lanningham-Foster et al., 2003). Urbanization and mechanization have dramatically impacted NEAT.

Although gender is biologically determined; there are gender-specific environmental cues that impact NEAT. Overall, adult men and women in the United States report similar levels of total physical activity (US Department of Health and Human Services [USDHHS], 1996; Caspersen and Merritt, 1995). In other

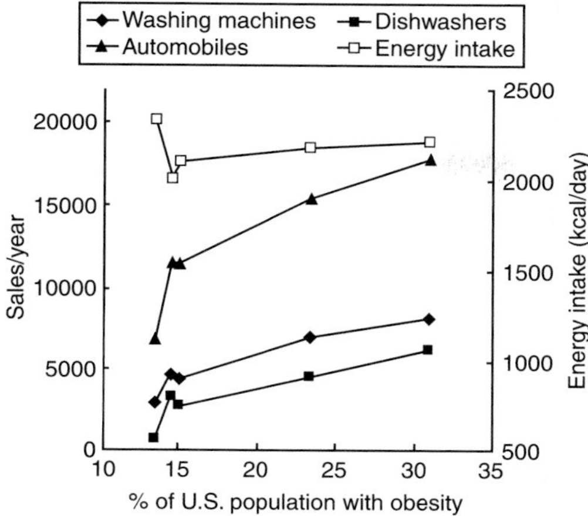

Figure 21-12 Sales of domestic machines and energy intake versus obesity rates for the U.S. population.

countries, such as Canada, England and Australia, men tend to be more active than women (Ford et al., 1991; Yeager et al., 1991). In children, there are consistent gender differences, with boys being more active than girls (Livingstone, 2000; Pratt et al., 1999). Gender may also influence physical activity in more subtle ways via societal and cultural expectations. Studies of daily activities of women living in rural areas of the Ivory Coast indicated that the total work burden of women was about 3 hours more per day that that of men in the same communities. These women had energy needs that were 30% greater than the World Health Organization/Food and Agriculture Organization standards suggest (Levine et al., 2001). There are likely to be environmental drives on NEAT that affect genders differently in many communities.

Groups with more education consistently report more leisure time physical activity than groups with less education. In the United States, high education groups are two to three times more likely to be active than low education groups (USDHHS, 1996; Caspersen and Merritt, 1995; Ford et al., 1991). In contrast, in low-income countries, where child labor is commonplace, poverty is predictive of greater child labor, and the most impoverished children have the highest NEAT levels (Levine et al., 2002; Grootaert, 1998).

Limited data are available regarding differences in NEAT during different seasons. Who volitionally walks to work in the rain? Data from Canada suggest wide differences in time spent in physical activity due to season. Time spent in activity was twice as high during the summer months compared to winter months (Katzmarzyk et al., 2001). Also, it is clear that occupation-associated NEAT is affected by season in agricultural communities where workloads vary cyclically (Pastore et al., 1993; Ferro-Luzzi et al., 1990; Singh et al., 1989).

Thus, a variety of geocentric environmental factors impact NEAT, although there are few data that quantify these effects or distinguish them from purposeful exercise. Regardless of these limitations, data strongly support the thesis that geocentric environmental factors promote sedentariness.

Biological Determinants of NEAT

Could NEAT be biologically regulated as well as environmentally influenced? Many important biological variables, such as appetite, are impacted by biological and environmental drives (de Castro, 2004). Several lines of evidence support the thesis that NEAT is biologically regulated. In humans, manipulation of energy balance is associated with changes in NEAT. With positive energy balance, NEAT increases. Moreover, the change in NEAT is predictive of fat gain (Fig. 21-13). Those who increase their NEAT in greatest measure in response to overfeeding gain the least fat, whereas those who do not increase their NEAT with overfeeding gain the most fat.

In humans, NEAT decreases substantially with profound negative energy balance (Dulloo, 2002). Data from a host of mammals suggest that the relationship between underfeeding and NEAT is complex. With negative energy balance, there is a short-term increase in physical activity that is regarded as a "foraging response" (Jones et al., 1990). With sustained negative energy balance, NEAT decreases as energy stores are depleted. This relationship appears to be consistent across biology from primates to rodents (Robin et al., 1998; Challet et al., 1997; Kemnitz et al., 1993; Masuda and Oishi, 1995; Jones et al., 1990; Mabry and Campbell, 1975). Interestingly, this foraging

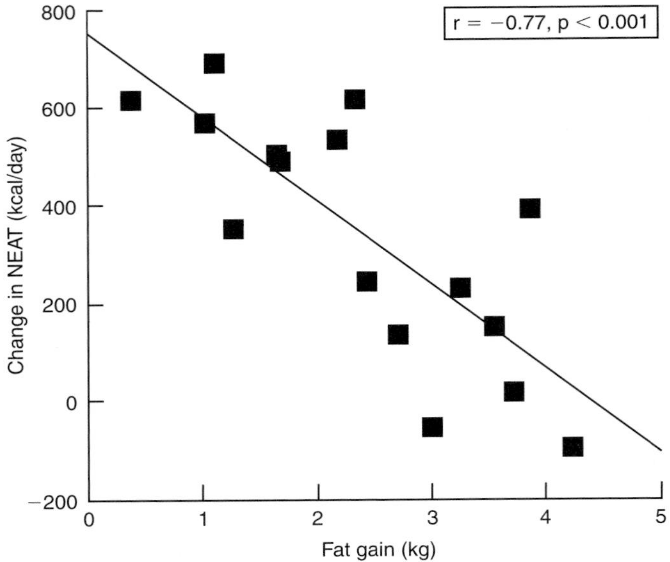

Figure 21-13 Changes in nonexercise activity thermogenesis (NEAT) with overfeeding. Healthy subjects (n = 16) were overfed by 1,000 kcal/day over baseline energy needs. Fat gain, on the *x* axis, was determined from dual x-ray absorptiometry. Change in NEAT was calculated from NEAT measured before and after overfeeding [NEAT = TEE − (BEE + TEF)]. *(Redrawn from Levine JA, Eberhardt NL, Jensen MD [1999] Role of nonexercise activity thermogenesis in resistance to fat gain in humans. Science 283:212-214.)*

response, which is normally potentiated by concurrent amphetamine administration, is blocked in rats following ablation of the mediobasal hypothalamus, suggesting that the hypothalamus plays a role in mediating this response (Mabry and Campbell, 1975). Furthermore, opioids, which interact with orexins, appear to be involved in the foraging response, as blockade of opioid receptors diminishes meal anticipatory locomotor activity (Thorburn and Proietto, 2000). Therefore, substantial evidence suggests that NEAT is biologically regulated and genetically determined (Thorburn and Proietto, 2000) and that NEAT is biologically or mechanistically impacted by shifts in energy balance.

How then might the relationship between fluxes in fuel availability and energy intake be linked to NEAT? There is good evidence that there is central regulation of NEAT. For example, orexin is a well-characterized protein that acts centrally in arousal and wakefulness. Orexin is well known to increase food intake, principally through activity on energy regulatory centers, including the rostral hypothalamus (Kotz et al., 2002). Orexin also increases NEAT when injected into this locus. However, when orexin is injected into the paraventricular nucleus there is an appetite-independent effect on NEAT, as illustrated in Figure 21-14 (Kiwaki et al., 2004). This supports the concepts that (1) there are central mediators of NEAT, (2) the NEAT circuit may interact with the appetite circuits, and (3) because the orexin–neuronally deplete mouse is obese (Hara et al., 2001) and because orexin-deficient narcoleptic humans may be overweight or obese (Kok et al., 2003; Dahmen et al., 2001), central mediation of NEAT might be important in obesity. It is, therefore, tenable that a hypothalamic integrator of NEAT exists.

There are other lines of indirect evidence that NEAT may be centrally modulated, and several loci in the central nervous system have been identified as mediating behaviors that influence NEAT (e.g., Cirulli et al., 2004). Humoral and peripheral signals are also likely to be important in NEAT. For example, thyroid hormone excess in animals increases NEAT (Levine et al., 2003), but its potential role in regulating NEAT in humans has not been defined. Leptin replacement in *Ob/Ob* mice is

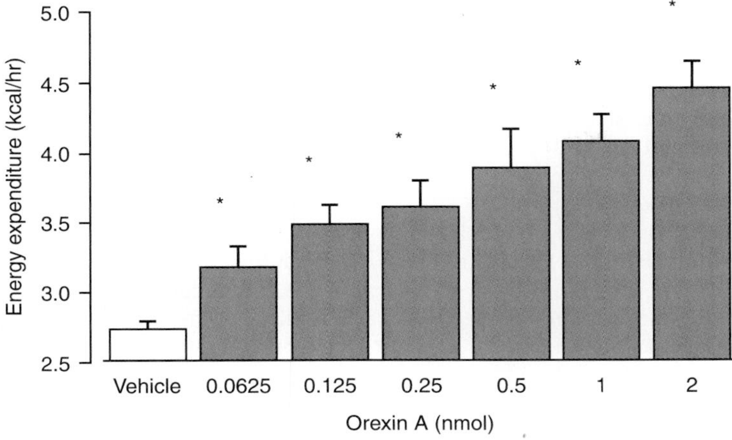

Figure 21-14 The effect of orexin on nonexercise activity thermogenesis (NEAT) when injected into the hypothalamic paraventricular nucleus of the rat. *(Redrawn from Kiwaki K, Kotz CM, Wang C, Lanningham-Foster L, Levine JA [2004] Orexin A (hypocretin 1) injected into hypothalamic paraventricular nucleus and spontaneous physical activity in rats. Am J Physiol Endocrinol Metab 286:E551-E559.)*

associated with increased physical activity (Pelleymounter et al., 1995). However, in human physiology, adipocyte leptin gene expression and blood levels track changes in adiposity but not changes in NEAT (Levine et al., 1999). The idea that the sympathetic nervous system may be involved in regulating NEAT is intriguing, but its role in human NEAT has not been defined (Ravussin and Tataranni, 1996). Therefore, humoral and peripheral signals may impact NEAT but their roles in NEAT regulation in humans have yet to be clarified.

We are learning more about the mechanism and regulation of human energy balance. As we do it is clear that energy expenditure is not simply passive heat loss associated with necessary mechanical inefficiency. In fact, energy expenditure, in particular NEAT, appears to be carefully modulated, and NEAT appears to play a crucial role in body weight regulation and in the genesis of obesity (Levine et al., 2005).

REFERENCES

Acheson KJ, Ravussin E, Wahren J, Jequier E (1984) Thermic effect of glucose in man, obligatory and facultative thermogenesis. J Clin Invest 74:1572-1580.

Adriaens MP, Schoffelen PF, Westerterp KR (2003) Intra-individual variation of basal metabolic rate and the influence of daily habitual physical activity before testing. Br J Nutr 90:419-423.

Argyropoulos G, Brown AM, Peterson R, Likes CE, Watson DK, Garvey WT (1998) Structure and organization of the human uncoupling protein 2 gene and identification of a common biallelic variant in Caucasian and African-American subjects. Diabetes 47:685-687.

Bell SC, Elborn JS, Nixon LE, Macdonald IA, Shale DJ (1999) Repeatability and methodology of resting energy expenditure in patients with cystic fibrosis. Respir Physiol 115:301-307.

Bielinski R, Schutz Y, Jequier E (1985) Energy metabolism during the postexercise recovery in man. Am J Clin Nutr 42:69-82.

Bogardus C, Lillioja S, Ravussin E, Abbott W, Zawadzki JK, Young A, Knowler WC, Jacobowitz R, Moll PP (1986) Familial dependence of the resting metabolic rate. N Engl J Med 315:96-100.

Bouchard C, Tremblay A, Nadeau A, Despres JP, Theriault G, Boulay MR, Lortie G, Leblanc C, Fournier G (1989) Genetic effect in resting and exercise metabolic rates. Metabolism 38:364-370.

Caspersen CJ, Merritt RK (1995) Physical activity trends among 26 states, 1986-1990. Med Sci Sports Exerc 27:713-720.

Challet E, Pevet P, Vivien-Roels B, Malan A (1997) Phase-advanced daily rhythms of melatonin, body temperature, and locomotor activity in food-restricted rats fed during daytime. J Biol Rhythms 12:65-79.

Cirulli F, Berry A, Chiarotti F, Alleva E (2004) Intrahippocampal administration of BDNF in adult rats affects short-term behavioral plasticity in the Morris water maze and performance in the elevated plus-maze. Hippocampus 14:802-807.

Coward WA (1998) Contributions of the doubly labeled water method to studies of energy balance in the Third World. Am J Clin Nutr 68:962S-969S.

Dahmen N, Bierbrauer J, Kasten M (2001) Increased prevalence of obesity in narcoleptic patients and relatives. Eur Arch Psychiatry Clin Neurosci 251:85-89.

D'Alessio DA, Kavle EC, Mozzoli MA, Smalley KJ, Polansky M, Kendrick ZV, Owen LR, Bushman MC, Boden G, Owen OE (1988) Thermic effect of food in lean and obese men. J Clin Invest 81:1781-1789.

Davis JR, Tagliaferro AR, Kertzer R, Gerardo T, Nichols J, Wheeler J (1983) Variations of dietary-induced thermogenesis and body fatness with aerobic capacity. Eur J Appl Physiol Occup Physiol 50:319-329.

de Castro JM (2004) Genes, the environment and the control of food intake. Br J Nutr 92: S59-S62.

Donahoo WT, Levine JA, Melanson EL (2004) Variability in energy expenditure and its components. Curr Opin Clin Nutr Metab Care 7:599-605.

Dulloo AG (2002) Biomedicine. A sympathetic defense against obesity. Science 297:780-781.

Dworatzek PD, Hegele RA, Wolever TM (2004) Postprandial lipemia in subjects with the threonine 54 variant of the fatty acid-binding protein 2 gene is dependent on the type of fat ingested. Am J Clin Nutr 79:1110-1117.

Elia M (2000) Hunger disease. Clin Nutr 19: 379-386.

Elia M (1992) Organ and tissue contribution to metabolic rate. In: Kinney JM, Tucker HN (eds) Energy Metabolism: Tissue Determinants and Cellular Corollaries. Raven Press Ltd., New York, pp 61-79.

Ferro-Luzzi A, Scaccini C, Taffese S, Aberra B, Demeke T (1990) Seasonal energy deficiency in Ethiopian rural women. Eur J Clin Nutr 44 Suppl 1:7-18.

Figueroa-Colon R, Franklin FA, Goran MI, Lee JY, Weinsier RL (1996) Reproducibility of measurement of resting energy expenditure in prepubertal girls. Am J Clin Nutr 64: 533-6.

Flatt JP (1985) Energetics of intermediary metabolism. In: Garrow JS, Halliday D (eds) Substrate and Energy Metabolism. John Libbey, London, pp 58-69.

Ford ES, Merritt RK, Heath GW, Powell KE, Washburn RA, Kriska A, Haile G (1991) Physical activity behaviors in lower and higher socioeconomic status populations. Am J Epidemiol 133:1246-1256.

Garrow JS (1986) Chronic effects of over- and under-nutrition on thermogenesis. Int J Vitam Nutr Res 56:201-204.

Gasic S, Schneider B, Waldhausl W (1997) Indirect calorimetry: variability of consecutive baseline determinations of carbohydrate and fat utilization from gas exchange measurements. Horm Metab Res 29:12-15.

Gibbons MR, Henry CJ, Ulijaszek SJ, Lightowler HJ (2004) Intra-individual variation in RMR in older people. Br J Nutr 91:485-489.

Granata GP, Brandon LJ (2002) The thermic effect of food and obesity: discrepant results and methodological variations. Nutr Rev 60:223-233.

Grootaert C (1998) Child labor in Cote d'Ivoire. The World Bank Social Development Department, Report No. 1905, Washington, DC.

Hara J, Beuckmann CT, Nambu T, Willie JT, Chemelli RM, Sinton CM, Sugiyama F, Yagami K, Goto K, Yanagisawa M, Sakurai T (2001) Genetic ablation of orexin neurons in mice results in narcolepsy, hypophagia, and obesity. Neuron 30:345-354.

Haugen HA, Melanson EL, Tran ZV, Kearney JT, Hill JO (2003) Variability of measured resting metabolic rate. Am J Clin Nutr 78:1141-1145.

Henry CJ, Lightowler HJ, Marchini J (2003) Intra-individual variation in resting metabolic rate during the menstrual cycle. Br J Nutr 89:811-817.

Hill JO, DiGirolamo M, Heymsfield SB (1985) Thermic effect of food after ingested versus tube-delivered meals. Am J Physiol 248: E370-E374.

Hill JO, Peters JC (1998) Environmental contributions to the obesity epidemic. Science 280:1371-4.

Hill JO, Wyatt HR, Reed GW, Peters JC (2003) Obesity and the environment: Where do we go from here? Science 299:853-855.

Jequier E, Schutz Y (1983) Long-term measurements of energy expenditure in humans using a respiration chamber. Am J Clin Nutr 38:989-998.

Jones LC, Bellingham WP, Ward LC (1990) Sex differences in voluntary locomotor activity of food-restricted and ad libitum-fed rats. Implications for the maintenance of a body weight set-point. Comp Biochem Physiol A 96:287-290.

Karst H, Steiniger J, Noack R, Steglich HD (1984) Diet-induced thermogenesis in man: thermic effects of single proteins, carbohydrates and fats depending on their energy amount. Ann Nutr Metab 28:245-252.

Katzmarzyk PT, Craig CL, Bouchard C (2001) Original article underweight, overweight and obesity: relationships with mortality in the 13-year follow-up of the Canada Fitness Survey. J Clin Epidemiol 54:916-920.

Kemnitz JW, Weindruch R, Roecker EB, Crawford K, Kaufman PL, Ershler WB (1993) Dietary restriction of adult male rhesus monkeys: design, methodology, and preliminary findings from the first year of study. J Gerontol 48: B17-B26.

Kinabo JL, Durnin JV (1990) Thermic effect of food in man: effect of meal composition, and energy content. Br J Nutr 64:37-44.

Kiwaki K, Kotz CM, Wang C, Lanningham-Foster L, Levine JA (2004) Orexin A (hypocretin 1) injected into hypothalamic paraventricular nucleus and spontaneous physical activity in rats. Am J Physiol Endocrinol Metab 286:E551-E559.

Kok SW, Overeem S, Visscher TL, Lammers GJ, Seidell JC, Pijl H, Meinders AE (2003)Hypocretin deficiency in narcoleptic humans is associated with abdominal obesity. Obes Res 11:1147-1154.

Kotz CM, Teske JA, Levine JA, Wang C (2002) Feeding and activity induced by orexin A in the lateral hypothalamus in rats. Regul Pept 104:27-32.

Kozak LP (2000) Genetic studies of brown adipocyte induction. J Nutr 130:3132S-3133S.

Lanningham-Foster L, Nysse LJ, Levine JA (2003) Labor saved, calories lost: the energetic impact of domestic labor-saving devices. Obes Res 11:1178-1181.

Leibel RL, Rosenbaum M, Hirsch J (1995) Changes in energy expenditure resulting from altered body weight. N Engl J Med 332:621-628.

Levine JA (2002) Non-exercise activity thermogenesis (NEAT). Best Pract Res Clin Endocrinol Metab 16:679-702.

Levine JA, Eberhardt NL, Jensen MD (1999) Leptin responses to overfeeding: relationship with body fat and nonexercise activity thermogenesis. J Clin Endocrinol Metab 84:2751-2754.

Levine JA, Lanningham-Foster LM, McCrady SK, Krizan AC, Olson LR, Kane PH, Jensen MD, Clark MM (2005) Interindividual variation in posture allocation: possible role in human obesity. Science 307:584-586.

Levine JA, Nygren J, Short KR, Nair KS (2003) Effect of hyperthyroidism on spontaneous physical activity and energy expenditure in rats. J Appl Physiol 94:165-170.

Levine JA, Schleusner SJ, Jensen MD (2000) Energy expenditure of nonexercise activity. Am J Clin Nutr 72:1451-1454.

Levine JA, Weisell R, Chevassus S, Martinez CD, Burlingame B (2002) Looking at child labor. Science 296:1025-1026.

Levine JA, Weisell R, Chevassus S, Martinez CD, Burlingame B, Coward WA (2001) The work burden of women. Science 294:812.

Livingstone B (2000) Epidemiology of childhood obesity in Europe. Eur J Pediatr 159:S14-S34.

Lucas AR, Beard CM, WM OF, Kurland LT (1988) Anorexia nervosa in Rochester, Minnesota: a 45-year study. Mayo Clin Proc 63:433-442.

Mabry PD, Campbell BA (1975) Potentiation of amphetamine-induced arousal by food deprivation: effect of hypothalamic lesions. Physiol Behav 14:85-88.

Marr JW, Heady JA (1986) Within- and between-person variation in dietary surveys: number of days needed to classify individuals. Hum Nutr Appl Nutr 40:347-364.

Masuda A, Oishi T (1995) Effects of restricted feeding on the light-induced body weight change and locomotor activity in the Djungarian hamster. Physiol Behav 58: 153-159.

McBride BW, Kelly JM (1990) Energy cost of absorption and metabolism in the ruminant gastrointestinal tract and liver: a review. J Anim Sci 68: 2997-3010.

Melanson KJ, Saltzman E, Vinken AG, Russell R, Roberts SB (1998) The effects of age on postprandial thermogenesis at four graded energetic challenges: findings in young and older women. J Gerontol A Biol Sci Med Sci 53:B409-B414.

Melanson KJ, Saltzman E, Russell R, Roberts SB (1996) Postabsorptive and postprandial energy expenditure and substrate oxidation do not change during the menstrual cycle in young women. J Nutr 126:2531-2538.

Merrill AL, Watt BK (1973) Energy values of foods ... basis and derivation. USDA Agriculture Handbook #74 (revised). US Department of Agriculture, Washington, DC.

Miles CW, Wong NP, Rumpler WV, Conway J (1993) Effect of circadian variation in energy expenditure, within-subject variation and weight reduction on thermic effect of food. Eur J Clin Nutr 47:274-284.

Morgan JB, York DA (1983) Thermic effect of feeding in relation to energy balance in elderly men. Ann Nutr Metab 27:71-77.

Murphy MP, Brand MD (1987) Variable stoichiometry of proton pumping by the mitochondrial respiratory chain. Nature 329:170-172.

Newsholme EA, Parry-Billings M (1992) Some evidence for the existence of substrate cycles and their utility in vivo. Biochem J 285(Pt 1): 340-341.

Pacy PJ, Webster J, Garrow JS (1986) Exercise and obesity. Sports Med 3:89-113.

Pastore G, Branca F, Demissie T, Ferro-Luzzi A (1993) Seasonal energy stress in an Ethiopian rural community: an analysis of the impact at the household level. Eur J Clin Nutr 47: 851-862.

Pelleymounter MA, Cullen MJ, Baker MB, Hecht R, Winters D, Boone T, Collins F (1995) Effects of the obese gene product on body weight regulation in ob/ob mice. Science 269:540-543.

Piers LS, Soares MJ, Makan T, Shetty PS (1992) Thermic effect of a meal. 1. Methodology and variation in normal young adults. Br J Nutr 67:165-175.

Poehlman ET, Melby CL, Badylak SF (1988) Resting metabolic rate and postprandial thermogenesis in highly trained and untrained males. Am J Clin Nutr 47:793-798.

Powanda MC, Beisel WR (2003) Metabolic effects of infection on protein and energy status. J Nutr 133:322S-327S.

Pratt M, Macera CA, Blanton C (1999) Levels of physical activity and inactivity in children and adults in the United States: current evidence and research issues. Med Sci Sports Exerc 31:S526-S533.

Ravussin E, Tataranni PA (1996)The role of altered sympathetic nervous system activity in the pathogenesis of obesity. Proceedings of the Nutrition Society 55:793-802

Reed GW, Hill JO (1996) Measuring the thermic effect of food. Am J Clin Nutr 63:164-169.

Robin JP, Boucontet L, Chillet P, Groscolas R (1998) Behavioral changes in fasting emperor penguins: evidence for a “refeeding signal” linked to a metabolic shift. Am J Physiol 274:R746-R753.

Romijn JA, Coyle EF, Sidossis LS, Rosenblatt J, Wolfe RR (2000) Substrate metabolism during different exercise intensities in endurance-trained women. J Appl Physiol 88:1707-1714.

Schoeller DA, Leitch CA, Brown C (1986) Doubly labeled water method: in vivo oxygen and hydrogen isotope fractionation. Am J Physiol 251:R1137-1143.

Segal KR, Edano A, Blando L, Pi-Sunyer FX (1990) Comparison of thermic effects of constant and relative caloric loads in lean and obese men. Am J Clin Nutr 51:14-21.

Singh J, Prentice AM, Diaz E, Coward WA, Ashford J, Sawyer M, Whitehead RG (1989) Energy expenditure of Gambian women during peak agricultural activity measured by the doubly-labelled water method. Br J Nutr 62:315-329.

Solomon SJ, Kurzer MS, Calloway DH (1982) Menstrual cycle and basal metabolic rate in women. Am J Clin Nutr 36:611-616.

Thorburn AW, Proietto J (2000) Biological determinants of spontaneous physical activity. Obes Rev 1:87-94.

Turley KR, McBride PJ, Wilmore JH (1993) Resting metabolic rate measured after subjects spent the night at home vs at a clinic. Am J Clin Nutr 58:141-144.

US Department of Health and Human Services (1996) Physical activity and health: A report of the Surgeon General. Atlanta, Georgia: US Department of Health and Human Services, Public Health Service, and CDC, National Center for Chronic Disease Prevention and Health Promotion, Washington, DC/Atlanta.

van Marken Lichtenbelt WD, Daanen HA (2003) Cold-induced metabolism. Curr Opin Clin Nutr Metab Care 6:469-475.

Vidal-Puig A, Solanes G, Grujic D, Flier JS, Lowell BB (1997) UCP3: an uncoupling protein homologue expressed preferentially and abundantly in skeletal muscle and brown adipose tissue. Biochem Biophys Res Commun 235:79-82.

Walston J, Andersen RE, Seibert M, Hilfiker H, Beamer B, Blumenthal J, Poehlman ET (2003) Arg64 beta3-adrenoceptor variant and the components of energy expenditure. Obes Res 11:509-511.

Westerterp-Plantenga MS, van Marken Lichtenbelt WD, Strobbe H, Schrauwen P (2002) Energy metabolism in humans at a lowered ambient temperature. Eur J Clin Nutr 56:288-296.

Weststrate JA (1993) Resting metabolic rate and diet-induced thermogenesis: a methodological reappraisal. Am J Clin Nutr 58:592-601.

Wolfe RR, George S (1993) Stable isotopic tracers as metabolic probes in exercise. Exerc Sport Sci Rev 21:1-31.

Yeager KK, Macera CA, Eaker E, Merritt RK (1991) Time trends in leisure-time physical activity: another perspective. Epidemiology 2:313-316.

Zurlo F, Schutz Y, Frascarolo P, Enzi G, Deriaz O, Jequier E (1986) Variability of resting energy expenditure in healthy volunteers during fasting and continuous enteral feeding. Crit Care Med 14(6):535-538.

RECOMMENDED READINGS

Bray G (1987) Overweight is risking fate: Definition, classification, prevalence, and risks. Ann NY Acad Sci 499:14-28.

Flatt JP (1985) Energetics of intermediary metabolism. In: Garrow JS, Halliday D (eds) Substrate and Energy Metabolism, John Libbey, London, pp 58-69.

Jequier E, Schutz Y (1988) Energy expenditure in obesity and diabetes. Diabetes Metab Rev 4:583-593.

Levine JA, Eberhardt NL, Jensen MD (1999) Role of nonexercise activity thermogenesis in resistance to fat gain in humans. Science 283:212-214.

Levine JA, Lanningham-Foster LM, McCrady SK, Krizan AC, Olson LR, Kane PH, Jensen MD, Clark MM. (2005) Interindividual variation in posture allocation: possible role in human obesity. Science 307:584-586.

Ravussin E, Bogardus C (1989) Relationship of genetics, age, and physical fitness to daily energy expenditure and fuel utilization. Am J Clin Nutr 49:968-975.

Chapter 22

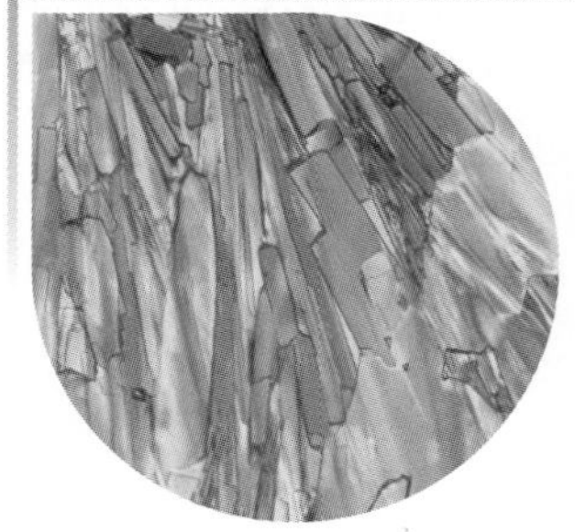

Control of Energy Balance

John C. Peters, PhD

OUTLINE

COMMON ABBREVIATIONS

EEPA	energy expenditure of physical activity
FFM	fat-free mass
RMR	resting metabolic rate
TEE	total energy expenditure
TEF	thermic effect of food

BASIC CONCEPTS

A typical adult human who consumes 2,500 kcal/day will ingest nearly 1 million kcal of energy in a single year. This energy is used to fuel obligatory metabolic processes (internal work) and to provide fuel for physical activity (external work). For an individual to maintain energy balance, therefore, the 1 million kcal ingested must be balanced by equivalent energy expenditure. Failure to achieve energy balance results in either an increase or decrease in body energy stores.

Given the widespread occurrence of obesity in developed countries, it might seem that the

This chapter is a revision of the chapter contributed by John C. Peters, PhD, Adamandia D. Kriketos, PhD, and James O. Hill, PhD, for the first edition.

precision of whatever system is operating to maintain energy balance is rather poor. On the contrary, even accounting for the prevalence of obesity, the precision is quite remarkable. A positive error of only 1% (considered respectable for most mechanical devices), 10,000 kcal/year, would represent the equivalent of 2.8 pounds of body fat. In fact, recent data indicate that the median weight gain in the adult population in the United States is 1.8 pounds per year (Hill et al., 2003). Therefore, the inherent error in the energy balance system is considerably less than 1%, and it is even smaller for those who gain less weight than average. Despite this relative precision, over a 10- to 20-year period this small error for the average person would lead to a weight gain of 18 to 36 pounds, which is enough to account for the "middle-age spread" that occurs in most adults.

How does the body balance energy intake and energy expenditure so precisely? Is energy balance itself controlled, or is the precision of energy balance a byproduct of precise control of something else? In this chapter, basic concepts of energy and nutrient balance are described and what is known about control of energy intake and expenditure and the way in which the two interact to influence energy balance is reviewed.

ENERGY BALANCE

Energy balance, by definition, is a condition in which energy intake and energy expenditure are equivalent over the time-period of observation. When energy intake exceeds energy expenditure, energy balance is positive and net body energy gain occurs. Conversely, when energy expenditure exceeds energy intake, negative energy balance occurs and net body energy is lost.

The Energy Balance Equation

Change in body energy stores
= Energy intake – Energy expenditure

Total body energy stores are substantial (Table 22-1). When an individual is at energy balance, these stores remain stable. Energy to fuel resting metabolism and everyday activity is provided by energy-yielding nutrients in food. Short-term energy needs (e.g., between meals) are met by utilization of liver and muscle glycogen reserves and some fat. Glycogen reserves and energy-yielding substrates in the circulation represent a very small storage depot and normally are exhausted within 24 hours during a fast. During prolonged fasting or during energy restriction for weight loss, significant protein is also degraded and used for energy in addition to substantial fat utilization. Although most of the triacylglycerol stored in adipose tissue is available to the body during a prolonged fast, not all energy contained in body protein is available for use as fuel. Body proteins serve important structural and functional purposes and, therefore, cannot be depleted without affecting survival of the organism.

The magnitude of change in body energy that occurs when there is an imbalance between energy intake and expenditure, of course, depends on the magnitude of the daily imbalance and the length of time over which the energy imbalance occurs. Because total daily energy needs in most individuals range between 1,500 and 3,000 kcal and because of the large size of body energy reserves,

Table 22-1
Energy Stores in a 30-kg Child and a 70-kg Adult Man

		30-kg Child*		70-kg Adult Man†	
Energy Form	**Storage Site**	**kg**	**kcal**	**kg**	**kcal**
Triglyceride	Adipose tissue	4.5	31,500	15	115,000
Protein	Muscle	1.5	6,250	6	25,000
Glycogen	Liver and muscle	0.13	500	0.35	1,400
Glucose or lipid	Body fluids	0.011	40	0.025	100

*Data from Rosenbaum M, Leibel RL (1988) Pathophysiology of childhood obesity. Adv Pediatr 35:73-137.
†Data from Cahill GF (1970) Starvation in man. N Engl J Med 282:668-675; and Frayn K (1996) Metabolic Regulation: A Human Perspective. Portland Press, London, pp 78-102.

short-term imbalances such as occur from meal to meal or from day to day would not be expected to lead to significant changes in body energy stores (body weight). Sustained imbalances that occur over several days, weeks, or months, however, can lead to substantial changes in body energy reserves and, hence, changes in body weight.

Gain or loss of significant amounts of body energy may, in turn, affect other components of the energy balance equation. Weight gain or loss is associated with gain or loss of active metabolic tissue mass, which itself results in an increase or decrease in total energy expenditure. Likewise, alterations in body mass usually affect energy intake, because food intake normally is proportional to energy expenditure. Therefore, when a prolonged imbalance occurs between energy intake (E_{in}) and energy expenditure (E_{out}), the resulting change in body energy (and body weight) is not a linear function of the energy excess or deficit, but depends on the composition of the tissue mass lost or gained and the effects of those specific changes on energy expenditure and energy intake.

NUTRIENT BALANCE

In a practical sense, people do not eat pure energy; they eat nutrients in the form of food and the nutrients are oxidized by the body to provide energy. The predominant energy-yielding nutrients in the human diet are the macronutrients: protein, carbohydrate, and fat. Alcohol, if ingested, is also a source of energy. Because there is little net conversion of either protein or carbohydrate into fat under most typical dietary conditions, achieving balance between energy intake and energy expenditure in an adult really requires achieving balance of each macronutrient (Flatt and Tremblay, 2004; Flatt, 1995). Nutrient and energy balance in the adult occurs when the intake of protein, carbohydrate, and fat (and alcohol) is equivalent to the body's oxidation of each.

When energy and nutrient balance are achieved, the following result:

- Protein intake = Protein oxidized
- Carbohydrate intake = Carbohydrate oxidized
- Fat intake = Fat oxidized
- Alcohol intake = Alcohol oxidized

If one of these energy-yielding nutrients is consumed in excess of the amount of that nutrient oxidized by the body in the short term, the excess is stored. As discussed in subsequent text of this chapter, the body appears to have metabolic priorities that dictate how much of a given nutrient is oxidized versus stored and the form in which the excess energy is stored. The form (i.e., glycogen or fat) in which the excess energy is stored in the short term, such as after a meal, can have an important influence on the long-term fate of that excess energy, which ultimately influences body weight and body composition.

IS ENERGY BALANCE OR NUTRIENT BALANCE REGULATED?

Body weight and body composition remain quite stable over long periods (years) in most individuals. This might suggest that body weight, body composition, or perhaps energy balance itself, is regulated, much like other homeostatic systems in biology, such as the regulation of blood glucose concentration. Indeed, research advances over the last decade have made it clear that a physiological system exists to maintain body energy homeostasis in response to variations in the supply of food energy and inconsistent patterns of energy expenditure.

Body Weight as a Set-Point

It has long been recognized that humans tend to maintain stable body weight over long periods, and they defend this weight against conditions that would otherwise promote weight gain or weight loss (Leibel et al., 1995). So, for example, when human subjects are overfed to force weight gain, upon cessation of overfeeding, they spontaneously lose weight and return toward the starting condition, although in many individuals the weight loss is not sufficient to return them to their exact starting point (Bouchard et al., 1996). Likewise, when individuals are subjected to a weight-reducing regimen for a prolonged period, they lose weight but rapidly regain lost body energy when the condition of negative energy balance is relieved (Sims and Horton, 1968).

These observations in humans have been the supportive basis for the concept of a body-weight "set-point," such that the energy balance system in an individual is programmed to defend a particular body weight. Studies in experimental animals have also provided strong evidence of a physiological mechanism that defends a particular body weight under a variety of conditions of energy deficit or energy surfeit (Keesey and Corbett, 1984). Numerous studies have shown that in order to alter this apparent body weight set-point under a given set of conditions, a change in the fundamental central nervous system mechanisms regulating food intake and energy expenditure is required (Keesey and Corbett, 1984; Stellar, 1954). For example, early studies in experimental animals showed that destruction of the ventromedial hypothalamus in the brain, the so-called satiety center, caused animals to overeat and reach a new higher body weight, which the animal then defended (i.e., a new set-point). Alternatively, destruction of the lateral hypothalamus, the so-called feeding center, resulted in reduced food intake, weight loss, and a new lower body weight or set-point that was defended. More recent studies have refined our understanding of the brain mechanisms affecting energy balance, and a number of specific hypothalamic brain structures and signaling systems that control different elements of energy intake, expenditure, and storage have been identified. These will be discussed in more detail later in this chapter.

Although the body defends body weight in response to challenges that either decrease or increase energy stores, this defense appears to be asymmetrical. The relative strength of the body's defense against a gain in body energy stores appears to be much weaker than that protecting against energy deficit (Schwartz et al., 2003), meaning that the physiological system controlling energy balance is biased toward preservation of existing weight and, when possible, toward weight gain. This is borne out by years of clinical experience in treating obese human subjects. Treatment of obese subjects using a myriad of therapeutic strategies has shown that, although a high percentage of subjects can successfully achieve weight loss, approximately 90% to 95% regain the weight once they discontinue the weight-management program.

The bias in the energy balance control system toward promoting weight gain is also apparent in the growing prevalence of obesity among both adults and children. Today, roughly one third of the U.S. population is obese, up from 25% just a decade ago, and an additional one third of the population is overweight (Flegal and Troiano, 2000; Kuczmarski et al., 1994). The relatively weak defense against positive energy balance appears to exist whether the energy gain is provoked by increased energy intake, decreased physical activity, or both. In experimental overfeeding studies, it has been shown that the body has a limited capacity to burn off excess energy, and most of the excess is stored (Horton et al., 1995). Furthermore, in population studies, decreases in physical activity are strongly associated with increases in body weight and fat content (Lissner and Heitmann, 1995). Considering that humans evolved largely in a subsistence environment, it should not be surprising that there is a bias toward efficiently storing excess dietary energy and defending body energy. Indeed, in evolutionary terms, a biological defense against storing excess energy when it is available would not appear to confer a natural selection advantage.

Body Weight as a Settling Point

Body weight and body composition do not remain fixed throughout the adult life of most individuals, despite periods of many years during which relative constancy is achieved. The general increase in body weight and body fat that occurs in most adults between the ages of 30 and 60 years and the frequent increase in body weight that occurs in many women following pregnancy and childbirth are two common situations in which a new stable higher body weight is achieved and defended. A substantial change in either the internal (e.g., hormonal) or external (e.g., activity level) environment can produce a substantial change in the level of body weight defended.

In view of the available evidence, it seems appropriate to refer to a particular body weight and composition that an individual might temporarily defend as a settling point, rather than a set-point. This concept seems more accommodating than the term set-point because it

Nutrition Insight

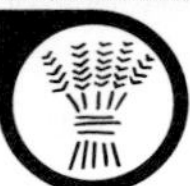

The Obesity Epidemic: Genetics Versus the Environment?

Over the last decade the prevalence of obesity (defined as a body mass index [BMI] ≥ 30) increased by nearly 40% from 23.3% in 1991 to 30.9% today (Flegal and Troiano, 2000). Among children, the increase was even more marked, rising by more than 50% such that 15% of children in the United States are now classified as obese (Ogden et al., 2002). It has long been recognized that obesity has strong genetic determinants, and several dozen candidate genes contributing to obesity have been identified (Barsh et al., 2000). However, the rise in the prevalence of obesity has happened too rapidly to be explained by changes in the gene pool within the population (Hill and Peters, 1998). A more likely explanation is that the individuals becoming obese possess some level of genetic susceptibility and that expression of these susceptibility genes is amplified in the obesity-promoting environment in which we live, causing phenotypic obesity (Hill and Peters, 2003).

The large variation in body weight within the population among people of similar age, sex, height, and socioeconomic status (a surrogate for some aspects of the environment) is direct evidence of the power of genetic influences on body weight. Close examination of the recent weight-gain trends for the population also highlights the power of genetic susceptibility. The figure below shows that the mean BMI of most U.S. adults in the lowest percentiles of body mass has not changed much over the last decade compared to the change of those individuals already at the upper range of BMI (Friedman, 2003). The disproportionate increase in the number of massively obese people in our commonly shared environment suggests that they may represent a subgroup that is particularly susceptible to obesity, whereas the people at the lowest BMIs in the population represent a subgroup whose genes confer some degree of obesity resistance. In any event, the steady increase in the mean body weight for the population highlights the strong push of the environment in promoting obesity. In effect, the environment is overwhelming the body-weight control system and is driving most individuals to gain some excess weight, with some gaining tremendous amounts of excess weight. This situation exemplifies the interaction between genes and the environment whereby the effects of high genetic susceptibility are amplified by a high-risk environment (Barsh et al., 2000).

takes into account that most people defend several different body weights over the course of a lifetime. These different settling points are determined by the different physiological, psychological, and environmental circumstances the individual may be experiencing during that period of life. For example, declining levels of physical activity, which in the United States are often associated with the transition from adolescence to adult life, encourage positive energy balance, weight gain, and a new, higher settling point (Hill et al., 2003; Hill and Peters, 1998).

The recent obesity epidemic exemplifies the power of environmental influences to increase the level at which body weight stability is reached and defended. Because the prevalence of obesity has risen so rapidly, the obesity epidemic cannot be explained by shifting genotypes and, hence, preprogrammed set-points within the population. Rather, changes in the food and physical activity environment acting on a background of genetic susceptibility have led to the high level of obesity seen in the population (Friedman, 2003; Peters et al., 2002). Regardless of whether the set-point or settling point construct seems more appealing, the existence of a physiological control system that defends body weight cannot be denied based on the available evidence.

Nutrition Insight

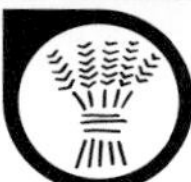

The Obesity Epidemic: Genetics Versus the Environment?—cont'd

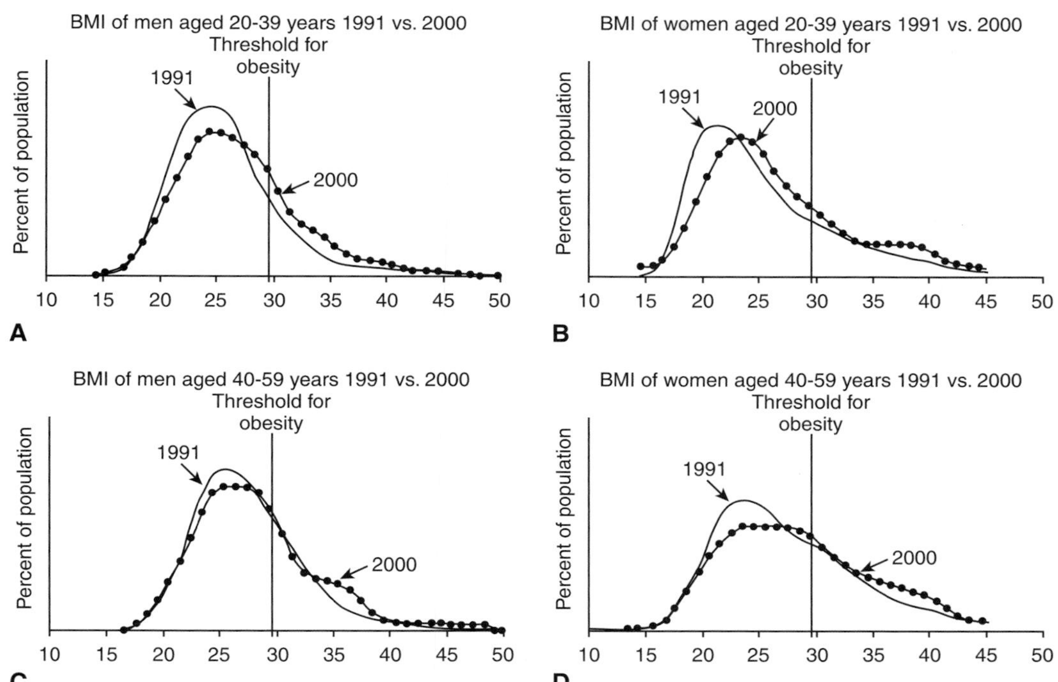

The smoothed distribution of BMI for men and women in the United States aged 20 to 39 years (**A** and **B**) and 40 to 59 years (**C** and **D**) is shown for the years 1991 and 2000. In both cases, the distributions have shifted to the right and become more skewed. For the 20-to-39 years age-group, the average BMI for males increased from 25.9 to 27.0, and the average BMI for females increased from 25.4 to 27.5. For the 40-to-59 years age-group, the average BMI for males increased from 27.5 to 28.3, and the average BMI for women increased from 27.6 to 29. In both cases, there was a marked increase in the number of individuals with a BMI greater than 30. At all ages, BMI is highly variable, with some individuals having a BMI greater than 45 and others having a BMI less than 20, a difference that in some cases corresponds to hundreds of pounds. *(Redrawn from Friedman JM [2003] A war on obesity, not the obese. Science 299:856-858.)*

CONTROL OF ENERGY INTAKE

Dietary energy is provided predominately by the macronutrients: protein, carbohydrate, and fat (and alcohol). Results from the first phase of the third National Health and Nutrition Examination Survey (McDowell et al., 1994) show that adult women and men consume, on average, between 1,500 and 3,000 kcal/day, depending on age and sex (Table 22-2). Of this total energy intake, the current typical American diet consists of approximately 15% of energy from protein, 49% from carbohydrate, and 34% from fat (see Table 22-2). An additional 2% of energy is consumed from alcohol. On a population basis, these values do not vary considerably as a function of age, sex, or ethnicity.

Energy intake is controlled by a complex system involving both behavioral and biological components. These components are interrelated in as much as food intake itself is a behavior and the biological components of

Table 22-2
Dietary Energy and Macronutrient Intakes in the United States

	Energy	Protein		Carbohydrate		Fat		Alcohol	
Sex and Age	kcal/day	g/day	% kcal	g/day	% kcal	g/day	% kcal	g/day	% kcal
FEMALES									
All ages	1,732	64	15.2	217	51.1	67	33.9	5	1.6
2-11 months	850	25	11.2	112	52.4	35	37.6	0	0.0
1-2 years	1,236	45	14.9	163	53.0	47	34.0	0	0.0
3-5 years	1,516	54	14.3	204	54.4	57	33.1	0	0.0
6-11 years	1,753	63	14.5	229	52.9	68	34.2	0	0.0
12-15 years	1,838	62	13.5	243	54.4	72	33.7	0	0.0
16-19 years	1,958	67	14.1	254	52.4	77	34.4	2	0.6
20-29 years	1,957	69	14.5	241	50.0	75	34.0	9	3.0
30-39 years	1,883	70	15.3	228	49.7	75	34.2	8	2.4
40-49 years	1,764	67	15.8	213	49.0	70	34.9	5	1.8
50-59 years	1,629	64	16.1	199	49.8	63	33.8	5	2.1
60-69 years	1,578	64	16.6	199	51.1	59	32.8	4	1.5
70-79 years	1,435	58	16.6	185	52.4	53	32.3	2	0.9
80 years+	1,329	52	15.9	179	54.5	47	31.3	1	0.6
MALES									
All ages	2,478	92	15.1	299	49.2	96	34.1	12	3.1
2-11 months	903	27	11.8	119	52.7	37	36.9	0	0.0
1-2 years	1,339	50	15.0	176	53.2	51	33.5	0	0.0
3-5 years	1,663	59	14.3	225	54.8	62	32.8	0	0.0
6-11 years	2,036	71	14.2	272	53.5	78	33.9	0	0.0
12-15 years	2,578	89	14.2	346	54.0	97	33.1	0	0.0
16-19 years	3,097	111	14.4	381	49.6	120	34.6	13	2.6
20-29 years	3,025	110	14.6	353	47.6	116	34.0	23	4.9
30-39 years	2,872	106	15.1	335	47.4	113	34.6	18	4.3
40-49 years	2,545	96	15.6	298	46.9	98	33.9	18	4.9
50-59 years	2,341	93	16.1	266	46.3	95	35.7	12	3.4
60-69 years	2,110	84	16.4	253	48.7	80	33.3	11	3.2
70-79 years	1,887	74	16.0	231	49.4	73	33.8	7	2.7
80 years+	1,776	69	16.0	225	51.2	67	33.3	4	1.5

Data from McDowell MA, Briefel RR, Alaimo K, Bischof AM, Caughman CR, Carroll MD, Loria CM, Johnson CL (1994) Energy and macronutrient intakes of persons ages 2 months and over in the United States: Third National Health and Nutrition Examination Survey, Phase 1, 1988-91. National Center for Health Statistics, Centers for Disease Control and Prevention, U.S. Department of Health and Human Services, Washington, DC, Publication No. 255.

the system must respond to, and indeed may be forced to adapt to, the consequences of this behavior. Ultimately, eating behavior involves the interaction and integration of genetics, neurobiology, metabolism, learning history, and the current context (e.g., physical, social, and emotional environment) in which eating is taking place.

BEHAVIORAL ASPECTS OF ENERGY INTAKE

Human eating behavior is a learned habitual behavior (Rodin, 1992). Food intake in any given circumstance is influenced by the learning history of the individual as it relates to that circumstance. Learning begins in early childhood, at which time the child develops food preferences through experience with different foods (Birch, 1999). Properties of the food itself (e.g., orosensory properties), energy content and density, as well as the social and cultural context in which the food is consumed, can be associated with the metabolic effects of the food to form the basis of a learned, conditioned response. This associative learning is important for controlling food and energy intake in a sociocultural environment in which food is typically eaten only at particular times. This is because there is a temporal separation between the orosensory stimulus and context in which food is eaten (which occur immediately) and the metabolic consequences of the food (which may take many hours to complete).

The taste (e.g., sweet, sour), energy density, and variety of foods offered to children have been found to shape children's food preferences (Birch, 1992). Infants and young children display an innate preference for the sweet taste (Drewnowski, 1997). In addition, studies in young children show that they will condition preferences for foods that are energy dense (Birch, 1999, 1992; Kern et al., 1993). Offering children a wide variety of foods to choose from increases the spectrum of foods they come to prefer. All of these factors appear to contribute to ensuring that the child consumes adequate energy and sufficient essential nutrients to support good growth and development. As the child grows older, learned food acceptance patterns and eating habits are continually reinforced and extended such that, by adulthood, there is a rich experiential background that affects eating behavior at any given meal.

At any given eating occasion, the amount and composition of food an individual consumes are affected by the immediate context of consumption superimposed on the underlying biology (i.e., mechanisms controlling food intake and energy balance) and the learning history. The cost of food acquisition, the variety of foods present, food packaging, serving size, the number of other people present, and the time of day are just a few of the factors that have been shown to affect short-term food intake and selection (Wansink, 2004; De Castro and De Castro, 1989; Rolls et al., 1981).

Much current research is focused on understanding the relative contribution of the modern food environment to the growing prevalence of obesity in both children and adults. Among the factors under investigation is the impact of portion size and food advertising on food selection and intake. Short-term food and energy intake is increased when there are many palatable foods from which to choose and when the food is served in large portions (Wansink, 2004). Likewise, aggressive advertising of high-calorie foods and increased participation in sedentary behaviors have been highlighted as environmental features that promote excessive eating, reduced energy expenditure, and, consequently, increased risk for excessive weight gain (Peters et al., 2002).

Beyond these immediate environmental and nutritional conditions, cognitive factors such as body awareness, self-image, and beliefs about particular foods can influence both short- and long-term food intake. The prevalence of eating disorders such as anorexia and bulimia nervosa among teenage girls is an example of how cognitive factors can override the biology and learning history, leading to inappropriate food and energy intake (Brownell and Fairburn, 1995).

BIOLOGICAL CONTROL OF ENERGY INTAKE

Underlying these complex behavioral elements are the biological mechanisms that control energy intake to meet energy needs. Control of energy intake is often viewed as part of a homeostatic system. In this homeostatic system, some aspect of body energy is the parameter considered to be maintained between some specified limits, and food intake and energy expenditure are considered as mechanisms for adding energy or removing energy from the body energy pool to maintain homeostasis (Bray and Tartaglia, 2000).

The homeostatic model assumes that what is being regulated is not energy intake per se, but rather body energy stores and potentially the distribution of energy within the various stores (e.g., glycogen or fat). Energy intake is controlled to maintain tissue energy stores, a scheme that also ensures that energy expenditure needs are met. The advantage of this system is that it does not rely on mechanisms that monitor short-term energy intake and expenditure, but it is more geared toward long-term integration of energy input and output and the net effect on body energy stores over time. Failure in the long-term to consume sufficient energy to meet energy expenditure needs would result in a change in tissue energy stores of the organism, which would in turn stimulate a response to restore energy stores.

The system that controls energy intake in relation to energy needs has several elements. It has a central controlling element, the brain, wherein all information about energy intake, expenditure, and adipose fuel stores is integrated and which directs a coordinated response to input stimuli. There are controlled systems for food ingestion, absorption, nutrient interconversion, metabolism, and storage. In addition, the system has both input (afferent) and output (efferent) signaling capabilities to and from the brain.

Afferent signals can be neural or humoral, and both serve as elements of a feedback loop that informs the brain about events in the periphery (e.g., sensory properties of available food or amount and composition of food eaten). Efferent signals are the output of the brain and are signals that drive motor function involved in food acquisition and ingestion, as well as signals that ensure that the appropriate hormonal environment exists to process incoming nutrients from the food ingested. These afferent and efferent signal pathways constitute the essential elements of a feedback scheme, conceptually similar to the functional elements of a common household heating system in which a temperature sensor is linked to a system that adjusts heat output in order to maintain temperature at a specified level.

Organization of the Systems Controlling Energy Balance

Control of energy balance is achieved through a coordinated system that involves central nervous system integration of short-term, meal-related afferent signals and long-term adiposity signals reflecting the content of body energy stores. These signaling pathways involve a variety of different neurotransmitter and neuropeptide systems. The central nervous system integration of these signals leads to efferent outputs that control a variety of systems affecting energy balance including appetite, energy expenditure and energy partitioning, reproduction, and growth (Fig. 22-1).

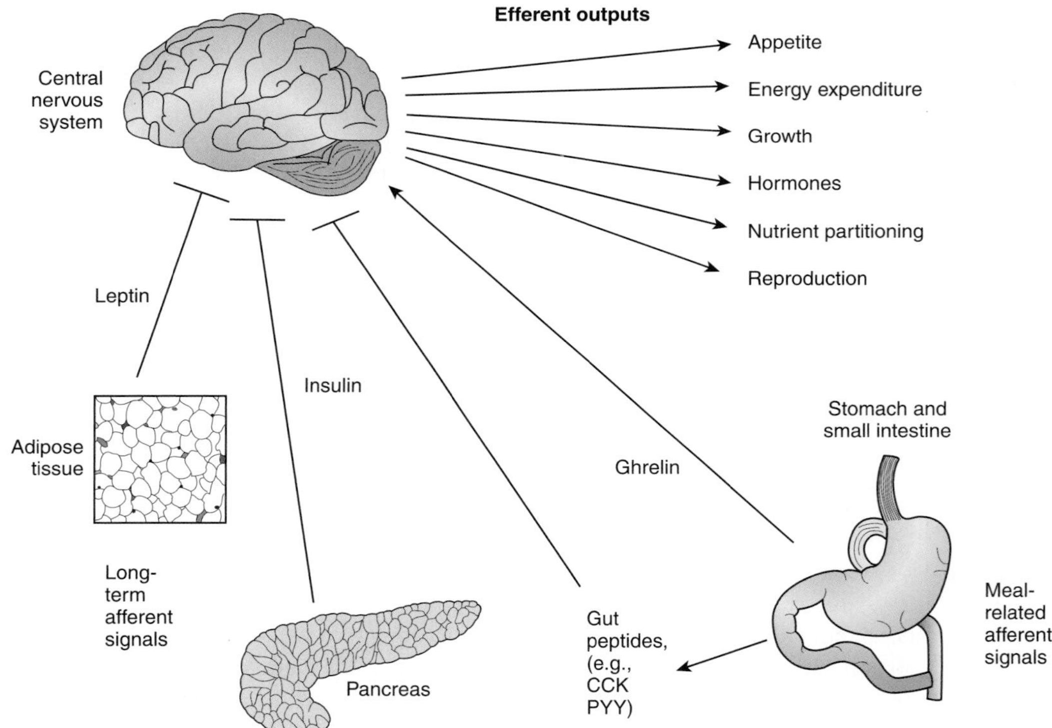

Figure 22-1 Organization of the systems controlling energy balance. Long-term adiposity signals, leptin and insulin, and meal-derived satiety signals act on brain mechanisms to inhibit food intake and increase energy expenditure. Ghrelin is the lone gut-derived peptide that stimulates feeding. Efferent brain outputs regulate a number of systems affecting energy homeostasis. *CCK*, Cholecystokinin; *PYY*, peptide YY. *(Modified from Flier JS [2004] Obesity wars: molecular progress confronts an expanding epidemic. Cell 116:337-350.)*

Meal-Related Afferent Signals

A variety of different meal-related signals have been identified; these signals serve to inform the brain about the quantity and quality of the food ingested. Signals derived from the absorbed nutrients themselves (e.g., glucose and amino acids) were some of the earliest suggested mechanisms by which the food consumed would inform the brain to influence control of appetite. The glucostatic (Mayer, 1953) and aminostatic (Mellinkoff, 1957) theories of food-intake control are based on the idea that either the blood or tissue concentration or rate of utilization of glucose or amino acids serves as a feedback signal to the brain to modulate food intake. Indeed, decades after the glucostatic theory was proposed, neurons in the hypothalamus have been shown to be sensitive to both high and low levels of glucose (Dunn-Meynell et al., 2002). Specific brain regions have been identified that sense amino acids (Blevins et al., 2004), and neurons in the hypothalamus involved in regulating food intake have been shown to sense fatty acids (Obici et al., 2002).

Gut Signals Affecting Energy Balance

When food comes into contact with the gastrointestinal (GI) tract, both mechanical and chemical signals are generated that influence food intake. Stretch receptors in the stomach signal the brain via neural pathways about meal size, while a variety of other signaling molecules play roles in meal initiation and termination (Kaplan and Moran, 2004; Woods, 2004). These signals are transmitted from the GI tract via the vagus nerve and other sympathetic nervous system afferents to the brainstem, where neurons of the nucleus of the solitary tract (NTS) integrate sensory information from the mouth, GI tract, and abdominal organs. Integrated output from the NTS is forwarded to hypothalamic brain centers where it is integrated with other signals relevant to long-term energy homeostasis (Schwartz et al., 2000).

Many of the meal-related signals originating in the GI tract are due to synthesis of a number of different gut peptides that have specific actions on brain centers involved in regulating energy balance (Box 22-1). Most of the peptides secreted by the GI tract are also synthesized in the brain (Woods, 2004). GI-derived signals act within the NTS primarily to reduce meal size and lengthen the inter-meal interval; their net effect is to act as a brake on eating. Most of the peptides listed reduce meal size and, therefore, are considered "satiety" peptides. It is important to note that these signals are neither generated individually nor do they act in isolation, but rather they are secreted in concert in response to meals in varying amounts that reflect the complex characteristics of the meal as well as the underlying state of energy balance of the organism (Woods, 2004).

Providing a complete overview of the numerous GI peptides and their specific functions is beyond the scope of this chapter. Brief descriptions of the actions of a few of these peptides are provided as examples of the kinds of roles played by these important signal molecules in the system controlling energy balance.

Among the gut peptides so far identified, ghrelin is unique in that it stimulates food intake (Cummings and Schwartz, 2003). This peptide may be involved in meal initiation, since ghrelin levels increase just prior to spontaneous eating

Box 22-1

GUT PEPTIDES THAT AFFECT FOOD INTAKE

Gut Peptides That Reduce Meal Size

Cholecystokinin (CCK)
Bombesin family (BBS, GRP, NMB)
Glucagon
Glucagon-like peptide 1, Glucagon-like peptide 2
Amylin
Somatostatin
Enterostatin
Apolipoprotein A-IV
Gastric inhibitory polypeptide (GIP)

Gut Peptide That Increases Meal Size

Ghrelin

Data from Woods SC (2004) Metabolic signals in the control of food intake. In: Stricker E, Woods SC (eds) Neurobiology of Food and Fluid Intake, 2nd ed. Vol. 14 of Handbook of Behavioral Neurobiology. Kluwer Academic/Plenum Publishers, New York, pp 241-272.

in animals (Cummings et al., 2001). In humans it appears that the decline in ghrelin levels that occurs following gastric bypass surgery in obese subjects may be, in part, responsible for the associated decline in appetite reported by these individuals (Cummings et al., 2002).

Cholecystokinin (CCK) is perhaps the best-studied of the so-called satiety peptides. CCK is released by the intestine into the circulation in response to certain amino acids and fatty acids in ingested food. It binds to receptors on peripheral vagal afferents, which send signals to the hindbrain to restrain meal size (Moran, 2000). Other key satiety peptides released after meal ingestion include gastric inhibitory polypeptide (GIP), glucagon-like peptide 1 (GLP-1) and peptide YY (PYY). For example, PYY is secreted into the circulation by the intestine in relation to meal size and binds to receptors in the brain to trigger a reduction in food intake. Postprandial levels of PYY appear to be reduced in obese individuals, and restoration of normal PYY levels in obese subjects reduces appetite.

GLP-1 is released in both gut and brain following meal ingestion, and it acts to reduce appetite as well as to stimulate the sympathetic nervous system (which increases energy expenditure) (Yamamoto et al., 2002). GIP is released from the duodenum, mainly in response to dietary fat ingestion. Animals deficient in the GIP receptor are resistant to obesity induced by high fat diets; therefore, this system may help mediate the obesity-promoting effects of diets high in fat (Miyawaki et al., 2002).

Long-Term Adiposity Signals

The concept that regulation of food intake may be tied to the size of the fat mass was first introduced by Kennedy (1953) several decades ago. It is only over the last 10 years that the nature of the signals that provide a link between the status of body fat depots and the brain, as well as the role of this system in controlling energy balance, has been elucidated.

Leptin and insulin are two key signals that inform the brain about the presence of excess metabolic fuel as well as the size of adipose fat stores (Campfield et al., 2004). Leptin, the protein product of the leptin or *ob* gene, is synthesized and secreted by adipose tissue in direct proportion to the size of fat stores (Flier, 1997). Animals lacking the *ob* gene display spontaneous obesity. Systemic or intracerebroventricular injection of leptin into genetically obese mice reduces food intake and increases energy expenditure, thereby resulting in reduction of body fat. Extremely high doses of leptin also reduce food intake in nonobese animals. Leptin exerts its effect on food intake and energy expenditure by binding to a specific leptin receptor present in brain and many other tissues (Tartaglia, 1997).

Circulating leptin concentrations and the protein itself are not abnormal in obese individuals, suggesting that any involvement in disordered energy balance (e.g., obesity) might involve decreased transport of leptin into the brain from the circulation or reduced sensitivity of the leptin receptor (Flier, 2004). Although a complete understanding of leptin's role in the control of energy homeostasis in humans is still emerging, from an evolutionary perspective the main function of leptin may be to signal the brain whether body fat stores are sufficient to support growth and reproduction (Takeda et al., 2003; Chehab et al., 1997; Rosenbaum et al., 1997).

Insulin, a hormone secreted by the β cells of the pancreas, regulates the disposition of metabolic fuels. Insulin is responsible for the profound metabolic shift between the fed and fasting states. Like leptin, circulating insulin levels reflect the energy state of the animal, falling in starvation and rising with increasing adiposity (Woods, 2004). Insulin is also transported into the brain and binds to a receptor (Woods, 2004). Large doses of insulin injected into the brain suppress food intake, and animals lacking the insulin receptor in brain become obese (Woods, 2004). There appears to be an interaction between insulin and leptin actions in brain, as animals with a mutated leptin receptor display a blunted action to insulin administered to the brain.

Leptin and insulin act in concert to affect brain centers that regulate energy balance. When adiposity is reduced (e.g., during weight loss), a drop in the circulating levels of leptin and insulin activate brain pathways that stimulate food intake and reduce energy expenditure. Conversely, these signals (circulating levels of leptin and insulin) are increased under conditions of positive energy balance, resulting in suppression of food intake and increased energy expenditure. Integration of adipose signals and meal-derived satiety signals occurs within specific neural circuits in the brain, the net effect being that adiposity signals increase or decrease the sensitivity of the brain to satiety signals. In this manner, the brain is constantly able to adjust food intake and energy expenditure based on signals reflecting short-term changes in energy status (satiety signals) and long-term alterations in energy stores (adiposity signals) (see Fig. 22-1). The integrated output of the brain centers receiving these inputs determines the nature and intensity of the efferent responses. These include efferent pathways determining hunger and food-seeking behaviors, the level of resting and activity-associated energy expenditure, and a variety of other neural and hormonal mechanisms involved in regulating growth and reproduction and energy partitioning within the body.

Central Nervous System Integration of Satiety and Adiposity Signals

Specialized centers within the brain integrate the various inputs encoding information about short-term and long-term energy utilization and stores, and coordinate efferent responses that serve to ensure there are sufficient energy stores for survival and reproduction. The hindbrain and hypothalamus are key structures involved in the control of food and energy intake (Berthoud, 2004; Stellar, 1954). Processing of meal-derived satiety signals occurs primarily within the NTS, a collection of neurons that integrate sensory information from the abdominal organs and GI tract and taste information from the mouth (Schwartz et al., 2000). Information from these various locations is communicated to the NTS by way of afferent fibers, predominately by the vagus nerve and spinal nerves carrying signals from the upper GI tract.

Early animal studies demonstrated that the ventromedial hypothalamus (VMH) is involved in suppression of feeding. More recently, the paraventricular nucleus (PVN), located within the VMH, has been identified as a key anatomic structure involved in processing both short-term and long-term satiety signals (Levine and Billington, 1997; Schwartz and Seeley, 1997). Conversely, the lateral hypothalamus (LH) is the brain center involved in stimulation of feeding. Damage or ablation of the VMH results in overeating and body weight gain, whereas destruction of the LH results in reduced food intake and body weight loss (Grossman, 1975).

One of the primary locations involved in interpreting long-term adiposity signals is in neurons of the arcuate nucleus within the hypothalamus. These neurons contain receptors for both insulin and leptin. Within this region of the hypothalamus are two subpopulations of neurons involved in energy homeostasis. The first of these neuron types is sensitive to negative energy balance (e.g., calorie restriction) and secretes neuropeptide Y (NPY) and agouti-related protein (AgRP) when activated. These peptides act within an adjacent brain region, the PVN, to stimulate food intake and reduce energy expenditure, and these effects are likely responsible for the hyperhpagia that occurs in response to body fat loss.

A second neuronal cell type opposes the actions of NPY neurons. These neurons synthesize and secrete melanocortins, which are peptides cleaved from a precursor molecule called proopiomelanocortin (POMC), as well as another peptide called cocaine-amphetamine–related transcript (CART). Therefore, these neuronal cells are called POMC or POMC/CART neurons. The net effect of activation of these POMC neurons is an increase in expression of α-melanocyte stimulating hormone (α-MSH), which acts to decrease food intake via activation of the melanocortin pathway, the major neural circuit inhibiting food intake (Seeley et al., 2004; Fan et al., 1997). The reciprocal regulation of the activity of these two types of neurons under conditions of energy surfeit or energy deficit is depicted in Figure 22-2. One of the remarkable aspects of this regulatory system is that when either NPY or POMC neurons are activated, they have dual actions that serve to amplify the strength of the signal-altering feeding behavior. For example, a decrease in fat mass reduces both leptin and insulin and activates NPY/AgRP neurons that stimulate feeding and simultaneously act to block α-MSH binding to melanocortin receptors, relieving inhibition of food intake (see Fig. 22-2, *A*). The net effect is to dramatically amplify the signal to eat.

Although integration of satiety information with long-term adiposity signals probably involves multiple brain areas, at least one key interconnection is between the NTS in the hindbrain, which receives and integrates satiety signals from the gut, and the PVN of the hypothalamus in the forebrain, which receives signals reflecting adipose stores. This integration is evidenced by the observation that both insulin and leptin (acting in the PVN) increase the satiating effect of CCK (which acts in the NTS).

Other Neuromodulators Involved in Energy Balance

It has long been recognized that the monoamine neurotransmitters, serotonin (5-hydroxytryptamine [5-HT]), norepinephrine (NE), and dopamine (DA) are involved in central nervous system control of feeding behavior. The monoamines are widely distributed throughout the central nervous system and act to enhance or diminish transmission via many pathways, affecting a variety of behaviors, including appetite and mood. For example, increased 5-HT neurotransmission appears to enhance the sensitivity of brain centers to the action of satiety peptides, whereas dopaminergic pathways appear to mediate some of the reward aspects of feeding (Liebowitz and Hoebel, 2004).

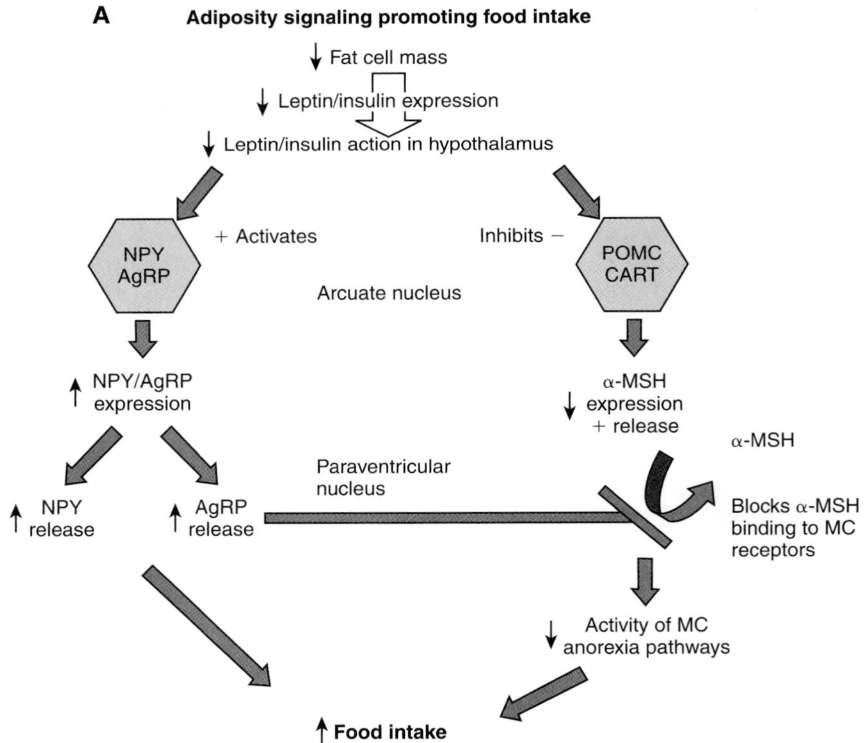

Figure 22-2 Central nervous system (*CNS*) adiposity signaling affecting food intake. **A,** CNS adiposity signaling promoting food intake. Decreased fat mass increases leptin and insulin signaling in the hypothalamic arcuate nucleus, which triggers release of neuropeptide Y *(NPY)* and agouti-related protein *(AgRP)* while simultaneously blocking α-melanocyte stimulating hormone (α-MSH) activation of melanocortin *(MC)* anorexia pathways. The net result is increased food intake (and decreased energy expenditure, not shown).

Finally, in addition to leptin, insulin, the monoamines, and the various neuropeptides already discussed, a number of other neuromodulators (Box 22-2) are involved in the central control of feeding behavior and energy balance in animals (Liebowitz and Hoebel, 2004; Blundell, 1991). The long list of involved neuromodulators underscores the complexity of the system controlling eating behavior and energy balance.

Efferent Signals Involved in Control of Energy Balance

Efferent signals include both the neuronal outputs that coordinate the various motor functions involved in food acquisition and ingestion and the signals that are associated with changes in food intake and body nutrient stores (Berthoud, 2004). Activity of the sympathetic and parasympathetic systems change in a reciprocal fashion with alterations in food intake and associated metabolism (Bray, 1991). The activity of the sympathetic nervous system appears to be inversely related to food intake, at least in animals. Administration of an appetite suppressant such as an amphetamine decreases food intake and increases sympathetic activity, which increases energy expenditure. Conversely, VMH lesions increase food intake and decrease sympathetic activity. Ingestion of food activates the parasympathetic nervous system, which stimulates the peripheral release of insulin, the predominant anabolic hormone associated with metabolic

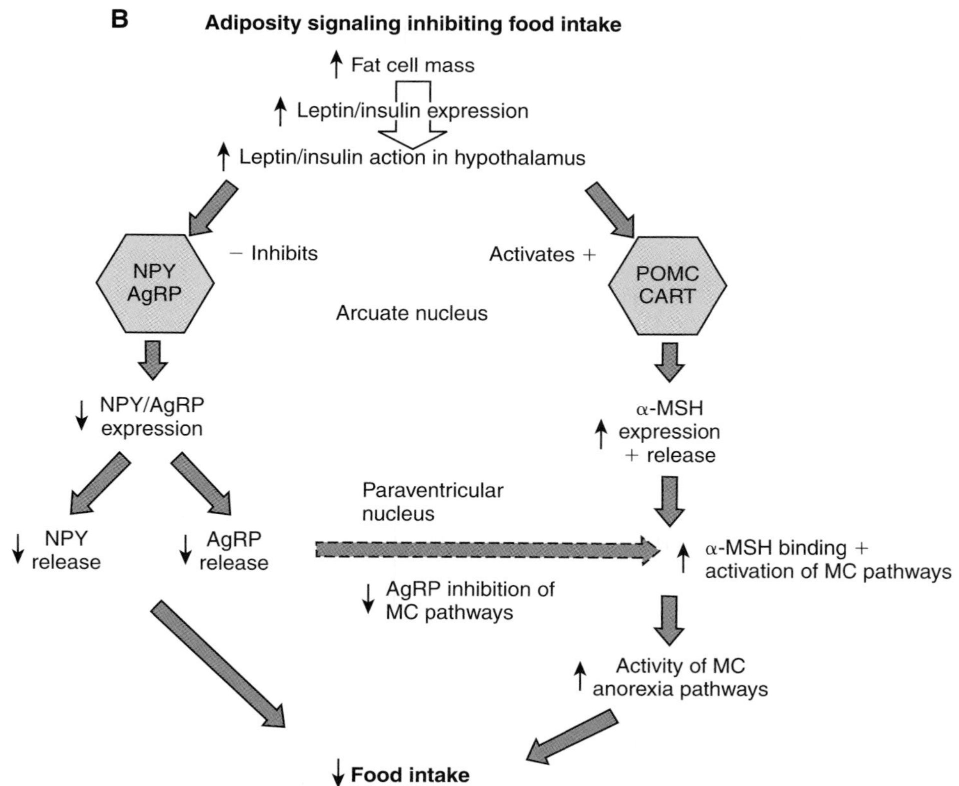

Figure 22-2, cont'd B, CNS adiposity signaling inhibiting food intake. Increased fat mass reduces leptin and insulin signaling in the hypothalamic arcuate nucleus, which inhibits release of NPY and AgRP while simultaneously increasing α-MSH activation of MC anorexia pathways. The net result is decreased food intake (and increased energy expenditure, not shown). *(Modified from Schwartz MW, Woods SC, Porte D Jr, Seeley RJ, Baskin DG [2000] Central nervous system control of food intake. Nature 404:661-671.)*

Box 22-2

NEUROMODULATORS THAT STIMULATE OR INHIBIT FOOD INTAKE

Neuromodulators That Stimulate Food Intake	Neuromodulators That Inhibit Food Intake
Neuropeptide (NPY)	Melanocortins (e.g., POMC, α-MSH)
Galanin, galanin-like peptides	Cytokines (e.g., TNF, IL-1, IL-6,)
Agouti-related protein (AgRP)	Cocaine-amphetamine–related transcript (CART)
Orexins A, B	Corticotropin-releasing hormone (CRH)
Melanin-concentrating hormone (MCH)	Neurotensin
Opioid peptides	Neuromedin U
Anandamide	Calcitonin
Growth hormone–releasing hormone (GHRP)	Acidic fibroblast growth factor
Beacon	Cyclo (His-Pro) dipeptide
VGF	Oxytocin and vasopressin
Prolactin	Prolactin-releasing peptide
	Ciliary neurotrophic factor (CNTF)

Data from Liebowitz SF, Hoebel BG (2004) Behavioral neuroscience and obesity. In: Bray GA, Bouchard C (eds) Handbook of Obesity, 2nd ed. Marcel Dekker, New York, pp 301-307.
IL-1, Interleukin-1; *IL-6,* interleukin-6; *MSH,* melanocyte-stimulating hormone; *POMC,* proopiomelanocortin; *TNF,* tumor necrosis factor.

processing of ingested nutrients. As outlined previously, the integration of leptin and insulin signals in the brain, which have reciprocal effects on food intake depending on the energy state of the animal, also have effects on energy expenditure that serve to restore energy homeostasis (Flier, 2004; Lowell and Spiegelman, 2000; Schwartz et al., 2000). For example, increased adiposity and increased leptin and insulin signaling in brain decreases food intake and at the same time stimulates energy expenditure. Reduced adiposity and diminished leptin and insulin signaling lead to increased food intake and reduced energy expenditure in order to protect energy stores.

CONTROL OF ENERGY EXPENDITURE

Total energy expenditure (TEE) reflects the total amount of heat produced plus work performed on the environment. For measurement purposes, TEE may be subdivided into the following three major components (Lowell and Spiegelman, 2000):

1. Resting metabolic rate (RMR), or, alternatively, basal energy expenditure (BEE)
2. The energy expended in physical activity (EEPA)
3. Adaptive thermogenesis, which includes the thermic effect of food (TEF)

These components and a further explanation of their contribution to the daily energy expenditure can be found in Chapter 21.

Energy expenditure is subject to the control of the central nervous system as noted previously. Two major components of TEE, RMR and much of adaptive thermogenesis, are regulated by efferent outputs of the brain centers involved in controlling energy balance. The energy expended in physical activity is not under autonomic control but is variable depending on the type and intensity of the activity chosen, the weight of the subject, and the mechanical efficiency of the activity performed.

The following sections describe how energy expenditure changes as a function of changes in the state of energy balance, body size and composition, aging, physical activity, and the composition of the fuel consumed and burned. Although these are predominantly descriptive rather than mechanistic aspects of energy expenditure, they are important from a practical sense in that they often represent variables that are measured in a medical or laboratory setting in an attempt to understand the causes of obesity and other disturbances in energy balance.

OVERFEEDING AND UNDERFEEDING

Overfeeding and underfeeding produce changes in TEE, which acts to oppose changes in body energy stores. The magnitude and duration of these changes is generally small in relation to the perturbation of energy balance and is not sufficient to prevent changes in body energy stores.

During food restriction, TEF and EEPA decline, as would be expected from reduced food intake and a reduction in total body mass. RMR, however, declines more rapidly than would be expected from the loss of body mass and from the decline in spontaneous physical activity due to general fatigue. In one study in which subjects were fed an energy-restricted diet for 24 weeks, subjects lost 23% of their initial body weight (Keys et al., 1950). Concurrent with this, RMR declined by 36% and muscle mass was reduced by 40%. In relative terms, RMR per unit of fat-free mass decreased by 14%, suggesting an increase in metabolic efficiency of the remaining body tissue. This adaptive reduction in RMR may be a defense against further loss of body energy stores. It has been suggested that this adaptive reduction in RMR may be mediated by altered neuroendocrine status (e.g., reduced circulating thyroid hormone) or reduced activity of the sympathetic nervous system (Danforth, 1984; Young and Landsberg, 1977).

During overfeeding, the adaptive increase in energy expenditure is generally modest and may be nutrient specific. For example, a 50% increase in total energy intake coming exclusively from carbohydrate has been observed to increase total daily energy expenditure by about 10%, owing to the energy cost of converting ingested carbohydrate to glycogen or fat and to an insulin-mediated increase in sympathetic nervous system activity. The response to fat is even more modest, whereby overfeeding to the same extent produced only a 3% increase in energy expenditure (Horton et al., 1995) reflecting mainly the fact that dietary fat can be stored as body fat with little or no metabolic processing required. As with underfeeding, these adaptive alterations in energy expenditure are believed to be mediated by changes in neuroendocrine status and the activity of the sympathetic nervous system.

CHANGES IN BODY COMPOSITION

Because RMR is influenced by body composition, changes in body composition can affect RMR. It has been suggested that one way to increase energy expenditure in order to combat obesity is to increase RMR by increasing muscle mass and decreasing fat mass. Although it is difficult to estimate the contribution of muscle mass per se to RMR, the contribution of fat-free mass (FFM) (which is largely muscle) can be estimated. Each one kilogram increase in FFM increases RMR by about 22 kcal/day. Therefore, it would be necessary to increase FFM by 4.5 kg in order to increase daily energy expenditure by 100 kcal. Increasing FFM, therefore, is not a practical means to increase energy expenditure in order to bring about a shift in energy balance.

Aging

Total daily energy expenditure declines with aging. FFM also declines with aging, and because RMR is highly correlated with FFM (see Chapter 21), a decline in RMR is expected. There is no convincing evidence that TEF changes with aging, and there is no strong theoretical reason why this would be expected. In addition, people often become more sedentary as they age, which reduces EEPA. Remaining physically active can prevent much of the decline in RMR with aging, largely due to preservation of lean tissue mass (Poehlman and Horton, 1990).

PHYSICAL ACTIVITY

The amount of physical activity performed is the factor most capable of modifying TEE, which can be increased by 100 kcal/day with only 20 to 30 minutes of walking at 2 to 3 miles/hour. With other moderate aerobic activities such as cycling, tennis, or swimming, the additional caloric expenditure above RMR can range from 125 to 350 kcal/30 minutes (Table 22-3).

Consequently, although total daily obligatory energy expenditure (i.e., RMR) can be altered in the short term by severe alterations in energy intake or in the longer term by changes in body composition, the magnitude of possible changes is relatively small. In contrast, substantial alterations in total daily energy expenditure can be produced by as little as 30 minutes of physical activity.

COMPOSITION OF ENERGY EXPENDITURE

The fuel for energy expenditure is supplied by protein, carbohydrate, and fat (and alcohol). This fuel can be supplied by the diet or by endogenous energy storage depots in the body. The relative contributions of these dietary fuels to the fuel mixture burned by the body appears to follow a hierarchy that is consistent with (1) the storage capacity of the body for each macronutrient in relation to its intake, (2) the energy cost of converting the ingested nutrient into a form with a greater storage capacity, and (3) the specific fuel needs of specific body tissues. In this metabolic hierarchy, the priorities for substrate oxidation are alcohol > protein > carbohydrate > fat.

Alcohol has highest priority for oxidation because there is no body storage pool and it can be toxic if it accumulates in body tissues. Amino acids are next in the oxidative hierarchy. Again, there is no specific storage pool in the body for excess amino acids; body proteins are functional in nature. Carbohydrate is third in the oxidative hierarchy. Carbohydrate can be stored as glycogen, but storage capacity is limited. Glycogen stores in a typical adult range from 200 to 500 g (predominantly in muscle and liver) and are only sufficient to supply a single day of energy needs. Conversion of carbohydrate to fat is energetically expensive, requiring investment of adenosine triphosphate (ATP) equivalent to 20% of the energy contained in the carbohydrate (Flatt, 1992); oxidation of excess glucose is more energetically efficient than is its conversion to fat. Carbohydrate is somewhat unique in that it is an obligatory fuel for certain tissues, including the central nervous system and red blood cells. In contrast to the other macronutrients, there is a virtually unlimited storage capacity for fat, largely in adipose tissue. Storage of dietary fat in adipose tissue is very efficient (97% to 98%) and, unlike carbohydrate, fat is not a unique fuel source for any body tissue.

Because of the high oxidative priority of alcohol and protein (amino acids), the body has an exceptional ability to maintain balances of these nutrients across a wide range of intakes of each. The amount of alcohol or amino acids that is oxidized is directly proportional to intake so that balance is achieved rapidly after ingestion of these fuels. In addition, because body carbohydrate stores are not significantly larger than daily carbohydrate intake and because net de novo lipogenesis from carbohydrate does

Table 22-3
Energy Cost of Various Forms of Physical Activity

Mild to Moderate Exercise	kcal burned per hour*
Walking (2-2.5 mph)	185-255
Bicycling or stationary cycling (5.5 mph)	245
Golf (walking with clubs)	270
Aerobic exercise (low-impact)	275
Ballroom dancing	300
Strength training	300
Hiking (3 mph, with 20-lb backpack)	400
Treadmill walking (4 mph)	345
Tennis	425
Rowing machine (easy)	300
Moderate to Intense Exercise	
Rope-jumping	660
Swimming	540
Walking (5 mph)	555
Bench-stepping class	610
Jogging (5.5 mph)	655
Bicycling or stationary cycling (13 mph)	655
Stair-climbing machine use	680
Running (7.2 mph)	700
Cross-country skiing (5 mph)	600
Rowing machine (higher-intensity)	655

Data calculated from Ainsworth BE, Haskell WL, Leon AS, Jacobs DR Jr, Montoye HJ, Sallis JF, Paffenbarger RS Jr (1993) Compendium of physical activities: classification of energy costs of human physical activities. Med Sci Sport Exerc 25:71-80.
*Values are kcal/hour above resting metabolic rate for an average 70-kg subject.
mph, Miles per hour.

not occur under normal circumstances, carbohydrate oxidation also closely matches carbohydrate intake, and carbohydrate balance is maintained across a wide range of carbohydrate intakes. By contrast, fat does not promote its own oxidation, and the amount of fat oxidized is not proportional to intake but comprises the difference between total energy needs and oxidation of the other fuels (Peters, 2003).

Fat oxidation = Total energy expenditure − (Protein oxidation + Carbohydrate oxidation + Alcohol oxidation)

The low metabolic priority for fat oxidation and the large storage capacity of the body for fat in relation to daily fat intake may weaken the precision of the body to regulate energy balance when the diet is rich in fat. The precision of regulation is likely to be poor under conditions of limited physical activity, because increased activity is the most efficient means to increase fat oxidation (Peters, 2003).

ACHIEVING STABLE BODY WEIGHT IN THE PREVAILING ENVIRONMENT: INTERACTION BETWEEN ENERGY INTAKE AND EXPENDITURE

It is evident from the preceding discussion that although we can consider energy and nutrient intake and expenditure as separate components of the energy-balance relationship, the two are inextricably linked, with each influencing the other. As described previously, the body has the ability to maintain energy and nutrient balance owing to the existence of a complex regulatory system involving integration of neural and humoral inputs and outputs from the brain centers that coordinately regulate energy intake and expenditure. Whether energy balance is reached at a healthy body weight is subject to a variety of other variables.

Despite the elegant neural control systems described earlier for defending body weight, it is possible to override these systems through

Nutrition Insight

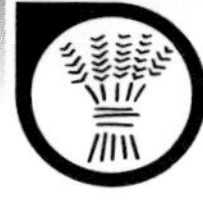

Energetic Equivalent of Body Tissues: Implications for Weight Loss

The energetic equivalent of a given amount of body mass either gained or lost depends on its composition. Lean tissue such as muscle is about 80% water, with the remaining 20% being largely protein with smaller amounts of fat and carbohydrate. In contrast, adipose tissue is only approximately 15% water, the remainder (85%) being storage lipid with a very small amount of protein contributing to the cell structure and intracellular enzymes. Given these differences in the composition of body tissues, the amount of energy represented by a kilogram of body weight will differ accordingly.

For example, the body energy lost when a kilogram of muscle is lost would be roughly 1,120 kcal (200 g × 5.6 kcal/g for protein). Only about 800 kcal of this energy would be net energy available to supply the body's fuel needs; the remaining 320 kcal would be required to metabolize the nitrogen derived from the breakdown of the amino acids in the protein to the excretory product, urea.

Loss of a kilogram of adipose tissue (85% lipid) represents a body energy loss of about 7,905 kcal (850 g × 9.3 kcal/g). In contrast to protein, essentially all of the energy represented by stored fat can contribute to net fuel energy. Therefore, a kilogram of body fat represents nearly 10 times (7,905 kcal/kg fat ÷ 800 kcal/kg lean) the energy for fuel represented by a kilogram of lean tissue.

These figures provide some perspective on weight loss claims appearing in the popular press. Take the example of a claim touting a 2.5-kg weight loss in a week by simply following a new diet (i.e., no exercise involved). If the weight loss were really adipose tissue, as hoped by the dieter, the loss would represent 41,995 kcal of body energy. For the average sedentary individual only about 2,500 kcal are needed each day to maintain body weight, or 17,500 kcal per week. It is, therefore, impossible to lose 2.5 kg of fat in a week by dieting alone—in order to lose 2.5 kg of fat, the individual would have to eat nothing for 16.5 days!

cognitive means. For example, many nonphysiological cues are involved in determining whether or not an individual chooses to eat; these cues range from the mere presence of food to complex social and cultural habits and circumstances. The amount eaten, while subject to the feedback systems described, can still be cognitively determined. Likewise, despite the body's ability to adjust resting and adaptive components of TEE, the amount of physical activity performed is still largely an individual cognitive choice. Therefore, the overall level of energy balance achieved is still subject to many nonphysiological factors. Indeed, the secular increase in body weight and the increase in the prevalence of obesity in the populations of most developed countries is testimony to the power of these external environmental and cognitive influences.

Although the average body weight in the population at which energy balance is achieved has risen over the years, most adults still maintain a relatively stable body weight and body composition over long periods and defend against major disruptions to the state of energy balance. For example, an increase in energy intake above TEE disrupts energy balance. If the increased energy intake is sustained, body weight increases and is accompanied by increases in TEE. Body weight stabilizes and energy balance is achieved when TEE is increased to the level of energy intake. Conversely, a decrease in energy intake disrupts energy balance and produces a loss of body weight, accompanied by a reduction in TEE. Body weight stabilizes when TEE declines to the level of energy intake.

Recent work highlighting the importance of achieving nutrient balance in addition to total energy balance has improved our understanding of how environmental factors, such as changes in the composition of food and changes in physical activity patterns, affect the body weight regulatory system (Flatt and Tremblay, 2004). As discussed in preceding text, acute changes in intake of alcohol, protein, or carbohydrate are rapidly balanced by changes in oxidation of each. In contrast, fat oxidation is not tightly linked to fat intake. As a consequence, positive or negative energy balances are largely conditions of positive or negative fat balance. The point at which a stable body weight and body composition is reached and defended, therefore, is that point at which fat balance is achieved (settling point).

For a given individual, the major factors that influence fat balance are the amount and composition of food eaten and the total amount of physical activity (Peters, 2003). Positive fat balance can be produced by overconsumption of energy or restriction of physical activity. Positive fat balance occurs when diets of any composition are overconsumed. This is because balances of protein, carbohydrate, and alcohol are preferentially achieved at the expense of fat oxidation. During carbohydrate overfeeding, for example, carbohydrate oxidation increases to maintain carbohydrate balance, but because carbohydrate is providing proportionately more fuel for oxidative needs, fat oxidation is providing less than usual, creating positive fat balance (Horton et al., 1995). Diets high in fat are particularly problematic: they increase the palatability and energy density of the food consumed, which contributes to overconsumption of total energy, and the excess energy does not increase fat oxidation and is efficiently stored. The best strategy for avoiding positive fat balance is to avoid overconsumption of energy. This may be facilitated by consuming a low-fat diet.

Restricting the habitual level of physical activity reduces fat oxidation because working muscle is a major contributor to the body's total oxidation of fat. Because fat intake and oxidation are not closely linked, positive fat balance results if the decline in fat oxidation is not offset by an equivalent reduction in fat intake.

Negative fat balance can be brought about by underconsumption of total energy or fat or by an increase in the level of habitual physical activity. During underconsumption of energy, the dietary supply of the priority metabolic fuels, carbohydrate and protein, is insufficient to meet the body's energy needs. The remaining energy needs must be met by fat oxidation, which comes largely from endogenous fat stores. Similarly, increased oxidation of fat is the predominant mechanism by which energy needs are met when the level of habitual physical activity is increased.

ENERGY BALANCE, FAT BALANCE, AND THE SETTLING POINT

In most individuals, in most environmental circumstances, maintenance of energy balance is largely a matter of achieving and maintaining fat balance. Given the preceding discussion, one might ask how a new steady state of body weight and body composition is achieved following a positive or negative perturbation in fat balance. There are two mechanisms by which this can occur. First, changes in behavior can lead to adjustments in either intake or oxidation of fat (e.g., altering total energy or fat intake and altering physical activity). Second, in the absence of sufficient behavioral changes, fat oxidation is altered following changes in the body fat mass. As an example of behavioral adjustments, the negative fat balance produced by reducing energy intake could be eliminated totally by a compensatory reduction in physical activity. However, this is not likely to be the typical response, and one would usually expect to see some loss of body mass and the accompanying reduction in energy expenditure. As an example of metabolic adjustments, overconsumption of total energy and fat produces positive energy balance. If the behavioral adjustments are absent or insufficient to subsequently offset the excess intake, increases in the body fat mass result. Increased body fat mass is associated with increased levels of circulating free fatty acids, which elevate total fat oxidation. Therefore, a stable body weight is reached at the point where the body fat mass has increased sufficiently so that fat oxidation equals fat intake (Peters, 2003).

The current environment in the United States is characterized by the wide availability of energy-dense foods, many of which are high in fat, coupled with an increasingly sedentary lifestyle (Hill et al., 2003; Peters et al., 2002). Under these circumstances, maintenance of a large body fat mass may be a necessary consequence in order to achieve fat balance and hence, energy balance.

REFERENCES

Barsh GS, Farooqi SI, O'Rahilly S (2000) Genetics of body-weight regulation. Nature 404:644-651.

Berthoud H-R (2004) The caudal brainstem and the control of food intake and energy balance. In: Stricker E, Woods SC (eds) Neurobiology of Food and Fluid Intake, 2nd ed. Vol 14 of Handbook of Behavioral Neurobiology. Kluwer Academic/Plenum Publishers, New York, pp 195-239.

Birch LL (1992) Children's preference for high-fat foods. Nutr Rev 50:249-255.

Birch LL (1999) Development of food preferences. Annu Rev Nutr 19:41-62.

Blevins JE, Truong GG, Gietzen DW (2004) NMDA receptor function within the anterior piriform cortex and lateral hypothalamus in rats on the control of intake of amino acid deficient diets. Brain Res 1019:124-133.

Blundell JE (1991) The biology of appetite. Clin Appl Nutr 1:21-31.

Bouchard C, Tremblay A, Despres JP, Nadeau A, Lupien PJ, Moorjani S, Theriault G, Kim SY (1996) Overfeeding in identical twins: 5-year postoverfeeding results. Metabolism 45:1042-1050.

Bray GA (1991) Obesity, a disorder of nutrient partitioning: The MONA LISA hypothesis. J Nutr 121:1146-1162.

Bray GA, Tartaglia LA (2000) Medicinal strategies in the treatment of obesity. Nature 404:672-677.

Brownell KD, Fairburn GC (eds) (1995) Eating Disorders and Obesity: A Comprehensive Handbook. Guilford Press, New York.

Campfield AL, Smith FJ, Jeanrenaud B (2004) Central integration of peripheral signals in the regulation of food intake and energy balance: role of leptin and insulin. In: Bray GA, Bouchard C (eds) Handbook of Obesity, 2nd ed. Marcel Dekker, New York, pp 461-479.

Chehab FF, Mounzih K, Lu R, Lim ME (1997) Early onset of reproductive function in normal female mice treated with leptin. Science 275:88-90.

Cummings DE, Purnell JQ, Frayo RS, Schmidova K, Wisse BE, Weigle DS (2001) A preprandial rise in plasma ghrelin levels suggests a role in meal initiation in humans. Diabetes 50: 1714-1719.

Cummings DE, Schwartz MW (2003) Genetics and pathophysiology of human obesity. Annu Rev Med 54:453-471.

Cummings DE, Weigel DS, Frayo RS, Breen PA, Ma M.K, Dellinger EP, Purnell JQ (2002) Plasma ghrelin levels after diet-induced weight loss or gastric bypass surgery. N Engl J Med 346: 1623-1630.

Danforth E Jr (1984) The role of thyroid hormones in the control of energy expenditure. Clin Endocrinol Metab 13:581-595.

De Castro J, De Castro E (1989) Spontaneous meal patterns in humans: influence of the presence of other people. Am J Clin Nutr 50:237-247.

Drewnowski A (1997) Taste preferences and food intake. Annu Rev Nutr 17:237-253.

Dunn-Meynell AA, Routh VH, Kang L, Gaspers L, Levin BE (2002) Glucokinase is the likely mediator of glucosensing in both glucose-exited and glucose-inhibited central neurons. Diabetes 51:2056-2065.

Fan W, Boston BA, Kesterson RA, Hruby VJ, Cone RD (1997) Role of melanocortinergic neurons in feeding and the agouti obesity syndrome. Nature 385:165-168.

Flatt JP (1992) The biochemistry of energy expenditure. In: Bjorntorp P, Brodoff B (eds) Obesity. JB Lippincott, Philadelphia, pp 100-116.

Flatt JP (1995) Diet, lifestyle, and weight maintenance. Am J Clin Nutr 62:820-836.

Flatt JP, Tremblay A (2004) Energy expenditure and substrate oxidation. In: Bray GA, Bouchard C (eds) Handbook of Obesity, 2nd ed. Marcel Dekker, New York, pp 705-731.

Flegal KM, Troiano RP (2000) Changes in the distribution of body mass index of adults and children in the US population. Int J Obes Relat Metab Disord 24:807-818.

Flier JS (1997) Leptin expression and action: new experimental paradigms. Proc Natl Acad Sci USA 94:4242-4245.

Flier JS (2004) Obesity wars: molecular progress confronts an expanding epidemic. Cell 116:337-350.

Friedman JM (2003) A war on obesity, not the obese. Science 299:856-858.

Grossman SP (1975) Role of the hypothalamus in the regulation of food and water intake. Psychol Rev 82:200-224.

Hill JO, Peters JC (1998) Environmental contributions to the obesity epidemic. Science 280:1371-1374.

Hill JO, Wyatt HR, Reed G, Peters JC (2003) Obesity and the environment: where do we go from here? Science 299:853-855.

Horton TJ, Drougas H, Brachey A, Reed GW, Peters JC, Hill JO (1995) Fat and carbohydrate overfeeding in humans: different effects on energy storage. Am J Clin Nutr 62:19-29.

Kaplan JM, Moran TH (2004) Gastrointestinal signaling in the control of food intake. In: Stricker E, Woods SC (eds) Neurobiology of Food and Fluid Intake, 2nd ed. Vol 14 of Handbook of Behavioral Neurobiology. Kluwer Academic/Plenum Publishers, New York, pp 273-303.

Keesey RE, Corbett SW (1984) Metabolic defense of the body weight set point. In: Stunkard AJ, Stellar E (eds) Eating and Its Disorders. Raven Press, New York, pp 87-96.

Kennedy GC (1953) The role of depot fat in the hypothalamic control of food intake in the rat. Proc R Soc Lond B Biol Sci 140:578-596.

Kern DL, McPhee L, Fisher J, Johnson S, Birch LL (1993) The postingestive consequences of fat condition preferences for flavors associated with high dietary fat. Physiol Behav 54:71-76.

Keys A, Brozek J, Henshel A, Michelson O, Taylor HL (1950) The Biology of Human Starvation. University of Minnesota Press, Minneapolis.

Kuczmarski RJ, Flegal KM, Campbell SM, Johnson CL (1994) Increasing prevalence of overweight among U.S. adults: The National Health and Nutrition Examination Surveys, 1960 to 1991. JAMA 272:205-211.

Leibel RL, Rosenbaum M, Hirsch J (1995) Changes in energy expenditure resulting from altered body weight. N Engl J Med 332:621-628.

Levine AS, Billington CJ (1997) Why do we eat? A neural systems approach. Annu Rev Nutr 17:597-619.

Liebowitz SF, Hoebel BG, (2004) Behavioral neuroscience and obesity. In: Bray GA, Bouchard C (eds) Handbook of Obesity, 2nd ed. Marcel Dekker, New York, pp 301-371.

Lissner L, Heitmann BL (1995) Dietary fat and obesity: evidence from epidemiology. Eur J Clin Nutr 49:79-90.

Lowell BB, Spiegelman BM (2000) Toward a molecular understanding of adaptive thermogenesis. Nature 404:652-660.

Mayer J (1953) Glucostatic mechanism of regulation of food intake. N Engl J Med 249:13-16.

McDowell MA, Briefel RR, Alaimo K, Bischof AM, Caughman CR, Carroll MD, Loria CM, Johnson CL (1994) Energy and macronutrient intakes of persons ages 2 months and over in the United States: Third National Health and Nutrition Examination Survey, Phase 1, 1988–91. National Center for Health Statistics, Centers for Disease Control and Prevention, U.S. Department of Health and Human Services, Washington, DC, Publication No. 255.

Mellinkoff S (1957) Digestive system. Annu Rev Physiol 19:175-204.

Miyawaki K, Yamada Y, Ban N, Ihara Y, Tsukiyama K, Zhou H, Fujimoto S, Oku A,

Tsuda K, Toyokuni S, Hiai H, Mizunoya W, Fushiki T, Holst JJ, Makino M, Tashita A, Kobara Y, Tsubamoto Y, Jinnouchi T, Jomori T, Seino Y (2002) Inhibition of gastric inhibitory polypeptide signaling prevents obesity. Nat Med 8:738-742.

Moran TH (2000) Cholecystokinin and satiety: current perspectives. Nutrition 16:858-865.

Obici S, Feng Z, Morgan K, Stein D, Karkanias G, Rossetti L (2002) Central administration of oleic acid inhibits glucose production and food intake. Diabetes 51:271-275.

Ogden CL, Flegal KM, Carroll MD, Johnson CL (2002) Prevalence and trends in overweight among US children and adolescents, 1999-2000. J Am Med Assoc 288:1728-1732.

Peters JC (2003) Dietary fat and body weight control. Lipids 38:123-127.

Peters JC, Wyatt HR, Donahoo WT, Hill JO (2002) From instinct to intellect: the challenge of maintaining healthy weight in the modern world. Obes Rev 3:69-74.

Poehlman ET, Horton ES (1990) Regulation of energy expenditure in aging humans. Annu Rev Nutr 10:255-275.

Rodin J (1992) Determination of food intake regulation in obesity. In: Bjorntorn P, Brodoff B, (eds) Obesity. J.B. Lippincott, Philadelphia, pp 220-230.

Rolls BJ, Rowe EA, Rolls ET, Kingston B, Megson A, Gunary R (1981) Variety in a meal enhances food intake in man. Physiol Behav 26:215-221.

Rosenbaum M, Leibel RL, Hirsch J (1997) Obesity. N Engl J Med 337:396-407.

Schwartz MW, Seely RJ (1997) The new biology of body weight regulation. J Am Diet Assoc 97:54-58.

Schwartz MW, Woods SC, Porte D Jr, Seeley RJ, Baskin DG (2000) Central nervous system control of food intake. Nature 404:661-671.

Schwartz MW, Woods SC, Seeley RJ, Barsh G S, Baskin DG, Leibel RL (2003) Is the energy homeostasis system inherently biased toward weight gain? Diabetes 52:232-238.

Seeley RJ, Drazen DL, Clegg DJ (2004) The critical role of the melanocortin system in the control of energy balance. Annu Rev Nutr 24:133-149.

Sims EA, Horton ES (1968) Endocrine and metabolic adaptation to obesity and starvation. Am J Clin Nutr 21:1455-1470.

Stellar E (1954) The physiology of motivation. Psychol Rev 61:5-11.

Takeda S, Elefteriou F, Karsenty G (2003) Common endocrine control of body weight, reproduction, and bone mass. Annu Rev Nutr 23:403-411.

Tartaglia LA (1997) The leptin receptor. J Biol Chem 279:6093-6096.

Wansink B (2004) Environmental factors that increase the food intake and consumption volume of unknowing consumers Annu Rev Nutr 24:455-479.

Woods SC (2004) Metabolic signals in the control of food intake. In: Stricker E, Woods SC (eds) Neurobiology of Food and Fluid Intake, 2nd ed. Vol 14 of Handbook of Behavioral Neurobiology. Kluwer Academic/Plenum Publishers, New York, pp 241-272.

Yamamoto H, Lee CE, Marcus JN, Williams TD, Overton JM, Lopez ME, Hollenberg AN, Baggio L, Saper CB, Drucker DJ, Elmquist JK, (2002) Glucagon-like peptide-1 receptor stimulation increases blood pressure and heart rate and activates autonomic regulatory systems. J Clin Invest 110:43-52.

Young JB, Landsberg L (1977) Suppression of sympathetic nervous system during fasting. Science 196:1473-1475.

RECOMMENDED READINGS

Flatt JP, Tremblay A (2004) Energy expenditure and substrate oxidation. In: Bray GA, Bouchard C (eds) Handbook of Obesity, 2nd ed. Marcel Dekker, New York, pp 705-731.

Flier JS (2004) Obesity wars: Molecular progress confronts an expanding epidemic. Cell 116:337-350.

Hill JO, Wyatt HR, Reed G, Peters JC (2003) Obesity and the environment: Where do we go from here? Science 299:853-855.

Liebowitz SF, Hoebel BG (2004) Behavioral neuroscience and obesity. In: Bray GA, Bouchard C (eds) Handbook of Obesity, 2nd ed. Marcel Dekker, New York, pp 301-371.

Rosenbaum M, Leibel RL, Hirsch J (1997) Obesity. N Engl J Med 337:396-407.

Schwartz MW, Woods SC, Porte D Jr, Seeley RJ, Baskin DG (2000) Central nervous system control of food intake. Nature 404:661-661.

Seeley RJ, Drazen DL, Clegg DJ (2004) The critical role of the melanocortin system in the control of energy balance. Annu Rev Nutr 24:133-149.

Woods SC (2004) Metabolic signals in the control of food intake. In: Stricker E, Woods SC (eds) Neurobiology of Food and Fluid Intake, 2nd ed. Vol 14 of Handbook of Behavioral Neurobiology. Kluwer Academic/Plenum Publishers, New York, pp 241-272.

Chapter 23

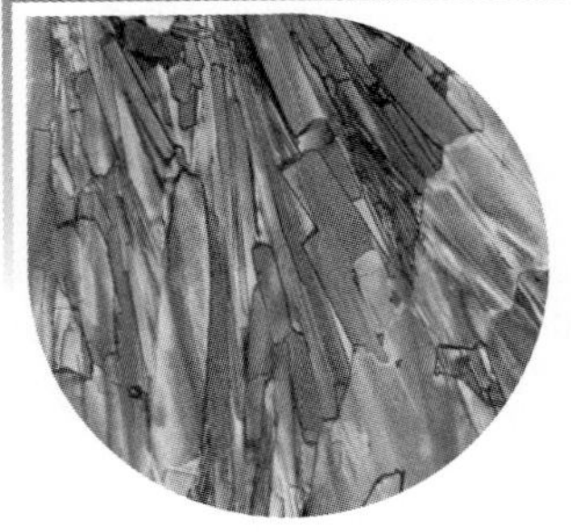

Disturbances of Energy Balance

Martha H. Stipanuk, PhD

OUTLINE

COMMON ABBREVIATIONS

BMI body mass index [weight in kg ÷ (height in m)^2]
EER energy expenditure requirement
PAL physical activity level
PEM protein-energy malnutrition
TEE total energy expenditure

This chapter is a revision of the chapter contributed by James O. Hill, PhD, Adamandia D. Kriketos, PhD, and John C. Peters, PhD, for the first edition.

OBESITY

Obesity is a disease in which the accumulation of body fat adversely affects health (Pi-Sunyer, 1993). Obesity is closely associated with other diseases, chiefly non–insulin-dependent diabetes mellitus (type 2 diabetes) and cardiovascular disease (Despres, 1993).

DEFINITION OF OBESITY

Although obesity specifically refers to having an abnormally high proportion of body fat, the body mass index (BMI) is most commonly used to define and to screen for obesity as well as overweight. The BMI, calculated as weight (kg) divided by height^2 (m^2), provides a more accurate indicator of obesity and overweight than does weight or weight for height. The World Health Organization (WHO), the United States, and most other countries, classify individuals with a BMI of 25 to 29.9 kg/m^2 as overweight and those with a BMI of 30 kg/m^2 or greater as obese. These categories are based on evidence that health risks increase more steeply in individuals with a BMI of 25 kg/m^2 or greater. The WHO classification is described in Table 23-1, which shows the BMI categories and the relative risk of comorbidities within each BMI category (WHO, 1997). A waist circumference of 39 inches or more for men and 35 inches or more for women indicates visceral obesity, a condition that further increases risk of comorbid conditions (WHO, 1997; Pi-Sunyer, 1993).

Table 23-1

Classification of Obesity Based on Body Mass Index and Risk of Comorbidities

Classification	BMI (kg/m^2)	Risk of Co-Morbidities
Underweight	<18.5	Low (but risk of other clinic problems increased)
Normal range	18.5-24.9	Average
Overweight	≥25	
Pre-obese	025.0-29.9	Increased
Obese class I	30.0-34.9	Moderate
Obese class II	35.0-39.9	Severe
Obese class III	≥40.0	Very severe

BMI, Body mass index.
Modified from World Health Organization (WHO) (1997) Obesity: Preventing and Managing the Global Epidemic: Report of a WHO Consultation on Obesity. Geneva, June 3-5.

BMI is very useful as a general guideline to monitor trends in the population, but by itself is not diagnostic of overweight or obesity. It should be noted that the BMI classification system will be correct for most, but not all, individuals; a person can be overweight without having an excess amount of fat if the excess weight comes from muscle, bone, and/or body water. Very muscular people may fall into the overweight category when they are actually healthy and fit. Elderly individuals who have lost body mass may be in the healthy weight category, according to their BMI, when they actually have reduced nutritional reserves.

In addition to high BMI values, the distribution of excess fat depots and the amount of weight gained during adulthood seem to be associated with increased risk of morbidity. Individuals who accumulate excess body fat in upper body adipose depots, particularly intraabdominal or visceral depots, may be at greater risk of developing negative health consequences of obesity than individuals who accumulate the same amount of excess body fat in the lower body (Pouliot et al., 1994). Data from many studies suggest that excess fat located in visceral depots is an independent risk factor for type 2 diabetes and cardiovascular disease (Despres, 1993). For any specific BMI, a larger waist circumference is associated with greater risk of impaired health than a smaller waist circumference, whereas a greater hip circumference appears to be protective (Lissner et al., 2001). The factors that determine the location of storage of excess fat are not well understood, but sex hormones and genetics seem to play important roles in regulating body fat distribution (Perissinotto et al., 2002; Lemieux, 1997; Zamboni et al., 1994). Regardless of BMI, a large weight gain after the age of 18 years is associated with a significantly greater risk of developing type 2 diabetes in both men and women (Colditz et al., 1995).

PREVALENCE OF OBESITY

Obesity is increasing at an alarming rate in both developed and developing countries and in both adults and children. The WHO monitors obesity on a worldwide basis. Obesity is a serious problem in the United States and nations in Western European, and is a growing problem in other countries such as China, India, and Australia. The worldwide prevalence of obesity ranges from less than 5% of the population in rural China, Japan, and some African countries to levels as high as 80% of the adult population in the South Pacific island nation of Nauru (WHO, 2003).

Prevalence rates for overweight and obesity in the United States are obtained from the National Health (and Nutrition) Examination Surveys (NHES or NHANES), which have provided prevalence data for obesity since 1960 (Fig. 23-1). Since 1999 NHANES has become a continuous survey in the United States. The prevalence of obesity has increased markedly during the past two or three decades, and current estimates indicate that one third of U.S. adults are obese and another one third are overweight. The age-adjusted prevalence of obesity among U.S. adults, ages 20 to 74 years, increased by 50% between the periods from 1976 to 1980 and 1988 to 1994 and by another 35% between the periods from 1988 to 1994 and 1999 to 2002. Therefore, the prevalence of obesity doubled between the periods from 1976 to 1980 and 1999 to 2002. Between the years from 1988 to 1994 and 1999 to 2002, the mean weight of non-Hispanic white adults increased by approximately 10 pounds and that of non-Hispanic black women by 13 pounds (Ogden et al., 2004). The 1999 to 2002 data indicated that 31% of U.S. adults, ages 20 to 74 years, are obese, whereas another 34% fall in the overweight category. Only 33.5% of U.S. adults have BMIs within the desirable range of greater than or equal to 18.5 to less than 25. Based on NHANES data, there are racial/ethnic and sex differences in the prevalence of obesity or overweight. Obesity and overweight prevalences are very high among non-Hispanic black women (~50% obese, ~75% overweight

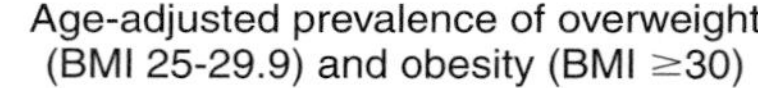

Age-adjusted prevalence of overweight
(BMI 25-29.9) and obesity (BMI ≥30)

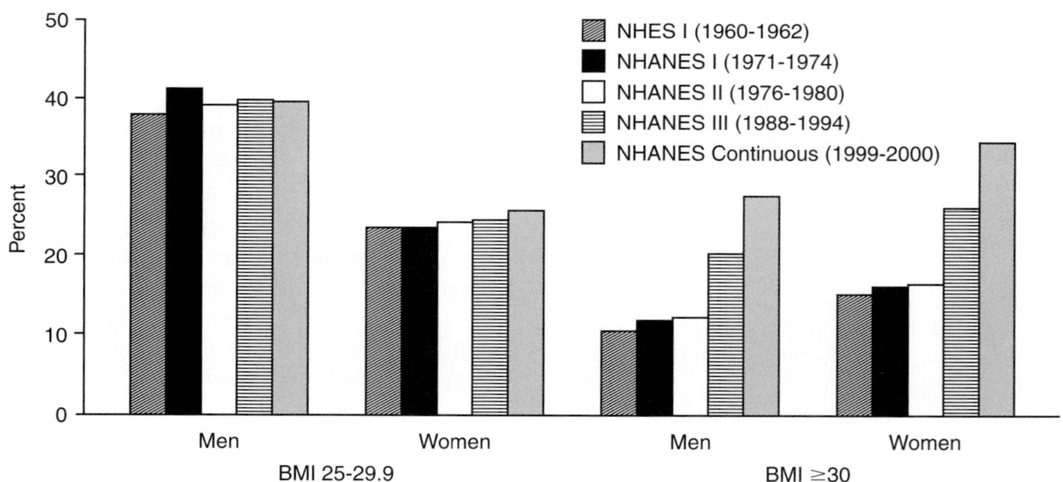

Figure 23-1 Prevalence of overweight and obesity in American adults. Overweight was defined as a body mass index (BMI) of 25.0 to 29.9 kg/m^2 and obesity as a BMI greater than or equal to 30 kg/m^2. *(Based on NHANES data as reported by Flegal KM, Carroll MD, Kuczmarski RJ, Johnson CL [1998] Overweight and obesity in the United States: prevalence and trends, 1960-1994. Int J Obesity 22:39-47; and Flegal KM, Carroll MD, Ogden CL, Johnson CL [2002] Prevalence and trends in obesity among U.S. adults, 1999-2000. JAMA 288:1723-1727.)*

based on 1999 to 2002 data) (Hedley et al., 2004). The prevalence of overweight and obesity is also higher among Hispanic women and American Indians, but lower among Asian Americans, than among non-Hispanic whites.

Overweight and obesity are more difficult to assess in children than in adults because children are constantly changing their height and weight. However, all indications are that overweight and obesity are also increasing in children. The Centers for Disease Control and Prevention Growth Charts for the United States (currently based on 1963 to 1994 data) are used to define overweight and at risk for overweight: "at risk for overweight" is defined as at or above the 85th percentile but less than the 95th percentile of the sex-specific BMI-for-age, and "overweight" is defined as at or above the 95th percentile of the sex-specific BMI-for-age. Based on the 1999 to 2002 data, 16% of children between the ages of 6 and 19 years had BMIs greater than or equal to the 95th percentile and 15% of children had BMIs between the 85th and 95th percentile levels. An analysis of age-adjusted prevalence of overweight in boys and girls in the periods from 1960 to 1962 through 1988 to 1991 indicates a marked increase in overweight in children since 1976 to 1980 (Troiano et al., 1995), and the 1999 to 2002 data demonstrate a further increase in incidence of BMI-for-age greater than or equal to 85% (overweight or risk of overweight) from approximately 22% in the period from 1988 to 1991 to 31% in 1999 to 2004.

HEALTH CONSEQUENCES OF OBESITY

Obesity is associated with many physiological and psychosocial risks. Box 23-1 lists the most frequently observed comorbidities associated with obesity. The risk of developing a comorbidity is influenced by the extent of obesity, the location of excess body fat, and the degree of weight gain over the adult years.

In general, obesity-associated morbidity and mortality increase in direct proportion to increases in BMI. This is shown in Figure 23-2, where all-cause mortality (risk of death from any cause) is plotted against BMI. It can be seen that all-cause mortality begins to increase at BMIs nearing 30 and continues to increase in

Box 23-1

FREQUENT COMORBIDITIES ASSOCIATED WITH OBESITY

Greatly Increased (relative risk >>3)

Diabetes
Gallbladder disease
Dyslipidemia
Insulin resistance
Breathlessness
Sleep apnea

Moderately Increased (relative risk ~2 to 3)

Coronary heart disease
Hypertension
Osteoarthritis (knees)
Hyperuricemia and gout

Slightly Increased (relative risk ~1 to 2)

Cancer (breast cancer in postmenopausal women, endometrial cancer, colon cancer)
Reproductive hormone abnormalities
Polycystic ovary syndrome
Impaired fertility
Low back pain due to obesity
Increased anesthetic risk
Fetal defects associated with maternal obesity

Modified from World Health Organization (WHO) (1997) Obesity: Preventing and Managing the Global Epidemic: Report of a WHO Consultation on Obesity. Geneva, June 3-5.

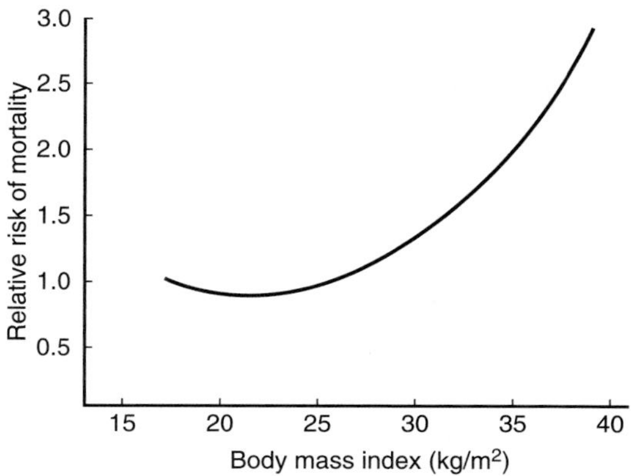

Figure 23-2 U-shaped relationship of body mass index to excess mortality in adults. Relative risk was defined as 1.0 for adults with body mass index (BMI) between 20 and 25.

a linear fashion at BMIs greater than 30. In a large prospective study of healthy individuals who had never smoked, the lowest mortality was found at BMIs (kg/m^2) between 22.0 and 26.4 in men and between 20.5 and 24.9 in women (Calle et al., 1999). Among subjects with the highest BMIs (>40.0), white men and women had a relative risk of death from all causes of 2.58 and 2.00, respectively, as compared with those with a BMI of 23.5 to 24.9. The major cause of obesity-associated death is cardiovascular disease (National Institutes of Health [NIH], 1998).

The prevalence of a number of specific medical conditions is strongly related to obesity in that they co-occur. Although obesity is considered a risk factor for many disease states, the causal mechanisms are not known for all associations. The data in Table 23-2 illustrate the strong relationship of BMI with the risk of type 2 diabetes, coronary heart disease, high blood pressure, and osteoarthritis (Mokdad et al., 2003). Significant associations were also found between BMI and the prevalence of hypercholesterolemia, asthma, and fair/poor general health. In addition, death rates from cancer are higher for overweight and obese men and women than for normal-weight men and women (Calle et al., 2003).

FACTORS INVOLVED IN DEVELOPMENT OF OBESITY

Obesity can occur only when energy ingested exceeds energy expended. However, because of the many genetic and environmental influences on both energy intake and energy expenditure, obesity must be considered to be a heterogeneous disorder with multiple causes. The gene × environment interaction is likely to explain the majority of variation in body weight, and separating the genetic from the environmental determinants of obesity presents a formidable challenge for scientists.

Genetic Factors

Some of the strongest evidence for a genetic component to body weight regulation, prior to the recent advances in genomics, came from studies of twins. Identical twins raised in different environments show similarities in body weight and body composition. Furthermore, when pairs of identical twins were overfed or subjected to long-term exercise training, the changes in body weight and body composition were more similar between identical twins than between fraternal twin pairs.

Major advances in the understanding of the genetic basis of obesity have occurred over the last few years. The 2003 update of the human obesity gene map contained more than 430 genes, markers, and chromosomal regions that have been associated or linked with human obesity phenotypes (Snyder et al., 2004). Among the candidate genes are several that have been supported by a number of positive studies: *ADRB2, ADRB3, INS, LDLR, LEP, LEPR, LIPE, PPARG, PPARGC1, NR3C1, TNF, UCP1, UCP2,* and *UCP3*. Mutations of several

Table 23-2
Prevalence of Medical Conditions by Body Mass Index (BMI) for Men and Women in the United States

		Body Mass Index			
		18.5-24.9	25-29.9	30-34.9	≥40
		Prevalence Ratio (%)			
Type 2 diabetes	Men	2.0	4.9	10.1	10.6
	Women	2.4	7.1	7.2	19.9
Coronary heart disease	Men	8.8	9.6	16.0	14.0
	Women	6.9	11.1	12.6	19.2
High blood pressure	Men	23.5	34.2	49.0	64.5
	Women	23.3	38.8	48.0	63.2
Osteoarthritis	Men	2.6	4.5	4.7	10.0
	Women	5.2	8.5	9.9	17.2

Data from NHANES III, 1988-1994.

genes have been associated with early onset and rather severe obesity in humans. The most common gene found to be involved with monogenic obesity syndromes is *MC4R*. Other cases involve *LEP, LEPR, POMC, PCSK1, PPARG,* and *PPP1R3A* (Farooqi and O'Rahilly, 2004; Snyder et al., 2004).These genes and the names of the encoded proteins are listed in Table 23-3. How the defects influence the balance of energy intake and energy expenditure to bring about obesity is largely unclear at this time. Whereas defects in *MC4R, POMC, PCSK1, LEP,* and *LEPR* affect regulation of energy intake, defects in genes such as *PPARG, PPARGC,* and the *UCP*s are predicted to result in defects in energy expenditure. Evidence to date indicates that most defects are associated with physiological perturbances in appetite and energy intake; measures of energy expenditure per unit of lean body mass are usually not different between obese and nonobese subjects.

Environmental Factors

There must be powerful environmental influences on the development of obesity. The large increase in the prevalence of obesity that has occurred in the United States over the last few decades cannot be attributed to genetic causes and suggests that changes in environmental factors are influencing the prevalence of obesity. Furthermore, when populations such as the Japanese or Chinese migrate to the United States, their BMIs increase (Fig. 23-3).

Increases in the proportion of fat, and consequently increases in the energy density of the diet, together with reductions in physical activity are thought to be major contributing factors to the increase in the prevalence of obesity (Pi-Sunyer, 1993). Americans consume diets with an average of 34% to 40% of total energy from fat. When similar diets are fed to laboratory rats, the majority of rats

Table 23-3
Candidate Genes That Have Been Associated or Linked With Human Obesity Phenotypes

	Gene	Name of Protein Encoded by Gene
Genes involved in monogenic obesity in humans	*MC4*	Melanocortin 4 receptor
	LEPR	Leptin receptor
	POMC	Proopiomelanocortin
	PCSK1	Proprotein convertase subtilisin/kexin type 1
	LEP	Leptin
	PPARG	Peroxisome proliferative activated receptor, gamma
	PPP1R3A	Protein phosphatase 1, regulatory (inhibitor) subunit 3A (glycogen and sarcoplasmic reticulum binding subunit, skeletal muscle)
Genes associated with human obesity phenotype in more than 5 studies	*ADRB2*	Adrenergic, beta-2, receptor, surface
	ADRB3	Adrenergic, beta-3, receptor
	INS	Insulin
	LDLR	Low density lipoprotein receptor
	LEP	Leptin
	LEPR	Leptin receptor
	LIPE	Hepatic lipase
	PPARG	Peroxisome proliferative activated receptor, gamma
	PPARGC1	Peroxisome proliferative activated receptor, gamma, coactivator 1
	NR3C1	Nuclear receptor subfamily 3, group C, member 1 (*GRL*, glucocorticoid receptor)
	TNF	Tumor necrosis factor, member 2
	UCP1	Uncoupling protein 1 (mitochondrial, proton carrier)
	UCP2	Uncoupling protein 2 (mitochondrial, proton carrier)
	UCP3	Uncoupling protein 3 (mitochondrial, proton carrier)

For other candidate genes see Snyder EE, Walts B, Perusse L, Chagnon YC, Weisnagel SJ, Rankinen T, Bouchard D (2004) The human obesity gene map: the 2003 update. Obes Res 12:369-439.

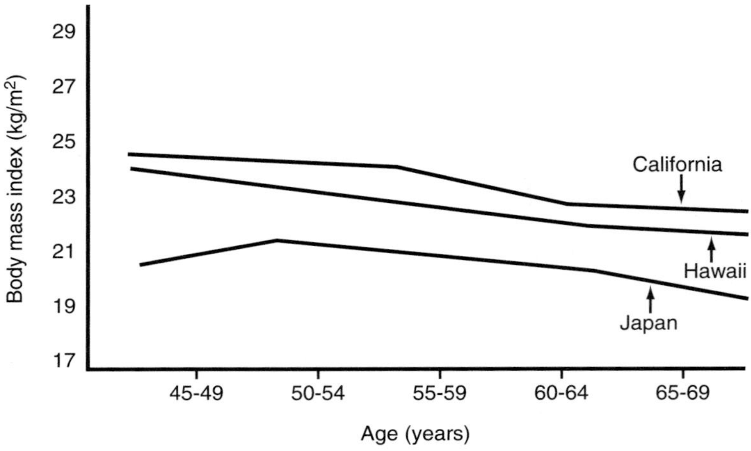

Figure 23-3 Mean body mass index in Japanese men aged 45 to 69 years in Hawaii, California, and Japan in 1965 to 1968. *(Modified from Curb JD, Marcus EB [1991] Body fat and obesity in Japanese Americans. Am J Clin Nutr 53:1552S-1555S. Copyright American Society for Clinical Nutrition.)*

become obese (Pagliassotti et al., 1997). Obesity appears to result both from an increased voluntary energy intake and from the fact that excess dietary fat is stored in the body more efficiently than is excess dietary carbohydrate or protein (Horton et al., 1995). This is discussed in more detail in Chapter 22.

Americans are becoming less physically active and more sedentary. Much of the decline in physical activity can be attributed to modernization, which has made it easier to be sedentary both at work and at home (WHO, 1997). The increased availability of automobiles and labor-saving devices has substantially reduced the amount of time spent being physically active. An increase in the time spent in sedentary activities such as watching television and playing video games is thought to play a role in reducing physical activity in children. The high attractiveness of these sedentary activities makes it difficult to promote more physically active behaviors (WHO, 1997).

It must be noted that, even in countries with a very high prevalence of obesity, not all individuals are overweight. Therefore, factors such as consumption of high-fat diets or physical inactivity should not be viewed as known causes of obesity but rather as factors that increase the probability of creating a mismatch between energy intake and energy expenditure. It is likely that an individual's genotype will help determine whether or not environmental variables such as high-fat diets and inactivity lead to positive energy balance and obesity.

Interactions of Genes and Environment

Obesity is most likely to occur when a genetically susceptible individual encounters an environment conducive to obesity. An example is provided by Pima Indians living in Arizona. This population shows an extremely high prevalence of obesity, which seems to occur as a result of relatively low energy requirements per unit of fat-free mass coupled with low levels of physical activity and high intake of an energy-dense diet. Researchers have identified a group of Pima Indians living in northern Mexico who are genetically similar to the Pima Indians living in southern Arizona (Fig. 23-4). The Mexican Pimas are farmers, consuming food that they grow and engaging in high levels of physical activity (Esparza et al., 2000). The Mexican Pimas are significantly less obese than the Arizona Pimas, demonstrating the importance of environmental factors on body weight. However, the mean BMI for the Mexican Pimas is still greater than might be expected for a highly active population consuming a low-fat diet, suggesting that Pima Indians have genes that favor high body weight.

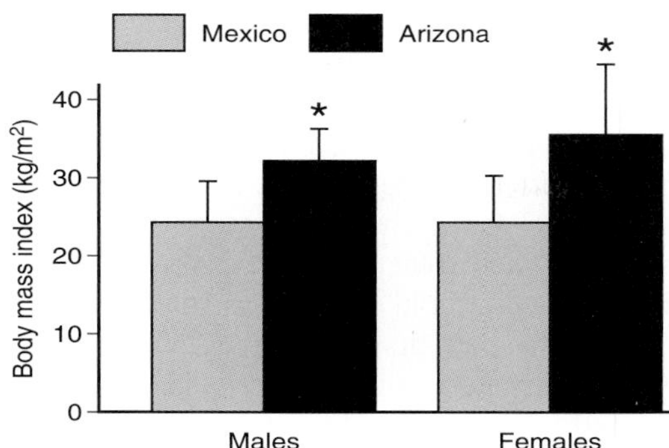

Figure 23-4 Mean body mass index (± standard deviation) of Pima Indians living in either a traditional lifestyle in Maycoba, Mexico, or a modern lifestyle in Arizona. *In both sexes, BMI was significantly higher ($P < 0.0001$) in Pimas living in Arizona compared with that of Pimas living in Mexico. *(Modified from Ravussin E, Tataranni PA [1997] Dietary fat and human obesity. J Am Diet Assoc 97:S42-S46. Copyright American Dietetic Association.)*

There is currently no consensus about the relative contribution of genetics versus environment to obesity. Some investigators have estimated that genes can explain 25% to 75% of the variation in body weight (Bouchard and Pérusse, 1993). However, the secular trend toward increased body weight in the United States highlights the importance of the interaction of the genotype with the environment. Because the genotype has not changed during the last decade, nongenetic factors, such as decreased physical activity and increased energy intake, must have made a major contribution to the increased body weight.

THERAPEUTIC APPROACHES TO THE TREATMENT OF OBESITY

Prevention of weight gain for both lean and obese individuals should be the first goal in obesity management. The second goal should be achievement of medically meaningful weight loss in overweight and obese individuals. Data from a number of studies have shown that modest weight loss (approximately 10%) is associated with substantial improvement in glycemic control (e.g., lower plasma insulin level) and lipid patterns (e.g., reduced low density lipoprotein [LDL] to high density lipoprotein [HDL] ratio) (Dansinger et al., 2005; Goldstein, 1992). Given the difficulty in maintaining large weight reductions, and data suggesting that more modest weight loss can improve health, it is important to set realistic goals for obesity treatment.

Compared to producing weight loss, maintaining a weight loss over a long period of time is difficult. Almost all "diets" work in the sense that they produce weight loss, but once the diet is discontinued the weight is usually regained over time (Dansinger et al., 2005). It is generally believed that the overall success rate in maintaining weight loss over 5 years is less than 5% to 10%. A great deal of research is aimed at understanding why maintaining a weight loss is so difficult and how to improve the success rate.

The current state-of-the-art program for obesity treatment consists of a behavioral treatment program aimed at modifying diet and physical activity. Such programs help overweight individuals make sustained changes in dietary and physical activity habits. Dietary modification usually involves some energy restriction, ranging from use of very low calorie diets to moderate energy restriction (Norris et al., 2004). Participants are also taught to increase physical activity. This has traditionally involved helping patients engage in regular aerobic activity, but in recent years, resistance training and the combination of aerobic and resistance training have been used. Better techniques for long-term maintenance of body weight after the conclusion of weight loss programs are greatly needed.

For obese adults (BMI ≥30 kg/m^2) who are unable to lose weight or maintain weight loss after diet or exercise alone, drug therapy may be recommended. Drug therapy may also be appropriate in persons with BMIs greater than 27 if they also have other significant conditions such as hypercholesterolemia. The available antiobesity drugs are either antiabsorptive drugs or antisatiety drugs. These prescription drugs are intended to be used in adults in conjunction with a weight loss program (reduced calorie diet, increased exercise) and are expected to result in modest weight loss.

Unfortunately, the choice of drugs for pharmacological treatment of obesity is very limited, and safety remains a concern. Amphetamines and amphetamine derivatives are no longer considered appropriate for use as appetite suppressants because they have a number of potentially dangerous side effects, including physical and psychological addiction, and can be used for only a few weeks. Two other appetite suppressants, fenfluramine and dexfenfluramine, were withdrawn from the market in 1997 after studies strongly suggested they could damage the heart's mitral valve. Herbal supplements that are marketed for weight loss often contain dangerous levels of ephedrine, an alkaloid present in some shrubs of the genus Ephedra (Chinese, Ma Huang). Use of these supplements has been associated with numerous deaths and injuries. The stimulant phenylpropanolamine, which was also used as a nasal decongestant in cough and cold products, was available as a nonprescription weight loss drug up until the year 2000 when the U.S. Food and Drug Administration (FDA) determined that phenylpropanolamine was associated with an increased risk of hemorrhagic stroke and withdrew its approval for sale in the United States.

Currently available drugs to treat obesity are orlistat and sibutramine. Orlistat (Xenical) is a lipase inhibitor that acts nonsystemically in the gut to inhibit pancreatic lipase, which is necessary for triglyceride digestion and absorption. In patients taking orlistat, approximately 30% of dietary fat passes through the bowel undigested and is excreted in the feces; this results in a loss of about 200 to 300 kcal/day. Fat-soluble vitamin supplements should be taken along with orlistat. Sibutramine (Meridia) is a norepinephrine and serotonin reuptake inhibitor that acts as an antisatiety drug. Serotonin and catecholamines affect mood and appetite; increasing the availability of these brain chemicals depresses appetite. Blood pressure should be carefully monitored in patients taking sibutramine because this drug can cause a significant elevation in blood pressure in some people. Safety and effectiveness have not been established for use of either orlistat or sibutramine for more than 12 months.

Surgical treatment is the only proven way to achieve long-term weight control for the severely obese. It is considered appropriate for those with BMIs greater than or equal to 40, or for those with BMIs greater than or equal to 35 who also have a life-threatening or disabling condition related to obesity, such as high blood pressure, cardiac illness, or type 2 diabetes. Gastrointestinal surgery (vertical banded gastroplasty or Roux-en-Y gastric bypass) is a viable option for many severely overweight patients (Sugerman, 1993). Most experts believe that patients should not be considered for surgery unless they have first tried more conventional treatments. Furthermore, potential patients should be selected only after careful examination by a multidisciplinary team with medical, surgical, psychiatric, and nutritional expertise. Lifelong medical surveillance after surgery is required. In appropriate patients, surgical treatment appears to produce substantial reductions in body weight, which in many patients are maintained over long periods and which often reduce the occurrence of comorbid conditions associated with obesity.

DIFFICULTIES INVOLVED IN THE MAINTENANCE OF A REDUCED BODY WEIGHT

Is the difficulty of maintaining a reduced body weight a problem with behavior or with physiology? Two metabolic changes that occur with weight loss and that may predispose to weight regain are a decrease in energy expenditure and a decrease in daily fat oxidation.

A lower body weight is associated with a lower energy requirement. If the level of physical activity does not change, all components of energy expenditure will decline with weight loss. The body mass lost by energy restriction consists of approximately 60% to 70% fat and 30% to 40% fat-free mass. Any decline in fat-free mass would be expected to produce a reduction in resting metabolic rate (RMR). In addition, a lower energy intake during or after weight loss would produce a decline in the thermic effect of food (TEF). Furthermore, as body mass declines, the energy cost of weight-bearing physical activity would decline. However, the declines in TEF and the energy cost of physical activity would be small in relation to the change in RMR.

A major question is whether the reductions in energy expenditure that occur with weight loss leave the reduced obese person with a lower level of energy expenditure than would be expected from the new body mass. Some, but not all, investigators have found this to be the case and suggest that this helps explain the high rate of relapse. Although there is debate about whether energy requirements of the reduced obese are lower than expected, it is clear that total energy expenditure declines with weight loss (assuming voluntary physical activity is constant). To maintain a reduced body weight, the reduced-obese individual must reduce energy intake and/or increase physical activity compared with before-weight-loss levels. The inability to make these permanent changes in lifestyle likely contributes to the high rate of weight regain. Again, gene × environment interactions are likely to be important, with some individuals probably showing greater declines in energy expenditure with weight loss than others. Those with greater declines in energy expenditure would be at higher risk for weight regain because they would be required to make and sustain greater lifestyle changes in order to maintain their reduced body weights.

Some investigators have reported that weight loss in obese individuals is associated with a reduced ability to oxidize fat. When compared with never-obese individuals consuming a similar diet, reduced, previously-obese individuals oxidize less fat in 24 hours. It has been suggested that this reduced ability to oxidize fat may involve reduced sympathetic nervous system activity. A reduced ability to oxidize fat may be a predisposing factor in body fat gain because any ingested fat that is not oxidized is stored as body fat. At present, fat oxidation has been studied in very few previously-obese subjects following weight loss. Whether a reduced ability to oxidize fat is a widespread characteristic of individuals who have lost weight and whether a low rate of fat oxidation contributes either to development of obesity or to an inability to maintain a weight reduction are questions that need to be addressed by further research.

The changes in energy expenditure and substrate oxidation that accompany weight loss make it essential to make permanent changes in lifestyle (e.g., diet and physical activity) in order to maintain a weight loss. Much of the poor success in weight maintenance could simply be because it is difficult for people to make permanent changes in behaviors that have been present for long periods. In support of this idea, when children and parents lose weight together, children are more successful in maintaining weight losses over time than their parents. This may be because it is easier for children to make and maintain the necessary lifestyle changes, having not practiced the predisposing lifestyle behaviors for as long a period as adults have.

METABOLIC SYNDROME

Along with the increase in the prevalence of obesity during the last decades, a new heterogeneous clinical disorder strongly associated with abdominal obesity and insulin resistance has been identified. This disorder has been called syndrome X and insulin-resistance syndrome and is now commonly known as metabolic syndrome (Moller and Kaufman, 2005). A joint conference of the American Heart Association (AHA), the National Heart, Lung and Blood Institute (NHLBI), and the American Diabetes Association (ADA) identified the major components of the syndrome as abdominal obesity, insulin resistance with or without glucose intolerance, atherogenic dyslipidemia, elevated blood pressure, a proinflammatory state, and a prothrombotic state (Grundy et al., 2004a). Individuals with this metabolic syndrome are at increased risk for development of type 2 diabetes, atherosclerotic cardiovascular disease, and cardiovascular death. Individuals with metabolic syndrome also seem to be more susceptible to some other conditions including polycystic ovary syndrome, fatty liver, cholesterol gallstones, asthma, sleep disturbances, and some forms of cancer.

DIAGNOSIS OF METABOLIC SYNDROME

Several schemes for the routine diagnosis of metabolic syndrome have been published. The National Cholesterol Education Program

(NCEP) Adult Treatment Panel III (ATP III) report (Grundy, 2001) states that three or more of the following must be present for a diagnosis of metabolic syndrome:

- Increased waist circumference: ≥102 cm (40 in.) in men and ≥88 cm (35 in.) in women
- Elevated triglycerides: ≥1.5 g/L (1.7 mmol/L)
- Reduced HDL cholesterol: <0.4g/L (1.0 mmol/L) in men and <0.5 g/L (1.3 mmol/L) in women
- Elevated blood pressure: ≥130/85 mm Hg or on treatment for hypertension
- Elevated fasting glucose: ≥1.1g/L (6.1mmol/L) [or ≥1.0 g/L (5.6 mmol/L), as established by American Diabetes Association]

The WHO criteria are similar (Alberti and Zimmet, 1998). WHO guidelines require the presence of impaired glucose regulation/insulin resistance, which is defined as type 2 diabetes mellitus *or* impaired fasting glycemia (>1.1 g/L) *or* impaired glucose tolerance *or* (for those with normal fasting glucose levels) glucose uptake below the lowest quartile for the background population under investigation under hyperinsulinemic/euglycemic conditions *plus* two of the following criteria:

- Elevated waist/hip ratio or elevated BMI: waist/hip ratio >0.90 in men and >0.85 in women; BMI >30 kg/m^2
- Elevated triglycerides: ≥1.5 g/L
- Reduced HDL cholesterol: <0.35 g/L (0.9 mmol/L) in men and <0.39 g/L (1.0 mmol/L) in women
- Elevated blood pressure: ≥140/90 mm Hg or on treatment for hypertension
- Excretion of albumin in urine: ≥20 μg/minute or albumin to creatine ratio ≥30 mg/g

Abnormal levels of various compounds that may serve as either markers or mediators of metabolic syndrome commonly aggregate with the major components listed in the preceding text. These include altered levels of plasma lipids (elevated serum triglycerides, elevated apolipoprotein B, elevated small dense low-density lipoprotein particles, and depressed levels of high-density lipoprotein cholesterol); altered levels of coagulation factors (elevated levels of plasminogen activator inhibitor-1 [PAI-1] and fibrinogen); elevated levels of cytokines (tumor necrosis factor–α and interleukin-6); and elevated levels of acute-phase proteins associated with inflammatory states (C-reactive protein [CRP]).

PREVALENCE OF METABOLIC SYNDROME

Characteristics of the metabolic syndrome occur in some children and adolescents, but the prevalence clearly increases with age so that the highest prevalence is observed in older persons. However, frequency rises rapidly in middle age and parallels, with some time lag, the development of obesity in the population. Aging is commonly accompanied by a loss of muscle mass and by an increase in body fat, particularly accumulation of fat in the abdomen.

By using the criteria of the NCEP ATP III and population statistics from 1988 to 1994, the overall prevalence of metabolic syndrome in adults in the United States was estimated to be approximately 24% (Ford et al., 2002). For adults older than 60 years of age, the prevalence was much higher at approximately 42%. Because the prevalence of both obesity and type 2 diabetes has increased markedly over the last 10 years, it is likely that these numbers underestimate the current prevalence of metabolic syndrome. About one third of obese individuals have the syndrome, and about three fourths of adults with type 2 diabetes have the syndrome.

Ethnic differences have been noted in the prevalence of metabolic syndrome and in the usefulness of the abdominal obesity measures. For example, Asians are less likely to exhibit the abdominal fat distribution pattern, and the prevalence of metabolic syndrome appears to be higher in Hispanic and South Asian populations.

ETIOLOGY OF METABOLIC SYNDROME

It is known that some monogenic disorders such as adipose tissue disorders cause severe metabolic syndrome, but these disorders are rare. Genetic forms of insulin resistance are a contributor to the metabolic syndrome in the general population. Polymorphisms in a variety of genes associate with the metabolic syndrome, but the contributions of these polymorphisms to the syndrome in the general public remain to be determined. The metabolic syndrome may also occur as a side effect of several commonly used drugs (e.g., corticosteroids, antidepressants, antipsychotics, and antihistamines), which can produce weight gain and, thus, predispose an individual to obesity and glucose intolerance.

There is little doubt, however, that the increasing prevalence of overweight/obesity is the main factor responsible for the rising prevalence of the metabolic syndrome in the United States and worldwide. Increases in the prevalence of metabolic syndrome follow increases in the prevalence of obesity/overweight in a population. Furthermore, a positive energy balance and increased adiposity are sufficient to initiate a cascade of events that result in all other aspects of metabolic syndrome.

Most commonly, the metabolic syndrome is associated with abdominal obesity, the form of obesity that often develops in middle age. An excess of visceral fat may be particularly pathogenic, but abdominal subcutaneous adipose tissue likely contributes as well, as can total body fat. Visceral adipose tissue may be particularly active in producing a number of these adipocyte-derived factors. In the presence of obesity, increased amounts of a number of compounds that may promote metabolic syndrome are released by adipocytes. These include nonesterified fatty acids, which can provoke peripheral insulin resistance and decreased peripheral glucose utilization; inflammatory cytokines (tumor necrosis factor–α and interleukin-6); resistin, an adipokine that can induce insulin resistance; and plasminogen activator inhibitor-1 (PAI-1), a protease inhibitor, which is also produced by the liver and endothelial cells, that acts to inhibit fibrinolysis (the breakdown of blood clots). Adiponectin and lectin are two other adipokines produced by white adipose tissue that play a role in metabolic syndrome. In obesity, adiponectin levels fall and leptin levels rise, but leptin insensitivity develops (Robinson and Graham, 2004). This leads to ectopic lipid accumulation and insulin insensitivity. Adiponectin has been shown to lower glucose levels, enhance insulin action, and reduce lipid accumulation in muscle and liver. Leptin acts as a satiety signal to the central nervous system and also has effects on peripheral tissues and functions as a cytokine that increases acutely during infection and inflammation (Faggioni et al., 2001). Leptin deficiency increases susceptibility to infectious and inflammatory stimuli and is associated with dysregulation of cytokine production. Although adipocyte-derived factors clearly appear to be involved in inducing insulin resistance and other features of the metabolic syndrome, the mechanism is likely very complex.

Most persons with multiple metabolic risk factors for metabolic syndrome are insulin resistant. Various schemes have been proposed to explain the connection between insulin resistance and metabolic risk factors. Insulin resistance is strongly associated with atherogenic dyslipidemia and a proinflammatory state, but it is less tightly associated with hypertension and the prothrombotic state. There is no doubt that insulin resistance leads to impaired glucose tolerance and type 2 diabetes, but a causal relationship between insulin resistance and the other risk factors is less certain owing to the complex interaction between obesity and defects in insulin signaling (i.e., it is not known if using drugs that reduce insulin resistance would substantially improve any of the components of the metabolic syndrome other than glucose intolerance). Therefore, the mechanistic links between insulin resistance and most of the components of the metabolic syndrome remain unclear.

The development of metabolic syndrome may be seen as an interaction between a genetic predisposition and lifestyle factors including overweight/obesity, physical inactivity, and intake of excess calories. Not all obese sedentary persons acquire metabolic syndrome, but metabolic syndrome is relatively uncommon in the absence of obesity and physical inactivity. For example, individuals with a family history of type 2 diabetes are at increased risk for metabolic syndrome, and this risk is further increased in those who become overweight or obese and adopt sedentary lifestyles. Also, women with a history of gestational diabetes or polycystic ovarian syndrome have an increased risk of metabolic syndrome. The subset of clinical features exhibited by individuals may also be strongly influenced by underlying genetic predisposition: whether dyslipidemia or glucose intolerance or visceral fat accumulation is the predominant phenotypic expression of metabolic syndrome may depend on an individual's genetic makeup.

Recent data suggest a link between malnutrition in utero (e.g., small-for-gestational age infants) with metabolic disturbances in later life. Reduced fetal growth is associated with an increased risk of the various components of metabolic syndrome in later life, and the initial development of insulin resistance appears to be a key component underlying the development of these metabolic complications (Levy-Marchal and Jaquet, 2004).

THERAPEUTIC APPROACHES TO THE TREATMENT OF METABOLIC SYNDROME

Two general approaches are used in the treatment of metabolic syndrome (Grundy et al., 2004b; Moller and Kaufman, 2005). The first strategy seeks to modify the root causes, including overweight/obesity and physical inactivity. Weight reduction and increased physical activity have been shown to improve lipid profiles, decrease blood pressure, and improve insulin sensitivity. The second strategy directly treats the metabolic risk. Although pharmacological modification of the associated risk factors may be more easily achieved in practice, the greatest potential for management of the syndrome clearly lies in reversing its root causes.

Dietary management and physical activity are considered first-line therapies in overweight and obese patients with metabolic syndrome. Emphasis should be on achievement of a medically beneficial weight loss (i.e., a reduction in obesity-associated risk factors) and prevention of weight regain. Modest reduced-energy diets (a reduction of 500 to 1,000 kcal/day) and a realistic goal for weight reduction (a loss of 7% to 10% of body weight over a 6- to 12-month period) are recommended. The standard exercise recommendation is a daily minimum of 30 minutes of moderate-intensity physical activity. Increasing the level of physical activity (i.e., 1 hour daily) is even more efficacious for weight control and improvement of clinical symptoms. Changes in diet composition, particularly the inclusion of unsaturated fat in the diet and the avoidance of very-high-carbohydrate diets, can reduce atherogenic dyslipidemia and may be beneficial, but the clinical significance of this is undetermined for patients with metabolic syndrome.

Weight loss lowers serum cholesterol and triglyceride levels, raises HDL cholesterol level, lowers blood pressure and glucose level, and reduces insulin resistance. Weight reduction can also decrease serum levels of CRP and PAI-1. Several clinical trials of subjects with prediabetes (impaired glucose tolerance or elevated fasting plasma glucose levels) showed that a combination of weight reduction and increased physical activity resulted in a marked reduction in the progression to new-onset diabetes (Norris et al., 2005).

In patients in whom lifestyle changes fail to reverse metabolic risk factors, consideration should be given to treating specific abnormalities with drugs. In the XENDOS trial, the use of orlistat (an intestinal lipase inhibitor indicated for the treatment of obesity) plus lifestyle modification reduced the incidence of type 2 diabetes in obese subjects 37% more than lifestyle modification alone (Torgerson et al., 2004).

Metformin and insulin sensitizers (such as thiazolidinediones) have been used in the treatment of type 2 diabetes. Statins and fibrates are used to reduce the risk for cardiovascular disease events in patients with metabolic syndrome. Lipid-lowering drugs may reduce the proinflammatory state. Antihypertensive drugs are used to treat hypertension. No drugs are available that target PAI-1 and fibrinogen, but antiplatelet therapy (low-dose aspirin) may be promising in patients with metabolic syndrome.

STARVATION AND PROTEIN ENERGY MALNUTRITION

In contrast to obesity, starvation can be induced by a reduction in energy intake leading to a decrease in body weight. An adequate energy intake is especially important in children in order to maintain a satisfactory growth rate. Reduced dietary intake leads to declines in growth velocity in the child and reductions in body weight in the adult. When compared with normal individuals of the same stature, age, and gender, undernourished subjects have a reduced lean body mass as well as less fat, whereas the obese have an increase in both.

DEFINITIONS OF UNDERNUTRITION

Graham Lusk in 1928 defined starvation as the deprivation of any element necessary for an organism's nutrition (Lusk, 1928). The term now usually refers to a chronic, inadequate intake of dietary energy, protein, or both. Adaptation to such a low-calorie diet typically includes a decrease in physical activity and a decrease in RMR. When these decreases do not lower the energy output sufficiently to bring energy expenditure into balance with the limited intake, endogenous fuels must be used to balance the equation, resulting in a net loss of body energy stores.

The term PEM, or protein-energy malnutrition, is applied to a group of related disorders. These include the clinical syndromes of marasmus, kwashiorkor, and intermediate states of marasmus-kwashiorkor along with milder forms of malnutrition. These typically are associated with poor weight gain or weight loss and a slowing of linear growth (stunting). Dietary energy and protein deficiencies usually occur together, but sometimes one predominates and, if severe enough, leads to the clinical syndrome of kwashiorkor or marasmus. Deficiencies of iron, vitamin A, iodine, zinc, and other micronutrients often occur simultaneously with PEM and are important causes of anemia, loss of night vision, blindness, goiter, brain damage, mental retardation, and skin lesions.

In general, marasmus is caused by an insufficient energy intake, resulting in emaciation. Kwashiorkor generally results from more adequate energy intake but an inadequate amount or quality of dietary protein, leading to decreased synthesis of visceral proteins. The term marasmus is derived from the Greek *marasmos,* which means "withering or wasting." The term *kwashiorkor,* taken from the Ga language of Ghana, means "first child–second child." The term referred to the sickness observed in children after weaning due to the birth of a second child, when breast milk was replaced by foods that are high in starch and low in protein (e.g., yam, cassava, sweet potato, or green banana). Children with marasmus appear emaciated with marked loss of subcutaneous fat and muscle wasting. Marasmic children have retarded growth and feel hungry. In addition to retarded growth, children with kwashiorkor typically have edema, a swollen abdomen, and a fatty liver, and often have characteristic skin changes and depigmentation of the hair. Children with kwashiorkor are usually apathetic and anorexic. Children with intermediate forms of marasmic kwashiorkor typically have some edema and more body fat than those with marasmus.

PREVALENCE AND CAUSES OF UNDERNUTRITION

Starvation affects many populations all over the world. Worldwide, the most common cause of malnutrition is inadequate food intake. At times, severe food shortages in poor, underdeveloped countries have led to overwhelming famine and starvation.

PEM is the most important nutritional disease in the developing countries because of its high prevalence and its relationship with child mortality rates, impaired physical growth, and inadequate social and economic development. The Food and Agriculture Organization (FAO, 2004) estimated that 852 million people worldwide were undernourished in 2000-2002. This number is made up of 815 million people in developing countries, 28 million in countries in transition, and 9 million in industrialized countries. More than 40 million preschool children in developing countries were classified as wasted, more than 112 million as underweight, and more than 135 million as stunted (≤2 standard deviations of the median value for weight-for-height, weight-for-age, or height-for-age values, respectively, of the NCHS/WHO international reference data; United Nations System, 2004). Of the total number of people affected by PEM, about 69% live in Asia and the Pacific, 10% in Latin American and the Caribbean, 8% in Near East and North Africa, and 13% in Sub-Saharan Africa. As a proportion of the total population, the prevalence of undernourishment is 16% in Asia and the Pacific, 10% in Latin American and the Caribbean, 10% in Near East and North Africa, and 33% in Sub-Saharan Africa. FAO lists 19 countries where 35% or more of the population is undernourished (FAO, 2004).

The clinical syndromes of marasmus and kwashiorkor most commonly occur in children younger than 5 years. This period is characterized by increased protein and energy requirements, dependence upon others for food, immature immune systems causing a greater susceptibility to infection, and exposure to nonhygienic conditions. Ineffective weaning secondary to ignorance, poor hygiene, economic factors, and cultural factors may also play a role. Gastrointestinal infections often precipitate clinical PEM because of associated diarrhea, anorexia, vomiting, increased metabolic needs, and decreased intestinal absorption. Parasitic infection plays a major role in many parts of the world. Maternal malnutrition prior to and/or during pregnancy also plays a role. Undernourished women are more likely to produce an underweight newborn baby; in some countries (e.g., India and Bangladesh) more than 30% of all children are born underweight. If intrauterine malnutrition is compounded after birth or after weaning by insufficient food to satisfy the infant's needs for catch-up growth, PEM can result. A high proportion of childhood deaths worldwide are due to being underweight.

When stunting occurs during the first 5 years of life, the damage to physical and cognitive development is usually irreversible. Malnourished people who survive childhood often have lifelong disabilities. In populations in which clinical PEM is observed, many older children and adults are stunted as a result of inadequate nutrition during periods of growth. Maternal stunting is a strong predictor for giving birth to a low-birth-weight infant, along with underweight and low weight gain during pregnancy, giving rise to a vicious cycle of deprivation. Interestingly, although low birth weight and undernutrition early in life are associated with an increased prevalence of PEM in environments with limited food resources, low birth weight and undernutrition early in life are associated with increased risk of obesity and diet-related diseases in adulthood in industrialized countries.

The origin of PEM can be secondary, when it is the result of other diseases that lead to low food ingestion, inadequate nutrient absorption or utilization, increased nutritional requirements, and/or increased nutrient losses. In contrast to the prevalence of primary PEM in developing countries, malnutrition more commonly is secondary to another disorder in industrialized countries. Secondary PEM may result from malabsorption, congenital defects, renal failure, endocrine disease, or emotional deprivation. Diseases such as cystic fibrosis, chronic renal failure, childhood malignancies, congenital heart disease, and neuromuscular diseases are associated with undernutrition. Fad diets, inappropriate management of food allergies, and psychiatric disease, such as anorexia nervosa, can also lead to severe PEM.

Undernutrition is present in many institutionalized and hospitalized patients (Hudson et al., 2000; Omran and Morley, 2000). These populations are susceptible to starvation due to the inability to eat or to the substantial increase in energy expenditure that results from severe trauma or infection. The elderly are particularly susceptible to PEM because of a higher incidence of dysphagia, lower muscle mass and body weight, and long-term residential care situations. Indications for a diagnosis of PEM in these populations is an unintentional loss of greater than 10% of usual body weight in less than 6 months and a serum albumin level of less than 36 g/L. Visceral protein depletion is also indicated by transferring less than 2 g/L and a total lymphocyte count of less than 1,500 per milliliter of blood. Weight loss in the elderly correlates with morbidity and mortality. Undernutrition increases the risk of respiratory and cardiac problems, infections, deep venous thrombosis and pressure ulcers, perioperative mortality, and multiorgan failure.

ADAPTATION TO SHORT-TERM OR PROLONGED STARVATION

The response to starvation can best be understood as a protective mechanism in which the body attempts to maintain energy balance and avoid loss of body mass. When energy intake is low, the body relies on endogenous fuel sources, which are mainly adipose tissue triacylglycerols and skeletal muscle proteins. The primary metabolic signals touching off these events are a fall in the plasma level of insulin and an increase in the concentration of glucagon, caused by limited intake of dietary carbohydrate and thus a low plasma glucose concentration. Hypoinsulinemia facilitates mobilization of free fatty acids, starvation ketosis, and net catabolism of skeletal muscle protein to maintain visceral protein synthesis.

The essential features of the metabolic response to starvation are altered rates and patterns of fuel utilization and protein metabolism, aimed at minimizing fuel needs and limiting lean tissue loss. The nature of the starvation diet determines the pattern of hormone levels and fuel consumption. In total fasting, the liver glycogen stores are rapidly depleted and the body turns to gluconeogenesis, mainly from amino acid side chains, to maintain plasma glucose levels. Therefore, starvation diets produce an alteration of overall protein metabolism that is characterized by an initial rapid loss of body protein, but this is followed by a prolonged period during which further protein losses are minimized to protect lean body mass. This is associated with a slowed rate of synthesis and breakdown of body protein.

In prolonged starvation, fat oxidation becomes the dominant fuel. Hepatic ketogenesis from fatty acids provides an additional fuel for most tissues. The brain switches from exclusively glucose to predominantly ketone body oxidation. The fuel of resting muscle switches from predominantly fatty acids to ketone bodies, finally returning, after weeks of total fasting, to fatty acid oxidation. The metabolic ketoacidosis of prolonged fasting induces a compensatory increase in renal production of ammonia in order to increase removal of hydrogen ions from the body as ammonium. This change is associated with augmented renal gluconeogenesis and a somewhat greater loss of body nitrogen than would occur without the acidosis. The body fat supply appears to determine the length of survival. Once fat is depleted, the body has no choice but to consume its functional protein reserves and death rapidly ensues. Loss of more than 40% of body weight is usually fatal, with death usually resulting from heart failure, electrolyte imbalance, or low body temperature. The survival of a nonobese fasting individual coincides roughly with the predicted time of depletion of fat, approximately 60 days. Obviously, obese individuals with their greater stores of fat have a survival advantage under starvation conditions.

ADAPTATION TO CHRONIC UNDERNUTRITION

Protein energy malnutrition develops gradually over many days or months in the face of inadequate sustained food intake. This process allows a series of metabolic and behavioral adjustments that result in decreased nutrient demands and alterations in fuel metabolism and body composition, similar to those seen in starvation.

As the cumulative energy deficit becomes more severe, subcutaneous fat is markedly reduced, and protein catabolism leads to muscular wasting. Visceral protein is preserved longer, especially in the marasmic patient. In marasmus, there is usually an increase in basal oxygen consumption, which then declines as the disease becomes more severe. In kwashiorkor, the severe dietary protein deficit leads to an earlier visceral depletion of amino acids that affects visceral cell function and reduces oxygen consumption. Thus in individuals with kwashiorkor, RMR decreases per unit of lean or total body mass. Because of a depletion of visceral protein and inadequate protein intake, individuals with kwashiorkor have hypoalbuminemia, which causes edema, and impaired apolipoprotein B synthesis, which causes fatty liver.

Blood glucose concentration usually remains normal, mainly at the expense of gluconeogenic amino acids, but it falls in severe PEM. The fall in blood glucose in severe PEM is not so much due to a reduction of total nitrogen or amino acid turnover but to an increase in the proportion of the amino acid pool that is used for resynthesis of protein and a corresponding reduction in the proportion of amino acids that are catabolized with nitrogen excretion and gluconeogenesis. The gradual and inevitable loss of body protein as a result of a long-term dietary protein deficit is primarily a loss of skeletal muscle protein. Some visceral protein is lost in the early development of PEM, but then the amount of visceral protein becomes stable until the nonessential tissue proteins are depleted. Once these less critical tissues are depleted, the loss of visceral protein increases; at this point death may be imminent unless nutritional therapy is successfully instituted.

If undernutrition is imposed early in life when growth is most rapid, complete recovery in size (height and weight) may never be possible, even though the undernutrition is temporary and plentiful food is supplied thereafter. Although undernutrition retards growth in all parts of the body, some parts are affected more than others. In severe undernutrition, adipocytes become unrecognizable as cells; the empty space between cells fills with an extracellular gel; and muscle fibers shrink. There is less change in the composition of the kidneys and heart, and the brain is the least affected. If undernutrition is imposed during adult life, mild-to-moderate PEM results in leanness, with reduction in subcutaneous tissue. The most common change in body composition is a reduction of adiposity below the average 12% and 20% expected in normal, well-nourished men and women, respectively.

TREATMENT OF PROTEIN ENERGY MALNUTRITION

The first step in the treatment of individuals with severe PEM is the correction of fluid and electrolyte abnormalities and the treatment of infections with antibiotics. The second step is oral feeding, which usually involves the introduction of a nutritious formula, with the daily amount being gradually increased over 1 to 3 weeks. The formula can be given through a tube, if necessary. Introduction of food may be delayed if diarrhea is severe. After several weeks, the formula can be replaced by solid foods.

RECOMMENDATIONS FOR ENERGY INTAKE AND EXPENDITURE

Recommendations for energy intake obviously must take energy expenditure for activity into account. Because of the strong evidence that a higher level of physical activity is beneficial in weight maintenance as well as having health benefits independent of weight regulation, a number of recommendations for activity level have been made in recent years.

DIETARY REFERENCE INTAKES: ESTIMATED ENERGY REQUIREMENTS

The Institute of Medicine (IOM, 2002) set estimated energy requirements (EERs) as part of the dietary reference intakes (DRIs). The EER is defined as the dietary energy intake that is predicted to maintain energy balance in a healthy adult of a defined age, gender, height, weight, and level of physical activity consistent with good health. In setting energy requirements, the IOM defined healthy weights as a BMI between 18.5 and 25 kg/m^2 for adults (which corresponds to 13% to 21% body fat in men and 23% to 31% body fat in women), as the 5th to 85th BMI percentiles for children aged 3 to 18 years, and as the 3rd to 97th weight-for-length percentiles for children aged 0 to 2 years. Equations were developed for prediction of TEE for normal-weight individuals based on data for total daily energy expenditure measured by the doubly labeled water technique. For children and pregnant and lactating women, an estimate of the needs associated with tissue deposition or secretion of milk were added to calculate the EER.

Recommendations for energy intake were established in terms of physical activity level (PAL), with PAL equal to total energy expenditure/basal energy expenditure (TEE/BEE). The following four categories were used:

1. Sedentary: PAL $\geq 1.0 < 1.4$;
2. Low active: PAL $\geq 1.4 < 1.6$
3. Active: PAL $\geq 1.6 < 1.9$
4. Very active: PAL $\geq 1.9 < 2.5$

For subjects in the doubly labeled water database used to estimate TEE, the mean PAL was in the low active/active range (1.5 to 1.8) for all age-sex groupings, except for the very young (those aged <8 years) and the elderly (those aged >71 years).

A fundamental difference between the DRIs for energy intake and other nutrients is that recommendations are not set with an allowance to provide for the needs of nearly all healthy individuals in the population. The sustained consumption of even small amounts of energy in excess or less than the amount expended can have consequences in terms of body weight and health, precluding the inclusion of an extra allowance to ensure adequate intakes for all individuals. Desirable energy intakes are those that support healthy body weights and composition and adequate levels of physical activity. In establishing estimates of energy requirements, the IOM's aim was to establish recommendations and requirements that allowed the maintenance of a stable weight within a healthy BMI range and level of physical activity consistent with long-term good health. Clearly, energy requirements need to be determined individually. Body weight provides a readily monitored indicator of the adequacy or inadequacy of habitual energy intake in each individual. Desirable intakes may be greater than energy expenditure for underweight individuals or less than energy expenditure for overweight individuals.

PREDICTIVE EQUATIONS FOR ESTIMATION OF TOTAL ENERGY EXPENDITURE AND ESTIMATED ENERGY REQUIREMENTS

The IOM (2002) developed the following predictive equations for TEE for various age and gender groups with adjustment for activity level:

- Children ages 0 through 2 years

$$\text{TEE (kcal/day)} = [89 \times \text{Wt}] - 100$$

- Boys ages 3 through 18 years

$$\text{TEE (kcal/day)} = 88.5 - [61.9 \times \text{Age}] + [\text{PA}] \times [(26.7 \times \text{Wt}) + (903 \times \text{Ht})]$$

- Girls ages 3 through 18 years:

$$\text{TEE (kcal/day)} = 135.3 - [30.8 \times \text{Age}] + [\text{PA}] \times [(10.0 \times \text{Wt}) + (934 \times \text{Ht})]$$

- Women age 19 years and older

$$\text{TEE (kcal/day)} = 354 - [6.91 \times \text{Age}] + [\text{PA}] \times [(9.36 \times \text{Wt}) + (726 \times \text{Ht})]$$

- Men aged 19 years and older

$$\text{TEE} = 662 - [9.53 \times \text{Age}] + [\text{PA}] \times [(15.9 \times \text{Wt}) + (540 \times \text{Ht})]$$

where

Wt = Weight (kg)
Ht = Height (m)
Age = Age (years)
PA = 1.00 if PAL is estimated to be $\geq 1.0 < 1.4$ (Sedentary)
PA = 1.11 if PAL is estimated to be $\geq 1.4 < 1.6$ (Low active)
PA = 1.25 if PAL is estimated to be $\geq 1.6 < 1.9$ (Active)
PA = 1.48 if PAL is estimated to be $\geq 1.9 < 2.5$ (Very active)

For adults with healthy body weights, the EER is equal to the TEE. For children up through age 18, an allowance for energy deposition was added to the TEE to calculate the EER. The amounts added (kcal/day) are 175, 56, 22, and 20 kcal/day for infants whose ages are 0 to 3 months, 4 to 6 months, 7 to 12 months, and 13 to 35 months, respectively; 20 kcal/day for boys and girls from 3 to 8 years of age; and 25 kcal/day for boys and girls from 9 to 18 years of age. An additional 180 kcal/day was added for pregnant women in the second and third trimesters of pregnancy. For lactating women, an additional 330 kcal/day was added for the first 6 months of lactation, which was calculated to be 170 kcal/day less than the 500 kcal/day needed for milk production so that weight gained during pregnancy can be lost. During the second 6 months of lactation, 400 kcal/day are added to provide for milk energy output, which on average is somewhat less than during the first 6 months.

RECOMMENDATIONS FOR PHYSICAL ACTIVITY

In 66% of the adult men and women with BMIs within the healthy range of 18.5 to 25, PALs were categorized as either active or very active. Based on this and on epidemiologic studies, the IOM recommends that adults get 60 minutes per day of physical activity of moderate intensity (e.g., brisk walking) in order to maintain a PAL greater than or equal to 1.6. Other organizations also recommend a PAL within the active range. The WHO (WHO, 1998) recommends a PAL of 1.75 (60 minutes of exercise per day). The International Association for the Study of Obesity recommends a similar amount of physical activity is necessary to prevent weight gain in adult populations: moderate intensity activity of approximately 45 to 60 minutes/day, or a PAL of 1.7.

Interestingly, reconstruction of the probable physical activity of ancestral humans living during the Stone Age yielded an average energy expenditure for physical activity as 1,240 kcal (5.4 MJ) per day, as contrasted with an estimated 555 kcal (2.3 MJ) per day for a hypothetical 64-kg contemporary American adult (Eaton and Eaton, 2003). Eaton and Eaton further proposed that the PAL for these ancestral humans was likely in the range of 1.74, which turns out to be very similar to the activity level currently recommended by the IOM, WHO, and other organizations.

How much exercise is required to obtain a particular PAL? The IOM estimated the amount of walking at a rate of 3 to 4 miles per hour that would be needed daily (on top of a sedentary lifestyle) to achieve various PAL levels. For example, a 70-kg individual would need to walk 2.2 miles per day for a PAL of 1.5 (low active), 7.3 miles per day for a PAL of 1.75 (active), or 16.7 miles per day for a PAL of 2.2 (very active) (Brooks et al., 2004; IOM, 2002).

The time needed in activity depends on effort. Health Canada (2003) suggests 60 minutes of light effort activity (e.g., light walking, volleyball); 30 to 60 minutes of moderate effort exercise (e.g., brisk walking, swimming); or 20 to 30 minutes of vigorous effort exercise (e.g., jogging, hockey). As an example for comparison purposes, the energy expended for activity is approximately the same for 45 to 60 minutes spent washing and waxing a car, washing windows, or playing volleyball as it is for 15 minutes spent shoveling snow, jumping rope, or running at a rate of 1 mile per 10 minutes. Physical activity is clearly helpful in maintenance of a desirable body weight and composition. Physical activity increases energy expenditure and allows greater food intake at a given body weight, which improves the intake of other essential nutrients. In addition to weight control, physical activity reduces risk of hypertension and type 2 diabetes, develops improvements in the cardiovascular system, improves lipoprotein profiles in older adults, slows bone loss associated with advancing age, lowers the risk of certain cancers, and helps reduce anxiety and depression.

REFERENCES

Alberti AG, Zimmet PZ (1998) Definition, diagnosis and classification of diabetes mellitus and its complications, I: diagnosis and classification of diabetes mellitus provisional report of a WHO consultation. Diabet Med 15: 539–553.

Bouchard C, Pérusse L (1993) Genetics of obesity. Annu Rev Nutr 13:337-334.

Brooks GA, Butte NF, Rand WM, Flatt J-P, Caballero B (2004) Chronicle of the Institute of Medicine physical activity recommendation: how a physical activity recommendation came to be among dietary recommendations. Am J Clin Nutr 79:921S-930S.

Calle EE, Rodriguez C, Walker-Thurmond K, Thun MJ (2003) Overweight, obesity, and mortality from cancer in a prospectively studied cohort of U.S. adults N Engl J Med 348:1625-1638.

Calle EE, Thun MJ, Petrelli JM, Rodriguez C, Heath CW Jr (1999) BMI and mortality in prospective cohort of U.S. adults. N Engl J Med 341:1097–105.

Colditz GA, Willett WC, Rotnitzky A, Manson JE (1995) Weight gain as a risk factor for clinical diabetes mellitus in women. Ann Intern Med 122:481-486.

Dansinger ML, Gleason JA, Griffith JL, Selker HP, Schaefer EJ (2005) Comparison of the Atkins, Ornish, Weight Watchers, and Zone diets for weight loss and heart disease risk reduction: a randomized trial. JAMA 293:43-53.

Despres J-P (1993) Abdominal obesity as an important component of insulin-resistance syndrome. Nutrition 9:452-459.

Eaton SB, Eaton SB (2003) An evolutionary perspective on human physical activity: implications for health. Comp Biochem Physiol Pt A 136:153-159.

Esparza J, Fox C, Harper IT, Bennett PH, Schulz LO, Valencia ME, Ravussin E (2000) Daily energy expenditure in Mexican and USA Pima Indians: low physical activity as a possible cause of obesity. Int J Obes Relat Metab Disord 24:55-59.

Faggioni R, Feingold KR, Grunfeld C (2001) Leptin regulation of the immune response and the immunodeficiency of malnutrition. FASEB J 15:2165-2171.

Farooqi IS, O'Rahilly S (2004) Monogenic human obesity syndromes. Recent Prog Horm Res 59:409-424.

Food and Agriculture Organization (FAO) (2004) The State of Food Insecurity in the World 2004: Monitoring Progress Towards the World Food Summit and Millennium Development Goals. FAO, Rome.

Ford E, Giles W, Dietz W (2002) Prevalence of the metabolic syndrome among U.S. adults. Findings from the Third National Health and Nutrition Examination Survey. JAMA 287:356-359.

Goldstein DJ (1992) Beneficial health effects of modest weight loss. Int J Obes 16:397-415.

Grundy SM (2001) United States Cholesterol Guidelines 2001: expanded scope of intensive low-density lipoprotein-lowering therapy. Am J Cardiol 88:23J-27J.

Grundy S, Brewer HB Jr, Cleeman JI, Smith SC Jr, Lenfant C (2004a) AHA/NHLBI/ADA conference proceedings: definition of metabolic syndrome. Report of the National Heart, Lung, and Blood Institute/American Heart Association conference on scientific issues related to definition. Circulation 109:433-438.

Grundy SM, Hansen B, Smith SC Jr, Cleeman JI, Kahn RA (2004b) AHA/NHLBI/ADA conference proceedings: clinical management of metabolic syndrome. Report of the American Heart Association/National Heart, Lung, and Blood Institute/American Diabetes Association conference on scientific issues related to management. Circulation 109:551-556.

Health Canada (2003) Canada's Physical Activity Guide to Healthy Active Living. Health Canada, Ottawa, Ontario, Canada. Retrieved November 12, 2005, from http://www.phac-aspc.gc.ca/pau-uap/paguide/

Hedley AA, Ogden CL, Johnson CL, Carroll MD, Curtin LR, Flegal KM (2004) Prevalence of overweight and obesity among US children, adolescents, and adults,1999-2002. JAMA 291:2847-2850.

Horton TJ, Drougas H, Brachey A, Reed G.W, Peters JC, Hill JO (1995) Fat and carbohydrate overfeeding in humans: different effects on energy storage. Am J Clin Nutr 62:19-29.

Hudson HM, Daubert CR, Mills RH (2000) The interdependency of protein-energy malnutrition, aging, and dysphagia. Dysphagia 15:31-38.

Institute of Medicine (2002) Dietary Reference Intakes: Energy, Carbohydrate, Fiber, Fat, Fatty Acids, Cholesterol, Protein, and Amino Acids. National Academy Press, Washington, DC.

Lemieux S (1997) Genetic susceptibility to visceral obesity and related clinical implications. Int J Obes Relat Metab Disord 21:831-838.

Levy-Marchal C, Jaquet D (2004) Long-term metabolic consequences of being born small for gestational age. Pediatr Diabetes 5:147-153.

Lissner L, Bjorkelund C, Heitmann BL, Deidell JC, Bengtsson C (2001) Large hip circumference independently predicts health and longevity in a Swedish female cohort. Obes Res 9:644-646.

Lusk G (1928) The Elements of the Science of Nutrition, 4th ed. W.B. Saunders, Philadelphia, pp 447-486.

Mokdad AH, Ford ES, Bowman BA, Dietz WH, Vinicor F, Bales VS, Marks JS (2003) Prevalence of obesity, diabetes, and obesity-related health risk factors, 2001. JAMA 289:76-79.

Moller DE, Kaufman KD (2005) Metabolic syndrome: a clinical and molecular perspective. Annu Rev Med 56:45-62.

National Institutes of Health (NIH) (1998) Clinical Guidelines on the Identification, Evaluation, and Treatment of Overweight and Obesity in Adults—The Evidence Report. Obes Res 6(Suppl 2):51S-209S.

Norris SL, Zhang X, Avenell A, Gregg E, Bowman B, Serdula M, Brown TJ, Schmid CH, Lau J (2004) Long-term effectiveness of lifestyle and behavioral weight loss interventions in adults with type 2 diabetes: a meta-analysis. Am J Med 117:762-774.

Norris SL, Zhang X, Avenell A, Gregg E, Schmid CH, Lau J (2005) Long-term non-pharmacological weight loss interventions for adults with prediabetes. Cochrane Database Syst Rev 2:CD005270.

Ogden CL, Fryar CD, Carroll MD, Flegal KM (2004) Mean body weight, height, and body mass index, United States 1960-2002. Adv Data 347:1-17.

Omran ML, Morley JE (2000) Assessment of protein energy malnutrition in older persons, Part I: History, examination, body composition, and screening tools. Nutrition 16:50-63.

Pagliassotti MJ, Gayles EC, Hill JO (1997) Fat and energy balance. Ann N Y Acad Sci 827:431-448.

Perissinotto E, Pisent C, Sergi G, Grigoletto F; ILSA Working Group (Italian Longitudinal Study on Ageing) (2002) Anthropometric measurements in the elderly: age and gender differences. Br J Nutr 87:177-186.

Pi-Sunyer FX (1993) Medical hazards of obesity. Ann Intern Med 119:655-660.

Pouliot M-C, Despres J-P, Lemieux S, Moorjani S, Bouchard C, Tremblay A, Nadeau A, Lupien PJ (1994) Waist circumference and abdominal sagittal diameter: Best simple anthropometric indexes of abdominal visceral adipose tissue accumulation and related cardiovascular risk in men and women. Am J Cardiol 73:460-468.

Robinson LE, Graham TE (2004) Metabolic syndrome, a cardiovascular disease risk factor: role of adipocytokines and impacts of diet and physical activity. Can J Appl Physiol 29:808-829.

Snyder EE, Walts B, Perusse L, Chagnon YC, Weisnagel SJ, Rankinen T, Bouchard C (2004) The human obesity gene map: the 2003 update. Obes Res 12:369-439.

Sugerman HJ (1993) Surgery for morbid obesity. Surgery 114:865-867.

Torgerson J, Hauptman J, Boldrin M. Sjostrom L (2004) XENical in the prevention of diabetes in obese subjects (XENDOS) study: a randomized study of orlistat as an adjunct to lifestyle changes for the prevention of type 2 diabetes in obese patients. Diabetes Care 27:155-161.

Troiano RP, Flegal KM, Kuczmarski RJ, Campbell SM, Johnson CL (1995) Overweight prevalence and trends for children and adolescents. Arch Pediatr Adolesc Med 149:1085-1091.

United Nations System (2004) Fifth Report on the World Nutrition Situation: Nutrition for Improved Development Outcomes. United Nations System Standing Committee on Nutrition Secretariat, Geneva.

World Health Organization (WHO) (2003) The WHO Global Database on Body Mass Index (BMI). Department of Nutrition for Health and Development (NHD), WHO, Geneva.

World Health Organization (WHO) (1998) Obesity: Preventing and Managing the Global Epidemic. WHO Technical Report Series 894. WHO, Geneva.

World Health Organization (WHO) (1997) Obesity: Preventing and Managing the Global Epidemic. Report of a WHO Consultation on Obesity. Geneva, June 3-5, 1997.

Zamboni M, Armellini F, Turcato E, de Pergola G, Todesco T, Bissoli L, Bergamo Andreis, IA, Bosello O (1994) Relationship between visceral fat, steroid hormones and insulin sensitivity in premenopausal obese women. J Intern Med 236:521-527.

RECOMMENDED READINGS

Institute of Medicine (IOM) (2002) Dietary Reference Intakes: Energy, Carbohydrate, Fiber, Fat, Fatty Acids, Cholesterol, Protein, and Amino Acids. National Academy Press, Washington, DC.

Moller DE, Kaufman KD (2005) Metabolic syndrome: a clinical and molecular perspective. Annu Rev Med 56:45-62.

Snyder EE, Walts B, Perusse L, Chagnon YC, Weisnagel SJ, Rankinen T, Bouchard C (2004) The human obesity gene map: the 2003 update. Obes Res 12:369-439.

World Health Organization (WHO) (1999) Management of Severe Malnutrition: A Manual for Physicians and Other Senior Health Workers. WHO, Geneva.

RECOMMENDED WEBSITES

Detailed advice for weight reduction can be obtained from obesity guidelines at websites maintained by:

National Heart, Lung and Blood Institute (NHLBI)
www.nhlbi.nih.gov

American Heart Association
www.americanheart.org

Centers for Disease Control and Prevention (CDC), National Center for Chronic Disease Prevention and Health Promotion
www.cdc.gov/nccdphp/dnpa/obesity/

American Obesity Association (AOA)
www.obesity.org/

Information about worldwide nutrition problems related to energy is available at websites maintained by:

United Nations System Standing Committee on Nutrition (SCN)
www.unsystem.org/scn/

Food and Agriculture Organization of the United Nations (FAO)
www.fao.org

World Health Organization (WHO)
www.who.int

Unit VI

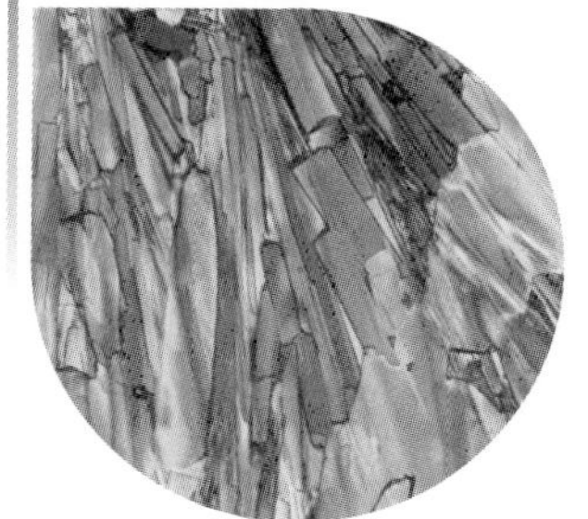

The Vitamins

Vitamins are defined as organic compounds that are required in the diet in only small amounts to maintain fundamental functions of the body (growth, metabolism, and cellular integrity). This definition distinguishes vitamins from the organic macronutrients because vitamins are neither catabolized to CO_2 and H_2O to satisfy part of the energy requirement nor used for structural purposes; hence, vitamins are required in much smaller amounts than are carbohydrates, proteins, and triacylglycerols. Vitamins are distinguished from the minerals (which also are required in relatively small amounts compared with nutrients used as sources of energy) by their organic rather than inorganic nature.

Well before the twentieth century, the curative effects of certain foods were recognized. An ancient Egyptian medical treatise recommended eating roast ox liver or black cock's liver to cure night blindness, and early reports indicate that writings as far back as 1500 BC stated that consumption of liver cured night blindness. It has been known for nearly three centuries that scurvy can be controlled by dietary means. In 1747, James Lind, a Scottish physician in the Royal Navy, hypothesized that various "acidic principles" might have antiscorbutic properties. Lind tested his theory by feeding a variety of acidic substances to sailors who had scurvy. The treatments included two oranges or one lemon per day, and these citrus fruits had miraculous curative powers. As early as 1855, beriberi, which was a common affliction among Japanese sailors, was found to be prevented or cured by using meat, milk, and vegetables to supplement the regular polished rice diet of Japanese seamen.

It was during the twentieth century, however, that the vitamins were isolated, identified, and chemically synthesized. The first of these essential dietary factors to be isolated and chemically identified was the anti-beriberi substance, which was isolated from rice polishings by Casimir Funk, a Polish biochemist who was working at the Lister Institute in London. Funk called this factor vitamine based on evidence that it was an "amine" that was "vital" for life. In 1912, Funk extended the use of this term and the "vitamine theory" to include those other trace dietary essentials that were missing in individuals with rickets, scurvy, and pellagra as well as in those with beriberi. The name vitamine was changed to vitamin later as the structures of additional essential organic factors were discovered and it became clear that most were not amines.

The first major subdivision of the vitamins stems from such work as was done by Wilhelm Stepp in Germany, Elmer McCollum and Margaret Davis at the University of Wisconsin, and Thomas Osborne and Lafayette Mendel at Yale University. By using different solvents to extract growth factors from foods, these investigators found one could separate "fat-soluble" and "water-soluble" factors. In around 1915, McCollum and Davis demonstrated a need for a fat-soluble factor "A" present in butterfat and egg yolk and a heat-labile, water-soluble factor "B" present in wheat germ for growth of young rats. The latter was found to cure beriberi. Ensuing efforts from a number of laboratories led to specific identification of the fat-soluble vitamins as belonging to groups now called A, D, E, and K. Other workers who concentrated on the effects of water-soluble vitamins came to realize that the factor that Axel Holst and Theodor Frolick in Oslo had shown in 1907 to be required for guinea pigs to avoid a scurvy-like condition was the antiscorbutic activity associated with lemon juice. Sylvester S. Zilva and others at the Lister Institute termed this factor vitamin C. In the search for factors that would prevent beriberi as well as pellagra, it became apparent that "water-soluble B" was not a single substance, as pointed out by Joseph Goldberger in the 1920s. The successive efforts of numerous investigators were required to unravel the "B complex." Most of the activity toward the certain identification of the individual B vitamins spanned about 25 years, from the isolation of B_1 (thiamin) in 1926 to the determination of the structure of vitamin B_{12} (cyanocobalamin) in 1955. The chemical synthesis of cyanocobalamin was not accomplished until 1970.

The identification of vitamins over the course of the twentieth century resulted in knowledge of 13 vitamins that are dietary essentials for humans. These include eight B vitamins (thiamin, niacin, riboflavin, folate, vitamin B_6, vitamin B_{12}, biotin, and pantothenic acid), vitamin C or ascorbic acid, and the fat-soluble vitamins A, D, E, and K. As vitamins were further characterized, it was found that the activity of a particular vitamin was often found in several closely related compounds known as vitamers. For example, vitamin B_6 is used to refer not only to pyridoxine (pyridoxol), but also to pyridoxal and pyridoxamine, and vitamin A is used to refer to retinol, retinal, and retinoic acid.

In addition, as more has been learned about the vitamins, it has become clear that some of the vitamins are not strictly dietary essentials. Vitamin D is synthesized in the skin from an endogenous precursor (7-dehydrocholesterol) upon exposure to sunlight. Niacin-containing coenzymes, and subsequently niacin, are synthesized from the amino acid tryptophan.

Most vitamins are not related chemically, and they differ in their biochemical/physiological roles. The historical water-soluble and fat-soluble classification distinguishes vitamins by their physical solubility in solvents, and this classification also broadly separates the vitamins by some of the types of processes involved in their digestion, absorption, and transport, as well as by some aspects of their functions.

The most common function of vitamins is as essential components of coenzymes. All of the B vitamins, vitamin C, and reduced vitamin K are required as coenzymes or as components of coenzymes that are synthesized from the vitamins. Coenzymes are defined as small, organic molecules that are required by an enzyme and that participate in the chemistry of catalysis. Most coenzymes shuttle back and forth between two (or more) different forms. Coenzymes include ascorbic acid, reduced vitamin K, biotin (covalently bound to enzyme), nicotinamide adenine dinucleotide (NAD) and nicotinamide adenine dinucleotide phosphate (NADP) (niacin-containing), flavin adenine dinucleotide (FAD) and flavin mononucleotide (FMN) (riboflavin-containing), thiamin pyrophosphate, several folate coenzymes, methyl-B_{12} and deoxyadenosyl-B_{12}, pyridoxal phosphate and pyridoxamine phosphate (vitamin B_6 coenzymes), and coenzyme A and enzyme-bound 4′–phosphopantetheine (derivatives of pantothenic acid). These coenzymes may be covalently attached to the enzyme protein (biotin, FAD in a few cases, and 4′–phosphopantetheine), tightly associated with specific apoenzymes to form the active holoenzyme (FAD and FMN, B_{12} coenzymes, most folate coenzymes, and B_6 coenzymes), or only weakly associated with their apoenzymes such that the cofactors behave in a manner similar to that of substrates (NAD and NADP, some folate coenzymes, coenzyme A, ascorbate, and reduced vitamin K). (It should be noted that not all coenzymes are formed from vitamins; for example, coenzyme Q, lipoic acid, dolichol phosphate, and biopterin are synthesized in the body.)

The other functions of vitamins are more varied. Two of the vitamins are required for synthesis of hormones: vitamin D is required for formation of 1,25-dihydroxyvitamin D, and vitamin A is required for formation of all-*trans*-retinoic acid. Vitamin A also acts as a visual pigment in the form of 11-*cis*-retinal. Vitamin E serves as a lipid-soluble antioxidant, and vitamin C also has antioxidant functions. The niacin-containing coenzyme NAD also serves as substrate for adenosine diphosphate (ADP)–ribosylation reactions.

In the following eight chapters, the vitamins are discussed. The details of coenzyme, hormone, and antioxidant function are discussed because these biochemical and physiological functions are the bases of the requirements for these vitamins, and clinical signs of deficiency result from impairment of these functions. Some of the B vitamins have been grouped because they play major roles in particular areas of metabolism. Niacin, riboflavin, and thiamin are grouped together because these three vitamins play critical roles in the central pathways of metabolism of energy-yielding nutrients. Folate, vitamin B_{12}, and vitamin B_6 are grouped together because amino acids are important substrates for reactions that require the coenzymes formed from these vitamins. Biotin and pantothenic acid are covered in a single chapter because these two vitamins are intimately (but not exclusively) involved in lipid metabolism. Vitamin C, vitamin A, vitamin D, vitamin E, and vitamin K are covered in individual chapters because of their specialized functions in the body.

Donald B. McCormick
Martha H. Stipanuk

Chapter 24

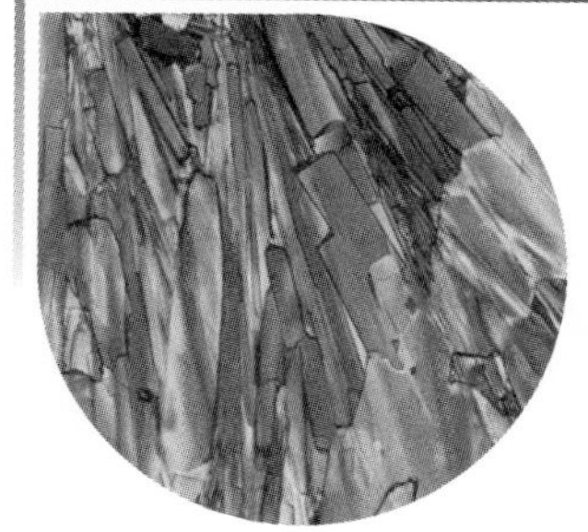

Niacin, Riboflavin, and Thiamin

Donald B. McCormick, PhD

OUTLINE

COMMON ABBREVIATIONS

FAD	flavin adenine dinucleotide
FMN	flavin mononucleotide
NAD	nicotinamide adenine dinucleotide
NADP	nicotinamide adenine dinucleotide phosphate
NaMN	nicotinate (nicotinic acid) mononucleotide
NMN	nicotinamide mononucleotide
TPP	thiamin pyrophosphate; also called TDP, thiamin diphosphate

NIACIN

Niacin (previously designated as vitamin B_3) is essential for formation of pyridine nucleotide coenzymes (nicotinamide adenine dinucleotide [NAD], nicotinamide adenine dinucleotide phosphate [NADP]) that function indispensably in oxidation–reduction reactions involved in the catabolism of glucose, fatty acids, ketone bodies, and amino acids. These coenzymes ultimately are coupled to electron-to-oxygen transfer systems, which are the terminal connections between energy-yielding metabolic events and molecular oxygen, and also are essential for reductive biosynthetic reactions. In addition, NAD, one of the coenzyme forms of niacin, also serves as the donor of adenosine diphosphate (ADP)–ribose moieties for ADP-ribosylation reactions. Niacin is the first of three B vitamins included in this chapter. The intimate involvement of the coenzymes formed from niacin, riboflavin, and thiamin in the intermediary metabolism of energy-yielding nutrients is the basis for grouping these three vitamins in a single chapter.

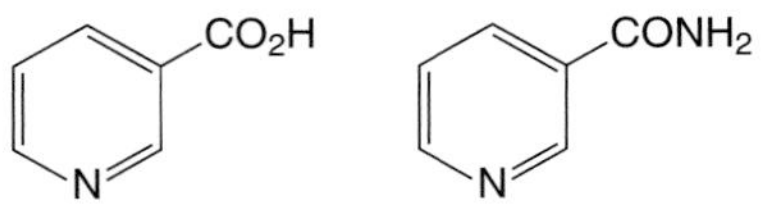

Figure 24-1 Structures of nicotinic acid and nicotinamide.

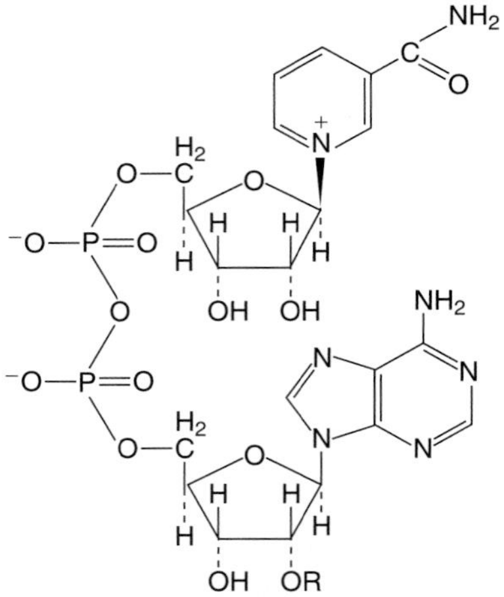

Figure 24-2 Structures of oxidized pyridine nucleotide coenzymes: NAD^+, R = H; $NADP^+$, R = PO_3^{-2}.

NIACIN AND PYRIDINE NUCLEOTIDE COENZYME STRUCTURE AND NOMENCLATURE

The term niacin is chemically synonymous with nicotinic acid (pyridine-3-carboxylic acid), which was prepared in 1867 by oxidation of nicotine, isolated in 1911 from rice polishings, and established in 1937 as a vitamin shown to cure black tongue in dogs. The word niacin now is used as the generic name for the specific compound, nicotinic acid or nicotinate, as well as for nicotinamide (pyridine-3-carboxamide or niacinamide). Because the amino acid tryptophan also may serve as a precursor for synthesis of pyridine nucleotide coenzymes, the term niacin equivalent (NE) is used for expression of niacin intakes and requirements. Niacin activity and niacin deficiency are used in the nutritional literature to refer collectively to nicotinic acid, nicotinamide, and NEs from tryptophan. Structures for the two vitaminic forms are shown in Figure 24-1.

The operational forms derived from these vitamers are pyridine nucleotide coenzymes. Because nicotinamide is a common constituent, current nomenclature for the biologically oxidized forms is nicotinamide adenine dinucleotide (NAD) and nicotinamide adenine dinucleotide phosphate (NADP). NAD was originally known as coenzyme I (CoI) and then diphosphopyridine nucleotide (DPN); NADP was first coenzyme II (CoII), then triphosphopyridine nucleotide (TPN). Structures for the oxidized forms of the two pyridine nucleotide coenzymes are shown in Figure 24-2.

The naming of the biologically reduced forms of pyridine nucleotides, wherein the nicotinamide ring bears an additional hydrogen at position 4, as illustrated in Figure 24-3, has followed two conventions. Because these coenzymes require two equivalents of hydrogen for their reduction, one earlier system was to add the prefix "dihydro" to the written name and indicate such forms with the abbreviations $NADH_2$ and $NADPH_2$. However, when substrate is oxidized and $NAD(P)^+$ is reduced (by two electrons), one hydrogen atom is abstracted from the substrate as a hydrid ion and the second hydrogen atom is released as a solvated proton. Because the reduced

Figure 24-3 Structure and numbering of the 1,4-dihydro-nicotinamide portion of reduced pyridine nucleotide coenzymes. *R*, Ribofuranosyl diphosphoadenosine.

coenzymes in neutral solution actually contain only one of the two hydrogens lost from the substrate during its oxidation, NADH and NADPH are now used as the abbreviations for the reduced coenzymatic forms. In addition, the oxidized forms are conventionally indicated with a plus, that is, NAD^+ and $NADP^+$, to reflect the charge on the quaternary pyridinium nitrogen, even though net charges on the coenzyme molecules in neutral or physiological solutions are negative because of pyrophosphoryl and phosphoryl ionizations (see Fig. 24-2). Hence, typical enzyme-catalyzed reactions, with a reduced substrate and an oxidized product, are written as follows:

$$\text{Substrate} + \text{NAD(P)}^+ \rightleftarrows \text{Product} + \text{NAD(P)H} + \text{H}^+$$

SOURCES, DIGESTION, AND ABSORPTION

Niacin, predominantly in covalently bound forms, is widely distributed in foods of both plant and animal origin. Good sources of preformed niacin include meats, poultry, fish, legumes, peanuts, and some cereals. Enrichment of grain products with niacin makes enriched flours and grain products good sources as well. In uncooked foods of animal origin, the major forms of niacin are the cellular pyridine nucleotides, NAD(H) and NADP(H). Although these are relatively stable to heat, some niacin undoubtedly is released during food processing by the action of tissue pyrophosphatases, phosphatases, and glycohydrolases. In uncooked foods of plant origin, there are even more diverse forms of bound niacin. Much of the niacin in cereals (largely in the bran) is not readily biologically available because it is esterified to complex carbohydrate (niacin) and to a lesser extent to peptides (niacinogens).

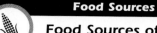

Food Sources

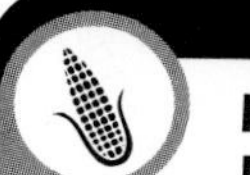

Food Sources of Preformed Niacin

Meats

- 14 mg per 3 oz beef liver
- 10 to 11 mg per 3 oz tuna, halibut, swordfish
- 7 mg per 3 oz rainbow trout
- 2 to 6 mg per 3 oz beef, lamb, pork, poultry, other fish

Cereals and Grain Products

- 2 to 10 mg per 1 cup ready-to-eat cereal
- 3 to 4 mg per 4-in. (3-oz) bagel
- 2 mg per 2-oz hard roll
- 1 mg per ½ cup noodles or pasta
- 2 mg per ½ cup graham crackers
- 1.5 mg per ½ cup barley, cooked
- 1.5 mg per ½ cup cooked rice

Vegetables

- 2 mg per ½ cup canned tomato product
- 1.5 mg per ½ cup mushrooms
- 1 mg per ½ cup corn
- 1 mg per ½ cup potatoes

Other

- 4 mg per 1 oz peanuts

Data from US Department of Agriculture/Agricultural Research Service (USDA/ARS) (2005) USDA National Nutrient Standard Database, Release 18. USDA/ARS, Washington, DC. Retrieved December 23, 2005, from www.ars.usda.gov/ba/bhnrc/ndl.

Pretreatment of corn with lime water (i.e., calcium hydroxide), as in the traditional preparation of tortillas in Mexico and Central America, releases much of the bound nicotinic acid. Roasting of green coffee beans converts some of the trigonelline (1-methyl nicotinic acid) to nicotinic acid. A portion of the L-tryptophan in proteins can be metabolized in some species (e.g., rats and humans) to produce nicotinate mononucleotide (NaMN), an intermediate in the pathway for synthesis of functional pyridine coenzymes from nicotinate (nicotinic acid) as shown in Figure 24-4.

Recommended dietary allowances (RDAs) or adequate intakes (AIs) for niacin now are given in terms of niacin equivalents (NEs) to include estimates of direct and indirect sources of the vitamin (Institute of Medicine [IOM], 1998). An estimated average conversion factor

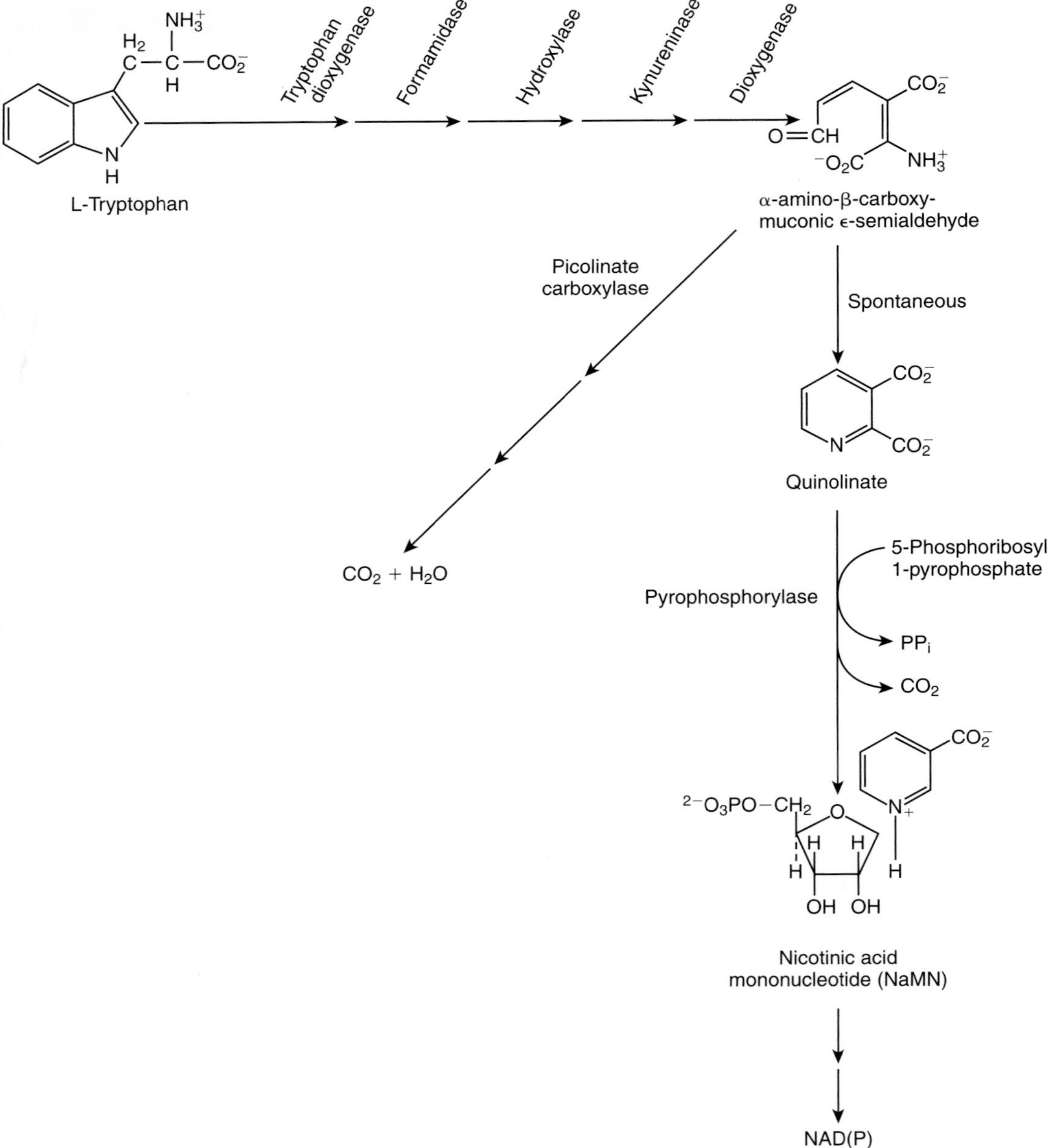

Figure 24-4 Metabolic conversion of L-tryptophan to nicotinate mononucleotide (NaMN).

of 60 mg tryptophan to yield 1 mg niacin is used to calculate the NEs available from tryptophan. Hence 1 NE is provided by 1 mg of nicotinic acid (nicotinate), 1 mg of nicotinamide, or 60 mg of tryptophan. The tryptophan content of proteins averages about 1%, and a diet for humans in excess of 100 g protein per day presumably could provide 16 mg NEs and meet the RDA without inclusion of preformed niacin.

The major pathway for tryptophan catabolism results in formation of CO_2 and H_2O, rather than quinolinate or NaMN, and humans convert only about 2.75% of the amino acid to NaMN. In the pathway for tryptophan degradation, the pathways for NaMN formation and complete oxidation diverge at the level of the intermediate α-amino-β-carboxymuconic ε-semialdehyde. The rate at which α-amino-β-carboxymuconic

Nutrition Insight

Enrichment of Grain Products With B Vitamins

Milling of grains results in loss of vitamins and minerals, which are concentrated in the outer layers of the kernels (bran and aleurone layer) and in the germ. Beginning in the early 1940s, the U.S. government established standards for enrichment of flour and other grain products. These standards are targeted at restoring the levels of thiamin, riboflavin, niacin, and iron to the levels found in whole-grain products. For example, the standards for enrichment of flour are 2.9 mg thiamin, 1.8 mg riboflavin, 24.0 mg niacin, and 20 mg iron per pound of flour. Beginning in 1998, enriched-grain products also have been fortified with folate. Hence, products labeled "enriched" are good sources of these four vitamins and iron. Whole-grain products are good sources of these nutrients as well as of a number of other vitamins and minerals that also are lost in milling but are not added as part of the enrichment program.

ε-semialdehyde undergoes the divergent decarboxylation reaction, which is catalyzed by a decarboxylase classically called picolinic carboxylase, determines the partitioning of this tryptophan metabolite to CO_2 versus NaMN. The product of the decarboxylation reaction, 2-aminomuconic semialdehyde, undergoes cyclization to picolinate (2-carboxypyridine), which is further oxidized to CO_2 and H_2O. The activity of this so-called carboxylase is relatively high in some animals, such as cats, which are dependent on preformed niacin in their diets. Picolinate carboxylase activity has been shown to be elevated, with an induced diabetic state in some species, such that the efficiency of conversion of tryptophan to NaMN and subsequently to NAD is impaired. A complementary DNA (cDNA) encoding the human enzyme has been cloned and characterized, and its expression, along with quinolate phosphoribosyltransferase (phosphorylase), was found in the brain (Fukuoka et al., 2002). Some steroid hormones (glucocorticoids and estrogens) elevate tryptophan dioxygenase and may increase the yield of pyridine coenzymes (Knox and Piras, 1967). The stress of cold exposure increases urinary output of niacin metabolites seemingly as a result of increased conversion of tryptophan to niacin (Okamoto et al., 2002). Sensitivity of the pathway to the status of micronutrients, especially B_6, riboflavin, Fe^{2+}, and perhaps Cu^{2+}, relates to the cofactor roles of these micronutrients with certain of the enzymes for tryptophan catabolism. (See Chapter 14 for further discussion of tryptophan metabolism.)

The coenzyme forms of niacin in the gastrointestinal tract are rapidly hydrolyzed to nicotinamide mononucleotide (NMN) by nonspecific pyrophosphatases in the intestinal lumen (Gross and Henderson, 1983). Alkaline phosphatase catalyzes further cleavage to nicotinamide riboside, from which nicotinamide slowly is released. In addition, NAD glycohydrolases (NADases) within mucosal cells may contribute to the breakdown of the coenzymes to nicotinamide.

Both nicotinic acid and its amide are absorbed from the small intestine by a sodium (Na^+)–dependent saturable process as well as by passive diffusion that continues to increase at higher nonphysiological concentrations of the vitamin (Bechgaard and Jespersen, 1977). Absorption of nicotinic acid also occurs by passive diffusion in the stomach.

TRANSPORT AND CONVERSION OF NIACIN TO ENZYMES

Facilitated and simple diffusion of niacin followed by formation and metabolic trapping of the nucleotides accounts for uptake of niacin from plasma by tissues. The facilitated diffusion of niacin into erythrocytes involves an anion transport protein as carrier. Both red cells and liver rapidly remove and convert niacin to NAD by the biosynthetic (Preiss-Handler) pathway. Intracellular NAD glycohydrolases then

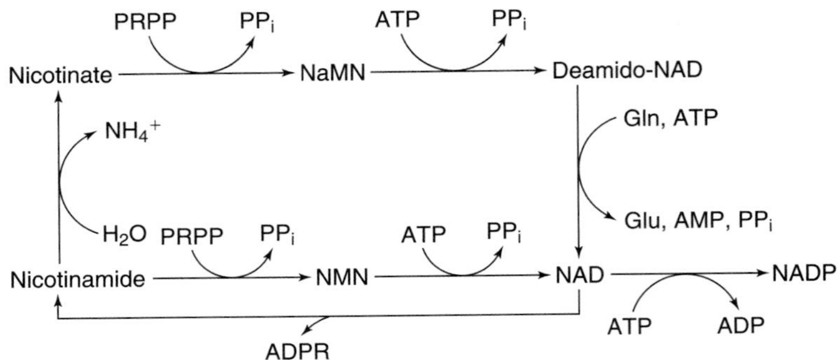

Figure 24-5 Interconnections of vitaminic and coenzymatic forms of niacin. *Glu*, Glutamate; *Gln*, glutamine; *NaMN*, nicotinate mononucleotide; *NAD(P)*, nicotinamide adenine dinucleotide (phosphate); *PP_i*, inorganic pyrophosphate; *PRPP*, phosphoribosyl-pyrophosphate.

release nicotinamide, which circulates to other tissues as precursor to pyridine nucleotide coenzymes.

Pyridine nucleotide formation from nicotinate and nicotinamide occurs widely in tissues, as summarized in Figure 24-5. The Preiss-Handler pathway involves a phosphoribosyl transferase–catalyzed conversion of nicotinate and phosphoribosylpyrophosphate (PRPP) to nicotinate mononucleotide (NaMN) with release of pyrophosphate. NaMN also arises from tryptophan metabolism via quinolinate, which undergoes decarboxylation during the phosphoribosyl transferase reaction. NaMN is adenylylated to form deamido-NAD in an ATP-requiring reaction catalyzed by NAD pyrophosphorylase. The conversion of the deamido intermediate to NAD is accomplished by an ATP-requiring NAD synthetase reaction in which the amide of glutamine is transferred to NaMN. Although nicotinamidase catalyzes hydrolysis of some nicotinamide to nicotinate that can be reutilized for NAD synthesis by the Preiss-Handler pathway, nicotinamide also is used directly for NAD synthesis. The Dietrich pathway couples PRPP with nicotinamide to form NMN, which with ATP directly forms NAD. Some NAD is phosphorylated by ATP and a kinase to form NADP.

NAD is turned over to regenerate nicotinamide and release the adenosine diphosphoribose (ADP-ribose) moiety in reactions catalyzed by glycohydrolases or ADP-ribosyl transferases. NAD glycohydrolases responsible for this can use water to catalyze a simple hydrolysis, or they can transfer the ADP-ribose to another base. ADP-ribosyl transferases can add the ADP-ribose moiety to specific protein bases. The poly-ADP-ribosylations that are catalyzed by poly(ADP-ribose) polymerase (synthetase) may account for the relatively rapid turnover of NAD in human cells (Rechsteiner et al., 1976).

NIACIN CATABOLISM AND EXCRETION

There is little loss of niacin into urine when intake is modest because both vitamers are actively reabsorbed from glomerular filtrates. Rather, several metabolites that are formed enzymatically, primarily in liver, appear in urine. The N^1-methyl derivatives result primarily from *S*-adenosylmethionine-dependent *N*-methyltransferase activity, but some N^1-methyl nicotinate also arises from food and bacterial methylation of niacytin (esterified nicotinic acid). The 2- and 4-pyridone oxidation products of N^1-methylnicotinamide arise from the action of aldehyde oxidase. Their quantities vary with species, as do such oxidation products as the *N*-oxide and 6-hydroxy compounds (McCreanor and Bender, 1986; Mrochek et al., 1976). Conjugation of nicotinic acid with glycine to form nicotinuric acid becomes increasingly significant as the quantity of nicotinic acid ingested increases toward pharmacological levels.

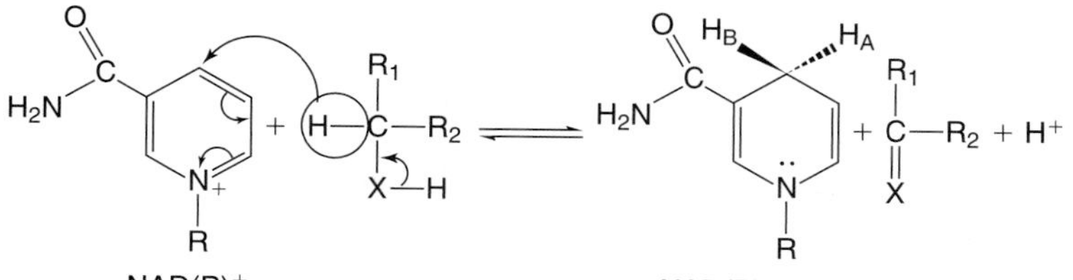

NAD(P)$^+$ NAD(P)H

Figure 24-6 Mechanism for substrate oxidation by pyridine nucleotide coenzymes. Typically, X is an electronegative atom (e.g., oxygen), and the subscripts A and B on prochiral hydrogens reflect stereospecificity.

FUNCTIONS OF PYRIDINE NUCLEOTIDE COENZYMES IN METABOLISM

The pyridine nucleotide coenzymes function in numerous oxidoreductase systems, usually of the dehydrogenase/reductase type, which include such diverse reactions as the conversion of alcohols (often sugars and polyols) to aldehydes or ketones, hemiacetals to lactones, aldehydes to acids, and certain amino acids to keto acids. The common mechanism of operation (generalized in Figure 24-6) involves the stereospecific abstraction of a hydride ion (H^-) from the substrate, with *para* addition to one (A) or the other (B) side of carbon 4 in the pyridine ring of the nucleotide coenzyme (Creighton and Murthy, 1990). The second hydrogen of the substrate group being oxidized is concomitantly removed as a proton (H^+), which in solution exists as the hydronium ion.

Most dehydrogenases that use NAD or NADP function reversibly. Glutamate dehydrogenase, for example, favors the oxidative direction, whereas others, such as glutathione reductase, catalyze preferential reduction. A further generality is that most NAD-dependent enzymes are involved in catabolic reactions, whereas NADP-dependent systems are more common to biosynthetic reactions. For example, NAD-dependent enzymes (e.g., 3-hydroxyacyl CoA dehydrogenase, 3-hydroxybutyrate dehydrogenase, glyceraldehyde 3-phosphate dehydrogenase, and branched-chain keto acid dehydrogenase) catalyze steps in the β-oxidation of fatty acyl CoAs, the oxidation of ketone bodies, the degradation of carbohydrates, and the catabolism of amino acids. NADPH serves as an important reducing agent for the synthesis of fats and steroids (e.g., reactions catalyzed by 3-ketoacyl reductase, enoyl reductase, and 3-hydroxy-3-methylglutaryl coenzyme A [HMG CoA] reductase). See Chapters 12, 14, 16, and 17 for more examples of NAD- and NADP-dependent reactions in carbohydrate, amino acid, and lipid metabolism.

For the pyridine nucleotide coenzymes to continue to react catalytically, they must cycle by coupling with oxidation–reduction sequences. This may occur by coupling dehydrogenation reactions with hydrogenation reactions (e.g., the coupling of glyceraldehyde 3-phosphate dehydrogenase with lactate dehydrogenase in anaerobic glycolysis or the coupling of NADPH production by the pentose phosphate pathway with fatty acid synthesis) or by coupling the dehydrogenation reactions with electron transport as found in mitochondria.

Both NAD and NADP serve as parts of the intracellular respiratory mechanism of all cells; they assist in the stepwise transfer of electrons or reducing equivalents from various energy substrates to the cytochromes, which in turn transfer the electrons (and H^+) to oxygen to form water. NADH (reduced NAD) usually donates its electrons to a flavin coenzyme in the mitochondrial electron transport chain responsible for ATP production. These reactions are outlined in Figure 24-7. The role of NADPH and cytochrome P450 in the hydroxylation of steroids (for biosynthesis of steroid hormones from cholesterol) is illustrated in Figure 24-8. Cytochrome P450 hydroxylase (monooxygenase) systems also exist in the endoplasmic reticulum (ER) of cells. These monooxygenase systems in the ER use reducing equivalents of NADH and NADPH and are involved in metabolism of drugs such as phenobarbital.

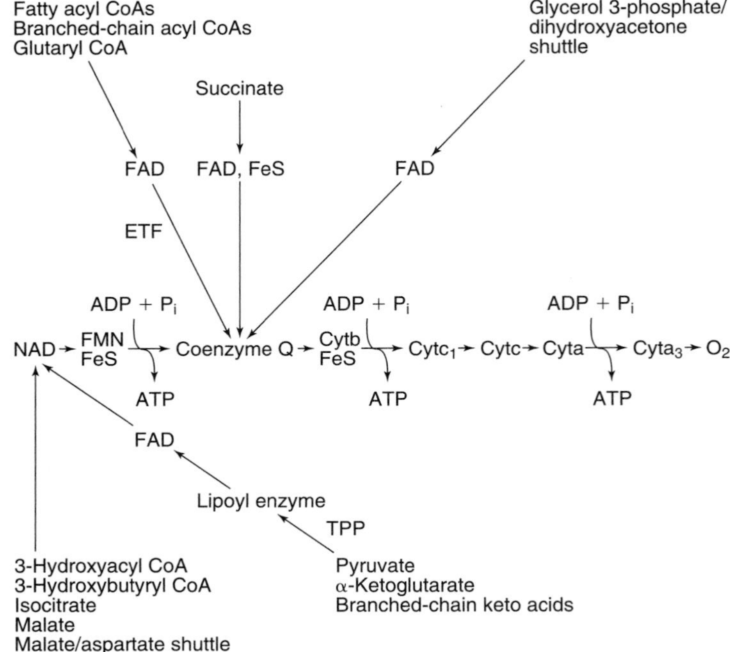

Figure 24-7 Role of pyridine nucleotides and flavocoenzymes in the funneling of reducing equivalents to the mitochondrial respiratory chain. Major sources of reducing equivalents generated in the mitochondria are shown. The main extramitochondrial source is NADH formed in glycolysis; these reducing equivalents are carried into the mitochondria by the malate–aspartate or the glycerol phosphate–dihydroxyacetone shuttles. *Cyt*, Cytochrome; *ETF*, electron transfer flavoprotein; *FAD*, flavin adenine dinucleotide; *FeS*, iron-sulfur protein; *FMN*, flavin mononucleotide; *TPP*, thiamin pyrophosphate.

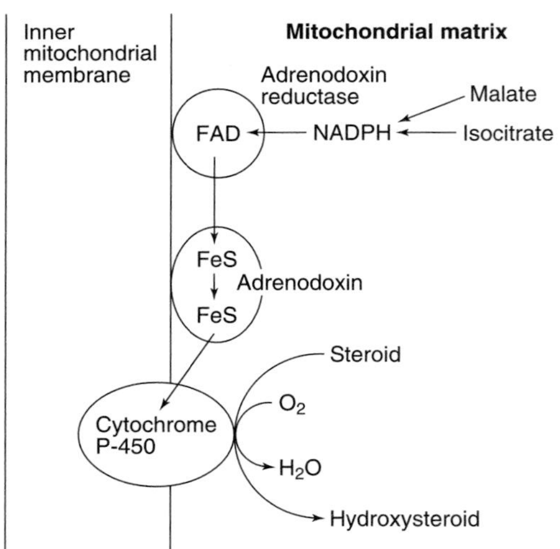

Figure 24-8 Mitochondrial cytochrome P450 monooxygenase system. *FeS*, iron-sulfur protein (adrenodoxin). Note that because NADP(H) cannot penetrate the mitochondrial membrane, sources of reducing equivalents are confined to substrates such as malate and isocitrate for which there are intramitochondrial NADP-specific dehydrogenases. *FAD*, Flavin adenine dinucleotide.

Because NAD and NADP do not cross the inner mitochondrial membrane, the cytosolic and mitochondrial pools do not mix. However, tissues that have mitochondria have systems capable of "shuttling" reducing equivalents across the inner mitochondrial membrane from the cytosol to the mitochondrial compartment. Reducing equivalents from NADH formed during oxidative metabolism in the cytosol are carried into the mitochondria by the glycerol phosphate and malate–aspartate shuttles (see Chapter 12). In addition, reducing equivalents may be carried out of the mitochondria during periods of active fatty acid biosynthesis (via citrate, which can be dehydrogenated by cytosolic NADP-linked isocitrate dehydrogenase to generate NADPH) or during active gluconeogenesis (via aspartate, which involves conversion of aspartate to fumarate by the urea cycle, fumarate to malate by cytosolic fumarase, and malate to oxaloacetate by NAD-dependent malate dehydrogenase with generation of NADH). The sequential actions of cytosolic citrate lyase, NAD-dependent malate dehydrogenase, and NADP-dependent malic enzyme can convert cytosolic NADH to cytosolic NADPH for use in lipid synthesis (see Chapter 16).

NONCOENZYMATIC FUNCTIONS OF NIACIN

Nicotinamide coenzymes also participate in other (nonredox) biological reactions that involve ADP-ribosylations. In these reactions, NAD serves as a substrate rather than as a coenzyme. The ADP-ribose moiety of NAD is transferred to the acceptor molecule, and free nicotinamide is released. In mammals, poly-ADP-ribosylated proteins appear to function in deoxyribonucleic acid (DNA) repair, DNA replication, and cell differentiation. Increased activity of poly(ADP-ribose) polymerase in mammalian cells appears to be a response to DNA fragmentation in the nucleus (increased excision–repair activity in response to DNA-damaging agents) (Junod et al., 1989; Schraufstatter et al., 1986). This enzyme adds mostly mono(ADP-ribose) to chromatin proteins, but also it can add homopolymeric chains of ADP-ribose. The activity of poly(ADP-ribose) polymerase is sufficiently large to cause a depletion of intracellular NAD following environmentally induced DNA damage. Studies in rats showed that niacin deficiency decreased bone marrow poly(ADP-ribose) and increased the risk of nitrosourea-induced leukemias (Boyonoski et al., 2002).

Pharmacological doses of nicotinic acid (but not nicotinamide) reduce serum cholesterol and triacylglycerol concentrations in man, decrease the concentrations of very low density lipoproteins (VLDLs) and low density lipoproteins (LDLs) but increase the concentration of high density lipoproteins (HDLs) in plasma, and reduce the recurrence rate of nonfatal myocardial infarction (DiPalma and Thayer, 1991). These metabolic changes appear to result from an antilipolytic effect, which involves the inhibition of cyclic adenosine monophosphate (cAMP) accumulation in adipose tissue through a G_i-protein–mediated inhibition of adenylate cyclase (Tunaru et al., 2003). The orphan G-protein–coupled receptor, human HM74 (mouse PUMA-G), is highly expressed in adipose tissue, where it appears to act as a nicotinic acid receptor. Furthermore, the nicotinic acid–induced decrease in free-fatty acid and triacylglycerol plasma levels was abrogated in mice lacking PUMA-G.

Use of large doses of nicotinic acid, but not large doses of nicotinamide, causes release of the vasodilator histamine and prostaglandins. Hence, flushing of the face is a common side effect of nicotinic acid administration, although this effect is attenuated in individuals with schizophrenia (Messamore et al., 2003). Long-term use may cause gastrointestinal irritation, possible liver damage, and other adverse effects. Large doses of either nicotinic acid or nicotinamide have stimulatory effects on the central nervous system. These effects are clearly unrelated to the vitamin function of niacin.

NIACIN DEFICIENCY

Pellagra ("rough skin") is a niacin-deficiency disease. Its occurrence has been associated with diets in which corn or sorghum was a staple item, including diets in the United States and Southern Europe in the early 1900s. Pellagra is still encountered in India and in parts of China and Africa.

The reasons for the association of pellagra with corn-based diets have been the subject of much research over the years and still are not completely understood. Much of the niacin in corn is bound in an unavailable form, but the tryptophan content of corn is also low, and corn products are relatively more deficient in tryptophan than in niacin. Degermination of corn could have played a role in the occurrence of pellagra in the past, because the milling removed much of the niacin and tryptophan in the corn. The fact that traditional Central American diets do not cause pellagra, even though they contain a large amount of corn, has been attributed to the cooking in lime that the corn receives in tortilla preparation; this alkaline treatment makes niacin more available, but also results in substantial loss of niacin in the washings. The absence of pellagra in Central and South American countries where the staple is maize has also been attributed to widespread consumption of coffee. Although the occurrence of pellagra also has been related to the presence of high levels of leucine in foods, a clear role of leucine in the cause of

Clinical Correlation

Case Study of Pellagra in an Adult Woman

Oakley and Wallace (1994) reported a case involving a young woman in New Zealand who presented with pellagra. She had a variety of neurological and dermal symptoms consistent with a diagnosis of pellagra. She did not have diarrhea. Her symptoms were precipitated by prolonged lactation and increased activity. She had breast-fed her daughter for 3 years and had been particularly active while building her own home. Dietary intake of niacin equivalents was within a normal range. Her total excretion of urinary amino acids was abnormally high (77 mmol/L compared with a reference range of 2 to 36 mmol/L). Chromatography of urinary amino acids revealed elevated loss of tryptophan and other large neutral amino acids (alanine, serine, threonine, valine, methionine, isoleucine, tyrosine, and phenylalanine). Taurine, glycine, ornithine, lysine, arginine, and aspartate were present in urine in normal amounts. Her symptoms resolved with oral nicotinamide plus other B vitamins.

Thinking Critically

1. From the information given, what underlying metabolic abnormality was probably responsible for the development of pellagra in this woman with a normal intake of niacin?
2. Pellagra secondary to inherited disorders usually presents in childhood. Why would periods of rapid growth or of prolonged lactation, as in this case, precipitate the appearance of pellagra? Why might increased activity precipitate the appearance of pellagra?

pellagra has not been supported by most recent studies.

Development of pellagra is often associated with poor diets and increased energy requirements. Pellagra also can develop in patients who are receiving certain drugs (e.g., isoniazid used in treatment of tuberculosis, which depletes the pyridoxal phosphate coenzyme essential for tryptophan conversion to NAD), in patients with malignant carcinoid in whom tryptophan is diverted mainly to serotonin with a reduction in its conversion to quinolinate or NAD, in individuals with chronic alcoholism, and in individuals with certain genetic disorders (e.g., those with Hartnup's disease, which affects intestinal transport and renal tubular reabsorption of tryptophan and other neutral amino acids, or individuals with a defect in the hydroxylation of kynurenine). See Chapters 9 and 14 for further discussion of Hartnup's disease and serotonin synthesis.

Symptoms of pellagra or niacin deficiency include (1) functional changes in the gastrointestinal tract that are manifested as an absence of normal response to histamine, diminished secretion of hydrochloric acid in the gastric juice, and an impaired absorption of vitamin B_{12}, fat, glucose, and D-xylose; and (2) nonspecific lesions of the central nervous system. The first symptoms of pellagra usually are weakness, lassitude, anorexia, and indigestion. These are followed by the classic "three Ds": (1) *dermatitis*, (2) *diarrhea*, and (3) *dementia*. The dermatitis has a characteristic appearance on those parts of the body exposed to sunlight, heat, or mild trauma (such as mechanical stress), such as the face, neck, hands, feet, and elbows. These lesions usually are bilaterally symmetrical. Diarrhea does not develop in all cases; it may be accompanied by vomiting, dysphagia, and a severe inflammation of the mouth and other mucous membranes. The mental symptoms develop in untreated cases and include irritability, headaches, sleeplessness, loss of memory, and emotional instability.

BIOCHEMICAL ASSESSMENT OF NIACIN NUTRITURE

Biochemical assessment of niacin nutritional status is usually based on measurement of urinary metabolites (McCormick and Greene, 1999). Measurements of *N*-methylnicotinamide, the 2-pyridone, the sum of these two metabolites, and the ratio of these two metabolites have been used as indicators of niacin

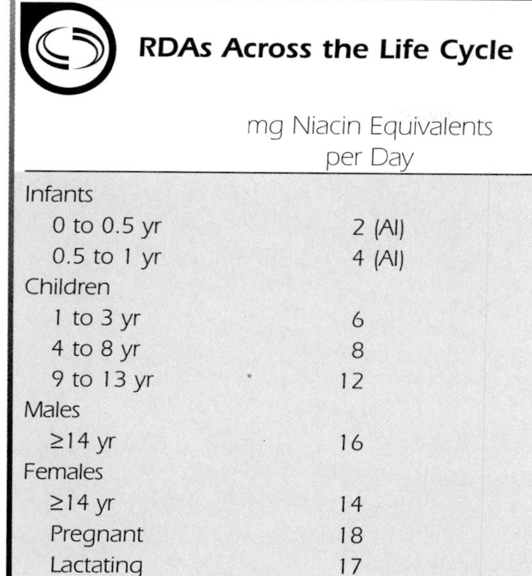

RDAs Across the Life Cycle

	mg Niacin Equivalents per Day
Infants	
0 to 0.5 yr	2 (AI)
0.5 to 1 yr	4 (AI)
Children	
1 to 3 yr	6
4 to 8 yr	8
9 to 13 yr	12
Males	
≥14 yr	16
Females	
≥14 yr	14
Pregnant	18
Lactating	17

Data from Institute of Medicine (1998) Dietary Reference Intakes for Thiamin, Riboflavin, Niacin, Vitamin B_6, Folate, Vitamin B_{12}, Pantothenic Acid, Biotin, and Choline. National Academy Press, Washington, DC.
AI, Adequate intake.

status. Results usually are better when determinations are made following administration of a test dose of nicotinate or nicotinamide.

NIACIN REQUIREMENTS

Because both the availability of niacin from bound niacin and the conversion of tryptophan to niacin vary, it is difficult to predict the niacin status of populations on the basis of analysis of diets for tryptophan and niacin. The IOM based current estimates of average niacin requirements primarily on the intakes that corresponded to urinary excretion of the niacin metabolite N′-methylnicotinamide at levels greater than 1.0 mg/day (IOM, 1998). The estimated average requirement (EAR) is 12 mg of NEs per day for men and 11 mg of NEs per day for women. The RDAs were set using a coefficient of variation of 15% (EAR + 30%) and are 16 mg NEs per day for men and 14 mg NEs per day for women.

Approximately 75 g of high-quality protein will provide about 15 mg of NEs from its tryptophan content, and most mixed diets supply more than 5 mg of preformed niacin. The RDA is relatively easy to meet, with typical intakes in the United States of 25 to 40 mg of NEs per day, but it should be recognized that tryptophan rather than niacin is the major source of NEs in typical diets. The tryptophan content of proteins ranges from about 0.6% for corn to 1.5% for animal products. One should note that niacin values given in food composition tables usually do not take into account the bioavailability of niacin (e.g., from cereals) and do not include an estimate of NEs available from tryptophan in the food.

Pregnant women and women taking contraceptive steroids or steroid hormones appear to have some differences in tryptophan metabolism as compared with nonpregnant females. There is some question of whether the increased urinary excretion of tryptophan degradation products represents increased flux through the pathway leading to increased NAD synthesis, or a decrease in kynureninase activity that results in increased excretion of tryptophan catabolites (and less NAD synthesis) as does a vitamin B_6 deficiency (see Chapter 14). Despite the lack of consensus about changes in tryptophan metabolism in pregnant women, an increased intake of NEs is recommended during pregnancy and lactation because of the increased energy requirements and needs for growth in maternal and fetal compartments and for secretion in the milk (IOM, 1998). The RDAs for pregnant and lactating women are 18 mg of NEs per day and 17 mg of NEs per day, respectively.

The EARs and RDAs for children were extrapolated from adult values. For infants, AIs were established based on intake. Breast milk contains an average of 1.8 mg of niacin and 210 mg of tryptophan per liter, but the AI is based on preformed niacin only. The AI for infants up to 6 months of age is 2 mg of preformed niacin per day. For infants from 7 to 12 months of age, the AI was extrapolated from adult values and is 4 mg of NEs per day.

Based on data from the Third National Health and Nutrition Examination Survey (NHANES III), the median intake of preformed niacin by adults is 24 mg/day for men and 19 mg/day for women. The 5th and 95th percentile ranges are 15 to 43 mg/day for men and 13 to 33 mg/day for women. If niacin intake were reported in NEs, taking the contribution of tryptophan into account, intakes of NEs in the United States would far exceed the established EARs and RDAs. For comparison, the niacin intake of adults in Quebec were assessed as NE, and mean or median intake of NEs was 35 to 54 mg for various age-groups of men and 25 to 30 mg for various age-groups of women (see IOM, 1998).

The upper tolerable intake level (UL) for adults is 35 mg/day of niacin (IOM, 1998). This is based on the dose of nicotinic acid that is associated with flushing effects. Flushing is the first observed adverse effect of nicotinic acid intake, and the UL is considered to be protective against potential adverse effects of nicotinamide.

RIBOFLAVIN

Like niacin, riboflavin (also known as vitamin B_2) is essential for synthesis of coenzymes that function indispensably in oxidation–reduction reactions involved in the catabolism of glucose, fatty acids, ketone bodies, and amino acids. These flavocoenzymes (FAD, FMN) are coupled ultimately to electron-to-oxygen transfer systems, which are the terminal connections between energy-yielding metabolic events and molecular oxygen and also are essential for reductive biosynthetic reactions.

RIBOFLAVIN AND FLAVOCOENZYME STRUCTURE AND NOMENCLATURE

Riboflavin is the common name for vitamin B_2, which is chemically specified as 7,8-dimethyl-10-(1′-D-ribityl)isoalloxazine. "Ribo" refers to the ribityl side chain, and "flavin" is now synonymous with any substituted isoalloxazine. The structure for this yellow, fluorescent, water-soluble compound is shown in Figure 24-9.

The physiologically functional flavocoenzymes derived from the vitamin are riboflavin 5′-phosphate, commonly called flavin mononucleotide (FMN), and flavin-adenine dinucleotide (FAD). This latter, most widespread coenzyme is shown with its component parts of FMN and 5′-adenylate (AMP) in Figure 24-10.

Although most flavin coenzymes are noncovalently associated (ionic, hydrophobic) with the apoenzymic proteins, some are covalently bound. In the case of humans, only a few covalent flavoproteins are known. These are the 8α-*N*(3)-histidyl(peptide)-FADs of the

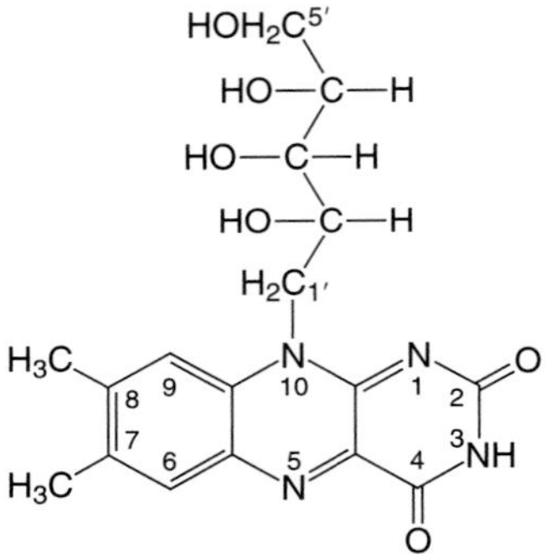

Figure 24-9 Structure with numbering of riboflavin.

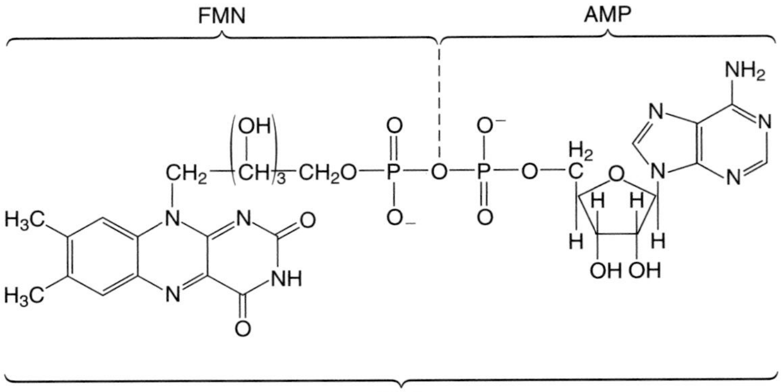

Figure 24-10 Structure of common flavocoenzymes, indicating that flavin adenine dinucleotide (FAD) comprises flavin mononucleotide (FMN) plus an AMP moiety.

dehydrogenases for succinate, sarcosine (*N*-methylglycine) and *N*,*N*-dimethylglycine that are in mitochondrial inner membranes, and the 8α-*S*-cysteinyl(peptide)-FAD of monoamine oxidase found in mitochondrial outer membranes. Structures for these mammalian types of covalent flavins are illustrated in Figure 24-11. Another covalently bound flavocoenzyme of uncertain linkage occurs in lysosomal pipicolate oxidase.

Flavocoenzymes are involved in oxidation–reduction reactions in which the ring portion of the flavocoenzyme involving nitrogens 1 and 5 and carbon 4α undergoes sequential addition or loss of hydrogens and electrons. Of nine chemically discernible forms (three levels of redox and three species for acidic, neutral, and basic conditions), five have biological relevance because of pH considerations. These biological forms are summarized in Figure 24-12.

8α-Substituted FAD where X =

N-Histidyl and *S*-Cysteinyl

Figure 24-11 Representative covalent flavins in mammals where 8α-attachment is to such electronegative atoms as *N* or *S* within amino acid residues of enzymes.

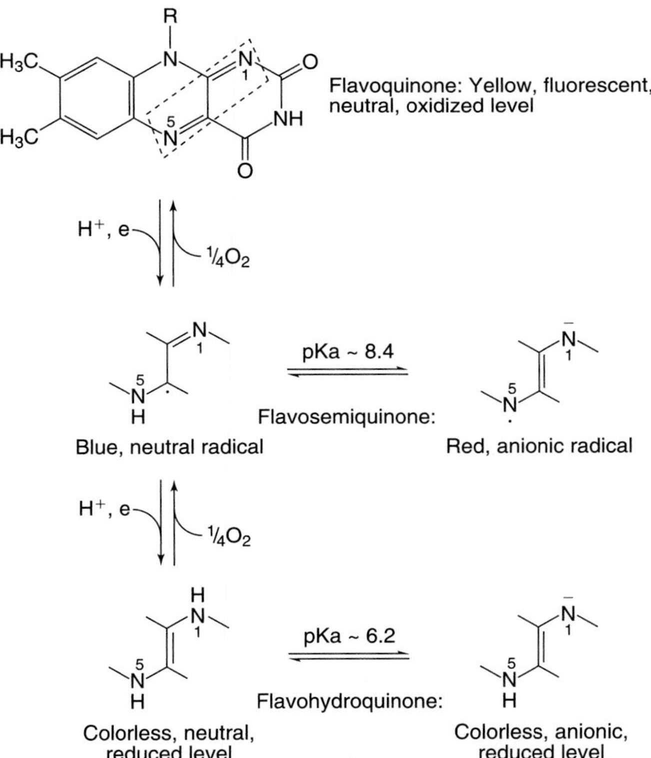

Figure 24-12 Physiologically relevant states of flavocoenzymes.

SOURCES, DIGESTION, AND ABSORPTION

Riboflavin within foods is mainly in coenzymatic forms, with over two thirds typically as FAD, except for milk and eggs, in which relatively large amounts of riboflavin per se occur. It has been estimated that at least one third of the adult RDA for riboflavin is supplied in the American diet by milk and dairy products (Block et al., 1985). Certainly meats, especially liver, and green vegetables supply much of the rest. Although cereals are rather poor sources, enriched flour and breakfast cereals contribute significant amounts of riboflavin. Covalently bound flavins present in food (~5% to 10% of total naturally occurring flavocoenzymes) are unavailable as nutritional sources of the vitamin, because the 8α-(amino acid)-riboflavins obtained from digestion cannot be used for resynthesis of coenzymes (Chia et al., 1978).

Food Sources

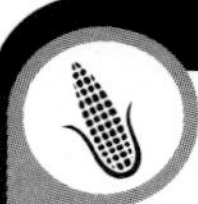

Food Sources of Riboflavin

Dairy Products

- 0.5 mg per 8 oz yogurt
- 0.45 mg per 1 cup milk
- 0.2 mg per ½ cup cottage cheese

Cereals and Grain Products

- 0.4 to 1.0 mg per 1 cup ready-to-eat cereal
- 0.3 mg per 4-in. (3-oz) bagel
- 0.1 mg per ½ cup graham crackers

Meats and Eggs

- 0.3 mg per 3 oz pork
- 0.25 mg per egg

Vegetables

- 0.15 mg per ½ cup spinach
- 0.15 mg per ½ cup mushrooms
- 0.15 mg per ½ cup soybeans

Data from US Department of Agriculture/Agricultural Research Service (USDA/ARS) (2005) USDA National Nutrient Standard Database, Release 18. USDA/ARS, Washington, DC. Retrieved December 23, 2005, from www.ars.usda.gov/ba/bhnrc/ndl.

Although riboflavin and its phosphate (FMN) are relatively stable to heat in slightly acidic and neutral conditions, they become more labile in base. Cleavage of the ribityl side chain with loss of vitaminic activity occurs when solutions that contain riboflavin are exposed to light. Such photo-products as lumichrome and lumiflavin are the result. Use of riboflavin for photo-inactivation of pathogens in blood components that contain no nucleic acids, namely erythrocytes, thrombocytes, and plasma, is due to the ability of light-excited flavin to photo-oxidize bases, especially guanyl residues, in the nucleic acids of bacterial and viral pathogens (Goodrich, 2000).

After ingestion, flavocoenzymes are released from noncovalent attachment to proteins during gastric acidification and subsequent proteolysis. Nonspecific action by pyrophosphatases (nucleotidohydrolases) and phosphomonoesterase (alkaline phosphatase) on the coenzyme forms occurs in the upper small intestine. A small amount of 8α-(amino acid)-riboflavins and traces of other ring and side-chain substituted flavins also are released during digestion.

Riboflavin and traces of other free flavins are absorbed primarily in the proximal small intestine by a saturable, Na^+-dependent transport process. The uptake that occurs with physiological levels of riboflavin intake is facilitated transport with internalization due to receptor-mediated endocytosis (Huang et al., 2003), but passive diffusion also occurs up to the limits imposed by the modest solubility of this vitamin. In the adult human, intake and apparent absorption increase proportionately up to about 27 mg in a single dose, but there is little or no further absorption at higher intakes (Zempleni et al., 1996a). Bile salts appear to facilitate uptake. There is very little enterohepatic circulation of riboflavin in humans.

TRANSPORT AND CONVERSION OF RIBOFLAVIN TO COENZYMES

Some of the riboflavin circulating in blood plasma is loosely associated with albumin, although significant amounts complex with other proteins, notably immunoglobulins (Whitehouse et al., 1991). Estrogen induction of distinct plasma riboflavin-binding proteins in mammals suggests sequestration for fetal uptake in a manner that corresponds to the role of elevated levels of riboflavin-binding protein in plasma and eggs of laying hens.

As with most water-soluble vitamins, uptake of riboflavin from plasma by tissues involves facilitated and simple diffusion with subsequent metabolic trapping. The facilitated diffusion may well involve a carrier, and a protein that binds riboflavin has been identified in the plasma membrane of hepatocytes (Nokubo et al., 1989). Metabolic trapping as riboflavin 5′-phosphate (FMN) reflects the role of flavokinase (Bowers-Komro and McCormick, 1987; Aw et al., 1983). There is an active, Na^+-dependent efflux of riboflavin from the choroid plexus in the brain and from renal tubular cells.

Flavocoenzymes are formed by a sequential pathway that involves two cytosolic enzymes, flavokinase and FAD synthetase, which are widely distributed in tissues. This two-step process is shown in Figure 24-13. Both steps require ATP, with Zn^{2+} being preferred as the metal ion in the γ-phosphate exchange catalyzed by flavokinase (Nakano and McCormick, 1991) and Mg^{2+} being used in the adenylylation catalyzed by the FAD synthetase (Oka and McCormick, 1987). Production of flavocoenzymes is sensitive to changes in flavokinase activity, which decreases during a deficiency of riboflavin (Lee and McCormick, 1983) and is induced by riboflavin repletion (Merrill et al., 1978). Thyroid hormone increases flavokinase activity by conversion of the enzyme from a less-active to a more-active form (Lee and McCormick, 1985). The FAD synthetase step may serve to downregulate flavocoenzyme formation in that FAD synthetase is inhibited by its product, FAD (Yamada et al., 1990). In the covalent attachment of FAD, the apoenzyme itself catalyzes the flavinylation (Decker, 1993).

$$\text{Riboflavin} \xrightarrow[\text{Flavokinase}]{\text{ATP} \searrow Zn^{2+} \nearrow \text{ADP}} \text{FMN} \xrightarrow[\text{FAD Synthetase}]{\text{ATP} \searrow Mg^{2+} \nearrow PP_i} \text{FAD}$$

Figure 24-13 Enzymatic steps in flavocoenzyme formation.

RIBOFLAVIN CATABOLISM AND EXCRETION

There is varied but not extensive catabolism of riboflavin in mammalian species, and many of the products that have been found in excreta, particularly urine, reflect the action of microflora in the gut and the effects of photodegradation (Chastain and McCormick, 1991). Because there is little storage of riboflavin as such, the urinary excretion of flavins (~0.3 mg/day in normal adults) reflects dietary intake. For normal adults eating varied diets, riboflavin accounts for 60% to 70% of urinary flavin. Other urinary flavins are the 7-hydroxymethyl metabolite, 10% to 15%; 8α-sulfonylriboflavin, 5% to 10%; 8-hydroxymethylriboflavin, 4% to 7%; riboflavinyl peptide ester, 4% to 5%; 10-(2′-hydroxyethyl)-flavin, 1% to 3%; traces of lumiflavin and varyingly 10-formylmethylflavin and the carboxymethylflavins (Roughead and McCormick, 1991; Chastain and McCormick, 1988; 1987). Both 7- and 8-hydroxymethylriboflavin are the result of the action of microsomal mixed-function oxidases. Side-chain degradation products, such as lumichrome, 10-formylmethylriboflavin, and the 10-hydroxyethylflavin, may result largely from the action of intestinal microorganisms. Both lumichrome and lumiflavin are photodecomposition products. The 8α-flavin peptides and their catabolites are formed from dietary and endogenous covalently linked flavins. Traces of 5′-riboflavinyl glucoside also have been found.

Secretion of flavin into milk is a significant process, and milk is a very important food source of riboflavin. In milk from cows (Roughead and McCormick, 1990a) and humans (Roughead and McCormick, 1990b), the flavin in highest concentration other than the free vitamin is FAD, which can account for more than one third of total flavin. Much of the FAD in cow's milk is hydrolyzed to FMN during pasteurization. Significant quantities of 10-(2′-hydroxyethyl)flavin and the 10-formylmethylflavin from which it is derived are secreted in milk, and 10-(2′-hydroxyethyl)flavin may reach 10% to 12% of the flavin in cow's milk. Because these catabolites have antivitaminic activities, as reflected in competitive inhibition both of cellular uptake and subsequent flavokinase-catalyzed phosphorylation of riboflavin, the presence of 10-(2′-hydroxyethyl)flavin in cow's milk subtracts from the biological activity of this food. Several percent of both 7- and 8-hydroxymethylriboflavins are also present, with more of the former. The 7-hydroxymethyl compound, also named 7α-hydroxyriboflavin, is the major flavin catabolite that appears in human plasma after oral administration of riboflavin (Zempleni et al., 1996b). Smaller amounts of other catabolites, including the 10-formylmethylflavin and lumichrome, account for most of the rest of the flavin in milk.

FUNCTIONS OF FLAVOCOENZYMES IN METABOLISM

Flavocoenzymes participate in oxidation–reduction reactions in numerous pathways and in energy production via the respiratory chain (see Figs. 24-7 and 24-8). Flavoproteins function in either one- or two-electron transfer reactions. Those involved in one-electron transfers cycle through the radical semiquinone, which can exist as either a neutral or anionic species (see Fig. 24-12). A further electron can lead to a fully reduced hydroquinone, again either neutral or anionic. The FMN portion of the microsomal NADPH-cytochrome P450 reductase uses reduced FAD as a one-electron donor and cytochrome P450 as an acceptor; it cycles between neutral semiquinone and fully reduced hydroquinone. The FAD in the electron-transferring flavoprotein, which mediates electron flow from fatty acyl CoA to the mitochondrial electron transport chain, cycles between oxidized quinone and anionic semiquinone. In addition, a single-step, two-electron transfer from substrate can occur in nucleophilic reactions. Such cases as hydride ion transfer from reduced pyridine nucleotide (e.g., with dihydroorotate dehydrogenase) or the carbanion generated by base abstraction of a substrate proton (e.g., with D-amino acid oxidase) may lead to attack at the flavin N-5 position; some species such as activated molecular oxygen add at the C-4α position to generate a transient hydroperoxide (e.g., with microsomal FAD-containing monooxygenase). These and other examples have been summarized along with a discussion of putative mechanisms (Merrill et al., 1981).

In these oxidation–reduction reactions, the ring portion of the flavocoenzyme involving nitrogens 1 and 5 and carbon 4α undergoes sequential addition or loss of hydrogens and electrons as shown in Figure 24-14. Flavocoenzymes are varyingly able to catalyze both one- and two-electron redox reactions. In some cases an enzyme (e.g., NADPH-cytochrome P450 reductase that contains both FAD and FMN) can catalyze both one and two-electron redox reactions. In most cases, however, a given flavoprotein probably catalyzes its natural reaction, not fully understood for all cases, by a one- or a two-electron transfer mechanism.

In a manner analogous to that of the pyridine nucleotide-dependent dehydrogenases, the transfer of hydrogen can take place at either face (*re* or *si*) of the isoalloxazine ring system. A number of flavoproteins have now been categorized on this steric basis (Creighton and Murthy, 1990).

Flavoprotein-catalyzed dehydrogenations include both pyridine nucleotide-dependent and independent reactions in which the pyridine nucleotides act as electron donors or acceptors, reactions with sulfur-containing compounds, hydroxylations, oxidative decarboxylations, dioxygenations, and reduction of O_2 to hydrogen peroxide. The intrinsic abilities of flavins to be

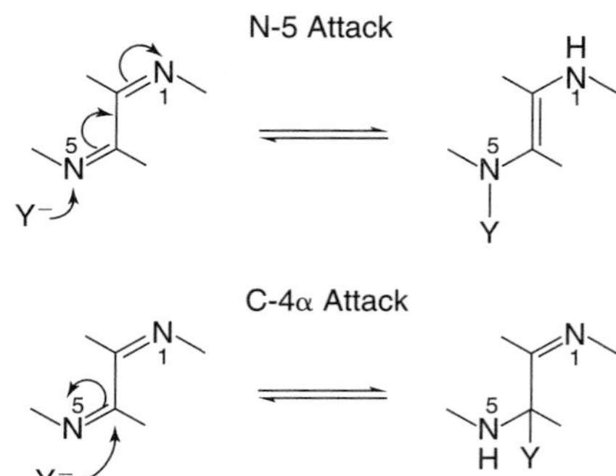

Figure 24-14 Reaction types encountered with flavoquinone coenzymes and natural nucleophiles (Y^-).

Clinical Correlation

Multiple Acyl CoA Dehydrogenase Disorders and Riboflavin

Multiple acyl CoA dehydrogenase disorders or glutaric acidemia type II results in excretion of a variety of organic acids (including glutaric, 2-hydroxyglutaric, adipic, suberic, ethylmalonic, and other dicarboxylic acids; and isovaleric, 2-methylbutyric, isobutyric, and other metabolites of branched-chain amino acids) along with esters of fatty acids with glycine or carnitine in the urine. The ω-oxidation of fatty acids to dicarboxylic acids and the transesterification of acyl groups with carnitine and glycine are the result of alternative pathways of metabolism for substrates that accumulate because they cannot be catabolized by their normal catabolic pathways..

Cultured skin fibroblasts from patients with multiple acyl CoA dehydrogenase deficiency have a severely reduced capacity for oxidation of a variety of organic acyl CoAs, including short-, medium-, and long-chain fatty acyl CoAs; glutaryl CoA (from lysine or tryptophan); isovaleryl CoA (from leucine); 2-methylbutyryl CoA (from isoleucine); and isobutyryl CoA (from valine). Although the oxidation of these metabolites requires several different dehydrogenases, each specific for its substrate, this group of dehydrogenases shares a common oxidizing agent, an electron transfer flavoprotein (ETF) that contains tightly bound flavin adenine diphosphate (FAD). The ETF-$FADH_2$ is reoxidized by ETF dehydrogenase with reduction of coenzyme Q (ubiquinone); this connects the flow of electrons to the electron transport chain and eventually to oxygen, with formation of water and generation of ATP. Multiple acyl CoA dehydrogenase deficiency has been attributed to a defect of either ETF or ETF dehydrogenase.

Multiple acyl CoA dehydrogenation disorders usually present in infancy with failure to thrive and repeated episodes of vomiting, lethargy, and coma with dicarboxylic aciduria and hypoketotic hypoglycemia. Mild or late-onset forms of multiple acyl CoA dehydrogenase disorders are rarer, and the clinical picture is variable.

Diagnosis of multiple acyl CoA dehydrogenase deficiency was made in a 62-year-old man who was admitted to the hospital because of easy fatigue in his legs during walking (Araki et al., 1994). He had also experienced fatigue of his neck muscles from holding his head erect. Biopsied muscle samples showed excessive lipid accumulation. The muscle free carnitine concentration was at the lower end of the normal range, and the acylcarnitine to free carnitine ratio in skeletal muscle was elevated to greater than the normal range. The concentrations of lactate and pyruvate in the blood were within the normal range in the resting state, but were markedly increased after a 7.5-minute walk. Riboflavin therapy resulted in a dramatic improvement in both clinical and biochemical parameters.

Thinking Critically

1. In this adult patient, how could you explain the excessive lipid storage in muscle? How would you explain muscle fatigue?
2. In this adult patient, a defect in FAD binding to ETF dehydrogenase was suspected. Why?
3. What dietary recommendations would you make for children with multiple acyl CoA dehydrogenase deficiency in terms of fat, carbohydrate, and protein intake? Would energy production via aerobic oxidation of glucose be affected in these patients? Explain.
4. Secondary carnitine deficiency has been diagnosed in a number of cases, as in this adult patient. Plasma free carnitine is typically low or undetectable, but acylcarnitine is present in plasma. Marked clinical improvements have been observed in patients following carnitine supplementation. What is a possible basis for the carnitine deficiency or the accumulation of acylcarnitine?

altered in their oxidation–reduction potentials upon differential binding to proteins, to participate in both one- and two-electron transfers, and in reduced (1,5-dihydro) form to react rapidly with oxygen permit them to function in a wide range of reactions.

RIBOFLAVIN DEFICIENCY

The physiological responses to inadequate dietary intake of riboflavin are numerous and can be severe. In ariboflavinosis, growth typically is stunted, and a variety of skin lesions appear. Clinical features of riboflavin deficiency include seborrheic dermatitis; soreness and burning of the lips, mouth, and tongue; photophobia; burning and itching of the eyes; superficial vascularization of the cornea; cheilosis; angular stomatitis; glossitis; anemia; and neuropathy. The similar skin lesions observed in riboflavin and vitamin B_6 deficiencies appear to reflect impaired collagen formation and, in the case of riboflavin, may be due to decreased activity of pyridoxine (pyridoxamine) 5′-phosphate oxidase, which requires FMN as a cofactor for the conversion of pyridoxine 5′-phosphate (PNP) and pyridoxamine 5′-phosphate (PMP) to pyridoxal 5′-phosphate (PLP). Riboflavin and its coenzyme derivatives are light sensitive. Newborn infants with hyperbilirubinemia who are treated with phototherapy commonly require additional riboflavin during treatment.

Enzymatic alterations occur in riboflavin deficiency. Flavokinase, which is unstable in the absence of its riboflavin substrate, decreases in activity, and there is an increase in FAD synthetase activity. These changes may explain the relatively greater decrease in hepatic FMN than in FAD levels that occurs in riboflavin deficiency. Marked decreases in the activities of FMN- and FAD-requiring enzymes, such as xanthine oxidase and glutathione reductase, occur in tissues from riboflavin-deficient animals.

Negligible amounts of riboflavin are excreted in the urine during riboflavin deficiency; this suggests that the body may be capable of reutilizing much of the riboflavin released by its own catabolic processes. Despite an apparent ability to conserve some riboflavin, the daily need to replace tissue turnover in the adult appears to remain greater than 0.5 mg.

BIOCHEMICAL ASSESSMENT OF RIBOFLAVIN NUTRITURE

Currently, the most commonly used method for assessing riboflavin status is the determination of glutathione reductase activity in freshly lysed erythrocytes (McCormick and Greene, 1999). The augmentation in activity after incubation with FAD in vitro has been used to assess riboflavin nutrition both in experimental animals and in humans. Both a low absolute activity of erythrocyte glutathione reductase and an elevated fractional stimulation of that activity by addition of FAD are indicative of riboflavin deficiency. Urinary riboflavin excretion (24 hours) of less than 10% of that ingested also may reflect inadequate nutrition. The red blood cell concentration of riboflavin also has been used as an indicator of riboflavin status, with values less than 0.15 mg/L of erythrocytes considered as low or deficient.

RIBOFLAVIN REQUIREMENTS

Riboflavin requirements have been related to protein allowances, lean body mass, metabolic body size, and energy intake. All of these are in themselves related; not surprisingly, allowances calculated by the various methods do not differ significantly. Urinary excretion of riboflavin is low in adults and children who consume less than 0.5 mg/1,000 kcal, and rises sharply as dietary riboflavin is increased to 0.75 mg/1,000 kcal and higher. Lesions of riboflavin deficiency have been seen in individuals receiving approximately 0.35 mg/1,000 kcal. FAD stimulation of erythrocyte glutathione reductase activity was in a normal range in adults with riboflavin intakes of 0.6 mg or more per 1,000 kcal.

Based on intakes that prevent clinical and biochemical signs of deficiency, the IOM (1998) set the EAR for riboflavin at 1.1 mg/day for men and 0.9 mg/day for women. The RDA was set as the EAR + 20% and is 1.3 mg/day for men and 1.1 mg/day for women (IOM, 1998). Increments of +0.3 mg/day and +0.5 mg/day were added to the RDAs for pregnant women and lactating women, respectively. EARs and RDAs for children were estimated by extrapolation from adult values on the basis of metabolic body weight plus an allowance for growth. The IOM (1998) established AIs for infants from birth to 6 months of age based on the average intake of riboflavin by breast-fed infants (0.35 mg riboflavin/L milk × 0.78 L milk/day + 0.3 mg/day). The AI for older infants was extrapolated from values for younger infants and adults.

Based on data from NHANES III, the median intake of riboflavin from food in the United States is 2.0 mg/day for men and 1.6 mg/day for women. The range of intakes (5th to 95th percentile levels) was 1.2 to 3.6 mg/day for men and 1.0 to 2.8 mg/day for women. Therefore, intakes for nearly all adults in the United States exceed the RDA.

Riboflavin has a low toxicity. No cases of riboflavin toxicity in humans have been reported. This may be due to its low solubility or to the ready excretion of unbound riboflavin in the urine.

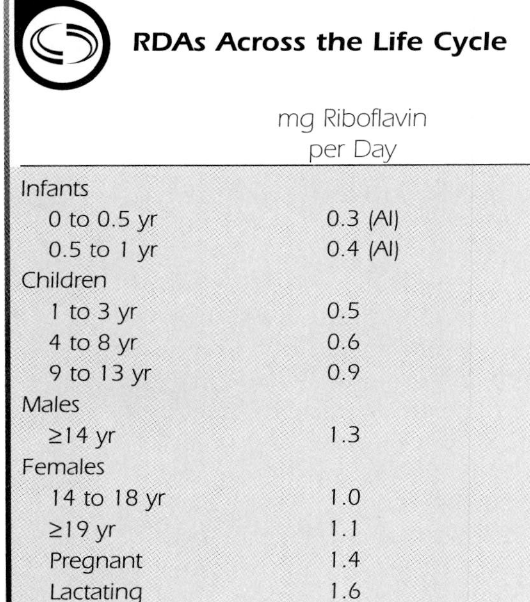

RDAs Across the Life Cycle

	mg Riboflavin per Day
Infants	
0 to 0.5 yr	0.3 (AI)
0.5 to 1 yr	0.4 (AI)
Children	
1 to 3 yr	0.5
4 to 8 yr	0.6
9 to 13 yr	0.9
Males	
≥14 yr	1.3
Females	
14 to 18 yr	1.0
≥19 yr	1.1
Pregnant	1.4
Lactating	1.6

Data from Institute of Medicine (1998) Dietary Reference Intakes for Thiamin, Riboflavin, Niacin, Vitamin B_6, Folate, Vitamin B_{12}, Pantothenic Acid, Biotin, and Choline. National Academy Press, Washington, DC.
AI, Adequate intake.

THIAMIN

Thiamin (also known as vitamin B_1) is required for formation of its coenzyme, thiamin pyrophosphate (TPP). TPP functions in prime interconversions of sugar phosphates and in decarboxylation reactions with energy production from α-keto acids and their acyl CoA derivatives, which are catabolically derived from carbohydrates and amino acids. TPP also functions in α-oxidation of 3-methyl-substituted fatty acids (Casteels et al., 2003).

THIAMIN AND THIAMIN COENZYME STRUCTURE AND NOMENCLATURE

Thiamin is a pyrimidyl-substituted thiazole (3-[2-methyl-4-aminopyrimidinyl]methyl-4-methyl-5-[β-hydroxyethyl]thiazole), as illustrated in Figure 24-15. The vitamin usually is isolated or synthesized and handled as a solid thiazolium salt (e.g., thiamin chloride hydrochloride).

The principal if not sole coenzyme form of thiamin is the pyrophosphate ester called TPP or thiamin diphosphate (TDP), also shown in Figure 24-15. Monophosphate and triphosphate esters occur naturally as well, and the triphosphate has been implicated in nerve function.

SOURCES, DIGESTION, AND ABSORPTION

Thiamin occurs in natural foods mainly as the phosphorylated derivatives. More abundant sources are unrefined cereal germs and whole grains, meats (especially pork), nuts, and legumes. Enriched flours and grain products in the United States contain added thiamin, as well as niacin and riboflavin (Gubler, 1991).

Elevation of temperature, especially in aqueous media above neutral pH, leads to rapid loss of thiamin activity. The thiazole ring

R = H Thiamin
R = P(O)(O⁻)—O—P(O)(O⁻)—O⁻ Thiamin pyrophosphate

Figure 24-15 Structures and numbering of thiamin and its pyrophosphate coenzyme.

is subject to base attack at carbon 2, followed by ring opening to an acyclic sulfide. Under oxidizing conditions, thiamin can form disulfides intermolecularly or thiochrome intramolecularly. Rupture of the methylene bridge to the thiazole nitrogen also occurs readily when thiamin is exposed to sulfite, which is formed during preservation of foods with sulfur dioxide.

Following release of thiamin during digestive hydrolysis catalyzed by pyrophosphatase and phosphatase in the upper small intestine, the vitamin is readily absorbed by a carrier-mediated process (McCormick and Greene, 1999). This high-affinity thiamin transporter is encoded by human gene *SLC19A2*, and it is expressed in all tissues of the human gastrointestinal tract and in liver, with liver, stomach, duodenum, and jejunum having higher levels of expression than the ileum and colon (Reidling et al., 2002). The thiamin transporter is homologous to the reduced-folate transporter. Although carrier-mediated transport predominates at intakes of thiamin up to 5 mg/day, passive diffusion increasingly contributes to absorption at higher intakes. Pyrophosphorylation catalyzed by thiamin pyrophosphokinase (thiaminokinase) takes place in the jejunal mucosal cells to yield TPP, a process of metabolic trapping that seemingly relates to the facilitation of uptake. The exit of thiamin from the mucosal cell on the basolateral side is a proton gradient–dependent specialized carrier-mediated transport that exchanges thiamin and H^+ with a 1:1 stoichiometry (Dudeja et al., 2003).

The saturable (specific) component of thiamin transport is missing in patients with the rare disease known as thiamin-responsive megaloblastic anemia (Rindi and Laforenza, 2000). All known patients with this disease who have been studied to date have mutations in the *SLC19A2* gene, which codes for the plasma membrane thiamin transporter. These patients have a general disturbance of thiamin transport, resulting in thiamin deficiency. In addition to thiamin-responsive megaloblastic anemia, this autosomal recessive disorder is associated with development of sensorineural deafness and diabetes mellitus; some patients develop cardiomyopathy, optic nerve atrophy, and retinal atrophy. Pharmacological doses of thiamin are able to reverse the anemia and diabetes mellitus in most patients.

Similarly to the brush-border membrane of the small intestine, the renal brush-border membrane appears to reabsorb thiamin by a saturable carrier-mediated transport system. Thiamin uptake by renal brush-border membrane vesicles was also stimulated by an outwardly directed H^+ gradient, allowing accumulation of thiamin inside the vesicles against a concentration gradient (Gastaldi et al., 2000).

Food Sources

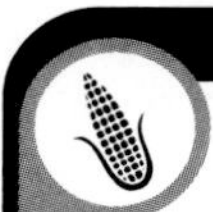

Food Sources of Thiamin

Meats

0.4 to 1.0 mg per 3 oz pork or ham

Cereals and Grain Products

0.3 to 0.9 mg per 1 cup ready-to-eat cereals
0.4 mg per 4-in. (3-oz) bagel
0.3 mg per 2-oz hard roll
0.15 mg per ½ cup noodles or pasta
0.1 mg per ½ cup cooked rice

Legumes

0.2 mg per ½ cup black beans, green peas
0.15 mg per ½ cup lentils or beans (pinto, kidney, great northern, limas)

Fruits

0.3 mg per 6 oz grapefruit juice
0.3 mg per 1 cup orange juice

Data from US Department of Agriculture/Agricultural Research Service (USDA/ARS) (2005) USDA National Nutrient Standard Database, Release 18. USDA/ARS, Washington, DC. Retrieved December 23, 2005, from www.ars.usda.gov/ba/bhrnc/ndl.

TRANSPORT AND CONVERSION OF THIAMIN TO COENZYME

Thiamin is carried by the portal circulation to the liver and from there to the general circulation. The free vitamin occurs in the plasma, but TPP predominates in the cellular components.

Leukocytes have a 10-fold higher concentration than erythrocytes. Thiamin transport into cells seems to occur by a similar saturable carrier in various tissues, but there is a marked variation of transport capacity among tissues. For example, transport capacity is high in hepatocytes as in enterocytes, but much lower in erythrocytes. This suggests that the number or efficiency of carrier sites may differ according to the type of tissue or its function (Rindi, 1992). There is a thiamin transporter in both the plasma and mitochondrial membranes of cells. The mitochondria also have a high-affinity transporter for TPP that may be important in supplying phosphorylated thiamine for certain mitochondrial enzymes (Song and Singleton, 2002).

Only a small amount, perhaps 30 mg, of this water-soluble vitamin and its phosphates are stored in the body. About half is in muscle and the rest in heart, liver, kidneys, and nervous tissues. Approximately 80% is as the pyrophosphate, 10% as the triphosphate, and the rest as thiamin and its monophosphate.

The three main enzymes that participate in the formation and interconversions of thiamine and its phosphate esters are noted in Figure 24-16. A pyrophosphokinase (diphosphokinase) catalyzes formation of the coenzyme TPP. Some of this is routed to the monophosphates and triphosphates by a TPP–ATP phosphoryltransferase activity shown to be attributable to cytosolic adenylate kinase (Kawasaki, 1992). This enzyme can reversibly catalyze the conversion of two moles of the diphosphate (ADP or TPP) to form one of triphosphate (ATP or TTP) and one of monophosphate (AMP or TMP). There are tissue phosphatases that can hydrolyze TMP to release thiamin. A membrane-associated triphosphatase, mainly in nervous tissue, and pyrophosphatases also contribute to the interconversions of free and phosphorylated forms of thiamin (Ogawa and Sakai, 1982).

THIAMIN CATABOLISM AND EXCRETION

Thiamin much in excess of tissue needs is rapidly excreted in the urine. At least 50 metabolites have been reported to occur in the urine from rats and humans (Neal, 1970), but six of these have been identified to reflect the main catabolic events. These major urinary catabolites of thiamin are thiamin acetic acid, 2-methyl-4-amino-5-formylaminomethylpyrimidine, 4-methyl-5-(2-hydroxyethyl)thiazole, 2-methyl-4-amino-pyrimidine-5-carboxylic acid, 2-methyl-4-amino-5-hydroxymethylpyrimidine, and 4-methylthiazole-5-acetic acid. In addition, small amounts of thiamin disulfide and thiochrome have been identified. Thiaminase II, present in intestinal bacteria, leads to formation of the pyrimidine and thiazole portions that are in part further oxidized in their hydroxymethyl functions to yield substituted pyrimidine carboxylates and thiazole carboxylates. Cleavage into the rings also occurs, as noted from the formation of the formylmethylaminopyrimidine. As with some urinary flavins, several of the numerous metabolites of thiamin arise from action of symbiotic microflora in the gut.

FUNCTIONS OF COENZYMATIC THIAMIN IN METABOLISM

There are two general types of reactions in which TPP functions as the Mg^{2+}-coordinated coenzyme for so-called active aldehyde transfers, which involve attack of carbonyl metabolites by the carbanion generated at carbon 2 on the thiazole moiety of TPP, as shown in Figure 24-17. First, in decarboxylation of α-keto acids, the condensation of the thiazole moiety of TPP with the α-carbonyl carbon on the acid leads to loss of CO_2 and production of a resonance-stabilized carbanion. Protonation and

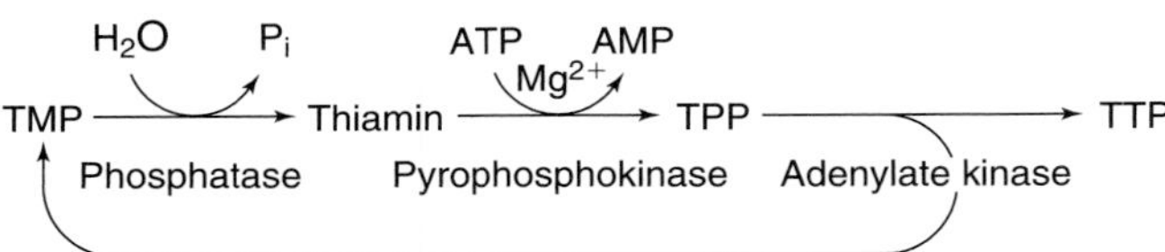

Figure 24-16 Interconversions of thiamin and its monophosphates (TMP), diphosphates (TPP), and triphosphates (TTP).

release of aldehyde (acetaldehyde from pyruvate) occur in fermentative organisms such as yeast, which have only the TPP-dependent decarboxylase. However, in higher eukaryotes, including humans, the TPP-dependent decarboxylases exist as part of multienzymic dehydrogenase complexes. These enzyme complexes transfer the α-hydroxyalkyl group from TPP to a covalently linked lipoic acid prosthetic group with oxidation of the hydroxyalkyl carbanion to an acyl group with the concomitant reduction of the lipoyl disulfide bond, transfer of the acyl group from the lipoyl prosthetic group to coenzyme A to form the respective acyl CoA, the reduction of FAD to $FADH_2$ with reoxidation of the dihydrolipoyl group to its disulfide form, and the oxidation of $FADH_2$ back to FAD by conversion of NAD^+ to NADH. These TPP-dependent (and FAD- and NAD-dependent) α-ketoacid dehydrogenase complexes are used to catalyze the oxidative decarboxylation of pyruvate to acetyl CoA, α-ketoglutarate to succinyl CoA, and the α-ketoacids from branched-chain amino acids to their respective acyl CoAs. The pyruvate and branched-chain amino acid dehydrogenase complexes also convert α-ketobutyrate to propionyl CoA.

Another general reaction involving TPP is the transformation of α-ketols (ketose phosphates). Although specialized phosphoketolases in certain bacteria and higher plants can split ketose phosphates to simpler, released products, the reactions of importance to humans and most animals are transketolations. Transketolase is a TPP-dependent enzyme found in the cytosol of many tissues, especially liver and blood cells, in which the pentose phosphate pathway (also called the hexose monophosphate shunt or 6-phosphogluconate pathway) of glucose metabolism exists. Transketolase catalyzes the reversible transfer of a glycoaldehyde moiety (α,β-dihydroxyethyl-TPP) from the first two carbons of a donor ketose phosphate (D-xylulose 5-phosphate or D-sedoheptulose 7-phosphate) to the aldehyde carbon of an aldose phosphate (D-ribose 5-phosphate or D-erythrose 4-phosphate). These sugar rearrangements are essential for synthesis of ribose and for funneling the 5-carbon sugar phosphate back into the glycolytic and gluconeogenic pathways as triose or hexose phosphates.

There are interconnecting pathways from metabolism of carbohydrates and amino acids that have steps critically dependent upon TPP, as summarized in Figures 24-17

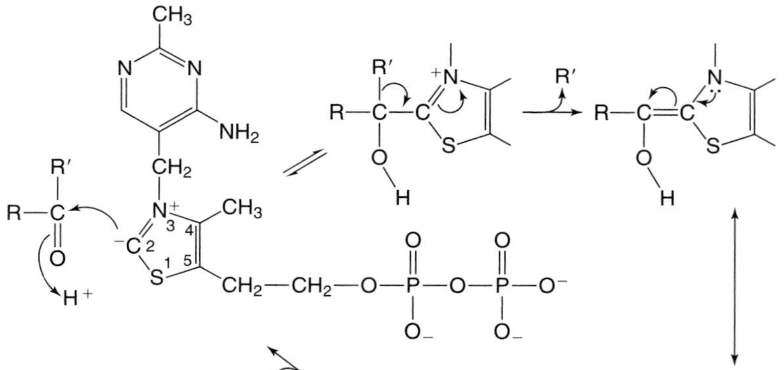

Figure 24-17 Function of the thiazole moiety of TPP in α-keto acid decarboxylations (where *R′* is a carboxylate lost as CO_2 and *R″* is a proton generating an aldehyde) and in ketolations (where *R′* is a carbohydrate moiety releasing a glycose and *R″* is a different glycose generating a new carbohydrate).

and 24-18. Additional discussion of reactions requiring TPP can be found in Chapters 12 and 14 (see Figs. 12-18, 12-20, 14-19, 14-21, and 14-28). An important role of TPP is in the α-oxidation of 3-methyl-branched fatty acids, such as phytanic acid, which undergo shortening by one carbon in a process that includes activation, 2-hydroxylation, a TPP-dependent cleavage, and aldehyde dehydrogenation. Failure of this system, mostly linked to the second enzyme of the sequence, phytanoyl CoA hydroxylase, results in Refsum's disease (Casteels et al., 2003).

Although thiamin as its pyrophosphate contributes to nervous system function in such essential reactions as energy production and biosynthesis of lipids and acetylcholine, it appears that there is another incompletely understood role, particularly for the triphosphate (Bender, 1992; Haas, 1988). Electrical stimulation of nerves leads to hydrolysis and release of both di- and triphosphates of thiamin from axonal membranes, which also have relatively high activities of enzymes that cause formation and breakdown of TTP.

THIAMIN DEFICIENCY

Beriberi is the name (Indonesian) given to the disease resulting from thiamin deficiency (McCormick and Greene, 1999). The causes for deficiency include inadequate intake due

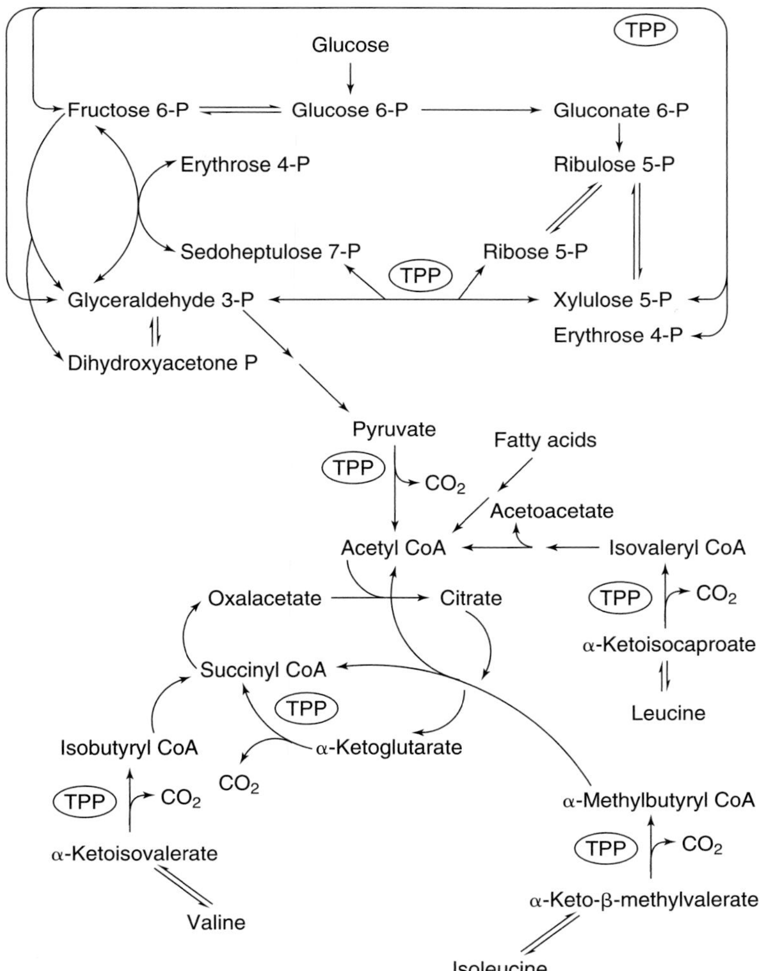

Figure 24-18 Pathways dependent on coenzymatic thiamin pyrophosphate (TPP).

to diets largely dependent on milled, non-enriched grains such as rice and wheat, or to the ingestion of raw fish that contain microbial thiaminases, which hydrolytically destroy the vitamin in the gastrointestinal tract. Tea may contain antithiamin factors that also have been detected in certain other plant extracts. Chronic alcoholism is a common contributor to deficiency in that there is not only a low intake of thiamin (and other B vitamins), but also impaired absorption and storage. There are several thiamin-responsive inborn errors of metabolism; these include a megaloblastic anemia attributable to lack of thiamin transporter, lactic acidosis due to low or defective pyruvate decarboxylase, branched-chain keto-aciduria with poor activity of the branched-chain keto acid dehydrogenase system, and subacute necrotizing encephalomyelopathy associated with a lack of thiamin triphosphate in neural tissues. Therapeutic doses of 5 to 20 mg of thiamin daily have proved beneficial in some cases. Finally, other at-risk patients are those undergoing long-term renal dialysis or intravenous feeding and even those with chronic febrile infections.

Clinical signs primarily involve the nervous and cardiovascular systems. In the adult, symptoms most frequently observed are mental confusion, anorexia, muscular weakness, ataxia, peripheral paralysis, paralysis of the motor nerves of the eye, edema (wet beriberi), muscle wasting (dry beriberi), tachycardia, and an enlarged heart. In infants, symptoms appear suddenly and severely, often involving cardiac failure and cyanosis (bluish coloration of skin and mucous membranes due to deficient oxygenation of the blood). Commonly, the distinction between wet (cardiovascular) and dry (neuritic) manifestations of beriberi relate to duration and severity of the deficiency, the degree of physical exertion, and caloric intake. The wet or edematous condition results from severe physical exertion and high carbohydrate intake, whereas the dry or polyneuritic form stems from relative inactivity with caloric restriction along with chronic thiamin deficiency. The three major physiological derangements that involve the cardiovascular system are peripheral vasodilation that leads to a high cardiac output state, biventricular myocardial failure, and retention of sodium and water that leads to edema. Nervous system involvement includes peripheral neuropathy, Wernicke's encephalopathy, and the amnesic psychosis of Korsakoff's syndrome.

BIOCHEMICAL ASSESSMENT OF THIAMIN NUTRITURE

Numerous methods have been used to assess the state of thiamin nutrition in man (McCormick and Greene, 1999). The most common of these are (1) the measurement of the activity of erythrocyte transketolase, a thiamin pyrophosphate-requiring enzyme; (2) the measurement of blood or urinary levels of thiamin using various chemical, microbiological, and chromatographic techniques; and (3) the measurement of blood levels of pyruvate and α-ketoglutarate. The measurement of whole blood or erythrocyte transketolase activity (basal level) and the enhancement of basal enzymatic activity by the addition of TPP are considered to be the most reliable methods; TPP stimulation of greater than 16% indicates possible deficiency. Symptoms of beriberi (such as peripheral neuropathy and cardiac abnormalities) usually do not appear until the TPP stimulation of erythrocyte transketolase activity is about 40%.

THIAMIN REQUIREMENTS

The RDA for thiamin is 1.2 mg of thiamin per day for men and 1.1 mg/day for women. EARs for thiamin are based on the relation between thiamin intake and appearance of clinical signs of deficiency, on excretion of thiamin and its metabolites, and on erythrocyte tranketolase and TPP effects; these estimates are 1.0 mg/day for men and 0.9 mg/day for women (IOM, 1998). RDAs were set assuming a coefficient of variation of 10% (i.e., EAR + 20%).

The RDAs have been increased by 0.3 mg/day for pregnant women and by 0.4 mg/day for lactating women to cover the estimated requirements for growth in maternal and fetal compartments, secretion in the milk, and small increases in energy utilization. Recommendations for infants are based on the thiamin content of human breast milk and on caloric intake; the AI for infants from birth to 6 months of age is 0.03 mg/kg/day or 0.2 mg/day. Recommendations for older infants and children are extrapolated from adult values with consideration of body size and needs for growth.

No UL was set by the IOM (1998) due to a lack of reports of adverse effects from consumption of excess thiamin by ingestion of food and supplements. Supplements that contain up to 50 mg/day are widely available.

Based on NHANES III, the median intake of thiamin by adults is about 1.7 mg/day for men and 1.4 mg/day for women. The 5th and 95th percentile intakes are about 1.0 to 3.2 mg/day for men and 0.9 to 2.4 mg/day for women. Therefore, most individuals in the United States have intakes greater than the EAR. The highest intakes of thiamin observed were for pregnant women taking supplements; the 95th percentile level for these women was 11 mg/day.

Thiamin requirements appear to be elevated in individuals with elevated caloric intakes, especially when calories are derived primarily from carbohydrates, in individuals consuming ethanol, in renal patients undergoing long-term dialysis, in patients fed intravenously for long periods, and in patients with chronic febrile infections. Folate deficiency appears to depress thiamin absorption. The depression of thiamin absorption observed in alcoholics may be secondary to a folate deficiency. Individuals deplete body stores of thiamin rapidly during starvation or semistarvation.

RDAs Across the Life Cycle

	mg Thiamin per Day
Infants	
0 to 0.5 yr	0.2 (AI)
0.5 to 1 yr	0.3 (AI)
Children	
1 to 3 yr	0.5
4 to 8 yr	0.6
9 to 13 yr	0.9
Males	
≥14 yr	1.2
Females	
14 to 18 yr	1.0
≥19 yr	1.1
Pregnant	1.4
Lactating	1.4

Data from Institute of Medicine (1998) Dietary Reference Intakes for Thiamin, Riboflavin, Niacin, Vitamin B_6, Folate, Vitamin B_{12}, Pantothenic Acid, Biotin, and Choline. National Academy Press, Washington, DC.
AI, Adequate intake.

Nutrition Insight

Alcoholism and Genetics as Factors in Thiamin Deficiency Disorders

In industrialized countries, symptomatic thiamin deficiency is usually associated with alcoholism. The majority of individuals with Wernicke-Korsakoff syndrome have a history of chronic alcohol abuse. Wernicke's encephalopathy is characterized by disturbances in ocular motility and by ataxia with tremors. Korsakoff's psychosis is characterized by confusion and severe impairment of memory, especially for recent events. A poor diet with low thiamin intake, sustained caloric intake from alcohol, and possible impairments in thiamin absorption and utilization play a role in the development of Wernicke-Korsakoff disease. It also appears that an inborn error or genetic variant predisposes some individuals to thiamin deficiency diseases. Fibroblast cultures from patients with Wernicke-Korsakoff disease show an elevated K_m of the transketolase enzymes for thiamin pyrophosphate (TPP) or, in other words, poor binding of coenzyme TPP to the apoenzyme transketolase to form active holoenzyme. Hence, alcohol consumption and genetic predisposition both may be factors in the development of thiamin deficiency diseases. Symptoms respond to parenterally administered thiamin, but not all patients recover completely.

Thiamin requirements and metabolism may be altered by various thiaminases and thiamin antagonists such as caffeic acid, tannic acid, and heme-containing animal tissues. Thiaminases are found in viscera of some freshwater fish and shellfish and in several microorganisms. Thiamin antagonists may be found in coffee, tea, rice bran, and other sources. Thiamin deficiency has been associated with consumption of large amounts of raw fish or large amounts of tea.

Some thiamin-responsive inborn errors of metabolism can be treated with pharmacological doses of thiamin. Some patients with inborn errors that result in low activity of the branched-chain keto acid dehydrogenase complex respond to treatment with 10 to 1,000 times the RDA for thiamin. Another thiamin-responsive inborn error is thiamin-responsive lactic acidosis, which is due to low activity of the pyruvate dehydrogenase complex in the liver.

Thiamin produces a variety of pharmacological effects and even death due to depression of the respiratory center when administered in doses thousands of times larger than those required for optimal nutrition. No toxic effects of thiamin administered by mouth have been reported in man. Thiamin is readily cleared by the kidneys. Injection of doses up to 200 times the daily maintenance dose generally has not led to toxic effects, but some individuals appear to develop a hypersensitivity to thiamin.

REFERENCES

Araki E, Kobayashi R, Kohtake N, Goto I, Hashimoto T (1994) A riboflavin-responsive lipid storage myopathy due to multiple acyl CoA dehydrogenase deficiency: an adult case. J Neurol Sci 126:202-205.

Aw TY, Jones DP, McCormick DB (1983) Uptake of riboflavin by isolated rat liver cells. J Nutr 113:1249-1254.

Bechgaard H, Jespersen S (1977) Gastrointestinal absorption of niacin in humans. J Pharm Sci 66:871-872.

Bender DA (1992) Vitamin B_1: thiamin. In:Bender DA (ed) Nutritional Biochemistry of the Vitamins. Cambridge University Press, Cambridge, pp 128-155.

Block G, Dresser CM, Hartman AH, Carroll MD (1985) Nutrient sources in the American diet: Quantitative data from the NHANES survey. Am J Epidemiol 122:13-26.

Bowers-Komro, DM, McCormick DB (1987) Riboflavin uptake by isolated rat kidney cells. In: Edmondson DE, McCormick DB (eds) Flavins and Flavoproteins. Walter de Gruyter, Berlin, pp 449-453.

Boyonoski AC, Spronck JC, Gallacher LM, Jacobs RM, Shah GM, Poirier GG, Kirkland JB (2002) Niacin deficiency decreases bone marrow poly(ADP-ribose) and the latency of ethylnitrosourea-induced carcinogenesis in rats. J Nutr 132:108-114.

Casteels M, Foulon V, Mannaerts GP, Van Beldhoven PP (2003) Alpha-oxidation of 3-methyl-substituted fatty acids and its thiamine dependence. Eur J Biochem 270:1619-1627.

Chastain JL, McCormick DB (1991) Flavin metabolites. In: Müller F (ed) Chemistry and Biochemistry of Flavins. Vol. I. CRC Press, Boca Raton, FL, pp 195-200.

Chastain JL, McCormick DB (1988) Characterization of a new flavin metabolite from human urine. Biochem Biophys Acta 967:131-134.

Chastain JL, McCormick DB (1987) Flavin catabolites: identification and quantitation in human urine. Am J Clin Nutr 46:830-834.

Chia CP, Addison R, McCormick DB (1978) Absorption, metabolism, and excretion of 8α-(amino acid)riboflavins in the rat. J Nutr 108:373-381.

Creighton DJ, Murthy NSRK (1990) Stereochemistry of enzyme-catalyzed reactions at carbon. In: Sigmon DS, Boyer PD (eds) The Enzymes. Vol. 19. Academic Press, San Diego, pp 323-421.

Decker KF (1993) Biosynthesis and function of enzymes with covalently bound flavin. Annu Rev Nutr 13:17-41.

DiPalma JR, Thayer WS (1991) Use of niacin as a drug. Annu Rev Nutr 11:169-187.

Dudeja PK, Tyagi S, Gill R, Said HM (2003) Evidence for a carrier-mediated mechanism for thiamine transport to human jejunal basolateral membrane vesicles. Dig Dis Sci 48:109-115.

Fukuoka S, Ishiguro K, Yanagihara K, Tanabe A, Egashira Y, Sanada H, Shibata K (2002) Identification and expression of a cDNA encoding human α-amino-β-carboxymuconate-ε-semialdehyde decarboxylase (ACMSD). A key enzyme for the tryptophan-niacin pathway and "quinolinate hypothesis." J Biol Chem 277:35162-35167.

Gastaldi G, Cova E, Verri A, Laforenza U, Faelli A, Rindi G (2000) Transport of thiamin in rat renal brush border membrane vesicles. Kidney Int 57:2043-2054.

Goodrich RP (2000) The use of riboflavin for the inactivation of pathogens in blood products. Vox Sanguinis 78, Suppl 2:211-215.

Gross CJ, Henderson LM (1983) Digestion and absorption of NAD by the small intestine of the rat. J Nutr 113:412-420.

Gubler CJ (1991) Thiamin. In: Machlin LH (ed) Handbook of Vitamins, 2nd ed. Marcel Dekker, New York, pp 233-281.

Haas RH (1988) Thiamin and the brain. Annu Rev Nutr 8:483-515.

Huang SN, Phelps MA, Swaan PW (2003) Involvement of endocytic organelles in the subcellular trafficking and localization of riboflavin. J Pharmacol Exp Ther 306: 681-687.

Institute of Medicine (1998) Dietary Reference Intakes for Thiamin, Riboflavin, Niacin, Vitamin B_6, Folate, Vitamin B_{12}, Pantothenic Acid, Biotin, and Choline. National Academy Press, Washington, DC.

Junod AJ, Jornot L, Petersen H (1989) Differential effects of hyperoxia and hydrogen peroxide on DNA damage, polyadenosine diphosphate-ribose polymerase activity, and nicotinamide adenine dinucleotide and adenosine triphosphate contents in cultured endothelial cells and fibroblasts. J Cell Physiol 140:177-185.

Kawasaki T (1992) Thiamin triphosphate synthesis in animals. In: Kobayashi T (ed) Proceedings of the 1st International Congress on Vitamins and Biofactors in Life Sciences. Center for Academic Publications Japan, Tokyo, pp 383-386.

Knox WE, Piras MM (1967) Tryptophan pyrrolase of liver. J Biol Chem 242:2959-2965.

Lee S-S, McCormick DB (1985) Thyroid hormone regulation of flavocoenzyme biosynthesis. Arch Biochem Biophys 237:197-201.

Lee S-S, McCormick DB (1983) Effect of riboflavin status on hepatic activities of flavin-metabolizing enzymes in rats. J Nutr 113:2274-2279.

McCormick DB, Greene HL (1999) Vitamins. In: Burtis CA, Ashwood ER (eds) Tietz Textbook of Clinical Chemistry, 3rd ed. W.B. Saunders, Philadelphia, pp 999-1029.

McCreanor GM, Bender DA (1986) The metabolism of high intakes of tryptophan, nicotinamide and nicotinic acid in the rat. Br J Nutr 56: 577-586.

Messamore E, Hoffman WE, Jankowsky A (2003) The niacin skin flush abnormality in schizophrenia: a quantitative dose-response study. Schizophr Res 62:251-258.

Merrill AH Jr, Addison R, McCormick DB (1978) Induction of hepatic and intestinal flavokinase after oral administration of riboflavin to riboflavin-deficient rats. Proc Soc Exp Biol Med 158:572–574.

Merrill AH Jr, Lambeth JD, Edmondson DE, McCormick DB (1981) Formation and mode of action of flavoproteins. Annu Rev Nutr 1:281-317.

Mrochek JE, Jolley RL, Young DS, Turner WJ (1976) Metabolic responses of humans to ingestion of nicotinic acid and nicotinamide. Clin Chem 22:1821-1827.

Nakano H, McCormick DB (1991) Stereospecificity of the metal·ATP complex in flavokinase from rat small intestine. J Biol Chem 266: 22125-22128.

Neal RA (1970) Isolation and identification of thiamin catabolites in mammalian urine; isolation and identification of some products of bacterial catabolism of thiamin. In: McCormick DB, Wright LD (eds) Methods in Enzymology. Vol. 18, part A. Academic Press, New York, pp 133-140.

Nokubo M, Ohta M, Kitani K, Zs-Nagy I (1989) Identification of protein-bound riboflavin in rat hepatocyte plasma membrane as a source of autofluorescence. Biochim Biophys Acta 931:303-308.

Oakley A, Wallace J (1994) Hartnup disease presenting in an adult. Clin Exp Dermatol 19:407-408.

Ogawa K, Sakai M (1982) Recent findings on ultra cytochemistry of thiamin phosphatases. In: Sable HZ, Gubler CJ (eds) Thiamin: Twenty Years of Progress. Vol. 378. Ann NY Acad Sci, New York, pp 188-214.

Oka M, McCormick DB (1987) Complete purification and general characterization of FAD synthetase from rat liver. J Biol Chem 262:7418-7422.

Okamoto H, Ishikawa A, Nishimuta M, Kodama N, Yoshitake Y, Fukuwatari T, Shibata K (2002) Effects of stress on the urinary excretion pattern of niacin catabolites, the most reliable index of niacin status, in humans. J Nutr Sci Vitaminol 48:417-419.

Rechsteiner M, Hillyard D, Olivera BM (1976) Turnover of nicotinamide adenine dinucleotide in cultures of human cells. J Cell Physiol 88:207-218.

Reidling JC, Subramanian VS, Dudeja PK, Said HM (2002) Expression and promoter analysis of SLC19A2 in the human intestine. Biochim Biophys Acta 1561:180-187.

Rindi G (1992) Some aspects of thiamin transport in mammals. In: Kobayahsi T (ed) Proceedings of the 1st International Congress on Vitamins and Biofactors in Life Sciences. Center for Academic Publications Japan, Tokyo, pp 379-382.

Rindi G, Laforenza U (2000) Thiamine intestinal transport and related issues: recent aspects. Proc Soc Exp Biol Med 224:246-255.

Roughead ZK, McCormick DB (1991) Urinary riboflavin and its metabolites: effects of riboflavin supplementation in healthy residents of rural Georgia (USA). Eur J Clin Nutr 45:299-307.

Roughead ZK, McCormick DB (1990a) Qualitative and quantitative assessment of flavins in cow's milk. J Nutr 120:382-388.

Roughead ZK, McCormick DB (1990b) Flavin composition of human milk. Am J Clin Nutr 52:854-857.

Schraufstatter IU, Hinshaw DB, Hyslope PA, Spragg RG, Cochrane CG (1986) Oxidant injury of cells. J Clin Invest 777:1312-1320.

Song Q, Singleton CK (2002) Mitochondria from cultured cells derived from normal and thiamine-responsive megaloblastic anemia individuals efficiently import thiamine diphosphate. BCM Biochem 3:8.

Tunaru S, Kero J, Schaub A, Wufka C, Blaukat A, Pfeffer K, Offermans S (2003) PUMA-G and HM74 are receptors for nicotinic acid and mediate its anti-lipolytic effect. Nat Med 9:352-355.

Whitehouse WSA, Merrill AH Jr, McCormick DB (1991) Riboflavin-binding protein. In: Müller F (ed) Chemistry and Biochemistry of Flavins. Vol. I. CRC Press, Boca Raton, FL, pp 287-292.

Yamada Y, Merrill AH Jr, McCormick DB (1990) Probable reaction mechanisms of flavokinase and FAD synthetase from rat liver. Arch Biochem Biophys 278:125-130.

Zempleni J, Galloway JR, McCormick DB (1996a) Pharmacokinetics of orally and intravenously administered riboflavin in healthy humans. Am J Clin Nutr 63:54-66.

Zempleni J, Galloway JR, McCormick DB (1996b) The identification and kinetics of 7α-hydroxyriboflavin (7-hydroxymethylriboflavin) in blood plasma from humans following oral administration of supplements. Int J Vitam Nutr Res 66:151-157.

RECOMMENDED READINGS

Bender DA (1992) Niacin. In: Bender DA (ed) Nutritional Biochemistry of the Vitamins. Cambridge University Press, Cambridge, pp 184-222.

Bender DA (1992) Vitamin B_1: Thiamin. In: Bender DA (ed) Nutritional Biochemistry of the Vitamins. Cambridge University Press, Cambridge, pp 128-155.

Gubler CJ (1991) Thiamin. In: Machlin LH (ed) Handbook of Vitamins, 2nd ed. Marcel Dekker, New York, pp 233-281

McCormick DB (1989) Two interconnected B vitamins: riboflavin and pyridoxine. Physiol Rev 69:1170-1198.

Chapter 25

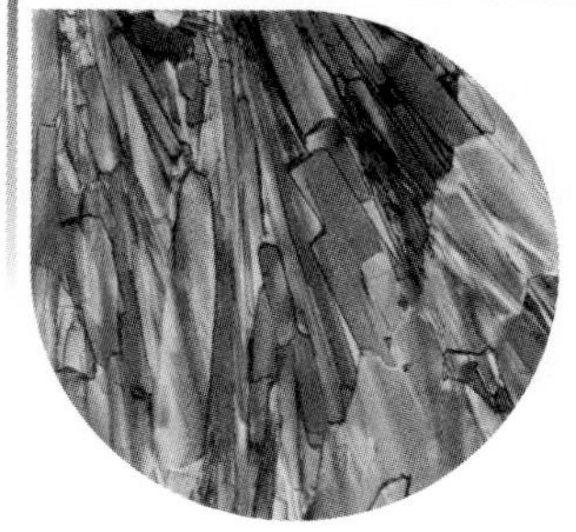

Folic Acid, Vitamin B_{12}, and Vitamin B_6

Barry Shane, PhD

OUTLINE

COMMON ABBREVIATIONS

AdoHcy	*S*-adenosylhomocysteine
AdoMet	*S*-adenosylmethionine
Cbl	cobalamin, vitamin B_{12}
H_4PteGlu	tetrahydropteroylglutamate
H_4PteGlu$_n$	tetrahydropteroylpolyglutamate, with n indicating the number of glutamyl residues
IF	intrinsic factor
PL	pyridoxal
PLP	pyridoxal 5′-phosphate
PM	pyridoxamine
PMP	pyridoxamine 5′-phosphate
PN	pyridoxine or pyridoxol
PNP	pyridoxine 5′-phosphate
PteGlu	pteroylmonoglutamate or folic acid
TC	transcobalamin

FOLATE

Folate was initially investigated as a dietary factor that prevented megaloblastic anemia of pregnancy and as a growth factor present in green leafy vegetables (foliage), hence its name. Folate and vitamin B_{12} deficiency lead to an identical and indistinguishable megaloblastic anemia in which blood cells are enlarged due to a derangement of DNA synthesis, and it has been known for many years that the pernicious anemia that results from defects in vitamin B_{12} availability is caused by induction of a secondary folate deficiency. Because of the role of folate coenzymes in the synthesis of DNA precursors, folate antagonists have found widespread clinical use as anticancer and antimicrobial agents. More recently, the observation that periconceptional supplementation with folate reduces the incidence of neural tube defects and possibly other birth defects has generated considerable clinical and public health interest and has led to fortification of the American food supply with folate.

CHEMISTRY OF FOLATE

Folic acid (pteroylmonoglutamate, PteGlu) consists of a 2-amino-4-hydroxy-pteridine (pterin) moiety linked via a methylene group at the C-6 position to a *p*-aminobenzoylglutamic acid moiety (Fig. 25-1). Folate metabolism involves the reduction of the pyrazine ring of the pterin moiety to the coenzymatically active tetrahydro form, the elongation of the glutamate chain by the addition of L-glutamate residues in an unusual γ-peptide linkage, and the acquisition and oxidation or reduction of one-carbon units at the N-5 and/or N-10 positions (see Fig. 25-1). Folate is the generic name for all these derivatives, whereas folic acid is usually used to refer specifically to either pteroylmonoglutamic acid or its ionized form. Folate coenzymes function as acceptors and donors of one-carbon moieties in reactions involving nucleotide and amino acid metabolism, which is known as one-carbon metabolism. More than 95% of tissue folates are polyglutamate species, primarily with glutamate chain lengths between 5 and 8. With most folate-dependent enzymes, the polyglutamates are more effective than pteroylmonoglutamates as substrates, and polyglutamates usually exhibit greatly increased affinities for these enzymes. The polyanionic nature of the polyglutamate chain, coupled with binding of folate polyglutamates by intracellular proteins, allows tissues to retain and concentrate polyglutamate forms of the vitamin, whereas the monoglutamate species are the transport forms.

SOURCES OF FOLATE

Folates are synthesized by microorganisms and plants as the 7,8-dihydrofolate form, and all naturally occurring folates are reduced derivatives. Fully oxidized folic acid is found in the diet only when foodstuffs are fortified with folic acid or when dietary folates are oxidized. Fully oxidized folic acid is also the common form of folate found in vitamin supplements. Reduced folates are less stable than folic acid, and their stability varies depending on the one-carbon substitution. Large losses of food folate can occur during food processing or preparation, especially due to heating under

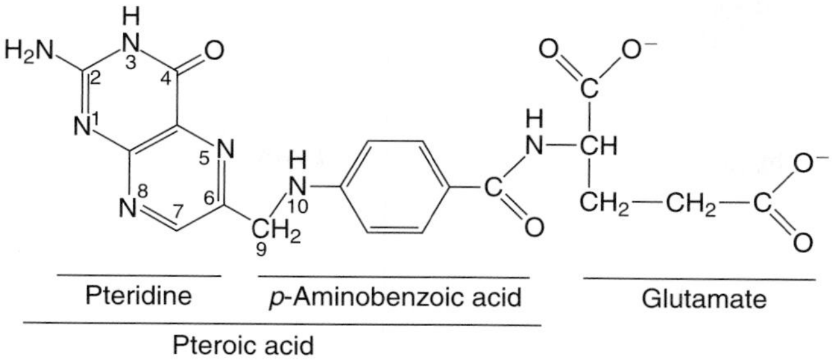

Pteridine p-Aminobenzoic acid Glutamate

Pteroic acid

Folic acid, pteroylglutamate (PteGlu)

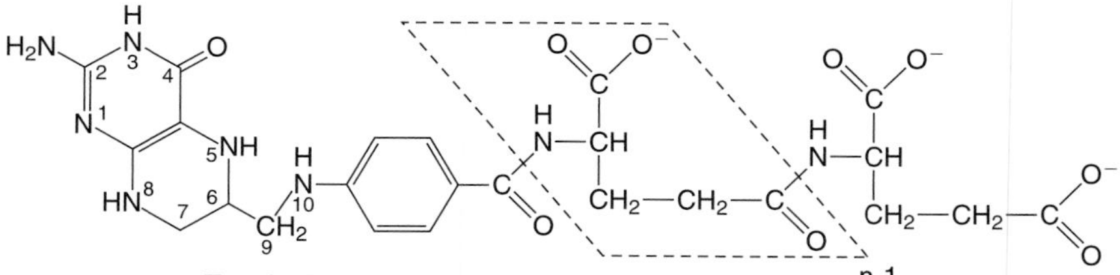

Tetrahydropteroylpoly-γ-glutamate ($H_4PteGlu_n$)

One Carbon Substituent		Position	Oxidation State
Methyl	$—CH_3$	N-5	Methanol
Methylene	$—CH_2—$	N-5, N-10	Formaldehyde
Methenyl	—CH=	N-5, N-10	Formate
Formyl	—CHO	N-5 or N-10	Formate
Formimino	HN=CH—	N-5	Formate

Figure 25-1 Structure of folic acid (PteGlu) and tetrahydropteroylpoly-γ-glutamate ($H_4PteGlu_n$). One-carbon substituents can be at the N-5 and/or N-10 positions of the reduced folate molecule.

oxidative conditions. Additional losses can occur by the leaching of folate from food into the cooking water.

BIOAVAILABILITY AND ABSORPTION OF FOLATE

Most dietary folates are polyglutamate derivatives and are hydrolyzed by a brush-border membrane γ-glutamylhydrolase (glutamate carboxypeptidase II, GCPII) activity in the small intestine to monoglutamate forms prior to absorption across the intestinal mucosa. The GCPII complementary DNA (cDNA) has recently been cloned and it expresses a protein identical to prostate-specific membrane antigen (PSMA), a marker for prostate cancer, and to *N*-acetylated α-linked acidic dipeptidase (NAALADase), a brain enzyme that regulates glutamate neurotransmission. As far as is known, the functions of PSMA and NAALADase are unrelated to folate metabolism.

Absorption of folate monoglutamate is via a saturable carrier-mediated process, but a diffusion-like process also occurs at high folate concentrations. The intestinal transporter, which is encoded by the reduced folate carrier gene (*RFC-1*), is a transmembrane protein that is expressed in most, if not all, tissues; the specificity of this transporter for various folates differs among tissues and between the apical and basolateral membranes of cells such as enterocytes. Affinities for reduced folates are in the low micromolar range. Affinities for folic acid are similar in some tissues such as the intestine but can be 100-fold lower in

Food Sources

Food Sources High in Dietary Folate Equivalents

Cereals and Grains

650 μg per ½ cup Kellog's All-Bran cereal
177 μg per 1 cup cream of wheat
150 to 400 μg per 1 cup ready-to-eat cereal
75 to 100 μg per ½ cup cooked rice
140 μg per 10 pretzels
120 μg per 3½-in. plain bagel

Legumes

180 μg per ½ cup lentils
110 to 150 μg per ½ cup pinto, black, navy, kidney beans
60 to 80 μg per ½ cup lima beans, kidney beans, split peas

Vegetables

120 to 130 μg per ½ cup okra, spinach, asparagus
80 to 85 μg per ½ cup broccoli, brussels sprouts
50 to 70 μg per ½ cup beets, corn

Data from US Department of Agriculture/Agricultural Research Service (USDA/ARS) (2005) USDA Nutrient Database for Standard Reference, Release 18. USDA/ARS, Washington, DC. Retrieved November 15, 2005, from www.ars.usda.gov/ba/bhnrc/ndl.

other tissues. These differences may reflect tissue-specific differences in posttranslational modification of the reduced folate carrier protein.

The mechanism by which folate crosses the mucosal cell and is released across the basolateral membrane into the portal circulation is not well understood. Some metabolism of folate, primarily to 5-methyl-H_4PteGlu, can occur during this process, but metabolism is not required for transport. The degree of metabolism in the intestinal mucosa is dependent on the folate dose given. When pharmacological doses of various folates are given, most of the transported vitamin appears unchanged in the portal circulation and in the peripheral circulation.

The bioavailability of folic acid when given as a supplement or in fortified food is high (Gregory, 1997a). However, the bioavailability of food folate is less than 50% and may be significantly lower than this because recent studies have suggested that methods commonly used for the analysis of folate in foodstuffs may have underestimated the folate content. Pharmacological doses of folate are well absorbed, but most of the vitamin is not retained in the body due to a limited capacity of tissues to retain large amounts of folate.

TRANSPORT AND TISSUE ACCUMULATION OF FOLATE

Pteroylmonoglutamates, primarily 5-methyl-H_4PteGlu, are the circulating forms of folate in plasma, and mammalian tissues cannot transport polyglutamates with chains of more than two glutamyl residues. After folate absorption into the portal circulation, much of this folate can be taken up by the liver via the reduced folate carrier. In the liver, it is metabolized to polyglutamate derivatives and retained, or it may be released into blood. Some folate is secreted in bile, but this can be reabsorbed in the intestine via an enterohepatic circulation. The plasma folate concentration in humans is usually in the 10 to 30 nmol/L range in unfortified populations. The predominance of 5-methyl-H_4PteGlu in plasma probably reflects that this is the major cytosolic folate in mammalian tissues. The extent of release of short-chain folylpolyglutamates from tissues is unknown. Plasma contains a soluble γ-glutamylhydrolase activity, and any polyglutamate released into plasma would be hydrolyzed to the monoglutamate.

Some plasma folate is bound to low-affinity protein binders, primarily albumin. Plasma also contains low levels of a high-affinity folate-binding protein. The levels of the high-affinity binder are increased in pregnancy and are very high in some leukemia patients, although the physiological significance of these elevated levels is unclear. The high-affinity binder is a soluble form of a second membrane-associated folate transporter known as folate-binding protein, or the folate receptor, which has particularly high affinity for folic acid. There are at least three distinct genes that code for the folate-binding protein, and the encoded protein is usually attached to the plasma membrane of cells via a glycosylphosphatidylinositol anchor. High levels of folate-binding protein are expressed in the choroid plexus, kidney proximal tubes, erythropoietic cells, and placenta, and in a number of human tumors, whereas lower levels have been found in a variety of other tissues. The presence of this high affinity transporter in the choroid plexus is thought to protect the brain from the effects of folate deficiency. Folate levels in the cerebral spinal fluid are considerably higher than in the peripheral circulation. Folate-binding protein effects reabsorption of folate in the kidney by a receptor-mediated endocytotic process and is believed to play a similar role in folate transport in other tissues. The function of the soluble form of folate-binding protein, which is expressed at high levels in milk, is not understood, but it may also play a role in folate transport.

Red blood cells contain higher levels of folate (normally 0.5 to 1 μmol/L) than are found in plasma (0.01 to 0.03 μmol/L). Mature red cells do not transport or accumulate folate; their folate stores are formed during erythropoiesis and are retained, probably due to binding to hemoglobin, through the 120-day lifespan of the human red cell. Red cell folate levels are often used as a measure of long-term folate status. Fasting plasma folate levels also are an indicator of status, but plasma levels also can be influenced by recent dietary intake.

INTRACELLULAR METABOLISM AND TURNOVER OF FOLATE

The interconversion of folate one-carbon forms is intertwined with the metabolic roles of folate and is outlined later. Folate coenzymes are found primarily in the mitochondria and cytosol of the cell, and accumulation of folate in these compartments requires the conversion of folates to polyglutamates, which is catalyzed by the enzyme folylpolyglutamate synthetase (Shane, 1989):

$$\text{MgATP} + \text{Folate(glu}_n) + \text{Glutamate} \rightarrow \text{MgADP} + \text{Folate(glu}_{n+1}) + \text{P}_i$$

Folylpolyglutamate synthetase is encoded by a single human gene, and cytosolic and mitochondrial isozymes are generated by alternative transcription start sites for the gene and by alternative translational start sites for its mRNA. Tetrahydrofolate and its polyglutamate forms are the preferred substrates for folylpolyglutamate synthetase, whereas 5-substituted folates such as 5-methyl-H_4PteGlu are poor substrates. Because 5-methyl-H_4PteGlu is the major folate transported into most tissues, the extent of folate accumulation is dependent on a tissue's ability to metabolize 5-methyl-H_4PteGlu to H_4PteGlu via the methionine synthase reaction (Figs. 25-2 and 25-3). Rapid efflux of unmetabolized 5-methyl-H_4PteGlu from the tissue to plasma occurs.

The mitochondrial folate transporter, which has recently been cloned and is encoded by the *mft* gene, shares no homology with the plasma membrane transporters. It has not been well characterized but is specific for reduced folates. The major hepatic mitochondrial folates are 10-formyl-H_4PteGlu$_n$ and H_4PteGlu$_n$, and much of the latter is bound to two folate enzymes, dimethylglycine dehydrogenase and sarcosine dehydrogenase. A large proportion of the major cytosolic folate in liver, 5-methyl-H_4PteGlu$_n$, is bound to glycine *N*-methyltransferase, whereas much of the cytosolic H_4PteGlu$_n$ is bound to 10-formyltetrahydrofolate dehydrogenase.

Tissues contain a soluble lysosomal γ-glutamylhydrolase activity, sometimes called folate conjugase, which may be involved in the hydrolysis of folylpolyglutamates with their subsequent release from the tissue. However, the major route of folate turnover and catabolism appears to involve the degradation of folate coenzymes to pterin derivatives and aminobenzoylpolyglutamates via oxidative cleavage at the C-9, N-10 bond. Recent studies suggest that methenyltetrahydrofolate synthetase, the normal enzymatic function of which is the conversion of the 5-formyl-H_4PteGlu$_n$ to 5,10-methenyl-H_4PteGlu$_n$, is responsible for some of this cleavage. The aminobenzoylpolyglutamates generated are hydrolyzed to aminobenzoylglutamate by lysosomal γ-glutamylhydrolase and are partly *N*-acetylated, at least in liver, and the *N*-acetyl-aminobenzoylglutamate is excreted in

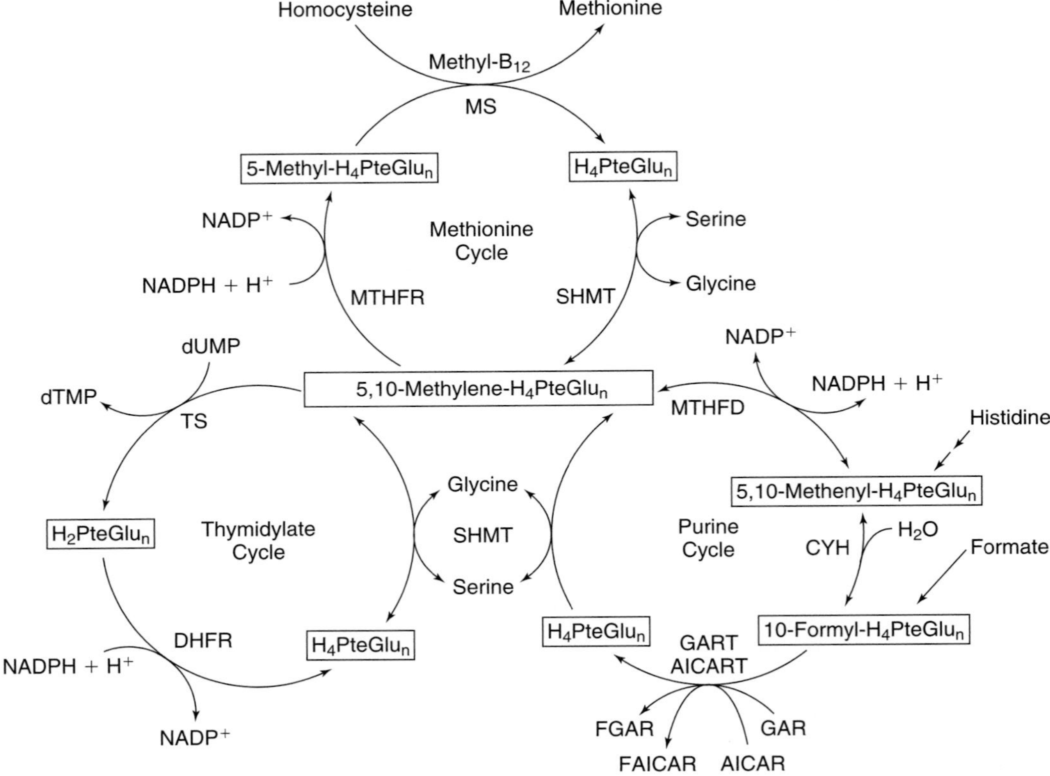

Figure 25-2 The major metabolic cycles of folate-dependent one-carbon metabolism in the cytoplasm of cells. *AICAR,* 5-amino-4-imidazolecarboxamide ribonucleotide; *AICART,* AICAR formyltransferase; *CYH,* methenyltetrahydrofolate cyclohydrolase; *DHFR,* dihydrofolate reductase; *dTMP,* 2-deoxythymidine 5′-monophosphate; *dUMP,* 2-deoxyuridine 5′-monophosphate; *GAR,* glycinamide ribonucleotide; *GART,* GAR formyltransferase; *MS,* methionine synthase; *MTHFD,* methylenetetrahydrofolate dehydrogenase; *MTHFR,* methylenetetrahydrofolate reductase; *SHMT,* Serine hydroxymethyltransferase; *TS,* thymidylate synthase.

the urine. In humans, only very small amounts of intact folate are found in urine, and cleavage products represent the bulk of the excretion. Under normal conditions of dietary intake and status, whole-body folate stores turn over slowly with a half-life in excess of 100 days.

METABOLIC FUNCTIONS OF FOLATE

Folate coenzymes act as acceptors or donors of one-carbon units in a variety of reactions involved in amino acid and nucleotide metabolism in mammalian tissues. The various metabolic cycles of one-carbon metabolism in the cytosol and mitochondria of mammalian tissues are shown in Figures 25-2, 25-3, and 25-4.

FOLATE AND ONE-CARBON METABOLISM

Although the major pathways of methionine, thymidylate, and purine synthesis occur in the cytosol, extensive folate metabolism occurs in the mitochondria; mitochondrial folate metabolism plays an important role in glycine metabolism and in providing one-carbon units for cytosolic one-carbon metabolism. Folate coenzymes act as co-substrates in these reactions. Consequently, folate metabolism and its regulation are interwoven with the regulation of the synthesis of products of one-carbon metabolism, and factors that regulate any one cycle of one-carbon metabolism would be expected to influence folate availability for the other cycles of one-carbon metabolism. The C-3 of serine

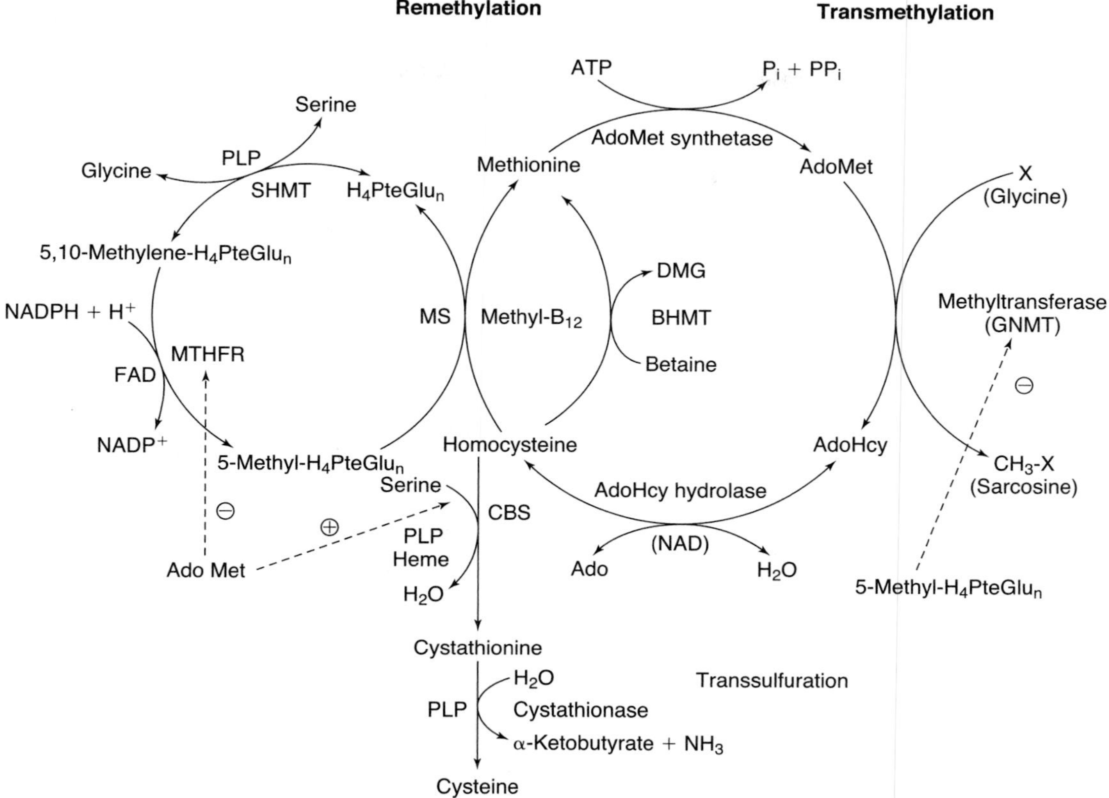

Figure 25-3 The folate-dependent methionine resynthesis cycle and its relationship to transmethylation and transsulfuration cycles in tissues. *AdoHcy, S*-adenosylhomocysteine; *AdoMet, S*-adenosylmethionine; *BHMT,* betaine homocysteine methyltransferase (liver-specific); *CBS,* cystathionine β-synthase; *DMG,* dimethylglycine; *GNMT,* glycine *N*-methyltransferase (primarily liver and kidney); *MS,* methionine synthase; *MTHFR,* methylenetetrahydrofolate reductase; *SHMT,* Serine hydroxymethyltransferase; *X,* methyl acceptor.

is the major source of one-carbon units for folate metabolism. Additional sources include formate, much of which is derived from serine metabolism in the mitochondria, and the imidazole ring C-2 of histidine.

Folates in mammalian tissues are metabolized to polyglutamates of chain lengths considerably longer than the triglutamate form required for folate retention. For most folate-dependent enzymes, the major kinetic advantages are achieved by elongation of the glutamate chain to the triglutamate. Longer polyglutamate forms are required for the enzymes involved in the methionine resynthesis cycle. Many of the enzymes involved in folate metabolism are multifunctional, with multiple catalytic sites on a single protein, or are part of multiprotein complexes. For some of these complexes, the longer polyglutamate derivatives allow channeling of substrates between active sites without release of intermediate products from the complex. The polyglutamate tail is believed to be "anchored" to a site on the complex. Channeling of substrates between active sites prevents the accumulation of intermediate products in bulk cell water and increases the efficiency of metabolic pathways.

AMINO ACID METABOLISM

Interconversion of Serine and Glycine

Serine hydroxymethyltransferase, a PLP-containing enzyme, catalyzes the reversible transfer of formaldehyde from serine to $H_4PteGlu_n$

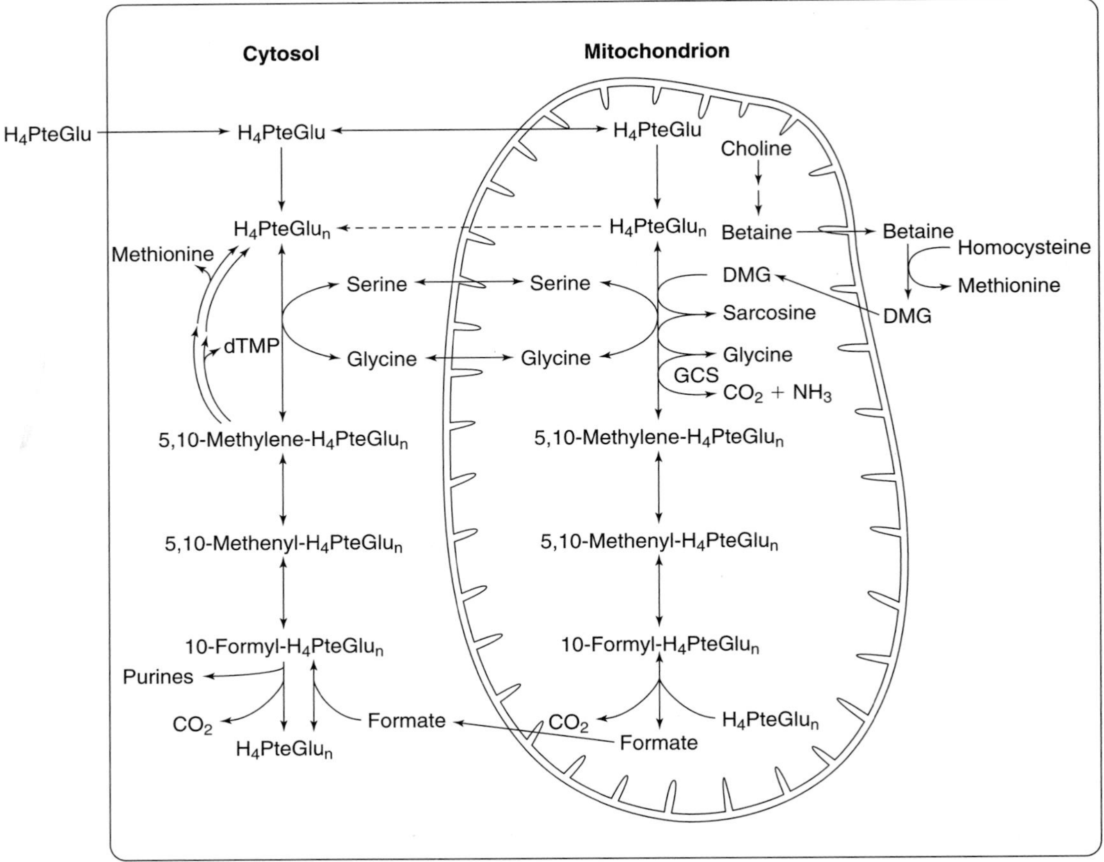

Figure 25-4 Compartmentalization of folate-dependent one-carbon metabolism. Mitochondrial choline degradation is restricted primarily to liver, whereas the mitochondrial glycine cleavage system (GCS) is primarily present in liver and kidney. *DMG,* Dimethylglycine.

to generate 5,10-methylene-$H_4PteGlu_n$ and glycine (see Fig. 25-2; also described in Chapter 14, Fig. 14-18):

$$\text{Serine} + H_4PteGlu_n \leftrightarrow \text{Glycine} + 5,10\text{-Methylene-}H_4PteGlu_n$$

Mammalian cells contain two serine hydroxymethyltransferase isozymes, one cytosolic and one mitochondrial, encoded by separate genes. The cytosolic enzyme is the predominant species in liver, although the mitochondrial form predominates in cultured cells. Serine hydroxymethyltransferase is an abundant protein in liver, and the C-3 of serine is the major source of one-carbon units for folate metabolism. The 5,10-methylene-$H_4PteGlu_n$ formed in this reaction plays a central role in one-carbon metabolism because its one-carbon moiety can be directed into any of the three cytosolic one-carbon cycles (methionine resynthesis, de novo purine synthesis, or thymidylate synthesis) as shown in Figure 25-2.

The directionality of the serine hydroxymethyltransferase reactions in the cytosol and mitochondria is not well understood. Serine, a nonessential amino acid, may be derived from glucose or obtained from the diet. Some tissues are net producers of glycine, whereas others, such as kidney, are net producers of serine from glycine. Mammalian cell mutants that lack mitochondrial serine hydroxymethyltransferase activity but have normal levels of cytosolic activity require exogenous glycine for growth. Serine and glycine are rapidly transported across the mitochondrial membrane, whereas transport of reduced folate occurs at a much slower rate. Although this suggests that the mitochondrial isozyme is required for net glycine synthesis, it is possible that the cytosolic enzyme is associated with the enzymes of cytosolic one-carbon metabolism and that the serine-to-glycine flux in the cytosol is regulated by the needs for one-carbon units for the various cycles of one-carbon metabolism. Glycine is a gluconeogenic amino acid, which suggests that, in liver and kidney at least, the net flux through one of the hydroxymethyltransferase isozymes will be in the direction of serine synthesis under normal conditions of net gluconeogenesis (see Chapter 14, Fig. 14-10). The major pathway of glycine catabolism is via the glycine cleavage system (see Fig. 25-4), a reaction in which an additional one-carbon moiety is supplied to the folate pool:

$$\text{Glycine} + H_4\text{PteGlu}_n + NAD^+ \rightarrow 5,10\text{-Methylene-}H_4\text{PteGlu}_n + NADH + CO_2 + NH_4^+$$

The mitochondrial glycine cleavage system, which is present in high concentrations in liver and kidney, is a multienzyme complex with four components (P-, H-, T-, and L-proteins). P-protein, which contains pyridoxal 5′-phosphate (PLP), catalyzes glycine decarboxylation and transfer of methylamine to lipoic acid on H-protein. The lipoic acid is reduced, and the carbon moiety from glycine is oxidized to the level of formaldehyde. T-protein catalyzes the transfer of formaldehyde to H_4PteGlu$_n$, and the reduced lipoate on H-protein is reoxidized by NAD^+ in a reaction catalyzed by L-protein. Although potentially reversible, the glycine cleavage system does not appear to play a role in the synthesis of glycine. Coupling of the serine hydroxymethyltransferase and glycine cleavage systems provides a mechanism for the synthesis of serine from glycine. One molecule of serine can arise by reversal of the hydroxymethyltransferase, with the 5,10-methylene-H_4PteGlu$_n$ required arising from oxidative decarboxylation of an additional molecule of glycine via the cleavage system.

Serine hydroxymethyltransferase also catalyzes the conversion of 5,10-methenylH_4-PteGlu$_n$ to 5-formyl-H_4PteGlu$_n$. 5-Formyl-H_4PteGlu$_n$ is a potent inhibitor of some folate-dependent enzymes, including serine hydroxymethyltransferase, and is the substrate for the folate catabolism enzyme; it is not used directly as a substrate in one-carbon transfer reactions. 5-Formyl-H_4PteGlu$_n$ can be reconverted to 5,10-methenyl-H_4PteGlu$_n$ by methenyltetrahydrofolate synthetase:

$$5\text{-Formyl-}H_4\text{PteGlu}_n + \text{MgATP} \rightarrow [5,10\text{-Methenyl-}H_4\text{PteGlu}_n]^+ + \text{MgADP} + P_i$$

5-Formyl-H_4PteGlu is used clinically and experimentally as a source of reduced folate because it is more stable than other reduced folates.

Methionine Cycle

A major cytosolic cycle of one-carbon utilization involves the reduction of 5,10-methylene-H_4PteGlu$_n$ to 5-methyl-H_4PteGlu$_n$, followed by the transfer of the methyl group to homocysteine to form methionine and regenerate H_4PteGlu$_n$ (see Fig. 25-3). 5,10-Methylene-H_4PteGlu$_n$ reduction is catalyzed by the flavoprotein methylenetetrahydrofolate reductase:

$$5,10\text{-Methylene-}H_4\text{PteGlu}_n + NADPH + H^+ \rightarrow 5\text{-Methyl-}H_4\text{PteGlu}_n + NADP^+$$

The reaction is irreversible under in vivo conditions and is the committed step in the flux of one-carbon units to the methionine resynthesis cycle.

The next enzyme in this cycle, methionine synthase, is one of only two B_{12}-dependent mammalian enzymes, and it catalyzes the transfer of the methyl group from 5-methyl-H_4PteGlu$_n$ to homocysteine:

$$5\text{-Methyl-}H_4\text{PteGlu}_n + \text{Homocysteine} \rightarrow H_4\text{PteGlu}_n + \text{Methionine}$$

The methionine synthase reaction is the only reaction in which the methyl group of 5-methyl-H_4PteGlu$_n$ can be metabolized in mammalian tissues. Although methionine is an essential amino acid, the methionine synthase reaction plays a major role in methyl group metabolism because it allows the reutilization of the homocysteine backbone as a carrier of methyl groups derived primarily from the C-3 of serine. The enzyme contains tightly bound cob(I)alamin, and the reaction proceeds via a methylcob(III)alamin intermediate, described in subsequent text of this chapter.

Homocysteine is not found in the diet but arises from hydrolysis of *S*-adenosylhomocysteine (AdoHcy), the product of *S*-adenosylmethionine (AdoMet)–dependent methylation reactions (see Fig. 25-3). Homocysteine can be metabolized to cysteine in reactions catalyzed by two PLP-dependent enzymes, cystathionine β-synthase and cystathionase. This transsulfuration pathway is described in Chapter 14. Alternatively, homocysteine can be converted back to methionine via the folate-dependent methionine synthase reaction described previously or by betaine-homocysteine methyltransferase, which catalyzes the transfer of one of the methyl groups of betaine to homocysteine to generate methionine and dimethylglycine. Betaine arises from choline oxidation in liver mitochondria (see Fig. 25-4). The cytosolic betaine methyltransferase does not contain bound cobalamin and does not use a folate coenzyme as a substrate. It is present in high concentrations in liver, and limited studies in humans indicate that up to 30% of homocysteine remethylation may occur through this reaction. In rodents, which have a more active choline degradation pathway, the betaine methyltransferase may be responsible for the majority of homocysteine remethylation under physiological conditions. The dimethylglycine product of the methyltransferase reaction is converted to glycine in the mitochondria. The folate-dependent mitochondrial flavoproteins dimethylglycine dehydrogenase and sarcosine dehydrogenase catalyze the oxidative demethylation of dimethylglycine to sarcosine and sarcosine to glycine, respectively, with the generation of 5,10-methylene-$H_4PteGlu_n$ in each of the dehydrogenase reactions.

The extent of homocysteine remethylation or transsulfuration is tissue-dependent, and many tissues export homocysteine and cystathionine into the circulation. Tissue levels of homocysteine are normally low; increased homocysteine levels cause increased levels of AdoHcy, an inhibitor of many methylation reactions. Kidney and liver are thought to be important organs for homocysteine remethylation and for transsulfuration.

Remethylation is also dependent on the methyl group status of the tissue. The major regulator of the folate-dependent methionine cycle is AdoMet, which is a potent allosteric inhibitor of methylenetetrahydrofolate reductase (see Fig. 25-3). Liver contains a high K_m AdoMet synthetase, and hepatic levels of AdoMet reflect methionine status. High levels of AdoMet inhibit the reductase, reducing synthesis of 5-methyl-$H_4PteGlu_n$ and, hence, remethylation of homocysteine. At the same time, the high levels of AdoMet activate cystathionine β-synthase, stimulating transsulfuration of homocysteine to cysteine. Conversely, when AdoMet is low, remethylation of homocysteine is favored and transsulfuration is inhibited.

Liver and kidney also contain a major cytosolic protein, glycine *N*-methyltransferase, which acts as a sink for excess methyl groups. This enzyme catalyzes the AdoMet-dependent methylation of glycine to sarcosine. Although folate is not a substrate for this enzyme, 5-methyl-$H_4PteGlu_n$ is a potent inhibitor, and the protein is a major cytosolic folate-binding protein. When AdoMet levels are high, methylenetetrahydrofolate reductase is inhibited, reducing 5-methyl-$H_4PteGlu_n$ formation and relieving inhibition of glycine *N*-methyltransferase, and consequently allowing removal of excess methyl groups. At low AdoMet concentrations, methylenetetrahydrofolate reductase is more active, 5-methyl-$H_4PteGlu_n$ accumulates, and glycine methyltransferase is inhibited. Excess methionine, which can be toxic, results in an elevated level of sarcosine, some of which is excreted in urine.

Several cases of glycine *N*-methyltransferase deficiency have been recently described. These cases were identified in a subset of infants with elevated plasma methionine levels after routine newborn screening of amino acid levels. This condition appears to be generally asymptomatic, provided methionine intakes are kept at a moderate level. At high methionine intakes, blood methionine levels increase dramatically.

Although methylenetetrahydrofolate reductase is the major regulatory enzyme in the methionine cycle, the significant proportion of methylfolates in tissues suggests that the methionine synthase reaction is also an important rate-limiting step in the metabolic cycles of one-carbon metabolism. Both methylenetetrahydrofolate reductase and methionine synthase are low-abundance proteins and are present at considerably lower concentrations than most of the other enzymes involved in the metabolism of folate coenzymes.

5-Methyl-H_4PteGlu is the major form of folate taken up by tissues. Removal of the methyl group, via the methionine synthase reaction, is required before the entering folate can be utilized in other reactions of one-carbon metabolism or metabolized to polyglutamates that are retained by cells. Because the entering monoglutamate has to compete with the preferred 5-methyl-H_4PteGlu$_n$ substrates, incorporation of exogenous folate by tissues is repressed by high intracellular folate (i.e., by expansion of the 5-methyl-H_4PteGlu$_n$ pool).

Histidine Catabolism

The C-2 of the imidazole ring of histidine provides one-carbon units at the oxidation level of formate for one-carbon metabolism. Cytosolic formiminoglutamate formiminotransferase catalyzes the transfer of a formimino group from formiminoglutamate, an intermediate in the histidine catabolism pathway, to H_4PteGlu$_n$, as follows:

$$\text{Formiminoglutamate} + H_4\text{PteGlu}_n \rightarrow \text{5-Formimino-}H_4\text{PteGlu}_n + \text{Glutamate}$$

The formimino moiety is converted to 5,10-methenyl-H_4PteGlu$_n$ in a formiminotetrahydrofolate cyclodeaminase catalyzed reaction:

$$\text{5-Formimino-}H_4\text{PteGlu}_n + H^+ \rightarrow [\text{5,10-Methenyl-}H_4\text{PteGlu}_n]^+ + NH_3$$

Formiminotransferase and cyclodeaminase activities reside on a single bifunctional protein. In folate deficiency, formiminoglutamate catabolism is impaired, and formiminoglutamate is excreted in elevated amounts in urine.

Nutrition Insight

New Recommendations for Choline Intake

Choline is formed in vivo by the synthesis and degradation of phosphatidylcholine, which occurs mainly in the liver. Adenosylmethionine serves as the methyl group donor for the three methylations involved in the conversion of phosphatidylethanolamine to phosphatidylcholine. Degradation of phosphatidylcholine gives rise to free choline. The free choline, which can also come from the diet, can be reconverted to phosphatidylcholine via formation of phosphocholine and cytidine 5′-diphosphate-choline and addition of phosphocholine to diacylglycerol, but this is a quantitatively less important pathway than the pathway for phosphatidylcholine synthesis from phosphatidylethanolamine. In addition to being a component of phospholipids, choline is required for synthesis of acetylcholine, a neurotransmitter, and serves as a precursor of betaine, which can donate a methyl group to homocysteine to reform methionine. Clearly, choline metabolism is related to overall methyl group metabolism and requirements because adenosylmethionine is a donor of methyl groups in the endogenous synthesis of choline and because betaine, derived from choline, can be a source of preformed methyl groups for synthesis of methionine and hence adenosylmethionine.

Choline is present as part of phospholipids in foods such as eggs, liver, and soybeans and as free choline in certain vegetables such as cauliflower. In addition, lecithin (phosphatidylcholine) is added to some processed foods as an emulsifying agent. Betaine is also present in some foods such as beets. Average daily intake of choline in the United States is estimated to be approximately 400 to 900 mg. Choline is usually added to infant formulas in amounts that approximate the choline content of human milk.

Continued

Nutrition Insight

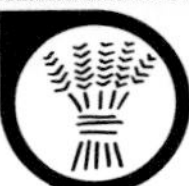

New Recommendations for Choline Intake—cont'd

Although dietary choline has been considered an important component of animal diets for a number of years, human needs for dietary choline are not well defined. Choline needs can be met at least partially by endogenous synthesis, and it is not clear whether a dietary supply of choline is needed at all stages of the life cycle. Dietary depletion studies in healthy humans have demonstrated increases in plasma alanine aminotransferase levels, which may suggest altered liver function. The Food and Nutrition Board of the National Academy of Sciences, IOM (IOM, 1998) recently set adequate intakes (AIs) for choline based on or extrapolated from the intakes required to maintain normal aminotransferase levels in subjects in these studies.

Adequate Intakes for Choline Across the Life Cycle

	mg Choline per day
Infant	
0 to 0.5 yr	125
0.5 to 1 yr	150
Children	
1 to 3 yr	200
4 to 8 yr	250
9 to 13 yr	375
Males	
>13 yr	550
Females	
14 to 18 yr	400
>18 yr	425
Pregnant	450
Lactating	550

Data from Institute of Medicine (1998) Dietary Reference Intakes for Thiamin, Riboflavin, Niacin, Vitamin B_6, Folate, Vitamin B_{12}, Pantothenic Acid, Biotin, and Choline. National Academy Press, Washington, DC.

NUCLEOTIDE SYNTHESIS

Thymidylate Cycle

Folates are not involved in the de novo synthesis of the pyrimidine ring (described in Chapter 14; see Fig. 14-15). However, folate is required for the synthesis of thymidylate (see Fig. 25-2). Thymidylate synthase catalyzes the transfer of formaldehyde from folate to the 5-position of deoxyuridine monophosphate (dUMP) for the formation of deoxythymidine monophosphate (dTMP):

$$5,10\text{-Methylene-}H_4PteGlu_n + dUMP \rightarrow H_2PteGlu_n + dTMP$$

The $H_4PteGlu_n$ of 5,10-methylene-$H_4PteGlu_n$ provides the reducing component for reduction of the transferred methylene moiety to a methyl group of dTMP and is oxidized to $H_2PteGlu_n$ in the process. $H_2PteGlu_n$ is inactive as a coenzyme and has to be reduced back to $H_4PteGlu_n$, in a reaction catalyzed by dihydrofolate reductase, before it can play a further role in one-carbon metabolism:

$$H_2PteGlu_n + NADPH + H^+ \rightarrow H_4PteGlu_n + NADP^+$$

The major role of dihydrofolate reductase is the reduction of $H_2PteGlu_n$ formed during thymidylate synthesis. Dihydrofolate reductase also reduces dietary $H_2PteGlu$ and catalyzes the reduction of pharmaceutical folic acid to dihydrofolate, although folic acid is a poorer substrate than dihydrofolate.

Thymidylate synthase activity is expressed only in replicating tissues, and expression of the synthase and dihydrofolate reductase messenger RNA (mRNA) is highest during the S phase of the cell cycle. Folate antagonists that inhibit these enzymes have been used extensively as anticancer agents. Methotrexate, a 4-aminofolic acid analog, is a potent inhibitor of dihydrofolate reductase. Treatment of rapidly growing cells with this drug causes trapping of folate in the nonfunctional dihydrofolate form. Slowly growing tissues, which have negligible or low levels of thymidylate synthase activity, do not convert reduced folate to the dihydrofolate form as rapidly, so are less affected by a dihydrofolate reductase inhibitor. Clinical resistance to drugs such as methotrexate often develops. Mechanisms for resistance include a decrease in the level of, or a mutation in, the reduced folate carrier resulting in decreased methotrexate uptake; amplification of the dihydrofolate reductase gene resulting in an increase in the level of dihydrofolate reductase activity; and a decrease in folylpolyglutamate synthetase activity, which reduces accumulation of the drug by the tissue.

Purine Cycle

10-Formyl-H_4PteGlu$_n$ is used in two steps of de novo cytosolic purine biosynthesis (see Chapter 14, Fig. 14-14). The C-8 and C-2 positions of the purine ring are derived from 10-formyl-H_4PteGlu$_n$ in reactions catalyzed by glycinamide ribonucleotide (GAR) transformylase and 5-amino-4-imidazolecarboxamide ribonucleotide (AICAR) transformylase (see Fig. 25-2):

$$\text{10-Formyl-}H_4\text{PteGlu}_n + \text{GAR} \rightarrow H_4\text{PteGlu}_n + \text{Formyl-GAR}$$

$$\text{10-Formyl-}H_4\text{PteGlu}_n + \text{AICAR} \rightarrow H_4\text{PteGlu}_n + \text{Formyl-AICAR}$$

10-Formyl-H_4PteGlu$_n$ is formed by the oxidation of 5,10-methylene-H_4PteGlu$_n$, which is catalyzed reversibly by methylenetetrahydrofolate dehydrogenase and methenyltetrahydrofolate cyclohydrolase (see Fig. 25-2):

$$\text{5,10-Methylene-}H_4\text{PteGlu}_n + \text{NADP}^+ \leftrightarrow [\text{5,10-Methenyl-}H_4\text{PteGlu}_n]^+ + \text{NADPH}$$

$$[\text{5,10-Methenyl-}H_4\text{PteGlu}_n]^+ + H_2O \leftrightarrow \text{10-Formyl-}H_4\text{PteGlu}_n + H^+$$

Alternatively, 10-formyl-H_4PteGlu$_n$ can be obtained by the direct formylation of H_4PteGlu$_n$ (see Fig. 25-4), catalyzed by formyltetrahydrofolate synthetase:

$$\text{Formate} + \text{MgATP} + H_4\text{PteGlu}_n \rightarrow \text{10-Formyl-}H_4\text{PteGlu}_n + \text{MgADP} + P_i$$

The dehydrogenase, cyclohydrolase, and synthetase are associated on a single trifunctional protein in mammalian tissues that is called C_1 tetrahydrofolate synthase. The synthase consists of two separate domains: one contains the dehydrogenase and cyclohydrolase activities and the other the synthetase activity.

Mitochondria can also interconvert 5,10-methylene-H_4PteGlu$_n$ and 10-formylH_4PteGlu$_n$, and this is thought to be catalyzed by a mitochondrial C_1 tetrahydrofolate synthase (see Fig. 25-4). The mitochondrial isoform has recently been cloned. Although the encoded mitochondrial protein is highly homologous to the cytosolic C_1 tetrahydrofolate synthase, the expressed protein appears to lack dehydrogenase activity, although it does have formyltetrahydrofolate synthetase activity.

A separate bifunctional 5,10-methylenetetrahydrofolate dehydrogenase–cyclohydrolase that uses NAD$^+$ rather than NADP$^+$ as the acceptor has also been described. One suggested role for this enzyme is to increase the one-carbon flux into purine biosynthesis and away from other one-carbon cycles such as methionine synthesis. This mitochondrial enzyme activity is found in embryonic, undifferentiated, and transformed tissues and cells but not in adult tissues. This has led to the suggestion that the mitochondrial pathway for the conversion of the folate one-carbon derived from serine to formate, which can then leave the mitochondria and be used for cytosolic purine biosynthesis, may be limited to development and to transformed cells. However, purified hepatic mitochondria from adult rodents metabolize serine to formate, indicating that adult mitochondria possess a functional methylenetetrahydrofolate dehydrogenase activity, although the nature of the protein that catalyzes this reaction remains unclear. The recent demonstration that disruption of the cytosolic serine hydroxymethyltransferase gene in mice does not lead to embryonic or adult lethality also indicates that mitochondrial generation of one-carbons for cytosolic pathways functions in the adult.

DISPOSAL OF ONE-CARBON UNITS

One-carbon moieties are oxidized to CO_2 in a reaction catalyzed by 10-formyltetrahydrofolate dehydrogenase (see Fig. 25-4):

$$\text{10-Formyl-}H_4\text{PteGlu}_n + \text{NADP}^+ + H_2O \rightarrow H_4\text{PteGlu}_n + CO_2 + \text{NADPH} + H^+$$

The purified enzyme also catalyzes the hydrolysis of 10-formyl-H_4PteGlu$_n$ to H_4PteGlu$_n$ and formate. The H_4PteGlu$_n$ product of the reaction has high affinity for the enzyme and is a potent inhibitor. In liver, the metabolic flux through this reaction may be regulated by the 10-formyl-H_4PteGlu$_n$/H_4PteGlu$_n$ ratio, rather than by the tissue concentration of 10-formyl-H_4PteGlu$_n$. The physiological role of this protein would appear to be to regulate the proportion of folate present in the $H_4PteGlu_n$ form, presumably to make it available for other reactions of one-carbon metabolism.

FOLATE DEFICIENCY: SYMPTOMS AND METABOLIC BASES

Folate deficiency is usually caused by a dietary insufficiency, although it can arise from other causes such as malabsorption syndromes or drug treatment. A number of cases of increased requirement due to genetic heterogeneity have been recently identified, including some individuals who require increased folate in early pregnancy to reduce the risk of birth defects. As might be expected from its metabolic roles, the clinical effects of deficiency are related to defects in DNA synthesis, particularly in fast-growing tissues, and in methyl group metabolism. The classic symptom is a megaloblastic anemia reflecting deranged DNA synthesis in erythropoietic cells. Folate deficiency is also associated with increased risk for vascular disease (Rimm et al., 1998) and an increased incidence of some cancers. Depression and polyneuropathy have also been reported, although the evidence linking folate deficiency to neurological disease is not conclusive. However, in frank genetic diseases involving rare cases of severe defects in various folate-dependent enzymes, neurological symptoms have been clearly documented, with many cases of mental retardation.

MEGALOBLASTIC ANEMIA

Megaloblastic anemia is characterized by enlarged red cells and hypersegmentation of the nuclei of circulating polymorphonuclear leukocytes with reduced cell number. Megaloblastic changes also occur in other tissues, but the condition is usually detected clinically by the anemia. The megaloblastic anemia of folate deficiency is identical to that observed in vitamin B_{12} deficiency. Folate deficiency anemia was not observed in a single study (Henriquez et al., 2004) in subjects with red cell folate levels greater than 140 μg/L (0.32 μmol/L). Megaloblastic cells have almost twofold the normal content of DNA, and the cells are arrested in the G2 phase of the cell cycle just prior to mitosis, preventing cell division. The DNA contains breaks suggesting a defect in DNA synthesis or repair. If cell division occurs, the cells undergo apoptosis (programmed cell death).

These defects are thought to be caused by defective thymidylate synthesis coupled with an enlarged deoxyuridine triphosphate (dUTP) pool that results in uracil misincorporation into DNA. Damaged reticulocytes and red cells are normally removed by the spleen. Splenectomized subjects with low red cell folate levels have an increased uracil content and double-strand breaks in their DNA, and folate supplementation reverses these abnormal findings (Blount et al., 1997). Uracil in DNA normally arises from deamination of cytosine, which constantly occurs at a slow rate. Because uracil behaves exactly as thymine in DNA, cytosine deamination to uracil can lead to a mutagenic change from a cytosine-guanine (C-G) base pair to a uracil (thymine)-adenine [U(T)-A] base pair during replication. Normally, this potential damage is repaired by uracil-DNA glycosylase, which removes the uracil base. A few additional bases are removed on either side of the damage, and the DNA is repaired by complementary base pairing, with a C being reinserted opposite the G.

Tissues also contain a dUTPase, which hydrolyzes dUTP to dUMP and keeps dUTP levels very low. Uridine misincorporation in place of thymidine during DNA synthesis or repair is normally minimized by competition between the small dUTP pool and the larger deoxythymidine triphosphate (dTTP) pool. If U is misincorporated in place of T (opposite an A), the glycosylase removes the U and a T is reinserted. In folate deficiency, dTTP pools are depressed and dUTP pools are increased, leading to increased incorporation of dUTP instead of dTTP. Increased repair by glycosylase would lead to more transient single-strand breaks. In addition, repair of the damage by reinsertion of T is inefficient due to the lower dTTP pools, and the probability of U being reinserted by mistake is higher, which leads to prolongation of the single-strand breaks. If U is misincorporated on both DNA strands in proximity, a double-strand break, which cannot be repaired, can occur during the uracil–DNA glycosylase-mediated repair.

CANCER

Epidemiological studies have suggested that folate deficiency is associated with increased risk for certain types of cancer, including colon cancer. The underlying mechanism has not been ascertained, but uracil misincorporation arising from defective thymidylate synthesis has been hypothesized as one possibility. In many genes transcription is turned off during development by methylation of the promoter regions, and epigenetic changes in DNA methylation play important roles in chromosome stability, X chromosome inactivation, and imprinting. Changes in gene expression and DNA methylation are early events in the progression of many human cancers and, in some cases, involve methylation-dependent inactivation of tumor suppressor genes. Because folate deficiency impairs the remethylation of homocysteine to methionine and alters AdoMet–AdoHcy ratios, it has been proposed that the increased cancer risk in folate deficiency may be due to hypomethylation of DNA.

The increased cancer risk in folate-deficient subjects is reduced in subjects homozygous for a common polymorphism in methylenetetrahydrofolate reductase (Ma et al., 1997). This polymorphism causes decreased enzyme activity and presumably impaired conversion of 5,10-methylene-H_4PteGlu$_n$ to 5-methyl-H_4PteGlu$_n$. It is thought that this impaired conversion of 5,10-methylene-H_4PteGlu$_n$ to 5-methyl-H_4PteGlu$_n$ allows a redirection of more of the folate one-carbons into the cycles of nucleotide biosynthesis in these subjects. However, this impairment would also reduce the one-carbon flux into methionine and could potentially influence the extent of DNA methylation. Methionine deficiency causes hypomethylation of DNA and the results of one study (Stern et al., 2000) have shown that global DNA methylation is reduced in subjects homozygous for the methylenetetrahydrofolate reductase polymorphism but only when their folate status was poor. In the same study, there was no effect of folate status on DNA methylation in subjects homozygous for the "wild type" allele. DNA hypomethylation has been reported in mice that are heterozygous and homozygous for deletion of the methylenetetrahydrofolate reductase gene (Chen et al., 2001). Common polymorphisms in other folate genes, including thymidylate synthase and cytosolic serine hydroxymethyltransferase, have been reported to influence cancer risk in human populations.

CANCER TREATMENT

Folate antagonists that are inhibitors of thymidylate synthase, dihydrofolate reductase, and de novo purine biosynthetic enzymes have been used extensively for the treatment of a variety of cancers. These metabolic poisons, which cause a functional folate deficiency, generally show a selective toxicity for rapidly growing tumors because of the increased rates of DNA synthesis in these tumors. In experimental animals, toxicity and drug effectiveness are reduced by the provision of purines and thymidine. Uracil misincorporation and apoptosis have been demonstrated as the mechanism for cell death. Uracil misincorporation is also potentially mutagenic, and successful treatment with antifolates, or with many other drugs used for cancer chemotherapy, for that matter, carries the risk of further cancers after 10 to 20 years. Although improved folate status may be beneficial in reducing cancer risk, supplementation with additional folate may be contraindicated in the cancer patient as some studies have suggested that high folate accelerates the growth of preexisting tumors.

HYPERHOMOCYSTEINEMIA AND VASCULAR DISEASE

It has long been known that severe genetic conditions that result in homocystinuria and a very marked hyperhomocysteinemia are associated with a variety of clinical symptoms, including early onset occlusive cardiovascular and cerebrovascular disease. These genetic diseases include deficiencies of methylenetetrahydrofolate reductase and cystathionine β-synthase, enzymes involved in the homocysteine remethylation and transsulfuration pathways, respectively. Elevated homocysteine increases proliferation of smooth muscle cells and inhibits proliferation of endothelial cells by a mechanism that is not understood. Many potential reasons for the adverse effects of homocysteine have been described. These include effects on transcription factors involved in regulation of cell growth, disulfide bond formation with proteins such as apolipoprotein B-100, modulation of nitric oxide (NO) synthase activity, and increased cellular AdoHcy levels. It has not been established whether any of these potential adverse changes are responsible for vascular disease.

Recently, it has been recognized that chronic mild hyperhomocysteinemia is a major risk factor for occlusive vascular disease (Refsum et al., 1998). Plasma homocysteine concentrations in patients with vascular disease are about 30% higher than in controls, and carotid artery stenosis is positively correlated with plasma homocysteine concentrations over the entire range of normal and abnormal homocysteine values (Selhub et al., 1995). Prospective assessment of vascular disease risk in men with higher homocysteine concentrations indicated that plasma homocysteine levels only 12% greater than the upper limit of normal levels are associated with a threefold increase in acute myocardial infarction (Stampfer et al., 1992).

Elevated plasma homocysteine levels are responsive to increased folate intake. Fasting homocysteine levels have been correlated inversely with both plasma folate and food folate intake. Increased folate intake lowers the mean plasma homocysteine of groups, with the greatest effect on those with the highest plasma homocysteine levels. A common polymorphism (alanine [ala] to valine [val]) in methylenetetrahydrofolate reductase that results in a "heat-labile" enzyme and decreased enzyme activity in tissues has been implicated as one reason for the folate-responsiveness of a subset of hyperhomocysteinemic subjects (Frosst et al., 1995). The incidence of the val/val homozygous genotype (approximately 10% in most populations) is significantly greater in groups of subjects with higher homocysteine levels. Although the contribution of this polymorphism to elevated homocysteine levels has varied from study to study, and the incidence of the polymorphism varies among different population groups, the val/val polymorphism may at most contribute to or be associated with 30% of the cases of hyperhomocysteinemia. Approximately 50% of the general population is heterozygous or homozygous for this polymorphism, and it is particularly interesting that a simple nutritional intervention may ameliorate at least some of the adverse effects of a potentially deleterious genetic trait. Although elevated homocysteine levels increase vascular disease risk, and increased folate intake decreases plasma homocysteine levels (Selhub et al., 1993), it remains to be determined whether increased folate intake reduces vascular disease risk.

B_{12}- and PLP-dependent enzymes are also involved in homocysteine metabolism. Impaired vitamin B_{12} status also has been associated with higher concentrations of fasting plasma homocysteine in the general population. Prior to fortification of the food supply with folic acid, B_{12} was found to be quantitatively a less important risk factor than was folate for hyperhomocysteinemia (Selhub et al., 1993). Improved vitamin B_6 status has little effect on fasting homocysteine levels but attenuates the increase in plasma homocysteine following a methionine load or a meal. The locus of the B_6 effect is believed to be the PLP-dependent cystathionine β-synthase, but a role for the PLP-dependent serine hydroxymethyltransferase cannot be excluded.

Therefore, folate status was the major nutritional determinant of the population-based risk for elevated fasting homocysteine in the United States population prior to folate fortification. Fortification of the American food supply since 1998 has resulted in a reduction in homocysteine levels with a halving of the incidence of elevated homocysteine, and vitamin B_{12} status has now become the major determinant of the population-based risk for elevated fasting homocysteine in the United States (Quinlivan and Gregory, 2003).

BIRTH DEFECTS

Neural tube defects, including most forms of spina bifida, are the most common types of birth defect in humans, affecting about 0.1% of births. The recurrence rate for this condition is about 4%. The observation that periconceptual folate supplementation with folic acid reduced the incidence of these defects by about two thirds led to fortification of the United States food supply with folic acid

Nutrition Insight

Genetic Heterogeneity and Vitamin Requirements: Methylenetetrahydrofolate Reductase Polymorphism and Homocysteinemia as an Example

Subjects who are homozygous for a common polymorphism in the methylenetetrahydrofolate reductase gene (C677T in the gene, resulting in an alanine to valine substitution in the protein) have lower lymphocyte methylenetetrahydrofolate reductase levels, higher plasma homocysteine levels, and a higher risk for vascular disease. Depending on the population, anywhere from 5% to 25% is homozygous and up to 50% heterozygous for this polymorphism, but the adverse effects are seen only in individuals who are homozygous for the val variant. The ala to val change in the protein lowers the affinity of the enzyme for its flavin adenine diphosphate (FAD) cofactor but does not affect the affinity of the enzyme for its substrates. Apoprotein that is lacking FAD is unstable, and the metabolic effects of this polymorphism are due to lower amounts of enzyme rather than abnormal enzyme activity. Folate stabilizes the enzyme by decreasing the rate of loss of FAD.

Among subjects with poor folate status, homozygotes for this polymorphism would be expected to display lower enzyme activity. Improved folate status would stabilize the protein, thereby reducing the difference in enzyme level compared with control subjects. Although it is expected that metabolic and adverse effects of this polymorphism would primarily affect people with poorer folate status, the level of folate intake at which differences between the val/val and ala/ala variants become insignificant currently is not known. In addition, elevated homocysteine levels in val/val subjects are observed only in individuals with relatively poor folate and riboflavin status, although the levels of the vitamins in these individuals are not necessarily as low as those that have traditionally been considered indicative of deficiency. An important question that remains to be answered is whether the present recommended dietary allowance (RDA) for folate is sufficient to normalize enzyme levels in val/val subjects or whether these individuals have a requirement that is higher than the RDA as set for the general population. Riboflavin deficiency is considered rare in the United States (see Chapter 24). However, levels that are normally considered adequate may be insufficient for val/val subjects. It is likely that genetic polymorphisms, particularly common ones such as this, are responsible for much of the variation in nutrient requirements among individuals. As more information becomes available, RDAs may eventually be set based on key informative genotypes of individuals.

A genetic defect in an enzyme complicates the interpretation of normal measures of nutrient status. Although a general folate deficiency can be detected by impairments in a variety of folate status indicators, not all indicators will suggest impaired status when the impairment is due to a genetic change. The val/val variant in methylenetetrahydrofolate reductase impairs homocysteine remethylation but may redirect more of the folate one carbon flux into nucleotide synthesis; this may explain why some studies have demonstrated a reduced risk of colon cancer in subjects with this polymorphism. Although inadequate folate status may be indicated in val/val subjects by higher plasma homocysteine levels, the deoxyuridine suppression test, which measures folate dependent thymidylate synthesis, may suggest improved folate status.

(Scott et al., 1990). The neural tube closes in the fourth week of gestation, and supplementation is useful only if given very early in pregnancy, at a time when many women do not realize they are pregnant. Although folate status affects the risk for neural tube defects, this condition is not thought to be a result of folate deficiency per se. It appears to be a genetic disease, possibly multigenetic, with a phenotype that can be modified by increased folate in the subset of individuals who are folate-responsive. As the mechanism behind the disease is not known, there is currently no screening technique to identify individuals at risk.

A defect in homocysteine metabolism has been proposed as a mechanism, although the evidence supporting this proposal can be considered only very preliminary. Plasma homocysteine levels are slightly higher in affected mothers, and homocysteine can cause teratogenic effects in cultured mouse embryos (Greene et al., 2003). An increased incidence of the homozygous ala to val polymorphism in methylenetetrahydrofolate reductase in affected mothers was reported that could account for at most 15% of neural tube defects (Volcik et al., 2003). An epidemiological study suggested that vitamin B_{12} status is an independent risk factor for neural tube defects (Groenen et al., 2004), which would implicate methionine synthase as a possible locus of the defect. However, no polymorphisms or mutations in the methionine synthase gene that track with neural tube defects have been identified to date.

A common variant in the formyltetrahydrofolate synthetase domain of the C1 tetrahydrofolate synthase gene has been reported to be a maternal risk factor for neural tube defects (Brody et al., 2002). Disruption of various folate genes in the mouse can lead to neural tube defects. Elimination of one of the two mouse folate binding protein genes (*FBP1*) leads to neural tube defects and embryonic loss, both of which can be prevented by supplying the mother with high doses of folate (Spiegelstein et al., 2004). However, no variants in the equivalent human gene have been found in human birth defects. A recent preliminary report presented evidence for the presence of circulating blocking antibodies to the folate receptor in women who had given birth to a neural tube–defect child (Rothenberg et al., 2004). If this is substantiated, it could explain why supplemental folic acid reduces the incidence of this condition.

The folate intervention trials that established the protective effect of folic acid, coupled with other surveys, have indicated that 400 μg of supplemental folic acid, in addition to customary dietary folate intake, is sufficient to provide the maximum benefit in reducing the incidence of folate-responsive birth defects. It is not known whether lower levels of supplementation would be as effective, nor whether disease risk could be reduced by dietary folate alone, as food folate is less bioavailable than folic acid. Preliminary studies have suggested that folate supplementation may also have a beneficial effect on other pregnancy outcomes, although one of the intervention trials that demonstrated the protective effect of folate for neural tube defects also noted an increased spontaneous abortion rate in supplemented subjects.

The recent implementation of fortification of the American food supply with folic acid was designed to provide an average daily intake of 100 μg of supplemental folic acid in addition to normal dietary folate intake. This represented a compromise between the needs of the relatively small population at risk for birth defects and the relatively larger population at risk for masking of the symptoms of vitamin B_{12} deficiency by high folate (see section on vitamin B_{12} later in this chapter). In fact, the legislated fortification of the food supply with folic acid has resulted in increased intakes of about 220 μg of supplemental folic acid per day, which are about twice those anticipated. Because folic acid added to food is more bioavailable than dietary folate, this would be equivalent to an extra 380 μg of food folate. Unsurprisingly, plasma and red cell folate levels have greatly increased in the United States population, and the proportion of the population with folate levels indicative of deficiency has dropped from approximately 20% to less than 1%. An additional potential benefit has been the reduction of plasma homocysteine levels in the United States population. It remains to be seen whether this has a positive effect on vascular disease incidence.

MALABSORPTION SYNDROMES

Some diseases of the intestinal tract, such as tropical sprue and nontropical sprue (gluten enteropathy), lead to general malabsorption syndromes, including folate deficiency. Folate is normally absorbed in the jejunum. In some sprue cases, the malabsorption in the jejunum is partially alleviated by increased absorption farther down in the small intestine.

ASSAY AND DETECTION OF DEFICIENCY

Folate status is most commonly assessed by plasma or red cell folate levels. This can be measured by microbiological assay using *Lactobacillus casei* as the test organism, but this test result can be confounded if the subject is receiving antibiotic treatment. The most widely used clinical test is a competitive radioassay procedure for plasma or red cell

Life Cycle Considerations

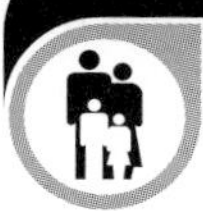

Folate and Birth Defects

The initial observation that periconceptual supplementation with folic acid reduced the incidence of neural tube defects—the major type of birth defects in humans—by greater than 70% was quite remarkable. Further studies confirmed this 70% reduction in populations with an underlying high incidence of birth defects and a lower, but still impressive, reduction in populations where the underlying incidence was low. Research in this area has focused on potential genetic causes, such as polymorphisms in genes encoding folate-dependent enzymes, and on potential environmental causes, such as reduced folate status, but the mechanism for the efficacy of increased folate intake is currently unknown. It is likely that these birth defects result from a combination of genetic and environmental factors. Experimental animals do not develop neural tube defects when placed on a folate-deficient diet during pregnancy. Although a number of mouse models of neural tube defects have been described and the causative genetic defect is known for some of these, none of the known defects appears to be responsible for human birth defects.

The risk of human neural tube defects is minimized by 400 μg/day of supplemental folic acid in addition to normal dietary folate intake. Lower levels of folic acid may be as effective, but this is not known. The additional folic acid is required in the first 3 weeks of pregnancy, a period when many women would not realize that they are pregnant. Furthermore, many women at risk may not be aware of, or be responsive to, the need for additional folate. Consequently, the American food supply is now fortified with folic acid with the intention to provide, on average, an additional 100 μg of folate, as folic acid, per day (i.e., 170 DFE/day). This level of fortification was chosen to balance the potential benefits of increased folic acid on prevention of birth defects with the potential adverse effects of increased folate intake on masking symptoms of vitamin B_{12} deficiency. The actual level of fortification has turned out to be approximately 200 μg/day (i.e., 340 DFE/day). Women of child-bearing age would need to take an additional 200 μg of folic acid daily, either as a supplement or as increased intake of fortified food, to meet current recommendations for 400 μg of supplemental non-food folic acid.

Fortification of the American food supply with folic acid was instigated in 1998 and has had a major impact on the folate status of the U.S. population. Significant elevations of plasma folate and decreases in plasma homocysteine levels have been observed, and birth defect rates have declined by about 20%. Whether higher levels of fortification would reduce rates even further is not known. The one third of the population that takes vitamin supplements is unlikely to receive any benefit from food fortification, and the relatively low incidence of birth defects in the United States had been declining for many years prior to folate fortification. A 20% decrease in birth defect rates may be close to the maximum achievable. Information on the extent to which this level of fortification protects against other conditions such as coronary disease and cancer should be obtained in the next few years in this grand experiment on 250 million Americans.

folate that uses milk folate-binding protein as the protein binder. Although simpler than the microbiological method, it is less precise. The levels of metabolites such as urinary formiminoglutamate and plasma homocysteine can also be used to assess folate status, but, as indicated in subsequent text, the levels of these metabolites are also abnormal under conditions of vitamin B_{12} deficiency, and in some cases, vitamin B_6 deficiency.

FOLATE REQUIREMENTS

Because folic acid added to food is more bioavailable than food folate, folate requirements are now stated as dietary folate equivalents (DFEs); 1 μg of folic acid is equivalent to 0.6 μg of folate from food:

$$\mu g \text{ of DFEs} = \mu g \text{ of Food folate} + (1.7 \times \mu g \text{ of Folic acid})$$

The Institute of Medicine ([IOM] 1998) set the estimated average requirement (EAR) for adults as 320 μg of DFEs per day, based mainly on controlled studies in which subjects received a folate-deplete diet supplemented with various levels of folic acid (O'Keefe et al., 1995). Assuming a 10% coefficient of variation, the recommended dietary allowance (RDA) for adults was set as the EAR + 20%, or 400 μg of DFEs per day. An intake of 600 μg of DFEs per day is recommended for pregnant women, but higher levels may be required to minimize the risk of birth defects. To reduce the risk of neural tube defects, it is recommended that women of child-bearing age, who are capable of becoming pregnant, consume 400 μg of folic acid per day from supplements and/or fortified food in addition to their food folate intake. The recommended intake for lactation is based on an increase in the EAR to cover the amount of folate secreted in milk; the RDA is 500 μg of DFEs per day. Recommendations for children were based on extrapolation from adult EARs on the basis of metabolic body weight ($kg^{0.75}$). Adequate intakes (AIs) for infants were based on the folate content of milk of well-nourished mothers. The AI of folate for infants during the first 6 months after birth (65 μg/day of DFE) was based on a mean daily intake of 0.78 L of milk that contains 85 μg/L of folate. The AI for infants ages 7 through 12 months was extrapolated from that for other age groups. Increases in dietary intake of folate do not affect maternal milk folate levels. As no information is available on the bioavailability of milk folate in infants compared to that of folic acid added to formula, the use of DFEs to calculate how much folic acid to add to formula would be inappropriate.

RDAs Across the Life Cycle

	μg DFEs per Day
Infants	
0 to 0.5 yr	65 (AI)
0.5 to 1.0 yr	80 (AI)
Children	
1 to 3 yr	150
4 to 8 yr	200
9 to 13 yr	300
14 to 18 yr	400
Adults	
19 to >70 yr	400*
Pregnant women	600
Lactating women	500

Data from Institute of Medicine (1998) Dietary Reference Intakes for Thiamin, Riboflavin, Niacin, Vitamin B_6, Folate, Vitamin B_{12}, Pantothenic Acid, Biotin, and Choline. National Academy Press, Washington, DC.

*To minimize the risk of neural tube defects, it is recommended that all women capable of becoming pregnant consume 400 μg of folic acid per day (from supplements and/or fortified foods) in addition to normal food folate intake. This is equivalent to an intake of 670 μg DFE as folic acid in addition to food folate intake and, as such, exceeds the RDA for women not capable of becoming pregnant.

DFEs, Dietary folate equivalents.

1 μg DFE = 1 μg food folate = 0.5 μg of folic acid taken on an empty stomach = 0.6 μg of folic acid with meals.

FOLATE TOXICITY

No toxicity of high doses of folate has been reported. However, large doses of folic acid can produce a hematological response in subjects with megaloblastic anemia caused by vitamin B_{12} deficiency. When folate was first isolated, and prior to the isolation of vitamin B_{12}, many patients with pernicious anemia were treated with large quantities of folic acid. Folate does not correct the severe neurological symptoms of vitamin B_{12} deficiency, and some studies suggested that folate treatment of vitamin B_{12}-deficient subjects may have exacerbated the development of neurological defects. Because large doses of folate may mask the development and diagnosis of anemia in vitamin B_{12}-deficient subjects and increase the risk that these subjects are recognized only when they develop irreversible neurological symptoms, megadose levels of folate should be avoided. The IOM (1998) set the tolerable upper intake level (UL) at 1 mg per day of folic acid from fortified food or supplements. There is no evidence of any adverse effect of high intakes of food folate per se.

VITAMIN B_{12}

A megaloblastic anemia was described in the nineteenth century that appeared to be associated with degenerative disease of the stomach. It was called pernicious anemia because of its invariably fatal outcome. In the 1920s George Minot and William Murphy described the first effective treatment of this disease, 1 pound of raw liver a day, for which they received a Nobel Prize. It soon became apparent that normal gastric juice contained a factor (intrinsic factor) that was required for the utilization of a dietary component (extrinsic factor, vitamin B_{12}) that was needed to prevent the anemia. Because of the identical anemia that arises from folate or B_{12} deficiency, it was originally thought that extrinsic factor was folic acid, and folic acid was used to treat pernicious anemia patients when it was isolated in the 1940s. With the isolation of vitamin B_{12} a few years later, it became clear that pernicious anemia was due to B_{12} deficiency.

CHEMISTRY OF VITAMIN B_{12}

Vitamin B_{12} (cobalamin) consists of a central cobalt atom surrounded by a heme-like planar corrin ring structure (Fig. 25-5), with the four pyrrole nitrogens coordinated to the cobalt. It contains a phosphoribo-5,6-dimethylbenzimidazolyl side group, with one of the nitrogens linked to the cobalt by coordination at the "bottom" position. When bound to enzymes, this lower axial ligand is usually replaced by an active-site histidine residue. The "upper" axial position can be occupied by a number of different ligands, including methyl, hydroxyl, and 5′-deoxyadenosyl groups (Fig. 25-6). In what is commonly known as vitamin B_{12}, the upper ligand is a cyano group (cyanocobalamin); cyanocobalamin is rarely found naturally but arises as an artifact formed by extraction of trace amounts of cyanide during purification of the vitamin from natural sources. Vitamin B_{12} is a complex molecule, and Nobel Prizes were awarded to Dorothy Hodgkin in 1964 for the determination of its

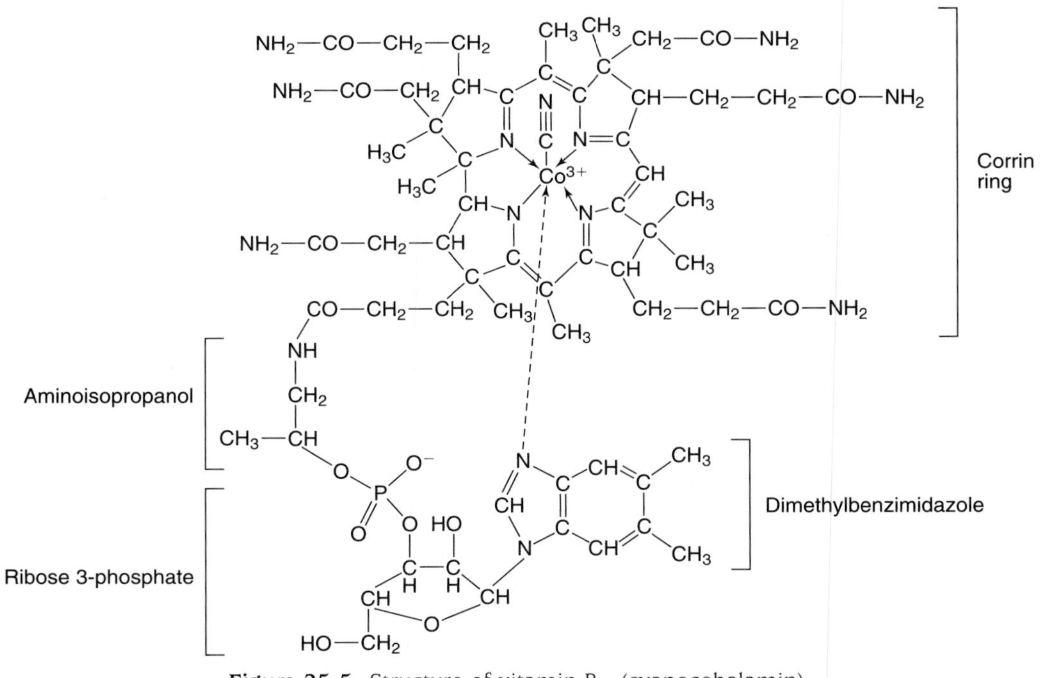

Figure 25-5 Structure of vitamin B_{12} (cyanocobalamin).

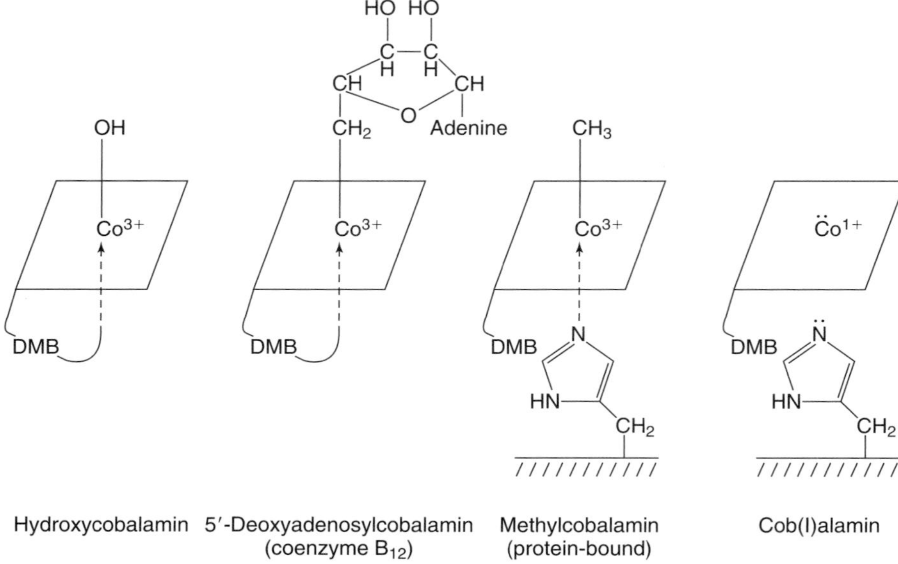

Figure 25-6 Intracellular forms of vitamin B_{12}. In vitamin B_{12} enzymes, the ligand to the lower axial position of the cobalt atom is an imidazole nitrogen of a histidyl residue on the protein instead of the dimethylbenzimidazolyl (DMB) side group of B_{12}; this is shown for methylcobalamin bound to methionine synthase. The lower axial position is unliganded (base-off form) in the cob(I)alamin-enzyme derivative.

structure and to Robert Woodward in 1965 for its synthesis. Metal–carbon bonds are rare in nature, and this molecule is the only example of a cobalt–carbon bond.

In cyanocobalamin and the naturally occurring hydroxy (or aqua) cobalamin forms, the cobalt atom is trivalent Co^{3+}, the most oxidized form. Cob(III)alamin is an electrophile, cob(II)alamin is a radical, and cob(I)alamin is a very strong nucleophile (Glusker, 1995). The coenzyme forms of the vitamin are the unliganded, fully reduced Co^{1+} derivative or cob(I)alamin; 5′-deoxyadenosylcob(III)alamin, also known as coenzyme B_{12}; and methylcob(III)alamin. These forms of the vitamin are very sensitive to oxidation and photolysis.

SOURCES OF VITAMIN B_{12}

Vitamin B_{12} is synthesized by some anaerobic microorganisms. Most higher organisms do not use vitamin B_{12} as a coenzyme and neither have a requirement for it nor synthesize the vitamin. Except for some algae, such as seaweed, plant sources do not contain vitamin B_{12}. The major dietary sources for humans are meat, dairy products, and some seafoods. B_{12} can also be obtained from fortified cereals and supplements. A strictly vegetarian diet provides very low levels of the vitamin, which can come from algal sources and possibly bacterial contamination associated with plant roots. Vegetarians tend to have low plasma vitamin B_{12} levels. Despite this, nutritional deficiency of vitamin B_{12} due to inadequate intake is rare. Instead, most problems of inadequate vitamin B_{12} status arise from defects in vitamin absorption.

BIOAVAILABILITY AND ABSORPTION OF VITAMIN B_{12}

The bioavailability of food vitamin B_{12} varies depending on the amount of B_{12} in the diet but normally averages around 50%. The mechanism of absorption is complex and is outlined in Figure 25-7. Vitamin B_{12} in food is bound to protein and is released in the stomach by the acidic environment and by proteolysis of binders by pepsin. The released vitamin B_{12} initially binds to R-binders, which are dietary proteins that have affinity for vitamin B_{12}. The stomach contains specialized parietal cells that contain the H^+, K^+-ATPase that produces gastric acid. In humans, these

Food Sources

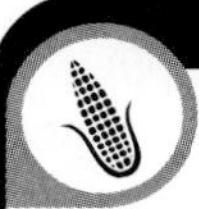

Food Sources High in Vitamin B_{12}

Mollusks and Crustaceans

42 to 84 µg per 3 oz clams
13 µg per 3 oz oysters
9 µg per 3 oz crab
2.6 µg per 3 oz lobster
1 µg per 3 oz shrimp

Fish

8 µg per 3 oz sardines
5 µg per 3 oz canned salmon
1-2 µg per 3 oz flounder, sole, swordfish, roughy, catfish

Meats

1.4 to 2.5 µg per 3 oz beef
2 to 2.2 µg per 3 oz lamb
0.5 to 0.6 µg per 3 oz pork

Dairy

1.0 to 1.3 µg per 1 cup milk
1.3 to 1.4 µg per 8 oz yogurt
0.6 to 0.8 µg per ½ cup cottage cheese
0.6 µg per 1 oz mozzarella cheese

Other

0.6 µg per 1 large egg
1.5 µg per ½ cup soy milk

Data from U.S. Department of Agriculture/Agricultural Research Service (USDA/ARS) (2005) USDA Nutrient Database for Standard Reference, Release 18. USDA/ARS, Washington, DC. Retrieved November 15, 2005, from www.ars.usda.gov/ba/bhnrc/ndl.

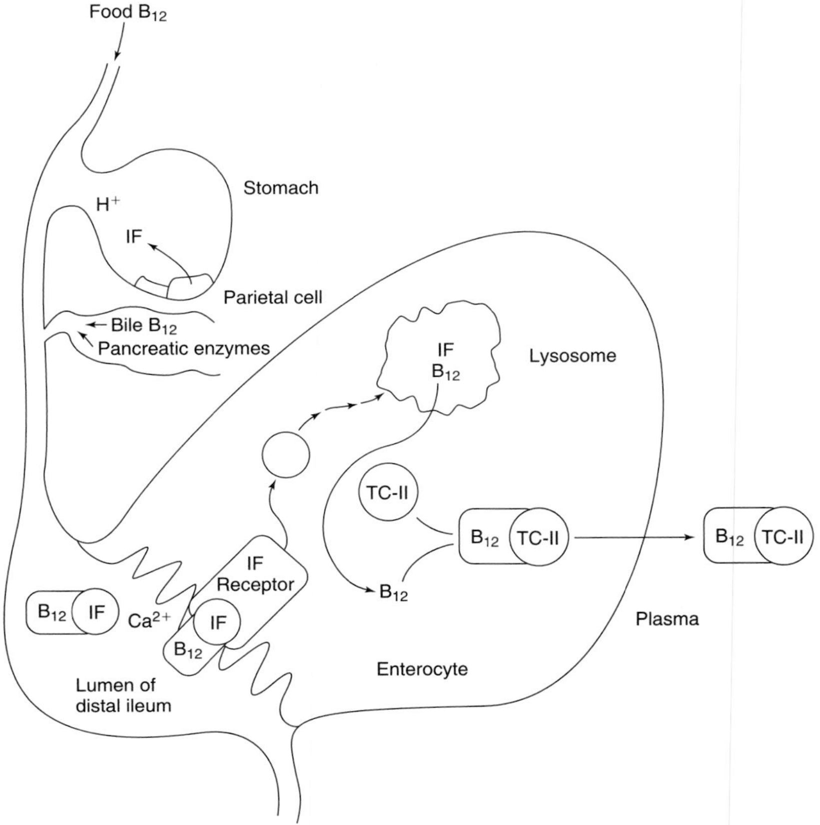

Figure 25-7 Absorption and processing of dietary B_{12}. *IF,* Intrinsic factor; *TC-II,* transcobalamin II.

cells also secrete a 50-kDa glycoprotein called intrinsic factor (IF) that can bind vitamin B_{12}. As the vitamin B_{12}–R-binder complexes pass through the small intestine, the R-binders are hydrolyzed by pancreatic proteases, and the freed vitamin B_{12} binds to IF. Sufficient IF is released following a meal to bind 2 to 4 μg of vitamin B_{12}. Vitamin B_{12} is absorbed via receptors located at the distal ileum at the end of the small intestine. The IF-receptor (cubilin) recognizes the IF–B_{12} complex, not vitamin B_{12} or unligated IF. In the presence of Ca^{2+}, the IF–B_{12} complex binds to the IF receptor, and the complex is internalized by a receptor-mediated endocytotic process. The endosomes fuse with lysosomes, and the IF is degraded and the vitamin B_{12} is released into the cytosol. Vitamin B_{12} is released from the gut epithelial cells as a complex bound to a 38-kDa protein called transcobalamin II (TC-II). This process of absorption across the gut epithelium takes about 3 to 4 hours. The 460-kDa IF receptor (cubulin) is also expressed in the kidney and in the yolk sac surrounding the developing embryo; the reason that this receptor is expressed in the kidney is not clear but may be related to its wide specificity for ligands. Additional ligands for the cubulin receptor include apolipoprotein A-II, immunoglobulin G (IgG) light chain and transferrin. Cubulin interacts with a second protein, amnionless (AMN), which shows a similar tissue distribution and appears to be required for the apical localization of cubulin in polarized cells.

Vitamin B_{12} can also be absorbed by a diffusion-like process, but this is very inefficient; less than 1% of a vitamin B_{12} dose can be absorbed by this process.

TRANSPORT OF VITAMIN B_{12}

The TC-II–B_{12} complex carries newly absorbed vitamin B_{12} around the body and provides tissues with vitamin B_{12}. TC-II is found in intestinal cells and in liver, kidney, and lymphoid tissues. Its site(s) of synthesis is not well understood, but it may be derived from the vascular epithelium. TC-II–B_{12} is transported into tissues by receptor-mediated endocytosis, in this case via a receptor that recognizes TC-II. The nature of the TC-II receptor is controversial, as a number of different-sized proteins have been reported in the literature as the putative receptor. In the kidney, a very large protein (megalin) is responsible for the reabsorption of TC-II-bound B_{12}. Megalin is also found in the yolk sac and, like cubulin, shows a wide specificity for ligands. However, the TC-II–B_{12} receptor in liver and most other tissues is not thought to be megalin. Once endocytosed, the TC-II–B_{12} complex is degraded in the lysosome, and the free vitamin B_{12} is transported from the lysosome to the cytosol (Fig. 25-8). The lysosomal vitamin B_{12} transporter has not been characterized. A rare human genetic disease involving a defect in this transporter has been described in which vitamin B_{12} accumulates in the lysosome.

The half-life of the TC-II–vitamin B_{12} complex in plasma is approximately 6 minutes. Plasma contains two additional vitamin B_{12}–binding glycoproteins or R-binders called haptocorrin (transcobalamin I, TC-I) and transcobalamin III (TC-III). They are less specific than TC-II and also bind B_{12} analogs. Plasma turnover of these transcobalamins is much slower than that of TC-II. Although newly absorbed vitamin B_{12} is associated with TC-II, about 75% of the plasma vitamin B_{12}, mainly methylcobalamin, is associated with TC-I. In healthy individuals, total TC-II protein levels (about 1 nmol/L serum) are twofold to threefold higher than TC-I levels. However, TC-I is about 90% saturated with B_{12}, whereas only about 10% of TC-II is holo-TC-II. Because of its much faster turnover, TC-II delivers about 4 nmoles of vitamin B_{12} to tissues per day, with a maximum capacity of approximately 6 nmol/day, whereas TC-I turnover accounts for only 0.1 nmol/day. Although the role of TC-I is not entirely clear, this 70-kDa glycoprotein transfers vitamin B_{12} to the liver. Liver contains a nonspecific asialoglycoprotein receptor that can mediate uptake of TC-I and TC-III.

Most of the body store of vitamin B_{12}, estimated at about 2 to 3 mg, is in the liver. 5′-Deoxyadenosylcobalamin is the major form of the vitamin in liver, whereas methylcobalamin is the major form in plasma. The vitamin is excreted via the urine and via the bile. Normally, the enterohepatic circulation results in effective reuptake of biliary vitamin B_{12}, via

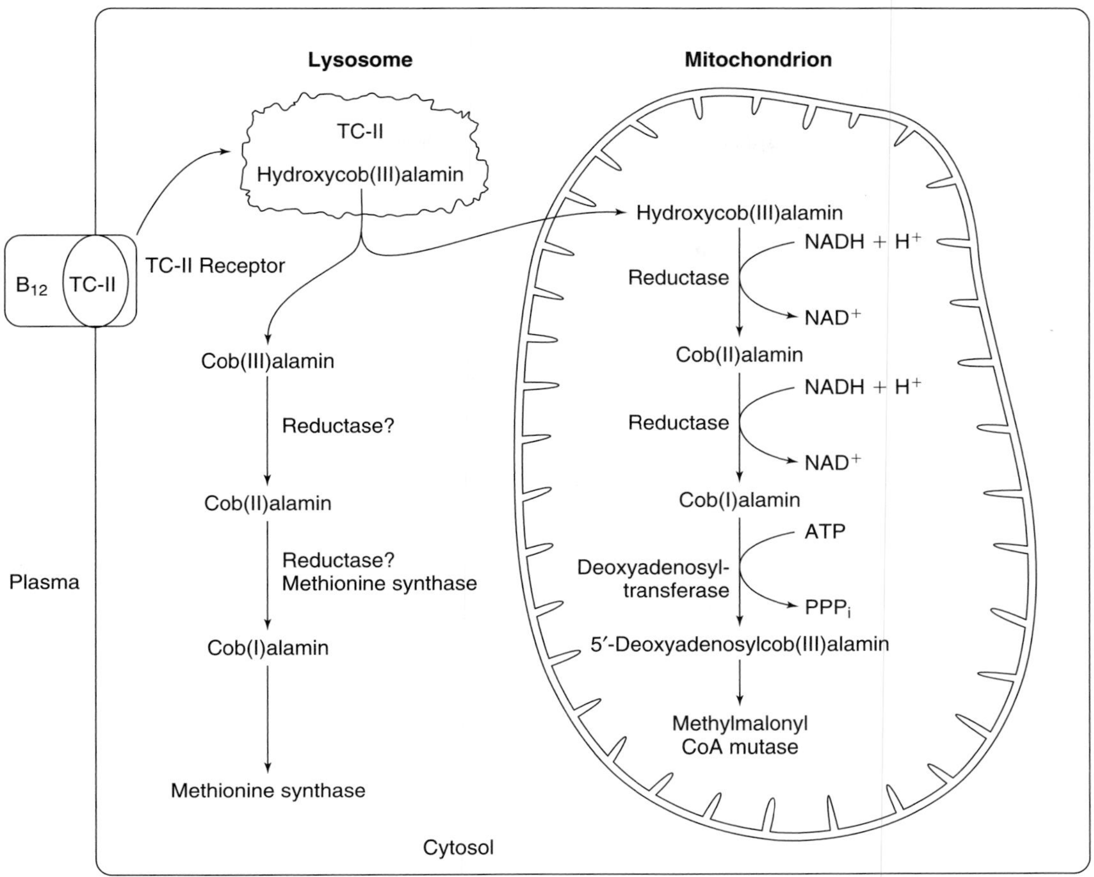

Figure 25-8 Tissue uptake and metabolism of B_{12}. *TC-II,* Transcobalamin II.

the IF receptor. Turnover rates of whole-body vitamin B_{12} have been estimated at approximately 0.1 %/day.

INTRACELLULAR METABOLISM OF VITAMIN B₁₂

Mammals need vitamin B_{12} as a cofactor for two enzymes, cytosolic methionine synthase, which utilizes methylcob(III)alamin as the cofactor, and mitochondrial methylmalonyl CoA mutase, which uses 5′-deoxyadenosylcob(III)alamin as its cofactor. Vitamin B_{12} is released into the cytosol of cells as hydroxycob(III)alamin and is reduced to cob(I)alamin. Cob(I)alamin is then methylated to methylcob(III)alamin after binding to methionine synthase. Alternatively, vitamin B_{12} can be transported into the mitochondria and reduced, and the 5′-deoxyadenosyl ligand added from ATP in a reaction catalyzed by a deoxyadenosyltransferase (see Fig. 25-8). Rare human genetic defects in many of these steps in vitamin B_{12} metabolism have been described.

METABOLIC FUNCTIONS OF VITAMIN B₁₂

The reduced vitamin B_{12} coenzymes are highly reactive and are capable of catalyzing very aggressive chemistry. Bacteria use 5′-deoxyadenosylcob(III)alamin as a cofactor for many reactions in which carbon–carbon bonds are cleaved by a mechanism that involves free radicals. During catalysis, the cobalt–carbon bond of the coenzyme is split, and a free radical is formed on the coenzyme, which can be transferred to an amino acid residue on the enzyme and then to the substrate.

METHIONINE SYNTHASE

Methylcobalamin is a cofactor for the previously described folate-dependent methionine synthase involved in homocysteine remethylation (see Figs. 25-2, 25-3, and 25-9). Methionine synthases are large, monomeric Zn metalloproteins (about 140 kDa) and consist of three domains: a catalytic domain containing the binding sites for 5-methyl-$H_4PteGlu_n$ and homocysteine, a B_{12} domain in which the B_{12} cofactor binds, and an accessory protein domain. Most of the methionine synthase in mammalian tissues is normally present as the holoenzyme form, containing a tightly bound B_{12} cofactor. The cob(I)alamin cofactor is methylated by 5-methyl-$H_4PteGlu_n$, generating enzyme-bound methylcob(III)alamin and releasing $H_4PteGlu_n$, and then methylcob(III)-alamin transfers its methyl group to homocysteine to generate methionine. Heterolytic cleavage of the cobalt–carbon bond regenerates the enzyme-bound cob(I)alamin cofactor. The cofactor is occasionally oxidized to the nonfunctional cob(II)alamin form during catalysis. The enzyme is reactivated by methionine synthase reductase, an accessory protein that catalyzes the AdoMet and NADPH-dependent reductive methylation of enzyme-bound cob(II)-alamin to methylcob(III)alamin. Bacteria possess two methionine synthase accessory proteins: one is a flavodoxin that uses NADH, FAD, and FMN as cofactors. The gene (*MTRR*) for a single human methionine synthase reductase protein that contains binding sites for NADPH, FAD, and FMN has been cloned. It belongs to the P450 reductase protein family. Human mutations that result in loss of methionine synthase activity and early onset megaloblastic anemia fall into two complementation groups. It has recently been shown that the *cbl*G complementation group results from mutations in the structural gene for methionine synthase (*MTR*), whereas mutations in methionine synthase reductase are responsible for the *cbl*E complementation group.

Methionine synthase can also catalyze the reduction of the anesthetic gas nitrous oxide

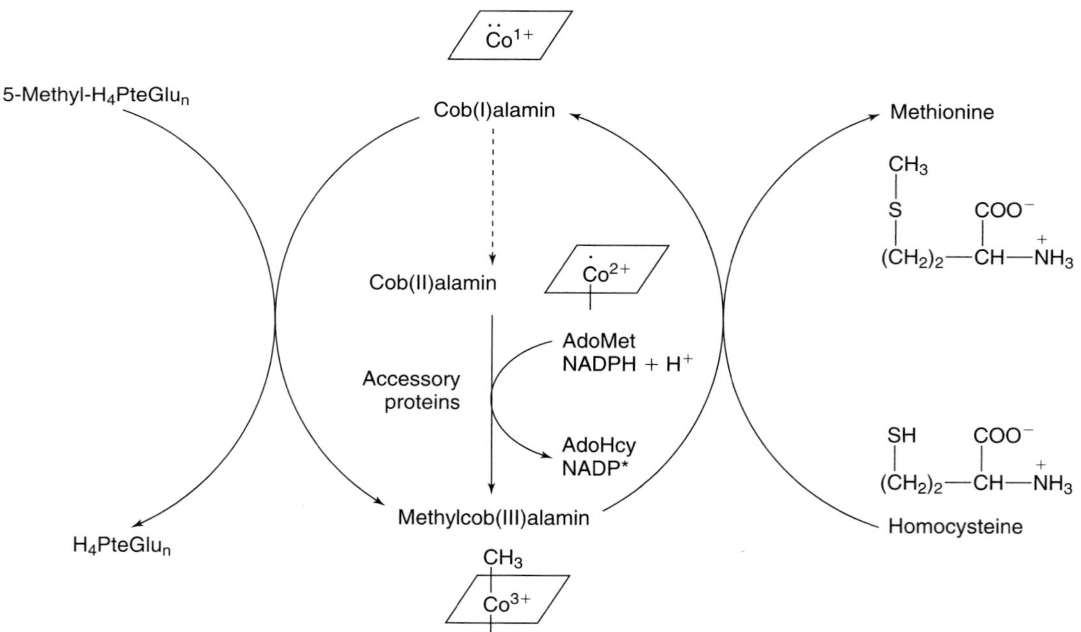

Figure 25-9 Remethylation of homocysteine via the methionine synthase reaction. Enzyme-bound cob(I)alamin can be methylated by 5-methyl-$H_4PteGlu_n$ to generate the methylcob(III)alamin intermediate, or it can be oxidized to the nonfunctional cob(II)alamin form. Cob(II)alamin is reduced and methylated via the action of methionine synthase reductase, a protein that interacts with methionine synthase.

to nitrogen. During this process, a hydroxyl radical is formed, which can lead to destruction of the polypeptide backbone of the protein and inactivation of the enzyme. Nitrous oxide is sometimes used to inactivate methionine synthase in experimental animals to generate a model for the metabolic effects of vitamin B_{12} deficiency.

The many organisms that do not use B_{12} cofactors possess a B_{12}-independent methionine synthase that catalyzes the 5-methyl-H_4-$PteGlu_n$–dependent methylation of homocysteine to methionine. This enzyme, which is not found in mammalian tissues, is absolutely specific for a folylpolyglutamate substrate. Many bacteria express the vitamin B_{12}–dependent enzyme when cultured in the presence of cobalamin, whereas the vitamin B_{12}–independent enzyme is induced in the absence of cobalamin. A question that arises is why have some organisms, such as mammals, retained the vitamin B_{12}–dependent enzyme, which necessitates a very complex process for vitamin B_{12} transport and metabolism and makes the organism susceptible to all the problems that can be caused by defects in these processes (see subsequent text of this chapter), rather than simply using the B_{12}-independent methionine synthase expressed by many other organisms? The answer is not obvious but may be related to the very poor catalytic activity of the B_{12}-independent enzyme. In organisms such as yeast, or bacteria cultured in the absence of cobalamin, the vitamin B_{12}–independent enzyme is induced to very high levels to compensate for its poor catalytic activity, and it is one of the major proteins expressed by these organisms. The more catalytically effective vitamin B_{12}–dependent enzyme is a low-abundance protein.

METHYLMALONYL CoA MUTASE

Mitochondrial β-oxidation of dietary odd-chain fatty acids produces propionyl CoA in addition to acetyl CoA. Propionyl CoA is converted to D-methylmalonyl CoA in a reaction catalyzed by the biotin-dependent propionyl CoA carboxylase. Propionyl CoA and methylmalonyl CoA can also arise during catabolism of isoleucine, valine, methionine, and threonine (see Chapter 14, Figs. 14-19, 14-21, and 14-28). A racemase converts D-methylmalonyl CoA to L-methylmalonyl CoA, and the 5′-deoxyadenosylcobalamin–dependent methylmalonyl CoA mutase catalyzes the conversion of L-methylmalonyl CoA to succinyl CoA (Fig. 25-10). The mutase reaction involves the breakage and migration of a carbon–carbon bond. All these reactions occur in the mitochondria, and the succinyl CoA that is formed has several potential fates, including entry into the citric acid cycle and heme biosynthesis. In liver, conversion of propionyl CoA to succinyl CoA allows the carbon skeletons of some amino acids, as well as propionyl CoA from odd-chain fatty acid metabolism, to be used for gluconeogenesis.

VITAMIN B_{12} DEFICIENCY: SYMPTOMS AND METABOLIC BASES

Vitamin B_{12} deficiency is rarely caused by a dietary insufficiency and most commonly arises from a defect in vitamin B_{12} absorption. The classical manifestations are pernicious anemia, which is a megaloblastic anemia identical to that observed with folate deficiency, and a severe and often irreversible neurological disease called subacute combined degeneration of the spinal cord, which is characterized

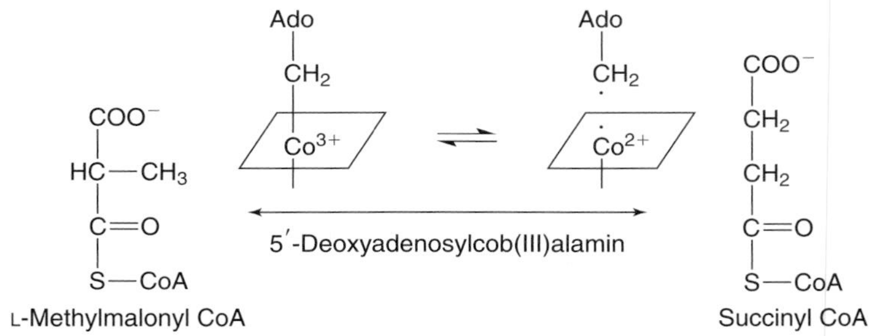

Figure 25-10 The methylmalonyl CoA mutase reaction. The mutase catalyzes the homolytic cleavage of coenzyme B_{12} to generate an adenosyl radical, which interacts with the substrate, and a B_{12} cofactor radical.

by demyelination and peripheral neuropathy. Memory loss and dementia have also been observed. Although the development of anemia often precedes the neurological disease and allows the detection and treatment of B_{12} deficiency prior to the development of neurological damage, this is not always the case, and some patients present with neurological disease in the absence of anemia. Neurological symptoms occur in 75% to 90% of patients with clinical B_{12} deficiency and may be the only symptom in 25%. The reason for this is not clear. Because the anemia is due to induction of a functional folate deficiency, it has been speculated that B_{12}-deficient subjects who have high folate intakes, such as vegetarians or individuals taking folate supplements, may be more likely to develop neurological symptoms without developing anemia, but firm evidence in support of this hypothesis is lacking.

VITAMIN B_{12} MALABSORPTION

Defects in vitamin B_{12} absorption affect a significant proportion of elderly people. Classical pernicious anemia is caused by an inability to absorb vitamin B_{12} as a result of lack of production of IF. The disease is age-related and is usually due to destruction of the parietal cells in the stomach, which is caused by an autoimmune disease in which antibodies to the H^+,K^+-ATPase or to IF are produced. Because body vitamin B_{12} stores are usually ample at the onset of the disease and the turnover of body stores is slow, it can take many years before deficiency symptoms become apparent. Whole-body turnover is increased, owing to an inability to reabsorb biliary vitamin B_{12} as well as dietary vitamin B_{12}. The destruction of the parietal cells decreases acid production, which also impairs release of dietary vitamin from protein binders. The prevalence of untreated pernicious anemia in elderly people has been estimated to be about 2%. About 3% of elderly people test positive for IF autoantibodies, which may suggest a somewhat higher incidence of untreated pernicious anemia (Carmel, 1996). The Schilling test is sometimes used clinically to verify a diagnosis of pernicious anemia. In this test, the absorption of labeled vitamin B_{12}, as measured by its appearance in urine, is defective in pernicious anemia patients but becomes normal if IF is given together with the labeled vitamin B_{12} dose.

Although absorption of vitamin B_{12} by diffusion potentially could overcome the loss of the IF-mediated transport of dietary vitamin B_{12}, this would require extremely high intakes of vitamin B_{12} because diffusion is very inefficient (<1%), and additional high doses would be required to make up for the failure to reabsorb biliary losses. Pernicious anemia is easily treated by monthly intramuscular injections of 1 mg of vitamin B_{12}.

Malabsorption of dietary vitamin B_{12} also can arise from any condition of decreased acid production or pancreatic insufficiency. The prevalence of atrophic gastritis in subjects 50 years and older has been estimated at 10% to 30%, and many elderly people have *Helicobacter pylori* infection. These conditions result in an impairment of food vitamin B_{12} absorption because of an impaired ability to release the vitamin from protein binders, while absorption of vitamin B_{12} in the absence of food is unimpaired. This condition can be detected by a modified Schilling test in which the absorption of food B_{12} is compared with that of crystalline vitamin B_{12}. Bacterial overgrowth in the gut also can compete for vitamin B_{12} and reduce the amount of vitamin available for absorption. Problems with bacterial overgrowth can be treated with antibiotics. Surgical stomach resection, a procedure that is sometimes used for the treatment of obesity, can also lead to decreased acid and IF production. Vitamin B_{12} absorption also can be impaired in general malabsorption syndromes, such as sprue and ileitis. Many vitamin B_{12}–deficient patients can be treated with daily oral supplements of 1 to 2 mg, particularly if these are started prior to vitamin B_{12} depletion.

MEGALOBLASTIC ANEMIA

The reason for the identical megaloblastic anemia that results from folate and vitamin B_{12} deficiency is best explained by the methyl trap hypothesis (Shane and Stokstad, 1985). The two vitamins are cofactors for the methionine synthase reaction. In patients with pernicious anemia, methionine synthase activity in bone marrow is reduced by more than 85%, and most of the protein is present in the apoenzyme form. This causes an accumulation of cellular folate in the 5-methyl-H_4PteGlu$_n$ form, and this is essentially the only form of folate found in the cytosol of experimental animals in which methionine synthase has been inactivated. 5-Methyl-H_4PteGlu$_n$ can be metabolized only via the methionine synthase reaction and is functionally unavailable unless converted to H_4PteGlu$_n$. The trapping of folate in this form results in lack of folate coenzymes for other reactions of one-carbon metabolism, including thymidylate and purine synthesis. Consequently, the symptoms are identical to those seen in folate deficiency: megaloblastic anemia. Megaloblastic changes occur in the blood profiles of subjects treated with the anesthetic nitrous oxide due to destruction of methionine synthase. After treatment, enzyme levels gradually return to normal owing to synthesis of new protein.

Tissue accumulation of folate is also grossly impaired. Because 5-methyl-H_4PteGlu is the major form of folate transported into tissues, and because its conversion to polyglutamates and retention by tissues requires its metabolism to H_4PteGlu, the block in methionine synthase activity results in an inability of tissues to accumulate exogenous folate such that most of the transported 5-methyl-H_4PteGlu is released back into the circulation. This reduction in the ability of tissues to accumulate folate, coupled with turnover of tissue folate pools, leads to a reduction in tissue folate levels, and an absolute tissue folate deficiency ensues on top of the functional deficiency caused by the methyl trap. In experimental animals placed on a vitamin B_{12}–deficient diet, or in animals treated with nitrous oxide to inhibit methionine synthase activity, plasma folate levels initially increase because of the inability of tissues to retain entering folate but then eventually drop to low levels because of an inability to retain folate in the body.

The complex regulation of the folate and vitamin B_{12}–dependent methionine resynthesis cycle has been discussed previously. It appears that no mechanisms exist that can compensate for impaired B_{12} availability.

Clinical Correlation

Megaloblastic Anemia: A Common Complication of Folate and Vitamin B_{12} Deficiency

Megaloblastic anemia, a manifestation of defective DNA synthesis in hematopoietic cells, can arise from impaired folate or vitamin B_{12} status. Folate-deficiency megaloblastic anemia is almost always a nutritional disease caused by inadequate folate in the diet, and its incidence is increased in pregnancy. Vitamin B_{12}–deficiency megaloblastic anemia, which is more common than that due to folate deficiency in the American population, is rarely due to inadequate dietary vitamin B_{12} but usually arises from malabsorption of the vitamin, a condition that affects a significant proportion of elderly people. An elevated folate intake can correct the anemia due to depressed B_{12} status but not the other symptoms of vitamin B_{12} deficiency. As a result of concerns about this masking effect of folate, the amount of folic acid added to fortified foods in the United States has been restricted.

Although rare, many cases of inborn errors of B_{12} metabolism have been described. Studies with cultured skin fibroblasts from patients with these inborn errors have indicated seven complementation groups that may correspond to defects in seven different genes. Some patients exhibiting megaloblastic anemia have defects in proteins involved in B_{12} transport or coenzyme synthesis, whereas others have defects in methionine synthase. Recently, several patients with functionally null mutations in methionine synthase were described in whom enzyme activity was completely lacking (Wilson et al., 1998). One infant had very severe megaloblastic anemia. The ability of these patients to survive gestation was surprising as the methionine synthase gene knockout in the mouse is embryonically lethal (Swanson et al., 2001), which again illustrates that experimental animal models for human disease do not always faithfully mimic the human condition.

SUBACUTE COMBINED DEGENERATION

The mechanism underlying the neurological symptoms of vitamin B_{12} deficiency is not understood. Most experimental animals do not develop neurological symptoms when placed on a vitamin B_{12}–deficient diet, in part because it is difficult to eliminate gut bacterial synthesis of vitamin B_{12} as a source of the vitamin. Although rarely used as a model, the South African fruit bat does display neurological abnormalities when made vitamin B_{12}–deficient, as do nonhuman primates.

Because mammals have only two B_{12}-dependent enzymes and methionine synthase is the locus of the defect causing anemia, attention has been focused on the role of methylmalonyl CoA mutase in the etiology of the neurological defects. Vitamin B_{12} deficiency causes accumulation of methylmalonyl CoA in the mitochondria, an elevation in circulating methylmalonate, acidosis, and elevated methylmalonate excretion. The accumulation of mitochondrial methylmalonyl CoA depletes the CoA pool available for other mitochondrial enzymes and metabolites, and the increased propionyl CoA can be incorporated into long-chain fatty acids in place of acetyl CoA. A role for the accumulation of unusual fatty acids in myelin as a reason for the demyelination has been proposed, but evidence for this is not convincing. In any case, demyelination is not caused by a block in methylmalonyl CoA mutase activity. Humans with severe genetic impairment of the *mut* locus encoding the mutase have a variety of severe clinical conditions and metabolic abnormalities but do not develop subacute combined degeneration of the spinal cord or megaloblastic anemia.

Monkeys treated with nitrous oxide develop neurological disease similar to that observed in humans, and these symptoms are prevented by methionine supplementation, suggesting that the neurological disease of B_{12} deficiency may also result from a defect in methionine synthase (in this case, because of the impairment in methionine synthesis). In the few known cases of genetic defects in methionine synthase or in the enzymes responsible for methylcobalamin synthesis, the patients exhibit the expected megaloblastic anemia and some also exhibit demyelination. Similarly, some patients with defects in methylenetetrahydrofolate reductase exhibit the same neurological symptoms as are observed in B_{12} deficiency. These patients do not exhibit megaloblastic anemia, because a defect in the reductase prevents the formation of 5-methyl-$H_4PteGlu_n$ and thus increases folate coenzyme availability for nucleotide synthesis. Although the mechanism responsible for the neurological disease of B_{12} deficiency is not understood, current evidence supports the hypothesis that it is related to defective methionine synthesis and that the locus of the defect is methionine synthase. A mouse "knockout" model for methionine synthase has recently been developed (Swanson et al., 2001). The homozygous deletion is embryonically lethal, as might be predicted because of the expected derangement in DNA synthesis. The heterozygote may prove to be a useful animal model for elucidating the development of neurological disease resulting from B_{12} deficiency.

A new model for B_{12} deficiency in the rat, involving the totally gastrectomized animal, has recently been described (Brunaud et al., 2003). Removal of the stomach induces severe B_{12} deficiency, and the rats develop neurological abnormalities similar to those observed in humans, including vacuolation, intramyelinic and interstitial edema of the white matter of the central nervous system, and astrogliosis. This accompanied by overproduction of tumor necrosis factor-alpha (TNF-α) and the reduced synthesis of two neurotrophic agents, epidermal growth factor (EGF) and interleukin-6 (IL-6), has led to the hypothesis that dysregulation of these agents is induced by B_{12} deficiency and is responsible for the subacute combined degeneration (SCD) condition. It remains to be established how B_{12} deficiency affects TNF-α and EGF levels and whether the dysregulation in these agents is causative of the SCD condition or results from it in this rather extreme animal model.

HYPERHOMOCYSTEINEMIA

The relationship of hyperhomocysteinemia to vascular disease risk was described in preceding text. Plasma homocysteine is elevated in pernicious anemia because of the block in methionine synthase activity. In population studies, subjects with the lowest deciles of plasma vitamin B_{12} had the highest plasma homocysteine values (Selhub et al., 1993). Although a slight correlation was observed between dietary vitamin B_{12} and homocysteine levels, it was weaker than that for plasma homocysteine and plasma B_{12}, reflecting that defects in absorption rather than dietary content play a greater role in the development of impaired vitamin B_{12} status. As indicated previously, with the improvement of the folate status of the U.S. population following food fortification, B_{12} status has become the major nutritional determinant of fasting homocysteine levels.

ASSAY AND DETECTION OF VITAMIN B_{12} DEFICIENCY

Total plasma vitamin B_{12} can be measured by microbiological assay. These tests sometimes also measure B_{12} analogs that have no vitamin activity in humans. The most widely used clinical test is a competitive radioassay procedure for plasma vitamin B_{12} that uses IF as the protein binder. IF will not bind B_{12} analogs, and this test is specific for biologically active forms of the vitamin. A plasma level of less than 200 pmol/L (about 250 ng/L) is considered indicative of deficiency. However, plasma levels greater than 250 ng/L are often seen in subjects who, by other criteria, such as vitamin malabsorption tests, are at risk for developing deficiency symptoms. Because plasma B_{12} is not a very sensitive indicator of status, other tests, such as the degree of saturation of TC-II by vitamin B_{12} or the level of holo TC-II are becoming more routinely used and appear to be more sensitive indicators of status.

Because B_{12} deficiency induces a folate deficiency, many of the biochemical effects of B_{12} deficiency are identical to those seen in folate deficiency. Although plasma folate level is initially elevated, as the deficiency progresses plasma and red cell folate concentrations are reduced, plasma homocysteine is elevated, and urinary formiminoglutamate excretion is increased. By using these biochemical tests it is not possible to distinguish whether an individual is folate- or vitamin B_{12}–deficient or both. A low plasma B_{12} level would be indicative of B_{12} deficiency, whereas a normal plasma B_{12} coupled with low plasma or red cell folate would suggest folate deficiency. An increase in plasma or urinary methylmalonate would also be a specific indicator of impaired vitamin B_{12} status and this test is becoming more extensively used clinically. Although folate status does not affect methylmalonate levels, a high-fiber diet may result in elevated methylmalonate levels. Fermentation of fiber in the colon can generate propionate, which is absorbed and metabolized to methylmalonate.

A diagnosis of megaloblastic anemia can be confirmed by the appearance and size of blood cells. Because of the severe and sometimes irreversible nature of the neurological disease in untreated B_{12} deficiency, early detection of neurological impairment is critical. The use of a tuning fork to check for an absent vibration sensation is a simple neurological test that can detect early stages of impairment.

VITAMIN B_{12} REQUIREMENTS

The IOM (1998) estimated the adult EAR on the basis of hematological evidence and serum B_{12} values. The current EAR is 2 μg/day of vitamin B_{12} for adults, and the RDA was set at 2.4 μg of vitamin B_{12} per day (EAR + 20%). An intake of 2.6 μg/day is recommended for pregnant women to allow for fetal deposition of 0.1 to 0.2 μg/day, and an intake of 2.8 μg/day is recommended for lactating women to allow for secretion of vitamin B_{12} in milk. Because of the high incidence of malabsorption of food vitamin B_{12} in elderly people, it is recommended that individuals older than 50 years meet the RDA by ingesting foods fortified with B_{12} or by taking a supplement. EARs for children were extrapolated from adult values based on body weight ($kg^{0.75}$), and the RDAs were set as 1.2 times the EARs. AIs for infants are based on the vitamin B_{12} content of milk of well-nourished mothers (0.42 μg/L).

Based on NHANES III (1988-1994), mean intakes of vitamin B_{12} by adults in the United States are approximately 5.1 μg/day for men and approximately 4.8 μg/day for women. The range of intakes for various population groups is about 3.3 μg/day (5th percentile) to 7.1 μg/day (95th percentile).

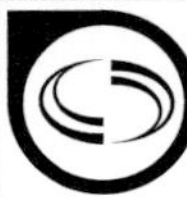

RDAs Across the Life Cycle

	μg Vitamin B_{12} per Day
Infants	
0 to 0.5 yr	0.4 (AI)
0.5 to 1.0 yr	0.5 (AI)
Children	
1 to 3 yr	0.9
4 to 8 yr	1.2
9 to 13 yr	1.8
14 to 18 yr	2.4
Adults	
19 to 50 yr	2.4
51 to >70 yr	2.4*
Pregnant women	2.6
Lactating women	2.8

Data from Institute of Medicine (1998) Dietary Reference Intakes for Thiamin, Riboflavin, Niacin, Vitamin B_6, Folate, Vitamin B_{12}, Pantothenic Acid, Biotin, and Choline. National Academy Press, Washington, DC.
*Adults older than 50 years of age are advised to obtain most of the recommended dietary allowance (RDA) for vitamin B_{12} from foods fortified with B_{12} or a B_{12}-containing supplement.
AI, Adequate intake.

VITAMIN B_{12} TOXICITY

No toxicity associated with high doses of vitamin B_{12} has been reported, and milligram doses are used to treat pernicious anemia with no apparent side effects.

VITAMIN B_6

Vitamin B_6 was originally isolated as an antidermatitis and antianemia factor for animals. The classical clinical symptoms of vitamin B_6 deficiency are a seborrheic dermatitis, microcytic anemia, epileptiform convulsions, and depression and confusion. Microcytic anemia is a reflection of decreased hemoglobin synthesis. More recently, interest in vitamin B_6 status has centered on its role in decreasing circulating homocysteine, a risk factor for vascular disease.

CHEMISTRY OF VITAMIN B_6

Vitamin B_6 compounds are 4-substituted 2-methyl-3-hydroxy-5-hydroxymethylpyridine compounds (Fig. 25-11). There are six major derivatives with vitamin activity: pyridoxal (PL), the 4-formyl derivative; pyridoxine (PN), the 4-hydroxymethyl derivative; pyridoxamine (PM), the 4-aminomethyl derivative; and their respective 5′-phosphate derivatives (PLP, PNP, and PMP). The major forms in animal tissues are the coenzyme species PLP and PMP. PN is usually the major form in plant foods, and a large proportion of the PN in plants can be present as a glucoside derivative. PN is the form of the vitamin normally present in supplements or fortified foods. The major excretory form of vitamin B_6 is the 4-carboxylate derivative known as 4-pyridoxic acid.

Vitamin B_6 compounds, and in particular PL and PLP, are light sensitive. Large losses of food vitamin B_6 can occur during heating and by leaching of the vitamin during food preparation.

SOURCES OF VITAMIN B_6

Cereals, meat, fish, poultry, and noncitrus fruits are the major contributors of vitamin B_6 in the American diet. Rich sources are highly fortified cereals, beef liver, and other organ meats.

BIOAVAILABILITY AND ABSORPTION OF VITAMIN B_6

Vitamin B_6 is absorbed in the small intestine by a nonsaturable passive diffusion mechanism. The 5′-phosphate derivatives are hydrolyzed by a phosphatase prior to transport. PN glucoside is normally deconjugated by a mucosal glucosidase. In humans, some PN glucoside is absorbed intact and can be hydrolyzed to PN in various tissues.

The bioavailability of vitamin B_6 supplements is greater than 90%. Bioavailability of nonglucoside forms of the vitamin in foods is greater than 75%, whereas the bioavailability of PN glucoside in food is about half as much. Vitamin B_6 in a mixed diet, which would typically contain approximately 15% PN glucoside, is about 75% bioavailable (Gregory, 1997b). Pharmacological doses of vitamin B_6 compounds are well absorbed, but most of the absorbed vitamin is eliminated in the urine at high doses.

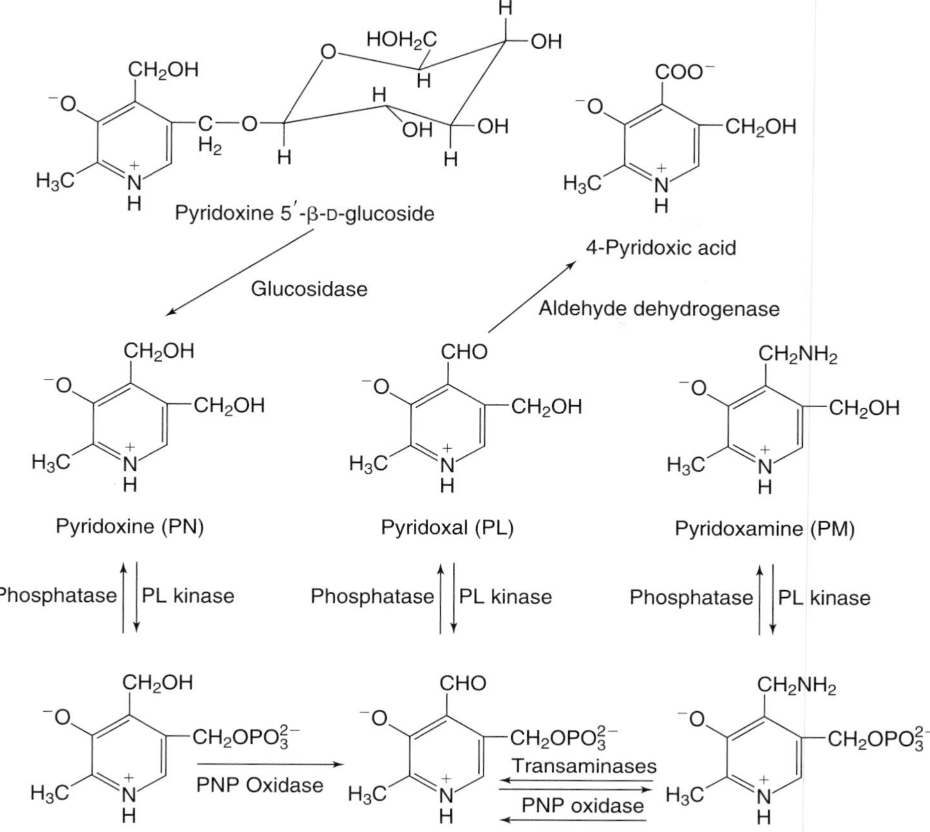

Figure 25-11 Vitamin B_6 compounds and their interconversion and metabolism.

Food Sources

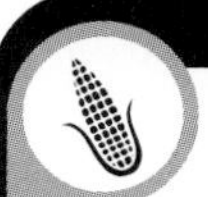

Food Sources High in Vitamin B_6

Cereals and Grains

- 0.3 to 1.0 mg per 1 cup ready-to-eat cereal
- 0.3 mg per ½ cup cooked enriched rice
- 0.15 mg per ½ cup brown rice

Vegetables

- 0.15 to 0.2 mg per ½ cup pinto beans, lentils, lima beans
- 0.1 mg per ½ cup lima beans, kidney beans, chickpeas
- 0.15 to 0.2 mg per ½ cup brussels sprouts, spinach, sweet red peppers, broccoli, sauerkraut, winter squash
- 0.25 mg per ½ cup carrot juice

Meat, Poultry, and Fish

- 0.4 mg per 3 oz turkey
- 0.3 to 0.4 mg per 3 oz pork
- 0.2 to 0.4 mg per 3 oz fish
- 0.25 to 0.5 mg per 3 oz beef

Other

- 0.3 mg per ½ cup prunes
- 0.2 mg per 1 cup orange juice
- 0.35 mg per 1 oz pistachio nuts
- 0.2 mg per 1 oz sunflower seeds

Data from U.S. Department of Agriculture/Agricultural Research Service (USDA/ARS) (2005) USDA Nutrient Database for Standard Reference, Release 18. USDA/ARS, Washington, DC. Retrieved November 15, 2005, from www.ars.usda.gov/ba/bhnrc/ndl.

TRANSPORT, METABOLISM, AND TISSUE ACCUMULATION OF VITAMIN B_6

Most of the absorbed nonphosphorylated B_6 is taken up by the liver and metabolized to PLP, the major coenzymatic form (see Fig. 25-11). PN, PL, and PM are converted to their respective 5′-phosphate derivatives by the enzyme PL kinase. PL kinase is present in all tissues, including red blood cells. PNP, which is normally found only at very low concentrations in tissues, and PMP are oxidized to PLP by the flavoprotein PNP oxidase. PMP can also be converted to PLP by transamination reactions. PLP is distributed in various subcellular compartments, but most is in the cytosol and mitochondria. Most of the PL kinase activity is found in the cytosol, and the mechanism by which PLP gets into the mitochondria is unclear.

PLP binds to proteins and PLP-dependent enzymes via Schiff base formation with the α-amino group of specific lysine residues (Fig. 25-12). PLP itself is not thought to cross membranes. However, protein-bound PLP is in equilibrium with free PLP, and free PLP can be hydrolyzed to PL by various phosphatases and released by the tissue; protein binding protects PLP from the action of these phosphatases. Conditions of increased phosphatase

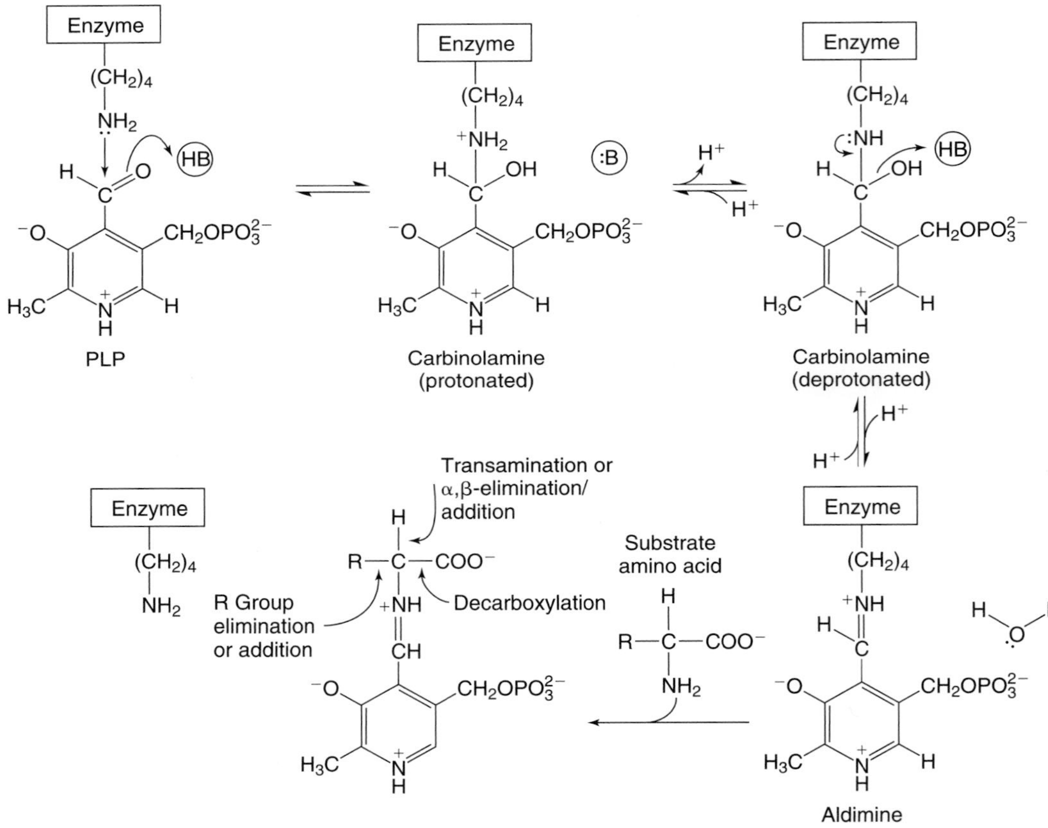

Figure 25-12 Schiff base formation between pyridoxal 5′-phosphate (PLP) and the ε-amino group of a lysine residue at the active site of an enzyme (*HB*, residue on the enzyme that acts as an acid–base catalyst). An entering amino acid substrate displaces the lysine residue and forms a Schiff base with the coenzyme. The coenzyme remains tightly bound to the protein via electrostatic interactions through its 5′-phosphate. Labilization of the various bonds around the α-carbon of the amino acid can result in elimination, addition, transamination, or decarboxylation reactions.

activity, both in tissues and in plasma, can lead to increased hydrolysis of PLP. Tissue protein capacity for binding PLP limits tissue accumulation of vitamin B_6. At high intakes of vitamin B_6, tissue-binding capacity is exceeded, and the free PLP is rapidly hydrolyzed to the nonphosphorylated PL, which is released by the liver and other tissues into the circulation. At pharmacological doses of B_6, the high PLP-binding capacities of proteins in muscle (phosphorylase), plasma (albumin), and red blood cells (hemoglobin) allow them to accumulate high levels of PLP even when other tissues are saturated.

PL in liver can be oxidized to the inactive excretory metabolite pyridoxic acid by a flavoprotein aldehyde dehydrogenase. In normal diets, urinary pyridoxic acid excretion accounts for about half the vitamin B_6 compounds excreted. With large doses of vitamin B_6, the proportion of unmetabolized vitamin excreted increases, and, at very high doses of PN, much of the dose is excreted unchanged in the urine. Vitamin B_6 is also excreted in feces, but this may be due to biosynthesis in the lower gut.

Plasma PLP, a major form of the vitamin in plasma, is derived from liver as a PLP-albumin complex. Because plasma PLP reflects liver PLP levels (and stores), plasma PLP is a sensitive indicator of tissue vitamin B_6 status. Circulating nonphosphorylated forms of the vitamin can be transported into tissues and blood cells. Plasma PLP is also a source of tissue vitamin, but it must dissociate from albumin and be hydrolyzed to PL before it is available.

Estimates of total body vitamin B_6 stores in healthy adults range from approximately 400 μmol to 1000 μmol (60 to 170 mg), and 80% to 90% of this is in muscle, primarily bound to phosphorylase. The overall body half-life of vitamin B_6 has been estimated to be approximately 25 days, with a daily fractional turnover rate of less than 3%. However, because the large pool bound to phosphorylase may turn over very slowly, the half-life may be significantly longer.

METABOLIC FUNCTIONS OF VITAMIN B_6

PLP serves as a coenzyme for more than 100 enzymes, which include primarily enzymes involved in amino acid metabolism, such as aminotransferases, decarboxylases, aldolases, racemases, and dehydratases (see Chapter 14). The carbonyl group of PLP binds to proteins as a covalent Schiff base with the ε-amine of a lysine residue in the active site. For practically all PLP enzymes, the initial step in catalysis involves displacement of the protein lysine residue by the amino group of the entering amino acid, which forms a new Schiff base with the coenzyme (see Fig. 25-12). The coenzyme is no longer covalently attached to the enzyme, but the aldimine derivative remains tightly bound. Electron movement and labilization of the different bonds around the α-carbon of the amino acid can result in transamination, decarboxylation, racemization, α,β-elimination/addition, or R-group elimination/addition. The catabolism of nearly all amino acids involves transfer of their amino groups to α-keto acids. The major amino group acceptors are α-ketoglutarate and pyruvate; transamination with these keto acids results in formation of glutamate and alanine, respectively, whereas the amino acid substrate is converted to its respective keto acid (see Chapter 14).

These transamination (aminotransferase) reactions proceed via a ketimine intermediate and initially generate the keto acid of the amino acid and PMP (Fig. 25-13). Reversal of this reaction using α-ketoglutarate or pyruvate as the entering keto acid generates glutamate or alanine. Aminotransferase reactions normally result in the transfer of the α-amino group of an amino acid to a keto acid. However, the PMP that is formed in the first part of the reaction sometimes dissociates from the enzyme before the keto acid can interact, which results in a slow conversion of PLP to PMP. A PMP-enzyme intermediate is not formed in other PLP-enzyme–catalyzed reactions.

Decarboxylases are involved in many areas of metabolism, including the formation of a number of hormones and neurotransmitters, such as epinephrine, serotonin, and dopamine. Elimination of CO_2 from a compound results in a large drop in free energy, and decarboxylase reactions are essentially irreversible.

PLP is a cofactor for mitochondrial δ-aminolevulinate synthase, which catalyzes the first and rate-limiting step in heme biosynthesis in

Amino acid

Enzyme—PLP Schiff base (aldimine)

$Enzyme—(CH_2)_4—NH_2$

Amino acid—PLP Schiff base (aldimine)

$-H^+, +H^+$

$Enzyme—(CH_2)_4—NH_2$

Keto acid—PMP Schiff base (ketimine)

H_2O H^+ H_2O H^+

$Enzyme—(CH_2)_4—NH_2$

Keto acid

PMP

liver (Fig. 25-14). Labilization of the R group of glycine and addition of succinate generates the transient intermediate α-amino-β-ketoadipate, which is rapidly decarboxylated to δ-aminolevulinate. Two molecules of aminolevulinate condense to form porphobilinogen, and further condensation and metabolism yields heme. The synthesis of δ-aminolevulinate synthase is regulated by heme.

As described previously, PLP is a cofactor for serine hydroxymethyltransferase, cystathionine β-synthase, and cystathionase, which are enzymes involved in the metabolism of homocysteine (see Fig. 25-3).

PLP enzymes are also involved in lipid and carbohydrate metabolism. PLP is a cofactor in the muscle glycogen phosphorylase reaction, but in this reaction the 5′-phosphate group, rather than the 4-carbonyl group, is directly involved in catalysis. Most of the PLP in the body is associated with muscle phosphorylase. PLP is a cofactor for serine palmitoyl transferase, an enzyme involved in sphingolipid synthesis.

Some recent studies have shown that PLP modifies the properties of the glucocorticoid receptor, and it has been suggested that PLP may play a role in steroid hormone action. Similarly, PLP has been shown to affect the transcription rate of some genes. High levels of PLP were used in both studies, and it has not been established that these observations have physiological relevance. PLP at high levels can form Schiff bases with nonspecific lysine residues on proteins.

VITAMIN B_6 DEFICIENCY: SYMPTOMS AND METABOLIC BASES

Vitamin B_6 deficiency can lead to seborrheic dermatitis, microcytic anemia, convulsions, depression, and confusion. Electroencephalographic abnormalities have also been reported in controlled studies of B_6 depletion. With the

Figure 25-13 Intermediates in the transamination of an amino acid to a keto acid. Reversal of these steps converts a second keto acid to an amino acid and regenerates the PLP cofactor bound to the enzyme.

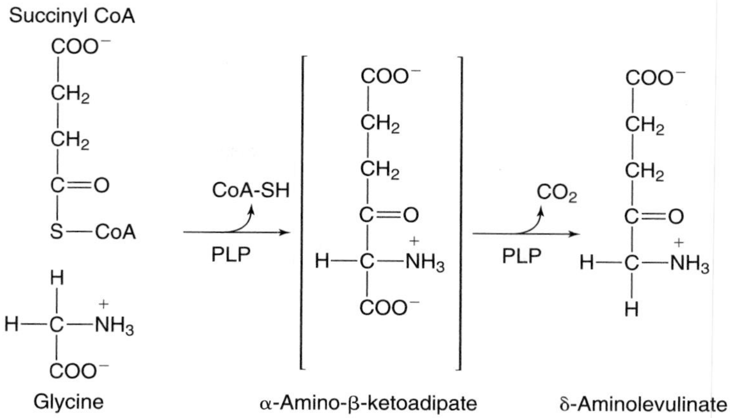

Succinyl CoA

Glycine

α-Amino-β-ketoadipate

δ-Aminolevulinate

Figure 25-14 The δ-aminolevulinate synthase reaction.

exception of the anemia, the exact mechanisms underlying these clinical abnormalities have not been established.

MICROCYTIC ANEMIA

Microcytic anemia is a reflection of decreased hemoglobin synthesis. Replication of the erythroid cell is regulated by its heme content, and reticulocyte cell division stops when the hemoglobin protein concentration reaches approximately 20%. Cells that are defective in heme biosynthesis continue to replicate; cell number can increase, but the cells are small (microcytic) and total blood concentration of hemoglobin is reduced (anemia). The role of PLP as a cofactor for δ-aminolevulinate synthase, the first enzyme in heme biosynthesis, can entirely explain this vitamin B_6–deficiency syndrome.

CONVULSIONS AND ELECTROENCEPHALOGRAPHIC ABNORMALITIES

PLP is a cofactor for decarboxylases that are involved in synthesis of neurotransmitters such as serotonin and dopamine, and vitamin B_6 status has been shown to influence biogenic amine levels in the brain. Reduced activity of some of these decarboxylases could reasonably explain the convulsions and electroencephalographic abnormalities, but the particular biogenic amine most responsible has not been established. It has also been proposed that the convulsions are caused by abnormal tryptophan metabolites that accumulate in the brain in vitamin B_6 deficiency. A widespread outbreak of convulsions occurred in the 1950s in infants who were fed a formula that contained very low vitamin B_6 content, and these convulsions did respond to PN administration. Although occasional cases of convulsions in breast-fed infants of mothers with poor vitamin B_6 status have been reported since then, these are quite rare, and the possibility that other factors were responsible for the convulsions has not been eliminated.

HYPERHOMOCYSTEINEMIA

As described earlier, plasma concentrations of homocysteine are influenced by vitamin B_6, folate, and vitamin B_{12} intakes. The increase in plasma homocysteine following a methionine load or a meal is responsive to, and primarily affected by, vitamin B_6 status, reflecting the ability of PLP-dependent cystathionine β-synthase to catalyze the transsulfuration and removal of homocysteine (see Fig. 25-3).

ALCOHOL

Alcoholics tend to have low plasma PLP levels and a decreased vitamin B_6 status that is independent of poor diet and of defects in metabolism caused by liver damage. Acetaldehyde, the oxidation product of ethanol, decreases cellular PLP levels and is thought to displace PLP from proteins, making PLP more susceptible to hydrolysis by phosphatases.

ASSAY AND DETECTION OF DEFICIENCY

A variety of biochemical indicators have been used to assess vitamin B_6 status. Plasma PLP is a reflection of liver PLP and thus tissue stores, and it generally correlates with other indices of B_6 status. Plasma PLP level is normally measured by an enzymatic assay using apotyrosine decarboxylase. A plasma PLP level of less than 20 nmol/L is considered to reflect adverse vitamin status in the adult, although some support a threshold of 30 nmol/L for assessing sufficiency. Clinical symptoms of vitamin B_6 deficiency and abnormal electroencephalographic patterns have been observed in some vitamin-depleted subjects when their plasma PLP levels fall to 10 nmol/L. Plasma PLP values decrease slightly with increased protein intake. They are high in the fetus and the neonate and decrease gradually throughout the lifespan.

The stimulation of red blood cell aspartate aminotransferase or alanine aminotransferase activities by PLP has been used to evaluate vitamin B_6 status. These tests assess the amount of enzyme in the apoenzyme versus holoenzyme form, the proportion of which increases with B_6 depletion. The excretion of tryptophan catabolites following a loading dose of tryptophan has also been used to assess vitamin B_6 status. The urinary excretion of xanthurenate, which is normally a minor tryptophan catabolite, is increased in vitamin B_6 deficiency. Although tryptophan is catabolized primarily to CO_2 (see Chapters 14 and 24), a number of branch-points in this pathway can lead to the synthesis of quantitatively minor metabolites such as NAD and xanthurenate. The activity of one of the enzymes in tryptophan catabolism, the PLP-dependent kynureninase, is reduced in vitamin B_6 deficiency, which causes a diversion of the metabolic flux into the xanthurenate synthesis pathway. Urinary excretion of xanthurenate can be a nonspecific test, however, because the first enzyme in the tryptophan catabolic pathway, tryptophan dioxygenase, may be induced by steroid hormones and the level of kynureninase itself is decreased during pregnancy. Xanthurenate, as well as other tryptophan catabolites, is elevated in pregnancy and in high-dose oral contraceptive users, in the absence of a vitamin B_6 deficiency. An increase in plasma homocysteine levels following a methionine challenge dose is a fairly specific test of vitamin B_6 status.

VITAMIN B_6 REQUIREMENTS

The primary criterion used in setting the EAR for vitamin B_6 was a plasma PLP value of at least 20 nmol/L (IOM, 1998). The EAR for vitamin B_6 is 1.1 mg/day for adults from 19 to 50 years, and the RDA is 1.3 mg/day or 20% more than the EAR to allow for variance in need. The estimated EARs were higher for adults older than 50 years, and higher for men than women in this older age group. Therefore, the EARs for women and men older than 50 years are 1.3 and 1.4 mg/day, respectively, and the RDAs are 1.5 and 1.7 mg/day, respectively. The RDAs for pregnant and lactating women were increased to 1.9 and 2.0 mg/day, respectively, to ensure adequate intake for the infant. AIs for infants are based on the vitamin B_6 content of milk of well-nourished mothers and the mean volume of milk consumed (0.13 mg/L × 0.78 L/day = 0.1 mg/day). Recommendations for older infants and children were estimated by extrapolation.

Clinical symptoms of vitamin B_6 deficiency have never been observed in experimental subjects receiving intakes of 0.5 mg/day. Because of the role of PLP as a coenzyme for many enzymes involved in amino acid metabolism, it has been proposed that vitamin B_6 requirements are influenced by protein intake and that the RDA should be based on protein intake. However, not all studies have demonstrated a relationship between protein intake and requirement. The median intake in the United States of vitamin B_6 from food sources is about 2 mg/day for men and about 1.5 mg/day for women; intakes are higher in supplement users. Based on NHANES III (1988-1994), the daily intakes of vitamin B_6 range from 1 mg (5th percentile) to 3 mg (95th percentile).

VITAMIN B_6 TOXICITY

A severe sensory neuropathy has been described in subjects taking very large doses of PN (1 to 6 g/day) for the treatment of conditions such as carpal tunnel syndrome, premenstrual

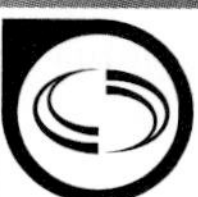

RDAs Across the Life Cycle

	mg Vitamin B_6 per Day
Infants	
0 to 0.5 yr	0.1 (AI)
0.5 to 1.0 yr	0.3 (AI)
Children	
1 to 3 yr	0.5
4 to 8 yr	0.6
9 to 13 yr	1.0
Males	
14 to 18 yr	1.3
19 to 50 yr	1.3
51 to >70 yr	1.7
Females	
14 to 18 yr	1.2
19 to 50 yr	1.3
51 to >70 yr	1.5
Pregnant	1.9
Lactating	2.0

Data from Institute of Medicine (1998) Dietary Reference Intakes for Thiamin, Riboflavin, Niacin, Vitamin B_6, Folate, Vitamin B_{12}, Pantothenic Acid, Biotin, and Choline. National Academy Press, Washington, DC.
AI, Adequate intake.

syndrome, asthma, and sickle cell disease. The reason for the sensory neuropathy is not known, but modification of proteins by PLP may be involved in the development of this condition. Although the efficacy of PN megadoses for treatment of these conditions has little scientific rationale, the toxic effects of megadoses have been clearly demonstrated. Because few studies have specifically looked for adverse effects of high doses of vitamin B_6, the highest safe dose is not known. Some evidence for toxicity has been reported for daily doses of 500 mg, whereas the absence of adverse effects has been rigorously documented in subjects taking daily doses of 100 mg or 300 mg of PN. A safe UL of 100 mg/day has been recommended by the IOM (1998); 100 mg of PN is approximately equal to total body stores in healthy individuals.

REFERENCES

Blount BC, Mack MM, Wehr CM, MacGregor JT, Hiatt RA, Wang G, Wickramasinghe SN, Everson RB, Ames BN (1997) Folate deficiency causes uracil misincorporation into human DNA and chromosomal breakage: Implications for cancer and neuronal damage. Proc Natl Acad Sci USA 94:3290-3295.

Brody LC, Conley M, Cox C, Kirke PN, McKeever MP, Mills JL, Molloy AM, O'Leary VB, Parle-McDermott A, Scott JM, Swanson DA (2002) A polymorphism, R653Q, in the trifunctional enzyme methylenetetrahydrofolate dehydrogenase/methenyltetrahydrofolate cyclohydrolase/formyltetrahydrofolate synthetase is a maternal genetic risk factor for neural tube defects: report of the Birth Defects Research Group. Am J Hum Genet 71:1207-1215.

Brunaud L, Alberto JM, Ayav A, Gerard P, Namour F, Antunes L, Braun M, Bronowicki JP, Bresler L, Gueant JL (2003) Vitamin B12 is a strong determinant of low methionine synthase activity and DNA hypomethylation in gastrectomized rats. Digestion 68:133-140.

Carmel R (1996) Prevalence of undiagnosed pernicious anemia in the elderly. Arch Intern Med 156:1097-1100.

Chen Z, Karaplis AC, Ackerman SL, Pogribny IP, Melnyk S, Lussier-Cacan S, Chen MF, Pai A, John SW, Smith RS, Bottiglieri T, Bagley P, Selhub J, Rudnicki MA, James SJ, Rozen R (2001) Mice deficient in methylenetetrahydrofolate reductase exhibit hyperhomocysteinemia and decreased methylation capacity, with neuropathology and aortic lipid deposition. Hum Mol Genet 10:433-443.

Frosst P, Blom HJ, Milos R, Goyette P, Sheppard CA, Matthews RG, Boers GJ, den Heijer M, Kluitmans LA, van den Heuvel LP, Rozen R (1995) A candidate genetic risk factor for vascular disease: a common mutation in methylenetetrahydrofolate reductase. Nat Genet 10:111-113.

Glusker JP (1995) Vitamin B_{12} and the B_{12} coenzymes. Vitam Horm 50:1-76.

Greene ND, Dunlevy LE, Copp AJ (2003) Homocysteine is embryotoxic but does not cause neural tube defects in mouse embryos. Anat Embryol (Berl) 206:185-191.

Gregory JF 3rd (1997a) Bioavailability of folate. Eur J Clin Nutr 51:S54-S59.

Gregory JF 3rd (1997b) Bioavailability of vitamin B-6. Eur J Clin Nutr 51:S43-S48.

Groenen PM, van Rooij IA, Peer PG, Gooskens RH, Zielhuis GA, Steegers-Theunissen RP (2004) Marginal maternal vitamin B_{12} status increases the risk of offspring with spina bifida. Am J Obstet Gynecol 191:11-17.

Henriquez P, Doreste J, Diaz-Cremades J, Lopez-Blanco F, Alvarez-Leon E, Serra-Majem L (2004) Folate status of adults living in the Canary Islands (Spain). Int J Vitam Nutr Res 74:187-192.

Institute of Medicine (IOM) (1998) Dietary Reference Intakes for Thiamin, Riboflavin, Niacin, Vitamin B_6, Folate, Vitamin B_{12}, Pantothenic Acid, Biotin, and Choline. National Academy Press, Washington, DC.

Ma J, Stampfer MJ, Giovannucci E, Artigas C, Hunter DJ, Fuchs C, Willett WC, Selhub J, Hennekens CH, Rozen R (1997) Methylenetetrahydrofolate reductase polymorphism, dietary interactions, and risk of colorectal cancer. Cancer Res 57:1098-1102.

O'Keefe CA, Bailey LB, Thomas EA, Hofler SA, Davis BA, Cerda JJ, Gregory JF III (1995) Controlled dietary folate affects folate status in nonpregnant women. J Nutr 125:2717-2729.

Quinlivan EP, Gregory JF III (2003) Effect of food fortification on folic acid intake in the United States. Am J Clin Nutr 77:221-225.

Refsum H, Ueland PM, Nygard O, Vollset SE (1998) Homocysteine and vascular disease. Annu Rev Med 49:31-62.

Rimm EB, Willett WC, Hu FB, Sampson L, Colditz GA, Manson JE, Hennekens C, Stampfer MJ (1998) Folate and vitamin B_6 from diet and supplements in relation to risk of coronary heart disease among women. JAMA 279:359-364.

Rothenberg SP, da Costa MP, Sequeira JM, Cracco J, Roberts JL, Weedon J, Quadros EV (2004) Autoantibodies against folate receptors in women with a pregnancy complicated by a neural-tube defect. N Engl J Med 350:134-142.

Scott JM, Kirke PN, Weir DG (1990) The role of nutrition in neural tube defects. Annu Rev Nutr 10:277-295.

Selhub J, Jacques PF, Wilson PWF, Rush D, Rosenberg IH (1993) Vitamin status and intake as primary determinants of homocysteinemia in an elderly population. JAMA 270:2693-2698.

Selhub J, Jacques PF, Bostom AG, D'Agostino RB, Wilson PWF, Belanger AJ, O'Leary DH, Wolf PA, Schaefer EJ, Rosenberg IH (1995) Association between plasma homocysteine concentrations and extracranial carotid-artery stenosis. N Engl J Med 332: 286-291.

Shane B (1989) Folylpolyglutamate synthesis and the regulation of one carbon metabolism. Vitam Horm 45:263-335.

Shane B, Stokstad ELR (1985) Vitamin B_{12}–folate interrelationships. Annu Rev Nutr 5:115-141.

Spiegelstein O, Mitchell LE, Merriweather MY, Wicker NJ, Zhang Q, Lammer EJ, Finnell RH (2004) Embryonic development of folate binding protein-1 (Folbp1) knockout mice: effects of the chemical form, dose, and timing of maternal folate supplementation. Dev Dyn 231:221-231.

Stampfer MJ, Malinow MR, Willett WC, Newcomer LM, Upson B, Ullmann D, Tishler PV, Hennekens CH (1992) A prospective study of plasma homocyst(e)ine and risk of myocardial infarction in US physicians. JAMA 268:877-881.

Stern LL, Mason JB, Selhub J, Choi SW (2000) Genomic DNA hypomethylation, a characteristic of most cancers, is present in peripheral leukocytes of individuals who are homozygous for the C677T polymorphism in the methylenetetrahydrofolate reductase gene. Cancer Epidemiol Biomarkers Prev 9:849-853.

Swanson DA, Liu ML, Baker PJ, Garrett L, Stitzel M, Wu J, Harris M, Banerjee R, Shane B, Brody LC (2001) Targeted disruption of the methionine synthase gene in mice. Mol Cell Biol 21:1058-1065.

Volcik KA, Shaw GM, Lammer EJ, Zhu H, Finnell RH (2003) Evaluation of infant methylenetetrahydrofolate reductase genotype, maternal vitamin use, and risk of high versus low level spina bifida defects. Birth Defects Res A Clin Mol Teratol 67:154-157.

Wilson A, Leclerc D, Saberi F, Campeau E, Hwang HY, Shane B, Phillips JA 3rd, Rosenblatt DS, Gravel RA (1998) Functionally null mutations in patients with the cblG-variant form of methionine synthase deficiency. Am J Hum Genet 63:409-414.

RECOMMENDED READINGS

Bailey LB (ed) (1995) Folate in Health and Disease. Marcel Dekker, New York.

Blakley RL, Benkovic SJ (eds) (1984) Folates and Pterins. Vol. 1. Chemistry and Biochemistry of Folates. Wiley, New York.

Blakley RL, Whitehead VM (eds) (1986) Folates and Pterins. Vol. 3. Nutritional, Pharmacological, and Physiological Aspects. Wiley, New York.

Rucker RB, Suttie JW, McCormick DB, Machlin LJ (eds.) (2001) Handbook of the Vitamins, 3rd ed. Marcel Dekker, New York.

Scriver CR, Sly SS, Childs B, Beaudet AL, Valle D, Kinzler KW, Vogelstein B (eds) (2001) The Metabolic and Molecular Bases of Inherited Disease, 8th ed. McGraw-Hill, New York.

Chapter 26

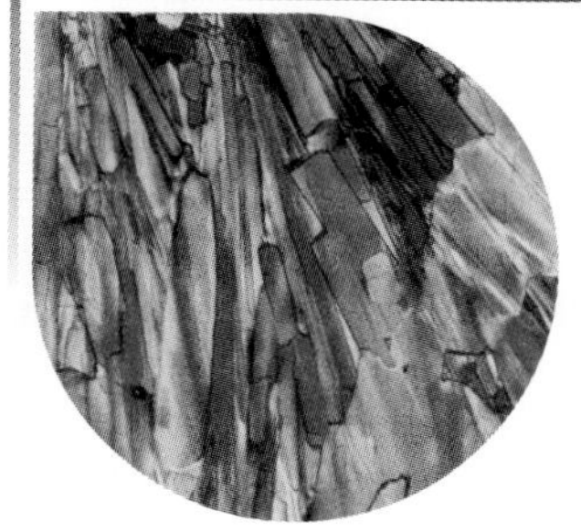

Pantothenic Acid and Biotin

Lawrence Sweetman, PhD

OUTLINE

COMMON ABBREVIATIONS

CoA coenzyme A
ACP acyl carrier protein
CPT carnitine palmitoyltransferase

PANTOTHENIC ACID

Pantothenic acid (vitamin B_5) was discovered in the 1930s as a factor in tissue extracts that prevented an experimental deficiency disease in fowl that was characterized by skin lesions. Pantothenic acid (pantothenate) is metabolized to two major enzyme cofactors: coenzyme A (CoA) and the 4′-phosphopantetheine prosthetic group of the acyl carrier protein (ACP) domain of fatty acid synthase. These cofactors contain a sulfhydryl group (–SH) that is directly involved in biochemical reactions, forming "high-energy" thioesters with carboxylic acids. CoA forms thioesters with a very wide range of metabolic intermediates and has been estimated to be a cofactor for about 4% of all known enzymes (Begley et al., 2001). ACP and CoA both are essential for the synthesis of fatty acids, and CoA has additional important roles in fatty acid oxidation, in ketone body metabolism, in oxidative metabolism of pyruvate via pyruvate dehydrogenase, in the citric acid cycle, and in the metabolism of a wide variety of organic acids, including those formed in the catabolism of many amino acids. Figure 26-1 outlines the cellular location and the interrelationships of these major areas of metabolism. These reactions include the formation of CoA thioesters, the transfer or condensation of the acyl group of the acyl CoA with another compound with the release of CoA, the requirement for CoA thioesters as substrates and products of dehydrogenation and dehydration reactions, and acyl group exchange reactions that do not involve the release of free CoA.

MICROBIAL AND PLANT BIOSYNTHESIS AND STRUCTURE OF PANTOTHENIC ACID

Microorganisms and plants synthesize pantoate (pantoic acid) from α-ketoisovalerate, the keto acid derived from the amino acid valine. A hydroxymethyl group is attached to α-ketoisovalerate, and the keto group is reduced to a hydroxy group to form pantoate. Pantoate is condensed with β-alanine to form pantothenate (pantothenic acid). In bacteria, β-alanine is produced by decarboxylation of the amino acid aspartate and is condensed with pantoate to form pantothenate (Begley et al., 2001). In plants, which are a more important dietary source of pantothenate, β-alanine is not derived from aspartate, but the precursor has not yet been determined. The synthesis of pantothenate does not occur in humans or other animals. Pantothenic acid is fairly widely distributed in foods, giving rise to its name (from Greek *pant-*, meaning "all" or "every"). Liver, milk, and legumes are good sources. Pantothenic acid is contained in foods in various bound forms, including CoA and CoA esters, ACP, and as a glucoside in tomatoes.

ABSORPTION, TRANSPORT, AND EXCRETION OF PANTOTHENIC ACID

CoA and ACP from the diet are enzymatically degraded in the intestine to release free pantothenic acid. Uptake of pantothenic acid is mediated by a saturable sodium (Na^+)-dependent multivitamin transporter, which uses the Na^+ electrochemical gradient to drive transport. The highest rate of transport occurs in the jejunum (Fenstermacher and Rose, 1986). This multivitamin transporter, which also transports biotin and lipoic acid, has been cloned from human intestinal cells (Prasad et al., 1999). Pantetheine also is absorbed by the intestine, but it is hydrolyzed to pantothenic acid in the intestinal cells. CoA, dephospho-CoA, and phosphopantetheine are not absorbed by the intestine and must be digested to pantothenic acid before absorption (Shibata et al., 1983). The absorbed pantothenic acid is transported by the blood, primarily as bound forms in red blood cells. How this is made available to tissues is unclear, and it may be that the low concentration of free pantothenic acid in plasma (0.06 to 0.08 mg/L as compared with 1.0 to 1.8 mg/L in whole blood) is the form that is available for uptake by tissues.

The transport of pantothenic acid (pantothenate) from the extracellular fluid into cells also occurs via a saturable Na^+-dependent mechanism by the mammalian Na^+-dependent multivitamin transporter (Prasad and Ganapathy, 2000). The transport across the blood-brain

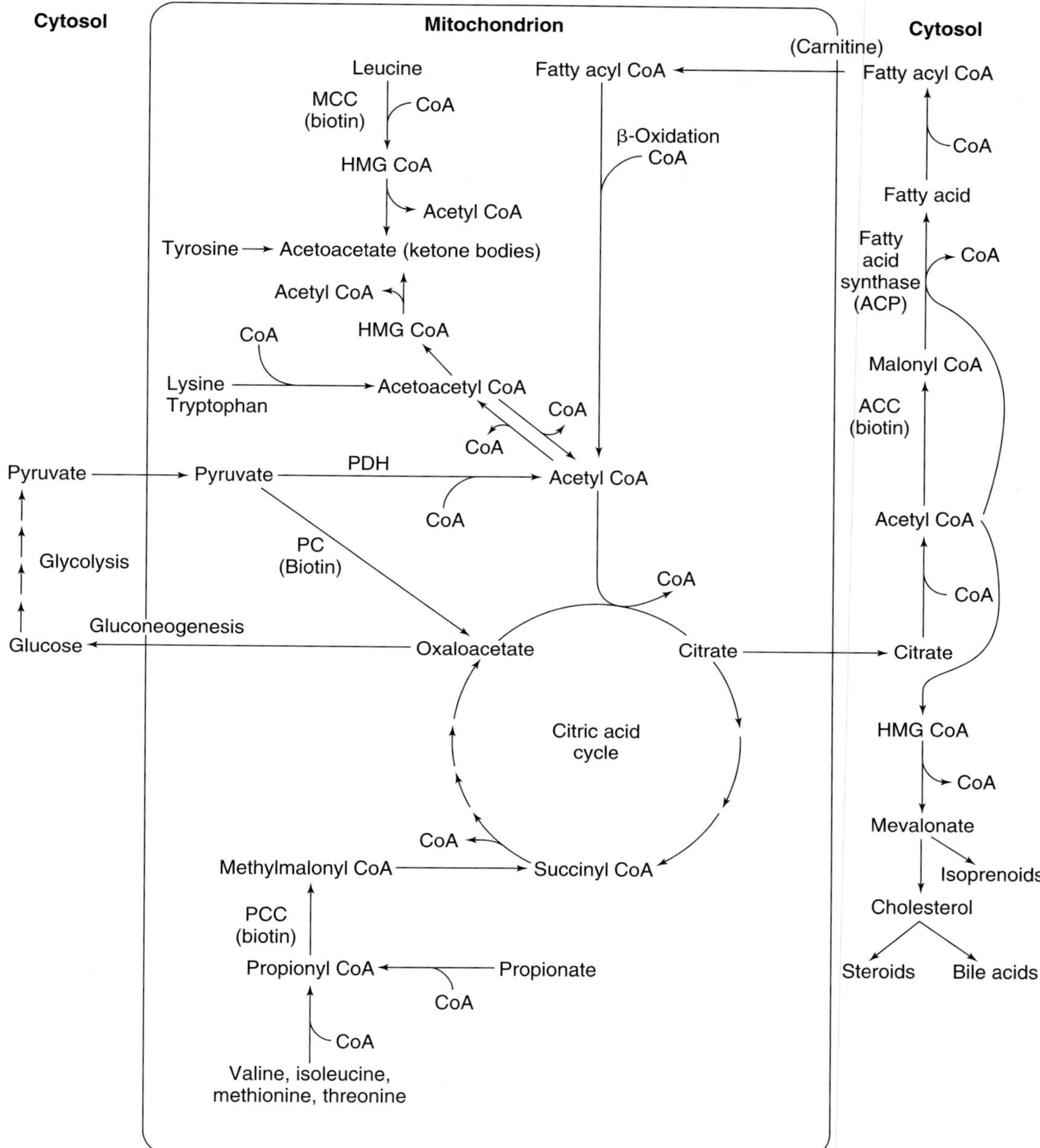

Figure 26-1 Roles of coenzyme A (CoA), acyl carrier protein (ACP), and biotin in cellular metabolism. The major steps of cellular metabolism in which pantothenic acid is involved as ACP in fatty acid synthase and as CoA in other reactions are summarized. The steps catalyzed by the four biotin-containing carboxylases (ACC, PCC, MCC, and PC) also are shown. *ACC,* Acetyl CoA carboxylase; *HMG CoA,* 3-hydroxy-3-methylglutaryl CoA; *MCC,* 3-methylcrotonyl CoA carboxylase; *PC,* pyruvate carboxylase; *PCC,* propionyl CoA carboxylase; *PDH,* pyruvate dehydrogenase.

barrier also is saturable but does not appear to be Na^+-dependent. In the kidney tubules, pantothenic acid largely is reabsorbed at physiological concentrations by a Na^+-dependent process (Tahiliani and Beinlich, 1991). At higher plasma concentrations not all pantothenic acid is reabsorbed from the renal filtrate and there is loss of pantothenic acid into the urine. As a result, there is a positive correlation between dietary intake of pantothenic acid and its excretion in the urine. There are no known catabolites of pantothenic acid; only pantothenic acid is excreted in urine.

COENZYME A AND ACYL CARRIER PROTEIN SYNTHESIS AND DEGRADATION

COENZYME A SYNTHESIS

Within cells, CoA is synthesized from pantothenic acid in five steps (Fig. 26-2). The initial reaction is phosphorylation of the hydroxyl group of the pantoic acid portion of pantothenic acid with adenosine triphosphate (ATP) catalyzed by pantothenate kinase to form 4′-phosphopantothenate. This is the rate-limiting step for synthesis of CoA, and regulation of pantothenate kinase activity controls the rate of CoA synthesis (Rock et al., 2000). The activity of pantothenate kinase is inhibited by the intermediates 4′-phosphopantothenate and dephospho-CoA, by the end product CoA, and by the acetyl-, propionyl-, and malonyl-esters of CoA (acyl CoAs). Carnitine protects pantothenate kinase from the inhibition by CoA and acyl CoA by competing with them for the same binding site on pantothenate kinase (Fisher et al., 1985).

The next step in the synthesis of CoA is catalyzed by 4′-phosphopantothenoylcysteine synthetase, which couples ATP hydrolysis with formation of an amide bond between the carboxyl group of 4′-phosphopantothenate and the amino group of the sulfur amino acid, cysteine. The product, 4′-phosphopantothenoylcysteine is decarboxylated by a specific decarboxylase to form 4′-phosphopantetheine. The final two steps of CoA synthesis are catalyzed by a bifunctional enzyme (CoA synthase) possessing both 4′-phosphopantetheine adenylyltransferase and dephospho CoA kinase activities (Zhyvoloup et al., 2003). The adenylyltransferase domain adds the adenosine monophosphate (AMP) group of ATP to the 4′-phospho group of 4′-phosphopantetheine to form dephospho-CoA; the dephospho-CoA kinase domain then uses ATP to phosphorylate the 3′-hydroxyl of dephospho-CoA. The human genes for the enzymes of CoA synthesis have been identified only recently. Genes encoding pantothenate kinase were identified in conjunction with the mapping of a hereditary neurodegenerative disorder (Zhou et al., 2001). Candidate genes for the enzymes catalyzing the subsequent steps were identified by a comparative genomics approach, and the encoded proteins were then expressed, purified, and reconstituted in vitro to synthesize CoA (Daugherty et al., 2002). All of the enzymes in the CoA biosynthetic pathway are present in the cytosol. The PanK2 isoform of human pantothenate kinase localizes to the mitochondria, but evidence for a complete CoA synthetic pathway in the mitochondria is lacking. The bifunctional CoA synthase contains an N-terminal domain that targets the enzyme to the cytosolic face of the mitochondria outer membrane but not to the inside of the organelle. CoA synthase is activated by phospholipids in the membrane.

Notable features of the structure of CoA are the 3′-phosphoadenosine 5′-diphosphate (3′-phospho-ADP) moiety linked with the pantoate portion, and the reactive sulfhydryl group at the end of the long, flexible chain derived from β-alanine and decarboxylated cysteine. Coenzyme A is often abbreviated as CoASH (instead of CoA) to illustrate this reactive sulfhydryl group, and thioesters of organic acids with CoASH are often abbreviated as acyl-SCoA (instead of acyl CoA).

The majority of the CoA in cells is found within the mitochondria, with about 75% of liver CoA in mitochondria and 95% of heart CoA in mitochondria. This is consistent with the mitochondria being the major cellular organelle involved in fatty acid oxidation and in the final oxidative steps in the catabolism of all fuels; CoA plays a major role in these processes. Because the mitochondria represent only a small fraction of the cellular volume, the concentration of CoA in mitochondria (2.2 mmol/L)

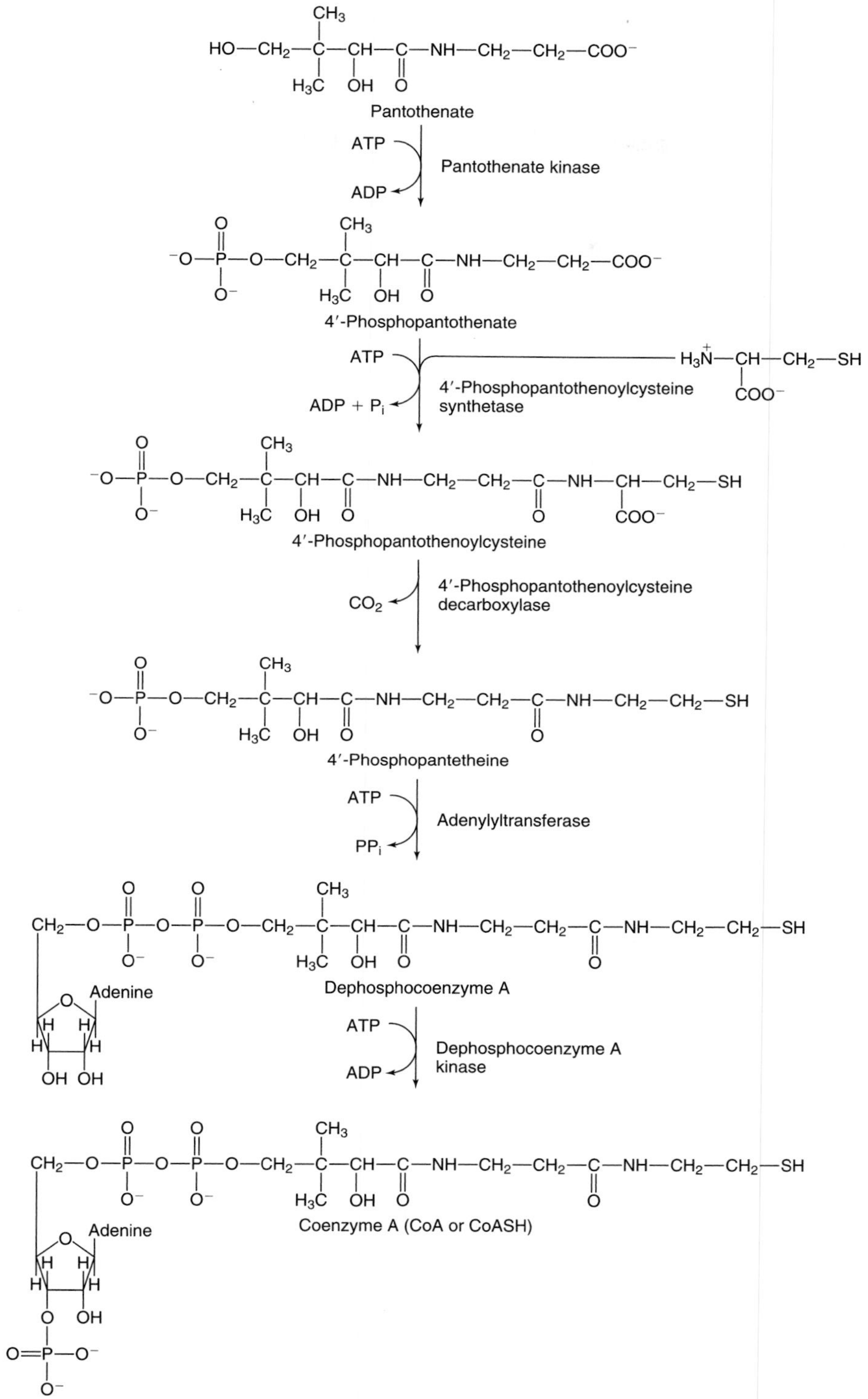
Pantothenate
ATP
ADP
Pantothenate kinase
4′-Phosphopantothenate
ATP
ADP + P$_i$
4′-Phosphopantothenoylcysteine synthetase
4′-Phosphopantothenoylcysteine
CO_2
4′-Phosphopantothenoylcysteine decarboxylase
4′-Phosphopantetheine
ATP
PP$_i$
Adenylyltransferase
Adenine
Dephosphocoenzyme A
ATP
ADP
Dephosphocoenzyme A kinase
Adenine
Coenzyme A (CoA or CoASH)

Figure 26-2 Coenzyme A synthesis and structure. CoA is synthesized from pantothenic acid, the amino acid cysteine, and ATP in mammalian cells.

is 40 to 150 times the concentration of CoA in the cytosol (0.015 to 0.05 mmol/L). This large concentration difference is maintained by the transport of the negatively charged CoA into the mitochondria, which is driven by the membrane electrical gradient (Tahiliani, 1989). CoA is also involved in the oxidation of very-long-chain fatty acids in peroxisomes, but little is known about how CoA enters these organelles. In the cytosol, CoA also is used for the synthesis of the ACP domain of the fatty acid synthase enzyme that catalyzes fatty acid synthesis.

ACYL CARRIER PROTEIN SYNTHESIS

There are several ACPs known in yeast and bacteria, but the ACP domain of fatty acid synthase is the most important and best studied. Fatty acid synthase is the only mammalian enzyme complex containing the ACP domain that has been well characterized. Fatty acid synthase is a single homodimeric multifunctional protein with seven enzymatic activities required for fatty acid synthesis (Smith et al., 2003). The ACP domain of fatty acid synthase is synthesized as an enzymatically inactive apoprotein that lacks the prosthetic group. Covalent attachment of the phosphopantetheine group coverts apo-ACP into the active functional holo-ACP (Joshi et al., 2003). This attachment reaction, catalyzed by 4′-phosphopantetheinyl transferase, transfers the 4′-phosphopantetheine portion of CoA to a specific serine residue of the ACP, forming a phosphoester bond and releasing the 3′-phospho-AMP moiety of CoA as a byproduct (Fig. 26-3). Note that, as in CoA, the reactive sulfhydryl group of ACP is at the end of the long chain derived

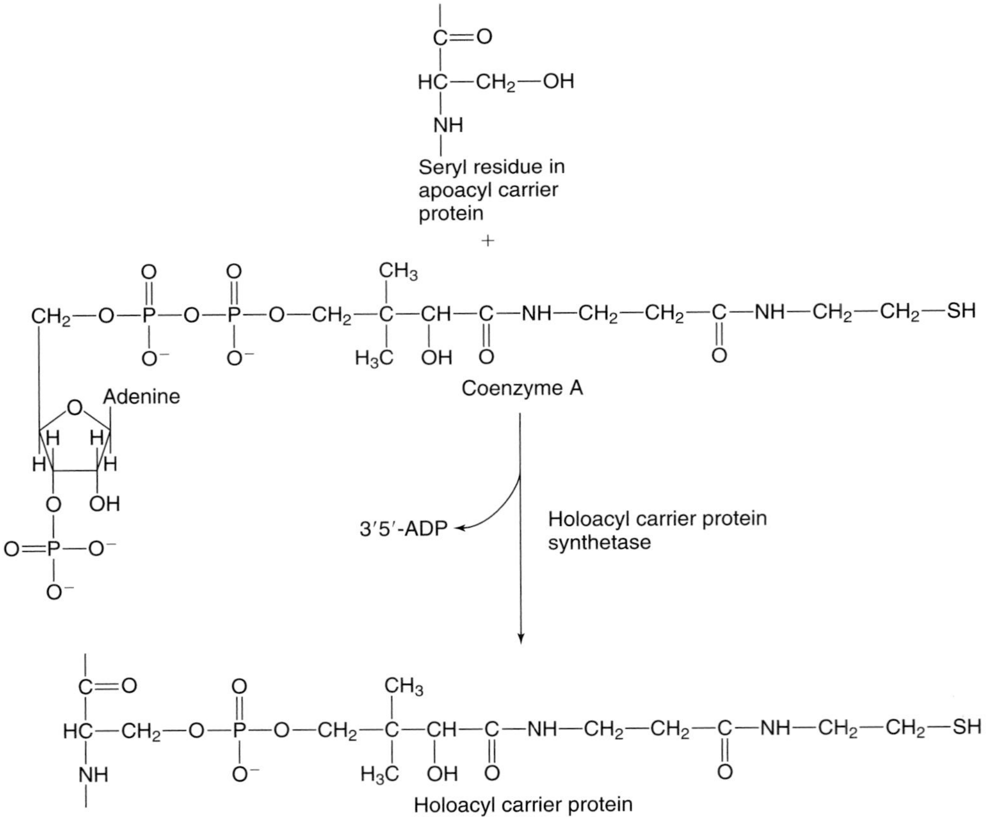

Figure 26-3 Acyl carrier protein (ACP) synthesis. CoA is cleaved to form 3′, 5′-ADP with attachment of 4′-phosphopantetheine, as a phosphate ester, to the hydroxyl group of a serine residue in apoACP to form holoACP, a component of fatty acid synthase.

from β-alanine and cysteine. There is an ACP hydrolase that releases 4′-phosphopantetheine from the holo-ACP domain to reform the apo-ACP domain. Interestingly, the combined action of the ACP hydrolase and synthetase results in the rapid turnover of the 4′-phosphopantetheine of ACP with a half-life measured in hours compared to the half-life of the fatty acid synthase, which is measured in days in rat tissues (Tweto et al., 1971).

COENZYME A AND 4′-PHOSPHOPANTETHEINE DEGRADATION

The intermediates in the degradation of CoA are similar to those formed in its synthesis except that the cysteine moiety is now a cysteamine moiety. Coenzyme A degradation is catalyzed by different enzymes than is its synthesis, but relatively little is known about CoA degradation. CoA does not appear to be degraded in the mitochondria. The 3′-phosphate group of CoA can be removed by nonspecific lysosomal phosphatases to form dephospho-CoA, and dephosphoCoA can be degraded to 4′-phosphopantetheine and AMP by a nucleotide pyrophosphatase located in the plasma membrane fraction. These reactions appear to be nonspecific, however, because of their broad substrate selectivities and their low affinities for CoA (Skrede, 1973). Surprisingly, acyl CoAs also are readily degraded to 4′-phosphopantetheine. Whether 4′-phosphopantetheine is derived from the degradation of CoA or the turnover of ACP, the phosphate is removed by phosphatases to give pantetheine. Pantetheine is then hydrolyzed to pantothenic acid and cysteamine by pantetheinases. The pantothenic acid can be excreted or used for resynthesis of CoA or ACP. Pantothenate kinase will also use pantetheine as a substrate, but it is not known if pantetheine is recycled back into CoA.

PANTETHEINASE–VANIN GENE FAMILY

Studies of thymus colonization by bone marrow precursor cells in mice following irradiation led to the identification of vanin-1, a membrane-anchored protein (Aurrand-Lions et al., 1996). The mouse genes for vanin-1 and vanin-3 were shown to encode different isoforms of the enzyme pantetheinase. Homologous human vanin genes (*VNN1*, *VNN2*, and *VNN3*) have been identified (Martin et al., 2001). Pantotheinase is an amidohydrolase that cleaves pantetheine to pantothenic acid and cysteamine. Interestingly, these Vanin genes are also homologous with the *BTD* gene for biotinidase, which is an amidohydrolase that cleaves biocytin to biotin and lysine, as is described in subsequent text.

The mouse vanin-3 is secreted by cells, and the mouse vanin-1 is a glycosylphosphatidyl inositol-anchored ectoenzyme that is expressed in all tissues but with particularly high levels in kidney (Pitari et al., 2000). vanin-1-deficient (knockout) mice, which develop normally, were shown to have low pantetheinase activity and low levels of cysteamine in liver and kidney compared to wild type mice. Induction of intestinal inflammation was reduced in the vanin-1-deficient mice compared to wild-type mice, but oral administration of cystamine restored the inflammatory response. This unexpected result suggests that one role for cysteamine may be the upregulation of the inflammatory response. The homologous vanins in humans would be expected to have functions similar to those in mice.

ROLES OF COENZYME A AND ACYL CARRIER PROTEIN IN METABOLISM

CoA has many functions in metabolism, including its role in the formation of ACP. Both CoA and ACP are used to form thioesters with carboxylic acid groups of fatty acids and other compounds, as shown in Figure 26-4. Many steps in the metabolism of fatty acids and certain amino acid derivatives, as well as a number of amphibolic steps in metabolism, occur using CoA thioester substrates and producing CoA thioester products.

COENZYME A AND ACYL CARRIER PROTEIN IN FATTY ACID SYNTHESIS

Both CoA and ACP are essential for the synthesis of fatty acids in the cytosol (see Fig. 26-1; see also Chapter 16). Acetyl CoA, the substrate for fatty acid synthesis in the cytosol, is generated in the mitochondria from the oxidative

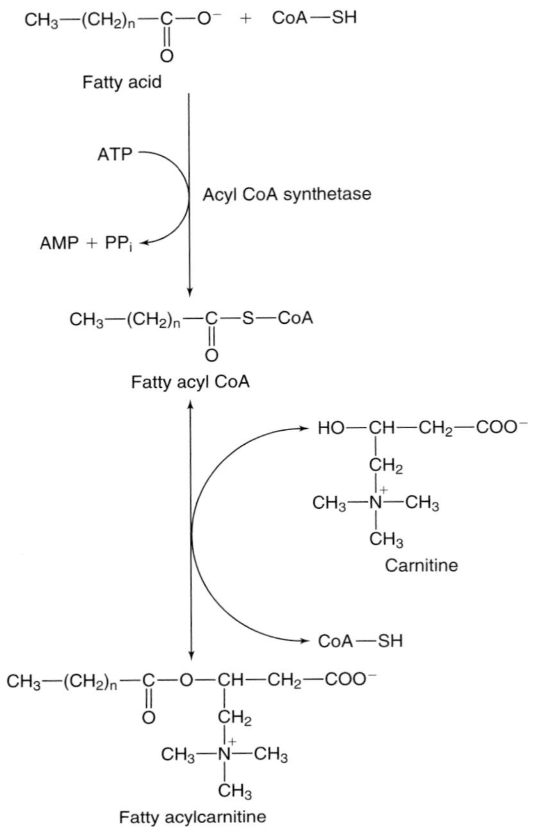

$CH_3—(CH_2)_n—C(=O)—O^- + CoA—SH$

Fatty acid

ATP → AMP + PP_i (Acyl CoA synthetase)

$CH_3—(CH_2)_n—C(=O)—S—CoA$

Fatty acyl CoA

$HO—CH(CH_2—N^+(CH_3)_3)—CH_2—COO^-$

Carnitine

CoA—SH

$CH_3—(CH_2)_n—C(=O)—O—CH(CH_2—N^+(CH_3)_3)—CH_2—COO^-$

Fatty acylcarnitine

Figure 26-4 Formation of fatty acyl CoA thioester and exchange with carnitine. Fatty acids are converted by acyl CoA synthetases in the cytosol to acyl CoA thioesters in reactions coupled with the hydrolysis of ATP. The acyl CoA thioesters are in equilibrium with acylcarnitine esters; the transesterification is catalyzed by carnitine acyl CoA transferases.

decarboxylation of pyruvate by pyruvate dehydrogenase. Pyruvate itself is generated from cytosolic metabolism of glucose or gluconeogenic substrates and then is transported into the mitochondria. Because the acetyl CoA generated in the mitochondria cannot cross the mitochondrial membrane, the carbon for fatty acid synthesis leaves the mitochondria in the form of citrate, which is formed by condensation of acetyl CoA with oxaloacetate. Citrate is transported to the cytosol, where it is cleaved by citrate lyase (in an ATP- and CoA-requiring reaction) to regenerate oxaloacetate and acetyl CoA; the cytosolic acetyl CoA then serves as substrate for fatty acid synthesis. Acetyl transacylase transfers the acetyl group from acetyl CoA to the phosphopantetheine sulfhydryl of ACP, releasing free CoA in the process; these two carbons from acetyl CoA form the methyl end of the fatty acid that will be synthesized. A biotin-containing enzyme, acetyl CoA carboxylase, uses bicarbonate and ATP to convert acetyl CoA to malonyl CoA. Fatty acid synthase utilizes this malonyl CoA to sequentially add 2-carbon units to the acetyl- or acyl-ACP, with the liberation of the third carbon of malonyl CoA as CO_2. This process results in the synthesis of even-numbered fatty acids, mainly palmitate. When the synthesis of a fatty acid is complete, a thioesterase hydrolyzes the ACP–fatty acid thioester, releasing the fatty acid and regenerating the ACP sulfhydryl. The rate of fatty acid synthesis is regulated primarily by the concentration of malonyl CoA, which is determined by regulation of the activity of acetyl CoA carboxylase.

COENZYME A IN OXIDATIVE DECARBOXYLATION REACTIONS CATALYZED BY α-KETO ACID DEHYDROGENASE COMPLEXES

A key role for CoA in fuel metabolism is its function in α-keto acid dehydrogenase complexes that catalyze the oxidative decarboxylation of keto acids. In the metabolism of carbohydrates, the end product of the glycolytic pathway for glucose is the simple, 3-carbon α-keto acid pyruvate. In order for pyruvate to be completely oxidized via the citric acid cycle and oxidative phosphorylation, pyruvate is oxidatively decarboxylated to acetyl CoA (with release of CO_2 and reduction of NAD^+) by the pyruvate dehydrogenase complex. This complex reaction involves five coenzymes (four of them derived from vitamins): thiamin pyrophosphate (TPP), NAD^+, FAD^+, lipoate, and CoA (see Chapters 12 and 24, specifically Fig. 12-18). In the decarboxylation of pyruvate, the 2-carbon aldehyde unit is attached to TPP, oxidized, transferred to a lipoyl enzyme, and then transferred to CoA to form acetyl CoA. Acetyl CoA is a central compound in metabolism, having several catabolic as well as anabolic fates. The CoA eventually is released as free CoA as further metabolism of acetyl CoA progresses (see Chapter 12, Figs. 12-17 and 12-19).

Two other enzyme complexes that catalyze the oxidative decarboxylation of keto acids with formation of acyl CoA products include the α-ketoglutarate dehydrogenase complex and the branched-chain α-keto acid dehydrogenase complex. The α-ketoglutarate dehydrogenase complex converts α-ketoglutarate to succinyl CoA. This reaction is part of the citric acid cycle and is required for the oxidation of the carbon chains of several amino acids, including glutamate, proline, arginine, and histidine. The CoA is released from succinyl CoA in the next step of the citric acid cycle. The branched-chain α-keto acid dehydrogenase complex, again in a series of reactions analogous to those of pyruvate dehydrogenase, catalyzes the first committed step in the catabolic pathway for the branched-chain amino acids. The α-keto acids from transamination of valine, isoleucine, and leucine are oxidatively decarboxylated to form branched-chain acyl CoA products with one less carbon in the chain. These are metabolized in a number of different steps as CoA esters and ultimately yield simple acyl CoA products such as acetyl CoA and propionyl CoA, which enter central pathways of metabolism. (See Chapter 14 for details of amino acid metabolism, including the role of coenzyme A.)

COENZYME A IN FATTY ACID β-OXIDATION

CoA plays a major role in the β-oxidation of fatty acids in the mitochondria, which may result in the complete degradation of fatty acids to acetyl CoA, which can be further oxidized in the citric acid cycle (see Fig. 26-1; see Chapter 12, Fig. 12-19). Most of the fatty acids consumed in dietary triacylglycerols or obtained from adipose stores are long-chain fatty acids with 16 or more carbon atoms. These long-chain fatty acids require a carrier system for their transport from the cytosol into the mitochondria. In the cytosol, the free, long-chain fatty acids are activated to CoA thioesters by acyl CoA synthetases that couple ATP hydrolysis with thioester formation. These fatty acyl CoAs are transesterified to carnitine to form "energy-equivalent" acylcarnitines, which are transported across the mitochondrial inner membrane. On the outer mitochondrial membrane, the enzyme carnitine palmitoyltransferase-I (CPT-I) converts the fatty acyl CoA to acyl carnitine and free CoA. A carnitine acylcarnitine–translocase moves the acylcarnitine into the mitochondria and free carnitine out of the mitochondria. Carnitine palmitoyltransferase-II (CPT-II) on the inner mitochondrial membrane regenerates fatty acyl CoA in the mitochondria.

In β-oxidation, 2-carbon segments of the fatty acyl CoA are sequentially removed as acetyl CoA. The series of reactions for each cycle are dehydrogenation to the unsaturated acyl CoA, hydration to 3-hydroxyacyl CoA, dehydrogenation to the 3-ketoacyl CoA, and thiolytic cleavage by CoA to release acetyl CoA and a fatty acyl CoA with two less carbons. There are multiple dehydrogenases with overlapping chain-length specificities that favor acyl CoAs with very long, long, medium, or short chains. Reducing equivalents generated in the various dehydrogenation steps are funneled into the electron transport chain. Most tissues use fatty acids as a fuel. Cardiac muscle is particularly dependent on fatty acid oxidation for energy, and many abnormalities of fatty acid oxidation can cause cardiomyopathy.

The rate of fatty acid oxidation is controlled by the rate of transport of fatty acids into the mitochondria. The rate of transport is controlled largely by the activity of CPT-I, which is strongly inhibited by malonyl CoA. When fatty acid synthesis is increased by activation of acetyl CoA carboxylase to produce more malonyl CoA as substrate for fatty acid synthase, the increased malonyl CoA inhibits CPT-I, decreasing fatty acid transport into the mitochondria and thus preventing the reoxidation of newly synthesized fatty acids (see Chapter 16, Figs. 16-2 and 16-9). When the plasma concentration of free fatty acids is elevated, as in the starved state, acetyl CoA carboxylase is inhibited, decreasing the synthesis of malonyl CoA and, hence, decreasing malonyl CoA inhibition of CPT-I by malonyl CoA so that fatty acids enter the mitochondria for β-oxidation.

COENZYME A IN KETONE BODY SYNTHESIS AND OXIDATION

Ketone bodies are an important source of fuel derived from fat metabolism when glucose is limited, as in starvation (see Fig. 26-1; also see Chapter 16, Figs. 16-14 and 16-15). Acetoacetate and its reduction product, 3-hydroxybutyrate, are called ketone bodies, although 3-hydroxybutyrate, unlike acetoacetate and its spontaneous decarboxylation product (acetone), is not a ketone. Ketone bodies are synthesized in the liver from acetoacetyl CoA and acetyl CoA derived from the β-oxidation of fatty acids (see Fig. 26-1). Acetoacetyl CoA is condensed with acetyl CoA to form 3-hydroxy-3-methylglutaryl CoA and free CoA by mitochondrial 3-hydroxy-3-methylglutaryl CoA (HMG CoA) synthetase. This is then cleaved by HMG CoA lyase to form free acetoacetate and acetyl CoA. The net result of this cycle is the conversion of acetoacetyl CoA to acetoacetate and free CoA, but there is no enzyme that directly catalyzes this hydrolysis. Acetoacetate and 3-hydroxybutyrate are interconverted by NAD(H)-dependent 3-hydroxybutyrate dehydrogenase, but 3-hydroxybutyrate is the major form found in the plasma.

Acetoacetate and 3-hydroxybutyrate are released from the liver into the blood and then are taken up by other tissues that are able to use them as fuels. In the extrahepatic tissues, the acetoacetate is converted to a CoA ester using succinyl CoA as the CoA donor. The acetoacetyl CoA can then be metabolized to acetyl CoA (i.e., the last step of β-oxidation), and the acetyl CoA can be further oxidized by the citric acid cycle and oxidative phosphorylation.

ADDITIONAL ROLES OF COENZYME A IN AMINO ACID AND ORGANIC ACID CATABOLISM

In addition to its major role in fatty acid synthesis and oxidation, in oxidative decarboxylation of α-keto acids, and in the citric acid cycle, CoA also is involved in the mitochondrial metabolism of a large number of other carboxylic acids as CoA thioesters. The catabolism of many amino acids involves the removal of the amino group, leaving a carboxyl group that can be esterified to CoA for further metabolism. As described in the preceding text, the branched-chain α-keto acids derived from valine, isoleucine, and leucine are decarboxylated to form acyl CoA derivatives. These are oxidized to unsaturated acyl CoAs in the same manner as the fatty acid acyl CoAs. 3-Methylcrotonyl CoA derived from leucine is carboxylated by a biotin-containing carboxylase and is eventually converted to HMG CoA, which is cleaved to acetoacetate (a ketone body) and acetyl CoA by the lyase involved in ketone body synthesis. Valine and isoleucine are metabolized via pathways involving acyl CoAs to form propionyl CoA and propionyl CoA plus acetyl CoA, respectively. In addition, the amino acids threonine and methionine also are metabolized via oxidative decarboxylation of α-ketobutyrate to propionyl CoA intermediates. Propionyl CoA is then carboxylated by a biotin-containing enzyme, as will be described later in this chapter, to form methylmalonyl CoA, which is then converted to succinyl CoA. The amino acids lysine, hydroxylysine, and tryptophan are catabolized to α-ketoadipate, which is oxidatively decarboxylated to form glutaryl CoA and ultimately two molecules of acetyl CoA.

OTHER METABOLIC ROLES OF COENZYME A

Acyl CoAs are involved in many synthetic reactions. The CoA ester, HMG CoA, formed in the cytosol, is the starting material for the synthesis of isoprenoids, cholesterol, steroid hormones, and bile acids. Isoprenoids include ubiquinone (which functions as coenzyme Q in the electron transport chain of mitochondria) and dolichol (which is involved in glycoprotein synthesis). Steroids include cholesterol, the steroid hormones derived from cholesterol, and the bile acids derived from cholesterol. Acetyl CoA is a substrate for the acetylation of amino and hydroxyl groups of many compounds (e.g., N-terminal amino acid residues of some proteins, sugar residues in glycosaminoglycans, and glycoproteins). Another role for CoA is the detoxification of drugs and other exogenous compounds. A well-known example is the conversion of benzoate to hippurate, which is excreted in the urine. Benzoyl CoA is synthesized in an ATP-requiring reaction, and the benzoyl group is then transferred to the amino group of glycine to form hippurate (benzoylglycine). Aspirin similarly is metabolized via a CoA ester to form the acylglycine salicylurate for excretion.

COENZYME A AND CARNITINE INTERRELATIONS

(See Chapter 16, Figs. 16-2 and 16-9.) The esters of CoA and carnitine have very similar energy contents. They are maintained in equilibrium by carnitine acyl CoA transferases. The carnitine palmitoyl CoA transferases and their role in transporting long-chain fatty acids into mitochondria for β-oxidation have already been described in this chapter and also in Chapter 16. In addition, carnitine acetyl CoA transferase catalyzes the interconversion of a number of short-chain carnitine esters and CoA thioesters. Additional transferases are involved in the interconversion of acylcarnitines and acyl CoAs of medium-chain fatty acids. Free carnitine and carnitine esters act as a buffer to maintain free CoA and acyl CoA levels. If acyl CoAs accumulate, as occurs in inherited disorders of fatty acid oxidation or inborn errors of metabolism of some organic acids, free CoA could be depleted below the levels needed for its essential roles in metabolism. The conversion of some acyl CoAs to acylcarnitines frees up CoA and maintains a more normal ratio of free to esterified CoA. In addition, acyl CoAs are inhibitors of a number of enzymes, and decreasing their concentration by converting them to acylcarnitines reduces this inhibition. The acylcarnitines also can be translocated out of the mitochondria, enter the blood circulation, and be excreted by the kidneys as a means of removing accumulated esters of CoA that may be toxic. A side effect of this is that, in inherited disorders in which acylcarnitines are excreted in large amounts, carnitine itself may become depleted in tissues, which, in turn, decreases the transport of fatty acids into the mitochondria (see Chapters 12 and 24).

PANTOTHENATE KINASE DEFICIENCY

An inherited disorder, pantothenate kinase–associated neurodegeneration (PKAN), formerly called Hallervorden-Spatz syndrome, has been shown to be caused by mutations in a pantothenate kinase gene, *PANK2* (Zhou et al., 2001). This is an autosomal recessive neurodegenerative disorder with iron accumulation in the basal ganglia of the brain and retinal degeneration, which manifests in childhood with a progressive course leading to early death. There are four different *PANK* genes in humans, with different expressions in different tissues.

Clinical Correlation

Carnitine Treatment of Fatty Acid Oxidation Disorders

A secondary deficiency of carnitine can occur in patients with inherited deficiencies of dehydrogenases involved in the β-oxidation of fatty acids (Roe and Coates, 1995). An example is medium-chain acyl CoA dehydrogenase (MCAD) deficiency, in which the oxidation of the medium-chain length octanoyl CoA is decreased. MCAD deficiency is a relatively common inherited disorder with a frequency as high as 1 in 10,000 in populations of Irish, English, or German descent. With a deficiency of MCAD, octanoyl CoA accumulates and is converted to octanoylcarnitine, resulting in increased plasma levels of octanoylcarnitine and increased excretion of octanoylcarnitine in the urine. Over a period of time, this increased loss of carnitine from the body as octanoylcarnitine in the urine can result in abnormally low levels of free carnitine in plasma and tissues. Administration of oral carnitine, usually 100 mg/kg body weight daily in four divided doses, raises the blood carnitine levels to normal and leads to increased excretion of octanoylcarnitine. This may help to dispose of the toxic accumulations of octanoate.

PANK1 is highly expressed in heart, liver, and kidney; *PANK3* is highly expressed in liver; *PANK4* is highly expressed in muscle; and *PANK2* is expressed in most tissues, including basal ganglia. A mutation in *PANK2* that resulted in low activity of pantothenate kinase in those tissues where it is the major expressed form of pantothenate kinase, would be expected to affect CoA levels because this enzyme is rate-limiting for the synthesis of CoA. In a study of patients with PKAN, all patients with the classic syndrome showing early onset with rapid progression had mutations in *PANK2*, most often resulting in protein truncation (Hayflick et al., 2003). Only about a third of patients with atypical disease (often with prominent speech-related and psychiatric symptoms) had *PANK2* mutations, and these mutations generally resulted in only an amino acid substitution. Some of these patients with residual activity of pantothenate kinase might benefit from treatment with large doses of pantothenic acid. PANK2 is the only pantothenate kinase that has an N-terminal mitochondrial targeting sequence, and it is found mainly in the mitochondria with a small cytosolic pool (Johnson et al., 2004). Localization is dependent on use of alternative translational start sites. Interestingly, there is a common variant that gives cytosolic localization of PANK2 due to mutation of the translational start site for synthesis of PANK2 with a mitochondrial targeting sequence; about 5% of the population are heterozygous for this variant and have cytosolic localization of PANK2. The mitochondrial localization of PANK2 as well as its relatively abundant expression in brain may help explain the role of PANK2 in susceptibility to neurodegenerative disorders. Knockout mice with PANK2 deficiency show retinal degeneration, and the homozygous males are infertile due to azoospermia (Kuo et al., 2005).

DIETARY SOURCES, RECOMMENDED INTAKES, AND DEFICIENCY SYMPTOMS

Pantothenic acid is widely distributed in plant and animal sources, existing both free and as ACP and CoA. Total pantothenic acid in foods is determined by hydrolysis of the bound and coenzyme forms to free pantothenic acid and quantitation of the released pantothenic acid by microbiological growth assays, radioimmunoassay, or, more recently, stable isotope dilution mass spectrometric assays. There is considerable loss of pantothenic acid in highly processed food. The average dietary intake of pantothenic acid in the composite Canadian diet is about 5 to 6 mg/day, with somewhat lower intake in the elderly and young children (Hoppner et al., 1978). A study of mixed total diet composites for young adults in the United States found a mean daily pantothenic acid intake of 5.9 mg with a standard deviation of 0.5 mg (Iyengar et al., 2000). From studies of dietary intake and urinary excretion, it is estimated that only about 50% of dietary pantothenic acid is available for absorption. Pantothenic acid is included in most multivitamin supplements, generally in the amount of 10 mg.

Food Sources

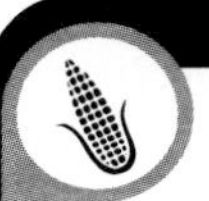

Food Sources of Pantothenic Acid

Fish and Poultry

0.7 to 1 mg per 3 oz fish
0.7 to 1 mg per 3 oz turkey or chicken
0.7 mg per large egg

Milk and Yogurt

1 to 1.5 mg per 8 oz container
0.9 mg per 1 cup milk

Legumes and Seeds

0.6 mg per ½ cup lentils or split peas, cooked
0.4 mg per ½ cup limas
2 mg per ¼ cup sunflower seed kernels

Other Vegetables

2.6 mg per ½ cup shitake mushrooms
0.5 to 1.7 mg per ½ cup mushrooms
0.7 per ½ cup sweet corn
0.5 to 0.6 mg per ½ cup peas or broccoli
0.4 per ½ cup potatoes

Data from US Department of Agriculture/Agricultural Research Service (USDA/ARS) (2005) USDA National Nutrient Standard Database, Release 18. USDA/ARS, Washington, DC. Retrieved December 23, 2005, from http://www.ars.usda.gov/ba/bhnrc/ndl.

The Institute of Medicine (IOM) did not establish estimated average requirements (EARs) or recommended dietary allowances (RDAs) for pantothenic acid because of lack of sufficient data. Adequate intakes (AIs) for pantothenic acid were set based primarily on amounts needed to replace urinary excretion with an assumed bioavailability of 50% (IOM, 1998). Urinary excretion for adults consuming typical American diets is approximately 2.6 mg/day, and the AI for adults is 5 mg/day. The AIs for children and adolescents were extrapolated from the adult value and are also consistent with the limited data for urinary excretion of pantothenic acid. AIs were set at 6 and 7 mg/day for pregnant and lactating women, respectively, to cover the increased physiological needs. The AI for infants during the first 6 months of life was based on the pantothenic acid intake of breast-fed infants (2.2 mg/L × 0.78 L/day) and is 1.7 mg/day; the AI for 7- to 12-month-old infants is 1.8 mg/day of pantothenic acid. No tolerable upper intake level (UL) was set for pantothenic acid because no reports of adverse effects of pantothenic acid in humans or animals were found.

AIs Across the Life Cycle

	mg Pantothenic Acid per Day
Infants	
0 to 0.5 yr	1.7
0.5 to 1 yr	1.8
Children	
1 to 3 yr	2
4 to 8 yr	3
9 to 13 yr	4
14 to 18 yr	5
Males	
≥ 19 yr	5
Females	
≥ 19 yr	5
Pregnant	6
Lactating	7

Data from Institute of Medicine (IOM) (1998) Dietary Reference Intakes for Thiamin, Riboflavin, Niacin, Vitamin B_6, Folate, Vitamin B_{12}, Pantothenic Acid, Biotin, and Choline. National Academy Press, Washington DC. *AI*, Adequate intake.

Because of the wide distribution of pantothenic acid in foods, no spontaneous deficiency has been reported. Pantothenic acid deficiency has been induced in a small number of human volunteers via a pantothenic acid–free diet. There were no clinical symptoms at 9 weeks, even though urinary excretion of pantothenic acid had decreased by 75%, but the volunteers appeared listless and complained of fatigue (Fry et al., 1976). Other volunteers fed a diet deficient in pantothenic acid together with an antagonist (ω-methylpantothenic acid) to block pantothenic acid utilization developed headaches, fatigue, and a sensation of weakness (Hodges et al., 1958; Bean and Hodges, 1954). Additional symptoms included personality changes, sleep disturbances, impaired motor coordination, and gastrointestinal disturbances. All symptoms were reversed by stopping the antagonist and giving pantothenic acid.

PANTOTHENIC ACID DIETARY SUPPLEMENTATION

There are broad health claims for supplementation with very large amounts of pantothenic acid of 500 to 1,000 mg, which is hundreds of times the AI level of 5 mg per day for adults. There are no reports of toxicity of pantothenic acid in humans at these or higher doses, although minor gastrointestinal effects can occur. The health claims for clinical benefits include increased energy and athletic ability, a cure for acne, decreased symptoms of arthritis, increased immunity, prevention of hair loss and graying, anti-aging, activation of the adrenal glands, synthesis of the neurotransmitter acetylcholine, lowering cholesterol and triglyceride levels, and improved wound healing. The claims are often based on a single or a few old studies with a small number of subjects. Well-controlled double-blind studies with a larger number of subjects have rarely been done to validate most of the claims. The effect of supplementation with very high levels of derivatives of pantothenic acid and thiamin on physiology and performance of trained cyclists was compared to placebo in a randomized double-blind study (Webster, 1998). There was no difference in any of the physiological parameters or in time trial performance.

BIOTIN

Biotin was discovered in 1927 as a factor that prevented dermatitis, hair loss, and neurologic abnormalities caused by feeding a diet high in raw egg whites to rats (Boas, 1927). The protein avidin in raw egg whites binds biotin with a very high affinity and prevents the intestinal absorption of biotin, causing a deficiency of biotin that leads to the clinical symptoms. Biotin is covalently attached as a coenzyme to form several holoenzymes that function as carboxylases. Three of the four enzymes that contain biotin are carboxylases that act on CoA ester substrates in fatty acid metabolism and amino acid catabolism, as shown in Figure 26-1. The fourth enzyme carboxylates pyruvate.

BIOTIN SYNTHESIS

Biotin contains two, 5-membered rings made from an ureido group attached to a tetrahydrothiophene ring. A side chain (valeric acid) of five carbons ending with a carboxyl group is attached to the tetrahydrothiophene ring (Fig. 26-5). Biotin is synthesized by bacteria, yeast, algae, and plants from the CoA thioester of pimelate, a 7-carbon dicarboxylic acid (which ends up forming the 5-carbon side chain plus 2 carbons of the ring structure). The subsequent reactions involve addition of decarboxylated alanine, transamination of the resulting keto compound to introduce another amino group, ATP-dependent addition of CO_2 to form the ureido group and, thus, desthiobiotin. The final step involves the insertion of sulfur to form the tetrahydrothiophene ring and, hence, biotin (Marquet et al., 2001). The natural isomer has the D-(+) configuration. Because biotin functions as a cofactor covalently bound to proteins called carboxylases, the biotin in the cell and in food sources may be attached in an amide bond to the ε-amino group of a lysine residue in enzyme proteins.

BIOTIN ABSORPTION, TRANSPORT, EXCRETION, AND DEGRADATION

In the digestion of dietary proteins and peptides that contain covalently bound biotin, the proteolytic enzymes and peptidases do not cleave

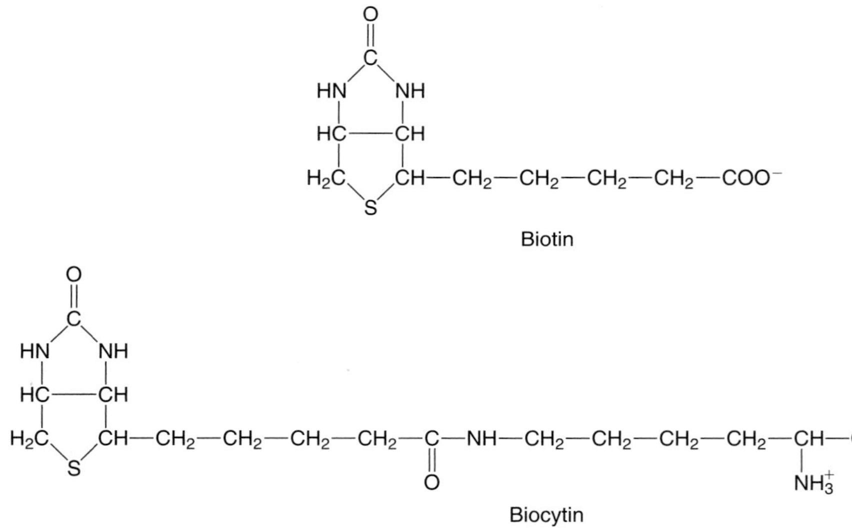

Biotin

Biocytin

Figure 26-5 Biotin and biocytin structures. Biotin has a 5-carbon valeric acid side chain attached to a five-membered ring containing a ureido group and a second ring of tetrahydrothiophene. The ureido group is involved in the reactions of carboxylases and is the portion of the molecule to which the protein avidin binds. In biocytin (*N*-biotinyl-L-lysine), the carboxyl group of biotin is linked by an amide bond to the ε-amino group of lysine. Biocytin is derived from the proteolytic degradation of biotin-containing carboxylase enzymes.

the biotinyl-lysine amide bond. Upon digestion, the lysine and small lysine-containing peptides with covalently attached biotin are released. The released lysine with biotin covalently attached is called biocytin (see Fig. 26-5). Biocytin and biotinyl-lysyl peptides are hydrolyzed, with release of free biotin and lysine or lysine-containing peptides, by a specific hydrolase called biotinidase, which is present in the pancreatic digestive secretions.

Free biotin from the diet or that produced by digestion of proteins plus the action of biotinidase is transported across the intestine by the Na^+-dependent multivitamin transporter that also transports pantothenic acid and lipoic acid (Prasad et al., 1999). Biocytin is not actively transported and, although it can be absorbed from the intestine by passive diffusion, its uptake is much slower than the active transport of biotin (Said et al., 1993).

In the blood, 80% of biotin is free in the plasma, with the rest bound reversibly or covalently to plasma proteins (Mock and Malik, 1992). Biotin enters cells by the multivitamin Na^+-dependent transporter (Prasad and Ganapathy, 2000). Biotin is actively transported across the blood-brain barrier, with cerebrospinal fluid concentrations being about 2.5 times plasma concentrations (Lo et al., 1991). In the kidney, biotin is reabsorbed by a carrier-mediated, Na^+-dependent transport system; the renal clearance is about 40% of that of creatinine.

Most early studies of biotin excretion assumed that the assays for biotin, either the microbiological growth assays or avidin-binding assays, were specific for biotin. Using chromatographic separations followed by avidin-binding assays, it was shown that a number of biotin degradation products are excreted and that biotin accounts for about 43% of the total excretion (Mock et al., 1993). The major metabolic degradation product (about 30% of the avidin-binding material) is bisnorbiotin (the biotin ring structure with a 3-carbon side chain) formed by shortening, via β-oxidation, of the 5-carbon valerate side chain by two carbons. The other degradation product (about 11% of the total) is biotin sulfoxide, in which the thiophene ring sulfur has been oxidized to a sulfoxide. Similarly, biotin was found to account for only about half of the avidin-binding material in serum (Mock et al., 1995). Small amounts of three additional metabolites of biotin, biotin sulfone, bisnorbiotin methylketone, and tetranorbiotin sulfoxide, were identified in urine (Zempleni et al., 1997).

HOLOCARBOXYLASE SYNTHETASE

The only known function of biotin in humans and other mammals is as a prosthetic group in four carboxylases. These enzymes are synthesized as enzymatically inactive apocarboxylase proteins that become active holocarboxylases after the covalent attachment of biotin. Holocarboxylase synthetase attaches the biotin to the apocarboxylases in two sequential reactions (Fig. 26-6). First, biotin is activated with ATP to form biotinyladenylate. This then reacts with the ε-amino group of a specific lysine residue, which is flanked by methionine residues, in the active site of the apocarboxylases to form an amide bond between the carboxyl of the biotin side chain and the ε-amino group of the lysine residue (i.e., the linkage present in biotinyl-lysine or biocytin); the AMP moiety of the biotinyladenylate is released. Note that the side chain of biotin coupled to the side chain of lysine puts the reactive ring portion of biotin at the end of a long, flexible chain in the holocarboxylase proteins.

Holocarboxylase synthetase is present in both the cytosol and the mitochondria. Acetyl CoA carboxylase is a cytosolic enzyme, and the apocarboxylase is biotinylated in the cytosol. The other three carboxylases are present in the mitochondria. It is not known whether their apoenzymes normally are biotinylated by cytosolic holocarboxylase synthetase and then transported into the mitochondria as holoenzymes, or whether the carboxylases are transported into the mitochondria as apoenzymes and then biotinylated to form the holocarboxylases. In experimental biotin deficiency in rats or cultured human fibroblasts, the apocarboxylases do accumulate in the mitochondria, and these mitochondrial apocarboxylases are converted rapidly to holocarboxylases when biotin is added to the diet or culture media, demonstrating that biotinylation can occur in the mitochondria.

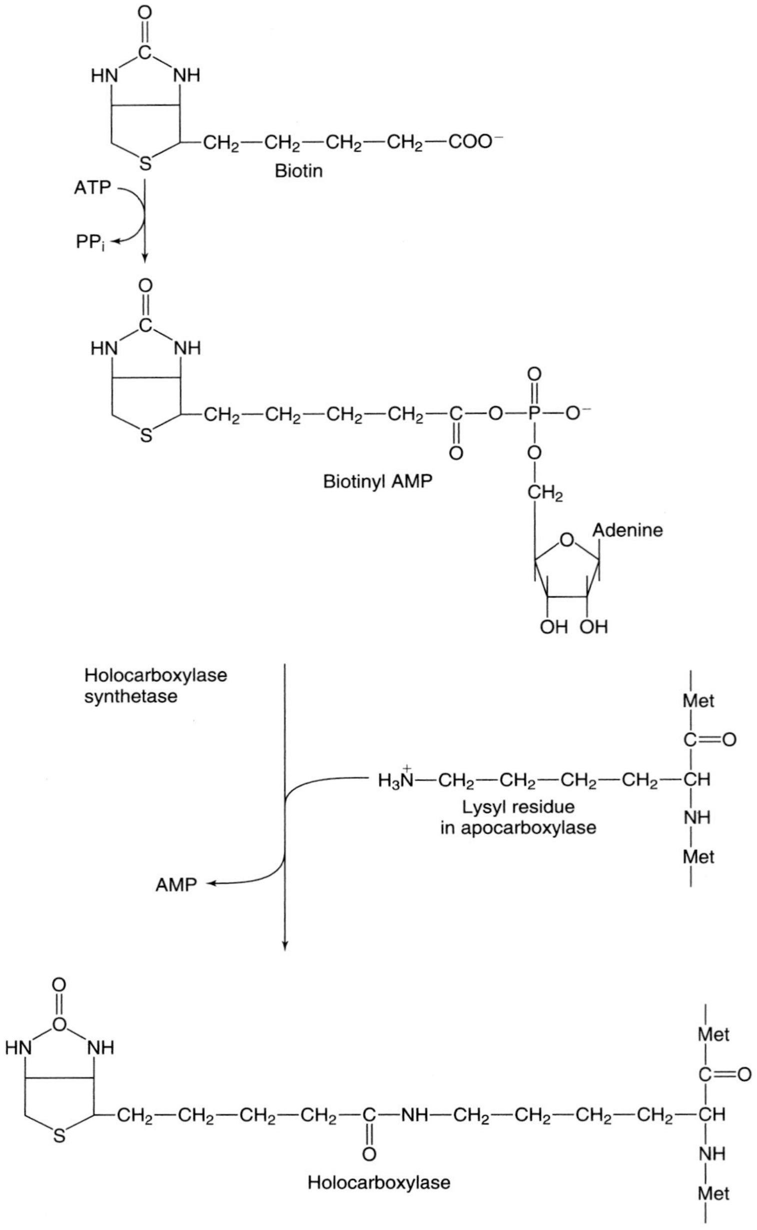

Figure 26-6 Holocarboxylase synthetase reaction. The formation of holocarboxylase involves two sequential reactions that are catalyzed by holocarboxylase synthetase: formation of biotinyl-AMP from biotin and ATP, followed by formation of an amide bond of biotin with a specific lysine residue in an apocarboxylase to form a holocarboxylase with release of AMP.

BIOTIN-CONTAINING CARBOXYLASES

The role of biotin in the carboxylases is to serve as a CO_2 carrier and carboxyl donor to substrates. There are four unique biotin-containing carboxylases in mammalian tissues, which are summarized in Figure 26-7. These carboxylases are acetyl CoA carboxylase, pyruvate carboxylase, propionyl CoA carboxylase, and 3-methylcrotonyl CoA carboxylase.

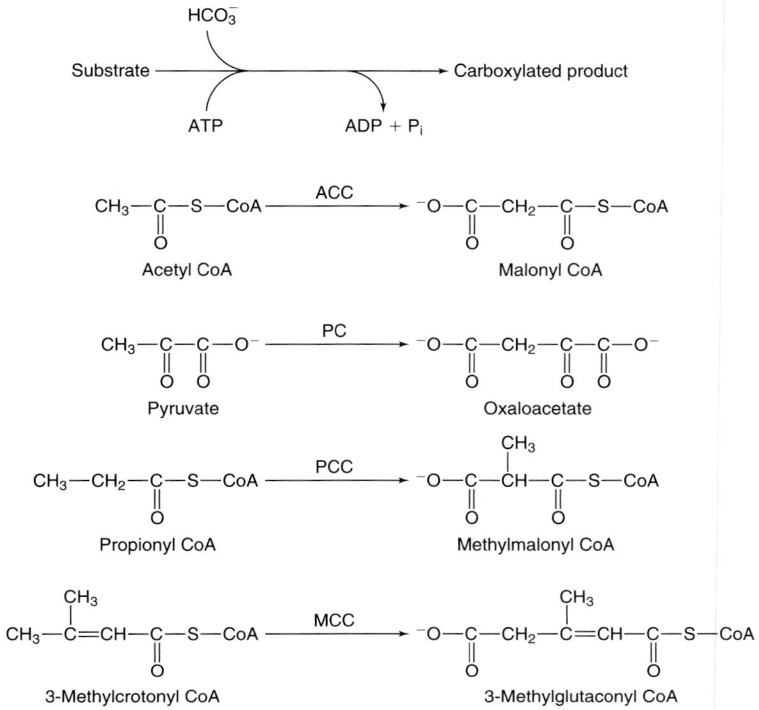

Substrate + HCO_3^- + ATP → Carboxylated product + ADP + P_i

$CH_3-C(=O)-S-CoA$ —ACC→ $^-O-C(=O)-CH_2-C(=O)-S-CoA$

Acetyl CoA → Malonyl CoA

$CH_3-C(=O)-C(=O)-O^-$ —PC→ $^-O-C(=O)-CH_2-C(=O)-C(=O)-O^-$

Pyruvate → Oxaloacetate

$CH_3-CH_2-C(=O)-S-CoA$ —PCC→ $^-O-C(=O)-CH(CH_3)-C(=O)-S-CoA$

Propionyl CoA → Methylmalonyl CoA

$CH_3-C(CH_3)=CH-C(=O)-S-CoA$ —MCC→ $^-O-C(=O)-CH_2-C(CH_3)=CH-C(=O)-S-CoA$

3-Methylcrotonyl CoA → 3-Methylglutaconyl CoA

Figure 26-7 Carboxylase substrates and products. The substrates and products of the four mammalian biotin-containing carboxylases are shown. Bicarbonate becomes a carboxyl group of the products, and the reaction is driven by energy released from the coupled hydrolysis of ATP. *ACC,* Acetyl CoA carboxylase; *MCC,* 3-methylcrotonyl CoA carboxylase; *PC,* pyruvate carboxylase; *PCC,* propionyl CoA carboxylase.

CARBOXYLASE MECHANISM

The carboxylases use energy from the hydrolysis of ATP to dehydrate HCO_3^- (bicarbonate) to CO_2 (carbon dioxide), forming ADP and carboxyphosphate. As shown in Figure 26-8, the carboxyphosphate then carboxylates the N-1 of biotin, with release of phosphate, to form N-1 carboxybiotinyl-enzyme, which then acts as the CO_2 carrier and donor. These two steps allow HCO_3^-, which is present at a higher concentration in the cell fluid than is CO_2, to be used for formation of bound CO_2, which is more chemically reactive than HCO_3^- in the nucleophilic attack of the substrate in carboxylation reactions (Knowles, 1989).

In carboxylation reactions, the carboxyl group of carboxy-biotinyl-enzyme is transferred via abstraction of a proton from an enolizable carbon of the acceptor to form a nucleophile that attacks the CO_2, resulting in the carboxylated product (see Fig. 26-8). The reaction also involves the metal ions magnesium and potassium. In the carboxylases, the active site for carboxylation of biotin (using HCO_3^- and ATP) and the active site for the transfer of the carboxyl group to the substrate are adjacent. The side chain of biotin provides the necessary flexibility to allow the biotinyl coenzyme to be carboxylated in one site and used as a CO_2 donor at a second site.

The substrates for all four mammalian carboxylases are monocarboxylic acids, and the products are dicarboxylic acids. Pyruvate, the substrate for pyruvate carboxylase, has an α-keto group that is easily enolized to activate the 3-carbon of pyruvate for participation in the carboxylation reaction to form oxaloacetate (which could also be called 3-carboxypyruvate). 3-Methylcrotonyl CoA, derived from leucine catabolism, is the substrate for 3-methylcrotonyl CoA carboxylase. It has an α,β-double bond conjugated with the thioester bond of

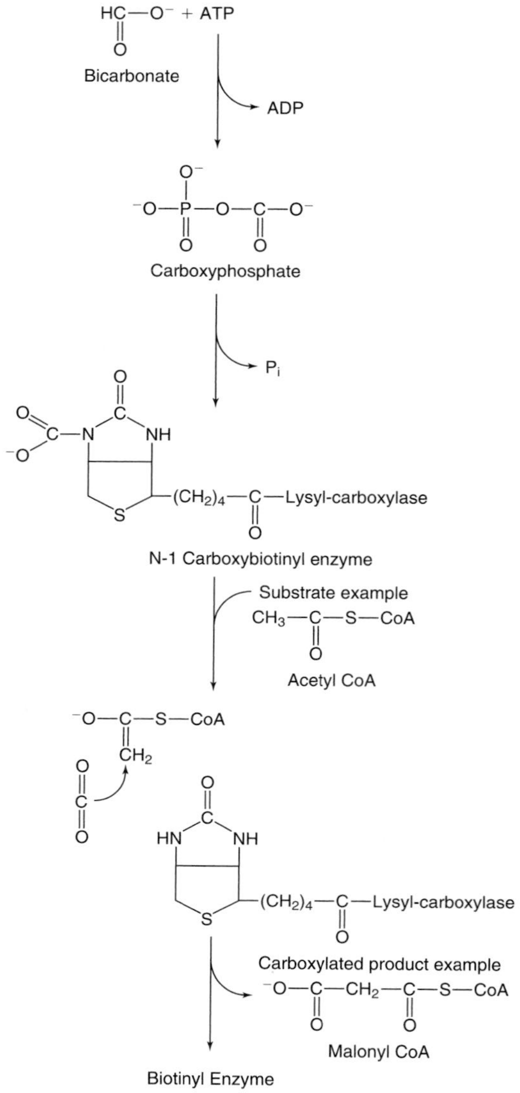

Bicarbonate

ADP

Carboxyphosphate

P_i

N-1 Carboxybiotinyl enzyme

Substrate example

Acetyl CoA

Carboxylated product example

Malonyl CoA

Biotinyl Enzyme

Figure 26-8 Mechanism of carboxylation by biotinyl enzymes. With energy provided by the hydrolysis of ATP, bicarbonate is attached to biotin to form N-1 carboxybiotin. The carboxyl group is then transferred to an enolizable carbon in the substrate to form the carboxylated product. The carboxylation of acetyl CoA to malonyl CoA is shown as an example.

CoA, making it reactive for carboxylation at the C-4 position to form the product 3-methylglutaconyl CoA. The other two acids that are substrates for carboxylases do not have an easily enolizable carbon, but the 2-carbon of these short-chain fatty acids is made more reactive by employing their CoA thioester derivatives. Therefore, acetyl CoA is carboxylated at the 2-carbon by acetyl CoA carboxylase to form malonyl CoA, and propionyl CoA is carboxylated at the 2-carbon by propionyl CoA carboxylase to form methylmalonyl CoA.

No inherited genetic deficiency of acetyl CoA carboxylase has been documented, probably reflecting the very essential role of this enzyme in fatty acid synthesis such that its absence would be incompatible with life. In contrast, cases of rare, inherited genetic deficiencies of each of the three mitochondrial carboxylases are known, and studies of the perturbed biochemistry in these patients has contributed to our knowledge of the important roles of biotin-containing carboxylases in normal metabolism. Patients with any one of these isolated carboxylase deficiencies do not respond biochemically or clinically to treatment with large doses of biotin because their defects are in the apocarboxylase protein rather than in the holocarboxylase synthetase that attaches biotin to the carboxylases. Even if a patient had a defect in an apocarboxylase at the site of attachment for biotin, higher concentrations of biotin would not be expected to increase the ability of normal holocarboxylase synthetase to covalently attach biotin to the apocarboxylase.

ACETYL CoA CARBOXYLASE

The role of acetyl CoA carboxylase in catalyzing the formation of malonyl CoA, which is the rate-limiting step for synthesis of fatty acids, has been described. The reaction catalyzed is shown in Figure 26-7. This cytosolic enzyme exists as a very large polymer with a molecular mass in the millions of daltons when it is active, and the enzyme is inactivated by dissociation into its protomer units. Citrate activates acetyl CoA carboxylase by increasing polymerization. CoA itself activates acetyl CoA carboxylase by lowering the K_m for acetyl CoA. The enzyme is inhibited by the products of fatty acid synthesis, the long-chain acyl CoAs, which act to depolymerize the enzyme. In addition, acetyl CoA carboxylase activity is regulated by covalent modification (phosphorylation) in response to the hormones insulin and glucagon. A high insulin-to-glucagon ratio favors dephosphorylation of the enzyme to an active form, whereas a low insulin-to-glucagon ratio favors phosphorylation to the inactive form. The amount of acetyl CoA carboxylase protein also is affected by dietary and hormonal changes. Therefore, the regulation of acetyl CoA carboxylase activity is complex, as might be expected for an enzyme that catalyzes the rate-limiting step of fatty acid synthesis and the production of a compound (malonyl CoA) that regulates fatty acid oxidation by controlling the transport of fatty acids into the mitochondria.

PYRUVATE CARBOXYLASE

Pyruvate carboxylase is a mitochondrial enzyme that catalyzes the synthesis of the citric acid cycle intermediate, oxaloacetate, from pyruvate, as shown in Figure 26-7. In all tissues, pyruvate carboxylase has an important anaplerotic role in maintaining the levels of oxaloacetate and other intermediates of central pathways of fuel metabolism, including the citric acid cycle. Anaplerosis refers to the replenishment of intermediates in a metabolic cycle that may be depleted by removal from the cycle. Carboxylation of pyruvate to oxaloacetate is an essential step in the utilization of precursors such as pyruvate, lactate, and many amino acids for gluconeogenesis. (See Chapters 12 and 14 for more details of these pathways.) Pyruvate carboxylase undergoes allosteric activation by its substrate pyruvate and also by the allosteric activator acetyl CoA, which is a product of pyruvate dehydrogenase and of fatty acid oxidation and an indicator of fuel availability in the mitochondria. In addition, the amount of pyruvate carboxylase protein in liver is increased in diabetes and in hyperthyroidism.

A genetic deficiency of pyruvate carboxylase results in accumulation of pyruvate. Pyruvate is reduced to lactate, resulting in elevated levels of lactate in blood. Pyruvate is also transaminated, resulting in an elevated concentration of alanine in the blood. In the more severe B form of pyruvate carboxylase deficiency, symptoms occur shortly after birth with severe lactic acidemia and elevated blood ammonia concentrations; death usually occurs before 3 months of age. In the A form of pyruvate carboxylase deficiency, patients present in the first few months of life with mild or moderate lactic acidemia and psychomotor retardation. Most children die within the first few years, and the survivors have severe mental retardation. Interestingly, the A form of pyruvate carboxylase deficiency occurs predominantly in Native Americans from the Algonkian linguistic group.

PROPIONYL CoA CARBOXYLASE

Propionyl CoA carboxylase catalyzes the carboxylation of propionyl CoA to methylmalonyl CoA in the mitochondria, as shown in Figure 26-7. The methylmalonyl CoA is isomerized by a vitamin B_{12} coenzyme-containing mutase to succinyl CoA, and succinyl CoA then can be metabolized by the citric acid cycle enzymes. Sources of propionyl CoA include the propionyl CoA formed from catabolism of the amino acids valine, isoleucine, threonine, and methionine; the propionyl CoA formed in the final step in the β-oxidation of odd-numbered or branched-chain fatty acids; the propionyl CoA released as a byproduct of bile acid synthesis from cholesterol; and a significant amount of propionate produced by the intestinal microflora. The sequential reactions of propionyl CoA carboxylase and methylmalonyl CoA mutase provide a path for the conversion of these propionate precursors to succinyl CoA and, hence, to oxaloacetate, a central intermediate in glucose and amino acid metabolism. Propionyl CoA carboxylase is not rate-limiting in the metabolism of propionyl CoA, the enzyme activity is not subject to regulation by effector molecules, and the levels of propionyl CoA carboxylase protein are not altered by dietary or hormonal changes.

Propionic acidemia is caused by an inherited deficiency of propionyl CoA carboxylase. Patients have repeated, life-threatening episodes of severe ketosis and metabolic acidosis, often beginning in the neonatal period. Symptoms include vomiting, dehydration, and lethargy, progressing to coma and death if not treated. Frequent neurological complications include developmental delay, seizures, cerebral atrophy, and electroencephalographic (EEG) abnormalities. The elevated concentrations of propionyl CoA result in formation of elevated levels of metabolites of propionate that are diagnostically characteristic of propionic acidemia.

These include methylcitrate, which is continuously elevated in urine, and 3-hydroxypropionate, propionylglycine, and a variety of other metabolites that are elevated during severe metabolic decompensation. A severe secondary elevation of blood ammonia also occurs during episodes. Propionyl CoA is in equilibrium with propionylcarnitine, which is excreted in the urine; loss of propionylcarnitine can lead to a secondary deficiency of carnitine. Therefore, treatment includes giving carnitine to prevent a carnitine deficiency and to promote the conversion of propionyl CoA to propionylcarnitine, which restores CoA concentrations and facilitates excretion of the nonmetabolizable propionate.

The most important treatment for propionic acidemia is the restriction of dietary protein in order to limit the amino acid precursors of propionate along with the use of special formulas that have very low levels of isoleucine, valine, methionine, and threonine, which are the amino acid precursors of propionate. The required intake of these essential amino acids is met by the addition of natural proteins with careful calculation of the intake of each amino acid. Clinical management requires continuous careful nutritional assessment because the amino acids that are restricted in these diets are essential amino acids that must be given in amounts sufficient for protein synthesis and normal growth.

3-METHYLCROTONYL CoA CARBOXYLASE

3-Methylcrotonyl CoA carboxylase has a single function, which is catalysis of a step in the catabolic pathway for leucine. It catalyzes the carboxylation of 3-methylcrotonyl CoA to 3-methylglutaconyl CoA, as shown in Figure 26-7. 3-Methylglutaconyl CoA subsequently is hydrated to 3-hydroxy-3-methylglutaryl CoA, which is cleaved to acetoacetate and acetyl CoA by the same lyase involved in ketone body metabolism. 3-Methylcrotonyl CoA carboxylase is not regulated by small molecules or by dietary or hormonal factors.

The inherited deficiency of 3-methylcrotonyl CoA carboxylase usually presents with episodes of vomiting, severe metabolic acidosis, extremely low plasma glucose concentrations, and very low levels of carnitine in plasma. The elevated 3-methylcrotonyl CoA is metabolized to relatively nontoxic metabolites, with the major one being 3-hydroxyisovalerate. The abnormal metabolites, 3-methylcrotonylglycine and 3-hydroxyisovalerylcarnitine, also are excreted. Treatment with carnitine to correct and prevent carnitine deficiency plus moderate restriction of protein in the diet to limit leucine intake generally result in normal development. A few relatives of affected patients have been found to have the same enzyme deficiency but no clinical symptoms. Newborn screening for inherited metabolic disorders by tandem mass spectrometry of acylcarnitines in dried blood spots has identified a much higher incidence of asymptomatic 3-methylcrotonyl-CoA carboxylase deficiency than expected from the number of patients ascertained by clinical symptoms, suggesting most patients may have a benign clinical course. Interestingly, newborn screening has detected babies with elevated 3-hydroxyisovalerylcarnitine levels who do not have the enzyme deficiency, but whose asymptomatic mothers are enzyme deficient (Koeberl et al., 2003).

HOLOCARBOXYLASE SYNTHETASE DEFICIENCY

The inherited deficiency of holocarboxylase synthetase activity results in decreased activities of all four of the biotin-containing carboxylases: acetyl CoA, pyruvate, propionyl CoA, and 3-methylcrotonyl-CoA carboxylases. The occurrence of multiple carboxylase deficiencies due to a genetic error in coding for one protein, the holocarboxylase, is strong evidence for the role of a single holocarboxylase in the formation of all four holocarboxylases. Multiple carboxylase deficiency results in clinical symptoms related to the roles of all four carboxylases in metabolism. Symptoms usually occur shortly after birth in patients with a more severe enzyme deficiency and include severe ketoacidosis, seizures, lethargy, and coma. Death can occur if these symptoms are not treated. Some patients, who have a milder form of holocarboxylase deficiency and who usually present at several months of age, also show symptoms of hair loss (alopecia) and an erythematous skin rash, which are typical symptoms of biotin deficiency in experimental animals. Elevated urinary excretion of the metabolites characteristic of each of the individual deficiencies are seen collectively in the urine of individuals with multiple carboxylase deficiency. The most elevated metabolite is 3-hydroxyisovalerate from deficiency of 3-methylcrotonyl CoA carboxylase. Also elevated are methylcitrate due to propionyl CoA carboxylase deficiency and lactate from the deficiency of pyruvate carboxylase. Treatment with large oral doses of biotin, ranging from 10 to 60 mg/day, usually gives dramatic normalization of the biochemical abnormalities, clearing of any skin rash, and regrowth of hair. Biotin treatment also results in neurological improvement, provided irreversible neurological damage had not occurred during an acute episode. Many patients who were diagnosed during their first episode and subsequently maintained on pharmacological doses of biotin are clinically well, although some continue to excrete moderately elevated amounts of abnormal metabolites. Because of the biotin-responsiveness, dietary protein restriction generally is unnecessary.

The structure of the human holocarboxylase synthetase gene has been determined and a variety of mutations identified (Dupuis et al., 1999; Sakamoto et al., 1999). When the kinetic properties of the mutant holocarboxylase synthetase in fibroblasts from patients were determined, the K_m for biotin generally was found to be highly elevated. In addition, the enzyme activity usually was significantly greater than zero, approaching normal levels for some patients, when activity was assayed at high concentrations of biotin. The mechanism by which treatment with pharmacological doses of biotin is believed to operate is the elevation of tissue levels of biotin far above normal and into the range of the K_m of the mutant holocarboxylase synthetase. Therefore, even with levels of holocarboxylase synthetase activity that are considerably lower than normal, elevated levels of biotin can result in adequate conversion of apocarboxylases to active holocarboxylases, effectively correcting the multiple carboxylase deficiencies. A complete absence of holocarboxylase synthetase activity, which would mean no activity of any of the four carboxylases, would probably be incompatible with life.

Holocarboxylase synthetase deficiency has been diagnosed prenatally and treated in utero by giving pregnant women 10 mg of biotin per day. The newborns had no biochemical abnormalities and no clinical symptoms and remained healthy on biotin therapy of 20 mg per day (Thuy et al., 1999; Suormala et al., 1998).

BIOTINIDASE DEFICIENCY

Another inherited disorder of biotin metabolism is the deficiency of biotinidase, the enzyme required to release biotin from biocytin or biotinyl-lysine–containing peptides derived from the proteolytic digestion of holocarboxylases in the normal turnover of the carboxylases and in the digestion of foods. Biotinidase is present in most cells, in plasma, and in pancreatic secretions. Patients generally do not present with symptoms for some time after birth, because sufficient biotin had been available in utero from the mother for full biotinylation of their carboxylases. The concentration of biotin in the cord blood of normal babies is higher than in the maternal blood, and normal newborns have higher plasma biotin levels than do older children. The plasma biotin concentration decreases after the second week of life, even though the biotin content of breast milk usually is increasing at this time. Biotinidase-deficient patients develop a clinically observable deficiency of biotin after weeks, months, or even years of life. Because of the failure to cleave biocytin, they develop symptoms of seizures, hypotonia, ataxia, developmental delay, hearing loss, optic atrophy, skin rash, and hair loss. The variable age of onset of symptoms probably is related to the relative amounts of available free biotin in the diet compared to the unusable protein-bound biotin (biocytin) and also to the amount of residual biotinidase activity found in a particular patient. The excretion of abnormal metabolite is similar to that of patients with holocarboxylase synthetase (multiple carboxylase) deficiency, but the concentrations of these metabolites in the urine generally are less elevated.

The effect of treatment of biotinidase deficiency with pharmacological doses of biotin

(10 mg per day) is dramatic, with prompt correction of the metabolic acidosis and disappearance of abnormal metabolites, followed by clearing of the skin rash and regrowth of hair. There may be a catch up in development, but the hearing loss and optic atrophy are not reversible. The rapid response to treatment results from the fact that biotinidase deficiency basically results in a deficiency of biotin. As soon as biotin is administered, the already synthesized inactive apocarboxylases are converted rapidly to active holocarboxylases, leading to normalization of metabolism. Although the usual treatment is with large doses of biotin, typically 10 mg/day, a more moderate intake of free biotin would probably be sufficient once the tissue levels of biotin have been raised to normal. However, there appears to be increased renal loss of biotin in biotinidase deficiency, as well as increased excretion of biocytin and biotinyl-peptides, so several hundred micrograms of biotin per day may be required.

Because of the wide variability of the symptoms among patients, biotinidase deficiency can be difficult to diagnose clinically. The incidence of biotinidase deficiency of 1 in 112,000 newborns is relatively high for an inborn error of metabolism, and treatment with biotin is very effective and inexpensive. Therefore, inexpensive screening tests have been developed to determine biotinidase deficiency in newborn screening programs using the same filter papers with dried blood spots that are used for screening for phenylketonuria (PKU) and other inherited disorders. In the United States, however, relatively few states perform routine newborn screening for biotinidase deficiency. Administration of the vitamin biotin to patients who are identified by newborn screening as deficient in biotinidase prevents all clinical symptoms.

DIETARY SOURCES, RECOMMENDED INTAKES, AND DEFICIENCY SYMPTOMS

Biotin is widely distributed in foods, existing both as free biotin and as biotin covalently bound to lysine residues in biotinyl-proteins. Total biotin generally has been determined by microbiological growth assays or avidin-binding assays after hydrolysis of bound forms to free biotin. There is very little information about the relative amounts of free biotin, biocytin, and protein-bound biotin in foods. Because biotin contents have been determined for relatively few foods, biotin is ordinarily not included in food composition tables. Liver, egg yolks, baker's yeast, and wheat bran are rich sources.

The daily intake of biotin in Canadian diets was calculated to be 60 μg per day (Hoppner et al., 1978). A similar analysis of biotin in mixed total diet composites in the United States found a somewhat lower mean intake of 35 μg (±7 μg SD) per day (Iyengar et al., 2000). Biotin also is produced by intestinal flora, but this appears to be relatively unavailable for absorption because the urinary excretion of biotin approximates that of the dietary intake, whereas fecal excretion is much higher. Multivitamin preparations generally contain 20 to 40 μg of biotin.

Because of insufficient information about biotin requirements, the IOM (1998) set only AIs for biotin. The AI for infants in the first 6 months of life was based on mean intake of breast-fed infants (6 μg/L × 0.78 L/day) and is 5 μg/day. The AIs for older infants (6 μg/day), children (8 to 12 μg/day), adolescents (25 μg/day), and adults (30 μg/day) were all extrapolated from the values for young infants, although this approach would be expected to overestimate the requirement for adults. No increment was added to the adult AI for pregnant women, but the AI for lactating women was increased to 35 μg/day to cover the amount of biotin secreted in the milk. The IOM did not establish a UL for biotin; no adverse effects of biotin in humans or animals have been reported. Use of up to 200 mg orally or up to 20 mg intravenously on a daily basis for treatment of patients with biotin-responsive inborn errors of metabolism has not produced any signs of toxicity.

Because of the wide distribution of biotin in foods, a dietary deficiency is very rare. However, with an abnormal diet low in biotin and high in raw egg whites, a deficiency with clinical symptoms of hair loss, dermatitis, and neurologic symptoms can occur. Raw egg whites contain the protein avidin, which binds biotin with a very high affinity, preventing its uptake from the intestine. A diet high in avidin has been given to human volunteers for 11 weeks to induce biotin deficiency (Sydenstricker et al., 1942). All subjects developed dermatosis, muscle pains, localized loss of sensation, anorexia, nausea, and weight loss. All symptoms were reversed rapidly by treatment with biotin.

Biochemical abnormalities and clinical symptoms of biotin deficiency can occur even when plasma biotin levels are in the normal range. A better indicator of biotin deficiency appears to be the elevation of 3-hydroxyisovalerate in urine, which is a measure of the low activity of 3-methylcrotonyl CoA carboxylase caused by abnormally low levels of intracellular biotin. A study of indicators of biotin deficiency involved 10 volunteers given a diet high in raw egg whites for 20 days (Mock et al., 1997). The mean urinary excretion of 3-hydroxyisovalerate was significantly elevated by 3 days and greater than normal for all subjects by 14 days, continuing to increase until 20 days when the study ended. Mean urinary

AIs Across the Life Cycle

	μg Biotin per Day
Infants	
0 to 0.5 yr	5
0.5 to 1 yr	6
Children	
1 to 3 yr	8
4 to 8 yr	12
9 to 13 yr	20
14 to 18 yr	25
Males	
≥19 yr	30
Females	
≥19 yr	30
Pregnant	30
Lactating	35

Data from Institute of Medicine (IOM) (1998) Dietary Reference Intakes for Thiamin, Riboflavin, Niacin, Vitamin B_6, Folate, Vitamin B_{12}, Pantothenic Acid, Biotin, and Choline. National Academy Press, Washington DC. *AI*, Adequate intake.

Clinical Correlation

Total Parenteral Nutrition and Biotin Deficiency

In the 1980s, a number of infants with intestinal malabsorption problems who received total parenteral nutrition (TPN) for extended periods developed clinical signs of biotin deficiency, including hypotonia, developmental delay, hair loss, and skin rash (Mock et al., 1985). The skin rash resembled that caused by zinc deficiency, and zinc deficiency was the initial diagnosis for these patients. Although plasma zinc was low in several patients, supplementation with zinc did not correct the rash. A deficiency of essential fatty acids also can cause a similar skin rash, but the patients were receiving adequate fatty acids in the parenteral feedings. When investigated biochemically, the patients were found to have abnormal excretions of urinary organic acids characteristic of biotin deficiency or of the inherited disorders of biotin metabolism, holocarboxylase synthetase and biotinidase deficiencies. Urinary excretion of biotin was below normal, but several patients had normal levels of biotin in plasma. Treatment with biotin dramatically corrected the clinical and biochemical symptoms, confirming that the patients were deficient in biotin. This disorder resulted from not including biotin among the vitamins given with the long-term TPN. These findings indicating biotin deficiency in infants and other patients on long-term TPN have led to the inclusion of biotin in the current vitamin therapy for long-term TPN.

Thinking Critically

1. Would you expect the amount of 3-hydroxyisovalerate to be normal or elevated in urine of patients receiving long-term TPN that lacked biotin? Would the amount change with biotin treatment?
2. What would be the expected clinical and biochemical response to treatment of biotin deficiency due to TPN with either large pharmacological amounts or smaller, normal intake amounts of biotin?

excretion of biotin was significantly decreased by 3 days. In contrast, the mean level of biotin in the plasma did not decrease significantly, even after 20 days on the diet.

Marginal biotin deficiency produced by feeding various amounts of raw egg whites to mice was found to be teratogenic, causing cleft palate, micrognathia, microglossia, and skeletal hypoplasia in a dose-dependent manner (Mock et al., 2003). A marginal biotin deficiency has been found in women during normal pregnancies, but it is not known whether this has consequences regarding congenital malformations (Mock et al., 2002).

More information about indicators of biotin deficiency has resulted from the chronic use of anticonvulsants. Patients with epilepsy who received long-term therapy with the anticonvulsants phenytoin, primidone, phenobarbital, or carbamazepine, either alone or in combinations, had reduced plasma biotin levels and excreted elevated amounts of 3-hydroxyisovalerate and other organic acids characteristic of biotin deficiency in their urine (Koeberl et al., 1984). Patients who received sodium valproate did not have these abnormalities. The mechanism by which the anticonvulsants affect biotin status is unclear.

Severe protein-energy malnutrition can result in marasmus or kwashiorkor. Many patients with severe malnutrition have clinical symptoms similar to those of biotin deficiency: dermatitis, alopecia, hypotonia, ataxia, and developmental delay. In studies of children with marasmus or kwashiorkor, Velazquez et al. (1989) found significantly lower levels of biotin in plasma, even though the urinary biotin concentration expressed relative to creatinine was elevated. Assays of the carboxylases in lymphocytes obtained from these patients showed they had partial deficiencies of propionyl CoA carboxylase and pyruvate carboxylase and a more severe deficiency of 3-methylcrotonyl CoA carboxylase, indicating biotin deficiency. Supplementation with biotin increased the carboxylase levels (Velazquez et al., 1995). It was concluded that decreased activities of the carboxylases in lymphocytes was a better indicator of biotin deficiency in malnutrition than were plasma levels of biotin. The biotin deficiency in malnutrition could result from a dietary deficiency of biotin, impaired intestinal absorption, or increased renal losses of biotin. In patients recovering from severe malnutrition, the biotin and carboxylase levels returned to normal.

BIOTIN AND GENE REGULATION

Holocarboxylase synthetase is required for the biotin-stimulated increase of the level of its own mRNA, the mRNA for acetyl CoA carboxylase, and the mRNA for the α-subunit of propionyl CoA carboxylase (Solorzano-Vargas et al., 2002). Fibroblasts from patients with holocarboxylase synthetase deficiency were unable to increase holocarboxylase synthetase mRNA in response to biotin unless the vitamin concentration was increased 100-fold. Addition of the cGMP analog, 8-Br-cGMP, restored holocarboxylase synthetase and carboxylase mRNA levels in the deficient fibroblasts. The mechanism for biotin-mediated regulation of the expression of holocarboxylase synthetase and biotin-dependent carboxylase genes appears to be via a signaling cascade that includes holocarboxylase synthetase-dependent production of biotinyl-AMP, guanylate cyclase, and cGMP-dependent protein kinase.

In addition to its role as a cofactor for carboxylase enzyme activity, it has been proposed that biotin may play a role in regulation of cell proliferation and gene expression via biotinylation of histones. Holocarboxylase synthetase, which synthesizes the activated form of biotin, biotinyl-AMP, for attachment of biotin to apocarboxylases, is largely localized in the nucleus and is associated with chromatin and the nuclear lamina (Narang et al., 2004). This nuclear holocarboxylase synthetase can biotinylate histones. Fibroblasts from patients with a genetic deficiency of holocarboxylase synthetase show very low biotinylation of histones as well as low activity of the carboxylases. Biotin can be removed from histones by biotinidase, the enzyme that hydrolyzes biocytin to biotin and lysine, and debiotinylation of histones is decreased in samples from biotinidase-deficient patients (Ballard et al., 2002). Additional studies are required to determine if biotinylation of histones has a regulatory function.

REFERENCES

Aurrand-Lions M, Galland F, Bazin H, Zakharyev V (1996) Vanin-1, a novel GPI-linked perivascular molecule involved in thymus homing. Immunity 5:391-405.

Ballard TD, Wolff J, Griffin JB, Stanley JS, van Calcar S, Zempleni J (2002) Biotinidase catalyzes debiotinylation of histones. Eur J Nutr 41:78-84.

Bean WB, Hodges RE (1954) Pantothenic acid deficiency induced in human subjects. Proc Soc Exp Biol Med 86:693-698.

Begley TP, Kinsland C, Strauss E (2001) The biosynthesis of coenzyme A in bacteria. Vitam Horm 61:157-171.

Boas MA (1927) The effect of desiccation upon the nutritive properties of egg white. Biochem J 21:712-724.

Daugherty M, Polanuyer B, Farrell M, Scholle M, Lykidis A, de Crecy-Lagard V, Osterman A (2002) J Biol Chem 277: 21431-21439.

Dupuis L, Campeau E, Leclerc D, Gravel RA (1999) Mechanism of biotin responsiveness in biotin-responsive multiple carboxylase deficiency. Mol Genet Metab 66:80-90.

Fenstermacher DK, Rose RC (1986) Absorption of pantothenic acid in rat and chick intestine. Am J Physiol 250:G155-G160.

Fisher MN, Robishaw JD, Neely JR (1985) The properties and regulation of pantothenate kinase from rat heart. J Biol Chem 260:15745-15751.

Fry PC, Fox HM, Tao HG (1976) Metabolic response to a pantothenic acid deficient diet in humans. J Nutr Sci Vitaminol 22:339-346.

Hayflick SJ, Westaway SK, Levinson B, Zhou B, Johnson MA, Ching KHL, Gitschier J (2003) Genetic, clinical and radiographic delineation of Hallervorden-Spatz syndrome. N Engl J Med 348:33-40.

Hodges RE, Ohlson MA, Bean WB (1958) Pantothenic acid deficiency in man. J Clin Invest 37:1642-657.

Hoppner K, Lampi B, Smith DC (1978) An appraisal of the daily intakes of vitamin B_{12}, pantothenic acid and biotin from a composite Canadian diet. Can Inst Food Sci Technol J 11:71-74.

Institute of Medicine (1998) Dietary Reference Intakes for Thiamin, Riboflavin, Niacin, Vitamin B_6, Folate, Vitamin B_{12}, Pantothenic Acid, Biotin, and Choline. National Academy Press, Washington, DC.

Iyengar GV, Wolf WR, Tanner JT, Morris ER (2000) Content of minor and trace elements, and organic nutrients in representative mixed total diet composites from the USA. Sci Total Environ 256:215-226.

Johnson MA, Kuo YM, Westeway SK, Parker SM, Ching KHL, Gitschier J, Hayflick SJ (2004) Mitochondrial localization of human PANK2 and hypotheses of secondary iron accumulation in pantothenate kinase-associated neurodegeneration. Ann N Y Acad Sci 1012:282-298.

Joshi AK, Zhang L, Rangan VS, Smith S (2003) Cloning, expression, and characterization of human 4′-phosphopantetheinyl transferase with broad substrate specificity. J Biol Chem 278:33142-33149.

Kishnani PS, McDonald MT, Chaing S, Boney A, Moore E, Frazier DM (2003) Evaluation of 3-methylcrotonyl-CoA carboxylase deficiency detected by tandem mass spectrometry newborn screening. J Inherit Metab Dis 26:25-35.

Knowles JR (1989) The mechanism of biotin-dependent enzymes. Annu Rev Biochem 58:195-221.

Koeberl DD, Millington DS, Smith WE, Weavil SD, Muenzer J, McCandless SE, Krause KH, Kochen W, Berlit P, Bonjour JP (1984) Excretion of organic acids associated with biotin deficiency in chronic anticonvulsant therapy. Int J Vitam Nutr Res 54:217-222.

Kuo YM, Duncan JL, Westaway SK, Yang H, Nune G, Yujun Xu E, Hayflick SJ, Gitschier J (2005) Deficiency of pantothenate kinase 2 (Pank2) in mice leads to retinal degeneration and azoospermia. Hum Mol Gen 14:49-57.

Lo W, Kadlecek T, Packman S (1991) Biotin transport in the rat central nervous system. J Nutr Sci Vitaminol 37:567-572.

Marquet A, Bui BTS, Florentin D (2001) Biosynthesis of biotin and lipoic acid. Vitam Horm 61:51-101.

Martin F, Malergue F, Pitari G, Phillipe JM, Phillips S, Chabret C, Graqnjeaud S, Mattei MG, Mungall AJ, Naquet P, Galland F (2001) Vanin genes are clustered (human 6q22-24 and mouse 10A2B1) and encode isoforms of pantetheinase ectoenzymes. Immunogenetics 53:296-306.

Martin F, Penet MF, Malergue F, Lepidi H, Desein A, Galland F, de Reggi M, Naquet P, Gharib B (2004) Vanin-1(–/–) mice show decreased NSAID- and Schistosoma-induced intestinal inflammation associated with higher glutathione stores. J Clin Invest 113:591-597.

Mock DM, Baswell DL, Baker H, Holman RT, Sweetman L (1985) Biotin deficiency complicating parenteral alimentation: diagnosis, metabolic repercussions, and treatment. J Pediatr 106:762-769.

Mock DM, Lankford GL, Mock NI (1995) Biotin accounts for only half of the total avidin-binding substances in human serum. J Nutr 125:941-946.

Mock DM, Lankford GL Cazin J Jr. (1993) Biotin and biotin analogs in human urine: Biotin accounts for only half of the total. J Nutr 123:1844-1851.

Mock DM, Malik M (1992) Distribution of biotin in human plasma: Most of the biotin is not bound to protein. Am J Clin Nutr 56:427-432.

Mock NI, Malik MI, Stumbo PJ, Bishop WP, Mock DM, (1997) Increased urinary excretion of 3-hydroxyisovaleric acid and decreased urinary excretion of biotin are sensitive early indicators of decreased biotin status in experimental biotin deficiency. Am J Clin Nutr 65:951-958.

Mock DM, Mock NI, Stewart CW, LaBorde JB, Hansen DK (2003) Marginal biotin deficiency is teratogenic in ICR mice. J Nutr 133: 2519-2525.

Mock DM, Quirk JG, Mock NI (2002) Marginal biotin deficiency during normal pregnancy. Am J Clin Nutr 75:295-299.

Narang MA, Dumas R, Ayer LM, Gravel RA (2004) Reduced histone biotinylation in multiple carboxylase deficiency patients; a nuclear role for holocarboxylase synthetase. Hum Mol Genetics 13:15-23.

Pitari G, Malergue F, Martin F, Phillipe JM, Massucci MT, Chabret C, Maras B, Dupre S, Naquet P, Galland F (2000) Pantetheinase activity of membrane-bound Vanin-1: lack of free cysteamine in tissues of vanin-1 deficient mice. FEBS Lett 483:149-154.

Prasad PD, Ganapathy V (2000) Structure and function of mammalian sodium-dependent multivitamin transporter. Curr Opin Clin Nutr Metab Care 3:263-266.

Prasad PD, Wang H, Huang W, Fei YJ, Leibach FH, Devoe LD, Ganapathy V (1999) Molecular and functional characterization of the intestinal Na^+-dependent multivitamin transporter. Arch Biochem Biophys 366:95-106.

Rock CO, Calder RB, Karim MA, Jackowski S (2000) Pantothenate kinase regulation of intracellular concentration of coenzyme A. J Biol Chem 275:1377-1383.

Roe CR, Coates PM (1995) Mitochondrial fatty acid oxidation disorders. In: Scriver CR, Beaudet AL, Sly WS, Valle D (eds) The Metabolic and Molecular Bases of Inherited Disease, 7th ed., Vol. I, McGraw-Hill, New York, pp 1501-1533.

Said HM, Thuy LP, Sweetman L, Schatzman B (1993) Transport of the biotin derivative biocytin (N-biotinyl-L-lysine) in rat small intestine. Gastroenterology 104:75-80.

Sakamoto O, Suzuki Y, Li X, Aoki Y, Hiratsuka M, Suormala T, Baumgartner ER, Gibson KM, Narisawa K (1999) Relationship between kinetic properties of mutant enzyme and biochemical and clinical responsiveness to biotin in holocarboxylase synthetase deficiency. Pediatr Res 46:671-676.

Shibata K, Gross CJ, Henderson LM (1983) Hydrolysis and absorption of pantothenate and its coenzymes in the rat small intestine. J Nutr 113:2207-2215.

Skrede S (1973) The degradation of CoA: subcellular localization and kinetic properties of CoA- and dephospho-CoA pyrophosphatase. Eur J Biochem 38:401-407.

Smith S, Witkowski A, Joshi AK (2003) Structural and functional organization of the animal fatty acid synthase. Prog Lipid Res 42:289-317.

Solorzano-Vargas RS, Pacheco-Alvarez D, Leon-Del-Rio A (2002) Holocarboxylase synthetase is an obligate participant in biotin-mediated regulation of its own expression and of biotin-dependent carboxylase mRNA levels in human cells. PNAS 99:5325-5330.

Suormala T, Fowler B, Jakobs C, Duran M, Lehnert W, Raab K, Wick H, Baumgartner ER (1998) Late-onset holocarboxylase synthetase-deficiency: pre- and post-natal diagnosis and evaluation of effectiveness of antenatal biotin therapy. Eur J Pediatr 157:570-575.

Sydenstricker VP, Singal SA, Briggs AP, DeVaughn NM, Isbell H (1942) Observations on the "egg white injury" in man. JAMA 118:1199-1200.

Tahiliani AG (1989) Dependence of mitochondrial coenzyme A uptake and the membrane electrical gradient. J Biol Chem 264:18426-18432.

Tahiliani AG, Beinlich CJ (1991) Pantothenic acid in health and disease. Vitam Horm 46:165-228.

Thuy LP, Jurecki E, Nemzer L, Nyhan WL (1999) Prenatal diagnosis of holocarboxylase synthetase deficiency by assay of the enzyme in chorionic villus material followed by prenatal treatment. Clin Chim Acta 284:59-68.

Tweto J, Liberati M, Larrabee AR (1971) Protein turnover and 4-phosphopantetheine exchange in rat liver fatty acid synthetase. J Biol Chem 246:2468-2471.

Velazquez A, Martin-del-Campo C, Baez A, Zamudio S, Quiterio M, Aguilar JL, Perez-Ortiz B, Sanchez-Ardines M, Guzman-Hernandez J,

Casanueva E (1989) Biotin deficiency in protein-energy malnutrition. Eur J Clin Nutr 43:169-173.

Velazquez A, Teran M, Baez A, Gutierrez, J, Rodriguez R (1995) Biotin supplementation affects lymphocyte carboxylases and plasma biotin in severe protein-energy malnutrition. Am J Clin Nutr 61:385-391.

Webster MJ (1998) Physiological and performance responses to supplementation with thiamine and panthothenic acid derivatives. Eur J Appl Physiol 77:486-491.

Zempleni J, McCormick DB, Mock DM (1997) Identification of biotin sulfone, bisnorbiotin methyl ketone and tetranorbiotin-1-sulfoxide in human urine. Am J Clin Nutr 65:508-511.

Zhou B, Westaway SK, Levinson B, Johnson MA, Gitschier J, Hayflick SJ (2001) A novel pantothenate kinase gene (PANK2) is defective in Hallervorden-Spatz syndrome. Nat Genet 28:345-349.

Zhyvoloup A, Nemazanyy I, Panasyuk G, Valovka T, Fenton T, Rebholz H, Wang ML, Foxon R, Lyzogubov V, Usenko V, Kyyamova R, Gorbenko O, Matsuka G, Filonenko V, Gout IT (2003) Subcellular localization and regulation of coenzyme A synthase. J Biol Chem 278:50316-50321.

RECOMMENDED READINGS

Leonardi R, Zhang YM, Rock CO, Jackowski S (2005) Coenzyme A; back in action. Prog Lipid Res 44:125-153.

Mock DM (1996) Biotin. In: Ziegler EE, Filer JLJ (eds) Present Knowledge in Nutrition, 7th ed. International Life Sciences Institutes—Nutrition Foundation, Washington, DC, pp 220-235.

Wolf B (2001) Disorders of biotin metabolism. In: Scriver CR, Beaudet AL, Sly WS, Valle D (eds) The Metabolic and Molecular Bases of Inherited Disease, 8th ed. Vol. III. McGraw-Hill, New York, pp 3935-3962.

Chapter 27

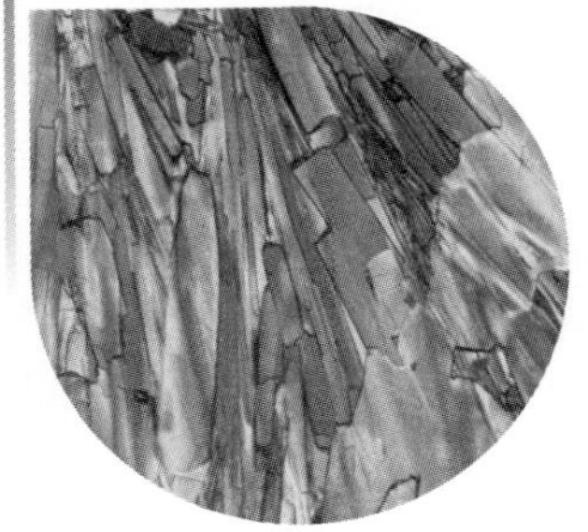

Vitamin C

Mark Levine, MD, Sebastian J. Padayatty, MD, FFARCS, MRCP, PhD, Yaohui Wang, MD, Christopher P. Corpe, PhD, Je-hyuk Lee, PhD, Jin Wang, PhD, Qi Chen, PhD, and Liqun Zhang, MD, PhD

OUTLINE

COMMON ABBREVIATION

SVCT sodium-dependent vitamin C transporter

NOMENCLATURE, STRUCTURE, FORMATION, CHEMICAL CHARACTERISTICS, AND DEGRADATION

Ascorbic acid (ascorbate, vitamin C) is a 6-carbon lactone synthesized from glucose by many animals (Fig. 27-1). Most mammals synthesize ascorbate in liver, and synthesis occurs in kidney in reptiles and some birds (Chatterjee, 1973). However, several species are unable to synthesize ascorbate, including humans, nonhuman primates, guinea pigs, Indian fruit bats, bulbuls, capybara, and some fish. Humans and primates lack gulonolactone oxidase, the terminal enzyme in the biosynthetic pathway. The DNA encoding the enzyme in these species has undergone substantial mutation so that no protein is produced (Nishikimi et al., 1994). Animals unable to synthesize ascorbate must ingest it to survive, and hence ascorbic acid is a vitamin.

Ascorbic acid is an electron donor (reducing agent) (Fig. 27-2), and its known biochemical and molecular functions are accounted for by this function. Two electrons from the double

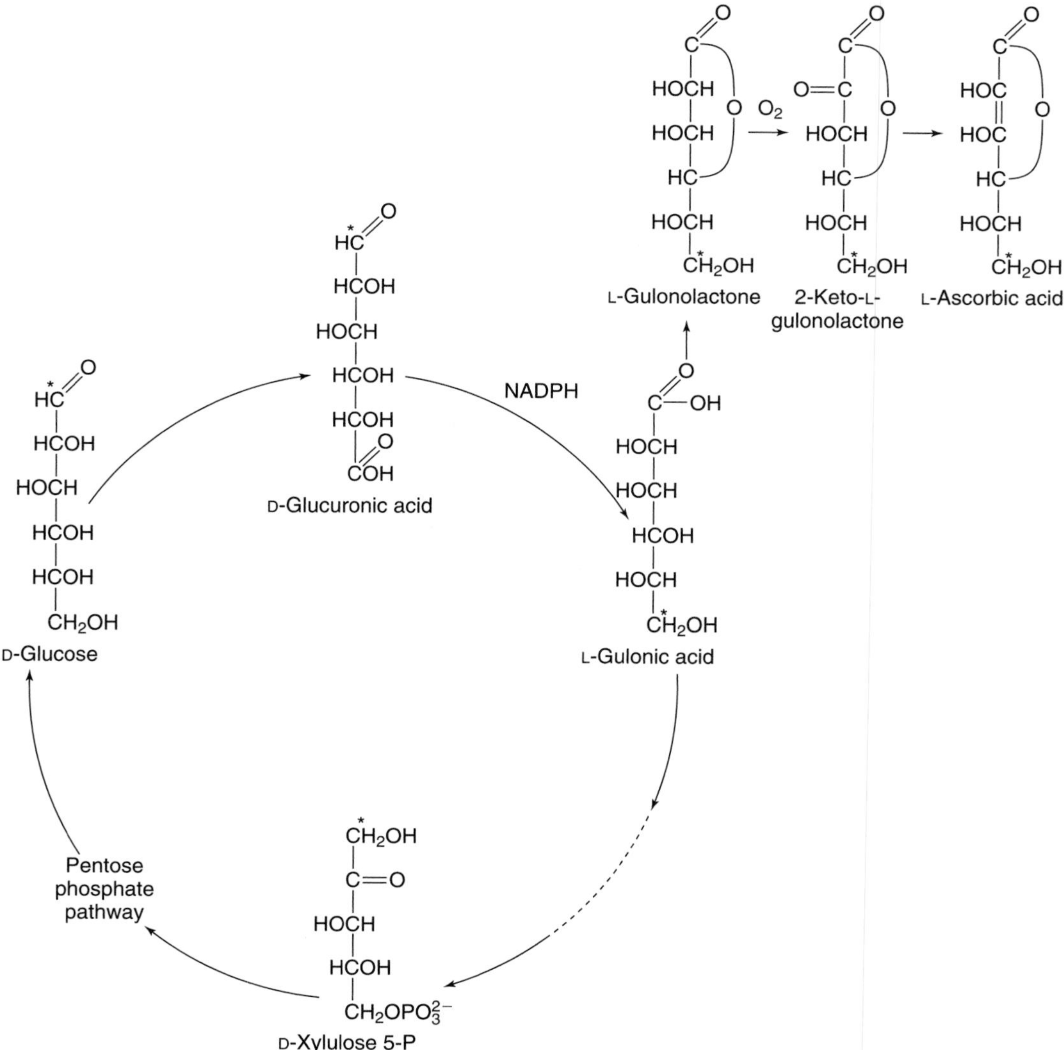

Figure 27-1 Pathway for biosynthesis of ascorbic acid from glucose in mammals. Humans lack gulonolactone oxidase and cannot convert L-gulonolactone to 2-keto-L-gulonolactone.

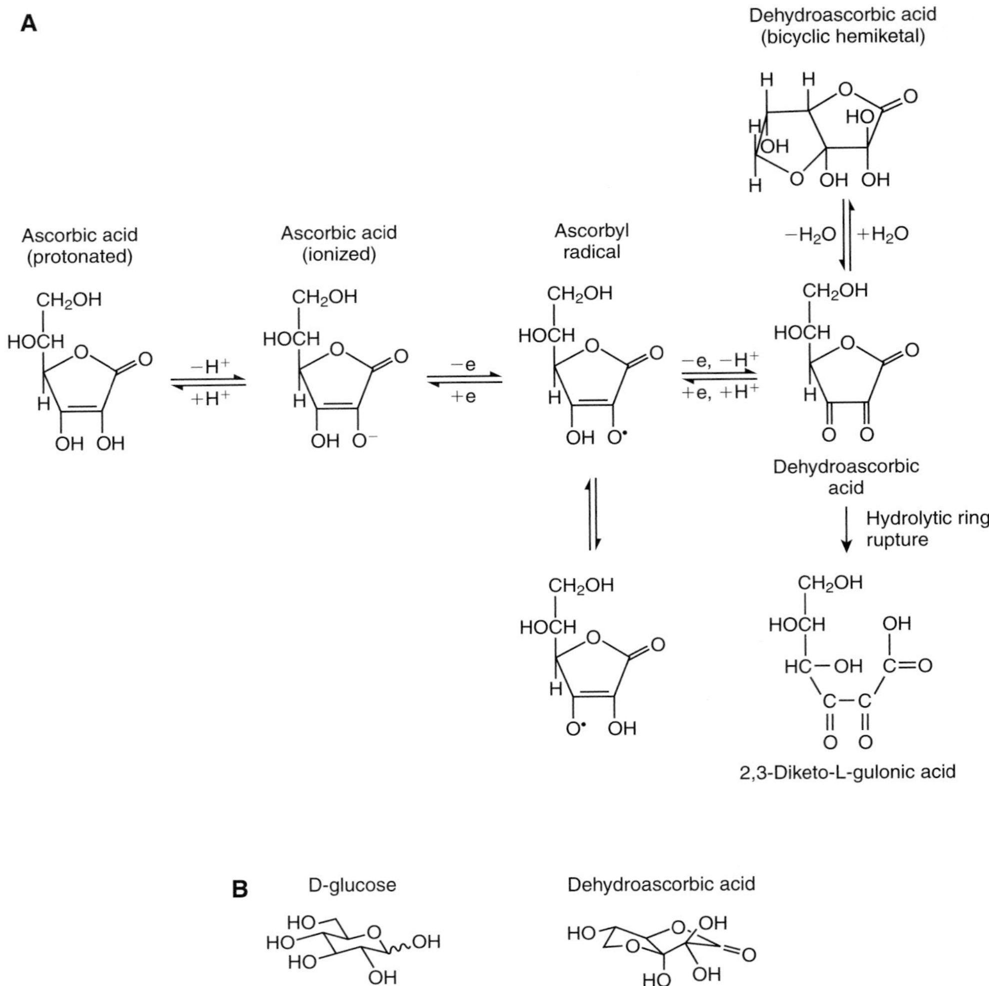

Figure 27-2 **A,** Ascorbic acid and its oxidation products. Ascorbic acid at physiological pH is present as the ascorbate anion. Dehydroascorbic acid exists in more than one form, and only two are shown here for simplicity. The hydrated hemiketal is believed to be the favored form in aqueous solutions (Tolbert and Ward, 1982; Corpe et al., 2005), but it is uncertain which form is present in biological systems. Semidehydroascorbic acid may also have other configurations, which are omitted for simplicity (Lewin, 1976). Formation of 2,3-diketogulonic acid by hydrolytic ring rupture is probably irreversible. **B,** Structural similarity between glucose and dehydroascorbic acid is shown (Corpe et al., 2005). *(Modified from Washko PW, Welch RW, Dhariwal KR, Wang Y, Levine M [1992] Ascorbic acid and dehydroascorbic acid analyses in biological samples. Anal Biochem 204:1-14.)*

bond at C-2–C-3 are available. The redox couple dehydroascorbic acid/ascorbate is approximately +0.06 volt under standard conditions (Lewin, 1976). The standard redox potential is based on the following relationship:

Electron acceptor + Electron(s) → Electron donor

The redox couple dehydroascorbic acid/ascorbic acid reflects donation of two electrons by ascorbate. However, it is likely that electrons from ascorbate are lost sequentially, with formation of the intermediate free radical called ascorbyl radical (sometimes also termed semidehydroascorbic acid, monodehydroascorbic acid, or ascorbate free radical). The half-life of ascorbyl radical is dependent on buffer components, and it can be less than 1 second in some media to as long as many minutes in metal-free buffers. Compared with other free radicals, ascorbyl radical is relatively stable, does not react well with other compounds to form potentially harmful free radicals, and can be reversibly reduced to ascorbate (Buettner and Moseley, 1993). Taken together, these properties suggest that ascorbate may be an ideal electron donor.

The redox potential of ascorbyl radical/ascorbate is approximately +0.3 volt under standard conditions. Based only on standard redox potentials, ascorbate would not appear to be a good electron donor. However, the overall propensity of redox couples to donate or accept electrons is the reduction potential. In addition to standard redox potential, the reduction potential as defined by the Nernst equation accounts for the concentrations of electron acceptor and electron donor. Standard conditions assume that concentrations are equal at 1 mol/L. However, the reduction potential can vary substantially when there are different concentrations of electron donor and acceptor. Under conditions in which ascorbate concentration is in excess of that of ascorbyl radical, ascorbate acts as an electron donor and ascorbyl radical is formed. In fact, the expected physiological condition is that ascorbate will be in great excess relative to ascorbyl radical. Once ascorbyl radical forms, the Nernst equation also predicts that the second electron will also be lost to form dehydroascorbic acid. Therefore, the redox potential for the dehydroascorbic acid/ascorbic acid couple reflects the sum of the dehydroascorbic acid/ascorbyl radical and ascorbyl radical/ascorbate couples. Thus, under physiological conditions, ascorbate actually is an excellent electron donor.

Dehydroascorbic acid is the first stable product formed from ascorbate oxidation (see Fig. 27-2). Dehydroascorbic acid is formed from ascorbate by a wide variety of oxidants found in biological systems, such as molecular oxygen, molecular oxygen plus trace metal (iron, copper), superoxide, hydroxyl radical, and hypochlorous acid. Although dehydroascorbic acid is more stable than ascorbyl radical, dehydroascorbic acid stability at physiological pH is measured in minutes rather than hours. At more acidic pH, especially less than pH 4, dehydroascorbic acid stability improves markedly. Dehydroascorbic acid may exist in one of multiple forms, and it is likely that the dominant form in vivo is the bicyclic hemiketal (Corpe et al., 2005). Although the term dehydroascorbic acid is used widely in the scientific literature, dehydroascorbic acid is probably not an acid in vivo, and the designation "dehydroascorbate" is incorrect.

Dehydroascorbic acid has two fates (see Fig. 27-2). One is hydrolysis, with irreversible rupture of the ring to yield 2,3-diketogulonic acid. Although 2,3-diketogulonic acid metabolism is not well characterized, its metabolic products may include oxalate, threonate, xylose, xylonic acid, and lynxonic acid (Lewin, 1976). It was reported that carbons from vitamin C were expired as carbon dioxide in animals, but this probably does not occur in humans (Baker et al., 1975). Of all known dehydroascorbic acid metabolites, oxalate is the one end product with clinical relevance. Excessive oxalate excretion in urine, or hyperoxaluria, can result in oxalate kidney stones in some people (Levine et al., 1999). Whether gram doses of vitamin C contribute to oxalate kidney stones remains a matter of debate.

The second fate of dehydroascorbic acid is reduction, either with one electron to ascorbyl radical or directly to vitamin C with two electrons. Dehydroascorbic acid reduction in biological systems can be mediated chemically or by protein-dependent pathways (Arrigoni and De Tullio, 2002; Rumsey and Levine, 1998; Winkler et al., 1994). It is unknown whether chemical- or protein-mediated reduction is the dominant process that occurs in vivo. Dehydroascorbic acid reduction chemically is mediated in vivo by glutathione, with formation of glutathione disulfide. Enzymatic reduction of dehydroascorbic acid is mediated in vivo by various proteins that require another electron donor. Two proteins use NADPH as the electron donor; these proteins are 3-alpha hydroxysteroid dehydrogenase and thioredoxin reductase. Three other proteins, glutaredoxin (thioltransferase), protein disulfide isomerase, and dehydroascorbate [sic] reductase, use glutathione as the electron donor.

These proteins have different K_ms for dehydroascorbic acid, ranging from approximately 250 μmol/L to several millimoles per liter. When compared to chemical reduction alone, at least some of these proteins with their respective reducing agents mediate reduction substantially faster. As described for glutaredoxin, protein-mediated reduction can involve ascorbate formation without ascorbyl radical as an intermediate (Yang et al., 1998).

Ascorbyl radical can also be reduced to vitamin C. Although the enzymes that catalyze this reduction have not been purified, several ascorbyl radical reducing activities have been reported in membranes of mitochondria, microsomes, and erthyrocytes (May et al., 2001). Ascorbyl radical can also be reduced by the cytosolic enzyme thioredoxin reductase (May et al., 1998).

Reduction of both dehydroascorbic acid and ascorbyl radical in humans is inefficient. If reduction were completely efficient, humans would not get scurvy if vitamin C ingestion suddenly stopped. Reduction efficiencies in vivo reflect sums of reduction rates and oxidation rates. Currently, there are no means to measure these rates separately in humans. What can be measured is ascorbate disappearance as a function of time and ascorbate dose. Such data show that when vitamin C ingestion ceases, healthy humans become vitamin C deficient after approximately 30 days (Levine et al., 2001; Levine et al., 1996).

Food Sources

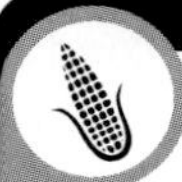

Food Sources of Vitamin C

Fruits

- 70 mg per 1 medium kiwi fruit
- 45 to 55 mg per ½ cup fresh or frozen strawberries, fresh papaya, or fresh orange sections
- 20 to 30 mg per ½ cup fresh cantaloupe or pineapple cubes, grapefruit or mandarin orange sections, or fresh mango
- 15 to 20 mg per ½ cup fresh or frozen raspberries or honeydew melon cubes

Juices

- 90 mg per ¾ cup fresh orange juice
- 70 mg per ¾ cup fresh grapefruit juice
- 60 to 70 mg per ¾ cup canned or frozen orange or grapefruit juice
- 70 to 180 mg per ¾ cup vitamin C–fortified fruit juice

Vegetables

- 120 to 140 mg per ½ cup sweet red pepper
- 50 to 60 mg per ½ cup sweet green pepper
- 35 to 60 mg per ½ cup broccoli or brussels sprouts
- 15 to 35 mg per ½ cup cauliflower, collards, kale, asparagus, red cabbage, edible-podded peas, sauerkraut, spinach, or sweet potato

Vegetable Juices

- 35 mg per ¾ cup canned tomato juice

Data from U.S. Department of Agriculture/Agricultural Research Service (USDA/ARS) (2005) USDA Nutrient Database for Standard Reference, Release 18. USDA/ARS, Washington, DC. Retrieved November 15, 2005, from www.ars.usda.gov/ba/bhnrc/ndl.

FOOD SOURCES, ABSORPTION, AND BIOAVAILABILITY

Ascorbate is found in many fruits and vegetables. Fruits high in vitamin C include cantaloupe, kiwi, strawberries, lemons, and oranges. Good vegetable sources are broccoli, red pepper, cauliflower, spinach, tomatoes, brussels sprouts, and asparagus. Fruit and vegetable juices that are good sources of the vitamin are orange, grapefruit, and tomato juices. Many foods, such as breakfast cereals and fruit drinks, are fortified with vitamin C. Foods low in vitamin C include meat, poultry, eggs, dairy products, and unfortified grains.

Both ascorbate and dehydroascorbic acid are present in foods. Ascorbate predominates, accounting for 80% to 90% of the total vitamin content, with dehydroascorbic acid accounting for 10% to 20% (Vanderslice and Higgs, 1991). There is little information concerning the relationship between food aging and progressive ascorbate oxidation and/or dehydroascorbic acid formation, but increased oxidation is expected as food ages.

The ascorbate epimer erythorbic acid (also called D-isoascorbic acid and D-araboascorbic acid), a food additive, is added as a preservative to smoked or cured meats and some beverages. Erythorbic acid has no antiscorbutic activity. There is potential for erythorbic acid to give false elevations of plasma ascorbate concentrations, however. For this to occur, plasma samples would have to be taken within a few hours after erythorbate-containing foods were eaten. Because erythorbic acid is cleared from plasma within 12 hours, potential interference from erythorbic acid is easily avoided by taking plasma samples after an overnight fast (Sauberlich et al., 1996).

In guinea pigs, ascorbic acid is absorbed in the ileum and probably in the jejunum of the small intestine. In animal intestine experimental systems, ascorbate absorption is Na^+-dependent, and ascorbate absorption in humans probably occurs by a similar mechanism (Stevenson, 1974). Guinea pigs specifically have been studied because, like humans, they must obtain ascorbate from the diet.

Bioavailability is a measure of the amount of substance absorbed. The absolute amount of a dose absorbed is its true bioavailability. True bioavailability is determined from oral and intravenous administration of a dose when a subject is at steady state (equilibrium for the dose). Once a subject is at steady state for the dose under study, that dose is administered orally, and the change in plasma concentration from the dose is measured by serial blood sampling. When the data are displayed as a function of time, an area under the curve and above baseline reflects the increment from the oral dose. The same dose is then administered intravenously, the change in plasma concentration is again determined by serial sampling, and the area under this curve is calculated. True bioavailability is the area under the curve from oral absorption divided by the area under the curve from intravenous administration, expressed as a percentage. One hundred percent bioavailability represents complete absorption. Because of the necessity for steady-state conditions and repeated serial sampling, true bioavailability data for vitamin C are limited. The available data indicate that true bioavailability is greater than 80% for vitamin C doses between 15 and 100 mg (Graumlich et al., 1997; Levine et al., 1996). Bioavailability declines for higher doses and is slightly less than 50% for a dose of 1,250 mg.

We know from studies with guinea pigs that dehydroascorbic acid, as well as ascorbic acid, is absorbed in the jejunum of the small intestine (Rose et al., 1988). Dehydroascorbic acid absorption is Na^+-independent. Once absorbed, dehydroascorbic acid is probably reduced to ascorbate. In animals that are unable to synthesize vitamin C, ingested dehydroascorbic acid prevents scurvy but much higher doses are needed when compared to ascorbate (Ogiri et al., 2002; Otsuka et al., 1986). Although dehydroascorbic acid might be absorbed by humans and reduced to ascorbate, the data are difficult to interpret because of assay imprecision and artifacts. There are no true bioavailability studies for dehydroascorbic acid in humans.

ASCORBATE (VITAMIN C) ACCUMULATION IN CELLS

Ascorbate is found in plasma of humans and animals. Because it is water soluble and not protein bound, it is likely that ascorbate distributes easily into the extracellular space. Ascorbate concentrations in almost all tissues are 5- to 100-fold higher than that of plasma. Ascorbate is accumulated by adrenal cortex, adrenal medulla, pituitary, white blood cells, endothelial cells, and many other tissues (Rumsey and Levine, 1998). Indeed, there probably is only one major cell type that does not concentrate ascorbate: the red blood cell.

Until relatively recently, mechanisms of ascorbate accumulation were unclear. Two major possibilities were identified, but were unresolved and were assumed to be mutually exclusive. One was transport of ascorbate as such, so that ascorbate was transported against its concentration gradient. The other possibility was transport of oxidized ascorbate as dehydroascorbic acid, with subsequent reduction within cells to ascorbate. Before 1980, ascorbate and dehydroascorbic acid measurements were often difficult to interpret because the methods were insensitive, nonspecific, subject to interference and artifacts, and could not account for the instability of the substances measured (Washko et al., 1992). Two fundamental developments in biomedical sciences were responsible for solving these problems. The first was widespread use of high performance liquid chromatography (HPLC) as a measurement technique. HPLC was first applied to ascorbate measurement in 1976 (Pachla and Kissinger, 1976). Although dehydroascorbic acid measurement remains difficult, subsequent refinement of HPLC assays for ascorbate have overcome assay problems (Levine et al., 1999). The second groundbreaking development was part of the revolution in molecular biology, with application of techniques to solving problems in cell biology. Expression cloning with the *Xenopus laevis* (frog) oocyte expression system was a key tool for identifying ascorbate and dehydroascorbic acid transporters (Daruwala et al., 1999; Tsukaguchi et al., 1999; Rumsey et al., 1997; Vera et al., 1993). By using these newer approaches, separate distinct mechanisms of ascorbate and dehydroascorbic acid transmembrane transport were identified.

Ascorbic acid is accumulated intracellularly both by ascorbate transport and by dehydroascorbic acid transport and reduction. Ascorbate itself is transported by one of two known Na^+-dependent transporters, termed SVCT 1 and 2 (sodium-dependent vitamin C transporters 1 and 2) (Daruwala et al., 1999; Tsukaguchi et al., 1999). These two transporters are in the nucleobase transporter superfamily (de Koning and Diallinas, 2000) and are unlike other Na^+-dependent transporters. SVCT1 is found in intestine, liver, and kidney and is an epithelial cell transporter. SVCT1 has a K_m of approximately 100 to 200 µmol/L and achieves a velocity approaching V_{max} at a concentration of approximately 1 mmol/L. SVCT2 is the widely distributed tissue transporter, with a K_m of approximately 5 to 10 µmol/L. SVCT2 achieves a velocity approaching V_{max} at a concentration of approximately 60-100 µmol/L. The K_m values for SVCT1 and 2 are within the range of ascorbate concentrations observed in the intestinal luminal contents or in human plasma, respectively. The SVCTs do not transport dehydroascorbic acid (Corpe et al, 2005; Takanaga et al., 2004; Daruwala et al., 1999).

The second mechanism for ascorbate accumulation in cells such as neutrophils is termed ascorbate recycling (Fig. 27-3). In this pathway, external ascorbic acid is oxidized to dehydroascorbic acid. Dehydroascorbic acid is then transported by facilitated glucose transporters into cells and immediately reduced to ascorbic acid (Rumsey et al., 1997; Vera et al., 1993; Washko et al., 1993). Glucose transporters 1, 3, and 4 (GLUT 1, 3, and 4) transport dehydroascorbic acid with high affinity, equal to or higher than that for glucose (Rumsey et al., 2000; Rumsey et al., 1997). There is structural similarity between dehydroascorbic acid and glucose, as shown in Figure 27-2, *B*. Dehydroascorbic acid reduction may be mediated intracellularly by glutathione and/or reducing proteins described in the preceding text.

Data from SVCT2 knockout mice show that Na^+-dependent transport is the dominant mechanism of ascorbate accumulation in mice (Sotiriou et al., 2002). The dominant pathway of ascorbate accumulation in humans is not clear, and some investigators propose that ascorbate recycling, the process of dehydroascorbic acid transport with intracellular reduction, may be the dominant pathway (Huang et al., 2001).

Ascorbate is most likely the predominant, if not exclusive, form of ascorbic acid in the human circulation under nonoxidizing conditions (Dhariwal et al., 1991b). If dehydroascorbic acid were to form in blood, it would be expected to be transported immediately into red blood cells or neutrophils and trapped by reduction, and plasma levels should remain very low. Outside the circulation, ascorbate is the expected extracellular substrate under nonoxidizing conditions. Under such conditions, it is likely that most ascorbate accumulation is mediated by the SVCTs. Therefore, ascorbate transport can be considered constitutive because the substrate ascorbate is continuously available. Once oxidants are generated, however, it is likely that these oxidants oxidize some ascorbate to dehydroascorbic acid. With dehydroascorbic acid formation, ascorbate recycling occurs: dehydroascorbic acid is transported into cells and reduced to ascorbate. As part of ascorbate recycling, dehydroascorbic acid transport can be considered substrate-induced transport, because the substrate is present only when oxidants cause its

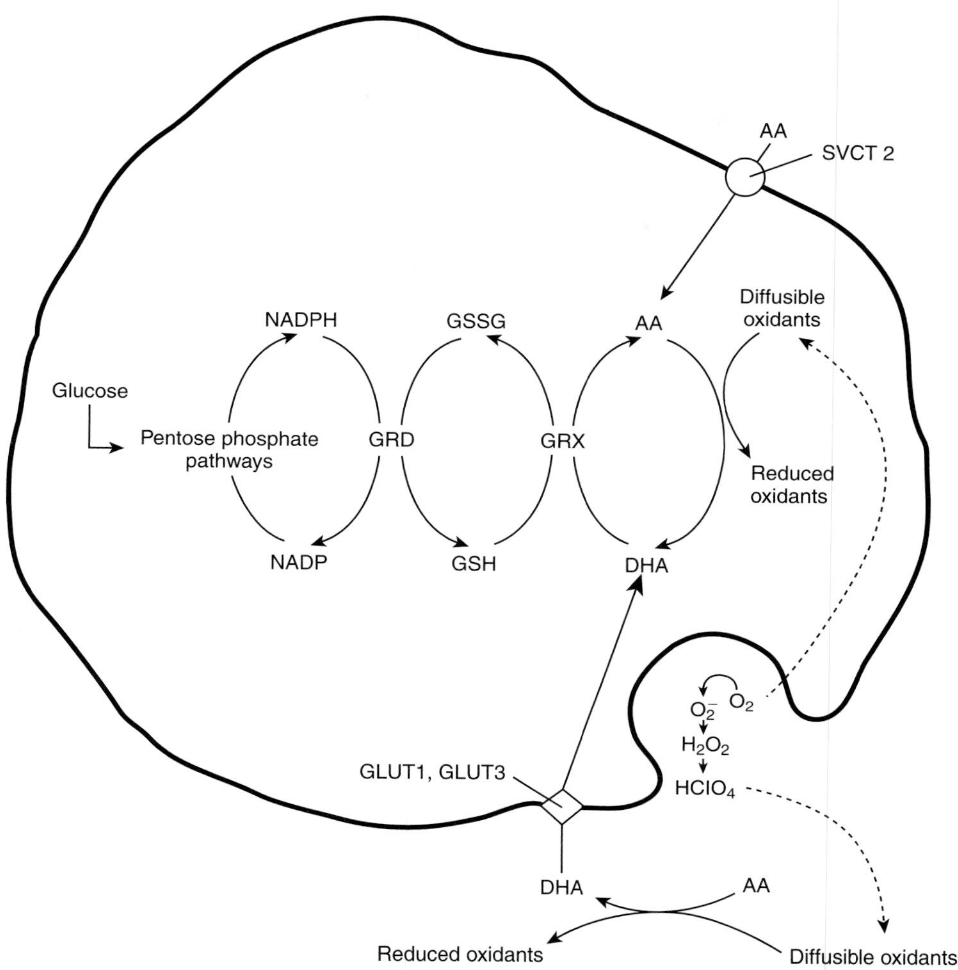

Figure 27-3 Mechanisms of vitamin C accumulation in human neutrophils. Vitamin C accumulation in neutrophils occurs by ascorbic acid transport and ascorbic acid recycling. Ascorbic acid (AA) as a substrate is transported by a sodium-dependent vitamin C transporter (SVCT2). This mechanism maintains millimolar concentrations inside resting neutrophils. Vitamin C recycling occurs when bacteria, yeast, or pharmacological agents activate neutrophils. Activated neutrophils secrete reactive oxygen species that oxidize extracellular AA to dehydroascorbic acid (DHA). DHA is rapidly transported into neutrophils by glucose transporters (i.e., GLUT1, GLUT3) and is then immediately reduced to AA by the glutathione-dependent protein glutaredoxin (GRX). Glutathione (GSH) utilized during DHA reduction is regenerated from glutathione disulfide (GSSG) by glutathione reductase (GRD) and NADPH. NADPH is a product of glucose metabolism through the pentose phosphate pathway. Although the figure shows DHA uptake by glucose transporters 1 and 3, different cell types might utilize other glucose transporters. *(Modified from Padayatty SJ, Levine M [2001] New insights into the physiology and pharmacology of vitamin C. Can Assoc Med J 164:353-355.)*

formation from ascorbate (see Fig. 27-3). Ascorbate recycling is most likely to occur during the time that diffusible oxidants are present and increased intracellular ascorbate could be utilized for oxidant quenching. By allowing cells in the presence of oxidants to increase intracellular ascorbate concentrations rapidly, ascorbate recycling is, therefore, a potentially protective mechanism. Dehydroascorbic acid transport by GLUTs under oxidizing conditions and constitutive ascorbate transport by SVCTs together provide a comprehensive explanation of ascorbate accumulation in tissues (see Fig. 27-3). Analog compounds that are accumulated only by one but not by both mechanisms may be very useful in the elucidation of the mechanisms of vitamin C accumulation in vivo (Corpe et al., 2005).

ENZYMATIC FUNCTIONS OF ASCORBATE

Vitamin C acts as an electron donor for 11 enzymes (Englard and Seifter, 1986; Levine, 1986) (Fig. 27-4). Three enzymes are found in fungi and are involved in reutilization pathways for pyrimidines or the deoxyribose moiety of deoxynucleosides (Stubbe, 1985; Wondrack et al., 1979). Because they are not known to be involved in mammalian reactions, they will not be discussed further here. Of the eight mammalian enzymes, three enzymes participate in collagen hydroxylation and two in carnitine biosynthesis. Of the remaining three enzymes, one is necessary for biosynthesis of the catecholamine norepinephrine, one is

Monooxygenases

Dopamine β-hydroxylase

3,4-Dihydroxyphenylethylamine (dopamine)

Norepinephrine

Peptidylglycine α-amidating monooxygenase

Peptide with C-terminal glycine

C-Terminal amidated peptide

Glyoxylate

Dioxygenases

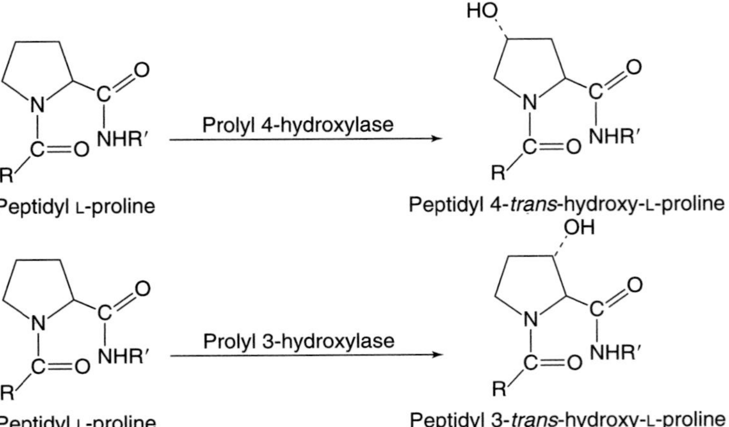

Figure 27-4 Classification of enzymatic reactions that utilize ascorbate. All the dioxygenase reactions shown except the one catalyzed by 4-hydroxyphenylpyruvate dioxygenase require α-ketoglutarate as a co-substrate (see also Figs. 27-7 and 27-10). (*Modified from Englard S, Seifter S [1986] The biochemical functions of ascorbic acid. Annu Rev Nutr 6:365-406. Copyright 1986 Annual Reviews.*)

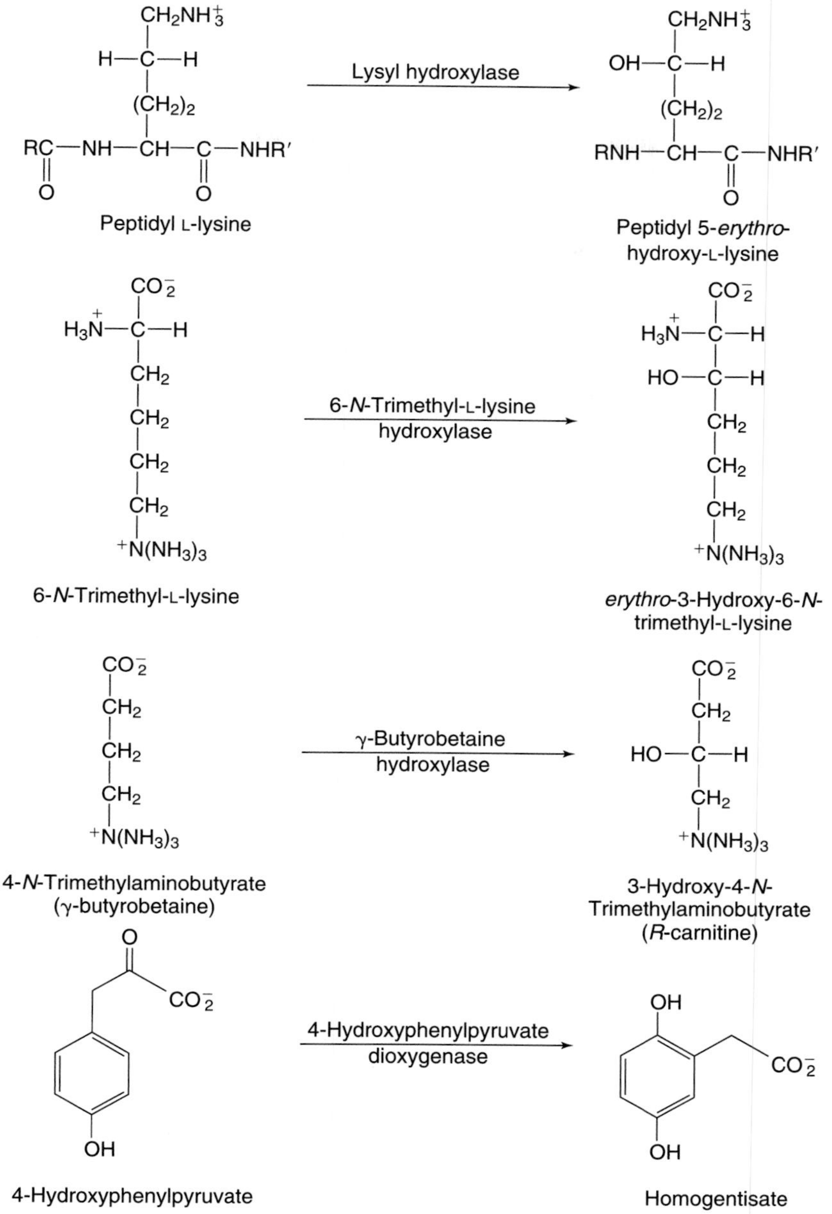

Peptidyl L-lysine → (Lysyl hydroxylase) → Peptidyl 5-*erythro*-hydroxy-L-lysine

6-*N*-Trimethyl-L-lysine → (6-*N*-Trimethyl-L-lysine hydroxylase) → *erythro*-3-Hydroxy-6-*N*-trimethyl-L-lysine

4-*N*-Trimethylaminobutyrate (γ-butyrobetaine) → (γ-Butyrobetaine hydroxylase) → 3-Hydroxy-4-*N*-Trimethylaminobutyrate (*R*-carnitine)

4-Hydroxyphenylpyruvate → (4-Hydroxyphenylpyruvate dioxygenase) → Homogentisate

Figure 27-4, cont'd

necessary for amidation of peptide hormones, and one is involved in tyrosine metabolism.

Enzymes that require ascorbate have either monooxygenase or dioxygenase activity. The monooxygenases dopamine β-hydroxylase and peptidyl-glycine α-monooxygenase incorporate a single oxygen atom into a substrate, either dopamine or a peptide with a terminal glycine. The remaining enzymes are dioxygenases, which incorporate molecular oxygen (O_2), with each oxygen atom being incorporated in a different way. The enzyme 4-hydroxyphenylpyruvate dioxygenase incorporates two oxygen atoms into different locations of one product. The other dioxygenases incorporate one atom of oxygen into α-ketoglutarate to form succinate and the other atom of oxygen into the enzyme-specific substrate.

MONOOXYGENASES

Dopamine β-Hydroxylase

Dopamine β-hydroxylase is necessary for hydroxylation of dopamine for synthesis of the catecholamine norepinephrine in peripheral neurons, central neurons, and adrenal medulla. Because of its abundance, enzyme from the adrenal medulla has been characterized in the most detail. The enzyme is a tetrameric glycoprotein, with subunits arranged as pairs of disulfide-linked monomeric species. There are both membrane-bound and soluble enzyme forms, which probably differ in subunit composition (Fleming and Kent, 1991). The enzyme is believed to contain two copper atoms per subunit.

The isolated enzyme requires molecular oxygen, a substrate to be hydroxylated, and ascorbate as the preferred electron donor. Catalase is added to isolated enzyme assays to scavenge the hydrogen peroxide that forms. Under these conditions, enzyme activity is easily measured, and ascorbate is consumed stoichiometrically 1:1 in relation to consumption of oxygen and to formation of product. The enzyme receives single electrons sequentially from two ascorbate molecules, with formation of ascorbate free radical as an intermediate (Fleming and Kent, 1991; Stewart and Klinman, 1988).

In intact tissue, dopamine β-hydroxylase is found in both soluble and membrane-bound enzyme forms that are localized exclusively in neurosecretory vesicles of neurons and in secretory vesicles (chromaffin granules) of the adrenal medulla (Levine et al., 1991) (Fig. 27-5).

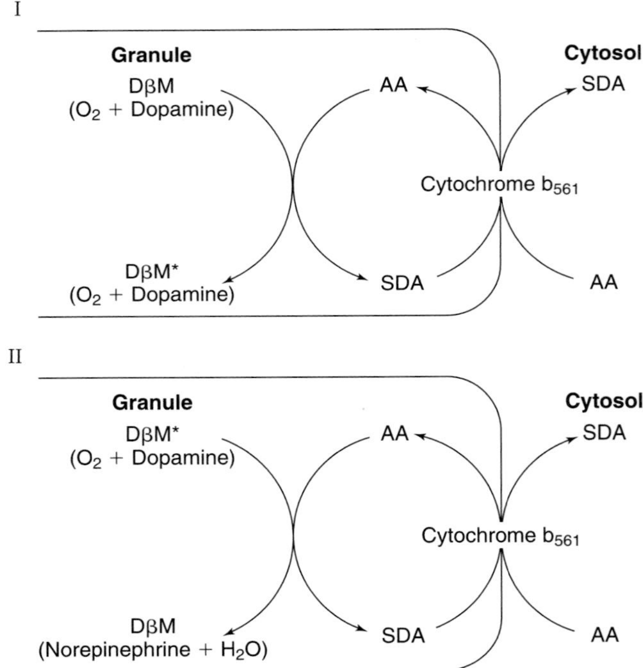

Figure 27-5 Transmembrane electron transfer and dopamine β-hydroxylase reduction in chromaffin granules. Intragranular ascorbic acid reduces dopamine β-hydroxylase by single electron transfer, with formation of semidehydroascorbic acid. In the presence of external (cytosolic) ascorbic acid, intragranular semidehydroascorbic acid is reduced by transmembrane electron transfer via cytochrome b_{561}. There are two steps, indicating that dopamine β-hydroxylase is reduced twice, each time by a single electron. Although oxygen and dopamine are shown associated with the enzyme during its reduction, the precise interaction is unknown. The enzyme catalyzes the hydroxylation of dopamine and the reduction of ½ O_2 to H_2O. *AA*, Ascorbate; *DβM*, dopamine β-monooxygenase (-hydroxylase); *DβM**, reduced dopamine β-monooxygenase (-hydroxylase); *SDA*, semidehydroascorbic acid.

Ascorbate is found within vesicles and in cell cytosol, but ascorbate itself is not transported across vesicles. Instead, electrons from cytosolic ascorbate are transferred in sequential one-electron steps to cytochrome b_{561} in the vesicle membrane (Fleming and Kent, 1991; Kent and Fleming, 1987). Single electrons accepted by cytochrome b_{561} undergo transmembrane electron transfer. Within vesicles, semidehydroascorbic acid accepts these electrons from membrane cytochrome b_{561} to form ascorbate (Dhariwal et al., 1991a). The intravesicular semidehydroascorbic acid is formed by action of dopamine β-hydroxylase. To summarize, semidehydroascorbic acid generated by enzyme action within vesicles is reduced to ascorbate by transmembrane electron transfer from external ascorbate. Without extravesicular (cytosolic) ascorbate, intact vesicles will synthesize norepinephrine from dopamine using intravesicular ascorbate until it is consumed (Levine et al., 1991). With extravesicular ascorbate, intravesicular ascorbate is maintained by transmembrane electron transfer.

The kinetics for ascorbate in norepinephrine biosynthesis were determined in situ, meaning in intact animal tissue (Levine et al., 1991). The K_m of dopamine β-hydroxylase for intravesicular ascorbate was approximately 0.5 mmol/L, which is similar to that of isolated enzyme (Kaufman, 1974). Just as for isolated enzyme, the stoichiometry of the overall reaction in intact tissue is 1:1 for ascorbate consumption to norepinephrine biosynthesis. Intact vesicles contain 10 to 15 mmol/L of ascorbate, which is sufficient to saturate dopamine β-hydroxylase with ascorbate. The K_m of transmembrane electron transfer for cytosolic ascorbate is approximately 0.3 mmol/L. Because cytosolic ascorbate is at least 10 times this value, transmembrane electron transfer should also proceed at the maximal transport rate. The corresponding kinetic parameters in human tissue are not known.

Why is ascorbate utilization by dopamine β-hydroxylase coupled to transmembrane electron transfer? One possibility is that this is a protective mechanism for synthesis of an essential hormone in the event of vitamin C deficiency. If deficiency occurs, intravesicular ascorbate will remain until it is consumed. Because intravesicular ascorbate concentrations permit hydroxylation to proceed at V_{max}, and cytosolic concentrations allow electron transfer to proceed at V_{max}, dopamine hydroxylation should continue even as cytosolic concentrations decline in the event of deficiency. It is unknown how intragranular ascorbate enters secretory vesicles. Because cytosolic ascorbate is also at millimolar concentration, it is possible that cytosolic ascorbate is trapped in vesicles during vesicle formation.

Peptidylglycine α-Amidating Monooxygenase

Biologically active peptides act as hormones or paracrine signaling agents and are often synthesized from inactive precursors by post-translational modification. To confer activity to many bioactive peptides, a carboxy-terminal α-amide group must be added by a process called α-amidation. α-Amidation is mediated by peptidylglycine α-amidating monooxygenase (PAM) (Prigge et al., 2000; Eipper et al., 1993a). Amidated peptide hormones include thyrotropin-releasing hormone, gonadotropin-releasing hormone, oxytocin, vasopressin, cholecystokinin, gastrin, calcitonin, substance P, and neuropeptide Y. Precursors to α-amidated peptides have a glycine residue that immediately follows the residue to be α-amidated. Unless the site is at the extreme carboxyl terminus of the precursor peptide, the α-amidation site must be exposed by endoproteolytic cleavage; the signal for cleavage is either x–glycine–basic amino acid–basic amino acid or x–glycine–basic amino acid. In α-amidation, the signal carboxy-terminal glycine is cleaved to release glyoxylate, leaving the amino acid residue "x" as "x-NH_2." Alpha-amidated peptides have been isolated with x represented by every amino acid except aspartic acid.

PAM is actually a bifunctional enzyme that contains two distinct monofunctional domains connected by a linker region (Prigge et al., 2000; Eipper et al., 1993a) (Fig. 27-6, *bottom*). The two domains are peptidylglycine α-hydroxylating monooxygenase (PHM) and peptidyl-α-hydroxyglycine α-amidating lyase (PAL). Although PHM and PAL make up the N-terminal and C-terminal domains, respectively, of the bifunctional protein, there are two intervening regions between the catalytic domains. After the PHM catalytic core, there is a protease-sensitive region (termed exon 15), followed by a non-catalytic region (termed exon A) that is sometimes excluded due to alternative splicing. PAL then follows exon A. The amidation reaction is a two-step reaction, with each reaction mediated by one of the component monofunctional subunits (see Fig. 27-6, *top*). The first-step reaction, mediated by PHM, results in hydroxylation of the peptidylglycine residue with formation of peptidylhydroxyglycine. In the second step, the peptidylhydroxyglycine moiety is cleaved into glyoxylate and the amidated peptide, as mediated by PAL.

PAM is localized to secretory vesicles. A transmembrane tail close to the carboxyl terminus anchors PAM to the vesicle membrane, and the carboxyl terminus itself is on the cytosolic or extravesicular side of the vesicle membrane (Prigge et al., 2000; Eipper et al., 1993a). The monofunctional domains PHM and PAL are localized to the intravesicular space.

The first-step reaction mediated by PHM is rate-limiting. PHM is similar to dopamine β-hydroxylase in several respects. Both enzymes are monooxygenases. As does dopamine β-hydroxylase, PHM requires ascorbate, oxygen, and copper (Prigge et al., 2000; Eipper et al., 1993a). As shown in Figure 27-6, two ascorbate molecules form two semidehydroascorbate (ascorbyl radical) molecules. Subsequently, these react spontaneously to form one ascorbic acid molecule and one dehydroascorbic

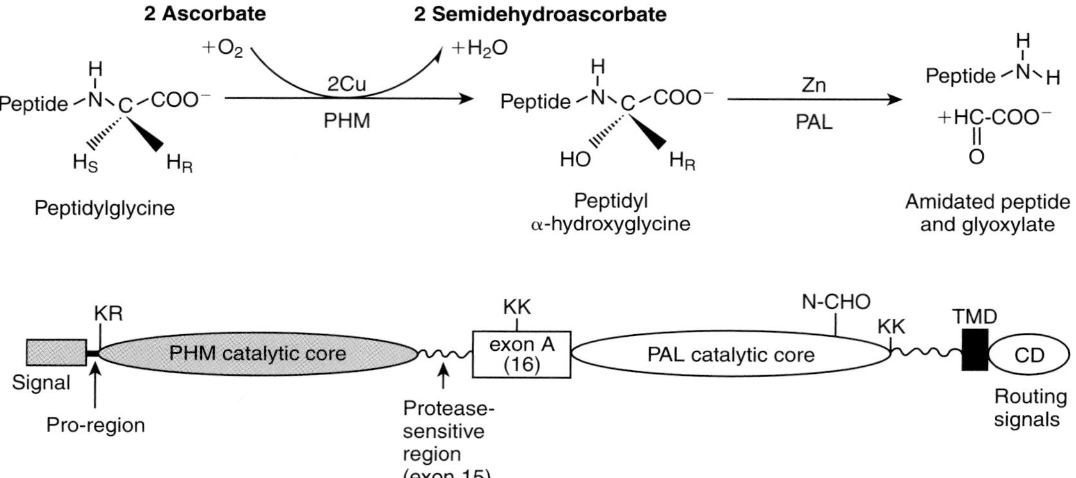

Figure 27-6 The PAM Reaction and the PAM Protein. The two-step conversion of peptidylglycine substrates into products is shown *(top)*. Peptidylglycine α-hydroxylating monooxygenase, PHM, has also been referred to as peptidylglycine α-amidating monooxygenase and peptidylglycine hydroxylase; peptidyl-α-hydroxyglycine α-amidating lyase, PAL, has also been referred to as peptidylamidoglycolate lyase and peptidyl α-hydroxyglycine lyase. The structure of a bifunctional membrane PAM protein is shown *(bottom)*. The hydrophobic signal sequence is removed in the ER. The 10-residue proregion is removed in a post-Golgi compartment in neuroendocrine cells; its presence facilitates exit from the endoplasmic reticulum (ER) but does not affect catalytic activity. A protease-sensitive region, termed exon 15, separates the end of the PHM catalytic core from exon A. Tissue-specific endoproteolytic cleavage in exon A can generate soluble PHM and membrane PAL. The PAL enzyme contains a single *N*-glycosylation site (N-CHO) and terminates just before Lys821-Lys822. Endoproteolytic cleavage can occur between PAL and the transmembrane domain (TMD), but the cleavage sites are not well characterized. The cytosolic region (cytosolic domain, CD) contains signals important to the localization of PAM in the distal *trans*-Golgi network and to its endocytosis from the plasma membrane. *(Modified from Prigge ST, Mains RE, Eipper BA, Amzel LM [2000] New insights into copper monooxygenases and peptide amidation: structure, mechanism and function. Cell Mol Life Sci 57:1236-1259.)*

acid molecule. The overall stoichiometry is that one molecule of ascorbic acid is consumed as one molecule of peptidylglycine is converted to product. Copper in PHM is essential for activation of molecular oxygen. PHM and dopamine β-hydroxylase share significant amino acid sequence similarity, indicating that these enzymes are evolutionarily linked. The enzymes have 28% identity extending through a common catalytic domain of approximately 270 residues (Prigge et al., 2000; Eipper et al., 1993a).

Ascorbate utilization by dopamine β-hydroxylase and PAM (PHM) are similar (Prigge et al., 2000; Eipper et al., 1993a). Ascorbic acid within vesicles is utilized by PHM with formation of semidehydroascorbic acid. Cytochrome b_{561} accepts single electrons from cytosolic ascorbate, with reduction of intravesicular semidehydroascorbic acid produced during peptide amidation (Prigge et al., 2000; Kent and Fleming, 1987). Therefore, as for dopamine β-hydroxylase, cytosolic ascorbate maintains intravesicular ascorbate concentrations. Just as for catecholamine-containing vesicles, it is unknown how ascorbate enters peptide secretory vesicles.

In contrast to dopamine β-hydroxylase, which requires ascorbate in situ (Levine et al., 1991), PAM can accept electrons from alternate donors other than ascorbate (Prigge et al., 2000; Eipper et al., 1993a). Some amidation occurs in the complete absence of ascorbate. For example, catecholamines can provide electrons in some cell systems to support peptide amidation.

DIOXYGENASES

Prolyl 4-Hydroxylase, Prolyl 3-Hydroxylase, and Lysyl Hydroxylase

Vitamin C plays a role in prolyl- and lysyl-reactions, which are involved in collagen synthesis as well as in regulation of at least one transcription factor. A cardinal symptom of vitamin C deficiency is poor wound healing, which provided an early clue that vitamin C may be involved in collagen biosynthesis (Crandon et al., 1940; Lind, 1753). The involvement of vitamin C in collagen synthesis is complex, involving both regulation of collagen synthesis at a pretranslational level and distinct regulation of posttranslational processing. These issues will be discussed separately.

Proteins of the collagen family are major components of the extracellular matrix or connective tissues that provide support for the organs and other structures of the body. Collagens are found in skin, bone, cartilage, tendons, and basement membranes of epithelial and smooth muscle cells.

Effects of vitamin C on posttranslational modification of procollagen are believed to be enzymatically mediated (Peterkofsky, 1991). Collagen is formed from precursor polypeptides, preprocollagen and procollagen, which must be processed for secretion and stability (Prockop and Kivirikko, 1995; Kivirikko and Myllyla, 1985). Preprocollagen is synthesized on polysomes bound to the rough endoplasmic reticulum (ER). The preprocollagen N-terminal signal sequence is essential for targeting the nascent preprocollagen to the lumen of the ER where the signal peptide is cleaved to yield procollagen. The procollagen polypeptide (except for the N-terminal and C-terminal sequences) is composed of repeats of the sequence Gly-X-Y, where *Gly* represents glycine and *X* or *Y* represents any other amino acid. Many (approximately one third) of the X and Y residues are proline. The basic amino acids, lysine and arginine, are also commonly found, and lysine is more common in some types of collagen than in others.

Procollagen undergoes modification in the ER prior to its secretion. Hydroxylation of certain prolyl and lysyl residues of the newly synthesized collagen polypeptide chain occurs along the length of procollagen polypeptides. Approximately half of the proline residues in the Y position of the Gly-X-Y triplet are converted to 4-hydroxyproline, and a few proline residues in the X position may be converted to 3-hydroxyproline. Hydroxylation of the prolyl or lysyl residues in the Y position is influenced by the amino acid in the X position. Once hydroxylation has occurred, a unique triple-helical structure forms, aided by the formation of disulfide bonds among the C-terminal sequences of three propeptide chains. The presence of glycine as every third amino acid residue is critical because it is the only amino acid that allows tight packing at the center of the triple helix. Hydroxylation of the proline residues in the Y position is important because this greatly increases the stability of collagen under physiological conditions. Some of the hydroxylysyl residues undergo further modification, with *O*-galactosyl or *O*-galactosyl-β-glycosyl substitution. The resulting procollagen is transported through the Golgi apparatus and is packaged into secretory vesicles that are moved to the cell surface for release of the procollagen. Transport of procollagen through the Golgi apparatus is accompanied by modification of the oligosaccharide groups. After secretion, procollagen peptidases remove peptides at the N- and C-terminal ends of the procollagen chains to form tropocollagen. Tropocollagen then forms fibrils spontaneously, and these fibrils are enzymatically modified for formation of stable intermolecular cross-links. The fibrils associate to form the collagen fibers found in connective tissues. (See Chapter 5 for further discussion of the posttranslational modification and crosslinking of tropocollagen.)

Vitamin C acts with prolyl 3-hydroxylase, prolyl 4-hydroxylase, and lysyl hydroxylase for procollagen hydroxylation (Myllyharju, 2003; Prockop and Kivirikko, 1995; Peterkofsky, 1991). These enzymes are α-ketoglutarate–dependent dioxygenases that require reduced (ferrous) iron. The enzymes require a reducing agent in vitro, and ascorbate is most effective. With isolated prolyl hydroxylase, ascorbate was observed to be consumed nonstoichiometrically. The reaction continued for several cycles in the absence of ascorbate but eventually ceased, and ascorbate was necessary to regenerate enzyme activity. These data are accounted for by the action of ascorbate with enzyme-bound iron. When hydroxylation of prolyl or lysyl residues occurs coupled with the oxidative decarboxylation of α-ketoglutarate to succinate, the enzyme-bound iron is believed to remain reduced as ferrous iron (Fe^{2+}) (Fig. 27-7, *A*). However, an uncoupled reaction can occur in which α-ketoglutarate and oxygen form succinate and carbon dioxide without hydroxylation of the prolyl or lysyl

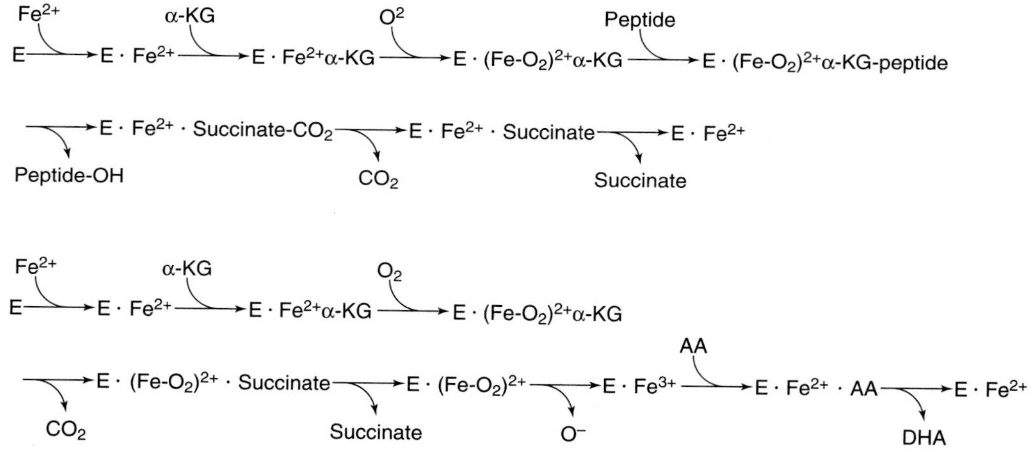

E —(Fe^{2+})→ E · Fe^{2+} —(α-KG)→ E · Fe^{2+}α-KG —(O^2)→ E · $(Fe\text{-}O_2)^{2+}$α-KG —(Peptide)→ E · $(Fe\text{-}O_2)^{2+}$α-KG-peptide

→ E · Fe^{2+} · Succinate-CO_2 (+ Peptide-OH) → E · Fe^{2+} · Succinate (+ CO_2) → E · Fe^{2+} (+ Succinate)

E —(Fe^{2+})→ E · Fe^{2+} —(α-KG)→ E · Fe^{2+}α-KG —(O_2)→ E · $(Fe\text{-}O_2)^{2+}$α-KG

→ E · $(Fe\text{-}O_2)^{2+}$ · Succinate (+ CO_2) → E · $(Fe\text{-}O_2)^{2+}$ (+ Succinate) → E · Fe^{3+} (+ O^-) —(AA)→ E · Fe^{2+} · AA → E · Fe^{2+} (+ DHA)

Figure 27-7 Mechanisms of prolyl 4-hydroxylase and lysyl hydroxylase. **A,** The probable mechanism for the complete hydroxylation reaction. The order of binding of O_2 and the peptide substrate are uncertain as is the order of release of the hydroxylated peptide and CO_2. **B,** The reaction in the absence of the peptide, in which the enzymes catalyze an uncoupled decarboxylation of α-ketoglutarate. Some peptides that do not become hydroxylated can increase the rate of the uncoupled decarboxylation. In the uncoupled reaction, the reactive iron-oxo complex is probably converted to Fe^{3+} and O^- and ascorbate is needed to reactivate the enzyme by reducing Fe^{3+} to Fe^{2+}. *α-KG,* α-Ketoglutarate; *AA,* ascorbate (ascorbic acid); *DHA,* dehydroascorbic acid; *E,* enzyme; *peptide-OH,* hydroxylated peptide. (*Modified from Kivirikko KI, Myllyla R [1985] Post-translational processing of procollagens. Ann N Y Acad Sci 460:187-201.*)

residue (see Fig. 27-7, *B*). In this case the iron moiety is oxidized to Fe^{3+}, and ascorbate is required as the specific reducing agent to reduce the iron moiety to Fe^{2+}.

Data concerning stoichiometry of ascorbate and enzymatic hydroxylation reactions are limited. In studies with cells, procollagen secretion declined in the absence of ascorbate (Peterkofsky, 1991). Procollagen is probably degraded more rapidly in the absence of hydroxylation. However, a few reports indicate that substantial residual prolyl residue hydroxylation occurred in the complete absence of ascorbate, which was as much as 50% of that seen with ascorbate. The alternative electron donors in the cell systems used in these studies are not known. In some cells a microsomal (ER) protein with a cysteinyl–cysteine active site may act as an alternative electron donor so that ascorbate is not required for prolyl hydroxylation (Peterkofsky, 1991).

There are other effects of ascorbate on collagen synthesis independent of procollagen hydroxylation. Collagen biosynthesis is decreased in scorbutic animals, but this is independent of hydroxylation reactions (Peterkofsky, 1991). This effect is mediated by an effect of scurvy on insulin-like growth factor-I (IGF-I). When scurvy occurs, excess IGF-I-binding proteins are synthesized. As a consequence of excess IGF-I-binding sites, free IGF-I is decreased in scorbutic animals compared with normal controls and IGF-I binding sites are unsaturated. Therefore, decreased free IGF-I mediates reduced collagen biosynthesis independently of hydroxylation (Gosiewska et al., 1994).

Other data also indicate that ascorbate stimulates collagen synthesis independently of hydroxylation (Sullivan et al., 1994; Geesin et al., 1988). In cell culture systems, ascorbate oxidation, or consequent lipid peroxidation, increases collagen mRNA levels. Because α-tocopherol prevents the ascorbate-mediated increase in collagen production, lipid peroxidation is thought to be involved. The lipid peroxidation product malondialdehyde stimulates collagen production and increases procollagen mRNA, mimicking the effect of ascorbate (Houglum et al., 1991). The physiological relevance of these studies is uncertain. Conversely, collagen itself can be denatured by oxidants such as superoxide (Mukhopadhyay and Chatterjee, 1994). There is animal and clinical evidence that topical ascorbate might protect collagen from oxidant damage (Darr et al., 1992).

Independent of a role in collagen biology, prolyl 4-hydroxylation has recently been described as a regulatory mechanism for the transcription factor hypoxia inducible factor alpha (HIFα). HIFα is synthesized continuously. Under ambient oxygen concentrations (normoxia), a key proline residue in a Leu-X-X-Leu-Ala-Pro sequence is hydroxylated by a distinct family of HIF prolyl 4-hydroxylases (Myllyharju, 2003; Bruick and McKnight, 2001). Hydroxylation of this proline residue is essential for HIFα to bind to other complexes, and this results in proteosomal degradation (Fig. 27-8). Hydroxylation of this proline does not occur under some conditions, such as low oxygen concentrations (hypoxia). Without hydroxylation, HIFα binds with HIFβ to form a stable dimer, which then induces hypoxia responsive genes that may play a central role in cancer growth. Several human HIF prolyl 4-hydroxylases have been identified. They show no clear sequence similarity to the collagen prolyl 4-hydroxylases, except for general conservation of the critical catalytic residues (Myllyharju, 2003). Similar to collagen prolyl 4-hydroxylases, HIF prolyl 4-hydroxylase activity in cells is regulated by ascorbate under normoxic conditions (Knowles et al., 2003; Myllyharju, 2003; Bruick and McKnight, 2001).

Trimethyllysine Hydroxylase and γ-Butyrobetaine Hydroxylase

Ascorbic acid participates in two hydroxylation reactions that are part of the pathway for carnitine synthesis. L-Carnitine, a zwitterionic quaternary amino acid, is required as part of fatty acid metabolism for formation of acyl carnitine derivatives (Rebouche, 1991; Englard and Seifter, 1986). Acylcarnitines are needed for transport of long-chain fatty acids into mitochondria for subsequent oxidation and ATP formation, as described in Chapter 16 (see Fig. 16-9). Carnitine palmitoyltransferase and carnitine palmitoylcarnitine translocase also can be involved in the disposal of short-chain organic acids from mitochondria, particularly

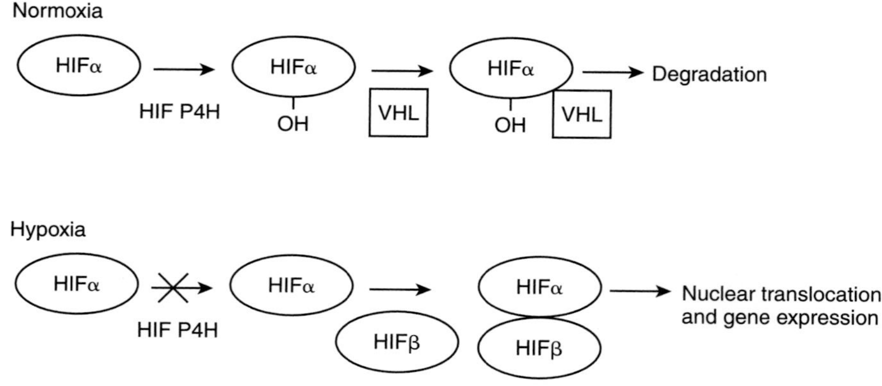

Figure 27-8 Regulation of the hypoxia inducible transcription factor HIFα by oxygen dependent prolyl 4 hydroxylation. With normoxia [*upper panel*], HIFα can undergo prolyl 4 hydroxylation by HIF prolyl 4 hydroxylases (HIF P4H). Hydroxylation is necessary for subsequent binding of the von Hippel Lindau (VHL) E3 ubiquitin ligase complex, which results in proteosomal degradation. With hypoxia, there is no prolyl hydroxylation [lower panel]. In this case HIFα is not degraded and instead forms a stable dimer with HIFβ. This dimer is then translocated into the nucleus, where it binds to HIF-responsive elements and induces expression of hypoxia-inducible genes. *(Modified from Myllyharju J [2003] Prolyl 4-hydroxylases, the key enzymes of collage biosynthesis. Matrix Biol 22:15-24.)*

when blocks in the complete metabolism of these organic acids are present. The formation of acylcarnitines presumably helps maintain a supply of nonesterified coenzyme A.

Human needs for carnitine are met by dietary intake and by synthesis from amino acid precursors. Dietary sources of carnitine include poultry, meat, fish, and dairy products. Free carnitine is absorbed almost completely. Carnitine is synthesized de novo from the essential amino acids lysine and methionine. The proportion of total carnitine accounted for by de novo synthesis is dependent on many factors, especially dietary carnitine and the coexistence of disease states such as renal failure, diabetes mellitus, malignancy, alcohol abuse, and myocardial ischemia.

In the pathway for de novo carnitine synthesis, the 4-carbon chain of carnitine is derived from carbons 3 to 6 of lysine, and the methyl groups of carnitine are provided by *S*-adenosylmethionine (Fig. 27-9). In mammals, certain peptide-bound lysine residues are methylated by protein-lysyl methyltransferases that use *S*-adenosylmethionine as the methyl donor. The methylated product is a 6-*N*-trimethyllysyl residue, and this residue has been found in calmodulin, histones, myosin, and cytochrome c. 6-*N*-Trimethyllysine released by proteolytic cleavage undergoes a four-step reaction sequence to form carnitine. The first reaction is a hydroxylation resulting in β-hydroxy-*N*-trimethyllysine and is mediated by trimethyllysine hydroxylase. In the second reaction, glycine is released with formation of γ-trimethylaminobutyraldehyde. This substrate undergoes dehydrogenation in the third reaction to form γ-butyrobetaine. In the fourth reaction, γ-butyrobetaine is hydroxylated by γ-butyrobetaine hydroxylase, with carnitine as the product (Rebouche, 1991; Englard and Seifter, 1986; Dunn et al., 1984).

The two hydroxylation reactions in the carnitine synthesis pathway are catalyzed by dioxygenases that require iron, α-ketoglutarate, and a reductant (Dunn et al., 1984). The best reductant in vitro is ascorbate. Of the two enzymes, γ-butyrobetaine hydroxylase has been studied more extensively. Its K_m for ascorbate is approximately 5 mmol/L (Englard and Seifter, 1986). It is likely that the mechanism of ascorbate action is to reduce iron, which is oxidized nonstoichiometrically over the course of repeated reactions, as occurs for prolyl and lysyl hydroxylases (Englard and Seifter, 1986).

Although the two enzyme activities for carnitine biosynthesis are most active in vitro

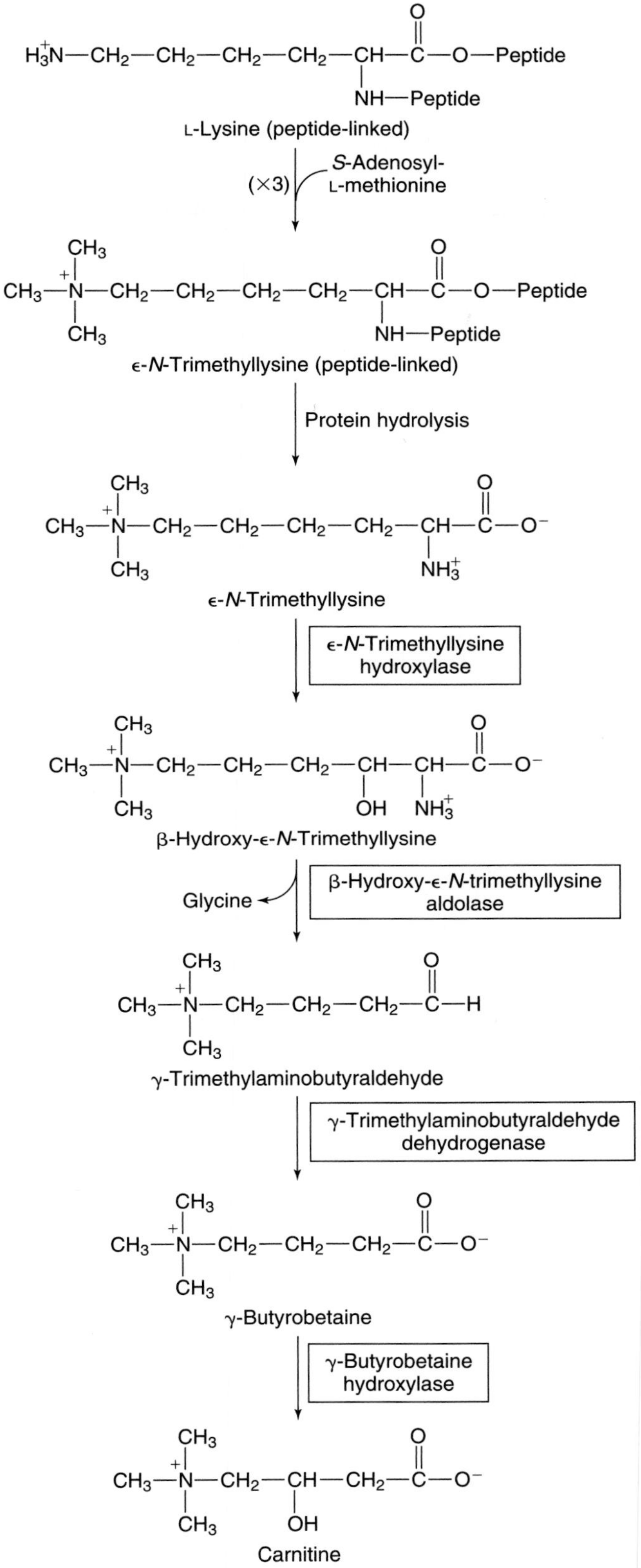

$H_3\overset{+}{N}{-}CH_2{-}CH_2{-}CH_2{-}CH_2{-}CH(NH{-}Peptide){-}C(=O){-}O{-}Peptide$

L-Lysine (peptide-linked)

↓ (×3) *S*-Adenosyl-L-methionine

$(CH_3)_3\overset{+}{N}{-}CH_2{-}CH_2{-}CH_2{-}CH_2{-}CH(NH{-}Peptide){-}C(=O){-}O{-}Peptide$

ε-*N*-Trimethyllysine (peptide-linked)

↓ Protein hydrolysis

$(CH_3)_3\overset{+}{N}{-}CH_2{-}CH_2{-}CH_2{-}CH_2{-}CH(NH_3^+){-}C(=O){-}O^-$

ε-*N*-Trimethyllysine

↓ ε-*N*-Trimethyllysine hydroxylase

$(CH_3)_3\overset{+}{N}{-}CH_2{-}CH_2{-}CH_2{-}CH(OH){-}CH(NH_3^+){-}C(=O){-}O^-$

β-Hydroxy-ε-*N*-Trimethyllysine

↓ β-Hydroxy-ε-*N*-trimethyllysine aldolase (→ Glycine)

$(CH_3)_3\overset{+}{N}{-}CH_2{-}CH_2{-}CH_2{-}C(=O){-}H$

γ-Trimethylaminobutyraldehyde

↓ γ-Trimethylaminobutyraldehyde dehydrogenase

$(CH_3)_3\overset{+}{N}{-}CH_2{-}CH_2{-}CH_2{-}C(=O){-}O^-$

γ-Butyrobetaine

↓ γ-Butyrobetaine hydroxylase

$(CH_3)_3\overset{+}{N}{-}CH_2{-}CH(OH){-}CH_2{-}C(=O){-}O^-$

Carnitine

Figure 27-9 Pathway of carnitine biosynthesis in mammals. Trimethyllysine hydroxylase and γ-butyrobetaine hydroxylase are the enzymes that utilize ascorbate (AA). *(Redrawn from Rebouche CJ [1991] Ascorbic acid and carnitine biosynthesis. Am J Clin Nutr 54:1147S-1152S.)*

with ascorbate as a reductant, the effects of ascorbate on carnitine biosynthesis in vivo are more complex and confusing (Rebouche, 1991; Englard and Seifter, 1986). In guinea pigs, ascorbate deficiency results in a variable decrease in the carnitine content of several tissues. Ascorbate-deficient guinea pigs have decreased activity of liver γ-butyrobetaine hydroxylase that can be restored by ascorbate injection (Dunn et al., 1984). Ascorbate deficiency decreases the activity of trimethyllysine hydroxylase in kidney but not liver.

The second ascorbic-acid–dependent step, hydroxylation of γ-butyrobetaine, occurs primarily in liver and kidney. γ-Butyrobetaine hydroxylase activity in liver would be expected to be decreased in ascorbate deficiency, because the hepatic ascorbate concentration in deficient animals falls to less than 20% of that of normal animals. However, there is probably a great excess of γ-butyrobetaine hydroxylase in liver and/or kidney because carnitine excretion can be increased by about 30-fold when γ-butyrobetaine is provided in the diet. Therefore, the activity of γ-butyrobetaine hydroxylase is not likely to limit carnitine synthesis in vivo unless ascorbate deficiency is extremely severe.

The effect of ascorbate deficiency on substrate utilization for carnitine biosynthesis is difficult to study in mammals because the precursor trimethyllysine is not transported from extracellular fluid into tissues. For any given tissue, the likely substrate for trimethyllysine hydroxylase is trimethyllysine synthesized within that particular tissue. The major site in animals for the initial steps, at least, in the conversion of trimethyllysine to carnitine is probably skeletal muscle, because this site is the major reservoir for free and peptide-bound trimethyllysine.

Furthermore, with vitamin C deficiency, it is unknown what percentage of carnitine deficiency is due to decreased biosynthesis versus increased urinary excretion. Results from guinea pig and human experiments indicate that vitamin C depletion has complex effects on carnitine biology in vivo (Johnston, 1999; Jacob and Pianalto, 1997; Johnston et al, 1996; Rebouche, 1995). In vitamin C–deficient guinea pigs, excessive urinary excretion of carnitine contributes to carnitine depletion. When vitamin C–deficient guinea pigs were provided with excess substrate as trimethyllysine or γ-butyrobetaine, their rate of carnitine synthesis was restored nearly to normal. (These data also indicate that there is excess capacity for carnitine synthesis, which is dependent on precursor availability.) Urinary carnitine excretion also increased in humans who were made vitamin C–deficient (Jacob and Pianalto, 1997).

Human experimentation has been difficult because carnitine is present in many foods and carnitine-containing foods have not been restricted in most clinical experiments done to date. Plasma carnitine values are not reliable indicators of carnitine status (Jacob and Pianalto, 1997; Johnston et al., 1996). One of the first clinical effects of vitamin C deprivation is fatigue (Levine et al., 2001; Levine et al., 1996; Crandon et al., 1940; Lind, 1753). Investigators have assumed that the mechanism of fatigue in scurvy is in part due to decreased carnitine biosynthesis or increased carnitine excretion. Decreased carnitine synthesis could lead to decreased oxidation of fatty acids in muscle and liver, with fatigue as a consequence. However, it is still not clear whether carnitine deficiency is the underlying explanation of the fatigue that occurs in patients with scurvy.

4-Hydroxyphenylpyruvate Dioxygenase

As part of tyrosine catabolism, 4-hydroxyphenylpyruvate dioxygenase catalyzes conversion of 4-hydroxyphenylpyruvate to homogentisate (Moran, 2005). The enzyme uses molecular oxygen to catalyze coupled oxidations. In the first oxidation, one oxygen atom is utilized for oxidative decarboxylation of the pyruvyl moiety, with formation of an acetyl moiety. The second oxygen atom is incorporated into a hydroxyl group replacing the acetyl group, which is shifted to the adjacent carbon (Lindblad et al., 1970) (Fig. 27-10). This latter reaction mechanism is sometimes called the "NIH shift" because it was first characterized by scientists at the National Institutes of Health. Hydroxyphenylpyruvate dioxygenase has been isolated from bacteria and animals, including humans. It appears to be a true dioxygenase and is similar to other keto acid–dependent

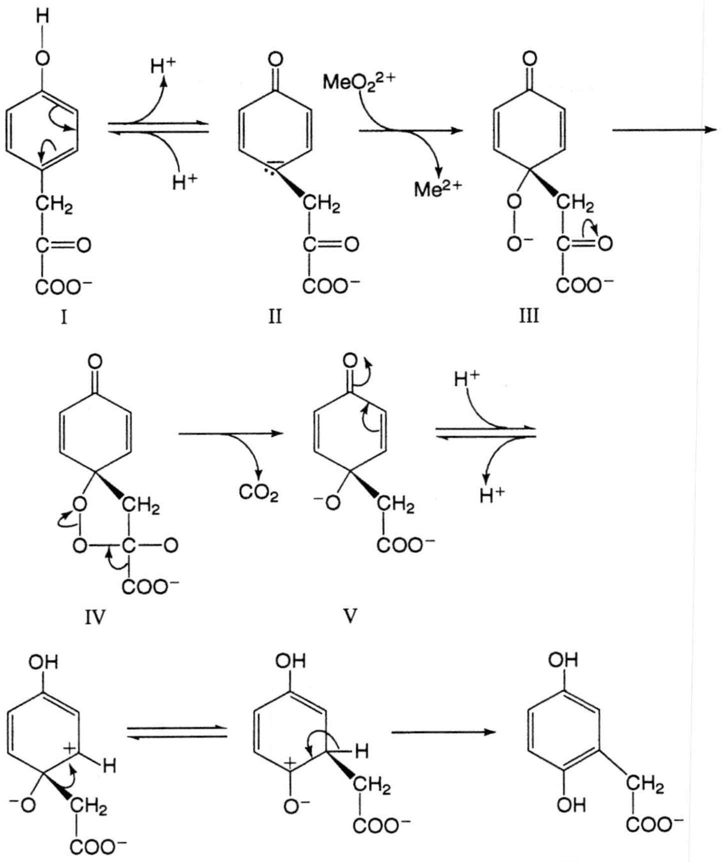

Figure 27-10 Proposed reaction mechanism for the enzymatic formation of homogentisate from *p*-hydroxyphenylpyruvate. The reaction of intermediate VI to VII represents the "NIH shift," and Me stands for metal (probably Fe^{2+}). (*Redrawn from Lindblad B, Lindstedt G, Lindstedt S [1970] The mechanism of enzymic formation of homogentisate from p-hydroxyphenylpyruvate. J Am Chem Soc 92:7446-7249. Copyright 1970 American Chemical Society.*)

dioxygenases, such as the α-ketoglutarate-dependent dioxygenases described previously that are involved in prolyl and lysyl hydroxylation and carnitine synthesis. However, in the hydroxyphenylpyruvate reaction the "α-keto acid" is part of the same molecule that is hydroxylated (Englard and Seifter, 1986). Iron is required by 4-hydroxyphenylpyruvate dioxygenase, and iron chelators decrease enzyme activity.

Ascorbate is utilized by hydroxyphenylpyruvate dioxygenase as a reducing agent (Lindblad et al., 1970). However, it is not certain whether the requirement for a reducing agent is similar to that of the collagen-synthesizing enzymes, described in the preceding text, where ascorbic acid reduces enzyme-bound iron that is oxidized in an uncoupled reaction. The stoichiometry for homogentisate formation and ascorbate consumption is not apparent. In addition, other reducing agents are effective in vitro for enzyme activity.

Animal studies and clinical trials support a relationship between ascorbate deficiency and tyrosine metabolism (Englard and Seifter, 1986; Levine et al., 1941). Scorbutic guinea pigs have excess tyrosine in the circulation (tyrosinemia) and excrete 4-hydroxyphenylpyruvate.

Premature human infants display the same pattern. In both guinea pigs and premature infants, ascorbate administration eliminates tyrosinemia and hydroxyphenylpyruvate excretion. Nevertheless, it remains possible that the effect of ascorbate is indirect (Englard and Seifter, 1986). In studies with enzyme isolated from bacteria, the enol form of 4-hydroxyphenylpyruvate is a noncompetitive inhibitor of hydroxyphenylpyruvate dioxygenase. Inhibition is relieved by ascorbate and other reducing agents. It is possible that enol-hydroxyphenylpyruvate interacts with enzyme-bound autoxidized iron, resulting in enzyme inhibition. Ascorbate could keep iron in its reduced form, thereby preventing inhibition. If this were the case, the mechanism of ascorbate action on homogentisate formation would be indirect.

NONENZYMATIC FUNCTIONS

VITAMIN C AS AN ANTIOXIDANT

Because it is an electron donor, vitamin C may also have nonenzymatic reductive functions (Table 27-1). Studies done in vitro suggest that vitamin C may have a role as a chemical reducing agent within cells and outside cells. In theory, these reactions may involve either sequential electron transfer from ascorbate, with ascorbyl radical formation as an intermediate, or simultaneous two electron loss, forming dehydroascorbic acid with no intermediate. Reactions involving metal intermediates, especially iron and copper, almost certainly proceed via ascorbyl radical formation.

Table 27-1
Vitamin C: Nonenzymatic Antioxidant/Prooxidant Functions

	Antioxidant Function
Site/Evidence	**Action**
KNOWN	
Human stomach	Prevention of formation of *N*-nitroso compounds
Human small intestine	Promotion of iron absorption
POSSIBLE	
Intracellular/studies done in vivo	DNA transcription (gene expression)
	mRNA stability and translation
	Prevention of protein oxidation
	Tetrahydrobiopterin stabilization
	Regulation of apoptosis
Extracellular/studies done in vitro	Quenching of aqueous peroxyl radicals and lipid peroxidation products
	Decrease in monocyte adhesion and platelet aggregation
	Quenching of reactive oxygen species generated by cells
Human plasma	Quenching of aqueous peroxyl radicals and lipid peroxidation products
	Prevention of LDL oxidation
	Conjugation of electrophilic lipid peroxidation products
	Prooxidant Function
Site/Evidence	**Action**
POSSIBLE	
Human cell nuclei	Mutagenesis (DNA damage)
Lipid hydroperoxides/studies done in vitro	Lipid peroxidation, causing DNA damage
Cell membrane, cell cytosol/studies done in vitro	Cell damage

DNA, Deoxyribonucleic acid; *LDL*, low-density lipoprotein; *RNA*, ribonucleic acid.

Intracellular Functions

Vitamin C achieves millimolar concentrations in many tissues and under physiological conditions is an excellent reducing agent as discussed in the preceding text. Independent of enzymatic function, its role has been studied as an intracellular electron donor in the following reaction types: DNA transcription, DNA repair, mRNA translation, protein stability, and apoptosis. Data show that vitamin C regulates gene transcription or mRNA stabilization for the following genes: collagen types I and III; elastin; acetylcholine receptor; fra-1; AP-1; some forms of cytochrome P-450; tyrosine hydroxylase; collagen integrins; and some ubiquitins (Arrigoni and De Tullio, 2002). Mechanisms of these effects are controversial. For example, the effect on collagen gene transcription and/or acetylcholine receptor may occur in vitro but not in vivo, and may be a consequence of vitamin C–mediated generation of lipid hydroperoxides in cell culture media (Houglum et al., 1991). DNA damage as a result of oxidative metabolism has been postulated to be a contributor to aging, cancer, and other degenerative diseases (Ames et al., 1995). Oxidant damage is repaired efficiently by DNA repair enzymes, but they do not repair all lesions. Other antioxidant defenses include proteins, lipid-soluble antioxidants, and vitamin C. It is controversial whether vitamin C specifically protects against oxidant-damaged DNA in vitro, or actually has prooxidant properties as discussed in subsequent text. Vitamin C may regulate translation of some specific mRNAs such as that for ferritin (Toth and Bridges, 1995). Vitamin C chemically stabilizes intracellular tetrahydrobiopterin and can enhance endothelial nitric oxide synthesis (Heller et al., 2001). As a posttranslational action, vitamin C has been proposed to prevent intracellular protein oxidation (Stadtman, 2004). Protection conferred by vitamin C could be significant in tissues with high oxidant production and/or oxygen concentration, such as neutrophils, monocytes, macrophages, lung, and eye tissues that have substantial light exposure (Padayatty et al., 2003). Vitamin C was able to inhibit cell death via apoptosis in some myeloid cells (Perez-Cruz et al., 2003), but other reports indicate vitamin C induces apoptosis (Park et al., 2004)

Extracellular Functions

Extracellular vitamin C could protect against oxidants and oxidant-mediated damage. In vitro studies imply that vitamin C could be the primary antioxidant in plasma for quenching aqueous peroxyl radicals as well as lipid peroxidation products (Polidori et al., 2004; Carr and Frei, 1999). Vitamin C in vitro is oxidized before other plasma antioxidants, including uric acid, tocopherols, and bilirubin. As expected, in vitro data show that vitamin C is a potent water soluble antioxidant in biological systems, perhaps as a consequence of the relative stability of the intermediate ascorbyl radical under physiological conditions.

As shown in vitro, extracellular vitamin C affects several pathways involved in atherogenesis. Vitamin C can decrease lipid peroxidation and protect extracellular low density lipoprotein (LDL) from metal catalyzed oxidation (Polidori et al., 2004; Carr and Frei, 1999; Jialal and Fuller, 1995) As described in the oxidative modification hypothesis, oxidized LDL has been proposed to be an initiating factor in atherogenesis (Steinberg, 2002). Metal catalyzed LDL oxidation in vitro is inhibited at vitamin C concentrations greater than 40 μmol/L (Carr and Frei, 1999; Jialal and Fuller, 1995). As an aqueous antioxidant, vitamin C can regenerate lipid soluble α-tocopherol (vitamin E) when it is oxidized in liposomes (Niki, 1987). Because LDL oxidation in vitro is also prevented by tocopherol (Jialal and Fuller, 1995), reduction of membrane oxidized tocopherol by aqueous vitamin C was hypothesized to play a pivotal role in preventing atherosclerosis. Animal and clinical evidence has not supported this relationship between tocopherol and vitamin C (Burton et al., 1990), perhaps because tocopherol reduction is maximal at very low vitamin C concentrations (Jacob et al., 1996).

As an antioxidant, extracellular vitamin C could have other effects. Adhesion of monocytes to endothelium and aggregation of platelets and leukocytes are decreased by vitamin C (Lehr et al., 1997). Extracellular vitamin C may quench oxidants that leak from activated neutrophils (Wang et al., 1997) or macrophages that may otherwise damage surrounding fibroblasts and collagen (Mukhopadhyay and Chatterjee, 1994). Vitamin C has recently been described to act as a nucleophile, forming conjugates with electrophilic lipid peroxidation products that were detected in human plasma (Sowell et al., 2004). This phenomenon, vitamin C conjugation or ascorbylation, may be a pathway to eliminate harmful lipid peroxidation products.

Nonenzymatic Functions of Vitamin C: Interpret Carefully

Antioxidant effects demonstrated in vitro do not automatically confer relevance in vivo for several reasons (Padayatty et al., 2003). Reaction specificity is a primary reason. Vitamin C–dependent antioxidant reactions may not be specific for vitamin C as an antioxidant, either in vitro or in vivo. Other potent antioxidants are present in cells; glutathione is present at higher concentrations than vitamin C and may have similar effects. In addition, the type or concentration of the oxidant selected for use in vitro, the presence of metals or other contaminants in vitro, and other aspects of the experimental conditions may not accurately mimic the conditions in vivo. For example, metals may be present in trace amounts as contaminants in cell culture media and thereby initiate oxidation, whereas metals are tightly bound to proteins and may not be available as vitamin C oxidizers in vivo.

Standard culture media do not contain vitamin C, because it is labile and oxidizes within 24 hours even when added. For this reason, cultured cells lack vitamin C unless the cells are primary cells that are freshly isolated or the culture media is regularly supplemented with freshly prepared vitamin C. For experimental simplicity, effects of intracellular vitamin C on cellular events are usually tested in cells cultured either with or without vitamin C addition. However, this often has little physiological meaning because in vivo, even in the presence of severe deficiency, most cells still contain vitamin C, as a consequence of the transport mechanisms described previously. Therefore, it would be more appropriate to the in vivo situation if comparisons were made between cells that have either low or high intracellular concentrations of vitamin C, but this has not usually been done.

Finally, extracellular and intracellular antioxidant actions of vitamin C must ultimately be considered from a clinical point of view. Unfortunately, there is little or no human evidence to date supporting clinical utility of vitamin C as an antioxidant (Padayatty et al., 2003).

Actions in Stomach and Duodenum

Vitamin C is secreted into gastric juice, where concentrations are about three times higher than those of plasma in healthy people (Rathbone et al., 1989). Vitamin C concentrations are lower in gastric juice of patients with gastric cancer, and for this reason it was hoped that vitamin C would be useful in preventing this serious cancer (Correa, 1992). A large epidemiological study indicated that vitamin C supplement use was not related in incidence of death from stomach cancer (Jacobs et al., 2002), although a smaller case control study suggested there was a protective relationship (Mayne et al., 2001).

Vitamin C quenches reactive oxygen metabolites in the stomach and duodenum and prevents formation of mutagenic *N*-nitroso compounds. Foods high in vitamin C reduce formation of nitrosamines in the gastrointestinal tract; this effect may be due to vitamin C itself or to other components of the food. It is uncertain whether reducing nitroso compounds has clinical benefit (Helser et al., 1992). Reduced risk of gastric and other cancers is correlated with high vitamin C dietary intake, meaning from foods (Mayne et al., 2001). However, it is unknown whether the protective effect is due to vitamin C itself or to other components in plant-derived foods that happen to contain vitamin C. Therefore, it is uncertain whether antioxidant action of vitamin C is important in vivo for preventing gastric cancer. What is clearly important is consumption of a variety of fruits and vegetables.

Iron Absorption

In the small intestine, vitamin C increases absorption of iron, probably by keeping it reduced (Fe^{2+}). Vitamin C increases soluble nonorganic iron absorption by 1.5- to 10-fold, depending on iron status, vitamin C dose, and the test meal studied. Amounts of vitamin C that enhance iron absorption are 20 to 60 mg, amounts commonly found in foods that are good sources of the vitamin (Hallberg, 1995). Vitamin C supplementation increased iron absorption in most studies (Hallberg, 1995). The final clinical outcome of increasing iron is to increase hemoglobin in anemic patients. The effect of vitamin C was modest on raising hemoglobin concentration, at least in the short term (Cook and Reddy, 2001). Nevertheless, vitamin C supplements are used clinically to increase iron absorption, especially in pregnancy, and should be avoided in patients with iron overload.

POTENTIAL FUNCTIONS AS A PROOXIDANT

Vitamin C as a cofactor or cosubstrate with enzymes has specific actions as a required electron donor. Vitamin C at physiological concentrations does not have prooxidant actions in healthy people (Levine et al., 2001). In vitro, vitamin C can behave as a prooxidant with pharmacological concentrations, which are achieved in humans only by intravenous administration (Padayatty et al., 2004; Clement et al., 2001). In vivo, pharmacological concentrations of vitamin C might produce prooxidant effects via the ascorbyl radical (Padayatty et al., 2004). It is also possible that nonspecific, nonenzymatic reduction of substrates by vitamin C can produce prooxidant compounds. Vitamin C has been shown to have prooxidant actions in vitro, either by decomposition of lipid hydroperoxides or by increasing 8-oxo-adenine in DNA (Chen et al., 2005; Lee et al., 2001; Podmore et al., 1998). Potential prooxidant properties of physiological and especially pharmacological concentrations of vitamin C require further study.

ASCORBATE FUNCTION AND TISSUE DISTRIBUTION

Based on the enzymology presented earlier, functions of ascorbate are reasonably clear in some tissues, such as adrenal medulla, pituitary, fibroblasts, osteoblasts, and chondrocytes. For other tissues or cells that concentrate ascorbate, potential roles of ascorbate have been suggested but not proved. These sites include neutrophils, monocytes/macrophages, lens, retina, cornea, peripheral and central neurons, liver, and endothelial cells. Still other tissues or cells, such as lymphocytes, platelets, pancreas, spleen, adrenal cortex, testis, and ovary, contain millimolar concentrations of ascorbate but have no known specific functions of ascorbate.

Once foods are ingested and digested, vitamin C is absorbed in the small intestine and then enters the mesenteric vein and hepatic portal venous system. Some of the vitamin C in the portal blood passes directly through the liver sinusoidal system into the hepatic vein, and some is transported into hepatocytes before it is resecreted and leaves the liver via the hepatic vein. The circulating vitamin C distributes into the general circulation and extravascular space. Vitamin C is not bound to any proteins. The best evidence indicates that dehydroascorbic acid is found either in trace amounts or not all, except locally under oxidizing conditions as discussed in the preceding text. As noted in the section on transport, ascorbic acid is concentrated by many cells and tissues to concentrations greater than 1 mmol/L (Rumsey and Levine, 1998).

When vitamin C in blood reaches the kidneys, vitamin C is freely filtered through the glomeruli and is reabsorbed in the proximal convoluted renal tubule by SVCT1. When tubular uptake of ascorbate is saturated due to high concentrations of ascorbate in the luminal fluid, the excess vitamin C that has not been taken up by the tubular cells is excreted in urine.

ASCORBATE DEFICIENCY

Scurvy, which was not attributed to vitamin C deficiency until the twentieth century, was first described several thousand years ago. The Scottish physician James Lind noted in 1753 that the disease could be prevented by a diet with limes (Lind, 1753). The active protective compound, ascorbic acid, was isolated in 1932 by the laboratories of Albert Szent-Gyorgyi and Charles King (King and Waugh, 1932; Svirbely and Szent-Gyorgyi, 1932). Once the vitamin was identified, its deficiency state was studied more systematically. Based on data gathered during World War II, the British Medical Research Council concluded that healthy men have body stores of vitamin C that are adequate to prevent scurvy for at least 160 days when a diet devoid of vitamin C is consumed (Bartley et al., 1953). This early estimate is clearly incorrect, however, and the actual vitamin C intakes of the subjects were almost certainly higher than those calculated at the time of the study (Hodges, 1971).

Subsequently, two studies of the clinical manifestations of severe vitamin C deficiency were conducted in prisoners housed in a metabolic ward (Baker et al., 1971; Baker et al., 1969). In the first study, other nutrients in addition to vitamin C were probably absent from the diet. This problem was corrected in the second study, and the symptoms and signs of scurvy are based on findings from this latter study of five men. Symptoms are what the patient tells the physician subjectively and signs are what the physician finds objectively on examination. The first sign of scurvy was petechial hemorrhage, or small areas of bleeding under the skin. Other signs included coiled hairs, bleeding gums, ecchymoses (larger areas of bleeding under the skin), hyperkeratosis (increased skin cells around hair follicles), arthralgias (joint pain), joint effusions (abnormal amounts of fluid in joints), and shortness of breath. All five men developed the sicca syndrome, or Sjögren's syndrome, with symptoms of dry eyes, dry mouth, scaly skin, dental caries, and gum tenderness (Hood et al., 1970). These men also had evidence of hypochondriasis and depression on psychological tests (Baker et al., 1971; Hodges et al., 1971; Kinsman and Hood, 1971).

Fatigue is an important early symptom in vitamin C deficiency. Although fatigue was not described as a symptom of vitamin C deficiency in the second prisoner study, it was mentioned in the first study and in Lind's classic work (Lind, 1753). Fatigue was the first symptom experienced by a researcher who purposely gave himself scurvy to study the disease course (Crandon et al., 1940). In an inpatient study using a wide dose range at the National Institutes of Health, which is described in more detail in subsequent text, healthy volunteers were made vitamin C–deficient but did not develop signs of scurvy. The majority of subjects had fatigue as their only symptom (Levine et al., 1996). Fatigue was reversed when plasma concentrations exceeded 20 μmol/L of ascorbate. Taken together, the findings show that fatigue is the first symptom of vitamin C deficiency and precedes all other symptoms and signs. A simple mnemonic to remember signs and symptoms of scurvy is "EFGH," representing ecchymoses, fatigue, gum bleeding and tenderness, and hyperkeratosis.

Overt vitamin C deficiency in the United States today is seen in malnourished populations, including those with cancer cachexia, poor intake, malabsorption, alcoholism, or chemical dependency. Because a substantial fraction of the population ingests less than one serving of fruit or vegetable daily, subclinical vitamin C deficiency may be much more common than overt deficiency. It may be much more difficult for health professionals to recognize because its only symptom, fatigue, is nonspecific and has myriad causes.

ADVERSE EFFECTS OF EXCESS VITAMIN C

As much as 400 mg daily of vitamin C can be consumed from food sources rich in this vitamin. Higher doses can be obtained only from supplements. Whether vitamin C supplements have benefit is controversial (Padayatty et al., 2003). However, doses from 400 mg to 1 g are generally safe and well tolerated. There is general acceptance that doses up to 1 or 2 g are safe in healthy people, although patients with hyperoxaluria may be at risk. Higher doses may produce other side effects, especially gastrointestinal ones (Levine et al., 1999; Cameron and Campbell, 1974). Adverse effects of excess vitamin C on various organ systems have been described. Other adverse effects and potential harms are usually patient population specific.

STOMACH AND INTESTINES

At doses of less than 2 g, vitamin C usually does not cause gastrointestinal side effects. Ingestion of 3 to 5 g as a single dose causes bloating and diarrhea in some people (Levine et al., 1999; Cameron and Campbell, 1974). As described previously, vitamin C promotes iron absorption from the small intestine. In theory, long-term vitamin C use could increases risk of iron overload in susceptible patients (Gerster, 1999), such as those with hemochromatosis, thalassemia major, sickle cell disease, sideroblastic anemia, and those who require frequent red blood cell transfusions. Patients with these conditions should not take large doses of vitamin C, but they should not avoid eating fruits and vegetables (Barton et al., 1998). In healthy subjects, intake of daily 2-g doses of vitamin C over a 1½-year period did not cause overabsorption of iron (Cook et al., 1984).

BLOOD

Glucose 6-phosphate dehydrogenase deficiency is an X-linked inherited disease that can cause hemolytic crises, sometimes precipitated as a consequence of oxidant stress. In subjects with glucose 6-phosphate dehydrogenase deficiency, hemolysis was a consequence of vitamin C given intravenously or as single oral doses greater than 6 g (Levine et al., 1999). Patients with glucose 6-phosphate dehydrogenase deficiency should avoid gram doses of vitamin C.

KIDNEY

Under certain conditions, vitamin C may increase excretion in urine of uric acid (hyperuricosuria) and oxalate (hyperoxaluria) (Levine et al., 1999). Hyperuricosuria can be induced by daily vitamin C doses of 3 g but does not occur at doses of less than 1 g (Levine et al., 1999). In some healthy subjects, oxalate excretion may increase at daily doses of 1 g or more of vitamin C, with unknown clinical significance. In some subjects with known hyperoxaluria, vitamin C doses greater than 1 g increase oxalate excretion and might cause oxalate kidney stones. In healthy people who at study entry never had kidney stones, increased vitamin C consumption from food and supplements was not associated with kidney stone formation.

Patients with end-stage renal disease are often treated using hemodialysis, which is performed several times per week. Because hemodialysis removes vitamin C, many patients who receive this treatment have low plasma and tissue vitamin C concentrations and require supplementation. In patients with renal failure who received maintenance hemodialysis, excess blood oxalate (hyperoxalemia) was induced by repeated intravenous vitamin C doses of greater than 500 mg. Optimum vitamin C intake for patients with end-stage renal disease on dialysis is not known. The concern on the one hand is to prevent deficiency in the face of predictable losses from hemodialysis, and on the other hand to prevent hyperoxalemia. Vitamin C intake for patients treated with hemodialysis probably should not exceed 200 mg daily (Levine et al., 1999).

MISCELLANEOUS

Vitamin C, at doses of 250 mg and greater may cause false-negative results for stool occult blood with guaiac-based tests. Intake of vitamin C should be reduced to less than 250 mg for several days prior to such testing (Levine et al., 1999). Several harmful effects have been erroneously attributed to vitamin C. These include hypoglycemia, rebound scurvy, infertility, mutagenesis, and destruction of vitamin B_{12}. None of these, however, are in reality caused by vitamin C.

RECOMMENDED INGESTION

DIETARY REFERENCE INTAKES FOR VITAMIN C

The earliest recommendations for vitamin C intake of 10 mg daily were based on the studies conducted by the British Royal Air Force during World War II (Bartley et al., 1953). Recommendations derived from these studies were based on the estimated amount of vitamin C that was needed to prevent scurvy, with an added safety margin. When it was recognized that the Royal Air Force data probably underestimated vitamin C intake, depletion–repletion studies were conducted using prisoners in Iowa, as mentioned in the preceding text. Results of these studies were used to set the 1980 and 1989 recommended dietary allowance (RDA) of vitamin C at 60 mg daily, using three criteria (National Research Council, 1980, 1989; Baker et al., 1971; Hodges, 1971; Baker et al., 1969). First, a steady state intake of 60 mg daily was believed to be adequate to protect against signs and symptoms of scurvy for at least 1 month if vitamin C ingestion suddenly stopped. Second, a sharp increase in vitamin C excretion greater than flat basal values was believed to indicate that body stores were close to saturation. The dose at which increased excretion began was estimated to be 60 mg daily. Third, 60 mg daily was proposed to provide adequate body stores of vitamin C and to compensate for metabolic losses. Because these studies were done with male adult subjects, recommendations were extrapolated for women and across age ranges of both sexes.

Nevertheless, there were a number of limitations to the Iowa studies. There was poor precision in the vitamin C assay, especially at lower concentrations; a narrow dose range was used; data analyses were incomplete; and there were few subjects at the doses selected (Baker et al., 1971; Hodges et al., 1971). In one of the depletion–repletion studies, subjects were fed a diet that was deficient in more nutrients than just vitamin C (Baker et al., 1969). The conclusion that 60 mg daily would compensate for metabolic losses was based on data obtained in deficient patients (Hodges et al., 1971). Because vitamin C metabolism changes as a function of depletion or repletion, use of data from deficient subjects to calculate metabolism for the general population is questionable. Perhaps most important, the 1980 and 1989 RDAs were based on the amount needed to prevent deficiency and not on a functional measure of vitamin status or on the amount needed to maintain optimal health (Levine, 1986). Indeed, at that time vitamin function was not considered as a basis for establishing RDAs for any of the vitamins.

In establishing the dietary reference intakes (DRIs) for vitamin C, the Institute of Medicine (IOM) included consideration of functional data in setting the DRIs and also based recommendations on the newly published depletion–repletion data from studies conducted at the National Institutes of Health. Data from healthy men (Levine et al., 1996) were used to determine the DRIs for vitamin C (IOM, 2000), and data from healthy women were published subsequently (Levine et al., 2001). Data from both men and women provided comprehensive concentration and pharmacokinetic data over a wide dose range (Levine et al., 2001; Graumlich et al., 1997; Levine et al., 1996). Both male and female subjects consumed a diet that was deficient in only vitamin C, without any other nutrient deficiencies. Subjects were vitamin C–depleted in approximately 4 weeks on this diet, and then were repleted stepwise, with vitamin C administered so that accurate pharmacokinetics could be determined at every dose. Steady-state fasting plasma concentrations were defined for each of seven doses, which ranged from 30 to 2,500 mg daily. At steady state for each dose, vitamin C concentrations were determined in circulating cells, vitamin C excretion in urine was measured, and bioavailability was determined.

The IOM set estimated average requirement (EAR) values for vitamin C based on neutrophil vitamin C concentrations in men (Levine et al., 1996); putative vitamin C antioxidant action in neutrophils (Anderson and Lukey, 1987; Halliwell et al., 1987); and urinary vitamin C excretion in men (Levine et al., 1996). Neutrophils accumulate vitamin C against a concentration gradient, and such accumulation is more avid in the presence of extracellular oxidants, when it is also mediated by ascorbate recycling as described earlier (Wang et al., 1997). Extracellular vitamin C may protect neutrophils from oxidants, and protection was assumed to be dependent on vitamin C accumulated intracellularly. An EAR was selected to achieve near-maximal neutrophil vitamin C concentration for oxidant protection, while at the same time minimizing urinary loss of vitamin C. Oxidant protection of neutrophils by vitamin C in vitro has been shown, using superoxide-mediated lucigenin-enhanced chemiluminescence in neutrophils activated with cytochalasin B and *N*-formyl-methionyl-leucyl-phenylalanine (Anderson et al., 1987; Anderson and Lukey, 1987).

The plasma and neutrophil vitamin C concentrations obtained from the NIH depletion–repletion study in seven healthy young men (Levine et al., 1996) are shown in Figures 27-11 and 27-12. At the 100-mg oral vitamin C dose, mean neutrophil vitamin C concentrations

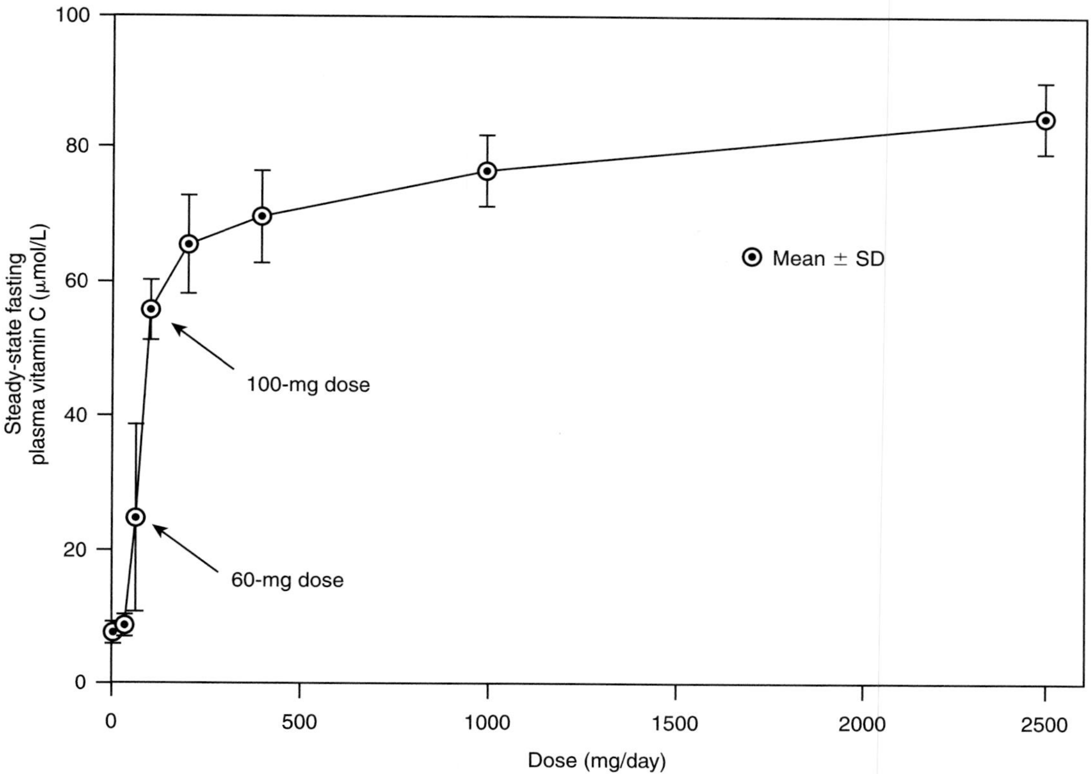

Figure 27-11 Steady-state fasting plasma vitamin C concentrations (mean ± SD) as a function of dose for 7 healthy men. Volunteers (ages 20-26 years) were studied as inpatients (study duration 146 ± 23 days, mean ± SD) and consumed a vitamin C deficient diet throughout the study, resulting in plasma and tissue vitamin C depletion at the beginning of the study. Vitamin C in solution was then administered by mouth at the doses shown until steady state was reached for each dose. Plasma vitamin C concentrations achieved by 60 mg/day and 100 mg/day oral vitamin C are indicated in the figure. *(Data from Levine M, Conry-Cantilena C, Wang Y, Welch RW, Washko PW, Dhariwal KR, Park JB, Lazarev A, Graumlich JF, King J, Cantilena LR [1996] Vitamin C pharmacokinetics in healthy volunteers: evidence for a recommended dietary allowance. Proc Natl Acad Sci U S A 93:3704-3709.)*

were nearly at the saturation level [1.25 ± 0.12 mmol/L (mean ± SD)] and urinary loss of the dose of vitamin C was approximately 25% (Fig. 27-13). At a dose of 60 mg, neutrophil vitamin C concentrations were only 0.81 ± 0.2 mmol/L, and there was no urinary loss at a 50-mg dose (Levine et al., 1996). A dose that would achieve 80% neutrophil saturation was chosen by the IOM to provide antioxidant protection with minimal urinary loss. By regression analysis, the dose corresponding to 80% saturation was found to be approximately 75 mg (IOM, 2000). This value was selected as the EAR for adult males ages 19 to 50 years, and EARs for other age and sex groups were derived by extrapolation from this value based on relative body weights. The EAR for pregnant women was increased by an estimate of that needed to ensure adequate transfer of vitamin C to the fetus, and the EAR for lactating women was increased by the average amount secreted in the milk. RDAs were set as the EAR + 20%, with rounding. Therefore, the RDA for men is 90 mg (75 mg × 1.2) per day and that for women is 75 mg (60 mg × 1.2).

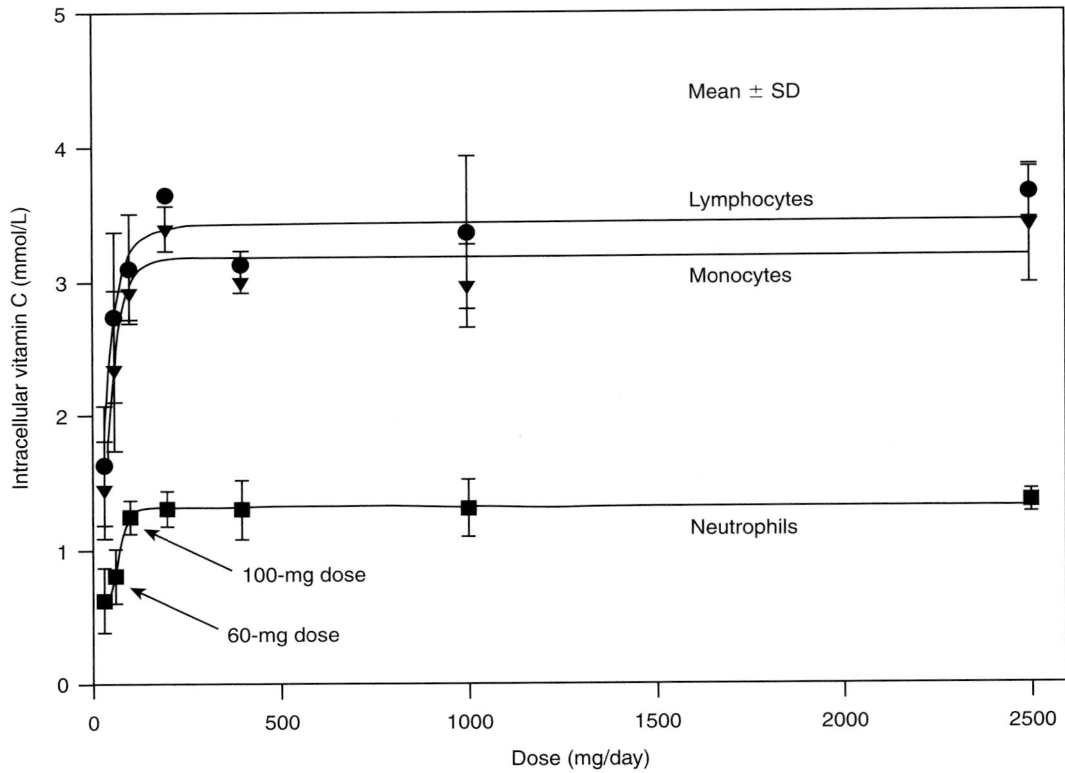

Figure 27-12 Intracellular vitamin C concentrations (mean ± SD) in circulating cells as a function of dose in 7 healthy men. Cells were isolated when steady-state was achieved for each dose. Note that neutrophil vitamin C concentrations did not increase appreciably after the 100 mg/day dose. Eighty percent neutrophil saturation was achieved between 60 mg/day and 100 mg/day dose, and the neutrophil vitamin C concentrations at these doses are indicated in the figure. *Closed squares,* neutrophils; *closed triangles,* monocytes; *closed circles,* lymphocytes. *(Data from Levine M, Conry-Cantilena C, Wang Y, Welch RW, Washko PW, Dhariwal KR, Park JB, Lazarev A, Graumlich JF, King J, Cantilena LR [1996] Vitamin C pharmacokinetics in healthy volunteers: evidence for a recommended dietary allowance. Proc Natl Acad Sci USA 93:3704-3709.)*

As for other nutrients, adequate intakes (AIs) were set for infants. That for infants up to 6 months of age was calculated as the average intake of vitamin C from human milk during the first 6 months of life (50 mg vitamin C per L milk × 0.78 L milk per day); the AI is 40 mg/day. For infants from 7 through 12 months of age, the AI is based on intake from human milk plus complementary foods and is 50 mg/day.

More recent data from depletion–repletion studies in 15 healthy young women suggest a higher EAR, and hence RDA, for vitamin C for women than that set by the IOM (Levine et al., 2001). As of this writing, these data have not been incorporated by the IOM into revised guidelines. An in depth analysis of the EAR and RDA values for vitamin C can be found elsewhere (Levine et al., 2004).

In the depletion–repletion studies used to calculate the EARs, the vitamin C dose was given as pure vitamin C in a solution that was administered in the fasting state. It is not known whether vitamin C in food sources is bioavailable to the same extent as pure vitamin C given during the fasting state. Therefore, the intake of vitamin C from foods may need to be higher than the present DRIs if the bioavailability of vitamin C from foods turns out to be less than that from the pure solutions used in the depletion–repletion studies.

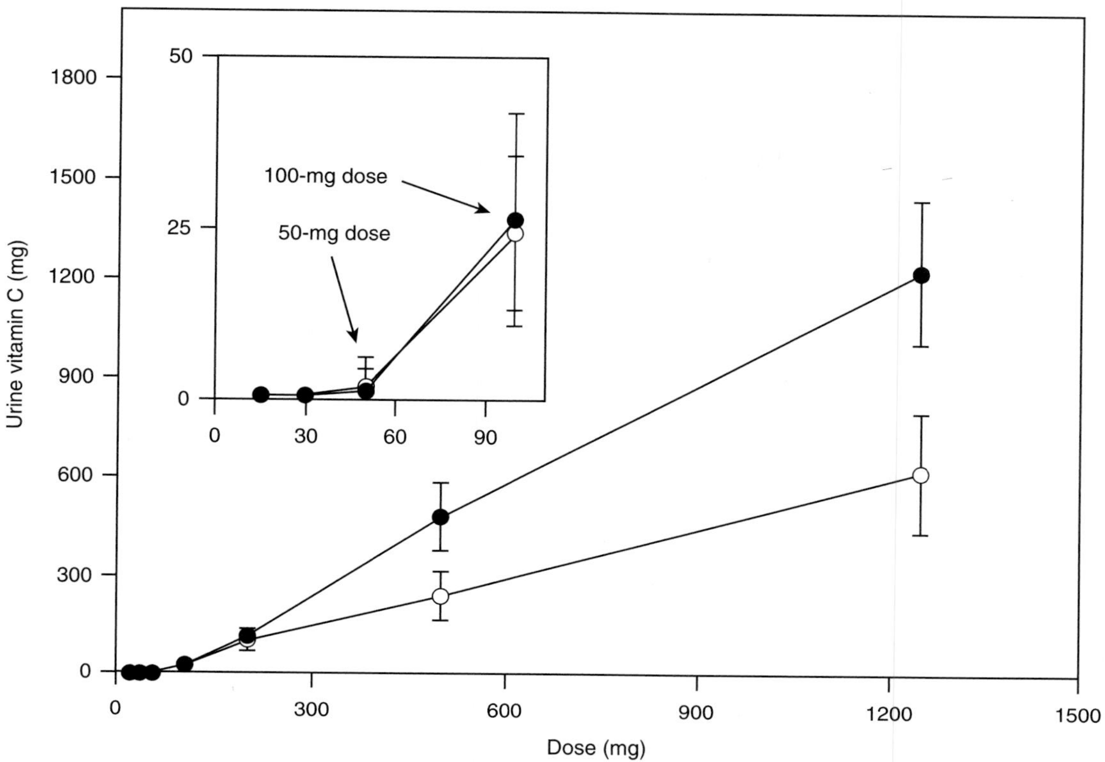

Figure 27-13 Urinary vitamin C excretion as a function of single vitamin C doses at steady-state. Vitamin C excretion over 24 hours was determined after administration of single doses given either orally *(open circles)* or intravenously *(filled circles)*. Data shown are mean values ± SD. *Inset*, Vitamin C excretion for single oral *(open circles)* or intravenous *(filled circles)* doses of 15 to 100 mg is shown enlarged for clarity. X-axis indicates dose (mg); Y-axis indicates amount (mg) excreted in urine in the 24 hours after a single dose of vitamin C. Note that approximately 25 mg of vitamin C is excreted in the urine at the 100-mg dose, while very little is excreted at the next lower dose of 50 mg. Urinary vitamin C excretion at the 50-mg and 100-mg vitamin C doses are indicated. (*Data from Levine M, Conry-Cantilena C, Wang Y, Welch RW, Washko PW, Dhariwal KR, Park JB, Lazarev A, Graumlich JF, King J, Cantilena LR [1996] Vitamin C pharmacokinetics in healthy volunteers: evidence for a recommended dietary allowance. Proc Natl Acad Sci USA 93:3704-3709.*)

Based on dietary intake data from NHANES III, 1988 to 1994, the median vitamin C intake from foods was about 100 mg/day for individuals in the United States; the 5th to 95th percentile range was 58 mg to 167 mg/day (IOM, 2000). When supplement use was included, median intake was estimated at 116 mg/day and the 5th- and 95th-percentile range was 61 mg to 430 mg/day. However, 14% of men and 10% of women had plasma vitamin C concentrations less than 11 µmol/L, which is close to deficiency. Other specific groups, such as smokers, also had lower values than the general population (Hampl et al., 2004).

BENEFITS OF FRUIT AND VEGETABLE INTAKE

Many studies have shown benefit associated with consumption of vitamin C–rich foods, meaning fruits and vegetables. Higher fruit and vegetable consumption and plasma vitamin C concentrations were inversely related to risk of acute myocardial infarction (heart attack), ischemic heart disease, angina pectoris, stroke, diabetic complications, blood

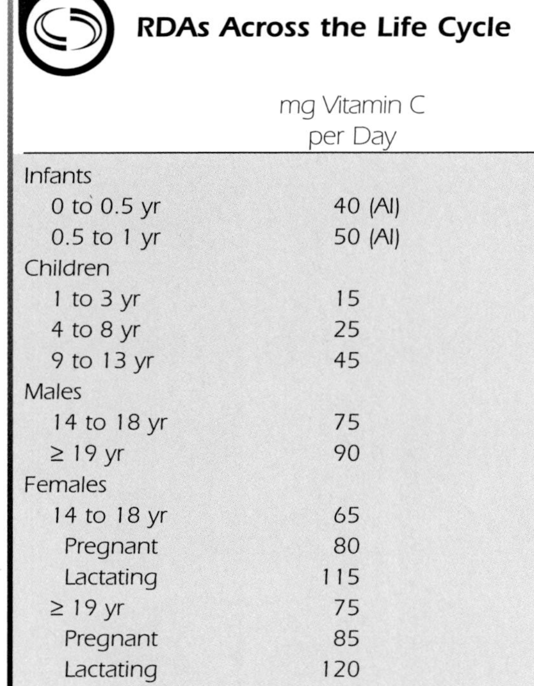

RDAs Across the Life Cycle

	mg Vitamin C per Day
Infants	
0 to 0.5 yr	40 (AI)
0.5 to 1 yr	50 (AI)
Children	
1 to 3 yr	15
4 to 8 yr	25
9 to 13 yr	45
Males	
14 to 18 yr	75
≥ 19 yr	90
Females	
14 to 18 yr	65
Pregnant	80
Lactating	115
≥ 19 yr	75
Pregnant	85
Lactating	120

Data from Institute of Medicine (IOM) (2000) Dietary Reference Intakes for Vitamin C, Vitamin E, Selenium, and Carotenoids. National Academy Press, Washington, DC. *AI*, Adequate intake.
NOTE: An additional intake of approximately 40 mg vitamin C per day is recommended for smokers.

pressure in hypertensive patients, and overall death (Voko et al., 2003; Gale et al., 2001; Khaw et al., 2001; Joshipura et al., 2001; Joshipura et al., 1999; Bates et al., 1998; Simon et al., 1998; Sahyoun et al., 1996). Intake of 200 mg or more vitamin C from fruits and vegetables was associated with lower risk of cancer (especially cancers of the oral cavity, esophagus, stomach, colon, and lung) (Key et al., 2004; Mayne et al., 2001; Ames et al., 1995; Byers and Guerrieri, 1995). These studies correlate fruit and vegetable intake with outcome. U.S. Department of Agriculture and National Cancer Institute recommendations that individuals consume at least five fruit and vegetable servings (at least 2½ cups of fruits and vegetables) daily are based on the extensive evidence of the potential benefits of such a diet (USDHHS/USDA, 2005). It is unknown whether benefits of fruits and vegetables are due to vitamin C itself, vitamin C plus other components of fruits and vegetables, or fruit and vegetable components independent of vitamin C (Khaw et al., 2001; Joshipura et al., 1999; Levine et al., 1999). Vitamin C may be only a surrogate marker for fruit and vegetable consumption or, perhaps, for other healthy lifestyle practices. Nevertheless, vitamin C–intake recommendations should be met by food intake, from fruits and vegetables. Intake of five or more varied fruits and vegetables will provide vitamin C intake of approximately 200 to 300 mg. Therefore, the best advice for obtaining adequate vitamin C and also optimizing health is to eat five or more varied servings daily of fresh fruits and vegetables.

UPPER LIMIT

The IOM set the tolerable upper intake level (UL) for vitamin C ingestion at 2 g daily, based on gastrointestinal intolerance at higher doses (IOM, 2000; Cameron and Campbell, 1974). There is no evidence for benefit of such doses and therefore no indications for such large oral doses exist.

REFERENCES

Ames BN, Gold LS, Willett WC (1995) The causes and prevention of cancer. Proc Natl Acad Sci USA 92:5258-5265.

Anderson R, Lukey PT (1987) A biological role for ascorbate in the selective neutralization of extracellular phagocyte-derived oxidants. Ann N Y Acad Sci 498:229-247.

Anderson R, Lukey PT, Theron AJ, Dippenaar U (1987) Ascorbate and cysteine-mediated selective neutralisation of extracellular oxidants during N-formyl peptide activation of human phagocytes. Agents Actions 20:77-86.

Arrigoni O, De Tullio MC (2002) Ascorbic acid: much more than just an antioxidant. Biochim Biophys Acta 1569:1-9.

Baker EM, Halver JE, Johnsen DO, Joyce BE, Knight MK, Tolbert BM (1975) Metabolism of ascorbic acid and ascorbic-2-sulfate in man and the subhuman primate. Ann N Y Acad Sci 258:72-80.

Baker EM, Hodges RE, Hood J, Sauberlich HE, March SC (1969) Metabolism of ascorbic-1-14C acid in experimental human scurvy. Am J Clin Nutr 22:549-558.

Baker EM, Hodges RE, Hood J, Sauberlich HE, March SC, Canham JE (1971) Metabolism of 14C- and 3H-labeled L-ascorbic acid in human scurvy. Am J Clin Nutr 24:444-454.

Bartley W, Krebs HA, O'Brien JRP (1953) Vitamin C requirement of human adults. Vol. 280. Medical Research Council, H.M. Stationery Office, London.

Barton JC, McDonnell SM, Adams PC, Brissot P, Powell LW, Edwards CQ, Cook JD, Kowdley KV (1998) Management of hemochromatosis. Hemochromatosis Management Working Group. Ann Intern Med 129:932-939.

Bates CJ, Walmsley CM, Prentice A, Finch S (1998) Does vitamin C reduce blood pressure? Results of a large study of people aged 65 or older. J Hypertens 16:925-932.

Bruick RK, McKnight SL (2001) A conserved family of prolyl-4-hydroxylases that modify HIF. Science 294:1337-1340.

Buettner GR, Moseley PL (1993) EPR spin trapping of free radicals produced by bleomycin and ascorbate. Free Radic Res Commun 19:S89-S93.

Burton GW, Wronska U, Stone L, Foster DO, Ingold KU (1990) Biokinetics of dietary RRR-alpha-tocopherol in the male guinea pig at three dietary levels of vitamin C and two levels of vitamin E. Evidence that vitamin C does not spare vitamin E in vivo. Lipids 25:199-210.

Byers R, Guerrieri N (1995) Epidemiologic evidence for vitamin C and vitamin E in cancer prevention. Am J Clin Nutr 62: 1385S-1392S.

Cameron E, Campbell A (1974) The orthomolecular treatment of cancer. II. Clinical trial of high-dose ascorbic acid supplements in advanced human cancer. Chem Biol Interact 9:285-315.

Carr AC, Frei B (1999) Toward a new recommended dietary allowance for vitamin C based on antioxidant and health effects in humans. Am J Clin Nutr 69:1086-1107.

Chatterjee IB (1973) Evolution and the biosynthesis of ascorbic acid. Science 182:1271-1272.

Chen Q, Espey MG, Cherukuri MK, Mitchell JB, Corpe CP, Buettner GR, Shacter E, Levine M (2005) Pharmacologic ascorbic acid concentrations selectively kill cancer cells: action as a pro-drug to deliver hydrogen peroxide to tissues. Proc Natl Acad Sci USA. 102:13604-13609.

Clement MV, Ramalingam J, Long LH, Halliwell B (2001) The in vitro cytotoxicity of ascorbate depends on the culture medium used to perform the assay and involves hydrogen peroxide. Antioxid Redox Signal 3:157-163.

Cook JD, Reddy MB (2001) Effect of ascorbic acid intake on nonheme-iron absorption from a complete diet. Am J Clin Nutr 73:93-98.

Cook JD, Watson SS, Simpson KM, Lipschitz DA, Skikne BS (1984) The effect of high ascorbic acid supplementation on body iron stores. Blood 64:721-726.

Corpe CP, Lee JH, Kwon O, Eck P, Narayanan J, Kirk KL, Levine M (2005) 6-Bromo-6-deoxy-L-ascorbic acid: an ascorbate analog specific for Na+-dependent vitamin C transporter but not glucose transporter pathways. J Biol Chem 280:5211-5220.

Correa P (1992) Human gastric carcinogenesis: a multistep and multifactorial process—First American Cancer Society Award Lecture on Cancer Epidemiology and Prevention. Cancer Res 52:6735-6740.

Crandon JH, Lund CC, Dill DB (1940) Experimental human scurvy. N Engl J Med 223:353-369.

Darr D, Combs S, Dunston S, Manning T, Pinnell S (1992) Topical vitamin C protects porcine skin from ultraviolet radiation-induced damage. Br J Dermatol 127:247-253.

Daruwala R, Song J, Koh WS, Rumsey SC, Levine M (1999) Cloning and functional characterization of the human sodium-dependent vitamin C transporters hSVCT1 and hSVCT2. FEBS Lett 460:480-484.

de Koning H, Diallinas G (2000) Nucleobase transporters (review). Mol Membr Biol 17:75-94.

Dhariwal KR, Black CD, Levine M (1991a) Semidehydroascorbic acid as an intermediate in norepinephrine biosynthesis in chromaffin granules. J Biol Chem 266:12908-12914.

Dhariwal KR, Hartzell WO, Levine M (1991b) Ascorbic acid and dehydroascorbic acid measurements in human plasma and serum. Am J Clin Nutr 54:712-716.

Dunn WA, Rettura G, Seifter E, Englard S (1984) Carnitine biosynthesis from gamma-butyrobetaine and from exogenous protein-bound 6-N-trimethyl-L-lysine by the perfused guinea pig liver. Effect of ascorbate deficiency on the in situ activity of gamma-butyrobetaine hydroxylase. J Biol Chem. 259:10764-10770.

Eipper BA, Milgram SL, Husten EJ, Yun HY, Mains RE (1993a) Peptidylglycine alpha amidating monooxygenase: a multifunctional protein with catalytic, processing, and routing domains. Prot Sci 2:489-497.

Eipper BA, Bloomquist BT, Husten EJ, Milgram SL, Mains RE (1993b) Peptidyl alpha amidating monooxygenase and other processing enzymes in the neurointermediate pituitary. Ann N Y Acad Sci 680:147-60.

Englard S, Seifter S (1986) The biochemical functions of ascorbic acid. Annu Rev Nutr 6:365-406.

Fleming PJ, Kent UM (1991) Cytochrome b561, ascorbic acid, and transmembrane electron transfer. Am J Clin Nutr 54:1173S-1178S.

Gale CR, Ashurst HE, Powers HJ, Martyn CN (2001) Antioxidant vitamin status and carotid atherosclerosis in the elderly. Am J Clin Nutr 74:402-408.

Geesin JC, Darr D, Kaufman R, Murad S, Pinnell SR (1988) Ascorbic acid specifically increases type I and type III procollagen messenger RNA levels in human skin fibroblast. J Invest Dermatol 90:420-424.

Gerster H (1999) High-dose vitamin C: a risk for persons with high iron stores? Int J Vitam Nutr Res 69:67-82.

Gosiewska A, Wilson S, Kwon D, Peterkofsky B (1994) Evidence for an in vivo role of insulin-like growth factor binding proteins 1 and 2 as inhibitors of collagen gene expression in vitamin C deficient and fasted guinea pigs. Endocrinology 134: 1329-1339.

Graumlich JF, Ludden TM, Conry-Cantilena C, Cantilena LR Jr, Wang Y, Levine M (1997) Pharmacokinetic model of ascorbic acid in healthy male volunteers during depletion and repletion. Pharm Res 14:1133-1139.

Hallberg L (1995) Iron and vitamins. Bibl Nutr Dieta 52:20-29.

Halliwell B, Wasil M, Grootveld M (1987) Biologically significant scavenging of the myeloperoxidase-derived oxidant hypochlorous acid by ascorbic acid. Implications for antioxidant protection in the inflamed rheumatoid joint. FEBS Lett 213:15-17.

Hampl JS, Taylor CA, Johnston CS (2004) Vitamin C deficiency and depletion in the United States: the Third National Health and Nutrition Examination Survey, 1988 to 1994. Am J Public Health. 94:870-875.

Heller R, Unbehaun A, Schellenberg B, Mayer B, Werner-Felmayer G, Werner ER (2001) L-Ascorbic acid potentiates endothelial nitric oxide synthesis via a chemical stabilization of tetrahydrobiopterin. J Biol Chem 276:40-47.

Helser MA, Hotchkiss JH, Roe DA (1992) Influence of fruit and vegetable juices on the endogenous formation of N-nitrosoproline and N-nitrosothiazolidine-4-carboxylic acid in humans on controlled diets. Carcinogenesis 13:2277-2280.

Hodges RE (1971) What's new about scurvy? Am J Clin Nutr 24:383-384.

Hodges RE, Hood J, Canham JE, Sauberlich HE, Baker EM (1971) Clinical manifestations of ascorbic acid deficiency in man. Am J Clin Nutr 24:432-443.

Hood J, Burns CA, Hodges RE (1970) Sjogren's syndrome in scurvy. N Engl J Med 282:1120-1124.

Houglum KP, Brenner DA, Chojkier M (1991) Ascorbic acid stimulation of collagen biosynthesis independent of hydroxylation. Am J Clin Nutr 54:1141S-1143S.

Huang J, Agus DB, Winfree CJ, Kiss S, Mack WJ, McTaggart RA, Choudhri TF, Kim LJ, Mocco J, Pinsky DJ, Fox WD, Israel RJ, Boyd TA, Golde DW, Connolly ES Jr (2001) Dehydroascorbic acid, a blood-brain barrier transportable form of vitamin C, mediates potent cerebroprotection in experimental stroke. Proc Natl Acad Sci USA 98:11720-11724.

Institute of Medicine (2000) Dietary Reference Intakes for Vitamin C, Vitamin E, Selenium, and Carotenoids. National Academy Press, Washington, DC.

Jacob RA, Kutnink MA, Csallany AS, Daroszewska M, Burton GW (1996) Vitamin C nutriture has little short-term effect on vitamin E concentrations in healthy women. J Nutr 126:2268-2277.

Jacob RA, Pianalto FS (1997) Urinary carnitine excretion increases during experimental vitamin C depletion of healthy men. J Nutr Biochem 8:265-269.

Jacobs EJ, Connell CJ, McCullough ML, Chao A, Jonas CR, Rodriguez C, Calle EE, Thun MJ (2002) Vitamin C, vitamin E, and multivitamin supplement use and stomach cancer mortality in the Cancer Prevention Study II cohort. Cancer Epidemiol Biomarkers Prev 11:35-41.

Jialal I, Fuller CJ (1995) Effect of vitamin E, vitamin C, and beta-carotene on LDL oxidation and atherosclerosis. Can J Cardiol 11:97G-103G.

Johnston CS (1999) Biomarkers for establishing a tolerable upper intake level for vitamin C. Nutr Rev 57:71-77.

Johnston CS, Solomon RE, Corte C (1996) Vitamin C depletion is associated with alterations in blood histamine and plasma free carnitine in adults. J Am Coll Nutr 15:586-591.

Joshipura KJ, Ascherio A, Manson JE, Stampfer MJ, Rimm EB, Speizer FE, Hennekens CH, Spiegelman D, Willett WC. (1999) Fruit and vegetable intake in relation to risk of ischemic stroke. JAMA 282:1233-1239.

Joshipura KJ, Hu FB, Manson JE, Stampfer MJ, Rimm EB, Speizer FE, Colditz G, Ascherio A, Rosner B, Spiegelman D, Willett WC (2001) The effect of fruit and vegetable intake on risk for coronary heart disease. Ann Intern Med 134:1106-1114.

Kaufman S (1974) Dopamine-beta-hydroxylase. J Psychiatr Res 11:303-316.

Kent U, Fleming PJ (1987) Purified cytochrome b561 catalyzes transmembrane electron transfer for dopamine beta-hydroxylase and peptidyl glycine alpha-amidating monooxygenase in reconstituted systems. J Biol Chem 262:8174-8178.

Key TJ, Schatzkin A, Willett WC, Allen NE, Spencer EA, Travis RC (2004) Diet, nutrition and the prevention of cancer. Public Health Nutr 7:187-200.

Khaw KT, Bingham S, Welch A, Luben R, Wareham N, Oakes S, Day N (2001) Relation between plasma ascorbic acid and mortality in men and women in EPIC-Norfolk prospective study: a prospective population study. European Prospective Investigation into Cancer and Nutrition. Lancet 357:657-663.

King CC, Waugh WA (1932) The Chemical Nature of vitamin C. Science 75:357-358.

Kinsman RA, Hood J (1971) Some behavioral effects of ascorbic acid deficiency. Am J Clin Nutr 24:455-464.

Kivirikko KI, Myllyla R (1985) Post-translational processing of procollagens. Ann N Y Acad Sci 460:187-201.

Knowles HJ, Raval RR, Harris AL, Ratcliffe PJ (2003) Effect of ascorbate on the activity of hypoxia-inducible factor in cancer cells. Cancer Res 63:1764-1768.

Lee SH, Oe T, Blair IA (2001) Vitamin C–induced decomposition of lipid hydroperoxides to endogenous genotoxins. Science 292: 2083-2086.

Lehr HA, Weyrich AS, Saetzler RK, Jurek A, Arfors KE, Zimmerman GA, Prescott SM, McIntyre TM (1997) Vitamin C blocks inflammatory platelet-activating factor mimetics created by cigarette smoking J Clin Invest 99:2358-2564.

Levine M (1986) New concepts in the biology and biochemistry of ascorbic acid. N Engl J Med 314:892-902.

Levine M, Conry-Cantilena C, Wang Y, Welch RW, Washko PW, Dhariwal KR, Park JB, Lazarev A, Graumlich JF, King J, Cantilena LR (1996) Vitamin C pharmacokinetics in healthy volunteers: evidence for a Recommended Dietary Allowance. Proc Natl Acad Sci USA 93:3704-3709.

Levine M, Dhariwal KR, Washko PW, Butler JD, Welch RW, Wang YH, Bergsten P (1991) Ascorbic acid and in situ kinetics: a new approach to vitamin requirements. Am J Clin Nutr 54:1157S-1162S.

Levine M., Padayatty S., Katz A., Kwon O, Eck P, Corpe C., Lee J-H., Wang Y (2004) Dietary allowances for vitamin C: Recommended Dietary Allowances and optimal nutrient ingestion. In: Asard H, May JM, Smirnoff N (eds) Vitamin C: Functions and Biochemistry in Animals and Plants. BIOS Scientific Publishers, London.

Levine M, Rumsey SC, Daruwala R, Park JB, Wang Y (1999) Criteria and recommendations for vitamin C intake. JAMA 281:1415-23.

Levine M, Wang Y, Padayatty SJ, Morrow J (2001) A new recommended dietary allowance of vitamin C for healthy young women. Proc Natl Acad Sci USA 98: 9842-9846.

Levine M, Wang Y, Rumsey SC (1999) Analysis of ascorbic acid and dehydroascorbic acid in biological samples. Methods Enzymol 299: 65-76.

Levine SZ, Gordon HH, Marples E (1941) A defect in the metabolism of tyrosine and phenylalanine in premature infants: Spontaneous occurrence and eradication by vitamin C. J Clin Invest 20:209-219.

Lewin S (1976) Vitamin C: Its Molecular Biology and Medical Potential. Academic Press, London.

Lind J (1753) A Treatise on the Scurvy. A. Millar, London.

Lindblad B, Lindstedt G, Lindstedt S (1970) The mechanism of enzymic formation of homogentisate from p-hydroxyphenyl pyruvate. J Am Chem Soc 92:7446-7449.

May JM, Cobb CE, Mendiratta S, Hill KE, Burk RF (1998) Reduction of the ascorbyl free radical to ascorbate by thioredoxin reductase. J Biol Chem 273:23039-23045.

May JM, Qu Z, Cobb CE (2001) Recycling of the ascorbate free radical by human erythrocyte membranes. Free Radic Biol Med 31:117-124.

Mayne ST, Risch HA, Dubrow R, Chow WH, Gammon MD, Vaughan TL, Farrow DC, Schoenberg JB, Stanford JL, Ahsan H, West AB, Rotterdam H, Blot WJ, Fraumeni JF Jr (2001)

Nutrient intake and risk of subtypes of esophageal and gastric cancer. Cancer Epidemiol Biomarkers Prev 10:1055-1062.

Moran GR (2005) 4-Hydroxyphenylpyruvate dioxygenase. Arch Biochem Biophys 433: 117-128.

Mukhopadhyay CK, Chatterjee IB (1994) Free metal ion-independent oxidative damage of collagen. Protection by ascorbic acid. J Biol Chem 269:30200-30205.

Myllyharju J (2003) Prolyl 4-hydroxylases, the key enzymes of collagen biosynthesis. Matrix Biol 22:15-24.

National Research Council (1980) Recommended Dietary Allowances, 9th ed., National Academy Press, Washington, DC.

National Research Council (1989) Recommended Dietary Allowances, 10th ed., National Academy Press, Washington, DC.

Niki E (1987) Interaction of ascorbate and alpha-tocopherol. Ann N Y Acad Sci 498: 186-199.

Nishikimi M, Fukuyama R, Minoshima S, Shimizu N, Yagi K (1994) Cloning and chromosomal mapping of the human nonfunctional gene for L-gulono-gamma-lactone oxidase, the enzyme for L-ascorbic acid biosynthesis missing in man. J Biol Chem 269:13685-13688.

Ogiri Y, Sun F, Hayami S, Fujimura A, Yamamoto K, Yaita M, Kojo S (2002) Very low vitamin C activity of orally administered L-dehydroascorbic acid. J Agric Food Chem 50:227-229.

Otsuka M, Kurata T, Arakawa N (1986) Antiscorbutic effect of dehydro-L-ascorbic acid in vitamin C–deficient guinea pigs. J Nutr Sci Vitaminol (Tokyo) 32:183-190.

Pachla LA, Kissinger PT (1976) Determination of ascorbic acid in foodstuffs, pharmaceuticals, and body fluids by liquid chromatography with electrochemical detection. Anal Chem 48:364-367.

Padayatty SJ, Katz A, Wang Y, Eck P, Kwon O, Lee JH, Chen S, Corpe C, Dutta A, Dutta SK, Levine M (2003) Vitamin C as an antioxidant: Evaluation of its role in disease prevention. J Am Coll Nutr 22:18-35.

Park S, Han SS, Park CH, Hahm ER, Lee SJ, Park HK, Lee SH, Kim WS, Jung CW, Park K, Riordan HD, Kimler BF, Kim K, Lee JH (2004) L-Ascorbic acid induces apoptosis in acute myeloid leukemia cells via hydrogen peroxide-mediated mechanisms. Int J Biochem Cell Biol 36:2180-2195.

Perez-Cruz I, Carcamo JM, Golde DW (2003) Vitamin C inhibits FAS-induced apoptosis in monocytes and U937 cells. J Clin Invest 102:336-343.

Peterkofsky B (1991) Ascorbate requirement for hydroxylation and secretion of procollagen: Relationship to inhibition of collagen synthesis in scurvy. Am J Clin Nutr 54:1135S-1140S.

Podmore ID, Griffiths HR, Herbert KE, Mistry N, Mistry P, Lunec J (1998) Vitamin C exhibits pro-oxidant properties. Nature 392:559.

Polidori MC, Mecocci P, Levine M, Frei B (2004) Short-term and long-term vitamin C supplementation in humans dose-dependently increases the resistance of plasma to ex vivo lipid peroxidation. Arch Biochem Biophys 423:109-115.

Prigge ST, Mains RE, Eipper BA, Amzel LM (2000) New insights into copper monooxygenases and peptide amidation: structure, mechanism and function. Cell Mol Life Sci 57:1236-1259.

Prockop DJ, Kivirikko KI (1995) Collagens: molecular biology, diseases, and potential for therapy. Annu Rev Biochem 64:403-434.

Rathbone BJ, Johnson AW, Wyatt JI, Kelleher J, Heatley RV, Losowsky MS (1989) Ascorbic acid: a factor concentrated in human gastric juice. Clin Sci 76:237-241.

Rebouche CJ (1991) Ascorbic acid and carnitine biosynthesis. Am J Clin Nutr 54:1147S-1152S.

Rebouche CJ (1995) The ability of guinea pigs to synthesize carnitine at a normal rate from Epsilon-N-Trimethyllysine or gamma-butyrobetaine in vivo is not compromised by experimental vitamin C deficiency. Metabolism 44:624-629.

Rose RC, Choi JL, Koch MJ (1988) Intestinal transport and metabolism of oxidized ascorbic acid (dehydroascorbic acid). Am J Physiol 254:G824-G828.

Rumsey SC, Daruwala R, Al-Hasani H, Zarnowski MJ, Simpson IA, Levine M (2000) Dehydroascorbic acid transport by GLUT4 in Xenopus oocytes and isolated rat adipocytes. J Biol Chem 275:28246-28253.

Rumsey SC, Kwon O, Xu GW, Burant CF, Simpson I, Levine M (1997) Glucose transporter isoforms GLUT1 and GLUT3 transport dehydroascorbic acid. J Biol Chem 272:18982-18989.

Rumsey SC, Levine M (1998) Absorption, transport, and disposition of ascorbic acid in humans. J Nutr Biochem 9:116-130.

Sahyoun NR, Jacques PF, Russell RM (1996) Carotenoids, vitamins C and E, and mortality in an elderly population. Am J Epidemiol 144:501-511.

Sauberlich HE, Tamura T, Craig CB, Freeberg LE, Liu T (1996) Effects of erythorbic acid on vitamin C metabolism in young women. Am J Clin Nutr 64:336-346.

Simon JA, Hudes ES, and Browner WS (1998) Serum ascorbic acid and cardiovascular disease prevalence in U.S. adults. Epidemiology 9:316-321.

Sotiriou S, Gispert S, Cheng J, Wang Y, Chen A, Hoogstraten-Miller S, Miller GF, Kwon O, Levine M, Guttentag SH, Nussbaum RL (2002) Ascorbic acid transporter slc23a1 is essential for vitamin C transport into the brain and for perinatal survival. Nat Med 8:514-517.

Sowell J, Frei B, Stevens JF (2004) Vitamin C conjugates of genotoxic lipid peroxidation products: Structural characterization and detection in human plasma. Proc Natl Acad Sci USA 101:17964-17969.

Stadtman ER (2004) Role of oxidant species in aging. Curr Med Chem 11:1105-1112.

Steinberg D (2002) Atherogenesis in perspective: hypercholesterolemia and inflammation as partners in crime. Nat Med 8:1211-1217.

Stevenson NR (1974) Active transport of L-ascorbic acid in the human ileum. Gastroenterology 67:952-956.

Stewart LC, Klinman JP (1988) Dopamine beta hydroxylase of adrenal chromaffin granules: structure and function. Annu Rev Biochem 57:551-592.

Stubbe J (1985) Identification of two alpha-ketoglutarate-dependent dioxygenases in extracts of Rhodotorula glutinis catalyzing deoxyuridine hydroxylation. J Biol Chem 260:9972-9975.

Sullivan TA, Uschmann B, Hough R, Leboy PS (1994) Ascorbate modulation of chondrocyte gene expression is independent of its role in collagen secretion. J Biol Chem 269: 22500-22506.

Svirbely JL, Szent-Gyorgyi A (1932) The chemical nature of vitamin C. Biochem J 26:865-870.

Takanaga H, Mackenzie B, Hediger MA (2004) Sodium-dependent ascorbic acid transporter family SLC23. Pflugers Arch 447:677-682.

Tolbert BM, Ward JB (1982) Dehydroascorbic Acid. In: Seib PA, Tolbert BM (eds) Ascorbic Acid: Chemistry, Metabolism, and Uses. American Chemical Society, Washington, DC.

Toth I, Bridges KR (1995) Ascorbic acid enhances ferritin mRNA translation by an IRP/aconitase switch. J Biol Chem 270:19540-19544.

Tsukaguchi H, Tokui T, Mackenzie B, Berger UV, Chen XZ, Wang Y, Brubaker RF, Hediger MA (1999) A family of mammalian Na^+-dependent L-ascorbic acid transporters. Nature 399:70-75.

U.S. Department of Health and Human Services, U.S. Department of Agriculture (USDHHS/USDA) (2005) Dietary Guidelines for Americans, 6th ed. U.S. Government Printing Office, Washington, DC.

Vanderslice JT, Higgs DJ (1991) Vitamin C content of foods: sample variability. Am J Clin Nutr 54(6 Suppl):1323S-1327S.

Vera JC, Rivas CI, Fischbarg J, Golde DW (1993) Mammalian facilitative hexose transporters mediate the transport of dehydroascorbic acid. Nature 364:79-82.

Voko Z, Hollander M, Hofman A, Koudstaal PJ, Breteler (2003) Dietary antioxidants and the risk of ischemic stroke: the Rotterdam Study. Neurology 61:1273-1275.

Wang Y, Russo TA, Kwon O, Chanock S, Rumsey SC, Levine M (1997) Ascorbate recycling in human neutrophils: Induction by bacteria. Proc Natl Acad Sci USA 94: 13816-13819.

Washko PW, Wang Y, Levine M (1993) Ascorbic acid recycling in human neutrophils. J J Biol Chem 268:15531-15535.

Washko PW, Welch RW, Dhariwal KR, Wang Y, Levine M (1992) Ascorbic acid and dehydroascorbic acid analyses in biological samples. Anal Biochem 204:1-14.

Winkler BS, Orselli SM, Rex TS (1994) The redox couple between glutathione and ascorbic acid: a chemical and physiological perspective. Free Radic Biol Med 17:333-349.

Wondrack LM, Warn BJ, Saewert MD, Abbott MT (1979) Substitution of nucleoside triphosphates for ascorbate in the thymine 7-hydroxylase reaction of Rhodotorula glutinis. J Biol Chem 254:26-29.

Yang Y, Jao S, Nanduri S, Starke DW, Mieyal JJ, Qin J (1998) Reactivity of the human thioltransferase (glutaredoxin) C7S, C25S, C78S, C82S mutant and NMR solution structure of its glutathionyl mixed disulfide intermediate reflect catalytic specificity. Biochemistry 37:17145-17156.

RECOMMENDED READINGS

Asard H, May JM, Smirnoff N (eds) (2004) Vitamin C: Functions and biochemistry in animals and plants. BIOS Scientific Publishers, London.

Carr AC, Frei B (1999) Toward a new recommended dietary allowance for vitamin C based on antioxidant and health effects in humans. Am J Clin Nutr 69:1086-1107.

Englard S, Seifter S (1986) The biochemical functions of ascorbic acid. Annu Rev Nutr 6:365-406.

Levine M, Katz A, Padayatty SJ (2005) Vitamin C. In: Shils ME, Shike M, Ross AC, Caballero B, Cousins RJ (eds) Modern Nutrition in Health and Disease, 10th ed. Lippincott, Williams, and Wilkins, Baltimore, pp. 507-524.

Levine M, Rumsey SC, Daruwala R, Park JB, Wang Y (1999) Criteria & recommendations for vitamin C intake. JAMA 281:1415-1423.

Rumsey SC, Levine M (1998) Absorption, transport, and disposition of ascorbic acid in humans. J Nutr Biochem 9:116-130.

Chapter 28

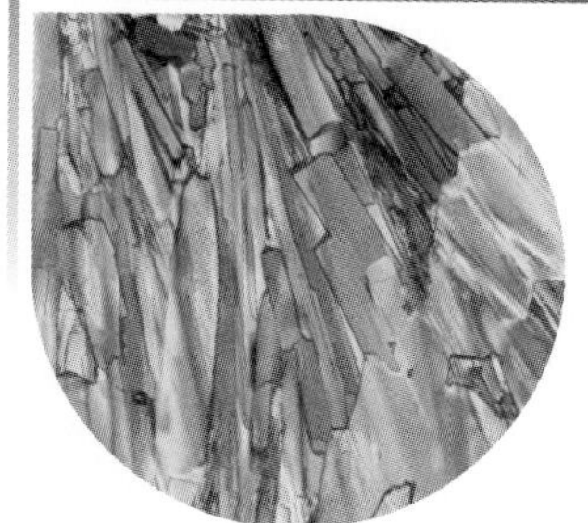

Vitamin K

Reidar Wallin, PhD, and Susan M. Hutson, PhD

OUTLINE

COMMON ABBREVIATIONS

ER	endoplasmic reticulum
Gla	γ-carboxyglutamic acid
Glu	glutamic acid
MK	menaquinone
VKOR	vitamin K 2,3-epoxide reductase
KH_2	reduced vitamin K, or vitamin K hydroquinone
K>O	vitamin K 2,3-epoxide

VITAMIN K: AN ANTIHEMORRHAGIC FACTOR

In the early 1930s Danish nutritional biochemist Henrich Dam was attempting to demonstrate that cholesterol was a dietary essential. He fed chicks a diet he had formulated to be low in fat and deficient in cholesterol, and noted that the chicks developed a hemorrhagic syndrome. Addition of cholesterol to the diet did not cure the syndrome, and Dam (1934) soon realized that, in removing cholesterol from the diet, he had also removed another essential factor. The hemorrhagic condition could be cured by

This chapter is a revision of the chapter contributed by John Suttie, PhD, for the first edition.

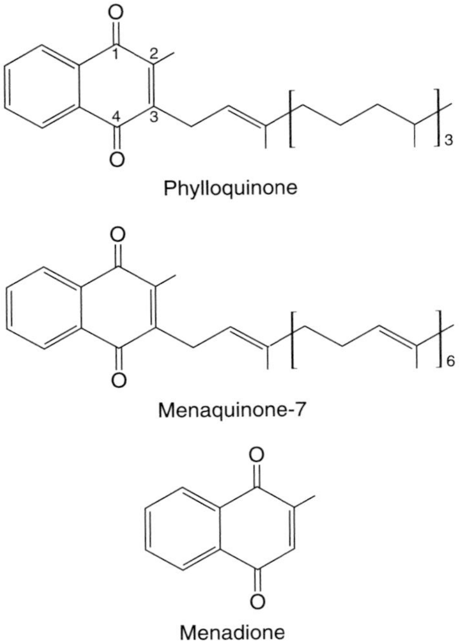

Phylloquinone

Menaquinone-7

Menadione

Figure 28-1 Structures of compounds with vitamin K activity. Phylloquinone synthesized in plants is the main dietary form of vitamin K. Menaquinone-7 is one of a series of menaquinones produced by intestinal bacteria, and menadione is a synthetic compound that can be converted to menaquinone-4 by animal tissues.

the addition of alfalfa meal to the diet or by the administration of a lipid extract of green plants. Efforts were then directed toward isolating and characterizing the active factor. By 1939 a series of investigations led by Dam in Denmark, Herman J. Almquist at Berkeley, and Edward Doisy at St. Louis University had established that the form of vitamin K found in alfalfa, later called vitamin K_1 or phylloquinone, was 2-methyl-3-phytyl-1,4-naphthoquinone. Bacterial forms of the vitamin, a series of multiprenyl menaquinones with an unsaturated side chain that were originally called vitamin K_2, subsequently were characterized. The 1943 Nobel Prize in Physiology or Medicine was awarded to Henrik Dam and Edward Doisy for their characterization of vitamin K, so named because a lack of this vitamin causes a defect in blood *koagulation*. The structures of vitamin K_1 and vitamin K_2 are shown in Figure 28-1.

NOMENCLATURE OF VITAMIN K ACTIVE COMPOUNDS

Compounds with vitamin K activity are 2-methyl-1,4-naphthoquinones with a hydrophobic substituent at the 3-position (see Fig. 28-1). Phylloquinone, originally called vitamin K_1, is the form of vitamin K that is isolated from green plants. Phylloquinone has a phytyl group at the 3-position of the naphthoquinone ring. The bacterially synthesized forms of the vitamin originally were called vitamin K_2 and are now more properly designated as menaquinones. These forms of the vitamin have an unsaturated multiprenyl group at the 3-position. Although a wide range of menaquinones (abbreviated as MK-n) are synthesized by bacteria, long-chain menaquinones with 6 to 10 isoprenoid groups in the side chain (MK-6 to MK-10) are the most common. The synthetic compound menadione (2-methyl-1,4-naphthoquinone) was shown very early to have vitamin K activity and commonly is used as a source of the vitamin in animal feeds. Menadione itself is now known not to be a substrate for the vitamin K–dependent carboxylase, but it is alkylated to an active form, MK-4, in mammalian tissues, preferentially in the extrahepatic tissues. Phylloquinone, available as a tablet or dispersed in a detergent for parenteral use, is the form of the vitamin available for human use.

MECHANISM OF ACTION OF VITAMIN K

DISCOVERY OF THE PHYSIOLOGICAL MECHANISM OF VITAMIN K ACTION

The discovery of vitamin K as an antihemorrhagic factor directed focus on the blood coagulation system as the physiological system targeted by the vitamin. The initial models of the system proposed by Macfarlane (1965) and Davie and Ratnof (1964) involve a "cascade" of activations of blood coagulation factors that result in conversion of the soluble plasma protein fibrinogen into the blood clot–forming protein fibrin. These first models have been modified extensively, and the currently accepted model of blood coagulation is shown in Figure 28-2. The cascade involves two pathways,

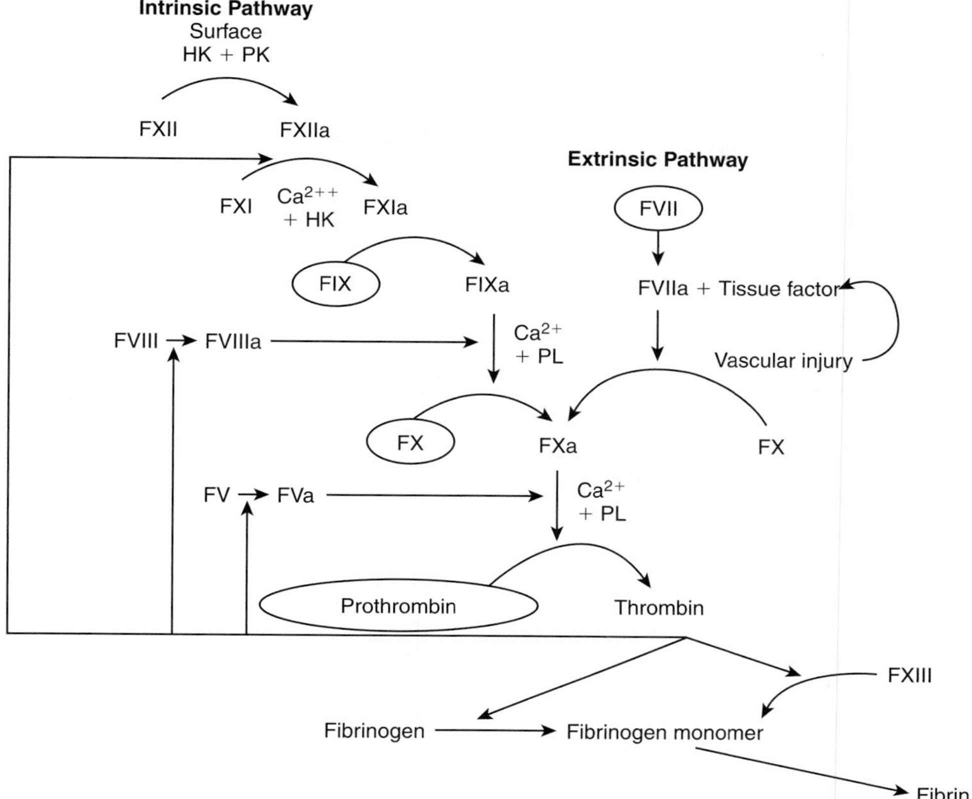

Figure 28-2 Vitamin K–dependent proteins involved in coagulation of blood. The figure shows a simplified version of the blood coagulation system. The system consists of an intrinsic and an extrinsic pathway. Each pathway consists of inactive proenzymes of coagulation factors that are converted to active proteases in a cascade of proteolytic reactions. Both pathways convert the proenzyme factor X to the active protease factor Xa. Factor Xa activates the proenzyme prothrombin to thrombin, and thrombin converts the plasma protein fibrinogen to fibrin. Fibrin is an insoluble polymer involved in arrest of blood loss at the site of vessel injury. Several proteins of the blood coagulation system are dependent upon a vitamin K–dependent posttranslational modification converting these proteins into γ-carboxyglutamic acid (Gla) containing proteins. These proteins are circled in the figure. *HK,* High-molecular-weight kinogen; *PK,* prekallikrein; *PL,* phospholipid.

the intrinsic and the extrinsic, which converge at the formation of active factor Xa (FXa) from its inactive proenzyme factor X (FX) form. The blood coagulation system is described in great detail by Furie and Furie (1992). The general theme underlying activation of the system is the sequential activation of proenzymes (zymogens) to become active enzymes in an amplifying cascade of reactions with the goal of converting prothrombin to thrombin, leading ultimately to fibrin clot formation (see Fig. 28-2).

Early on, the hemorrhagic condition that resulted from the dietary lack of vitamin K was thought to be due solely to a lowered concentration of the plasma clotting factor prothrombin, but it was later shown that the levels of clotting factors VII, IX, and X were also depressed in the deficient state. Because the synthesis of the functional zymogens is dependent on vitamin K, these four clotting factors are known as the vitamin K–dependent clotting factors. The vitamin K–dependent clotting factors are circled in Figure 28-2. These proteins were shown to bind calcium ions (Ca^{2+}) and to bind to negatively charged phospholipid surfaces.

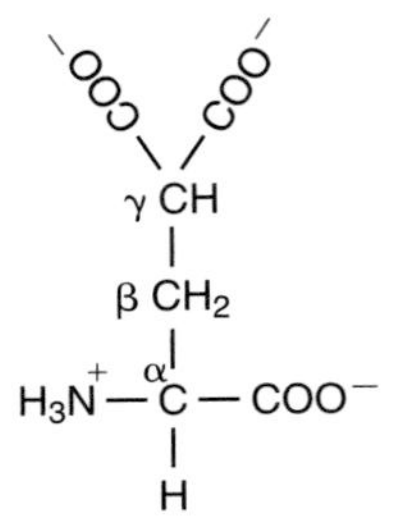

Figure 28-3 Structure of γ-carboxyglutamic acid (Gla). Gla is a Ca^{+2} binding amino acid.

Studies of prothrombin production became the key to determining the mechanism of action of vitamin K. Experiments with whole animals carried out in the mid-1960s strongly suggested that vitamin K was involved in converting an inactive hepatic precursor of plasma prothrombin to biologically active prothrombin. This hypothesis was strengthened by clinical observations that an immunochemically similar, but biologically inactive, form of prothrombin was present in increased concentrations in the plasma of patients treated with anticoagulants that antagonized vitamin K action. The inactive proteins were called PIVKA factor (proteins induced in vitamin K absence) (Hemker and Reekers, 1974). Characterization of this "abnormal prothrombin" isolated from the plasma of cows fed the anticoagulant dicoumarol revealed that it lacked the specific Ca^{2+}-binding sites present in normal prothrombin and it did not demonstrate a Ca^{2+}-dependent association with negatively charged phospholipid surfaces. These findings suggested that the function of vitamin K was to modify a liver precursor of this plasma protein to facilitate calcium binding. The action of the vitamin was, therefore, not at the level of gene transcription, but occurred after messenger RNA (mRNA) translation. By comparing peptides obtained from proteolytic digests of normal bovine prothrombin and abnormal prothrombin obtained from cows treated with dicumarol, Stenflo and colleagues (1974) identified the vitamin K modification as γ-carboxylation of glutamic acid residues in newly formed vitamin K–dependent protein precursors. The structure of γ-carboxyglutamic acid (Gla), a previously unrecognized acidic amino acid (Nelsestuen et al., 1974; Stenflo et al., 1974) is shown in Figure 28-3. It was found that that all 10 of the glutamic acid residues in the first 42 residues of bovine prothrombin were converted to Gla. The discovery of Gla in vitamin K–dependent coagulation factors revealed, for the first time, the role of Ca^{2+} in blood clotting. Calcium-binding by the Gla residues is essential for anchoring these coagulation factors to negatively charged lipids at the site of injury (Furie and Furie, 1992).

VITAMIN K: A SUBSTRATE FOR A γ-CARBOXYLASE

The discovery of Gla residues in prothrombin led to the demonstration (Esmon et al., 1975) that crude rat liver microsomal preparations (vesicles derived from the endoplasmic reticulum [ER] when cells are disrupted) contained an enzymatic activity that promoted a vitamin K–dependent incorporation of $^{14}CO_2$ into endogenous precursors of vitamin K–dependent proteins present in these preparations. Subsequent studies established that the $^{14}CO_2$ was present in Gla residues. Small peptides containing adjacent Glu-Glu residues such as Phe-Leu-Glu-Glu-Val were shown to be substrates for the enzyme present in detergent-solubilized microsomal preparations, and they were used to study the properties of this unique vitamin K–dependent γ-carboxylase. It is now well established that vitamin K–dependent γ-carboxylation of glutamate residues in proteins is a posttranslational modification reaction that occurs on the luminal side of the rough ER.

Vitamin K–dependent proteins are secretory proteins that migrate through the ER and the Golgi apparatus before the proteins are secreted from the cells as mature proteins (Stanton et al., 1991). As shown in Figure 28-4, the vitamin K–dependent proteins are equipped with a signal peptide for penetration into the ER lumen. Upon entering the lumen the N-terminal signal peptide is removed by signal peptidase. In addition, all precursors of vitamin K–dependent proteins are equipped with a unique propeptide which, in most of the proteins, constitutes the N-terminal part of the precursor after the signal peptide is removed (see Fig. 28-4). These propeptides are recognized by the γ-carboxylase in the ER membrane. They anchor the vitamin K–dependent protein precursors to the enzyme for γ-carboxylation of glutamic acid residues in a reaction where reduced vitamin K (KH_2) is the

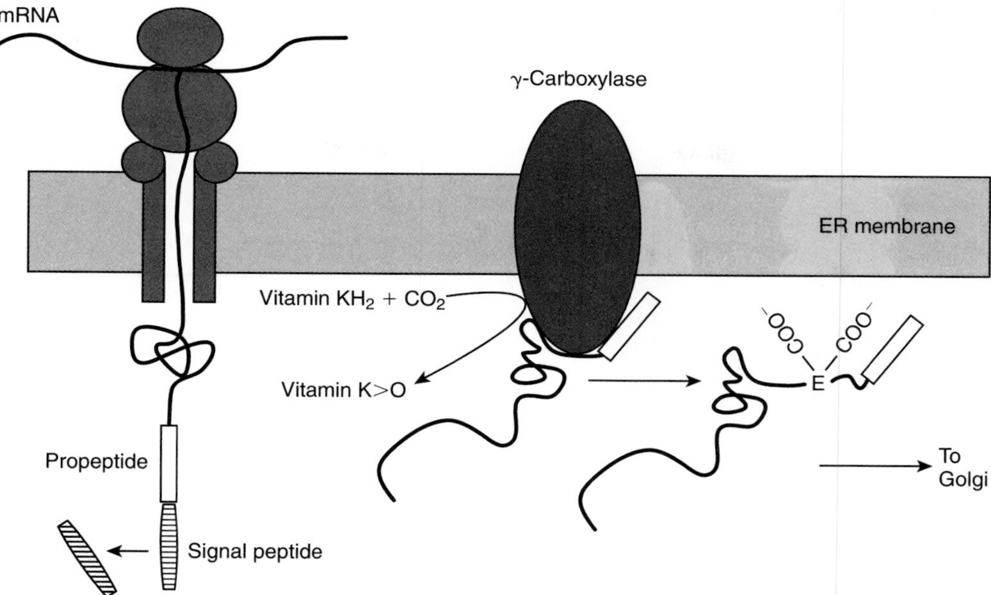

Figure 28-4 Posttranslational vitamin K–dependent modification of vitamin K–dependent protein in the endoplasmic reticulum (ER). Vitamin K–dependent proteins are secretory glycoproteins. They are equipped with a signal peptide for translocation into the ER lumen and a propeptide that serves as the recognition signal that destines these proteins for vitamin K–dependent γ-carboxylation of glutamate (E) residues by the γ-carboxylase, which is an integral protein in the ER membrane. Reduced vitamin K (KH_2) is cofactor for the modification reaction and vitamin K epoxide (K>O) is a product.

active cofactor for the modification reaction. Upon completion of γ-carboxylation, the vitamin K–dependent proteins are released from the γ-carboxylase and exit the ER in secretory vesicles for transport to the Golgi apparatus for additional modifications. The major modifications the proteins undergo in the Golgi apparatus are glycosylations. The proteins move through the *cis*, medial, and *trans* Golgi compartments (Fig. 28-5). Because of the addition of sialic acid residues, the vitamin K–dependent proteins become more acidic in the Golgi apparatus. The propeptide stays attached to the protein throughout its migration through the Golgi apparatus but is proteolytically released from the protein in the *trans*-Golgi apparatus by the protease furin (Stanton et al., 1991). Release of the propeptide is essential for the coagulation factors to function as zymogens in the blood coagulation system. Bleeding disorders have been shown to result in the appearance, in blood, of vitamin K–dependent coagulation factors with the propeptide still attached (Diuguid et al., 1986).

THE VITAMIN K CYCLE AND THE VITAMIN K–DEPENDENT γ-CARBOXYLATION SYSTEM

As indicated in Figure 28-4, reduced vitamin K (KH_2 or vitamin K hydroquinone) is the γ-carboxylase cofactor. When one Glu residue is converted to one Gla residue, the cofactor KH_2 is converted to vitamin K 2,3-epoxide (K>O) (Fig. 28-6). The epoxide is reduced back to the hydroquinone cofactor by the enzyme vitamin K 2,3-epoxide reductase (VKOR). VKOR is inhibited by warfarin, a coumarin anticoagulant drug. The oxidation of vitamin KH_2 in the γ-carboxylation reaction and the reduction of K>O back to KH_2 by VKOR constitute the vitamin K cycle. The complete set of biochemical reactions shown in Figure 28-6 constitutes the vitamin K–dependent γ-carboxylation system. In the system, VKOR regenerates the reduced vitamin K cofactor used by the γ-carboxylase.

CHEMISTRY OF VITAMIN K ACTION

The vitamin K–dependent carboxylation reaction does not require adenosine triphosphate

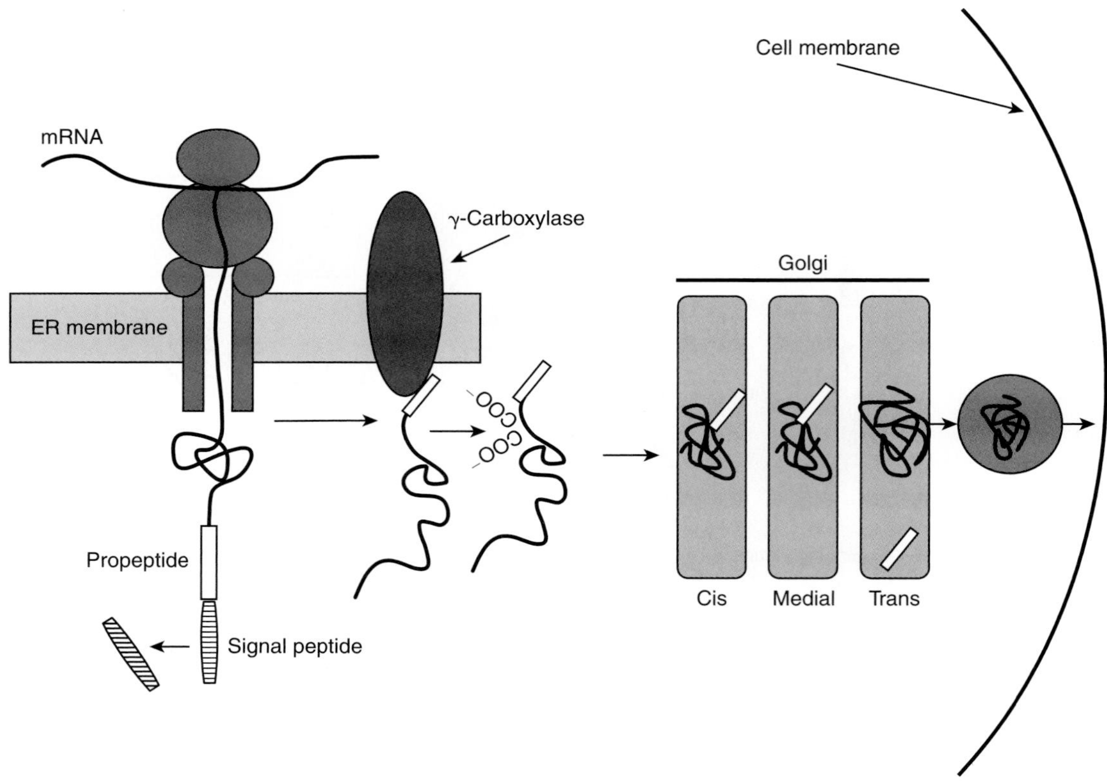

Figure 28-5 Transport of vitamin K–dependent protein precursors through the secretory pathway of the cell. Gamma-carboxylated precursors of vitamin K–dependent proteins exit the ER in secretory vesicles and migrate through the *cis*, medial and *trans* compartments of the Golgi apparatus. The major modifications the proteins undergo in the Golgi apparatus are glycosylations. The propeptide is released from the precursor in the *trans*-Golgi apparatus by the protease furin. Release of the propeptide is required for synthesis of functional vitamin K–dependent proteins.

(ATP), and the available data are consistent with the view that the energy to drive this carboxylation reaction is derived from the oxidation of the reduced form of vitamin K by O_2 to form vitamin K 2,3-epoxide (Fig. 28-7). The lack of a biotin cofactor requirement and direct studies of the CO_2/HCO_3^- requirement led to the knowledge that CO_2 rather than HCO_3^- is the active species in the carboxylation reaction. Studies of substrate specificity at the vitamin K–binding site of the enzyme have shown that the only important structural feature of this substrate is a 2-methyl-1,4-naphthoquinone substituted at the 3-position with a rather hydrophobic group (see Fig. 28-1). The 2-ethyl and desmethyl analogs of the vitamin have little activity, and methyl substitution of the benzenoid ring has little effect on or decreases substrate binding.

Early studies of the mechanism of action of the γ-carboxylation reaction indicated that the mechanistic role of vitamin K was to abstract the hydrogen on the γ-carbon of the glutamyl residue to allow attack of CO_2 at this position. This was established by using substrates tritiated at the γ-carbon of each Glu residue to demonstrate that the enzyme catalyzed a vitamin KH_2–dependent and O_2-dependent, but CO_2-independent, release of tritium from the substrate. At saturating concentrations of CO_2, there is an apparent equivalent stoichiometry between vitamin K 2,3-epoxide formation and Gla formation. It has been established that γ-carboxylation and vitamin K epoxidation are

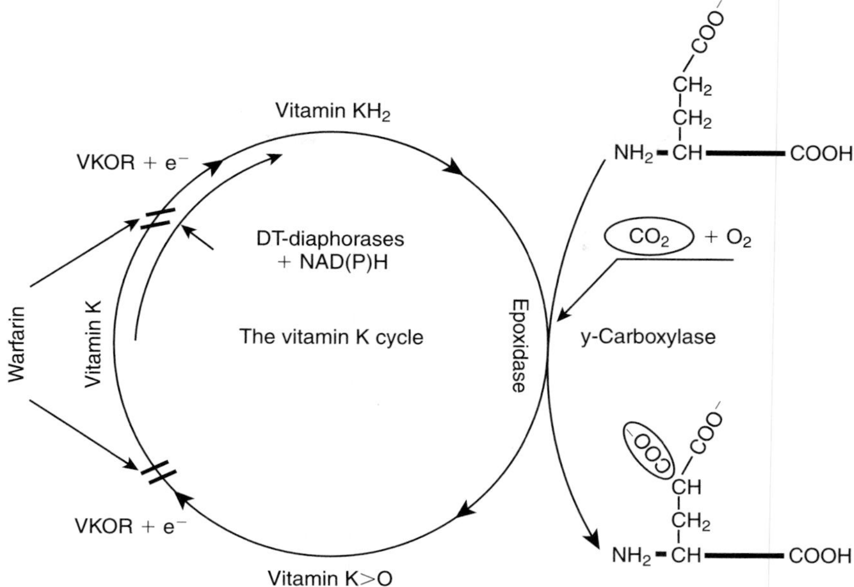

Figure 28-6 The vitamin K–dependent γ-carboxylation system. Reduced vitamin K (Vit.KH_2) is cofactor for γ-carboxylase. Concomitant with γ-carboxylation, Vit.KH_2 is converted to vitamin K 2,3-epoxide (Vit.K>O). Vit.K>O is reduced back to the Vit.KH_2 cofactor by vitamin K 2,3-epoxide reductase (VKOR). These enzyme activities constitute the vitamin K cycle. VKOR is inhibited by warfarin and other coumarin anticoagulant drugs. DT-Diaphorases are flavoproteins that can reduce vitamin K quinone (Vit.K) but not the vitamin K epoxide. The complete set of enzyme reactions shown in the figure constitutes the vitamin K–dependent γ-carboxylation system.

carried out by the same enzyme. However, the enzyme is inactive as an epoxidase until a protein or peptide substrate for γ-carboxylase is bound to the enzyme (Sugiura et al., 1997). Therefore, epoxidase activity is turned off, and no highly reactive vitamin K intermediate is generated unless the carboxylase is associated with a substrate.

The manner in which epoxide formation is coupled to γ-hydrogen abstraction has been an important mechanistic question. One possibility is through the action of an oxygenated vitamin K intermediate that would also be a logical intermediate on the pathway to epoxide formation (see Fig. 28-7). Hydrogen abstraction is known to be stereospecific, and it is the pro S hydrogen at the γ-position of the Glu residue that is removed. The fate of the activated Glu residue in the absence of CO_2 has been shown to be protonation rather than formation of an adduct. The enzyme has been shown to catalyze a vitamin KH_2 and oxygen-dependent exchange of ^3H from ^3H_2O into the γ-position of a Glu residue, and this exchange reaction is decreased as the concentration of HCO_3^- in the medium is increased. There is a close association between epoxide formation, Gla formation, and γ-C–H bond cleavage. The efficiency of the γ-carboxylation reaction, defined as the ratio of Gla residues formed to γ-C–H bonds cleaved, is independent of Glu substrate concentration, and the data suggest that this ratio approaches unity at high CO_2 concentrations.

A major gap in an understanding of the mechanism of action of this enzyme has been the assumption that abstraction of a hydrogen from the γ-carbon of glutamic acid would require a strong base (presumably formed from the vitamin), and the lack of evidence for such an intermediate. More recent data (Dowd et al., 1995) suggest that an initial attack of O_2 at the naphthoquinone carbonyl carbon adjacent to the methyl group results in the formation of a

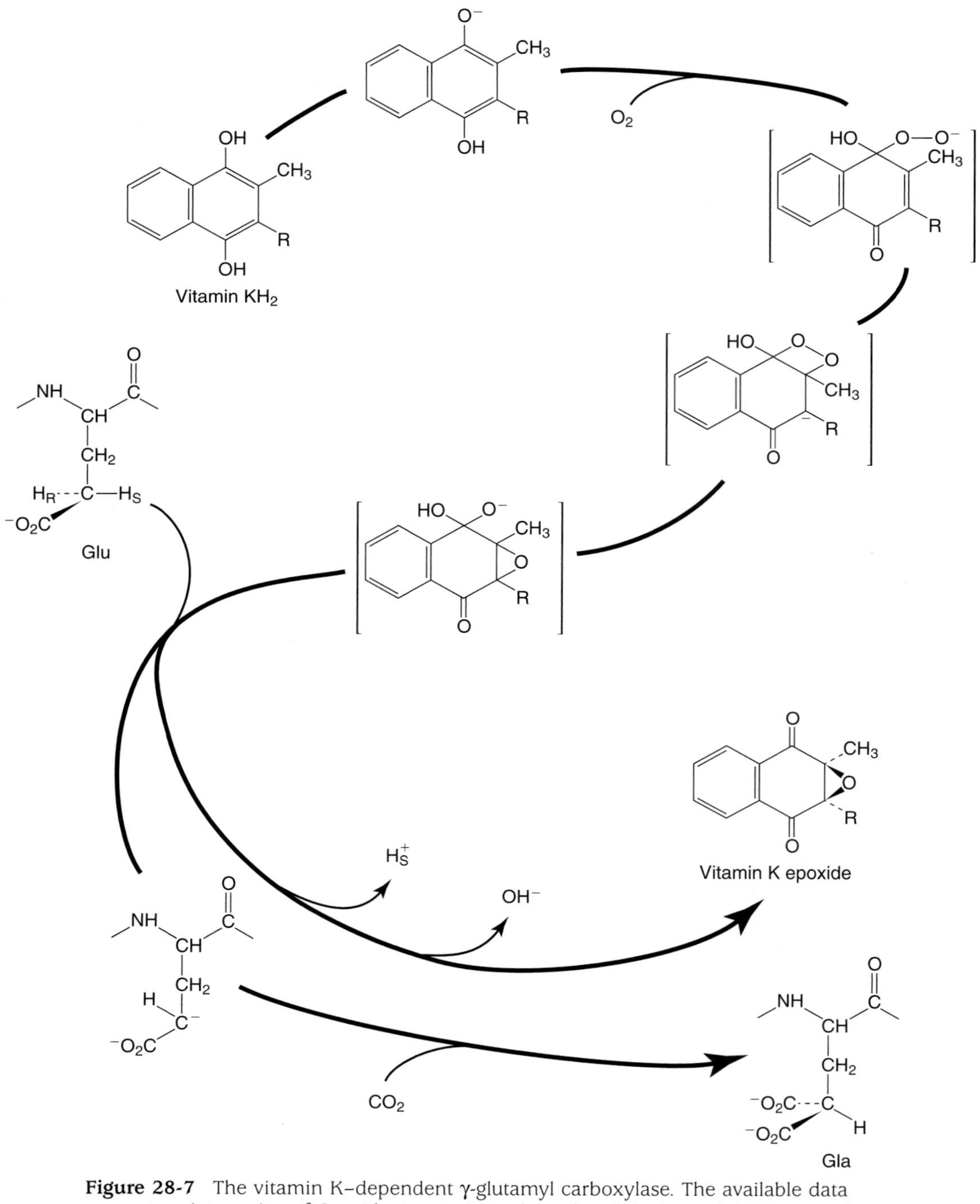

Vitamin KH_2

Glu

Vitamin K epoxide

Gla

Figure 28-7 The vitamin K–dependent γ-glutamyl carboxylase. The available data support an interaction of O_2 with vitamin KH_2, the reduced (hydronaphthoquinone) form of vitamin K, to form an oxygenated intermediate that is sufficiently basic to abstract the γ-hydrogen of the glutamyl residue (Glu). The products of this reaction are vitamin K 2,3-epoxide and a glutamyl carbanion. Attack of CO_2 on the carbanion leads to the formation of a γ-carboxyglutamyl residue (Gla). The bracketed peroxy, dioxetane, and alkoxide intermediates have not been identified in the enzyme-catalyzed reaction but are postulated based on model organic reactions.

dioxetane ring that generates an alkoxide intermediate. This intermediate is hypothesized to be the strong base that abstracts the γ-methylene hydrogen and leaves a carbanion that can interact with CO_2 (see Fig. 28-7). This pathway leads to the possibility that a second atom of molecular oxygen can be incorporated into the carbonyl group of the epoxide product; this activity can be followed by utilization of $^{18}O_2$ in the reaction. Although this general scheme is consistent with all of the available data, the mechanism remains a hypothesis at this time.

γ-CARBOXYLATION OF PROTEIN GLU RESIDUES

The physiological role of the vitamin K–dependent γ-carboxylase poses an interesting question in terms of enzyme-substrate recognition. This microsomal enzyme recognizes a small fraction of the total hepatic secretory protein pool and then carboxylates 9 to 12 Glu sites in the first 45 N-terminal residues of the vitamin K-dependent plasma proteins. The propeptide regions of these proteins show sequence homology. The propeptide region appears to be both a docking and recognition site for the γ-carboxylase and a modulator of the activity by decreasing the apparent K_m of the γ-carboxylase for the Glu-containing protein substrates. The propeptide domain is undoubtedly of major importance in directing the efficient γ-carboxylation of the multiple Glu sites in these substrates, but it is not known if the enzyme starts at one end of the Gla region and sequentially carboxylates all Glu sites or if the enzyme carboxylates randomly within this region. Reduction of KH_2 levels by anticoagulant therapy results in the production of a complex mixture of partially carboxylated forms of prothrombin, and the available data suggest that the most amino-terminal potential Gla residue of these under-γ-carboxylated forms is preferentially carboxylated (Malhotra, 1972). A more recent model for Glu γ-carboxylation has been proposed by Stenina and colleagues (2001). Their data are consistent with a model of tethered processivity of γ-carboxylation, which, in short, means that the vitamin K–dependent precursor protein will not leave the γ-carboxylase before the Gla region has been completed.

PURIFICATION AND CHARACTERIZATION OF γ-CARBOXYLASE

Early studies of γ-carboxylation were hampered by the lack of purified γ-carboxylase. By using an affinity approach, where the ligand was a large peptide containing the propeptide region and the Gla region of factor IX (residues −18 to 41 of the precursor), Wu and colleagues (1991) purified a microsomal protein of molecular weight 94 kDa that exhibited γ-carboxylase activity and that required lipid for activity. Data from a topological study carried out by Tie and colleagues (2000) predict that γ-carboxylase spans the ER membrane at least five times. Therefore, γ-carboxylase is considered a true integral protein of the ER membrane.

WARFARIN RESISTANCE AND THE VITAMIN K–DEPENDENT γ-CARBOXYLATION SYSTEM

As shown in Figure 28-6, the anticoagulant warfarin inhibits VKOR (vitamin K 2,3-epoxide reductase) of the vitamin K cycle. Warfarin resistance is a problem in prophylactic medicine and also in rodent pest control. The problem can be pharmacological, nutritional, or genetic. Pharmacological resistance is associated with high turnover of the drug in the liver by the cytochrome P450 system where Cyp2C9 is the most active cytochrome involved in metabolism of warfarin (Hanatani et al., 2003). Nutritional resistance results from high intake of vitamin K. Vitamin K is an antidote to warfarin, and patients undergoing warfarin therapy need to be careful with green vegetables in their diets because these vegetables can contain high concentrations of vitamin K (Suttie, 1978). The mechanism by which vitamin K works as an antidote to warfarin has been established (Wallin and Martin, 1987). When the liver concentration of vitamin K is elevated, vitamin K can be reduced by an alternative pathway in the liver and provide the γ-carboxylase with cofactor. This pathway is catalyzed by

DT-diaphorases, enzymes that are able to use either NADH or NADPH for vitamin K reduction (Wallin and Martin, 1987). Warfarin does not inhibit some of these enzymes. Therefore, if the VKOR pathway for vitamin K reduction is blocked by warfarin, the alternative pathway can "drive" vitamin KH_2 cofactor production and maintain a normally functioning blood coagulation system if vitamin K levels are elevated. Indeed, this is the standard procedure used to treat warfarin intoxication in patients and animals. This bypass pathway is depicted in Figure 28-6. The DT-diaphorases cannot reduce vitamin K 2,3-epoxide, however, so vitamin K cannot be effectively recycled for participation in a second carboxylation reaction.

Genetic warfarin resistance has been described in humans (Vermeer and Schurgers, 2000) and was a major problem in rodent pest control before the second generation anticoagulants (superwarfarins) were introduced as poisons (Meehan, 1984). These poisons are hydrophobic derivatives of dicumarol, the parent compound of warfarin, but they cannot be used in humans because of their toxicity. Genetic resistance to some of the second-generation anticoagulants has been described in rodents.

Most biochemical data on VKOR and genetic warfarin resistance attributed to vitamin K 2,3-epoxide and vitamin K quinone reduction by VKOR have been derived from experiments with crude rat liver microsomes. Consistent findings from these experiments have been (1) genetic warfarin resistance, attributed to VKOR, is associated with low VKOR activity in

Clinical Correlation

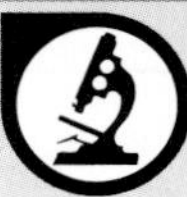

Warfarin: Rat Poison and an Effective Clinical Drug

Following discovery of dicoumarol and the synthesis of a large number of analogs, the initial use of these vitamin K antagonists was as a rodenticide. Rats and other rodents can be killed by a large number of toxic agents, but they rapidly become "bait shy." That is, if they ingest a nonlethal dose of a poison, they will refuse to eat bait containing that compound in the future. The turnover time of the circulating vitamin K–dependent clotting factors in plasma is such that they are present at a level that will prevent hemorrhage for 2 or 3 days after their synthesis has been blocked by warfarin ingestion. During this period the rats continue to eat the poisoned bait and eventually die of internal hemorrhage. These are, therefore, very effective rodenticides. As might be expected, the widespread use of rodenticides containing warfarin has led to the selection of mutant strains that are resistant to this toxic agent. These warfarin-resistant "super rats" are, however, susceptible to other 4-hydroxycoumarins, and the rat poisons commonly available at the present time contain these compounds as the active anticoagulant.

Much lower doses of 4-hydroxycoumarins will not result in hemorrhage but will decrease the rate at which blood clots, and they are prescribed widely as antithrombotic drugs. The oral anticoagulant used in the United States is warfarin, but some of the other 4-hydroxycoumarins, which have somewhat different pharmacokinetic properties, are used widely in other countries. They are used to treat patients who have been diagnosed with deep vein thrombosis, pulmonary embolism, and myocardial infarction in order to prevent the recurrence of thrombosis. They also are given to patients after the insertion of prosthetic heart valves in order to prevent systemic arterial embolism.

There is a rather wide variation in warfarin sensitivity from one patient to another, and the appropriate dose for each individual must be determined by careful monitoring of the "prothrombin time" as the dose is gradually increased to the therapeutic level. Plasma is obtained from blood treated with a Ca^{2+} chelator to prevent coagulation. This test measures the time it takes for the plasma to clot after it has been recalcified and after clotting has been initiated by the addition of a crude tissue factor and phospholipid preparation.

liver and (2) resistant rats require high intake of vitamin K to avoid excessive bleeding (Hermodson et al., 1969). Collectively these observations led to the consensus that warfarin resistance is linked to a genetically altered VKOR enzyme. Kohn and colleagues (2003) were able to map warfarin resistance to the *Rw* locus on chromosome 1 in the rat. Members of two families with familial multiple coagulation factor deficiency (FMFD), a disease in which patients have a deficiency in all of the vitamin K–dependent coagulation factors, were investigated by Fregin and colleagues (2002), who mapped the disease to the 16p12-q21 region on chromosome 16. They noted that a linkage group of genes on 16p11 is orthologous to genes around warfarin resistance loci *Rw* in rats (Kohn et al., 2003; Greaves and Ayres, 1967) and *War* in mice (Wallace and MacSwiney, 1976). This homology led the investigators to propose that FMFD and warfarin resistance may be caused by allelic mutations in the same gene. DNA sequencing of genes in the region resulted in identification of missense mutations in a gene of unknown function from all of the FMFD patients studied. The wild-type gene in unaffected individuals codes for an 18-kDa ER membrane protein, now known as VKOR complex subunit 1 (VKORC1); overexpression of this gene yielded a protein that exhibited warfarin-sensitive VKOR activity. Furthermore, it was shown that certain missense mutations in the gene resulted in significant warfarin resistance to the host (Rost et al., 2004). Using synthetic short interfering RNAs (siRNAs) to silence genes in the warfarin-resistant region on chromosome 16, Li and colleagues (2004) identified the same gene as that responsible for expression of warfarin-sensitive VKOR activity.

It has been proposed that additional forms of genetic warfarin resistance exist. One form has been shown to be associated with overexpression of the chaperone protein calumenin in rat liver (Wallin et al., 2001a). Calumenin belongs to the CREC (Cab45, reticulocalbin, ERC-45, calumenin) subfamily of Ca^{2+} binding proteins (Honore and Vorum, 2000). The CREC proteins are found in the secretory pathways of cells, and most of the proteins have been shown to have chaperone functions. Despite being a hydrophilic water-soluble acidic protein, calumenin appears to be associated with ER membrane proteins. Data supporting this concept include immunocytochemical studies of the ER membrane (Honore and Vorum, 2000) and the demonstration that calumenin is strongly associated with lipid-detergent micelles, derived from the ER membrane, which also carry the VKOR enzyme complex (Wallin et al., 2001a). Expression of calumenin in cell lines has been shown to inhibit VKOR activity and confer warfarin resistance to the VKOR enzyme complex. In addition, calumenin has been shown to be associated with the γ-carboxylase and to inhibit γ-carboxylase activity (Wajih et al., 2004). Therefore, calumenin appears to be a chaperone that regulates the capacity of the vitamin K–dependent γ-carboxylation system for production of functional vitamin K–dependent proteins. This regulatory role puts calumenin in a central position regarding maintenance of a normal blood coagulation system.

CHARACTERIZATION OF VKOR OF THE VITAMIN K CYCLE

The discoveries in the 1970s of vitamin K_1 2,3-epoxide as a metabolite of vitamin K_1 in liver (Matschiner et al., 1970) and of the warfarin-sensitive vitamin K cycle (Whitlon et al., 1978) led to numerous attempts to characterize VKOR at the biochemical level. From these early studies it became clear that thiols (–SH groups) are involved in the catalytic mechanism of vitamin K_1 2,3-epoxide reduction by VKOR and that warfarin binds to a thiol redox center in VKOR. The most plausible model for the mechanism of inhibition of VKOR by warfarin came from work in Fasco's laboratory (Fasco et al., 1983). Their experimental data, which was confirmed by others, led to the proposal that warfarin binds to an oxidized thiol redox center and prevents reduction of the center by an unknown electron donor. The identity of the physiological electron donor has not been established.

Analysis of the recently discovered VKORC1 is likely to provide additional support for Fasco's model. This 18-kDa protein with 163 amino acid residues is a hydrophobic protein with three predicted trans-membrane domains (Li et al., 2004). Cys132 and Cys135 occur in a CXXC

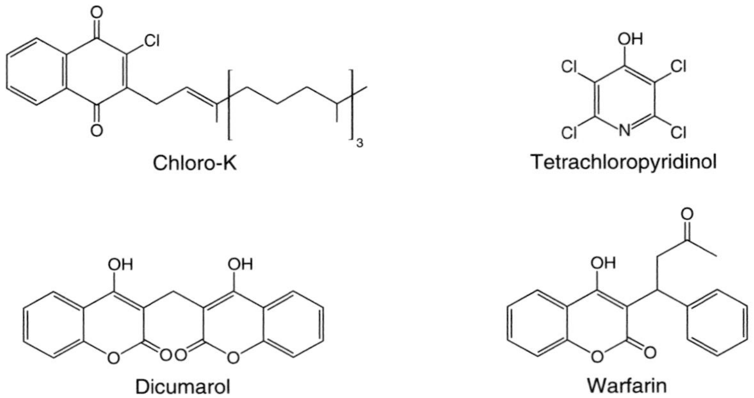

Figure 28-8 Vitamin K antagonists. Chloro-K and tetrachloropyridinol are inhibitors of the vitamin K–dependent γ-glutamyl carboxylase. The 4-hydroxycoumarins, dicoumarol and warfarin, do not inhibit the carboxylase enzyme but prevent recycling of vitamin K–epoxide to the enzymatically active form of the vitamin.

motif located at the N-terminal side of the third α-helix trans-membrane domain. This is a typical location for thiol redox centers in proteins with thioredoxin-like redox domains. The CXXC center is embedded in a hydrophobic environment, which is consistent with the finding that hydrophobic, but not hydrophilic, thiol-reducing trialkylphosphines will reach the center and trigger VKOR activity (Wallin et al., 2002). Mutation of the cysteine residues in the center would be expected to produce an inactive enzyme. Because the wild-type VKORC1 cDNA, when transfected into mammalian and insect cells, generates warfarin-sensitive VKOR activity, transfection experiments with cDNAs containing a mutant CXXC center have provided data in support of Fasco's redox model of VKOR (Wajih et al., 2005).

ANTAGONISM OF VITAMIN K ACTION BY VARIOUS INHIBITORS

The vitamin K analog 2-chloro-3-phytyl-1, 4-naphthoquinone (chloro-K) is an effective inhibitor of γ-glutamyl carboxylase, and the reduced form of this analog has been shown to be competitive with reduced vitamin KH_2 as an inhibitor of γ-carboxylase activity (Fig. 28-8). Chloro-K also has been shown to be an antagonist in vivo, and administration of this compound to animals results in a hemorrhagic condition. Substitution of a trifluoromethyl group, a hydroxymethyl group, or a methoxymethyl group for the 2-methyl group of vitamin K also results in analogs that are inhibitory compounds. Some compounds not structurally related to vitamin K are also vitamin K antagonists, and tetrachloropyridinol and other polychlorinated phenols have been shown to be strong inhibitors of γ-glutamyl carboxylase.

The most widely used antagonists of vitamin K are the 4-hydroxycoumarins (see Fig. 28-8). Dicoumarol [3,3′-methylene bis-(4-hydroxycoumarin)] originally was isolated from moldy sweet clover as the factor responsible for a hemorrhagic disease of cattle that was common in the midwestern United States in the early 1930s. A large number of compounds based on this structure have been synthesized, and the most widely used is warfarin [3-(α-acetonylbenzyl)-4-hydroxycoumarin] (see Fig. 28-8). These compounds are "indirect" vitamin K antagonists in that they do not inhibit the γ-carboxylase (Hildebrandt and Suttie, 1982), but rather inhibit VKOR and, therefore, the regeneration of vitamin KH_2 from vitamin K 2,3-epoxide.

SOURCES OF VITAMIN K

The major form of vitamin K in the diet is phylloquinone of plant origin. Prior to the development of methodology for analysis of foods for their vitamin K content by lipid extraction followed by high-performance liquid chromatography (HPLC), the vitamin K content of foods was estimated based on chick biological assays. Tables of vitamin K content of foods that were compiled prior to the mid-1990s were based on the chick bioassay and generally reported higher values for vitamin K than have been obtained with the HPLC method; in particular, most animal products including liver, cheeses, and whole eggs are not good sources of phylloquinone. A large number of foods and edible oils has been analyzed by these modern methods, and good estimates of the phylloquinone content of a wide range of foods are now available and are in the U.S. Department of Agriculture (USDA) nutrient database (USDA/ARS, 2005) and other publications (Dismore et al., 2003; Booth and Suttie, 1998). In general, green vegetables are the major source of phylloquinone in the diet, and foods such as kale, collards, spinach, parsley, broccoli, brussels sprouts, cabbage, and lettuce are excellent sources of the vitamin. Green leafy vegetables can provide as much as 400 to 500 μg per ½-cup serving. Plant oils and margarine are the second major source of phylloquinone in the diet. The phylloquinone content of plant oils is variable, with soybean and canola oils containing greater than 100 μg phylloquinone per 100 g (7.4 Tbsp), cottonseed oil and olive oil containing about 50 μg per 100 g, and corn oil containing less than 5 μg per 100 g. Fruits and nuts are not very important sources of vitamin K, but a few fruits (e.g., blueberries, blackberries, grapes, kiwi fruit, avocado, and prunes) provide on the order of 10 to 30 μg per ½-cup serving.

The bioavailability of phylloquinone to humans has not been studied extensively. The plasma level of deuterium-labeled phylloquinone was extensively enriched after intake of broccoli or collards grown hydroponically with deuterium oxide in order to label vitamin K within the food matrix (Erkkila et al., 2004; Dolnikowski et al., 2002). Based on the appearance of vitamin K in plasma following a single meal, the absorption of food-bound phylloquinone appeared to be much slower than that of pure phylloquinone or food-bound menaquinones (Booth et al., 2002; Schurgers and Vermeer, 2000; Garber et al., 1999). However, in a longer-term metabolic study involving 36 subjects and a cross-over design, no difference in the relative bioavailability of phylloquinone from broccoli or fortified oil was observed. Supplementation of a mixed diet, which contained 100 μg of phylloquinone, with 400 μg of phylloquinone from either broccoli or fortified oil for a 5-day period yielded similar increases in the plasma phylloquinone concentration and similar decreases in the percentage of osteocalcin that was undercarboxylated (Booth et al., 1999). However, because of the uncertain bioavailability of food phylloquinone, the Institute of Medicine (IOM, 2002) recommends that phylloquinone from vegetable sources not be considered to be more than 20% as available as phylloquinone consumed as a supplement.

Hydrogenation of phylloquinone-rich vegetable oils results in some conversion of phylloquinone to 2′,3′-dihydrophylloquinone (Booth et al., 1996). These hydrogenated vegetable oils are widely used by the food industry, and

Food Sources

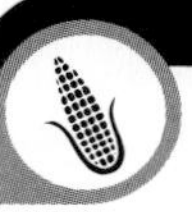

Food Sources of Phylloquinone

Vegetables

- 400 to 500 μg per ½ cup kale, collards, or spinach
- 75 to 150 μg per ½ cup brussels sprouts, broccoli, or asparagus
- 30 to 50 μg per ½ cup leaf lettuce, cabbage, or rhubarb
- 5 to 20 μg per ½ cup green peas, tomato sauce, soybeans, carrots, cauliflower, or green beans

Fruits

- 30 μg per medium kiwi fruit
- 15 μg per ½ cup blueberries or blackberries
- 13 μg per ½ cup seedless grapes

Plant Oils

- 15 to 25 μg per 1 Tbsp soybean or canola oil
- 5 to 20 μg per 1 Tbsp (oil-based) salad dressings
- 5 to 15 μg per 1 Tbsp margarine
- 7 μg per 1 Tbsp olive oil

Data from U.S. Department of Agriculture/Agricultural Research Service (USDA/ARS) (2005) USDA Nutrient Database for Standard Reference, Release 18. USDA/ARS, Washington, DC. Retrieved November 15, 2005, from www.ars.usda.gov/ba/bhnrc/ndl.

dihydroquinone is found in margarines, infant formulas, and many prepared foods. The estimated intake of 2′,3′-dihydrophylloquinone is 12 to 24 μg/day for older children and adults (Booth et al., 1996). Administration of the dihydrophylloquinone to rats counteracted warfarin-induced prolonged blood coagulation and decreased the effects of warfarin on serum total osteocalcin levels (Sato et al., 2003). Dihydrophylloquinone was absorbed and detected in tissues of the rats, but it was not converted to MK-4 as is phylloquinone. In humans, dihydrophylloquinone was less well-absorbed than phylloquinone and had no measurable biological effect on measures of bone formation and resorption (Booth et al., 2001).

Animal products are not rich sources of vitamin K. Limited amounts of MK-4 and higher menaquinones (i.e., MK-5–MK-10) have been found in some animal products including eggs, butter, various cheeses, beef and porcine liver, and fermented soybean products (Koivu-Tikkanen et al., 2000). A high amount of MK-4 was found in chicken meat. Although the higher menaquinones were found to be essentially absent in the milk of several species, MK-4 has been measured in the milk of various species and in a range of infant formulas (Indyk and Woollard, 1997). The total vitamin K content calculated from the sum of phylloquinone, MK-4, and higher menaquinones in animal products was in general low in terms of total dietary phylloquinone content.

Clinical Correlation

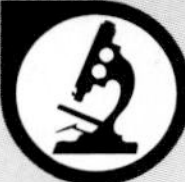

Vitamin K and Osteoporosis

Vitamin K_2 (MK-4) has been approved for treatment of osteoporosis in Japan (Iwamoto et al., 2003). MK-4 administration has been shown to increase γ-carboxylation of plasma osteocalcin indicating increased uptake of MK-4 by bone tissue. The mechanism underlying MK-4 prevention of osteoporosis is believed to be similar to the effect of the extensively used antiosteoporotic drugs bisphosphonates.

Intestinal anaerobes such as *Escherichia coli* and *Bacteroides fragilis* produce menaquinones, and the human gut contains large quantities of bacterially produced vitamin K. Early studies indicated that germ-free animals had an increased vitamin K requirement, but the nutritional significance of menaquinones produced in the lower bowel is not yet clear. The extent of, or mechanism of, absorption of menaquinones from the lower bowel has not been clearly established, although human liver does contain significant quantities of menaquinones. Cases of patients exhibiting a vitamin K–responsive hypoprothrombinemia after antibiotic administration have been reported. These episodes usually have been assumed to be the result of an influence of the antibiotic on menaquinone synthesis, but the limited data available indicate that most antibiotics do not negatively influence menaquinone production. Many of the case reports may simply reflect very low dietary intakes of vitamin K due to limited food intake in severely ill patients or, perhaps, hematological responses to various underlying illnesses.

The historical difficulty in producing a vitamin K deficiency in human subjects has been a second factor that suggests to investigators that menaquinones synthesized in the lower bowel are of nutritional importance. The total hepatic pool of menaquinones in humans is approximately 10 times that of phylloquinone, and this source of vitamin K appears to be at least to some extent utilizable. The high concentration in liver may reflect a slow turnover of this form of the vitamin. Limited data obtained from a rat model suggest that when a typical long-chain bacterial menaquinone (MK-9) is present in liver at concentrations similar to those of phylloquinone, it is not as effectively used as phylloquinone. The current data, therefore, suggest that menaquinones provide only a minor portion of the vitamin K needed to satisfy the human requirement.

VITAMIN K_1 CONVERSION TO MK-4 IN EXTRAHEPATIC TISSUES

In studies with germ-free rats, Ronden and colleagues (1998) found that phylloquinone was converted into MK-4 in extrahepatic tissues. The exact enzymatic pathway leading to the conversion has not yet been established. A physiological function for extrahepatic MK-4 has been the theme behind several studies. The studies have elucidated new functions for vitamin K and the potential of MK-4 as a prophylactic agent in treatment of osteoporosis (Iwamoto et al., 2003), arterial calcification (Spronk et al., 2003), and liver cancer (Habu et al., 2004). MK-4 has also been found to be the major form of vitamin K in the brain, where it is concentrated in myelinated regions (Carrie et al., 2004). These findings indicate a physiological role for MK-4 in the brain. In support of this hypothesis is the observation that mothers who use warfarin during pregnancy have an increased risk of damage to the central nervous system of the fetus (Pati and Helmbrecht, 1994). Interestingly, Sunderam and Lev (1988) found that warfarin administration reduces synthesis of sulfatides and other sphingolipids in mouse brain. MK-4 has also been shown to be a ligand for the steroid and xenobiotic receptor SXR and can affect gene expression of alkaline phosphatase, osteoprotegerin, osteopontin, and matrix Gla protein (Tabb et al., 2003). These proteins are involved in bone formation and regulation of bone formation (Wallin et al., 2001b).

ABSORPTION, TRANSPORT, AND METABOLISM OF VITAMIN K

Dietary phylloquinone is absorbed from the gut into the lymphatic system, and any conditions that result in a general impairment of lipid absorption will also adversely influence vitamin K absorption. Following incorporation into chylomicrons in the mucosa of the duodenum and jejunum, the vitamin is secreted into the lymph and ultimately enters the liver in association with the chylomicron remnant particles. Circulating phylloquinone is found in the high density (HDL), low density (LDL), and very low density (VLDL) lipoprotein fractions, and its concentration is increased in hyperlipidemic patients. The apolipoprotein E (apo E) genotype is known to influence plasma lipoprotein clearance and has also been demonstrated to influence circulating phylloquinone concentrations.

Circulating phylloquinone concentrations are highly dependent on recent dietary intake, and even postabsorptive values cover a wide range. Plasma phylloquinone concentrations in the healthy population appear to be about 1 nmol/L, with a range from 0.3 to 2.5 nmol/L (0.15 to 1.15 μg/L) (Sadowski et al., 1989). The plasma phylloquinone concentration of the healthy newborn is only approximately 0.05 nmol/L. Early studies did not detect circulating menaquinones in plasma, but, more recently, measurable concentrations of some of the long-chain menaquinones, mainly MK-7 and MK-8, have been reported (Suttie, 1995).

Measurements of human liver vitamin K content also are available. Values reported have been in the range of 2 to 20 ng of phylloquinone per gram of liver (Usui et al., 1990). A broad spectrum of bacterially produced long-chain menaquinones (MK-7 through MK-10) also is found in human liver, and the total concentration of menaquinones appears to be about 10-fold higher than that of phylloquinone (Suttie, 1995). Both forms of the vitamin are rapidly concentrated in liver of experimental animals following ingestion. In contrast to the other fat-soluble vitamins, which have a significant tissue storage pool, phylloquinone has a very rapid turnover in liver. The relatively high concentration of menaquinones found in human liver compared to the main dietary source of vitamin K, phylloquinone, may reflect a slower turnover of long-chain menaquinones relative to phylloquinone as has been demonstrated in animal models.

Phylloquinone is excreted predominantly in feces via the bile, but significant amounts also are excreted in the urine. Very little dietary phylloquinone is excreted unmetabolized, but the major metabolites are not well characterized. They appear to represent the stepwise oxidation of the side chain at the 3-position followed by formation of conjugates with glucuronic acid. The 2,3-epoxide, which is formed as the result of the biochemical role of vitamin K as substrate for the liver microsomal γ-glutamyl carboxylase, appears to be subject to the same general pathways of oxidative degradation as is the parent vitamin. Very limited information suggests that the pathway of degradative metabolism of menaquinones is similar to that of phylloquinone.

PHYSIOLOGICAL ROLES OF VITAMIN K–DEPENDENT PROTEINS

The vitamin K–dependent formation of Gla is old on an evolutionary scale, and some sea snails have Gla peptides that are used as potent neurotoxins (Bush et al., 1999). Vitamin K–dependent proteins are produced ubiquitously in the body. The most studied and best understood of these are the vitamin K–dependent plasma proteins involved in blood clotting, which are synthesized in the liver. These proteins include the coagulation cascade zymogens: prothrombin, factor VII, factor IX, and factor X (see Fig. 28-2). Vitamin K–dependent plasma proteins involved in anticoagulation are protein C, protein S, and protein Z (Broze, 2001; Furie and Furie, 1992).

The first extrahepatic vitamin K–dependent protein to be discovered was isolated from bone and contained three Gla residues. It is the second most abundant protein in bone and is called osteocalcin or bone Gla protein (BGP). Osteocalcin is a small 8-kDa protein synthesized by the bone-forming cells (osteoblasts). A small amount of this bone protein circulates in plasma, and the degree of γ carboxylation of plasma osteocalcin is sensitive to vitamin K nutritional status. Osteocalcin is believed to play a regulatory role in bone formation, and mice without functional osteocalcin characteristically acquire increased bone density (Ducy et al., 1996). Matrix Gla protein (MGP) is a 14-kDa vitamin K–dependent protein synthesized by chondrocytes, osteoblasts, vascular smooth muscle cells, and other cell types (Wallin et al., 2001b; Loeser et al., 1993). MGP is unique among the members of the vitamin K–dependent protein family by having the propeptide as part of the mature protein sequence (Sweatt et al., 2003). MGP null mice show extensive calcification of the arterial wall and cartilage, and MGP is believed to be an important calcification inhibitor (Luo et al., 1997). One hypothesis for MGP's mechanism of action as a calcification inhibitor is its binding to bone morphogenetic protein-2 (BMP-2), a potent growth factor that transforms preosteoblastic cells into bone-forming cells (Abedin et al., 2004). It has been demonstrated that the Gla modification of MGP is essential for the protein to bind BMP-2. This finding leads to the prediction that vitamin K deficiency may trigger the pathology of arterial calcification. Reports supporting this hypothesis are emerging (Schori and Stungis, 2004).

The vitamin K–dependent protein Gas6 (growth arrest gene 6), a homolog of the anticoagulation factor protein S, is a ligand for the Axl receptor, which is a member of a family of cell adhesion molecule–related tyrosine kinase receptors (Stitt et al., 1995). Gas6 has been shown to induce Axl tyrosine phosphorylation and promote cell survival, migration, and growth (Fridell et al., 1998). Gas6 is expressed extensively in the brain (Prieto et al., 1999). γ-Carboxylation of Gas6 is a prerequisite for the protein to promote growth of Schwann cells and smooth muscle cells in the central nervous system, and under-γ-carboxylation of Gas6 has been proposed as a possible mechanism underlying the pathology of Alzheimer's disease (Li et al., 1996). Four vitamin K–dependent putative membrane proteins—PRGP1, PRGP2, TmG3, and TmG4—some of which are located in the brain, have also been described, but the functions of these proteins are unknown (Kulman et al., 2001; 1997).

VITAMIN K DEFICIENCY

Although a primary vitamin K deficiency is uncommon in the adult human population, a vitamin K–responsive hemorrhagic disease of the newborn is also a rare but long-recognized syndrome. Vitamin K stores of the newborn are low because of poor placental transfer of the vitamin, and the sterile gut precludes any possible production and utilization of menaquinones during early life. These conditions are complicated by a general hypoprothrombinemia in infants caused by the inability of immature liver to synthesize normal levels of clotting factors.

The breast-fed infant is at particular risk. The vitamin K content of breast milk is less than that of cow's milk, and a low intake of phylloquinone by nursing infants has been shown to be a strong contributing factor in the development of vitamin K deficiency in the newborn.

Plasma vitamin K concentrations in a group of exclusively breast-fed infants averaged 1.2 μg/L at 2 weeks of age and had decreased to 0.2 μg/L by 6 weeks of age (Greer, 2001). (The lower limit of adult normal levels is 0.5 μg/L.) Commercial infant formulas are now routinely supplemented with vitamin K. Nursing mothers can increase vitamin K levels in their milk by taking phylloquinone supplements (Thijssen et al., 2002). The American and Canadian pediatric societies recommend intramuscular administration of phylloquinone at birth as routine prophylaxis, and such prophylaxis is required by law in some other countries. The practice of oral or intramuscular administration of vitamin K to the newborn is almost universal in developed countries, but hemorrhagic disease remains a potential problem for breast-fed infants in some areas of the world.

The most common condition known to result in a vitamin K–responsive hemorrhagic event in the adult is a low dietary intake of vitamin K by a patient who also is receiving antibiotics. These cases are numerous, which suggests that patients with restricted food intake who also are receiving antibiotics should be closely observed for signs of vitamin K deficiency. These episodes historically have been attributed to an interference of antibiotics with the microbial synthesis of menaquinones in the gut, but evidence to substantiate this effect is lacking.

Vitamin K deficiency also has been reported in patients subjected to long-term total parenteral nutrition, and supplementation of the vitamin is advised in these circumstances. Supplementation in the case of biliary obstruction also is advisable because the impairment of lipid absorption resulting from the lack of bile salts adversely affects vitamin K absorption. Depression of the plasma levels of vitamin K–dependent coagulation factors frequently has been found in patients with malabsorption syndromes and other gastrointestinal disorders (e.g., cystic fibrosis, sprue, celiac disease, ulcerative colitis, regional ileitis, Ascaris infection, and short-bowel syndrome), and patients usually respond to vitamin K administration with an increase in the level of plasma coagulation factors.

ASSESSMENT OF VITAMIN K STATUS

Although recent advances in methodology have made it possible to routinely measure the plasma or serum phylloquinone concentration, the factors influencing these concentrations and their relationship to dietary intake have not yet been clarified. Alteration of plasma phylloquinone by dietary restriction of the vitamin now has been reported in a number of studies (Braam et al., 2004). However, because of the close relationship of plasma phylloquinone to recent dietary intake, these measurements lack utility for assessing vitamin K status. The clinical "prothrombin time," which is a measure of the rate of thrombin generation in a small sample of plasma, historically has been used to assess the activities of the vitamin K–dependent clotting factors. A major problem in determining a dietary requirement for vitamin K has been the relative insensitivity of the commonly used prothrombin time as a measure of the activity of the vitamin K–dependent plasma proteins. Assessment of vitamin K status by use of the relatively insensitive clinical prothrombin time has meant that a rather large decrease in vitamin K–dependent clotting factor synthesis was needed to produce an apparent deficiency.

More-sensitive clotting assays and the ability to immunochemically detect circulating forms of prothrombin that lack some or all of the normal content of Gla residues now permit monitoring of much milder forms of vitamin K deficiency. The plasma concentration of under-γ-carboxylated prothrombin is a sensitive measure of vitamin K status, with low intakes of phylloquinone being associated with elevated concentrations. There are a number of reports that vitamin K status may be important in maintaining skeletal health, and the extent of under-γ-carboxylation of circulating osteocalcin has been considered as a possible criterion of vitamin K sufficiency. Although it is clear that vitamin K intake affects the degree of osteocalcin γ-carboxylation, technical problems with current assays, as well as the uncertain physiological significance of the measure, limit the current usefulness of the degree of carboxylation of osteocalcin for assessment of vitamin K status. Nevertheless, it is clear that there is a preferential utilization of vitamin K by the liver to support hepatic γ-carboxylation functions, and nonhepatic functions may be important for adequate monitoring of vitamin K status.

RECOMMENDATIONS FOR VITAMIN K INTAKE

The IOM (2002) in setting the DRIs, did not set a recommended dietary allowance (RDA) for vitamin K because of the lack of adequate data to estimate the average requirement. Adequate intakes (AIs) were set based on representative dietary intake data from healthy individuals. The AI for infants is based on the average intake of milk (0.78 L/day) and the average phylloquinone concentration in human milk (2.5 μg/L), which yields an AI of 2.0 μg/day after rounding for infants up to 6 months of age. This AI determination assumes that infants receive the recommended 1 mg of prophylactic vitamin K at birth. Because infant formulas typically provide 50 to 100 μg/L of phylloquinone, formula-fed infants have much higher intakes. The AI for 6- to 12-month-old infants was set at 2.5 μg/day by extrapolating up from the AI for younger infants because an intake of 2.5 μg/day has not been associated with adverse clinical outcomes. The AI would have been much higher if it had been extrapolated down from the typical intakes of older children, and the intake of the older infant will generally be much higher than the AI due to intake of complementary foods.

The AIs for children were determined on the basis of the median intake for each age group reported by the Third National Health and Nutrition Examination Survey (NHANES III) and rounding up to the nearest 5 μg/day. The AIs for men and women of all ages were set according to the highest median intake value observed among the four adult age groupings used in NHANES III. These AIs are 120 μg/day for men and 90 μg/day for women. No additional intake was recommended for pregnant or lactating women.

The AI values set by the IOM (2002) would be judged adequate by the criteria used previously to set the 1989 RDAs, which was 1 μg per kg body weight per day based on limited studies indicating that the vitamin K requirement of humans was in the range of 0.5 to 1.5 μg/kg/day.

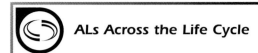

ALs Across the Life Cycle

	μg Vitamin K per Day
Infant	
0 to 0.5 yr	2.0
0.5 to 1 yr	2.5
Children	
1 to 3 yr	30
4 to 8 yr	55
9 to 13 yr	75
14 to 18 yr	75
Pregnant females	75
Males	
≥ 19 yr	120
Females	
≥ 19 yr	90
Pregnant	90
Lactating	90

Data from Institute of Medicine (IOM) (2002) Dietary Reference Intakes for Vitamin A, Vitamin K, Arsenic, Boron, Chromium, Copper, Iodine, Iron, Manganese, Molybdenum, Nickel, Silicon, Vanadium, and Zinc. National Academy Press, Washington, DC.
AI, Adequate intake.

No tolerable upper intake level (UL) was established because ingestion of high doses of phylloquinone, the natural form of the vitamin, has no toxic effect. Menadione, a synthetic form of the vitamin, was administered to infants at one time but was shown to be associated with hemolytic anemia and liver toxicity and is no longer used.

REFERENCES

Abedin M, Tintut Y, Demer LL (2004) Vascular calcification: mechanisms and clinical ramifications. Arterioscler Thromb Vasc Biol 24:1161-1170.

Booth SL, Lichtenstein AH, Dallal GE (2002) Phylloquinone absorption from phylloquinone-fortified oil is greater than from a vegetable in younger and older men and women. J Nutr 132:2609-2612.

Booth SL, Lichtenstein AH, O'Brien-Morse M, McKeown NM, Wood RJ, Saltzman E, Gundberg CM. (2001) Effects of a hydrogenated form of vitamin K on bone formation and resorption. Am J Clin Nutr 74:783-790.

Booth SL, O'Brien-Morse ME, Dallal GE, Davidson KW, Gundberg CM (1999) Response of vitamin K status to different intakes and sources of phylloquinone-rich foods: comparison of younger and older adults. Am J Clin Nutr 70:368-377.

Booth SL, Pennington JA, Sadowski JA (1996) Dihydro-vitamin K_1: primary food sources and estimated intakes in the American diet. Lipids 31:715-720.

Booth, SL, Suttie JW (1998) Dietary intake and adequacy of vitamin K. J Nutr 128:785-788.

Braam L, McKeown N, Jacques P, Lichtenstein A, Vermeer C, Wilson P, Booth S (2004) Dietary phylloquinone intake as a potential marker for a heart-healthy dietary pattern in the Framingham Offspring cohort. J Am Diet Assoc 104:1410-1414.

Broze GJ Jr (2001) Protein Z dependent regulation of coagulation. Thromb Haemostas 86:8-13.

Bush KA, Stenflo J, Roth DA, Czerwiec E, Harrist A, Begley GS, Furie BC, Furie B (1999) Hydrophobic amino acids define the carboxylation recognition site in the precursor of the gamma-carboxyglutamic-acid-containing conotoxin epsilon-TxIX from the marine cone snail Conus textile. Biochemistry 38:14660-14466.

Carrie I, Portaulalian J, Vicaaretti R, Rochford J, Potvin S, Ferland G (2004) Menaquinone-4 concentration is correlated with sphingolipid concentration in rat brain. J Nutr 134:167-172.

Dam H (1934) Haemorrhages in chicks reared on artificial diets: a new deficiency disease. Nature 133:909-910.

Davie EW, Ratnof OD (1964) Waterfall sequence for intrinsic blood clotting. Science 145:1310-1311.

Dismore ML, Haytowitz DB, Gebhardt SE, Peterson JW, Booth SL (2003) Vitamin K content of nuts and fruits in the US diet. J Am Diet Assoc. 103:1650-1652.

Diuguid DL, Rabiet MJ, Furie BC, Liebman HA, Furie B (1986) Molecular basis of hemophilia B: defective enzyme due to an unprocessed propeptide is caused by a point mutation in the factor IX precursor. Proc Natl Acad Sci U S A 83:5803-5807.

Dolnikowski GG, Sun Z, Grusak MA, Peterson JW, Booth SL (2002) HPLC and GC/MS determination of deuterated vitamin K (phylloquinone) in human serum after ingestion of deuterium-labeled broccoli. J Nutr Biochem 13:168-174.

Dowd P, Hershline R, Ham SW, Naganathan S (1995) Vitamin K and energy transduction: a base strength amplification mechanism. Science 269:1684-1691.

Ducy P, Desbois C, Boyce B, Pinero G, Story B, Dunstan C, Smith E, Bonadio J, Goldstein S, Gundberg C, Bradley A, Karsenty G (1996) Increased bone formation in osteocalcin-deficient mice. Nature 382:448-452.

Erkkila AT, Lichtenstein AH, Dolnikowski GG, Grusak MA, Jalbert SM, Aquino KA, Peterson JW, Booth SL (2004) Plasma transport of vitamin K in men using deuterium-labeled collard greens. Metabolism 53:215-221.

Esmon CT, Sadowski JA, Suttie JW (1975) A new carboxylation reaction: the vitamin K–dependent incorporation of $H^{14}CO_3^-$ into prothrombin. J Biol Chem 250:4744-4748.

Fasco MJ, Principe LM, Walsh WA, Friedman PA (1983) Warfarin inhibition of vitamin K 2,3-epoxide reductase in rat liver microsomes. Biochemistry 22:5655-5660.

Fregin A, Rost S, Wolz W, Krebsova A, Muller CR, Oldenburg J (2002) Homozygosity mapping of a second gene locus for hereditary combined deficiency of vitamin K–dependent clotting factors to the centromeric region of chromosome 16. Blood 100:3229-3232.

Fridell YW, Villa J Jr, Attar EC, Liu ET (1998) GAS6 induces Axl-mediated chemotaxis of vascular smooth muscle cells. J Biol Chem 273: 7123-7126.

Furie B, Furie B (1992) Molecular and cellular biology of blood coagulation. N Engl J Med 326:800-806.

Garber AK, Binkley NC, Krueger DC, Suttie JW (1999) Comparison of phylloquinone bioavailability from food sources or a supplement in human subjects. J Nutr 129:1201-1203.

Greaves JH, Ayres P (1967) Heritable resistance to warfarin in rats. Nature 215: 877-878.

Greer FR (2001) Are breast-fed infants vitamin K deficient? Adv Exp Med Biol 501:391-395.

Habu D, Shiomi S, Tamori A, Takeda T, Tanaka T, Kubo S, Nishiguchi S (2004) Role of vitamin K_2 in the development of hepatocellular carcinoma in women with viral cirrhosis of the liver. JAMA 292:358-361.

Hanatani T, Fukuda T, Onishi S, Funae Y, Azuma J (2003) No major difference in inhibitory susceptibility between CYP2C9.1 and CYP2C9.3. Eur J Clin Pharmacol 59:233-235.

Hemker HC, Reekers PPM (1974) Isolation and purification of proteins induced by vitamin K absence. Thromb Diath Haemorrhag Suppl 57:83-85.

Hermodson MA, Suttie JW, Link KP (1969) Warfarin metabolism and vitamin K requirement in the warfarin-resistant rat. Am J Physiol 217:1316-1319.

Hildebrandt EF, Suttie JW (1982) Mechanism of coumarin action: sensitivity of vitamin K metabolizing enzymes of normal and warfarin-resistant rat liver. Biochemistry 21:2406-2411.

Honore B, Vorum H (2000) The CREC family, a novel family of multiple EF-hand, low-affinity Ca^{2+}-binding proteins localized to the secretory pathway of mammalian cells. FEBS Lett 466:11-18.

Indyk HE, Woollard DC (1997) Vitamin K in milk and infant formulas: determination and distribution of phylloquinone and menaquinone-4. Analyst 122:465-469.

Institute of Medicine (IOM) (2002) Dietary Reference Intakes for Vitamin A, Vitamin K, Arsenic, Boron, Chromium, Copper, Iodine, Iron, Manganese, Molybdenum, Nickel, Silicon, Vanadium and Zinc. National Academy Press, Washington, DC.

Iwamoto J, Takeda T, Ichimura S (2003) Combined treatment with vitamin K_2 and bisphosphonate in postmenopausal woman with osteoporosis. Yonsei Med J 44:751-756.

Kohn MH, Pelz HJ, Wayne RK (2003) Locus-specific genetic differentiation at *Rw* among warfarin resistant rat (Rattus norvegicus) populations. Genetics 164:1055-1070.

Koivu-Tikkanen TJ, Ollilainen V, Piironen VI (2000) Determination of phylloquinone and menaquinones in animal products with fluorescence detection after postcolumn reduction with metallic zinc. J Agricl Food Chem 48:6325-6333.

Kulman JD, Harris JE, Haldeman BA, Davie EW (1997) Primary structure and tissue distribution of two novel proline-rich γ-carboxyglutamic acid proteins. Proc Natl Acad Sci U S A 94:9058-9062.

Kulman JD, Harris JE, Xie L, Davie EW (2001) Identification of two novel transmembrane gamma-carboxyglutamic acid proteins expressed broadly in fetal and adult tissues. Proc Natl Acad Sci U S A 98:1370-1375.

Li T, Chang CY, Jin DY, Lin PJ, Khvorova A, Stafford DW (2004) Identification of the gene for vitamin K epoxide reductase. Nature 437:541-544.

Li R, Chen J, Hammonds G, Phillips H, Armanini M, Wood P, Bunge R, Godowski PJ, Sliwkowski MX, Mather JP (1996) Identification of Gas6 as a growth factor for human Schwann cells. J Neurosci 16:2012-2019.

Loeser RF, Wallin R, Sadowski J (1993) Vitamin K and vitamin K-dependent proteins in the elderly: implications for bone and cartilage biology. In: Watson RR (ed) Handbook of Nutrition in the Aged, 2nd ed. CRC Press, Boca Raton, FL, pp 263-280.

Luo G, Ducy P, McKee MD, Pinero GJ, Loyer E, Behringer RR, Karsenty G (1997) Spontaneous calcification of arteries and cartilage in mice lacking matrix Gla protein. Nature 386:78-81.

Macfarlane RG (1965) The basis of the cascade hypothesis of blood coagulation. Thromb Diath Haemorrhag 15:591-602.

Malhotra OP (1972) Terminal amino acids of normal and dicumarol-treated prothrombin. Life Sci 11:445-454.

Matschiner JT, Bell RG, Amelotti JM, Knauer TE (1970) Isolation and characterization of a new metabolite of phylloquinone in the rat. Biochim Biophys Acta 201:309-315.

Meehan AP (ed) (1984) Rats and Mice: Their Biology and Control. Rentokil Limited, Felcourt, East Grinstead, W. Sussex.

Nelsestuen GL, Zytkovicz TH, Howard JB (1974) The mode of action of vitamin K: identification of γ-carboxyglutamic acid as a component of prothrombin. J Biol Chem 249:6347-6350.

Pati S, Helmbrecht GD (1994) Congenital schizencephaly associated with in utero warfarin exposure. Reprod Toxicol 8:115-120.

Prieto AL, Weber JL, Tracy S, Heeb MJ, Lai C (1999) Gas6, a ligand for the receptor protein-tyrosine kinase Tyro-3, is widely expressed in the central nervous system. Brain Res 816:646-661.

Ronden JE, Drittij-Reijnders MJ, Vermeer C, Thijssen HH (1998) Intestinal flora is not an intermediate in the phylloquinone-menaquinone-4 conversion in the rat. Biochem Biophys Acta 1379:69-75.

Rost S, Fregin A, Ivaskevicius V, Conzelmann E, Hortnagel K, Pelz HJ, Lappegard K, Seifried E, Scharrer I, Tuddenham EG, Muller CR, Stron TM, Oldenburg J (2004) Mutations in VKORC1 cause warfarin resistance and multiple coagulation factor deficiency type 2. Nature 437:537-541.

Sadowski JA, Hood SJ, Dallal GE, Garry PJ (1989) Phylloquinone in plasma from elderly and young adults: Factors influencing its concentration. Am J Clin Nutr 50:100-108.

Sato T, Ozaki R, Kamo S, Hara Y, Konishi S, Isobe Y, Saitoh S, Harada H (2003) The biological activity and tissue distribution of 2′,3′-dihydrophylloquinone in rats. Biochem Biophys Acta 1622:145-150.

Schori TR, Stungis GE (2004) Long-term warfarin treatment may induce arterial calcification in humans: case report. Clin Invest Med 27:107-109.

Schurgers LJ, Vermeer C (2002) Differential lipoprotein transport pathways of K-vitamins in healthy subjects. Biochim Biophys Acta 1570:27-32.

Spronk HM, Soute BA, Schurgers LJ, Thijssen HH, De Mey JG, Vermeer C (2003) Tissue-specific utilization of menaquinone-4 results in the prevention of arterial calcification in warfarin-treated rats. J Vasc Res 40:531-537.

Stanton C, Taylor R, Wallin R (1991) Processing of prothrombin in the secretory pathway. Biochem J 277:59-65.

Stenflo J, Fernlund P, Egan W, Roepstorff P (1974) Vitamin K dependent modifications of glutamic acid residues in prothrombin. Proc Natl Acad Sci U S A 71:2730-2733.

Stenina O, Pudota BN, McNally BA, Hommema EL, Berkner KL (2001) Tethered processivity of the Vitamin K-dependent carboxylase: Factor IX is efficiently modified in a mechanism which distinguishes Gla's from Glu's and which accounts for comprehensive carboxylation in vivo. Biochemistry 40:10301-10309.

Stitt TN, Conn G, Gore M, Lai C, Bruno J, Radziejewski C, Mattsson K, Fisher J, Gies DR, Jones PF, Masiakowski P, Ryan TE, Tobkes NJ, Chen OH, DiStefano PS, Long GL, Basilico C, Goldfarb MP, Lemke G, Glass DJ, Yancopoulos GD (1995) The anticoagulation factor protein S and its relative, Gas6, are ligands for the Tyro 3/Axl family of receptor tyrosine kinases. Cell 24:661-670.

Sugiura I, Furie B, Walsh CT, Furie BC (1997) Propeptide and glutamate-containing substrates bound to the vitamin K-dependent carboxylase convert its vitamin K epoxidase function from an inactive to an active state. Proc Natl Acad Sci USA 94:9069-9074.

Sundaram KS, Lev M (1988) Warfarin administration reduces synthesis of sulfatides and other sphingolipids in mouse brain. J Lipid Res 29:1475-1479.

Suttie JW (1978) Vitamin K. In: Deluca HF (ed) Handbook of Lipid Research. Plenum Press, New York, pp 211-277.

Suttie JW (1995) The importance of menaquinones in human nutrition. Annu Rev Nutr 15:399-417.

Sweatt A, Sane DC, Hutson SM, Wallin R (2003) Matrix Gla protein (MGP) and bone morphogenetic protein-2 in aortic calcified lesions of aging rats. J Thromb Haemost 1:178-185.

Tabb MM, Sun A, Zhou C, Grun F, Errandi J, Romero K, Pham H, Inoue S, Mallick S, Lin M, Forman BM, Blumberg B (2003) Vitamin K_2 regulation of bone homeostasis is mediated by the steroid and xenobiotic receptor SXR. J Biol Chem 7:278:43919-43927.

Tie J, Wu SM, Jin D, Nicchitta CF, Stafford DW (2000) A topological study of the human gamma-glutamyl carboxylase. Blood 96:973-978.

Thijssen HH, Drittij MJ, Vermeer C, Schoffelen E (2002) Menaquinone-4 in breast milk is derived from dietary phylloquinone. Br J Nutr 87:219-226.

U.S. Department of Agriculture, Agricultural Research Service (USDA/ARS) (2005) USDA National Nutrient Database for Standard Reference, Release 18. USDA/ARS, Washington, DC. Retrieved November 15, 2005, from www.ars.usda.gov/ba/bhnrc/ndl.

Usui Y, Tanimura H, Nishimura N, Kobayashi N, Okanoue T, Ozawa K (1990) Vitamin K concentrations in the plasma and liver of surgical patients. Am J Clin Nutr 51:846-852.

Vermeer C, Schurgers LJ (2000) A comprehensive review of vitamin K and vitamin K antagonists. Hematol Oncol Clin North Am 14:339-353.

Wajih N, Sane DC, Hutson SM, Wallin R (2004) The inhibitory effect of calumenin on the vitamin K-dependent γ-carboxylation system: characterization of the system in normal and warfarin resistant rats. J Biol Chem 279:25276-25283.

Wajih N, Sane DC, Hutson SM, Wallin R (2005) Engineering of a recombinant vitamin K-dependent gamma-carboxylation system with enhanced gamma-carboxyglutamic acid forming capacity: evidence for a functional CXXC redox center in the system. J Biol Chem 280:10540-10547.

Wallace ME, MacSwiney FJ (1976) A major gene controlling warfarin-resistance in the house mouse. J Hyg (Lond) 76:173-181.

Wallin R, Martin LF (1987) Warfarin poisoning and vitamin K antagonism in rat and human liver. Design of a system in vitro that mimics the system in vivo. Biochem J 241:389-396.

Wallin R, Hutson SM, Cain D, Sweatt A, Sane DC (2001a) A molecular mechanism for genetic warfarin resistance in the rat. FASEB J 15:2542-2544.

Wallin R, Wajih N, Greenwood GT, Sane DC (2001b) Arterial calcification: a review of mechanisms, animal models, and the prospects for therapy. Med Res Rev 21: 274-301.

Wallin R, Sane DC, Hutson SM (2002) Vitamin K 2,3-epoxide reductase and the vitamin K-dependent gamma-carboxylation system. Thromb Res 108:221-226.

Whitlon DS, Sadowski JA, Suttie JW (1978) Mechanism of coumarin action: significance of vitamin K epoxide reductase inhibition. Biochemistry 17:1317-1317.

Wu S-M, Morris DP, Stafford DW (1991) Identification and purification to near homogeneity of the vitamin K-dependent carboxylase. Proc Natl Acad Sci U S A 88:2236-2240.

RECOMMENDED READINGS

Dowd P, Ham S-W, Naganathan S, Hershline R (1995) The mechanism of action of vitamin K. Annu Rev Nutr 15:419-440.

Link KP (1959) The discovery of dicumarol and its sequels. Circulation 19:97-107.

Suttie JW (1992) Vitamin K and human nutrition. J Am Diet Assoc 92:585-590.

Wallin R, Hutson SM (2004) Warfarin and the vitamin K-dependent gamma-carboxylation system. Trends Mol Med 10:299-302.

Chapter 29

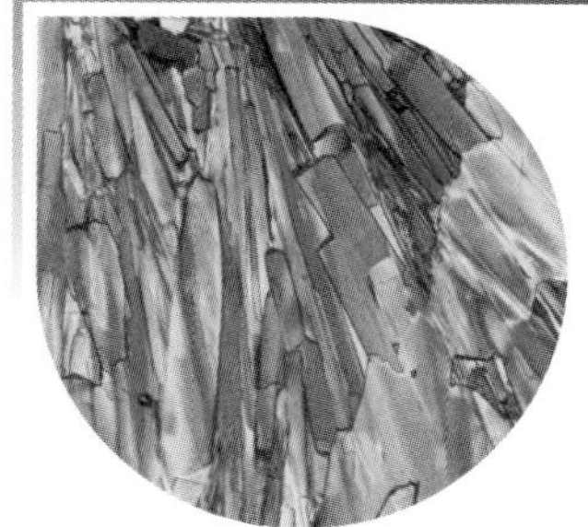

Vitamin E

Robert S. Parker, PhD

OUTLINE

NOMENCLATURE AND STRUCTURE OF VITAMIN E

Vitamin E was discovered more than 80 years ago as a lipid-soluble substance necessary for the prevention of fetal death and resorption in rats that had been fed a rancid lard diet (Evans and Bishop, 1922). Vitamin E is the collective term for all of the structurally related tocopherols and tocotrienols (collectively termed tocochromanols, or the "vitamers" of vitamin E) and their derivatives that qualitatively exhibit the biological activity of RRR-α-tocopherol in prevention of rat fetal resorption. Therefore, the term vitamin E is not synonymous with α-tocopherol. Tocopherol is derived from the Greek words *tokos* (childbirth), *phero* (to bring forth), and *ol* (alcohol), and relates to the role of vitamin E in reproduction in animals.

Four tocopherols and four tocotrienols occur naturally. All consist of a chromanol head group and a phytyl side chain and differ in the number and position of methyl groups on the phenol ring of the chromanol head group (Fig. 29-1). The structure of a tocotrienol is similar to that of a tocopherol, except that the hydrophobic phytyl side chain of the tocotrienols contains double bonds at the 3′, 7′, and 11′ positions. In addition to these eight naturally occurring vitamers, synthetic α-tocopherol, as either free or ester forms, is available commercially. The tocopherol molecule has three chiral centers in its phytyl tail, making a total of eight stereoisomeric forms possible.

This chapter is a revision of the chapter contributed by Ching K. Chow, PhD, for the first edition.

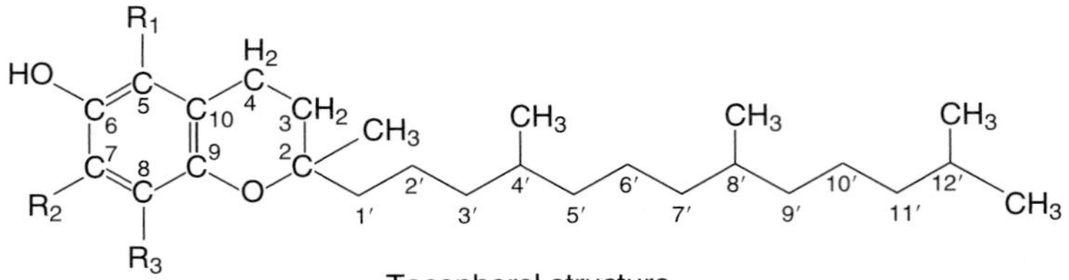

Tocopherol structure

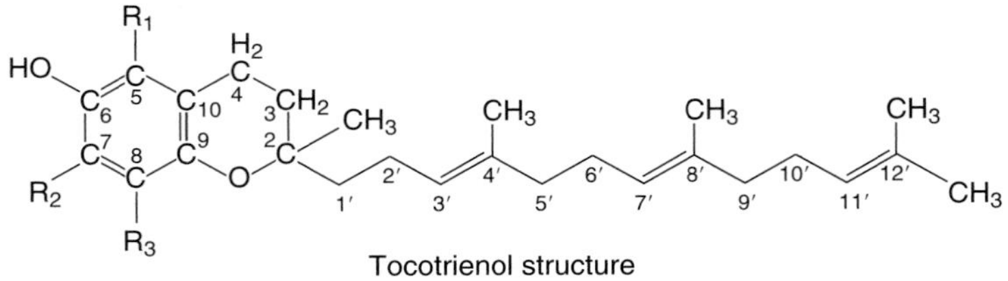

Tocotrienol structure

Position of methyls	Tocopherol structure	Tocotrienol structure
R_1,R_2,R_3	α-Tocopherol (α-T)	α-Tocotrienol (α-T-3)
R_1,R_3	β-Tocopherol (β-T)	β-Tocotrienol (β-T-3)
R_2,R_3	γ-Tocopherol (γ-T)	γ-Tocotrienol (γ-T-3)
R_3	δ-Tocopherol (δ-T)	δ-Tocotrienol (δ-T-3)

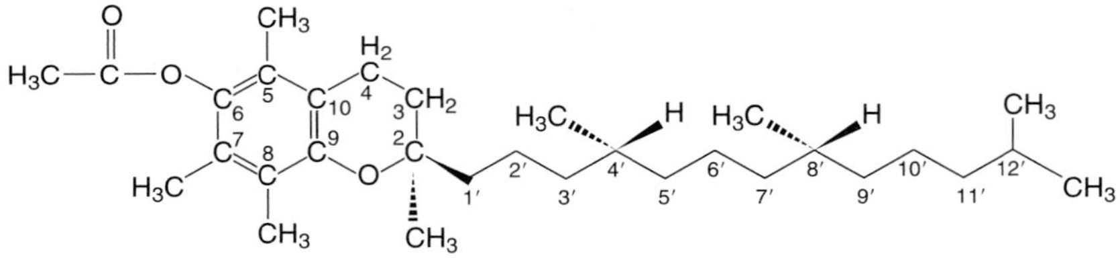

2R, 4′R, 8′R-α-Tocopherol acetate

Figure 29-1 Chemical structures of tocopherols, tocotrienols, and α-tocopheryl acetate.

The naturally occurring isomer of α-tocopherol (formerly known as d-α-tocopherol) biosynthesized by plants is the 2R, 4′R, 8′R stereoisomer, whereas synthetic α-tocopherol consists of a mixture of all eight possible stereoisomers. The tetrahedral arrangement of substituents around each asymmetric chiral center is designated R (from the Latin *rectus,* meaning "right") or S (from the Latin *sinister,* meaning "left"). To distinguish the naturally occurring stereoisomer of α-tocopherol from the synthetic mixture, naturally occurring α-tocopherol is designated as RRR-α-tocopherol, and the synthetic mixture of α-tocopherol stereoisomers (previously known as dl-α-tocopherol) is designated as all-racemic (all-rac)-α-tocopherol. Naturally occurring tocopherols in foods exist as the free (unesterified) forms. Synthetic ester forms of α-tocopherol are produced by forming ester linkages between the 6-hydroxyl group of the phenolic ring of α-tocopherol and the carboxylate group of acetic acid (see Fig. 29-1) or succinic acid. The acetate or succinate ester forms of α-tocopherol are more chemically stable and are, therefore, more suitable for food fortification or vitamin supplement formulations than unesterified α-tocopherol.

ABSORPTION, TRANSPORT, AND METABOLISM OF VITAMIN E

The absorption and transport of vitamin E follows to a large extent the paths of cholesterol absorption and transport. Vitamin E is absorbed with other lipids, incorporated into chylomicrons, and eventually transported by other circulating lipoproteins. The tocochromanols are metabolized to water-soluble metabolites that are excreted primarily via the urine.

ABSORPTION

The process of intestinal absorption of vitamin E is similar to that of other lipid components of the diet. Tocopheryl esters, when present, first are hydrolyzed to free tocopherol by pancreatic esterases in the proximal lumen of the small intestine. Tocopherols and toco-trienols, as constituents of bile-salt micelles, are taken up, apparently by passive diffusion, into enterocytes lining the small intestine. Within the enterocyte, tocochromanols are incorporated, along with other lipids, into nascent triglyceride-rich chylomicrons. The chylomicrons are secreted into the intercellular space, from which they enter the lymphatics and, eventually, the bloodstream. Estimates of the absorption efficiency of tocopherol vary widely, but it appears that roughly half of the tocopherols consumed in foods is absorbed, with the remainder excreted in the feces. There appear to be no major differences in the rates of intestinal absorption of the various forms of vitamin E (Kayden and Traber, 1993).

TRANSPORT AND TISSUE UPTAKE

Because of its virtual insolubility in water, vitamin E requires special transport mechanisms in the aqueous milieu of the body. As described, dietary tocopherols taken up by the small intestine are incorporated into triacylglycerol-rich chylomicrons, secreted into the intestinal lymph, and eventually delivered to the liver in the chylomicron remnants. Newly absorbed vitamin E taken up by parenchymal cells of the liver is either incorporated into nascent very low density lipoproteins (VLDLs) and secreted back into the bloodstream or metabolized within the liver to water-soluble metabolites. Endogenous vitamin E in other tissues appears to be released to high density lipoproteins (HDLs) and other plasma lipoproteins and recirculated to the liver or other tissues. Tocopherols undergo exchange between lipoproteins, facilitated by a phospholipid transfer protein found in plasma (Kostner et al., 1995). Therefore, in the fasting state tocopherols are approximately equally distributed between low density lipoproteins (LDLs) and HDLs.

Tocopherols circulating in lipoproteins can be taken up by tissues via various receptor-mediated processes. Chylomicron remnants are taken up by the parenchymal cells of the liver via an apolipoprotein E receptor–mediated mechanism, and LDL particles are taken up by liver and other tissues via the LDL receptor pathway. Other mechanisms of cell uptake may involve selective uptake from HDLs via scavenger receptors, as is the case with cholesterol. In addition, some of the vitamin E in association with chylomicrons and VLDLs may be transferred to peripheral cells during the lipolysis of these triglyceride-rich lipoproteins by lipoprotein lipase. Recent studies of vitamin E delivery to tissues in transgenic mice overexpressing human lipoprotein lipase in muscle demonstrated enhanced vitamin E uptake by skeletal muscle but not by adipose tissue or brain (Sattler et al., 1996). (See Chapter 17 for an overview of lipoprotein metabolism.)

The process of secretion of α-tocopherol from the liver via VLDLs is critical to maintaining normal plasma vitamin E levels. A tocopherol-binding protein, called α-tocopherol transfer protein (α-TTP) plays an important role in this process. This protein is found predominantly in liver, and preferentially binds RRR-α-tocopherol relative to other forms of vitamin E (Hosomi et al., 1997). In the liver, α-TTP facilitates the secretion of α-tocopherol into the plasma lipoprotein pool (Traber et al., 1993) via a non–Golgi-dependent mechanism that has not been fully elucidated (Kaempf-Rotzoll et al., 2003). This results in the preferential enrichment of LDLs and HDLs with α-tocopherol compared with the other forms of vitamin E. The critical role

Clinical Correlation

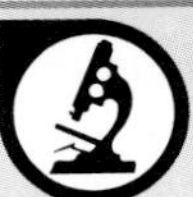

Familial Isolated Vitamin E Deficiency

Secondary vitamin E deficiency occurs in patients with generalized fat malabsorption caused by disorders such as abetalipoproteinemia, cystic fibrosis, short-bowel syndrome, and cholestatic liver disease. In these patients, prolonged deficiency of vitamin E eventually causes a decrease in the tocopherol content of nervous tissues and results in spinocerebellar dysfunction with progressive ataxia. In contrast, over the last 2 decades, a number of patients have been documented as having specific inherited forms of vitamin E deficiency. These cases have been described as familial isolated vitamin E deficiency or ataxia with isolated vitamin E deficiency. Patients with this autosomal recessive neurodegenerative disease develop symptoms that resemble those of Friedreich's ataxia. These patients have normal gastrointestinal absorption of dietary lipids and α-tocopherol, with normal incorporation of lipids and vitamin E into chylomicrons. They have, however, an impaired ability to secrete α-tocopherol from the liver, a function that apparently allows healthy individuals to efficiently reincorporate α-tocopherol obtained from lipoprotein remnants back into the plasma lipoprotein pool (Traber et al., 1993). Therefore, in patients with familial isolated vitamin E deficiency, the absorption and transport of vitamin E to the liver are normal, but the hepatic incorporation of α-tocopherol into VLDL is impaired; this results in a low or undetectable plasma vitamin E concentration and insufficient delivery of vitamin E to tissues.

The α-tocopherol transfer protein (α-TTP) is a cytosolic liver protein with high binding affinity for RRR-α-tocopherol. The physiological function of this protein had remained unclear until 1995, even though it was known that this protein transferred α-tocopherol between membranes in vitro. The cDNA for α-TTP was isolated from rats and humans, and the human α-TPP gene was shown to be located at chromosome 8q13 (Arita et al., 1995). Familial vitamin E deficiency mutations had previously been mapped to this same location. Ouahchi and colleagues (1995) demonstrated α-TTP gene mutations in patients with familial isolated vitamin E deficiency, confirming that mutations of the gene for α-TTP are responsible for isolated vitamin E deficiency. The degree of functionality of the mutant α-TTP seems to be associated with the degree of severity of the neurological damage and age of onset as well as with plasma vitamin E concentration (Gotoda et al., 1995). High doses of vitamin E can prevent or mitigate the neurological course of this disease. Serum vitamin E concentrations in patients increase when they are treated with large doses of vitamin E, presumably because of the direct transfer of tocopherol from chylomicrons or their remnants to tissues or to other circulating lipoproteins.

Thinking Critically

1. The affinity of α-TTP for various forms of vitamin E varies and is highest for RRR-α-tocopherol. There seems to be a linear relationship between the relative binding affinity (RRR-α-tocopherol, 100%; RRR-β-tocopherol, 38%; SRR-α-tocopherol, 11%; RRR-γ-tocopherol, 9%; and RRR-δ-tocopherol, 2%) and the known biological activity obtained from the rat resorption–gestation assay (Hosomi et al., 1997). How might α-TTP and the tocopherol-ω-oxidation pathway work together to determine the biological potency of the various forms of vitamin E? Explain. Do you think the type of tocopherol used as supplements for patients with familial isolated vitamin E deficiency would matter? Explain.
2. Many animal studies have shown that certain vitamin E deficiency symptoms can be partially reversed by other antioxidant compounds, raising questions about the specificity of the vitamin E requirement. What information was obtained from the studies of patients with familial isolated vitamin E deficiency with regard to specific functions of vitamin E?

of α-tocopherol transfer protein in regulating plasma tocopherol concentration has been demonstrated in patients with familial isolated vitamin E deficiency (Gotoda et al., 1995; Ouahchi et al., 1995; Kayden and Traber, 1993). These patients have clear signs of vitamin E deficiency (extremely low plasma vitamin E and neurological abnormalities) but have no fat malabsorption or lipoprotein abnormalities. Absence of functional α-TTP in these patients impairs secretion of α-tocopherol from liver into the bloodstream, resulting in the very low concentration of plasma vitamin E. The plasma vitamin E level of these patients can be normalized with high-dose vitamin E supplementation.

METABOLISM OF VITAMIN E

Tocopherols and tocotrienols other than α-tocopherol undergo extensive postabsorptive metabolism to water soluble metabolites that are excreted primarily in the urine. This catabolic process involves severe truncation of the hydrophobic phytyl side chain, the moiety responsible for the fat-solubility of vitamin E. The metabolic pathway is depicted in Figure 29-2 and involves an initial hydroxylation of a terminal methyl group (ω-hydroxylation) of the phytyl side chain. In the human, the enzyme cytochrome P450-4F2, an endoplasmic reticulum enzyme that requires NADPH and is expressed primarily in the liver, has been implicated in this reaction (Sontag and Parker, 2002). This hydroxylated intermediate is further oxidized, apparently by an NAD^+-dependent dehydrogenase, to the corresponding carboxychromanol. Truncation of the phytyl side chain subsequently occurs by sequential removal of 2- or 3-carbon units, ultimately yielding the 3′-carboxychromanol (see Fig. 29-2). Despite the relatively high water solubility of these short chain metabolites, they appear to be largely conjugated with glucuronic acid, presumably at the phenolic hydroxyl group, prior to their excretion in urine. α-Tocopherol is a relatively poor substrate for this catabolic pathway. Therefore, the tocopherol-ω-oxidation process is considered to play a central role in the selective retention and tissue deposition of α-tocopherol that results from the preferential elimination of the other forms of vitamin E via this pathway. α-Tocopherylquinone, an oxidation product of α-tocopherol (Fig. 29-3), also undergoes phytyl side-chain truncation to yield tocopheronic acid (Chow et al., 1967), which is also excreted in the urine as a glucuronide conjugate. It is not known what proportion of urinary α-tocopheronic acid is derived from dietary versus endogenous α-tocopherolquinone.

PLASMA CONCENTRATION OF VITAMIN E AND RELATIONSHIP WITH DIETARY INTAKE

Usual plasma vitamin E concentrations in humans range from 20 to 30 μmol of α-tocopherol per liter or about 5 to 8 mmole α-tocopherol per mole of cholesterol. Plasma concentrations of γ-tocopherol are typically about one tenth those of α-tocopherol, and smaller amounts of δ-tocopherol are usually present. The relative proportions of tocopherols in plasma (and tissues) lie in stark contrast to those found in foods, and dietary intakes of γ-tocopherol, and occasionally even δ-tocopherol, exceed those of α-tocopherol. This difference is brought about by the actions of α-tocopherol transfer protein and the tocopherol-ω-oxidation pathway described in the preceding text.

With respect to α-tocopherol, plasma concentrations appear to be linearly related to intake over the range of intakes possible from foods (i.e., up to approximately 20 mg/day). At greater intakes (from supplements) plasma concentrations are nonlinearly related to intake such that only relatively small increases in plasma α-tocopherol are achieved even with a 10-fold increase in intake over that from diet. A supplemental intake of α-tocopherol of roughly 400 mg/day is usually needed to achieve a doubling of the plasma α-tocopherol concentration, and the maximal plasma α-tocopherol concentration achievable is roughly 50 to 60 μmol/L (Princen et al., 1995). The reason for this nonlinearity at high intakes of α-tocopherol is not clear. A consequence of supplementation with α-tocopherol is suppression of the plasma concentrations of γ- and δ-tocopherols. The mechanism

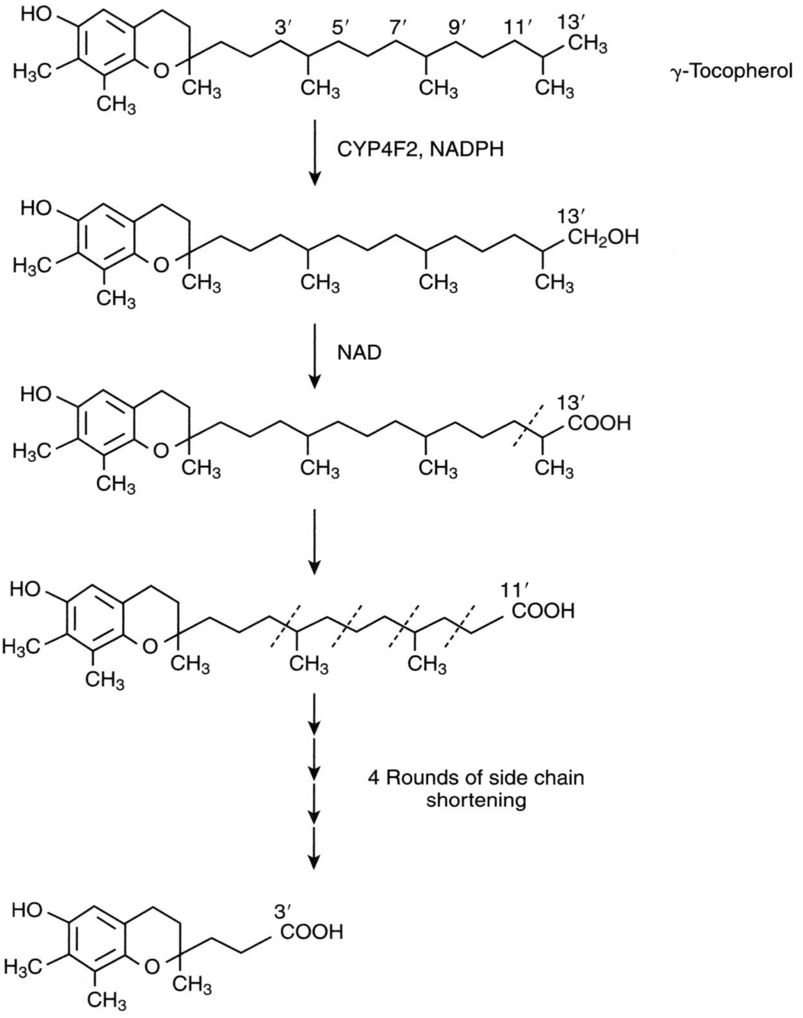

Figure 29-2 The ω-oxidation pathway of vitamin E metabolism. The pathway of ω-oxidation of the phytyl tail of tocopherols and tocotrienols, shown here with γ-tocopherol as substrate, involves an initial ω-hydroxylation at a terminal methyl group catalyzed by cytochrome P450-4F2 (CYP4F2). Subsequent reactions involve oxidation to the terminal carboxylic acid and sequential removal of 2- or 3-carbon moieties (Sontag and Parker, 2002) in a process analogous to the oxidation of fatty acids. The final products, 3-carboxychromanols, are conjugated with glucuronic acid and excreted in the urine. Among the various forms of vitamin E, α-tocopherol is a poor substrate for this pathway. Therefore, ω-oxidation contributes to the selective tissue enrichment with α-tocopherol via postabsorptive catabolism and elimination of the other forms of the vitamin.

responsible for this suppression is not known. Supplementation with γ-tocopherol does not suppress concentrations of α-tocopherol.

Because tocopherols are transported by plasma lipoproteins, individuals with higher plasma cholesterol levels typically have higher plasma tocopherol concentrations. In disorders causing lipid malabsorption (such as in individuals with cystic fibrosis or abetalipoproteinemia), plasma lipid, lipoprotein, and vitamin E concentrations frequently are all reduced concurrently (Machlin, 1991).

Figure 29-3 Reactions of α-tocopherol with peroxyl radicals. α-Tocopherol can scavenge two lipid peroxyl radicals (ROO•) as shown with the reaction of one peroxyl radical converting α-tocopherol to α-tocopheroxyl radical, which can react with a second peroxyl radical to form an adduct that is subsequently degraded to α-tocopheryl quinone.

Nutrition Insight

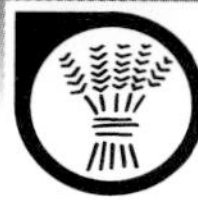

Are Non–α-Tocopherols Also Important for Health?

RRR-γ-tocopherol is the major form of vitamin E consumed in the diet, whereas the current dietary intake recommendations consider only RRR-α-tocopherol. Most supplements contain only α-tocopherol, and their use is associated with suppression of plasma levels of other tocopherols. RRR-α-tocopherol has traditionally been the focus of study because of its superior potency in bioassays for prevention of deficiency symptoms. However, results of several recent studies suggest that other forms of vitamin E may have beneficial biological effects, perhaps not involving antioxidant activity (Hensley et al., 2004; Jiang et al., 2001). Some have suggested that vitamin E supplements be composed of a mixture of tocopherols similar to that in a typical diet.

There are differences in the chemical reactivities of α-tocopherol and γ-tocopherol with respect to chemical activity. In vitro, γ-tocopherol traps potentially mutagenic electrophiles, such as reactive nitrogen oxide species including peroxynitrite. The 5-position of γ-tocopherol is highly nucleophilic and reactive toward electrophiles such as $NO^•$ and $NO_2^•$. In peroxynitrite-induced lipid peroxidation studies, α-tocopherol was converted to α-tocopheryl quinone (a 2 electron oxidation product), whereas γ-tocopherol was converted to 5-NO_2-γ-tocopherol and its orthoquinone tocored (Christen et al., 1997). This ability is not shared by α-tocopherol, which is methylated at C-5 on the phenol ring; α-tocopherol may trap the electrophile but is likely to remain chemically reactive. Supplementation with γ-tocopherol inhibited protein nitration and ascorbate oxidation in rats with inflammation (Jiang et al., 2002). Other studies in rats demonstrate that dietary supplementation with γ-tocopherol, but not α-tocopherol, reduced inflammation by suppressing the synthesis of various proinflammatory substances produced by cells of the immune system (Jiang and Ames, 2003). The 3′-carboxychromanol metabolite of γ-tocopherol has been shown to exhibit natriuretic activity in bioassays (Wechter et al., 1996), but its function in humans is currently uncertain.

Several human studies have reported an inverse association between serum or plasma concentrations

Continued

Nutrition Insight

Are Non–α-Tocopherols Also Important for Health?—cont'd

of γ-tocopherol and risk for a variety of diseases. For example, in a Swedish study of male patients with coronary heart disease and healthy age-matched reference subjects, the serum α-tocopherol concentrations did not differ significantly between the groups (Ohrvall et al., 1996). However, the coronary heart disease group had a lower mean serum concentration of γ-tocopherol and a higher α- to γ-tocopherol ratio. The findings suggested that γ-tocopherol may be important, either itself or as a marker for another protective dietary factor. Another study found that men in the highest quartile of plasma γ-tocopherol concentration had a fivefold lower cancer incidence compared to men in the lowest quartile (Helzlsouer et al., 2000). Conversely, serum γ-tocopherol concentrations have been reported to be positively related to risk of cervical and oral and pharyngeal cancers (Zheng et al., 1993; Potischman et al., 1991).

Thinking Critically

1. Based on what is known or not known about the functions or effects of various forms of vitamin E, do you agree with the 2000 DRI recommendation to consider only α-tocopherol as meeting nutrition needs?
2. Based on the experimental data used to establish the 2000 RDA values and observational studies of vitamin E status, do you think most individuals need to consume more vitamin E?
3. Given that all tocochromanols are effective antioxidants, how might the preferential accumulation of α-tocopherol be explained?

BIOLOGICAL FUNCTIONS OF VITAMIN E

Although many biochemical abnormalities are associated with vitamin E deficiency, some species-specific, the mechanism(s) by which vitamin E prevents these various metabolic and pathologic lesions have not yet been elucidated. The tocopherols and tocotrienols have long been recognized to be superior free radical antioxidants when tested in vitro, and it is this characteristic that is most often ascribed to their essentiality in vivo. Vitamin E (primarily α-tocopherol) is the major lipid-soluble, free radical chain-breaking antioxidant found in plasma, red blood cells, and tissues, and it plays an essential role in maintaining the integrity of biological membranes (Burton and Traber, 1990; Chow, 1985).

VITAMIN E AS A FREE RADICAL–SCAVENGING ANTIOXIDANT

Vitamin E is present in all cellular membranes, where it is thought to act to protect membrane lipids and perhaps proteins from free radical–induced oxidative damage. The reaction of α-tocopherol with polyunsaturated fatty acid peroxyl radicals to prevent uncontrolled lipid peroxidation is the best-understood action of vitamin E. A variety of carbon- and oxygen-centered free radicals are generated during the course of normal metabolism in vivo. These include the superoxide, lipid alkoxyl, and peroxyl radicals. Among them, peroxyl radicals derived from polyunsaturated fatty acids have special significance because of their involvement in lipid peroxidation. Lipid peroxidation is the most common indicator of free radical production in living systems. (See Chapter 18 for more information on polyunsaturated fatty acids and lipid peroxidation.)

The process of lipid peroxidation (or autoxidation) can be divided into three phases: initiation, propagation, and termination. In the initiation phase (reaction I), carbon-centered lipid radicals ($R^\bullet$) can be produced by proton abstraction from a polyunsaturated fatty acid (RH) when a free radical initiator ($I^\bullet$) is present.

Transition metal ions (Fe^{2+}, Cu^{2+}), ultraviolet light, and ionizing radiation have been implicated as initiators of lipid peroxidation. This lipid radical reacts readily with molecular oxygen to form a peroxyl radical (ROO•) (reaction II). In the propagation phase, the peroxyl radical formed can react with another polyunsaturated fatty acid to form a fatty acid hydroperoxide (ROOH) and a new carbon-centered radical (reaction III). The propagative process can continue until all substrate fatty acids are oxidized or the chain reaction is broken (termination phase). Free radicals can be scavenged and the chain reaction terminated by self-quenching (reaction IV) or by the action of an antioxidant (AH) (reaction V), which generates an antioxidant free radical, A•. Of the free radical process inhibitors or antioxidants that are known, tocopherols are among the most effective chain-breakers.

$$RH \xrightarrow{I^*} R^\bullet \qquad \text{(Reaction I)}$$

$$R^\bullet + O_2 \rightarrow ROO^\bullet \qquad \text{(Reaction II)}$$

$$ROO^\bullet + R'H \rightarrow ROOH + R'^\bullet \qquad \text{(Reaction III)}$$

$$R^\bullet \text{ (or } ROO^\bullet) + R'^\bullet \rightarrow R\text{-}R' \text{ (or } ROOR') \qquad \text{(Reaction IV)}$$

$$R^\bullet \text{ (or } ROO^\bullet) + AH \rightarrow RH \text{ (or } ROOH) + A^\bullet \qquad \text{(Reaction V)}$$

The action of α-tocopherol in quenching lipid peroxyl radicals is shown in Figure 29-3; the 6-hydroxyl group of the chroman ring is the reactive portion of the tocochromanols. The phenolic hydrogen atom is donated to a free radical, resulting in the quenching of the free radical and the formation of the tocopheroxyl radical. Tocopherols react more rapidly with peroxyl radicals than do polyunsaturated fatty acids, and the tocopherol radical is relatively unreactive. These two features conspire to render the tocopherols and tocotrienols extremely effective as free radical chain-breaking antioxidants. The tocopheroxyl radical has been shown in vitro to be reduced back to tocopherol by a variety of low-molecular-weight, water-soluble reducing substances such as ascorbic acid (Packer et al., 1995; Chow, 1991). The extent to which this regenerative process resulting from the interaction of these two vitamins occurs in vivo remains uncertain. Although the nature and extent of the vitamin E regenerative process in vivo remains speculative, it provides a working rationale for the observation that it is very difficult to deplete vitamin E in adult animals or humans. Although the oxidation of α-tocopherol to α-tocopheroxyl radical is reversible, further oxidation of the tocopheroxyl radical to α-tocopheryl quinone is not reversible.

Antioxidant activity of tocopherols is experimentally determined by their chemical reactivity with radicals or by their ability to inhibit autoxidation of fats and oils. The relative antioxidant activity of tocopherols varies considerably depending on the experimental conditions and the assessment method employed (Kamal-Eldin and Appelqvist, 1996). Efforts have also been made to compare the antioxidant efficacy of tocopherols and tocotrienols in living cells. In cells made selenium deficient, and therefore susceptible to adverse oxidation events (see Chapter 39 for discussion of the antioxidant function of selenium), tocopherols and tocotrienols exhibit different capacities to prevent cell death (Saito et al., 2003). However, the observed differences between the vitamers was mostly attributable to their ability to become associated with cell membranes, rather than to intrinsic differences in their chemical antioxidant activity. Tocopherol esters, which lack the critical free phenolic hydroxyl group, cannot function as antioxidants and must be hydrolyzed to free tocopherols in vivo before they can perform this function.

Vitamin E is not the only means by which cells are protected from oxidative damage. Other major cellular antioxidant mechanisms include a variety of low-molecular-weight reducing agents such as ascorbic acid and reduced glutathione (GSH), several enzymes including superoxide dismutase, GSH peroxidase and catalase, and transition-metal binding proteins such as ferritin, transferrin, ceruloplasmin, and albumin (Chow, 1991). These various antioxidant systems act at different stages and cellular locations. However, vitamin E occupies a unique position in the overall antioxidant picture owing to its localization in cell membranes and its efficacy at remarkably dilute concentrations. Cell membranes typically contain only one molecule of α-tocopherol per several hundred phospholipid molecules.

OTHER FUNCTIONS OF VITAMIN E

Several nonantioxidant functions of vitamin E have been proposed. α-Tocopherol, for example, has been reported to influence protein kinase C activity and cell proliferation as well as synthesis of arachidonic acid metabolites involved in the immune response. Among these and other biological functions proposed for vitamin E, prevention of free radical–initiated lipid peroxidation and the resulting tissue damage is most widely accepted by investigators.

DEFICIENCY, HEALTH EFFECTS, TOXICITY, AND BIOPOTENCY OF VITAMIN E

Much of what is known about the physiological consequences of vitamin E deficiency and toxicity has come from animal studies. Recent studies of patients with familial vitamin E deficiency have enhanced our understanding of the consequences of vitamin E deficiency in humans. Epidemiological studies and clinical intervention trials have provided new insights into the effect of vitamin E status on human health.

DEFICIENCY SYMPTOMS

A number of species-dependent, tissue-specific vitamin E deficiency symptoms have been reported. In some instances the development and severity of vitamin E deficiency symptoms are associated with the status of other nutrients, including selenium and sulfur-containing amino acids (Machlin, 1991). For example, the most common deficiency sign is necrotizing myopathy, which occurs in almost all species in the skeletal muscle and in some heart and smooth muscles. Myopathy primarily results from selenium deficiency in domestic animals, but rabbits and guinea pigs develop severe debilitating myopathy when fed a diet deficient in vitamin E but adequate in selenium. On the other hand, rats manifest a relatively benign myopathy when fed a vitamin E–deficient diet, and chickens do not develop myopathy unless the diet is depleted of both vitamin E and sulfur-containing amino acids. The reason for the species-dependent and tissue-specific vitamin E deficiency symptoms remains to be delineated.

In humans, lower plasma/serum levels of vitamin E (<12 μmol/L) are associated with a shorter lifespan of red cells and their increased susceptibility to hemolysis when exposed to an oxidizing agent. Vitamin E deficiency is rarely observed in adults. When it occurs, it is usually a result of lipoprotein deficiencies or lipid malabsorption syndromes. Low plasma vitamin E levels have been observed in patients with a variety of fat malabsorption conditions. Recent studies of children and adults with specific causes of fat/vitamin E malabsorption (such as abetalipoproteinemia, chronic cholestatic hepatobiliary disorder, and cystic fibrosis) have clearly shown that neurological abnormalities do occur in association with malabsorption syndromes of various etiologies (Kayden and Traber, 1993; Machlin, 1991). The similarity of the neurological abnormalities to those that occur in patients with familial isolated vitamin E deficiency suggests that the neurological symptoms are related specifically to the lack of adequate vitamin E in neural tissues.

Unlike the case of vitamin A, there is apparently no storage organ for vitamin E. Tocopherols accumulate in adipose tissue, but their mobilization from this tissue is slow and insufficient to prevent vitamin E deficiency in animals. Transfer of vitamin E across the placenta is inefficient, and the concentration of tocopherols in fetal blood and tissues is considerably lower than that of the maternal system. Infants born prematurely are susceptible to lung and ocular abnormalities that have been linked to insufficient antioxidant protection of these tissues.

HEALTH EFFECTS OF VITAMIN E

Increased intake of vitamin E has been associated with enhanced immune response and reduced risk of cardiovascular disease, certain cancers, and other degenerative diseases.

Several indexes of immune response, including measures of delayed-type hypersensitivity, antibody production, lymphocyte proliferation and cytokine production are influenced by the status of essential nutrients, including vitamin E. Vitamin E supplementation is associated with enhanced production of the cytokine interleukin 2, enhanced lymphocyte proliferation, and decreased production of immunosuppressive prostaglandin E_2 (Meydani et al., 1990).

Several diet-related factors, including low vitamin E status, have been implicated in the increased incidence of coronary heart disease. In recent years, some, but not all, epidemiological studies have shown that a higher dietary intake or a higher plasma level of α-tocopherol is associated with decreased risk of cardiovascular diseases (Stampfer et al., 1993). The ability of vitamin E to prevent LDL oxidation, platelet adhesion, or both, may be responsible for the reduced risk of cardiovascular disease. Increased vitamin E intake from foods has been associated with reduced risk for a variety of cancers (Byers and Guerrero, 1995). Vitamin E may reduce disease risk by inactivating environmental mutagens/carcinogens, altering metabolic activation processes, enhancing the immune system, inhibiting cell proliferation, or other mechanisms that may or may not be related to its antioxidant activity. Paradoxically, clinical intervention trials using high doses of α-tocopherol have yielded no consistent protective effects on prevention of cardiovascular disease (Vivekananthan et al., 2003; Stocker, 1999).

TOXICITY OF VITAMIN E

Vitamin E is a relatively nontoxic nutrient, probably due in part to the inability to accumulate concentrations more than about three times that resulting from usual intake from foods, as discussed in the preceding text. The most well-established symptom of high α-tocopherol intake is increased blood coagulation time and, therefore, increased risk of hemorrhage. The most recent recommendations of the Institute of Medicine (IOM, 2000) for vitamin E intake established tolerable upper intake levels (ULs) for vitamin E. This value was set for adults at 1,000 mg/day of any form of vitamin E, based on the risk of hemorrhage.

BIOPOTENCY

The tocochromanols differ in their antioxidant and biological activities when examined in living organisms. The comparative biological activity of tocopherols is assessed in bioassays by determining their relative ability to prevent deficiency symptoms such as fetal resorption or erythrocyte hemolysis in rats. Another measure, the curative myopathy test, is based on the ability of tocopherol to suppress the release of pyruvate kinase from skeletal muscle into the serum of vitamin E–deficient rats. The biological activity of various forms of vitamin E has been expressed as units of activity in relation to that of all-rac-α-tocopheryl acetate, which is a common form of vitamin E used in vitamin supplements or for food fortification. The relative values in USP reference standard units (USP Vitamin E unit) or international units (IUs) per milligram of compound assign 1 unit to 1.00 mg of all-rac-α-tocopheryl acetate. Vitamin E activity is also expressed as α-tocopherol equivalents (α-TE), and 1 α-TE is equivalent to 1.00 mg of RRR-α-tocopherol or 1.49 mg all-rac-α-tocopheryl acetate.

Forms of Vitamin E	Relative USP or IU Units per mg	α-Tocopherol Equivalents per mg
All-rac-α-tocopheryl acetate	1.00	0.67
All-rac-α-tocopherol	1.10	0.74
RRR-α-tocopheryl acetate	1.36	0.91
RRR-α-tocopherol	1.49	1.00

The relative activity of various tocopherols and tocotrienols based on bioassay methods is shown in Table 29-1.

FOOD SOURCES AND INTAKE OF VITAMIN E

FOOD SOURCES

Tocopherols occur ubiquitously in plant and animal foods, but some foods are particularly rich sources. Oilseeds and their food products such as salad dressings, mayonnaise, margarines,

Table 29-1
Activity of Different Forms of Vitamin E

Form	Resorption–Gestation* (%)	Erythrocyte Hemolysis† (%)
RRR-α-tocopherol	100	100
RRR-β-tocopherol	25 to 50	15 to 27
RRR-γ-tocopherol	8 to 19	3 to 20
RRR-δ-tocopherol	0.1 to 3	0.3 to 2
RRR-α-tocotrienol	21 to 50	17 to 25
RRR-β-tocotrienol	4 to 5	1 to 5
RRR-α-tocopheryl acetate	91	—
All-rac-α-tocopherol‡	74	—
All-rac-α-tocopheryl acetate‡	67	—

Data from Machlin L J (1991) Vitamin E. In: Machlin L J (ed) Handbook of Vitamins, 2nd ed. Marcel Dekker, New York, pp 99-144; and Pryor WA (1995) Vitamin E and Carotenoid Abstracts, VERIS, La Grange, IL, pp. vii-xi.
*Based on the fetal development and/or prevention of fetal loss in rats.
†Based on the prevention of hemoglobin release from red blood cells exposed to hydrogen peroxide.
‡A mixture of eight stereoisomers.

Food Sources

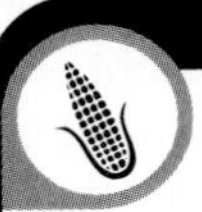

Food Sources of α-Tocopherol

Vegetable Oils

5 to 6 mg per Tbsp sunflower or safflower oil
2 mg per Tbsp canola, peanut, corn, or olive oil
1 mg per Tbsp soybean oil

Nuts

7.3 mg per oz almonds
4.3 mg per oz hazelnuts
2.6 mg per oz pinenuts
2.2 mg per oz peanuts

Vegetables

1.3 mg per ½ cup pumpkin or sweet potato
1.2 mg per ½ cup broccoli or red pepper
1.1 mg per ½ cup asparagus
0.8 mg per ½ cup carrots
0.7 mg per ½ cup kidney beans

Fruits

0.9 mg per ½ cup mangos or papayas
0.7 mg per ½ cup peaches or apricots
0.6 mg per ½ cup raspberries

Data from U.S. Department of Agriculture/Agricultural Research Service (USDA/ARS) (2005) USDA Nutrient Database for Standard Reference, Release 18. USDA/ARS, Washington, DC. Retrieved November 15, 2005, from www.ars.usda.gov/ba/bhnrc/ndl.

and spreads are the best sources. The majority of the tocopherols consumed in the United States are not α-tocopherol. γ-Tocopherol, the predominant form of tocopherols present in soybean oil and corn oil, accounts for more than half the estimated total tocopherol intake (Chow, 1985). Conversely, the major form in sunflower oil, safflower oil, and olive oil is α-tocopherol. Some foods and oils also contain β- and δ-tocopherols. Vitamin E–fortified breakfast cereals, peanut butter, eggs, potato chips, whole milk, and tomato products represent other major sources of vitamin E based on food consumption data. Tocotrienols are less widely distributed and are found in barley and rice brans and in palm oil.

DIETARY INTAKE OF VITAMIN E

Vitamin E intake is assessed by the combined use of food intake data and information on the tocopherol content of foods. These assessments are generally considered as rough estimates due to the inherent difficulty in obtaining accurate and complete food intake data coupled with incomplete food composition data. Most nutrient databases and nutrition labels do not distinguish among the various forms of tocopherols in foods. Estimates, based on NHANES III (1988-1994), place the median intake of α-tocopherol alone from the diet at about 8 mg/day for men and 6 mg/day for women (IOM, 2000; Alaimo et al., 1994). The ranges of α-tocopherol intake for adult men and women are about (1st to 99th percentiles) 2 to 31 mg/day for men and 1.5 to 25 mg/day for women. If supplement intake is included, median estimates of α-tocopherol intake are increased by approximately 0.4 mg per day.

RECOMMENDED INTAKE OF VITAMIN E AND ASSESSMENT OF VITAMIN E STATUS

Vitamin E was not officially recognized as an essential nutrient in the United States until 1968 when a daily intake of 30 international units (IU, or the biological equivalent of 30 mg all-rac-α-tocopheryl acetate) was recommended for adult men by the National Research Council of the National Academy of Sciences. In 1974 the recommended dietary allowance (RDA) was reduced to 15 IU for adult men. In 1980 the RDA was redefined to take into account the dietary contribution of non–α-tocopherols, and the requirement was expressed as α-tocopherol equivalents (α-TEs). One α-TE was set as the biological equivalent of 1 mg RRR-α-tocopherol using the relative biopotency values for the different vitamers established in the rat fetal gestation–resorption assay. The 1989 RDA for vitamin E was set at 10 α-TE for adult men and 8 α-TE for adult (nonpregnant, nonlactating) women (NRC, 1989). The most recent set of recommendations was established in 2000 by the IOM. The 2000 RDA was based only on the α-tocopherol form of vitamin E and represents a change from the 1989 recommendations. Other forms of vitamin E (e.g., γ-tocopherol) were not considered to contribute to the RDA on the basis of poor binding to the α-tocopherol transfer protein, despite their demonstrated value (albeit lower than α-tocopherol) in animal models of curative vitamin E deficiency. Only the 2R stereoisomers of α-tocopherol are considered to satisfy the current RDA for vitamin E, based on their much higher affinity for α-tocopherol transfer protein.

The nutritional status of vitamin E in humans is most commonly assessed on the basis of the concentration of α-tocopherol in serum (or plasma), often normalized to plasma cholesterol. The only bioassay of vitamin E status conducted in humans is the susceptibility of isolated red blood cells to hemolysis upon exposure to hydrogen peroxide. The RDA is based largely on red blood cell hemolysis data obtained using erythrocytes from a small group of human subjects who were intentionally depleted of vitamin E and then repleted to varying extents (Horwitt et al., 1963). In that study, erythrocytes isolated from subjects with plasma α-tocopherol concentrations less than 12 μmol/L exhibited increased hemolysis (release of hemoglobin) when exposed to hydrogen peroxide. Based on experimental data from these repletion studies with vitamin E deficient subjects, the relationship between α-tocopherol intake and plasma α-tocopherol concentration was determined (Horwitt, 1960). The IOM (2000) used the intake needed to achieve a plasma concentration of 12 μmol/L as the basis for setting an estimated average requirement (EAR) for adults of 12 mg α-tocopherol per day. The current RDA was set at two standard deviations (20%) greater than the EAR and is 15 mg α-tocopherol per day for all adults. No increment was added for pregnant women except for a 1 mg increase for pregnant adolescents. For lactating women, the RDA was increased to 19 mg α-tocopherol per day to compensate for secretion in milk.

EARs and RDAs were set for children by extrapolation from adult values based on lean body mass and need for growth. Adequate intakes (AIs) for infants from birth to 6 months of age were established based on α-tocopherol intake from human milk. Therefore, the AI for infants during the first 6 months is 4 mg α-tocopherol/day (0.78 L milk/day × 4.9 mg α-tocopherol/L of milk). The AI for infants from 7 to 12 months of age is 5 mg/day and was extrapolated from that for younger infants.

Consequently, according to estimates of average daily intake of α-tocopherol of 6 to 8 mg, most individuals in the United States are not meeting the current recommendations (Maras et al., 2004). Individuals consuming low fat diets tend to have lower intakes of

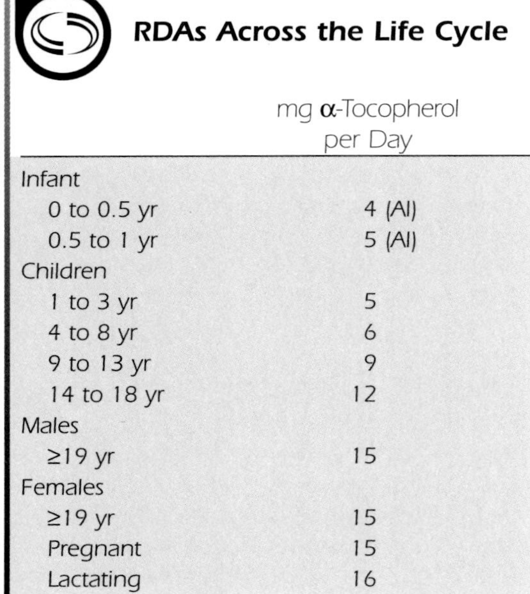

RDAs Across the Life Cycle

	mg α-Tocopherol per Day
Infant	
0 to 0.5 yr	4 (AI)
0.5 to 1 yr	5 (AI)
Children	
1 to 3 yr	5
4 to 8 yr	6
9 to 13 yr	9
14 to 18 yr	12
Males	
≥19 yr	15
Females	
≥19 yr	15
Pregnant	15
Lactating	16

Data from Institute of Medicine (2000) Dietary Reference Intakes for Vitamin C, Vitamin E, Selenium, and Carotenoids. National Academy Press, Washington, DC.
AI, Adequate intake.

vitamin E, because the richest sources of vitamin E are vegetable oils and their products. Conversely, the mean plasma α-tocopherol concentration of adults in the United States is approximately 26 μmol/L, and the concentration of the 25th percentile is 20 μmol/L (Ford and Sowell, 1999), well above the 12 μmol/L concentration considered sufficient to prevent hydrogen peroxide–induced hemolysis.

REFERENCES

Alaimo K, McDowell M, Briefel R, Bischof A, Caughman C, Loria C, Johnson C (1994) Dietary intake of vitamins, minerals, and fiber of persons ages 2 months and over in the United States: Third National Health and Nutrition Examination Survey, Phase 1, 1988-91. Adv Data 14:1-28.

Arita M, SatoY, Miyata A, Tanabe T, Takahashi E, Kayden HJ, Arai H, Inoue K (1995) Human α-tocopherol transfer protein: cDNA cloning, expression and chromosomal localization. Biochem J 306:437-443.

Burton GW, Traber MG (1990) Vitamin E: antioxidant activity, biokinetics, and bioavailability. Annu Rev Nutr 10:357-382.

Byers T, Guerrero N (1995). Epidemiologic evidence for vitamin C and vitamin E in cancer prevention. Am J Clin Nutr 62: 1385S-1392S.

Chow CK (1991) Vitamin E and oxidative stress. Free Radic Biol Med 11:215-232.

Chow CK (1985) Vitamin E and blood. World Rev Nutr Diet 45:133-166.

Chow CK, Draper HH, Csallany AS, Chiu M (1967) The metabolism of C14-α-tocopheryl quinone and C14-α-tocopheryl hydroquinone. Lipids 2:390-397.

Christen S, Woodall AA, Shigenaga MK, Southwell-Keely PT, Duncan MW, Ames BN (1997) γ-Tocopherol traps mutagenic electrophiles such as NO_x and complements α-tocopherol: physiological implications. Proc Natl Acad Sci U S A 94:3217-3222.

Evans HM, Bishop KS (1922) On the existence of a hitherto unrecognized dietary factor essential for reproduction. Science 56: 650-651.

Ford ES, Sowell A (1999) Serum alpha-tocopherol status in the United States population: findings from the Third National Health and Nutrition Examination Survey. Am J Epidemiol 150:290-300.

Gotoda T, Arita M, Arai H, Inoue K, Yokota T, Fukuo Y, Yazaki Y, Yamada N (1995) Adult-onset spinocerebellar dysfunction caused by a mutation in the gene for the α-tocopherol-transfer protein. N Engl J Med 333:1313-1318.

Helzlsouer K, Huang H, Alberg A, Hoffman S, Burke A, Norkus E, Morris J, Comstock G (2000) Association between alpha-tocopherol, gamma-tocopherol, selenium, and subsequent prostate cancer. J Natl Cancer Inst 92: 2018-2023.

Hensley K, Benaksas E, Bolli R, Comp P, Grammas P, Hamdheydari L, Mou S, Pye Q, Stoddard M, Wallis G, Williamson K, West M, Wechter W, Floyd R (2004) New perspectives on vitamin E: γ-tocopherol and carboxyethylhydroxychroman metabolites in biology and medicine. Free Radic Biol Med 36:1-15.

Horwitt M (1960) Vitamin E and lipid metabolism in man. Am J Clin Nutr 8:451-461.

Horwitt M, Century B, Zeman A (1963) Erythrocyte survival time and reticulocyte levels after tocopherol depletion in man. Am J Clin Nutr 12:99-106.

Hosomi A, Arita M, Sato Y, Kiyose C, Ueda T, Igarashi O, Arai H, Inoue K (1997) Affinity for α-tocopherol transfer protein as a determinant of the biological activities of vitamin E analogs. FEBS Lett 409:105-108.

Institute of Medicine (2000) Dietary Reference Intakes for Vitamin E, Vitamin E, Selenium and Carotenoids. National Academy Press, Washington, DC.

Jiang Q, Ames B (2003) Gamma-tocopherol, but not alpha-tocopherol, decreases proinflammatory eicosanoids and inflammation damage in rats. FASEB J 17: 816-822.

Jiang Q, Christen S, Shigenaga M, Ames B (2001) γ-Tocopherol, the major form of vitamin E in the U.S. diet, deserves more attention. Am J Clin Nutr 74:714-722.

Jiang Q, Lyddesfeld J, Shigenaga M, Shigeno E, Christen S, Ames B (2002) Gamma-tocopherol supplementation inhibits protein nitration and ascorbate oxidation in rats with inflammation. Free Radic Biol Med 33:1534-1542.

Kaempf-Rotzoll D, Traber M, Arai H (2003) Vitamin E and transfer proteins. Curr Opin Lipidol 14:249-254.

Kamal-Eldin A, Appelqvist LA (1996) The chemistry and antioxidant properties of tocopherols and tocotrienols. Lipids 31: 671-701.

Kayden HJ, Traber MG (1993) Absorption, lipoprotein transport, and regulation of plasma concentrations of vitamin E in humans. J Lipid Res 34:343-358.

Kostner GM, Oettl K, Jauhiainen M, Ehnholn C, Esterbauer H (1995) Human plasma phospholipid transfer protein accelerates exchange/transfer of α-tocopherol between lipoproteins and cells. Biochem J 305:659-667.

Machlin L J (1991) Vitamin E. In: Machlin LJ (ed) Handbook of Vitamins, 2nd ed. Marcel Dekker, New York, pp 99-144.

Maras J, Bermudez O, Qiao N, Bakun P, Boody-Alter E, Tucker K (2004) Intake of α-tocopherol is limited among U.S. adults. J Am Diet Assoc 104:567-575.

Meydani SN, Barklund MP, Liu S, Miller RA, Cannon JG, Morrow FD, Rocklin R, Blumberg JB (1990) Vitamin E supplementation enhances cell-mediated immunity in healthy elderly subjects. Am J Clin Nutr 52:557-563.

National Research Council (1989) Recommended Dietary Allowances, 10th ed. National Academy Press, Washington, DC.

Ohrvall M, Sundlof G, Vessby B (1996) Gamma, but not alpha, tocopherol levels in serum are reduced in coronary heart disease patients. J Intern Med 239:111-117.

Ouahchi K, Arita M, Kayden H, Hentati F, Hamida MB, Sokol R, Arai H, Inoue K, Mandel J-L, Koenig M (1995) Ataxia with isolated vitamin E deficiency is caused by mutations in the α-tocopherol transfer protein. Nat Genet 9:141-145.

Packer L, Witt EH, Trischler HJ (1995) Alpha-lipoic acid as a biological antioxidant. Free Radic Biol Med 19:227-250.

Potischman N, Herrero R, Brinton A, Reeves W, Stacewicz-Sapuntzakis M, Jones C, Brenes M, Tenorio F, de Britton R, Gaitan E (1991) A case-control study of nutrient status and invasive cervical cancer. II. Serological indicators. Am J Epidemiol 134: 1347-1355.

Princen H, van Duyvenvoorde W, Buytenhek R, van der Laarse A, van Poppel G, Gevers Leuven J, van Hinsbergh V (1995) Supplementation with low doses of vitamin E protects LDL from lipid peroxidation in men and women. Arterioscler Thromb Vasc Biol 15:325-333.

Saito Y, Yoshida Y, Adazawa T, Takahashi D, Niki E (2003) Cell death caused by selenium deficiency and protective effect of antioxidants. J Biol Chem 278: 39428-39434.

Sattler W, Levak-Frank S, Radner H, Kostner GM, Zechner R (1996) Muscle-specific overexpression of lipoprotein lipase in transgenic mice results in increased α-tocopherol levels in skeletal muscle. Biochem J 318:15-19.

Sontag TJ, Parker RS (2002) Cytochrome P450 omega-hydroxylase pathway of tocopherol catabolism. Novel mechanism of regulation of vitamin E status. J Biol Chem 28: 25290-25296.

Stampfer MJ, Henneckens CH, Ascherio A, Giovannucci E, Colditz GA, Rosner B, Willett WC (1993) Vitamin E consumption and the risk of coronary disease in men. N Engl J Med 328:1450-1456.

Stocker R (1999) The ambivalence of vitamin E in atherogenesis. Trends Biol Sci 24: 219-223.

Traber MG, Sokol RJ, Kohlschuetter A, Yokota T, Muller DPR, Dufour R, Kayden HJ (1993) Impaired discrimination between stereoisomers of α-tocopherol in patients with familial isolated vitamin E deficiency. J Lipid Res 34:201-210.

Vivekananthan D, Penn M, Sapp S, Hsu A, Topol E (2003) Use of antioxidant vitamins for the prevention of cardiovascular disease: Meta-analysis of randomized trials. Lancet 361:2017-2023.

Wechter WJ, Kantoci D, Murray ED Jr, D'Amico DC, Jung ME, Wang W-H (1996) A new endogenous natriuretic factor: LLU-α. Proc Natl Acad Sci U S A 93:6002-6007.

Zheng W, Blot W, Diamond E, Norkus E, Spate V, Morris J, Comstock G (1993) Serum micronutrients and the subsequent risk of oral and pharyngeal cancer. Cancer Res 53:795-798.

RECOMMENDED READING

Packer L, Fuchs J (eds) (1993) Vitamin E in Health and Disease. Marcel Dekker, New York.

Chapter 30

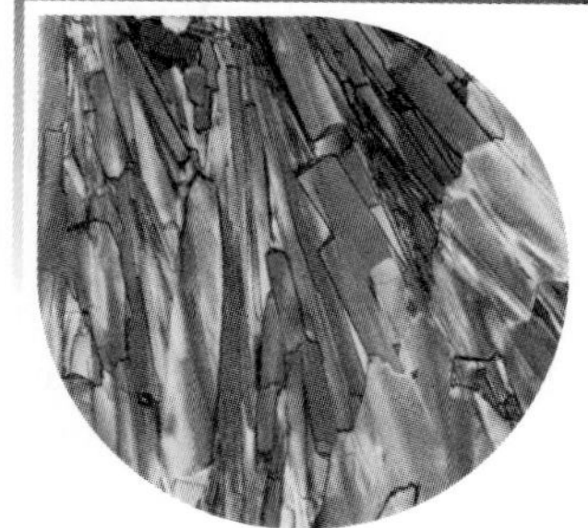

Vitamin A

Noa Noy, PhD

OUTLINE

COMMON ABBREVIATIONS

RBP	retinol-binding protein
CRBP	cellular retinol-binding protein
CRABP	cellular retinoic acid–binding protein
CRALBP	cellular retinal-binding protein
IRBP	interphotoreceptor retinoid-binding protein
RAR	retinoic acid receptor
RXR	retinoid X receptor
ARAT	acyl-CoA:retinol acyltransferase
LRAT	lecithin:retinol acyltransferase
RPE	retinal pigment epithelium
IPM	interphotoreceptor matrix
RAE	retinol activity equivalent

CHEMISTRY AND PHYSICAL PROPERTIES OF VITAMIN A AND CAROTENOIDS

Vitamin A was initially recognized as an essential growth factor present in foods of animal origin such as animal fats and fish oils, and this factor was called fat-soluble A (Osborn and Mendel, 1919; McCollum and Davis, 1915). It was also observed that some plants displayed the activity of this fat-soluble A factor. Subsequently, in the early 1930s, it became clear that some of the plant-derived compounds known as carotenoids display vitamin A activity due to the ability of animals to convert them to retinol.

NOMENCLATURE

Vitamin A nomenclature has undergone various changes since the discovery of this fat-soluble vitamin. Currently, the term vitamin A is used to generically describe compounds that exhibit the biological activity of retinol, the alcoholic form of vitamin A. The term can thus be applied to many naturally occurring and synthetic derivatives of retinol. Of the more than 600 carotenoids that are known to exist in nature, about 50 display vitamin A activity and are termed provitamin A. More recently, the term retinoids has been coined to describe compounds that share structural similarities with retinol regardless of their biological activity.

LABILITY AND LIMITED SOLUBILITY OF RETINOIDS IN WATER

The structures of some physiologically important retinoids as well as the most active provitamin A carotenoid, all-*trans*-β-carotene, are shown in Figure 30-1.

In general, retinoids comprise three distinct structural domains: they contain a β-ionone ring, a spacer of a polyunsaturated chain, and a polar end group. The polar end group of naturally occurring retinoids can exist at several oxidation states varying from the low oxidation state of retinol, to retinal, and to the even higher oxidation state in retinoic acid. Vitamin A is stored in vivo in the form of retinyl esters in which the retinyl moiety is esterified with a long-chain fatty acid with concomitant loss of the polar end group (see Fig. 30-1). Retinol can also be converted in vivo to conjugated species with larger, more polar, end groups (e.g., retinoyl β-glucuronide; see Fig. 30-1).

In recent years, a wide array of synthetic analogs of retinoids has been developed. The β-ionone ring has been replaced systematically by multiple hydrophobic groups, the spacer chain has been derivatized to a variety of cyclic and aromatic rings, and the polar end group has been converted into derivatives or precursors of active species. Active synthetic analogs, similarly to naturally occurring retinoids, retain an amphipathic nature typified by a hydrophobic moiety and a polar terminus.

The large hydrophobic moiety of retinoids results in a limited solubility of these compounds in water. In addition, the multiple double-bonds of the spacer chain render retinoids susceptible to photodegradation, isomerization, and oxidation. Therefore, vitamin A and its analogs are stable in a crystalline form or when dissolved in organic solvents under nonoxidizing conditions, but they are labile when exposed to light or in aqueous solutions in the presence of oxygen. The poor solubility and the lability of retinoids in aqueous phases raise important questions regarding their physiology: How do these insoluble compounds transfer across aqueous spaces between different organs, cells, and subcellular locations? How is their structural integrity retained in vivo when they traverse the aqueous phases of serum and cytosol?

OPTICAL PROPERTIES OF RETINOIDS AND CAROTENOIDS

Physical methods that have been used to study retinoids include ultraviolet, visible, infra-red, and fluorescence spectroscopy, nuclear magnetic resonance spectroscopy, electron spin resonance spectroscopy, and mass spectroscopy. Retinoids have absorption spectra with characteristic maxima in the 320- to 380-nm range. The absorption spectra of carotenoids center in the visible range at around 450 nm. Some retinoids, most notably retinols, are highly fluorescent and display fluorescence emission maxima in the range of 460 to 500 nm. Conversely, carotenoids do not display significant fluorescence at physiologically relevant temperatures. The optical properties of retinoids

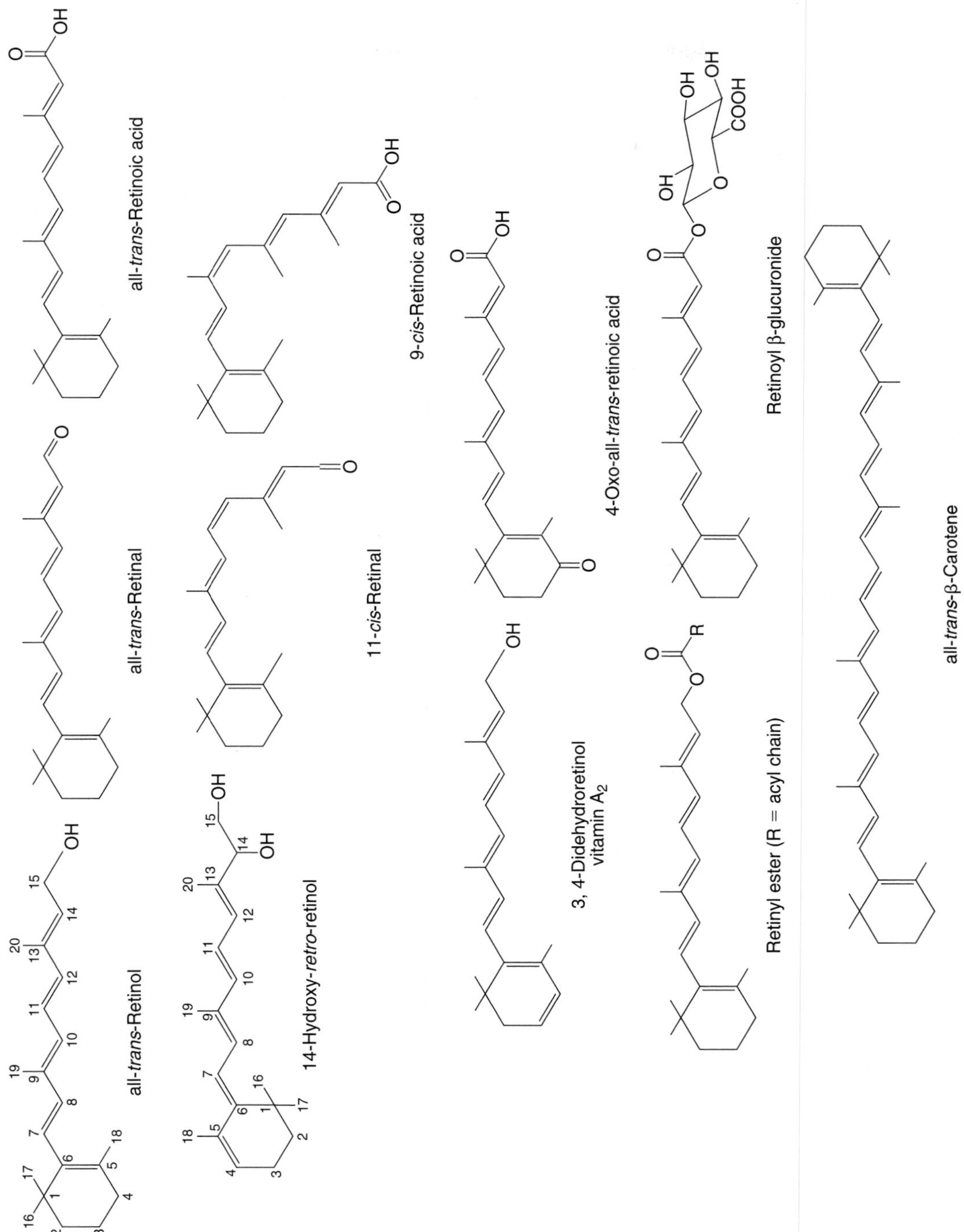

all-*trans*-Retinol

all-*trans*-Retinal

all-*trans*-Retinoic acid

14-Hydroxy-*retro*-retinol

11-*cis*-Retinal

9-*cis*-Retinoic acid

3, 4-Didehydroretinol
vitamin A_2

4-Oxo-all-*trans*-retinoic acid

Retinyl ester (R = acyl chain)

Retinoyl β-glucuronide

all-*trans*-β-Carotene

Figure 30-1 Structures of vitamin A, β-carotene, and some of their biologically active derivatives.

and, in particular, the environmental sensitivity of the fluorescence of retinols, have been widely used to probe their interactions within the cell, such as within the cell membrane and at the binding sites of specific binding proteins.

PHYSIOLOGICAL FUNCTIONS OF VITAMIN A

Vitamin A and its metabolites participate in a wide spectrum of biological functions. They are essential for vision, reproduction, and immune function, and they play important roles in cellular differentiation, proliferation, and signaling. The diverse effects of vitamin A are exerted by several types of retinoids that function via a variety of mechanisms. The 11-*cis*-isomer of retinal participates in visual transduction; retinoic acid and possibly other retinoids are responsible for the effects of vitamin A on gene transcription; and it has also been suggested that *retro*-derivatives of retinol are important for proliferation and activation of lymphocytes. Other retinoid derivatives that are known to be present endogenously display biological activities, but the mechanisms of actions of these compounds are not uniformly understood.

ROLE OF 11-*Cis*-RETINAL IN THE VISUAL FUNCTION

Light is sensed in the vertebrate eye by rhodopsin, a membrane protein located in the outer segments of photoreceptor cells. Rhodopsin utilizes 11-*cis*-retinal as its chromophore. Two types of photoreceptor cells exist in the human retina: (1) rods, which are stimulated by weak light of a broad range of wavelengths, and (2) cones, which are responsible for color vision and function under bright light. Absorption of a photon by the 11-*cis*-retinal moiety of rhodopsin triggers a chain of events that culminates in hyperpolarization of the plasma membrane of the cell. As photoreceptor cells form synapses with secondary neurons, the hyperpolarization is communicated further until the visual signal is transmitted to the brain.

The process of the visual signal transduction is a classical example of a signaling cascade and is well characterized (Fig. 30-2) (Saari, 1994; Dowling, 1987). Absorption of a photon by rhodopsin-bound 11-*cis*-retinal results in isomerization of the chromophore to the all-*trans*-form, a process that induces the protein to undergo several conformational changes through a series of short-lived intermediates. One of the protein intermediates (metarhodopsin II, R* in Fig. 30-2) interacts with another membrane protein named transducin. Transducin is a so-called G-protein; its interaction with R* leads to an exchange of a transducin-bound guanosine diphosphate (GDP) with a guanosine triphosphate (GTP). In the GTP-bound state, transducin activates an enzyme called phosphodiesterase.

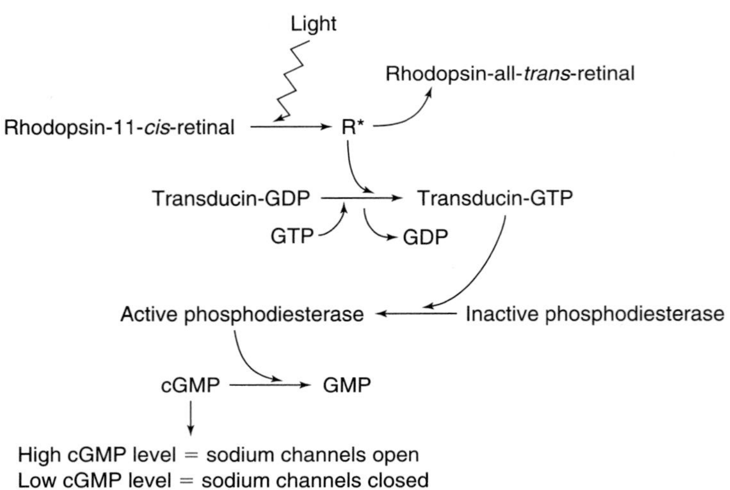

Figure 30-2 Early events in transduction of the visual signal.

Phosphodiesterase catalyzes the breakdown of cyclic guanosine monophosphate (cGMP), which acts to keep the sodium channels of the plasma membranes of rod outer segments in the open state, to an inactive product, GMP. Because the level of cGMP in rod outer segments in the dark is high (~0.07 mM), the sodium channels are open and the membranes of the cells are depolarized. Activation of phosphodiesterase following illumination results in lower levels of cGMP and leads to closing of the sodium channels and to hyperpolarization of the plasma membrane. The process of visual transduction is regulated further at several levels including phosphorylation of rhodopsin intermediates, enzymatic hydrolysis of retinal from metarhodopsin II, and the ability of a protein known as arrestin to block the interaction of the activated rhodopsin with transducin.

Bleached rhodopsin can be regenerated in the dark by 11-*cis*-retinal freshly supplied to the photoreceptors from retinal pigment epithelium cells (Fig. 30-3), where vitamin A is stored in the form of all-*trans*-retinyl esters. These storage species are enzymatically converted in the pigment epithelium to 11-*cis*-retinal, which is then transported across the interphotoreceptor matrix to photoreceptors. The metabolism and transport of retinoids in the eye are discussed later in this chapter.

REGULATION OF CELL PROLIFERATION AND DIFFERENTIATION BY RETINOIC ACIDS

Retinoids have profound effects on the differentiation and growth of a variety of normal and neoplastically transformed cells (Gudas, 1994). One striking example is the differentiation pattern of HL-60 cells, which originated from a human promyelocytic leukemia. These cells differentiate into macrophages when treated with 1,25-dihydroxyvitamin D_3 or with phorbol esters. In contrast, when treated with retinoic acid, HL-60 cells differentiate into granulocytes, and this is followed by an arrest in cell proliferation (Breitman et al., 1980). Other examples include retinoic acid–induced inhibition of the differentiation of fibroblasts into adipocytes and enhancement of differentiation in neuronal cells. Retinoids have also been shown to control the formation of particular patterns such as digit development during embryogenesis (Hofmann and Eichele, 1994). In addition, studies in isolated cells, in

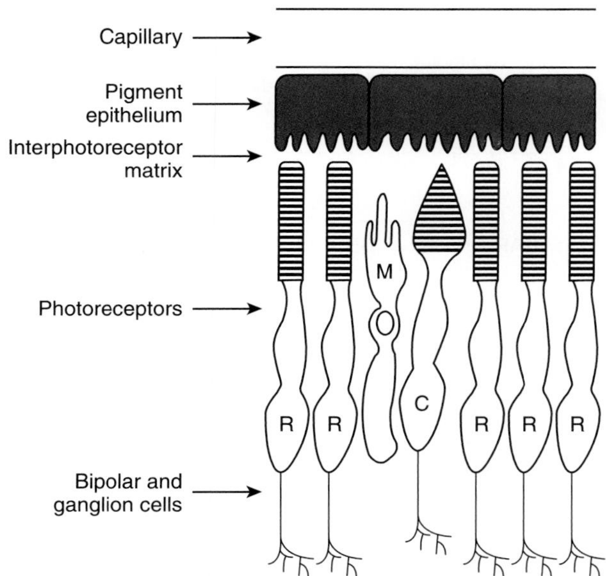

Figure 30-3 Schematic drawing of cells in the retina that are active in utilization and metabolism of retinoids. *C*, Cone; *M*, Müller cell; *R*, rod.

animal models, and in human subjects have demonstrated that retinoids can inhibit the process of carcinogenesis and, in some cases, induce transformed cells to revert to normal phenotype. This last point is well exemplified by the successful treatment of human acute promyelocytic leukemia by retinoic acid (Warrel et al., 1993).

Many of the effects of retinoids on cells are due to the ability of retinoic acid, a vitamin A metabolite, to modulate the expression of genes that encode many types of proteins including growth factors, transcription factors, enzymes, extracellular matrix proteins, protooncogenes, and binding proteins. Retinoic acid therefore regulates a complex array of metabolic pathways and cellular responses.

RETINOID NUCLEAR RECEPTORS

The mechanisms by which retinoic acid regulates gene transcription have become increasingly clear as a result of the identification of transcription factors that are specifically activated by these compounds. These proteins, termed retinoid receptors, bind to DNA recognition sequences (called retinoic acid response elements, RAREs) in the promoter region of target genes, and upon binding of retinoic acid, enhance the rate of transcription of these genes (Chambon, 1994; Giguère, 1994; Glass, 1994). Retinoid receptors, which have a molecular weight of about 50 kDa, are members of a super-family of ligand-inducible transcription factors termed nuclear hormone receptors. Similar to the other proteins in this family, retinoid receptors comprise several functional domains (Fig. 30-4). The N-terminal region of the receptors (A/B domain) is responsible for the basal, that is, the ligand-independent, activation function. The DNA-binding domain (domain C) contains zinc-fingers responsible for the association of the receptor with DNA. (See Chapter 37 for more information on the role of zinc-finger motifs in DNA-binding by proteins.) Domain D is a hinge region that confers flexibility to the protein molecule. Domain E, termed the ligand-binding domain, contains the ligand-binding pocket and is responsible for ligand-induced transcriptional activation by the receptors. The ligand-binding domain also contains regions that mediate the interactions of retinoid receptors with a variety of accessory proteins (see subsequent text). The C-terminal region of retinoid receptors is termed F, and its function is unknown at present.

Two classes of retinoid receptors, the retinoic acid receptor (RAR) and the retinoid X receptor (RXR), and several subtypes of each

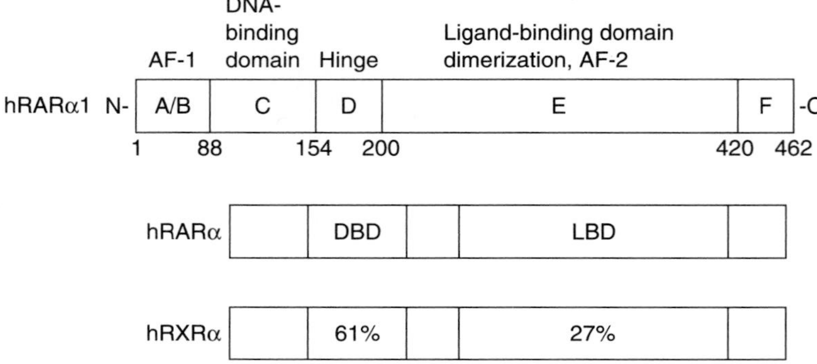

Figure 30-4 Structure of retinoid nuclear receptors. The amino acid sequence of the human RARα1 is represented by bars and residue numbers (Leid et al., 1992). The receptor contains five domains. These include the N-terminal domain, A/B, which contains a basal transactivation function; domain C, which is the DNA-binding region and also participates in dimerization; domain D, which is a hinge region; and domain E, which contains the ligand-binding and dimerization functions. Domain E is also important for ligand-dependent transcriptional activation. The function of the carboxyl terminal domain F is not completely clear. Homology between the DNA-binding domain and the ligand-binding domains of RARα and RXRα is shown; percentage values represent the percentage of identical amino acid residues in these domains of RARα and RXRα.

have been identified. RARs can be activated by both the all-*trans*- and the 9-*cis*-isomers of retinoic acid. RXRs are activated by 9-*cis*-retinoic acid, which is currently believed to be the major physiological ligand for this receptor, although it has also been reported that RXR can be activated by the long-chain polyunsaturated fatty acid docosahexaenoic acid.

Like other nuclear hormone receptors, RAR and RXR bind to their DNA response elements as dimers. Dimerization, which is stabilized by strong interactions between the ligand-binding domains and by weaker interactions between the DNA-binding domains of the two monomers, serves to increase the specificity of binding of receptors to particular DNA sequences as well as the strength of their interactions with response elements. Mirroring dimer formation by the proteins, DNA response elements for retinoid receptors are usually arranged as two repeats of the same hexanucleotide sequence. RXR can bind to DNA and regulate the transcription of target genes as a homodimer (RXR-RXR). In contrast, RAR homodimers do not form readily. Instead, RAR associates with RXR with a high affinity to form heterodimers, and these RXR-RAR heterodimers serve as the transcriptionally active species of RAR (Durand et al., 1992). In addition to heterodimerization with RAR, RXRs can also interact with other members of the hormone receptor family. For example, they can form heterodimers with the vitamin D_3 receptor (VDR), with the thyroid hormone receptor (TR), with the peroxisome proliferator–activated receptor (PPAR), which is activated by long-chain fatty acids and some of their metabolites, and with liver X receptor (LXR), which responds to cholesterol metabolites. (See Chapters 18 and 31 for more information of transcriptional control by vitamin D and fatty acids.) RXR has also been reported to form active heterodimers with a few nuclear receptors termed orphan receptors, which are proteins that belong to the super-family of nuclear receptors but for which the ligand is unknown. Heterodimers of RXR with other nuclear receptors can respond to the individual ligands of the two partners and, consequently, the transcriptional activities of RXR-heterodimers are regulated by more than one type of ligand. Therefore, RXRs function as "master regulators" of several signaling nutrients and hormones as they converge at the genome to regulate gene expression (Fig. 30-5).

Activation of gene transcription by nuclear receptors depends critically on binding of activating ligands. In the absence of ligands, the receptors associate with accessory proteins that function as transcriptional corepressors. These proteins display enzymatic activities that catalyze deacetylation of histones, resulting in a more compact chromatin structure and leading to repression of transcriptional rates (Jenster, 1998). Upon ligand-binding, nuclear receptors undergo a dramatic conformational change that leads to dissociation of corepressors and to the recruitment of transcriptional coactivators. Some coactivators catalyze histone acetylation, thereby loosening the chromatin, whereas others interact with components of the general transcription machinery (Westin et al., 2000; Yuan et al., 1998). Consequently, ligand-binding results in enhancement of transcriptional rates of target genes for particular receptors. Unlike other receptors, the association of RXR with corepressors is weak, suggesting that ligand-dependent activation of this receptor might operate via a different mechanism. Indeed, it was demonstrated that RXR is unique in that, in the absence of its ligand, it exists as a homotetramer, and that binding of 9-*cis*-retinoic acid results in rapid dissociation of these tetramers to the active

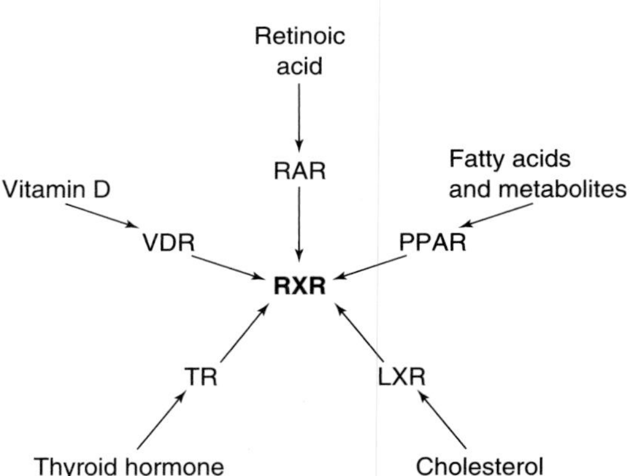

Figure 30-5 Heterodimerization partners of retinoid X receptor (RXR) and their respective ligands.

Clinical Correlation

Potential Therapeutic Uses of Ligands for Retinoid Nuclear Receptors

By virtue of their ability to modulate the rate of transcription of a variety of genes, retinoids can be potent therapeutic agents. Retinoic acid and synthetic ligands that activate RAR are currently used in therapy and chemoprevention of several types of cancer including promyelocytic leukemia and head and neck cancers. The ability of retinoid X receptor (RXR) to serve as a common partner for several nuclear receptors, such as retinoid acid receptor (RAR), vitamin D_3 receptor (VDR), thyroid hormone receptor (TR), liver X receptor (LXR), and peroxisome proliferator–activated receptor (PPAR), suggests that retinoid derivatives that are selective toward RXR might be useful in treating a variety of disorders. Indeed, RXR-selective retinoids enhance sensitivity to insulin and decrease hypertriglyceridemia in mouse models of noninsulin-dependent diabetes and obesity (Mukherjee et al., 1997). It was suggested that this antidiabetic activity is mediated by heterodimers of RXR with PPAR. It was also reported that retinoids increase the expression of apolipoproteins A-I and A-II in a human hepatoblastoma cell line, an activity that was ascribed to RXR-RAR heterodimers (Vu-Dac et al., 1996). Because apo-A-containing HDL is known to have a protective effect against coronary artery disease, these observations suggest that RXR ligands potentially are of clinical use in protecting against cardiovascular disease.

species—dimers and monomers (Kersten et al., 1998, 1995a, 1995b). Ligand-induced dissociation of tetramers therefore seems to be the initial step in activation of RXR.

OTHER RETINOIDS

In addition to retinal and retinoic acid, other retinoids have been shown to be endogenously present in a variety of tissues. The functions of these derivatives are not completely understood, but some of them have been shown to be biologically active. For example, retinol itself has been implicated in regulating lymphocyte physiology. Vitamin A deficiency in animals and in humans is associated with impaired immune function and results in changes in mass, distribution, morphology, and properties of lymphocytes. Lymphocyte survival and proliferation were shown to critically depend on the presence of retinol. This activity apparently cannot be replaced by retinoic acid but could be sustained by *retro*-retinoids, a class of vitamin A derivatives in which the polyene tail is rigidly attached to the β-ionone ring by a double bond with the remaining double bonds retaining the conjugated system and extending it to the 3,4 double bond within the ring (Ross and Hammerling, 1994). The mechanisms by which retinol and *retro*-retinoids support lymphocyte growth are not known. These compounds do not associate with any of the known retinoid nuclear receptors, and they seem to function by signaling pathways that operate at levels other than regulating gene transcription.

Another biologically active retinoid is 3,4-didehydroretinol, also known as vitamin A_2. It is abundant in freshwater fish, where its metabolite 11-*cis*-dehydroretinal can serve as a ligand for visual pigments. In the human, 3, 4-didehydroretinol was reported to accumulate in tissues of individuals with psoriasis and several other disorders of keratinization (Vahlquist and Torma, 1988). 3,4-Didehydroretinoic acid was found in chick limb buds, where it can affect development, presumably by activating retinoid nuclear receptors (Thaller and Eichele, 1990). Oxidized retinoid metabolites such as 4-oxo-retinoic acid were reported to be highly active in determining the positions at which particular digits develop in early embryos and to avidly bind to RARβ (Pijnappel et al., 1993). In addition, it has been demonstrated that some proteins are modified by covalent retinoylation (Takahashi and Breitman, 1991). The addition of a retinoate moiety to proteins

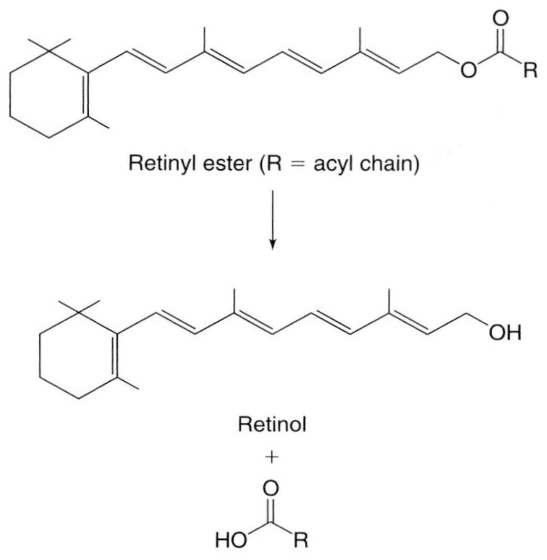

Retinyl ester (R = acyl chain)

Retinol

+

Fatty acid

Figure 30-6 Reaction catalyzed by retinyl ester hydrolase.

seems to represent a novel mechanism by which retinoids can affect cellular physiology. At present, however, the effects of retinoylation on the functions of proteins modified in this fashion are not known.

ABSORPTION, TRANSPORT, STORAGE, AND METABOLISM OF VITAMIN A AND CAROTENOIDS

ABSORPTION AND METABOLISM OF VITAMIN A IN THE INTESTINES

Two major forms of vitamin A are present in the diet: retinyl esters that are derived from animal sources, and carotenoids, mainly β-carotene, that originate from plant food (see Fig. 30-1). Retinyl esters are hydrolyzed in the intestinal lumen to yield free retinol and the corresponding fatty acid (Fig. 30-6). After hydrolysis, retinol is taken up by the enterocytes. Retinyl ester hydrolysis requires the presence of bile salts that serve to solubilize the retinyl esters in mixed micelles and to activate the hydrolyzing enzymes. Several enzymes that are present in the intestinal lumen may be involved in the hydrolysis of dietary retinyl esters. Cholesterol (nonspecific) esterase is secreted into the intestinal lumen from the pancreas and has been shown in vitro to display retinyl ester hydrolase activity. In addition, a retinyl ester hydrolase that is intrinsic to the brush-border membrane of the small intestine has been characterized in the rat as well as in the human (Rigtrup and Ong, 1992). The different hydrolyzing enzymes are activated by different types of bile salts and have distinct substrate specificities. For example, whereas the pancreatic esterase is selective for short-chain retinyl esters, the brush-border membrane enzyme preferentially hydrolyzes retinyl esters containing a long-chain fatty acid such as palmitate or stearate. The latter enzyme is of greater importance in hydrolyzing dietary retinyl esters.

Retinol, produced by retinyl ester hydrolysis, enters the absorptive cells of the small intestine. It has been shown that these cells preferentially take up retinol in the all-*trans* configuration, and that uptake can be inhibited by the sulfhydryl reagent *N*-ethyl maleimide (Dew and Ong, 1994). These observations were interpreted to reflect the presence of a plasma membrane transporter that specifically mediates the uptake of all-*trans* retinol from the intestinal lumen into the absorptive cells.

Carotenoids are absorbed by enterocytes at a lower efficiency than that for the absorption of free retinol. Formation of vitamin A from β-carotene entails its central cleavage into two molecules of retinal, a reaction catalyzed by the cytosolic enzyme β-carotene-15,15′-monooxygenase (Fig. 30-7). This enzyme, which was recently cloned, is most highly expressed in the intestinal mucosa but is also found in liver, kidney, lungs, retina, and the brain. In addition, activities that catalyze eccentric cleavage have been reported and, recently, an enzyme that cleaves β-carotene at the 9′,10 double bond to produce apo-carotenal and retinoic acid has been cloned and characterized. The amounts of carotenoids that can pass intact from intestinal cells into blood vary considerably between different species. In the rat, very limited amounts of carotenoids pass into the circulation. Conversely, in humans, 60% to 70% of absorbed β-carotene is cleaved in the intestine with the remainder transferred intact into blood and deposited in several tissues such as liver and adipose tissue. The serum level of

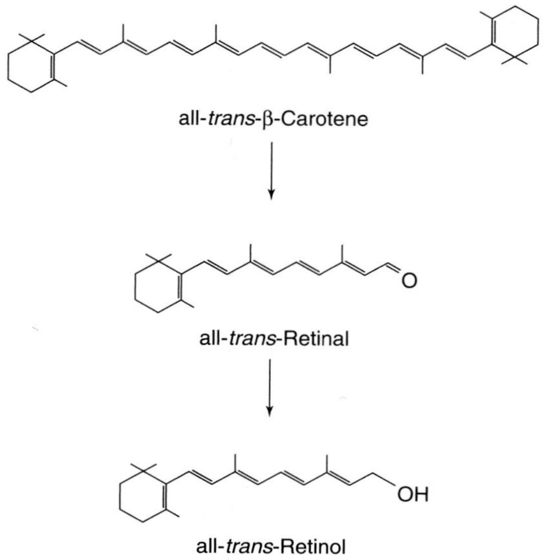

all-*trans*-β-Carotene

all-*trans*-Retinal

all-*trans*-Retinol

Figure 30-7 Cleavage of β-carotene in intestinal epithelium.

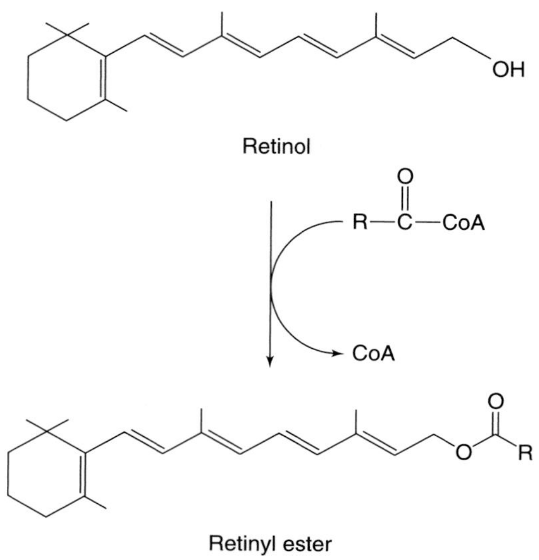

Retinol

R—C(=O)—CoA

CoA

Retinyl ester

Figure 30-8 Reaction catalyzed by acyl CoA: retinol acyltransferase (ARAT).

carotenoids reflects dietary intake, suggesting that a significant fraction of newly absorbed carotenoids is exported from enterocytes into blood without being metabolically converted within these cells.

It has been suggested that carotenoids may have function(s) other than to serve as precursors for retinol. For example, it has been shown that, under some circumstances, β-carotene associated with biological membranes displays an antioxidant activity and can protect membrane lipids from oxygen radical damage (Pacifici and Davies, 1991). It should be noted, however, that there is no evidence to suggest that carotenoids are an essential nutrient.

STORAGE AND MOBILIZATION OF VITAMIN A

Vitamin A is stored in the form of retinyl esters in which retinol is esterified with a long-chain fatty acid. Esterification is accompanied by loss of the polar end groups of both the retinyl and the fatty acyl moieties and results in exceedingly hydrophobic species, which accumulate within lipid droplets in storage cells. Two classes of enzymes that can catalyze the formation of retinyl esters have been identified (MacDonald and Ong, 1988; Ross, 1982). One of these utilizes activated fatty acids in the form of fatty acyl CoAs and is termed acyl coenzyme A:retinol acyltransferase (ARAT) (Fig. 30-8).

A second type of retinol-esterifying enzyme that functions independent of the presence of exogenous fatty acyl CoAs is known as lecithin:retinol acyltransferase (LRAT) (Fig. 30-9). This enzyme synthesizes retinyl esters by catalyzing the *trans*-esterification of a fatty acyl moiety from the *sn*-1 position of phosphatidylcholine to retinol.

Both ARAT and LRAT are integral membrane proteins and are associated with the microsomal fractions of cells of various tissues. Retinyl esters in plasma and in the liver mainly contain the fatty acyl moieties of palmitate and stearate, regardless of the composition of fatty acids in the diet. The composition of the acyl chains in retinyl esters thus corresponds to the primary species of fatty acids found in the *sn*-1 position of phosphatidylcholines, implicating LRAT as the predominant enzyme in esterification of retinol in the intestine and in liver. The cDNA coding for LRAT has been cloned, and tissue distribution analysis showed that LRAT mRNA is present in intestines, liver, testes, retina, and other tissues known for high activities of vitamin A processing. It is worth noting, however, that it has also been reported that retinol esterification in lactating mammary

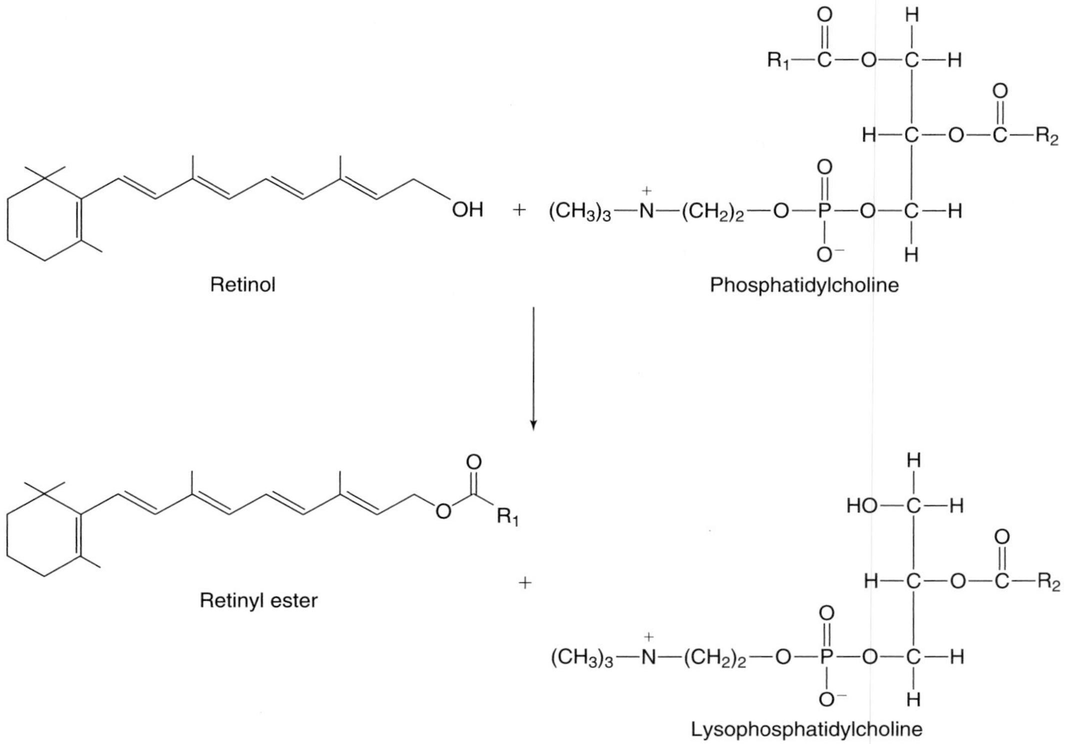

Figure 30-9 Reaction catalyzed by lecithin:retinol acyltransferase (LRAT).

gland is catalyzed mainly by ARAT (Randolph et al., 1991). Hence, the relative contributions of the two enzymes to retinyl ester synthesis may be tissue-specific.

ESTERIFICATION OF RETINOL IN THE INTESTINE

Formation of retinyl esters is the final step of vitamin A absorption in the intestine. Retinyl esters, along with other lipids, are then packaged in chylomicrons and secreted into the lymphatic system, which serves to deliver them to tissues for storage or use. Activities of both ARAT and LRAT have been noted in intestinal mucosa: the LRAT activity predominates, and ARAT activity contributes significantly to esterification only upon intake of large amounts of retinol.

Delivery of Retinyl Esters to the Liver

The major site of vitamin A storage in the body is the liver. It has been reported that retinyl esters in chylomicrons may be hydrolyzed by a lipoprotein lipase at the adipocyte surface, and it was suggested that this activity may facilitate uptake of retinol by these cells (Blaner et al., 1994). However, a significant fraction of retinyl esters is retained in chylomicron remnants and these are cleared from plasma into liver parenchymal cells by receptor-mediated endocytosis.

Hydrolysis and Re-Formation of Retinyl Esters

Following uptake of retinyl esters from the circulation by hepatic parenchymal cells, vitamin A is transferred to hepatic stellate cells where it is stored. Although the mechanism by which vitamin A is transported between the two cell types is not completely understood, it has been shown that chylomicron retinyl esters are hydrolyzed in the parenchymal cells and that new retinyl esters are formed in the stellate cells, suggesting that vitamin A is transported between the two cell types in the form of free retinol (Blaner and Olson, 1994).

The distribution of retinoids between stellate and parenchymal cells has been shown in the rat to depend on the vitamin A status. Under normal dietary conditions, the main fraction of retinyl esters in the liver is found in the stellate cells where they accumulate in lipid droplets. In vitamin A–deficient animals, retinoids are re-distributed into parenchymal cells in a process that, again, seems to involve hydrolysis of retinyl esters. Therefore, absorption and mobilization of vitamin A between different tissues and cells requires continuous hydrolysis and re-formation of retinyl esters (Fig. 30-10).

Several distinct enzymatic activities catalyzing the hydrolysis of retinyl esters have been described in different membrane fractions of both parenchymal and stellate cells of the liver. Some of the retinyl ester hydrolases are activated by bile salts, but the activities of others are independent of bile salts. Re-formation of retinyl esters is catalyzed in the liver by both LRAT and ARAT, with the former pathway predominating under physiological concentrations of retinol.

Although previously little appreciated, it is becoming increasingly clear that, in addition to the liver, extrahepatic tissues play an important role in the overall metabolism and storage of vitamin A. Retinoids are found in extrahepatic organs including adipose depots, kidney, testis, lung, bone marrow, and the eye. These tissues contain significant amounts of retinol and retinyl esters and display esterification as well as retinyl ester hydrolase activities (Blaner and Olson, 1994).

SYNTHESIS OF RETINAL AND RETINOIC ACID FROM RETINOL

Retinoic acid is produced from retinol by two sequential oxidation steps: retinol is converted to retinal, which is then oxidized into retinoic acid. These metabolic conversions are catalyzed, respectively, by retinol dehydrogenases and retinal dehydrogenases in reactions that entail the dehydrogenation of the substrates using the electron acceptors NAD^+ or $NADP^+$. Two classes of enzymes can function as retinol dehydrogenases in vitro: (1) cytosolic medium-chain alcohol dehydogenases and (2) members of the family of short-chain dehydrogenases/reductases (SDRs) that are associated with the membranes of the endoplasmic reticulum (ER) of various cells. In contrast to soluble alcohol dehydrogenases, it has been reported that some SDR-type retinol dehydrogenases are able to metabolize retinol when bound to the cellular retinol-binding protein (CRBP). Hence, while the relative contributions of soluble versus microsomal activities to retinal synthesis in various tissues has not been completely established, it is currently believed that retinal formation in vivo

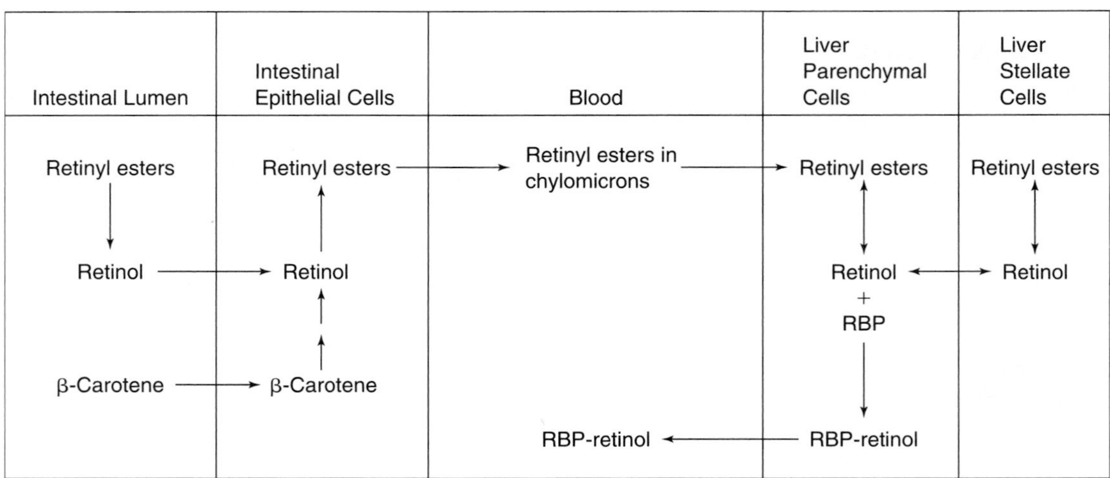

Figure 30-10 Movement of retinol between different organs and cells involves hydrolysis and formation of retinyl esters.

occurs mainly by microsomal SDRs. The first such enzymes to be cloned were the hepatic all-*trans*-retinol dehydrogenase and the bovine *cis*-retinol dehydrogenase, which is highly expressed in the retinal pigment epithelium of the eye (Simon et al., 1996; Chai et al., 1995). Subsequently, multiple isozymes have been identified in various tissues. Some of these display a dual specificity toward *cis*- and all-*trans*-retinol, whereas others are more selective for particular isomeric configurations.

To date, four mammalian cytosolic retinal dehydrogenases (RalDHs) that catalyze the NAD^+-dependent oxidation of all-*trans* retinal to all-*trans*-retinoic acid have been identified. Recent studies utilizing genetically manipulated mouse models indicated that these enzymes indeed play critical roles in retinoic acid synthesis in vivo. It was shown that genetic ablation of RalDH2 results in lethality on about embryonic day 9.5 because of severe trunk, hindbrain, and heart defects resembling those of vitamin A–deficient embryos (Niederreither et al., 1999). Homozygous RalDH1 "knockout" mice are viable and exhibit no gross malformations. However, it has been reported that RA synthesis in liver of these mice is greatly reduced, suggesting that RalDH1 participates in RA synthesis in vivo (Fan et al., 2003). Mice in which RalDH3 has been "knocked-out" display suppressed RA synthesis and ocular and nasal malformations similar to those observed in vitamin A–deficient fetuses (Dupe et al., 2003). It is important to note that these defects can be prevented by maternal treatment with retinoic acid, demonstrating the importance of the enzyme in retinoic acid synthesis. Less is known about the physiological function of RalDH4, which was recently cloned and shown to display a selectivity toward 9-*cis*-retinal suggesting that it may play a role in synthesis of 9-*cis*-retinoic acid (Lin et al., 2003).

Other potential pathways for formation of retinoic acid include oxidation of retinal by microsomal cytochrome P450 and direct production of retinoic acid by cleavage of β-carotene in a process that might not involve retinol or retinal as intermediates. Retinoic acid is also found in plasma at a concentration on the order of 10 nmol/L, and circulating retinoic acid originating from dietary intake may be a source for retinoic acid in some tissues.

METABOLISM OF RETINOIC ACID

Retinoic acid is converted in vivo into several metabolites. The functional significance of these metabolites is incompletely understood.

Retinoic Acid Isomers

The most stable isomer of retinoic acid and the predominant species of this compound in vivo is the all-*trans* form. Another isomer, 13-*cis*-retinoic acid has been reported to be present in blood and in the small intestine. This isomer comprises a significant fraction of retinoic acid at equilibrium and may be present in vivo as a result of nonspecific isomerization. As discussed in the preceding text, another isomer, 9-*cis*-retinoic acid, binds to nuclear retinoid receptors with high affinity and is a powerful modulator of gene transcription.

Polar and Oxidized Metabolites of Retinoids

Several types of polar metabolites of retinoids are formed by the action of "detoxifying" enzymes, which catalyze the conjugation of polar groups onto hydrophobic substrates, thereby enhancing the solubility of the substrate.

Retinoid β-glucuronides are synthesized from either retinoic acid or retinol in a variety of tissues including liver, kidney, and intestine. These compounds are also found in blood at concentrations that are comparable to those of retinoic acid. Retinoid glucuronides are formed by microsomal UDP-glucuronyl transferases, which catalyze the conjugation of glucuronic acid to hydrophobic substrates. Retinoyl β-glucuronide can be hydrolyzed back to yield retinoic acid, a reaction that is catalyzed by the lysosomal β-glucuronidase. Retinoyl β-glucuronide has been shown to act as a competent inducer of cell differentiation (Zile et al., 1987), but it does not bind to retinoid nuclear receptors and its mechanisms of action are not known.

Retinoic acid, retinol, and retinal can be metabolized by several forms of the microsomal cytochrome P450 system. Cytochrome P450 reactions, which require NADPH and molecular oxygen, convert these substrates to multiple oxidized metabolites, which are found in various tissues. Several isotypes of cytochrome P450s that are highly specific in converting retinoic acid to 4-oxo-retinoic acid (e.g., CYP26) have been identified (Haque and Anreola, 1998). These enzymes are usually considered to function in catalyzing the degradation of retinoic acid, thereby downregulating retinoid signaling. It may be worth noting, however, that some oxidized retinoids, such as 4-oxo-retinoic acid, can activate retinoid receptors and thus may be directly involved in affecting cellular physiology (Nikawa et al., 1995; Pijnappel et al., 1993).

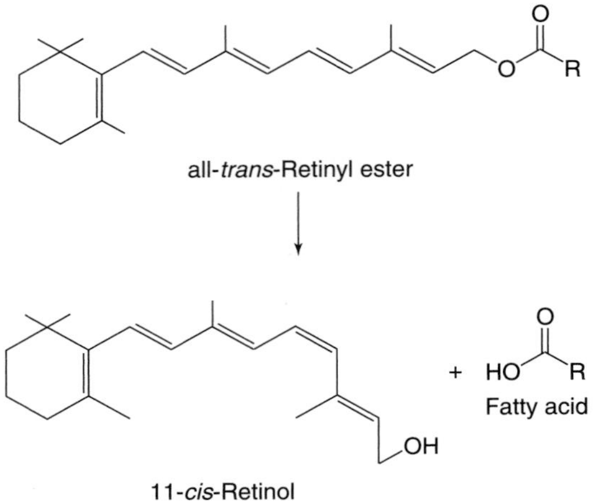

RETINOID METABOLISM IN THE EYE

Synthesis of Retinyl Esters in Retinal Pigment Epithelium

The main vitamin A form that circulates in blood is all-*trans*-retinol. This species is taken up into the eye by retinal pigment epithelium (RPE) (see Fig. 30-3). RPE cells contain an unusually high level of enzymatic activity for conversion of retinol to retinyl esters. The esterification activity is catalyzed by an LRAT and results in formation of all-*trans* retinyl esters, which serve as storage species as well as precursors to the 11-*cis*-retinoids that participate in the visual cycle. LRAT of the RPE cells displays a broad substrate specificity and in the presence of 11-*cis*-retinol can form 11-*cis*-retinyl ester. High levels of these esters have been shown to accumulate in RPE cells in the dark (Saari, 1994).

Formation of 11-*Cis*-Retinoids

Conversion of all-*trans*-retinoids to the 11-*cis* configuration in the eye is a critical part of the visual cycle. In the RPE, this reaction is catalyzed by a microsomal isomerase termed all-*trans*-retinyl ester isomerohydrolase. This enzyme utilizes the energy stored in the ester bond of all-*trans*-retinyl esters to produce the 11-*cis* species. Retinyl ester hydrolysis is thus coupled with an isomerization reaction to produce 11-*cis*-retinol (Canada et al., 1990) (Fig. 30-11).

all-*trans*-Retinyl ester

\+ HO–C(=O)–R
Fatty acid

11-*cis*-Retinol

Figure 30-11 Reaction catalyzed by all-*trans*-retinyl ester isomerohydrolase.

In RPE cells, 11-*cis*-retinol can also be produced by hydrolysis of 11-*cis*-retinyl esters, a reaction that is catalyzed by a microsomal retinyl ester hydrolase. This enzyme can also hydrolyze retinyl esters in the all-*trans* configuration, but displays a significantly higher specific activity toward the 11-*cis* substrates (Blaner et al., 1987).

The retinoid that supports visual function, 11-*cis*-retinal, is formed in the RPE by oxidation of 11-*cis*-retinol, a reaction catalyzed by a microsomal *cis*-retinol dehydrogenase. Several enzymes that function as *cis*-retinol dehydrogenases are expressed in the RPE. This redundancy might suggest that loss-of-function mutations in any one of the genes that encode for these enzymes would result in only minor aberrations. Indeed, mutation of the 11-*cis*-retinol dehydrogenase RDH5 in humans leads to a non-progressive night blindness without retinal dystrophy (Yamamoto et al., 1999). In contrast, it was recently reported that mutations in RDH12 are associated with a childhood-onset severe retinal dystrophy, suggesting that this isotype plays a more important role in the visual cycle (Janecke et al., 2004). Following its formation, 11-*cis*-retinal is exported from the RPE to photoreceptor cells where it serves to regenerate bleached rhodopsin.

It was recently suggested that, unlike rod photoreceptor cells that obtain 11-*cis*-retinal from the RPE, 11-*cis*-retinoids necessary for rhodopsin regeneration in cone cells originate in Müller cells (see Fig. 30-3). By studying retinas from animals that have mainly cones

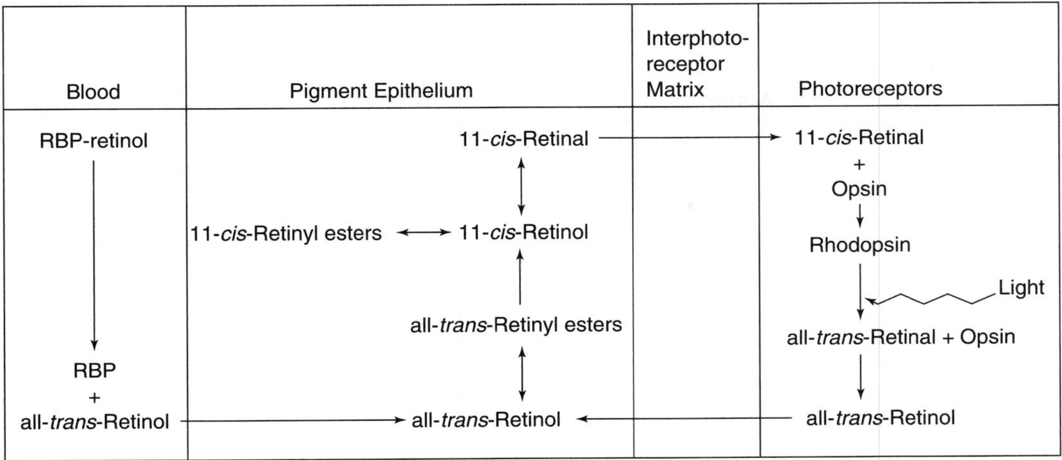

Figure 30-12 Major metabolic conversions of retinoids in the eye.

(chicken and ground squirrel), Mata and colleagues (2002) demonstrated an enzymatic activity in Müller cells that catalyzes direct isomerization of free (unesterified) all-*trans*-retinol. They suggested that the resulting 11-*cis*-retinol is transported to cone cells where it is converted to 11-*cis*-retinal. It was further proposed that this novel pathway for synthesis of 11-*cis*-retinal is significantly faster than that afforded by the RPE retinyl ester isomerohydrolase and can support the higher rhodopsin turnover that characterizes bright-light vision mediated by cones.

Metabolism of Retinal in Photoreceptor Cells

The absorption of a photon by rhodopsin in photoreceptor cells leads to isomerization of rhodopsin-bound 11-*cis*-retinal to the all-*trans*-retinal. Photoisomerization initiates visual transduction and also results in the hydrolysis of the retinal–rhodopsin complex. Free all-*trans*-retinal is then converted by a retinol dehydrogenase into all-*trans*-retinol. All-*trans*-retinol produced in photoreceptor cells is transported to the RPE where it can be converted back to 11-*cis*-retinal. The major metabolic conversions of retinoids in photoreceptor and pigment epithelial cells are shown in Figure 30-12.

RETINOID-BINDING PROTEINS

Because of its amphipathic nature and its poor solubility in water, vitamin A efficiently dissolves in the hydrophobic core of cellular membranes. However, the presence of excess vitamin A in membranes results in disruption of membrane structure and function. In addition, in order to reach their target cells and their sites of action inside cells, retinoids must traverse the oxygen-rich aqueous spaces of plasma and cytosol. Therefore, in considering retinoid biology it is important to understand how these poorly soluble compounds are transported through aqueous phases without loss of structural integrity, and how their concentrations in cellular membranes are retained below membranolytic levels. Answers to these questions were provided by the identification of multiple water-soluble proteins that specifically bind different vitamin A derivatives (Table 30-1). Retinol circulates in blood bound to serum retinol-binding protein (RBP). In cells, there exist proteins that selectively bind retinol, retinal, and retinoic acid. In addition, the interphotoreceptor matrix, which is the extracellular space between the photoreceptors and retinal pigment epithelium (RPE) cells in the eye (see Fig. 30-3), contains a protein that displays a broad specificity for retinoids. Recently, a protein in the RPE cells was reported to function as a retinyl ester–binding protein. Cellular retinol-, retinal-, and retinoic acid–binding proteins are highly conserved across species that utilize vitamin A, implying that they play critical roles in the biology of retinoids. The interactions of retinoids with these proteins

Table 30-1
Retinoid-Binding Proteins

	M_r (kDa)	Major Ligand(s)	Major Location
Retinol-binding protein (RBP)	21.2	All-*trans*-retinol	Blood
Cellular retinol-binding protein (CRBP)	15.7	All-*trans*-retinol All-*trans*-retinal	Most tissues
Cellular retinol-binding protein II (CRBPII)	15.6	All-*trans*-retinol All-*trans*-retinal	Small intestine; fetal liver
Cellular retinoic acid-binding protein (CRABP)	15.5	All-*trans*-retinoic acid	Most tissues
Cellular retinoic acid-binding protein II (CRABPII)	15.0	All-*trans*-retinoic acid	Skin, ovary, uterus
Cellular retinal-binding protein (CRALBP)	36.0	11-*cis*-retinal 11-*cis*-retinol	Retina
Interphotoreceptor retinoid-binding protein (IRBP)	136.0	11-*cis*-retinal All-*trans*-retinol	Interphotoreceptor matrix
RPE65	65.0	All-*trans*-retinyl esters	Retinal pigment epithelium

M_r, Molecular mass.

retard their degradation, decrease their concentrations in membranes, and increase their concentrations in aqueous spaces. In addition to these general roles, particular retinoid-binding proteins have specific functions in regulating the metabolism and action of their respective ligands.

RETINOL-BINDING PROTEIN AND TRANSPORT OF RETINOL IN BLOOD

Retinol circulates in blood bound to a plasma protein named retinol-binding protein (RBP), which is a single polypeptide with a molecular weight of 21 kDa, and it contains one binding site for retinol. The main site of synthesis and secretion of this protein is the liver, which is also the main storage site for vitamin A. Secretion of retinol-binding protein (RBP) from the liver is tightly regulated by the availability of retinol (Soprano and Blaner, 1994). During vitamin A deficiency, RBP secretion is inhibited and the protein accumulates in the ER. Upon an increase in retinol levels, RBP moves to the Golgi apparatus and is secreted into blood in the form of the holo-protein. Some extrahepatic tissues including adipose tissue, kidney, testis, brain, and the digestive tract were found to synthesize and secrete RBP. Interestingly, it was reported that RPE cells in the eye synthesize RBP and secrete it, not into the blood, but toward the retina into the interphotoreceptor matrix (Ong et al., 1994a). This suggests that RBP may serve as a carrier protein for retinol in compartments other than plasma.

In plasma, RBP is bound to another protein called transthyretin (TTR), a 56-kDa protein that, in addition to associating with RBP, functions as a carrier for thyroid hormones. It is believed that binding of RBP to TTR serves to prevent the loss of the smaller protein from the circulation by filtration in the glomeruli. Although TTR is a tetrameric protein made up of four equivalent subunits, it is usually found bound to only one molecule of RBP. Therefore, the protein complex responsible for the plasma transport of retinol contains TTR-RBP-retinol at a molar ratio of 1:1:1. The concentration of this complex in plasma is kept constant at 1 to 2 μmol/L except in extreme cases of vitamin A deficiency or in disease states.

The retinol-binding site of RBP is a hydrophobic β-barrel that encapsulates the retinol molecule with its β-ionone ring buried deep in the barrel, the isoprene chain stretched along the barrel axis, and the hydroxyl end group lying almost at the surface of the protein (Fig. 30-13) (Newcomer et al., 1984).

Because most of the physiologically important retinoids differ from retinol only in the composition of their head groups, the structure

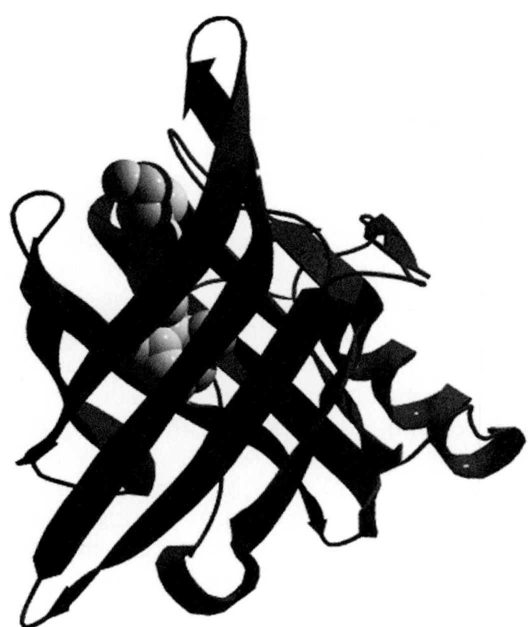

Figure 30-13 Retinol binding protein. Retinol (depicted in light gray) is bound with the β-ionone ring deep in the pocket and the head group positioned near the protein surface.

of the RBP binding site suggests that it may bind other retinoids. Indeed, RBP displays a broad specificity for retinoids. However, in the presence of ligands with polar end groups larger than a hydroxyl, such as the carboxyl group of retinoic acid, the interactions of RBP with TTR are hindered. Consequently, the only retinoid that is found to be associated with RBP in plasma is retinol. In contrast, retinoic acid circulates in plasma bound to serum albumin.

The tight interaction of retinol with the TTR–RBP complex allows this poorly soluble vitamin to circulate in the aqueous plasma. However, target tissues for vitamin A, except for perhaps the liver, do not take up the protein complex. Therefore, in order to reach the interior of cells, retinol must dissociate from RBP prior to uptake. There are currently two opposing views of how this process is accomplished.

It has been proposed that a specific receptor for RBP exists in the plasma membranes of target cells. This putative receptor is postulated to recognize and bind circulating RBP and to mediate the release of retinol from the protein and its transfer across the plasma membrane to the cytosol. This hypothesis is based on the observations that uptake of radiolabeled retinol by some cells can be inhibited in the presence of RBP complexed with nonlabeled retinol, and that plasma membranes of some target cells seem to possess a RBP-binding activity.

In contrast, because the association of retinol with RBP is reversible, the ligand can spontaneously dissociate from the protein. Because of the hydrophobic nature of retinol, it can also spontaneously associate with cellular membranes. Therefore, there might not be a need to postulate the existence of specialized receptors to facilitate the dissociation of the RBP–retinol complex or the movement of retinol across membranes. The rates by which retinol spontaneously dissociates from the TTR–RBP complex and traverses membranes were found to be faster than the rates by which retinol is taken up by several target cells, suggesting that the rate of uptake is not limited by the rate of release of retinol from RBP or by events at the plasma membrane (Noy and Xu, 1990; Fex and Johannesson, 1987). It was thus proposed that retinol spontaneously and rapidly equilibrates between binding proteins in plasma and in cytosol and that the rate of uptake is regulated by the rate of retinol metabolism. This hypothesis is supported by the observations that the uptake of retinol from RBP into target cells proceeded rapidly and did not seem to be a saturable process (Soprano and Blaner, 1994).

CELLULAR RETINOL- AND RETINOIC ACID–BINDING PROTEINS

Cellular retinol-binding proteins (CRBPs) and cellular retinoic acid–binding proteins (CRABPs) belong to the family of intracellular lipid binding proteins (iLBPs), the members of which include proteins that bind lipophilic ligands such as retinoids and long-chain fatty acids. The iLBPs are characterized by their low molecular weight (~15 kDa) and by a shared β-clam structure composed of two 5-stranded orthogonal β-sheets that form a ligand binding pocket. A helix-loop-helix forms a "lid" over the entrance to the ligand-binding pocket of these proteins, raising the question of how respective ligands enter or exit the pocket (Fig. 30-14) (Gutierrez-Gonzalez et al., 2002; Veerkamp

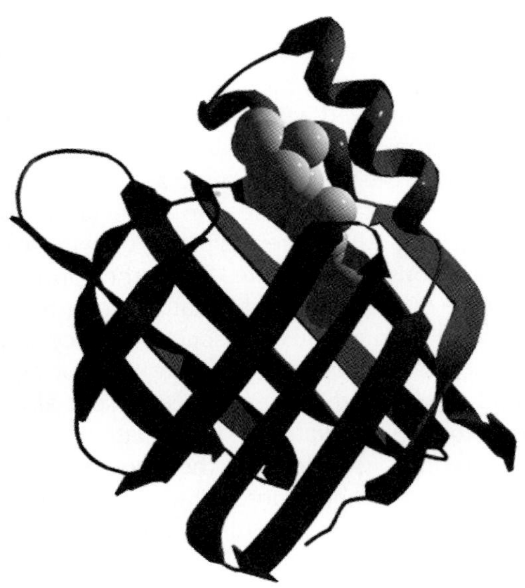

Figure 30-14 Cellular retinoic acid–binding protein II. Retinoic acid (depicted in light gray) is bound with the carboxyl head group directed inward and the β-ionone ring near the entrance to the ligand binding pocket.

and Maatman, 1995; Kleywegt et al., 1994). Although similar in their three-dimensional structures, iLBPs are less homologous in their primary sequences and they bind lipophilic molecules with distinct selectivities. Recent studies have begun to identify the specific functions of CRBPs and CRABPs in the biology of their respective ligands.

Cellular Retinol-Binding Proteins

Four isotypes of cellular retinol-binding proteins (CRBP-I, II, III and IV) have been identified to date, with the best characterized ones being CRBP-I and CRBP-II. CRBP-I is present in many tissues including liver, kidney, ovary, testis, lung, eye, spleen, and the small intestine. CRBP-II is found almost exclusively in the mucosal epithelium of the small intestine (Ong et al., 1994b). Although they are named for their interactions with retinol, both CRBP-I and CRBP-II also bind retinal. The affinity of CRBP-I for retinol was reported to be significantly stronger as compared with CRBP-II (Li et al., 1991). In contrast, the two proteins bind retinal with a similar affinity. The evolutionary conservation of the two proteins and their characteristic organ and cellular distribution suggest that they play important and distinct roles in the physiology of vitamin A.

Both CRBP-I and CRBP-II were shown to protect their ligands from the activity of some enzymes while allowing them to be metabolized by others. CRBP-II regulates such a selectivity in the intestine. In intestinal cells, free retinal is reduced efficiently to retinol by a soluble retinol dehydrogenase, but the reaction is inhibited when the substrate is presented to the enzyme bound to CRBP-II. In contrast, an intestinal microsomal dehydrogenase (associated with the ER) can reduce retinal both in the absence and the presence of the binding protein (Kakkad and Ong, 1988). Similarly, esterification of retinol by ARAT of the small intestine is inhibited in the presence of CRBP-II, but intestinal LRAT can metabolize both free and CRBP-II–bound retinol (Herr and Ong, 1992). Because most of the retinol in intestinal cells is bound to CRBP-II, these findings provide an explanation for the predominance of the LRAT- over the ARAT-catalyzed reaction in formation of retinyl esters in small intestine.

Similarly to the ability of intestinal LRAT to access retinol when bound to CRBP-II, hepatic LRAT can metabolize retinol bound to CRBP-I. Interestingly, it was also reported that this enzyme is inhibited by the addition of apo-CRBP-I (Herr and Ong, 1992) and that apo-CRBP-I activates liver retinyl ester hydrolase (Boerman and Napoli, 1991). The observations that apo-CRBP-I inhibits the LRAT reaction but activates the hydrolase suggest the following scenario: when the concentration of retinol, and thus the level of holo-CRBP-I, is high, retinyl ester formation will proceed at a fast rate. Conversely, when the availability of retinol decreases, apo-CRBP-I levels will increase, leading to lower rates of esterification and an enhanced retinyl ester hydrolysis. The notion that CRBP-I regulates the maintenance of vitamin A storage is supported by studies of mice in which the CRBP-I gene has been disrupted. This work revealed that CRBP-I deficiency is accompanied by a 50% reduction of retinyl ester pools in hepatic stellate cells, a reduction that appears to stem from decreased retinyl ester synthesis accompanied by an accelerated rate of clearance of hepatic retinyl esters (Ghyselinck et al., 1999).

A question that arises from the observations that retinol bound to CRBPs can serve as substrate for particular enzymes relates to the mechanism by which the enzymes access this ligand. This question is especially intriguing as retinol is bound to CRBP with the polar end group buried deeply inside the binding pocket (Cowan et al., 1993). It is therefore difficult to envision how any enzyme could gain access to the ligand's end group in such a location. It has been suggested in regard to this that protein–protein interactions between the binding protein and specific enzymes may result in a conformational change in the CRBP region that covers the binding site, allowing for direct diffusion of retinol from the binding protein into the enzyme's active site (Jamison et al., 1994).

Cellular Retinoic Acid–Binding Proteins

The transcriptional activities of retinoic acid are mediated by the nuclear hormone receptors known as RARs as discussed in the preceding text. In addition to RAR, retinoic acid binds to two intracellular lipid-binding proteins, CRABP-I and CRABP-II, which have sub-nanomolar affinities for retinoic acid. These proteins are highly conserved among species, and they are expressed differentially across tissues and developmental stages. In the adult, CRABP-I is expressed almost ubiquitously, whereas CRABP-II is expressed in the skin, ovary, uterus, and the choroid plexus of the brain.

It has been reported that increased expression of CRABP-I in cells enhances the rate of formation of polar metabolites of retinoic acid and decreases the transcriptional activity of RAR. It was also shown that sensitivity of F9 teratocarcinoma cells to retinoic acid–induced differentiation is correlated inversely with the cellular level of CRABP-I (Boylan and Gudas, 1992, 1991). Although the molecular mechanism underlying these effects remains to be clarified, available information suggests that CRABP-I dampens cellular response to RA, perhaps by facilitating retinoic acid degradation.

In contrast to CRABP-I, recent studies revealed that CRABP-II sensitizes cells to retinoic acid. This activity stems from the ability of the binding protein to directly deliver retinoic acid from the cytosol to RAR in the nucleus. It was reported that CRABP-II, which is predominantly cytosolic in the absence of retinoic acid, translocates to the nucleus upon ligand-binding, and it was demonstrated that CRABP-II associates directly with RAR to form a complex that mediates "ligand-channeling" from the binding protein to the receptor. Hence, CRABP-II facilitates transfer of the retinoic acid ligand to RAR and potentiates RAR's ability to upregulate gene expression (Dong et al., 1999). In agreement with these observations, it was reported that CRABP-II significantly enhances the retinoic acid–induced, RAR-mediated, inhibition of cancer cell growth in cultured cells as well as in mouse models of breast cancer (Manor et al., 2003; Budhu and Noy, 2002).

CELLULAR RETINOL-BINDING PROTEIN

The eye and the pineal gland contain a binding protein that is highly specific toward the 11-*cis* isomers of retinal and retinol. Cellular retinal-binding protein (CRALBP), a 36-kDa protein, is a member of the Sec14 lipid-binding/transfer protein family. This family currently encompasses approximately 20 members in mammals including CRALBP and α-tocopherol transfer protein (see Chapter 29). The location of CRALBP in the retina and its specificity toward retinoids that function in vision suggest that its roles are similar to those of the retinoid-binding proteins discussed in the preceding text (i.e., it functions in transport and metabolism of 11-*cis*-retinoids). Indeed, it has been shown that CRALBP can influence the metabolic fate of 11-*cis*-retinol in pigment epithelium cells (Saari et al., 1994). In these cells, 11-*cis*-retinol can be either oxidized by retinol dehydrogenase to 11-*cis*-retinal and exported to photoreceptor cells for regeneration of rhodopsin or esterified by LRAT to form 11-*cis*-retinyl esters (see Fig. 30-12). The presence of CRALBP inhibits the esterification reaction, most likely as a result of sequestration of 11-*cis*-retinol by the protein. In contrast, CRALBP stimulates the reaction catalyzed by 11-*cis*-retinol dehydrogenase, suggesting that direct interactions exist between the binding protein and this enzyme. Recently, CRALBP was also implicated in supporting the isomerization of all-*trans*- to 11-*cis*-retinol in Müller cells in the eye (Mata et al., 2002).

INTERPHOTORECEPTOR RETINOID-BINDING PROTEIN

Regeneration of active visual pigments in the eye requires a continuous flux of retinoids between different cell types via the aqueous interphotoreceptor matrix space that separates them (see Fig. 30-12). The low solubility of retinoids in water and the physiological requirement for their rapid transfer across an aqueous space raise questions regarding the mechanism by which the transport is accomplished.

The main soluble protein component of the interphotoreceptor matrix (IPM) is a 136 kDa, highly glycosylated protein that binds retinoids and other hydrophobic ligands such as long-chain fatty acids. It is believed that this protein, termed the interphotoreceptor retinoid-binding protein (IRBP), serves as a carrier for retinoids between the various cells that participate in the visual cycle (i.e., photoreceptors, RPE cells, and, perhaps, Müller cells). In contrast with other known retinoid-binding proteins, IRBP possesses three distinct sites for retinoids (Shaw and Noy, 2001). Participation of IRBP in shuttling of retinoids in the IPM is implied by the observations that the composition of retinoids associated with the protein in the IPM is modulated by light and that binding of retinoids to IRBP stabilizes them against degradation. It was also reported that IRBP can take up 11-*cis* retinal from RPE and that it can efficiently deliver 11-*cis*-retinal to bleached-rod outer segments (Saari, 1994; Pepperberg et al., 1993). However, the exact role of IRBP in the transport process is not known. Theoretically, IRBP could serve simply as a storage compartment for retinoids in the IPM, with the ability to bind and release these ligands according to their concentration gradients. Alternatively, IRBP could function to selectively target specific retinoids to particular locations in the eye by a yet unidentified mechanism. It has been reported that docosahexaenoic acid (DHA), which is a polyunsaturated fatty acid that is highly enriched in photoreceptor cells, specifically inhibits binding of the visual chromophore 11-*cis*-retinal to one of the IRBP retinoid binding sites. The following scenario was thus suggested: while IRBP is in the vicinity of the RPE, where the concentration of DHA is low, it will possess a high affinity for 11-*cis*-retinal and associate with it. Movement to the vicinity of photoreceptor cells will expose IRBP to high levels of DHA resulting in rapid release of 11-*cis*-retinal from the regulated binding site (Chen et al., 1996). This and other models for the function and mechanism of action of IRBP are under investigation.

BINDING OF RETINYL ESTERS BY RPE65

RPE65, a protein that is highly expressed in RPE cells, plays a critical role in generation of 11-*cis*-retinoids in the eye. Such a role is demonstrated by the observations that RPE cells of mice lacking functional RPE65 accumulate high levels of all-*trans*-retinyl esters but completely lack 11-*cis*-retinoids and thus are unable to generate visual pigments. In addition, mutations in the *RPE65* gene in humans result in a severe recessive blinding disease called Leber's congenital amaurosis. It was recently reported that RPE65 serves as a shuttling protein for all-*trans*-retinyl esters in RPE cells (Mata et al., 2004; Gollapalli et al., 2003). Specifically, it was demonstrated that this protein selectively binds all-*trans*-retinyl but not 11-*cis*-retinyl esters, that it efficiently extracts all-*trans*-retinyl esters from phospholipid membranes, and that it strongly stimulates the enzymatic conversion of all-*trans*-retinyl esters to 11-*cis*-retinol by RPE microsomal fractions, although it does not display an isomerase activity on its own. It was, therefore, suggested that RPE65 participates in 11-*cis*-retinol synthesis by presenting retinyl esters as a substrate to isomerohydrolase, which, in turn, catalyzes their isomerization to the visual chromophore.

NUTRITIONAL CONSIDERATIONS OF VITAMIN A

DIETARY REFERENCE INTAKES FOR VITAMIN A AND CAROTENOIDS

In establishing the DRIs, the Institute of Medicine (IOM, 2001) chose a new basis for expressing vitamin A requirements: retinol activity equivalents (RAEs). One μg RAE is equivalent to 1 μg of retinol, 12 μg of β-carotene, 24 μg of α-carotene, and 24 μg of β-cryptoxanthin. New data have demonstrated that dietary carotenoids are less available than carotenoids in oil, which were used previously for establishing the retinol equivalents (National Research Council [NRC], 1989). This correction of bioconversion efficiencies means that vitamin A intake has been overestimated in the past and that more carotene-rich foods than previously thought are needed to meet the vitamin A requirement.

The IOM set DRIs for vitamin A in terms of RAE. Adequate intakes (AIs) were set for infants based on their intake from human milk and, in the case of older infants, from complementary foods. These are 0.40 mg RAE (0.485 mg/L × 0.78 L milk/day) and 0.50 mg RAE (0.3 mg/day from milk + 0.2 mg/day from complementary food) per day for infants 0 to 6 months of age and 7 to 12 months of age, respectively. An estimated average requirement (EAR) for vitamin A was estimated for adults based on the amount of dietary vitamin A required to maintain a given body-pool size in well-nourished subjects (IOM, 2001; Olson, 1987). The EAR was set at 0.627 mg RAE/day for men and 0.503 mg RAE/day for women. The recommended dietary allowances (RDAs) were set as the EAR + 40%, with rounding to the nearest 0.100 mg, and are 0.90 mg RAE/day for men and 0.70 mg RAE/day for women. DRIs for children were extrapolated from the adult EARs/RDAs, using metabolic weight ($kg^{0.75}$) as a basis for extrapolation. An increment of 0.050 mg RAE/day was added to the EAR for pregnant women, based on the accumulation of vitamin A in the liver of the fetus during gestation and an assumption that the liver contains approximately half of the fetus's vitamin A stores. An increment of 0.040 mg/day was added to the EAR for lactating women, based on the average secretion of vitamin A in human milk during the first 6 months of lactation. Therefore, the RDAs (EAR + 40%) are 0.77 mg RAE/day for pregnant women and 1.30 mg RAE/day for lactating women.

Food intake data indicate that approximately 26% and 34% of the RAEs consumed by men and women, respectively, are in the form of provitamin A carotenoids. The median intake of adult men (ages 19 to 70 years) from foods is approximately 0.77 mg RAE/day, with the 5th- and 95th-percentile range being 0.31 to 1.76 mg RAE/day (NHANES III, 1988-1994). For women, the median intake is approximately 0.60 mg RAE/day, with a range of 0.27 to 0.90 mg RAE/day.

Recommendations regarding daily intake of vitamin A also have been put forward by Expert Committees of the Food and Agriculture Organization and the World Health Organization (FAO/WHO, 2002). The FAO/WHO recommendations are given as retinol equivalents (REs), and likely overestimate the vitamin A activity of plant carotenoids. One μg RE is equal to 1 μg retinol, 6 μg β-carotene, or 12 μg of other provitamin A carotenoids. The recommended safe intakes are 0.375 mg RE/day for infants

RDAs Across the Life Cycle

	mg Retinol Equivalents (RAEs) per Day
Infants	
0 to 6 mo	0.40 (AI)
7 to 12 mo	0.50 (AI)
Children	
1 to 3 yr	0.30
4 to 8 yr	0.40
9 to 13 yr	0.60
Males	
14 to 18 yr	0.90
19 to >70	0.90
Females	
14 to 18 yr	0.70
Pregnant	0.75
Lactating	1.20
19 to >70 yr	0.70
Pregnant	0.77
Lactating	1.30

From Institute of Medicine (IOM) (2001) Dietary Reference Intakes for Vitamin A, Vitamin K, Arsenic, Boron, Chromium, Copper, Iodine, Iron, Manganese, Molybdenum, Nickel, Silicon, Vanadium, and Zinc. National Academy Press, Washington, DC.
1 μg RAE = 1 μg retinol, 12 μg β-carotene, 24 μg α-carotene, or 24 μg β-cryptoxanthin.

Food Sources

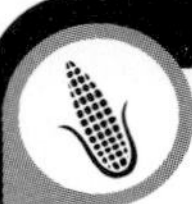

Food Sources of Retinol Activity Equivalents (RAE)*

Meats, Fish, Eggs

9.0 mg per 3 oz turkey giblets
6.5 mg per 3 oz beef liver
0.06 to 0.07 mg per 3 oz fish
0.08 to 0.09 mg per egg

Vegetables and Fruits

0.30 to 0.90 mg per ½ cup pumpkin
0.20 to 0.27 mg per ½ cup winter squash
0.50 mg per ½ cup sweet potatoes
0.33 to 0.60 mg per ½ cup carrots
0.27 to 0.55 mg per ½ cup spinach, collards, kale
0.19 mg per ½ cup red peppers
0.19 mg per ½ cup cantaloupe
0.08 mg per ½ cup romaine lettuce

Dairy Products/Fortified Products†

0.13 to 0.15 mg per ½ cup ricotta cheese
0.14 to 0.15 mg per 1 cup milk (vitamin A added)
0.12 mg per 1 Tbsp margarine
0.11 to 0.16 mg per 1 cup ready-to-eat cereal

Data from U.S. Department of Agriculture/Agricultural Research Service (USDA/ARS) (2005) USDA Nutrient Database for Standard Reference, Release 18. USDA/ARS, Washington, DC. Retrieved November 15, 2005 from www.ars.usda.gov/ba/bhnrc/ndl/.
*1 μg RAE = 1 μg retinol, or 12 μg β-carotene, or 24 μg α-carotene, or 24 β-cryptoxanthin.
†Vitamin A in fortified foods and vitamin supplements is in the form of retinyl ester (e.g., retinyl acetate or retinyl palmitate).
RAE, Retinal activity equivalents.

from birth to 6 months of age, 0.40 mg RE/day for children from 7 months to 3 years of age, 0.45 mg RE/day for children 4 to 6 years of age, 0.50 mg RE/day for children from 7 to 10 years of age, 0.60 mg RE/day for adolescents, 0.50 mg RE/day for female adults, 0.60 mg RE/day for male adults, 0.60 mg RE/day for all adults older than age 65, 0.80 mg RE/day for pregnant women, and 0.85 mg/day for lactating women. The safe level of intake is defined as the average continuing intake of vitamin A required to permit adequate growth and other vitamin A–dependent functions and to maintain an acceptable total body reserve of the vitamin. These FAO/WHO safe levels of intake appear to be similar to the EARs established by the IOM (2001) for the U.S. and Canadian populations. However, the use of RE instead of RAE, in fact, yields average safe intakes that are substantially lower than those estimated by the IOM for the North American population. This factor needs further consideration, particularly because diets in most developing countries are low in preformed vitamin A and populations are dependent largely upon provitamin A carotenoids in plants as a source of retinol equivalents.

VITAMIN A DEFICIENCY

Vitamin A deficiency is manifested by a number of symptoms, the most serious being ocular problems and a depressed immune function. Vitamin A deficiency is rare in developed countries, where the mean daily intake usually exceeds the RDA. However, in many developing countries in Southern and Southeastern Asia, in Africa, and in Central and South America, vitamin A deficiency is a serious nutritional problem that especially affects preschool-age children. Vitamin A deficiency is most common in populations consuming mainly plant-based diets with little dietary fat.

Children younger than 6 years of age are particularly affected by vitamin A deficiency. Vitamin A deficiency–related blindness is most prevalent in children younger than 3 years of age. It has been estimated that 1.5 million children worldwide are blind and that vitamin A deficiency is the cause of approximately 70% of these cases (Underwood, 1994). The initial signs of vitamin A deficiency are night blindness and impaired epidermal integrity manifested by hyperkeratosis. These conditions can be reversed upon supplementation of vitamin A. If left untreated, night blindness is followed by xerophthalmia, a disease associated with structural changes in the cornea. The first visible structural change is drying of the conjunctiva and the cornea (xerosis) and the development of an opaque area called Bitot's spot. This is followed by development of keratomalacia, which involves irreversible damage to the cornea and leads to blindness (Sommer, 1982).

In addition to keratinization of the cornea, deficiency of vitamin A results in keratinization of tracheal epithelium and in thinning of the intestinal epithelium. Xerophthalmia was reported to be accompanied by upper respiratory infection and diarrhea and to be exacerbated by protein-energy malnutrition. Vitamin A deficiency is also associated with a lower resistance to infections and with increased mortality in young children (Sommer et al., 1983). Mortality rates in children with night blindness or Bitot's spots (white foamy patches on the conjunctiva) were reported to be three- to eight-fold greater as compared with children with no visible signs of vitamin A deficiency (Sommer, 1983), and supplementation of vitamin A in children in vitamin A–deficient areas was shown to significantly reduce the incidence of mortality (Underwood, 1994). The increased susceptibility to infection associated with vitamin A deficiency has been shown both by epidemiological evidence and by studies with laboratory animals to stem from compromised immune function (Ross and Hammerling, 1994).

It should be noted that although ocular symptoms are the most specific indicators of vitamin A deficiency, ocular manifestations occur only after other tissues have impaired functions that are less specific and less easily assessed. Low serum levels of retinol (less than 0.70 μmol/L) indicate subclinical vitamin A deficiency, but subclinical deficiency can be present with serum retinol levels as high as 1.05 μmol/L. Assessment of the response of persons to vitamin A supplementation can be used to identify individuals with critically depleted body stores.

VITAMIN A AND THE MAINTENANCE OF HEALTH

A diet rich in vitamin A and carotenoids can play a protective role against several physiological abnormalities. It was reported in early studies that epithelium of vitamin A–deficient organs are histologically similar to that of neoplastic tissues (Wolbach and Howe, 1925), and a number of epidemiological studies have indicated that consumption of vitamin A and carotenoids is inversely correlated with development of several types of cancer. In addition, results of some studies have suggested that retinoids and carotenoids can reverse precancerous oral lesions (Hong and Itri, 1994). Conclusive evidence for the efficacy of dietary preformed vitamin A or of carotenoids in prevention of cancer is still being sought. Dietary vitamin A also plays an important role in enhancing immune responses. It has been reported that even mild vitamin A deficiency can lead to impaired immune response and lymphocyte function and that vitamin A supplementation of children with no apparent deficiency results in significant reduction in disease mortality (Gerster, 1997). Vitamin A, via its metabolite retinoic acid, is also essential for embryogenesis. Vitamin A deficiency during gestation has been shown to induce fetal malformations in animals and is likely to have similar outcomes in humans. However, specific effects of vitamin A deficiency on fetal development in humans are difficult to discern because vitamin A deficiency is usually accompanied by general protein-energy malnutrition. Interestingly, the vitamin A–induced malformations that have been observed in animals with vitamin A deficiency are similar to those that are found in animals given excess vitamin A (Gerster, 1997).

VITAMIN A EXCESS

Acute vitamin A toxicity has been reported to occur following consumption of polar bear and seal liver by Eskimos and Arctic explorers. Chronic toxicity can occur following routine intake of smaller, but still large, doses of vitamin A over a period of several months and has been observed following daily ingestion exceeding 15.0 mg retinol. Higher sensitivity is observed in infants and young children in whom toxic manifestation can occur following daily ingestion of more than 6.0 mg retinol. Both acute and chronic forms of vitamin A toxicity are rare occurrences and are easily reversed following cessation of excessive intake. A third type of vitamin A toxicity can occur with ingestion of even lower doses of excess vitamin A during early pregnancy: during pregnancy, vitamin A can have teratogenic effects leading to fetal abnormalities. The teratogenic effects of vitamin A most likely stem from the higher levels of retinoic acid formed upon excessive intake.

In establishing tolerable upper intake levels (ULs) for vitamin A intake, the IOM considered

Life Cycle Consideration

Vitamin A Supplements in Pregnancy

Studies in animals have shown that retinol can be teratogenic in early pregnancy and lead to fetal abnormalities including craniofacial, cardiac, thymic, and central nervous system malformations. In humans, the synthetic retinoid isotretinoin, which is used in treatment of severe acne, results in similar malformations. The period of sensitivity in humans is the second to the fifth week of pregnancy. The incidence of birth defects associated with cranial neural crest tissue in babies born to women who consumed more than 4.50 mg retinol per day was reported to be 3.5-fold higher as compared to babies born to women whose daily consumption of vitamin A was 1.50 mg or less (Rothman et al., 1995). The increased incidence of defects was concentrated among babies born to women who consumed high levels of vitamin A prior to the seventh week of gestation. These observations suggest that intake of vitamin A at doses that are only several-fold higher than the recommended dietary allowance (RDA) during early pregnancy is associated with a marked increase in the incidence of birth defects. Conversely, it was recently reported that vitamin A supplements at a total dose exceeding 3.0 mg retinol did not result in a higher incidence of neural crest defects (Lammer et al., 1996). As pointed out by Gerster (1997), it seems prudent at the present time to follow the recommendations of the Teratology Society of the United States that the daily vitamin A dose for women should never exceed 3.0 mg RE (retinol equivalents), and that it is reasonable to replace part of the vitamin A supplement for pregnant women with β-carotene, which has never been shown to be teratogenic, either in animals or in humans.

teratogenicity as the critical adverse effect on which to base a UL for women of childbearing age and liver abnormalities (i.e., liver pathology characteristic of vitamin A intoxication) as the critical adverse effect for setting ULs for other adults. Adverse effects have been observed due to intake of preformed vitamin A, so the ULs are stated in terms of vitamin A or retinol intake. The UL for adult men and women is 3.0 mg/day of preformed vitamin A. The UL, although based on different criteria, was the same for women 19 to 50 years of age and women older than 51 years of age.

REFERENCES

Blaner WS, Das SR, Gouras P, Flood MT (1987) Hydrolysis of 11-*cis* and all-*trans* retinyl palmitate by homogenates of human retinal epithelial cells. J Biol Chem 262:53-58.

Blaner WS, Obunike JC, Kurlandsky SB, Al-Haideri M, Piantedosi R, Deckelbaum RJ, Goldberg IJ (1994) Lipoprotein lipase hydrolysis of retinyl esters: possible implications for retinoid uptake by cells. J Biol Chem 269:16559-16565.

Blaner WS, Olson JA (1994) Retinol and retinoic acid metabolism. In: Sporn MB, Roberts AB, Goodman DS (eds) The Retinoids: Biology, Chemistry, and Medicine, 2nd ed. Raven Press, New York, pp 229-255.

Boerman MHEM, Napoli JL (1991) Cholate-independent retinyl ester hydrolysis. J Biol Chem 266:22273-22278.

Boylan JF, Gudas LJ (1992) The level of CRABP-I expression influences the amounts and types of all-*trans*-retinoic acid metabolites in F9 teratocarcinoma stem cells. J Biol Chem 267:21486-21491.

Boylan JF, Gudas LJ (1991) Overexpression of the cellular retinoic acid binding-I results in a reduction in differentiation-specific gene expression in F9 teratocarcinoma cells. J Cell Biol 112:965-980.

Breitman TR, Selonick SE, Collins SJ (1980) Induction of differentiation of the human promyelocytic leukemia cell line (HL-60) by retinoic acid. Proc Natl Acad Sci U S A 77:2936-2940.

Budhu AS, Noy N (2002) Direct channeling of retinoic acid between cellular retinoic acid- binding protein II and retinoic acid receptor sensitizes mammary carcinoma cells to retinoic acid-induced growth arrest. Mol Cell Biol 22:2632-2641.

Canada FJ, Law WC, Rando RR, Yamamoto T, Derguini F, Nakanishi K (1990) Substrate specificities and mechanism in the enzymatic processing of vitamin A into 11-*cis* retinol. Biochemistry 29:9690-9697.

Chai X, Boerman MHEM, Zhai Y, Napoli JL (1995) Cloning of a cDNA for liver microsomal retinol dehydrogenase. J Biol Chem 270: 3900-3904.

Chambon P (1994) The retinoid signaling pathway: molecular and genetic analysis. Semin Cell Biol 5:115-125.

Chen Y, Houghton LA, Brenna JT, Noy N (1996) Docosahexaenoic acid modulates the interactions of the interphotoreceptor matrix retinoid-binding protein with 11-*cis*-retinal. J Biol Chem 271:20507-20515.

Cowan SW, Newcomer ME, Jones TA (1993) Crystallographic studies on a family of cellular lipophilic transport proteins: the refinement of P2 myelin protein and the structure determination and refinement of cellular retinol-binding protein in complex with all-*trans* retinol. J Mol Biol 230:1225-1246.

Dew SE, Ong DE (1994) Specificity of the retinol transporter of the rat small intestine brush border. Biochemistry 33:12340-12345.

Dong D, Ruuska SE, Levinthal DJ, Noy N (1999) Distinct roles for cellular retinoic acid-binding proteins I and II in regulating signaling by retinoic acid. J Biol Chem 274:23695-23698.

Dowling JE (1987) The Retina: An Approachable Part of the Brain. Harvard University Press, Cambridge, MA.

Dupe V, Matt N, Garnier JM, Chambon P, Mark M, Ghyselinck NB (2003) A newborn lethal defect due to inactivation of retinaldehyde dehydrogenase type 3 is prevented by maternal retinoic acid treatment. Proc Natl Acad Sci U S A 100:14036-14041.

Durand B, Saunders M, Leroy P, Leid M, Chambon P (1992) All-*trans* and 9-*cis* retinoic acid induction of CRABPII transcription is mediated by RAR-RXR heterodimers bound to DR1 and DR2 repeated motifs. Cell 71:73-85.

Fan X, Molotkov A, Manabe S, Donmoyer CM, Deltour L, Foglio MH, Cuenca AE, Blaner WS, Lipton SA, Duester G (2003) Targeted disruption of Aldh1a1 (Raldh1) provides evidence for a complex mechanism of retinoic acid synthesis in the developing retina. Mol Cell Biol 23: 4637-4648.

Fex G, Johannesson G (1987) Studies of the spontaneous transfer of retinol from retinol:retinol binding protein complex to unilamellar liposomes. Biochim Biophys Acta 901:255-264.

Food and Agriculture Organization/World Health Organization (2002) Vitamin A. In: Human Vitamin and Mineral Requirements. Report of a joint FAO/WHO expert consultation, FAO/WHO, Rome.

Gerster H (1997) Vitamin A—Functions, dietary requirements and safety in humans. Int J Vit Res 67:71-90.

Ghyselinck NB, Bavik C, Sapin V, Mark M, Bonnier D, Hindelang C, Dierich A, Nilsson CB, Hakansson H, Sauvant P, Azais-Braesco V, Frasson M, Picaud S, Chambon P (1999) Cellular retinol-binding protein I is essential for vitamin A homeostasis. EMBO J 18:4903-4914.

Giguère V (1994) Retinoic acid receptors and cellular binding proteins: complex interplay in retinoid signaling. Endocrinol Rev 15:61-77.

Glass CK (1994) Differential recognition of target genes by nuclear receptor monomers, dimers and heterodimers. Endocrinol Rev 15:391-407.

Gollapalli DR, Maiti P, Rando RR (2003) RPE65 operates in the vertebrate visual cycle by stereospecifically binding all-*trans*-retinyl esters. Biochemistry 42:11824-11830.

Gudas LJ (1994) Retinoids and vertebrate development. J Biol Chem 269:15399-15402.

Gutierrez-Gonzalez LH, Ludwig C, Hohoff C, Rademacher M, Hanhoff T, Ruterjans H, Spener F, Lucke C (2002) Solution structure and backbone dynamics of human epidermal-type fatty acid-binding protein (E-FABP). Biochem J 364:725-737.

Haque M, Anreola F (1998) The cloning and characterization of a novel cytochrome P450 family, CYP26, with specificity toward retinoic acid. Nutr Rev 56:84-85.

Herr F, Ong DE (1992) Differential interaction of lecithin:retinol acyltransferase with cellular retinoid binding proteins. Biochemistry 31:6748-6755.

Hofmann C, Eichele G (1994) Retinoids in development. In: Sporn MB, Roberts AB, Goodman DS (eds) The Retinoids: Biology, Chemistry, and Medicine, 2nd ed. Raven Press, New York, pp 387-441.

Hong WK, Itri LM (1994) Retinoids and human cancer. In: Sporn MB, Roberts AB, Goodman DS (eds) The Retinoids: Biology, Chemistry, and Medicine, 2nd ed. Raven Press, New York pp 597-630.

Institute of Medicine (2001) Dietary Reference Intakes for Vitamin A, Vitamin K, Arsenic, Boron, Chromium, Copper, Iodine, Iron, Manganese, Molybdenum, Nickel, Silicon, Vanadium, and Zinc. National Academy Press, Washington, DC.

Jamison RS, Newcomer ME, Ong DE (1994) Cellular retinoid-binding proteins: limited proteolysis reveals a conformational change upon ligand-binding. Biochemistry 33: 2873-2879.

Janecke AR, Thompson DA, Utermann G, Becker C, Hubner CA, Schmid E, McHenry CL, Nair AR, Ruschendorf F, Heckenlively J, Wissinger B, Nurnberg P, Gal A (2004) Mutations in RDH12 encoding a photoreceptor cell retinol dehydrogenase cause childhood-onset severe retinal dystrophy. Nat Genet 36:850-854.

Jenster G (1998) Coactivators and corepressors as mediators of nuclear receptor function: an update. Mol Cell Endocrinol 143:1-7.

Kakkad B, Ong DE (1988) Reduction of retinaldehyde bound to cellular retinol-binding protein (type II) by microsomes from rat small intestine J Biol Chem 263:12916-12919.

Kersten S, Dong D, Lee W, Reczek PR, Noy N (1998) Auto-silencing by the retinoid X receptor. J Mol Biol 284:21-32.

Kersten S, Kelleher D, Chambon P, Gronemeyer H, Noy N (1995a) The retinoid X receptor forms tetramers in solution. Proc Natl Acad Sci U S A 92:8645-8649.

Kersten S, Pan L, Chambon P, Gronemeyer H, Noy N (1995b) On the role of ligand in retinoid signaling: 9-*cis* retinoic acid modulates the oligomeric state of the retinoid X receptor. Biochemistry 34:13717-13721.

Kleywegt GJ, Bergfors T, Senn H, Le Motte P, Gsell B, Shudo K, Jones TA (1994). Crystal structures of cellular retinoic acid binding proteins I and II in complex with all-*trans*-retinoic acid and a synthetic retinoid. Structure 2:1241-1258.

Lammer EJ, Shaw GM, Wasserman CR, Block G (1996) High vitamin A intake and risk for major abnormalities involving structures with an embryological cranial neural crest cell component. Teratology 53:91-92.

Leid M, Kastner P, Chambon P (1992) Multiplicity generates diversity in the retinoic acid signaling pathways. TIBS 17:427-433.

Li E, Qian SJ, Winter NS, d'Avignon A, Levin MS, Gordon JI (1991) Fluorine nuclear magnetic resonance analysis of the ligand-binding properties of two homologous rat cellular retinol binding proteins expressed in *E. coli*. J Biol Chem 266:3622-3629.

Lin M, Zhang M, Abraham M, Smith SM, Napoli JL (2003) Mouse retinal dehydrogenase 4 (RALDH4), molecular cloning, cellular expression, and activity in 9-*cis*-retinoic acid biosynthesis in intact cells. J Biol Chem 278:9856-9861.

MacDonald PN, Ong DE (1988) A lecithin: retinol acyltransferase activity in human and rat liver. Biochem Biophys Res Commun 156:157-163.

Manor D, Shmidt EN, Budhu A, Flesken-Nikitin A, Zgola M, Page R, Nikitin AY, Noy N (2003) Mammary carcinoma suppression by cellular retinoic acid binding protein-II. Cancer Res 63:4426-4433.

Mata NL, Moghrabi WN, Lee JS, Bui TV, Radu RA, Horwitz J, Travis GH (2004) Rpe65 is a retinyl ester binding protein that presents insoluble substrate to the isomerase in retinal pigment epithelial cells. J Biol Chem 279:635-643.

Mata NL, Radu RA, Clemmons RC, Travis GH (2002) Isomerization and oxidation of vitamin a in cone-dominant retinas: a novel pathway for visual-pigment regeneration in daylight. Neuron 36:69-80.

McCollum EV, Davis M (1915) The essential factors in the diet during growth. J Biol Chem 23:231-246.

Mukherjee R, Davies PJA, Crombie DL, Bischoff ED, Cesario RM, Jow L, Hamann LG, Boehm MF, Mondon CE, Nadzan AM, Paterniti JR, Heyman RA (1997) Sensitization of diabetic and obese mice to insulin by retinoid X receptor agonists. Nature 386:407-410.

National Research Council (1989) Recommended Dietary Allowances, 10th ed. National Academy Press, Washington, DC.

Newcomer ME, Jones TA, Aqvist J, Sundelin J, Rask L, Peterson PA (1984) The three-dimensional structure of retinol-binding protein EMBO J 3:1451-1454.

Niederreither K, Subbarayan V, Dolle P, Chambon P (1999) Embryonic retinoic acid synthesis is essential for early mouse post-implantation development. Nat Genet 21:444-448.

Nikawa T, Schulz WA, van den Brink CE, Hanusch M, van der Saag P, Stahl W, Sies H (1995) Efficacy of all-*trans*-β-carotene, canthaxanthin, and all-*trans*-, 9-*cis*, and 4-oxoretinoic acids in inducing differentiation of an F9 embryonal carcinoma RARβ-lacZ reporter cell line. Arch Biochem Biophys 316:665-672.

Noy N, Xu Z-J (1990) The interactions of retinol with binding proteins: implications for the mechanism of uptake by cells. Biochemistry 29:3878-3883.

Olson, JA (1987) Recommended dietary intake of vitamin A in humans. Am J Clin Nutr 45:704.

Ong DE, Davis JT, O'Day WT, Bok D (1994a) Synthesis and secretion of retinol-binding protein and transthyretin by cultured retinal pigment epithelium. Biochemistry 33: 1835-1842.

Ong DE, Newcomer ME, Chytil F (1994b) Cellular retinoid binding proteins. In: Sporn MB, Roberts AB, Goodman DS (eds) The Retinoids: Biology, Chemistry, and Medicine, 2nd ed. Raven Press, New York, pp 283-318.

Osborne TB, Mendel LB (1919) The vitamins in green foods. J Biol Chem 37:187-200.

Pacifici RE, Davies KJA (1991) Protein, lipid, and DNA repair systems in oxidative stress: the free-radical theory of aging revisited. Gerontology 37:166-180.

Pepperberg DR, Okajima TL, Wiggert B, Ripps H, Crouch RK, Chader G J (1993) The interphotoreceptor retinoid binding protein. Mol Neurobiol 7:61-85.

Pijnappel WWM, Hendriks HFJ, Folkers GE, van den Brink CE, Dekker EJ, Edelenbosch C, van der Saag PT, Durston AJ (1993) The retinoid ligand 4-oxo-retinoic acid is a highly active modulator of positional specification. Nature 366:340-344.

Randolph RK, Winkler KE, Ross AC (1991) Fatty acyl coenzyme A dependent and fatty acyl coenzyme A independent retinol esterification by rat liver and mammary gland microsomes. Arch Biochem Biophys 288:500-508.

Rigtrup KM, Ong DE (1992) A retinyl ester hydrolase activity intrinsic to the brush border membrane of rat small intestine. Biochemistry 31:2920-2926.

Ross CA (1982) Retinol esterification by rat liver microsomes. J Biol Chem 257:2453-2459.

Ross CA, Hammerling U (1994) Retinoids and the immune system. In: Sporn MB, Roberts AB, Goodman DS (eds) The Retinoids: Biology, Chemistry, and Medicine, 2nd ed. Raven Press, New York, pp 532-543.

Rothman KJ, Moore LL, Singer MR, Nguyen US, Mannino S, Milunsky A (1995) Teratogenicity of high vitamin A intake. N Engl J Med 333:1369-1415.

Saari JC (1994) Retinoids in the photosensitive systems. In: Sporn MB, Roberts AB, Goodman DS (eds) The Retinoids: Biology, Chemistry, and Medicine, 2nd ed. Raven Press, New York, pp 351-385.

Saari JC, Bredberg DL, Noy N (1994) Control of substrate flow at a branch in the visual cycle. Biochemistry 33:3106-3112.

Shaw NS, Noy N (2001) Interphotoreceptor retinoid-binding protein contains three retinoid binding sites. Exp Eye Res 72:183-190.

Simon A, Lagercrantz J, Bajalica-Lagercrantz S, Eriksson U (1996) Primary structure of human 11-*cis* retinol dehydrogenase and organization and chromosomal localization of the corresponding gene. Genomics 36:424-430.

Sommer A (1982) Field Guide to the Design and Control of Xerophthalmia, 2nd ed. World Health Organization, Geneva.

Sommer A, Tarwotjo I, Hussaini G, Susanto D (1983) Increased mortality in children with mild vitamin A deficiency. Lancet 2:585-588.

Soprano DR, Blaner WS (1994) Plasma retinol-binding protein. In: Sporn MB, Roberts AB, Goodman DS (eds) The Retinoids: Biology, Chemistry, and Medicine, 2nd ed. Raven Press, New York, pp 257-281.

Takahashi N, Breitman TR (1991) Retinoylation of proteins in leukemia, embryonal carcinoma, and normal kidney cell lines: differences associated with differential responses to retinoic acid. Arch Biochem Biophys 285:105-110.

Thaller C, Eichele G (1990) Isolation of 3,4-didehydroretinoic acid, a novel morphogenetic signal in the chick wing bud. Nature 345:815-819.

Underwood BA (1994) Vitamin A in human nutrition: public health considerations. In: Sporn MB, Roberts AB, Goodman DS (eds) The Retinoids: Biology, Chemistry, and Medicine, 2nd ed. Raven Press, New York, pp 211-217.

Vahlquist A, Torma H (1988) Retinoids and keratinization, current concepts. Int J Dermatol 27:81-95.

Veerkamp J H, Maatman RG (1995) Cytoplasmic fatty acid-binding proteins: their structure and genes. Prog Lipid Res 34:17-52.

Vu-Dac N, Schoonjans K, Kosykh V, Dallongeville J, Heyman RA, Staels B, Auwerk J (1996) Retinoids increase human lipoprotein A-II expression through activation of the retinoid X receptor but not the retinoic acid receptor. Mol Cell Biol 16:3350-3360.

Warrel RP Jr, de The H, Wang ZY, Degos L (1993) Acute promyelocytic leukemia. N Engl J Med 329:177-189.

Westin S, Rosenfeld MG, Glass CK (2000) Nuclear receptor coactivators. Adv Pharmacol 47:89-112.

Wolbach SB, Howe P (1925) Tissue changes following deprivation of fat-soluble A vitamin. J Exp Med 42:753-778.

Yamamoto H, Simon A, Eriksson U, Harris E, Berson E L, Dryja T P (1999) Mutations in the gene encoding 11-*cis* retinol dehydrogenase cause delayed dark adaptation and fundus albipunctatus. Nat Genet 22:188-191.

Yuan CX, Ito M, Fondell JD, Fu ZY, Roeder RG (1998) The TRAP220 component of a thyroid hormone receptor-associated protein (TRAP) coactivator complex interacts directly with nuclear receptors in a ligand-dependent fashion. Proc Natl Acad Sci USA 95:7939-7944.

Zile MH, Cullum ME, Simpson RU, Barua AB, Swartz DA (1987) Induction of differentiation of human promyelocytic leukemia cell line HL-60 by retinoyl glucuronide, a biologically active metabolite of vitamin A. Proc Natl Acad Sci USA 84:2208-2212.

Chapter 31

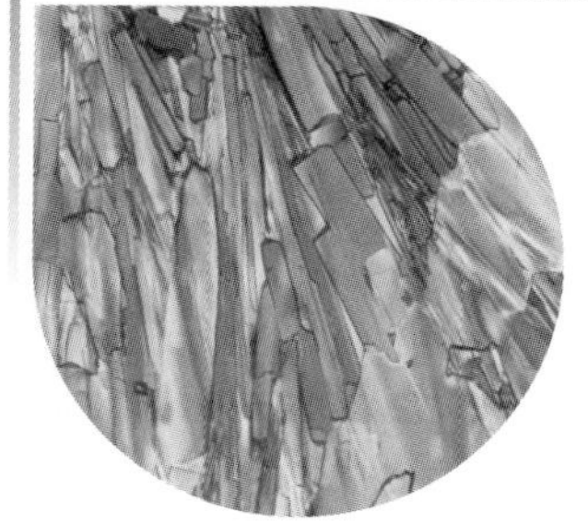

Vitamin D

Michael F. Holick, MD, PhD

OUTLINE

COMMON ABBREVIATIONS

7-DHC	7-dehydrocholesterol
25(OH)D	25-hydroxyvitamin D; also known as calcidiol
1,25(OH)$_2$D	1,25-dihydroxyvitamin D; also known as calcitriol
VDR	vitamin D receptor
VDRE	vitamin D response element

PHOTOBIOLOGY OF VITAMIN D_3

Vitamin D is not by strict definition a vitamin because it can be synthesized in the skin by the action of sunlight. Factors that limit exposure of the skin to sunlight may play a major role in determining a person's vitamin D status. Intake from supplements and fortified foods, as well as a few natural sources, is also important for many populations.

PHOTOSYNTHESIS OF PREVITAMIN D_3 IN HUMAN SKIN

7-Dehydrocholesterol (7-DHC, provitamin D_3), the immediate precursor of cholesterol, is present in the viable epidermis and dermis.

During exposure to sunlight, 7-DHC absorbs sunlight (photons) with energies of between 290 and 315 nm (ultraviolet B radiation, UVB). This process causes a transformation of 7-DHC to previtamin D_3 (Fig. 31-1) (Holick, 1994). After previtamin D_3 is made, it undergoes an internal transformation of its double bonds, which is stimulated by the body's temperature, to form vitamin D_3 over a period of a few hours (see Fig. 31-1). As previtamin D_3 is converted to vitamin D_3, its three-dimensional structure changes, facilitating the translocation of vitamin D_3 from the skin cell into the bloodstream. Once in the bloodstream, vitamin D_3 is bound to a specific vitamin D–binding protein that is an α_1-globulin.

SUNLIGHT-MEDIATED REGULATION OF VITAMIN D_3 SYNTHESIS IN THE SKIN

It is not possible to make an intoxicating amount of vitamin D_3 in the skin from prolonged exposure to sunlight. The reason for this is that once previtamin D_3 is photosynthesized in the skin, it can either be converted to vitamin D_3 or, if the skin is exposed to more sunlight, be degraded into biologically inert photoproducts known as lumisterol and tachysterol (see Fig. 31-1) (Holick, 1994). Similarly, vitamin D_3 is also sensitive to photodegradation by sunlight (Webb et al., 1989). Therefore, if vitamin D_3 does not exit from the skin into the circulation before being exposed to sunlight, it is degraded by sunlight into supersterol I, supersterol II, and 5,6-*trans*-vitamin D_3 (see Fig. 31-1).

EFFECT OF MELANIN PIGMENTATION ON THE CUTANEOUS PRODUCTION OF PREVITAMIN D_3

Loomis (1967) popularized the theory that melanin pigmentation in humans evolved to protect people who lived at or near the equator from producing excessive, intoxicating amounts of vitamin D_3. He further speculated that as peoples migrated north and south of the equator they lost their skin pigmentation in order to promote an adequate amount of vitamin D_3 synthesis in their skin to protect their bones from developing rickets and osteomalacia. Melanin is an excellent sunscreen that absorbs the ultraviolet radiation from sunlight. Therefore, melanin competes with 7-DHC in the skin for the UVB photons. As a result, increased skin pigmentation decreases the production of previtamin D_3 in the skin (Clemens et al., 1982).

A black person with very dark skin pigmentation will require about 10-fold longer exposure to simulated sunlight to make the same amount of vitamin D_3 in their skin as does a light-skinned white person (Clemens et al., 1982). Because sunlight prevents an excessive production of either previtamin D_3 or vitamin D_3 in the skin, by causing the photodegradation of excessive amounts of these compounds, it is unlikely that melanin pigmentation evolved for the purpose of preventing vitamin D_3 intoxication due to excessive exposure to sunlight of peoples who live near the equator. It is, however, intriguing to consider the possibility that skin pigmentation gradually disappeared in peoples that migrated north and south of the equator in order to promote an adequate production of vitamin D_3 in the skin. This concept remains a theory and has not been proved. However, it should be noted that blacks who live in Northern Europe, where food is not fortified with vitamin D as it is in the United States, do not have a higher incidence of rickets and osteomalacia caused by vitamin D deficiency than Northern European whites.

ENVIRONMENTAL EFFECTS ON THE PRODUCTION OF VITAMIN D_3

The time of day, season of the year, and latitude have dramatic effects on the amount of solar UVB radiation that reaches the earth's surface. In winter, vitamin-producing UVB photons pass through the ozone layer at an oblique angle and are absorbed by the ozone in great numbers. More UVB photons are able to penetrate the ozone layer in the spring, summer, and fall months because the sun is directly overhead. At latitude 42° N (Boston), sunlight is incapable of producing vitamin D_3 in the skin from November through February. Ten degrees north of Boston (52° N, Edmonton, Canada), this period is extended to include October and March (Fig. 31-2) (Webb et al., 1988).

Because casual exposure to sunlight provides most of our vitamin D requirement, the inability of the sun to produce vitamin D_3 in

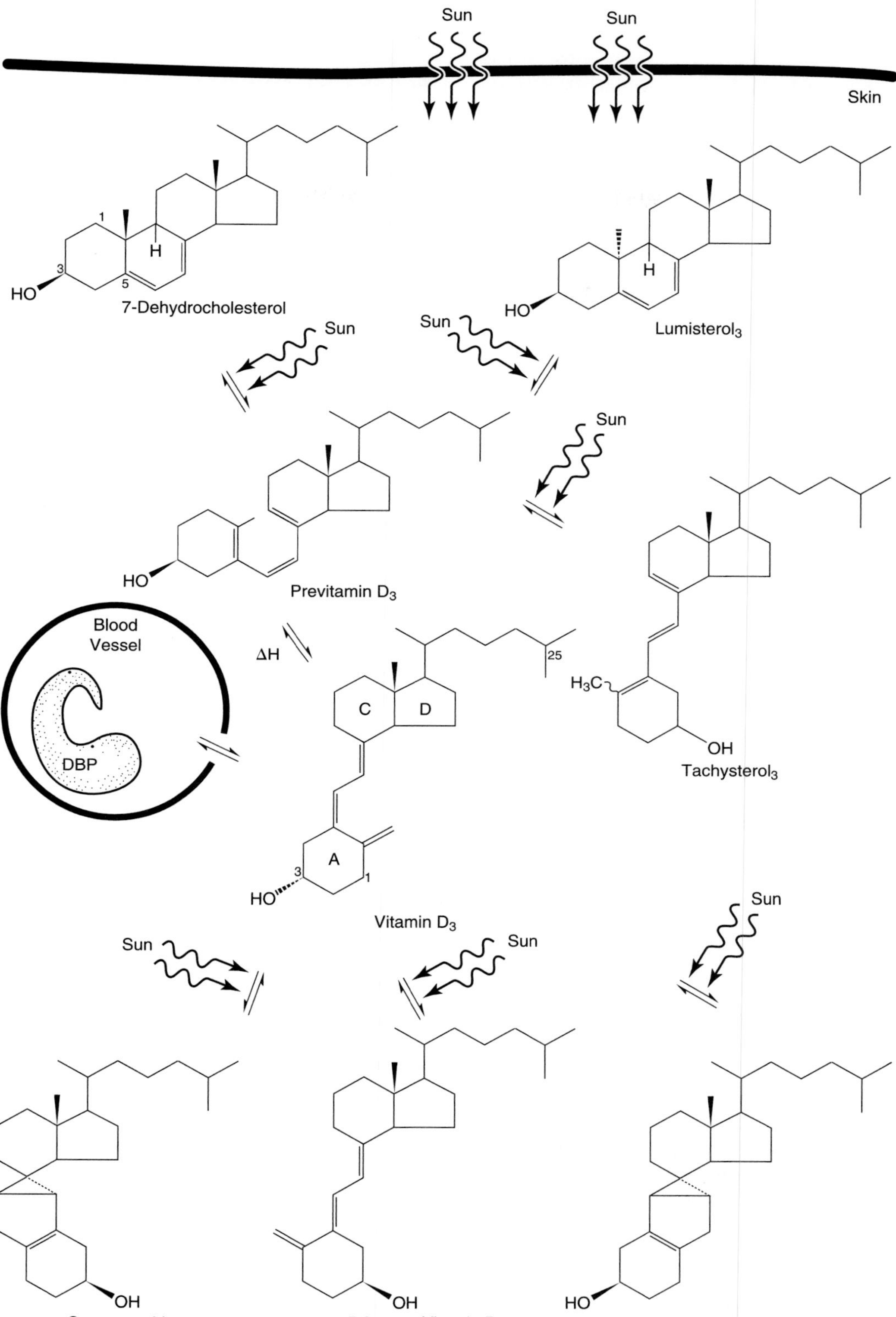

Figure 31-1 Photochemical events that lead to the production of vitamin D_3 and the regulation of vitamin D_3 in the skin. *DBP*, Vitamin D binding protein. *(Modified from Holick MF [1994] Vitamin D: new horizons for the 21st century. Am J Clin Nutr 60:619-630. Used with permission of the American Society for Clinical Nutrition.)*

northern and southern latitudes during the winter may necessitate supplementation of vitamin D by the elderly to prevent vitamin D deficiency. For children and young adults, the cutaneous production of vitamin D_3 during the spring, summer, and fall is adequate to produce enough for storage in the fat for use during the winter months.

Exposure to sunlight at lower latitudes, such as in Los Angeles (24° N), Puerto Rico (18° N), and Buenos Aires (34° S), results in the cutaneous production of vitamin D_3 during the entire year. During the summer in Boston, exposure to sunlight from the hours of 9 AM to 5 PM Eastern Standard Time (EST) results in sufficient UVB photons to produce previtamin D_3 in the skin. In the spring and fall months, vitamin D production commences at approximately 10 AM and ceases after 3 PM EST.

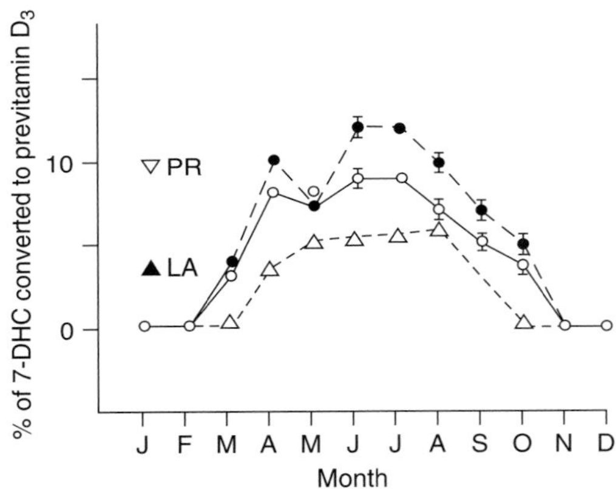

Figure 31-2 Photosynthesis of previtamin D_3 after exposure of a solution of 7-dehydrocholesterol (7-DHC) to sunlight in Boston (42° N) for 1 hour *(open circles)* or 3 hours *(closed circles)*; in Edmonton, Canada, (52° N) for 1 hour *(open triangles)*; in Los Angeles (34° N) for 1 hour *(closed triangle)*; and in Puerto Rico for 1 hour (18° N) *(inverted triangle)*. Measurements were made in the middle of the indicated month on a cloudless day, either from 12 to 1 PM (1 hour) or from 11 AM to 2 PM (3 hours). Measurements in Los Angeles and Puerto Rico were made only in January. *(Modified from Webb AR, Kline L, Holick MF [1988] Influence of season and latitude on the cutaneous synthesis of vitamin D_3: exposure to winter sunlight in Boston and Edmonton will not promote vitamin D_3 synthesis in human skin. J Clin Endocrinol Metab 67:373-378. Copyright The Endocrine Society.)*

EFFECT OF AGING ON THE CUTANEOUS PRODUCTION OF VITAMIN D_3

Aging affects many different metabolic processes. Therefore, it is not surprising that aging also decreases the capacity of human skin to produce vitamin D_3. Aging decreases the concentration of 7-DHC in the epidermis and thereby reduces the capacity of the skin to produce vitamin D_3 by approximately 75% by age 70 years compared with younger adults (Fig. 31-3) (Holick et al., 1989).

EFFECTS OF SUNSCREEN USE AND CLOTHING ON THE CUTANEOUS PRODUCTION OF VITAMIN D_3

The public is now very much aware that chronic excessive exposure to sunlight can increase the risk of skin cancer and cause photoaging of the skin. This knowledge has led to the general recommendation that people with minimal skin pigment should always wear sunscreen when outdoors (Gilchrest, 1993). Commercial sunscreens work by absorbing solar UVB radiation, and some products also absorb some or all of the solar ultraviolet A (320 to 400 nm) radiation.

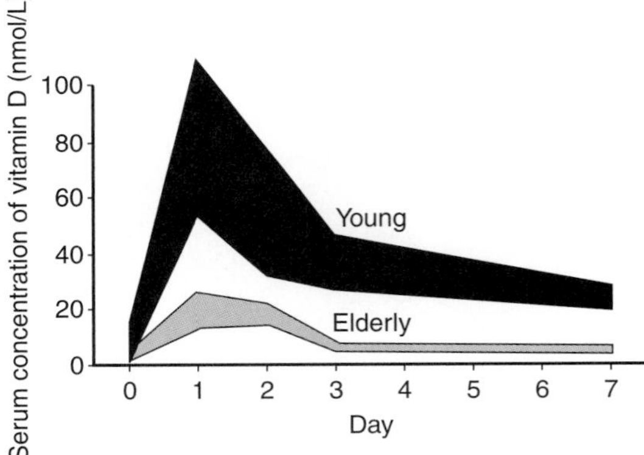

Figure 31-3 Circulating concentrations of vitamin D in healthy young (20 to 30 years of age) and elderly (62 to 80 years of age) subjects in response to a whole-body exposure (at time zero) to 1 minimal erythemal dose of simulated sunlight. The shaded areas on the graph represent the mean ± 1 SEM for the serum vitamin D concentrations for the two subject groups. *(Modified from Holick MF, Matsuoka LY, Wortsman J [1989] Age, vitamin D, and solar ultraviolet. Lancet 2: 1104-1105.)*

Therefore, sunscreens act like melanin and prevent these high-energy photons from having adverse effects on the skin. Sunscreen use has been proven to decrease the risk of some forms of skin cancer, including squamous cell carcinoma, and to reduce photodamage that causes photoaging of the skin. However, because the solar radiation that is responsible for causing the damaging effects to the skin is the same radiation that causes the cutaneous production of vitamin D_3, it is not surprising that the topical application of a sunscreen can diminish or completely prevent the vitamin D_3 production in the skin.

When a young adult exposes the whole body to simulated sunlight that causes a minimal sunburning (1 minimal erythemal dose [MED]), the amount of vitamin D_3 that is produced in the skin and enters the circulation is equivalent to taking between 10,000 and 25,000 IU (250 to 625 μg) of vitamin D orally. When healthy young adult volunteers applied a sunscreen preparation with a sun protection factor of 8 (SPF-8) before being exposed to a whole-body dose of 1 MED of simulated sunlight, plasma levels of vitamin D_3 did not rise above the baseline value (Fig. 31-4). To further investigate the impact of sunscreen use on the cutaneous production of vitamin D_3, 10 volunteers who wore typical clothing for a summer day (short-sleeved blouse or shirt and shorts) topically applied a sunscreen with an SPF of 25 only to the face or to unclothed areas with the exception of the face. Twenty-four hours after exposure to 0.9 MED of simulated sunlight, a small increase in the circulating concentration of vitamin D_3 (from a baseline of 3.0 ± 1.0 (mean ± SEM) to 4.4 ± 1.0 μg/L of serum) was noted in the volunteers who exposed only their faces. When the face was protected and the arms and legs were exposed, there was a significant increase in the serum vitamin D level—from 1.9 ± 0.3 to 4.4 ± 0.8 μg/L.

Clothing absorbs most ultraviolet radiation; therefore, covering the skin with most types of clothing will prevent the cutaneous production of vitamin D_3 (Matsuoka et al., 1992) (Fig. 31-5).

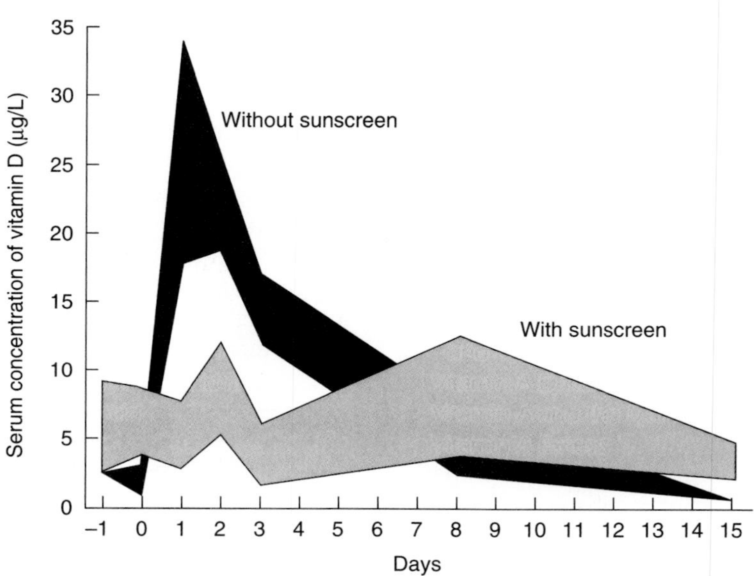

Figure 31-4 Circulating concentrations of vitamin D in young adults with (sun protection factor [SPF-8]) and without (topical placebo cream) sunscreen after a single exposure (at time zero) to 1 minimal erythemal dose of simulated sunlight. The shaded areas on the graph represent the mean ± 1 SEM for the serum vitamin D concentrations for the two treatment groups. *(Modified from Matsuoka LY, Ide L, Wortsman J, MacLaughlin JA, Holick MA [1987] Sunscreens suppress cutaneous vitamin D_3 synthesis. J Clin Endocrinol Metab 64:1165-1168. Copyright The Endocrine Society.)*

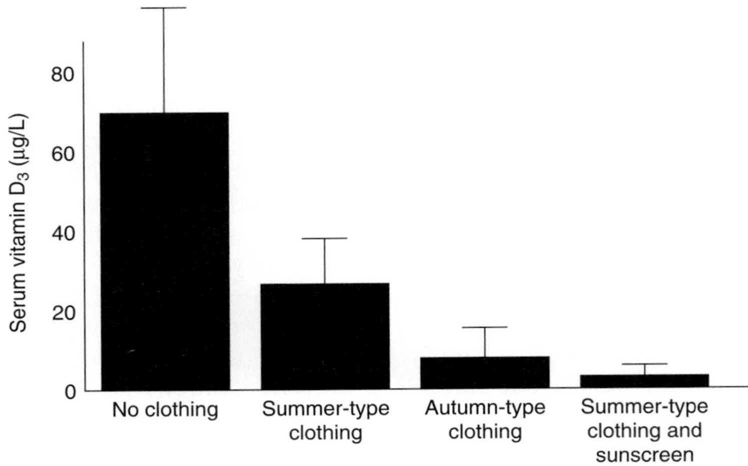

Figure 31-5 Circulating concentrations of vitamin D in human subjects who wore no clothing, summer-type clothing, or autumn-type clothing, or who wore summer clothing and also used a sunscreen. Serum vitamin D concentration was measured 24 hours after whole-body exposure to 1 minimal erythemal dose of ultraviolet B radiation. Bars represent the mean value, and error bars represent 1 SEM. *(Modified from Matsuoka LY, Wortsman J, Dannenberg MJ, Hollis BW, Lu Z, Holick MF [1992] Clothing prevents ultraviolet-B radiation-dependent photosynthesis of vitamin D. J Clin Endocrinol Metab 75:1099-1103. Copyright The Endocrine Society.)*

Populations such as Bedouins living in the Negev Desert in Israel, who are required to have most of the skin surface covered by clothing, are prone to develop vitamin D deficiency (Taha et al., 1984).

It is recommended that children and young adults always wear a sunscreen with an SPF of at least 15 to prevent the consequences of chronic excessive exposure to sunlight. There is no need to be concerned about the effect of sunscreen use on preventing the cutaneous production of vitamin D_3 in this population because it is unlikely that they will always wear a sunscreen or use the proper amount of the agent before going outdoors. However, there is reason for concern with regard to elderly people, who often depend on sunlight for their vitamin D requirement. If they limit their outdoor activities and apply a sunscreen properly before going out, they can substantially reduce or even prevent the production of vitamin D_3 and develop a subclinical vitamin D deficiency (Blok et al., 2000; Holick, 1994).

EFFECT OF OBESITY ON VITAMIN D BIOAVAILABILITY

Obesity is associated with vitamin D deficiency (Bell et al., 1985). To determine whether vitamin D deficiency in obese people could be because the large fat depot is acting as a sink for vitamin D, Wortsman and colleagues (2000) exposed obese and nonobese adults to the same amount of simulated ultraviolet radiation in a tanning bed. They observed that obese subjects were able to raise their blood levels of vitamin D_3 on average by no more than 45% of the increase achieved by normal weight individuals. When obese and nonobese volunteers were given 50,000 IU (1,250 µg) of vitamin D_2 a similar observation was made; that is, the blood level of vitamin D_2 increased by approximately 45% to 50% as much in obese volunteers as was observed in the nonobese volunteers.

FOOD SOURCES OF VITAMIN D AND THE RECOMMENDED DIETARY ALLOWANCES

Naturally occurring vitamin D is rare in foods. Vitamin D is used to refer to either vitamin D_2 or vitamin D_3, both of which can be converted to active vitamin D metabolites. Vitamin D_2 originates from the yeast and plant sterol ergosterol, whereas vitamin D_3 originates from 7-DHC in animals. The major structural difference between vitamin D_2 and vitamin D_3 is in the side chain. Unlike vitamin D_3, vitamin D_2

has a double bond between carbons 22 and 23 and a methyl group on carbon 24.

Originally it was thought that vitamin D_2 had the same biological activity as vitamin D_3 in humans. However, Vieth and colleagues (2001) and Armas and colleagues (2004) have reported that vitamin D_2 is only about 20% to 40% as effective as vitamin D_3 in raising blood levels of 25-hydroxyvitamin D [25(OH)D]. Furthermore, it may be that vitamin D_2 increases the catabolic pathway of vitamin D_2 and vitamin D_3 such that when a pharmacological dose of vitamin D_2 is given to a patient both $25(OH)D_2$ and $25(OH)D_3$ are rapidly catabolized leading to a lowering of levels of both $25(OH)D_2$ and $25(OH)D_3$ in the serum after 28 days of treatment.

The major natural sources of vitamin D_3 are fatty fish, such as mackerel and salmon, and fish oils, including cod and tuna liver oils. The major dietary sources of vitamin D are foods fortified with vitamin D_2 or D_3. Milk has been fortified with vitamin D (100 IU [2.5 μg] per 8 oz) in the United States since the 1930s. More recently, some cereals and breads have been fortified with vitamin D. Other dairy products, including ice cream and cheeses are not fortified with vitamin D, whereas some yogurts are.

Despite widespread fortification of milk with vitamin D, the measured vitamin D content in milk is quite variable. Several recent studies suggest that in the United States and western Canada, up to 80% of samples tested did not contain between 400 and 600 IU/quart (10 and 15 μg/quart) of vitamin D. Almost 50% of the samples did not contain 50% of the vitamin D stated on the label, and approximately 15% of the skim milk samples contained no detectable vitamin D (Holick, 1994). Multivitamin preparations containing vitamin D were found to be a good source of vitamin D and contained between 400 and 600 IU (10 and 15 μg) of vitamin D per tablet; pharmaceutical preparations labeled as 50,000 IU (1,250 μg) of vitamin D_2 contained the stated amount ± 10%.

The Institute of Medicine (IOM, 1997) used serum 25(OH)D concentration as the primary indicator for determining adequacy of vitamin D intake. Serum levels of 25(OH)D below 27.5 nmol/L (11 μg/L) are considered consistent with vitamin D deficiency. The serum 25(OH)D level reflects both total cutaneous production of vitamin D and oral ingestion of either vitamin D_2 or D_3. Because of variable synthesis of vitamin D from exposure to sunlight, accumulation of stored vitamin D in fat tissue during the summer months, and variable amounts of vitamin D in fortified food products, insufficient data were available to determine estimated average requirements (EARs) and recommended dietary allowances (RDAs) for vitamin D. Instead, the IOM (1997) set adequate intakes (AIs), based on the amount of dietary vitamin D needed to maintain normal serum 25(OH)D in populations exposed to limited sunlight.

The AI of vitamin D for infants and children was set at 5 μg/day (200 IU/day). For infants, this is more than would be obtained from breast milk (mean of less than 1 μg/day, or less than 40 IU/day) but less than that obtained from most formulas (10 μg/L or 400 IU/L). Because most children exposed to inadequate sunlight maintained normal serum 25(OH)D levels on intakes of 2.5 μg/day, an AI of 5 μg/day was considered to cover the needs of children of all ages regardless of exposure to sunlight. Similarly, the AI for adults from 19 through 50 years was largely based on studies of

Food Sources

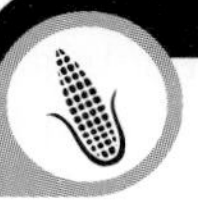

Food Sources of Vitamin D

Fatty Fish

- 30 to 35 μg per 1 Tbsp cod liver oil
- 8 to 13 μg per 3 oz pink salmon
- 5 to 9 μg per 3 oz sardines or mackerel
- 5 μg per 3 oz tuna fish, canned in oil

Other Natural Sources

- 0.5 μg per 1 medium egg yolk or egg
- 0.3 μg per 3 oz beef liver

Foods Fortified With Vitamin D (check label)

- 2.5 μg per 1 cup cow's milk
- 2.5 μg per 1 cup orange juice
- 1 μg per 1 cup ready-to-eat cereal
- 1.5 μg per 1 Tbsp margarine

Data from U.S. Department of Agriculture/Agricultural Research Service (USDA/ARS) (2005) USDA National Nutrient Database for Standard Reference, Release 18. USDA/ARS, Washington, DC. Retrieved November 15, 2005, from www.ars.usda.gov/ba/bhnrc.ndl/.

women in higher latitudes (higher than 40° N or higher than 40° S), which also indicated that an intake of 5 μg/day should be more than adequate for maintenance of an adequate 25(OH)D concentration during the winter months (Kinyamu et al., 1997). No increments in vitamin D intake were recommended for pregnant or lactating women.

Studies of older adults indicated that intakes greater than 5 μg/day of vitamin D are necessary to prevent seasonal variation in serum concentration of parathyroid hormone (PTH), and to prevent bone loss and low serum 25(OH)D levels. In the absence of sunlight, the actual requirement for vitamin D in adults may be as much as 15 to 20 μg/day (Holick, 2004; Heaney et al., 2003; Tanpricha et al., 2002; Holick, 1994; Dawson-Hughes et al., 1991). Therefore, the AI was set at 10 μg/day for adults 51 to 70 years of age and at 15 μg/day for adults older than 70 years of age. Most experts agree that these recommendations are only appropriate if some sunlight exposure is included. In the absence of adequate sunlight exposure, 25 μg/day (1000 IU/day) of dietary or supplemental vitamin D is desirable for both children and adults (Holick, 2004a, 2004b; Heaney et al., 2003).

Excessive intake of vitamin D leads to hypervitaminosis D, which is characterized by an elevated serum 25(OH)D level and hypercalcemia. Most adverse effects of excess vitamin D are thought to be mediated via hypercalcemia. The IOM (1997) set the tolerable upper intake levels (ULs) for vitamin D at 50 μg (2,000 IU)/day for children and adults and at 25 μg (1,000 IU)/day for infants. For most individuals, vitamin D intake from food and supplements is unlikely to reach the UL. Nevertheless, persons who use many supplements or who have very high intakes of fish or fortified milk, ingesting more than 125 μg (5,000 IU)/day, may be at risk for vitamin D toxicity.

AIs Across the Life Cycle

	μg Vitamin D per Day
Infants	
0 to 1 yr	5
Children	
1 to 18 yr	5
Adults	
19 to 50 yr	5
Pregnant	5
Lactating	5
51 to 70 yr	10
>70 yr	15

Data from Institute of Medicine (IOM) (1997) Dietary Reference Intakes for Calcium, Phosphorus, Magnesium, Vitamin D, and Fluoride. National Academy Press, Washington, DC.
AI, Adequate intake. 1 μg vitamin D = 40 IU vitamin D.

VITAMIN D IN BONE HEALTH

Vitamin D plays a critical role in mineralization of the bone, and bone disorders result from inadequate circulating levels of the biologically active metabolite of vitamin D. Vitamin D acts to maintain the plasma calcium and phosphorus concentrations so that skeletal mineralization occurs.

RICKETS AND OSTEOMALACIA

Vitamin D deficiency causes rickets in children (Holick, 2004b, 1994). Before the epiphyseal plates close, vitamin D deficiency causes a disorganization and hypertrophy of the chondrocytes at the mineralization front as well as a mineralization defect, resulting in short stature and bony deformities that are characteristic of vitamin D–deficiency rickets (Fig. 31-6). In adults, the epiphyseal plates are closed, and, hence, vitamin D deficiency in adults does not result in many of the bony deformities seen in vitamin D–deficient children. Vitamin D deficiency in adults causes osteomalacia. Osteomalacia is a very significant metabolic bone disease, especially in elderly people. Adults with vitamin D deficiency have a mineralization defect in the skeleton that results in poor mineralization of the collagen matrix (osteoid). Although this does not cause bony deformities, it can cause severe osteopenia (a decrease in the opacity of the skeleton as seen in radiographs). This mineralization defect can lead to increased risk of skeletal fractures (Aaron et al., 1974). In addition, osteomalacia can cause localized or generalized, unrelenting deep bone pain. This is thought to be due to the hydration of the unmineralized matrix in the periosteum, which exerts an outward pressure on the sensory fibers of the periosteal covering, giving the patient a throbbing bone pain (Holick, 2003).

CONSEQUENCES OF VITAMIN D DEFICIENCY

The major function of vitamin D in maintaining a healthy skeleton is to maintain the serum calcium and phosphorus concentrations within their physiological ranges to keep the calcium × phosphorus product [e.g., (serum Ca of 10.0 mg/100 mL) × (serum P of 4.0 mg/100 mL) = 40] high enough for skeletal mineralization. (See Chapter 32 for more information on calcium and phosphorus.)

As the body becomes vitamin D deficient, the efficiency of intestinal calcium absorption decreases from the usual 30% to 50% to no more than 10% to 15%. This results in a decrease in the ionized calcium concentration in the blood, which signals the calcium sensor in the parathyroid glands to increase the production and secretion of PTH (Fig. 31-7).

Figure 31-6 Child with rickets showing the characteristic bony deformities, including bowed legs and rachitic rosary of the rib cage. *(From Fraser D, Scriver CR [1994] Disorders associated with hereditary or acquired abnormalities of vitamin D function: hereditary disorders associated with vitamin D resistance or defective phosphate metabolism. In: DeGroot LJ [ed] Endocrinology. Grune and Stratton, New York, pp 797-808.)*

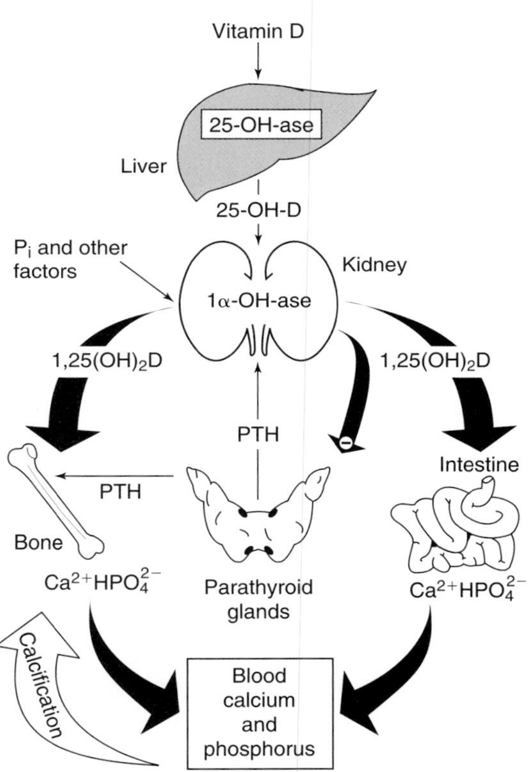

Figure 31-7 Metabolism of vitamin D and the biological actions of $1,25(OH)_2D$. *25-OH-ase,* Vitamin D 25-hydroxylase; *1α-OH-ase,* 25-hydroxyvitamin D 1α-hydroxylase. *(From Holick MF, Krane S, Potts JT [1994] Calcium, phosphorus, and bone metabolism: Calcium-regulating hormones. In: Isselbacher KJ, Braunwald E, Wilson JD, Martin JB, Fauci AS, Kasper DL [eds] Harrison's Principles of Internal Medicine, 13th ed. McGraw-Hill, New York, pp 2137-2151.)*

PTH, in turn, attempts to conserve calcium in the kidney by increasing renal tubular reabsorption of calcium. With vitamin D, PTH helps mobilize monocyte-like stem cells through the receptor activator of NFκB ligand (RANKL) (Holick, 2004b) to become active bone calcium-resorbing multinucleated giant cells known as osteoclasts, which can cause erosion of the skeleton, thereby causing or exacerbating osteoporosis (see Fig. 31-7). Although PTH performs an invaluable function in retaining calcium in the kidney, it also induces a leaking of phosphorus into the urine, which results in hypophosphatemia. Therefore, patients with subclinical vitamin D deficiency often have a normal serum calcium concentration with a low or low-normal serum phosphorus concentration. Patients with longstanding vitamin D deficiency have low serum concentrations of both calcium and phosphorus. This results in a substantial decrease in the calcium × phosphorus product, resulting in a defect in bone matrix mineralization that leads to rickets in children and osteomalacia in adults. The hallmarks for vitamin D insufficiency and deficiency are a low-normal (10 to 20 μg/L) and a low or undetectable (less than 10 μg/L) serum concentration of 25(OH)D, respectively.

There is ample clinical evidence that increasing dietary calcium intake to at least 1,000 mg/day, along with supplementation of at least 10 to 20 μg of vitamin D daily, will decrease vertebral and nonvertebral fractures and increase bone mineral density (Dawson-Hughes, 1997; Chapuy et al., 1992). During the winter in New England, when sunlight loses its ability to produce vitamin D_3 in the skin, there is marked loss of bone mineral density of the hip and spine that is related to a decrease in circulating levels of 25(OH)D and an increase in PTH levels (Fig. 31-8) (Rosen et al., 1994).

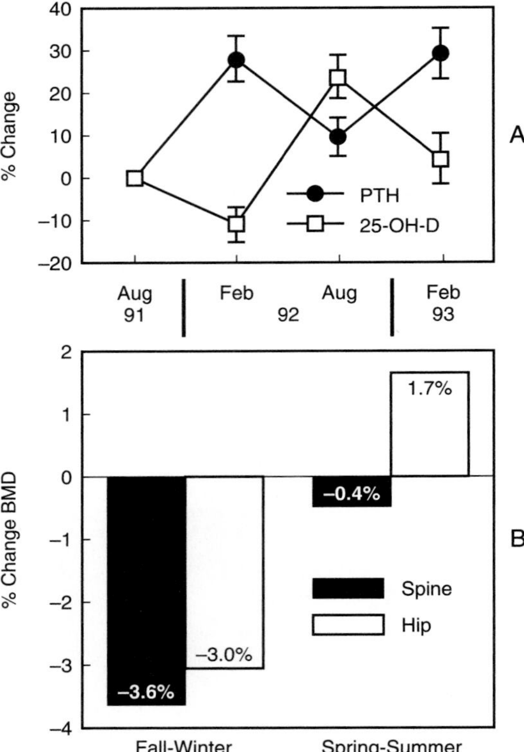

Figure 31-8 **A,** Seasonal changes (as percentage of previous measurement) in serum PTH and 25(OH)D. Measurements were made at 6-month intervals over an 18-month period in healthy women with a mean age of 77 years. Results are ± SEM. **B,** Percentage change in the bone mineral density (BMD) of the average L_2–L_4 spine and femoral neck (hip) of 15 older rural Maine women over a 6-month period consisting of fall and winter or of spring and summer. *(Data from Rosen CJ, Morrison A, Zhou H, Storm D, Hunter SJ, Musgrave K, Chen T, Wei W, Holick MF [1994] Elderly women in Northern New England exhibit seasonal changes in bone mineral density and calciotropic hormones. Bone Miner 25:83-92.)*

VITAMIN D METABOLISM AND FUNCTION

In the body, vitamin D undergoes two hydroxylation reactions that convert it to the biologically active form 1,25-dihydroxyvitamin D [$1,25(OH)_2D$]. This active form of vitamin D acts on target tissues, especially intestine and bone. It acts to regulate calcium absorption and bone mineral mobilization in order to maintain calcium homeostasis.

METABOLISM

Vitamin D_2 and vitamin D_3 that are used to fortify foods are ingested, mixed with other lipids, taken up by enterocytes, and incorporated into chylomicrons. Chylomicrons are released by the enterocytes and enter the lymphatic system, which drains into the venous bloodstream. Ultimately, this vitamin D (in chylomicron remnants) reaches the liver, where it is hydroxylated to 25(OH)D and again enters the circulation bound to vitamin D–binding protein. Vitamin D_3 that is synthesized in the skin enters the circulation and is bound to the vitamin D–binding protein.

Both vitamin D_2 and vitamin D_3 in the circulation are taken up by the liver and hydroxylated on C-25 to produce 25(OH)D (see Fig. 31-7). 25(OH)D is the major circulating form of vitamin D, and it is present in the circulation bound to the vitamin D–binding protein. It is 25(OH)D that is measured in the blood to determine the vitamin D status of a patient. The hepatic vitamin D 25-hydroxylase is not tightly regulated; therefore, any increase in vitamin D intake or in the cutaneous production of vitamin D_3 leads to an increase in the circulating concentration of 25(OH)D. That is why 25(OH)D is so valuable as a marker for determining the vitamin D status of a patient. Low or undetectable circulating concentrations of 25(OH)D are diagnostic of vitamin D deficiency, and 25(OH)D levels that are at least three times (~150 μg/L) the upper limit of the normal range (normal range, 10 to 55 μg/L of serum by most clinical laboratories) are diagnostic for vitamin D intoxication (Koutkia et al., 2001; Holick et al., 1994).

Once 25(OH)D is made, it enters the circulation, and most of it is bound to the vitamin D–binding protein (DBP). DBP is a ligand of cubilin and megalin, which are two membrane-associated proteins that act in concert to mediate endocytic uptake of various small proteins and vitamin–carrier complexes across absorptive epithelia. Delivery of 25(OH)D to the kidney, and thus its conversion to $1,25(OH)_2D$, is dependent upon the glomerular filtration of 25(OH)D/DBP complexes from the plasma, followed by megalin-mediated endocytic uptake of 25(OH)D/DBP from the glomerular filtrate into the proximal tubular cells of the kidney (Leheste et al., 2002). Therefore, these endocytic receptors in the renal tubules are the major means by which 25(OH)D is targeted to the kidney.

In the kidney, the 25(OH)D is hydroxylated on C-1 to form $1,25(OH)_2D$, which is then secreted into the circulation (see Fig. 31-7). $1,25(OH)_2D$ is considered to be the biologically active form of vitamin D that is responsible for carrying out most if not all of the biological functions of vitamin D. The major function of $1,25(OH)_2D$ is to increase the efficiency of intestinal calcium absorption, thereby increasing the utilization of dietary calcium (see Fig. 31-7). $1,25(OH)_2D$ can increase the efficiency of intestinal calcium absorption from a basal level of 10% to 15% up to a level of 30% to 80%.

REGULATION OF 25-HYDROXYVITAMIN D METABOLISM

The major factor that regulates the metabolism of 25(OH)D to $1,25(OH)_2D$ is PTH (see Fig. 31-6). The exact mechanism by which PTH stimulates the kidney's production of $1,25(OH)_2D$ is not well characterized. However, there is evidence that the hypophosphatemic effect of PTH on the kidney may be responsible for increasing the renal production of $1,25(OH)_2D$ (Holick, 2003; Holick et al., 1994). Indeed, hypophosphatemia and hyperphosphatemia are associated with increased and decreased circulating concentrations of $1,25(OH)_2D$, respectively (Portale et al., 1986). A variety of other hormones associated with growth and development of the skeleton or calcium regulation, including growth hormone and prolactin, indirectly increase the renal production of $1,25(OH)_2D$.

It is recognized that elderly people often lose their ability to adapt to a low calcium diet by increasing their efficiency of intestinal calcium absorption (Ireland and Fordtran, 1973). Although the exact mechanism is not fully understood, there is evidence that the ability of the kidney to upregulate the production of $1,25(OH)_2D$ by PTH is no longer operative (Riggs et al., 1981; Slovik et al., 1981). Furthermore, aging may also decrease the intestinal vitamin D receptor (VDR) responsiveness to $1,25(OH)_2D$ (Ebeling et al., 1992; Riggs et al., 1981).

EXTRARENAL PRODUCTION OF 1,25-DIHYDROXYVITAMIN D

Although the kidney is the major site for $1,25(OH)_2D$ production, the placenta of pregnant women also has the capacity to make it. This apparently is important during the last trimester of pregnancy, when circulating levels of $1,25(OH)_2D$ are increased to enhance the efficiency of intestinal calcium absorption in the mother to meet the increased need of the fetus for calcium to mineralize its skeleton.

BIOLOGICAL FUNCTIONS OF 1,25-DIHYDROXYVITAMIN D

The major biological function of vitamin D is to maintain calcium homeostasis in order to maintain cellular metabolic processes and neuromuscular functions. The principal biological function of $1,25(OH)_2D$ is to increase the efficiency of intestinal calcium absorption. $1,25(OH)_2D$ directly affects the entry of calcium through the plasma membrane by increasing the expression of the epithelial calcium channel protein (TRPV6, also called CaT1) of the intestinal absorptive cell (Bouillon, 2001). This enhances the movement of calcium through the cytosol and across the basolateral membrane of the enterocyte into the circulation. $1,25(OH)_2D$ alters the flux of calcium across the intestinal absorptive cell by increasing the production and activity of several proteins in the small intestine, including calcium-binding protein (calbindin D_{9K}), alkaline phosphatase, low-affinity calcium-dependent ATPase, calmodulin, brush-border actin, and brush-border proteins with molecular masses of 80 to 90 kDa. Although the exact function of calbindin is not well understood, it is specifically induced by $1,25(OH)_2D$ and is thought to be one of the major proteins responsible for alterations in the flux of calcium across the gastrointestinal mucosa. When $1,25(OH)_2D$ is given as a single intravenous dose to vitamin D–deficient animals, it causes a biphasic response. Within the first 2 hours there is a rapid increase in the flux of calcium across the gastrointestinal mucosa that peaks by 6 hours; another response begins after 12 hours and peaks after 24 hours (Norman, 1998).

$1,25(OH)_2D$ also increases the efficiency of the absorption of intestinal phosphorus in the jejunum and ileum of the small intestine. Because dietary phosphate is often plentiful and at least 40% to 60% of dietary phosphorus is absorbed passively, the role of $1,25(OH)_2D$ in enhancing phosphorous absorption is less critical. (See Chapter 32 for more discussion of the role of $1,25(OH)_2D$ in regulation of calcium and phosphate homeostasis.) Originally, it was thought that $1,25(OH)_2D_3$ stimulated monocytes, directly inducing them to become mature osteoclasts. However, it is now recognized that both $1,25(OH)_2D$ and PTH stimulate osteoclastic activity indirectly by interacting with specific receptors in mature osteoblasts. RANKL (receptor activator of NF-κB ligand) is a membrane protein in cells of the osteoblastic lineage that interacts with its receptor, RANK, on hemopoietic precursors to promote osteoclast formation and maintain osteoclast viability and activity. Both PTH and $1,25(OH)_2D$ upregulate the expression of RANKL on the surface of mature osteoblasts (Holick, 2003). Monocytic osteoclast precursor cells have the receptor RANK. Once the RANK on the monocytic cell interacts with the RANKL of the osteoblast, there is signal transduction inducing the monocyte to become a multinucleated osteoclast. Osteoblasts also produce osteoprotegerin, a soluble protein that acts as a decoy receptor for RANKL. Osteoprotegerin binds to RANKL and prevents its interaction with the receptor RANK on osteoclast precursor cells, which blocks stimulation of osteoclast formation. Thus RANKL stimulates while osteoprotegerin inhibits osteoclastogenesis. Once osteoclasts have matured, they release hydrochloric acid and collagenases, which dissolve the bone mineral and matrix, respectively, releasing calcium into the extracellular space. There also are a number of cytokines (including interleukin 1, interleukin 6, and interleukin 12) and hormones that directly interact with osteoclasts to increase bone calcium mobilization. (See Chapter 32, Fig. 32-4 for further discussion of the osteoprotegerin/RANKL/RANK system.)

Mature osteoblasts also respond to $1,25(OH)_2D$ by increasing their expression of alkaline phosphatase, osteopontin, and osteocalcin, as well as a variety of cytokines. 1,25(OH)$_2$D plays an important role in the bone remodeling process. However, 1,25(OH)$_2$D does not directly induce bone to mineralize. Instead, 1,25(OH)$_2$D promotes the mineralization of osteoid laid down by osteoblasts by maintaining extracellular calcium and phosphorous concentrations within the normal supersaturating range, which results in the passive deposition of calcium hydroxyapatite into the bone matrix (Holtrop et al., 1986).

METABOLISM OF 1,25-DIHYDROXYVITAMIN D

1,25(OH)$_2$D is metabolized in its target tissues—the intestine, bone, and kidney, as well as in the liver. Both 25(OH)D and 1,25(OH)$_2$D undergo a 24-hydroxylation to form 24,25-dihydroxyvitamin D and 1,24,25-trihydroxyvitamin D, respectively. These metabolites are considered to be biologically less active and are the first step in the biodegradation of 25(OH)D and 1,25(OH)$_2$D. These hydroxylated vitamin D metabolites undergo additional hydroxylations in the side chain, resulting in the cleavage of the side chain between C-23 and C-24, which forms the biologically inert, water-soluble calcitroic acid. More than 40 different metabolites of vitamin D have been identified to date, but 1,25(OH)$_2$D is believed to be responsible for most, if not all, of the biological actions of vitamin D on calcium and bone metabolism (Holick, 2004b; Bouillon et al., 1995; DeLuca, 1988).

MOLECULAR BIOLOGY OF VITAMIN D

Vitamin D is lipophilic, as is its active form. Therefore, the mechanism of action of 1,25(OH)$_2$D is similar to the action of other small hydrophobic hormones that act via nuclear receptors, such as retinoic acid, thyroid hormone, estrogen, and glucocorticoids. All target tissues for vitamin D contain a nuclear receptor for 1,25(OH)$_2$D, known as the VDR (vitamin D receptor), which recognizes 1,25(OH)$_2$D 1,000 times better than it recognizes 25(OH)D. It is the unbound (free) 1,25(OH)$_2$D that enters into the target cell where it is recognized by the VDR.

Nutrition Insight

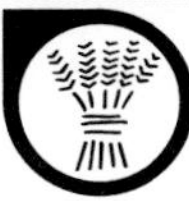

Cells Involved in Bone Formation and Resorption

The major cells in bone that are concerned with bone formation and resorption are the osteoblasts, the osteocytes, and the osteoclasts. Osteoblasts are the bone-forming cells that secrete collagen, forming a matrix around themselves that then calcifies. Osteoblasts have vitamin D receptors and are responsive to changes in circulating concentrations of 1,25(OH)$_2$D. Osteoblasts arise from osteoprogenitor cells that are of mesenchymal origin. The osteoblasts seem to form at least a partial membrane that separates bone fluid (the fluid in most immediate contact with hydroxyapatites) from the extracellular fluid of the rest of the body. In this way, the calcium and phosphate concentrations in bone fluid can be carefully regulated.

As osteoblasts become surrounded by new bone (calcified matrix), they become osteocytes. Osteocytes remain in contact with one another and with osteoblasts via tight junctions between long protoplasmic processes that run through channels in the bone.

Osteoclasts are multinuclear cells that erode and resorb previously formed bone. Osteoclasts are derived from monocytic stem cells in the bone marrow as a result of stimulation of these cells by 1,25(OH)$_2$D–induced RANKL on osteoblasts to promote their differentiation into osteoclasts. Osteoclasts appear to phagocytose and break down bone, resulting in a characteristic "chewed-out" edge on the bone surrounding an active osteoclast.

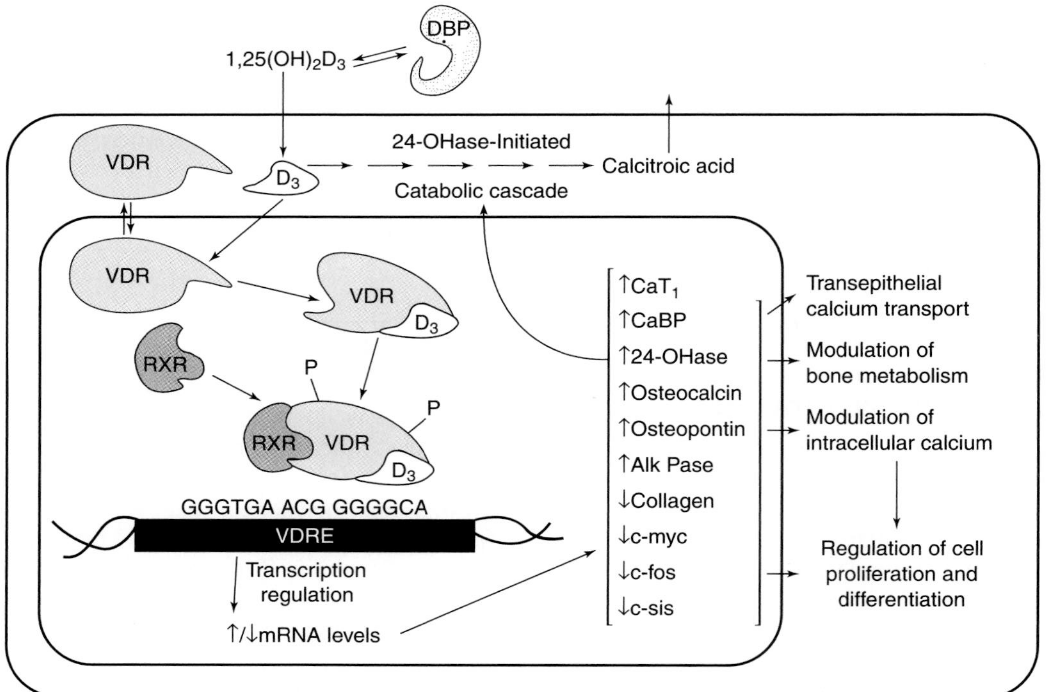

Figure 31-9 Proposed mechanism of action of 1,25$(OH)_2D_3$ in target cells resulting in a variety of biological responses. The free form of 1,25$(OH)_2D_3$ *(D_3)* enters the target cell and interacts with its nuclear vitamin D receptor *(VDR)*, which is then phosphorylated *(P)*. The 1,25$(OH)_2D_3$–VDR complex combines with the retinoic acid X-receptor *(RXR)* to form a heterodimer, which, in turn, interacts with the vitamin D response element *(VDRE)*, causing an enhancement or inhibition of transcription of vitamin D–responsive genes, such as the 25(OH)D-24-hydroxylase *(24-OHase)*. (*From Holick MF [1996] Vitamin D: photobiology, metabolism, mechanism of action, and clinical applications. In: Favus MJ [ed] Primer on the Metabolic Bone Diseases and Disorders of Mineral Metabolism, 3rd ed. Lippincott-Raven, Philadelphia, pp 74-81.)*

Although the exact mechanism by which 1,25$(OH)_2D$ interacts with its receptor and causes activation of transcription of specific genes is not completely understood, a sequence of events is required for 1,25$(OH)_2D$ to carry out its biological functions. Once 1,25$(OH)_2D$ enters the cell, it eventually finds its way to the nucleus, where it binds to the VDR. The VDR–1,25$(OH)_2D$ complex, in turn, binds a retinoic acid X receptor (RXR) to form a heterodimeric complex (Darwish and DeLuca, 1993; Pike, 1991). This heterodimeric complex interacts with a specific vitamin D–responsive element (VDRE) within the DNA. The DNA-binding motif of the VDR, which is present in the N-terminal part of the molecule, contains two zinc finger motifs that interact with the VDRE in the DNA (Fig. 31-9). The VDRE is composed of two tandemly repeated hexanucleotide sequences separated by three base pairs. This interaction of ligand-bound VDR-RXR with VDREs ultimately leads to an increase or a decrease in the transcription of the vitamin D–responsive genes and a change in the rate of synthesis of new messenger RNAs (mRNAs).

The best-characterized proteins that are induced by 1,25$(OH)_2D$ in osteoblasts are osteocalcin, osteopontin, and alkaline phosphatase. The major gene products induced in the small intestine by 1,25$(OH)_2D$ are the calcium-binding protein calbindin and the epithelial calcium channel (Bouillon et al., 1995; Wasserman et al., 1984).

BIOLOGICAL FUNCTIONS OF 1,25-DIHYDROXYVITAMIN D IN NONCALCEMIC TISSUES

A wide variety of tissues and cells, including the brain, gonads, breast, skin, mononuclear cells, and activated B and T lymphocytes, possess VDR. The first insight into the biological action of 1,25$(OH)_2$D in noncalcemic tissues was the observation that promyelocytic leukemic cells with VDR transformed into mature, functional macrophages after the cells were treated with 1,25$(OH)_2$D (Tanaka et al., 1982). It is now recognized that 1,25$(OH)_2$D can inhibit the proliferation and induce terminal differentiation of a variety of normal and tumor cells, possibly by directly or indirectly altering transcription of cell growth regulatory genes such as *c-myc*, *c-fos*, and *c-sis* (see Fig. 31-9).

In general, 1,25$(OH)_2$D has not been found useful for treating malignant disorders. It is possible that clones of cells that have a defective VDR could become the dominant tumor cell type, resulting in malignant cells that are no longer responsive to the antiproliferative activity of 1,25$(OH)_2$D (Koeffler et al., 1985). However, there is one clinical application for the antiproliferative activity of 1,25$(OH)_2$D and its analogs. Because epidermal cells possess a VDR, it was reasoned that patients with the skin disorder called psoriasis might benefit from either topical or oral 1,25$(OH)_2$D therapy. Psoriasis is a hyperproliferative disorder that causes redness, scaling, and raised lesions. A multitude of studies have now demonstrated the therapeutic efficacy of 1,25$(OH)_2$D and its analogs for treating psoriasis. This has led to the development of an analog, calcipotriene (Dovonex), which is highly effective when applied topically, for the treatment of psoriasis. Unlike other treatments for psoriasis, there is no evidence that the topical application of calcipotriene has any significant undesirable side effects (Perez et al., 1996; Kragballe, 1989).

As early as 1941, it was appreciated that a higher mortality due to cancer was associated with living at northern latitudes in the United States compared to living in the more southern states (Apperly, 1941). It is now recognized that living at higher latitudes increases the risk of colon, prostate, breast, ovarian, and a variety of other cancers (Grant, 2002; Hanchette and Schwortz, 1992; Garland et al., 1989; Apperly, 1941). It also has been observed that if serum 25(OH)D levels are at least 20 μg/L, there is marked reduction in risk of developing colon and prostate cancer (Ahonen et al., 2000; Garland et al., 1991). In addition, exposure to moderate sunlight has been reported to reduce the onset of prostate cancer by 3 to 5 years (Bodiwala et al., 2003; Luscombe et al., 2001). Although 1,25$(OH)_2$D was known to be a potent inhibitor of cancer cell growth in vitro, it was perplexing how exposure to more sunlight or ingesting more vitamin D could decrease risk of these serious common cancers. The kidney's production of 1,25$(OH)_2$D is tightly regulated so that increased exposure to sunlight or increased intake of vitamin D does not result in increased blood levels of 1,25$(OH)_2$D.

Nutrition Insight

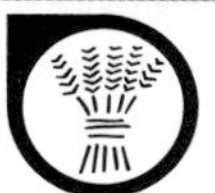

Role of Vitamin D for Health

Most tissues in the body not only have a vitamin D receptor (VDR) but also have the capacity to make 1,25$(OH)_2$D. Now that it is recognized that 1,25$(OH)_2$D is a potent modulator of cell growth, and that it stimulates insulin secretion and regulates the immune system and the production of renin in the kidneys, it can be appreciated that maintaining an adequate vitamin D status is not only important for bone health but important for the prevention for many chronic disease including various cancers, type 1 diabetes, multiple sclerosis, rheumatoid arthritis, hypertension, and cardiovascular heart disease. Without adequate sun exposure, children and adults need 25 μg (1,000 IU) of vitamin D_3 a day in order to satisfy their body's requirement for this vital vitamin/hormone.

There needed to be another explanation. Although it was known that, in addition to the kidney, the skin had the ability to convert $25(OH)D_3$ to $1,25(OH)_2D_3$ (Bikle et al., 1986), the observation in 1998 that the prostate also had the enzymatic machinery to make $1,25(OH)_2D_3$ was a significant advance (Schwartz et al., 1998). It was subsequently found that most other tissues including breast, bone cells, and brain make $1,25(OH)_2D$ (Holick, 2004b). Therefore, it is now hypothesized that increased vitamin D intake or increased exposure to sunlight raises blood levels of 25(OH)D to a level that allows these other organs to synthesize $1,25(OH)_2D$ (Cross et al., 2001; Tangpricha et al., 2001). Once formed, the $1,25(OH)_2D$ can act on a variety of genes that regulate cell proliferation and differentiation as well as apoptosis. Therefore, $1,25(OH)_2D$ may act as a regulator of cell growth, thereby decreasing the risk of some common cancers.

There is mounting evidence that $1,25(OH)_2D$ may be an important immunomodulator. It is also recognized that activated T and B lymphocytes and macrophages have a VDR. Vitamin D deficiency has been associated with increased risk of several autoimmune diseases including type 1 diabetes (Hypponen et al., 2001), multiple sclerosis (van der Mei et al., 2003), rheumatoid arthritis (Merlino et al., 2004), and Crohn's disease (Cantorna, 2000).

Vitamin D sufficiency may also decrease risk of hypertension and cardiovascular disease. Individuals living at latitudes farther from the equator have increased risk of hypertension and cardiovascular heart disease (Rostand et al., 1979). It is now recognized that the renal production of renin is downregulated by $1,25(OH)_2D$ (Li et al., 2002). This may be the explanation for why exposure to UVB in a tanning bed results in remission of hypertension (Krause et al., 1998). It has also been reported that vitamin D sufficiency decreases risk of cardiovascular heart disease and congestive heart failure (Holick, 2004b; Zitterman et al., 2003; Holick, 2002).

Clinical Correlation

Vitamin D–Dependent Rickets Type II

The vitamin D receptor (VDR) is a nuclear transcription factor that binds to the vitamin D response element (VDRE) of certain genes to regulate their expression. Vitamin D–dependent rickets type II (VDDRII) is a rare autosomal recessive disease that results from target organ resistance to the action of $1,25(OH)_2D$. Mutations in the gene for VDR result in an inability of VDR to bind $1,25(OH)_2D$ or of the receptor-hormone complex to bind to VDRE in DNA. Affected patients usually present early in childhood with severe rickets, hypocalcemia, and growth retardation. Cultured fibroblasts obtained from these patients fail to respond to $1,25(OH)_2D$ by increasing synthesis of 25(OH)D-24-hydroxylase; this is used as a test for a defect in the $1,25(OH)_2D$ receptor–effector system. In patients with VDDRII, physiological doses of $1,25(OH)_2D$ have no therapeutic effect. In some patients, high-dose calcium therapy or pharmacological doses of vitamin D metabolites have resulted in biochemical and radiological improvement.

Thinking Critically

1. What effect would you expect a defect in the $1,25(OH)_2D$ receptor–effector system to have on calcium absorption? Why?
2. Would high-dose calcium therapy (intravenous or oral) potentially improve bone growth in patients with defects in the $1,25(OH)_2D$ receptor–effector system? Why?
3. For pharmacological doses of $1,25(OH)_2D$ to be effective, would some residual VDR need to be present? Why?

RECOMMENDATIONS FOR SATISFYING THE VITAMIN D REQUIREMENT FOR MAXIMAL BONE HEALTH

Vitamin D evolved as a calciotropic hormone responsible for maintaining blood calcium and phosphorus within the normal physiological ranges. Only when the body's need for calcium to maintain metabolic functions is satisfied is any additional calcium that is absorbed through the intestine deposited into the skeleton.

Increasing vitamin D intake or increased exposure to a sensible amount of sunlight (usually no more that 5 to 10 minutes between 10 AM and 3 PM, or no more than approximately 25% of the amount of time that would be required to cause a mild pinkness to the skin) is often more than adequate to satisfy a person's vitamin D requirement. Vitamin D deficiency is a significant health problem, especially for elderly people. Because most of our vitamin D comes from casual exposure to sunlight, it is important to recognize that adults older than the age of 50 years should intentionally seek exposure of their skin to suberythemal (not causing sunburn) doses of sunlight. For example, for middle-aged and older adults who live in Boston, exposure of the hands, arms, and legs to suberythemal doses of sunlight (approximately 5 to 15 minutes a day depending on the skin's sensitivity to sunlight) two to three times a week is recommended for obtaining sufficient amounts of vitamin D_3.

Vitamin D_3 that is produced in the skin is stored in the body fat; therefore, vitamin D_3 that is produced in the spring, summer, and fall can be stored and is available during the winter when available sunlight is incapable of producing vitamin D_3 in the skin. This is why children and most adults do not become vitamin D–deficient during the winter months in far northern and southern latitudes. Because a topical application of a sunscreen can essentially prevent the production of vitamin D_3 in the skin, people who wish to stay outdoors for long periods should expose their skin only to suberythemal amounts of sunlight for their vitamin D_3 and then apply a sunscreen with a SPF of 15 or greater to prevent the consequences of chronic excessive exposure to sunlight. Children and young adults should always wear a sunscreen before going outdoors to help prevent skin damage and skin cancer. Because children and young adults generally do not always wear a sunscreen over all sun-exposed areas, they are still able to produce enough vitamin D from sun exposure to satisfy their body's requirement.

Although milk, some cereals, and bread products may contain vitamin D, this is highly variable and should not be depended on as the only source of vitamin D. A multivitamin tablet that contains 10 μg (400 IU) of vitamin D is an excellent source and will help maintain circulating concentrations of 25(OH)D. However, in the absence of any sunlight, a multivitamin may not be adequate to maintain normal vitamin D status because a total of 25 μg (1000 IU) of vitamin D/day is needed (Tangpricha et al., 2003; Holick, 1994). Adults 51 years and older who have little exposure to sunlight likely require at least 10 to 15 μg of dietary vitamin D daily to satisfy the body's requirement. Vitamin D deficiency can be corrected by administering an oral dose of 1,250 μg (50,000 IU) vitamin D_2 once a week for 8 weeks. The serum 25(OH)D level can be expected to increase from less than 15 μg/L to 25 to 40 μg/L. This treatment will maintain a normal vitamin D status for at least 2 to 4 months. After the 8 weeks, patients can be placed on a multivitamin containing 10 μg (400 IU) of vitamin D_3, or 1,250 μg (50,000 IU) of vitamin D_2 every other week, which should help maintain their vitamin D status. An adequate source of calcium in combination with vitamin D from sunlight and/or a multivitamin containing vitamin D is essential for guaranteeing a healthy skeleton throughout life. Not only is adequate vitamin D nutrition important for maximizing bone health, but there is mounting scientific evidence that vitamin D is important for overall health and well being (Holick, 2004b). By maintaining adequate vitamin D stores one could significantly decrease risk of many common cancers and serious autoimmune disease as well as prevent hypertension and cardiovascular heart disease (Fig. 31-10).

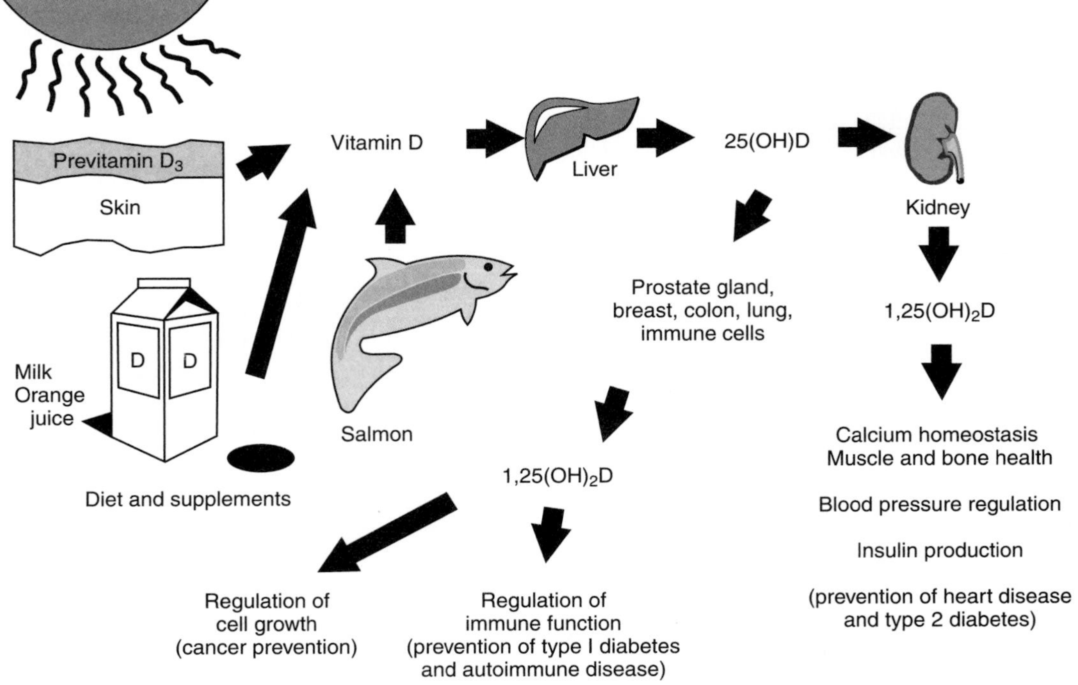

Figure 31-10 Photoproduction and sources of vitamin D. Vitamin D is metabolized in the liver to 25-hydroxyvitamin D [25(OH)D] which is responsible for maintaining calcium homeostasis. 25(OH)D is also converted to 1,25$(OH)_2$ D in a variety of other cells and tissues for the purpose of regulating cell growth, immune function, as well as a variety of other physiological processes that are important for the prevention of many chronic diseases.

Life Cycle Considerations

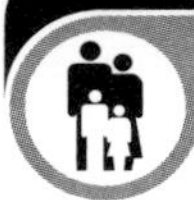

Vitamin D Deficiency in Elderly People

Elderly people are more prone to develop a vitamin D deficiency, which may cause osteomalacia, exacerbate osteoporosis, and increase the risk of fractures. A decrease in the capacity of human skin to produce vitamin D occurs with age because the concentration of 7-dehydrocholesterol in the skin decreases with age. In addition, production of vitamin D_3 may be restricted in elderly people as a result of limited exposure to sunlight through indoor confinement or use of sunscreen or protective clothing from concern about sun-induced cancer or wrinkles. In a study of sunlight-deprived elderly subjects, a large proportion of homebound elderly persons had below-normal serum 25(OH)D concentrations (Gloth et al., 1995). Vitamin D supplementation or increased exposure to sunlight may improve calcium absorption, suppress parathyroid hormone (PTH) levels, and decrease bone loss in elderly people. Calcium intake, hormonal status, exercise, and genetics also may be important factors in the development of osteomalacia and osteoporosis in elderly individuals.

REFERENCES

Aaron J E, Gallagher J C, Anderson J, Stasiak L, Longton E, Nordin B, Nicholson M (1974) Frequency of osteomalacia and osteoporosis in fractures of the proximal femur. Lancet 7851:230-233.

Ahonen M H, Tenkanen L, Teppo L, Hakama M, Tuohimaa P (2000) Prostate cancer risk and pre-diagnostic serum 25-hydroxyvitamin D levels (Finland). Cancer Causes Control 11:847-852.

Apperly FL (1941) The relation of solar radiation to cancer mortality in North America. Cancer Res 1:191-195.

Armas LA, Hollis BW, Heaney RP (2004) Vitamin D_2 is much less effective than vitamin D_3 in humans. J Clin Endocrinol Metab 89:5387-5391.

Bell NH, Greene A, Epstein S, Oexmann MJ, Shaw S, Shary J (1985) Evidence for alteration of the vitamin D-endocrine system in obese subjects. J Clin Invest 76:470-473.

Bikle DD, Nemanic MK, Gee E, Elias P (1986) 1,25-Dihydroxyvitamin D_3 production by human keratinocytes: kinetics and regulation. J Clin Invest 78:557-566.

Blok BH, Grant CC, McNeil AR, Reid IR (2000) Characteristics of children with florid vitamin D deficient rickets in the Auckland region in 1998. NZ Med J 113:374-376.

Bodiwala D, Luscombe CJ, Liu S, Saxby M, French M, Jones PW (2003) Prostate cancer risk and exposure to ultraviolet radiation: further support for the protective effect of sunlight. Cancer Lett 192:145-149.

Bouillon R (2001) Vitamin D: from photosynthesis, metabolism, and action to clinical applications. In: DeGroot LJ, Jameson JL (eds) Endocrinology. WB Saunders, Philadelphia, pp 1009-1028.

Bouillon R, Okamura WH, Norman AW (1995) Structure-function relationships in the vitamin D endocrine system. Endocr Rev 16:200-257.

Cantorna MT (2000) Vitamin D and autoimmunity: is vitamin D status an environmental factor affecting autoimmune disease prevalence? Proc Soc Exp Biol Med 223:230-233.

Chapuy MC, Arlot M, Duboeuf F, Brun J, Crouzet B, Arnaud S, Delmas P, Meuner P (1992) Vitamin D_3 and calcium to prevent hip fractures in elderly women. N Engl J Med 327:1637-1642.

Clemens TL, Henderson SL, Adams JS, Holick MF (1982) Increased skin pigment reduces the capacity of skin to synthesize vitamin D_3. Lancet 1:74-76.

Cross HS, Bareis P, Hofer H, Bischof MG, Bajna E, Kriwanek S (2001) 25-Hydroxyvitamin D_3-1α-hydroxylase and vitamin D receptor gene expression in human colonic mucosa is elevated during early cancerogenesis. Steroids 66:287-292.

Darwish H, DeLuca HF (1993) Vitamin D–regulated gene expression. Crit Rev Eukaryot Gene Expr 3:89-116.

Dawson-Hughes B, Dallal GE, Krall EA, Harris S, Sokoll, LJ, Falconer G (1991) Effect of vitamin D supplementation on wintertime and overall bone loss in healthy postmenopausal women. Ann Intern Med 115:505-512.

Dawson-Hughes B, Harris SS, Krall EA, Dallal GE (1997) Effect of calcium and vitamin D supplementation on bone density in men and women 65 years of age or older. N Engl J Med 337:670-676.

DeLuca H (1988) The vitamin D story: a collaborative effort of basic science and clinical medicine. FASEB J 2:224-236.

Ebeling PR, Sandgren ME, DiMagno EP, Lane AW, DeLuca HF, Riggs BL (1992) Evidence of an age-related decrease in intestinal responsiveness to vitamin D: relationship between serum 1,25-dihydroxyvitamin D_3 and intestinal vitamin D receptor concentration in normal women. J Clin Endocrinol Metab 75:176-182.

Garland CF, Comstock GW, Garland FC, Helsing KJ, Shaw EK, Gorham ED (1989) Serum 25-hydroxyvitamin D and colon cancer: eight-year prospective study. Lancet 18:1176-1178.

Garland CF, Garland FC, Gorham E D (1991) Can colon cancer incidence and death rates be reduced with calcium and vitamin D? Am J Clin Nutr 54:193S-201S.

Gilchrest BA (1993) Sunscreens—a public health opportunity. N Engl J Med 329:1193-1194.

Gloth FM III, Gundberg CM, Hollis BW, Haddad JG Jr., Tobin JD (1995) Vitamin D deficiency in homebound elderly persons. JAMA 274:1683-1686.

Grant WB (2002) An estimate of premature cancer mortality in the U.S. due to inadequate doses of solar ultraviolet-B radiation. Cancer 94:1867-1875.

Hanchette CL, Schwartz GG (1992) Geographic patterns of prostate cancer mortality. Cancer 70:2861-2869.

Heaney RP, Dowell MS, Hale CA, Bendich A (2003) Calcium absorption varies within the reference range for serum 25-hydroxyvitamin D. J Am Coll Nutr 22:142-146.

Holick MF (2004a) Vitamin D: importance in the prevention of cancers, type 1 diabetes, heart disease, and osteoporosis. Am J Clin Nutr 79:362-371.

Holick MF (2004b) Sunlight and vitamin D for bone health and prevention of autoimmune diseases, cancers, and cardiovascular disease. Am J Clin Nutr 80(suppl):1678S-1688S.

Holick MF (2003) Vitamin D: photobiology, metabolism, mechanism of action, and clinical applications. In: Favus MJ (ed) Primer on the Metabolic Bone Diseases and Disorders of Mineral Metabolism, 5th ed. American Society for Bone and Mineral Research, Washington, DC, pp 129-137

Holick MF (2002) Sunlight and vitamin D, both good for cardiovascular health. J Gen Intern Med (editorial) 17:733-735.

Holick MF (1994) Vitamin D: new horizons for the 21st century. Am J Clin Nutr 60:619-630.

Holick MF, Krane S, Potts JT (1994) Calcium, phosphorus, and bone metabolism: calcium-regulating hormones. In: Isselbacher KJ, Braunwald E, Wilson JD, Martin JB, Fauci AS, Kasper DL (eds) Harrison's Principles of Internal Medicine, 13th ed. McGraw-Hill, New York, pp 2137-2151.

Holick MF, Matsuoka LY, Wortsman J (1989) Age, vitamin D, and solar ultraviolet. Lancet 2:1104-1105.

Holtrop ME, Cox KA, Carnes DL, Holick MF (1986) Effects of serum calcium and phosphorus on skeletal mineralization in vitamin D–deficient rats. Am J Physiol 251:E234-E240.

Hypponen E, Laara E, Jarvelin M-R, Virtanen SM (2001) Intake of vitamin D and risk of type 1 diabetes: a birth-cohort study. Lancet 358:1500-1503.

Institute of Medicine (IOM) (1997) Dietary Reference Intakes for Calcium, Phosphorus, Magnesium, Vitamin D, and Fluoride. National Academy Press, Washington, DC.

Ireland P, Fordtran, JS (1973) Effect of dietary calcium and age on jejunal calcium absorption in humans studied by intestinal perfusion. J Clin Invest 52:2672-2681.

Kinyamu HK, Gallagher JC, Balhorn KE, Petranick KM, Rafferty KA (1997) Serum vitamin D metabolites and calcium absorption in normal young and elderly free-living women and in women living in nursing homes. Am J Clin Nutr 65:790-797.

Koeffler H P, Hirji K, Itri L and The Southern California Leukemia Group (1985) 1,25-Dihydroxyvitamin D_3: in vivo and in vitro effects on human preleukemic and leukemic cells. Cancer Treat Rep 69:1399-407.

Koutkia P, Chen TC, Holick MF (2001) Vitamin D intoxication with an over-the-counter supplement. N Engl J Med 345:66-67.

Kragballe K (1989) Treatment of psoriasis by the topical application of the novel vitamin D_3 analogue MC 903. Arch Dermatol 125: 1647-1652.

Krause R, Buhring M, Hopfenmuller W, Holick MF, Sharma AM (1998) Ultraviolet B and blood pressure. Lancet 352:709-710.

Leheste JR, Melsen F, Wellner M, Jansen P, Schlichting U, Renner-Muller I, Andreassen TT, Wolf E, Bachmann S, Nykjaer A, Willnow TE (2002) Hypocalcemia and osteopathy in mice with kidney-specific megalin gene defect. FASEB J 10:247-249.

Li Y, Kong J, Wei M, Chen ZF, Liu S, Cao LP (2002) 1,25-Dihydroxyvitamin D_3 is a negative endocrine regulator of the renin-angiotensin system. J Clin Invest 110:229-238.

Loomis F (1967) Skin-pigment regulation of vitamin D biosynthesis in man. Science 157:501-506.

Luscombe CJ, Fryer AA, French ME, Liu S, Saxby MF, Jones PW, Strange RC (2001) Exposure to ultraviolet radiation: association with susceptibility and age at presentation with prostate cancer. Lancet 358:641-642.

Matsuoka LY, Wortsman J, Dannenberg MJ, Hollis BW, Lu Z, Holick MF (1992) Clothing prevents ultraviolet-B radiation-dependent photosynthesis of vitamin D. J Clin Endocrinol Metab 75:1099-1103.

Merlino LA, Curtis J, Mikuls TR, Cerhan JR, Criswell LA, Saag KG (2004) Vitamin D intake is inversely associated with rheumatoid arthritis: results from the Iowa women's health study. Arthritis Rheum 50:72-77.

Norman AW (1998) Receptors for $1\beta,(OH)_2D_3$: past, present, and future. J Bone Miner Res 13:1360-1369.

Perez A, Chen T C, Turner A, Raab R, Bhawan J, Poche P, Holick MF (1996) Efficacy and safety of topical calcitriol (1,25-dihydroxyvitamin D_3) for the treatment of psoriasis. Br J Dermatol 134:238-246.

Pike JW (1991) Vitamin D_3 receptors: structure and function in transcription. Annu Rev Nutr 11:189-216.

Portale AA, Halloran BP, Murphy MM, Morris RC Jr (1986) Oral intake phosphorus can determine the serum concentration of 1,25-dihyroxy-vitamin D by determining its production rate in humans. J Clin Invest 77:7-12.

Riggs BL, Hamstra A, DeLuca HF (1981) Assessment of 25-hydroxyvitamin D 1α-hydroxylase reserve in postmenopausal osteoporosis by administration of parathyroid extract. J Clin Endocrinol Metab 53:833-835.

Rosen C J, Morrison A, Zhou H, Storm D, Hunter SJ, Musgrave K, Chen T, Wei W, Holick MF (1994) Elderly women in northern New England exhibit seasonal changes in bone mineral density and calciotropic hormones. Bone Miner 25:83-92.

Rostand SG (1979) Ultraviolet light may contribute to geographic and racial blood pressure differences. Hypertension 30:150-156.

Schwartz GG, Whitlatch LW, Chen TC, Lokeshwar BL, Holick MF (1998) Human prostate cells synthesize 1,25-dihydroxyvitamin D3 from 25-hydroxyvitamin D3. Cancer Epidemiol Biomarkers Prev 7:391-395.

Slovik DM, Adams JS, Neer RM, Holick MF, Potts JT (1981) Deficient production of 1,25-dihydroxyvitamin D in elderly osteoporotic patients. N Engl J Med 305:372-374.

Taha SA, Dost SM, Sedrani SH (1984) 25-Hydroxyvitamin D and total calcium: extraordinarily low plasma concentrations in Saudi mothers and their neonates. Pediatr Res 18:739-741.

Tanaka H, Abe E, Miyaura C, Kuribayashi T, Konno K, Nishi Y, Suda T (1982) 1,25-Dihydroxycholecalciferol and human myeloid leukemia cell line (HL-60): the presence of cytosol receptor and induction of differentiation. Biochem J 204:713-719.

Tangpricha V, Flanagan JN, Whitlatch LW, Tseng CC, Chen TC, Holt PR, Lipkin MS, Holick MF (2001) 25-Hydroxyvitamin D-1α-hydroxylase in normal and malignant colon tissue. Lancet 357:1673-1674.

Tangpricha V, Koutkia P, Rieke SM, Chen TC, Perez AA, Holick MF (2003) Fortification of orange juice with vitamin D: a novel approach to enhance vitamin D nutritional health. Am J Clin Nutr 77:1478-1483.

van der Mei IA, Ponsonby AL, Dwyer T, Blizzard L, Simmons R, Taylor BV, Butzkueven H, Kilpatrick T (2003) Past exposure to sun, skim phenotype, and risk of multiple sclerosis: case-control study. BMJ 327:316.

Vieth R, Chan PC, MacFarlane GD (2001) Efficacy and safety of vitamin D_3 intake exceeding the lowest observed adverse effect level. Am J Clin Nutr 73:288-294.

Wasserman RH, Fullmer CS, Shimura F (1984) Calcium absorption and the molecular effects of vitamin D_3. In: Kumar R (ed) Vitamin D: Basic and Clinical Aspects. Nijhoff, Boston, pp 233-257.

Webb AR, Kline L, Holick MF (1988) Influence of season and latitude on the cutaneous synthesis of vitamin D_3: exposure to winter sunlight in Boston and Edmonton will not promote vitamin D_3 synthesis in human skin. J Clin Endocrinol Metab 67:373-378.

Webb AR, DeCosta BR, Holick MF (1989) Sunlight regulates the cutaneous production of vitamin D_3 by causing its photodegradation. J Clin Endocrinol Metab 68:882-887.

Wortsman J, Matsuoka LY, Chen TC, Lu Z, Holick MF (2000) Decreased bioavailability of vitamin D in obesity. Am J Clin Nutr 72:690-693.

Zittermann A, Schleithoff SS, Tenderich G, Berthold HK, Körfe, R, Stehle P (2003) Low vitamin D status: a contributing factor in the pathogenesis of congestive heart failure? J Am Coll Cardiol 41:105-112.

RECOMMENDED READINGS

Ahonen MH, Tenkanen L, Teppo L, Hakama M., Tuohimaa P (2000) Prostate cancer risk and pre-diagnostic serum 25-hydroxyvitamin D levels (Finland). Cancer Causes Control 11:847-852.

Armas LA, Hollis BW, Heaney RP (2004) Vitamin D_2 is much less effective than vitamin D_3 in humans. J Clin Endocrinol Metab 89:5387-5391.

Grant WB (2002) An estimate of premature cancer mortality in the U.S. due to inadequate doses of solar ultraviolet-B radiation. Cancer 94:1867-1875.

Holick MF (2004) Vitamin D: importance in the prevention of cancers, type 1 diabetes, heart disease, and osteoporosis. Am J Clin Nutr 79:362-371.

Holick MF (2004) Sunlight and vitamin D for bone health and prevention of autoimmune diseases, cancers, and cardiovascular disease. Am J Clin Nutr 80(suppl):1678S-1688S.

Holick MF, Jenkins M (2004) The UV Advantage. ibooks, New York.

Malabanan A, Veronikis IE, Holick MF (1998) Redefining vitamin D insufficiency. Lancet 351:805-806.

Zittermann A, Schleithoff SS, Tenderich G, Berthold HK, Körfe, R, Stehle P (2003) Low vitamin D status: a contributing factor in the pathogenesis of congestive heart failure? J Am Coll Cardiol 41:105-112.

Unit VII

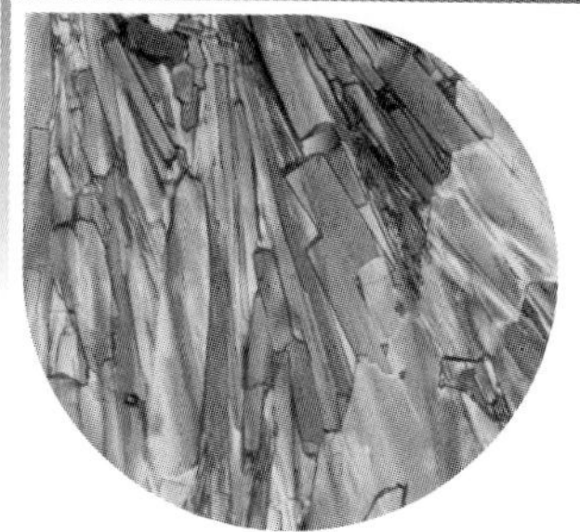

Minerals and Water

The organic components of the diet have been discussed in detail in the preceding chapters. In this unit, the biological roles of water and a number of essential elements that can be supplied in inorganic form are considered.

Water (H_2O) makes up the largest component of the body, accounting for about 73% of lean body mass in adults. As a percentage of total body weight, water content ranges from 75% of body weight in the neonate to 50% of body weight in older adults. Water serves as the principal fluid medium of the cell in which metabolic processes take place. The extracellular water bathing the cells serves as a medium for the transport of nutrients and oxygen to the cells and for removal of wastes from the body. In addition, water is necessary for organ form and plays an important role in the regulation of body temperature.

From the 90 or so elements that occur naturally in the environment, a limited number (perhaps 22) are essential for human life. The organic nutrients—the carbohydrates, proteins, lipids, and vitamins—are made up almost entirely of six relatively small elements: hydrogen, carbon, nitrogen, oxygen, phosphorus, and sulfur. Two rather common features of the elements discussed in this unit, as opposed to those that make up the organic nutrients, are that these minerals are required in smaller amounts and for very specialized functions. In addition, although some of these elements (e.g., selenium and iodine) are also capable of forming covalent bonds, weaker types of bonds are much more common. In contrast to the strong covalent bonds found in organic molecules, in which each atom donates one electron to form a pair of outer orbital electrons that are shared, the ionic bonds (salt bridges) found in salts are formed by a single electron donated by one of the paired atoms. The coordinate covalent bonds found in metal chelates (e.g., heme and vitamin B_{12}) possess properties of both the covalent bond and the ionic bond: two electrons from one atom are donated to form the bond to another atom.

Minerals or inorganic nutrients are sometimes grouped by the amount of each element that is required by the human body. Essential elements include those classified as macroelements; calcium, phosphorus, magnesium, sodium, potassium, chloride, and sulfur are required at levels of greater than 100 mg/day by adults. Because the sulfur requirement is met by intake of sulfur amino acids, sulfur usually is not considered with the macroelements. The microelements may be considered in two groups: trace elements required in amounts ranging between 1 mg and 100 mg/day and ultratrace elements required in amounts in the microgram per day range (less than 1 mg/day). Trace elements include iron, zinc, manganese, copper, and fluorine. Ultratrace elements include selenium, molybdenum, iodine, chromium, boron, and cobalt. Some evidence of a benefit of arsenic, nickel, vanadium, and silicon comes from animal studies, but these four ultratrace elements have not been proved to be essential or beneficial for humans. Sulfate is not considered in detail in this unit because requirements for sulfate are thought to be met if the sulfur amino acid requirement is met as is discussed in Chapter 14. Similarly, cobalt is not considered in this unit because the only requirement humans have for cobalt is as part of preformed vitamin B_{12}, which is discussed in Chapter 25.

Minerals serve a diverse range of functions in the body, and many of these functions are discussed in the chapters in this unit. The deposition of calcium and phosphate as hydroxyapatite is essential for bone formation. Calcium is considered to be a second messenger molecule; binding of calcium to various proteins acts as a cellular signaling event. Sodium, potassium, and chloride as well as calcium, magnesium, phosphate, and sulfate are important inorganic electrolytes involved in ionic and osmotic balance and electrical gradients. Many of the trace elements are found in association with enzymes and other proteins in which these metals serve structural, catalytic, or binding roles; examples include the role of zinc in the tertiary structure of various proteins, the catalytic role of copper or zinc at the active site of superoxide dismutase, and the role of iron in oxygen binding by hemoglobin. Some minerals are required solely for the synthesis of specialized organic compounds, as demonstrated by the incorporation of iodine into thyroid hormones, of selenium into selenocysteine for synthesis of selenoproteins, and of molybdenum into an organic cofactor required by several mammalian enzymes.

Martha H. Stipanuk

Chapter 32

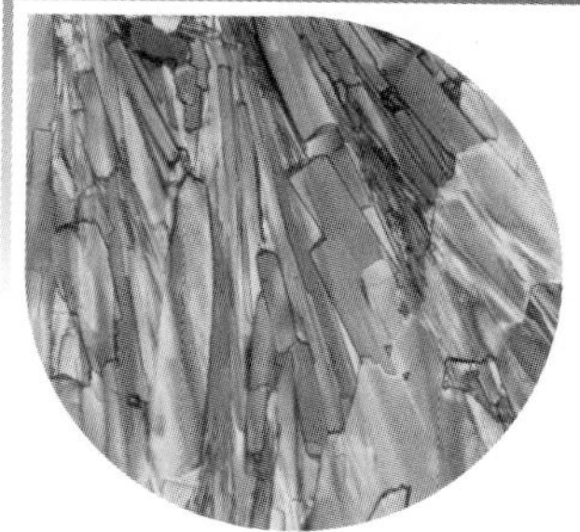

Calcium and Phosphorus

Richard J. Wood, PhD

OUTLINE

COMMON ABBREVIATIONS

Gla	γ-carboxyglutamate
IP_3	inositol 1,4,5-triphosphate
$1,25(OH)_2D$	1,25-dihydroxyvitamin D
P_i	inorganic phosphate, mainly HPO_4^{2-} and $H_2PO_4^-$ at physiological pH
PIP_2	phosphatidyl inositol 4,5-bisphosphate
PTH	parathyroid hormone
PTHrP	parathyroid hormone–related protein
TRPV	transient receptor potential (TRP) cation channel subfamily V

CHEMICAL PROPERTIES OF CALCIUM AND PHOSPHORUS

A consideration of the chemistry of calcium and phosphorus illustrates the unique biochemical niches filled by these elements. The important roles of these two elements in cell membrane function, cellular homeostasis, and the formation of the inorganic component of the skeleton and the intimate intertwining of the hormonal regulation of calcium and phosphorus homeostasis provide a functional basis for discussing calcium and phosphate in a single chapter.

CHEMICAL PROPERTIES OF CALCIUM

The chemical characteristics of the calcium atom are important in defining the function of this element in living organisms. Calcium belongs to the divalent metals in group IIA of the periodic table; this group of metals has two valence electrons that are lost when the metals ionize. Calcium gives up electrons readily and thus forms positive ions (Ca^{2+}) in solution. The double-positive charge on the Ca^{2+} nucleus pulls the outer electronic shells of the calcium ion into a tightly bound configuration. The relatively low ionic radius of calcium produces a high charge density or ionic potential. This electrostatic property of calcium has an important effect on the behavior of the ion in aqueous solution and on its participation in biological processes.

The biological activity of calcium is influenced by the concentration of the ionized or free Ca^{2+} in solution; the stability constant of Ca^{2+} with various ligands in solution; and the partition coefficient of Ca^{2+}, which defines the stability of Ca^{2+} binding in a nonaqueous phase such as cell membranes. The rate of movement of Ca^{2+} across cell membranes is limited by the permeability of the membrane to Ca^{2+}, as well as by the effect of Ca^{2+} itself on the membrane. The latter effect is due to an increase in rigidity and electrical resistance of the cell membrane when Ca^{2+} binds to membrane lipids. Moreover, binding of Ca^{2+} to the protein components of cell membranes can change the fluidity of the membrane by influencing the possibilities of cross-linking between proteins. These chemical properties of calcium have particular relevance to the development of specific channels in cell membranes that selectively allow passage of ions; for example, the latter effect is important in determining the permeability of cells to sodium (Na^+) and potassium (K^+) ions. The flow of ions through channels in the membrane creates an electrical circuit that requires energy to drive the flow. The currents generated are a major factor in the control of many cellular functions.

An additional factor that determines the biological activity of Ca^{2+} is related to the notion that the binding constant of Ca^{2+} for some large binding molecules can change under conditions in which the conformation of the binding anion changes. This conformational change can result in the development of a range of binding constants for the interaction of Ca^{2+} with the molecule. This phenomenon has important implications for regulation of cellular activities involving Ca^{2+} binding because a given response may occur progressively, rather than suddenly, in response to conformational stress at the binding site (Robertson, 1988). For example, calmodulin is a highly conserved, ubiquitous calcium-binding protein in cells, and calmodulin modulates a wide variety of cellular reactions. Calmodulin contains four calcium-binding ("EF-hand") domains that contain a high proportion of glutamate and aspartate (acidic) residues. These calcium-binding domains are highly conserved and consist of approximately 30 to 40 amino acid residues in a helix-loop-helix structure known as an EF-hand (Fig. 32-1). Calcium-binding domains usually occur in pairs and are also present in other cellular calcium-binding proteins, such as troponin C in muscle and calbindin D_{9K} in the intestine. Although many calcium-binding proteins contain calmodulin-like motifs, some other calcium-binding proteins, such as the vitamin K–dependent proteins that contain γ-carboxyglutamate (Gla) residues and the annexins, do not contain EF-hand domains.

In addition to the aforementioned electrostatic properties of Ca^{2+}, other properties of calcium ions in aqueous solution also influence their biological activity; these include the high electrical field associated with the Ca^{2+} ion, which causes it to become surrounded by water molecules that shield the charge. This so-called water of hydration depends partly on the charge density of the ion and partly on the number of interactions that can occur with other ions in solution. Ca^{2+} is capable of forming 6 to 12 coordination bonds. The shielding of Ca^{2+} by water molecules increases the effective ionic radius of Ca^{2+} by fivefold, from about 1 Å to 6 Å. The net effect of charge density and coordination number—the effective ionic radius of Ca^{2+}—influences the solution properties of the Ca^{2+} ion, including its chemical activity, its diffusion coefficients, and the ability of Ca^{2+} to traverse semipermeable membranes.

Another factor that influences chemical activity of Ca^{2+} is the electrical field produced by other ions in solution. Therefore, the effective concentration of Ca^{2+} in solution will differ from its actual chemical concentration by a factor that depends upon the ionic strength of the solution. Moreover, because Ca^{2+} is a divalent cation in solution, it also has the capacity to form soluble ion pairs or complexes with divalent anions based on mutual electrostatic attraction, which effectively reduces the concentration of free Ca^{2+}.

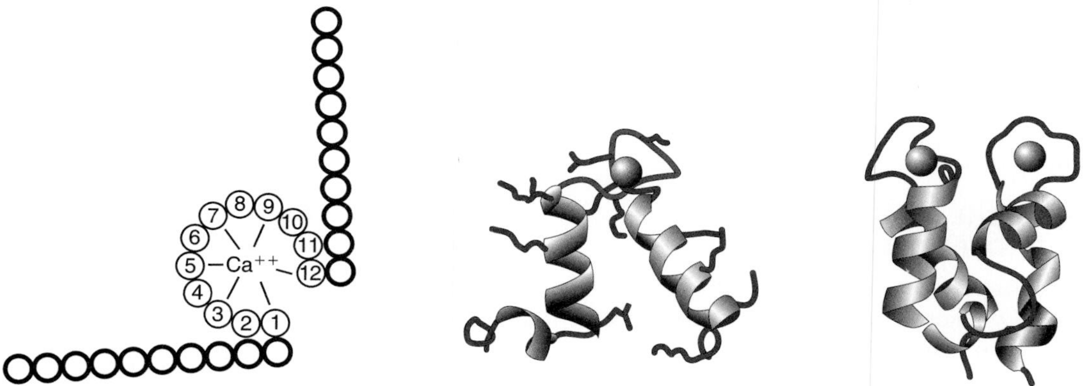

Figure 32-1 EF-hand calcium-binding motif. A commonly found calcium-binding motif in proteins is called the EF-hand structure. The EF-hand is composed of two perpendicular 10- to 12-amino-acid residue alpha helices with a 12-residue calcium binding loop region (helix-loop-helix). Calcium ions bind within the calcium binding loop to oxygen ligands provided by amino acids 1, 3, 5, 7, 9, and 12. In most EF-hand proteins the residue at position 12 is a glutamate, which contributes both of its side-chain oxygens for calcium coordination. EF-hand elements usually occur in pairs and are found in a large number of calcium-binding proteins, such as calmodulin and calbindin D.

Consequently, the selective binding chemistry of Ca^{2+} in biological systems is determined by its charge-to-size ratio and its ability to interact with chelating anions, weak acidic groups such as carboxylates and phosphates, and neutral oxygen donors such as carbonyl and hydroxyl groups. In addition, the high coordination number of Ca^{2+} and its ability to form irregular bond lengths allow it to interact with large molecules that have many possible coordination sites; this facilitates the rapid binding and release processes necessary for Ca^{2+} to act as a signaling messenger for the actions of various hormones and growth factors. However, in order for Ca^{2+} to function properly as a "second messenger" signaling molecule in mediating hormonal action, as a factor involved in motor nerve fiber function, and in mineralization of bone tissue via the formation of calcium phosphate complexes such as hydroxyapatite [$Ca_{10}(OH)_2(PO_4)_6$] crystals, the concentration of free Ca^{2+} in cells must be tightly regulated.

Two important energy-requiring membrane pump systems have evolved to help maintain calcium homeostasis in cells by ejecting calcium out of cells. These are the Na^+, Ca^{2+}-exchange system in excitable cells and the magnesium (Mg^{2+})-dependent Ca^{2+}-ATPase enzyme system in nonexcitable cells. In addition, various other strategies are employed by the cell to control intracellular free Ca^{2+} concentrations, including the binding of Ca^{2+} to various cytosolic Ca^{2+}-binding proteins and small chelating ions, such as citrate, phosphate, ADP, and ATP, and the sequestering of Ca^{2+} within various subcellular compartments.

CHEMICAL PROPERTIES OF PHOSPHATE

In biological systems, phosphorus is present as free phosphate, phosphate anhydrides, or phosphate esters. The major forms of phosphate in aqueous environments are $H_2PO_4^-$ and HPO_4^{2-}.These two orthophosphates are found at a ratio of 1:4 at a physiological pH of 7.4. Phosphate is an important anion in the body and is involved with a variety of biochemical and physiological functions. Mg^{2+} and other cations, including Ca^{2+}, are found associated with phosphate compounds. In anhydrides and esters, phosphate is always negatively charged, and the terminal phosphate group is always partially protonated.

Examples of anhydrides and esters of phosphate in the body include inositol 1,4, 5-trisphosphate (IP_3), an important regulator of calcium release from intracellular stores; ATP, the major energy currency of the body; and phosphatidylcholine, a constituent of cell membranes. DNA and RNA are polymers based on phosphate ester monomers. A variety of enzymatic activities are controlled by alternate phosphorylation and dephosphorylation of proteins by cellular kinases and phosphatases. The metabolism of all major metabolic substrates is dependent on the functioning of phosphate as a cofactor in a variety of enzymes and as the principal reservoir for metabolic energy in the form of ATP, creatine phosphate, and phosphoenolpyruvate.

Another important role of phosphate in the body is based on the fact that neutral molecules are soluble in lipid and will pass through membranes. Because phosphates are ionized at physiological pH, phosphorylation of molecules such as glucose causes the trapping of phosphorylated molecules within cells. The majority of phosphate in the body is found in bone where it combines with calcium to form hydroxyapatite, $Ca_{10}(OH)_2(PO_4)_6$, the principal inorganic compound found in the skeleton. Phosphate is also important in the control of acid–base balance in the body; the urinary excretion of phosphate as $H_2PO_4^-$ versus HPO_4^{2-} is one mechanism for regulation of acid–base balance.

PHYSIOLOGICAL OR METABOLIC FUNCTIONS OF CALCIUM AND PHOSPHORUS

Both calcium and phosphate serve numerous roles in the body. These include roles as diverse as their structural role in formation of bone mineral, the regulation of enzyme activity by reversible phosphorylation of specific amino acid residues in the protein, the role of calcium as a second messenger in the cell, and the formation and hydrolysis of energy-rich phosphate bonds in ATP to fuel muscle contraction.

CALCIUM AS A SECOND MESSENGER

Increased Cytosolic Ca^{2+}

Almost all the calcium within cells is bound within organelles such as the endoplasmic reticulum (ER), the nucleus, and other membrane-bound compartments. Consequently, the free calcium in cell cytosol is only about 10^{-7} mol/L, compared to an extracellular concentration of 10^{-3} mol/L, thereby creating a 10,000-fold chemical gradient for Ca^{2+} across cell membranes. A relatively large increase in cytosolic Ca^{2+} concentration can be caused by very small changes in the release of Ca^{2+} from intracellular sites or in its transport across the cell membrane. Changes in intracellular Ca^{2+} concentrations in response to cell-surface binding of peptide hormones or growth factors (first message) can act as a second messenger to elicit a variety of cellular phenomena, as summarized in Box 32-1.

Ligand binding to cell surface receptor proteins can result in the stimulation of the enzyme phospholipase C and in hydrolysis of phosphatidylinositol to diacylglycerol and inositol 1,4,5-triphosphate (IP_3) in the cell membrane. Increased cytosolic IP_3 causes the subsequent release of intracellular Ca^{2+} stores. Depolarization of excitable cells, such as heart muscle and nerve terminals, causes an opening of calcium-selective membrane channels, as well as the release of Ca^{2+} from internal sources, mainly from the ER. The subsequent rise in free cytosolic Ca^{2+} concentration triggers muscle contraction or secretion of neurotransmitters.

Box 32-1

REGULATION OF SELECTED CELLULAR ACTIVITIES BY INTRACELLULAR CALCIUM

- Excitation–contraction coupling in muscle
- Neurotransmitter release
- Microtubule assembly
- Membrane permeability to K^+ and Ca^{2+}
- Exocrine and endocrine gland secretion of hormones
- Cell division and reproduction
- Cell-to-cell communication
- Certain enzyme activities (e.g., phosphorylase kinase)
- Chromosome movement
- Initiation of DNA synthesis

Calcium-Dependent Trigger Proteins in Cells

Cytosolic Ca^{2+} can bind to cellular Ca^{2+}-binding proteins, including calmodulin, a ubiquitous cytosolic protein that can activate cellular kinases and other enzymes, and troponin C, a muscle protein that is bound to actinomycin contractile fibers. Binding of Ca^{2+} to Ca^{2+}-dependent proteins such as calmodulin causes a conformational change in the protein. This activation of the protein by Ca^{2+} binding causes subsequent activation of calmodulin-dependent enzymes that can then directly or indirectly alter cellular activity, as illustrated in Figure 32-2.

Removal of the Ca^{2+} Stimulus

Cell recovery following stimulation of cellular activity by increased cytosolic concentrations of Ca^{2+} can involve a variety of cellular mechanisms that work to remove the stimulus by lowering Ca^{2+} concentrations. This can be accomplished by buffering free Ca^{2+} via molecular sequestration involving calcium-binding proteins, by physical compartmentalization of Ca^{2+} through uptake into cellular organelles, and by removal of excess Ca^{2+} from the cell through pumping Ca^{2+} out of the cell via energy-dependent Ca^{2+} pumps found on the plasma membrane.

ROLE OF CALCIUM IN ACTIVATION OF OTHER PROTEINS

Ca^{2+} binding to some proteins can affect cellular activity without first causing a conformational change in the Ca^{2+}-dependent protein. For example, cellular Ca^{2+} concentrations can control biological activity by facilitating the conversion of inactive proenzymes to active enzymes. This process is illustrated by considering some of the enzymes involved in digestion and blood clotting.

Phospholipase A_2

This enzyme has a strong, predetermined fold that generates a rather immobile cavity for Ca^{2+} binding. Therefore, the binding of Ca^{2+} to phospholipase A_2 has little effect on the

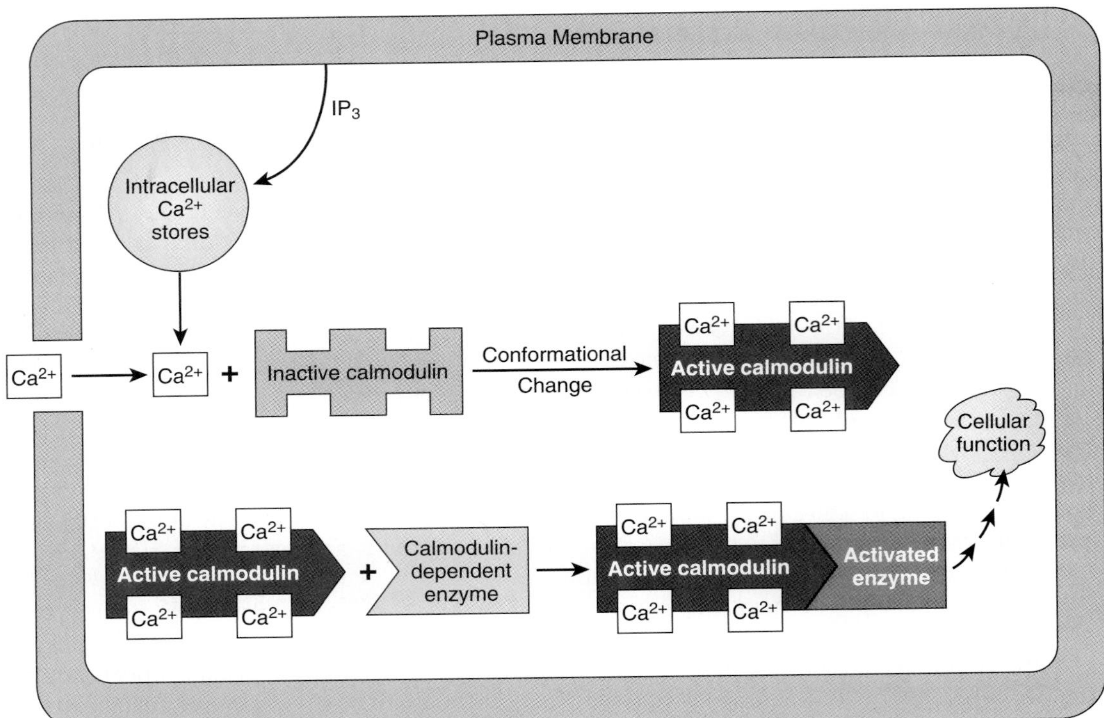

Figure 32-2 The general scheme for activation of Ca^{2+}-dependent enzymes by calcium binding to calmodulin. The concentration of free intracellular Ca^{2+} can be increased by inositol triphosphate (IP_3)–dependent release of Ca^{2+} from intracellular stores and/or increased influx of Ca^{2+} across the plasma membrane in response to a signal initiated in the plasma membrane by binding of a hormone or growth factor to its receptor. Calcium ions bind to calmodulin, a ubiquitous cellular calcium-binding protein, resulting in a conformational change in this protein. The Ca^{2+}-dependent alteration of calmodulin structure exposes a region of the protein that can now bind to and activate a calmodulin-dependent target enzyme. The activation of the enzyme subsequently results directly or indirectly in a change in cellular function. The Ca^{2+} signal is turned off by lowering the cytosolic Ca^{2+} concentration by sequestering free Ca^{2+} or pumping the Ca^{2+} out of the cell via plasma membrane Ca^{2+}-ATPase pumps.

conformation of the protein. In the case of phospholipase A_2, Ca^{2+} is needed to hold the phosphate group of the phospholipid substrate in a suitable location for hydrolysis of the *sn*-2 ester linkage. Arachidonic acid is derived from membrane phospholipids by the action of phospholipase A_2, and this reaction acts as the rate-limiting step in prostaglandin synthesis, as described further in Chapter 18.

Calpains

Calpains are Ca^{2+}-dependent proteinases that contain calmodulin-like domains with EF-hand binding sites. Calpains are nonlysosomal, intracellular proteases present in both the cytoplasm and nucleus of mammalian cells and are active at neutral pH. Calpain proteinase complexes consist of an approximate 80-kDa catalytic subunit and an approximate 30-kDa regulatory subunit. In the presence of a calpain activator protein, which also is a Ca^{2+}-binding protein, physiological concentrations of Ca^{2+} result in the dissociation and activation of the calpain complex. Progressive binding of Ca^{2+} to the calpain complex is linearly related to the dissociation of the two subunits, which reaches completion when all eight Ca^{2+}-binding sites of calpain (four per subunit) are occupied. Moreover, the activity of the catalytic subunit itself also is enhanced in the presence of physiological concentrations of Ca^{2+} (Reverter et al., 2001; Michetti et al., 1997).

Blood-Clotting Enzymes

In the case of the blood-clotting enzymes, Ca^{2+} has a dual role. Ca^{2+} binds to membrane phospholipids via the negative charge associated with the phospho moiety of the phospholipid and also plays a role in promoting cross-linking by binding to Gla or hydroxyaspartate residues in pro–blood-clotting enzymes.

Annexins

Annexins are a family of Ca^{2+}- and phospholipid-binding proteins. These proteins have a unique architecture that allows them to dock onto membranes in a Ca^{2+}-dependent reversible manner. Annexins are found both inside and outside of cells and act as membrane scaffold proteins involved in membrane–membrane and membrane–cytoskeleton interactions. They are involved in the mediation of Ca^{2+}-regulated exocytotic events, certain aspects of endocytosis, and in stabilization of specific domains of organelle and plasma membranes (Rescher and Gerke, 2004). For example, annexin A2 molecules in smooth muscle cell membranes organize lipid rafts, which are glycosphingolipid- and cholesterol-rich (detergent-insoluble) membrane microdomains. Annexin A2 in association with an S100A10 subunit may also be involved in mediating the transport of plasma membrane proteins (such as sucrase–isomaltase, an intestinal brush-border enzyme, and TRPV5 and TRPV6, which are transient receptor potential cation-channel subfamily V members that function as calcium transporters) to the cell surface, either within the biosynthetic pathway or upon recycling of the channels through an endosomal recycling organelle.

CALCIUM AND PHOSPHORUS AS COMPONENTS OF MINERALIZED TISSUE

Mineral Composition of Bone and Teeth

The skeleton is an important reservoir for minerals in the body. Approximately 99% of the body's calcium, 80% to 90% of the phosphates, 70% of magnesium, and 40% to 50% of sodium are found in bone (Driessens and Verbeeck, 1990). The mineral component of bone is largely calcium and phosphate. In the body, calcium is found mainly as the calcium phosphate compound hydroxyapatite. Forty-seven percent of skeletal weight is dry, fat-free bone, with 26% of the dry, fat-free bone weight contributed by calcium.

The skeleton is made up of two macroscopically recognizable types of bone tissue: cortical bone and trabecular bone. Approximately 80% of the skeleton is composed of dense cortical bone; the remainder is composed of sponge-like trabecular bone that is found mostly in the axial skeleton and the ends of long bones. Trabecular bone is a frequent site of osteoporotic bone fracture and is particularly sensitive to calcium deficiency due to its relatively high rate of turnover. Compact bone consists mainly of extracellular substance or matrix; about 40% of the weight of the bone matrix is due to the presence of organic (nonmineral) components, primarily of type I collagen. Degradation products of type I collagen that are present in plasma or excreted in urine (e.g., deoxypyridinium or N-telopeptide region of collagen) can be used as markers of the rate of bone resorption.

The hard outer layer of teeth is composed of enamel, which is 96% (by weight) inorganic matter, 3% water, and 1% organic matter. The inner dentine layer of the tooth is composed of 70% mineral, 20% organic matter, and 10% water. The major inorganic constituents of teeth are calcium and phosphate. The turnover of calcium in teeth is negligible.

Calcium-Binding Proteins in Bone

The most abundant noncollagenous protein (NCP) produced by bone cells is osteonectin, a 32-kDa phosphorylated glycoprotein, which accounts for approximately 2% of the total protein in developing bone and has a high affinity for binding calcium and hydroxyapatite (Termine, 1993). Its function in bone may be associated with proliferation of osteoblasts (bone-forming cells) and matrix mineralization. This protein can also be found in platelets and nonskeletal tissues that are rapidly proliferating. The best-studied Ca^{2+}-binding protein in bone is osteocalcin. Osteocalcin (also known as bone Gla-protein, BGP) is a 6-kDa, bone-specific, Gla-containing NCP protein in which Ca^{2+} binding occurs via the Gla side chains. Vitamin K is required for the posttranslational modification of glutamate residues of preosteocalcin to Gla residues. Another Gla-protein, matrix-Gla-protein (MGP), is a 9-kDa NCP found in bone and cartilage and also in other tissues in the body. Both osteocalcin and MGP are structurally similar, but the functions of these proteins are unknown. Osteocalcin and MGP production in bone is enhanced by 1, 25-dihydroxyvitamin D [$1,25(OH)_2D$], and serum osteocalcin is used as a biochemical marker of bone turnover.

IMPORTANT BIOLOGICAL FUNCTIONS OF PHOSPHATE

Oxidative Phosphorylation to Form ATP

ATP serves as a common intermediate between cellular processes that generate free energy, such as glycolysis and respiration, and processes that consume free energy. Important cellular processes that require free energy (such as biosynthesis, contraction and motility, and active transport) depend largely on the energy released from splitting the energy-rich phosphate bond of ATP. Most catabolic pathways appear to be regulated by the energy state or the phosphorylation potential of the cell. AMP and ADP often serve as stimulatory regulators of catabolic reactions, whereas ATP often acts as an inhibitor of regulatory enzymes controlling the rate of catabolic pathways. Biosynthetic reactions are also regulated by AMP, ADP, and ATP, particularly the pathways leading to fuel storage in the form of glycogen and fat.

HPO_4^{2-} and $H_2PO_4^-$ as an Acid–Base Buffer System

It is crucial for the body to maintain acid–base balance within narrow limits. One of the major ways in which large changes in H^+ concentration are prevented is by buffering. The body's buffers, which are primarily weak acids, are able to take up or release H^+ so that changes in pH are minimized. Phosphate is an effective buffer in the body. If H^+ ions are added to the extracellular fluid, they will combine with HPO_4^{2-} to form $H_2PO_4^-$ (Rose, 1984). Conversely, if H^+ ions are lost from the extracellular fluid, H^+ will be released from $H_2PO_4^-$.

DNA and RNA

The hidden plan for an organism's development lies within information-containing elements called genes that are carried by chromosomes in the nucleus of a cell. Genetic instructions are coded within the DNA of the genes and are transcribed into messenger ribonucleic acid (mRNA) molecules that can be translated in the extranuclear compartment into functional proteins. Ribosomal RNAs and transfer RNAs are also necessary for protein synthesis. Both DNA and RNA are linear polymers of nucleotides linked together by covalent phosphodiester linkages that join the 5′-carbon of one nucleotide to the 3′-carbon of the next to form a sugar-phosphate backbone.

Phospholipids

Phospholipids are small molecules that resemble triacylglycerols because they are composed of fatty acids and glycerol. However, in phospholipids the glycerol is joined to only two fatty acids and the remaining site on glycerol is joined to a phosphate group, which in turn is linked to another small hydrophilic compound such as ethanolamine, choline, or serine. The fatty acid chains provide a hydrophobic tail for phospholipid molecules, whereas the phosphate-linked polar head group provides a hydrophilic head. As ionic amphiphiles, phospholipids aggregate or self-assemble when mixed with water, but because of the two pendant alkyl chains present in phospholipids and the unusual mixed charges in their head groups, micelle formation is unfavorable relative to a bilayer structure. Phospholipid molecules spread out to form thin films on water, with the hydrophobic tails facing away from the water and the hydrophilic heads in contact with the water. The structural basis of cell membranes is based on two such phospholipid films aligned tail-to-tail in sandwich fashion, creating a lipid bilayer.

Metabolic Trapping of Substrates

Neutral molecules can pass more readily across cell membranes than charged molecules can. Phosphorylation of substrates can result in the metabolic trapping of the phosphorylated compounds within the cell. For example, vitamin B_6 vitamers are released from food during the process of digestion. Nonspecific phosphatases in the intestine hydrolyze the 5′-phosphate of these vitamers, allowing passage of the vitamin into the enterocyte via a nonsaturable, passive absorption process. After absorption, the vitamers can be phosphorylated and thus retained (Leklem, 1996).

Nucleotides, Creatine Phosphate, and Other Phosphoesters

The principal forms of purine and pyrimidine compounds in cells are nucleotides, which consist of nucleosides (purine or pyrimidine bases attached to β-D-ribose or β-D-2-deoxyribose) that have one or more phosphate groups esterified to the sugar moiety (usually to the 5′-carbon). The most abundant nucleotide in normal cells is adenosine 5′-triphosphate (ATP). The major purine derivatives in cells are the adenosine and guanosine triphosphates and diphosphates, certain coenzymes or "activated" compounds that contain adenosine phosphate moieties, nucleotide derivatives such as guanosine diphosphate (GDP)–mannose, and, of course, DNA and RNA, which are polymers synthesized from nucleotide precursors including ATP and guanosine triphosphate (GTP). The major pyrimidine derivatives in cells are the uridine, cytidine, and thymidine triphosphates and diphosphates, nucleotide derivatives [such as uridine diphosphate (UDP)-glucose and cytidine diphosphate (CDP)-choline] that act as substrates for various reactions, DNA (containing deoxycytidine and deoxythymidine residues), and RNA (containing uridine and cytidine residues).

Synthesis of purine and pyrimidine nucleotides is regulated by the concentrations of nucleotides in the cell. For example, the rate-limiting step in de novo purine synthesis is the reaction catalyzed by 5-phosphoribosyl pyrophosphate (PRPP) glutamyl aminotransferase (see Chapter 14, Fig. 14-14), which is strongly regulated by inosine 5′-monophosphate (IMP), guanosine monophosphate (GMP), and adenosine monophosphate (AMP).

Nucleotide triphosphates are required for synthesis of the active forms of a number of substrates and coenzymes for enzymatic reactions. These include synthesis of phosphate-containing "activated" metabolic intermediates such as 3′-phosphoadenosine 5′-phosphosulfate (PAPS) as well as a number of nucleotide diphosphate derivatives such as UDP-glucuronide. Phosphate esters of sugars and their derivatives play major roles as intermediates in metabolism of glucose and other carbohydrates. These phosphate esters are formed mainly by ATP-requiring reactions that transfer a phosphate group from ATP to the sugar with release of free ADP.

Coenzymes are molecules that are associated with enzymes and are essential for their catalytic functions. Coenzymes generally participate in reactions as carrier molecules that transfer chemical groups to other molecules. Some coenzymes contain AMP moieties contributed by ATP in the coenzyme synthetic pathway; these include nicotinamide adenine dinucleotide (phosphate) [NAD(P)], flavin adenine dinucleotide (FAD), and coenzyme A. Other coenzymes such as pyridoxal phosphate (PLP), flavin mononucleotide (FMN), and thiamine diphosphate (TPP) are phosphate esters of vitamin precursors. In addition to the AMP moiety, NADP and coenzyme A contain additional phosphate groups esterified to the 2′- and 3′-positions, respectively, of the adenosine moiety. The negatively charged phosphate groups present in these coenzymes are involved in interactions with their apoenzyme binding sites, and the 2′-phosphate of NADP allows enzymes to discriminate between NAD(H) and NADP(H) (Alberts et al., 1989). Coenzymes are discussed in more detail in Chapters 24, 25, and 26.

Creatine phosphate is a high-energy phosphate ester that plays a special role in muscle during work. The hydrolysis of ATP provides the energy for driving a large number of biochemical reactions. In addition, both ADP and ATP are powerful effectors of many enzymes. Therefore, the concentration and ratios of the adenine nucleotides are tightly controlled, and ATP cannot be increased to provide a reservoir of available energy. As an alternative, the muscle stores large amounts of high-energy phosphate as creatine phosphate. Creatine phosphate is used to replenish ATP levels by transfer of the phosphate group from creatine phosphate to ADP in a reaction catalyzed by

Nutrition Insight

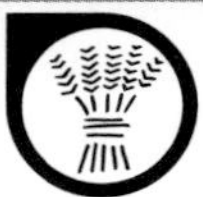

Sulfate: An Important Physiological Anion With Similarities to Phosphate

Sulfate is analogous to phosphate in many ways in that it forms esters with various organic compounds. Inorganic sulfate is converted to 3′-phosphoadenosine-5′-phosphosulfate (PAPS), which serves as the sulfate donor for synthesis of glycosaminoglycans (e.g., chrondroitin sulfate and heparin sulfate), sulfolipids (e.g., cerebroside sulfate), and sulfation of many endogenous compounds (e.g., catecholamines and hydroxysteroids) and exogenous compounds (dietary phenols and catechols) as a mechanism for enhancing their excretion. In addition, like phosphate, inorganic sulfate is an important electrolyte.

The major source of inorganic sulfate for humans is from degradation of sulfur amino acids, but significant amounts of sulfate may be present in foods and drinking water. Estimates of sulfate intake from various sources are approximately 2.8 g per day (29 mmol/day) from sulfur-containing compounds, mainly methionine and cyst(e)ine, in foods; approximately 0.8 g per day (8 mmol/day) from sulfate in drinking water and beverages; and approximately 0.85 g per day (9 mmol/day) from inorganic sulfate in food. Therefore, approximately 64% of the body's sulfate is derived from metabolism of sulfur amino acids, whereas about 36% comes from inorganic sulfate present in foods, beverages, and drinking water. It is assumed that sulfate requirements are met when recommended intakes of sulfur amino acids are met, and that no inorganic sulfate, per se, is required in the diet. Adverse effects of excess sulfate ingestion include osmotic diarrhea and ulcerative colitis. Because high concentrations of sulfate give water an odor and off taste, most people limit their intake of water with high levels of sulfate. The U.S. Environmental Protection Agency (EPA) recommends an upper limit of 250 mg/L for drinking water, but this is not enforced and some public water sources in the United States do have sulfate levels greater than 500 mg/L.

creatine kinase. (See Chapter 20 for more detail about the role of creatine phosphate in exercising muscle.)

Signaling Molecules: Cyclic AMP, Cyclic GMP, and Inositol Triphosphate

A more recently recognized function of nucleotides and their derivatives is their role as mediators of key metabolic processes. For example, 3′,5′-cyclic AMP (cAMP) functions as a second messenger in hormone-mediated control of glycogenolysis and glycogenesis. Cyclic 3′,5′-GMP (cGMP) also serves as an intracellular messenger by activating a specific protein kinase that phosphorylates target proteins in the cell. In the eye, cGMP acts directly on sodium channels in the plasma membrane of the rod cells. In the absence of a light signal, cGMP is bound to the sodium channel, keeping it open. In the presence of light, a series of reactions occur that lead to an increase in cGMP phosphodiesterase, which hydrolyzes cGMP to 5′-GMP. The drop in cGMP allows the sodium channel to close. In this way, the light signal is converted into an electrical signal.

GTP and GDP bound to G-proteins play a critical role in the signaling mechanism of G-protein-coupled receptors in the plasma membrane. The exchange of GDP for GTP in activation of the G-protein, or the hydrolysis of GTP to GDP in the inactivation of the G-protein, regulates activity of adenylate cyclase, which is also located on the inner surface of the plasma membrane (see Chapter 19, Fig. 19-10).

Inositol triphosphate (IP_3) couples receptor activation at the plasma membrane to Ca^{2+} release from a calcium-sequestering compartment in the cell interior. Phosphatidylinositol (PI) in the cell membrane is converted by a phosphorylation reaction (PI kinase) into the polyphosphatidylinositols: phosphatidylinositol 4-phosphate (PIP) and phosphatidylinositol 4, 5-bisphosphate (PIP_2). Activation of a cell-surface receptor activates a G-protein in the cell membrane that in turn activates phospholipase C, which cleaves PIP_2 to form IP_3 and diacylglycerol. IP_3 is a water-soluble molecule that stimulates the release of Ca^{2+} from intracellular stores. Diacylglycerol can be further cleaved to yield arachidonic acid, which can be used to synthesize prostaglandins and other signaling molecules, or it can activate protein kinase C, which is a Ca^{2+}-dependent enzyme. (See Chapters 18 and 19 for more detail about these signaling processes.)

Reversible Covalent Modification of Proteins

Many protein molecules have two or more slightly different conformations available to them, and, by shifting reversibly from one to the other, protein molecules can alter their function. A common mechanism employed by the cell to control the shape of certain proteins involves covalent modification by transfer of a phosphate group from ATP to a serine, threonine, or tyrosine residue in the protein, forming a covalent linkage. The alternate phosphorylation and dephosphorylation of proteins via protein kinases and phosphatases is an important cellular control mechanism. (See Chapters 12 and 19 for more discussion of the role of phosphorylation in the regulation of enzyme activities.) In addition, ATP-driven conformational changes in membrane-bound proteins can act as pumps to cause the influx or efflux of ions from a cell. For example, the Na^+,K^+-ATPase in the cell membrane pumps 3 Na^+ into the cell and 2 K^+ out of the cell during each cycle of conformational change driven by ATP-mediated phosphorylation (see Chapter 34, Fig. 34-2).

HORMONAL REGULATION OF CALCIUM AND PHOSPHATE METABOLISM

To maintain homeostasis and supply the mineral needs of the body, calcium and phosphate absorption by the intestine and reabsorption by the kidney, and bone mineral turnover are coordinately regulated by the hormones $1,25(OH)_2D$ (also called calcitriol), parathyroid hormone (PTH), and calcitonin, as summarized in Figure 32-3. A fourth hormone, parathyroid hormone–related protein (PTHrP), which is produced by several different cell types, has been identified recently and shown to cause hypercalcemia in patients with certain cancers. However, the physiological role of PTHrP is not well understood.

PARATHYROID HORMONE

PTH is a peptide hormone that is produced in the parathyroid gland and acts on certain cells through PTH receptors on the cell surface. The biologically active form of PTH is a single-chain polypeptide of 84 amino acids; however, only the first 31 amino acids of PTH are essential for biological activity. The parathyroid gland contains a membrane protein (extracellular calcium-sensing receptor) that acts as a sensor of plasma-ionized calcium levels (Chattopadhyay et al., 1996). A drop in ionized calcium in the blood is detected by the calcium sensor, leading to an increase in PTH secretion. The multiple actions of PTH ultimately lead to an increase in calcium in the extracellular fluid, creating a negative feedback regulatory loop.

Bone and kidney are the primary target organs for PTH. The peptide hormone interacts with specific receptors on the plasma membrane of bone cells (osteoblasts) and tubular kidney cells to stimulate cAMP production. Cyclic AMP acts as a second messenger to activate certain enzymes, such as protein kinases, which trigger a cascade of biochemical events that ultimately result in expression of the physiological actions of PTH. Increased plasma PTH concentrations are detected by renal PTH receptors, causing the kidneys to rapidly increase the rate of renal calcium reabsorption (which decreases urinary calcium loss) and decrease the rate of phosphate reabsorption (which increases urinary phosphate loss). PTH also increases the activity of the renal 25-hydroxyvitamin D 1α-hydroxylase that converts the biologically inactive vitamin D metabolite 25-hydroxyvitamin D [25(OH)D] into the active hormonal form of vitamin D, $1,25(OH)_2D$.

There are no PTH receptors in the intestine, but the PTH-mediated increase in circulating

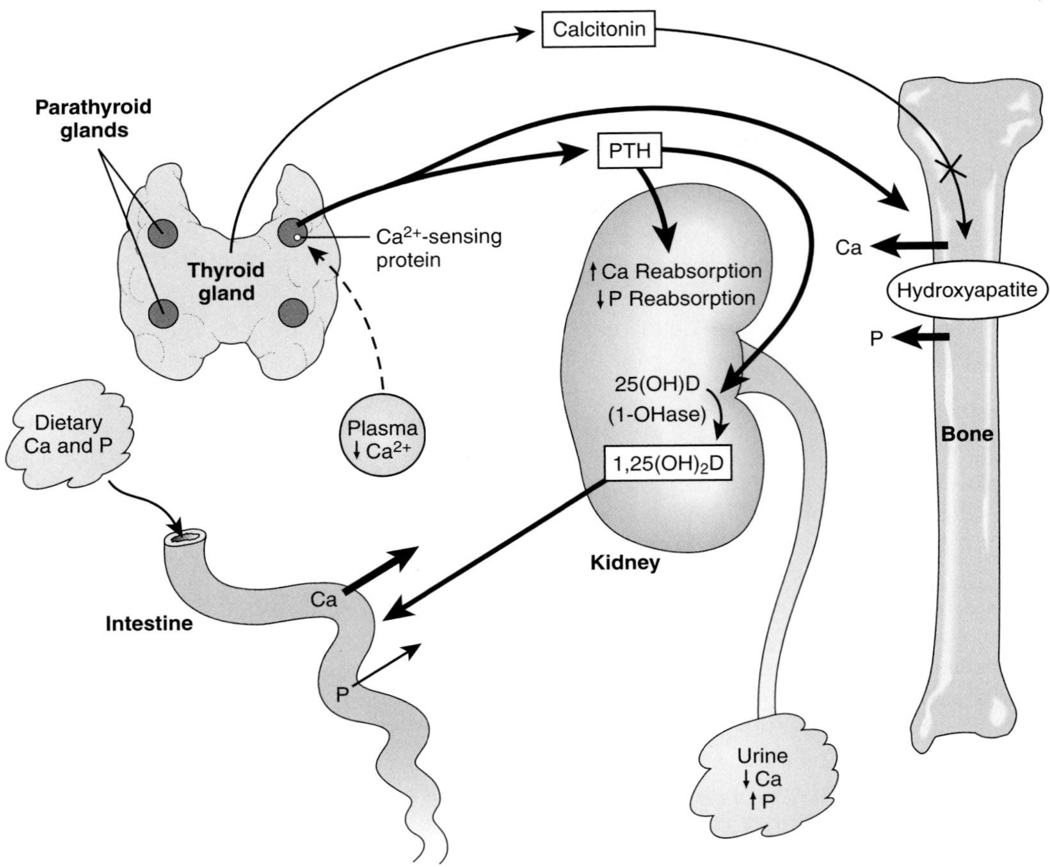

Figure 32-3 Hormonal control of calcium and phosphate metabolism. Calcium and phosphate homeostasis is maintained by the coordinated actions of three organ systems: intestine, kidney, and bone. A fall in plasma ionic Ca^{2+} level is detected by a calcium-sensor protein in the parathyroid glands that subsequently causes an increased secretion of the peptide hormone PTH from the parathyroid glands. Elevated levels of PTH in the plasma activate PTH receptors in the kidneys as well as in bone osteoblasts. The renal effect of PTH is to cause an immediate increase in renal calcium reabsorption and a decrease in renal phosphate reabsorption. PTH also has a delayed effect on calcium and phosphate metabolism by stimulating the activity of the renal 1α-hydroxylase (1-OHase) that converts inactive 25(OH)D to the active vitamin D metabolite $1,25(OH)_2D$. The primary action of $1,25(OH)_2D$ is to significantly increase intestinal calcium absorption and, to a lesser extent, phosphate absorption. In addition, $1,25(OH)_2D$ can also promote bone resorption by stimulating the production of osteoclasts.

Elevations of plasma ionic Ca^{2+} brought about by these changes in calcium flux serve as a signal to create a negative feedback loop by removing the stimulus to the calcium-sensing protein in the parathyroid gland and promoting a drop in PTH secretion. Hypercalcemia also stimulates the secretion of calcitonin from the thyroid gland. Calcitonin interacts with calcitonin receptors on osteoclasts and inhibits bone resorption.

25(OH)D, 25-Hydroxyvitamin D; *$1,25(OH)_2D$,* 1,25-dihydroxyvitamin D; *PTH,* parathyroid hormone.

$1,25(OH)_2D$ leads to a vitamin D receptor–dependent increase in intestinal calcium and phosphate absorption. Despite the fact that PTH plays an important role in bone resorption, no PTH receptors are found on bone-resorbing cells called osteoclasts (Mundy, 1993). PTH produces a bone-resorbing effect by stimulating expression of RANKL (RANK [receptor activator of NF-κB] ligand) and decreasing osteoprotegerin (OPG) production by preosteoblast cells

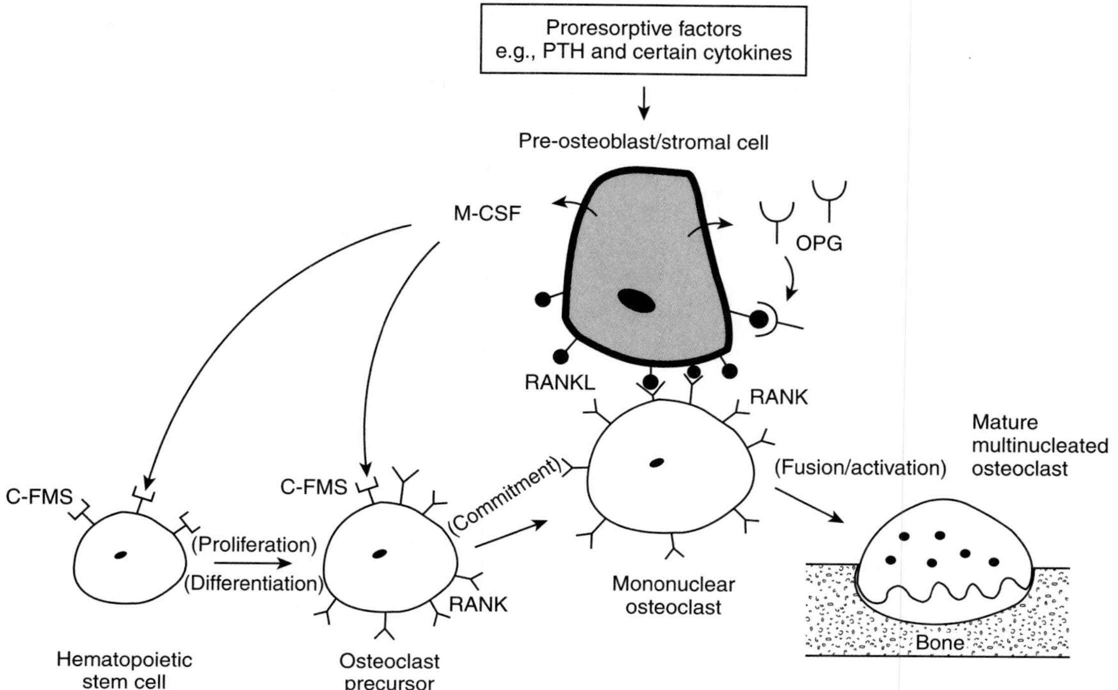

Figure 32-4 Osteoblast-mediated regulation of osteoclastogenesis. Various pro-resorptive factors (e.g., cytokines TNF-α and IL-1, PTH, and 1,25(OH)$_2$D) stimulate the production of macrophage-colony stimulating factor (M-CSF) by preosteoblast/stromal cells. M-CSF binds to its receptor (c-Fms) on osteoclast precursor cells leading to an expansion of this cell pool. M-CSF also directly increases the production of soluble and membrane-bound RANKL (receptor activator of NF-κB ligand) by osteoblasts. RANKL binds to its receptor (RANK) on osteoclasts and is critical for the differentiation, fusion into multinucleated cells, activation, and survival of osteoclasts. OPG (osteoprotegerin) is a soluble factor produced by pre-osteoblasts that acts as a receptor decoy by binding RANKL, thereby putting a brake on osteoclastogenesis. Hormones, such as PTH, 1,25(OH)$_2$D, glucocorticoids, TGF-β, and estrogen, variously regulate RANKL and OPG to affect bone resorption activity.

in bone (Fig. 32-4). These factors work in conjunction with RANK, a receptor for RANKL that is present on osteoclasts. Receptor activation by RANKL promotes osteoclast differentiation and activation into mature active bone-resorbing osteoclasts (Khosla, 2001). Therefore, PTH is secreted in response to low calcium levels and acts to restore steady-state calcium levels by stimulating an increased flux of calcium into the plasma compartment via increased calcium absorption from the intestine, increased calcium reabsorption in the kidney, and bone mineral resorption. Hyperphosphatemia, which would result from the accompanying increased intestinal absorption and skeletal release of phosphorus is prevented by the phosphaturic effect of PTH on the kidneys.

1,25-DIHYDROXYVITAMIN D

Vitamin D can enter the circulation after synthesis in the skin or absorption from the diet. Vitamin D is transported through the body bound to a vitamin D–binding protein. This complex binds to liver cells, allowing vitamin D to enter the hepatocytes. In the liver, the vitamin D molecule may either be stored or hydroxylated at C-25. The 25(OH)D that is formed by hydroxylation leaves the liver and is bound again in the blood by the vitamin D–binding protein. 25(OH)D can then be taken up by the kidney, where it can be further hydroxylated at the C-1 position to form $1,25(OH)_2D$, the active hormone form of vitamin D. The renal conversion of 25(OH)D to $1,25(OH)_2D$ is regulated primarily by PTH.

$1,25(OH)_2D$ likely plays many roles in the body and classically acts on cells through an intracellular receptor protein called the vitamin D receptor (VDR) that is found in many different tissues. In addition, a $1,25(OH)_2D$–membrane-associated rapid response to steroid-binding protein ($1,25D_3$-MARRS) has been found on plasma membranes, and it appears to regulate the rapid nongenomic aspects of $1,25(OH)_2D$ action (Nemere et al., 2004). However, the physiological importance of these rapid vitamin D–mediated effects on cells has yet to be determined. When activated by $1,25(OH)_2D$, the nuclear VDR interacts with specific gene promoter regions in DNA and affects transcription of these vitamin D–specific genes. In the mammalian enterocyte, $1,25(OH)_2D$ increases expression of a membrane calcium channel (TRPV6, also called CaT1) (Wood et al., 2001) and calbindin D_{9K}, a 9-kDa intracellular Ca^{2+}-binding protein that facilitates the absorption of calcium (Bronner, 1998), as well as a number of other proteins probably involved with the antiproliferative effects of $1,25(OH)_2D$ (Wood et al., 2004). In addition, $1,25(OH)_2D$ increases the apical membrane Na^+-dependent phosphate transporter (Npt2) that facilitates phosphate absorption in the brush-border membrane of the enterocyte.

Osteoblasts also have vitamin D receptors and produce vitamin D–regulated proteins, such as osteocalcin. However, many of the details of how $1,25(OH)_2D$ affects bone turnover and mineralization at the molecular level remain to be determined. One effect of $1,25(OH)_2D$ on bone is to increase production of RANKL by preosteoblasts (see Fig. 32-4), thereby promoting bone resorption (Khosla, 2001). However, in intact animals supraphysiological concentrations of $1,25(OH)_2D$ are necessary for this proresorptive effect to be observed; lower concentrations of $1,25(OH)_2D$ apparently inhibit PTH-induced RANKL expression, promoting bone formation (Suda et al., 2003). (See Chapter 31 for additional information about the hormonal actions of $1,25(OH)_2D$.)

CALCITONIN

Calcitonin, synthesized by the C cells of the thyroid gland, is a polypeptide containing 32 amino acid residues, almost all of which are needed for biological activity. A rise in plasma Ca^{2+} is the strongest calcitonin secretagogue. When blood Ca^{2+} increases acutely, there is a parallel increase in calcitonin secretion, whereas an acute drop in plasma Ca^{2+} causes a decrease in calcitonin secretion. Calcitonin acts in opposition to PTH and lowers blood calcium levels. The main biological function of calcitonin is to inhibit osteoclastic bone resorption. The plasma membrane of osteoclasts has calcitonin receptors that respond to calcitonin by increasing cAMP production, which in turn mediates the actions of calcitonin, including inhibition of the movement of the pseudopod-like extensions of osteoclasts. Inactivation of calcitonin occurs primarily in the kidney.

The role of calcitonin in calcium homeostasis and skeletal metabolism has not been well established in humans, and many questions remain unanswered about the physiological significance of the hormone (Deftos, 1993). Nevertheless, the hypocalcemic effect of calcitonin has led to the use of this hormone as a drug to treat diseases associated with high rates of bone resorption and concomitant hypercalcemia, such as Paget's disease, osteoporosis, and hypercalcemia of malignancy.

PARATHYROID HORMONE–RELATED PROTEIN

PTHrP is a family of protein hormones encoded by a single gene. PTHrP peptides bind to several PTHrP receptors to bring about their effects. The N-terminal segment of PTHrP is closely related to PTH, and PTHrP can activate the PTH receptor as well as PTHrP receptors. PTHrP can be produced in an unregulated manner by various types of tumors. This unregulated production of PTHrP in some cancer patients leads to the development of the so-called humoral hypercalcemia of malignancy (Burtis, 1993). PTHrP is normally synthesized in small amounts in many tissues in the body, including skin and other epithelia, the central nervous system, many endocrine glands, islet cells, breast, uterus, and urinary bladder. Physiologically, PTHrP probably acts locally as an autocrine or paracrine hormone. When PTHrP is produced in an unregulated fashion by tumors, it acts as a systemic hormone and causes hypercalcemia via its effect on the PTH/PTHrP receptors. A midregion fragment of PTHrP has been shown to stimulate the activity of a placental calcium pump, and the carboxy-terminal region of the molecule may inhibit osteoclastic bone resorption.

OTHER HORMONES AFFECTING CALCIUM AND PHOSPHATE METABOLISM

Although PTH, 1,25$(OH)_2$D, and calcitonin are the major calcium- and phosphate-regulating hormones, several other hormones, including glucocorticoids, thyroid hormone, growth hormone, insulin, and estrogen, can also affect bone turnover and mineral metabolism (Favus, 1996).

The main effect of glucocorticoids on bone is an inhibition of osteoblastic activity, although osteoclastic activity is also impaired. There is a reduced incorporation of sulfate into cartilage and of amino acids into collagen. Glucocorticoid treatment can reduce intestinal calcium absorption. An excess of glucocorticoids can lead to hypocalcemia and PTH stimulation, which causes a reduction in renal phosphate reabsorption and increased urinary phosphate losses. In Cushing's disease or when cortisol is used to treat arthritis, glucocorticoid excess can lead to bone loss, especially of trabecular bone, and result in osteoporosis. In children, excess glucocorticoid frequently causes delayed growth and skeletal maturation.

Thyroid hormone stimulates bone resorption, and both compact and trabecular bone are lost in hyperthyroidism. Increased urinary phosphate is observed in hyperthyroid patients in association with increased serum phosphate. In hypothyroidism, the bone-mobilizing effect of PTH is impaired, leading to secondary hyperparathyroidism.

Growth hormone can stimulate the growth of cartilage and bone through the trophic action of insulin-like growth factor (IGF). Growth hormone can also stimulate the 1α-hydroxylase enzyme in the kidney, causing increased serum 1,25$(OH)_2$D levels. Levels of growth hormone and IGF decline in the aged. In senescent rats, growth hormone administration can increase calcium and phosphate absorption independent of changes in serum 1,25$(OH)_2$D (Fleet et al., 1994).

Insulin, a pancreatic hormone involved primarily with regulating glucose metabolism, also stimulates the osteoblastic production of collagen. In addition, insulin can reduce the renal reabsorption of calcium and sodium and decrease urinary phosphate losses.

Estrogen receptors have been identified in bone, and gonadal hormones are known to play an important role in maintaining bone mass. Estrogen deficiency, which occurs in women after menopause, causes an increased loss of bone mineral and is an important factor in the development of postmenopausal osteoporosis. Estrogen hormone replacement therapy in postmenopausal women reduces the rate of bone loss and the incidence of bone fracture. Hypogonadism in adult men is a risk factor for osteoporosis, which may be related to the effects of testosterone on bone resorption.

CALCIUM AND PHOSPHATE HOMEOSTASIS

Mineral balance represents the equilibrium condition in which the amount of a mineral absorbed from the diet equals the sum of all the daily losses of the mineral from the body. Because 99% of the calcium in the body is found in the skeleton, changes in calcium balance are reflected in changes in bone mass. During growth, a positive calcium and phosphate balance must be maintained to supply sufficient amounts of these minerals for bone growth. In contrast, during periods of bone loss, as occur with immobilization and commonly during aging, loss of bone calcium causes a negative calcium balance. Coordination of calcium and phosphate fluxes across the intestine, kidney, and bone maintains calcium and phosphate homeostasis in the face of marked changes in daily intakes of these minerals and of longer-term metabolic changes associated with changing calcium and phosphate needs throughout the life cycle.

INTESTINAL ABSORPTION

The unidirectional absorption of calcium or phosphate from the diet is called "true" absorption. However, there is also some obligatory mineral loss into the gastrointestinal tract, as part of digestive secretions and sloughed intestinal cells. Loss of endogenous calcium is referred to as endogenous fecal loss. The difference between true intestinal absorption and endogenous fecal loss is called "net" absorption, which is thus always lower than true absorption. Net absorption of calcium and phosphate is the nutritionally important absorbed amount that is available to build new bone, to maintain steady-state plasma levels of these minerals, and to replace any skeletal and renal losses.

True Intestinal Absorption of Calcium

The unidirectional rate of intestinal calcium absorption is regulated primarily by the circulating level of $1,25(OH)_2D$. The efficiency of true calcium absorption varies in response to the dietary calcium intake and throughout the lifespan as a function of metabolic need. Fractional calcium absorption is highest in infancy (~60%) and decreases to about 25% in young adults, except for rises during early puberty and during the last two trimesters of pregnancy (Institute of Medicine [IOM], 1997). Aging is associated with a gradual decline in intestinal calcium absorption (Avioli et al., 1965), which may reflect both an age-dependent decline in the plasma $1,25(OH)_2D$ concentration and an intestinal resistance to the action of the active hormone (Pattanaungkul et al., 2000; Wood et al., 1998).

Mechanism of Calcium Transport in the Intestine

Kinetic studies of calcium transport suggest that there are two distinct pathways for calcium absorption in the intestine (Bronner, 1988). One pathway represents an active, energy-dependent, transcellular pathway, with limited capacity, that is under hormonal regulation. The second absorption pathway is a nonsaturable, energy-independent, concentration-dependent, paracellular transport pathway that is not regulated. The active, saturable, transcellular transport pathway is found mainly in the duodenum and proximal jejunum, is regulated by $1,25(OH)_2D$, and involves the vitamin D–dependent membrane channel protein TRPV6/CaT1, the cytosolic calcium-binding protein calbindin D, and the basolateral Ca^{2+}-ATPase. Quantitatively, the most important site of calcium absorption in the intestine is the ileum, due to the relatively long sojourn of calcium in this segment of the intestine. It has been shown in humans that removal of the ileum has a more devastating effect on calcium absorption than removal of the jejunum. Although calcium can also be absorbed by the colon, this segment of the intestine apparently plays a minor role in the overall economy of calcium absorption in humans. However, in rats, the cecum has a high rate of vitamin D–dependent calcium absorption, which increases during dietary calcium deficiency (Nellans and Goldsmith, 1983).

The paracellular calcium transport pathway is present throughout the intestine. In humans with normal serum $1,25(OH)_2D$ (~50 ng/L), 63% and 74% of calcium absorption from meals containing 120 and 300 mg (3 and 7.5 mmol) of calcium, respectively, occurred by the vitamin D–dependent transport route (Sheikh et al., 1988). However, three fourths of the observed increase in total calcium absorption that occurred due to ingestion of the higher calcium-containing meal was by way of a vitamin D–independent (passive) transport pathway. In other words, the vitamin D–responsive, saturable calcium absorption pathway is nearly saturated at relatively low dietary calcium intakes. Calcium absorption will continue to increase with higher calcium intakes due to the vitamin D–independent, concentration-dependent paracellular absorption pathway. The total amount of calcium absorbed from the intestine represents the sum of the saturable, carrier-mediated calcium transport process and the nonsaturable concentration-dependent process.

The molecular details of transcellular calcium transport are still not fully understood. A simplified model of the molecular details of calcium transport across the enterocyte is shown in Figure 32-5. Conceptually, the

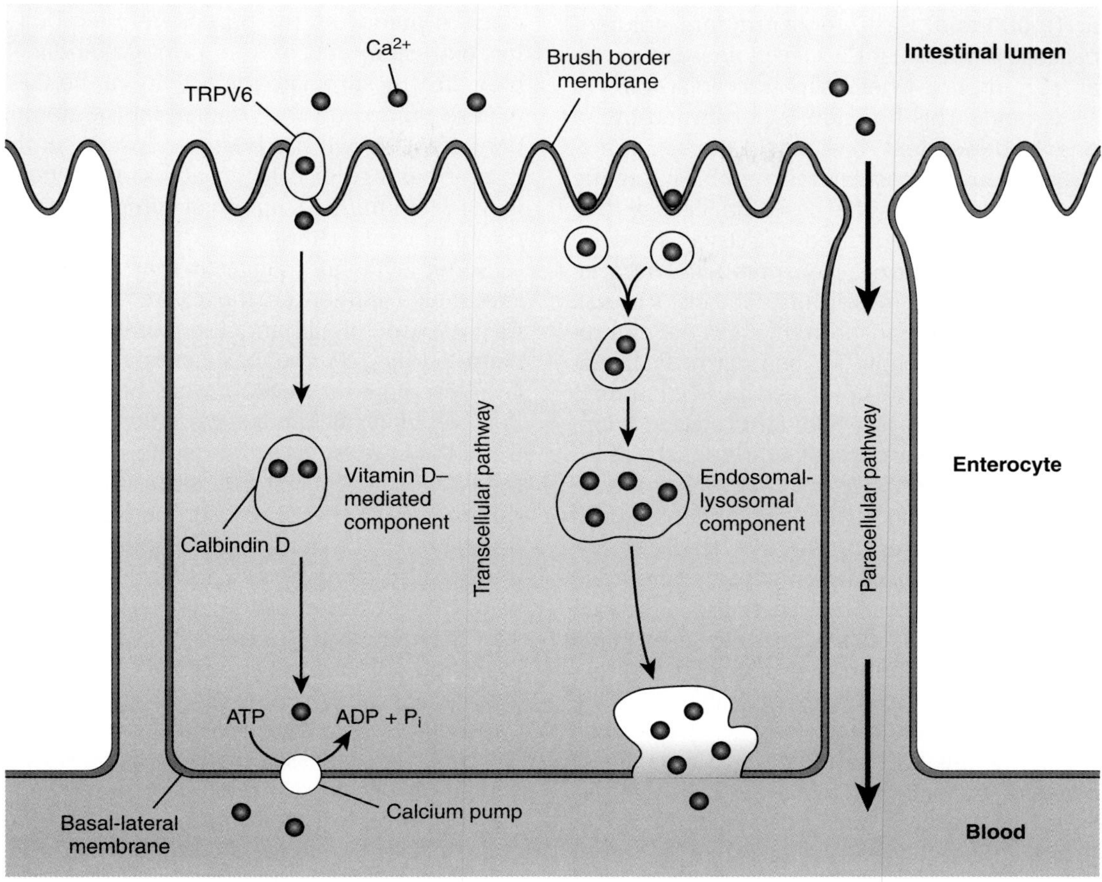

Figure 32-5 Model of calcium-transport pathways across the intestine. Calcium crosses the intestine by two possible routes. One pathway is the paracellular transport pathway, which is characterized by a nonsaturable, energy-independent, concentration-dependent mode of calcium transport. The paracellular calcium-transport pathway probably occurs between the absorptive cells and is not hormonally regulated. The second pathway is the transcellular transport pathway, which is characterized by a saturable, energy-dependent, limited capacity mode of transport across the enterocyte. The calcium transcellular transport pathway is regulated primarily by 1,25$(OH)_2$D via a genomic mechanism that regulates the production of the brush-border calcium channel TRPV6; the cytosolic mobile calcium buffer calbindin D; and the basolateral membrane Ca^{2+}-ATPase exporter pump. The coordinated vitamin D–regulated actions of TRPV6 as a gatekeeper to regulate cellular calcium influx and of calbindin D as a chaperone protein to deliver calcium for export to the ATP-dependent calcium pumps on the basolateral membrane efficiently increase the absorption of dietary calcium to help maintain serum calcium concentrations in the face of low dietary calcium intake or increased calcium need. Some evidence suggests that calcium may also be transported through the cell in endosomal and lysosomal vesicles and exit from the cell via the process of exocytosis. The relative quantitative importance of this putative transcellular calcium transport pathway process and the details of its regulation are unknown.

transport of any minerals across the intestinal cell must involve mechanisms that allow the ionic form of the mineral to traverse three formidable cellular barriers: (1) the brush-border membrane, (2) the aqueous cell cytosol, and (3) the basolateral membrane. In the case of calcium, two additional important constraints are present. First, the final step in the process of transport out of the enterocyte requires that calcium be transported "uphill" against a 10,000-fold Ca^{2+} concentration gradient because intracellular Ca^{2+} levels are maintained at 10^{-7} mol/L, whereas extracellular Ca^{2+} is 10^{-3} mol/L. This function is performed by an energy-dependent calcium pump (Ca^{2+}-ATPase) on the basolateral membrane of the enterocyte. Second, because intracellular free Ca^{2+} concentration is used by cells as a second messenger to control a large number of intracellular events vital to cell function and survival, Ca^{2+} vectorially transported across the enterocyte must somehow be compartmentalized. This function may be served by the vitamin D–dependent protein calbindin D. In addition, some evidence suggests that Ca^{2+} may be physically sequestered inside endosomal and lysosomal vesicles during its absorptive sojourn through the enterocyte (Nemere, 1992).

Studies in isolated brush-border membrane vesicle preparations have shown that the rate of calcium transport across the intestinal brush-border membrane is greater in vitamin D–replete compared with vitamin D–deplete animals (Fontaine et al., 1981). However, the molecular details of how vitamin D status alters calcium transport across the brush-border membrane are not well understood. According to the liponomic theory, which has been postulated to explain the effects of vitamin D on calcium transport across the brush-border membrane, vitamin D–dependent changes in membrane lipid composition and membrane fluidity are responsible for altering the rate of calcium transport across the membrane (Fontaine et al., 1981). The characteristics of calcium movement across the brush border are consistent with the notion of a vitamin D–regulated calcium carrier protein being present in the membrane. This putative brush-border membrane calcium carrier may be the calcium transporter TRPV6/CaT1 (Peng et al., 1999), which is regulated by 1,25$(OH)_2$D (Van Cromphaut et al., 2001; Wood et al., 2001).

The increased rate of calcium absorption observed in response to vitamin D treatment is associated with an increased synthesis of the vitamin D–dependent cytosolic protein calbindin D. Calbindin is believed to act as an intracellular calcium "ferry" that facilitates the diffusion of calcium across the aqueous cytosol and delivers ionic calcium to the ATP-dependent calcium pumps on the basolateral membrane for extrusion out of the cell. Calbindin D may directly stimulate the activity of the Ca^{2+}-ATPase pumps on the basolateral membrane (Walters, 1989). It has been proposed that the rate of passage of calcium across the cytosol is the rate-limiting step in calcium absorption (Bronner et al., 1986).

Some evidence suggests that vitamin D status also influences the expression of the Ca^{2+}-ATPase mRNA and the number of calcium pumps on the basolateral membrane (Wasserman et al., 1992). It has been argued, however, that calcium exit from the enterocyte is not the primary rate-limiting step controlling the efficiency of intestinal calcium absorption (Bronner et al., 1986). Part of the transcellular transport of calcium in the intestine may involve trafficking and compartmentalization of calcium by an endosomal–lysosomal pathway (Nemere and Norman, 1988). According to this theory, calcium enters the cell by endocytosis in primary endosomes formed at the cell surface. The calcium in these endosomal vesicles is then passed on to lysosomes from which the calcium can then exit from the cell via the process of exocytosis. However, there is little direct evidence as yet demonstrating that exocytosis of calcium accounts for the bulk of vectorially transported calcium across the enterocyte. Additional experiments based on modern molecular biological techniques will be necessary to demonstrate more definitively the important regulatory step(s) in intestinal calcium transport.

Intestinal Absorption of Phosphate

Phosphate absorption in humans has been shown to be linearly related to phosphate intake over a wide range of phosphate intakes (Lee et al., 1981a). Approximately 60% to 70% of phosphate is absorbed from a typical mixed diet, making phosphate absorption about twice as efficient as calcium absorption. Phosphate absorption is influenced by vitamin D status, although to a less marked degree than calcium absorption. Administration of 1,25$(OH)_2$D directly increases phosphate absorption in humans (Ramirez et al., 1986). In rats, 1,25$(OH)_2$D increases phosphate absorption in all segments of the small intestine but with the major effect in the jejunum (Lee et al., 1981b).

Little is known about the molecular details of intestinal phosphate absorption. The preferred transport form is HPO_4^{2-} (Lee et al., 1981a). The kinetics of phosphate uptake in vitro by isolated intestinal brush-border vesicle preparations is consistent with the suggestion that phosphate is transported across the apical membrane of the enterocyte by a carrier-mediated mechanism. Transport of phosphate into the intestinal cell is by an active, Na^+-dependent pathway mediated by the apical membrane phosphate transporter protein (Peerce et al., 1993). However, intestinal adaptation to a low phosphate diet in VDR knockout mice indicate that this process is independent of the action of $1,25(OH)_2D$ on the nuclear VDR (Segawa et al., 2004). Like calcium, phosphate is absorbed by both a saturable and a nonsaturable transport pathway.

Endogenous Fecal Loss of Calcium and Phosphate

Approximately 3.5 mmol/day (140 mg/day) of calcium enters the intestinal lumen in secretions, but about 29% of this is reabsorbed, so that the minimum endogenous fecal calcium is usually 2.5 mmol/day (100 mg/day) (Heaney and Recker, 1994). Reports of endogenous fecal losses of phosphate have been variable, but reported losses are usually lower than those observed for endogenous fecal calcium losses.

URINARY EXCRETION

Urinary Calcium

Because of the binding of plasma calcium to albumin, a significant portion of plasma calcium cannot enter the renal filtrate. Nevertheless, approximately 240 mmol (9.7 g) of calcium are filtered each day by the kidneys. Urinary calcium excretion is usually only 2.5 to 6 mmol/day (100 to 240 mg/day) for normal individuals; this represents only about 1% to 2.5% of the calcium filtered by the kidney. Approximately 50% of excreted calcium is in the free Ca^{2+} form, and the remainder is complexed with small anions such as sulfate, phosphate, citrate, and oxalate. Patients with renal stones (nephrolithiasis) frequently have

Clinical Correlation

Dietary Calcium Intake and Renal Calcium Stones

Many patients with calcium kidney stones (nephrolithiasis) have idiopathic hypercalciuria. In about 90% of these patients with excess urinary calcium losses the condition is characterized by elevated active calcium absorption by the intestine, normal serum calcium and parathyroid hormone (PTH) levels, and an elevated serum $1,25(OH)_2D$ level. The vitamin D hormone elevation may be the primary defect, and it is associated with a renal phosphate leak (Vosburgh and Peters, 1987). For reasons that are not completely understood, renal stone formers exhibit a lower bone mineral content. Possible explanations are the hypophosphatemia, hypercalciuria, and elevated serum $1,25(OH)_2D$ accompanied by a low calcium intake. Unfortunately, maintenance of stone formers on a low calcium diet may exacerbate bone loss. Epidemiological evidence suggests that low calcium diets are associated with an increased risk of nephrolithiasis, probably due to a greater degree of oxalate absorption from the intestine when diets are low in calcium (Curhan et al., 1993). Conversely, use of calcium supplements also has been shown to be associated with increased risk of stone formation.

hypercalciuria (urinary calcium greater than 250 mg/day) and kidney stones composed of calcium oxalate crystals.

Mechanisms of renal-tubular calcium transport are similar to those found in the intestinal epithelium. Active calcium transport is found in the distal convoluted tubule and possibly the distal proximal tubule, and it involves an apical membrane calcium channel protein (TRPV5) (Hoenderop et al., 2000) and a vitamin D–dependent, 28-kDa protein, calbindin D_{28K}. Paracellular calcium transport, by which most (70%) renal calcium reabsorption occurs, takes place in the proximal tubule, the thick ascending limb of the loop of Henle, and the connecting and collecting ducts. Urinary calcium and urinary sodium losses are frequently found to be positively associated because these two minerals share a common resorption mechanism in the proximal renal tubule; paracellular transport of calcium in the proximal tubule is mediated by solvent drag in parallel to the paracellular movement of water and sodium.

There are large diurnal fluctuations in the rate of urinary calcium excretion, due mainly to the calciuretic effect of various food components. Dietary calcium intake has a positive, but weak, relationship with urinary calcium excretion. Approximately 8% of the increment in dietary calcium intake over the usual range of dietary calcium intakes of 300 to 1,600 mg/day is lost in the urine (Lemann, 1993). Dietary intake of simple sugars and protein can increase urinary calcium losses. For example, it has been calculated that for each 50-g increment in daily protein intake, an additional 1.5 mmol (60 mg) of calcium is lost in the urine (Kerstetter and Allen, 1990). The mechanism of protein-induced hypercalciuria involves a reduction of renal calcium reabsorption mediated in part by the sulfur amino acid content of the protein. The metabolism of these amino acids causes the generation of an acid (fixed anion, SO_4^{2-}) load, which can inhibit renal calcium reabsorption.

Conversely, there is an inverse relationship between dietary phosphate intake and urinary calcium. Elevations in serum phosphate decrease serum ionic calcium and thereby cause an increase in PTH synthesis, which in turn increases calcium reabsorption in the kidney. In addition, phosphate can affect renal tubular calcium transport independent of PTH (Lau et al., 1982). This anticalciuretic effect of phosphate has practical implications, because the high phosphate content of meat causes a considerable blunting of the usual hypercalciuric effect of consuming a high-protein diet (Hegsted et al., 1981).

Urinary Phosphate

The kidneys provide the primary route for phosphate loss from the body and play an important role in the regulation of phosphate homeostasis (Lee et al., 1981a). The great majority of plasma inorganic phosphate is filtered at the renal glomerulus. The kidney can efficiently regulate plasma phosphate levels, and the fractional excretion of filtered phosphate by the kidneys varies from 0.1% to 20%. Approximately 40% of the total phosphate reabsorption in the kidney occurs within the first few convolutions of the proximal tubule, and 60% to 70% has occurred by the time the ultrafiltrate reaches the last segment of the cortical superficial nephrons.

The transport of phosphate in the renal tubules occurs by two processes: one is dependent on sodium and the other is not. In the proximal tubule, phosphate is reabsorbed by an active, Na^+-dependent phosphate transport system. Brush-border membranes from proximal tubule cells have a Na^+- and pH-dependent, saturable phosphate transport system mediated by the Npt2 phosphate transporter, whereas phosphate transport across the basolateral membranes is via a passive transport process only. The primary regulator of the rate of renal phosphate reabsorption is the plasma phosphate concentration. In vitro studies in porcine and monkey renal cell lines have shown that treatment of cells with a low-phosphate medium causes a two- to sevenfold increase in the rate of phosphate transport (Escoubet et al., 1989). This autoregulatory phenomenon is probably a widespread process that occurs in most, if not all, cell types.

The chief hormonal regulator of renal phosphate reabsorption is PTH. Plasma PTH is positively correlated with urinary excretion of phosphate and negatively affects reabsorption of phosphate by both the Na^+-dependent and Na^+-independent phosphate transport pathways. In addition, renal phosphate handling is also affected indirectly by PTH inhibition of proximal and distal bicarbonate reabsorption. The full molecular details of PTH action on renal phosphate transport are not precisely understood. Presumably, the steps involve transmembrane transduction of the cell-surface signal initiated by PTH binding to its receptor and induction of an intracellular second messenger.

BONE RESORPTION AND FORMATION

Bone is composed of collagen fibers, noncollagenous proteins, and deposited minerals—primarily as hydroxyapatite. Crystals of hydroxyapatite are found in and on the collagen fibers and in the ground substance (glycoproteins and proteoglycans) of bone. Longitudinal bone growth occurs in children until closure of the epiphyses during adolescence. However, bone mineral density continues to increase until about the age of 30 years (Recker et al., 1992), and bone tissue is continually remodeled throughout life. This remodeling process occurs at localized sites in both cortical and trabecular bone. Although the entire bone calcium pool turns over on average every 5 to 6 years, a given local bone surface on trabecular bone may undergo complete remodeling once every 2 years. However, the rate of remodeling varies greatly among specific bones, with the lumbar vertebral bone turning over most rapidly. Two important cell types in bone are the osteoblasts, involved in bone formation, and the osteoclasts, involved in bone resorption.

Bone Formation

The activity of osteoblasts in bone determines the rate of bone matrix (collagen and ground substance) deposition. Osteoblasts originate from a local-precursor mesenchymal stem cell that can be stimulated to undergo proliferation and differentiate into preosteoblasts and then into mature osteoblasts. Osteoblasts, which have cellular receptors for PTH, estrogen, and $1,25(OH)_2D$, regulate the flux of calcium and phosphate in bone and presumably mediate the deposition of hydroxyapatite in bone tissue. Osteoblasts are usually found in clusters of 100 to 400 cells per bone-forming site along the bone surface; osteoblasts lay down bone matrix that is initially unmineralized (Baron, 1993). During bone formation and mineralization, most of the osteoblasts differentiate into flattened cells that line or cover the bone surface. Some osteoblasts become trapped within the mineralized matrix and differentiate into osteocytes that are connected with each other and with the lining cells on the surface by cytoplasmic processes. Because the plasma membrane of the osteoblast is rich in the enzyme alkaline phosphatase, biochemical measures of bone-specific serum alkaline phosphatase are used as a convenient marker of bone formation rates. Osteoblasts also synthesize a vitamin D–dependent protein called osteocalcin, which is presumably important to the function of the skeleton. Serum osteocalcin also is used as a biochemical marker of bone formation.

In vitamin D deficiency there is a defect in mineralization of bone matrix. A cardinal feature of osteomalacia (adult vitamin D deficiency) is an overabundance of unmineralized bone matrix that is evident on histological staining of bone biopsies.

Bone Resorption

The activity of osteoclasts in bone determines the rate of bone breakdown. The osteoclast has a monocytic–phagocytic cell lineage and is characterized histologically as a giant multinucleated cell that is usually found in contact with a calcified bone surface within a lacuna (hole) that is the result of its own resorptive activity (Baron, 1993). Usually, only one to five osteoclasts are found associated with one of these resorptive cavities. The contact zone of the osteoclast with the bone is characterized by the presence of a ruffled border on the osteoclast. The ruffled border portion of the osteoclast plasma membrane is surrounded by a ring of contractile proteins, which serve to attach the cell to the bone surface and seal off the subosteoclastic bone-resorbing compartment.

The attachment of the cell to the bone matrix is performed by integrin receptors that bind to specific sequences in matrix proteins (Baron, 1993). Lysosomal enzymes are actively secreted via the ruffled border of the osteoclast into the sealed-off extracellular bone-resorbing compartment. The osteoclast also secretes collagenase as well as protons to acidify the bone-resorbing compartment. The acid environment dissolves the hydroxyapatite crystals, and the secreted enzymes break down the bone matrix. The dissolution of bone helps maintain calcium and phosphate concentrations in the plasma. End products of bone matrix breakdown, such as hydroxyproline and amino-terminal collagen peptides, are excreted in the urine and can be used as convenient biochemical measures of bone resorption rates.

The mode of regulation of osteoclast activity is complex. Osteoclasts have receptors for calcitonin, and their activity is decreased by calcitonin. However, osteoclasts also respond to other regulatory signals, such as

PTH, 1,25$(OH)_2$D, and prostaglandin E_2, via osteoblast mediation. Figure 32-4 illustrates the role of the OPG/RANKL/RANK system in the process of osteoclastogenesis (Khosla, 2001). In brief, various proresorptive cytokines (e.g., tumor necrosis factor alpha [TNF-α] and interleukin 1 [IL-1]) stimulate the production of macrophage-colony stimulating factor (M-CSF) by preosteoblast/stromal cells. M-CSF binds to its receptor (c-Fms) on osteoclast precursor cells leading to an expansion of these precursor cells. M-CSF also directly increases the production of soluble and membrane-bound RANKL (RANK ligand) by osteoblasts. RANKL binds to its receptor (RANK) on osteoclasts; ligand binding stimulates the differentiation, fusion into multinucleated cells, activation, and survival of osteoclasts. OPG (osteoprotegerin) is a soluble factor produced by pre-osteoblasts that acts as a receptor decoy and binds RANKL, thereby putting a brake on osteoclastogenesis. Hormones, such as PTH, 1,25$(OH)_2$D, glucocorticoids, TGF-β, and estrogen, variously regulate RANKL and OPG to affect bone resorption activity.

Bone-Remodeling Cycle: "Coupled" Bone Formation and Bone Resorption

After the osteoclasts have finished removing a certain amount of bone, they are replaced by bone-forming osteoblasts that then proceed to replace the excavated bone material. The total resorptive period at a given bone site takes approximately 40 days to complete. About 1 week after the resorptive phase, the formation activity of osteoblasts begins and continues for about 145 days (Melsen and Mosekilde, 1988). Therefore, the remodeling of bone involves a recurring cycle of skeletal events involving the coordinated activities of osteoblasts and osteoclasts. This process of bone remodeling can be divided into four phases: activation, resorption, formation, and a resting phase.

Activation is the process by which osteoclast precursor cells are transformed into osteoclasts. Prostaglandins or lymphokines produced by cells at the bone site probably act to attract osteoclasts to the specific area of bone destined to be resorbed. Bone resorption and formation are mediated by the activity of osteoclasts and osteoblasts. During the process of remodeling, a "coupling" is somehow established between bone resorption and bone formation that ensures the overall integrity of the skeleton despite the ongoing bone-remodeling process. Factors leading to the uncoupling of bone formation and bone resorption are important in the development of osteoporosis.

Because the process of bone remodeling is relatively long, clinical trials evaluating potential therapeutic agents (such as calcium supplementation) on bone mass need to be carried out for at least 2 to 3 years. Otherwise, simple transient effects on bone remodeling caused by the intervention and due to the temporary disruption of the normal remodeling process would not be distinguished from changes that would have a sustained long-term benefit on the skeleton (Heaney, 1994).

DIETARY SOURCES, BIOAVAILABILITY, AND RECOMMENDED INTAKES FOR CALCIUM AND PHOSPHORUS

DIETARY SOURCES OF CALCIUM AND PHOSPHATE

The great majority of calcium in American diets is supplied by dairy products. If milk-based products are excluded from the diet or used in limited amounts, then the relatively low calcium content of many foods makes it difficult to achieve recommended amounts of dietary calcium. Some relatively rich vegetarian sources of calcium include calcium-set tofu and certain green vegetables. More calcium-fortified foods, such as orange juice, have appeared on the market in response to recommendations to increase calcium intakes to prevent osteoporosis (National Institutes of Health [NIH], 1994).

Phosphate is found widely distributed in foodstuffs. In general, food sources high in protein (meats, milk, eggs, and cereals) are also high in phosphate. Dairy products, meat, fish, poultry, and eggs supply about 70% of typical phosphate intakes in the United States (Life Sciences Research Office, 1989). Phosphate in meat is found mainly as intracellular organic compounds, which are mostly hydrolyzed in the gastrointestinal tract to release inorganic

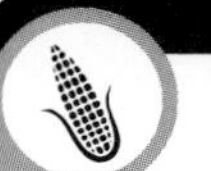

Food Sources

Food Sources of Calcium

Dairy Products

300 mg per ½ cup ricotta cheese
415 mg per 8-oz container yogurt, skim milk, plain
275 mg per 8-oz container yogurt, whole milk, plain
200 to 225 mg per 1 oz cheese (Swiss, provolone, mozzarella, cheddar)
275 mg per cup milk, whole
305 mg per cup milk, skim

Tofu

170 mg per 3 oz tofu (firm, prepared with calcium sulfate)
95 mg per 3 oz tofu (soft, prepared with calcium sulfate)

Vegetables

160 mg per ½ cup collards, cooked
130 mg per ½ cup spinach, cooked
90 mg per ½ cup kale, cooked
75 mg per ½ cup baked beans
60 mg per ½ cup beans (navy, great northern)
175 mg per ½ cup rhubarb, cooked

Leavening Agents

340 mg per 1 tsp baking powder, double-acting

Fish (with bones)

325 mg per 3 oz sardines, canned
180 mg per 3 oz salmon, canned

Data from U.S. Department of Agriculture/Agricultural Research Service (USDA/ARS) (2005) USDA Nutrient Database for Standard Reference, Release 18. USDA/ARS, Washington, DC. Retrieved November 15, 2005, from www.ars.usda.gov/ba/bhnrc/ndl.

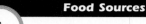

Food Sources

Food Sources of Phosphorus

Meats

200 to 220 mg per 3 oz pork, fresh, cooked
170 to 200 mg per 3 oz beef, lean, cooked
200 mg per 3 oz chicken breast, cooked
200 to 285 mg per 3 oz fish (halibut, haddock, swordfish, salmon, tuna), cooked
415 mg per 3 oz sardines, canned

Leavening Agents

456 mg per 1 tsp baking powder, double-acting

Dairy Products

200 to 225 mg per ½ cup cheese, ricotta
140 to 170 mg per ½ cup cheese, cottage
245 mg per cup milk, skim
220 mg per cup milk, whole
355 mg per 8-oz container yogurt, skim milk, plain
215 mg per 8-oz container yogurt, whole milk, plain

Legumes

180 mg per ½ cup lentils, cooked
140 mg per ½ cup chickpeas, cooked
105 to 125 mg per ½ cup beans (pinto, kidney, black, white, chickpeas), cooked

Grains

205 mg per ½ cup wheat flour, whole grain
145 mg per ½ cup cornmeal, whole grain
125 mg per ½ cup white rice, dry

Data from U.S. Department of Agriculture/Agricultural Research Service (USDA/ARS) (2005) USDA Nutrient Database for Standard Reference, Release 18. USDA/ARS, Washington, DC. Retrieved November 15, 2005, from www.ars.usda.gov/ba/bhnrc/ndl.

phosphate, which is available for intestinal absorption. Processed meat also contains various polyphosphates and pyrophosphates as additives.

CALCIUM AND PHOSPHATE BIOAVAILABILITY

Bioavailability refers to the fraction of a nutrient in food that is absorbed and metabolically available. Ideally, an evaluation of dietary calcium and phosphate adequacy should consider not only the quantitative aspects of consumption but also the relative bioavailability of these minerals from the diet. A variety of dietary factors have been considered to influence calcium bioavailability (Allen and Wood, 1994). From a practical perspective, however, the most important dietary factors influencing calcium absorption from food are the levels of dietary fiber, phytate, and oxalate.

Milk has long been considered to be the best dietary source of calcium. However, large segments of the population are lactose-intolerant (see Chapter 8) and may avoid milk or desire to consume only limited quantities. In recent years, investigators have utilized intrinsically incorporated, stable isotopes of calcium to study the bioavailability of calcium from various foodstuffs. Using this approach, the absorbability of calcium from several foods has been shown to be equivalent to or better than that of calcium from milk. Some low-oxalate green leafy vegetables have been shown to be sources of highly bioavailable calcium (Heaney and Weaver, 1990), but milk is clearly one of the richest sources of highly absorbable dietary calcium on a per serving basis (Fig. 32-6).

Phosphate from meat is well absorbed (greater than 70%) by humans. Little is known about the bioavailability of phosphate from different plant-based foods. Phosphate in grains is mostly in the form of phytate (myo-inositol hexaphosphate), an organophosphate compound used by plants to store phosphate. For example, more than 80% of the total phosphate in wheat, rice, and maize is found as phytate, and as much as 35% of the phosphate in mature potato tubers is in this chemical form.

DIETARY REFERENCE INTAKES FOR CALCIUM AND PHOSPHORUS

Many people in the United States do not consume recommended levels of dietary calcium (Fig. 32-7), although phosphate intakes appear quite adequate (Fig. 32-8). Recommended calcium and phosphate intakes throughout the life cycle for the American and Canadian populations were updated in 1997 by the IOM (IOM, 1997).

Adequate Intakes and Tolerable Upper Intake Levels for Calcium

With the exception of infants, current recommended intakes for calcium are based on the amount of dietary calcium that will result in maximum calcium retention, which has been determined from calcium balance studies. However, because of methodologic limitations in estimating precisely the dietary calcium intakes needed for maximal calcium retention in all age groups, an estimated average requirement (EAR) for calcium could not be derived with sufficient confidence. Therefore, rather

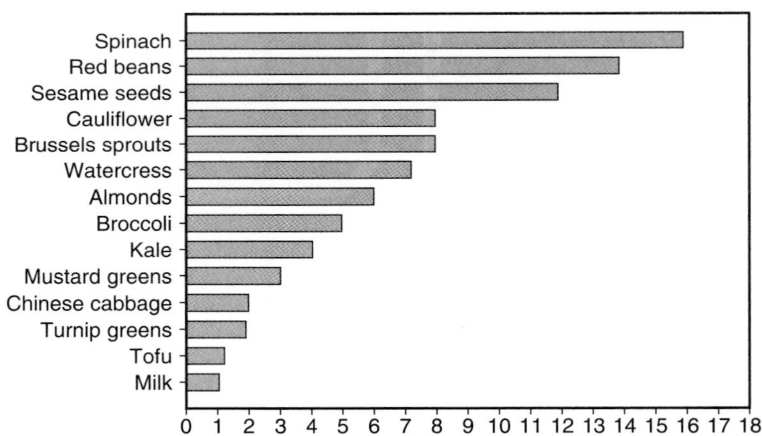

Figure 32-6 Relative bioavailability of calcium from various food sources. Shown are the estimated number of standard servings of a given food source that would need to be consumed to absorb an equivalent amount of calcium as derived from one serving of milk. The numbers of servings of each food are based on the calcium content of the food and the estimated bioavailability of calcium from that food source. Serving sizes are ½ cup, except for milk (1 cup), almonds (1 oz), and sesame seeds (1 oz). (*Data from Weaver CM, Plawecki KL [1994] Dietary calcium: adequacy of a vegetarian diet. Am J Clin Nutr 59[Suppl]:1238S-1241S.)*

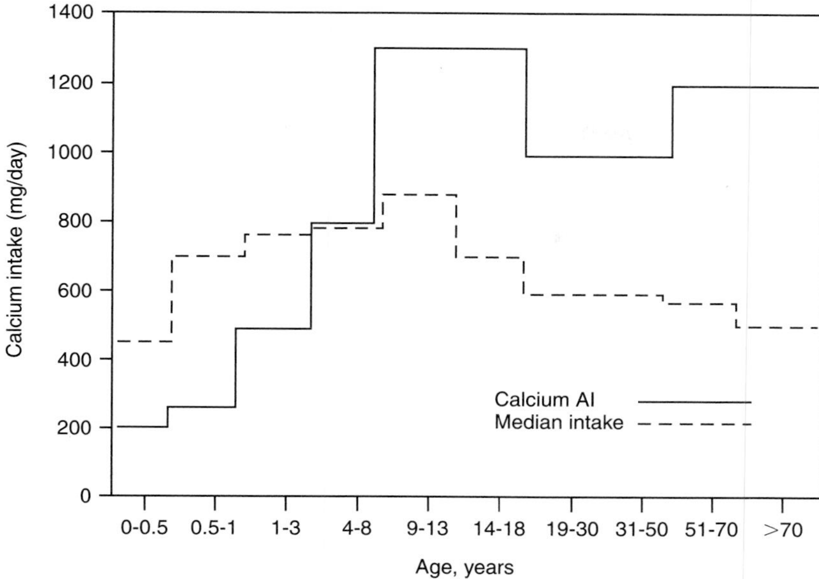

Figure 32-7 Median calcium intakes for girls and women in the United States compared with current recommended intakes for calcium. Shown are median (50th percentile) values for calcium intakes in girls and women of various ages, based on the Continuing Survey of Food Intake of Individuals (United States Department of Agriculture, 1994-1996), and the current recommended intakes of calcium (adequate intakes) for these populations, developed as dietary reference intakes (DRIs) by the Institute of Medicine (IOM, 1997).

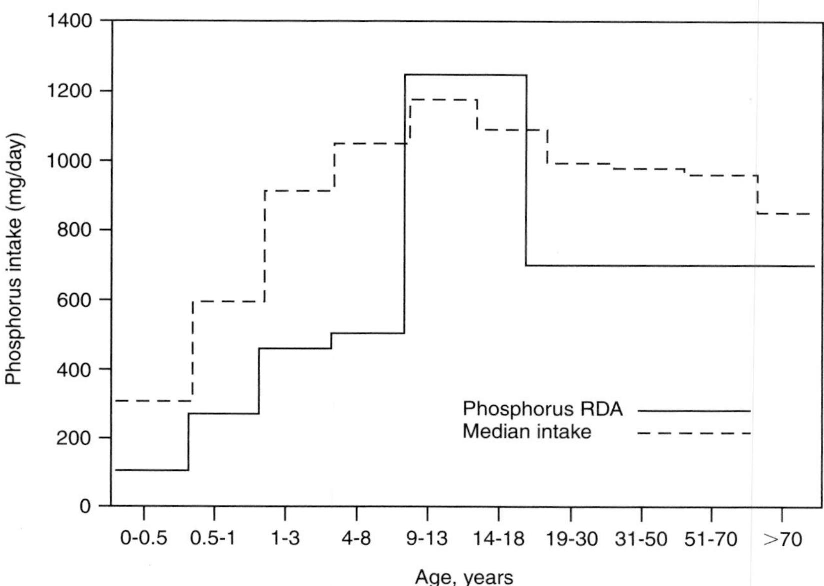

Figure 32-8 Median phosphorus intakes for girls and women in the United States compared with current recommended intakes for phosphorus. Shown are median (50th percentile) values for phosphorus intakes in girls and women of various ages, based on the NFCS Continuing Survey of Food Intake of Individuals (United States Department of Agriculture, 1994) and the current recommended intakes of phosphorus (recommended dietary allowances, RDAs) for these populations developed as dietary reference intakes (DRIs) by the Institute of Medicine (IOM, 1997).

AIs Across the Life Cycle

	mg Calcium per Day
Infants	
0 to 0.5 yr	210
0.5 to 1 yr	270
Children	
1 to 3 yr	500
4 to 8 yr	800
9 to 18 yr	1,300
Adults	
19 to 50 yr	1,000
51 to >70 yr	1,200

NOTE: No additional intake is recommended for pregnant and lactating women.
AI, Adequate intake.
Data from Institute of Medicine (IOM) (1997) Dietary Reference Intakes for Calcium, Phosphorus, Magnesium, Vitamin D, and Fluoride. National Academy Press, Washington, DC.

than the traditional calcium recommended dietary allowance (RDA), an adequate intake (AI) level was estimated for calcium pending the development of a more comprehensive database (IOM, 1997).

The AI levels of calcium for infants are based on the mean intake of calcium in breast-fed infants (IOM, 1997). The concentration of calcium in breast milk is relatively constant—approximately 264 mg/L during the first 6 months of lactation and 210 mg/L during the second 6 months of lactation. The average intake of breast milk during the first 6 months of life is 0.78 L/day; therefore, the AI was established as 210 mg of calcium per day (264 mg/L × 0.78 L/day) for up to 6 months. For the second 6 months of infancy, the AI was established based on an estimate of breast-milk intake (210 mg/day × 0.6 L/day) plus an estimate of solid food intake of calcium (140 mg/day) for a total AI of 270 mg/day. Special consideration is needed for infants fed infant formulas due to the lower bioavailability of calcium. Calcium intakes of 315 mg/day should be adequate to achieve maximal calcium retention in infants fed infant formulas during the first 6 months, and total calcium intakes of 335 mg/day are adequate for formula-fed infants who are 6 to 12 months of age.

The calcium AIs for children are 500 mg/day for 1- to 3-year-olds, 800 mg/day for 4- to 8-year-olds, and 1,300 mg/day for 9- to 18-year-olds (IOM, 1997). The AI for 4- to 8-year-old children was based on calcium balance studies in girls in this age group that showed that a mean intake of 800 to 900 mg/day resulted in mean calcium retention of 130 to 174 mg/day (~20% of intake). Because of a lack of data for young children, the AI for children 1 to 3 years of age was estimated on the basis of net accretion of approximately 100 mg calcium/day and using an estimate of 20% for the calcium absorption efficiency. During ages 9 through 18 years, calcium retention increases to a peak during the pubertal growth phase and then declines. Peak calcium accretion rates are approximately 212 mg/day in girls and 282 mg/day in boys. The AI for both males and females 9 through 18 years of age was based on balance studies showing that calcium intake in the range of 1,300 mg/day was sufficient to support the peak level of calcium retention. This peak level of recommended calcium intake is also supported by calcium supplementation trials in which maximal rates of increase in bone mineral content occurred at dietary calcium intakes near 1,300 mg/day.

The AIs for adults are 1,000 mg/day (25 mmol/day) for persons ages 19 to 50 years and 1,200 mg/day (30 mmol/day) for persons 51 years of age and older (IOM, 1997). In setting the AIs for adults, balance studies, bone mineral density, the need for calcium accretion, and calcium intake data were considered. Calcium requirements of women have been studied more extensively because women are more prone to osteoporosis, and data for women were largely used in setting the AIs for both genders. Although growth of long bones normally ceases before 19 years of age, accretion of bone mass continues for about 10 years after adult stature is achieved. The AI for adults at ages 19 to 30 years was based primarily on a limited number of calcium balance studies in women that indicated that a calcium intake of about 1,000 mg/day was adequate to allow retention of 10 mg Ca per day. Limited data were available for adults ages 31 to 50 years, but most

Life Cycle Considerations

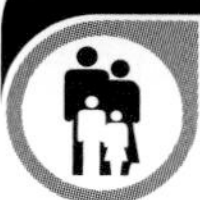

Calcium Supplementation and Osteoporosis

Osteoporosis is a multifactorial disease that is clinically characterized by low bone mass and bone pain and an increased risk of bone fracture. According to the National Health and Nutrition Examination Survey (NHANES) III, the prevalence of osteoporosis (defined as a bone mineral density that is more than 2.5 standard deviations below the mean for young adult women) in white, non-Hispanic women older than 50 years of age in the United States is between 17% and 20% (Looker et al., 1995). The prevalence of osteoporotic fracture is dramatically increased in elderly people. It has been estimated that osteoporotic bone fracture is found in about 7% of women by age 60 years and in 25% of women by age 80 years (Nordin, 1983). The age-associated increase in the occurrence of osteoporosis has enormous public health significance because of the increasing proportion of elderly individuals in the United States population; the fastest growing segment of the population are those older than 85 years old.

Several factors may be involved in the pathogenesis of postmenopausal osteoporosis, including reduced intestinal calcium absorption and increased urinary calcium loss. Some of the bone loss that is seen in elderly people can be ameliorated by calcium supplementation (Aloia et al., 1994; Reid et al., 1993; Dawson-Hughes et al., 1990). However, the role of dietary calcium in the causation and treatment of osteoporosis is still the focus of intense debate. Among the reasons for this debate is the complex nature of osteoporosis and, until recently, the low sensitivity with which bone mineral density could be measured. Certainly the rather abrupt changes in bone and calcium metabolism that accompany menopause in women cannot be attributed solely to an abrupt decrease in calcium intake or absorption.

Despite the fact that a number of investigators have noted a lack of association between current calcium intake and bone mineral density, a significant relation has been observed between an individual's lifetime history of calcium intake and peak bone mineral density. A higher bone mineral density delays the appearance of symptoms of bone loss but does not change the rate of loss (Matkovic et al., 1979). An important question, then, is to what extent high calcium intakes can maximize peak bone mass in younger adults or slow the rate of loss of bone mass with aging. In designing clinical trials to test the effects of dietary calcium or supplements on bone loss, it is essential to account for potential confounding factors such as age, menopausal status, serum estrogen levels, vitamin D status, smoking, parity, lactation history, history of oral contraceptive use, usual calcium intake, and usual level of physical activity.

data supported an intake of 1,000 mg/day or more as a plateau intake at which there is no net loss of calcium. The AI of calcium for adults ages 51 through 70 years was set at 1,200 mg/day based primarily on clinical trial data in women, which demonstrated a positive reduction of bone loss with calcium intakes greater than 1,000 mg/day, and on the assumption that needs would be somewhat higher than those of the 19- through 50-year age-group due to a fall in calcium absorption with advancing age. The AI for persons older than 70 years was also set at 1,200 mg/day because of a lack of sufficient data to estimate the intake consistent with a calcium balance plateau near zero. Overall, studies with older adults have indicated that the effectiveness of dietary calcium supplements to slow bone loss is greater for cortical-rich sites (e.g., proximal radius and femoral neck versus spine) and is greater when the usual calcium intake of the subjects is low. Menopause causes accelerated bone loss due to estrogen deficiency, but increases in calcium intake do not necessarily prevent this loss, and the IOM committee judged the evidence to be insufficient to support different AIs for women based on their menopausal or estrogen status.

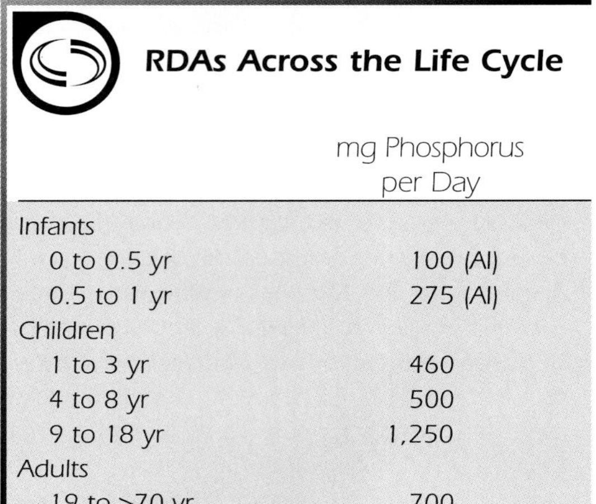

RDAs Across the Life Cycle

	mg Phosphorus per Day
Infants	
0 to 0.5 yr	100 (AI)
0.5 to 1 yr	275 (AI)
Children	
1 to 3 yr	460
4 to 8 yr	500
9 to 18 yr	1,250
Adults	
19 to >70 yr	700

NOTE: No additional intake is recommended for pregnant and lactating women.
AI, Adequate intake.
Data from Institute of Medicine (IOM) (1997) Dietary Reference Intakes for Calcium, Phosphorus, Magnesium, Vitamin D, and Fluoride. National Academy Press, Washington, DC.

The AIs for pregnant and lactating women were not increased for pregnancy and lactation. Approximately 25 to 30 g (625 to 750 mmol) of calcium is transferred by the mother to the fetus during pregnancy, and most of this occurs during the third trimester. However, the increased demand for calcium in pregnancy is compensated for by an increase in calcium absorption efficiency, which may be related to pregnancy-associated increases in circulating $1,25(OH)_2D$.

There is a very substantial demand for calcium during lactation to provide the approximately 210 mg of calcium needed daily for milk production. However, no evidence suggests that the calcium need of lactating women is increased above that of nonlactating women. The additional calcium needed for milk production is supplied by maternal skeletal stores. The loss of calcium from the skeleton is not prevented by increased dietary calcium. The loss of maternal bone mineral density that occurs during lactation is regained following weaning.

A tolerable upper intake level (UL) for calcium intake was set at 2,500 mg/day for children and adults. Very high intakes of calcium (greater than 4 g/day) have been associated with hypercalcemia and, consequently, calcium deposition in tissues and kidney failure. High calcium intakes may also increase the risk of mineral depletion in vulnerable populations due to adverse effects of calcium on iron and zinc bioavailability. The UL for calcium is a conservative estimate and provides protection for individuals who might be susceptible to adverse effects of high calcium intakes, such as patients with calcium renal stones or hyperabsorptive hypercalciuria.

Recommended Dietary Allowances and Tolerable Upper Intake Levels for Phosphorus

In contrast to the past procedure of setting recommendations for phosphorus intake to equal those for calcium on an equimass or equimolar basis, the most recent dietary reference intakes (DRIs) for phosphorus were set independent of recommended calcium intakes (IOM, 1997).

AIs were set for infants. An AI for phosphorus was set for infants in the first 6 months of life based on mean intake of phosphorus from human milk by breast-fed infants (0.78 L milk/day × 124 mg P/L milk) and is 1,200 mg/day. The AI for infants 6 to 12 months old is based on the average intake of phosphorus from human milk (75 mg/day) plus that obtained from infant foods (200 mg/day) and is 275 mg/day.

An EAR for phosphorus for children ages 1 through 3 years was based on a factorial approach and set at 380 mg/day. The sum of mean accretion of phosphorus in bone and soft tissue of growing children (54 mg/day) and an estimate of urinary excretion at intakes near the requirement (213 mg/day) was then divided by a conservative estimate of fractional phosphorus absorption (0.70) to arrive at an EAR of 380 mg/day. The RDA was calculated as the EAR + 20%, which is 460 mg/day. A similar factorial approach (summation of requirements for maintenance plus growth and correction for absorption efficiency) was used to set the EAR for children in the 4 to 8, 9 to 13, and 14 to 18-year age-groups. RDAs for these groups were set as the EAR + 20%. The RDAs are 500 mg/day for 4- to 8-year-old children and 1,250 mg/day for boys and girls who are 9 through 18 years of age.

In contrast to the factorial methodology used to derive an EAR for growing children, the EAR for adults (older than 19 years of age) was established as 580 mg/day (18.7 mmol/day) on the basis of the amount of ingested phosphorus needed to maintain serum phosphate at the lower limit of the normal range (0.87 mmol/L) (IOM, 1997). The RDA for phosphorus for adults was set as the EAR + 20% or 700 mg/day (22.6 mmol/day). Serum phosphate levels were used as the criterion of adequacy because it can be assumed that dietary phosphorus intakes are adequate to meet cellular and skeletal needs when serum phosphate levels are in the normal range. Conversely, phosphorus balance is not a good criterion of adequate intake of phosphorus because phosphate balance can be zero at an intake that is inadequate to maintain serum phosphate within a normal range.

No increase in the RDA for phosphorus was recommended for pregnant or lactating women. Although the content of phosphorus for the full-term infant (17.1 g) must be supplied by the pregnant mother, intestinal absorption of phosphorus increases during pregnancy and was judged to be adequate to offset the increased need. Likewise, increased bone resorption and decreased urinary excretion of phosphorus during lactation provide the phosphorus needed for milk production (~90 to 120 mg/day).

There is no evidence for adverse effects of high dietary phosphorus intakes in healthy humans, but a conservative estimate of the UL was made based on phosphorus intakes associated with the upper boundary of adult normal values for serum phosphate. The ULs for phosphorus are 3.0 g/day for young children (1 to 8 years of age), 4.0 g/day for older children and adults (9 to 70 years), 3.0 g/day for older adults (older than 70 years), 3.5 g/day for pregnant women, and 4.0 g/day for lactating women. The basis for setting lower ULs for older adults and pregnant women was an increased prevalence of impaired renal function in older adults and the increased absorption efficiency for phosphorus during pregnancy.

CALCIUM AND PHOSPHORUS DEFICIENCY AND ASSESSMENT OF STATUS

Calcium deficiency is difficult to assess, and many possible indicators of calcium deficiency are also indicators of vitamin D status, bone diseases, and hormonal imbalances. Phosphorus deficiency is rare and is seldom caused by a lack of phosphorus in the diet.

CALCIUM DEFICIENCY AND STATUS ASSESSMENT

In experimental animals that are severely restricted in dietary calcium (and that develop hypocalcemia), increased serum levels of PTH and 1,25$(OH)_2$D, higher fractional intestinal absorption of calcium and phosphate, and lower calcium but higher phosphate levels in urine are consistently observed. Bone resorption and turnover are also stimulated, and net loss of bone mineral ensues.

In humans, chronic calcium deficiency is difficult to assess. Measurement of serum total and ionic calcium levels is inadequate for assessment of calcium status because the plasma calcium level is tightly controlled. When observed, low total serum calcium levels are usually explainable by low levels of serum albumin, a protein that binds calcium in the plasma, rather than by a calcium deficiency. Moreover, abnormal levels of biochemical measures associated with calcium homeostasis are not necessarily proof of a dietary calcium deficiency, because vitamin D deficiency, bone diseases, and other hormonal imbalances can produce similar symptoms.

Calcium balance data provide useful information on whether the current level of calcium absorption is sufficient to replace calcium lost in urine and sweat and via endogenous intestinal secretions. Because 99% of the body's calcium store is found in bone, it is axiomatic that if an individual is in consistent negative calcium balance, then calcium is being lost from bone. However, balance studies provide no information on the extent to which bone calcium has been lost in the past. During growth, provision of sufficient dietary calcium in humans is necessary to achieve maximum levels of bone mineral density, but a positive calcium balance does not imply optimal bone mineralization (Bonjour et al., 1997).

Precise modern bone densitometric techniques can be used to monitor the response of bone mineral density to dietary intervention. The sensitivity of these techniques has improved dramatically in recent years, and use of these techniques has demonstrated the need for high calcium intakes to maximize bone growth in children and to retard bone loss in the elderly (NIH, 1994).

PHOSPHORUS DEFICIENCY AND STATUS ASSESSMENT

Dietary phosphorus deficiency is considered to occur very rarely because of the high phosphorus content of the diet, an efficient intestinal absorption of dietary phosphorus, and the ability of the kidneys to elaborate an essentially phosphorus-free urine in response to hypophosphatemia. An exception to this general rule is the premature infant who is fed human milk. Compared with the milk of other animals, human milk is relatively low in phosphorus. Despite similar caloric densities, human milk supplies only approximately 150 mg of P per L in comparison with the 1,000 mg/L supplied by cow's milk. Although human milk is a sufficient source of phosphorus for the full-term infant, the phosphorus content of mother's milk is inadequate to meet the phosphorus demand of premature infants, who have a higher rate of phosphorus deposition in the skeleton and soft tissues per unit of body size than do full-term infants. Inadequate phosphorus intake in the preterm infant causes hypophosphatemia and inadequate bone mineralization, and the symptoms of rickets develop despite an adequate vitamin D status.

Phosphorus depletion can also occur from overingestion of aluminum hydroxide antacids, which can inhibit phosphorus absorption by binding dietary phosphorus in the gut. Phosphate depletion has been induced experimentally in healthy individuals by feeding a very low phosphorus diet accompanied by antacids. Abnormalities of phosphorus homeostasis and phosphorus depletion can also occur in association with various disease states. The symptoms of phosphate depletion include a diminished concentration of intracellular organic phosphoric acid esters, such as 2,3-diphosphoglycerate (in erythrocytes) and ATP (in muscle and other cell types). In the red blood cell, 2,3-diphosphoglycerate interacts with hemoglobin to promote the release of oxygen from oxyhemoglobin. Tissue oxygen levels can be lowered as a consequence of depleted 2,3-diphosphoglycerate levels because of a shift in the equilibrium for oxyhemoglobin dissociation so that less oxygen is liberated. Additional symptoms of severe phosphorus depletion include hemolysis of red blood cells, diminished phagocytic function of granulocytes, severe muscle weakness, and markedly increased excretion of calcium in the urine.

The most commonly used index of phosphorus status is the serum phosphorus level. However, this measure of status can be an inadequate reflection of body phosphorus stores for a variety of reasons. Only 1 % of total body phosphorus is in the extracellular fluid, and plasma phosphorus is under some degree of physiological control. Plasma phosphorus is determined by the tubular reabsorptive capacity of the kidney, which in turn is regulated by the level of PTH, growth hormone, and other factors. The level of phosphorus in the plasma can be artificially elevated due to muscle and bone catabolism or acutely decreased due to rapid shifts of phosphorus into the intracellular compartment. Nevertheless, the plasma phosphate level is directly related to absorbed phosphorus and was used as a functional criterion to establish the EARs (and RDAs) for phosphorus for the adult population (IOM, 1997).

Other approaches to assessing phosphorus status are available. Intracellular phosphorus levels in red blood cells, leukocytes, and platelets have been investigated as possible indicators of phosphorus status and were found to correlate with circulating phosphorus. Urinary phosphorus levels reflect dietary phosphorus intake under normal conditions. Hypophosphaturia and hypercalciuria occur with phosphate depletion. Likewise, serum alkaline phosphatase and 1,25$(OH)_2$D may be elevated in phosphate deficiency, but these biochemical changes are not specific enough to predict body phosphorus stores accurately. Newer developments in nuclear magnetic resonance (NMR) techniques offer a powerful research tool for assessment in vivo of intracellular phosphorus levels, and whole body neutron activation analysis can be used to measure total body phosphorus in living subjects. However, these expensive and sophisticated methodologies have limited applicability, and additional approaches to the problem of assessing phosphorus status are needed.

CLINICAL DISORDERS INVOLVING ALTERED CALCIUM AND PHOSPHORUS HOMEOSTASIS

Several clinical disorders are associated with altered calcium and phosphorus homeostasis. Changes in calcium and phosphorus stores may be caused by an increase or a decrease in intestinal absorption or renal reabsorption. In addition, rapid shifts in serum phosphorus levels occur in response to several conditions that stimulate movement of phosphorus into or out of intracellular compartments.

Intestinal disorders, such as Crohn's disease and celiac disease, and intestinal resection or bypass can result in poor mineral and vitamin D absorption owing to fat malabsorption. In chronic liver disease, poor mineral absorption can occur secondary to vitamin D deficiency caused by impaired hydroxylation of vitamin D. In chronic renal failure, impairment of calcium and phosphate homeostasis is associated with the reduced renal synthesis of $1,25(OH)_2D$ and the development of secondary hyperparathyroidism.

Excessive intestinal absorption of calcium occurs in sarcoidosis, a chronic granulomatous disease, because of enhanced extrarenal $1,25(OH)_2D$ production. Elevated $1,25(OH)_2D$ also explains hyperabsorption of calcium in primary hyperparathyroidism and the hyperabsorption of calcium found in many patients with renal calcium stones (nephrolithiasis).

Hypercalcemia can be found in some cancer patients, owing to an excess production by the tumor of PTHrP. This protein is produced by some epithelial cancers and can act physiologically like PTH to increase renal calcium reabsorption and bone resorption, but its production is not under normal negative feedback control by elevated serum ionized calcium (Stewart, 1993).

Phosphate imbalance can occur in various disease states for a variety of reasons (Berner and Shike, 1988). In starvation, despite underlying phosphorus depletion, normal plasma phosphorus levels may be maintained because of increased muscle catabolism. Excessive amounts of phosphorus can be lost in the urine of uncontrolled diabetics, owing to polyuria and the development of metabolic acidosis. However, plasma phosphorus level can be normal or slightly elevated in ketotic patients due to the release of large amounts of phosphorus from intracellular sites. Recovering burn patients are at risk of hypophosphatemia due to massive diuresis. Likewise, excessive urinary phosphorus losses are also seen in patients with dysfunctions of the proximal renal tubule, such as seen in Fanconi's syndrome. In alcoholism, phosphate depletion can occur because of low dietary phosphorus, intestinal malabsorption, increased urinary losses, secondary hyperparathyroidism, hypomagnesemia, and hypokalemia.

The clinical sequel of chronic hyperphosphatemia is frequently ectopic calcification (Berner and Shike, 1988). In chronic renal failure, reduced renal function may cause hyperphosphatemia. Chronic hyperphosphatemia can be managed in these patients by limiting dietary phosphorus intake when possible and by administering oral phosphate binders containing aluminum, calcium, or magnesium salts. Hyperphosphatemia can also be seen with severe hemolysis and various endocrine dysfunctions, such as hypoparathyroidism, acromegaly, and severe hyperthyroidism.

REFERENCES

Alberts B, Bray D, Lewis J, Raff M, Roberts K, Watson JD (1989) Molecular Biology of the Cell. Garland Publishing, New York.

Allen LH, Wood RJ (1994) Calcium and phosphorus. In: Shils M, Olson J, Shike M (eds) Modern Nutrition in Health and Disease, 8th ed. Vol. 1. Lea & Febiger, Philadelphia, pp 144-163.

Aloia JF, Vaswani A, Yeh JK, Ross PL, Flaster E, Dilmanian FA (1994) Calcium supplementation with and without hormone replacement therapy to prevent postmenopausal bone loss. Ann Intern Med 120:97-103.

Avioli LV, McDonald JE, Lee SE (1965) Influence of aging on the intestinal absorption of ^{47}Ca in women and its relation to ^{47}Ca absorption in postmenopausal osteoporosis. J Clin Invest 44:1960-1967.

Baron R (1993) Anatomy and ultrastructure of bone. In: Favus MJ (ed) Primer on the Metabolic Bone Diseases and Disorders of Mineral Metabolism, 2nd ed. Raven Press, New York, pp 3-9.

Berner YN, Shike M (1988) Consequences of phosphate imbalance. Annu Rev Nutr 8: 121-148.

Bonjour J-P, Carrie A-L, Ferrari S, Clavien H, Slosman D, Theintz G, Rizzoli R (1997) Calcium-enriched foods and bone mass growth in prepubertal girls: a randomized, double-blind, placebo-controlled trial. J Clin Invest 99:1287-1294.

Bronner F (1998) Calcium absorption: a paradigm for mineral absorption. J Nutr 128:917-920.

Bronner F (1988) Gastrointestinal absorption of calcium. In: Nordin B (ed) Calcium in Human Biology. Springer-Verlag, New York, pp 93-124.

Bronner F, Pansu D, Stein WD (1986) An analysis of intestinal calcium transport across the rat intestine. Am J Physiol 250:G561-G569.

Burtis WJ (1993) Parathyroid hormone–related protein assays. In: Favus MJ (ed) Primer on the Metabolic Bone Diseases and Disorders of Mineral Metabolism, 2nd ed. Raven Press, New York, pp 99-102.

Chattopadhyay N, Mithal A, Brown EM (1996) The calcium-sensing receptor: a window into the physiology and pathophysiology of mineral ion metabolism. Endocrinol Rev 17:289-307.

Curhan GC, Willett WC, Rimm EB, Stampfer MJ (1993) A prospective study of dietary calcium and other nutrients and the risk of symptomatic kidney stones. N Engl J Med 328:833-838.

Dawson-Hughes B, Dallal G, Krall EA, Sadowski L, Sahyoun N, Tannenbaum S (1990) A controlled trial of the effect of calcium supplementation on bone density in postmenopausal women. N Engl J Med 323:878-883.

Deftos LJ (1993) Calcitonin. In: Favus MJ (ed) Primer on the Metabolic Bone Diseases and Disorders of Mineral Metabolism. Raven Press, New York, pp 70-76.

Driessens FCM, Verbeeck RMH (1990) Biominerals. CRC Press, Boca Raton, FL.

Escoubet B, Djabali K, Amiel C (1989) Adaptation to P_i deprivation of cell Na-dependent P_i uptake: a widespread process. Am J Physiol 256:C322-C328.

Favus MJ (ed) (1996) Primer on the Metabolic Bone Diseases and Disorders of Mineral Metabolism, 3rd ed. Lippincott-Raven Publishers, Philadelphia.

Fleet JC, Bruns ME, Hock JM, Wood RJ (1994) Growth hormone and parathyroid hormone stimulate intestinal calcium absorption in aged female rats. Endocrinology 134:1755-1760.

Fontaine O, Matsumoto T, Goodman DBP, Rasmussen H (1981) Liponomic control of Ca^{2+} transport: relationship to mechanism of 1,25-dihydroxyvitamin D_3. Proc Natl Acad Sci USA 78:1751-1754.

Heaney RP (1994) The bone-remodeling transient: Implications for the interpretation of clinical studies of bone mass change. J Bone Miner Res 9:1515-1523.

Heaney RP, Weaver CM (1990) Calcium absorption from kale. Am J Clin Nutr 51:656-657.

Heaney RP, Recker RR (1994) Determinants of endogenous fecal calcium in healthy women. J Bone Miner Res 9:1621-1627.

Hegsted M, Schuette SA, Zemel MB, Linkswiler HM (1981) Urinary calcium and calcium balance in young men as affected by level of protein and phosphorus intake. J Nutr 111:553-562.

Hoenderop JG, Willems PH, Bindels RJ (2000) Toward a comprehensive molecular model of active calcium reabsorption. Am J Physiol Renal Physiol 278:F352-F360.

Institute of Medicine (1997) Dietary Reference Intakes for Calcium, Phosphorus, Magnesium, Vitamin D, and Fluoride. National Academy Press, Washington, DC.

Kerstetter JE, Allen LH (1990) Dietary protein increases urinary calcium. J Nutr 120: 134-136.

Khosla S (2001) Minireview: the OPG/RANKL/RANK system. Endocrinology 142:5050-5055.

Lau K, Goldfarb S, Goldberg M, Agus ZS (1982) Effects of phosphate administration on tubular calcium transport. J Lab Clin Med 99:317-324.

Lee D, Brautbar N, Kleeman C (1981a) Disorders of phosphorus metabolism. In: Bronner F, Coburn J (eds) Disorders of Mineral Metabolism. Vol. III. Academic Press, New York, pp 284-423.

Lee DB, Walling MM, Levine BS, Gafter U, Silis V, Hodsman A, Coburn JW (1981b) Intestinal and metabolic effect of 1,25-dihydroxyvitamin D_3 in normal adult rat. Am J Physiol 240:G90-G96.

Leklem JE (1996) Vitamin B-6. In: Zeigler EE, Filer LJ Jr (eds) Present Knowledge in Nutrition. ILSI Press, Washington, DC, pp 174-183.

Lemann J (1993) Urinary excretion of calcium, magnesium, and phosphorus. In: Favus MJ (ed) Primer on the Metabolic Bone Diseases and Disorders of Mineral Metabolism, 2nd ed. Raven Press, New York, pp 50-54.

Life Sciences Research Office, Federation of American Societies for Experimental Biology (1989) Nutrition Monitoring in the United States—An Update Report on Nutrition Monitoring, DHHS Publication No. [PHS] 89-1255. U.S. Government Printing Office, Washington, DC.

Looker AC, Johnson CC Jr, Wahner HW, Dunn WL, Calvo MS, Harris TB, Heyse SP, Lindsay RL (1995) Prevalence of low femoral bone density in older U.S. women from NHANES III. J Bone Miner Res 10:796-802.

Matkovic V, Kostial K, Simonovic I, Buzina R, Brodarec A, Nordin BE (1979) Bone status and fracture rates in two regions of Yugoslavia. Am J Clin Nutr 32:540-549.

Melsen F, Mosekilde L (1988) Calcified tissues: Cellular dynamics. In: Nordin B (ed) Calcium in Human Biology. Springer-Verlag, London, pp 187-208.

Michetti M, Salamino F, Minafra R, Melloni E, Pontremoli S (1997) Calcium-binding properties of human erythrocyte calpain. Biochem J 325:721-726.

Mundy GR (1993) Bone resorbing cells. In: Favus MJ (ed) Primer on the Metabolic Bone Diseases and Disorders of Mineral Metabolism, 2nd ed. Raven Press, New York, pp 25-32.

National Institutes of Health (1994) Optimal calcium intake. NIH Consensus Development Panel on Optimal Calcium Intake. JAMA 272:1942-1948.

Nellans HN, Goldsmith RS (1983) Mucosal calcium uptake by rat cecum: identity with transcellular calcium absorption. Am J Physiol 244:G618-G622.

Nemere I (1992) Vesicular calcium transport in chick intestine. J Nutr 122:657-661.

Nemere I, Norman AW (1988) 1,25-Dihydroxyvitamin D_3-mediated vesicular transport of calcium in intestine: Time course studies. Endocrinology 122:2962-2969.

Nemere I, Farach-Carson MC, Rohe B, Sterling TM, Norman AW, Boyan BD, Safford SE (2004) Ribozyme knockdown functionally links a 1,25(OH)2D3 membrane binding protein (1,25D3-MARRS) and phosphate uptake in intestinal cells. Proc Natl Acad Sci USA 101:7392-7397.

Nordin BEC (1983) Osteoporosis with particular reference to the menopause. In: Avioli LV (ed) The Osteoporotic Syndrome. Grune and Stratton, New York, pp 13-43.

Pattanaungkul S, Riggs BL, Yergey AL, Vieira NE, O'Fallon WM, Khosla S (2000) Relationship of intestinal calcium absorption to 1, 25-dihydroxyvitamin D [1,25(OH)2D] levels in young versus elderly women: evidence for age- related intestinal resistance to 1,25(OH)2D action. J Clin Endocrinol Metab 85:4023-4027.

Peerce BE, Cedilote M, Seifert S, Levine R, Kiesling C, Clarke RD (1993) Reconstitution of intestinal Na(+)-phosphate cotransporter. Am J Physiol 264:G609-G616.

Peng JB, Chen XZ, Berger UV, Vassilev PM, Tsukaguchi H, Brown EM, Hediger MA (1999) Molecular cloning and characterization of a channel-like transporter mediating intestinal calcium absorption. J Biol Chem 274:22739-22746.

Ramirez JA, Emmett M, White MG, Fathi N, Santa Ana CA, Morawski SG, Fordtran JS (1986) The absorption of dietary phosphorus and calcium in hemodialysis patients. Kidney Int 30:753-759.

Recker RR, Davies KM, Hinders SM, Heaney RP, Stegman MR, Kimmel DB (1992) Bone gain in young adult women. JAMA 268:2403-2408.

Reid IR, Ames RW, Evans MC, Gamble GD, Sharpe SJ (1993) Effect of calcium supplementation on bone loss in postmenopausal women. N Engl J Med 328:460-464.

Rescher U, Gerke V (2004) Annexins—unique membrane binding proteins with diverse functions. J Cell Sci 117:2631-2639.

Reverter D, Strobl S, Fernandez-Catalan C, Sorimachi H, Suzuki K, Bode W (2001) Structural basis for possible calcium-induced activation mechanisms of calpains. Biol Chem 382:753-766.

Robertson WG (1988) Chemistry and biochemistry of calcium. In: Nordin BEC (ed) Calcium in Human Biology. Springer-Verlag, London, p 1-26.

Rose DB (1984) Clinical Physiology of Acid-Base and Electrolyte Disorders. McGraw-Hill, New York.

Segawa H, Kaneko I, Yamanaka S, Ito M, Kuwahata M, Inoue Y, Kato S, Miyamoto K (2004) Intestinal Na-P(i) cotransporter adaptation to dietary P(i) content in vitamin D receptor null mice. Am J Physiol Renal Physiol 287:F39-F47.

Sheikh MS, Ramirez A, Emmett M, Santa Ana C, Fordtran JS (1988) Role of vitamin D-dependent and vitamin D-independent mechanisms in absorption of food calcium. J Clin Invest 81:126-132.

Stewart AW (1993) Humoral hypercalcemia of malignancy. In: Favus MJ (ed) Primer on the Metabolic Bone Diseases and Disorders of Mineral Metabolism. Raven Press, New York, pp 169-172.

Suda T, Ueno Y, Fujii K, Shinki T (2003) Vitamin D and bone. J Cell Biochem 88:259-266.

Termine JD (1993) Bone matrix proteins and the mineralization process. In: Favus MJ (ed) Primer on the Metabolic Bone Diseases and Disorders of Mineral Metabolism, 2nd ed. Raven Press, New York, pp 21-24.

United States Department of Agriculture (1994) NFCS Continuing Survey of Food Intakes by Individuals, 1991. U.S. Department of Commerce, National Technical Information Service, Springfield, VA.

Van Cromphaut SJ, Dewerchin M, Hoenderop JG, Stockmans I, Van Herck E, Kato S, Bindels RJ, Collen D, Carmeliet P, Bouillon R, Carmeliet G (2001) Duodenal calcium absorption in vitamin D receptor-knockout mice: functional and molecular aspects. Proc Natl Acad Sci USA 98:13324-13329.

Vosburgh E, Peters TJ (1987) Pathogenesis of idiopathic hypercalciuria: A review. J R Soc Med 80:34-37.

Walters JRF (1989) Calbindin-D9k stimulates the calcium pump in rat enterocyte basolateral membranes. Am J Physiol 256:G124-G128.

Wasserman RH, Smith CA, Brindak ME, Talamoni ND, Fuller CS, Penniston JT, Kumar R (1992) Vitamin D and mineral deficiencies increase the plasma membrane calcium pump of chicken intestine. Gastroenterology 102:886-894.

Wood RJ, Fleet JC, Cashman K, Bruns ME, Deluca HF (1998) Intestinal calcium absorption in the aged rat: evidence of intestinal resistance to 1,25-dihydroxyvitamin D. Endocrinology 139:3843-3848.

Wood RJ, Tchack L, Taparia S (2001) 1,25-Dihydroxyvitamin D3 increases the expression of the CaT1 epithelial calcium channel in the Caco-2 human intestinal cell line. BMC Physiol 1:11.

Wood RJ, Tchack L, Angelo G, Pratt RE, Sonna LA (2004) DNA microarray analysis of vitamin D-induced gene expression in a human colon carcinoma cell line. Physiol Genomics 17:122-129.

RECOMMENDED READINGS

Bronner F (ed) (1990) Intracellular Calcium Regulation. Wiley-Liss, New York.

Favus MJ (ed) (2003) Primer on the Metabolic Bone Diseases and Disorders of Mineral Metabolism, 5th ed. American Society of Bone and Mineral Research, Washington, DC.

New SA, Bonjour J-P (eds) (2003) Nutritional Aspects of Bone Health. The Royal Society of Chemistry, Cambridge, UK.

Nordin BEC (ed) (1988) Calcium in Human Biology. Springer-Verlag, London.

Chapter 33

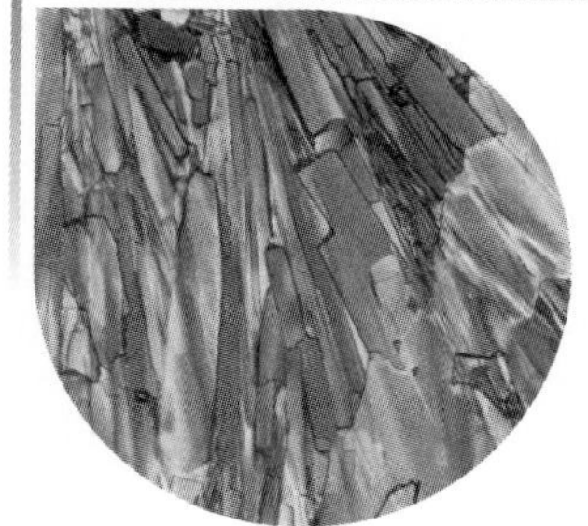

Magnesium

Martin Konrad, MD, and Karl-Peter Schlingmann, MD

OUTLINE

COMMON ABBREVIATIONS

CaSR	*Ca/Mg sensing receptor*
PTH	parathyroid hormone
TRP	transient receptor potential
TRPM	melastatin-related TRP cation channel

Magnesium (Mg^{2+}) plays an important role in numerous physiological processes. It is a cofactor for various enzymes that are involved in muscle contraction, neurotransmitter release, and the regulation of ion channels. The essential role of Mg^{2+} in fundamental cellular functions is mainly based on two important properties of Mg^{2+}: (1) its ability to chelate anionic ligands, especially adenosine triphosphate (ATP), and (2) its ability to compete with calcium (Ca^{2+}) for binding sites resulting in a modulation of intracellular and extracellular free Ca^{2+} concentrations.

CHEMISTRY OF MAGNESIUM

Mg^{2+} is a divalent metal ion with an atomic number of 12 and a molecular weight of 24. It is one of the most abundant elements in the earth's crust and is also prevalent in seawater.

This chapter is a revision of the chapter contributed by Robert R. Rude, MD, for the first edition.

In vertebrates, it is the fourth most abundant cation in the body (after calcium, Ca^{2+}; potassium, K^+; and sodium, Na^+) and the second most abundant intracellular cation (after K^+). Throughout evolution Mg^{2+} has come to be involved in numerous biological processes. Consideration of the basic chemical properties of Mg^{2+} that make it unique among biological cations allows insight into the biological properties of Mg^{2+}. Comparison of the size of a Mg^{2+} ion to K^+, Na^+, and Ca^{2+} reveals that the ionic radius of Mg^{2+} is considerably smaller, whereas its hydrated radius is substantially larger than that of the other cations. Therefore, the ionic radius of Mg^{2+} is among the smallest of all cations, while its hydrated radius is the largest. This difference is reflected by the enormous difference in volume between the hydrated and the ionic form of Mg^{2+}. Hydrated Mg^{2+} occupies 400 times the volume occupied by ionic Mg^{2+}. In comparison, hydration of Na^+ and Ca^{2+} results in only a 25-fold change in volume, and hydration of K^+ results in only a fourfold change in volume. This property of Mg^{2+} has an important influence on Mg^{2+} biology. For example, because transport proteins usually carry dehydrated cations, Mg^{2+} transport proteins must first recognize and interact with the hydrated cation and then remove the hydration shell in order to deliver the bare ion into the transport pathway. This represents an enormous challenge because of the volume change. The fact that Mg^{2+} transport proteins are quite different from other ion transporters probably reflects these peculiar chemical properties of Mg^{2+} (Maguire and Cowan, 2002; Shaul, 2002).

The coordination number and solvent exchange rate for Mg^{2+} also determine its biochemical functions. Like Na^+, Mg^{2+} is invariably hexacoordinate. In contrast, Ca^{2+} can adopt arrangements involving 6, 7, or 8 coordinate bonds. This allows a much greater flexibility in structures formed with Ca^{2+} than in structures formed with Mg^{2+}. This difference in rigidity might reflect the different roles of Ca^{2+} and Mg^{2+} in basic biochemical processes. As a signaling molecule, Ca^{2+} must bind to various proteins and induce a conformational change. Therefore, the Ca^{2+} binding site must exhibit some flexibility to allow Ca^{2+} binding to proteins in at least two different states. In contrast, the predominant role of Mg^{2+} is to bind nucleotide triphosphates (mainly ATP) in the catalytic pocket of a given enzyme. After Mg^{2+}-ATP binding in the active site of an enzyme, not all six coordination positions of Mg^{2+} are filled by interaction with either the protein or ATP. Several water molecules remain coordinated with Mg^{2+}. The purpose of Mg^{2+} binding to the phosphoryl moieties of ATP appears to be an activation of the phosphate ester toward hydrolysis. For those ATP-independent enzymes, the Mg^{2+} ion may serve to hold a water molecule in a specific position. The slow exchange rate of water in the hydration shell of Mg^{2+} may also play a role here. This may allow the formation of a structure containing water in a particular geometry. This ability of Mg^{2+} to position a water molecule for participation in the catalytic mechanism of an enzyme is an example of outer sphere complexation, a reaction mechanism exhibited by only a few metals. Therefore, the common role of Mg^{2+}, chelation of ATP as Mg^{2+}-ATP in a variety of enzymes, is not only a simple binding and neutralization of charge but also a functional part of enzyme catalysis (Cowan, 2002).

ABSORPTION AND EXCRETION OF MAGNESIUM

Mg^{2+} homeostasis in the body is obtained by balancing the intestinal absorption of Mg^{2+} with renal excretion.

INTESTINAL MAGNESIUM ABSORPTION

Intestinal Mg^{2+} absorption is inversely proportional to the amount ingested. Under normal dietary conditions in healthy individuals, approximately 30% to 50% of ingested Mg^{2+} is absorbed (Fine et al., 1991). Mg^{2+} is absorbed along the entire intestinal tract, including the large and small bowel, but the sites of maximal Mg^{2+} absorption appear to be the distal jejunum and the ileum. The colon absorbs only small amounts of Mg^{2+}, which may be important in the context of dietary restriction or compromised Mg^{2+} absorption in the small intestine. When dietary intake is restricted, fractional absorption of Mg^{2+} may increase up to 80%. Conversely, it may be reduced to 20% on high Mg^{2+} diets.

Intestinal absorption occurs through two different pathways as illustrated in Figure 33-1: a saturable active transcellular pathway and a nonsaturable paracellular passive transport pathway (Kerstan and Quamme, 2002; Fine et al., 1991). Saturation kinetics of the transcellular transport system are indicative of a limited active transport capacity. At a low intraluminal Mg^{2+} concentration, absorption occurs primarily via the active transcellular route. When Mg^{2+} concentrations are high, more absorption occurs via the paracellular pathway. This results in a curvilinear function for total Mg^{2+} absorption (Kayne and Lee, 1993).

Little is known about the hormonal regulation of intestinal Mg^{2+} transport. Vitamin D and its metabolites 25-hydroxyvitamin D and 1,25-dihydroxyvitamin D have been found to enhance intestinal Mg^{2+} absorption. It is likely that intestinal Mg^{2+} absorption is also influenced by other hormones, but these have not been extensively studied. A variety of hormones are involved in the regulation of Mg^{2+} transport via changes in both transepithelial and paracellular permeability in the kidney tubules, and one would predict that similar mechanisms for regulation of intestinal Mg^{2+} transport are likely to exist in the intestine (Kerstan and Quamme, 2002).

Bioavailability may be a factor in intestinal Mg^{2+} absorption because other nutrients can affect Mg^{2+} absorption. High levels of dietary

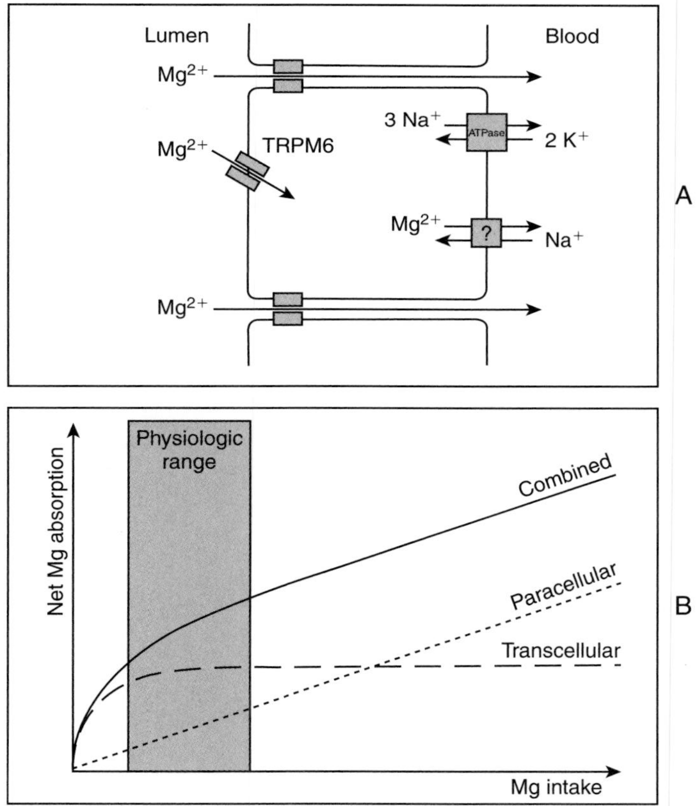

Figure 33-1 **A,** Proposed model of intestinal Mg^{2+} absorption by two independent pathways: passive paracellular absorption and active transcellular transport consisting of an apical entry through a Mg^{2+} channel and a basolateral exit through a putative Na^{+}-coupled exchange. **B,** Kinetics of intestinal Mg^{2+} absorption in humans. Paracellular transport linearly rising with intraluminal concentrations *(dotted line)* and saturable active transcellular transport *(dashed line)* together yield a curvilinear function for net Mg^{2+} absorption *(solid line).*

fiber from fruits, vegetables, and grains decrease fractional Mg^{2+} absorption (Siener and Hesse, 1995). However, diets high in vegetables are Mg^{2+}-rich, and the high Mg^{2+} content of these diets offsets decreased fractional absorption associated with the higher fiber intake. Many foods high in fiber also contain phytate, which may decrease intestinal Mg^{2+} absorption because Mg^{2+} binds to the phosphate groups on phytic acid (Franz, 1989). The ability of phosphate to bind Mg^{2+} may explain decreases in intestinal Mg^{2+} absorption in subjects on high-phosphate diets (Franz, 1989). Although dietary calcium has been reported to both decrease and increase Mg^{2+} absorption, human studies have shown no effect (Fine et al., 1991). Dietary protein may also influence intestinal Mg^{2+} absorption; Mg^{2+} absorption is lower when protein intake is less than 30 g/day (Hunt and Schofield, 1969).

RENAL MAGNESIUM HANDLING

The kidney is the principal organ involved in Mg^{2+} homeostasis (Quamme and Dirks, 1986). In the case of Mg^{2+} depletion, the kidney is able to achieve almost complete Mg^{2+} conservation by lowering excretion to less than 1% of the filtered load. In contrast, during excess intake, urinary Mg^{2+} excretion is high and may even exceed the filtered load. Under normal conditions, approximately 80% of the total plasma Mg^{2+} is filtered through the glomerulus, and most of this is reabsorbed (greater than 95%) as the filtrate passes through the nephrons as illustrated in Figure 33-2.

Approximately 5% to 15% of the filtered Mg^{2+} is reabsorbed in the proximal tubule. The major site of tubular Mg^{2+} reabsorption is the thick ascending limb of the loop of Henle, which accounts for 65% to75% of renal Mg^{2+} reabsorption. In the distal convoluted tubule,

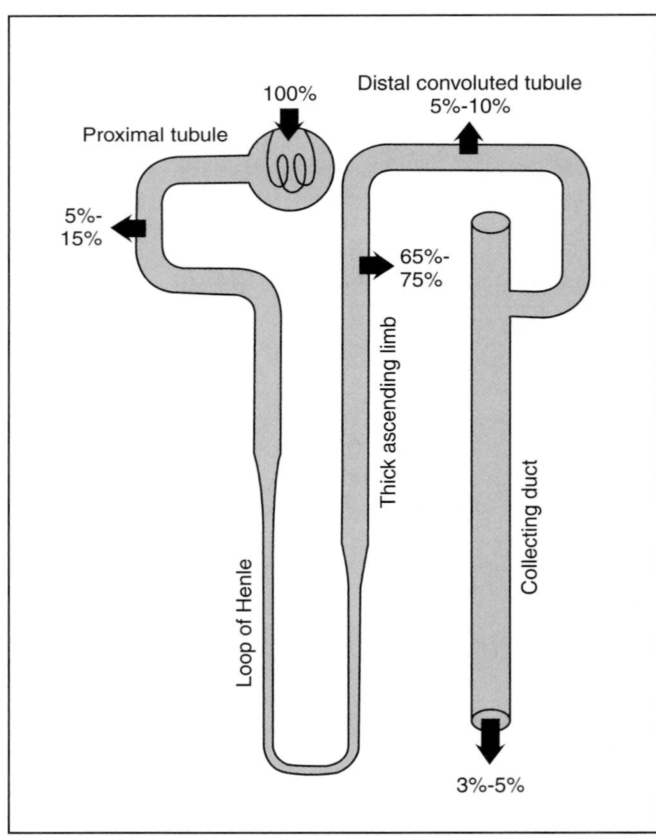

Figure 33-2 Summary of the tubular handling of Mg^{2+}. The 100% represents the total filtered load and the other percentage values represent the fraction of the filtered load absorbed at each tubular site.

Mg^{2+} reabsorption is about 5% to 10%. Absorption in the distal convoluted tubule may appear negligible, but as there is no evidence for Mg^{2+} reabsorption beyond this point, reabsorption in the distal convoluted tubule is of crucial importance for regulating the amount of Mg^{2+} that is excreted in the urine.

PROXIMAL TUBULE

As mentioned in the preceding text, only 5% to 15% of the filtered Mg^{2+} is reabsorbed by the proximal tubule in adults. In contrast, during the neonatal period, approximately 70% of Mg^{2+} is reabsorbed in this nephron segment. This difference is due to a higher Mg^{2+} permeability of the proximal tubules during early stages of development (Leliévre-Pegorier et al., 1983). The normal developmental maturation process in handling of Mg^{2+} involves a decrease in permeability of the proximal tubule to Mg^{2+}. This developmental difference must be considered when analyzing Mg^{2+} homeostasis in young infants compared to older individuals.

LOOP OF HENLE

As mentioned previously, the thick ascending limb of the loop of Henle is responsible for reabsorption of 65% to 75% of the filtered Mg^{2+}. All of this occurs in the cortical segment of the thick ascending limb, and no Mg^{2+} reabsorption occurs in the medullary segment of the thick ascending limb. Mg^{2+} reabsorption in the cortical thick ascending limb of the loop of Henle is passive, with movement from the tubular lumen to the interstitium driven by the lumen-positive transepithelial voltage (Fig. 33-3, *A*). The transepithelial voltage is determined by the transepithelial Na^+, K^+, Cl^- cotransport and active Na^+ reabsorption, and, along the nephron, the lumen-positivity is unique for the thick ascending limb of the loop of Henle. Therefore, any changes in these transport mechanisms affect the transepithelial voltage and consequently influence Mg^{2+} (and Ca^{2+}) reabsorption.

The molecular nature of paracellular absorption of Mg^{2+} (and also Ca^{2+}) was completely ignored until 1999, when Simon and coworkers, using a positional gene cloning approach, identified the first component of this reabsorption pathway (Simon et al., 1999). Genetic analysis of a rare human disease phenotype called familial hypomagnesemia with hypercalciuria and nephrocalcinosis (FHHNC) led to identification of mutations in gene *CLDN16* (formerly *PCLN-1*) as the underlying genetic

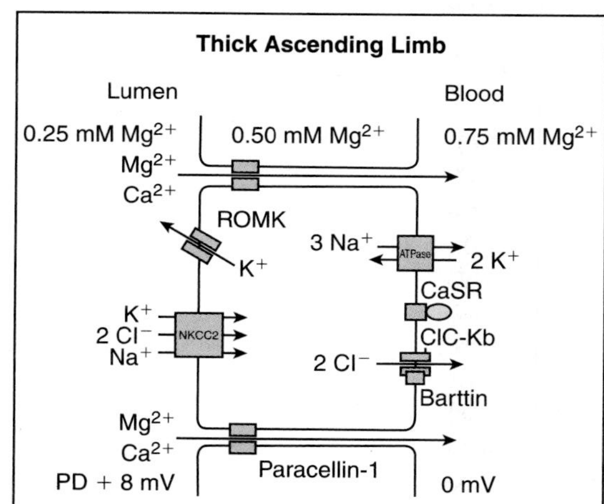

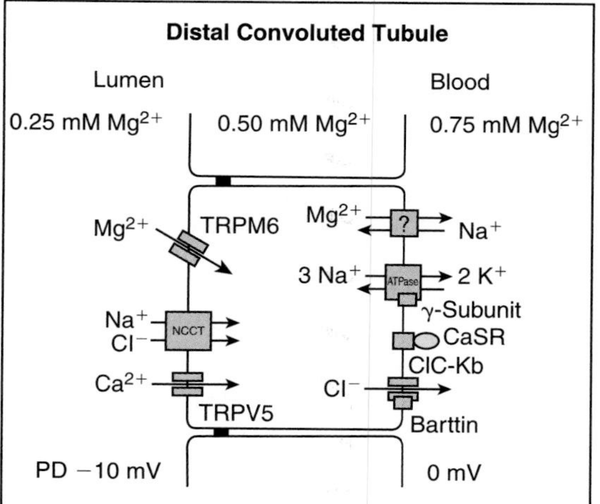

Figure 33-3 **A,** Mg^{2+} reabsorption in the thick ascending limb of Henle's loop. Lumen-positive transcellular potential difference (PD) generated by transcellular NaCl reabsorption drives the paracellular Mg^{2+} reabsorption. **B,** Mg^{2+} reabsorption in the distal convoluted tubule. Active transcellular transport involving an apical entry step probably through a Mg^{2+}-selective ion channel and a basolateral exit that presumably is mediated by a Na^+-coupled exchange mechanism. *Barttin,* β-subunit for ClC-Kb; *CaSR,* calcium-sensing receptor; ClC-Kb, chloride channel Kb; *ROMK,* renal outer medullary potassium channel; *TRPM6,* melastatin-related TRP cation channel 6; *TRPV5,* transient receptor potential cation channel V5.

defect in this disease. *CLDN16* encodes the tight junction protein paracellin-1 (claudin 16), which is a member of the claudin family of tight junction proteins. In kidney, paracellin-1 expression is restricted to tight junctions of the thick ascending limb of the loop of Henle. From the FHHNC disease phenotype, which represents a selective defect of paracellular reabsorption of Ca^{2+} and Mg^{2+} along with intact Na^+Cl^- reabsorption, it was speculated that paracellin-1 is involved in the control of Mg^{2+} and Ca^{2+} permeability in the cortical thick ascending limb of the loop of Henle by building a Ca^{2+}- and Mg^{2+}-selective paracellular pore. Tight junction proteins such as paracellin-1 are involved in the formation of junctional complexes that function as barriers between adjacent epithelial cells. Other claudins may also enable paracellular ion fluxes.

In a study of individuals with idiopathic hypercalciuria, a novel mutation of *CLDN16* was identified that caused inactivation of a PDZ-domain binding motif in paracellin-1 and thereby prevented the association of paracellin-1 with the tight junction scaffolding protein ZO-1 (Muller et al., 2003). Disruption of this interaction leads to mistargeting of paracellin-1 to lysosomes in kidney epithelial cells. Affected individuals exhibit a transient but severe hypercalciuria with nephrocalcinosis (without disturbance of Mg^{2+} metabolism). Ikari and colleagues (2004) confirmed the importance of the interaction between paracellin-1 and ZO-1 for localization of paracellin-1 to the tight junctions in studies with a canine kidney cell line. Paracellin-1 expression increased transepithelial resistance and paracellular permeability at the same time. This, as well as the FHHNC phenotype, might argue for the formation of a pore-like structure with channel properties by a protein complex that includes paracellin-1 and ZO-1, as was previously hypothesized based on the large number of negative residues in the first extracellular loop of paracellin-1 (Simon et al., 1999). Interestingly, cation transport was inhibited by Mg^{2+}. Whether this was caused by a direct effect of Mg^{2+} on the paracellin-1/ZO-1 complex remains unclear; inhibition via the Ca^{2+}/Mg^{2+}-sensing receptor (CaSR) represents an alternative explanation.

Mg^{2+} reabsorption in cortical thick ascending limb of the loop of Henle is regulated by a variety of hormones that act mainly by increasing the reabsorption rate. These hormonal responses are mediated by changes in both transepithelial voltage and paracellular permeability. For example, it has been shown that 1,25-dihydroxyvitamin D influences the Mg^{2+} transport in the cortical thick ascending limb of the loop of Henle by downregulating paracellin-1 expression at the transcriptional level (Efrati et al., 2005).

Micropuncture studies have also demonstrated that hypermagnesemia or hypercalcemia decreases Mg^{2+} reabsorption in the cortical thick ascending limb of the loop of Henle (Quamme and Dirks, 1986). Micropuncture studies performed in parathyroidectomized dogs showed that elevated filtered Mg^{2+} concentrations were initially associated with increased Mg^{2+} reabsorption until an apparent tubular reabsorptive maximum, Tm, was reached, beyond which any additional filtered Mg^{2+} was excreted with the urine (Massry et al., 1969). This is mediated by the extracellular Ca^{2+}/Mg^{2+}-sensing receptor (CaSR), which is expressed in the basolateral membrane. Activation of CaSR leads to inhibition of salt reabsorption and of paracellular Ca^{2+} and Mg^{2+} transport in the thick ascending limb of the loop of Henle (Di Stefano et al., 1997; Hebert, 1996).

Loop diuretics such as furosemide, which act to inhibit the Cl^- pump in the ascending loop of Henle and subsequently block Na^+ reabsorption, may lead to hypomagnesemia, as these drugs have a large effect on transepithelial voltage. However, long-term treatment with furosemide induces adaptive processes that lead to almost normal Mg^{2+} excretion rates. This adaptation probably occurs in nephron segments other than the thick ascending limb of the loop of Henle.

DISTAL CONVOLUTED TUBULE

Mg^{2+} reabsorption in the distal convoluted tubule is mediated by an active transcellular transport mechanism as shown in Figure 33-3 (Dai et al., 2001). Mg^{2+} enters the distal convoluted tubule cell across the apical membrane through ion channels. Uptake of Mg^{2+} is driven by the lumen-negative potential difference in this region of the tubule. Extrusion into the interstitium probably occurs by a Na^+-dependent exchange mechanism. The exact pathways involved in Mg^{2+} reabsorption in the distal tubule are still largely unknown, but a first component of this transport mechanism has been identified. Mutations in a member of the transient receptor potential (TRP) ion channel family, TRPM6, were identified in patients with primary hypomagnesemia with secondary hypocalcemia (Schlingmann et al., 2002; Walder et al., 2002). Functional studies demonstrated that TRPM6, as its closest homolog TRPM7, is permeable to Ca^{2+} and Mg^{2+} and is inhibited by intracellular levels of Mg^{2+} or Mg^{2+}-ATP (Voets et al., 2003; Nadler et al., 2001). There is also evidence for heteromultimerization between TRPM6 and TRPM7 and that these heteromultimers form Mg^{2+}/Ca^{2+} channels at the cell surface (Chubanov et al., 2004). By using immunohistochemistry, Voets and colleagues (2004) demonstrated the apical localization of TRPM6 in distal convoluted tubule cells. The clinical observation that patients with primary hypomagnesemia with secondary hypocalcemia have a renal Mg^{2+} leak at the level of the distal convoluted tubule (in addition to intestinal Mg^{2+} absorption failure) underscores the important role of TRPM6 in Mg^{2+} reabsorption in this segment of the nephron.

Different hormones regulate Mg^{2+} transport rates in the distal convoluted tubule as they do in the cortical thick ascending limb of the loop of Henle. Although the overall outcomes of hormonal regulation are similar in both nephron segments, the cellular mechanisms are completely different. There is a direct effect of hormones on active Mg^{2+} transport in the distal convoluted tubule, whereas variations in the transport rates are indirectly mediated by influences on the transepithelial voltage or the paracellular permeability in the thick ascending limb of the loop of Henle. Mg^{2+} transport rates in the distal convoluted tubule change rapidly upon a decrease in Mg^{2+} availability, which allows efficient Mg^{2+} conservation. Conversely, during hypermagnesemia (or hypercalcemia) fractional excretion rates for Mg^{2+} are increased via activation of the CaSR, which results in inhibition of Mg^{2+} (or Ca^{2+}) reabsorption.

Amiloride and chorothiazide both increase Mg^{2+} transport in the distal convoluted tubule. However, the effects on Mg^{2+} homeostasis are different. Amiloride is considered as a Mg^{2+}-sparing diuretic agent, whereas chronic thiazide administration often leads to Mg^{2+} wasting. The latter phenomenon is poorly understood but may involve hypokalemia, which often results from thiazide therapy.

BODY MAGNESIUM CONTENT

The normal adult total body Mg^{2+} content is approximately 25 g, or 1,000 mmol, and 50% to 60% of this total resides in bone, as shown in Figure 33-4 (Elin, 1987). One third of skeletal Mg^{2+} is on the surface of bone, and this fraction may serve as a reservoir for maintaining

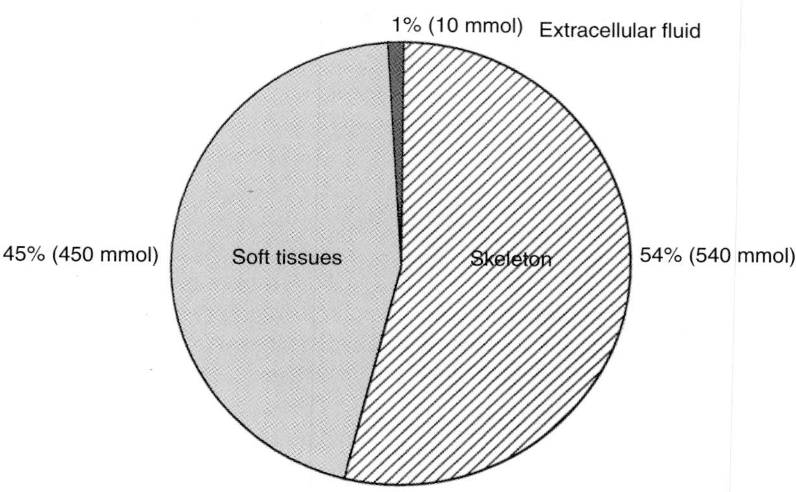

Figure 33-4 Distribution of Mg^{2+} in the body.

a normal extracellular Mg^{2+} concentration (Wallach, 1988).

Extracellular Mg^{2+} accounts for only about 1% of total body Mg^{2+}, as shown in Figure 33-4. The normal serum Mg^{2+} concentration is 0.7 to 1.0 mmol/L. Most of the plasma Mg^{2+}, approximately 60% to 65%, is ionized or free Mg^{2+} (Elin, 1997; Altura et al., 1992). Of the remaining 35% to 40%, 5% to 10% is complexed to anions such as phosphate, citrate, and sulfate, and 30% is bound to proteins (chiefly albumin), as shown in Figure 33-5 (Elin, 1987).

Mg^{2+} is present in higher concentrations inside cells than in the plasma. Soft tissue contains about one half of the total body Mg^{2+}, approximately 470 mmol. The Mg^{2+} content of soft tissues varies between 2.5 and 9 mmol/kg wet tissue weight (Elin, 1987). In general, the higher the metabolic activity of the cell, the higher the Mg^{2+} content. For example, the Mg^{2+} content of liver cells is about four times that of red blood cells.

Within the cell, significant amounts of Mg^{2+} are in the nucleus, mitochondria, and endoplasmic (or sarcoplasmic) reticulum as well as in the cytosol (Cowan, 1995; Birch, 1993). Most of the Mg^{2+} is bound to proteins and other negatively charged molecules such as nucleoside triphosphates and diphosphates (e.g., ATP and adenosine diphosphate [ADP]) and nucleic acids (e.g., ribonucleic acid [RNA] and deoxyribonucleic acid [DNA]); in the cytoplasm, about 80% of the Mg^{2+} is complexed with ATP (Frausto da Silva and Williams, 1991). Only 1% to 5% of the total intracellular Mg^{2+} is free ionized Mg^{2+} (Romani et al., 1993).

The concentration of free Mg^{2+} in the cytosol of mammalian cells has been reported to range from 0.2 to 1.0 mmol/L, but values vary with cell type and means of measurement (Romani et al., 1993). The free Mg^{2+} concentration in the cell cytosol is maintained relatively constant even when the Mg^{2+} concentration in the extracellular fluid is experimentally varied above or below the physiological range (Dai and Quamme, 1991). The relative constancy of the free Mg^{2+} concentration in the intracellular milieu is attributed to the limited permeability of the plasma membrane to Mg^{2+} and to the operation of specific Mg^{2+} transport systems that regulate the rates at which Mg^{2+} enters or leaves cells (Romani et al., 1993). Although the concentration differential between the cytosol and the extracellular fluid for free Mg^{2+} is minimal, Mg^{2+} enters cells down an electrochemical gradient owing to the relative electronegativity of the cell interior. Maintenance of the normal intracellular concentrations of free Mg^{2+} requires that Mg^{2+} be actively transported out of the cell.

Tissues vary in the rates at which Mg^{2+} exchange occurs and in the percentage of total Mg^{2+} that is readily exchangeable. The rate of Mg^{2+} exchange in heart, liver, and kidney appears to exceed that in skeletal muscle, red blood cells, brain, and testis (Romani et al., 1993). Increased cellular Mg^{2+} content has been reported for rapidly proliferating cells, indicating a possible relationship between the metabolic state of a cell and the relative rates of Mg^{2+} transport into and out of cells.

Cellular Mg^{2+} transport has been studied extensively. Physiological studies suggest a

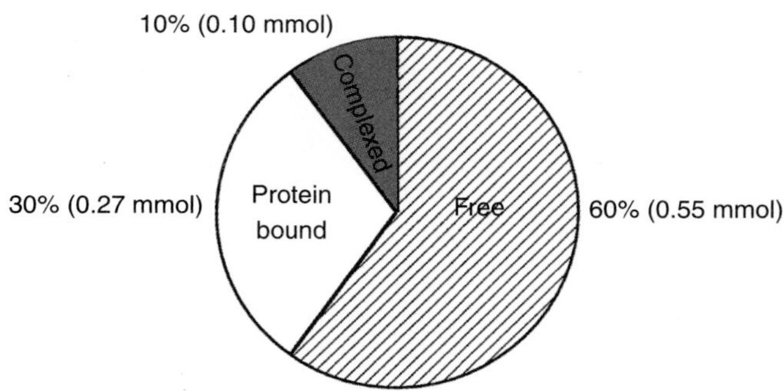

Figure 33-5 Physiochemical states of Mg^{2+} in normal plasma.

variety of Mg^{2+} transport proteins in different human tissues. Many investigations have pointed to the existence of functional Na^+/Mg^{2+} exchange mechanisms, with Mg^{2+} efflux being dependent on Na^+,K^+-ATPase activity. However, the molecular nature of cellular Mg^{2+} transporters remained unknown until the recent discovery of Mg^{2+} permeating properties of members of the TRP family. In 2001 two independent groups reported the functional characterization of TRPM7, although these reports used older nomenclatures for this protein—LTRPC7, ChaK1, or TRP-PLK (Nadler et al., 2001; Runnels et al., 2001). TRPM7 is a remarkable protein consisting of an ion channel with a covalently bound kinase domain at the C terminus. It was first cloned in an effort to characterize a family of atypical so-called α-kinases, with structural similarity to elongation factor-2 (EF-2) kinase, which do not display sequence similarity to conventional eukaryotic protein kinases.

These two initial reports presented conflicting data regarding TRPM7 channel permeation characteristics. One group described TRPM7 as a nonselective cation channel conducting Na^+ and Ca^{2+} (Runnels et al., 2001), whereas the other reported a complex permeation profile with selectivity toward divalent cations (Nadler et al., 2001). TRPM7 gating was reported to be controlled by intracellular Mg^{2+}, Mg^{2+}-nucleotide complexes, G proteins, and by phosphatidylinositol 4,5-bisphosphate (PIP_2) hydrolysis (reviewed in Fleig and Penner, 2004). Subsequent studies established that, in contrast to all previously characterized ion channels, TRPM7 exhibits the ability to permeate independently a variety of trace metal ions and is similarly permeable for both Ca^{2+} and Mg^{2+}. The ubiquitous expression pattern together with its constitutive activity rendered TRPM7 a promising candidate for a general mechanism for cellular entry of metal ions. The most exciting data concerning the role of TRPM7 for cellular Mg^{2+} handling originated from targeted gene deletion of TRPM7 in a genetically modified vertebrate cell line (Nadler et al., 2001). TRPM7 deletion resulted in intracellular Mg^{2+} depletion and growth arrest, which could be overcome by Mg^{2+} supplementation. Furthermore, patch clamp experiments after heterologous expression of TRPM7 clearly indicated that TRPM7 activity is suppressed by millimolar concentrations of intracellular Mg^{2+} and Mg^{2+}-ATP (Schmitz et al., 2003).

The exact role of the kinase domain of TRPM7 in modulating ion channel activity, however, is still not completely understood. Even though TRPM7 kinase activity is not required for channel activation and disruption of kinase activity resulted in a reduced sensitivity to intracellular Mg^{2+}, deletion of the kinase domain led to a complete suppression of channel activation at physiological intracellular Mg^{2+} levels (Schmitz et al., 2003). These findings clearly indicate a functional coupling between the channel gating mechanism and the kinase domain.

The important role of members of the TRPM ion channel family for Mg^{2+} metabolism was substantiated by the discovery of mutations in TRPM6, the closest relative of TRPM7, in patients affected with primary hypomagnesemia with secondary hypocalcemia as discussed in preceding text (Schlingmann et al., 2002; Walder et al., 2002). Affected individuals exhibit a combined intestinal/renal defect of Mg^{2+} absorption/reabsorption. TRPM6 and TRPM7 are able to form functional heteromultimers. Therefore, TRPM6 (or a TRPM6/TRPM7 heteromultimer) appears to be a key element in the transcellular (epithelial) transport of Mg^{2+} in intestine and kidney, whereas TRPM7 appears to be responsible for general cellular Mg^{2+} import in virtually every cell type (Fleig and Penner, 2004).

PHYSIOLOGICAL ROLES OF MAGNESIUM

The main biological role of Mg^{2+} in mammalian cells is involved with anion charge neutralization (Cowan, 1995; Frausto da Silva and Williams, 1991). Mg^{2+} is particularly found in association with organic polyphosphates such as nucleotide triphosphates and nucleotide diphosphates (e.g., $ATP^{4-} \cdot Mg^{2+}$ and $ADP^{3-} \cdot Mg^{2+}$). Mg^{2+} is also found associated with other highly anionic species, including multisubstituted phosphates of sugars such as inositol triphosphate, nucleic acids (RNA and DNA), and some carboxylates (e.g., isocitrate-Mg^{2+} as substrate for isocitrate lyase; carboxylate groups on proteins).

Mg^{2+} is normally bound between the β- and γ-phosphates of nucleotide triphosphates such as ATP and between the α- and β-phosphates of nucleotide diphosphates such as ADP, as shown in Figure 33-6. This arrangement serves to neutralize the negative charge density on the ATP or other nucleotide triphosphates or diphosphates and to facilitate binding of the nucleotide phosphate to the enzymes that use them as substrates. In most reactions in which Mg^{2+} is involved, it is present as a complex with a nucleotide triphosphate or diphosphate, which serves as substrate. The Mg^{2+} in these complexes does not interact directly with the enzyme in most cases but is linked by the substrate in an enzyme–substrate–metal type of substrate-bridged complex. Hence, Mg^{2+} plays a dominant role in all nucleotide triphosphate or diphosphate-dependent enzymatic reactions, which are widespread in metabolism. These reactions include those catalyzed by kinases, G-proteins, adenylate cyclase, ATP synthases, ATPases, and reactions coupled to ATP hydrolysis.

Mg^{2+} also is required for binding to some enzymes or other proteins to stabilize them in the active conformation or to induce the formation of a binding site or active site. Some enzymes known to require enzyme-bound Mg^{2+} are enolase and pyruvate kinase; the Mg^{2+} in these enzymes coordinates the binding of substrate to the active site. Mg^{2+} is also bound to the myosin regulatory light chain in the actin–myosin complex and is present in glutamine synthetase. Mg^{2+} also is required for the conformational regulation of the binding of some elongation factors.

In addition, Mg^{2+} is found in association with nucleic acids, which are negatively charged polymers due to the phosphate groups in the nucleotide chains. Mg^{2+} stabilizes bending of RNA or DNA into particular curved or folded structures. This presumably occurs because of the cross-linking of the oxyanion centers of the phosphate residues by the divalent cation.

CELLULAR ENERGY METABOLISM

Mg^{2+} is involved in numerous steps in central pathways of carbohydrate, lipid, and protein metabolism and in mitochondrial ATP synthesis. For example, many steps in the glycolytic pathway require Mg^{2+}, either in the form of a complex with the ATP or ADP substrate or as a part of the metalloenzyme itself. The steps catalyzed by hexokinase and phosphofructokinase require Mg^{2+}-ATP (i.e., $ATP^{4-} \cdot Mg^{2+}$) as substrate, whereas the steps catalyzed by phosphoglycerate kinase and pyruvate kinase require Mg^{2+}-ADP (i.e., $ADP^{3-} \cdot Mg^{2+}$) as substrate. Both enolase, which interconverts 2-phosphoglycerate and phosphoenolpyruvate, and pyruvate kinase, which converts phosphoenolpyruvate to pyruvate, require enzyme-bound Mg^{2+} · Mg^{2+} is bound to these enzymes through several carboxylate groups on the

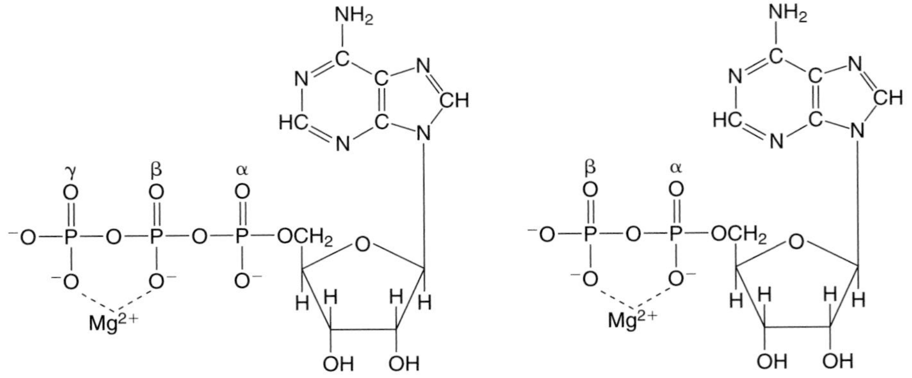

Adenosine 5′-triphosphate
$ATP^{4-} \cdot Mg^{2+}$

Adenosine 5′-diphosphate
$ADP^{3-} \cdot Mg^{2+}$

Figure 33-6 Physiological forms of Mg^{2+}-ATP and Mg^{2+}-ADP.

protein and forms an active complex with the enzyme before the substrate is bound. The bound Mg^{2+} in enolase may coordinate the hydroxyl group of 2-phosphoglycerate, making it a better leaving group. Pyruvate kinase requires both K^+ and Mg^{2+}. The K^+ plays a conformational role, whereas Mg^{2+} coordinates the binding of the substrate phosphoenolpyruvate to the enzyme active site.

Mg^{2+} is required for phosphorylation and dephosphorylation reactions. ADP phosphorylation by the mitochondrial ATP synthase (F_1F_0-ATPase) involved in oxidative phosphorylation utilizes Mg^{2+}-ADP as substrate. In cardiac and skeletal muscle, as well as other soft tissues, the creatine–phosphocreatine cycle acts as a reserve for high energy phosphate. Phosphocreatine can be used to convert ADP to ATP when the muscle is subjected to a heavy workload. This occurs via a reversible reaction catalyzed by creatine kinase. As is true for all kinases, Mg^{2+} is an activating ion functioning with ADP and ATP in the reversible reaction catalyzed by creatine kinase.

NUCLEIC ACID AND PROTEIN SYNTHESIS

The transcription, translation, and replication of nucleic acids (RNA and DNA) require enzymes that catalyze the hydrolysis and formation of phosphodiester bonds. Almost all these enzymes require Mg^{2+} for optimal activity. For example, DNA polymerase I is thought to require Mg^{2+} for stabilization of the conformation required for catalysis. RNA polymerases, which catalyze transcription (the synthesis of RNA using a DNA template) also require Mg^{2+}; the cation again is thought to effect a conformational change in the enzyme to produce a catalytically competent state.

Replicating cells must be able to synthesize new protein, and all cells must continually replace protein that is degraded. Protein synthesis has been reported to be highly sensitive to Mg^{2+} depletion. Mg^{2+} is required for virtually every step of protein biosynthesis: the formation of the aminoacyl–transfer RNA species (which requires Mg^{2+}-ATP) and the maintenance of its conformation (which is required for recognition by messenger RNA), as well as the maintenance of the ribosomes, require Mg^{2+}. Mg^{2+} is also required for structure and activity of elongation factor–guanosine triphosphate (GTP) complexes that allow protein synthesis to begin and for the GTPase activities that occur during elongation and termination of protein biosynthesis.

SECOND MESSENGER SYSTEMS

Many hormones, neurotransmitters, and other cellular effectors regulate cellular activity via the adenylate cyclase system. The hormone–receptor unit interfaces with adenylate cyclase via a guanine nucleotide-binding protein (G-protein). Activation or inhibition of adenylate cyclase involves the dissociation of a G-protein into α and β-γ subunits; this process requires the presence of GTP and Mg^{2+}. As is the case for other ATP-utilizing enzymes, the actual substrate for adenylate cyclase is Mg^{2+}-ATP. There is also evidence for a Mg^{2+}-binding site on adenylate cyclase through which Mg^{2+} directly increases enzyme activity. G-proteins, along with GTP and Mg^{2+}, are also required for many other signaling events in cells.

Another group of hormones and neurotransmitters exert their effects by raising the ionized calcium (Ca^{2+}) concentration in the cytosol of their target cells through the activation of the phosphoinositol cycle. One of the principal mechanisms by which this is thought to occur is by receptor-mediated activation of phospholipase C. Phospholipase C hydrolyzes a specific phospholipid present in the plasma membrane, PIP_2 (phosphatidylinositol 4,5-bisphosphate), to yield two biologically active products, diacylglycerol and inositol 1,4,5-triphosphate (IP_3). Diacylglycerol activates protein kinase C, and IP_3 triggers calcium release from the ER. The IP_3 is rapidly inactivated by dephosphorylation. It appears that Mg^{2+} is essential for the normal functioning of this phosphoinositol cycle because the kinase that forms the PIP_2 and also the enzymes that inactivate IP_3 require Mg^{2+} at concentrations that are physiological (Volpe et al., 1990; Connolly et al., 1985). In contrast, higher Mg^{2+} concentrations may decrease intracellular Ca^{2+} by two mechanisms: (1) noncompetitive inhibition of IP_3 binding to its receptor, and (2) inhibition of the release of Ca^{2+} via IP_3-gated channels (Volpe et al., 1990) (Fig. 33-7).

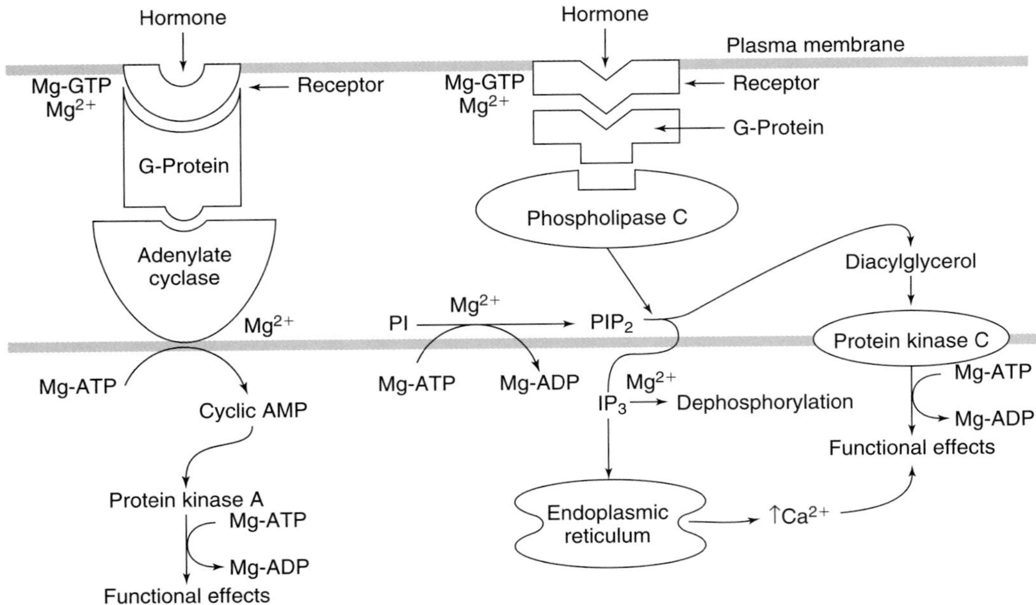

Figure 33-7 Schematic representation of the role of Mg^{2+} in two second messenger systems, adenylate cyclase and phosphatidylinositol. *GTP,* Guanosine triphosphate; *G-protein,* guanine nucleotide regulatory protein; *IP_3,* inositol 1,4,5-triphosphate; *PI,* phosphatidylinositol; *PIP_2,* phosphatidylinositol 4,5-bisphosphate.

ION CHANNELS

Ion channels are proteins that are responsible for generating electrical signals across the cell membrane. These proteins allow passage of ions into or out of cells when the channels are open. Ion channels are classified according to the type of ion they allow to pass, such as Na^+, K^+, or Ca^{2+} (Ackerman and Clapham, 1997; O'Rourke, 1993). Mg^{2+} plays an important role in the function of a number of ion channels.

Mg^{2+} deficiency results in cellular K^+ depletion. Several mechanisms may contribute to the K^+ loss. Mg^{2+} is necessary for the active transport of K^+ out of cells by the Na^+,K^+-ATPase pump. Mg^{2+}-depleted animals and humans have been found to have a reduction in the concentration of Na^+,K^+-ATPase pumps in skeletal muscle, and this reduction in number of transport systems may contribute to the decrease in cellular K^+ (Dorup, 1994). In addition, activity of the Na^+,K^+-ATPase pump is dependent on Mg^{2+}, as has been observed in heart, so Na^+ and K^+ transport activity may also be impaired during Mg^{2+} deficiency due to decreased activity of the Na^+,K^+-ATPase pump (Ryan, 1991). Another mechanism for K^+ loss is an increased efflux of K^+ from cells via other Mg^{2+}-sensitive K^+ channels, as has been seen in skeletal muscle (Dorup, 1994). Mg^{2+} is also involved in regulating a number of K^+ channels in heart muscle (Matsuda, 1991; White and Hartzell, 1989). Inwardly rectifying K^+ channels normally allow K^+ to pass more readily inward than outward, and intracellular Mg^{2+} appears to block the outward movement of K^+ through these channels in myocardial cells. In the absence of Mg^{2+}, K^+ is transported equally well in both directions, and a deficiency in Mg^{2+} may lead to a reduced amount of intracellular K^+. As the resting membrane potential of heart muscle cells is determined in part by the intracellular K^+ concentration, a decreased intracellular K^+ concentration will result, by a complex mechanism, in partial depolarization (i.e., a less negative resting membrane potential) of electrical tissues at rest. The arrhythmogenic effect of Mg^{2+} deficiency may therefore be related to its effect on maintenance of intracellular K^+, as discussed in subsequent text.

Mg^{2+} has been called "nature's physiological calcium channel blocker" (Iseri and

French, 1984). During Mg^{2+} depletion, intracellular Ca^{2+} rises. This may be caused by both uptake from extracellular Ca^{2+} and release from intracellular Ca^{2+} stores. Mg^{2+} has been demonstrated to decrease the inward Ca^{2+} flux through slow Ca^{2+} channels (O'Rourke, 1993; White and Hartzell, 1989). In addition, Mg^{2+} will decrease the transport of Ca^{2+} out of the endoplasmic reticulum (ER) into the cell cytosol. As discussed previously, the ability of IP_3 to release Ca^{2+} from intracellular stores is inversely related to Mg^{2+} concentrations, and, therefore, a fall in Mg^{2+} concentration may allow a greater rise in intracellular Ca^{2+}. Consequently, because Ca^{2+} plays an important role in skeletal and smooth muscle contraction, a state of Mg^{2+} depletion may result in muscle cramps, hypertension, and coronary and cerebral vasospasm (Altura and Altura, 1995).

FOOD SOURCES, RECOMMENDED INTAKES, AND TYPICAL INTAKES OF MAGNESIUM

Based primarily on limited balance study data, the Institute of Medicine (IOM, 1997) set estimated average requirements (EARs) for adults. For young adults, ages 19 to 30 years, the EAR was set at 330 mg/day for men and 255 mg/day for women. For adults older than 30 years of age, the EAR was set slightly higher at 350 mg/day and 265 mg/day for men and women, respectively. The recommended dietary allowances (RDAs) for adults were set as the EAR + 20%—400 or 420 mg/day (16.7 or 17.5 mmol/day) for men and 310 or 320 mg/day (12.9 or 13.3 mmol/day) for women, with the lower values being for adults between 19 and 31 years of age. An incremental intake of +40 mg per day was added to obtain RDAs for pregnant women. No increment was added for lactation. The magnesium requirements of children and adolescents for maintenance and growth were estimated from available balance study data or extrapolated from data for older children, and RDAs were set as the EAR + 20%. For infants, adequate intakes (AIs) were set based on the average intake from human milk during the first 6 months of life (AI = 30 mg/day) or from human milk plus complementary foods for infants from 7 to 12 months of age (AI = 75 mg/day).

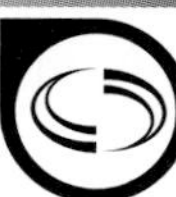

RDAs Across the Life Cycle

	mg Magnesium per Day
Infants	
0 to 6 mo	30 (AI)
7 to 12 mo	75 (AI)
Children	
1 to 3 yr	80
4 to 8 yr	130
9 to 13 yr	240
Males	
14 to 18 yr	410
19 to 30 yr	400
>30 yr	420
Females	
14 to 18 yr	360
19 to 30 yr	310
>30 yr	320
Pregnant	+40
Lactating	+0

Data from Institute of Medicine (IOM) (1997) Dietary Reference Intakes for Calcium, Phosphorus, Magnesium, Vitamin D, and Fluoride. National Academy Press, Washington, DC.
AI, Adequate Intake.

The current EAR and RDA values are still a matter of debate as they were based on balance studies, which are not ideal for estimating the RDA because Mg^{2+} absorption is inversely related to intake and body Mg^{2+} content.

Mg^{2+} is almost ubiquitous in foods. The primary dietary sources are whole grain cereals, legumes, nuts, and chocolate. Other vegetables, fruits, meats, and fish have an intermediate Mg^{2+} content, whereas dairy products and beverages have a low Mg^{2+} content (Elin, 1994). A number of reports indicate that an increasing proportion of the general population does not consume adequate magnesium and consequently develops hypomagnesemia. This is probably largely due to the refining and processing of food, which is known to considerably reduce the Mg^{2+} content. For example, processing of wheat to flour or brown rice to polished rice reduces the Mg^{2+} content by approximately 80%.

Dietary data suggest that the average Mg^{2+} intake has declined markedly over the last

100 years. This is at least partially due to the consumption of more refined foods. In fact, approximately 75% of subjects surveyed in the United States had dietary intakes of magnesium that fell below the RDA in 1986 (Marier, 1986). In more recent data from the Continuing Survey of Food Intakes by Individuals, 1994-1996, the median dietary intake of magnesium in the United States was estimated to be about 220 mg/day for women and 320 mg/day for men (IOM, 1997; Cleveland et al., 1996). These estimated median intakes are substantially below the current RDAs. In contrast to these studies of the U.S. population, a recent EPIC-Oxford study analyzing 65,000 people from Great Britain found a mean daily Mg^{2+} intake of 350 mg in females and 382 mg in males (Davey et al., 2002). As expected, vegans had a higher Mg^{2+} intake than vegetarians, fish-eaters, or meat-eaters (Davey et al., 2002).

The medical significance of marginal Mg^{2+} intakes on human health is not clear. Although low dietary Mg^{2+} intakes have not been unequivocally linked to chronic disease, epidemiological studies have suggested an inverse relationship between dietary Mg^{2+} intake and blood pressure (Altura and Altura, 1995), atherosclerotic vascular disease and sudden death

Food Sources

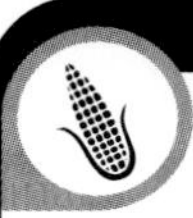

Food Sources of Magnesium

Legumes

- 60 to 75 mg per ½ cup soy, white, or black beans (cooked)
- 35 to 50 mg per ½ cup navy, lima, or kidney beans, or chickpeas, split peas, or lentils (cooked)
- 60 mg per 1 cup soy milk

Nuts

- 100 mg per 1 oz Brazil nuts
- 80 mg per 1 oz almonds or cashews
- 70 mg per 1 oz pine nuts
- 45 mg per 1 oz hazelnuts or walnuts

Vegetables and Fruits

- 80 mg per ½ cup cooked spinach
- 40 mg per ½ cup cooked okra
- 30 mg per ½ cup sweet potato
- 20 mg per ½ cup edible to pod peas, corn, or summer squash
- 20 mg per ½ cup bananas

Fish

- 40 to 90 mg per 3 oz serving (halibut, tuna, or haddock)
- 55 mg per 3 oz crab meat

Cereals and Grain Products

- 110 mg per ½ cup all bran cereal
- 40 mg per ¾ cup wheat bran flakes
- 40 mg per ½ cup brown rice
- 30 mg per ½ cup cooked bulgur
- 55 mg per 1 cup cooked oatmeal
- 25 to 30 mg per ½ cup white rice

Other

- 40 mg per 8 oz plain yogurt
- 40 mg per 1 Tbsp blackstrap molasses

Data from U.S. Department of Agriculture/Agricultural Research Service (USDA/ARS) (2005) USDA Nutrient Database for Standard Reference, Release 18. USDA/ARS, Washington, DC. Retrieved November 15, 2005, from www.ars.usda.gov/ba/bhnrc/ndl.

Clinical Correlation

Magnesium Deficiency in Chronic Alcohol Abuse

Chronic alcoholics are prone to Mg^{2+} depletion for several reasons. First, as blood alcohol levels rise, the kidney is less efficient at reabsorbing Mg^{2+} from the tubular fluid. Alcoholics also have frequent episodes of diarrhea, which result in loss of large amounts of Mg^{2+}. Lastly, these subjects are usually poorly nourished and have a low Mg^{2+} intake. Alcohol and refined foods have very low Mg^{2+} content. Mg^{2+} is not included in routine blood tests, but other measurements may provide clues that suggest a Mg^{2+} deficiency. Low blood calcium is one such clue.

Thinking Critically

1. What is the effect of Mg^{2+} deficiency on calcium metabolism?
2. Would high-dose calcium correct the adverse effects of Mg^{2+} deficiency on calcium homeostasis? Why?
3. What would be the correct therapy? Why?

(Altura and Altura, 1995), and osteoporosis (Freudenheim et al., 1986; Yano et al., 1985).

Adverse effects of magnesium ingestion as part of naturally occurring substances in foods has not been associated with any adverse effects. However, because nonfood sources of magnesium, such as various magnesium salts, are used for pharmacological purposes, a tolerable upper intake level (UL) was set by the IOM (1997). Diarrhea was used as the most sensitive indicator of excess magnesium intake from nonfood sources and, indeed, magnesium salts are used as cathartics. The UL for adolescents and adults is 350 mg (14.6 mmol) of supplementary magnesium.

MAGNESIUM DEPLETION

Mg^{2+} depletion is usually secondary to another disease process or to a therapeutic agent. Some disorders that can be associated with Mg^{2+} depletion are summarized in Box 33-1 (Rude, 1996; Whang et al., 1994).

CAUSES

Mg^{2+} may be lost via the gastrointestinal tract, either by excessive loss of secreted fluids or impaired absorption of both dietary and endogenous Mg^{2+}. The Mg^{2+} content of upper intestinal tract fluids is approximately 0.5 mmol/L, and vomiting or nasogastric suction may contribute to Mg^{2+} depletion from loss of these fluids. The Mg^{2+} content of diarrheal fluids and fistulous drainage is much higher (up to 7.5 mmol/L), and, consequently, Mg^{2+} depletion is common in patients with acute or chronic diarrhea, regional enteritis, ulcerative colitis, or an intestinal or biliary fistula. Malabsorption syndromes such as celiac sprue may result in Mg^{2+} deficiency. Steatorrhea and resection or bypass of the small bowel, particularly the ileum, often result in intestinal Mg^{2+} malabsorption and loss from the body. Lastly, acute severe pancreatitis may be associated with hypomagnesemia; this could be due to the clinical problem causing the pancreatitis (e.g., alcoholism) or to Mg^{2+} binding to necrotic fat surrounding the pancreas.

Excessive excretion of Mg^{2+} into the urine is another cause of Mg^{2+} depletion. Renal Mg^{2+} excretion is proportional to tubular fluid flow as well as to Na^+ and Ca^{2+} excretion. Therefore, both chronic intravenous fluid therapy with Na^+-containing fluids and disorders such as primary aldosteronism in which there is extracellular volume expansion may result in Mg^{2+} depletion. Hypercalcemia and hypercalciuria have been shown to decrease renal Mg^{2+} reabsorption and are probably the cause of the excessive renal Mg^{2+} excretion and the hypomagnesemia observed in many

Box 33-1

MAJOR CAUSES OF MAGNESIUM DEFICIENCY

Gastrointestinal Disorders

Prolonged nasogastric suction/vomiting
Acute and chronic diarrhea
Malabsorption syndromes (e.g., celiac sprue)
Extensive bowel resection
Intestinal and biliary fistulas
Acute hemorrhagic pancreatitis

Renal Loss

Chronic parenteral fluid therapy
Osmotic diuresis (e.g., due to presence of glucose in diabetes mellitus)
Hypercalcemia
Drugs
- Diuretics (e.g., furosemide, hydrochlorothiazide)
- Aminoglycosides
- Calcineurin inhibitors (cyclosporin A, tacrolimus)
- Amphotericin B
- Pentamidine
- Cisplatin
- Beta-mimetics
- Catecholamines

Alcohol
Metabolic acidosis (e.g., starvation, diabetic ketoacidosis, and alcoholism)
Renal diseases
- Chronic pyelonephritis, interstitial nephritis, and glomerulonephritis
- Diuretic phase of acute tubular necrosis
- Postobstructive nephropathy
- Renal tubular acidosis
- Postrenal transplantation
- Inherited tubular diseases

Endocrine disorders
- Hyperparathyroidism
- Hyperthyreosis
- Hyperaldosteronism
- Syndrome of inappropriate secretion of antidiuretic hormone (SIADH)

Clinical Correlation

Cardiac Dysrhythmia in Patients With Diabetes Mellitus

Cardiovascular disease is a common cause of morbidity and mortality in patients with diabetes mellitus. This is in part due to hyperlipidemia and hypertension leading to coronary heart disease. Mg^{2+} deficiency has been linked to hypertension, perhaps by altering Ca^{2+} channels resulting in increased Ca^{2+} in the vascular smooth muscle causing vasospasm. Patients with diabetes mellitus are at risk for Mg^{2+} depletion. Renal Mg^{2+} loss has been correlated with high blood glucose and high urine glucose excretion. It is thought that the osmotic diuresis due to the glucose causes the kidney to waste Mg^{2+}. Dietary Mg^{2+} intake in diabetics also tends to fall short of the recommended dietary allowance (RDA) (Schmidt et al., 1994). Other medications may also contribute to Mg^{2+} loss. Patients with high blood pressure and heart disease frequently receive diuretics such as furosemide. Furosemide blocks the reabsorption of Mg^{2+} in the thick ascending limb of the loop of Henle, the major site of renal Mg^{2+} reabsorption, and this causes marked urinary Mg^{2+} loss.

Thinking Critically

1. Does Mg^{2+} deficiency contribute to heart dysrhythmias? Why?
2. How does Mg^{2+} deficiency affect potassium homeostasis?
3. Will potassium therapy alone correct the potassium deficit in Mg^{2+}-deficient patients?

hypercalcemic states. An osmotic diuresis will result in increased renal Mg^{2+} excretion due to excessive urinary volume. Osmotic diuresis due to glucosuria can, thus, result in Mg^{2+} depletion, and diabetes mellitus is probably the most common clinical disorder associated with Mg^{2+} depletion. The degree of Mg^{2+} depletion in patients with diabetes mellitus has been related to the amount of glucose excreted into the urine and, hence, with the degree of osmotic diuresis.

A number of drugs can cause renal Mg^{2+} wasting and Mg^{2+} depletion. These include furosemide, aminoglycosides, amphotericin B, cisplatin, cyclosporine, and pentamidine (Shah and Kirschenbaum, 1991). An elevated blood alcohol level has been associated with hypermagnesuria, and increased urinary excretion of Mg^{2+} is one factor contributing to Mg^{2+} depletion in chronic alcoholism. Metabolic acidosis may also impair renal conservation of Mg^{2+}. Lastly, a number of inherited renal disorders may be associated with Mg^{2+} wasting because of impaired renal reabsorption of Mg^{2+}. In these disorders hypomagnesemia may either be a leading symptom or may be part of a complex phenotype resulting from tubular dysfunction (Schlingmann et al., 2004; Konrad and Weber, 2003; for review see Cole and Quamme, 2000).

MANIFESTATIONS

The biochemical and physiological manifestations of severe Mg^{2+} depletion are summarized in Box 33-2.

Hypokalemia

A common feature of Mg^{2+} depletion is hypokalemia (Whang et al., 1994). During Mg^{2+} depletion there is loss of potassium from the cell with intracellular potassium depletion, which is enhanced due to the inability of the kidney to conserve potassium. Attempts to replete the potassium deficit with potassium therapy alone are not successful without simultaneous Mg^{2+} therapy. This potassium depletion may be a contributing cause of the electrocardiographic findings and cardiac dysrhythmias discussed in subsequent text.

Hypocalcemia

Hypocalcemia is also a common manifestation of moderate to severe Mg^{2+} depletion (Rude, 1994). The hypocalcemia may be a major contributing factor to the increased neuromuscular excitability often present in Mg^{2+}-depleted patients. The pathogenesis of hypocalcemia is multifactorial. Impaired parathyroid hormone (PTH) secretion appears to be a major factor in hypomagnesemia-induced hypocalcemia. Serum PTH concentrations are usually low in these patients, and Mg^{2+} administration will immediately stimulate PTH secretion. Patients with hypocalcemia due to Mg^{2+} depletion also exhibit both renal and skeletal resistance to

Box 33-2

MAJOR MANIFESTATIONS OF MAGNESIUM DEPLETION

Biochemical

Hypokalemia

Excessive renal potassium excretion
Decreased intracellular potassium

Hypocalcemia

Impaired parathyroid hormone (PTH) secretion
Renal and skeletal resistance to PTH
Resistance to vitamin D

Neuromuscular

Positive Chvostek's and Trousseau's sign
Spontaneous carpal-pedal spasm
Seizures
Vertigo, ataxia, nystagmus, athetoid and choroform movements
Muscular weakness, tremor, fasciculation and wasting
Psychiatric: depression, psychosis

Cardiovascular

Electrocardiographic abnormalities

Prolonged PR- and QT-intervals
U-waves

Cardiac dysrhythmias

Atrial tachycardia, fibrillations, torsades de pointes

Gastrointestinal

Nausea, vomiting
Anorexia

exogenously administered PTH, as manifested by subnormal urinary cyclic AMP (cAMP) and phosphate excretion and a diminished calcemic response. All these effects are reversed following several days of Mg^{2+} therapy. The basis for the defect in PTH secretion and PTH end-organ resistance is not known. Because cAMP is an important second messenger in PTH secretion and is required for mediating PTH effects in kidney and bone, it has been postulated that there may be a defect in the activity of adenylate cyclase. As discussed previously, Mg^{2+} is both an essential part of the substrate (Mg^{2+}-ATP) for adenylate cyclase and essential for catalytic activity.

Vitamin D metabolism and action may also be abnormal in hypocalcemic Mg^{2+}-deficient patients. Resistance to vitamin D therapy has been reported in such cases. This resistance may be due to impaired metabolism of vitamin D because plasma concentrations of 1,25-dihydroxyvitamin D are low. Because PTH is a major stimulator of the synthesis of 1,25-dihydroxyvitamin D production, the decrease in PTH secretion observed in hypomagnesemia and hypocalcemia may also be a cause of the impaired metabolism of vitamin D (Rude, 1994).

Neuromuscular Manifestations

Neuromuscular hyperexcitability may be the presenting complaint of patients with Mg^{2+} deficiency. Tetany and muscle cramps may be present. Generalized seizures (convulsions) may also occur. Other neuromuscular signs may include dizziness, disequilibrium, muscular tremor, wasting, and weakness (Whang et al., 1994). Although hypocalcemia often contributes to the neurological signs, hypomagnesemia without hypocalcemia has been reported to result in neuromuscular hyperexcitability.

Cardiovascular Manifestations

Mg^{2+} depletion may also result in electrocardiographic abnormalities as well as in cardiac dysrhythmias (Hollifield, 1987), which may be manifested by a rapid heart rate (tachycardia), skipped heart beats (premature beats), or a totally irregular cardiac rhythm (fibrillation). Cardiac dysrhythmias are also known to occur during K depletion; therefore, the effect of Mg^{2+} deficiency on potassium loss from the body may be the cause of the dysrhythmias (Rude, 1996; Whang et al., 1994). Patients with myocardial infarction also commonly have cardiac dysrhythmias. Mg^{2+} administration to patients with acute myocardial infarction has been shown to decrease the mortality rate in some (Woods et al., 1992) but not all studies (ISIS-4 Collaborative Group, 1995).

DIAGNOSIS OF MAGNESIUM DEFICIENCY

Although Mg^{2+} is a relatively abundant cation in the body, more than 99% of it is either intracellular or in the skeleton. The less than

1% of total Mg^{2+} present in the body fluids is the most assessable for clinical testing, and the serum Mg^{2+} concentration is the most widely used measure of Mg^{2+} status. The total serum Mg^{2+} concentration is usually 17 to 22 mg/L (0.7 to 1.0 mmol/L). A serum concentration of less than 17 mg/L usually indicates some degree of Mg^{2+} depletion (Rude, 1996), but the measurement of serum Mg^{2+} concentration does not necessarily reflect the true total body Mg^{2+} content. Low intracellular Mg^{2+} has been documented in patients with serum levels greater than 17 mg/L. Intracellular levels of Mg^{2+} in muscle, red blood cells, and lymphocytes, as well as in bone, appear to reflect more accurately whole body Mg^{2+} status, but these tests have not been developed for clinical use (Rude, 1996). Recently, ion-specific electrodes have become available for determining ionized Mg^{2+} in the plasma. Some results suggest that the concentration of free ionized Mg^{2+} in the plasma may be a better index of Mg^{2+} status than the total serum Mg^{2+} concentration, but further evaluation is necessary (Altura et al., 1992).

In patients at risk for Mg^{2+} deficiency but with normal serum Mg^{2+} levels, Mg^{2+} status can be further evaluated by determining the amount of Mg^{2+} excreted in the urine following an intravenous infusion of Mg^{2+}. Normal subjects excrete at least 80% of an intravenous Mg^{2+} load within 24 hours, whereas patients with Mg^{2+} deficiency excrete much less. The Mg^{2+} load test, however, requires normal renal handling of Mg^{2+}. If excess Mg^{2+} is being excreted by the kidneys due to diuresis, the Mg^{2+} load test may yield an inappropriate negative result. Conversely, if renal function is impaired and less blood is being filtered, this test could give a false-positive result.

MAGNESIUM TOXICITY

Mg^{2+} intoxication is not a frequently encountered clinical problem, although mild-to-moderate elevations in the serum Mg^{2+} concentration may be seen in as many as 12% of hospitalized patients (Wong et al., 1983). Symptomatic hypermagnesemia is almost always caused by excessive intake or administration of Mg^{2+} salts (Mordes, 1978). Most patients with hypermagnesemia have concomitant renal failure, and hypermagnesemia is usually seen in patients with renal failure who are receiving Mg^{2+} as an antacid, enema, or infusion. Mg^{2+} infusions also are sometimes given for pregnancy-induced hypertension and for treatment of Mg^{2+} deficiency.

Neuromuscular symptoms are the most common presenting problem in Mg^{2+} intoxication. One of the earliest demonstrable effects of hypermagnesemia is the disappearance of the deep tendon reflexes at serum Mg^{2+} concentrations of 2 to 3 mmol/L. Depressed respiration and apnea due to paralysis of the voluntary musculature may be seen at serum Mg^{2+} concentrations in excess of 4 to 5 mmol/L. Cardiac arrest may occur at concentrations greater than 6 mmol/L. Moderate elevations in the serum Mg^{2+} concentration (increases of ~1.5 to 2.5 mmol/L) can result in a mild reduction in blood pressure. Other nonspecific manifestations of Mg^{2+} intoxication include nausea, vomiting, and cutaneous flushing at serum levels of 1.5 to 4 mmol/L (Mordes, 1978).

REFERENCES

Ackerman MJ, Clapham DE (1997) Ion channels—basic science and clinical disease. N Engl J Med 336:1575-1586.

Altura BM, Altura BT (1995) Role of magnesium in the pathogenesis of hypertension updated: relationship to its actions on cardiac, vascular smooth muscle, and endothelial cells. In: Laragh H, Brenner BM (eds) Hypertension: Pathophysiology, Diagnosis, and Management, 2nd ed. Raven Press, New York, pp 1214-1242.

Altura BT, Shirey TL, Young CC, Hiti J, Dell'Orfano K, Handwerker SM, Altura BM (1992) A new method for the rapid determination of ionized Mg in whole blood, serum and plasma. Methods Find Exp Clin Pharmacol 14:297-304.

Birch NJ (1993) Magnesium and the Cell. Academic Press, New York.

Chubanov V, Waldegger S, Mederos y Schnitzler M, Vitzthum H, Sassen MC, Seyberth HW, Konrad M, Gudermann T (2004) Disruption of TRPM6/TRPM7 complex formation by a mutation in the TRPM6 gene causes hypomagnesemia with secondary hypocalcemia. Proc Natl Acad Sci USA 101:2894-2899.

Cleveland LE, Goldman JD, Borrud LG (1996) Data tables: results from USDA's 1994 continuing survey of food intakes by individuals and 1994 diet and health knowledge survey. Agricultural Research Service, U.S. Department of Agriculture, Beltsville, MD.

Cole DE, Quamme GA (2000) Inherited disorders of renal magnesium handling. J Am Soc Nephrol 11:1937-1947.

Connolly TM, Bross TE, Majerus PW (1985) Isolation of a phosphomonoesterase from human platelets that specifically hydrolyzes the 5-phosphate of inositol 1,4,5-triphosphate. J Biol Chem 260:7868-7874.

Cowan JA (2002) Structural and catalytic chemistry of magnesium-dependent enzymes. Biometals. 2002:225-235.

Cowan JA (1995) The Biological Chemistry of Magnesium. VCH Publishers, New York.

Dai LJ, Quamme GA (1991) Intracellular Mg and magnesium depletion in isolated renal thick ascending limb cells. J Clin Invest 88:1255-1264.

Dai LJ, Ritchie G, Kerstan D, Kang HS, Cole DE, Quamme GA (2001) Magnesium transport in the renal distal convoluted tubule. Physiol Rev 81:51-84.

Davey GK, Spencer EA, Appleby PN, Allen NE, Knox KH, Key TJ (2002) EPIC-Oxford: lifestyle characteristics and nutrient intakes in a cohort of 33883 meat-eaters and 31546 non meat-eaters in the UK. Public Health Nut 6:259-268.

Di Stefano A, Desfleurs E, Simeone S, Nitschke R, Wittner M (1997) Ca^{2+} and Mg^{2+} sensor in the thick ascending limb of the loop of Henle. Kidney Blood Press Res 20:190-193.

Dorup I (1994) Magnesium and potassium deficiency: its diagnosis, occurrence and treatment in diuretic therapy and its consequences for growth, protein synthesis, and growth factors. Acta Physiol Scand 150:Suppl 618:7-46.

Efrati E, Arsentiev-Rozenfeld J, Zelikovic I (2005) The human paracellin-1 gene (hPCLN-1): renal epithelial cell-specific expression and regulation. Am J Physiol Renal Physiol: 288 F272-F283.

Elin R (1997) Evaluating the role of ionized magnesium in laboratory and clinical practice. In: Smetana R (ed) Advances in Magnesium Research: 1. John Libbey & Co., London, pp 525-531.

Elin R (1987) Assessment of magnesium status. Clin Chem 33:1965-1970.

Elin RJ (1994) Magnesium: the fifth but forgotten electrolyte. Am J Clin Pathol 102:616-622.

Fine KD, Santa Ana CA, Porter JL, Fordtran JS (1991) Intestinal absorption of magnesium from food and supplements. J Clin Invest 88:396-402.

Fleig A, Penner R (2004) The TRPM ion channel subfamily: molecular, biophysical and functional features. Trends Pharmacol Sci 25:633-639.

Franz KB (1989) Influence of phosphorus on intestinal absorption of calcium and magnesium. In: Itokawa Y, Durlach J (eds) Magnesium in Health and Disease. John Libbey & Co., London, pp 71-78.

Frausto da Silva JJR, Williams RJP (1991) The biological chemistry of magnesium:phosphate metabolism. In: The Biological Chemistry of the Elements. Oxford University Press, Oxford, pp 241-267.

Freudenheim JL, Johnson NE, Smith EL (1986) Relationships between usual nutrient intake and bone-mineral content of women 35–65 years of age: longitudinal and cross-sectional analysis. Am J Clin Nutr 44:863-876.

Hebert SC (1996) Extracellular calcium-sensing receptor: implications for calcium and magnesium handling in the kidney. Kidney Int 50:2129-2139.

Hollifield JW (1987) Magnesium depletion, diuretics, and arrhythmias. Am J Med 82:(Suppl 3A):30-37.

Hunt MS, Schofield FA (1969) Magnesium balance and protein intake level in adult human females. Am J Clin Nutr 22:367-373.

Ikari A, Hirai N, Shiroma M, Harada H, Sakai H, Hayashi H, Suzuki Y, Degawa M, Takagi K (2004) Association of paracellin-1 with ZO-1 augments reabsorption of divalent cations in renal epithelial cells. J Biol Chem: 279: 54826-54832.

Institute of Medicine (IOM) (1997) Dietary Reference Intakes for Calcium, Phosphorus, Magnesium, Vitamin D, and Fluoride. National Academy Press, Washington, DC.

Iseri LT, French JH (1984) Magnesium: nature's physiologic calcium blocker. Am Heart J 108:188-193.

ISIS-4 Collaborative Group (1995) Fourth International Study of Infarct Survival: a randomised factorial trial assessing early oral captopril, oral mononitrate, and intravenous magnesium sulphate in 58,050 patients with suspected acute myocardial infarction. Lancet 345:669-685.

Kayne LH, Lee DBN (1993) Intestinal magnesium absorption. Miner Electrolyte Metab 19:210-217.

Kerstan D, Quamme GA (2002) Intestinal absorption of magnesium. In: Massry SG, Morii H, Nishizawa Y (eds) Calcium in Internal Medicine. Springer-Verlag, London Berlin Heidelberg, pp 171-183.

Konrad M, Weber S (2003) Recent advances in molecular genetics of hereditary magnesium-losing disorders. J Am Soc Nephrol 14:249-260.

Leliévre-Pegorier M, Merlet-Bénichou C, Roinel N, de Rouffignac C (1983) Developmental pattern of water and electrolyte transport in the superficial nephron. Am J Physiol 244:F15-F21.

Maguire ME, Cowan JA (2002) Magnesium chemistry and biochemistry. Biometals 15:203-210.

Marier JR (1986) Magnesium content of the food supply in the modern-day world. Magnesium 5:1-8.

Massry SG, Coburn JW, Kleeman CR (1969) Renal handling of magnesium in the dog. Am J Physiol 216:1460-1467.

Matsuda H (1991) Magnesium gating of the inwardly rectifying K^+ channel. Annu Rev Physiol 53:289-298.

Mordes JP (1978) Excess magnesium. Pharmacol Rev 29:273-300.

Muller D, Kausalya PJ, Claverie-Martin F, Meij IC, Eggert P, Garcia-Nieto V, Hunziker W (2003) A novel claudin 16 mutation associated with childhood hypercalciuria abolishes binding to ZO-1 and results in lysosomal mistargeting. Am J Hum Genet 73:1293-1301.

Nadler MJ, Hermosura MC, Inabe K, Perraud AL, Zhu Q, Stokes AJ, Kurosaki T, Kinet JP, Penner R, Scharenberg AM, Fleig A (2001) LTRPC7 is a Mg.ATP-regulated divalent cation channel required for cell viability. Nature 411:590-595.

O'Rourke B (1993) Ion channels as sensors of cellular energy: mechanism for modulation by magnesium and nucleotides. Biochem Pharmacol 46:1103-1112.

Quamme GA, Dirks JH (1986) The physiology of renal magnesium handling. Renal Physiol 9:257-269.

Romani A, Marfella C, Scarpa A (1993) Cell magnesium transport and homeostasis: role of intracellular compartments. Miner Electrolyte Metab 19:282-289.

Romani A, Scarpa A (1992) Regulation of cell magnesium. Arch Biochem Biophys 298:1-12.

Rude RK (1996) Magnesium disorders. In: Kokko JP, Tannen RL (eds) Fluids and Electrolytes, 3rd ed. WB Saunders, Philadelphia, pp 421-445.

Rude RK (1994) Magnesium deficiency in parathyroid function. In: Bilezikian JP (ed) The Parathyroids. Raven Press, New York, pp 829-842.

Runnels LW, Yue L, Clapham DE (2001) TRP-PLIK, a bifunctional protein with kinase and ion channel activities. Science 291:1043-1047.

Ryan MF (1991) The role of magnesium in clinical biochemistry: an overview. Ann Clin Biochem 28:19-26.

Schlingmann KP, Konrad M, Seyberth HW (2004) Genetics of hereditary disorders of magnesium metabolism. Pediatr Nephrol 19:13-25.

Schlingmann KP, Weber S, Peters M, Niemann Nejsum L, Vitzthum H, Klingel K, Kratz M, Haddad E, Ristoff E, Dinour D, Syrrou M, Nielsen S, Sassen M, Waldegger S, Seyberth HW, Konrad M (2002) Hypomagnesemia with secondary hypocalcemia is caused by mutations in TRPM6, a new member of the TRPM gene family. Nat Genet 31:166-170.

Schmidt LE, Arfken CL, Heins JM (1994) Evaluation of nutrient intake in subjects with non-insulin-dependent diabetes mellitus. J Am Diet Assoc 94:773-774.

Schmitz C, Perraud AL, Johnson CO, Inabe K, Smith MK, Penner R, Kurosaki T, Fleig A, Scharenberg AM (2003) Regulation of vertebrate cellular Mg(2 +) homeostasis by TRPM7. Cell 114:191-200.

Shah GM, Kirschenbaum MA (1991) Renal magnesium wasting associated with therapeutic agents. Miner Electrolyte Metab 17:58-64.

Shaul O (2002) Magnesium transport and function in plants: the tip of the iceberg. Biometals 15:309-323.

Siener R, Hesse A (1995) Influence of a mixed and a vegetarian diet on urinary magnesium excretion and concentration. Br J Nutr 73:783-790.

Simon DB, Lu Y, Choate KA, Velazquez H, Al-Sabban E, Praga M, Casari G, Bettinelli A, Colussi G, Rodriguez-Soriano J, McCredie D, Milford D, Sanjad S, Lifton RP (1999) Paracellin-1, a renal tight junction protein required for paracellular Mg^{2+} resorption. Science 285:103-106.

Voets T, Nilius B, Hoefs S, van der Kemp AW, Droogmans G, Bindels RJ, Hoenderop JG (2004) TRPM6 forms the Mg^{2+} influx channel involved in intestinal and renal Mg^{2+} absorption. J Biol Chem 279:19-25.

Volpe P, Alderson-Lang BH, Nickols GA (1990) Regulation of inositol 1,4,5-triphosphate-induced Ca^{2+} release. I. Effect of magnesium ion. Am J Physiol 258:C1077-C1085.

Walder RY, Landau D, Meyer P, Shalev H, Tsolia M, Borochowitz Z, Boettger MB, Beck GE, Englehardt RK, Carmi R, Sheffield VC (2002) Mutation of TRPM6 causes familial hypomagnesemia with secondary hypocalcemia. Nat Genet 31:171-174.

Wallach S (1988) Availability of body magnesium during magnesium deficiency. Magnesium 7:262-270.

Whang R, Hampton EM, Whang DD (1994) Magnesium homeostasis and clinical disorders of magnesium deficiency. Ann Pharmacol 28:220-226.

White RE, Hartzell HC (1989) Magnesium ions in cardiac function: regulator of ion channels and second messengers. Biochem Pharmacol 38:859-867.

Wong ET, Rude RK, Singer FR, Shaw ST (1983) A high prevalence of hypomagnesemia and hypermagnesemia in hospitalized patients. Am J Clin Pathol 79:348-352.

Woods KL, Fletcher S, Roffe C, Haider Y (1992) Intravenous magnesium sulphate in suspected acute myocardial infarction: result of the second Leicester Intravenous Magnesium Intervention Trial (LIMIT-2). Lancet 339:1553-1558.

Yano K, Heilbrun LK, Wasnich RD, Hankin JH, Vogel JM (1985) The relationship between diet and bone mineral content of multiple skeletal sites in elderly women living in Hawaii. Am J Clin Nutr 42:877-888.

RECOMMENDED READINGS

Birch NJ (1993) Magnesium and the Cell. Academic Press, New York.

Cowan JA (1995) The Biological Chemistry of Magnesium. VCH Publishers, New York.

Frausto da Silva JJR, Williams RJP (1991) The biological chemistry of magnesium:phosphate metabolism. In: The Biological Chemistry of the Elements. Oxford University Press, Oxford, pp 241-267.

Rude RK (1996) Magnesium disorders. In: Kokka JP, Tannen RL (eds) Fluids and Electrolytes, 3rd ed. WB Saunders, Philadelphia, pp 421-445.

Chapter 34

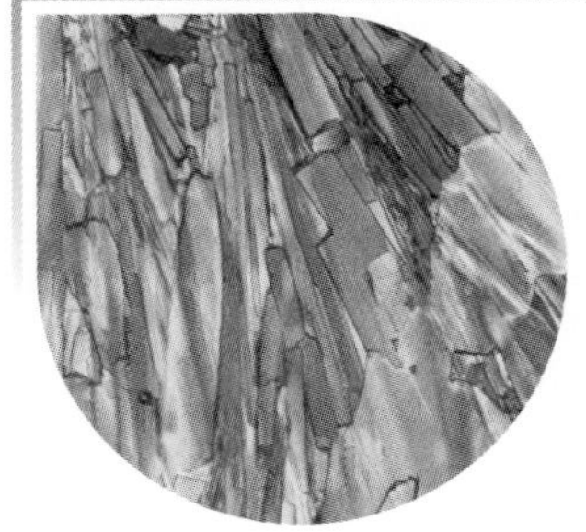

Sodium, Chloride, and Potassium

Hwai-Ping Sheng, PhD

OUTLINE

COMMON ABBREVIATIONS

AVP arginine vasopressin, also known as antidiuretic hormone (ADH)

ANP atrial natriuretic peptide

FUNCTIONS AND DISTRIBUTION OF SODIUM, CHLORIDE, AND POTASSIUM

Sodium, chloride, and potassium exist largely as free hydrated ions that bind only weakly to organic molecules. These three major ions are widely distributed in the body and are the principal electrolytes of body fluids.

DISTRIBUTION BETWEEN INTRACELLULAR AND EXTRACELLULAR FLUID COMPARTMENTS

In essence, the fluids in the body can be compartmentalized into an extracellular and an intracellular compartment. These two compartments are separated by membranes that surround the cells. Because of the properties of the cell membranes, these major ions or electrolytes, together with others in smaller quantities, are distributed unequally across the plasma membranes so that the composition of the extracellular fluid is very different from that of the intracellular fluid. The extracellular fluid contains high concentrations of sodium (Na^+), chloride (Cl^-), and bicarbonate (HCO_3^-) ions, and intracellular fluid contains high concentrations of potassium (K^+), magnesium (Mg^{2+}), and phosphate ions (HPO_4^{2-} and $H_2PO_4^-$) as illustrated in Figure 34-1. The concentration of Na^+ in the extracellular fluid is regulated at

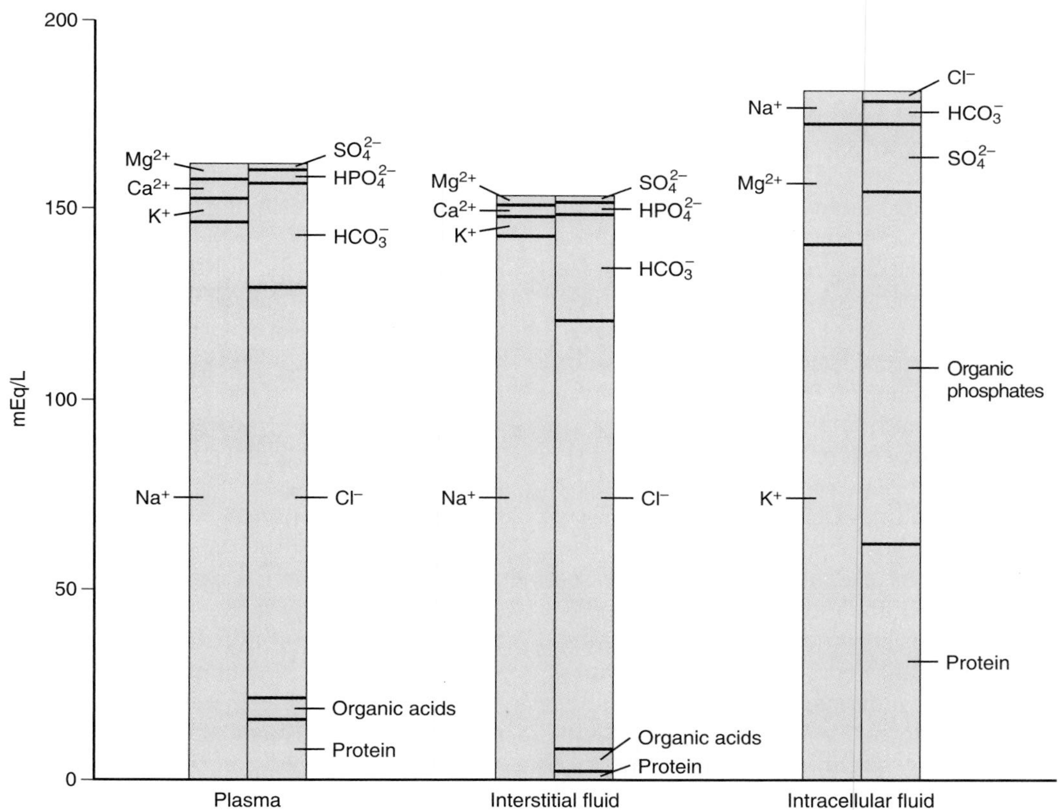

Figure 34-1 Ionic composition of plasma, interstitial, and intracellular compartments. Concentrations are expressed in milliequivalents (mEq) per liter.

approximately 145 mmol/L, whereas its concentration in the intracellular fluid is 12 mmol/L. The distribution of Cl^- generally follows that of Na^+ with an extracellular concentration of about 110 mmol/L and an intracellular concentration of about 2 mmol/L. The concentration of K^+ is 150 mmol/L inside the cells and 4 to 5 mmol/L in the extracellular fluid. Therefore, Na^+ and Cl^- are responsible for the osmolarity of the extracellular fluid, whereas K^+, being the principal intracellular cation, is responsible for the osmolarity of the intracellular fluid compartment (Rose and Post, 2001).

Movement of Sodium and Potassium Across Cell Membranes

Large differences in concentrations of ions across cell membranes are the result of the permeability characteristics of cell membranes as well as the activity of membrane transport proteins located on plasma membranes. Movements of ions across cell membranes can occur by passive diffusion along a concentration or electrical gradient through ion channels or by active transport ("pumping") against these gradients coupled to an energy-yielding process. The selective permeability of the cell membranes prevents the movement out of cells of proteins and phosphates, which are mostly organic metabolic intermediates. High concentrations of these intracellular organic anions require neutralization of the excess negative charges by cations, of which K^+ is the most important. The intracellular accumulation of K^+ in exchange for Na^+, against their concentration gradients, is achieved by the Na^+-K^+-pump of the plasma membrane.

The Mg^{2+}-dependent, Na^+- and K^+-activated ATPase (Na^+,K^+-ATPase) is the molecular basis of the Na^+-K^+-pump. Details of the structure of this membrane-bound protein became available in the 1980s, and this has permitted increased understanding of the mechanism of Na^+ and K^+ pumping by this enzyme. Structurally, the functional unit of this enzyme is a heterodimer of two subunit proteins, the α- and β-subunits (Blanco and Mercer, 1998). The α- and β-subunits are expressed in various isoforms in a variety of tissues, and the relative proportion of each subunit isoform varies among tissues.

At present, four α-subunit (α_1–α_4) and three β-subunit (β_1–β_3) isoforms have been identified. The α-subunit spans the membrane and has two large cytoplasmic domains. It is responsible for ATP hydrolysis and cation transport, as it contains sites for cation-binding (Na^+- and K^+-binding) and sites for binding ATP and phosphorylation in the intracellular portion. The β-subunit, with a large extracellular domain, is a glycoprotein that also spans the membrane. It modulates the Na^+ and K^+ affinity of the enzyme. As illustrated in Figure 34-2, three Na^+ from the cytosol bind to the inward facing cation-binding sites of the α-subunit. Binding of ATP on the cytoplasmic side of the transporter activates the catalytic site of the transporter, which then cleaves the ATP and phosphorylates the aspartate residue on the α-subunit. Phosphorylation of the aspartate residue causes the transport protein to change conformation, resulting in the release of three Na^+ from the transport protein into the extracellular fluid. The transporter is now in a conformation that allows binding of K^+ to the outward facing cation-binding sites. Binding of two K^+ results in dephosphorylation of the α-subunit. The transport protein then returns to its previous conformation and two K^+ are released into the cytosol in the process.

The overall stoichiometry of the Na^+,K^+-ATPase reaction is that, with the hydrolysis of one molecule of ATP, three Na^+ and two K^+ are translocated across the cell membrane to maintain or restore the normally high K^+ and low Na^+ concentrations inside the cells. The net movement of cations out of the cell creates a negative charge in the cell compared with the outside. Therefore, the Na^+,K^+-ATPase is an electrogenic pump. The maintenance of a differential gradient for Na^+ and K^+ across cell membranes is a prerequisite for the ionic homeostasis of the cells, for cell volume regulation, and for transport of other ions and secondary active transport of sugars, amino acids, neurotransmitters, and other solutes across cell membranes. Furthermore, in electrically excitable cells, creation and maintenance of Na^+ and K^+ gradients across cell membranes are required for the generation and maintenance of the resting potential and the generation and propagation of action potentials.

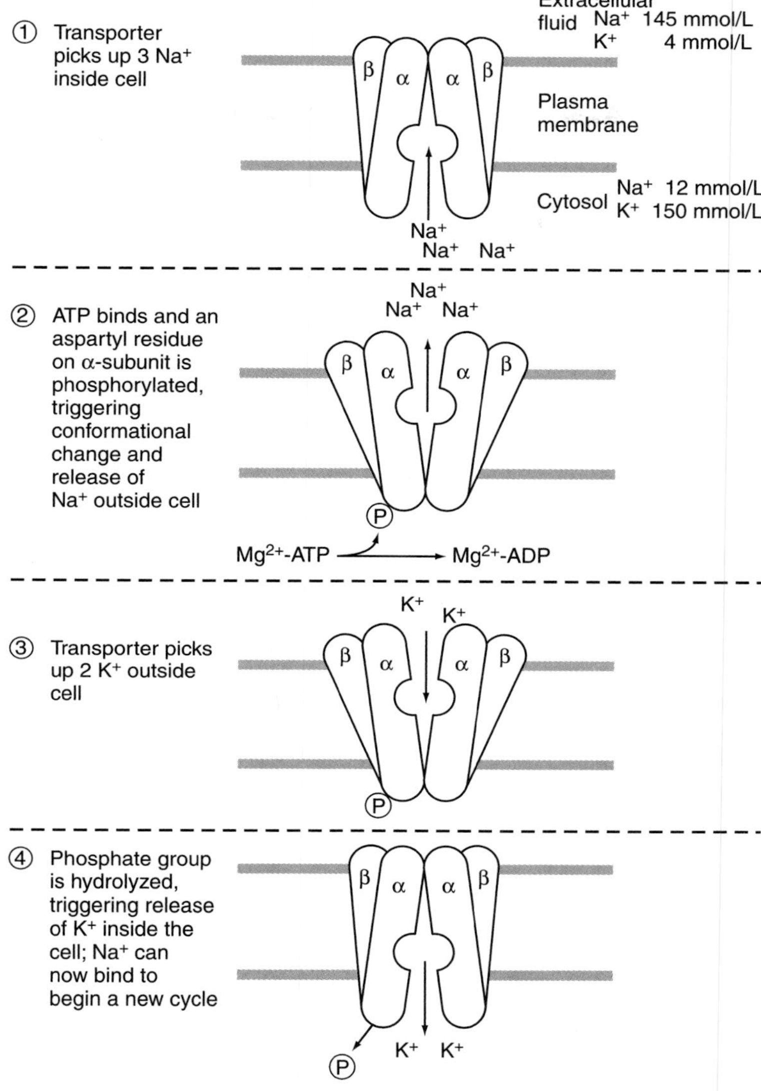
Extracellular fluid Na+ 145 mmol/L
K+ 4 mmol/L
① Transporter picks up 3 Na+ inside cell
β α α β
Plasma membrane
Cytosol Na+ 12 mmol/L K+ 150 mmol/L
Na+ Na+ Na+
② ATP binds and an aspartyl residue on α-subunit is phosphorylated, triggering conformational change and release of Na+ outside cell
Na+ Na+ Na+
P
Mg2+-ATP
Mg2+-ADP
③ Transporter picks up 2 K+ outside cell
K+ K+
④ Phosphate group is hydrolyzed, triggering release of K+ inside the cell; Na+ can now bind to begin a new cycle
K+ K+

Figure 34-2 Schematic representation of the enzyme Na^+,K^+-ATPase, which is responsible for primary active transport of Na^+ and K^+ in opposite directions across plasma membranes. The enzyme consists of two types of subunits (α and β) and is thought to have the subunit composition $(\alpha\beta)_2$ and to have one set of cation-binding sites. The α-subunit contains the K^+ and Na^+ binding sites; it also contains a site for binding ATP and a phosphorylation site in the intracellular portion. Binding of Na^+ and ATP intracellularly activates the enzyme ATPase, which cleaves one molecule of ATP to ADP and phosphorylates an aspartate residue on a subunit. Phosphorylation causes a conformational change in the carrier protein molecule, thereby extruding Na^+ on the extracellular surface and allowing extracellular K^+ to bind. K^+ binding activates intracellular hydrolysis of the bound phosphate group, resulting in a conformational change and release of K^+ inside the cell. The transporter is now ready to bind Na^+ for another transport cycle. For each ATP hydrolyzed, $3Na^+$ ions are moved out of the cell and $2K^+$ ions are moved into it. This accounts for the low intracellular Na^+ and high intracellular K^+ concentrations.

DISTRIBUTION BETWEEN VASCULAR AND INTERSTITIAL FLUID COMPARTMENTS

Collectively, the extracellular fluid in the vascular compartment (plasma) and spaces surrounding cells (interstitial fluid) is called extracellular fluid. In contrast to the vast differences in composition between the intracellular and extracellular fluid compartments, the composition of fluids in plasma and interstitial spaces is very similar. Similarities in composition between plasma and interstitial fluid are due to the permeability characteristics of the capillary endothelium that separates them. The capillary endothelium acts as a semipermeable barrier that allows free movement of solutes of low molecular weight while retaining proteins in the vascular compartment. The small amount of protein that diffuses into the interstitial space is returned to the circulation via the lymphatics. This accounts for the low concentration of protein, less than 10 g/L, in the interstitial fluid, compared with an average of 73 g/L in the plasma. The concentration difference of protein across the capillary endothelium affects the distribution of diffusible ions so that the concentration of any diffusible cation is higher and the concentration of any diffusible anion is lower in the plasma than in the interstitial fluid, in accordance with the Gibbs-Donnan equilibrium (see Chapter 35). This Gibbs-Donnan effect is small at the normal concentration of plasma protein. It causes a difference of approximately 5% in the concentrations of Na^+, K^+, and Cl^- across the capillary endothelium. For all practical purposes the ionic compositions of plasma and interstitial fluid are considered to be the same.

SODIUM: A MAJOR DETERMINANT OF EXTRACELLULAR FLUID VOLUME

The concentrations of the three major ions in body fluids are controlled within narrow limits in order for the body to function properly, as these ions play central roles in electrolytic balances and current, in osmotic control, and in transport of organic molecules by cells. The volume of the extracellular fluid compartment (interstitial fluid and plasma) is determined primarily by the total amount of osmotic particles present. Because of its abundance, Na^+, together with its accompanying anions Cl^- and HCO_3^-, is the major determinant of osmolarity of extracellular fluid. Hence, a rough estimate of the osmolarity of plasma can be obtained by doubling its Na^+ concentration. Because Na^+ concentration in the plasma is regulated at approximately 145 mmol/L, the osmolarity of plasma and body fluids is thus estimated to be 290 mmol/L.

Any disturbances in Na^+ balance will change the osmolarity, and hence volume, of the extracellular fluid compartment. This can be illustrated simply by the infusion of a hypertonic NaCl solution into the circulation. The added Na^+ distributes rapidly between the vascular and interstitial fluid compartments, causing increases in the Na^+ concentration and osmolarity of both of these compartments. Osmoreceptors present in the supraoptic and paraventricular nuclei in the hypothalamus are stimulated by the increased osmolarity of the fluid that bathes them (Baylis and Thompson, 1988). Stimulation of these cells activates the thirst mechanism and also causes the release of arginine vasopressin hormone (AVP) (also called antidiuretic hormone [ADH]) from the posterior pituitary. Drinking of water in response to thirst, together with the AVP-induced decrease in water excretion by the kidneys, restores the osmolarity toward normal and increases the volume of the extracellular fluid. Conversely, a decrease in the osmolarity of the extracellular fluid due to a loss of NaCl in excess of water from the body causes excretion of water by the kidneys. This will restore the osmolarity of the extracellular fluid compartment toward normal and decrease its volume. Therefore, any alteration in the concentrations of Na^+ and Cl^- in the extracellular fluid results in parallel changes in its volume when the mechanisms for thirst and secretion of AVP function normally.

MEMBRANE POTENTIALS IN NERVES AND MUSCLES

Resting Membrane Potential

Much of our understanding of the ionic mechanisms of membrane potentials comes from experiments on the giant squid axon and frog sartorius muscle preparations.

When a microelectrode of tip diameter less than 0.5 μm is inserted into a cell, a potential difference between the tip of the microelectrode inside the cell and a reference electrode placed outside the cell can be recorded. This potential difference under resting conditions is the resting membrane potential of the cell; the inside of the cell is negative with respect to the outside under resting conditions. The magnitude of this resting membrane potential differs among tissues and is determined by the differences in specific ion concentrations in the intracellular and extracellular fluids and the differences in membrane permeabilities to the different ions. Because Na^+ and K^+ are the major ions, they generally play the most important roles in generating the membrane potential.

The concentration differences of electrolytes across the cell membranes causes K^+ to diffuse out of the cell and Na^+ into the cell down their concentration gradients through the K^+-Na^+ leak channels. However, passive K^+ efflux is greater than passive Na^+ influx because the K^+-Na^+ leak channels are more permeable to K^+ than to Na^+ in the resting state. Because the membrane is impermeable to most of the organic anions in the cell, the K^+ efflux is not accompanied by an equal efflux of anions, and the membrane is maintained in a polarized state, with the inside negative relative to the outside (i.e., the resting membrane potential). The electrical potential developed begins to influence the efflux of K^+ and influx of Na^+ across the membrane. The negativity inside the cells attracts these cations and the positivity outside the cells repulses these cations. For K^+, as long as efflux due to its concentration gradient is greater than influx due to the electrical potential, there will be net efflux. The membrane potential at which efflux of K^+ is equal to its influx is called the equilibrium potential for K^+.

A K^+ equilibrium potential of approximately −95 mV is calculated from its concentrations in the intracellular and extracellular fluids. Similarly, an equilibrium potential of +60 mV for Na^+ is calculated from its concentration gradient. Because the membrane is more permeable to K^+ than to Na^+, the resting membrane potential is closer to the K^+ equilibrium potential, approximately −70 mV for many mammalian neurons and −90 mV for skeletal muscle fibers. At that resting membrane potential, there is a net influx of Na^+ and a net efflux of K^+ through their channels. However, the concentrations of intracellular Na^+ and K^+ remain relatively constant due to the activity of the Na^+,K^+-ATPase in the membrane. In the resting state, the number of ions moved by the Na^+,K^+-ATPase equals the number of ions that move in the opposite direction through the membrane channels down their concentration or electrical gradients.

In most cells, because of the absence of an active Cl^- pump, movements of Cl^- across membranes are passive through Cl^- channels. The negative membrane potential moves Cl^- out, and the concentration gradient moves Cl^- into the cell. Therefore, the Cl^- concentration gradient across the membrane adjusts until the equilibrium potential for Cl^- is equal to the resting membrane potential. Unlike K^+ and Na^+, Cl^- flux responds to the membrane potential and makes no contribution to its magnitude.

Action Potential

Membrane potentials can be depolarized (decreased in negativity) or hyperpolarized (increased in negativity) depending on the direction of current flow across the cell membrane. The magnitude of change in membrane potential depends on the intensity of current flow, which, in turn, is dependent on the strength of the stimulus. Depolarization of the cell membrane can be achieved by transient activation of nerve and muscle cells. A weak stimulus (subthreshold stimulus) decreases the resting membrane potential (depolarization), making it less negative, which leads to increased K^+ efflux that restores the membrane potential to its resting value. The size of this depolarization diminishes as the current moves along the membrane away from the point of stimulation. However, when a stronger stimulus is applied to the cell membrane, the size of potential change is larger. When depolarization reaches the threshold membrane potential, an action potential is triggered. This is characterized by a rapid large response in which the membrane potential actually reverses from a potential of −70 mV to +30 mV. After this rapid reversal, the potential repolarizes and returns toward its resting membrane potential. A transient hyperpolarization, known as hyperpolarizing afterpotential, occurs before the potential finally returns to its resting membrane potential of −70 mV. The action potential differs from the local response to a subthreshold stimulus in that its magnitude does not increase with an increase in stimulus strength, and, once the action potential is elicited, it is propagated without changes in size or shape as it travels along the length of the nerve or muscle fibers. Thus the action potential is described as an all-or-none response.

Both the voltage-gated Na^+ channels and voltage-gated K^+ channels play important roles in the events of the action potential. In the giant squid axon, when the membrane depolarizes by approximately 20 mV to 40 mV (i.e., from −70 mV to a value of −50 mV to −30 mV), successive increases in membrane conductance to Na^+ and K^+ occur. The voltage-gated Na^+ channels are activated during the early part of the action potential and begin to allow a rapid inflow of Na^+ into the cells. At the same time, the voltage-gated K^+ channels also open, but the K^+ channels open more slowly than the Na^+ channels so that more Na^+ ions enter the cell than K^+ ions leave the cell, and the membrane depolarizes. A rapid inflow of Na^+ causes further depolarization and opens more voltage-gated Na^+ channels. This process is a positive feedback cycle, which allows great influx of Na^+ along its inwardly directed concentration gradient so that at its peak conductance, which corresponds to the peak of the action potential, the concentration gradient dominates over the electrical gradient for Na^+ and the membrane potential moves toward +60 mV, the equilibrium potential of Na^+.

Immediately after the overshoot, the membrane potential returns rapidly to its resting potential. Several events allow for rapid repolarization: the rapid decrease of Na^+ conductance due to the rapid closure of the voltage-gated Na^+ channels, which prevents further entry of Na^+ ions, and the continued increase in K^+ conductance, which peaks at about the middle of the repolarization phase and then returns slowly to resting levels. Therefore, the decrease in Na^+ entry and the simultaneous exit of K^+ cause repolarization of the cell.

At the end of the action potential, the return of the membrane potential to the negative state causes the voltage-gated K^+ channels to close back to their original status, but again after a delay. This slight delay accounts for the slight hyperpolarization of the membrane potential after an action potential. Chloride permeability does not change during the action potential. Chloride distributes passively along its concentration and electrical gradients across the membrane. Therefore, depolarization is caused by Na^+ influx, whereas repolarization is a manifestation of K^+ efflux. Although Na^+ enters the nerve cell and K^+ leaves it during the action potential, the number of ions involved is minute relative to the total numbers present. In nerve and skeletal muscle cells, the alternation of K^+ steady-state potentials with pulsed sodium potentials due to opening and closing of voltage-gated Na^+ channels gives rise to a traveling wave of depolarization, which is the current message that is conducted along the nerve or muscle fiber.

Cardiac and smooth muscle cells also contain calcium (Ca^{2+})-transporting ATPase, which actively transports Ca^{2+} out of the cells, creating a Ca^{2+} concentration gradient. In addition, voltage-gated Ca^{2+} channels, which are highly permeable to Ca^{2+} but only slightly permeable to Na^+, are also present in cell membranes; these are called Ca^{2+}-Na^+ channels. In contrast to the Na^+ channels, which are fast channels, the Ca^{2+}-Na^+ channels are slow to activate. Opening of these channels during an action potential allows rapid inflow of mostly Ca^{2+} and some Na^+ into the cells. The increase in intracellular Ca^{2+} concentration plays an essential role in the signal transduction pathway that couples membrane excitability to events within the cells, such as contractile and secretory activities. In some types of smooth muscle cells, the fast Na^+ channels are absent so that the action potentials are caused almost entirely by activation of the slow Ca^{2+}-Na^+ channels.

Importance of Potassium Gradient

The high concentration gradient of K^+ between the intracellular fluid and the plasma is important for maintaining the normal resting membrane potential across cell membranes and for excitability of nerves and muscles. Changes in the concentration of K^+ in the plasma change this gradient and will adversely affect the aforementioned functions (Rodriguez-Soriano, 1995). For instance, in hyperkalemia, when the concentration of K^+ in the plasma exceeds 5.5 mmol/L, the membrane depolarizes, causing muscular weakness, flaccid paralysis, and cardiac dysrhythmias. Cardiac dysrhythmias associated with hyperkalemia range from sinus bradycardia to ventricular tachycardia, ventricular fibrillation, and, ultimately, cardiac arrest (asystole) when a plasma concentration of 8 mmol/L is reached. Because of the adverse effects of hyperkalemia on the heart, hyperkalemia constitutes a medical emergency. In contrast, in hypokalemia, when the concentration of K^+ in the plasma is less than 3.5 mmol/L, the membrane hyperpolarizes, and this can interfere with the normal functioning of nerves and muscles, resulting in muscle weakness and decreased smooth muscle contractility. Hypokalemia is also a risk factor for atrial and ventricular dysrhythmias (He and MacGregor, 2001). Severe hypokalemia can lead to paralysis, metabolic alkalosis, and death. Therefore, it is important to regulate the concentration of K^+ in the plasma within narrow limits.

ROLE OF THE ELECTROCHEMICAL SODIUM GRADIENT IN NUTRIENT TRANSPORT PROCESSES

Sodium is important in many nutrient transport processes (Kutchai, 2004). Transepithelial transport of Na^+ in the small intestine and in the kidney is similar and plays an important role in the absorption of Cl^-, amino acids, glucose, galactose, and water. The transport properties of the apical membrane (plasma membrane facing the gastrointestinal lumen and the renal tubular lumen) are different from those of the basolateral membrane (facing the interstitial space). The apical membranes contain very few, if any, Na^+,K^+-ATPase transporters, whereas the basolateral membranes of these cells contain a large amount of Na^+,K^+-ATPase. Active extrusion of Na^+ across the basolateral membrane by the Na^+,K^+-ATPase reduces the concentration of intracellular Na^+ and provides an electrochemical potential gradient for Na^+ to move across the apical membrane from the lumen into the cytosol to replace the Na^+ that is extruded. This transepithelial transport of Na^+ creates an electrochemical potential difference for Na^+ across the epithelial cells so that the epithelial cells are polarized, with the lumen slightly electronegative with respect to the interstitial fluid on the basal side of the epithelial cells.

Entry of Na^+ across the apical membrane is either through the voltage-dependent Na^+ channels or by carrier-mediated transport (facilitated diffusion) in which other solutes are cotransported (in the same direction) or countertransported (in the opposite direction). Entry of Na^+ down an electrochemical gradient results in either the entry of Cl^- in the same direction as Na^+ movement or the secretion of K^+ or H^+ in the opposite direction in exchange for Na^+, as illustrated in Figure 34-3. The Na^+ is then extruded actively from epithelial cells by the Na^+,K^+-ATPase in the basolateral membrane. An equivalent molar amount of Cl^- is also transported from the lumen into the intercellular and interstitial spaces, either through the paracellular space (junctions between the apical borders of adjacent epithelial cells) or across the epithelial cells via the apical and basal membranes. Transport of Na^+ and Cl^- across epithelial cells increases the concentrations of these two ions in the intercellular spaces and provides an osmotic gradient for the absorption of water. A large proportion of water uptake occurs by the paracellular route, and only a small proportion of water flux is through the epithelial cells.

Some of the carrier proteins in the apical membrane, such as the sodium–glucose transport protein 1 (SGLT1) and a number of the amino acid transport systems, have receptor sites for binding both Na^+ and a monosaccharide or an amino acid (see Fig. 34-3). Because Na^+ is coupled to either a monosaccharide or an amino acid on the carrier protein, entry of Na^+ down its electrochemical gradient across the apical membrane also brings in a monosaccharide or an amino acid. Therefore, these transporters use the entry of Na^+ to actively transport the monosaccharide or amino acid across the apical membrane

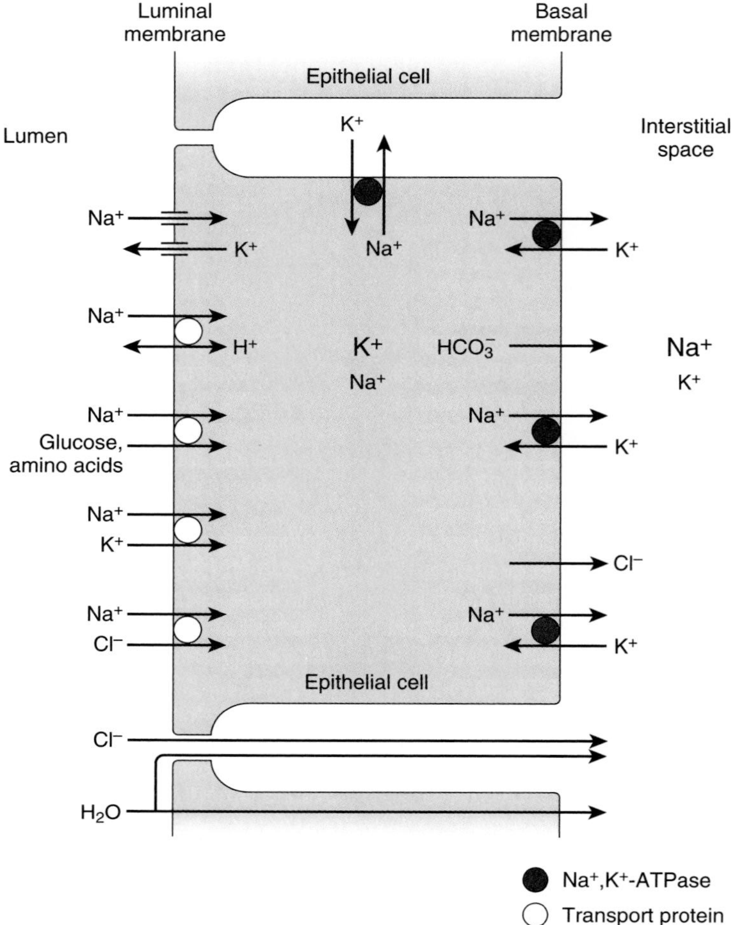

Figure 34-3 Schematic representation of how active extrusion of Na^+ via the enzyme Na^+,K^+-ATPase across the basal membrane of an epithelial cell creates an electrochemical gradient for the entry of Na^+ across the luminal membrane. Entry of Na^+ is by diffusion through ion channels or carrier-mediated transport (facilitated diffusion), which uses the electrochemical gradient created by the Na^+,K^+-ATPase as a driving force for cotransport or countertransport of other solutes. Only the most common types of transport are shown.

into the epithelial cells. This process of cotransport of organic solutes is frequently referred to as secondary active transport. The Na^+ gradient allows cotransport to occur against the concentration gradient for monosaccharides or amino acids. The increase in concentrations of these organic solutes inside the epithelial cells then allows the diffusion, usually facilitated by another carrier, of these nutrients across the basolateral membrane into the interstitial fluid.

OTHER FUNCTIONS OF ELECTROLYTES

Interactions With Macroions

Many macromolecules present in the extracellular and intracellular compartments contain multiple ionizing groups on their surfaces and are classed as macroions. Their behavior in solution depends on their surface charges, which either repel each other so that they remain separated in solution or attract each other so that they associate. Nucleic acids are large polyelectrolytes that carry multiple negative charges, whereas proteins are polyampholytes that contain both acidic and basic groups on their surfaces. Therefore, depending on the pH of the solution, proteins may carry substantial net positive or negative charges. Most plasma and intracellular proteins have net negative charges at a plasma pH of 7.4, but a few have net positive charges. Another important macroion is a group of polysaccharides, the glycosaminoglycans, which are of major structural importance and which carry carboxylate and sulfate groups. A major function of the glycosaminoglycans, such as chondroitin sulfates and keratan sulfates of connective tissue and dermatan sulfates of skin, is the formation of a matrix to hold together the protein components of connective tissue and skin. A very highly sulfated glycosaminoglycan is heparin, a natural anticoagulant produced by the mast cells that line the arterial walls. Heparan sulfate, which is less highly sulfated than is heparin, is linked to many cell surface proteins and matrix proteoglycans.

Macroion surfaces are modified by a counterion atmosphere enriched in oppositely charged small ions, mainly Na^+, K^+, and Cl^-. The counterion atmosphere is greatly affected by the ionic strength of the solution (i.e., a measure of the concentration and charge of ions in solution). At low ionic strength, the counterion atmosphere is diffuse, with minimal interference to interactions of macroions, whereas at high ionic strength, the counterion atmosphere is concentrated about the macroions and effectively reduces their interactions. This explains the observation that increasing salt concentration of a solution containing protein increases the solubility of the protein.

Activation of Enzymes

Activators of enzyme-catalyzed reactions are frequently metal ions such as Mg^{2+}, zinc (Zn^{2+}), manganese (Mn^{2+}), and Ca^{2+}, whereas only a limited number of enzymes require the presence of Na^+, K^+, or Cl^-. The most common and most widely distributed enzyme in the cell membrane is the Na^+,K^+-ATPase, the activation of which requires the presence of Na^+ and K^+. Enzymes that require the presence of Cl^- for activation include the angiotensin-converting enzyme (ACE) that catalyzes the conversion of angiotensin I to angiotensin II (Bunning and Riordan, 1987). Although the presence of Mg^{2+} is required for activation of a number of enzymes by K^+ in mammalian tissues, K^+ by itself is important for the activity of pyruvate kinase (Larsen et al., 1994).

SODIUM, CHLORIDE, AND POTASSIUM BALANCE

Total body sodium has been estimated at 100 g, chloride at 95 g, and potassium at 140 g for a 70-kg adult (Forbes, 1987). To achieve balance (maintain a stable content) of these elements in the body, the amount consumed must equal the amount lost from the body. In the growing child, a positive balance for these elements is important because of the accretion for tissue formation.

LOSS OF SODIUM, CHLORIDE, AND POTASSIUM

Obligatory loss of fluids through skin, feces, and urine invariably causes loss of sodium and chloride (see Chapter 35). Minimum obligatory loss of sodium in the absence of profuse sweating and gastrointestinal and renal diseases has been estimated to be approximately 40 to 185 mg/day (1.7 to 8.0 mmol/day), which consists of an obligatory loss of sodium in urine of 5 to 35 mg/day, in feces of 10 to 125 mg/day, and minimal dermal losses of 25 mg/day (Dahl, 1958). Studies over a 12-day period have shown that sweat and fecal excretion accounted for only 2% to 5% of total sodium excretion in adults consuming an average intake of salt; the remainder of the salt consumed was excreted in the urine (Sanchez-Castillo et al., 1987b). However, loss of sodium can increase greatly under certain circumstances, such as diarrhea, diabetes, and profuse sweating during strenuous physical activity in hot weather. Under most, but not all, circumstances, loss of sodium is accompanied by a similar molar loss of chloride.

Food Sources

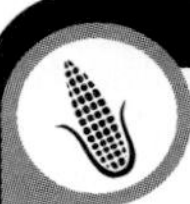

Food Sources High in Sodium

Soups

2.5 g per 1 cup miso soup
0.7 to 1.1 g per 1 cup canned soup

Condiments and Leavening Agents

2.3 g per 1 tsp table salt
0.9 g per 1 Tbsp soy sauce
0.8 g per 1 dill pickle (2 oz)
0.36 g per 1 tsp baking powder

Cured Meats

0.9 to 1.1 g per 3 oz ham
0.5 to 0.6 g per 1.7 oz hotdog
0.4 g per 3 medium slices cooked bacon
0.4 g per 2 slices (~2 oz) bologna

Cheese

0.4 g per ½ cup cottage cheese
0.4 g per 1 oz processed cheese
0.4 g per 1 oz blue cheese

Canned Vegetables and Tomato Sauce

0.8 g per ½ cup sauerkraut
0.6 g per ½ cup marinara/spaghetti sauce
0.2 g per ½ cup canned green peas

Data from U.S. Department of Agriculture/Agricultural Research Service (USDA/ARS) (2005) USDA Nutrient Database for Standard Reference, Release 18. USDA/ARS, Washington, DC. Retrieved November 15, 2005, from www.ars.usda.gov/ba/bhnrc/ndl.

As with sodium and chloride, obligatory loss of fluid through feces, sweat, and urine also causes loss of potassium via these routes. In the normal healthy adult, potassium loss via these routes is less than 800 mg/day, with less than 400 mg via fecal loss, 200 to 400 mg via urinary loss, and negligible amounts from sweat (National Research Council, 1989).

INTAKE OF SODIUM AND CHLORIDE

Dietary Intake

Dietary sodium is consumed mainly as sodium chloride, with small amounts as sodium bicarbonate, sodium glutamate, and sodium citrate. These sodium salts are low in fresh vegetables and fresh fruits but high in cured meat products, processed foods, and canned vegetables. Studies in a British population found that only 10% of sodium intake came from natural foods, 15% from table salt added during cooking and at the table, and 75% from salts added during manufacturing and processing (Sanchez-Castillo et al., 1987a). The amount of chloride consumed parallels the amount of sodium, as dietary chloride is consumed almost exclusively as a salt of sodium.

Daily salt consumption has been estimated by assessing salt intake or measuring urinary sodium excretion. Usually consumption far exceeds the needs of an individual, although it varies widely between individuals and cultures. Average Americans consume between 1.5 and 7 g/day of sodium or between 4 and 18 g/day of sodium chloride (Institute of Medicine [IOM], 2004). This wide range of reported intakes is due to the different methods of assessment and to the large variability of discretionary salt intake. Individuals consuming a diet high in processed foods have high salt intakes. In Japan, where consumption of salt-preserved fish and the use of salt for seasoning are customary, salt intake is high, ranging from 14 to 20 g/day (Kono et al., 1983). Conversely, salt consumption estimated from urinary sodium excretion of the Yanomamo Indians in Brazil is very low, 0.9 mmol or 53 mg of sodium chloride/day (Mancilha-Carvalho et al., 2003). Vegetarians typically consume an average of 760 mg/day of NaCl. Individuals with low or very low sodium intakes do not normally exhibit chronic deficiencies because of the efficiency of the mechanism of salt conservation.

Recommended Intake

Daily minimum requirements of sodium and chloride in the adult can be estimated from the amount needed to replace obligatory losses. This amounts to about 0.185 g/day of sodium (8 mmol/day) or less when substantial sweating does not occur (IOM, 2004). The IOM declined to define an estimated average requirement (EAR), and hence recommended dietary allowance (RDA), for sodium because of inadequate data from dose–response studies. Adequate intakes (AIs) were set based on a level that would meet the sodium needs and also allow intake of a diet made up of foods found in a Western-type diet and providing sufficient levels of other important nutrients. The AI for adult women and men who are 19 through 50 years of age is 1.5 g (65 mmol)/day of sodium. The AI for chloride was set to be equimolar to that for sodium and is 2.3 g (65 mmol)/day for adults through age 50 years. These AIs are equivalent to the intake of 3.8 g of sodium chloride (table salt) per day. The AIs for sodium and chloride are intended to be sufficient for excess sodium chloride loss in sweat by unacclimatized persons who are exposed to high temperatures or who are moderately physically active, but would not be appropriate for individuals engaged in extreme endurance activity or prolonged exposure to heat which would increase the loss of sodium chloride via sweat. It should be noted that, based on the Third National Health and Nutrition Examination Survey (NHANES III), the estimated median intake of sodium from foods (not including salt added at the table) is 3 g for women and 4 g for men in the United States and exceeds the AI for adults.

The AIs for older adults and for children were extrapolated from those for adults ages 19 to 50 years based on mean energy intakes for various age-sex groups. The AIs for sodium and chloride, respectively, are 1.0 g and 1.5 g/day for children 1 through 3 years of age and 1.2 g and 1.9 g/day for children 4 through 8 years of age. The AIs for boys and girls from 9 through 18 years of age are the same as those for young adults. The sodium and chloride AIs are lower for elderly adults due to their lower energy needs: 1.3 and 2.0 g/day, respectively, for adults from 51 through 70 years of age and 1.2 g and 1.8 g/day, respectively, for adults older than 70 years. No increase in sodium or chloride intake was deemed necessary during pregnancy or lactation. All AIs for chloride are equimolar to those for sodium.

The AIs for infants are based on typical intake from human milk and complementary foods. Therefore, the AI for sodium intake of infants from 0 through 6 months of age is 5 mmol/day or 0.12 g/day (0.78 L of milk/day × 0.16 g sodium/L of milk). For older infants, the AI is calculated as 0.08 g from human milk plus 0.29 g from complementary foods for a total of 0.37 g (16 mmol) sodium/day. AIs for chloride are equimolar to the AIs for sodium: 0.18 g and 0.57 g, respectively, per day for the first and second half of the first year of life.

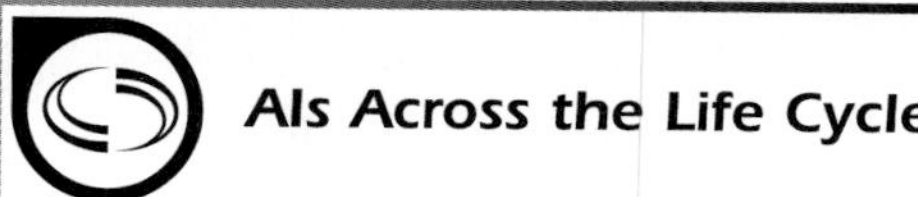

AIs Across the Life Cycle

	Sodium g per Day	Chloride g per Day
Infants		
0 to 6 mo	0.12	0.18
7 to 12 mo	0.37	0.57
Children		
1 to 3 yr	1.0	1.5
4 to 8 yr	1.2	1.9
9 to 18 yr	1.5	2.3
Adults		
19 to 50 yr	1.5	2.3
Pregnant	1.5	2.3
Lactating	1.5	2.3
51 to 70 yr	1.3	2.0
>70 yr	1.2	1.8

Data from Institute of Medicine (IOM) (2004) Dietary Reference Intakes for Water, Potassium, Sodium, Chloride, and Sulfate. National Academy Press, Washington, DC.
AI, Adequate Intake.

There is no apparent threshold level for sodium intake below which there is no increased risk for cardiovascular diseases across the range of blood pressures typically observed in the United States and Canada. Several trials have demonstrated that dietary sodium intake close to the AI (e.g., 1.2 g/day) was associated with lower blood pressure than higher intakes (e.g., 2.3 g/day) (Johnson et al., 2001; Sacks et al., 2001; MacGregor et al., 1989). Based on these studies, the IOM set a tolerable upper intake level (UL) for sodium intake at 2.3 g (100 mmol)/day of sodium and that for chloride at 3.6 g (100 mmol)/day for adults. The ULs for young children are somewhat lower.

INTAKE OF POTASSIUM

Dietary Intake

Potassium is widely distributed in foods, especially in vegetables and fruits. Intakes of potassium vary widely, depending on dietary habits.

Food Sources

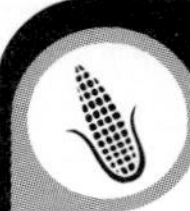

Food Sources High in Potassium

Vegetables

0.3 to 0.4 g per ½ cup beans (soy, pinto, kidney, navy, or lima)
0.35 g per ½ cup lentils
0.69 g per 1 cup carrot juice
0.55 g per 1 cup tomato juice
0.47 g per ½ cup marinara (spaghetti) sauce
0.4 to 0.5 g per ½ cup winter squash, sweet potato, or spinach
0.25 to 0.35 g per ½ cup cabbage, spinach, or pumpkin

Fruits

0.44 to 0.50 g per 1 cup orange juice
0.27 g per ¼ cup raisins
0.21 g per ½ cup melon
0.40 g per ½ cup plums
0.36 g per ½ cup plantains
0.27 g per ½ cup bananas

Fish

0.4 to 0.5 g per 3- oz serving (halibut, tuna, cod, or flounder)

Dairy Products

0.39 g per 1 cup milk
0.55 g per 1 cup plain yogurt

Leavening Agents

0.495 g per 1 tsp cream of tartar

Data from U.S. Department of Agriculture/Agricultural Research Service (USDA/ARS) (2005) USDA Nutrient Database for Standard Reference, Release 18. USDA/ARS, Washington, DC. Retrieved November 15, 2005, from www.ars.usda.gov/ba/bhnrc/ndl.

Based on the NHANES III data, the median intake of potassium in the United States is about 3.3 g/day for men and 2.2 g/day for women (IOM, 2004). These values do not include the use of salt substitutes or reduced-sodium salts. These salt substitutes contain from 0.4 to 2.8 g potassium per teaspoon as potassium chloride. Because of the growing evidence of the beneficial effects of potassium in the protection against cardiovascular diseases, concern of possible underconsumption of potassium has led to recommendations for increased intake of dietary fruits and vegetables.

Recommended Intake

To replace the loss of potassium in feces, sweat, and urine, an adult should consume not less than 0.8 g/day of potassium. The IOM (2004) did not set an EAR or RDA for potassium because of insufficient dose–response data to establish an EAR. Intakes higher than the median intake may reduce risk for some chronic diseases. The adult AI for potassium was set at 4.7 g (120 mmol)/day based upon the dietary level that blunted the severe salt sensitivity prevalent in African American men (Morris et al., 1999). This potassium intake is also associated with a lower risk of kidney stones, lower blood pressure, and decreased bone loss. No increment was added to the AI for pregnant women, but the AI for lactating women was increased to 5.1 g (130 mmol)/day to allow for the potassium content in human milk secreted during the first 6 months of lactation. Based on the NHANES III data, the percentage of adults in the United States who consume an amount of potassium that is equal to or greater than the AI is only 10% of men and less than 1% of women (IOM, 2004). A diet rich in fruits and vegetables is necessary to obtain the AI for potassium from natural foods.

The AIs for infants were based on typical intakes from human milk and complementary foods and are 0.4 g (10 mmol)/day of potassium for infants from birth through 6 months of age and 0.7 g (18 mmol)/day for infants from 6 through 12 months of age. AIs for children were extrapolated from the adult AI on the basis of median energy intake levels. The AIs for potassium are 3.0 g/day for 1- to 3-year-old children, 3.8 g/day for 4- to 8-year-old children, 4.5 g/day for boys and girls from 9 through 13 years of age, and 4.7 g/day for the 14- to 18-year-old group.

There is no evidence that a high level of potassium from foods has adverse effects, so a UL for potassium was not set by the IOM (2004). Chronic consumption of a high level of potassium can result in hyperkalemia in individuals with impaired urinary excretion of potassium, and supplemental potassium should be used only under medical supervision.

AIs Across the Life Cycle

	g Potassium g per Day
Infants	
0 to 6 mo	0.4
7 to 12 mo	0.7
Children	
1 to 3 yr	3.0
4 to 8 yr	3.8
9 to 13 yr	4.5
14 to 18 yr	4.7
Adults	
19 to 50 yr	4.7
Pregnant	4.7
Lactating	5.1
51 to 70 yr	4.7
>70 yr	4.7

Data from Institute of Medicine (IOM) (2004) Dietary Reference Intakes for Water, Potassium, Sodium, Chloride, and Sulfate. National Academy Press, Washington, DC.
AI, Adequate intake.

REGULATION OF SODIUM, CHLORIDE, AND POTASSIUM BALANCE

Maintenance of sodium and potassium balance is important from several aspects. Sodium, as a major extracellular cation, plays an important role in maintaining the extracellular fluid volume. Conversely, potassium is a major intracellular cation, and its high intracellular concentration is essential for cellular functions such as growth, protein synthesis, and control of intracellular volume. The high concentration gradient of K^+ across cell membranes is vital in maintaining the resting membrane potential, cell excitability, and muscle contraction. Therefore, to prevent disturbances in fluid distribution and disturbances in neuromuscular excitability, mechanisms exist to control the body balance of sodium and potassium within narrow limits.

The kidneys are the main site of regulation of sodium, chloride, and potassium balance; the intestines play a relatively minor role. The kidneys respond to a deficiency of these elements in the diet by decreasing their excretion, and they respond to an excess by increasing their excretion in the urine. The amount of Na^+ and K^+ excreted by the kidney can be adjusted either by changing the amount filtered at the glomerulus, which is accomplished by changing the glomerular filtration rate, or by changing the amount reabsorbed or secreted by tubular cells. For long-term regulation, the control of glomerular filtration rate, plays a relatively minor role. Urinary loss of Na^+ is controlled by varying the rate of sodium reabsorbed from the filtrate by tubular cells (Stanton et al., 2004), whereas urinary loss of potassium is controlled by varying the rate of secretion of potassium into the lumen by tubular cells in the distal tubules (Malnic et al., 2004).

RENAL EXCRETION OF SODIUM, CHLORIDE, AND POTASSIUM

The rate of renal excretion of Na^+, Cl^-, and K^+ depends on the tubular functions of the kidneys. These electrolytes are filtered freely from the glomerular capillaries across the glomerular membrane into the Bowman's space of the nephrons (functional units of the kidneys) so that their concentrations in the glomerular filtrate are similar to those in the plasma. As the filtrate flows along the renal tubules, reabsorption of Na^+, Cl^-, and K^+ and secretion of K^+ by renal tubular cells alter the final concentrations of Na^+, Cl^-, and K^+ in the urine. Figure 34-4 illustrates the basic renal processing of Na^+, Cl^-, and K^+. Net reabsorption of all three ions occurs in the proximal tubule, the thick ascending limb of the loop of Henle, and the distal convoluted tubule. Normally, 95% to 98% of the filtered load of these ions and water is reabsorbed by these segments. Reabsorption of the remaining 2% to 5% of the filtered Na^+, Cl^-, and water, and the secretion of K^+ in the cortical collecting tubule are variable and depend greatly on the needs of the individual.

In normal individuals, when there is a high dietary intake of Na^+, reabsorption of Na^+ from the cortical collecting tubule is low resulting in the excretion of the excess Na^+ in the urine. However, when sodium intake is low or when there is a sodium deficit from excessive loss via the skin or the gastrointestinal tract, much of the Na^+ in the filtrate is reabsorbed, resulting

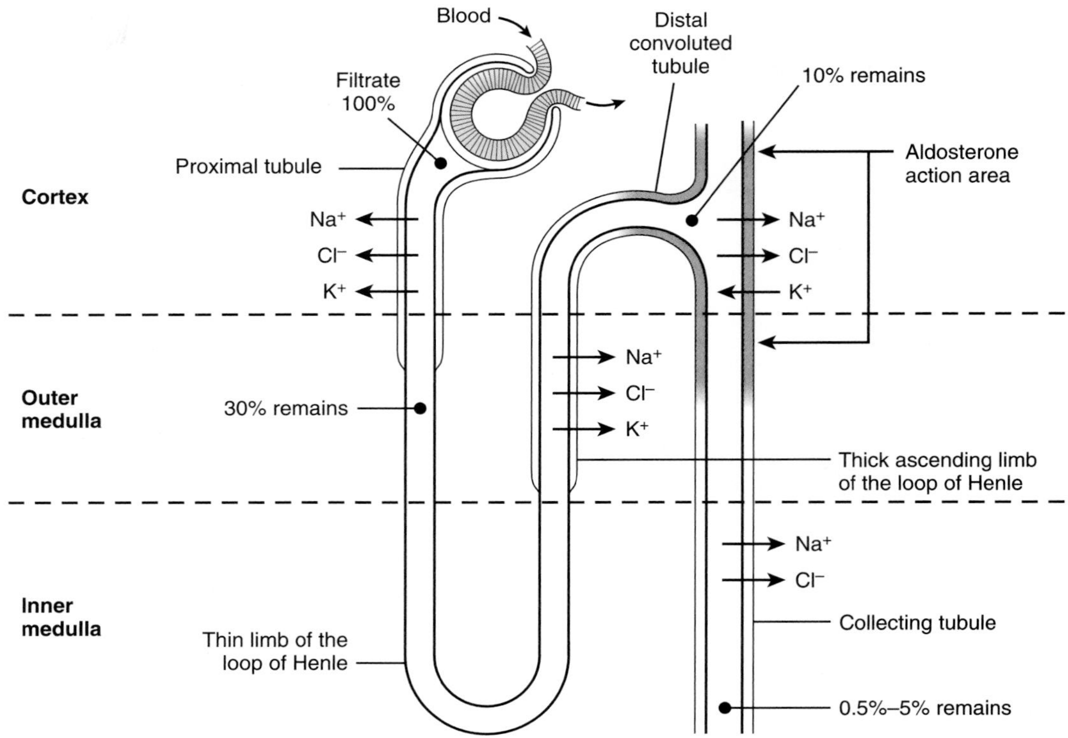

Figure 34-4 Resorption of Na^+, K^+, and Cl^+ and secretion of K^+ at different parts of the nephron. The nephron is the functional unit of the kidney; there are approximately 1 million nephrons in each human kidney.

in very low Na^+ concentration in the urine. In contrast to Na^+, K^+ is secreted by the tubular cells of the cortical collecting tubules (Rodriguez-Soriano, 1995). In the absence of disease, changes in K^+ excretion are not due to changes in reabsorption of K^+ in the proximal tubules but to changes in K^+ secretion by the cortical collecting tubules. During potassium depletion, most of the filtered K^+ is reabsorbed, and virtually no K^+ is secreted. The small amount of K^+ excreted comes from the filtered K^+ that escaped reabsorption. However, when potassium intake is high, secretion of K^+ is increased, thereby eliminating the excess potassium. A normal Western diet contains about 3 g/day of potassium and requires the renal tubular secretion of K^+ in order to maintain potassium balance. Reabsorption of Na^+ and Cl^-, and secretion of K^+ are under the control of various homeostatic regulatory mechanisms that effectively maintain a balance of these elements in the body despite a wide range of intakes and occasional large losses via the skin or the gastrointestinal tract.

CONTROL OF RENAL EXCRETION OF SODIUM AND CHLORIDE

No important receptors capable of detecting the amount of sodium in the body have been identified. However, because Na^+ is the main determinant of extracellular fluid volume, physiological mechanisms that control the volume of extracellular fluid effectively maintain a balance for sodium and chloride (Abassi et al., 2004). Changes in extracellular fluid volume lead to corresponding changes in the effective circulating volume. Any change in this effective circulating volume will affect the “fullness” or “pressure” in the circulation and will cause a change in cardiac filling pressure, cardiac output, and arterial pressure. Located throughout the vascular system are volume or pressure sensors (baroceptors) that detect these changes and send either excitatory or inhibitory signals to the central nervous system and/or the endocrine glands to effect appropriate responses by the kidneys to match the amount of Na^+ ingested. The three major mechanisms that participate in the regulation of sodium balance are as follows: (1) vascular pressure receptors: renal sympathetic and AVP pathways; (2) the renin–angiotensin–aldosterone system; and (3) natriuretic peptides.

Vascular Pressure Receptors: Renal Sympathetic and Arginine Vasopressin Pathways

In order to maintain a stable effective circulatory volume, barocepters are present in several sites within the vascular bed. These baroreceptors sense changes in a physical parameter, such as stretch or tension. Essentially two kinds of baroceptors are present: (1) the vascular low-pressure receptors located in the central venous portion of the circulation and (2) the vascular high-pressure receptors located in the arterial side of the vascular tree (Abassi et al., 2004). The low-pressure receptors respond primarily to distention of the walls of the cardiac atria and the pulmonary vein. These baroceptors send signals via afferent fibers in the vagus nerve to the hypothalamic and medullary centers of the central nervous system. The high-pressure receptors respond primarily to changes in blood pressure in the walls of the aortic arch and the carotid sinus. The aortic arch and carotid baroceptors send impulses via the vagus and the glossopharyngeal nerves to the hypothalamic and medullary regions of the central nervous system. Increases in vagal and glossopharyngeal nerve activities from both the low-pressure and high-pressure receptors inhibit secretion of AVP from the posterior pituitary and also inhibit the sympathetic outflow and renal sympathetic activity. In hypervolemia, the activities of the vagal and glossopharyngeal nerves are increased, resulting in a decrease in both the sympathetic outflow and secretion of AVP. In hypovolemia, there is a reflex increase in the renal sympathetic activity and in secretion of AVP (Quail et al., 1987).

The kidney is supplied by sympathetic adrenergic nerves that innervate all segments of the renal vasculature and tubule. Under normal arterial pressure, there is minimal sympathetic nerve activity to the kidneys. As part of a reflex response to a fall in systemic arterial pressure, the renal sympathetic nerves are activated to bring about a decrease in renal excretion of Na^+ and Cl^- (Abassi et al., 2004). Three major mechanisms are involved in the sympathetic effects on renal Na^+ and Cl^- transport. First, sympathetic nerve activity stimulates the α_1-adrenergic receptors of the afferent and efferent arterioles of the glomerulus. This increases the overall renal vascular resistance, resulting in a decrease in renal blood flow and the glomerular filtration rate. This in turn leads to an overall reduction in the filtered load of Na^+. Second, sympathetic nerve endings stimulate Na^+,K^+-ATPase activity and Na^+/H^+ exchange in the proximal tubular cells leading to an increased reabsorption of Na^+ and Cl^-. The stimulatory effect on Na^+,K^+-ATPase activity is mediated by stimulation of the α_1-adrenergic receptors, whereas that of Na^+/H^+ antiport is mediated by stimulation of α_2-adrenergic receptors. These two actions decrease renal excretion of Na^+ and Cl^-. Third, in addition to their effects on renal hemodynamics and reabsorption of Na^+, sympathetic nerves also stimulate the α_1-adrenergic receptors located on the juxtaglomerular cells of the afferent and efferent arterioles to release renin. Renin subsequently increases the circulating levels of angiotensin II and aldosterone, which are important in stimulating reabsorption of Na^+. Studies in rats have shown that the basal level of sympathetic nerve activity is sufficient to exert a tonic stimulation on renin release and tubular Na^+ and Cl^- reabsorption, whereas renal hemodynamics are affected only when sympathetic nervous activity is increased above the baseline level. All these adaptive responses restore the effective circulating volume and blood pressure toward their normal values.

AVP primarily increases the permeability of the collecting ducts to water so that water is reabsorbed from the tubular lumen into the hyperosmotic medullary interstitium. It also enhances reabsorption of Na^+ and Cl^- by the thick ascending limb of the loops of Henle and, to a lesser degree, by the collecting ducts (Canessa et al., 1994).

The regulation of volume via the vascular pressure receptors (i.e., renal sympathetic and

AVP reflex pathways) is effective during hypovolemia. When the effective circulating volume is low, the overall effect is a reflex increase in Na^+ and Cl^-, and water retention via the activation of renal sympathetic nerves and secretion of AVP. Conversely, sympathetic nerve activity has much less effect on renal excretion of Na^+ and Cl^- in hypervolemia because the sympathetic nerve activity to the kidneys is minimal in euvolemia and, hence, is not decreased substantially by hypervolemia.

Renin–Angiotensin–Aldosterone System

The renin–angiotensin–aldosterone system plays an important role in the regulation of renal hemodynamics and Na^+ transport. The baroceptors located in the afferent arterioles of the glomerulus of each nephron sense changes in perfusion pressure, whereas chemoreceptors located in the macula densa area of the thick ascending limb of the loop of Henle sense changes in the Na^+ load in the tubular fluid. These sensors respond to changes by influencing the synthesis and secretion of renin by the juxtaglomerular cells located at the afferent arterioles (Fig. 34-5) (Levens et al., 1981).

Renin, a proteolytic enzyme, is synthesized and stored in an inactive form called prorenin in the juxtaglomerular cells of the afferent arterioles in the kidneys (Candido et al., 2004). It is released in response to stimuli from the renal sympathetic nerves and by an intrarenal reflex mechanism via the juxtaglomerular apparatus when the effective circulating volume is decreased. The juxtaglomerular apparatus includes the high-pressure baroceptors in the afferent arterioles and in the macula densa of the thick ascending limb of the renal tubules of the kidneys. When perfusion pressure to the kidneys is decreased, or when delivery of NaCl to the macula densa is decreased, secretion of renin is stimulated. In the circulation,

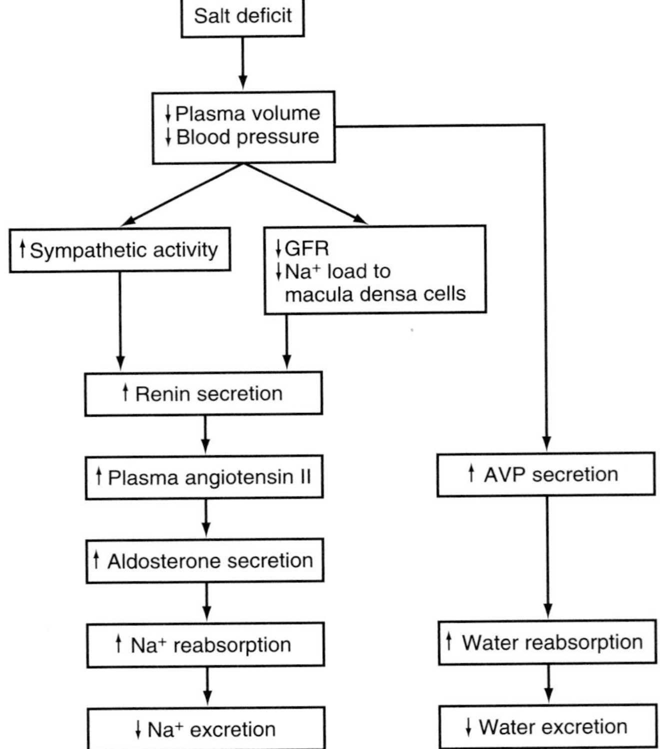

Figure 34-5 Schematic representation of the control of renal excretion of sodium and water during salt deficit.

renin acts as an enzyme to split off a small polypeptide, angiotensin I (a decapeptide), from angiotensinogen, a protein produced by the liver. Angiotensin I is biologically inactive and undergoes further cleavage to form angiotensin II (an octapeptide), a reaction catalyzed by antiotensin converting enzyme (ACE) that is present in large amounts on the luminal surface of the endothelium of blood vessels in the lungs and also of vessels in other organs including the liver and kidneys.

Angiotensin II has important physiological functions. It is an important circulating vasoactive hormone, which causes arteriolar constriction, thereby raising peripheral resistance and sustaining blood pressure in response to a decrease in blood volume. It stimulates secretion of AVP and thirst. Furthermore, it conserves body sodium indirectly via secretion of aldosterone and directly by influencing renal hemodynamics and tubular epithelial Na^+ reabsorption and K^+ secretion (Abassi et al., 2004). In its intrarenal effects, angiotensin II decreases renal plasma flow by its prominent vasoconstrictor effect on the efferent arteriole. The increase in arteriolar resistance causes a drop in hydrostatic pressure in the peritubular capillaries. This leads to an increase in Na^+ and fluid reabsorption in the proximal tubule in accordance to the Starling's forces (see Chapter 35). In addition, angiotensin II acts directly on the tubular transport system in both the proximal and distal tubules. In the proximal tubules, it stimulates the Na^+,K^+-ATPase and $Na^+/(3)HCO_3^-$ symporter in the basolateral membrane and the Na^+,H^+-exchanger in the apical membrane. The overall effect is an increase in reabsorption of NaCl and $NaHCO_3$ in the proximal tubule. In the distal tubules, angiotensin II stimulates Na^+,H^+-exchanger in the apical membrane, and it also directly stimulates the Na^+ channel activity. The overall effect is an increase in reabsorption of NaCl and $NaHCO_3$ in the kidney.

Aldosterone is a steroid hormone produced and secreted by the zona glomerulosa cells of the adrenal cortex. Its secretion is stimulated by a low plasma Na^+ concentration, a high plasma K^+ concentration, and angiotensin II. Aldosterone stimulates mainly the cells of the cortical collecting tubules, and to a lesser extent the distal convoluted and medullary collecting tubules, to reabsorb Na^+ and secrete K^+. Aldosterone activates the electrogenic Na^+ and K^+ channels in the apical membrane, increases synthesis of these electrogenic ion channels, and increases synthesis of the basolateral membrane Na^+,K^+-ATPase (O'Neil, 1990). These changes cause an increase in the rate of reabsorption of Na^+ by increasing the active transport of Na^+ out of the cells across the basolateral membrane and the passive influx of Na^+ across the apical membrane. At the same time, the rate of movement of K^+ into the cells across the basolateral membrane and out of the cells across the apical membrane into the tubular lumen is increased. The increased reabsorption of Na^+ also increases the potential difference across the tubular epithelial cells (the lumen becomes more negative), so that more K^+ is secreted into the lumen along the electrical gradient.

Natriuretic Peptides

A group of peptides found in different organs of the body, such as the heart, brain, kidney, adrenal gland, and liver, exhibit potent hypotensive, natriuretic, and diuretic activities. Because the natriuretic peptides were first found as membrane-bound secretory granules in the myocytes of the cardiac atria, they are called atrial natriuretic peptides (ANPs). The major stimulus to ANP secretion from the cardiac atria and ventricle is volume expansion, which stretches the myocytes, but neurohumoral factors such as AVP and angiotensin II can also modulate ANP release into the circulation (Candido et al., 2004). Other peptides, which are structurally similar but genetically distinct, include brain natriuretic peptide (BNP) and C-type natriuretic peptide (CNP). Both BNP and CNP were first isolated from porcine brain, but BNP was later found to be secreted predominantly from the heart, especially the cardiac ventricles. Although CNP is also found in the heart and kidney, abundant expression of CNP and its receptors in the brain suggests its role as a neuromodulator in the brain. Both ANP and BNP increase renal Na^+ excretion and also increase the excretion of water by inhibiting the secretion of AVP from the posterior pituitary (Zeidel, 1990).

Demonstration of the presence of natriuretic peptides in the kidney led to the postulation that these peptides form a renal natriuretic peptide system that regulates renal circulation and local transport of Na^+ and water. ANP acts predominantly in the glomeruli and inner medulla of the kidneys. It causes natriuresis via three different mechanisms. First, ANP causes vasodilation of the afferent and efferent arterioles of the glomerulus, with its actions on the afferent arterioles being predominant. The increase in renal blood flow and glomerular capillary hydrostatic pressure increases the glomerular filtration rate and filtered load of Na^+. Second, ANP also acts directly on the cells in the medullary portion of the collecting duct. It acts through its second messenger, cyclic guanosine monophosphate (cGMP), to inhibit reabsorption of Na^+ and Cl^-. Third, ANP inhibits secretion of aldosterone partly by its direct inhibitory action on the adrenal cortex and partly via its inhibition of the secretion of renin from the juxtaglomerular cells of the kidneys. Taking all these effects together, ANP increases renal excretion of Na^+, Cl^-, and water in hypervolemia. Hypothetically, a decrease in circulating levels of ANP would be expected to decrease renal excretion of Na^+, Cl^-, and water. However, there is no convincing evidence to indicate that circulating levels of ANP play an important role in hypovolemia.

CONTROL OF RENAL EXCRETION OF POTASSIUM

More than 90% of the potassium in the diet is absorbed by intestinal epithelial cells into the circulation and is distributed throughout the extracellular fluid. In the adult, the volume of extracellular fluid is about 20% of body weight, or 14 L. The rise in the concentration of K^+ in plasma immediately stimulates physiological mechanisms to promote rapid entry of K^+ into cells so that a rapid rise in the plasma concentration is prevented. If the potassium absorbed during a meal (~1.5 g, or 40 mmol) were to remain in the extracellular fluid compartment, the concentration of K^+ in the plasma would increase to 6.9 mmol/L, a potentially lethal concentration. Therefore, uptake of K^+ by cells is essential in preventing life-threatening hyperkalemia. However, in the long-term, to maintain K^+ balance, the excess K^+ from the diet must be excreted by the kidneys. The distal tubule and collecting tubule remove the excess K^+ from the plasma by secreting it into the tubular lumen.

Normally, approximately 67% of filtered K^+ is reabsorbed from the proximal tubule and a further 20% is reabsorbed from the loop of Henle. Further reabsorption of K^+ occurs in the distal tubules when dietary intake is low. However, when K^+ intake is high, the excess K^+ is removed from the plasma into the tubular fluid by the distal tubule and collecting tubule of the kidneys. The two most important homeostatic regulatory mechanisms for K^+ secretion are aldosterone and plasma K^+ concentration. In addition, other factors such as acid–base balance influence K^+ secretion by the distal and collecting tubules.

Aldosterone

The most important hormone regulating secretion of K^+ is aldosterone, the release of which is triggered by a high concentration of K^+ in plasma, by a low concentration of Na^+ in plasma, or by angiotensin II. These feedback loops regulate K^+ concentration in the plasma and provide a relatively large tolerance to changes in dietary K^+. Lack of aldosterone, for example in Addison's disease, causes a marked depletion of body Na^+ and retention of K^+ (Nerup, 1974). Conversely, excess aldosterone, for example in Conn's syndrome, is associated with depletion of K^+ and retention of Na^+ (Ganguly and Donohue, 1983).

Plasma Concentrations of Sodium and Hydrogen

Other factors that can directly affect secretion of K^+ by the distal nephrons are plasma concentrations of K^+ and H^+ (Rodriguez-Soriano, 1995). These ions act by changing the concentration of intracellular K^+ in tubular cells. When the concentration of intracellular K^+ is increased, the concentration gradient for K^+ across the apical membrane increases, thereby promoting diffusion of K^+ into the lumen. A decrease in the concentration of intracellular K^+ decreases the concentration gradient across the luminal membrane, and secretion of K^+ is reduced. Under normal circumstances, the concentration of intracellular K^+ in tubular cells reflects that of the plasma. This is because an increase in the concentration of plasma K^+ directly stimulates the Na^+,K^+-ATPase pump at the basolateral membrane of the distal nephrons. In addition, an increase in the concentration of K^+ in the plasma causes secretion of aldosterone, which further increases the uptake of K^+ by tubular cells and the excretion of K^+ in the urine.

Secretion of K^+ by the tubular cells in response to changes in acid–base balance is complex. In general, acute acidosis decreases secretion of K^+, causing retention of potassium, whereas acute alkalosis increases secretion and loss of potassium from the body (Adrogue and Madias, 1981). An increased concentration of H^+ in plasma probably acts by inhibiting the Na^+,K^+-ATPase activity at the basolateral membrane so that the intracellular K^+ concentration in the tubular cells is decreased, resulting in a decrease in secretion of K^+ by the tubular cells. However, with chronic acid–base disorders, the response of the kidney is varied. It depends on the etiology of the disorders and the presence of other factors that may influence secretion of K^+. Changes in pH alter other processes that influence secretion of K^+. Metabolic acidosis may be associated with an increase in secretion of K^+ and mild K^+ depletion, which may be explained by an acidosis-induced increase in secretion of aldosterone. Metabolic alkalosis is almost always accompanied by depletion of K^+.

CONTROL OF INTESTINAL ABSORPTION AND EXCRETION OF SODIUM, CHLORIDE, AND POTASSIUM

Under normal circumstances, about 99% of dietary Na^+, Cl^-, and K^+ is absorbed, and the remainder is excreted in the feces. Analogies may be drawn between the excretion of these ions in the kidneys and the intestines. Absorption of Na^+ and Cl^- occurs along the entire length of the intestines; 90% to 95% is absorbed in the small intestine and the rest in the colon. Absorption of K^+ occurs in the small intestine, but normally there is net secretion of K^+ in the colon. In the colon, net absorption occurs during K^+ deficit, and net secretion occurs in K^+ excess. Intestinal absorption and secretion of Na^+, K^+, and Cl^- are subject to regulation by the nervous system, hormones, and paracrine agonists released from neurons in the enteric nervous system in the wall of the intestines. The most important of these factors is aldosterone, which stimulates absorption of Na^+ and secretion of K^+, mainly by the colon and, to a lesser extent, by the ileum. The mechanism of aldosterone action is similar to that in the renal tubules.

ACTIVATION OF SALT APPETITE

Salt (NaCl) deficiency and hypovolemia have been shown to motivate the search for and ingestion of sodium-containing foods and fluids. The presence of salt appetite (or salt cravings) in animals, for example in ruminants, is to ensure that there is an adequate intake of salt to protect the body, and thus the extracellular fluid, from excessive loss of NaCl due to sweating, diarrhea, pregnancy, or lactation. Salt deficiency, for example, in patients with adrenal deficiency, may result in taste alterations such that the individual will have a strong desire for salty food.

Both neural and hormonal systems have been implicated in the control of salt appetite (Daniels and Fluharty, 2004). Behavioral studies in animals have shown the role of the gustatory neuraxis (which involves the facial nerves from the tongue to the brain) in their adaptive regulation of salt intake. Deprivation of this relay of sodium taste information to the brain abolishes the expression of sodium preferences and the ability of the animal to modify its behavior for sodium intake. Hypovolemia and hypotension, which activate baroceptors, are also implicated in the activation of salt appetite. Various hormones, such as aldosterone, AVP, oxytocin, and especially the renin–angiotensin system, stimulate drinking behavior and salt appetite. All components of the renin–angiotensin system (renin, angiotensinogen, ACE, and angiotensin receptors) are present in the neuronal centers in the hypothalamus. Evidence exists also that peripherally derived angiotensin II stimulates salt appetite in rats by its direct action on the brain. These neuronal centers also are important in the thirst mechanism. Stimulation of this region simultaneously creates a craving for salt and thirst.

INTERACTIONS AMONG SYSTEMS IN VOLUME REGULATION

The systems of feedback loops with their reinforcing (positive) and modulating (negative) pathways are highly integrated and effective in regulating circulating volume and blood pressure. The integrated pathways of the sympathetic nervous system, the renin–angiotensin–aldosterone system, ANP, and AVP, when acting together, provide multiple backup systems that permit the body to regulate the vasomotor tone and excretion of Na^+ and Cl^- in response to changes in volume, even when one of the regulatory systems fails. This regulatory feedback mechanism can best be examined by the following examples of changes in dietary NaCl.

To maintain a normal effective circulating volume, termed euvolemia, a precise balance of excretion of Na^+ and Cl^- to match their consumption is required. In euvolemic individuals, daily excretion of Na^+ and Cl^- equals the daily consumption. Excretion of Na^+ and Cl^- in the urine can vary over a wide range, from a very low level to as much as 23 g/day, depending on the diet.

In the case of positive salt balance, retention of sodium and chloride increases the volume of extracellular fluid and, hence, body weight. It is mainly this increase in fluid volume that triggers the homeostatic regulatory mechanisms to increase excretion of Na^+ and Cl^-. Expansion of volume causes excretion of Na^+ and Cl^- via the following mechanisms: (1) reflex suppression of the sympathetic nervous discharge to the kidneys, due to stimulation of the low-pressure stretch receptors and high-pressure baroreceptors; (2) suppression of the renin–angiotensin–aldosterone system; (3) stimulation of the secretion of ANP from the cardiac atria; and (4) suppression of the AVP system. The loss of Na^+, Cl^-, and water from the body returns the volume of extracellular fluid and body weight to their original levels.

The opposite occurs in negative salt balance, in which acute depletion of Na^+ and Cl^- decreases the volume of extracellular fluid. The various control systems act together to conserve body Na^+ and Cl^- by the following mechanisms: (1) reflex increase in sympathetic nervous discharge to the kidneys; (2) stimulation of the renin–angiotensin–aldosterone system; and (3) stimulation of the AVP system. These mechanisms act together to conserve Na^+ and Cl^- in the body during depletion (see Fig. 34-5).

FACTORS AFFECTING TRANSMEMBRANE DISTRIBUTION OF POTASSIUM

As mentioned previously, changes in the concentration gradient of K^+ between the intracellular fluid and plasma will adversely affect the normal resting membrane potential and excitability of nerves and muscles. Various mechanisms are present to effect either a rapid release of K^+ from the cells or an uptake of K^+ into the cells whenever there is a change in plasma K^+ concentration in order to maintain within narrow limits the concentration of K^+ in the plasma. These mechanisms involve responses to changes in the concentrations of catecholamines or insulin or changes in plasma pH. Although aldosterone enhances secretion of K^+ by the tubular cells of the distal nephrons, its effects on transmembrane distribution of K^+ are controversial.

Catecholamines

Catecholamines have dual effects on the movement of K^+ across cell membranes because they activate both the α-adrenergic and β-adrenergic receptors on cell membranes (Moratinos et al., 1993). Stimulation of α_1- and α_2-adrenergic receptors causes hyperkalemia due to the activation of hepatic Ca^{2+}-dependent K^+ channels, thus releasing K^+ from the liver. In contrast, stimulation of β-adrenergic receptors causes hypokalemia by promoting cellular uptake of K^+ in the liver, muscles, and myocardium through stimulation of Na^+,K^+-ATPase. Both adrenergic sympathetic activity and circulating catecholamines can influence cellular uptake and release of K^+. The opposing effects of α- and β-adrenergic fibers have important physiological consequences. During exercise the sympathetic nervous system is activated; epinephrine from the adrenal medulla and norepinephrine from the sympathetic nerve endings are released. The released epinephrine potentially causes an initial hyperkalemia owing to its action on the α-adrenergic receptors in the liver to release K^+, followed by sustained hypokalemia owing to its action on the β-receptors in the muscles to promote cellular K^+ uptake. However, norepinephrine released by the sympathetic nerve endings during exercise also stimulates release of K^+ from the liver, and the dual effects of the two catecholamines ensure that hypokalemia does not occur during exercise.

Insulin

During a meal, the high concentrations of glucose, amino acids, gastrointestinal hormones, and K^+ in the plasma cause insulin to be released from the β cells of the pancreas. Insulin promotes uptake of K^+ by the liver, skeletal muscles, cardiac muscles, and adipocytes, thereby attenuating the rapid postprandial rise in plasma K^+ concentration (Mount and Zandi-Nejad, 2004). This reflex regulatory feedback mechanism helps to maintain the concentration of K^+ in plasma and the concentration gradient between plasma and intracellular fluid. The mechanism of insulin-mediated uptake of K^+ by cells is independent of its effects on uptake of glucose. Insulin stimulates tissue uptake of K^+ by stimulating Na^+,K^+-ATPase activity in plasma membranes. Other electroneutral transport pathways, such as Na^+/H^+ exchange and $Na^+/K^+/2Cl^-$ cotransport in peripheral tissues, are also activated, but the roles of these in K^+ homeostasis is less clear.

Plasma pH

The effect of plasma pH on transmembrane distribution of K^+ is complex and depends on the presence of other physiological factors that affect distribution of K^+. In general, acute metabolic acidosis caused by accumulation of nonmetabolizable acids releases intracellular K^+ and increases plasma K^+ concentration. Acute metabolic alkalosis shifts K^+ into cells and decreases the concentration of K^+ in the plasma (Rodriguez-Soriano, 1995).

SODIUM AND CHLORIDE IMBALANCE AND ITS CONSEQUENCES

In general, sodium retention results in proportionate water retention, and sodium loss results in proportionate water loss due to osmoregulation involving AVP. Various situations can cause an isotonic expansion or contraction of the extracellular volume. Physiological regulatory mechanisms for conservation of sodium seem to be better developed in humans than are mechanisms for excretion of sodium, possibly because of an evolutionary history during which salt deficit was more common than salt excess. Because of the well-developed capacity for retention of sodium, pathological states characterized by inappropriate retention of sodium are much more common than salt-losing conditions.

SODIUM CHLORIDE RETENTION

Retention of Na^+ occurs when Na^+ intake exceeds renal Na^+ excretory capacity. This situation can occur with rapid ingestion of large amounts of salt (e.g., ingestion of seawater) or during too-rapid saline infusion. Hypernatremia and hypervolemia resulting in acute hypertension usually occur in these situations. The hypervolemia will initiate the Na^+ regulatory mechanisms causing natriuresis. Hypervolemia can occur also in pathological conditions such as congestive heart failure or renal failure and when there is excessive secretion of aldosterone in Conn's syndrome. In congestive heart failure, circulatory insufficiency stimulates the baroreceptors to reflexly increase renal retention of Na^+. This positive Na^+ balance, together with secondary water retention, causes accumulation of fluid in the vascular and interstitial spaces. Accumulation of fluid in the interstitial space is perceived as edema. In renal diseases and hyperaldosteronism, retention of sodium and water by the kidneys also causes hypervolemia and edema. In renal diseases, because retention of fluid is primarily due to failure of the kidneys, the retained fluid is less readily excreted. Therefore, although there is a sustained release of ANP, hypervolemia persists. Edema and ultimately heart failure are signs of excess Na^+ and Cl^- that exceed the upper limits of tolerance/regulation (Abassi et al., 2004).

SODIUM CHLORIDE DEFICIENCY

Loss of Na^+ can occur through either renal or nonrenal routes. Hypovolemia and hyponatremia may occur through increased renal loss of Na^+ owing to decreased reabsorption (Briggs et al., 1990). Administration of diuretics, which inhibit NaCl reabsorption, or the presence of an osmotic solute in excess of the renal reabsorptive capacity (e.g., in diabetes mellitus) causes diuresis and loss of Na^+. Chronic renal diseases that increase the permeability of the glomerular membranes or diseases that cause tubulointerstitial damage, thereby decreasing the tubular capacity for reabsorption of Na^+, result in Na^+ loss. Transient increases in loss of Na^+ also occur in tubular necrosis and in certain toxic nephropathies. Deficiency of aldosterone in Addison's disease results in a greatly enhanced excretion of Na^+ and retention of K^+ (Briggs et al., 1990).

The most common route for nonrenal loss of Na^+ is through the gastrointestinal tract from vomiting and diarrhea (Field et al., 1989).

Clinical Correlation

Diarrhea

Each day approximately 8 to 10 L of fluid passes through the gastrointestinal tract. About 2 L of these fluids is from the consumption of liquids and solid foods, and 6 to 8 L comprises secretions from the various parts of the gastrointestinal tract. The intestines absorb most of these fluids so that only 100 to 200 mL of fluid is lost daily in the stool of an adult. The average electrolyte contents of the stool are 35 to 50 mmol/L for Na^+, 75 to 90 mmol/L for K^+, 16 mmol/L for Cl^-, and 30 to 40 mmol/L for HCO_3^-.

Diarrhea is defined as an increase in stool liquidity and a fecal fluid volume of more than 200 mL/day in adults. Depending on the severity, several liters of fluid can be lost, leading to profound fluid and electrolyte imbalance. Although there are many causes of diarrhea, generally it can be classified pathogenically into (1) osmotic, (2) secretory, (3) structural, and (4) primary motility disorders. Clinically, the most common and important causes of diarrhea are osmotic and secretory.

Osmotic diarrhea can be caused either by ingestion of poorly absorbable solutes such as magnesium sulfate, sorbitol, and lactulose, or by malabsorption or maldigestion of specific solutes because of enzyme deficiencies (e.g., lactase deficiency). The presence of these solutes (and their fermentation products in the large intestine) increases the intestinal luminal osmolarity. This creates an osmotic gradient across the mucosal cells of the intestines, resulting in a diffusion of water from the interstitial fluid compartment into the lumen of the intestines. In addition, the water that would normally be absorbed or reabsorbed along with the solutes remains in the lumen. Osmotic diarrhea ceases once the aggravating factor is passed out of the lumen.

Secretory diarrhea is characterized by either an increased intestinal secretion or failure of distal reabsorption of normal secretions. Viral enteritis and bacterial infections are the most common causes of secretory diarrhea. Bacteria such as *Vibrio cholerae* and *Escherichia coli* release toxins that activate intestinal adenylate cyclase, resulting in increased secretion of sodium chloride and water, whereas enteroinvasive bacteria such as shigellae and salmonellae invade intestinal mucosa, producing ulceroinflammatory lesions.

The degree of dehydration due to diarrhea can range from mild to severe. This can be assessed clinically by examining the patient for skin turgor, mental status, blood pressure, urine output, and whether the eyeballs are sunken. Fluid replacement is of utmost importance to prevent circulatory collapse, especially in cases of severe dehydration such as those seen in patients with cholera. Diarrhea also causes electrolyte and acid–base imbalances, including hypokalemia, hyperchloremia, and metabolic acidosis.

Clinical Correlation

Diarrhea—cont'd

The World Health Organization (WHO) has recommended the use of oral rehydration therapy for treatment of mild-to-moderate cases of diarrhea, especially in developing countries. Because of the high cost of intravenous fluid therapy and the distance of some areas from medical facilities, the program has been very successful in reducing mortality from diarrheal diseases, particularly in infants. Oral rehydration fluid contains 3.5 g of NaCl, 2.5 g of $NaHCO_3$, 1.5 g of KCl, and 20 g of glucose in 1 L of water. An alternative household remedy is to mix three "finger pinches" of salt and a "fistful of sugar" with about 1 quart of water to make the solution.

Thinking Critically

Diarrhea is characterized by dehydration, electrolyte imbalance, and acid–base imbalance. Discuss why hypokalemia, hyperchloremia, and metabolic acidosis occur.

Severe and prolonged diarrhea causes hyponatremia, hypokalemia, and dehydration. Diseases causing diarrhea are among the leading sources of infant mortality and are a major world health problem. In an acute diarrheal episode in which an infant loses 5% of body weight, the infant is at risk for shock. A more gradual depletion of body fluid may not result in shock until the body weight has been reduced by about 10%. Although diarrhea causes losses of K^+ and HCO_3^- as well as of Na^+, the immediate concern in treating severe diarrhea is to replace Na^+ and water to restore the circulatory volume. Dehydration in diarrhea can be reversed by oral or, in emergencies, intravenous rehydration therapy.

Manifestations of hypovolemia are a result of diminished regional tissue perfusion and vary with the degree of volume contraction (Briggs et al., 1990). The loss of Na^+ and hypovolemia produce symptoms, including orthostatic hypotension and an increase in pulse rate. Orthostatic hypotension occurs when a person moves suddenly, either from a reclining to an upright position or from a sitting to a standing position. Vasoconstriction and decreased muscle perfusion during hypovolemia may also lead to muscular weakness and cramps. As hypovolemia becomes more severe, dizziness and syncope (fainting) may accompany the orthostatic hypotension. In severe forms of hypovolemia, the circulatory volume can be greatly compromised and circulatory shock may result. In hypovolemic individuals, mechanisms to conserve sodium are activated. If the loss is not of renal origin, the normal response is an immediate decrease in renal excretion of Na^+ to a very low level. In chronic sodium deficiency, the urine is virtually free of Na^+.

POTASSIUM IMBALANCE AND ITS CONSEQUENCES

HYPERKALEMIA

Retention of K^+ resulting in hyperkalemia occurs when K^+ consumption exceeds the capacity of the kidneys to excrete K^+. Hyperkalemia is diagnosed when the plasma K^+ concentration exceeds 5.5 mmol/L (Mount et al., 2004). This rarely happens when the kidneys are functioning normally because their capacity to excrete K^+ is substantial. A reduced capacity occurs when there is a defect in the secretory process in the distal nephrons, a lack of aldosterone secretion, or a lack of responsiveness of the renal tubules to aldosterone.

Hyperkalemia can also occur in the absence of retention of K^+. A shift of intracellular K^+ into the plasma to cause hyperkalemia can occur in metabolic acidosis or from tissue damage as in hemolysis, burns, major trauma, or lysis of tumor cells. In the treatment of hyperkalemia, consumption of K^+ is restricted, but, most importantly, the underlying causes of hyperkalemia must be treated.

An important clinical manifestation of hyperkalemia is cardiac dysrhythmias, which range from sinus bradycardia to ventricular tachycardia, ventricular fibrillation, and, ultimately, cardiac arrest (asystole) when a plasma concentration of 8 mmol/L is reached. Because of the adverse effects of hyperkalemia on the heart, hyperkalemia constitutes a medical emergency. Other symptoms include paresthesia, muscle weakness, and, eventually, flaccid paralysis.

HYPOKALEMIA

Hypokalemia is diagnosed when the plasma K^+ concentration is less than 3.5 mmol/L. It is usually associated with depletion of body K^+ (Mount et al., 2004), and the change in plasma K^+ concentration parallels the change in intracellular K^+ concentration. However, a low plasma K^+ concentration does not necessarily imply a depletion of body potassium or low intracellular concentrations because other factors may be present that cause a shift of K^+ from the extracellular to the intracellular compartment. This can occur in acute alkalosis or hyperinsulinemia. Depletion of K^+ rarely arises from insufficient consumption of K^+ because the normal amount consumed usually exceeds that required for the replacement of obligatory losses and maintenance of tissues. Depletion occurs only when intake is inadequate during prolonged fasting or when severe restriction of dietary K^+ occurs.

Depletion of K^+ and hypokalemia can occur through either renal or nonrenal routes. Renal K^+ loss can occur in endocrine and metabolic disorders such as hyperaldosteronism, metabolic alkalosis, and diuretic therapy. As with Na^+ depletion, the commonest route for nonrenal loss is vomiting and diarrhea; in these situations, the normal reflex response (increased renal and colon K^+ absorption) is prevented because of the hypovolemia that accompanies the vomiting and diarrhea. Hypovolemia initiates regulatory reflex responses to retain Na^+ and water by the kidneys. The enhanced reabsorption of Na^+ from the cortical collecting tubule under the influence of aldosterone further exacerbates the loss of K^+.

Manifestations of K^+ deficiency are due to alterations of cellular metabolism and hyperpolarization of cellular membranes. Symptoms include depressed neuromuscular functions, such as muscle weakness and cramps, and, in more severe hypokalemia, cardiac dysrhythmias, paralysis, metabolic alkalosis, and death.

NUTRITIONAL CONSIDERATIONS

Habitual high dietary salt intake has been implicated in the development of hypertension (Weinberger, 1996), gastric mucosal damage, and gastric cancer (Correa, 1992). High consumption of potassium, on the other hand, has a protective action against cardiovascular diseases (He and MacGregor, 2001).

Primary hypertension, or abnormally high blood pressure, is a significant risk factor for cardiovascular disease, stroke, and renal failure in industrialized societies. Although there is a genetic predisposition to hypertension, identification of reliable and specific genetic markers has been elusive. However, the recent finding of the association of blood pressure and the common T481S variant of the chloride channel ClC-Kb in the kidneys is promising (Jeck et al., 2004). This inherited susceptibility is expressed in the presence of other predisposing factors, such as obesity, consumption of alcohol, unbalanced diet, and stress (Folkow, 1982). Both epidemiological and experimental studies implicate a primary role for dietary factors in the control of blood pressure. Consumption of a high-fat, high-sodium (salt), low-potassium, low-calcium, or low-magnesium diet may contribute to the development of hypertension (Reusser and McCarron, 1994). Therefore, lifestyle modification, such as weight loss, increased physical activity, moderation of alcohol consumption, and an overall healthy dietary pattern, such as the DASH (Dietary Approaches to Stop Hypertension) diet, has been recommended to help reduce blood pressure (Sacks et al., 2001).

ASSOCIATION OF HIGH SALT INTAKE WITH HYPERTENSION

Although habitual high salt consumption and hypertension have been linked for more than a century, controversy remains regarding the mechanisms by which salt influences blood pressure, and in the relationship of sodium intake with cardiovascular morbidity and mortality. This is not surprising because individual differences are influenced by various dynamic variables, such as genetic susceptibility, body mass, cardiovascular factors, regulatory mechanisms mediated through the neural and hormonal systems, and the kidneys.

Implications of salt intake in hypertension come from observations that the highest incidence of hypertension occurs in northern Japan, where salt intake may be as high as 20 g/day (Kono et al., 1983). In the United States, where salt intake averages between 5 and 13 g/day, results from the NHANES III collected on 9,901 participants from age 18 through 74 years from 1988 to 1991, indicated that 24% of the adult population had hypertension this number did not include normotensive individuals who were being treated for hypertension (Burt et al., 1995). Conversely, societies with low salt intake, such as the Yanomami Indians, have a low incidence of hypertension (Oliver et al., 1975).

The most comprehensive population-based study on the relationship between dietary salt and blood pressure was carried out by The INTERSALT Cooperative Research Group (Stamler, 1997). This group studied the association between blood pressure and 24-hour excretion of Na^+ and K^+ in the urine in more than 10,000 men and women between 20 and 59 years of age from 52 geographically separate centers in 32 countries in Africa, the Americas, Asia, and Europe. Highly standardized procedures were used in this international collaborative study so that comparisons could be made between centers. The variables measured include age, sex, body mass index, alcohol consumption, arterial blood pressure, and 24-hour urine collection for the analysis of urinary Na^+ and K^+ excretion. Median daily urinary excretion of sodium ranged between 4.6 mg and 5.6 g, but the distribution within this range was uneven. Four centers had mean values of less than 1.3 g/day, none had values between 1.3 and 2.4 g/day, four had values between 2.4 g and 3.2 g/day, and 44 had values between 3.2 g and 5.6 g/day. Therefore, the bulk of the data on the association between blood pressure and excretion of sodium were for populations with high mean excretion (3.2-5.6 g/day) of sodium.

Cross-center analyses, which involved all 52 centers, showed that median systolic blood pressure, but not diastolic pressure, was significantly related to median values for excretion of sodium, after adjustments for age, sex, body mass index, and consumption of alcohol. However, when the four centers with very low median values of sodium excretion were excluded from the analyses, the correlation between systolic blood pressure and excretion of sodium was not significant. The INTERSALT study also showed that populations in the four centers with median values for sodium excretion that were less than 1.3 g/day had low blood pressure, rare or absent hypertension, and no age-related rise in blood pressure, as occurred in populations in other centers. In centers where the subjects' average excretion of sodium was more than 2.4 g/day, median values for excretion of sodium were related significantly to the age-related rise in blood pressure (Rodriguez et al., 1994). Although it was recognized that the association of blood pressure or prevalence of hypertension with median values for excretion of sodium was relatively weak, nonetheless the evidence supports the general contention that habitual intake of salt is an important factor in the occurrence of hypertension.

Dietary Salt Restriction

Intervention studies of dietary salt restrictions to lower blood pressure have produced mixed results. This may be explained by the fact that not all hypertensive patients are salt-sensitive, and many cases of hypertension are due to other causes. Nevertheless, the results of the DASH-Sodium trial and the Trials of Hypertension Prevention (Sacks et al., 2001; Cook et al., 1998) have demonstrated changes in blood pressure in response to dietary sodium reduction, thereby confirming the conclusions of the INTERSALT study (Jones, 2004). However, questions still remain on whether moderate dietary sodium restriction should be recommended to all individuals in general.

Moderate restriction of salt was found to decrease systolic and diastolic blood pressure over periods of several weeks to a few years in both hypertensive and normotensive patients. The response of blood pressure to salt restriction depended on age, the degree of restriction, and the initial blood pressure (Reusser and McCarron, 1994). Older patients seemed to have a greater response to salt restriction. The highest rate of success in reducing hypertension was obtained in nonoverweight, mildly hypertensive patients. There was some evidence that salt restriction may also decrease the incidence of stroke and ischemic heart disease.

Genetic Factors

Even though evidence suggests that genetic susceptibility contributes to the relationship between high intake of sodium salts and hypertension, the link between genetic polymorphism and hypertension remains unknown. Numerous studies involving genome-wide scans using polymorphism markers have identified regions of chromosomes relating to salt sensitivity in salt-sensitive rats (Garrett et al., 2000). Similar findings have been reported for humans. Cohort studies have linked regions on chromosome 12 (Mansfield et al., 1997) and 17 (Gu et al., 2004) to hypertension. However, the pathway that determines the genetic disposition to hypertension remains unclear. It has been proposed that because inherited and acquired forms of hypertension act via a final common pathway that involves alteration of renal sodium reabsorption, perturbations in this pathway may be an important determinant of salt sensitivity (Lifton et al., 2001).

Recently, Jeck and colleagues (2004) identified abnormalities in membrane transport systems that function as markers for genetic susceptibility to hypertension. Chloride channel ClC-Kb, named for its expression in kidney, is expressed in the basolateral membrane of the distal tubule of the kidney and participates in renal Na^+ and Cl^- reabsorption. Jeck and colleagues (2004) found an association between hypertension and carriers of ClC-Kb^{T481S}, the common T481S variant (threonine to serine mutant). In the white population studied, carriers of the T481S allele had significantly higher systolic and diastolic blood pressures and a significantly higher prevalence of hypertension. These individuals also had significantly higher plasma Na^+ levels. Thus the T481S is a gain-of-function mutation that may lead to increased renal salt retention and consequently blood pressure elevation.

ASSOCIATION OF HIGH SALT INTAKE WITH GASTRIC MUCOSAL DAMAGE

A high intake of salt from salted and smoked products has been associated with a high risk of atrophic gastritis and the development of gastric cancer (Correa, 1992). Based on evidence from case-control and epidemiological studies, a WHO/FAO Expert Consultation concluded that "salt-preserved foods and salt probably increase the risk of stomach cancer" (World Health Organization [WHO], 2003). Salt acts as an irritant that damages the stomach mucosa and makes the mucosal cells more susceptible to the polycyclic aromatic hydrocarbons and nitrosamines contained in most salted, smoked meat and fish products. These substances are gastric carcinogens that can induce glandular stomach tumors (Capoferro and Torgersen, 1974). Salt also enhances *Helicobacter pylori* colonization in the stomach, which acts as a gastric carcinogen in animals (Fox et al., 1999). A positive association between consumption of salty foods and increased *H. pylori* infection has been reported in a cross-sectional study of Japanese men (Tsugane et al., 1994). Therefore, a diet high in salt appears to enhance the initiation of cancer by damaging the gastric mucosal barrier, thereby facilitating the action of *H. pylori* and chemical carcinogens present in the diet.

PROTECTIVE ACTION OF DIETARY POTASSIUM AGAINST CARDIOVASCULAR DISEASES

The beneficial effect of K^+ on health has been of interest over the last few decades. Epidemiological studies, clinical intervention trials, and animal experiments have shown that high potassium intake protects against hypertension and cardiovascular diseases. Populations that ingest diets rich in potassium exhibit lower rates of hypertension and have a lower incidence of cardiovascular diseases, whereas those with diets habitually low in potassium (mainly industrialized cultures) appear to have an increased incidence of cardiovascular diseases (Young et al., 1995). In some studies in which no correlation was found between blood pressure and intake of sodium, an inverse relationship of potassium intake with blood pressure, incidence of stroke, and other cardiovascular diseases was found. These results were substantiated by the INTERSALT study, which also showed that the inverse relationship between blood pressure and potassium intake is independent of sodium intake (Stamler, 1997). The antihypertensive effect of potassium may be mediated by its effect on the heart, baroreflex sensitivity, vasodilation, and natriuresis (Barri and Wingo, 1997). Furthermore, there was a direct relationship between blood pressure and the ratio of Na^+ to K^+ excreted in the urine (Intersalt Cooperative Research Group, 1988).

High potassium intake also reduces the risk of stroke independent of its effect on blood pressure and prevents the development of renal vascular, glomerular, and tubular damage (He and MacGregor, 2001). Increasing intake of fruits and vegetables has been found to be associated with a 27% reduction in the risk of stroke, independent of blood pressure, although in this case, other nutrients found in fruits and vegetables may contribute to the effect (Bazzano et al., 2002). Despite evidence supporting the cardiovascular protective action of potassium, its mechanism of action is still unknown. It has been proposed that increased potassium consumption increases plasma K^+ concentration, which in turn inhibits free radical formation in vascular endothelial cells, vascular smooth muscle cell proliferation, and platelet aggregation such that the rate of formation of atherosclerotic lesions is decreased (Young et al., 1995).

Data on the usefulness of potassium supplementation to reduce blood pressure in hypertensive patients are mixed. As with the restriction of dietary sodium in the treatment of hypertension, the success of supplementation with potassium depends on the presence of other variables associated with hypertension (Krishna, 1994). In some clinical trials, supplementation with potassium or an increase in dietary potassium from natural foods reduced blood pressure and the incidence of stroke mortality (Young et al., 1995). In other trials, the beneficial effects of potassium were short-lived or nonexistent. Animal models of both salt-sensitive and non–salt-sensitive rats have shown that supplementation with potassium protects against hypertension, stroke, cardiac hypertrophy, and renal glomerular lesions.

REFERENCES

Abassi ZA, Winaver J, Skorecki KL (2004) Control of extracellular fluid volume and the pathophysiology of edema formation. In: Brenner BM (ed) Brenner & Rector's The Kidney, 7th ed. Elsevier Saunders, Philadelphia, pp 777-855.

Adrogue HJ, Madias NE (1981) Changes in plasma potassium concentration during acid-base disturbances. Am J Med 71:456-467.

Barri YM, Wingo CS (1997) The effects of potassium depletion and supplementation on blood pressure: a clinical review. Am J Med Sci 314:37-40.

Baylis PH, Thompson CJ (1988) Osmoregulation of vasopressin secretion and thirst in health and disease. Clin Endocrinol 29:549-576.

Bazzano LA, He J, Ogden LG, Loria CM, Vupputuri S, Myers L, Whelton PK (2002) Fruit and vegetable intake and risk of cardiovascular disease in US adults: the first National Health and Nutrition Examination Survey Epidemiologic Follow-up Study. Am J Clin Nutr 76:93-99.

Blanco G, Mercer RW (1998) Isozymes of the Na-K-ATPase: heterogeneity in structure, diversity in function. Am J Physiol Renal Physiol 275:F633-F650.

Briggs JP, Sawaya BE, Schnermann J (1990) Disorders of salt balance. In: Kokko JP, Tannen RL (eds) Fluids and Electrolytes, 2nd ed. WB Saunders, Philadelphia, pp 70-138.

Bunning P, Riordan JF (1987) Sulfate potentiation of the chloride activation of angiotensin-converting enzyme. Biochemistry 26:3374-3377.

Burt VL, Whelton P, Rocella EJ, Brown C, Cutler JA, Higgins M, Horan MJ, Labarthe D (1995) Prevalence of hypertension in the US adult population. Results from the Third National Health and Nutrition Examination Survey, 1988-1991. Hypertension 25:305-313.

Candido R, Burrell LM, Jandeleit-Dahm KA, Cooper ME (2004) Vasoactive peptides and the kidney. In: Brenner BM (ed) Brenner & Rector's The Kidney, 7th ed. Elsevier Saunders, Philadelphia, pp 663-726.

Canessa CM, Schild L, Buell G, Thorens B, Gautschi I, Horisberger JD, Rossier BC (1994) Amiloride-sensitive epithelial Na^+ channel is made of three homologous subunits. Nature 367:463-467.

Capoferro R, Torgersen O (1974) The effect of hypertonic saline on the uptake of tritiated 7,12-dimethylbenz[a]anthracene by gastric mucosa. Scand J Gastroenterol 9:343-349.

Cook NR, Kumanyika SK, Cutler JA (1998) Effect of change in sodium excretion on change in blood pressure corrected for measurement error. The Trials of Hypertension Prevention, Phase I. Am J Epidemiol 148:431-444.

Correa P (1992) Human gastric carcinogenesis: a multistep and multifactorial process. First American Cancer Society Award Lecture on Cancer Epidemiology and Prevention. Cancer Res 52:6735-6740.

Dahl LK (1958) Salt intake and salt need. N Engl J Med 258:1152-1156.

Daniels D, Fluharty SJ (2004) Salt appetite: a neurohormonal viewpoint. Physiol Behav 81:319-337.

Field M, Rao MC, Chang EB (1989) Intestinal electrolyte transport and diarrheal disease. N Engl J Med 321:800-806.

Folkow B (1982) Physiological aspects of primary hypertension. Physiol Rev 62:347-504.

Forbes GB (1987) Human Body Composition; Growth, Aging, Nutrition, and Activity. Springer-Verlag, New York, pp 169-195.

Fox JG, Dangler CA, Taylor NS, King A, Koh TJ, Wang TC (1999) High-salt diet induces gastric epithelial hyperplasia and parietal cell loss, and enhances *Helicobacter pylori* colonization in C57BL/6 mice. Cancer Res 59:4823-4828.

Ganguly A, Donohue JP (1983) Primary aldosteronism: pathophysiology, diagnosis and treatment. J Urol 129:241-247.

Garrett MR, Saad Y, Dene H, Rapp JP (2000) Blood pressure QTL that differentiate Dahl-sensitive and spontaneously hypertensive rats. Physiol Genomics 3:33-38.

Gu F, Ge D, Huang J, Chen J, Yang W, Gu D (2004) Genetic susceptibility loci for essential hypertension and blood pressure on chromosome 17 in 147 Chinese pedigrees. J Hypertens 22:1511-1518.

He FJ, MacGregor GA (2001) Beneficial effects of potassium. BMJ 323:497-501.

Institute of Medicine (2004) Dietary Reference Intakes for Water, Potassium, Sodium, Chloride, and Sulfate. National Academy Press, Washington, DC.

Intersalt Cooperative Research Group (1988) Intersalt: an international study of electrolyte excretion and blood pressure. Results for 24 hour urinary sodium and potassium excretion. BMJ 297:319-328.

Jeck N, Waldeffer S, Lampert A, Boehmer C, Waldegger P, Lang PA, Wissinger B, Friedrich B, Risler T, Moehle R, Lang UE, Zill P, Bondy B, Schaeffeler E, Asante-Poku S, Seyberth H, Schwab M, Lang F (2004) Activating mutation of the renal epithelial chloride channel ClC-Kb predisposing to hypertension. Hypertension 43:1175-1181.

Johnson AG, Nguyen TV, Davis D (2001) Blood pressure is linked to salt intake and modulated by the angiotensinogen gene in normotensive and hypertensive elderly subjects. J Hypertens 19:1053-1060.

Jones DW (2004) Dietary sodium and blood pressure. Hypertension 43:932-935.

Kono S, Ikeda M, Ogata M (1983) Salt and geographical mortality of gastric cancer and stroke in Japan. J Epidemiol Community Health 37:43-46.

Krishna GG (1994) Role of potassium in the pathogenesis of hypertension. Am J Med Sci 307(Suppl 1):S21-S25.

Kutchai HC (2004) The gastrointestinal system. Digestion and absorption. In: Berne RM, Levy MN, Koeppen BM, Stanton BA (eds) Physiology, 5th ed. Mosby, St. Louis, pp 595-620.

Larsen TM, Laughlin LT, Holden HM, Rayment I, Reed GH (1994) Structure of rabbit muscle pyruvate kinase complexed with Mn^{2+}, K^+, and pyruvate. Biochemistry 33:6301-6309.

Levens NR, Peach MJ, Carey RM (1981) Role of intrarenal renin–angiotensin system in the control of renal function. Circ Res 48:157-167.

Lifton RP, Gharavi AG, Geller DS (2001) Molecular mechanisms of human hypertension. Cell 104:545-556.

MacGregor GA, Markandu ND, Sagnella GA, Singer DRDJ, Cappuccio FP (1989) Double-blind study of three sodium intakes and long-term effects of sodium restriction in essential hypertension. Lancet 2:1244-1247.

Malnic G, Bailey MA, Giebisch G (2004) Control of renal potassium excretion. In: Brenner BM (ed)

Brenner & Rector's The Kidney, 7th ed. Elsevier Saunders, Philadelphia, pp 453-495.

Mancilha-Carvalho JJ, Souza e Silva NA (2003) The Yanomami Indians in the INTERSALT study. Arq Bras Cardiol 80:289-300.

Mansfield TA, Simon DB, Farfel S, Bia M, Tucci JR, Lebel M, Gutkin M, Vialettes B, Christofilis MA, Kauppinen-Makelin R, Mayan H, Risch N, and Lifton RP (1997) Multilocus linkage of familial hyperkalemia and hypertension, pseudoaldosteronism type II, to chromosomes Iq31-42 and 17p11-q21. Nature Genet 16: 202-205.

Moratinos J, Reverte M (1993) Effects of catecholamines on plasma potassium: the role of alpha- and beta-adrenoceptors. Fundam Clin Pharmacol 7:143-153.

Morris RC Jr, Sesbastian A, Forman A, Tanaka M, Schmidlin O (1999) Normotensive salt-sensitivity: effects of race and dietary potassium. Hypertension 33:18-23.

Mount DB, Zandi-Nejad K (2004) Disorders of potassium balance. In: Brenner BM (ed) Brenner & Rector's The Kidney, 7th ed. Elsevier Saunders, Philadelphia, pp 997-1040.

National Research Council (1989) Recommended Dietary Allowances, 10th ed. National Academy Press, Washington, DC, pp 247-261.

Nerup J (1974) Addison's disease—clinical studies: a report of 108 cases. Acta Endocrinol 76:127-141.

Oliver WJ, Cohen EL, Neel JV (1975) Blood pressure, sodium intake and sodium-related hormones in the Yanomamo Indians, a "no-salt" culture. Circulation 52:146-151.

O'Neil RG (1990) Aldosterone regulation of sodium and potassium transport in the cortical collecting duct. Semin Nephrol 10:365-374.

Quail AW, Woods R, Korner PI (1987) Cardiac and arterial baroreceptor influences in release of vasopressin and renin during hemorrhage. Am J Physiol 252:H1120-H1126.

Reusser ME, McCarron DA (1994) Micronutrient effects on blood pressure regulation. Nutr Rev 52:367-375.

Rodriguez BL, Labarthe DR, Huang B, Lopez-Gomez J (1994) Rise of blood pressure with age. New evidence of population differences. Hypertension 24:779-785.

Rodriguez-Soriano J (1995) Potassium homeostasis and its disturbance in children. Pediatr Nephrol 9:364-374.

Rose BD, Post TW (2001) Clinical Physiology of Acid-base and Electrolyte Disorders, 5th ed. McGraw-Hill Book Company, New York, pp 285-298.

Sacks FM, Svetkey LP, Vollmer WM, Appel LJ, Bray GA, Harsha D, Obarzanek E, Conlin PR, Miller ER, Simons-Morton DG, Karanja N, Lin PH (2001) Effects of blood pressure of reduced dietary sodium and the Dietary Approaches to Stop Hypertension (DASH) diet. N Engl J Med 344:3-10.

Sanchez-Castillo CP, Branch WJ, James WP (1987a) A test of the validity of the lithium-marker technique for monitoring dietary sources of salt in men. Clin Sci 72:87-94.

Sanchez-Castillo CP, Warrender S, Whitehead TP, James WP (1987b) An assessment of the sources of dietary salt in a British population. Clin Sci 72:95-102.

Stamler J (1997) The INTERSALT Study: Background, methods, findings, and implications. Am J Clin Nutr 65(Suppl): 626S-642S.

Stanton BA, Koeppen BM (2004) Solute and water transport along the nephron: tubular function. In: Berne RM, Levy MN, Koeppen BM, Stanton BA (eds) Physiology, 5th ed. Mosby, St. Louis, pp 643-658.

Tsugane S, Tei Y, Takahashi T, Watanabe S, Sugano K (1994) Salty food intake and risk of *Helicobacter pylori* infection. Jpn J Cancer Res 85:474-478.

Weinberger MH (1996) Salt sensitivity of blood pressure in humans. Hypertension 27:481-490.

World Health Organization (WHO) (2003) Diet, Nutrition and the Prevention of Chronic Diseases, WHO Technical Report Series 916. WHO, Geneva.

Young DB, Lin H, McCabe RD (1995) Potassium's cardiovascular protective mechanisms. Am J Physiol 268:R825-R837.

Zeidel ML (1990) Renal actions of atrial natriuretic peptide: regulation of collecting duct sodium and water transport. Annu Rev Physiol 52: 747-759.

RECOMMENDED READINGS

Abassi ZA, Winaver J, Skorecki KL (2004) Control of extracellular fluid volume and the pathophysiology of edema formation. In: Brenner BM (ed) Brenner & Rector's The Kidney, 7th ed. Elsevier Saunders, Philadelphia, pp 777-855.

Briggs JP, Sawaya BE, Schnermann J (1990) Disorders of salt balance. In: Kokko JP, Tannen RL (eds) Fluids and Electrolytes, 2nd ed. WB Saunders, Philadelphia, pp 70-138.

He FJ, MacGregor GA (2001) Beneficial effects of potassium. BMJ 323:497-501.

Jones DW (2004) Dietary sodium and blood pressure. Hypertension 43:932-935.

Rodriguez-Soriano J (1995) Potassium homeostasis and its disturbance in children. Pediatr Nephrol 9:364-374.

Stamler J (1997) The INTERSALT Study: background, methods, findings, and implications. Am J Clin Nutr 65(Suppl):626S-642S.

World Health Organization (WHO) (2003) Diet, Nutrition and the Prevention of Chronic Diseases, WHO Technical Report Series 916. WHO, Geneva.

Chapter 35

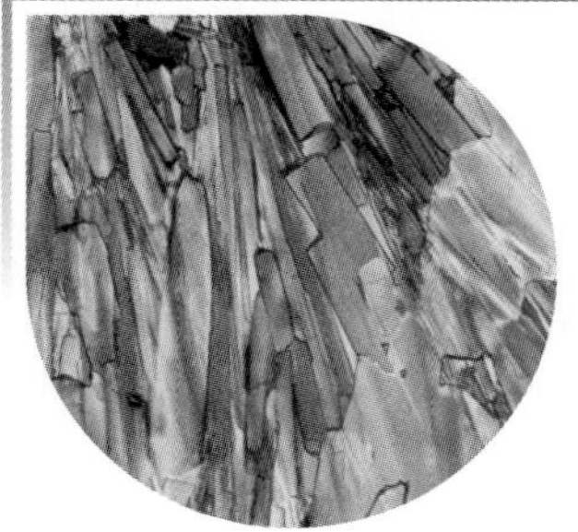

Body Fluids and Water Balance

Hwai-Ping Sheng, PhD

OUTLINE

COMMON ABBREVIATIONS

AVP	arginine vasopressin; also known as antidiuretic hormone (ADH)	C_{osm}	osmolar clearance
AQPs	aquaporins	C_{water}	free-water clearance

PHYSIOLOGICAL FUNCTIONS OF WATER

Water is an essential nutrient vital to the existence of both animals and plants. In the body, water is present inside and around the cells and within all blood vessels. Water performs several functions that are essential to life: it is the principal fluid medium in which nutrients, gases, and enzymes are dissolved; the extracellular water bathing the cells serves as a medium for the transport of nutrients and oxygen to the cells and for removing wastes from the cells; and intracellular water establishes the physicochemical medium that allows various metabolic processes to take place. Furthermore, the volume of the intracellular fluid provides turgor to the tissues, which is important for the tissue or organ form and, ultimately, the body form. Another important physiological function of water is its role in the regulation of body temperature. This is achieved by removing excess heat from the body by evaporative water loss from the skin.

BODY WATER COMPARTMENTS

BODY WATER CONTENT

Water makes up the largest component of the body; its content in the body varies with age, sex, and adiposity of the individual. In the neonate body water makes up approximately 75% of body weight, decreasing progressively to about 60% in the young adult, and continuing to decline to approximately 50% at about 50 years of age. The higher proportion of water in the neonate is, for the most part, the result of a larger fraction of body mass as extracellular fluid space in the infant. A combination of factors causes the proportion of extracellular fluid space to decrease gradually with an increase in age. These factors include an increase in the amount of cellular tissues, such as muscles, at the expense of extracellular space, and an increase in the proportion of body mass made up of adipose tissues and the supporting structures of skeleton, cartilage, and connective tissues, all of which contain a relatively low water content.

Adult women have lower water content when compared with men of comparable age, and obese individuals have lower water content than their leaner counterparts. These variations can be attributed to differences in the proportion of adipose tissue relative to lean tissue in the body. Fat cells have a relatively low content of water, about 10%, whereas other cellular tissues such as muscles contain an average of 70% water. Therefore, water content in the body varies inversely with the relative proportion of adipose tissue, and can explain the lower water content both in women and in obese individuals. However, when body water is calculated on a lean body weight basis, it constitutes a relatively constant proportion, 73.2% for adults and 82% for neonates.

DISTRIBUTION OF BODY WATER

Water in the body is distributed throughout the various body fluid compartments. As shown in Figure 35-1, the simplest subdivision is an intracellular and an extracellular compartment, with the two compartments separated by the cell membrane. In adults, the intracellular fluid compartment makes up approximately 40% of body weight, whereas the extracellular fluid compartment makes up about 20%; in other words, of the 42 L of body water in a 70-kg adult, about two thirds (28 L) is in the intracellular compartment and about one third (14 L) is in the extracellular compartment. The extracellular fluid is made up of the following subdivisions: interstitial fluid, including the lymph; plasma; and cavity or transcellular fluids, the largest volume of which is present as secretory fluids in the lumen of the gastrointestinal tract. Interstitial fluid (fluid bathing the cells) and plasma are the two largest components of the extracellular fluid

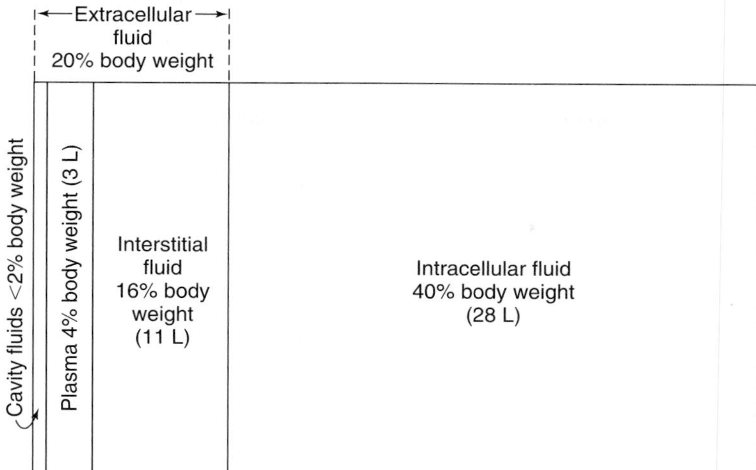

Figure 35-1 Major body fluid compartments of an adult. Intraluminal gastrointestinal water constitutes the largest fraction of the cavity fluids. In general, water moves freely between adjacent compartments along an osmotic gradient.

compartment, with the interstitial fluid constituting about four fifths of the extracellular fluid (11 L, or 16% of body weight) and plasma making up about one fifth of the extracellular fluid (3 L, or 4% of body weight).

The distribution of water in the various compartments determines the size of the compartments and is governed by solute particles and physical forces that maintain equilibrium across membranes separating these compartments. Osmotic forces and hydrostatic pressures are the prime determinants of water distribution in the body.

FLUID DISTRIBUTION BETWEEN EXTRACELLULAR AND INTRACELLULAR FLUID COMPARTMENTS

Osmosis and Osmotic Pressure

To understand the distribution and direction of water movement between cells and interstitium, it is important to understand the concept of osmotic forces. The concept of osmosis is explained simply in Figure 35-2. A membrane that is impermeable to solutes but permeable to water separates the two compartments—A and B—which contain the same volume of fluid but different numbers of solute particles. Water diffuses across the membrane in both directions, but more water molecules diffuse from compartment A, a region of higher water concentration (lower solute concentration), to compartment B, a region of lower water concentration (higher solute concentration). The process of net movement of water caused by a concentration difference of water or solutes is called osmosis. Osmosis of water results in the expansion of compartment B at the expense of compartment A. No further net diffusion of water occurs when the solute concentrations in both compartments are equal; that is, when osmotic equilibrium is established (Rose and Post, 2001a). To reach this state of equilibrium, changes in the volumes of the compartments have occurred. The volume of compartment B has increased at the expense of compartment A. This situation can occur only when the two compartments are flexible volumetrically so that the net flow of water from one compartment to another does not create a pressure difference across the membrane. However, if the walls of compartment B do not expand, the increase in hydrostatic pressure in compartment B due to influx of water will oppose further inflow of water. The amount of pressure to be applied in order to prevent the inflow of water into compartment B through the membrane is called osmotic pressure (Rose and Post, 2001a). The osmotic pressure of a solution, therefore, reflects the concentration of osmotically active particles in that solution.

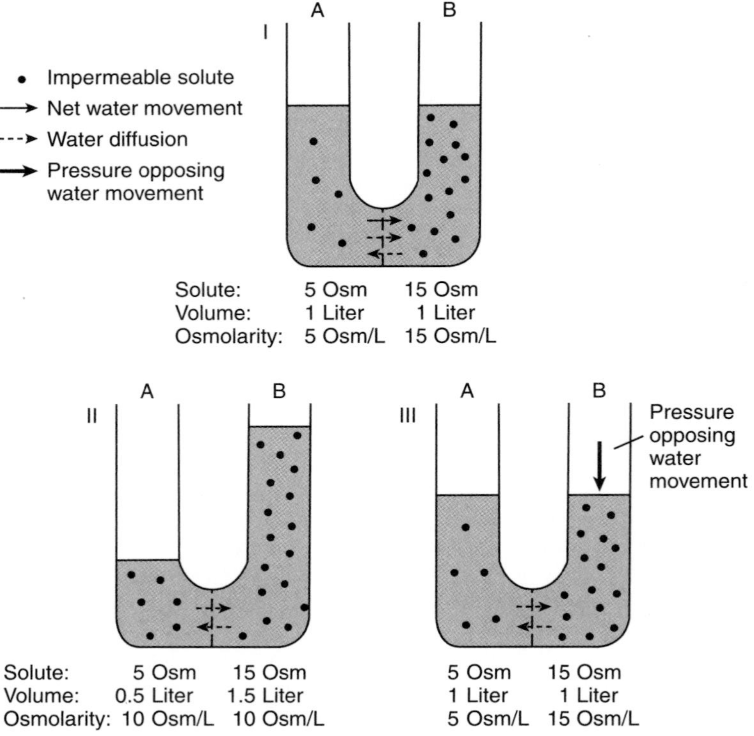

Figure 35-2 Osmosis and osmotic pressure can be illustrated by two compartments separated by a semipermeable membrane, permeable to water but not to solutes (*circles*). In *diagram I,* compartments A and B are shown filled with equal volumes of solution, but the solution in compartment A is hypo-osmotic with reference to the solution in compartment B. There is net movement of water from A to B until the solutions in the two compartments are iso-osmotic, as shown in *diagram II.* The movement of water across the semipermeable membrane leads to a change in the initial volumes at equilibrium. In this example, the volume of compartment B increased, whereas the volume of compartment A decreased. Because the volume of compartment B increased, there were no significant changes in hydrostatic pressure in the compartments. As shown in *diagram III,* application of a pressure can prevent osmotic movement of water across the semipermeable membrane. This pressure is called the osmotic pressure.

The process of osmosis also explains the movement of water across cell membranes. Most cell membranes are semipermeable; that is, relatively impermeable to most solutes but highly permeable to water. Although water is a polar molecule, it is able to penetrate the nonpolar lipid region of membranes through a group of membrane proteins called aquaporins (AQPs), which form water channels through which water can readily diffuse. The number of these AQP-water channels differs in membranes of different tissues, and, in some cells, the number of channels, and thus the permeability to water, can be altered in response to hormones. In the steady state, the volume of water that diffuses across the membrane in either direction is balanced precisely so that no net diffusion of water occurs and the volume of the cell remains unchanged. However, under certain conditions, when a concentration difference for water develops across the cell membrane by active transport of solutes, osmotic forces will develop across the cell membrane and water will move rapidly between these two compartments until an osmotic equilibrium is achieved. When this happens, net influx of water causes the cell to expand, whereas net efflux of water causes the cell to contract. Therefore, at equilibrium, the osmolarity of the intracellular and interstitial fluid compartments remains similar, at approximately 290 mOsm/L.

Osmolality and Osmolarity

As noted, a difference in the solute concentrations of two fluids separated by a semipermeable membrane causes osmotic movement of water. Therefore, it is useful to have a concentration term that refers to the total concentration of solute particles that cause osmotic movement of water. Because it is the number, and not the size or type, of solute particles that causes water movement, the term osmole (Osm) is used to describe the number of solute particles, regardless of their mass. One osmole is the number of particles (i.e., Avogadro's number, or 6.02×10^{23}) in 1 mole or 1 gram molecular weight of an undissociated solute. A solution containing either 1 mole of glucose (180 g) or 1 mole of albumin (70,000 g) in 1 kg of water has a concentration of 1 Osm/kg of water because neither glucose nor albumin dissociates in solution. If the solute in solution dissociates into 2 ions, then 1 mole of the dissociated solute will contain 2 osmoles. For example, 1 mole of sodium chloride (NaCl) dissociates to yield 1 mole each of sodium and chloride ions; therefore, 1 mole of NaCl in 1 kg of water will have an osmolal concentration of 2 Osm/kg of water. Likewise, a solution that contains 1 mole of a solute that dissociates into 3 ions (for example, $CaCl_2$) has an osmolal concentration of 3 Osm/kg.

Strictly speaking, ions in solutions exert interionic attraction to, or repulsion from, each other and can, therefore, cause a decrease or an increase in the actual number of osmotically active particles in the solution. Any deviations can be corrected for if the osmotic coefficient for the molecule is known. For example, the osmotic coefficient for NaCl is 0.93. Therefore, 1 mol of NaCl in 1 kg of water has an osmolal concentration of 1.86 rather than 2 mOsm/kg. In practice, the osmotic coefficients of different solutes are often disregarded when determining the osmolal concentrations of physiological solutions.

The concentration of body fluids can be expressed as osmole per kilogram of water (osmolality) or osmole per liter of fluid (osmolarity). Therefore, osmolarity, but not osmolality, is affected by the volume of solutes present in the body fluid. The normal osmolarity of plasma is approximately 290 mOsm/L. Solutes, mainly proteins, occupy about 5% of plasma volume. Therefore, the osmolality of plasma is about 5% higher, at approximately 305 mOsm/kg of water. Because body fluids are dilute solutions, differences between osmolality and osmolarity are small and the two terms are often used synonymously. In practice, it is easier to express solute concentrations of plasma in mOsm/L than in mOsm/kg.

Iso-osmotic, Hypo-osmotic, and Hyperosmotic Solutions

The terms iso-osmotic, hypo-osmotic, and hyperosmotic are used to describe the relation of osmolar concentrations between different solutions. When two solutions are of equal osmolarity, they are iso-osmotic. A solution is hypo-osmotic when its osmolarity is lower and hyperosmotic when its osmolarity is higher than that of the reference solution. When cells are suspended in a hypo-osmotic solution, water enters the cells, causing them to expand. Conversely, when cells are suspended in a hyperosmotic solution, water diffuses out of the cells, causing them to contract. When cells are suspended in an iso-osmotic solution, no net flux of water occurs, and cell size remains the same. However, this is not the case if cells are suspended in an iso-osmotic solution containing a highly permeant solute (e.g., urea). Urea diffuses into cells along its concentration gradient, causing an osmotic flow of water into cells, and the cells expand (Fig. 35-3). Therefore another term, tonicity, is used to describe the physiological osmolar concentration of a solution.

Isotonic, Hypotonic, and Hypertonic Solutions

The term tonicity refers not only to the osmolarity of a solution relative to plasma but also to whether the solution will affect cell volume. An isotonic solution has an osmolarity of 290 mOsm/L, and when cells are placed in this solution, no net diffusion of water occurs. Solutions in which suspended cells shrink are called hypertonic, and solutions in which suspended cells expand are called hypotonic. Sodium chloride solution at a concentration of 290 mOsm/L is an isotonic solution because sodium is kept out of cells by active

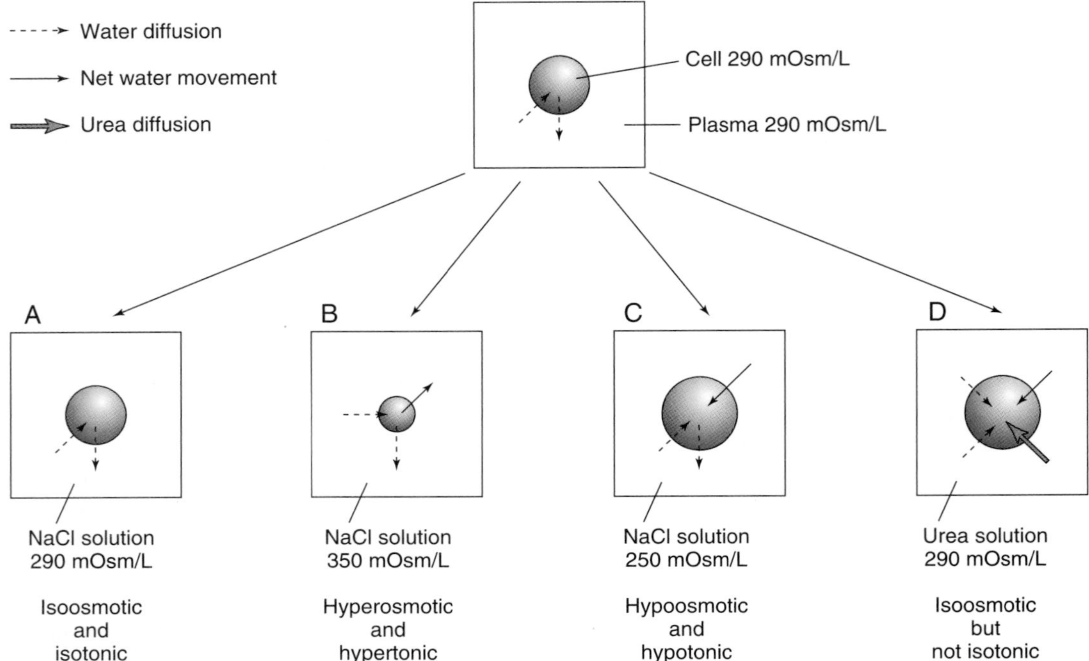

Figure 35-3 The concepts of osmolarity and tonicity can be illustrated by a red blood cell suspended in various media. In the body, red blood cells are suspended in plasma; because plasma is iso-osmotic and isotonic, the rate of water diffusion out of the cell is equal to that into the cell. No net movement of water occurs, and the cell volume remains the same. When a red blood cell is suspended in a 290-mOsm/L NaCl solution, no net movement of water occurs *(A)*. The solution is iso-osmotic and isotonic. When a red blood cell is suspended in a 350-mOsm/L NaCl solution, there is a net movement of water out of the cell along an osmotic gradient *(B)*. The cell will shrink. The solution is hyperosmotic and hypertonic. When a red blood cell is suspended in a 250-mOsm/L NaCl solution, there is a net movement of water into the cell, causing cell expansion and hemolysis *(C)*. The solution is hypo-osmotic and hypotonic. When a red blood cell is suspended in a 290-mOsm/L urea solution, urea diffuses into the cell along its concentration gradient and water follows, resulting in net entry of water, which causes the cell to hemolyze *(D)*. (The increased volume of water and solute in the cell causes the cell membrane to rupture.) The solution is iso-osmotic but not isotonic.

transport processes. Conversely, a solution of urea or glucose at a concentration of 290 mOsm/L is iso-osmotic to plasma but not isotonic. Red blood cells suspended in an iso-osmotic solution of urea or glucose will hemolyze. Urea diffuses readily into cells along its concentration gradient, causing an osmotic flow of water into the cells (see Fig. 35-3). Glucose, on the other hand, is taken up and metabolized by red blood cells, causing a progressive decrease in the osmolarity of the suspension fluid and causing water to move into the cells to maintain iso-osmolarity. It is important, therefore, to understand the difference between osmolarity and tonicity, especially in intravenous fluid therapy. A solution containing 0.9% NaCl (290 mOsm/L) is isotonic with plasma. This isotonic saline solution is commonly used as replacement fluid during the postoperative period.

Osmolarity and Volume of Extracellular and Intracellular Fluid Compartments

In contrast to movement of water across cell membranes, movement of solutes is more variable and depends on the presence of specific membrane transporters. Whereas cell membranes are relatively impermeable to proteins and organic phosphates, they selectively extrude sodium out of the cell in exchange for potassium. Therefore, sodium and its accompanying anions, mainly chloride, are the major solutes in the extracellular fluid. Inside the cells, the major cations are potassium and magnesium, and the major anions are proteins and organic phosphates. Water will distribute passively between the intracellular and extracellular compartments according to the osmolar concentrations, which are determined by the quantity of diffusible and nondiffusible solutes present in each of these compartments. Consequently, the volume of each of these compartments depends on the amount of solutes present and the total volume of body water. Whenever an inequality of osmolar concentration occurs across the cell membrane, water diffuses rapidly from the compartment of lower osmolarity to one of higher osmolarity so that any differences in osmolarity are corrected within a few minutes. In the steady state, the osmolarity of extracellular and intracellular fluids is equal.

FLUID DISTRIBUTION BETWEEN PLASMA AND INTERSTITIAL FLUID COMPARTMENTS

Plasma circulates throughout the body and provides the medium for transporting water, solutes, and gases from one part of the body to another. As the blood flows through the capillaries, interstitial fluid is delivered continuously to tissues by ultrafiltration near the arterial ends and returned to the circulation near the venous ends by forces across the capillary endothelium. In this way, the absorbed solutes and water from the gastrointestinal tract and dissolved oxygen from the lungs are carried to the tissues by plasma and by interstitial fluid to the cells. Similarly, metabolic waste products, including dissolved carbon dioxide, are carried by the same route, but in the opposite direction, from the tissues to the kidneys and lungs to be eliminated. Therefore, as first described by Claude Bernard (1813-1879) as the *milieu intérieur*, the interstitial fluid constitutes the immediate environment of the body cells.

The interstitial fluid protects the cells in the body from direct contact with the external environment and acts as a buffer for the cells from sudden changes in solute and water content caused by ingestion or loss from the body. The body possesses various physiological control systems that regulate the elimination of solutes and water from the body, so that the composition and volume of the plasma and, indirectly, the composition and volume of the interstitial and intracellular fluids are maintained relatively constant.

A small fraction of interstitial fluid is continuously drained away through lymphatic channels. This fluid, called lymph, drains into the thoracic duct, which returns the fluid to the circulation via the right subclavian vein. The total volume of lymph fluid is small, about 1 to 2 L. Transcellular, or cavity, fluids are generally considered to be specialized secretory fluids produced by active transport processes occurring across epithelial cells. These fluids differ from interstitial fluid in that they are not simple ultrafiltrates of plasma; their compositions differ markedly from that of plasma and are adapted specifically to the function of particular organs. Examples of transcellular fluids are fluids in the lumen of the gastrointestinal tract, the cerebrospinal fluid, and fluids in the intraocular, pleural, peritoneal, and synovial spaces. Of these, intraluminal gastrointestinal fluid constitutes the largest fraction. The total volume occupied by these fluids is small, about 1 to 2 L.

Two factors, the Gibbs-Donnan equilibrium and the Starling forces, affect the distribution of solutes and flow of protein-free plasma through fenestrations of the capillary endothelium. These fenestrations (20- to 100-nm diameter pores) are highly permeable to almost all solutes in the plasma except proteins, so that interstitial fluid and plasma have a similar composition except for the higher concentration of proteins in the plasma. Except in the brain, diffusion constitutes the most important means by which net movement of nutrients, gases, and metabolic end products occurs across the capillary walls. At the same time that diffusional exchange of the aforementioned solutes is occurring, another process also is taking place across the capillary wall—the bulk flow of protein-free plasma. The function of the bulk flow of protein-free plasma is the distribution of extracellular fluid from the blood vessels to the interstitium rather than the exchange of solutes and gases.

Gibbs-Donnan Equilibrium

On average, the concentration of proteins in the interstitial fluid is less than 10 g/L, compared with 73 g/L in the plasma. The differential concentration of protein affects the distribution of diffusible ions and osmotic pressures across the capillary endothelium. When two fluid compartments, A and B, are separated by a semipermeable membrane, the concentrations of any diffusible cation or anion are equal across the membrane so that no differences in concentration exist for any of the ions. On the basis of thermodynamic principles, Gibbs and Donnan showed that at equilibrium, the product of the concentrations of diffusible cations and anions in the two compartments are equal and electrical neutrality is maintained:

$$[\text{Cation}]_A \times [\text{Anion}]_A = [\text{Cation}]_B \times [\text{Anion}]_B$$

When a nondiffusible cation or anion is added to one of the compartments, the diffusible ions will redistribute themselves so that the concentration of each of the ions will no longer be equal across the cell membrane.

At normal plasma pH of 7.4, the majority of plasma proteins behave as negatively charged particles. Because proteins are confined to the vascular compartment, electrical neutrality in the plasma can be maintained only by an unequal distribution of the smaller diffusible ions, resulting in lower concentrations of each of the diffusible anions and higher concentrations of the diffusible cations in the plasma than in the interstitial fluid. At a normal concentration of plasma protein (73 g/L), this effect is small, with the concentration of monovalent anions (for example, chloride) about 5% lower and that of monovalent cations (for example, sodium and potassium) approximately 5% higher in the plasma than in the interstitial fluid. For all practical purposes, the concentrations of ions in the plasma and interstitial fluid can be considered to be about equal.

Colloid Osmotic Pressure

The concentration difference of proteins across capillary endothelium not only affects the distribution of diffusible ions, it also causes an osmotic gradient across the capillary endothelium. This osmotic gradient exerts a pressure that is called the colloid osmotic pressure, or oncotic pressure. Colloid osmotic pressure is of physiological importance in determining net water movement across the capillary endothelium.

Starling's Law

The capillary wall is permeable to almost all plasma solutes, except proteins, and it also is highly permeable to water. Therefore, in the presence of a hydrostatic pressure difference across it, the capillary wall behaves like a porous filter through which protein-free plasma moves by bulk flow from the capillaries to the interstitium. The magnitude of the bulk flow is determined by two opposing forces acting across the capillary endothelium.

Starling first proposed the concept that the two opposing forces that govern water movement across the capillary endothelium are created by the difference in hydrostatic pressure and the difference in colloid osmotic pressure across the capillary wall (Taylor, 1981). Therefore, the movement of fluid depends on four variables: hydrostatic pressures and protein concentrations in both the plasma and interstitial fluid. The following equations describe the forces responsible for net water movement across an idealized capillary endothelium:

$$\text{Net driving pressure} = (P_c - P_{if}) - (\pi_c - \pi_{if})$$

$$\text{Net volume of water flow} = K_f[(P_c - P_{if}) - (\pi_c - \pi_{if})]$$

where K_f is the product of water permeability and filtration surface area of the capillary endothelium, P_c is the capillary hydrostatic pressure, P_{if} is the interstitial fluid hydrostatic pressure, π_c is the capillary colloid osmotic pressure, and π_{if} is the interstitial fluid colloid osmotic pressure.

Under normal circumstances, as blood flows along the capillary, the balance of these forces results in a net pressure gradient favoring the movement of a small amount of fluid from the arterial end of the capillary into the interstitium. Because of a fall in capillary hydrostatic pressure along the length of the capillary, much of the fluid reenters the capillary at the

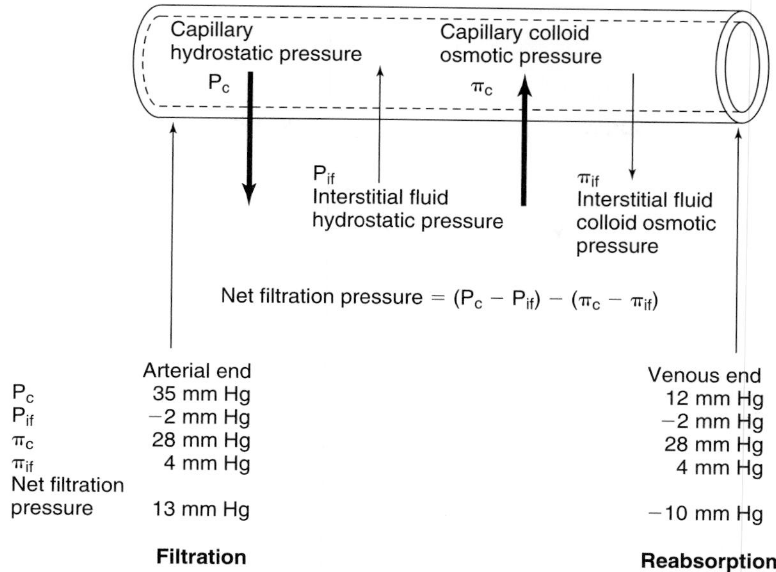

Figure 35-4 Illustration of the Starling forces across the capillary endothelium.

venous end (Fig. 35-4). The small amount of fluid that remains in the interstitium is returned to the circulation by the lymphatic vessels, which empty into the subclavian vein via the thoracic duct (Taylor, 1981).

Therefore, under normal circumstances, the difference in hydrostatic pressure between capillary blood and interstitial fluid favors filtration out of the capillary, and the difference in colloid osmotic pressure favors absorption of interstitial fluid into the capillary. An imbalance in any of these forces affects net movement of water across the capillary endothelium and ultimately will affect distribution of fluid between the plasma and interstitial compartments. For example, a decrease in plasma protein concentration in disease states, such as liver and kidney diseases, results in an accumulation of fluid in the interstitial spaces, causing edema.

Other factors that may affect the distribution of fluid across capillary endothelium include the integrity of the capillary endothelium and the lymphatic drainage system. An increase in capillary permeability allows plasma albumin to enter the interstitium to an abnormal extent, thereby reducing the difference in colloid osmotic pressure (i.e., $\pi_c - \pi_{if}$ in Starling's equation). This increase in permeability occurs in sepsis, venom shock, drug overdose, and anaphylactic reactions, and it can cause large volumes of fluids to leak from the vascular to the interstitial space. The lymphatic system can reduce the volume of edema fluid by returning the fluid to the intravascular system via the thoracic duct. Blockage of lymphatic drainage causes accumulation of fluid in the interstitial fluid compartment.

WATER BALANCE

For an individual to maintain water balance, the amount of water consumed must equal the amount lost from the body. This is illustrated in Table 35-1 for a 65-kg man in a temperate environment and consuming a balanced diet that provides adequately for his energy requirements. Even with the excretion of a maximally concentrated urine, water normally contained in the food (preformed water) and water produced by oxidation of food (metabolic water, or water of oxidation) are inadequate to provide for losses of water from the respiratory tract, skin, gastrointestinal tract, and kidneys. Therefore, an individual requires ingestion of free water to maintain water balance. The body possesses several homeostatic regulatory mechanisms capable of maintaining balance of water over a wide range of water

Table 35-1
Daily Water Balance in a 65-kg Man Calculated to Illustrate Minimal Required Drinking Water Intake

Water Intake		Water Loss	
Source	**Liters**	**Route**	**Liters**
Preformed water	0.85	Insensible—lungs	0.30
Metabolic water	0.37	Insensible—skin	0.40
Drinking—minimum	0.22	Feces	0.10
		Urine	0.64
Total	1.44	Total	1.44

intakes so that health remains unimpaired. An inequality between intake and loss of water ultimately alters the composition and osmolarity of body fluids.

LOSS OF WATER

Water is lost from the body by essentially four different routes: respiratory tract, skin, gastrointestinal tract, and kidneys. Of the four routes, water loss from kidneys is the most important because renal water excretion is regulated to maintain a constant osmolarity of the body fluids.

Insensible Water Loss

Water is lost continuously from the body by two routes: (1) passive evaporation from the upper respiratory tract during respiration and (2) passive evaporation from the skin. These passive evaporative losses from the respiratory tract and skin are termed "insensible losses" or "insensible perspiration" because they occur continuously and without our awareness. Insensible water loss from the skin, which occurs independent of sweating, averages between 0.3 and 0.5 L daily for an individual living in a temperate environment and doing minimal physical activity (Geigy Scientific Tables, 1981).

Evaporative water loss from the respiratory tract occurs during respiration because expired air is saturated with moisture to a vapor pressure of about 47 mm Hg, whereas the vapor pressure of inspired air is usually less than 47 mm Hg. An individual loses an average of between 0.14 and 0.47 L daily by this route; the amount of the loss depends on body size, the degree of physical activity, and environmental temperature and humidity. It is to be expected that evaporative water loss from the lungs is increased when the atmospheric vapor pressure decreases (i.e., in cold, dry climates).

On average, an individual will lose a total of 0.4 to 0.9 L of water daily from insensible loss through both the respiratory tract and skin. However, when body temperature rises to higher than 39°C, evaporative loss from the respiratory tract increases due to a significant increase in the respiratory minute volume (Reithner, 1981). Although the increase in water loss by this route can be by as much as 0.1 L daily, the dermal loss due to sweating at high body temperatures is of greater importance in increasing water loss. Cutaneous water loss due mainly to sweating was found to be increased up to 6 to 8 times the basal level when rectal temperature was above 39.5°C (Lamke et al., 1980). Therefore, water intake needs to be substantially increased in individuals with fever.

Water loss occurring through sweating is important in hyperthermia during which excess body heat is dissipated from the skin. The volume of water lost as sweat is highly variable, depending on the environment and the physical activity of the individual. Evaporation of sweat from the skin is an effective means of removing excess heat from the body. For every gram of water that evaporates from the skin, 0.58 kcal of heat is lost from the body. Water loss as sweat is substantially less in an environment of moderate temperature and humidity than in a warm, humid environment where loss through perspiration can be considerable.

Normally, the volume of sweat in a 65-kg adult doing light work at an ambient temperature of 29°C (84.2°F) amounts to about 2 to 3 L daily, but it can increase to a maximum of about 2 to 4 L per hour for a short time in an

Clinical Correlation

Heat Acclimatization

Humans have relatively efficient heat dissipation mechanisms, but the thermoregulatory mechanism may be overwhelmed in a number of conditions, resulting in the development of hyperthermia. The risk of hyperthermia occurs when individuals move from a cool temperate climate to a tropical climate and perform physical exertion, or when athletes perform in tropical conditions without prior conditioning to the hot, and particularly hot and humid, ambient conditions. The inability to adequately dissipate body heat leads to a steady rise in body core temperature with the consequence of heat-related illness, which ranges from heat cramps to heat stroke. Prompt transfer to a cooler environment with adequate ventilation to accelerate body heat dissipation, adequate fluid replacement, and cessation of physical activity are essential for treatment of an individual with heat-related illness.

Adaptation to heat, or heat acclimatization, will improve the individuals' thermoregulatory responses to heat stress. This adaptation process is obtained several days after exposure and is usually fully achieved after 14 days, although it has been found that, in well-trained athletes, the heat induced impairment of physiological responses and performances are still evident after 14 days (Voltaire et al., 2002). During acclimatization, a number of physiological adaptations to improve the individual's thermoregulatory ability occur. Typical physiological changes include heightened sweating response, reduced sodium concentration in the sweat, expanded plasma volume, and greater stability in cardiovascular function during exercise in the heat. Not only is sweating more profuse, it begins sooner and at a lower body temperature to improve dissipation of body heat. In addition, after adaptation, the greatly reduced sodium concentration in the sweat due to increased secretion of the adrenal mineralocorticoid hormone aldosterone is important, as it helps to conserve body sodium by minimizing sodium loss from the body. The resulting higher plasma osmolarity at a given sweat output will improve the thermoregulatory responses to heat stress (Takamata et al., 2001).

Heat stress, especially in competitive athletes, causes a spectrum of symptoms ranging from heat cramps to heat stroke (Squire, 1990). Heat cramps are an acute disorder of skeletal muscle characterized by brief, intermittent, and excruciating muscle cramps. Heat cramps often occur in people who are acclimatized to perform in hot climates and who consume a large amount of water to replace water losses without accompanying salt replacement. Although acclimatization is associated with diminished sodium concentration in the sweat, the loss of sodium in sweat can be considerable as the rate of sweat secretion increases. This condition can be prevented by adequate salt intake together with water replacement.

Continued

unacclimatized individual who is performing heavy physical activity in a hot, humid environment. This levels off to about 0.5 L per hour over a 24-hour period as the duration of perspiration increases (Geigy Scientific Tables, 1981). Even at maximal sweating, the rate of heat loss may not be rapid enough to dissipate the heat from the body. When the body temperature rises to a critical level, higher than 40.5°C (105°F), the individual is likely to develop heatstroke. However, after acclimatization to hot weather for a few weeks, an individual will have greater tolerance of the hot, humid environment, with as much as a doubling of the sweat rate capacity. Evaporation of this large volume of sweat effectively removes the excess heat from the body. Acclimatization also involves a decrease in the concentration of sodium chloride in the sweat, allowing for better conservation of sodium chloride (Takamata et al., 2001). The loss of several liters of sweat a day in a hot climate results in serious losses of both sodium chloride and water, which need to be replaced.

Clinical Correlation

Heat Acclimatization—cont'd

Heat exhaustion is caused by profuse sweating in a hot environment when the volume of water lost is not replaced by voluntary drinking and the plasma volume becomes depleted. There is dilation of blood vessels in the skin in an attempt to dissipate body heat. The resultant decrease in peripheral resistance together with depletion of plasma volume causes weakness and fainting. Body temperature in this individual is only moderately raised. The weakness and fainting is a safety mechanism, which, by the cessation of physical exertion in a hot and humid environment, prevents further rise in body temperature, thereby ensuring that the heat-loss mechanism is not overextended. Treatment by external cooling and adequate hydration should be instituted in heat exhaustion. Prolonged untreated heat exhaustion can lead to heat stroke in which body temperature increases steadily due to a complete breakdown in the heat-regulating system. When this happens, the individual fails to sweat even in the face of a rapidly rising body temperature. When the elevated body temperature reaches a critical level, collapse, delirium, seizures, or coma occurs.

Thinking Critically

Exercise in the heat places the athlete at risk for heat illness. Children are at even greater risk for heat illness because their thermoregulatory mechanism is less efficient. Therefore, it is important for the sports medicine team to be familiar with preventing and treating heat-related illness, especially in children and adolescents.

1. How does one prevent heat illness in athletes?
2. How does one treat heat illness when it occurs during sports competition?

Water Loss by the Gastrointestinal Tract

The volume of water loss in feces is small, about 0.1 L a day, and does not cause problems with water balance unless excessive loss occurs during diarrhea. The volume of fluid ingested varies among individuals but averages about 1.7 L daily. Added to this ingested volume, the small intestine receives an additional 7 L of secretory fluids, which are made up of salivary, gastric, biliary, pancreatic, and intestinal secretions. Normally, approximately 90% to 95% of these fluids is absorbed by the small intestine, and the remainder by the colon, leaving only approximately 0.1 L of water to be excreted in the feces. Absorption of water in the intestine is passive, along an osmotic gradient created by the absorption of nutrients from the lumen of the intestine into the plasma. In diseases of the gastrointestinal tract, large volumes of water can be lost in the feces, causing diarrhea. This occurs in gastroenteritis due to bacterial or viral infection or in any situation in which absorption of nutrients is compromised. Certain bacterial toxins, such as cholera toxin, can increase the secretion of sodium chloride from the crypt cells of the small intestinal mucosa into the lumen of the small intestine. The lumen becomes hyperosmotic, and diffusion of water occurs from the plasma into the lumen, causing diarrhea. Several liters of fluid, up to 10 to 20 L, can be lost, resulting in dehydration (Kutchai, 2004).

Water Loss by the Kidneys

As shown in Table 35-1, for a 65-kg reference man the minimal urine volume that an adult must produce, assuming a normal renal function, is approximately 0.64 L a day. Metabolism of 70 g dietary protein results in the production of about 21 g of urea, which cannot be utilized by the body and has to be excreted in the urine. This 21 g of urea contributes 350 mosmoles to the total osmotic load of substances presented to the kidneys. Added to this osmotic load is an additional 420 mosmoles from phosphates, sulfates, other waste products, and ions (especially sodium chloride and potassium salts). Therefore, the total load of osmotically active substances requiring excretion by the kidneys is approximately 770 mosmoles a day.

Because the human kidneys can maximally concentrate urine to an osmolar concentration of 1,200 mOsm/L, the minimal volume of urine at maximal attainable osmolarity for this individual is 0.64 L a day. This volume of urine is known as the obligatory water loss.

INTAKE OF WATER

The minimal amount of water required daily to replace obligatory water losses from the respiratory tract, skin, feces, and urine is about 1.44 L. Water consumed by an individual comes from beverages, preformed water in food, and water produced by oxidation of food. If the composition of the ingested food is known, the yield of metabolic water can be calculated. Oxidation of 1 g each of carbohydrate, fat, and protein will yield approximately 0.6 g, 1.0 g, and 0.4 g of water, respectively. Assuming that the 65-kg man used as an example in Table 35-1 consumes 400 g of carbohydrate, 100 g of fat, and 70 g of protein, the total yield of metabolic water from the food eaten amounts to 370 g. Preformed water in food can be calculated from the difference between wet and dry weights of food; however, usually it is assumed that water makes up 60% of the wet weight. Therefore, the weight of preformed water in the sample diet is about 850 g, and the total volume of water (preformed plus metabolic) derived from ingested food is about 1.22 L a day (1.22 kg/day). To remain in water balance, the individual has to drink a minimum of 0.22 L of additional water. The ingested volume of water and other beverages varies greatly among individuals depending on habit, custom, physical activity, and environment. On average, humans habitually drink between 1 and 2 L or more of water and beverages a day. The excess water is excreted by the kidneys.

A reasonable allowance for water intake based on recommended energy intake is 1 mL/kcal for adults and 1.5 mL/kcal for infants (National Research Council, 1989), or 35 mL/kg body weight in adults and 150 mL/kg in infants. Infants require more water on a body weight basis because of their relatively larger body surface area and metabolic rate, resulting in higher obligatory losses, and the relatively limited capacity of their kidneys to handle the renal solute load. This is especially important for infants on formula, as most formula has a higher solute load than does human milk. Water loss can be increased greatly in individuals doing heavy work; in athletes undergoing severe training in a hot climate; and in individuals with fever, vomiting, diabetes, or diarrhea. Under these circumstances, water need is increased.

RENAL EXCRETION OF WATER

As discussed in Chapter 34, the kidneys contribute significantly to homeostasis by stabilizing the volume and osmolarity of the body fluids. In their regulatory function, the kidneys process blood by removing substances that are in excess and conserving substances that are in deficit as these substances pass through the kidneys. In water excess, caused by drinking large volumes of fluid, a large volume of dilute urine (hypo-osmotic with respect to plasma) is excreted. Conversely, in water deficit, when there is a need to conserve body water, a smaller volume of concentrated (hyperosmotic) urine is excreted. Excretion of dilute urine involves the reabsorption of filtered solutes in excess of water, whereas the excretion of concentrated urine entails the reabsorption of water in excess of solutes (Knepper and Gamba, 2004).

To understand how the kidneys produce either dilute or concentrated urine, the following have to be considered:

- The transport and permeability properties of the various segments of the nephron
- The countercurrent multiplier system that generates a hyperosmolar medullary interstitium
- The countercurrent exchanger system of the vasa recta
- The change of the collecting tubules from a diuretic to an antidiuretic state under the influence of an antidiuretic hormone

TRANSPORT AND PERMEABILITY CHARACTERISTICS OF VARIOUS SEGMENTS OF THE NEPHRON

There are approximately 1 million nephrons in each kidney. Each nephron consists of an initial filtering component, called the renal corpuscle, and a tubular component that extends out from the renal corpuscle and is responsible for transporting solutes and water. The renal corpuscle is made up of the glomerular capillaries, which protrude into a fluid-filled capsule, the Bowman's capsule. Plasma is filtered across the glomerular membrane into the Bowman's capsule of the nephron. The ultrafiltrate formed is protein-free, and its ionic composition is similar to that of plasma except for the 5% difference due to the Gibbs-Donnan effect. As the filtrate flows along the nephrons, its volume and composition are altered so that normally only 1 % of the filtered load is excreted as urine, the composition of which differs markedly from that of the initial filtrate. The proximal tubules reabsorb 65% of the filtrate, and the loops of Henle reabsorb another 25%. The final reabsorption of solutes (especially sodium chloride and urea) and water in the distal nephron (distal convoluted and collecting tubules) is highly variable; it depends on the needs of the body and is under the influence of hormones (Knepper and Gamba, 2004). The alterations in the composition and volume of the filtrate are made possible by (1) the permeability characteristics of the various nephron segments and (2) the various transport processes that occur across the tubular cells of the nephrons. As discussed in subsequent text of this chapter, solutes are transported across tubular cells, resulting in the establishment of a concentration gradient in the medullary region of the kidneys. The establishment of a concentration gradient allows the kidneys to excrete concentrated urine.

Proximal Tubule

In the proximal tubule, active reabsorption of sodium ions results in cotransport of other solutes, the passive reabsorption of chloride ions, or the secretion of hydrogen ions. Active sodium reabsorption is dependent on Na^+,K^+-ATPase, the Na^+ pump. Water is reabsorbed passively along the osmotic gradient created. The rates of reabsorption of solutes and water are equal in the proximal tubule so that the osmolarity of the tubular fluid leaving the proximal tubule is similar to that of plasma, at 290 mOsm/L. This iso-osmotic reabsorption applies regardless of whether dilute or concentrated urine is produced. Therefore, segments distal to the proximal tubule must be responsible for the production of either concentrated or dilute urine.

Distal Tubule

The final production of concentrated or dilute urine is attributed to the water permeability of the latter part of the distal convoluted tubules and the cortical and medullary collecting tubules of the kidneys. This process is under the control of arginine vasopressin (AVP), a peptide hormone that is also known as antidiuretic hormone (ADH) and which is secreted by the posterior pituitary. In water deprivation, secretion of AVP is increased so that the collecting tubules are permeable to water; water diffuses out of the tubular lumen into the hyperosmotic interstitium resulting in the excretion of concentrated urine. This process is important for water conservation in conditions of water deprivation. In the absence of AVP, the water permeability of the collecting tubules is low; water remains in the tubular lumen resulting in the excretion of a large volume of dilute urine. This is termed water diuresis.

The establishment of an osmotic gradient from iso-osmotic in the corticomedullary region to hyperosmotic in inner medullary region is made possible by the anatomical arrangements and the functional characteristics of the various segments of the distal tubules. Anatomically, mammalian kidneys are characterized by having varying lengths of loops of Henle, which penetrate the medullary region to varying depths, the loops of Henle acting as a countercurrent multiplier system and the medullary blood vessels (i.e., the vasa recta) acting as a countercurrent diffusion system. This arrangement, together with the different transport and permeability characteristics of the various segments of the distal tubules to sodium chloride, urea, and water, enable the kidney to establish an osmotic gradient in the medulla with the highest osmolarity found in the inner medullary region near the papillary tip of the kidneys.

The transport of sodium chloride, urea, and water differs in different segments.

The descending and ascending thin limbs are relatively permeable to sodium chloride, and urea, thereby permitting these solutes to diffuse passively along their concentration gradient between the tubular and interstitial fluids. The thick ascending limb and the distal convoluted and collecting tubules can actively transport sodium chloride out of the tubular fluid. The ascending thick limb, distal convoluted tubules, and cortical and outer medullary collecting tubules are relatively impermeable to urea. Conversely, the inner medullary collecting tubule is very permeable to urea. The high urea permeability in the inner medullary collecting tubule is due to the presence of specialized urea transporters present in the apical and basolateral plasma membranes (Knepper and Star, 1990). In the presence of AVP, the permeability to urea rises to a very high level; this response is mediated by the intracellular production of cyclic AMP, which activates the apical urea transporter.

The descending thin limb is highly permeable to water, whereas the ascending thin limb, ascending thick limb, and first part of the distal convoluted tubules are relatively impermeable to water. The latter part of the distal convoluted tubule and the cortical and medullary collecting tubules are impermeable to water in the absence of AVP, but their permeability to water is increased in the presence of AVP.

COUNTERCURRENT MULTIPLIER SYSTEM OF THE LOOP OF HENLE

In mammals, the loops of Henle extend from the cortex for varying distances down into the medullary region. Each loop of Henle consists of two parallel limbs of small diameter, with the tubular fluid flowing in opposite directions (countercurrent flow) and in close proximity. The hairpin conformation of the loop of Henle is such that fluid flows from the corticomedullary region to the medullary region in the descending thin limb and in the opposite direction in the ascending thin and thick limbs. Because of the flow and permeability characteristics of these segments, the loops of Henle operate as a countercurrent multiplier system and establish and maintain an osmotic gradient between the fluids in the corticomedullary region and the inner medullary region (Knepper and Gamba, 2004). This osmotic gradient is made up of concentration gradients of mainly sodium chloride and urea and is essential for formation of concentrated urine in the collecting ducts. As illustrated in Figure 35-5, the osmolarity of the interstitial fluid increases steadily from 290 mOsm/L in the corticomedullary region to about 1,200 mOsm/L in the inner medullary region.

Active transport of sodium chloride out of the ascending thick limb of the loop of Henle is fundamental to the development of the osmotic gradient between the cortex and inner medulla. The highest levels of Na^+,K^+-ATPase are found in the thick ascending limbs, consistent with their role in powering countercurrent multiplication in the outer medulla. However, the passive movement of urea down its concentration gradient from the tubular fluid into the interstitium also plays an important role, especially when the kidney is maximally concentrating urine. The mechanisms that contribute to the buildup of solutes, especially sodium chloride and urea in the medullary region, are as follows.

The ascending thick limb actively transports sodium chloride from the tubular fluid to the interstitium. Because the ascending thin and thick limbs are impermeable to water, active movement of sodium chloride into the interstitium dilutes the fluid in the lumen and produces a hypo-osmotic tubular fluid but a hyperosmotic interstitial fluid. The early distal convoluted and collecting tubules contribute further to the kidney's diluting ability by reabsorbing more sodium chloride. In water diuresis, when circulating AVP levels are low, the hypo-osmolarity is maintained and dilute urine is excreted.

In antidiuresis, under the influence of AVP, water is removed from the late distal convoluted and the cortical and outer medullary portions of the collecting tubules, and, in the process, urea is concentrated in the tubular fluid. Because the inner medullary portion of the collecting tubule is permeable to urea and the permeability increases in the presence of AVP, urea moves from concentrated tubular

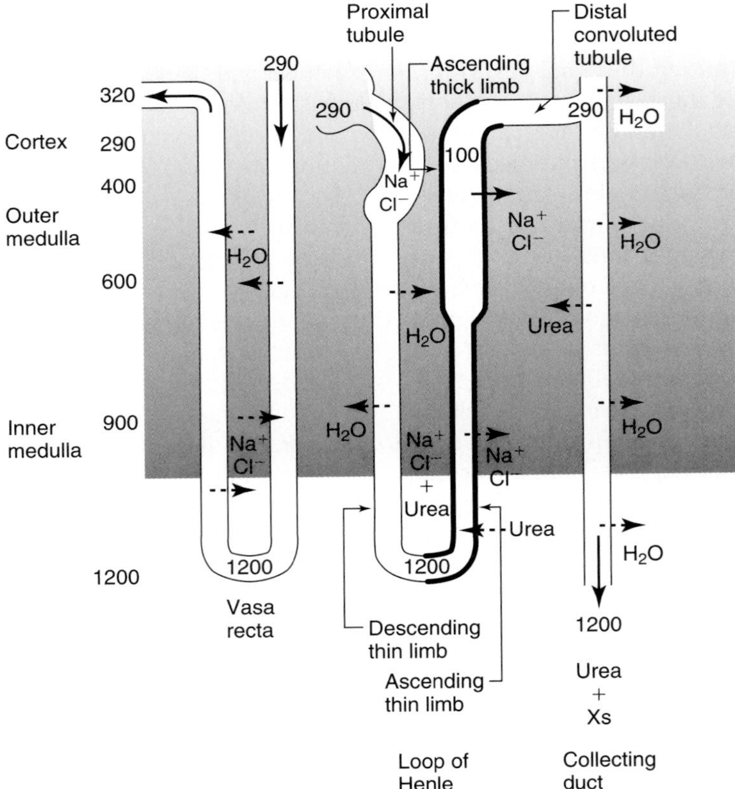

Figure 35-5 Establishment of an osmotic gradient in the medullary region of the kidney by the countercurrent multiplier system of the loop of Henle. Each human kidney contains approximately 1 million nephrons. The structures of only a single nephron with a long loop of Henle that penetrates into the inner medulla and of a single blood capillary are shown. Transport of NaCl out of the tubular fluid in the ascending limb and diffusion of water out of the tubular fluid in the descending limb create a small osmotic gradient that is multiplied by the counterflow of the tubular fluid. Tubular fluid is very dilute (hypo-osmotic) by the time it reaches the distal convoluted tubule. In the presence of arginine vasopressin (AVP), the late distal convoluted tubule and the collecting tubule are permeable to water. The tubular fluid equilibrates with the hypertonic interstitium, and concentrated urine is formed as shown. In the absence of AVP, the tubular fluid in the collecting tubule remains hypo-osmotic, and dilute urine is formed (see text for explanation). (*Xs*, Solutes other than urea.)

fluid down its concentration gradient into the interstitium, thereby increasing the osmolarity in the inner medullary region to a high level. Some of the urea in the interstitium diffuses passively into the lumen of both the descending and ascending thin limbs along its concentration gradient. Because the descending thin limb is very permeable to water but less so to sodium chloride and urea, water moves out of the tubule so that the osmolarity of the fluid flowing into this segment equilibrates with the surrounding hyperosmotic interstitial fluid. The fluid that enters the ascending limb has a higher concentration of sodium chloride because of the removal of water from the descending thin limb. Sodium chloride then moves passively from the tubular fluid in the ascending thin limb down its concentration gradient into the interstitium and adds further to the hyperosmolarity of the inner medullary region. There is more passive efflux of sodium chloride than passive influx of urea because the ascending thin limb is more permeable to sodium than urea, so there is a net efflux of osmotically active solutes. Because of low water permeability, luminal fluid in the ascending limb is hypo-osmotic relative to its surrounding interstitium. Therefore, both passive and active transport of sodium chloride out of the tubular fluid of the ascending limbs results in the formation of tubular fluid that is hypo-osmotic, with reference to plasma, when it enters the distal convoluted tubule. The establishment of this small osmotic gradient between the tubular fluid in the ascending and descending thin limbs of the loop of Henle with each pass of fluid can be multiplied by the continuous counterflow of fluid. Consequently, an osmotic gradient between the interstitial fluids in the corticomedullary region and the inner medullary region can be established and maintained.

The collecting tubules run parallel and in close vicinity to the loops of Henle through the area of high osmolarity to drain into the ureter (see Fig. 35-5). The fluid entering the collecting tubules is hypo-osmotic. In the absence of AVP, the collecting tubules are relatively impermeable to water and the tubular fluid remains hypo-osmotic; dilute urine is excreted. Under the influence of AVP, the collecting tubules are permeable to water, the tubular fluid in the collecting tubules equilibrates with the hyperosmotic interstitial fluid and concentrated urine is excreted. Therefore, the countercurrent multiplier of the loop of Henle provides the mechanism for excretion of either dilute or concentrated urine. The high osmolarity of the interstitial fluid provides the driving force for the absorption of water from the descending thin limb of the loop of Henle and from the outer, and finally, the inner medullary portions of the collecting tubule.

As discussed previously, urea contributes substantially to the establishment of the osmotic gradient in the renal medulla, and, hence, to the ability to form a concentrated urine. In the presence of AVP, the permeability of the inner medullary collecting tubules to water is increased. Further reabsorption of water by this segment results in an even higher concentration of urea to diffuse passively out of the tubule into the interstitium. The movement of urea and water out of the inner medullary collecting tubule maintains a high concentration of urea in the tubular fluid and the interstitium in this region. The contribution of urea to the osmotic gradient varies with the amount of urea filtered and, hence, with the dietary intake of protein. In antidiuresis, urea contributes about 600 mOsm/L to the osmolarity of the inner medullary region, with the majority of the remaining 600 mOsm/L contributed by sodium chloride.

The countercurrent multiplier system in the kidneys is an energy-efficient process. By its operation, a considerable osmotic gradient (~900 mOsm/L) is generated between the plasma (290 mOsm/L) and the tubular fluids in the inner medullary region (1,200 mOsm/L) during antidiuresis. The energy cost associated with the establishment of this large osmotic gradient of 900 mOsm/L represents only the energy expended in generating small osmotic gradients between adjacent segments of the descending and ascending limbs of the loops of Henle.

COUNTERCURRENT EXCHANGER OF THE VASA RECTA

It is essential that the osmotic gradient that is established by the countercurrent multiplier system in the medullary interstitium be maintained and not dissipated by the blood supply. This goal is achieved by the specialized anatomical arrangement of the medullary blood vessels, the vasa recta. The descending vasa recta receive blood from the efferent arterioles of the nephrons and supply blood to the capillary plexuses at each level of the medulla. Blood from the capillary plexuses drains into the ascending vasa recta (Plakke and Pfeiffer, 1964). As the ascending vasa recta pass from the inner medulla toward the cortical region, they come into proximity of the descending vasa recta at the outer medullary region. With this counterflow arrangement, the vasa recta permit a passive countercurrent exchange of solutes and water and provide a means of perfusion of the medullary area while maintaining the medullary interstitial osmotic gradient.

Because of the permeability of the capillary endothelium to both solutes and water, the osmolarity of the plasma in the vasa recta equilibrates with that of the medullary interstitial fluid at each level. The osmolarity of plasma in the descending vasa recta is 290 mOsm/L, which is similar to that of the systemic plasma. As the blood flows deeper into the medulla, it equilibrates with the surrounding hyperosmotic interstitial fluid by gaining solutes and losing water, so that by the time the plasma reaches the inner medullary region, its osmolar concentration is that of the surrounding interstitium (that is, 1,200 mOsm/L). The opposite process happens in the ascending vasa recta. As blood flows from a region of higher to lower osmolarity, it becomes less and less hyperosmotic by passive loss of solutes and passive uptake of water. As a result, the osmolarity of the plasma in the ascending vasa recta leaving the medulla is only slightly higher than that of systemic plasma. By this arrangement, the vasa recta remove the excess solutes and water that are added to the interstitial fluid by the various nephron segments in the medulla while at the same time preserving the osmotic gradient in the medullary interstitium.

EXCRETION OF DILUTE AND CONCENTRATED URINE

Human kidneys can dilute urine to one sixth the osmolarity of plasma or concentrate it up to four times that of plasma; that is, humans can excrete urine of osmolarity between 50 and 1,200 mOsm/L. Dilute urine is produced when the circulating level of plasma AVP is low. Under this condition the permeability to water in the more distal portion of the distal convoluted tubule and in the collecting tubule is low. As illustrated in Figure 35-5, tubular fluid leaving the ascending thick limb of the loop of Henle is hypo-osmotic, with an osmolarity of approximately 100 mOsm/L. In the production of this dilute fluid, the ascending thick limb of the loop of Henle plays an important role because of its large reabsorptive capacity. Because it is the major site of dilution of tubular fluid, the ascending thick limb is often referred to as the diluting segment of the kidney. Further reabsorption of solutes, especially sodium chloride, by the tubular cells of the distal nephron dilutes the tubular fluid to an osmolarity of 50 mOsm/L.

The production of concentrated urine occurs when the circulating AVP levels are high, the permeability to water is increased in the more distal portions of the distal convoluted tubules and collecting tubules, and the permeability to urea is increased in the inner medullary collecting tubule. As the collecting tubule passes from the corticomedullary to inner medullary region, the tubular fluid equilibrates with the hyperosmotic interstitial fluid and water is removed. Removal of water concentrates the urea in the collecting tubule. The high permeability of the inner medullary tubule to urea under the influence of AVP causes urea to move from the tubular fluid into the interstitium, thereby further increasing the osmolarity in the interstitium. In antidiuresis, concentrated urine of an osmolarity as high as 1,200 mOsm/L is excreted. Because a hyperosmotic medullary interstitium is essential for the concentration of urine, any process that reduces this hyperosmolarity will impair the ability of the kidneys to concentrate urine maximally.

CONCEPT OF FREE-WATER CLEARANCE

The fundamental process in the dilution and concentration of urine is the separation of solutes and water by both the ascending thin and thick limbs of the loop of Henle, which may be thought of as the generation of a volume of water that is free of solutes. When plasma osmolarity is low due to an excess of water in the body, the circulating level of AVP is low and the permeability of the collecting tubule to water is low, resulting in the excretion of solute-free water from the body. The clearance of this solute-free water by the kidney is called free-water clearance (C_{water}). Free-water clearance is sometimes calculated because it can provide a means to quantify the loss or gain of water from the kidneys by the excretion of dilute or concentrated urine; this will reflect the ability of the kidneys to maintain osmolarity of the body fluids (Rose and Post, 2001b).

Free-water clearance is calculated as the difference between the rate of urine flow and the rate of clearance of total solutes (in osmoles) from the plasma. The clearance of total solutes from the plasma by the kidneys is called osmolar clearance (C_{osm}) and can be defined as the volume of water necessary for the excretion of the osmotic load in the urine so that urine is iso-osmotic with plasma. The osmolar clearance, C_{osm}, can be calculated and has the unit of volume/unit time, or liters/day (L/day):

$$C_{osm} = (U_{osm} \times V)/P_{osm}$$

where U_{osm} is the osmolarity of urine (mOsm/L), V is the rate of urine flow (L/day), and P_{osm} is plasma osmolarity (mOsm/L):

$$C_{water} = V - C_{osm}$$

Therefore, when the rate of urine flow is greater than C_{osm} (i.e., when C_{water} is positive) relatively more water than solute is excreted in the urine; dilute or hypo-osmotic urine is excreted. Conversely, when the rate of urine flow is smaller than C_{osm} (i.e., when C_{water} is negative) relatively more solute is excreted in the urine, and urine is hyperosmotic.

The minimal urine volume (excretion of hyperosmotic urine) possible for a reference adult was calculated for Table 35-1 and was based on excretion in the urine of about 770 mosmoles of solutes per day. Excretion of the solute load can be accomplished by producing urine that is either iso-osmotic ($U_{osm}/P_{osm} = 1$), hyperosmotic ($U_{osm}/P_{osm} > 1$), or hypo-osmotic ($U_{osm}/P_{osm} < 1$) with respect to plasma. In the example used in Table 35-1, the urinary flow rate of the individual was 0.64 L/day and the osmolarity was 1,200 mOsm/L. C_{osm} can be calculated as follows:

$$C_{osm} = (1{,}200 \text{ mOsm/L} \times 0.64 \text{ L/day})/290 \text{ mOsm/L} = 2.6 \text{ L/day}$$

Because the urinary flow rate (0.64 L/day) is less than C_{osm} (2.6 L/day), a negative C_{water} is obtained. This negative C_{water} expresses the renal conservation of water in which solute-free water is reabsorbed by the kidneys and a concentrated urine is excreted. To excrete an iso-osmotic urine, the 770 mosmoles of solutes would need to be excreted in 2.6 L/day of urine, or about four times the minimum obligatory urine volume. In this case of iso-osmotic urine excretion, C_{osm} equals urinary flow rate, C_{water} is equal to zero, and no excretion of solute-free water occurs. The production of a dilute urine requires a flow rate of more than 2.6 L/day; in this case, solute-free water is excreted by the kidneys and C_{water} is positive.

The determination of C_{water} provides important information on the functions of the segments of the nephron involved in the production of dilute and concentrated urine. In the absence of AVP, the renal tubular structures (ascending thin and thick limbs of the loop of Henle, the distal convoluted tubule, and the collecting tubule) are involved in the dilution of luminal fluid by separating solutes from water in the lumen; quantitatively, the ascending thick limb is the most important in reabsorbing solutes. For the kidneys to excrete a maximal volume of solute-free water, AVP must be absent so that water reabsorption by the collecting tubules does not occur. Conversely, for the kidneys to excrete concentrated urine, solute-free water is reabsorbed by the collecting tubules, and this occurs only in the presence of AVP secretion.

REGULATION OF WATER BALANCE

Disturbances of water balance lead to a change in plasma osmolarity, whereas disturbances of sodium balance result in a change in the volumes of body fluids. For an individual to maintain a constant osmolarity of the body fluids at 290 mOsm/L, the ratio of sodium chloride to total body water has to be regulated within narrow limits. Water excess or water deficit will invariably affect the ratio of sodium chloride to water, thereby changing the plasma osmolarity. To maintain water balance, physiological feedback mechanisms are present to modify either water loss or water intake to bring plasma osmolarity back toward normal (Thompson et al., 1986). Feedback mechanisms that are sensitive to changes in blood volume and blood pressure are also present and these mechanisms affect thirst and renal excretion of water (Robertson, 1983) (Fig. 35-6).

RENAL EXCRETION OF WATER

Water excess results in the excretion of dilute urine, whereas water deficit results in the excretion of concentrated urine. This ability to excrete either concentrated or dilute urine depends on the circulating level of plasma AVP. In antidiuresis, when there is a need to conserve water, the circulating level of AVP is high. AVP increases the permeability to water

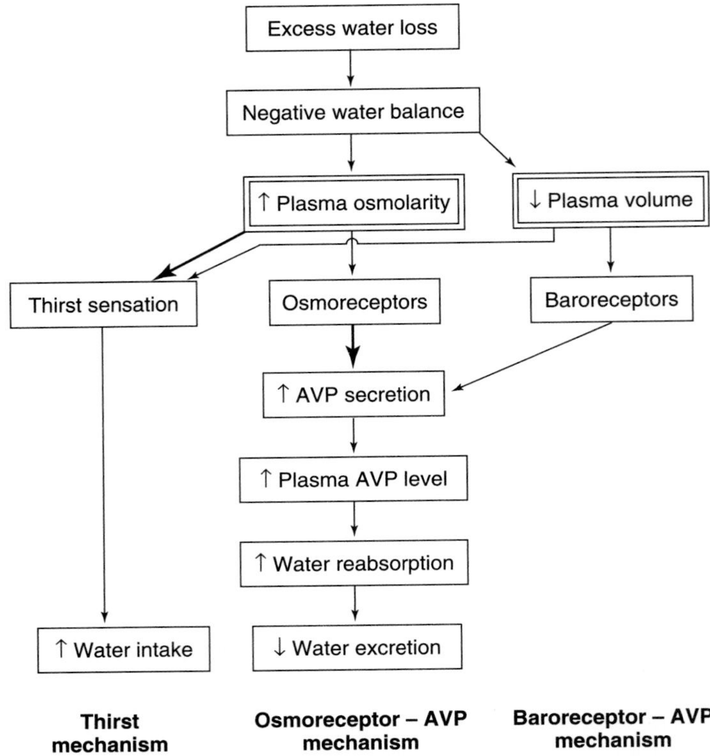

Figure 35-6 Integration of the osmoreceptor–AVP, baroreceptor–AVP, and thirst mechanisms in the regulation of water balance in water deficit.

in the collecting tubule, resulting in the reabsorption of water and excretion of concentrated urine. In water diuresis, the circulating level of AVP is low and the collecting tubule is impermeable is water, resulting in the excretion of large volumes of solute-free water.

Effects of AVP in the Kidney

Reabsorption of water across tubular epithelium can occur only if the epithelium is permeable to water. Water permeability depends largely on the presence of transporter proteins, called aquaporins, which function as water channels. To date, at least seven aquaporins (AQPs) have been shown to be expressed in different locations in the kidney tubules, but AQP-2 is the predominant AVP-regulated water channel. AQP-2 is present in abundance in the apical plasma membrane and in intracellular vesicles in the collecting tubular cells and is the chief target of AVP (Nielsen et al., 2002). Some AQP-2 water channels are also found in the basolateral plasma membrane of the inner medullary collecting tubular cells. When AVP binds to receptors located on the basolateral membrane of the tubular cell, adenylate cyclase is activated and the intracellular level of cyclic AMP increases. This activates the AQP-2 water channels to "shuttle" from intracellular vesicles to the apical plasma membrane, thereby providing areas of high water permeability in the membrane (Fig. 35-7). The time course for these reactions to occur is rapid, within 40 seconds. This process temporarily provides channels that allow free diffusion of water from the tubular fluid into the cells along an osmotic gradient. When AVP is removed, these AQP-2 water channels are reinternalized into the cell, and the luminal membrane becomes impermeable to water. The downregulation of AQP-2 in the apical membrane is rapid, occurring within minutes. Thus, the insertion and removal of membrane vesicles containing water channels provide a rapid mechanism for controlling the permeability of the luminal membrane to water.

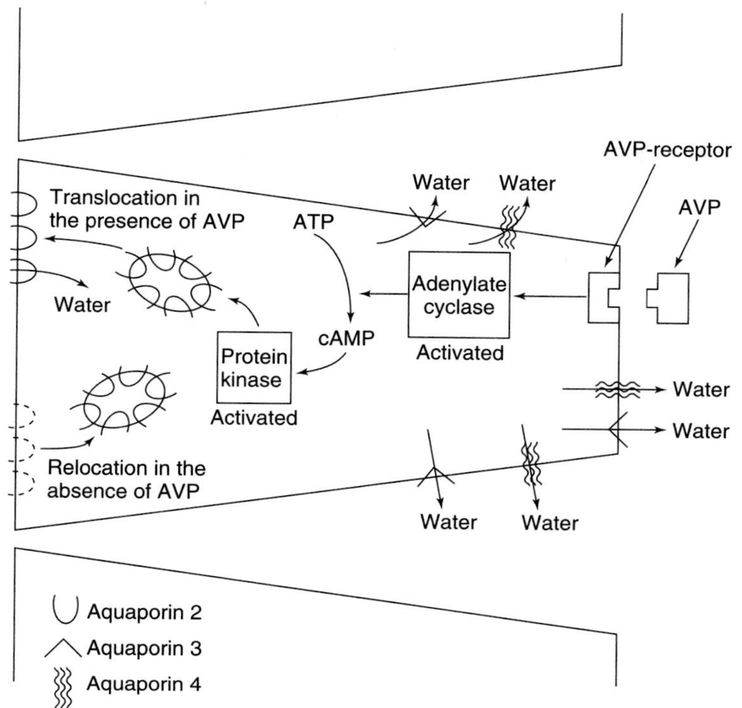

Figure 35-7 Proposed mechanism of some major events that result from the action of arginine vasopressin (AVP) on the collecting tubule to increase its water permeability.

Once water enters the cell, it exits across the highly permeable basolateral membrane to the interstitium. The water permeability of the basolateral membrane of the collecting tubule results from the presence of large numbers of AQP-3 water channels located mainly in the lateral membrane and to AQP-4 water channels located in both the basal and lateral membranes. AQP-3, but not AQP-4, water channels are affected by AVP. Therefore, when there is a need to conserve water, AVP is released to increase the permeability to water in the luminal brush border of the collecting tubule so that water moves from the tubular lumen into the collecting tubular cells and AQP-3 and AQP-4 act as exit channels for the water. By this route, water moves from the lumen of the collecting tubules to the hyperosmotic interstitium of the medullary region. The presence of AQP-2 in the inner medullary collecting tubule increases further the permeability to water in the inner medullary region resulting in the excretion of concentrated urine. In water excess, the collecting tubules are impermeable to water as a consequence of the absence of AVP, and a large volume of solute-free water is excreted.

Synthesis of AVP

Arginine vasopressin, is a small peptide, 9 amino acids in length. It is synthesized by the magnocellular neurons located within the supraoptic and paraventricular nuclei of the hypothalamus; synthesis in the supraoptic nuclei is more important quantitatively (Baylis and Thompson, 1988). The synthesized hormone is packaged as granules in vesicles in the neurons; transported in combination with a carrier protein, neurophysin, down the axons of these neurons; and stored as secretory granules in the nerve endings located in the posterior pituitary gland (neurohypophysis) until released. When the supraoptic and paraventricular nuclei are stimulated, nerve impulses are transmitted along the hypothalamic–hypophysial tract to the nerve endings at the neurohypophysis to release the secretory granules by exocytosis. After release, the neurophysin and AVP separate, and the AVP enters the circulation. Although AVP causes vessel constriction, its vasopressor effect is less potent than its antidiuretic effect.

Release of AVP

Secretion of AVP is influenced by many different stimuli, but the primary physiological factors are changes in plasma osmolarity and changes in effective circulating volume and pressure of the vascular system (Menninger, 1985) (see Fig. 35-6). In addition, secretion of AVP can be changed by other stimuli to the central nervous system as well as by various hormones and drugs. The most prominent stimulus is nausea. Stimulation of the chemoreceptor zone in the area postrema of the brainstem by nausea-producing agents such as morphine and nicotine increases AVP secretion (Verbalis et al., 1987). Secretion of AVP is also stimulated by angiotensin II (Keil et al., 1975) and inhibited by ethanol (Carney et al., 1995).

Osmoreceptor Control of AVP Secretion

The most potent stimulus that influences the secretion of AVP is a change in plasma osmolarity (see Fig. 35-6). Sodium chloride, the major contributor to osmotic pressure in the plasma, is the most potent solute in stimulating the secretion of AVP. When a hypertonic sodium chloride solution is injected into the artery supplying the hypothalamus, the neurons in the supraoptic and paraventricular nuclei immediately send nerve impulses to the nerve endings in the neurohypophysis to release AVP into the circulation. Conversely, injection of a hypotonic sodium chloride solution into the same artery inhibits the secretion of AVP (Zerbe and Robertson, 1983).

Normally, the plasma osmolarity is set at 290 mOsm/L. An increase in plasma osmolarity above this set point by as little as 0.5% is sufficient to stimulate AVP secretion (Thompson et al., 1986). A group of cells that acts as osmoreceptors and is sensitive to changes in osmolarity of the extracellular fluid is thought to be located in the vicinity of the magnocellular neurons that synthesize AVP. The most sensitive osmoreceptor cells are located in the organum vasculosum in the anteroventral wall of the third ventricle (Zimmerman et al., 1987). These osmoreceptors respond to changes in osmolarity of the extracellular fluid and send appropriate signals to the supraoptic and paraventricular nuclei of the hypothalamus that either increase or decrease the secretion of AVP from their nerve endings in the neurohypophysis. When the extracellular fluid bathing these osmoreceptor cells is hypertonic, water diffuses out of the cells along an osmotic gradient, which causes the cells to decrease in size. Transmission of nerve impulses to the neurohypophysis increases, and the secretion of AVP is stimulated. Conversely, a hypotonic extracellular fluid causes water to move into these cells, leading to a decrease in transmission of nerve signals to the neurohypophysis and the inhibition of secretion of AVP. Therefore, these cells act as osmometers; they respond to osmotically induced changes in their water content. Stimulatory potency of the solutes depends on the permeability of the osmoreceptor to the solutes involved. For example, the plasma membrane of these osmometer cells is not permeable to sodium, and an osmotic gradient can be set up when plasma concentration of sodium changes. In contrast, urea, which penetrates cell membranes easily, is a noneffective solute in causing a change in AVP secretion. Because the half-life of the released AVP is short, less than 20 minutes, the circulating levels of AVP can decrease or increase rapidly within minutes in response to changes in the osmolarity of the plasma.

Baroreceptor Control of AVP Secretion

A decrease in effective circulating volume or arterial pressure stimulates secretion of AVP from the neurohypophysis (see Fig. 35-6). However, the sensitivity of this system is less than that of the osmoreceptors; compared to sensitivity of AVP secretion to as little as a 0.5% change in plasma osmolarity, a decrease of about 5% to 10% in blood volume or blood pressure is required before AVP secretion is stimulated (Menninger, 1985).

The receptors or sensors activated by this response are located in the central venous portion of the circulation (right atrium and pulmonary vein) and in the arterial side (aortic arch and carotid sinus) of the vascular system. The low-pressure receptors in the venous side of the circulation respond to overall vascular volume, and the high-pressure receptors in the arterial side of the circulation respond to arterial pressure. Both groups of receptors are sensitive to stretch and are termed baroreceptors. In hypervolemia, excitation of the baroreceptors sends signals to the brainstem (solitary tract nucleus of the medulla oblongata), which is part of the center that regulates heart rate and blood pressure. Signals are then relayed from the brainstem to hypothalamus to inhibit AVP secretion. In hypovolemia, these baroreceptors are not stimulated, and the secretion of AVP is increased.

THIRST MECHANISM IN CONTROL OF WATER INTAKE

In addition to the increase in secretion of AVP during water deficit to minimize water loss by the kidneys, an increase in plasma osmolarity or a decrease in blood volume or arterial pressure also alters the desire for drinking water. Therefore, the subjective feeling of thirst, which leads to increase in fluid intake necessary to counterbalance fluid loss, helps maintain a relatively constant plasma osmolarity.

Thirst Center

The neural centers for thirst have not been defined completely. It appears that two areas are involved in the perception of thirst and thus regulation of water intake. Osmoreceptors for thirst similar to those that control osmotically stimulated AVP release are present in the area along the anteroventral wall of the third ventricle, and these receptors respond to changes in plasma osmolarity (Thrasher et al., 1982). Whether these osmoreceptors are the same cells that stimulate AVP release or distinct cells is not known. Another small area that promotes drinking is located anterolaterally in the preoptic nucleus (Zimmerman et al., 1987). Very little is known about the pathways involved in the response of thirst to decreased blood volume or arterial pressure, but it is believed that both the baroreceptor–AVP pathway and renin–angiotensin system are involved. Angiotensin II may stimulate thirst by a direct effect on the brain. The evidence comes primarily from studies in experimental animals. Therefore, the renin–angiotensin system may help regulate not only sodium balance but water balance as well, constituting one of the pathways by which thirst is stimulated when the extracellular volume is decreased.

Osmotic and Hypovolemic Stimulation of Thirst

Many stimuli alter the perception of thirst, but the most important ones are changes in plasma osmolarity and changes in effective circulating volume or blood pressure (Andersson, 1978). When plasma osmolarity is increased or when the blood volume or pressure is reduced, the individual perceives thirst. As for AVH secretion, the most potent of these stimuli is hypertonicity; an increase of only 2% to 3% above basal level in plasma osmolarity produces a strong desire to drink (Phillips et al., 1985). In contrast, the threshold for stimulating thirst by hypovolemia is significantly higher. A decrease of about 5% to 10% in blood volume or blood pressure is required before a similar thirst response is produced (Zimmerman et al., 1987; Thompson et al., 1986). Another factor that influences drinking is dryness of the mucosa of the mouth and esophagus.

A person finds relief from thirst by the act of drinking even before water is absorbed from the gastrointestinal tract to have an effect on the plasma osmolarity. Receptors in the pharynx, esophagus, and stomach probably are involved in this response (Thrasher et al., 1981). However, these mechanisms provide relief only temporarily. The increase in plasma osmolarity has to be corrected before the desire to drink is satisfied.

INTEGRATION OF OSMORECEPTOR–AVP, BARORECEPTOR–AVP, AND THIRST MECHANISMS

The osmoreceptor–AVP, baroreceptor–AVP, and thirst systems work in concert to regulate the osmolarity of body fluids and maintain water balance. Under normal physiological conditions, the plasma osmolarity is maintained within narrow limits by the very sensitive osmoregulatory system for AVP secretion to adjust the renal water excretion to small changes in osmolarity. In water deficit, plasma osmolarity increases and blood volume contracts. This stimulates the release of AVP to increase water reabsorption from the kidneys. However, the volume of water reabsorbed may be insufficient to correct fully for the water deficit. Stimulation of the thirst sensation to promote drinking leads to water intake, and the plasma osmolarity and blood volume are returned to normal. Conversely, when the plasma osmolarity is decreased and blood volume is increased in water excess, thirst sensation is suppressed, AVP is not secreted, and any unregulated water intake in excess of body need is excreted in the urine.

ABNORMAL STATES OF OSMOLARITIES AND VOLUMES

Disturbances of water balance consist of either depletion or excess of water and are manifested by alterations in the body fluid osmolarity. Because the major determinant of plasma osmolarity is sodium ions, these disorders alter the plasma concentration of sodium ions. To understand the disturbances in volume, osmolarity, and distribution of body fluids, the following two fundamental physiological facts must be kept in mind:

1. Fluid compartments are in osmotic equilibrium because water permeates the cell membrane and diffuses freely between the extracellular and intracellular fluid compartments.
2. When the extracellular fluid becomes hypertonic, water diffuses out of cells until the osmolarities of the extracellular and intracellular fluids are equal; the reverse is true when extracellular fluid becomes hypotonic.

Changes in the osmolarity of the extracellular compartment will invariably affect the volume of the intracellular compartment. Water deficit is usually associated with hypernatremia (high plasma sodium concentration) and water excess with hyponatremia (low plasma sodium concentration). Under normal circumstances, if the disturbances are not of renal origin, the kidneys compensate for the deficit or excess by appropriately adjusting urine volume and composition, thereby ensuring that the osmolarity of the body fluids is stabilized within narrow limits.

HYPONATREMIA IN POSITIVE WATER BALANCE

Ingestion of an excessive amount of water will dilute all the body fluid compartments; the volumes of both the intracellular and extracellular compartments increase and their osmolarities decrease (hyponatremia and hypervolemia). The excess water will distribute throughout the body in proportion to the initial volumes of the intracellular and extracellular compartments. Under normal circumstances, secretion of AVP is inhibited and the excess water excreted. However, in conditions in which the low plasma osmolarity fails to inhibit secretion of AVP (such as in severe low-output congestive heart failure [Uretsky et al., 1985]), cell expansion, hypervolemia, and hyponatremia occur. Acute water intoxication caused by too rapid parenteral fluid replacement will cause expansion of brain cells, leading to symptoms of headache, nausea, vomiting, muscle twitching, convulsion, and finally death.

HYPERNATREMIA IN NEGATIVE WATER BALANCE

In general, water is never lost without ions, nor ions without water, although the relative proportions of ions and water lost vary in different circumstances. When loss of water exceeds loss of ions, the osmolarity of the extracellular fluid increases. Water diffuses out of the cells until the osmolarities across the cell membrane are equal. The volumes of both compartments will decrease and their osmolarities will increase. Secretion of AVP is stimulated, the kidneys conserve water, and concentrated urine is excreted. Excessive sweating during heavy physical exertion in a hot and humid climate causes loss of both electrolytes and water, but water loss exceeds that of electrolytes, leading to hypernatremia and hypovolemia (Randall, 1976). Although the kidney will conserve both electrolytes and water during dehydration by excreting concentrated urine low in sodium, fluid loss ultimately has to be replaced by fluid intake.

Inadequate replacement of water loss leads to pronounced thirst, fatigue, decreased urine output, and fever.

ACCUMULATION OF EXCESS FLUID IN TISSUES: EDEMA

In edema, there is an accumulation of excess fluid in body tissues. Edema occurs when there is an imbalance of forces governing the diffusion of water across either the cell membrane or the capillary endothelium or when the permeability of these membranes is increased. The most common edema occurs in the interstitial fluid compartment, but intracellular edema may occur also.

Edema commonly involves expansion of the interstitial space. Edema formation may be a result of an increase in filtration of plasma into the interstitial space or a failure of the lymphatics to return the filtered fluid to the circulation. An increase in filtration of plasma can result from an imbalance in any of the factors that affect net movement of water across the capillary endothelium. Examples include an increase in permeability of the capillary endothelium that results from endothelial cell contraction elicited by chemical mediators of inflammation, such as histamine and bradykinin, and the decrease in plasma oncotic pressure that results from a decrease in plasma protein concentration in individuals with liver cirrhosis, kidney diseases, or protein malnutrition. An increase in filtration pressure due to venous congestion secondary to congestive heart failure is another common cause of edema (Mitchell and Cotran, 2003).

Intracellular edema can also occur when the permeability of the cell membrane to solutes is increased, when the concentration of a permeable solute in the plasma is increased, or in hyponatremia. Both the increase in membrane permeability and the increase in plasma concentration of a permeable solute cause an influx of solutes into the cells. Water diffuses passively along the osmotic gradient into the cells, and the cells expand. In tissue inflammation, permeability of the cell membrane increases, and this causes an influx of sodium and other ions and, subsequently, water into the cells. In hyponatremia, water enters the cells along the osmotic gradient, causing the cells to expand.

Clinical Correlation

Edema Formation

Edema is the accumulation of an excessively large amount of fluid in the interstitial space. The extent of edema depends on the pathological states that affect lymphatic drainage or one or more of the Starling's forces regulating the movement of fluid between the intravascular and interstitial compartments. Therefore, any condition that increases filtration rate across the capillary wall at a rate faster than the rate at which the lymphatics can drain will cause edema.

Edema can be localized or generalized. Localized edemas are restricted to a discrete vascular area or tissue, such as the swelling that accompanies injury or inflammation. Chemicals, such as histamine, are released locally in response to injury and they cause vasodilation and thus elevate capillary pressure and filtration. In addition, these chemicals increase permeability of capillary endothelial cells to proteins leading to the leakage of plasma proteins into the interstitial spaces in the injured tissues. This increases the oncotic pressure in the interstitial fluid, which then adds to the force for filtration, with the consequence of edema.

Generalized edema exists when an abnormally large amount of fluid accumulates in the interstitial spaces throughout the body. Some common causes of generalized edema are congestive heart failure, nephrotic syndrome, liver disease, and nutritional or "hunger" edema. In congestive heart

Continued

Clinical Correlation

Edema Formation—cont'd

failure, impaired cardiac emptying results in a rise in ventricular end-diastolic pressure with the consequence of elevated venous pressure and elevated capillary hydrostatic pressure, which in turn promote transudation of fluids out of the vascular channel into the interstitial spaces. The loss of fluid from the vascular tree diminishes the effective blood volume, and the kidneys respond by retaining salt and water in an effort to increase intravascular fluid volume. However, because the cardiac output remains low, this leads to a vicious cycle that is self-perpetuating unless treatment to increase cardiac output is instituted. Treatment consists of reducing sodium and fluid retention through use of diuretics, improving cardiac output with inotropic agents such as digitalis, and reducing vascular resistance through use of vasodilating drugs. Edema can occur in either the pulmonary or systemic capillary beds. The systemic edema due to congestive heart failure is usually most prominent in the lower extremities when the patient is standing or sitting, and the edema shifts to the sacral area when the patient is lying down. Because gravity influences the distribution of the edema, it is termed dependent edema.

A decrease in plasma oncotic pressure due to an abnormally low plasma protein concentration increases net capillary filtration pressure causing edema. Plasma protein concentration can be reduced when protein production is decreased in liver disease or when there is a loss of protein in urine. Although very little protein is lost in the urine of healthy individuals, large quantities of protein are filtered and excreted in the urine of patients with nephrotic syndrome because of the increase in glomerular capillary-wall permeability such as which occurs in membranous glomerulonephritis and focal segmental glomerulosclerosis. Nephrotic syndrome is characterized by massive proteinuria, hypoalbuminemia, generalized edema, hyperlipidemia, and lipiduria. The shift of fluid from the intravascular to extravascular compartment causes a compensatory increase in the secretion of aldosterone, which further aggravates the condition by reabsorption of filtered sodium from the renal tubules. Therefore, therapies consist of treatment of the underlying cause, sodium restriction, and judicious use of diuretics. Edema due to renal dysfunction tends to be massive and more equally distributed than is edema of cardiac origin. Generalized massive edema is termed anasarca. When finger pressure is applied to the edematous area, temporary displacement of fluid leaves a pitted depression, hence the term pitting edema.

Another cause of edema is impaired lymphatic drainage. In filariasis, a parasitic worm infestation of the lymphatic system, lymphatic flow is obstructed. Obstruction to lymphatic flow is also seen following radical surgery for breast cancer in which axillary lymph nodes are removed. This edema is usually located distal to the point of obstruction.

Thinking Critically

Children with kwashiorkor, a form of protein-energy malnutrition, often present with signs of inanition and edema. Kwashiorkor is usually characterized by a diet poor in protein and relatively more adequate in total energy.

1. Why does edema develop in these children?
2. Discuss the occurrence of edema with regard to the Starling forces that determine fluid movement in and out of the vascular and interstitial spaces.

REFERENCES

Andersson B (1978) Regulation of water intake. Physiol Rev 58:582-603.

Baylis PH, Thompson CJ (1988) Osmoregulation of vasopressin secretion and thirst in health and disease. Clin Endocrinol 29:549-576.

Carney SL, Gillies AH, Ray CD (1995) Acute effect of ethanol on renal electrolyte transport in the rat. Clin Exp Pharmacol Physiol 22:629-634.

Geigy Scientific Tables (1981) In: Lintner C (ed) Geigy Scientific Tables, 8th ed. Vol. 1. Ciba-Geigy Limited, Basel, Switzerland, p 108.

Keil LC, Summy-Long J, Severs WB (1975) Release of vasopressin by angiotensin II. Endocrinology 96:1063-1065.

Knepper MA, Gamba G (2004) Urine concentration and dilution. In: Brenner BM (ed) Brenner & Rector's The Kidney, 7th ed. Vol. 1. Saunders, Philadelphia, pp 599-636.

Knepper MA, Star RA (1990) The vasopressin-regulated urea transporter in renal inner medullary collecting duct. Am J Physiol 259:F393-F410.

Kutchai HC (2004) Digestion and absorption. In: Berne RM, Levy MN, Koeppen BM, Stanton BA (eds) Physiology, 5th ed. Mosby, St. Louis, pp 595-620.

Lamke LO, Nilsson G, Reithner L (1980) The influence of elevated body temperature on skin perspiration. Acta Chir Scand 146: 81-84.

Menninger RP (1985) Current concepts of volume receptor regulation of vasopressin release. Fed Proc 44:55-58.

Mitchell RN, Cotran RS (2003) Hemodynamic disorders, thrombosis, and shock. In: Kumar V, Cotran RS, Robbins SL (eds) Robbins Basic Pathology,7th ed. WB Saunders, Philadelphia, pp 79-102.

National Research Council (1989) Recommended Dietary Allowances, 10th ed. National Academy Press, Washington, DC.

Nielsen S, Frøkaer J, Marples D, Kwon T-H, Agre P, Knepper MA (2002) Aquaporins in the kidney: from molecules to medicine. Physiol Rev 82:205-244.

Phillips PA, Rolls BJ, Ledingham JG, Forsling ML, Morton JJ (1985) Osmotic thirst and vasopressin release in humans: a double-blind crossover study. Am J Physiol 248: R645-R650.

Plakke RK, Pfeiffer EW (1964) Blood vessels of the mammalian renal medulla. Science 146:1683-1685.

Randall HT (1976) Fluid, electrolyte, and acid-balance. Surg Clin North Am 56: 1019-1058.

Reithner L (1981) Insensible water loss from the respiratory tract in patients with fever. Acta Chir Scand 147:163-167.

Robertson GL (1983) Thirst and vasopressin function in normal and disordered states of water balance. J Lab Clin Med 101:351-371.

Rose BD, Post TW (2001a) The total body water and the plasma sodium concentration. In: Clinical Physiology of Acid-Base and Electrolyte Disorders, 5th ed. McGraw-Hill, New York, pp 241-257.

Rose BD, Post TW (2001b) Regulation of plasma osmolality. In: Clinical Physiology of Acid-Base and Electrolyte Disorders, 5th ed. McGraw-Hill, New York, pp 285-298.

Squire DL (1990) Heat illness. Fluid and electrolyte issues for pediatric and adolescent athletes. Pediatr Clin North Am 37:1085-1109.

Takamata A, Yoshida T, Nishida N, Morimoto T (2001) Relationship of osmotic inhibition in thermoregulatory responses and sweat sodium concentration in humans. Am J Physiol Regul Integr Comp Physiol. 280:R623-R629.

Taylor AE (1981) Capillary fluid filtration; Starling forces and lymph flow. Circ Res 49:557-575.

Thompson CJ, Bland J, Burd J, Baylis PH (1986) The osmotic thresholds for thirst and vasopressin release are similar in healthy man. Clin Sci 71:651-656.

Thrasher TN, Keil LC, Ramsay DJ (1982) Lesions of the organum vasculosum of the lamina terminalis (OVLT) attenuate osmotically-induced drinking and vasopressin secretion in the dog. Endocrinology 110:1837-1839.

Thrasher TN, Nistal-Herrera JF, Keil LC, Ramsay DJ (1981) Satiety and inhibition of vasopressin secretion after drinking in dehydrated dogs. Am J Physiol 240:E394-E401.

Uretsky BF, Verbalis JG, Generalovich T, Valdes A, Reddy PS (1985) Plasma vasopressin response to osmotic and hemodynamic stimuli in heart failure. Am J Physiol 248:H395-H402.

Verbalis JG, Richardson DW, Stricker EM (1987) Vasopressin release in response to nausea-producing agents and cholecystokinin in monkeys. Am J Physiol 252:R1138-1142.

Voltaire B, Galy O, Coste O, Recinais S, Callis A, Blonc S, Hertogh C, Hue O (2002) Effect of fourteen days of acclimatization on athletic performance in tropical climate. Can J Appl Physiol 27:551-562.

Zerbe RL, Robertson GL (1983) Osmoregulation of thirst and vasopressin secretion in human subjects: Effect of various solutes. Am J Physiol 244:E607-E614.

Zimmerman EA, Ma LY, Nilaver G (1987) Anatomical basis of thirst and vasopressin secretion. Kidney Int 32:S14-S19.

RECOMMENDED READINGS

Baylis PH (1987) Osmoregulation and control of vasopressin secretion in healthy humans. Am J Physiol 253:R671-78.

Berl T, Verbalis J (2004) Pathophysiology of water metabolism. In: Brenner BM (ed) Brenner &

Rector's The Kidney, 7th ed. Vol. 1. Saunders, Philadelphia, pp 857-919.

Knepper MA, Gamba G (2004) Urine concentration and dilution. In: Brenner BM (ed) Brenner & Rector's The Kidney, 7th ed. Vol. 1. Saunders, Philadelphia, pp 599-636.

Menninger RP (1985) Current concepts of volume regulation of vasopressin release. Fed Proc 4:55-58.

Rose BD, Post TW (2001) The total body water and the plasma sodium concentration. In: Clinical Physiology of Acid-Base and Electrolyte Disorders, 5th ed. McGraw-Hill, New York, pp 241-257.

Rose BD, Post TW (2001b) Regulation of plasma osmolality. In: Clinical Physiology of Acid-Base and Electrolyte Disorders, 5th ed. McGraw-Hill, New York, pp 285-298.

Chapter 36

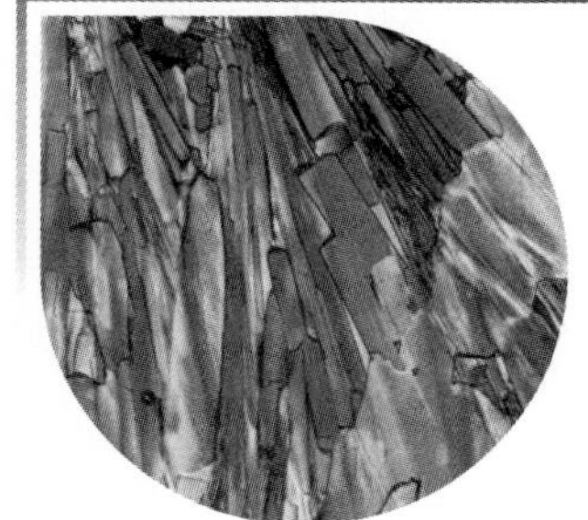

Iron

Robert R. Crichton, PhD, FRSC

OUTLINE

This chapter is a revision of the chapter contributed by Roy D. Baynes, MD, PhD, and Martha H. Stipanuk, PhD, for the first edition.

COMMON ABBREVIATIONS

IRE	iron regulatory element
IRP	iron regulatory protein
IREG-1	iron regulated gene/transporter-1 (also known as metal transporter protein-1 and as ferroportin)
DCT-1	divalent cation transporter-1
HFE	hereditary hemochromatosis gene

BIOLOGICAL FUNCTIONS OF IRON

It is doubtful that life on earth would be possible in the absence of iron. Iron is a transition element that is redox active, is a good Lewis acid, and is capable of forming bonds with electronegative elements (oxygen, nitrogen, and sulfur). The biological importance of iron resides to a great extent in its capacity to exist in several oxidation states, the principal ones being ferrous [Fe^{2+} or Fe(II)] and ferric [Fe^{3+} or Fe(III)], although higher valent Fe^{4+} or Fe^{5+} is generated during the catalytic cycle of a number of enzymes such as catalases, peroxidases, and cytochrome P450s.

Iron is a constituent of numerous proteins, particularly those involved in the transport and metabolism of oxygen, as can be seen from the partial list of iron-containing proteins shown in Box 36-1. Iron proteins can be classified according to the coordination chemistry

Box 36-1

TYPES AND EXAMPLES OF IRON-CONTAINING PROTEINS

I. Heme Proteins

- A. O_2 carriers (globins)
  - a. Hemoglobin
  - b. Myoglobin
- B. NO binding
  - a. Guanylate cyclase
- C. Mitochondrial electron transport chain
  - a. Cytochrome b_{560} in succinate dehydrogenase/Complex II
  - b. Cytochrome b_{562}, b_{566}, and c_1 in the cytochrome *c* reductase/Complex III
  - c. Cytochrome *c*
  - d. Cytochrome *a* in cytochrome *c* oxidase/Complex IV
- D. Mini-electron transport systems
  - a. Cytochrome b_{561} in adrenal chromaffin granules
  - b. Cytochrome b_5 in fatty acyl CoA desaturases
  - c. Cytochrome b_5 in sulfite oxidase
- E. Monooxygenases, dioxygenases, and oxidases
  - a. Cytochrome P450 systems that are involved in synthesis of steroid hormones, the oxygenation of eicosanoids, heme oxygenase, and the oxidation of a variety of lipophilic xenobiotics
  - b. Nitric oxide (NO) synthase
  - c. Sulfite oxidase
  - d. Tryptophan 2,3-dioxygenase
  - e. Cytochrome a_3 of cytochrome *c* oxidase
- F. Peroxidases
  - a. Catalase
  - b. Secretory peroxidases (lactoperoxidase)
  - c. Thyroid peroxidase
  - d. Peroxidase active site of PGH_2 (prostaglandin H_2) synthase
  - e. Chloroperoxidases (myeloperoxidase)

II. Iron-Sulfur Cluster Proteins

- A. Mitochondrial electron transport chain
  - a. NADH dehydrogenase/Complex I: one or more 2Fe-2S clusters; three 4Fe-4S clusters
  - b. Succinate dehydrogenase/Complex II: one 2Fe-2S cluster, two 4Fe-4S clusters
  - c. Cytochrome *c* reductase/Complex III: one 2Fe-2S cluster (Rieske protein)
  - d. ETF dehydrogenase: one 4Fe-4S cluster
- B. Mini-electron transport systems
  - a. Adrenodoxin component of cytochrome P450 systems: two 2Fe-2S clusters

Box 36-1

TYPES AND EXAMPLES OF IRON-CONTAINING PROTEINS—cont'd

b. Xanthine oxidase: two different Fe-S clusters
c. Dihydropyrimidine dehydrogenase (uracil and thymine degradation): two 4Fe-4S clusters

C. Nonredox enzymes containing iron-sulfur clusters
a. Aconitase (mitochondrial; interconverts citrate and isocitrate): one 4Fe-4S center; the 4Fe-4S center is essential for enzyme activity because one Fe^{2+} of the cluster coordinates the –OH group of citrate so as to facilitate its elimination, followed by rehydration to form isocitrate
b. Aconitase (cytosolic; iron regulatory protein-1): one 4Fe-4S center; the apoprotein (without the Fe-S cluster) is the active iron regulatory protein, which can bind iron-responsive elements (IREs) on mRNAs.
c. Ferrochelatase (heme synthesis): one 2Fe-2S center

III. Mononuclear Nonheme Iron Proteins

A. Monooxygenases that contain Fe^{2+} and require tetrahydrobiopterin as a cofactor; hydroxylation of aromatic amino acids
a. Phenylalanine hydroxylase (tyrosine synthesis)
b. Tyrosine hydroxylase (DOPA/dopamine synthesis)
c. Tryptophan hydroxylase (5-hydroxytryptamine/serotonin synthesis)

B. Dioxygenases that require a keto acid co-substrate (usually α-ketoglutarate), Fe^{2+}, and a reducing agent (ascorbic acid); the substrate is hydroxylated, and the keto acid co-substrate is oxidatively decarboxylated (i.e., α-ketoglutarate is converted to succinate)
a. Prolyl 3-hydroxylase and prolyl 4-hydroxylase
b. Lysyl hydroxylase
c. ε-*N*-Trimethyllysine hydroxylase and γ-butyrobetaine β-hydroxylase (carnosine synthesis)
d. Hydroxyphenylpyruvate dioxygenase (tyrosine metabolism—homogentisate formation; in this example, the keto acid that is oxidatively decarboxylated is the pyruvyl side chain of the same molecule that is hydroxylated)
e. Hypoxia inducible factor α (HIF-α)–specific prolyl 4-hydroxylase
f. Asparaginyl β-hydroxylase (factor inhibiting HIF)
g. Phytanoyl CoA 2-hydroxylase

C. Dioxygenases that add O_2 to a single substrate and require Fe^{2+}
a. Lipoxygenases (forms ROOH product; e.g., arachidonate 15-lipoxygenase)
b. Cysteine dioxygenase (forms RSO_2^- product)
c. 3-Hydroxyanthranilate 3,4-dioxygenase (cleaves aromatic ring)
d. Homogentisate 1,2-dioxygenase (cleaves aromatic ring)

IV. Dinuclear Nonheme Iron Proteins

A. Ribonucleotide reductase (Fe–O–Fe is required for formation of the catalytically essential tyrosyl free radical)
B. Fatty acyl CoA desaturases (responsible for the introduction of a double bond into long-chain fatty acids)
C. Purple acid phosphatases (type 5 acid phosphatases)
D. Ferroxidase (ferritin heavy subunit)

---

of their iron: heme proteins, iron-sulfur (Fe-S) proteins, and nonheme, non–iron-sulfur proteins. This latter group includes proteins that contain single Fe atoms and di-iron μ-oxygen-bridged centers as well as proteins involved in iron transport and storage. Iron most often has a coordination number of 6, which gives octahedral stereochemistry; however, tetracoordinate iron (e.g., Fe-S clusters), and five-coordinate complexes are also occasionally found (Crichton, 2001).

HEME PROTEINS

Heme is Fe^{2+}-protoporphyrin IX or an Fe^{2+}-derivative thereof (Fig. 36-1), and many proteins contain heme prosthetic groups. The corresponding

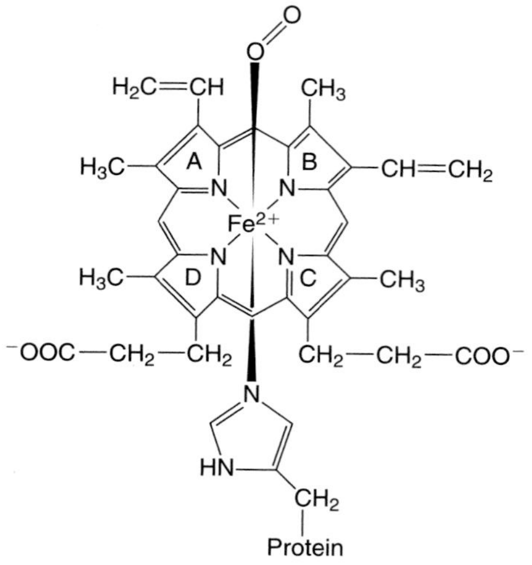

Figure 36-1 An example of heme iron. Ferroprotoporphyrin IX is shown; the proximal ligand for the ferrous atom is a histidine residue on the protein and the sixth ligand (distal ligand) is to oxygen as it is in oxygenated hemoglobin or myoglobin. In deoxyhemoglobin or deoxymyoglobin, the ferrous atom is 5-coordinate. In contrast, in many of the heme-containing cytochromes, the heme iron is 6-coordinate with no substrate binding site; both the distal and proximal ligands are contributed by side chains from the protein (e.g., imidazole nitrogen of histidine or sulfur of methionine). Protoporphyrin IX has 4 methyl, 2 propionate, and 2 vinyl substituents on the porphyrin structure; other forms of heme are derived from protoporphyrin IX. The b-type cytochromes contain ferroprotoporphyrin IX, as does hemoglobin. In the c-type cytochromes, the vinyl substituents on the A and B pyrrole rings are attached to the protein via thioether linkages. In the a-type cytochromes, the vinyl substituent on the A ring is modified, and a hydrophobic isoprenoid tail is attached to it; in addition, the methyl substituent on the D ring is replaced by a formyl group.

Fe^{3+}-protoporphyrin IX complex is defined as hemin. Heme Fe^{2+} is always coordinated to the four nitrogen atoms of the tetrapyrrole structure, with the 5th, and, in some cases the 6th, coordination position occupied by amino acid residues of the protein. In some heme proteins, such as cytochrome *c*, the protoporphyrin is covalently linked to amino acid residues of the protein. Many heme-containing enzymes, including cytochrome oxidase, peroxidases, catalases, and cytochrome P450s, are involved in the activation of O_2 or in the metabolism of peroxides (ROOH). They possess an unoccupied sixth coordination site that serves as the oxygen binding site in proteins that bind O_2 or as the binding site for organic ligands (e.g., through carbon–iron bonds in cytochrome P450s) or inorganic ligands (e.g., NO binding to guanylate cyclase) (Crichton, 2001). Examples of such heme-containing enzymes are listed in Box 36-1 and include monooxygenases (hydroxylases), dioxygenases, oxidases, and peroxidases.

Most cytochromes (e.g., cytochromes *b, c*) do not bind oxygen, and the 6th coordinate position of the Fe^{2+} of the heme in these cytochromes is occupied by an amino acid residue of the protein (often a histidine or methionine residue). In contrast to cytochrome a_3 and P450, which both bind oxygen and transfer electrons, most cytochromes only transfer electrons with the iron in the heme alternating between Fe^{2+} and Fe^{3+}. Although the cytochromes in electron transport chains all catalyze single electron oxidations–reductions of the heme iron, they may be involved in reactions that require two or more electrons. For example, in the mitochondrial respiratory chain, complex IV (cytochrome *c* oxidase) is able to catalyze the four-electron reduction of one O_2 molecule (to form two H_2O molecules). It contains two type *a* hemes, *a* and a_3, and two Cu-containing centers, Cu_A and Cu_B. Oxygen binds to the dinuclear complex of heme a_3 and Cu_B and is reduced to H_2O.

PROTEINS WITH IRON-SULFUR CENTERS

The most common types of iron-sulfur centers are 2Fe-2S and 4Fe-4S clusters, which consist of equal numbers of iron and sulfide ions; the iron atoms of each cluster are also coordinated to four protein cysteinyl sulfhydryl groups, as shown in Figure 36-2. When both the sulfide and cysteine residues are considered, one can see that each Fe atom is coordinated by 4 sulfur atoms; these 4 sulfur atoms are tetrahedrally located around the Fe atom.

Most Fe-S cluster proteins are involved in electron transfer reactions. These include proteins of the mitochondrial electron transport chain as well as various mini-electron transport systems, such as the adrenodoxin component of mitochondrial cytochrome P450 systems

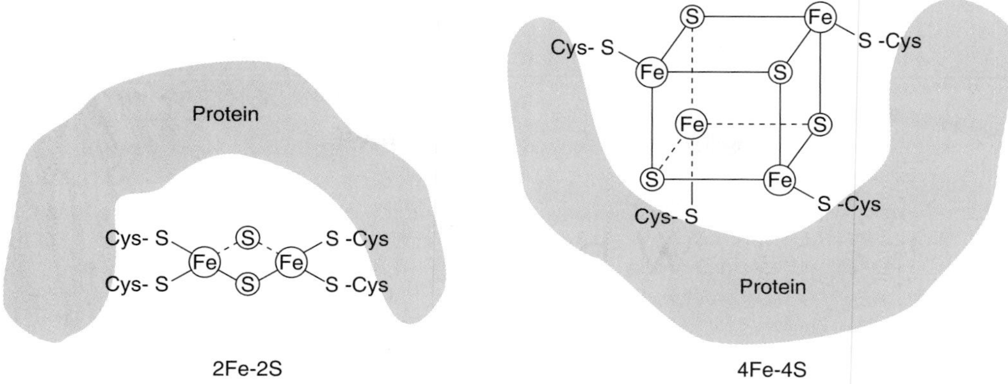

Figure 36-2 The two most common types of iron-sulfur clusters, namely 2Fe-2S and 4Fe-4S, consisting of equal numbers of iron and sulfide ions coordinated to 4 cysteinyl sulfhydryl groups of the protein.

(Beinert et al., 1997). However, a number of Fe-S proteins have functions other than electron transfer, including catalysis and acting as biological sensors for iron, oxygen, and superoxide (Flint and Allen, 1996). The mitochondrial enzyme, aconitase contains a 4Fe-4S center that acts as a Lewis acid in the dehydration reaction by which citrate is converted to isocitrate. As is discussed in a subsequent section of this chapter, there is a cytosolic isozyme of aconitase known as an iron regulatory protein (IRP) that acts as a biosensor for iron levels within the cell.

MONONUCLEAR NONHEME IRON PROTEINS

A number of enzymes contain iron as a single Fe atom, which is coordinately bound to imidazole (histidine) or carboxylate (glutamate and aspartate) ligands on the protein. Generally, the Fe does not form a very stable complex with the protein when in the reduced Fe^{2+} oxidation state, and exchange of iron can occur. These enzymes are involved in reactions that use O_2 as substrate. One subgroup of these iron metalloenzymes requires a keto acid substrate (usually α-ketoglutarate) and a reducing agent. In these reactions, one of the oxygen atoms from O_2 is transferred to the substrate, which is hydroxylated, and the other oxygen atom is transferred to the keto acid co-substrate, which undergoes oxidative decarboxylation. (See Chapter 27, especially Fig. 27-7, for examples and an explanation of the role of ascorbic acid in these reactions.) Another subgroup of iron-containing metalloenzymes is the aromatic amino acid hydroxylases that require tetrahydrobiopterin as a cofactor. Some other Fe^{2+}-containing enzymes add both oxygen atoms from O_2 to a single substrate; these dioxygenases include the 15-lipoxygenase involved in eicosanoid synthesis (see Chapter 18).

DINUCLEAR NONHEME IRON PROTEINS

A family of proteins containing carboxylate-bridged dinuclear iron sites are involved in functions as diverse as mediating reversible oxygen binding (haemerythrin), the oxidation of Fe^{2+} to Fe^{3+} (ferritins), the catalysis of hydroxylation, epoxidation, and desaturation reactions, and the conversion of ribonucleotides into deoxyribonucleotides (Kurtz, 1997; Nordlund and Eklund, 1995). The common link in all of these dinuclear iron proteins is that they react with dioxygen and they all contain a four helical bundle protein fold, which surrounds a (μ-carboxylato)di-iron core with the two iron atoms separated by 0.4 nm or less (Kurtz, 1997). An example of this class of proteins is ribonucleotide reductase (nucleotide 5′-diphosphate reductase), and the structure of the Fe^{3+}-O^{2-}-Fe^{3+} complex is represented in Figure 36-3 (Nordlund et al., 1990). Each Fe^{3+} ion is octahedrally coordinated by the O^{2-} ion (the oxo bridge), by four carboxylate or imidazole groups on the protein, and by coordination with

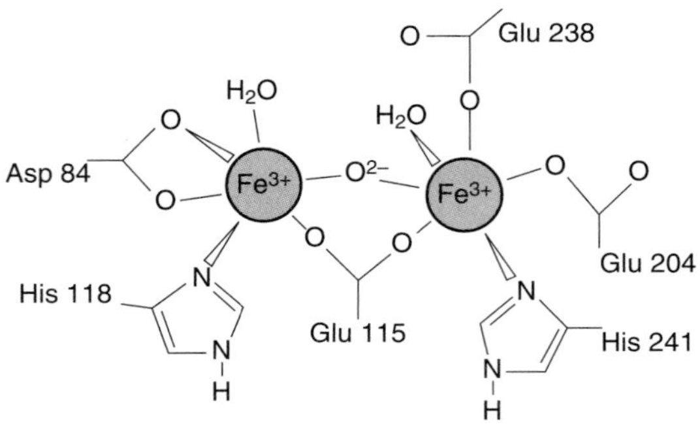

Figure 36-3 The structure and active site of ribonucleotide reductase. *(Modified from Nordlund P, Sjoberg B-M, Eklund H [1990] Three-dimensional structure of the free radical protein of ribonucleotide reductase. Nature 345:593-598. Copyright 1990 Macmillan Magazines Limited.)*

a H_2O molecule. The cytoplasmic ribonucleotide reductase enzyme system participates in the reduction of the four common ribonucleotides to their corresponding deoxyribonucleotides, which are essential for deoxyribonucleic acid (DNA) synthesis. The reaction of the apoenzyme with Fe^{2+} and O_2 results in formation of the Fe^{3+}-O^{2-}-Fe^{3+} bridge and of a tyrosyl free radical in the protein, which plays an essential role in catalysis.

PROTEINS OF IRON TRANSPORT AND IRON STORAGE

Given the many essential functions of iron in oxygen-requiring processes, electron transport, and deoxyribonucleotide synthesis, it is not surprising that efficient mechanisms have developed for iron assimilation and storage. The properties of iron that are so essential for cellular metabolism also make it possible for iron to participate in the generation of highly cytotoxic free radicals, notably the hydroxyl radical. In the aerobic extracellular environment, ferrous ions are readily oxidized to ferric ions; ferric ions can rapidly form complexes with hydroxide ions or water to form polyhydroxides, which are relatively insoluble. If these polyhydroxides form in body fluids, this results in the iron becoming unavailable for cellular uptake, and precipitation of these iron aggregates in tissues could have pathological consequences. Consequently, the mechanisms of iron exchange, transport, and storage must also serve to maintain an extremely low free iron concentration. A list of proteins involved in iron transport, storage, and recycling is in Box 36-2.

Box 36-2

PROTEINS THAT BIND IRON OR IRON-CONTAINING MOIETIES

Iron-Binding Proteins

Transferrin (Fe^{3+})
Lactoferrin (Fe^{3+})
Ferritin (Fe^{3+})
Hemosiderin (Fe^{3+})

Proteins That Use Iron as a Substrate

Ferroxidase (Fe^{2+}/Fe^{3+})
Ferrochelatase (Fe^{2+})

Heme-Binding Protein

Hemopexin (heme or hematin)

Protein That Uses Heme as a Substrate

Heme oxygenase

Hemoglobin-Binding Protein

Haptoglobins (oxyhemoglobin dimers)

Transferrin-Binding Protein

Transferrin receptor

PROTEINS OF IRON TRANSPORT

Transferrin

The major plasma protein involved in the transport of iron is transferrin (Crichton, 2001; Wessling-Resnick, 2000; Lindley, 1996; Baker and Lindley, 1992). Transferrin is a glycoprotein synthesized principally in the liver. It is composed of a single polypeptide chain of about 680 amino-acid residues with two iron-binding sites, encoded on chromosome 3. The protein is made up of two similar amino- and carboxy-terminal lobes, each organized into two distinct domains; each lobe contains an iron-binding site (Fig. 36-4). The affinity of transferrin for Fe^{3+} is high (K_d 10^{-19} to 10^{-20}). Four of the six atoms required to coordinate the Fe^{3+} are provided by the protein (an aspartate, a histidine, and two tyrosine residues), and the remaining two by a carbonate anion (CO_3^{2-}), which is essential for

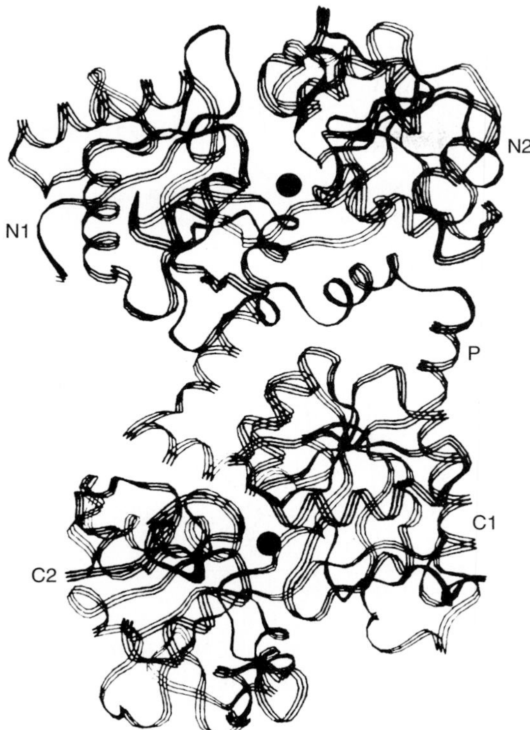

Figure 36-4 A ribbon diagram showing the characteristic folding of transferrins into two lobes (N-lobe above and C-lobe below) and four domains (N1, N2, C1, and C2). Iron atoms are shown as filled circles. The interlobe connecting peptide (P) is helical in lactoferrin but irregular in transferrin. *(From Baker EN, Lindley PF [1992] New perspectives on the structure and function of transferrins. J Inorg Biochem 47:147-160. Copyright 1992 Elsevier Science.)*

iron binding. Binding and release of iron by transferrin results in striking conformational changes in each of the two lobes. In the absence of bound Fe^{3+}, the two domains of each lobe are free to swing apart and adopt an open conformation. In the presence of Fe^{3+} and carbonate they take up a pincerlike closed position around the iron atom.

The mean normal plasma iron concentration is approximately 20 μmol/L, and the mean normal plasma transferrin concentration is approximately 30 μmol/L (with each molecule of transferrin containing two iron-binding sites). Consequently, plasma transferrin is normally only about one third saturated with iron, and, therefore, the plasma has significant excess iron-binding capacity. Transferrin is distributed throughout most of the extracellular fluids of the body, with a continuous circulation from blood to interstitial fluid. The delivery of transferrin-bound iron to cells is dependent upon the expression of transferrin receptors.

Transferrin Receptor

Transferrin receptors are involved in the cellular uptake of iron from the circulation, and they have highest affinity for saturated (diferric) transferrin. The transferrin receptor is a transmembrane glycoprotein composed of two identical 95-kDa monomers linked by a pair of disulfide bridges; each monomer consists of 760 amino-acid residues organized into an amino-terminal cytoplasmic domain of 61 amino acids, a membrane-spanning segment of 28 amino acids, and a large extracellular domain of 671 amino acids. The cytoplasmic domain is required for appropriate intracellular trafficking of the transferrin–transferrin receptor complex. The peptide sequence tyrosine-threonine-arginine-phenylalanine in the cytoplasmic domain has been identified as the signal for endocytosis via coated pits, and the serine residue at position 24 is a phosphorylation site. The three-dimensional structure of the transferrin-binding extracellular domain has been determined (Fig. 36-5), but the details of the transferrin-binding site are not yet elucidated (Lawrence et al., 1999). The transmembrane domain, consisting largely of hydrophobic amino acid residues, functions as a signal peptide for translocation across the endoplasmic reticulum during synthesis and as a membrane anchor for the protein. A cysteine residue at position 62 is the major site of post-translational fatty acid acylation; the significance of this is uncertain.

Several sites of *N*- and *O*-linked glycosylation have been identified in the extracellular domain. These glycan chains may play a role in translocation of the receptor to the cell surface and in facilitating the interaction between the receptor and transferrin. Cysteinyl residues at positions 89 and 98 in the extracellular domain of each polypeptide form a pair of disulfide bridges that hold the homodimer together. The extracellular domain has serine protease–sensitive sites at arginine 100 and

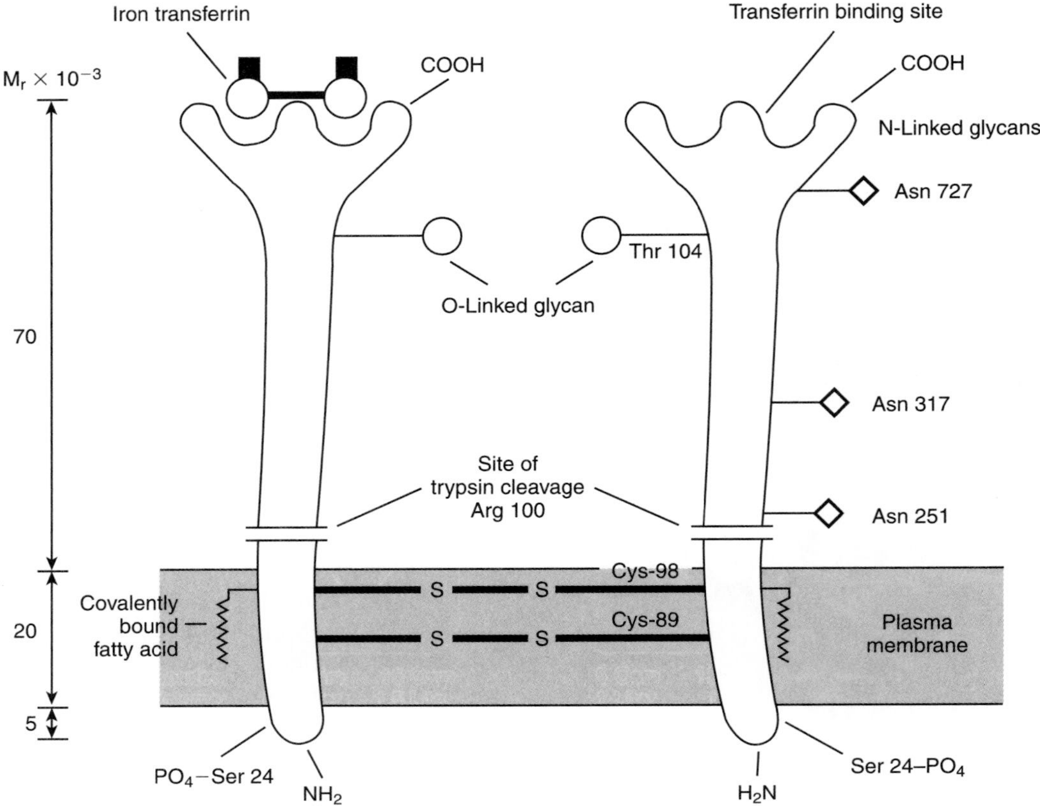

Figure 36-5 Diagramatic representation of the transferrin receptor. *(Redrawn from Crichton RR [2001] Inorganic Biochemistry of Iron Metabolism: From Molecular Mechanisms to Clinical Consequences, 2nd ed. John Wiley and Sons, New York, p 117.)*

arginine 121. Each receptor dimer can bind two transferrin molecules, one to each subunit. The receptor is fundamental to the cellular binding and uptake of iron-bearing transferrin; the pathway of internal iron exchange is discussed more comprehensively in a subsequent section of this chapter. The transferrin receptor is encoded on chromosome 3 (Testa et al., 1993).

Other Transport Proteins

A number of other proteins present in plasma may play a role in iron transport. This is particularly likely in iron overload, hemolytic anemia, and conditions of ineffective erythropoiesis during which free hemoglobin or heme may be present in the plasma compartment. These transport proteins include haptoglobin, hemopexin, ferritin, lactoferrin, and albumin. The amount of iron carried by each of these proteins is uncertain but usually is relatively trivial in comparison with that carried by transferrin.

Haptoglobin binds free oxyhemoglobin dimers, and hemopexin and albumin bind free heme and hematin. All three proteins are synthesized and secreted by the liver, and the bound forms are also taken up by the liver. Haptoglobin is an 85-kDa α-2 glycoprotein encoded on chromosome 16, and hemopexin is a 70-kDa β glycoprotein encoded on chromosome 11. Hepatocytes have a specific receptor for the haptoglobin–hemoglobin complex, and this complex is internalized by receptor-mediated endocytosis. Both receptor and ligand are degraded. The haptoglobin receptor is as yet incompletely understood, as is the mapping of its gene. In addition, the hemopexin–heme complex is internalized by hepatocytes via receptor-mediated endocytosis. The receptor and the hemopexin molecule both appear to be recycled. The hemopexin receptor is known to be an 85-kDa molecule composed of a 20-kDa and a 65-kDa subunit. The mapping of its gene is as yet undetermined. The mechanism by which heme in association with albumin makes its way into hepatocytes is uncertain.

The iron-storage protein ferritin is primarily an intracellular protein. Minor amounts are present in the circulation in proportion to iron stores. In contrast to cellular ferritin, the plasma ferritin is glycosylated and relatively iron-poor. Consequently, ferritin is unlikely to play a major role in iron transport under normal circumstances. However, in situations of iron overload and tissue injury, the plasma ferritin concentration is increased, and some of the plasma ferritin is the nonglycosylated tissue ferritin, which has a higher iron content. Ferritin in these circumstances is taken up in the liver both by putative specific ferritin receptors and, in the case of tissue ferritin, by the asialoglycoprotein receptor. In these circumstances, ferritin may contribute modestly to iron transport. A more subtle role for ferritin in iron transport has been suggested by observations that macrophages may release ferritin directly and that this ferritin can be taken up by specific hepatic ferritin receptors. This pathway has been suggested to be of significance in iron transport within the liver. Precise quantitative data, however, are still lacking.

Lactoferrin is an iron-binding protein found predominantly in neutrophils, secretory epithelium, and secretions, including milk. It is structurally similar to transferrin. Amounts on the order of 2 to 3 mg/L (25 to 40 nmol/L) have been reported in human plasma. This concentration is several orders of magnitude lower than that of transferrin (30 μmol/L). Lactoferrin binds iron much more tightly than transferrin, particularly at acidic pH. This, together with kinetic data, indicates that the role of lactoferrin in iron transport is probably negligible. Its functional significance in neutrophils and in secretions appears to relate to its antibacterial properties. This antibacterial activity is thought to be partially due to the ability of lactoferrin to sequester iron and, thus, reduce iron availability in infectious conditions.

Nontransferrin-Bound Iron

Under normal circumstances, there is virtually no iron in the systemic circulation that is not bound to heme, transferrin, or ferritin: the normal level of nontransferrin-bound iron is less than 1 μmol/L (less than 0.056 mg/L). Much higher levels may be detected in conditions of iron overload (hereditary hemochromatosis) or hemolytic anemia (e.g., thalassemia major). This iron is not dialyzable and can be detected either by the addition of chelators or by the bleomycin assay, which is based on the ability of bleomycin to degrade DNA only in the presence of free iron. The nature of this nondialyzable, but available, iron is incompletely understood, but candidates for formation of this nontransferrin-bound iron include nonspecific interaction of free iron with other plasma proteins and/or interactions with citrate, ascorbate, histidine, or other amino acids. Regardless of the specific form, this nontransferrin-bound iron is rapidly cleared from the circulation by the liver by a passive carrier-mediated process, and its uptake may contribute significantly to the deposition of iron in parenchymal cells of the liver in conditions of iron overload (Breuer et al., 2000).

PROTEINS OF IRON STORAGE

Ferritin

Iron is delivered to the cells of the body by one of the transport mechanisms outlined in the previous section. Certain specialized cells obtain additional iron by other pathways. The cells of the reticuloendothelial system acquire significant amounts of iron from phagocytized and catabolized red blood cells. Mucosal cells of the gastrointestinal tract procure food iron by the process of iron absorption. These aspects of iron exchange are more fully delineated in subsequent sections of this chapter. Most of the iron delivered to or acquired by cells is believed to cross the cell membrane as Fe^{2+} or Fe^{3+} and to enter a poorly characterized intracellular transit pool, usually referred to as labile iron, which has been described as somewhat like the Loch Ness monster—only to disappear from view before its presence, or indeed its nature, can be confirmed (Crichton, 1984). The labile iron pool represents iron in transit between extracellular supplies and intracellular demands, both functional as well as storage. Although its exact chemical nature remains uncertain, it is thought to represent approximately micromolar concentrations of iron (Breuer et al., 1995). This pool reflects the readily available iron within the cell and is believed to be the key regulator of internal and external iron exchange.

To prevent the unwanted effects of iron-catalyzed free radical generation or iron oxidation and precipitation, it is imperative that the cell safely store excess iron. Hence, the iron-storage proteins ferritin and hemosiderin fulfill a cellular "housekeeping" function in all cells in addition to their role as an iron reservoir in specialized cells (macrophages of the reticuloendothelial system and parenchymal cells of the liver) from which body iron pools can be replenished as iron is utilized or lost. The major storage sites of ferritin in normal subjects are liver, spleen, and skeletal muscle. The half-life of ferritin in the liver is about 60 hours. Hemosiderin represents a very small fraction of normal body iron stores, mostly in macrophages, but increases dramatically in iron overload.

The apoferritin molecule (iron-free) has a molecular mass of approximately 500 kDa and is composed of 24 subunits of molecular weight in the vicinity of 20 kDa. These subunits form a hollow protein shell (Fig. 36-6) with

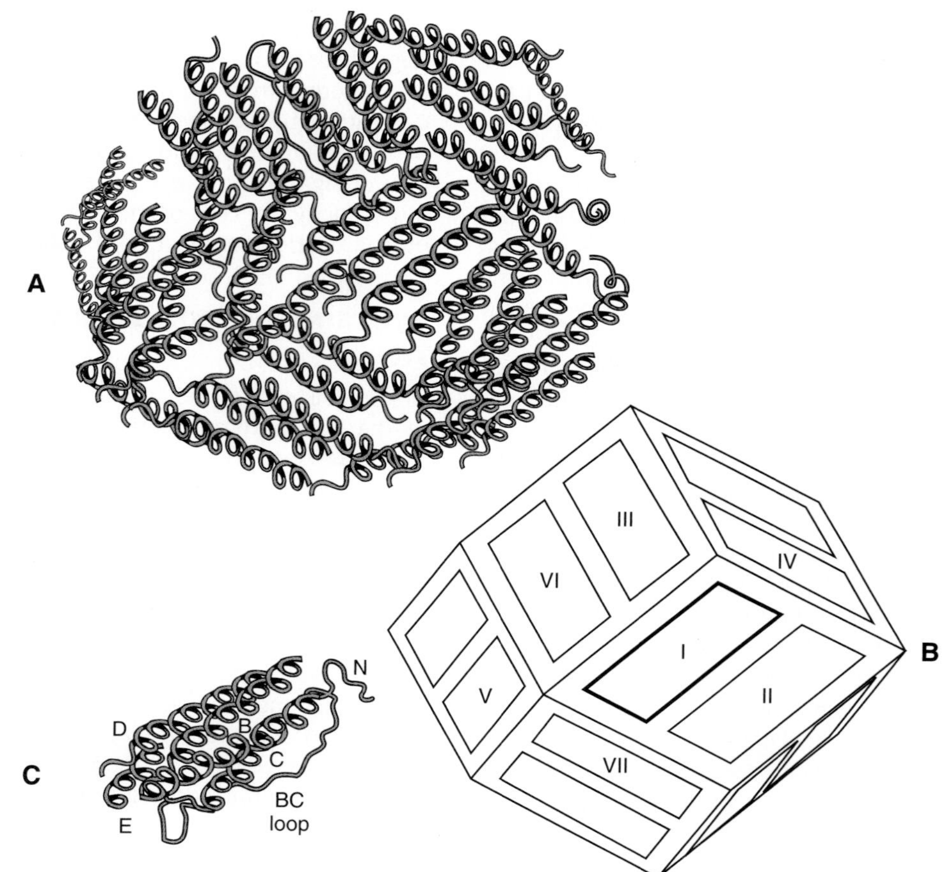

Figure 36-6 Structure of recombinant horse L-chain apoferritin. **A,** An overview of a ferritin molecule showing the relative positions and interfaces between symmetry related subunits. **B,** The labeling scheme of the symmetry-related subunits. Subunits I/II constitute a dimer related by a twofold symmetry axis; subunits I, III, and IV together form a threefold axis, whereas subunits I, VI, V, and VII are positioned around a fourfold axis of symmetry. **C,** A ribbon diagram of the α-carbon backbone. (*Redrawn from Crichton RR [2001] Inorganic Biochemistry of Iron Metabolism: From Molecular Mechanisms to Clinical Consequences, 2nd ed. John Wiley and Sons, New York, p 139.*)

an external diameter of 12 to 13 nm, delimiting a cavity of 7 to 8 nm in diameter within which up to 4,500 atoms of iron are stored in a nontoxic, water-soluble, yet bioavailable form. In mammalian ferritins the iron core resembles the mineral known as ferrihydrite. The protein shell has a high degree of symmetry, with fourfold, threefold and twofold axes of symmetry. In Figure 36-6, an overview of a ferritin molecule showing the relative positions and interfaces between symmetry related subunits is shown. The labeling scheme of the symmetry related subunits is shown in Figure 36-6, *B*. Therefore subunits I/II constitute a dimer related by a twofold symmetry axis; subunits I, III, and IV surround a threefold axis, whereas subunits I, VI, V, and VII are positioned around a fourfold axis of symmetry. A ribbon diagram of the α-carbon backbone is shown in Figure 36-6, *C*. The subunit is roughly cylindrical, a little more than 5 nm long and 2.5 nm wide, with approximately 80% of the amino acid sequence present in five α-helices. Each of the 24 subunits consists of a long central bundle of four parallel and antiparallel helices, A, B, C, and D, with a fifth short helix E (163-174) butting onto one end of this α-helical bundle, and a long extended loop joining the B and C helices (see Fig. 36-6, *C*).

The subunits in mammalian ferritins are of two biochemically distinct types. The heavier H subunit has a molecular mass of approximately 21 kDa, is encoded by a gene on chromosome 11, and has a more acidic isoelectric point. The lighter L subunit has a molecular mass of approximately 19 kDa, is encoded by a gene on chromosome 19, and has a more basic isoelectric point. Different proportions of H and L subunits make up the 24-subunit apoferritin, leading to distinct isoferritins with various tissue specificities. The L-rich basic isoferritins predominate in tissues such as liver and spleen. Iron administration tends to enhance predominantly L subunit synthesis. These observations indicate a predominant role for the L ferritin subunit in iron storage. The H-rich, more acidic isoferritins are found in tissues such as the heart, erythrocytes, and mononuclear leukocytes, which are not major sites of iron storage.

The ferritin molecule is ideally suited to serve both the housekeeping and storage functions because its structure allows for the deposition of large amounts of iron in a soluble and nontoxic, yet biologically available form (Crichton, 2001; Harrison and Arosio, 1996). Human H and L subunits are less similar to each other than are human H subunits to other mammalian H subunits, or human L chains to other L chains. This underscores the complementary role of the two subunit types, which play different roles in storing, detoxifying, and maintaining Fe^{3+} in a soluble form. In the first step of iron incorporation, Fe^{2+} penetrates the apoferritin shell through channels at the surface of the protein and is oxidized at dinuclear iron centers (known as ferroxidase centers) localized in the H subunits. Fe^{3+} then migrates to nucleation centers within L subunits, in the interior of the protein shell. Once a nucleus of iron core has formed at the nucleation sites, deposition of iron on this inorganic core, essentially in the form of the mineral ferrihydrite, drives the further incorporation of iron. The maximum storage capacity of each ferritin molecule is approximately 4,500 iron atoms. The mechanism of iron release from ferritin is not at all well understood, although it appears to be facilitated by reducing conditions and by a more acidic pH.

As mentioned, ferritin is also found in serum, and its concentration is a useful indication of body iron status. The origin of serum ferritin is not well established; it is usually glycosylated, suggestive of an active secretory pathway, and animal studies suggest that it is mostly derived from liver. In severe iron loading, larger amounts of the nonglycosylated form are found, suggestive of leakage from damaged cells.

Hemosiderins

Hemosiderin is also a storage form of iron. Hemosiderins are observed predominantly in conditions of iron overload, such as hereditary hemochromatosis and transfusion-dependent hemoglobinopathies. The hemosiderins are thought to be the product of lysosomal degradation of ferritin (Ward et al., 1994) but are less well characterized. They are more abundant when there is iron overload. The iron in hemosiderin is less available to chelation than is that in ferritin, and when it is present in the goethite form it is even less labile and chelatable than when in the ferrihydrite form (Ward et al., 2000)

REGULATION OF CONCENTRATIONS OF PROTEINS OF IRON TRANSPORT AND STORAGE

Given the key role played by iron in cellular metabolism and proliferation, the concentrations of the proteins of iron transport and storage must be highly regulated. The mechanisms involved in the regulation of the levels of these proteins are beginning to be understood.

TRANSCRIPTIONAL REGULATION OF SYNTHESIS OF FERRITIN, TRANSFERRIN RECEPTORS, AND TRANSFERRIN

Tissue differences in the expression of H and L ferritins exist and are in part due to differences in transcriptional activity. Changes in expression of ferritin in response to cellular iron content also differ for the H and L ferritin subunits. Transcriptional control of ferritin expression has been documented in a number of human cells and cell lines. Factors such as cellular differentiation and inflammatory cytokines (such as tumor necrosis factor-α and interleukin-1) may bring about differential subunit expression (Harrison and Arosio, 1996).

Changes in expression of the transferrin receptor have been observed in response to different phases of the cell cycle, to cellular differentiation, and to cytokines, including α- and γ-interferons. These responses in transferrin receptor expression appear to be predominantly mediated by changes in transcription.

The expression of transferrin also appears to be transcriptionally regulated. Transferrin is expressed predominantly in the liver, and transcription rates are increased in the presence of functional iron deficiency or increased steroid hormone levels (e.g., in pregnancy and in individuals taking exogenous estrogen). Transcription of transferrin is also modulated in relation to inflammatory cytokines; although these cytokines enhance transferrin transcription, catabolism of the molecule is also increased such that the net effect is a reduction in the circulating concentration of transferrin.

The specific mechanisms by which transcription of ferritin, transferrin receptor, or transferrin is altered have not been clearly defined, although it has been suggested that a number of nuclear transcription factors may be modulating factors in the regulation of the transcription of the ferritin and transferrin receptor genes. Several DNA-binding proteins have been identified that interact with the transferrin promoter region.

POSTTRANSCRIPTIONAL REGULATION OF FERRITIN AND TRANSFERRIN RECEPTOR SYNTHESIS

Iron-Responsive Elements

It has long been appreciated that ferritin biosynthesis can be regulated in response to changes in cellular iron content, even when transcription has been inhibited, and that this regulation involves a sequence of approximately 30 nucleotides in the 5′-untranslated region (5′-UTR) of the ferritin mRNA. This sequence is highly conserved through all the ferritin genes studied. Biosynthesis of the transferrin receptor is also regulated in the presence of transcriptional inhibition, but in this case the regulation involves nucleotide sequences in the 3′-untranslated portion of the transferrin receptor mRNA. These sequences all show significant homology and have been termed iron-responsive elements or IREs (Eisenstein, 2000; Hentze and Kühn, 1996).

These IREs can be fitted to a consensus motif, as shown in Figure 36-7. They consist of a lower stem of variable length made up of complementary pairs of ribonucleic acid (RNA) bases; the lower stems of the IREs in the ferritin H and L subunit mRNAs are guanine-cytosine (GC)–rich, whereas they tend to be adenine-uracil (AU)–rich in the transferrin receptor messenger RNAs (mRNAs). Above the lower stem is an unpaired cytosine base, which produces a characteristic bulge in the stem structure. Above this is an upper stem that consists of five complementary base pairs. A 6-base loop is found on top of the upper stem; 5 of the 6 bases forming this loop are almost always CAGUG.

In the mRNAs for ferritin L and H, there is a single stem-loop IRE in the 5′-UTR. In contrast,

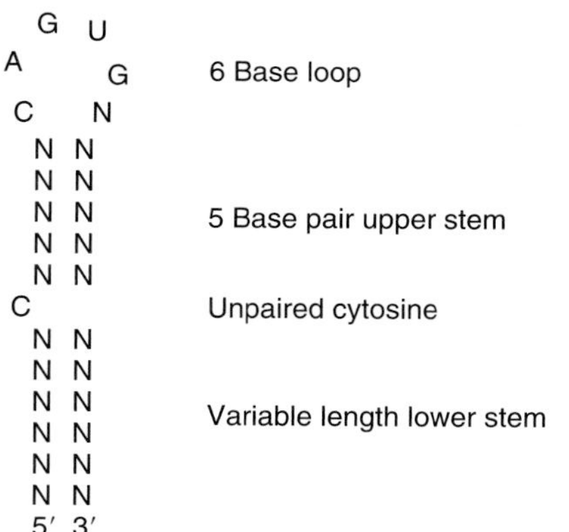

Figure 36-7 Consensus sequence for iron-responsive elements (IREs).

transferrin receptor mRNA contains as many as five tandem IREs in the 3′-UTR. The binding of the 5′- and 3′-flanking IREs results in different effects on translation, as will be discussed in subsequent text. In addition to the ferritin H, ferritin L, and transferrin receptor mRNAs, the mRNAs for several other proteins have been found to contain IREs or IRE-resembling sequences. The mRNA for the erythroid form of δ-aminolevulinate synthase (the first enzyme in the heme biosynthetic pathway), the mRNA for the mitochondrial form of aconitase, and the putative basolateral iron transport protein of the small intestine, iron regulated transporter-1 (IREG-1), also contain a single IRE in the 5′-UTP. The divalent cation transporter protein, DCT-1, involved in transport of Fe^{2+} across the apical membrane of the small intestine and in the transport of iron out of the endosome during the transferrin uptake cycle, has a single IRE in the 3′-UTR of its mRNA.

Iron Regulatory Proteins

Two cytosolic proteins have been identified that interact directly with the IREs to modulate mRNA translation, and these are designated iron regulatory proteins (IRPs). IRP-1 and IRP-2 have a molecular mass of approximately 90 kDa and 105 kDa, respectively, the difference being due to a 73-residue inclusion in the latter protein. IRP-1 is encoded by a gene on chromosome 9. When iron is in adequate amounts, IRP-1 exists in a 4Fe-4S form, has aconitase activity, and lacks IRE-binding activity. When the cellular iron concentration is low, the protein no longer has an Fe-S cluster. This apoprotein form of IRP-1 no longer has aconitase activity, but acquires IRE-binding activity. IRP-2 is less abundant than IRP-1 in most cells, with greatest expression in intestine and brain, and has around 80% homology with IRP-1. However, whereas the apo form of IRP-2 binds to IREs in iron-replete cells, the holo-IRP-2 is ubiquitinated in its 73-residue inclusion and is subsequently degraded by the proteosome. Although the cysteine residues that coordinate the iron-sulfur cluster in IRP-1 are conserved in IRP-2, IRP-2 has no detectable aconitase activity.

The specific mechanisms by which IRE–IRP interactions modulate protein biosynthesis are still incompletely understood, but they are clearly different for ferritin than for transferrin receptor synthesis. Interaction of IRPs with the 5′ stem-loop IRE of the ferritin mRNA prevents the formation of ferritin-mRNA polysomes. Hence, when the iron supply is low, IRPs are active and they bind to the IRE on ferritin mRNAs and block ferritin synthesis. Conversely, when iron is abundant, the IRP is inactive, does not bind to the IRE, and does not restrict ferritin synthesis.

In contrast, when active IRPs bind to the stem-loop structures on the 3′-end of the transferrin receptor mRNA, the transferrin receptor mRNA is stabilized against degradation. It appears that there is a determinant for rapid mRNA turnover within this 3′-UTR and that IRP binding to the stem-loop structure in some way masks the rapid turnover determinant. Consequently, when cytoplasmic iron levels are low, transferrin receptor mRNA concentrations increase and more transferrin receptor is synthesized, resulting in higher concentrations of transferrin receptors in cell membranes. When iron is in excess, the IRPs no longer bind to the IREs, and the transferrin receptor mRNA, which is no longer protected by the IRPs, is degraded.

Therefore, when iron supplies are limiting, transferrin receptors are expressed, which allows the cell to take up more iron, whereas the synthesis of ferritin is blocked. When the cellular levels of iron are adequate, ferritin is synthesized and the storage of potentially

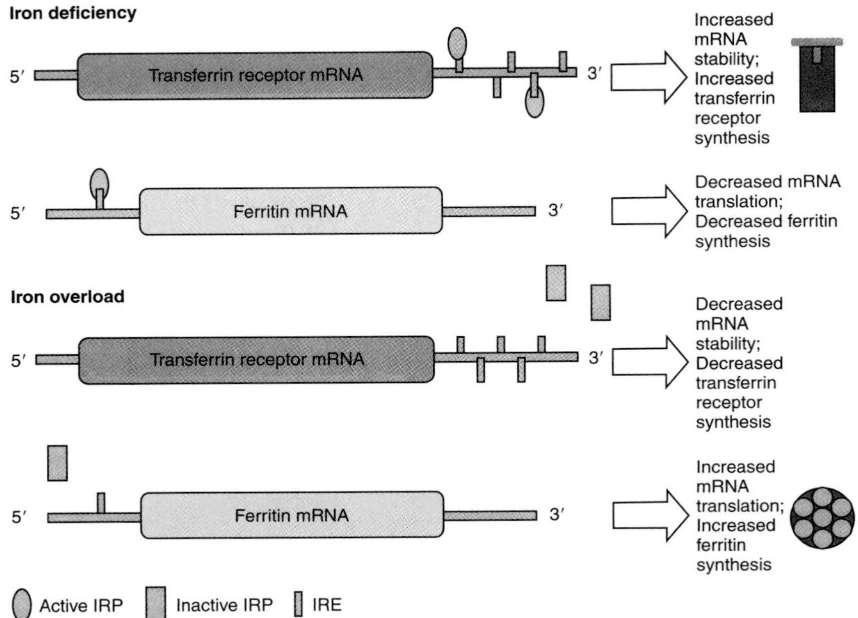

Figure 36-8 Reciprocal regulation of ferritin and transferrin receptor production at the level of their mRNAs by iron responsive proteins (IRPs) and iron responsive elements (IREs) in iron deficiency and excess. In the iron-deficient state, IRPs are active and bind to IREs, which stabilizes transferrin receptor mRNA against degradation, thus increasing transferrin receptor synthesis, and blocks ferritin mRNA translation, thus decreasing ferritin synthesis. When iron is abundant, the opposite situation occurs: IRPs do not bind to IREs, due to their inactivation or degradation, and transferrin receptor mRNA is degraded while ferritin mRNA is translated to produce ferritin.

toxic iron in ferritin is thus facilitated, whereas the transferrin receptor mRNA is destroyed by ribonucleases so that less transferrin receptor is synthesized.

This IRE–IRP regulatory mechanism is one of the first examples of how a single protein can coordinately regulate distinct mRNAs, thereby decreasing the translation of one (ferritin) by inhibiting polysome formation while simultaneously increasing translation of the other (transferrin receptor) by limiting degradation of its mRNA (Binder et al., 1994). Although the major determinant of IRP activity is the cytosolic content of exchangeable iron, recent data indicate that nitric oxide, a metabolite of L-arginine, is also able to modulate iron removal from iron-sulfur proteins (Hentze and Kühn, 1996). Clearly this could also result in modulation of high-affinity IRP and might be one of the factors involved in posttranscriptional regulation of proteins of iron metabolism in situations of inflammation and stimulated cytokine production.

BODY IRON COMPARTMENTS

Understanding the disorders of iron metabolism is greatly facilitated by the consideration of body iron (approximately 40 mg/kg in women and 50 mg/kg in men) as two major compartments, namely functional and storage iron, as summarized in Table 36-1. Functional iron is composed predominantly of the iron in hemoglobin of red blood cells and erythroid tissues (28 mg/kg body weight in women and 32 mg/kg body weight in men), iron in myoglobin in the muscle (4 mg/kg in women and 5 mg/kg in men), and iron-containing enzymes in all cells of the body (1 to 2 mg/kg body weight). The storage iron compartment is an intrinsically more variable compartment, accounting for between 0 and 20 mg of iron per kg of body weight. This storage iron is held in association with the protein complexes called ferritin and hemosiderin; storage iron is located predominantly in macrophages of the reticuloendothelial system and in parenchymal

Table 36-1
Typical Iron Distribution in Adults

	Men	Women
	mg Iron/kg Body Weight	
Functional iron		
Hemoglobin	32	28
Myoglobin	5	4
Iron-containing enzymes	1-2	1-2
Storage iron		
Ferritin (and hemosiderin)	~11	~6
Transport iron		
Transferrin	0.04	0.04

cells of the liver. These storage proteins serve as a repository for dietary iron absorbed in excess of that needed to replace losses from the functional compartment; this provides a mechanism to prevent accumulation of free iron ions, which would be toxic, and to provide an emergency reserve supply from which sudden deficits in the functional compartment may be replenished.

A much smaller third compartment can be thought of as the transport system interfacing between the storage and functional compartments. This transport compartment consists of iron bound to transferrin and accounts for approximately 0.04 mg of iron per kg. Although the amount of iron in this compartment at any given time is quantitatively small, flux of iron through this compartment is relatively large on a daily basis (40 mg of Fe per day, or approximately 0.6 mg/kg/day), and measurements of this transport compartment provide important and clinically useful information for defining the stage of iron deficiency or excess.

INTERNAL IRON EXCHANGE AND IRON DELIVERY TO CELLS

Transferrin is the major iron-transport molecule. Although the total amount of plasma transferrin-bound iron is only about 50 μmol (i.e., 2.8 mg in 2.5 L of plasma), the rate of plasma iron turnover determined by ferrokinetic evaluation is approximately 700 μmol/day in an adult. Hence, the plasma iron pool is turned over 10 or more times daily. This estimate of iron turnover is much greater than would be predicted from the rate of transferrin synthesis, catabolism, or lymphatic circulation, indicating that transferrin is significantly reutilized, with only limited catabolism during iron delivery (Aisen, 1998).

THE TRANSFERRIN CYCLE

The apotransferrin molecule binds iron released from cells of iron storage (i.e., macrophages of the reticuloendothelial system and parenchymal cells of the liver) and iron procurement (i.e., enterocytes of the intestine). The iron released from cells crosses the plasma membrane in all likelihood as ferrous iron, but during this process or shortly thereafter the iron is oxidized to the ferric form. The likely oxidase is plasma ceruloplasmin, which has ferroxidase activity (Harris et al., 1995). The ferric iron is rapidly bound by transferrin, which has two Fe^{3+}-binding sites. In plasma, the iron-free (apo) form, the two single-iron (monoferric) forms, with iron in either the N- or C-terminal lobe, and the two-iron (diferric) form of transferrin are all normally found, with an average overall iron saturation of about one third. At physiological pH, the affinity of transferrin for its receptor correlates directly with its degree of iron occupancy; the apo form of transferrin has negligible affinity for transferrin receptor, whereas the diferric form has highest affinity.

Because transferrin uptake is mediated by transferrin receptor, transferrin iron is delivered to tissues in proportion to their surface expression of transferrin receptors. In practical terms, this means that approximately 80% of transferrin iron is routinely delivered to erythroid precursors. (The transferrin cycle is illustrated in Fig. 36-9.) After binding to the transferrin receptor, the receptor ligand complexes tend to aggregate within clathrin-coated pits. Thereafter they are internalized by the process of receptor-mediated endocytosis. The vesicles lose their clathrin coats, and, then, within the endocytic vesicles, an ATP-dependent proton pump in the endosomal membrane pumps protons into the lumen of the endosome from the cytosol. The combined effects of transferrin binding to its receptor and the acidic environment that is produced results in iron release from transferrin, probably subsequent to protonation of the carbonate anion. The released iron probably then undergoes a reduction step, and the resulting

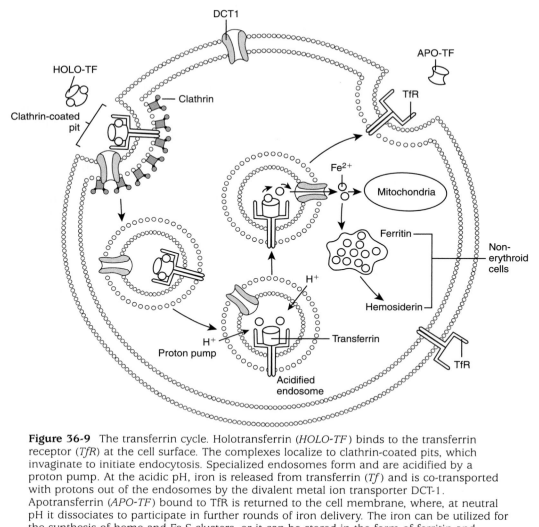

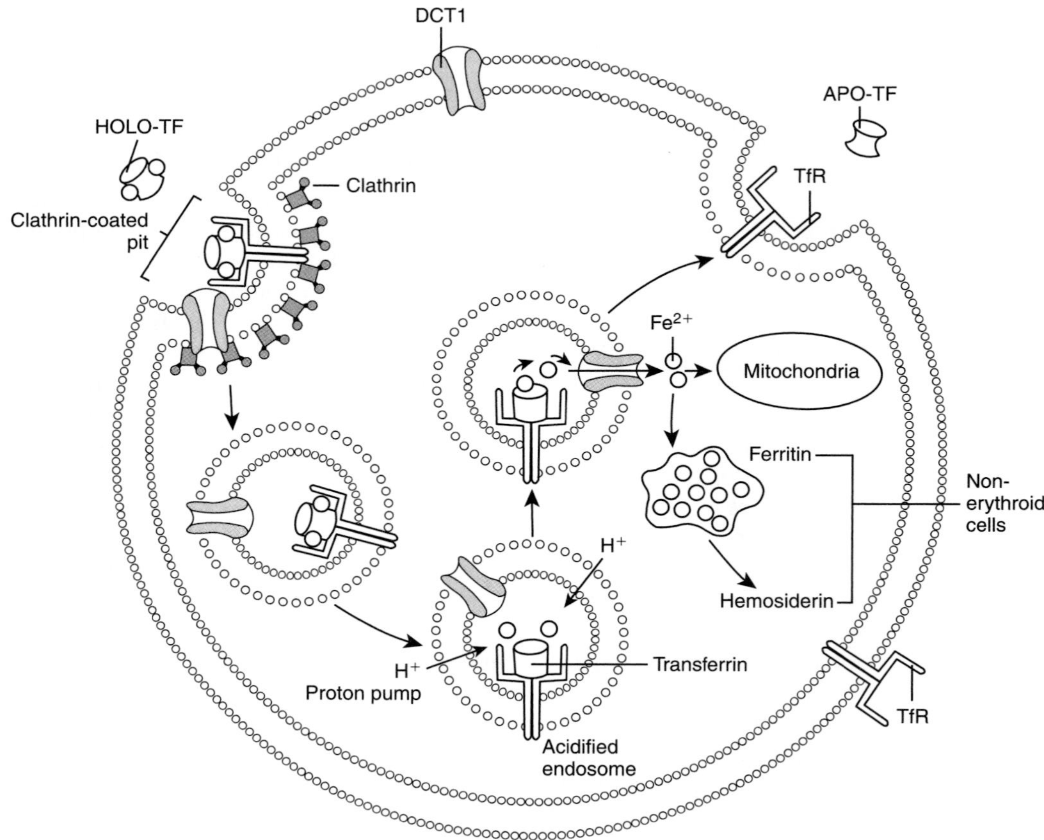

Figure 36-9 The transferrin cycle. Holotransferrin (*HOLO-TF*) binds to the transferrin receptor (*TfR*) at the cell surface. The complexes localize to clathrin-coated pits, which invaginate to initiate endocytosis. Specialized endosomes form and are acidified by a proton pump. At the acidic pH, iron is released from transferrin (*Tf*) and is co-transported with protons out of the endosomes by the divalent metal ion transporter DCT-1. Apotransferrin (*APO-TF*) bound to TfR is returned to the cell membrane, where, at neutral pH it dissociates to participate in further rounds of iron delivery. The iron can be utilized for the synthesis of heme and Fe-S clusters, or it can be stored in the form of ferritin and hemosiderin. *(Modified from Zecca L, Youdim MBH, Riederer P, Connor JR, Crichton RR [2004] Iron, brain ageing and neurodegenerative diseases. Nat Rev Neurosci 5:863-873.)*

ferrous iron is transported across the endocytic membrane into the cytosol by DCT-1 (divalent cation transporter-1).

The apotransferrin molecule produced upon iron release has an extremely high affinity for the transferrin receptor in the more acidic environment of the endosome. By remaining bound to the receptor, apotransferrin largely escapes degradation when the endosome delivers its soluble contents into secondary lysosomes, and the majority of the apotransferrin–transferrin receptor complexes are returned to the cell surface after iron release has occurred. The rapidly recycling endosome passes through the Golgi apparatus prior to fusing with the plasma membrane at the cell surface. After fusion has occurred, the transferrin–transferrin receptor complex is exposed to physiological pH, at which the apotransferrin dissociates from the receptor and is returned to the interstitial fluid. From the interstitial fluid, the apotransferrin returns to the circulation where it is again able to bind iron and participate in additional cycles of iron delivery. The membrane-bound transferrin receptor is able to participate in further cycles of receptor-mediated endocytosis. This cellular transferrin recycling pathway is extremely rapid; one complete cycle for uptake of the transferrin–transferrin receptor complex, release of the iron, return of the apotransferrin–transferrin receptor complex to the plasma membrane, and return of transferrin to the circulation requires only 3 to 10 minutes.

TRANSFERRIN-RECEPTOR DEGRADATION

A minor portion of the endocytosed transferrin and transferrin receptor is processed via an alternative pathway. In this pathway the endocytic vesicle membrane undergoes internal outpouching. The internal blebs formed are then pinched off in a process that forms a larger vesicle containing numerous small 50-nm-diameter vesicles called exosomes. These exosomes carry the transferrin receptor on their surfaces with the extracellular domain directed into the cavity of the greater vesicle and the cytoplasmic domain into the interior of the exosome. This whole structure is referred to as the multivesicular endosome or body. By a much slower process, the multivesicular body fuses with the plasma membrane to release its contents (i.e., the exosomes) to the exterior by the process of exocytosis. This process represents a transferrin-receptor degradative pathway. It appears that the receptors attached to the exosomes undergo proteolytic cleavage, probably within the multivesicular body, such that a soluble proteolytic product of the intact receptor is released to the circulation (Baynes et al., 1994b). Little, if any, exosomally bound transferrin receptor is detectable in the circulation.

NONTRANSFERRIN-BOUND IRON

As indicated previously, iron can also be internalized into cells by other pathways that do not involve transferrin. These include the haptoglobin–hemoglobin complex, the hemopexin–heme complex, the iron–albumin complex, ferritin iron, and non–protein-bound iron. The organ most involved in clearing these forms of iron from the circulation is the liver. In most of these mechanisms the iron is delivered primarily into an endocytic vesicle, as with transferrin. Only in the case of the non–protein-bound form of iron does it appear that the iron is taken up directly across the plasma membrane.

POSTENDOCYTIC TRANSMEMBRANE IRON TRANSPORT

After the iron has been freed from its carrier protein by processes within the endocytic vesicle, the iron is still separated from the cytosol by the vesicle membrane. The process of transport across this membrane is becoming better understood. It appears likely that the iron, either after liberation from its carrier or during the transport process, undergoes reduction, which is possibly mediated by a membrane-associated ferrireductase. Current data suggest that the ferrous iron is then transported across the vesicle membrane into the cytoplasm by the DCT-1. This transport protein, also involved in uptake of ferrous iron and other divalent cations at the apical surface of the intestinal absorptive cells, acts as a symport, transporting both a divalent cation like Fe^{2+} together with a proton across the endosomal membrane into the cytosol.

CYTOSOLIC TRANSPORT

Once iron has successfully crossed the endosomal vesicle membrane into the cytosol, it enters the low-molecular-weight pool from which it is transported to sites where it is incorporated into heme, ferritin, and nonheme-iron proteins. The nature of the cytosolic transporters is unclear, as is the mechanism by which iron is delivered to such organelles as mitochondria.

THE RED CELL CYCLE

As shown in Table 36-1, the majority of body iron is present in hemoglobin in red blood cells and erythroid tissues; typically, hemoglobin iron represents about two thirds of the total body iron. Each day in the normal adult approximately 2×10^{11} red blood cells are produced, and this requires more than 2×10^{20} atoms, or almost 24 mg, of iron. The majority of this (~17 mg) is incorporated into hemoglobin. Clearly hemoglobin synthesis and red blood cell turnover dominate the events of iron homeostasis, and the daily turnover of body iron is more than 10 times the daily amount absorbed from the diet.

Iron is incorporated into red blood cells during their synthesis in the bone marrow.

Erythroblasts (nucleated, developing red blood cells) are synthesized by the bone marrow from stem cells. An erythroblast eventually loses its nucleus to become a reticulocyte and ultimately a mature red blood cell called an erythrocyte. Transferrin-bound iron is taken up by erythroblasts and is transported into the mitochondria to form heme. The incorporation of iron into protoporphyrin IX is catalyzed by the mitochondrial enzyme, ferrochelatase. The supply of iron to the erythroblast for hemoglobin synthesis is regulated in a feedback manner by heme, which inhibits release of iron from transferrin.

Once released from the bone marrow, mature erythrocytes circulate for approximately 120 days. As erythrocytes circulate in the blood, a number of physicochemical changes occur. These include oxidative damage with modification of membrane lipids and proteins, loss of surface sialic acid and electrostatic charge, the generation of advanced glycation end products, decreases in ion gradients, and metabolic depletion of glycolytic and other enzymes. Which of these changes or combinations is responsible for recognition of senescence is uncertain, but intact senescent cells are removed from the circulation by specialized macrophages of the liver, spleen, and bone marrow. Although quantitatively less significant, a fraction of red blood cell precursors will be removed during erythropoiesis by apoptotic processes, often described as "ineffective erythropoiesis."

Within the macrophage, hemoglobin iron is liberated by the action of the enzyme heme oxygenase (Fig. 36-10). Heme oxygenase is a substrate-inducible enzyme that catalyzes the cleavage of the α-methene bridge that joins the two pyrrole residues containing the vinyl substituents in the protoporphyrin; action of heme oxygenase releases Fe^{2+} from the tetrapyrrole structure, forming biliverdin, which is converted into bilirubin. The liberated iron enters the low-molecular-weight pool from which it is either incorporated into stores in the form of ferritin or is released into the interstitial fluid and circulation for recycling via transferrin. Iron is thought to be transported across the macrophage membrane as ferrous iron bound to the protein variously designated as IREG-1 (McKie et al., 2000), ferroportin (Donovan et al., 2000), or metal transport protein-1 (MTP1; Abboud and Haile, 2000). The iron, now in the plasma, undergoes oxidation by a ferroxidase (possibly ceruloplasmin) prior to uptake by circulating apoferric or monoferric transferrin. The macrophage system returns an almost equivalent amount of iron (approximately 22 mg Fe per day) to the plasma as is cleared from the circulation by the transferrin receptor mechanism.

Therefore, the iron in hemoglobin is scavenged and returned to the circulation where it exists as transferrin-bound iron. The process of transferrin iron delivery to erythroid bone marrow accounts for at least 80% of transferrin iron turnover. Most of this iron is used for synthesis of hemoglobin for new red blood cells. The other 20% of transferrin iron turnover is accounted for by delivery of iron to other cells, primarily to the liver.

If red blood cells are destroyed in the bloodstream and heme or hemoglobin is released into the bloodstream, these iron-containing compounds are bound by haptoglobin (which binds oxyhemoglobin dimers) or hemopexin and albumin (which bind heme and hematin). Normally, little free heme or hemoglobin exists in plasma, and these binding proteins are largely free of ligand. Nevertheless, these hemoglobin and heme-binding proteins do serve to remove and recycle any iron present in the plasma as free hemoglobin or heme, and they may be quantitatively important in conserving iron in hemolytic disease states. Because the protein complexes of heme and hemoglobin are too large to be filtered through the renal glomeruli, heme and hemoglobin are scavenged as long as sufficient ligand-free haptoglobin or hemopexin is present in the circulation. The haptoglobin–hemoglobin and hemopexin–heme complexes are taken up by the liver by receptor-mediated processes, and the iron is released by the action of heme oxygenase.

EXTERNAL IRON EXCHANGE AND IRON ABSORPTION

External iron exchange is concerned with the processes by which iron is either lost from or added to the body. Normally only approximately 0.05% (2 to 2.5 mg) of body iron is lost each day. This iron loss must be replaced by absorption of a similar amount of iron

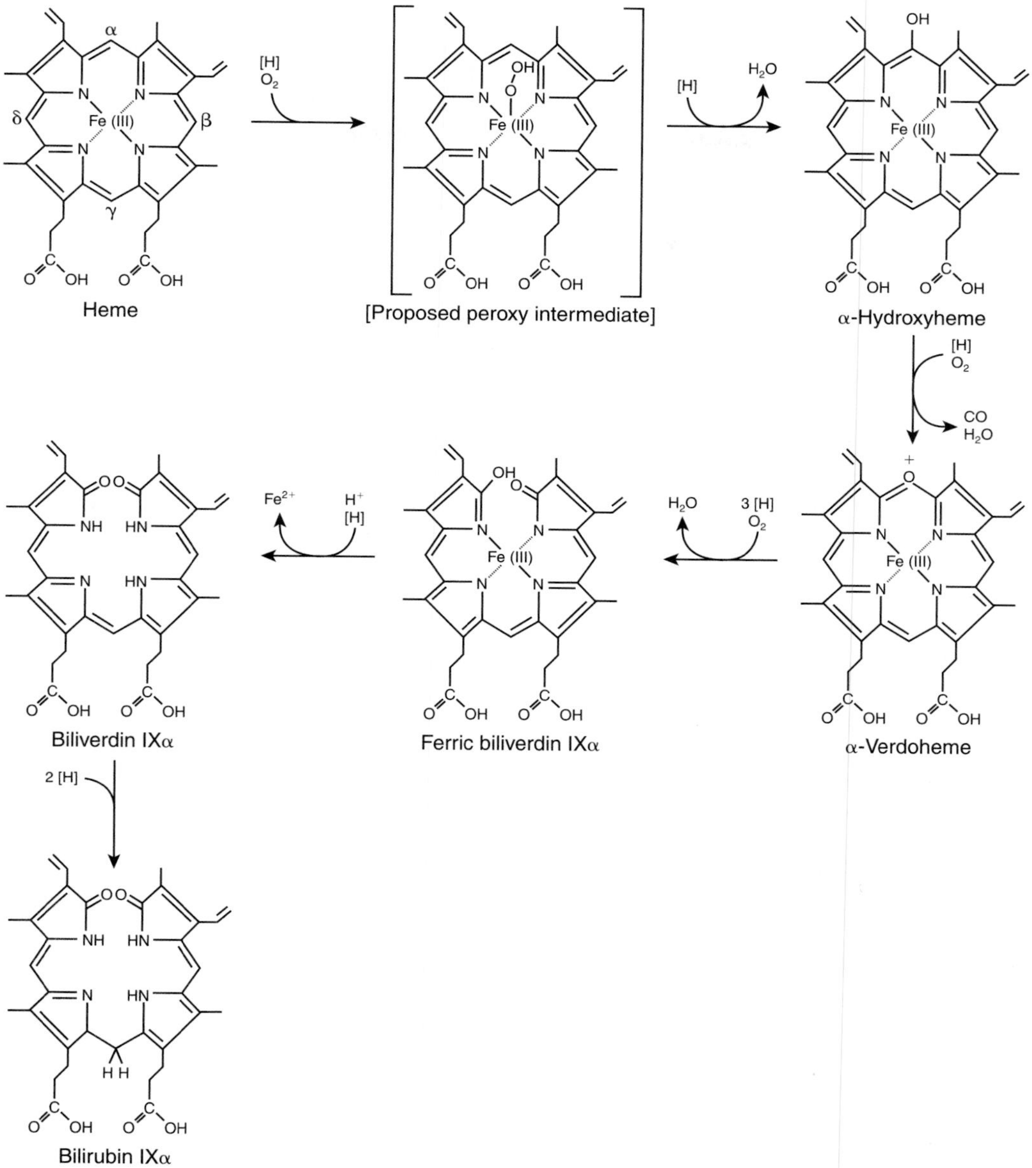

Figure 36-10 The sequence of reactions catalyzed by heme oxygenase in mammals. *(Modified from Crichton RR [2001] Inorganic Biochemistry of Iron Metabolism: From Molecular Mechanisms to Clinical Consequences, 2nd ed. John Wiley and Sons, New York, p 175.)*

from dietary sources. Net negative balance results when losses exceed absorption. When iron absorption is less than that needed to replace losses and to meet demands for growth, this ultimately results in a depletion of the functional iron compartment. When absorption exceeds losses, positive balance occurs as a result of growth or an increase in iron in the storage compartment. If positive iron balance is sustained in an adult, it may ultimately lead to iron overload.

IRON LOSSES AND REQUIREMENTS FOR ABSORBED IRON

In the basal state, iron is lost passively in cells that are shed from the skin surface or the epithelial lining of internal organs. Small amounts of red blood cells are also lost via the gastrointestinal tract. The normal amount of iron lost in men is on the order of 14 μg/kg/day. These losses are distributed among gastrointestinal tract, skin, and urinary tract in a ratio of 6:3:1. In a 70-kg man, this basal loss would average 0.98 mg/day. For a nonmenstruating 55 kg-woman, this would be 0.77 mg/day. The coefficient of variance for these estimates is calculated to be approximately 15%. In iron deficiency these losses may be reduced by 50%, whereas in iron overload these losses are slightly increased. Menstruation increases the amount of iron loss, and absorption of 1.36 mg of iron is the median requirement for maintenance of iron balance in normal menstruating women. To maintain balance in 95% of women, absorption of 2.84 mg/day of iron is required.

The other physiological cause of increased iron loss is pregnancy. Although a pregnant woman should be in positive iron balance during the course of the pregnancy, it is not unusual for the course of pregnancy and parturition to result in a net loss of iron from the mother's body. The iron requirements specific to pregnancy over the 9-month gestational period, for a 55-kg woman, are calculated to be 320 mg for basal losses, 360 mg for the products of conception (fetus, 270 mg; placenta and umbilical cord, 90 mg), and approximately 150 mg as peripartum blood loss. An additional 450 mg of iron is required for expanded maternal red cell mass; however, this iron will not be lost with parturition but will be returned to the mother during postpartum contraction of red cell mass. The greatest increases in total requirements (up to 6 mg of iron per day) are for fetal growth and erythroid expansion during the second and third trimesters, which are only slightly offset by the diminished loss of iron as a result of the amenorrhea of pregnancy. Lactation results in a further iron loss of 0.3 to 0.6 mg/day postpartum due to secretion in the milk, but this additional loss is largely balanced by the accompanying amenorrhea.

Growth markedly increases iron requirements for formation of both erythroid and nonerythroid tissues. Because of more-efficient oxygen delivery to tissues, the newborn infant initially experiences a decrease in hemoglobin concentration, with a shift of iron into stores. Growth and erythropoiesis exhaust this supply of iron within 6 months, so that in the first year of life the infant must absorb 0.3 mg of iron per day to maintain iron homeostasis. In the second year of life, growth causes this figure to rise to 0.4 mg/day. Slow growth from this time until puberty results in a gradual increase in requirements to 0.5 to 0.8 mg/day. Puberty and adolescent growth spurts increase iron requirements to 1.6 mg/day in young men and to 2.4 mg/day in young women. The higher requirement in young women reflects concomitant menarche.

Basal iron losses and physiologically enhanced losses as in menstruation, pregnancy, and lactation are normal iron losses. Iron loss may be increased in situations of pathological and nonpathological blood loss. Pathological losses occur in such situations as bleeding from the urinary, genital, and gastrointestinal tracts. The gastrointestinal tract is the most common site of pathological bleeding, secondary to conditions such as esophagitis, gastritis, varices, peptic ulcers, neoplasms, diverticulosis, angiodysplasia, and inflammatory bowel disease. In developing regions of the world, infection with parasites such as hookworm may increase iron loss. Heavy infestation may cause bleeding of sufficient magnitude to increase requirements of iron by as much as 3 to 5 mg/day. Nonpathological increases in blood loss may be secondary to the effects of aspirin or nonsteroidal antiinflammatory drugs, which may cause gastric bleeding, or to voluntary blood donation.

Stimulation of erythropoiesis by administered erythropoietin, which is used to treat various disease states (e.g., renal failure), or by endogenous erythropoietin, which is elevated in hemolytic states related to abnormalities in hemoglobin formation (e.g., thalassemia or sickle cell disease), further increases iron requirements. Endogenous erythropoietin production by the kidney is stimulated when oxygen delivery to the kidney is reduced, as in anemia.

IRON ABSORPTION

Intestinal iron absorption reflects a composite of three determinants: the iron content of the diet, the bioavailability of the dietary iron, and the capacity of the mucosal cells to absorb the iron. In terms of the iron content of the diet, Western diets have remarkably consistent iron contents, averaging 6 mg/1,000 kcal. Iron in Western diets tends to be highly bioavailable, with an estimated iron availability in the range of 14% to 17%. Therefore, a 2,000-kcal diet should provide about 1.8 mg of absorbed iron/day. Clearly, it is difficult for many women with normal activity levels to obtain sufficient iron from the diet alone.

Methods Used to Assess Iron Absorption

A number of in vitro and animal models have been evaluated in an attempt to predict iron absorption in humans. In vitro methods generally simulate in vivo digestive processes, including acid hydrolysis, proteolytic digestion, and the addition of bile acids. The amount of released soluble low-molecular-weight iron is then determined. Such methods give a crude prediction of food iron bioavailability. These in vitro techniques are at best indicators of trends in bioavailability rather than indicators of absolute levels of iron absorption.

A variety of experimental animals have been used as models for studying iron absorption, and a number of important proteins involved in iron absorption have been recently identified in animal studies. Absorption of radioisotopes of iron has been evaluated in whole animals and in isolated gut loops. The most widely used animals for these studies have been the rat and the mouse, but significant disparities in nonheme iron absorption have been well documented between rodents and humans. This makes the rodent model unsuitable as a predictor of human iron absorption (Reddy and Cook, 1993). However, once genes involved in iron absorption have been identified in rodents, their presence in the human genome makes their involvement in the absorption process highly probable. Other animals have been evaluated only partially as models for studying human iron absorption, but studies of human iron absorption ultimately must be done in humans.

Prior to the ready availability of radioisotopes, iron balance techniques were employed to evaluate human iron bioavailability. Prolonged stool collections make this a cumbersome method, and the small amounts of iron absorbed each day (i.e., the small difference between intake and fecal excretion) result in this approach being highly inaccurate. Likewise, measurements of increases in plasma iron concentration with iron intake also are of marginal value for assessing food iron bioavailability, given variable absorption and the multicompartmental kinetics involved. Changes in plasma iron levels following pharmacological doses of iron, however, are useful as a crude screening test for gastrointestinal malabsorption of iron.

Progress in defining iron bioavailability and iron absorption was facilitated in past decades by the use in humans of radioisotopes. Absorption was estimated from the amount of radioiron (either ^{59}Fe or ^{55}Fe) incorporated into circulating erythrocytes 2 to 3 weeks after ingestion of the radioactive label, or whole-body counters were used to assess whole-body retention of radioiron. Foods under study could be labeled either intrinsically or by extrinsic tagging. Intrinsic labeling relies on either hydroponic cultivation of vegetable material or biosynthetic labeling of animal material. Extrinsic tagging is a simpler and valid indicator of bioavailability and absorption because the extrinsic iron enters a common pool with intrinsic iron; enhancing and inhibitory influences affect the common pool in aggregate, and neither affect the intrinsic or extrinsic pool selectively. It was initially observed that when a small amount of soluble inorganic iron was added to a food item of vegetable origin just before it was eaten, the added iron was absorbed in an identical manner to the food iron. This is the principle of extrinsic tagging: When a number of foodstuffs are eaten together, their nonheme iron forms a common pool within the gastrointestinal tract, and this is the pool that is labeled by the extrinsic radioactive tag.

To facilitate comparison of different iron absorption studies, it is desirable to factor out the effect of variations in body iron status on absorption. This has been done by administering a standard reference dose of radiolabeled inorganic iron containing 3 mg of iron as ferrous ascorbate. The ratio of absorption from a given meal to that from the reference dose can be used to measure the relative bioavailability of the nonheme iron in the meal. Clear disadvantages of this method are that additional isotope must be ingested and that day-to-day variability in individual absorption may affect the results. Serum ferritin concentration, an excellent marker of body iron stores, provides as useful a correction and comparison factor as does the reference iron absorption and may be used instead.

Because of general concern about radioisotopes in human subjects, particularly in children and pregnant women, stable isotopes of iron including ^{54}Fe, ^{56}Fe, ^{57}Fe, and ^{58}Fe have been evaluated as alternative tracers. These techniques are still in their infancy, are extremely costly, and require highly sophisticated laboratory facilities. However, it is very likely that, as the technology is refined, use of stable isotopes will replace the ^{55}Fe and ^{59}Fe methodologies.

Much of what is known of iron bioavailability in the diet and iron absorption is based upon single-meal studies in which the single meal was isotopically labeled. The study protocol, however, is not reflective of the usual conditions pertaining during the absorptive process because the test includes a protracted fast, the meal administration, and a subsequent period of fasting. Significant discrepancies have recently been documented between putative promotory ligands (e.g., ascorbic acid) and inhibitory factors (e.g., soy protein) as documented by single-meal studies when compared with a lack of effect of these factors over the course of longitudinal studies of iron absorption. Data comparing results of long-term studies of labeled diets with results of single-meal studies have clearly established that single-meal studies tend to grossly exaggerate enhancing or inhibitory influences (Cook et al., 1991). Although single-meal studies are very useful for evaluation of iron absorption in populations consuming simple diets that consist largely of a single staple, they are relatively unhelpful in the evaluation of more complex diets as consumed in the developed world.

Heme Iron Absorption

Hemoglobin and myoglobin are the major protein sources from which heme iron is derived, and foods derived from animal tissues are the predominant sources of heme iron. Heme iron in meat is an important source of dietary iron, not only because of its intrinsic high bioavailability but also because a "meat factor" enhances the bioavailability of the nonheme iron present in the diet. Consequently, in developed regions where heme iron accounts for approximately 10% to 15% of total dietary iron, heme iron accounts for 35% of the iron actually absorbed. In population studies in developed communities, meat ingestion is the major determinant of iron status.

Heme is released from hemoglobin during digestion in the small intestine. This is a rapid process, with 70% of a specific hemoglobin dose being converted to heme within 30 minutes of ingestion in a dog model. Heme fed by itself is poorly absorbed, possibly due to the formation of relatively nonabsorbable heme polymers, but this is largely only of mechanistic interest because heme is not usually consumed in its free form. The globin moiety and other proteins present in the diet appear, during digestion, to yield residues that inhibit heme polymerization and maintain it in free, absorbable form. The heme is thought to bind to a specific receptor and to be taken up by enterocytes via endocytosis. The heme moiety is then catabolized within the mucosal cell by heme oxygenase. The release of iron from heme by heme oxygenase appears to be the rate-limiting step in absorption of heme iron. After heme degradation, the liberated iron appears to enter a common iron pool that also includes absorbed nonheme iron; further transport either into mucosal cellular stores of ferritin or across the basolateral membrane of the enterocyte into the interstitial fluid occurs from this common iron pool.

When physiological amounts of heme iron, ranging from 0.25 mg to 6 mg, are ingested with food, a linear increase in the amount of heme iron absorbed occurs, reflecting a constant percentage absorption of heme iron over this range. Luminal factors other than the presence of proteins to protect against heme polymerization do not appear to influence heme iron absorption. Although heme iron absorption is inversely correlated with body iron status, this relationship is much less pronounced than in the case of nonheme iron. Indeed, the slopes of the regression lines describing the relationship have been calculated to be −0.358 for heme iron as compared with −0.936 for nonheme iron. This has two obvious ramifications. First, iron deficiency is least likely in areas of significant meat consumption. Second, iron overload is most likely in these same areas. These data all suggest that heme iron absorption is less regulated in response to iron status than is nonheme iron absorption.

Nonheme Iron Absorption

Nonheme iron is the largest component of dietary iron. Its absorption, as determined in single-meal studies, is influenced by the balance between a large number of potentially enhancing and inhibitory influences. These influences, however, appear to be more important in the setting of diets consisting of a single staple or only a few foods, as consumed in certain less-developed regions of the world, than in developed regions where multicomponent mixed diets are the rule.

Nonheme iron compounds are found in foods of both plant and animal origin. Iron in plants is present in three major forms: as metalloproteins, with the predominant example being plant ferritin; as soluble iron in the sap of xylem, phloem, and plant vacuoles; and as nonfunctional iron complexed either to plant structural components or to storage compounds predominantly in the form of phytates (inositol hexaphosphates or pentaphosphates). A large amount of dietary nonheme iron is present as contaminant ferric oxides and hydroxides. Nonheme iron in animal-derived food is found in many forms, including ferritin and hemosiderin in meat products, iron bound to the phosphoprotein phosphovitin in egg yolk, and iron in milk bound to lactoferrin or associated with fat globule membranes and low-molecular-weight compounds such as citrate. Nonheme iron in the form of ferritin, hemosiderin, contaminating oxides, and hydroxides, as well as certain formulations of iron added in food fortification or enrichment or taken as supplements, enter the common iron pool poorly and may contribute little, if at all, to the overall iron economy.

Once nonheme food iron enters the alimentary canal, it is acted upon by the gastric juices containing pepsin and hydrochloric acid. Because the acid appears to be important in reducing ferric to ferrous iron, the effect of achlorhydria (lack of hydrochloric acid in the gastric juice) is most pronounced on absorption of ferric rather than ferrous iron salts. As iron enters the duodenum and pH rises, the ferric iron is rapidly precipitated as ferric oxyhydroxides, whereas the ferrous iron remains relatively soluble as pH rises. Uptake into the mucosal cell occurs rapidly, with the greatest proportion being taken up within the first 5 minutes after the digesta enters the duodenum, and with ferrous salts being better absorbed than ferric salts. The solubility of iron in the duodenum can be greatly modified by the presence of various ligands.

Molecular Mechanisms of Nonheme Iron Absorption

The mechanisms by which luminal nonheme iron crosses the mucosal cell membrane to enter the enterocyte and is then transferred to the circulation have become much more clearly understood in the last few years, largely as a result of the identification of a number of new proteins that appear to be involved in mucosal iron absorption (Fig. 36-11). Nonheme dietary iron seems to be taken across the brush-border membrane of the enterocyte, after reduction of any Fe^{3+} to Fe^{2+} by an apical membrane–bound ferri-reductase, by DCT-1. Within the intestinal cell, Fe^{2+} derived from both heme and nonheme Fe^{2+} enters a low-molecular-weight pool. This iron can either be stored in ferritin in the mucosal cell or it can be transported across the basolateral membrane by the transmembrane transporter protein, IREG-1, to reach the interstitial fluid/plasma. The incorporation of iron into the apotransferrin of plasma may be facilitated by the oxidation of Fe^{2+} to Fe^{3+}, either by hephaestin, a membrane-bound protein, or by ceruloplasmin, the principal copper-containing protein of serum.

The first Fe^{2+} transport protein to be discovered was DCT-1. In microcytic anemia (*mk*) mice, which have an autosomal recessive inherited defect in intestinal iron transport, the transport defect was shown by positional cloning to be due to a missense mutation (G185R) in the murine natural resistance–associated macrophage protein gene *Nramp2*

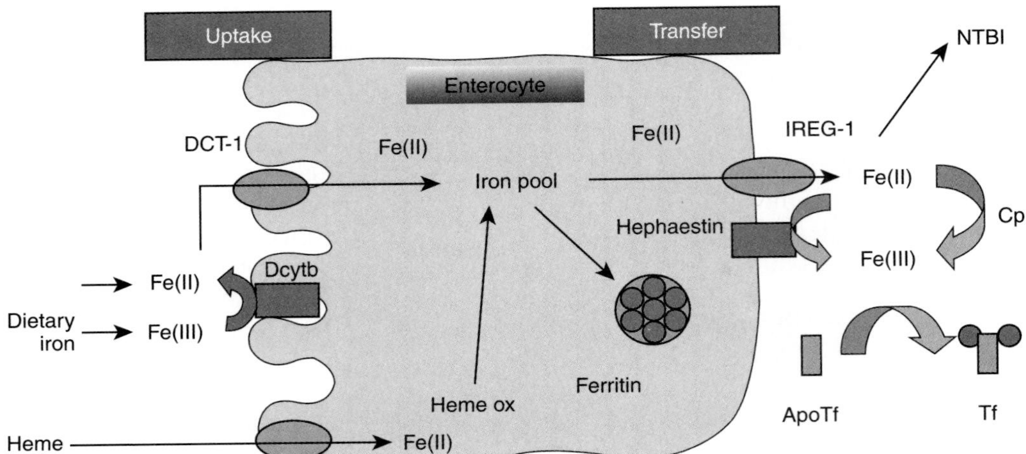

Figure 36-11 Schematic representation of iron absorption in normal subjects. Iron is taken up from the gastrointestinal tract either as heme or nonheme iron. The former is degraded to release Fe(II) by heme oxygenase, whereas the latter is reduced by DcytB and transported across the apical membrane by DCT-1. Within the enterocyte the iron pool can equilibrate with the intracellular storage protein ferritin. At the basolateral membrane, iron is transported out of the cell by IREG-1; its incorporation into apotransferrin may be aided by the ferroxidase activity of hephaestin. *Dcytb,* Duodenal cytochrome b; *DCT1,* divalent cation transporter protein 1; *IREG-1,* iron-regulated transporter-1; *Heme ox,* heme oxygenase; *Cp,* ceruloplasmin; *Tf,* transferrin; *NTBI,* non–transferrin-bound iron. *(Redrawn from Crichton RR [2001] Inorganic Biochemistry of Iron Metabolism: From Molecular Mechanisms to Clinical Consequences, 2nd ed. John Wiley and Sons, New York, p 213.)*

(now designated as *DCT1*) (Fleming et al., 1997). At around the same time DCT-1 was identified as a new metal-ion transporter in the rat (Gunshin et al., 1997), with broad substrate specificity. DCT-1 is not specific for Fe^{2+} and transports other divalent metal ions, including cobalt, copper, manganese, nickel, and zinc (Gunshin et al., 1997). The metal ion transport is coupled to cotransport of a proton and depends on the cell membrane potential. The DCT-1 protein has 12 putative membrane-spanning domains, is expressed at the highest levels in the proximal duodenum, and is upregulated by dietary iron deficiency (Gunshin et al., 1997). The Belgrade rat, which has an autosomal recessively inherited anemia, associated with both abnormal reticulocyte iron uptake and abnormal gastrointestinal iron absorption, has the same missense mutation in *DCT-1* as the *mk* mouse (Fleming et al., 1998). There are two mRNAs for DCT-1, one of which has an IRE in its 3′-UTR; expression of this DCT-1 mRNA with the IRE is upregulated in the proximal duodenum during dietary iron starvation (Canonne-Hergaux et al., 1999). DCT-1 is localized in the apical membrane of the cultured human intestinal epithelial Caco-2 cells, where it functions as a proton-dependent iron transport mechanism with a marked preference for iron over other divalent cations (Tandy et al., 2000).

Evidence for a duodenal ferric reductase has been around for some time, but the gene for this enzyme has been identified only recently. Dcytb (for duodenal cytochrome *b*) encodes a plasma membrane di-heme protein (McKie et al., 2001). The amino acid sequence encoded by Dcytb has around 50% similarity to the cytochrome b_{561} family of plasma membrane reductases, and Dcytb is highly expressed in the brush-border membrane of duodenal enterocytes. When Dcytb cDNA is expressed in *Xenopus* oocytes and cultured cells, ferric reductase activity is found. The expression of both Dcytb mRNA and protein in the duodenum are regulated by changes in physiological modulators of iron absorption, indicating that Dcytb represents an important component of the iron absorption pathway.

Once nonheme iron enters the enterocyte, it enters a low-molecular-weight pool. From this pool, the iron may be rapidly transported across the basolateral membrane into the interstitial fluid from where it enters the systemic circulation by a mechanism that is discussed in subsequent text. Alternatively, the iron taken up from the lumen of the gastrointestinal tract can be stored within enterocytes in the iron storage protein ferritin. There appears to be little release of iron from ferritin in the enterocyte once it has been stored; the majority of enterocyte ferritin is apparently destined for excretion via the process of shedding of mucosal cells.

Other proteins have been recently identified that are involved in iron transfer across the basolateral membrane into the circulation, where the natural acceptor is assumed to be apotransferrin. These are hephaestin and IREG-1. The first of these was discovered in sex-linked anemia (sla) mice, which have a genetically inherited block in intestinal iron transport and develop a severe anemia; iron uptake from the intestinal lumen is normal in these mice, but they fail to transfer it to the circulation. Hence, iron accumulates in the enterocytes and is lost during the subsequent turnover of the intestinal epithelium. The mutant gene in sla mice was identified and designated *Heph*; it encodes hephaestin, a transmembrane-bound ceruloplasmin homolog that is highly expressed in intestine (Vulpe et al., 1999). Hephaestin is a multicopper ferroxidase that is inserted into the basolateral membrane by a GPI (glycophosphoinositol)-anchor. Hephaestin may act, together with the basolateral iron transporter IREG-1, to load iron onto apotransferrin.

The basolateral ferrous iron transporter IREG-1 was found almost simultaneously by three groups (Abboud and Haile, 2000; Donovan et al., 2000; McKie et al., 2000). The iron-regulated gene *IREG-1* was identified by subtractive cloning techniques and isolated from duodenal mucosa of homozygous atransferrinemic mice, which have high levels of iron absorption (McKie et al., 2000). IREG-1 is a transmembrane protein, with 10 potential membrane-spanning regions, that localizes to the basolateral membrane of polarized epithelial cells. Both IREG-1 mRNA and IREG-1 protein levels are increased under conditions of increased iron absorption, although, curiously, the 5′-UTR of IREG-1 mRNA contains a functional IRE. Ferroportin a multiple transmembrane–domain protein, was identified as the gene product responsible for hypochromic anemia in zebrafish (Donovan et al., 2000); and MTP-1 (metal transporter protein), expressed in the reticuloendothelial system, the duodenum, and the uterus of pregnant mice, was also reported at about the same time (Abboud and Haile, 2000). The nucleotide sequences coding for ferroportin, MTP-1, and IREG-1 were all found to be identical, however, demonstrating that IREG-1, MTP-1, and ferroportin all refer to the same gene product.

Practical Considerations Concerning Nonheme Iron Absorption

After iron enters the common luminal pool, it is subject to interactions with a number of ligands contained in the food, as well as other food constituents that affect its absorption. Based on a large number of predominantly single food studies, foods can be classified as having low, intermediate, or high iron bioavailability, as shown in Box 36-3. These data are based largely on single-meal studies (Bothwell et al., 1989), which in all likelihood exaggerate the effects on iron bioavailability over those likely to be observed from a normal mixed diet. The tabulation reflects the net effect of the composite of both enhancing and inhibitory ligands consumed as part of the single food under test.

The major ligands in foods that enhance nonheme iron absorption appear to be the organic acids, including ascorbic, citric, malic, and lactic acids. These organic acids are particularly found in citrus and deciduous fruits. These organic acids, when tested in single-meal studies, all appear to increase nonheme iron absorption, but their significance in mixed diets is less clear. Studies of the effects of chronic ingestion of high doses of vitamin C or multivitamin supplements failed to show any effects of ascorbic acid on long-term iron status in subjects consuming mixed diets. This may reflect the importance of duodenal iron reduction in the mechanism of iron absorption.

A large number of inhibitory ligands are found in ingested foods. These include phytates, polyphenols, calcium, and fiber. Phytates are widely distributed in various grains and

Box 36-3

RELATIVE BIOAVAILABILITY OF NONHEME IRON IN A NUMBER OF FOODS

Foods	Low	Intermediate	High
Cereals	Maize	Corn flour	
	Oatmeal	White flour	
	Rice		
	Sorghum		
	Whole wheat flour		
Fruits	Apple	Cantaloupe	Guava
	Avocado	Mango	Lemon
	Banana	Pineapple	Orange
	Grape		Papaw
	Peach		Tomato
	Pear		
	Plum		
	Rhubarb		
	Strawberry		
Vegetables	Eggplant	Carrot	Beetroot
	Legumes	Potato	Broccoli
	Soy flour		Cabbage
	Isolated soy protein		Cauliflower
			Pumpkin
			Turnip
Beverages	Tea	Red wine	White wine
	Coffee		
Nuts	Almond		
	Brazil		
	Coconut		
	Peanut		
	Walnut		
Animal proteins	Cheese		Fish
	Egg		Meat
	Milk		Poultry

vegetable foods and particularly limit iron absorption by the formation of diferric and tetraferric phytate complexes. Polyphenols are also widely distributed in various vegetables and are found in beverages such as tea and coffee. In single-meal studies, polyphenols and phytate are profoundly inhibitory of iron absorption, but their impact on iron nutrition when consumed as part of a mixed diet is not well-defined. Calcium may also inhibit nonheme iron absorption. The effect of calcium is most prominent when the basal meal is one of relatively poor iron bioavailability. Finally, certain components of dietary fiber cause a modest reduction in nonheme iron absorption.

Nonheme iron absorption from meals containing significant amounts of vegetable-derived protein, such as soybeans, other legumes, and nuts, tends to be inhibited. Although these foods contain a number of other inhibitory ligands, including phytates and polyphenols, there appears to be a close relationship between the presence of intact vegetable protein and the degree of inhibition of iron absorption. Indeed, the inhibitory effect of soy protein is progressively reduced by increasing the extent of protein hydrolysis (e.g., as produced by fermentation) to the point at which products such as miso and soy sauce actually act as promoters of iron absorption in single-meal studies. Vegetable protein products may also bind to polyphenols and reduce their inhibitory effects on nonheme iron absorption. Consequently, nonheme iron absorption reflects not only iron–ligand interactions but also ligand–ligand interactions.

Animal tissue protein is a rich source of highly absorbable heme iron and also has a marked enhancing effect on nonheme iron absorption. The nature of this "meat factor" that enhances nonheme iron absorption is the subject of much current investigation. Various mechanisms have been suggested, including an interaction of cysteine residues or carboxylate groups of the proteins with luminal nonheme iron to maintain iron in a soluble form, enhanced gastric acid production in response to meat ingestion, and interactions between phytates and meat-derived peptides that reduce the inhibitory effects of phytate.

Regulation of Mucosal Iron Absorption

Nonheme iron absorption is regulated both at the luminal brush-border membrane absorptive site and the basolateral membrane transfer sites, whereas the regulation of heme iron absorption appears to reside predominantly at the transcellular and basolateral transmembrane transfer sites. Mucosal conditioning appears to occur in the crypts of the intestinal villus, with a delay on the order of 24 to 48 hours before this is reflected in altered absorption by the enterocytes. This delay corresponds to the time for migration of cells from crypt to villous apex. Regulation at the level of the mucosal cell is reflected in reduced absorption on a high-iron diet, but the most significant regulatory determinants of mucosal iron absorption are the amount of iron in the body iron stores and the level of erythropoiesis (red cell development) (Finch, 1994). There is a reciprocal relationship between body iron stores and iron absorption: as stores decline, absorption increases (Finch, 1994).

Two key regulators of iron absorption that reflect the level of iron stores have recently been identified, namely hepcidin, an antimicrobial peptide synthesized in the liver (Ganz, 2003), and hemojuvelin, a 426-residue protein that shows homology to a molecule involved in axonal guidance in the central nervous system (Papanikolaou et al., 2004). Hepcidin is an antimicrobial peptide synthesized in the liver (Ganz, 2003), which was shown in animal studies to be involved in the regulation of iron homeostasis (Nicolas et al., 2001; Pigeon et al., 2001). The mRNA for murine hepcidin is upregulated in dietary or parenteral iron overload as well as by immune stimuli (treatment with lipopolysaccharide). Hepcidin is a negative regulator of iron uptake in the small intestine and of iron release from macrophages. Thus, a deficiency of hepcidin in mice leads to iron overload in liver (due to hyperabsorption of iron in the small intestine) but not in spleen (due to unregulated iron release from macrophages leading to the presence of iron-depleted macrophages in the spleen). In contrast, transgenic mice that constitutively overexpressed hepcidin died within a few hours of birth of severe anemia (Nicolas et al., 2002). In a study of two patients with hepatic adenomas and severe iron refractory anemias, similar to the mouse overexpression model, Weinstein and colleagues (2002) showed that removal of the tumor fully reversed the hematological abnormalities. The resected tumors were shown to overexpress hepcidin mRNA, suggesting that overproduction of hepcidin in these patients was the cause of their anemia. It has been suggested that hepcidin is the long awaited iron regulatory hormone (Fleming and Sly, 2001). In the absence of hepcidin, there is both hyperabsorption of iron from the gut, causing iron overload, and unregulated release of iron from macrophages, causing splenic iron depletion.

Subsequent studies have confirmed that infection and inflammation induce hepcidin synthesis. Up to a 100-fold increase in urinary hepcidin excretion was observed in patients with anemia of chronic infection (Nemeth et al., 2003), and studies in human liver cell cultures, in mice, and in human volunteers showed that interleukin-6 (IL-6) is the necessary and sufficient cytokine for the induction of hepcidin during inflammation

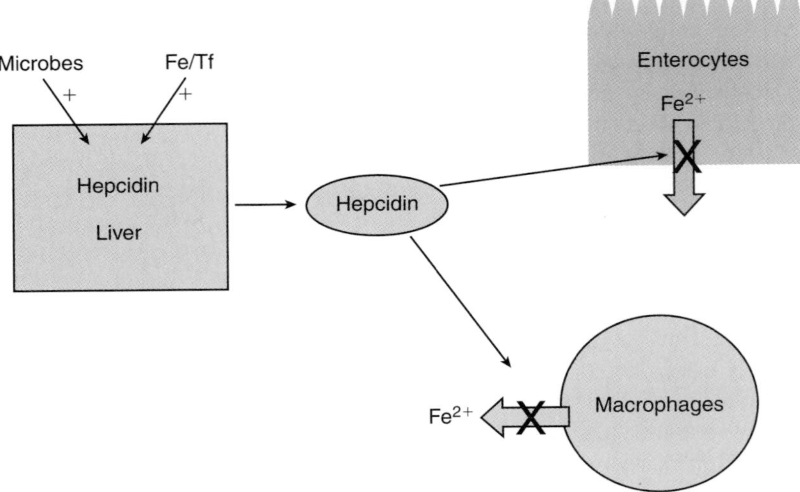

Figure 36-12 Hepcidin synthesis in the liver and its effects on iron metabolism. Hepatic sinusoids are lined by endothelial cells and Kupffer cells. Exposure of these cells to microbes or highly iron-saturated transferrin (Fe/Tf) causes the release of interleukin-6 (IL-6) and possibly other signals *(arrows)* that act on hepatocytes to induce the synthesis and secretion of hepcidin. Plasma hepcidin inhibits iron uptake from enterocytes in the duodenum into the circulation and inhibits iron release from macrophages in the spleen and elsewhere.

(Nemeth et al., 2004). Our current thinking on the role of hepcidin in iron metabolism is illustrated in Figure 36-12 (Ganz, 2003). Exposure of the cells lining the hepatic sinusoids to microbes or highly iron-saturated transferrin causes release of IL-6, and possibly of other signals, which induces the synthesis and secretion of hepcidin into the circulation. The plasma hepcidin binds IREG-1 (ferroportin) and blocks iron uptake from villous cells of the duodenum and prevents iron release from macrophages in the spleen and elsewhere.

Although little is known at present concerning the way in which hemojuvelin functions, it has become clear that its action involves the regulation of hepcidin expression in an as-yet-unidentified manner. This iron-dependent signalling pathway requires the presence of hemojuvelin, HFE, and probably also transferrin receptor-2 (TFR2, a member of the transferrin receptor family of unknown function).

Iron absorption is also increased by an enhanced erythropoietic activity. The rate of erythropoiesis is regulated by the concentration of erythropoietin, produced by the kidneys.

RECOMMENDED DIETARY INTAKES OF IRON

The Institute of Medicine (IOM, 2001) based the estimated average requirements (EARs) and recommended dietary allowances (RDAs) for iron on factorial modeling of iron needs. The components of iron requirements included basal iron losses, menstrual losses, and iron accretion during pregnancy and growth. An adequate intake was set for infants from 0 to 6 months of age; this was calculated as the average iron concentration of human milk (0.35 mg/L) times the average intake of breast milk (0.78 L), and is 0.27 mg/day of iron.

The EAR for infants from 7 to 12 months of age, 6.9 mg/day, was based on the sum of the average requirements for absorbed iron for iron deposition (0.43 mg/day) and for replacement of basal iron losses (0.26 mg/day) corrected for a moderate bioavailability of 10%. The RDA was similarly calculated, but based on the requirement of the 97.5th percentile group, and is 11 mg/day of iron. EARs and RDAs were similarly calculated for growing children and adolescents except that a bioavailability of 18% was applied to convert the need for absorbed iron to the need for dietary iron. Replacement of menstrual iron losses was also considered for adolescent girls aged 14 to 18. The EARs range from 3.0 mg/day for children 1 to 3 years of age to 7.9 mg/day for girls aged 14 to 18 years; the RDAs range from 7 mg/day to 15 mg/day, respectively.

For adult men and postmenopausal women, the basal loss (0.014 mg/kg/day) was the only component used to estimate total needs for absorbed iron, and the need for absorbed iron was modeled at the 50th percentile for the EAR and at the 97.5th percentile for the RDA. A bioavailability of 18% was assumed. This approach yielded EARs of 6 mg/day for men of all ages and 5 mg/day of iron for women over 50 years of age. The RDA was set at 8 mg/day of iron for men and postmenopausal women. For women aged 19 to 50 years, menstrual losses were calculated to average 0.51 mg/day over a 28-day cycle. The need for iron to replace menstrual losses was added to the basal loss to yield an EAR and RDA of 8.1 mg/day and 18 mg/day, respectively, for women of child-bearing age.

For pregnant women, an additional allowance was added to allow for iron deposition in the fetus and related tissues and for expansion of hemoglobin mass; these amounted to 2.0 mg/day and 2.7 mg/day, respectively, during the third trimester of pregnancy. Iron bioavailability was considered to be 25% during pregnancy. The EAR and RDA for pregnant women (aged 19-50 years) are 22 mg/day and 27 mg/day, respectively. Similarly, for lactating women, an additional allowance was added to cover the replacement of the iron secreted in human milk (0.27 mg/day). The EAR and RDA for lactating women (aged 19-50 years) are 6.5 mg/day and 9 mg/day, respectively.

Based on the third National Health and Nutrition Examination Survey (NHANES III) (1988-1994), the median intake of iron from food is about 17.5 mg/day for adult men (aged 19-70 years) and 12.1 mg/day for adult women; the 5th and 95th percentile intakes were 10 to 31 mg/day for men and 7 to 21 mg/day for women (IOM, 2001). When iron intake from both food and supplements are considered,

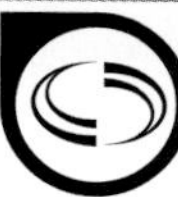

RDAs Across the Life Cycle

	mg Iron per Day
Infants	
0 to 0.5 yr	0.27 (AI)
0.5 to 1 yr	11
Children	
1 to 3 yr	7
4 to 8 yr	10
9 to 13 yr	8
Males	
14 to 18 yr	11
19 to >70 yr	8
Females	
14 to 18 yr	15
Pregnant	27
Lactating	10
19 to 50 yr	18
Pregnant	27
Lactating	9
>50 yr	8

Data from Institute of Medicine (IOM) (2001) Dietary Reference Intakes for Vitamin A, Vitamin K, Arsenic, Boron, Chromium, Copper, Iodine, Iron, Manganese, Molybdenum, Nickel, Silicon, Vanadium, and Zinc. National Academy Press, Washington, DC.
AI, Adequate intake.

median intake is 18.4 mg/day for men and 13 mg/day for women.

Recommendations for iron intake deserve careful consideration. Iron deficiency severe enough to result in anemia is associated with significant morbidity, whereas uncontrolled iron absorption, as in hemochromatosis, causes multiorgan failure. The prevalence of iron deficiency anemia in the United States is very low. The implication is that current iron consumption is adequate, because iron deficiency without anemia is not associated with any proven liability. The data, however, indicate that, along with a reduction in iron deficiency anemia, a rise has occurred in the iron stores in American men and postmenopausal women. The epidemiological data indicating potential liabilities of such a modest increase in body iron have resulted in the recommended daily iron intake becoming a highly controversial

Food Sources

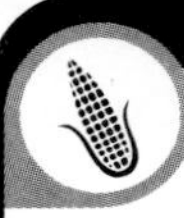

Food Sources of Iron

Meats and Fish

12 to 24 mg per 3 oz clams
6 mg per 3 oz oysters
5 mg per 3 oz beef liver
2 to 3 mg per 3 oz beef chuck or round
2 mg per 3 oz turkey
2 mg per 3 oz lamb

Legumes

4.5 mg per ½ cup soybeans
3 mg per ½ cup lentils
2.5 mg per ½ cup kidney or garbanzo beans
2 mg per ½ cup limas, navy, great northern, or black beans

Other Vegetables and Fruits

2 to 3 mg per ½ cup spinach
2 mg per ½ cup pumpkin
1 to 2 mg per ½ cup tomatoes
1.5 mg per ½ cup sour cherries
1.8 mg per ½ cup raisins
1 mg per ½ cup green peas
1 mg per ½ cup sweet potatoes

Cereal and Grain Products (whole grain, enriched, or fortified)

4 to 18 mg per cup ready-to-eat cereals
3 to 3.5 mg per 3 oz bagel
3 mg per 3 oz graham crackers
2.5 mg per 10 pretzels (2 oz)
1 mg per ½ cup egg noodles
1 mg per ½ cup rice
1 mg per ½ cup couscous

Miscellaneous

2.6 mg per 3 oz semisweet chocolate
3.5 mg per 1 Tbsp blackstrap molasses

Data from U.S. Department of Agriculture/Agricultural Research Service (USDA/ARS) (2005) USDA Nutrient Database for Standard Reference, Release 18. USDA/ARS, Washington, DC. Retrieved December 16, 2005 from www.ars.usda.gov/ba/bhnrc/ndl/.

area, with the debate ranging over such areas as whether the recommendations for intake should factor in positive storage balance, how best to define the iron status of a population, whether a safe upper limit rather than a recommended daily allowance should be the guideline for all groups not at high risk for iron deficiency, and whether the diet is excessively fortified (Lynch and Baynes, 1996). In regions where the diet is less varied and its iron content is less bioavailable, a higher recommended daily iron intake is needed to meet the requirement for absorbed iron.

ASSESSMENT OF IRON STATUS

Much of the confusion relating to prevalence of iron deficiency is a function of the mechanisms used to evaluate iron status of either individuals or populations. To evaluate optimally a population or individual, it is important to define which iron compartment is being assessed and which test is being used to evaluate the compartment in question.

MEASUREMENTS OF IRON STATUS

The single best measure to assess stores noninvasively is the serum ferritin concentration, because in the range of 20 to 200 μg/L, it bears a quantitative relationship to iron stores, with each 1 μg/L being indicative of 8 mg of storage iron. Careful phlebotomy studies (in which blood was slowly and systematically removed from the volunteer to deplete the stores without rendering the person anemic) have shown that serum ferritin concentrations decrease until stores are exhausted, which is indicated by a serum ferritin of 12 μg/L. Beyond this point, the functional compartment becomes depleted. Serum ferritin concentration shows little, but somewhat erratic, further reduction as the functional compartment becomes depleted. It should be noted, however, that alcohol consumption, infection, inflammation, neoplasia, and hepatic dysfunction may all spuriously raise the serum ferritin concentration relative to stores and, therefore, result in a misleadingly high serum ferritin concentration. The size of stores also can be assessed invasively by measurements of the iron content of bone marrow or liver biopsies or by quantitative phlebotomy as just outlined. These latter methods, however, are unsuitable for routine use. Recent developments in magnetic resonance imaging may allow iron stores to be assessed noninvasively.

At the point when stores are exhausted, the transport compartment begins to become depleted. This is best evaluated by measurements of serum iron, transferrin, and the percentage saturation of transferrin. Once the percent iron saturation of transferrin drops below 16%, iron supply becomes limited for tissue needs and erythropoietic requirements. At this point, functional depletion commences.

To assess functional compartment depletion of iron, the useful measurements include the mean red blood cell volume and the red blood cell free erythrocyte protoporphyrin. These, however, become abnormal relatively late in the development of functional depletion because red blood cells survive in the circulation for a relatively long period (~120 days). A better measure of functional iron depletion is the soluble form of the transferrin receptor (Baynes et al., 1994b); this soluble form of transferrin receptor is the extracellular domain released by proteolytic cleavage at the surface of the exosome. The cleavage occurs between arginine 100 and leucine 101 and is mediated by a membrane-associated serine protease (Baynes et al., 1994a). The concentration of this cleavage product of transferrin receptor remains relatively constant until stores and the transport compartment are both depleted. Thereafter, the cleavage product of transferrin receptor shows a highly predictable increase with functional compartment depletion and, indeed, has been shown to be the single best measure of functional compartment depletion. The circulating concentration of the cleavage product of transferrin receptor appears to reflect the body's cellular pool of transferrin receptor, which is upregulated in iron deficiency.

Ultimately functional depletion can become severe enough and of sufficient duration for anemia to develop. Anemia can be quantified by measuring the hemoglobin concentration in the blood. These compartment depletions correlate well with the clearly defined stages of storage iron depletion, iron-deficient erythropoiesis, and iron deficiency anemia, as shown in Figure 36-13.

Iron excess is best evaluated noninvasively: an elevated serum ferritin concentration and a percent transferrin saturation in excess of normal both indicate iron excess. When percent saturation exceeds 62%, the risk of nonprotein-bound iron being present in the circulation and contributing to parenchymal tissue injury becomes very high. The degree of tissue iron overload can be invasively assessed by quantifying the iron content of a liver biopsy.

EVALUATION OF INDIVIDUALS

To evaluate the iron status of an individual, the results of the combination of tests just discussed can accurately define the precise stage of iron nutrition (Baynes, 1996). The importance of defining this in individuals relates to appropriate diagnosis and treatment of iron deficiency in the early stages and to the distinction of anemias due to iron deficiency from those due to other causes. In addition, a diagnosis of iron deficiency mandates a search for the underlying cause because serious pathology might be present. Because of concern about relationships between iron and heart disease and cancer, iron supplements should be used only when there is a definitive iron deficiency.

Early diagnosis of iron excess in an individual and early intervention are also important uses of measures of iron status. If iron excess is not diagnosed and treated in its early stages, serious long-term organ damage may occur.

EVALUATION OF POPULATIONS

Accurate determination of the iron nutritional status of a population is crucial for determining national and international nutritional priorities. Once a problematic area is defined and an intervention is initiated, repeat population evaluation is essential to evaluate the response. The choice of measurements is to some extent dependent upon whether the highest prevalence is expected to be depleted stores, depleted transport compartment, or functional depletion. The best portrayal of iron status will be provided by combined measurements of serum ferritin (stores), serum transferrin receptor (transport compartment), and hematocrit (degree of anemia) (Cook et al., 1996). Formal evaluation of this combination approach in a large field setting was provided by a study in which pregnant women in the Caribbean were given iron supplements (Simmons et al., 1993).

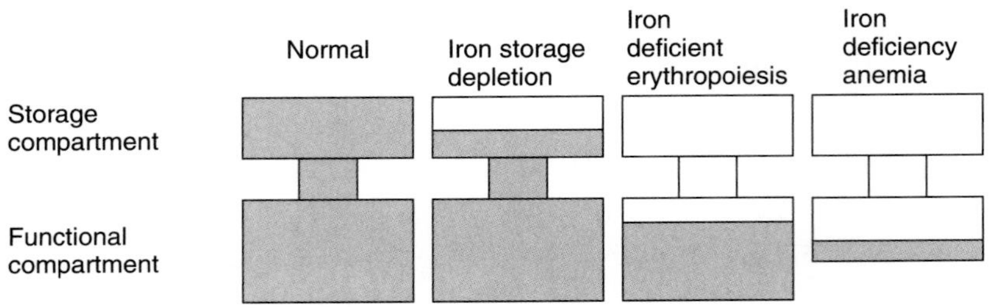

Measurement	Normal	Iron storage depletion	Iron deficient erythropoiesis	Iron deficiency anemia
Storage compartment				
Functional compartment				
Marrow iron* (stainable)	1-3+	0	0	0
Red cell distribution width†	<15	<15	>15	>15
Serum ferritin (μg/L)	>12	<12	<12	<12
Mean cell volume (fL)†	>80	>80	<80	<80
% Transferrin saturation‡	35±15	>16	<16	<16
Free erythrocyte protoporphyrin (μg/100 mL RBC)†	<70	<70	>70	>70
Transferrin receptor (mg/L)¶	<8.5	<8.5	≥8.5	>>8.5
Hemoglobin (g/100 mL) Male	>13	>13	>13	<13
Hemoglobin (g/100 mL) Female	>12	>12	>12	<12

*Invasive test; †insensitive and late marker of functional depletion; ‡lacks sensitivity and specificity; ¶Kansas City Monoclonal ELISA.

Figure 36-13 Sequential compartment depletions, stages of iron depletion, and the accompanying changes in iron-related measurements. *(Modified from Bothwell TH, Charlton RW, Cook JD, Finch CA [1979] Iron Metabolism in Man. Blackwell Scientific Publications, Oxford, UK, p 45.)*

In the light of increasing concerns over risks of excess iron nutrition, it has become important to also assess degrees of iron overload. This is particularly important in regions where the diet is heavily fortified with iron.

IRON DEFICIENCY

Precise data on the prevalence of iron deficiency on a global basis are not readily available. However, much can be inferred from the global prevalence of anemia. Clearly not all anemia is due to iron deficiency, but a crude correction can be arrived at by assuming that anemia in adult men is an estimate of anemia due to causes other than iron deficiency and that anemia due to these other causes will occur at rates similar in women. Therefore, it can be calculated that roughly 0.5 billion people in the world have iron-deficiency anemia. Because anemia reflects the endpoint of functional iron deficiency, two to three times this number of people must be afflicted by depleted iron stores or lesser degrees of functional compartment depletion. In developed areas of the world, only about 8% of the population are anemic. Conversely, approximately 36% of the population of underdeveloped and developing regions of the world are anemic. Consequently, the iron nutritional imperatives are clearly different between developed and developing regions. The preliminary data from NHANES III suggest that iron-deficiency anemia is currently an unusual finding in the United States (Centers for Disease Control and Prevention, 1998).

Life Cycle Considerations

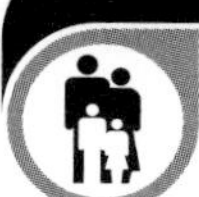

Iron Deficiency and Low Iron Stores in Infants, Children, and Women of Child-Bearing Age

Iron deficiency affects a large number of infants, children, and women of child-bearing age in both developed nations and the developing world. Estimates of the prevalence of iron deficiency among women and children in developing countries are as high as 60%. Data from the third National Health and Nutrition Examination Survey (NHANES III), which was conducted during 1988 to 1994, indicated a low rate of iron deficiency in the United States (Centers for Disease Control and Prevention, 1998). Approximately 3% of children ages 12 to 36 months in the United States had iron deficiency anemia, and an additional 6% had low iron stores (based on elevated erythrocyte protoporphyrin concentration, low serum ferritin concentration, and low transferrin saturation). The NHANES III results indicated that 11% of nonpregnant women ages 16 to 49 years in the United States had low iron stores, and 3% to 5% also had iron deficiency anemia. The NHANES III data also indicated that the prevalence of iron deficiency is higher among children and women living at or below the poverty level than among those living above the poverty level.

Iron deficiency is of nutritional concern during infancy and childhood, especially among children less than 24 months of age. The iron stores of full-term infants are estimated to be adequate to meet iron requirements for 4 to 6 months, whereas those of preterm infants are smaller and may be depleted sooner. A rapid rate of growth, along with frequently inadequate intake of dietary iron, places young children at particular risk. Breast milk provides iron in a highly available form and is sufficient to meet an infant's needs during the first 6 months of life, but other sources of iron are recommended after 6 months. Iron-fortified formula and iron-fortified cereals are important sources of iron for infants in the first year of life. Risk for iron deficiency drops after 24 months of age because of the slower rate of growth and more diversified diet.

Adolescent girls and women of child-bearing age (12 to 49 years) are also at some risk of iron deficiency. Most women in this age-group have high iron requirements due to menstrual blood losses and do not meet their needs for iron from dietary intake, partly because of relatively low energy expenditure and food intake. During pregnancy, iron requirement is high due to an increase in blood volume and the growth of fetal and maternal tissues. The requirement for absorbed iron during pregnancy (4.5 mg/day) is three times higher than during nonpregnancy (1.5 mg/day) and is only partially compensated for by increased iron absorption and decreased menstrual loss throughout pregnancy. Because most women enter pregnancy with low iron stores, routine iron supplementation during pregnancy has been the standard practice in many countries to prevent the development of iron deficiency anemia during the later part of pregnancy.

Consequences of iron deficiency include adverse developmental outcomes and greater risk of lead poisoning in children, reduced work capacity in adults, and possibly an increased risk of poor pregnancy outcomes, such as preterm delivery and higher maternal mortality.

LIABILITIES OF IRON DEFICIENCY

The liabilities of iron deficiency correlate with functional iron depletion. Storage iron depletion has not been shown to carry any adverse liabilities. Of the adverse health effects of functional depletion, the demonstration that iron deficiency in infants appears to result in abnormalities of psychomotor development is of major concern. These abnormalities appear to be a consequence of altered dopamine metabolism, and there is some evidence that these abnormalities may be reversible only to a limited extent. That reductions in work performance, effort tolerance, and peak effort output result from iron deficiency is well documented. Where people depend upon manual labor for their livelihood, these impairments clearly translate into significant economic disadvantage. It now appears clear that iron deficiency contributes to adverse pregnancy outcomes, with higher rates of premature delivery and perinatal mortality in iron-deficient populations. Impaired immune responses, gastrointestinal abnormalities, changes in the hair and nails, impaired thermogenesis, altered thyroid metabolism, and changes in catecholamine turnover have also been observed in subjects with iron deficiency (Baynes, 1994).

TREATMENT AND PREVENTION

Treatment of the individual subject with iron deficiency is obviously appropriate, but a search for the cause of the iron deficiency should also be undertaken (Baynes and Cook, 1995). In populations with a low incidence of iron deficiency, identification and treatment of individuals are most appropriate. In most cases, the problem of iron deficiency is correctable with orally administered ferrous iron salts. Side effects of iron supplement ingestion frequently limit compliance, but these side effects may be dramatically reduced by a formulation of iron that allows for slow release of iron over a number of hours within the stomach. This formulation relies on the use of a matrix that keeps the iron close to the surface of the gastric contents (Simmons et al., 1993).

In populations with a very high prevalence of iron deficiency, the appropriate prevention strategy involves a pilot unscreened therapeutic supplementation trial. If the program is shown to be successful, then it should be rapidly translated into a regional or national program. The possibility that a weekly supplement may facilitate better compliance and obtain reasonable efficacy compared with daily supplementation has been suggested; this suggestion is predicated in part on the notion, derived from rat data, that continuous intake is inhibitory to absorption (Viteri et al., 1995; Fairweather-Tait et al., 1985). However, human absorption data refute this suggestion and confirm the advantage of daily supplementation (Cook and Reddy, 1995).

In regions of intermediate prevalence, one or two intervention strategies appear appropriate. These should take the form of either a pilot fortification trial or a pilot prophylactic supplementation program. If successful, these should be extended regionally. Surveillance of population iron status should be undertaken to guard against the production of excessive positive iron balance.

In populations in which the prevalence of iron deficiency is low, a public health initiative aimed at improving overall iron nutrition is inappropriate. The only appropriate activity should be the screening of high-risk groups, such as infants, pregnant women, and trained athletes, and therapeutic supplementation of individuals who are identified as being iron-deficient. Indeed, if it appears that population iron status is increasing to levels higher than putative normal values, consideration should be given to reducing the levels of iron fortification and supplementation.

IRON EXCESS

The very limited ability of the human body to excrete iron led to the conclusion that iron balance in man is essentially determined by

Life Cycle Considerations

Iron Overload

Iron overload can result in the impairment of organ structure and function from the excessive deposition of iron in parenchymal cells of the organ. Hereditary hemochromatosis results from homozygosity for a recessive HLA-linked gene on chromosome 6 and is limited largely to people of European origin. Homozygote frequencies are estimated to be between 1 in 100 and 1 in 1,000, with about 5% to 20% of the population being heterozygous for the HLA-linked iron-loading gene. This abnormality

Life Cycle Considerations

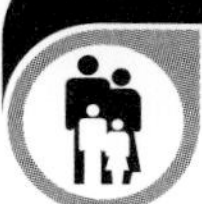

Iron Overload—cont'd

leads to absorption of more iron than is required (a greater rate of iron absorption than is appropriate, given the body stores); the amount of iron absorbed in excess of requirements is only a few milligrams per day, but over a number of years, this can result in an increase in iron stores to 20 to 50 times the normal levels, representing the accumulation of 20 to 40 g of surplus iron.

Because of interactions of genetics with iron supply and needs, phenotypic expression of this disorder is rare in populations where iron deficiency is prevalent (due to lack of bioavailable iron in the diet), is encountered about 10 times more frequently in men than in women (owing to greater losses by women due to menstruation and pregnancy), and is typically diagnosed after the age of 40 years, with age at onset being younger in men than in women (Bothwell et al., 1995).

The earliest biochemical signs of iron overload are elevations in the plasma iron concentration, a high plasma transferrin saturation, and elevated plasma ferritin concentrations. As iron stores enlarge, hemosiderin deposits become more prominent in the liver; examination of liver biopsy specimens from patients with hereditary hemochromatosis reveals that the hepatocytes (parenchymal cells) are loaded with hemosiderin, whereas the Kupffer cells are relatively free of stored iron. Organ damage occurs only after the concentrations of stored iron are grossly elevated, but this damage is largely irreversible. Early diagnosis and treatment are essential to avoid tissue damage. Repeated phlebotomy (e.g., the removal of 500 mL of blood, which contains 200 to 250 mg of iron, each week over a period of 2 to 3 years) to remove the excess iron, followed by less frequent removal of blood to prevent reaccumulation, is the usual treatment.

A picture resembling hemochromatosis may also be caused by iron-loading anemias. These iron-loading anemias include thalassemia major and certain other hereditary anemias in which erythropoiesis is ineffective. Thalassemia major occurs in patients who are homozygous for mutations that lead to a decrease in β-globin synthesis, which in turn leads to deficient hemoglobin synthesis and the accumulation of α-globin chains in the bone marrow. Iron overload occurs in these patients as a consequence of enhanced absorption of iron and of essential treatment of the anemia with multiple blood transfusions. In these chronic hyperplastic anemias, the iron deposition occurs in both reticuloendothelial and parenchymal cells, and organ damage tends to develop as parenchymal cell loading proceeds. Treatment of iron overload in these patients is by chelation therapy.

Another cause of iron overload is largely of dietary origin and has been observed only in sub-Saharan Africa. This unique type of iron overload is related to the consumption of indigenous beers that are brewed in iron containers and that contain approximately 15 to 40 mg of iron per L. Large quantities of this beer are consumed by many men; it is estimated that an additional 50 to 100 mg of iron in a highly available form are ingested each day. This type of iron overload results in hemosiderin deposits in reticuloendothelial cells throughout the body and, with advanced disease, in the parenchymal cells of the liver. More recent data have suggested that a genetic component also contributes to this form of iron overload (Gordeuk et al., 1992).

Thinking Critically

1. What effect would blood removal or chelation therapy over an extended period (~1 year) have on plasma iron concentration, transferrin saturation, total iron binding capacity, and plasma ferritin levels?
2. Would you expect the prevalence of symptomatic hemochromatosis to increase or decrease with introduction of an iron-fortification program or an increase in the intake of bioavailable iron? Why?

iron absorption (McCance and Widdowson, 1937). The consequence is that, if we absorb a little more iron than we excrete, or if we receive a parenteral iron burden in the form of blood transfusions, we can become "iron-loaded." In hemochromatosis, iron is absorbed in excess of requirements, leading to transferrin hypersaturation and the accumulation of significant concentrations of nonprotein-bound iron in the circulation. This leads to progressive parenchymal cell iron loading, resulting in the well-recognized clinical complications of cardiomyopathy, diabetes mellitus, various other endocrine abnormalities (particularly of pituitary and sex hormones), arthritis, cutaneous pigmentation, liver cirrhosis, and liver cancer. The mechanism by which iron causes organ damage is uncertain, but lipid peroxidation and fibrogenesis appear to be important contributory factors. The frequency of hereditary hemochromatosis in white populations is roughly 3 per 1,000, with a high heterozygous carrier rate of about 10% to 15% of the population. Iron overload is more likely to be manifested in areas of high iron intake and particularly when the dietary iron is highly bioavailable. The disease is in large measure treatable by removal of body iron by therapeutic phlebotomy (removal of blood over time).

There are a number of well-recognized situations of iron overload, which are presented in Box 36-4. The best defined of these is the autosomally recessively inherited disorder, hereditary hemochromatosis, now designated as HFE-1. The hemochromatosis gene has been localized to chromosome 6 and shown to encode a major histocompatibility complex class I–like molecule, called HFE (Feder et al., 1996). HFE inhibits binding of the transferrin molecule to the transferrin receptor (Feder et al., 1998; Gross et al., 1998). The mutation of cysteine 282 to tyrosine (C282Y) of the *HFE* gene is very common; approximately 15% of the northern European population is heterozygous, and more than 0.5% of the population are homozygous. Although the homozygous state is relatively common, it is only rarely associated with illness, with a clinical penetrance (defined as the extent to which a phenotypic effect is exerted in individuals carrying the mutation) estimated to be of the order of only 1% (Beutler et al., 2003). The second most frequent mutation in the *HFE* gene is histidine 63 to aspartate (H63D), and since the H63D mutation is very common, the compound heterozygous C282Y/H63D is also very common in the population. It appears that the penetrance of this compound heterozygous genotype is only about 1% of that of the homozygous C282Y genotype (Beutler, 1997).

Box 36-4

CLASSIFICATION OF IRON-LOADING DISORDERS

Primary Iron Overload

(Hemochromatosis)
Classic congenital hemochromatosis, mutations in HFE (HFE-1)
Juvenile hemochromatosis, mutations in hemojuvelin, or in hepcidin (HFE-2)
Transferrin receptor-2 mutations (HFE-3)
IREG-1 (ferroportin) mutations (HFE-4)

Secondary Iron Overload

(Usually associated with transfusion treatment of anemia)
Thalassemias
Pyruvate kinase deficiency
Dyserythropoietic anemia
Glucose 6-phosphate dehydrogenase deficiency
Hereditary spherocytosis
Sideroblastic anemia (deficiency of δ-aminolevulinic acid synthase)
Other anemias treated by multiple blood transfusions

Although most cases of hereditary hemochromatosis are due to mutations in HFE, some 20% of patients in the United States who are diagnosed with hereditary hemochromatosis do not have mutations in *HFE* (Beutler et al., 1996). In the southern European population, the proportion is even larger (Carella et al., 1997). Over the last few years a number of other causes of hemochromatosis have been described (see Table 36-1), which involve mutations in some of the genes that have been shown to play a key role in iron metabolism. Juvenile, or type 2 hemochromatosis (HFE-2), is transmitted as a recessive trait, and leads to severe iron overload and organ damage before 30 years of age.

Most patients with juvenile hemochromatosis have mutations that map to the centromeric region of chromosome 1q. Recent elegant positional cloning studies (Papanikolaou et al., 2004) showed that the causal gene encodes a 426 residue protein called hemojuvelin, which shows homology to a molecule involved in axonal guidance in the central nervous system. Analysis of Greek, Canadian, and French families with hemochromatosis showed that one mutation, G320V, was found in all three populations and accounted for two-thirds of the mutations found. A number of other mutations of hemojuvelin have been identified in 1q-linked juvenile hemochromatosis (Lanzara et al., 2004; Lee et al., 2004). It is assumed that hemojuvelin plays a crucial role in iron metabolism, although what that role might be is not clear. A rarer form of juvenile hematochromatosis, with clinical expression identical to the 1q-linked form, maps to chromosome 19 and is due to mutations in hepcidin (Roetto et al., 2003). Patients with juvenile hemochromatosis associated with mutations in either hepcidin or hemojuvelin have low or absent urinary hepcidin levels, as do patients with hemochromatosis due to the C282Y mutation in *HFE* (C282Y) and those with hemochromatosis associated with mutations in transferrin receptor-2 (Nemeth et al., 2005).

In addition to HFE-1 and HFE-2, two other forms of hemochromatosis, HFE-3 and HFE-4, result from mutations in TFR2 and IREG-1, respectively. HFE-3 is linked to chromosome 7q, and is associated with mutations in the *TFR2* gene, which encodes a protein of unknown function that is a member of the transferrin receptor family (Roetto et al., 2002, 2001; Camaschella et al., 2000). An autosomal dominant form of iron storage disease, HFE-4, is caused by mutations in the *IREG-1* (i.e., the ferroportin/*MTP1*) gene (reviewed in Pietrangelo, 2004). The clinical features of HFE-4 are quite characteristic, with an early increase in serum ferritin despite low-normal transferrin saturation, progressive iron accumulation that is predominantly in reticuloendothelial macrophages, marginal anemia, and often low tolerance to phlebotomy (Pietrangelo et al., 1999). Mutations in *IREG-1* are widespread in the population, and it has been shown that a common polymorphism (Q248H) in *IREG-1* associates with a tendency to low hemoglobin and high ferritin in African and African American populations (Gordeuk et al., 2003).

Iron overload with similar organ damage is well recognized in patients with such hemoglobinopathies as β-thalassemia major and who are generally dependent upon frequent blood transfusions. The blood transfusions, along with the increased iron absorption observed in these conditions, lead to a massive increase in body iron content. This increase in iron content eventually leads to saturation of the normal iron carrier proteins and the presence of non–transferrin-bound iron in the circulation and, ultimately, to iron loading of tissues and consequent tissue damage. Tissue iron levels can be estimated by determination of serum ferritin levels (as long as there is no inflammatory-associated condition) or measured by a liver biopsy or noninvasively by the superconducting quantum interference device (SQUID), where this is available, or by magnetic resonance imaging (MRI) (Beutler et al., 2003). Cardiac iron measurement, using the MRI T2* technique (magnetic resonance imaging with measurement of the relaxation time T2*), has proved extremely useful in diagnosis of cardiac dysfunction (Anderson et al., 2001) and in monitoring changes in cardiac iron during intensive chelation therapy (Anderson et al., 2002).

The ravages of iron overload can be reversed by such treatment modalities as allogenic bone marrow transplantation. In this treatment, the hematopoietic stem cells of the patient are destroyed and replaced with normal stem cells from a suitable donor. However, secondary iron overload is more usually treated by iron chelation therapy (Fig. 36-14), which up until recently used the well-established hexadentate chelator desferrioxamine B (Desferal) or a more recently available orally administered bidentate chelator (Deferiprone) (Beutler et al., 2003). The denticity of a chelator refers to the number of bonds that it forms with the metal ion. Because Fe^{3+} prefers to be hexacoordinate, three molecules of a bidentate chelator are required to chelate one Fe^{3+} ion, whereas only one molecule of a hexadentate chelator suffices. Iron removal by Desferal is inefficient (i.e., typically only 5% or less of the drug

Deferoxamine

Hexadentate

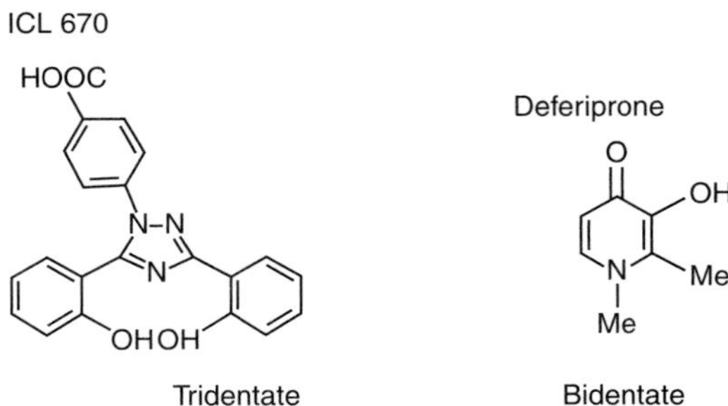

Figure 36-14 The structures of the iron chelators Desferal (Deferoxamine), ICL 670 and Deferiprone.

administered promotes iron excretion) and, because of poor gastrointestinal absorption and rapid elimination from the circulation, effective therapy usually requires subcutaneous or intravenous administration by a portable infusion pump for 9 to 10 hours for 5 to 6 days per week. This cumbersome and unpleasant regimen poses serious problems of patient compliance and increases the cost of treatment. Deferiprone, which is now licensed in 25 countries, causes the serious problem of agranulocytosis in approximately 1 % of patients. However, because of its ability to cross cellular membranes, this agent appears to have superior cardioprotective properties, and it may yield better cardioprotective results when used in tandem therapy with Desferal (Hershko et al., 2004). A new orally active tridentate (forming a 2:1 chelator-to-iron complex) iron chelator, ICL 670, developed by Novartis from the screening of more than 700 candidate drugs, has been shown in preclinical studies to be excreted predominantly by the fecal route and to be extremely promising.

A number of publications have suggested that even relatively modest increases in iron status may place subjects at risk for development of occlusive coronary artery disease. The initial hypothesis was that poor iron status might be protective against coronary heart disease. This was related to the observation that premenopausal women had a lower incidence of coronary heart disease as well as low iron stores, whereas both iron stores (as measured by serum ferritin) and risk of coronary heart disease increased following menopause. The first convincing evidence of a relationship between coronary heart disease and body iron stores was a study of men by Salonen and colleagues (1992), which showed evidence of a higher risk of coronary heart disease associated with high stored iron levels (plasma ferritin, greater than 200 μg/L) after adjustment for a number of other risk factors including smoking, serum high density lipoprotein level, and blood pressure. Nevertheless, it must be remembered that increased ferritin levels may be associated with increases in the acute phase response. Elevated fibrinogen levels and high white blood cell counts are both indicators of a stimulated acute phase response and are associated with an increased risk of heart disease. Analysis of transferrin saturation in conjunction with ferritin levels would be a more pertinent marker of body iron stores.

Although at least seven epidemiological studies have reported a positive correlation between iron status and ischemic heart disease, more than 18 studies have failed to confirm a relationship (Meyers, 1996). If iron played a substantial role in coronary heart disease, patients who are homozygous or heterozygous for genetic hemochromatosis might show an increased risk for the disease. This has not been found to be the case, and a recent study found no consistent association between either *HFE* mutations or serum iron indicators and the prevalence of coronary heart disease (Waalen et al., 2002). Furthermore, analysis of serum or cardiac muscle from these patients showed no relationship between iron content and coronary heart disease. Increased cardiac iron content is present in some thalassemic patients and is associated with cardiac dysfunction; myocardial siderosis occurs when serum ferritin exceeds 1,800 μg/L.

Aside from iron overload due to genetic disease, and of even greater concern, the appearance of a progressive increase in the iron nutritional status of the American population is indicated by comparison of data from the National Health and Nutrition Examination Surveys (NHANES) II, Hispanic HANES, and NHANES III. The increase in iron status over time appears to be greater than can be accounted for by methodological differences among studies. At this time, the prudent course appears to be a very conservative approach to the use of iron fortification and supplementation in developed regions of the world.

High-dose iron supplements are frequently associated with constipation and other gastrointestinal side effects including nausea, vomiting, and diarrhea. Although these gastrointestinal symptoms are not serious side effects when compared with other possible risks, the Institute of Medicine (IOM, 2001) used gastrointestinal side effects as the critical adverse effect on which to base the upper tolerable intake level (UL) for iron. The UL of iron for adults is 45 mg/day; the UL for infants and children younger than age 14 is 40 mg/day. The IOM (2001) noted that homozygotes for hereditary hemochromatosis and individuals with other iron-loading disorders may not be protected by this UL.

REFERENCES

Abboud S, Haile DJ (2000) A novel mammalian iron-regulated protein involved in intracellular iron metabolism. J Biol Chem 275:19906-19912.

Aisen P (1998) Transferrin, the transferrin receptor, and the uptake of iron by cells. Met Ions Biol Syst 35:585-631.

Anderson LJ, Holden S, Davis B, Prescott E, Charrier CC, Bunce NH, Firmin DN, Wonke B, Porter J, Walker JM, Pennell DJ (2001) Cardiovascular T2-star (T2*) magnetic resonance for the early diagnosis of myocardial iron overload. Eur Heart J 22:2171-2179.

Anderson LJ, Wonke B, Prescott E, Holden S, Walker JM, Pennell, DJ (2002) Comparison of effects of oral deferiprone and subcutaneous desferrioxamine on myocardial iron levels and ventricular function in beta thalassaemia. Lancet 360:516-520.

Baker EN, Lindley PF (1992) New perspectives on the structure and function of transferrins. J Inorg Biochem 47:147-160.

Baynes RD (1996) Assessment of iron status. Clin Biochem 29:209-215.

Baynes RD (1994) Iron deficiency. In: Brock JH, Halliday JW, Pippard MJ, Powell LW (eds) Iron Metabolism. WB Saunders, London, pp 198-218.

Baynes RD, Cook JD (1995) Iron deficiency anemia. In: Brain MC, Carbone PO (eds) Current Therapy in Hematology-Oncology, 5th ed. Mosby Press, Philadelphia, pp 57-61.

Baynes RD, Shih YJ, Cook JD (1994a) Mechanism of production of the serum transferrin receptor. Adv Exp Med Biol 356:61-68.

Baynes RD, Skikne BS, Cook JD (1994b) Circulating transferrin receptors and assessment of iron status. J Nutr Biochem 5:322-330.

Beinert H, Holm RH, Munck E (1997) Iron-sulfur clusters: Nature's modular, multipurpose structures. Science 277:653-659.

Beutler E (1997) Genetic irony beyond haemochromatosis: Clinical effects of HLA-H mutations. Lancet 349:296-297.

Beutler E, Gelbart T, West C, Lee P, Adams M, Blackstone R, Pockros P, Kosty M, Venditti CP, Phatak PD, Seese NK, Chorney KA, Ten Elshof AE, Gerhard GS, Chorney M (1996) Mutation analysis in hereditary hemochromatosis. Blood Cells Mol Dis 22:187-194.

Beutler E, Hoffbrand AV, Cook JD (2003) Iron deficiency and overload. Hematology (Am Soc Hematol Educ Program), pp 40-61.

Binder R, Horowitz JA, Basilion JP, Koeller DM, Klausner RD, Harford JB (1994) Evidence that the pathway of transferrin receptor mRNA degradation involves an endonucleolytic cleavage within the 3′ UTR and does not involve poly (A) tail shortening. EMBO J 13:1969-1980.

Bothwell TH, Baynes RD, MacFarlane BJ, MacPhail AP (1989) Nutritional iron requirements and food iron absorption. J Intern Med 226:357-365.

Bothwell TH, Charlton RW, Motulsky AG (1995) Hemochromatosis. In: Scriver CR, Beaudet AL, Sly WS, Valle D (eds) The Metabolic and Molecular Bases of Inherited Disease, 7th ed. Vol. II. McGraw-Hill, New York, pp 2237-2269.

Breuer W, Epsztejn S, Cabantchik ZI (1995) Iron acquired from transferrin by K562 cells is delivered into a cytoplasmic pool of chelatable iron (II). J Biol Chem 270:24209-24215.

Breuer W, Hershko C, Cabantchik ZI (2000) The importance of non-transferrin bound iron in disorders of iron metabolism. Transfus Sci 23:185-192.

Camaschella C, Roetto A, Cali A, De Gobbi M, Garozzo G, Carella M, Majorano N, Totaro A, Gasparini P (2000) The gene TFR2 is mutated in a new type of haemochromatosis mapping to 7q22. Nat Genet 25:14-15.

Canonne-Hergaux F, Gruenheid S, Ponka P, Gros P (1999) Cellular and subcellular localization of the Nramp2 iron transporter in the intestinal brush border and regulation by dietary iron. Blood 93:4406-4417.

Carella M, D'Ambrosio L, Totaro A, Grifa A, Valentino MA, Piperno A, Girelli D, Roetto A, Franco B, Gasparini P, Camaschella C (1997) Mutation analysis of the HLA-H gene in Italian hemochromatosis patients. Am J Hum Genet 60:828-832.

Centers for Disease Control and Prevention (1998) Recommendations to Prevent and Control Iron Deficiency in the United States. MMWR Recomm Rep 47:1-29.

Cook JD, Dassenko SA, Lynch SR (1991) Assessment of the role of nonheme iron availability in iron balance. Am J Clin Nutr 54:717-722.

Cook JD, Reddy MB (1995) Efficacy of weekly compared with daily iron supplementation. Am J Clin Nutr 62:117-120.

Cook JD, Skikne B, Baynes R (1996) The use of the serum transferrin receptor for the assessment of iron status. In: Hallberg L, Nils-Georg A (eds) Iron Nutrition in Health and Disease. John Libbey, London, pp 49-58.

Crichton RR (2001) Inorganic Biochemistry of Iron Metabolism: From Molecular Mechanisms to Clinical Consequences, 2nd ed. John Wiley and Sons, New York.

Crichton RR (1984) Iron uptake and utilization by mammalian cells II. Intracellular iron utilization. Trends Biochem Sci 9:283-286.

Donovan A, Brownlie A, Zhou Y, Shepard J, Pratt SJ, Moynihan J, Paw BH, Drejer A, Barut B, Zapata A, Law TC, Brugnara C, Lux SE, Pinkus GS, Pinkus JL, Kingsley PD, Palls J, Fleming MD, Andrews NC, Zon LI (2000) Positional cloning of zebrafish *ferroportin1* identifies a conserved vertebrate iron exporter. Nature 403:776-781.

Eisenstein RS (2000) Iron regulatory proteins and the molecular control of mammalian iron metabolism. Annu Rev Nutr 20:627-662.

Fairweather-Tait SJ, Swindell TE, Wright AJ (1985) Further studies in rats on the influence of previous iron intake on the estimation of bioavailability of Fe. Br J Nutr 54:79-86.

Feder JN, Gnirke A, Thomas W, Tsuchihashi Z, Ruddy DA, Basava A, Dormishian F, Domingo R, Ellis MC, Fullan A, Hinton LM, Jones NL, Kimmel BE, Kronmal GS, Lauer P, Lee VK, Loeb DB, Mapa FA, McClelland E, Meyer NC, Mintier GA, Moeller N, Moore T, Morikang E, Wolff RK (1996) A novel MHC class I-like gene is mutated in patients with hereditary hemochromatosis. Nat Genet 13:399-408.

Feder JN, Penny DM, Irrinki A, Lee VK, Lebron JA, Watson N, Tsuchihashi Z, Sigal E, Bjorkman PJ, Schatzman RC (1998) The haemochromatosis gene product complexes with the transferrin receptor and lowers its affinity for ligand binding. Proc Natl Acad Sci U S A 95:1472-1477.

Finch C (1994) Regulators of iron balance in humans. Blood 84:1697-702.

Fleming MD, Trenor CCI, Su MA, Foernzler D, Beier DR, Dietrich WF, Andrews NC (1997) Microcytic anemia mice have a mutation in Nramp2, a candidate iron transporter. Nat Genet 16:383-386.

Fleming MD, Romano MA, Su MA, Garrick LM, Garrick MD, Fleming NC (1998) *Nramp2* is mutated in the anemic Belgrade (b) rat: evidence of a role for Nramp2 in endosomal iron transport. Proc Natl Acad Sci U S A 95:1148-1153.

Fleming RE, Sly WS (2001) Hepcidin: a putative iron-regulatory hormone relevant to hereditary hemochromatosis and the anemia of chronic disease. Proc Natl Acad Sci U S A 98:8160-8162.

Flint DH, Allen RM (1996) Iron-Sulfur Proteins with Nonredox Functions. Chem Rev 96:2315-2334.

Ganz T (2003) Hepcidin, a key regulator of iron metabolism and mediator of anemia of inflammation. Blood 102:783-788.

Gordeuk V, Mukiibi J, Hasstedt SJ, Samowitz W, Edwards CQ, West G, Ndambire S, Emmanual J, Neal N, Chapanduka Z, Randall M, Boone P, Romano P, Martell RW, Yamashita T, Effler P, Brittenham G (1992) Iron overload in Africa. Interaction between a gene and dietary iron content. N Engl J Med 326:95-100.

Gordeuk VR, Caleffi A, Corradini E, Ferrara F, Jones RA, Castro O, Onyekwere O, Kittles R, Pignatti E, Montosi G, Garuti C, Gangaidzo IT, Gomo ZA, Moyo VM, Rouault TA, MacPhail P, Pietrangelo A (2003) Iron overload in Africans and African-Americans and a common mutation in the SCL40A1 (ferroportin 1) gene. Blood Cells Mol Dis 31:299-304.

Gross CN, Irrinki A, Feder JN, Enns CA (1998) Co-trafficking of HFE, a nonclassical major histocompatability complex class 1 protein, with the transferrin receptor implies a role in intracellular iron regulation. J Biol Chem 273:22068-22074.

Gunshin H, Mackenzie B, Berger UV, Gunshin Y, Romero MF, Boron WF, Nussberger S, Gollan JL, Hediger MA (1997) Cloning and characterization of a mammalian proton-coupled metal-ion transporter. Nature 388:482-488.

Harris ZL, Takahashi Y, Miyajima J, Serizawa M, MacGillivray RTA, Gitlin JD (1995) Aceruloplasminemia: Molecular characterization of this disorder of iron metabolism. Proc Natl Acad Sci U S A 92:2539-2543.

Harrison PM, Arosio P (1996) The ferritins: molecular properties, iron storage function, and cellular regulation. Biochim Biophys Acta 1275:161-203.

Hentze MW, Kühn LC (1996) Molecular control of vertebrate iron metabolism: mRNA-based regulatory circuits operated by iron, nitric oxide and oxidative stress. Proc Natl Acad Sci U S A 93:8175-8182.

Hershko C, Cappellini MD, Galanello R, Piga A, Tognoni G, Masera G (2004) Purging iron from the heart. Br J Haematol 125:545-551.

Institute of Medicine (2001) Dietary Reference Intakes for Vitamin A, Vitamin K, Arsenic, Boron, Chromium, Copper, Iodine, Iron, Manganese, Molybdenum, Nickel, Silicon, Vanadium, and Zinc. National Academy Press, Washington, DC.

Kurtz DM Jr (1997) Structural similarity and functional diversity in diiron-oxo proteins. J Biol Inorg Chem 2:159-167.

Lanzara C, Roetto A, Daraio F, Rivard S, Ficarella R, Simard H, Cox TM, Cazzola M, Piperno A, Gimenez-Roqueplo AP, Grammatico P, Volinia S, Gasparini P, Camaschella C (2004) Spectrum of hemojuvelin gene mutations in 1q-linked juvenile hemochromatosis. Blood 103:4317-4321.

Lawrence CM, Ray S, Babyonyshev M, Galluser R, Borhani DW, Harrison SC (1999) Crystal structure of the ectodomain of human transferrin receptor. Science 286:779-782.

Lee PL, Beutler E, Rao SV, Barton JC (2004) Genetic abnormalities and juvenile hemochromatosis: mutations of the HJV gene encoding hemojuvelin. Blood 103:4669-4671.

Lindley PF (1996) Iron in biology: a structural viewpoint. Rep Prog Phys 59:867-933.

Lynch SR, Baynes RD (1996) Deliberations and evaluations of the approaches, endpoints, and paradigms for iron dietary recommendations. J Nutr 126(Suppl):2404S-2409S.

McCance RA, Widdowson EM (1937) Absorption and Excretion of Iron. Lancet 230:680-684.

McKie AT, Barrow D, Latunde-Dada GO, Rolfs A, Sager G, Mudaly E, Mudaly M, Richardson C, Barlow D, Bomford A, Peters TJ, Raja KB, Shirali S, Hediger MA, Farzaneh F, Simpson RJ (2001) An iron-regulated ferric reductase associated with the absorption of dietary iron. Science 291:1755-1759.

McKie AT, Marciani P, Rolfs A, Brennan K, Wehr K, Barrow D, Miret S, Bomford A, Peters TJ, Farzaneh F, Hediger MA, Hentze MW, Simpson RJ (2000) A novel duodenal iron-regulated transporter, IREG1, implicated in the basolateral transfer of iron to the circulation. Mol Cell 5:299-309.

Meyers DG (1996) The iron hypothesis—does iron cause atherosclerosis? Clin Cardiol 19:925-929.

Nemeth E, Rivera S, Gabayan V, Keller C, Taudorf S, Pedersen BK, Ganz T (2004) IL-6 mediates hypoferremia of inflammation by inducing the synthesis of the iron regulatory hormone hepcidin. J Clin Invest 113:1271-1276.

Nemeth E, Roetto A, Garozzo G, Ganz T, Camaschella C (2005) Hepcidin is decreased in TFR2-hemochromatosis. Blood 105:1803-1806

Nemeth E, Valore EV, Territo M, Schiller G, Lichtenstein A, Ganz T (2003) Hepcidin, a putative mediator of anemia of inflammation, is a type II acute-phase protein. Blood 101:2461-2463.

Nicolas G, Bennoun M, Devaux I, Beaumont C, Grandchamp B, Kahn A and Vaulont S (2001) Lack of hepcidin gene expression and severe tissue iron overload in upstream stimulatory factor 2 (USF2) knockout mice. Proc Natl Acad Sci U S A 98:8780-8785.

Nicolas G, Bennoun M, Porteu A, Mativet S, Beaumont C, Grandchamp B, Sirito M, Sawadogo M, Kahn A and Vaulont S (2002) Severe iron deficiency anemia in transgenic mice expressing liver hepcidin. Proc Natl Acad Sci U S A 99:4596-4601.

Nordlund P, Eklund H (1995) Di-iron-carboxylate proteins. Current Opin Struct Biol 5:758-766.

Nordlund P, Sjoberg B-M, Eklund H (1990) Three-dimensional structure of the free radical protein of ribonucleotide reductase. Nature 345:593-598.

Papanikolaou G, Samuels ME, Ludwig EH, MacDonald ML, Franchini PL, Dube MP, Andres L, MacFarlane J, Sakellaropoulos N, Politou M, Nemeth E, Thompson J, Risler JK, Zaborowska C, Babakaiff R, Radomski CC, Pape TD, Davidas O, Christakis J, Brissot P, Lockitch G, Ganz T, Hayden MR, Goldberg YP (2004) Mutations in HFE2 cause iron overload in chromosome 1q-linked juvenile hemochromatosis. Nat Genet 36:77-82.

Pietrangelo A (2004) The ferroportin disease. Blood Cells Mol Dis 32:131-138.

Pietrangelo A, Montosi G, Totaro A, Garuti C, Conte D, Cassanelli S, Fraquelli M, Sardini C, Vasta F, Gasparini P (1999) Hereditary hemochromatosis in adults without pathogenic mutations in the hemochromatosis gene. N Engl J Med 341:725-732.

Pigeon C, Ilyin G, Courselaud B, Leroyer P, Turlin B, Brissot P, Loreal O (2001) A new mouse liver-specific gene, encoding a protein homologous to human antimicrobial peptide hepcidin, is overexpressed during iron overload. J Biol Chem 276:7811-7819.

Reddy MB, Cook JD (1993) Absorption of nonheme iron in ascorbic acid–deficient rats. J Nutr 124:882-887.

Roetto A, Daraio F, Alberti F, Porporato P, Cali A, De Gobbi M, Camaschella C (2002) Hemochromatosis due to mutations in transferrin receptor 2. Blood Cells Mol Dis 29:465-470.

Roetto A, Papanikolaou G, Politou M, Alberti F, Girelli D, Christakis J, Loukopoulos D, Camaschella C (2003) Mutant antimicrobial peptide hepcidin is associated with severe juvenile hemochromatosis. Nat Genet 33:21-22.

Roetto A, Totaro A, Piperno A, Piga A, Longo F, Garozzo G, Cali A, De Gobbi M, Gasparini P, Camaschella C (2001) New mutations inactivating transferrin receptor 2 in hemochromatosis type 3. Blood 97:2555-2560.

Salonen JT, Nyyssonen K, Korpela H, Tuomilehto J, Seppanen R, Salonen R (1992) High stored iron levels are associated with excess risk of myocardial infarction in Eastern Finnish men. Circulation 86:803-811.

Simmons WK, Cook JD, Bingham KC, Thomas M, Jackson J, Jackson M, Ahluwalia M, Khan S G, Patterson AW (1993) Evaluation of a gastric delivery system for iron supplementation in pregnancy. Am J Clin Nutr 58:622-626.

Tandy S,Williams M, Leggett A, Lopez-Jimenez M, Dedes M, Ramesh B, Srai SK, Sharp P (2000) Nramp2 expression is associated with pH-dependent iron uptake across the apical membrane of human intestinal Caco-2 cells. J Biol Chem 275:1023-1029.

Testa U, Pelosi E, Peschle C (1993) The transferrin receptor. Crit Rev Oncogen 4:241-276.

United States Department of Agriculture/ Agricultural Research Service (USDA/ARS) (2004) USDA Nutrient Database for Standard Reference, Release 17. USDA/ARS, Washington, DC. Retrieved April 13, 2005, from http://www.nal.usda.gov/fnic/foodcomp/.

Viteri FE, Xunian L, Tolomei K, Martin A (1995) True absorption and retention of supplemental iron is more efficient when iron is administered every three days rather than daily to iron-normal and iron-deficient rats. J Nutr 125:82-91.

Vulpe CD, Kuo YM, Murphy TL, Cowley L, Askwith C, Libina N, Gitschier J, Anderson GJ (1999) Hephaestin, a ceruloplasmin homologue implicated in intestinal iron transport, is defective in the sla mouse. Nat Genet 21:195-199.

Waalen J, Felitti V, Gelbart T, Ho NJ, Beutler E (2002) Prevalence of coronary heart disease associated with HFE mutations in adults attending a health appraisal center. Am J Med 113:472-479.

Ward RJ, Legssyer R, Henry C, Crichton RR (2000) Does the haemosiderin iron core determine its potential for chelation and the development of iron-induced tissue damage? J Inorg Biochem 79:311-317.

Ward RJ, Ramsey M, Dickson DP, Hunt C, Douglas T, Mann S, Aouad F, Peters TJ, Crichton RR (1994) Further characterisation of forms of haemosiderin in iron-overloaded tissues. Eur J Biochem 225:187-194.

Weinstein DA, Roy CN, Fleming MD, Loda MF, Wolfsdorf JI, Andrews NC (2002) Inappropriate expression of hepcidin is associated with iron refractory anemia: implications for the anemia of chronic disease. Blood 100:3776-3781.

Wessling-Resnick M (2000) Iron Transport. Annu Rev Nutr 20:129-151.

Zecca L, Youdim MBH, Riederer P, Connor JR, Crichton RR (2004) Iron, brain ageing and neurodegenerative diseases. Nature Rev Neurosci 5:863-873.

RECOMMENDED READINGS

Bothwell TH, Charlton RW, Cook JD, Finch CA (1979) Iron Metabolism in Man. Blackwell Scientific Publications, Oxford, UK.

Crichton RR (2001) Inorganic Biochemistry of Iron Metabolism: From Molecular Mechanisms to Clinical Consequences, 2nd ed. John Wiley and Sons, New York.

Beutler E, Hoffbrand AV, Cook JD (2003) Iron Deficiency and Overload. Hematology (Am Soc Hematol Educ Program), pp 40-61.

Chapter 37

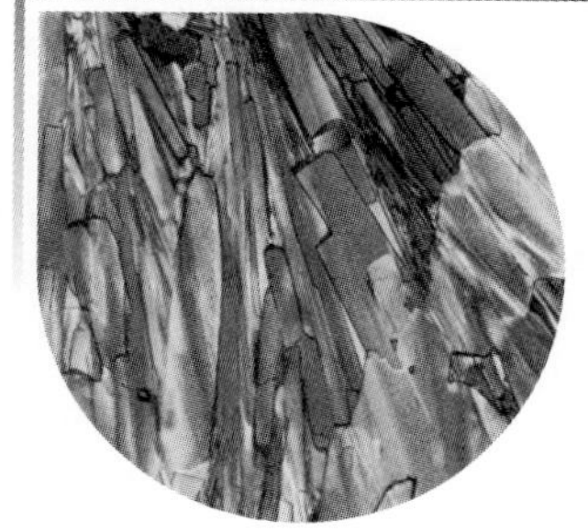

Zinc, Copper, and Manganese

Arthur Grider, PhD

OUTLINE

This chapter is a revision of the chapter contributed by James C. Fleet, PhD, for the first edition.

ZINC, COPPER, AND MANGANESE IN ENZYME SYSTEMS

Zinc (Zn), copper (Cu), and manganese (Mn) are found within the periodic table as transition metals, defined as those elements containing *d* or *f* orbitals that are progressively filled with electrons. Manganese and copper contain partially filled *d* orbitals, whereas the *d* orbitals of zinc are completely filled. Zinc, copper, and manganese function as electron-pair acceptors (Lewis acids). In biological systems, the electron-pair donors (Lewis bases) are amino acids or water (Fig. 37-1). A partial list of enzymes dependent on these minerals is contained in Table 37-1. Because more than 200 zinc-containing metalloenzymes with at least 20 distinct biological functions have been identified in various species, the metalloenzyme function is particularly associated with zinc. However, the metalloenzyme function is central to our understanding of the biology of copper and manganese as well as of zinc, and the loss of specific metalloenzyme function may account for the symptoms associated with deficiencies of these three metals.

Simplest Terms: Acid + Base --------→ Complex

Generalized: e^- Acceptor + e^- Donor ---→ Complex
Lewis acid **Lewis base**

Specific: Metal Ion + Ligand ------→ Metal ligand complex
Zn^{2+} **Amino acid**

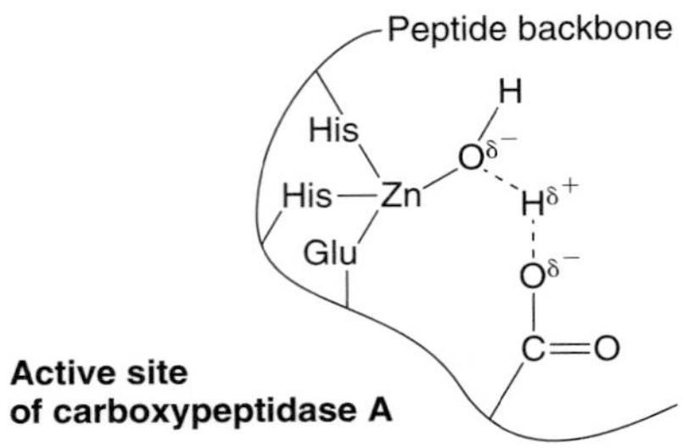

Figure 37-1 Metal–ligand complex formation. The biological roles of minerals like copper, zinc, or manganese frequently depend on their interaction with biological ligands such as amino acids in proteins. These interactions are defined by the chemistry of the mineral. This is illustrated in the figure using the general chemical principles of Lewis acid–base theory.

There are four biological roles in which metals function: signaling, structural, catalytic, and regulatory. The last three roles relate directly to the functions of metals in proteins and enzyme systems. What makes zinc, copper, and manganese so useful in enzyme systems? Some general guidelines that one can follow to assess the likelihood that a mineral will fit a particular biological role include (1) the charge of the ion (determines the stability and reactivity of the metal in an enzyme), (2) the size of the atom (limits the sites a metal can fit), and (3) the natural abundance of a metal and its natural location within a cell (e.g., cytosolic versus extracellular localization will define the likelihood of incorporation into specific enzymes) (Glusker, 1991).

When the chemical features of zinc are examined, it becomes apparent why this metal is so prevalent in proteins and enzyme systems. First, with the exception of potassium (K^+) and magnesium (Mg^{2+}), zinc is the most common intracellular metal ion. It is found in the cytosol, in vesicles and organelles, and in the nucleus. Therefore, it is in the correct proximity to be incorporated into many cellular enzymes. Next, zinc's flexible coordination geometry makes it ideal for the active site of enzymes. One hypothesis regarding metalloenzymes is that the active site of metalloenzymes is "poised for catalysis," a condition called the entatic state (Vallee and Galdes, 1984).

Researchers have defined the entatic state as the condition in which the geometry of the metal binding site in an enzyme is distorted and asymmetrical (Fig. 37-2). When this strain is released by allowing the metal binding site to return to a less distorted form, the energy released may contribute to lowering the energy of activation of the enzymatic reaction. Theoretically, this permits a faster, more efficient enzymatic reaction. Zinc can sit in this entatic state because it has several possible coordination geometries, and because the coordination geometry is easily distorted. In addition, zinc is a strong Lewis acid (only copper is better), and the presence of a strong Lewis acid like zinc at an active site can supply a hydroxyl group (OH^-), which is important

Table 37-1
Vertebrate Enzymes Containing or Activated by Copper, Zinc, or Manganese

Enzyme	Function	Role of Metal
COPPER		
Lysyl oxidase	Collagen synthesis	Catalytic
Peptidylglycine α-amidating monoxygenase	Neuropeptide synthesis	Catalytic
Superoxide dismutase (cytosolic and extracellular)	O_2^- to H_2O_2	Catalytic
"Ferroxidase"/ceruloplasmin	Release of stored iron	Catalytic
Cytochrome *c* oxidase	Oxidative phosphorylation	Catalytic
Dopamine β-hydroxylase	Neurotransmitter synthesis	Catalytic
Tyrosine oxidase	Melanin synthesis	Catalytic
ZINC		
Alcohol dehydrogenase	Alcohol metabolism	Catalytic, noncatalytic
Superoxide dismutase (cytosolic)	O_2^- to H_2O_2	Noncatalytic
Superoxide dismutase (extracellular)	O_2^- to H_2O_2	Noncatalytic
Terminal deoxynucleotide transferase	Add dNTPs to 3′ end of DNA	?
Alkaline phosphatase	Bone formation	Catalytic, noncatalytic
5′-Nucleotidase	Hydrolysis of 5′-nucleotides	?
Fructose 1,6-bisphosphatase	Glycolysis	Regulatory
Aminopeptidase	Protein digestion	Catalytic, regulatory
Angiotensin-converting enzyme	Angiotensin I to II	Catalytic
Carboxypeptidase A and B	Protein digestion	Catalytic
Neutral protease	Protein digestion	Catalytic
Collagenase	Collagen breakdown	Catalytic
Carbonic anhydrase	$CO_2 \rightarrow HCO_3^-$	Catalytic
δ-Aminolevulinic acid dehydratase	Heme biosynthesis	Catalytic
MANGANESE		
Arginase	Urea formation	Catalytic
Pyruvate carboxylase	Gluconeogensis	Catalytic
Superoxide dismutase (mitochondrial)	O_2^- to H_2O_2	Catalytic
Farnesyl pyrophosphate synthetase	Cholesterol synthesis	Catalytic
Glycosyltransferases	Cartilage formation	Regulatory
Phosphoenolpyruvate carboxylase	Gluconeogenesis	Regulatory
Xylosyltransferase	Cartilage formation	Regulatory

for many enzymatic reactions (see Fig. 37-1). In this instance zinc uses water as a fourth ligand (the other three being amino acid residues in the enzyme). The hydroxyl group results when the water molecule forms a partial dipole that is loosely associated with zinc and with a negatively charged group in the enzyme (e.g., a carboxyl group from an aspartate residue).

Like zinc, manganese and copper can supply the hard base, OH^-, for enzymatic reactions when they are present in the active sites of enzymes. However, they have the advantage over zinc when redox reactions are required. Whereas manganese (Mn^{2+}, Mn^{3+}, and Mn^{7+}) and copper (Cu^{1+} and Cu^{2+}) have multiple valence states and can cycle between them as part of an enzymatic reaction, zinc has only one common valence state (Zn^{2+}) and cannot function in these situations. For example, Zn^{2+} serves a structural role in cytosolic and extracellular Cu/Zn superoxide dismutase (SOD), whereas the catalytic reaction of SOD in detoxifying superoxide involves a redox reaction that utilizes either copper (cytosolic and extracellular Cu/Zn-SODs) or manganese (mitochondrial Mn-SOD).

Understanding the central role of zinc, copper, and manganese in association with proteins and enzymes also serves as a framework to explain how researchers have tried to develop functional status assessment tools that can be utilized in defining optimal dietary requirements.

ABSORPTION, TRANSPORT, STORAGE, AND EXCRETION OF ZINC, COPPER, AND MANGANESE

Humans or animals must effectively obtain and retain zinc, copper, and manganese so that these minerals may be utilized for their primary roles in enzyme systems or in other interactions with proteins and biological ligands. Despite the importance of these minerals in mammalian biology, there are still considerable gaps in our knowledge about their metabolism. Of the three metals, the most is known about the metabolism of zinc and copper, whereas very little is known about manganese.

ABSORPTION

Zinc, copper, and manganese are each absorbed throughout the length of the small intestine. Copper may also be absorbed in the stomach. Because of its length and the relatively long period that the digest spends in it, the jejunum is probably where the greatest total amounts of these minerals are absorbed. Absorption is regulated at the intestinal level for copper and zinc; this is probably also true for manganese, although evidence is limited. Absorption can be separated into a saturable, regulated portion and a nonregulated, diffusional component (Fig. 37-3). Because of the existence of both carrier-mediated and nonregulated diffusional absorption of these minerals, the efficiency of absorption falls (lower fractional absorption), although the total amount of mineral entering the body increases as the dietary level of the mineral increases. Some information is known regarding the specific mechanisms of zinc and copper absorption and is described here. Little is known about the mechanism of manganese absorption, but there is some evidence that it competes with iron for a common absorption mechanism. (See Chapter 36 for a discussion of iron absorption.)

Zinc Absorption

There are two mechanisms for the intestinal transport of minerals from the lumen of the intestine to the portal circulation: transcellular and paracellular transport. Transcellular transport, the movement of zinc across the apical

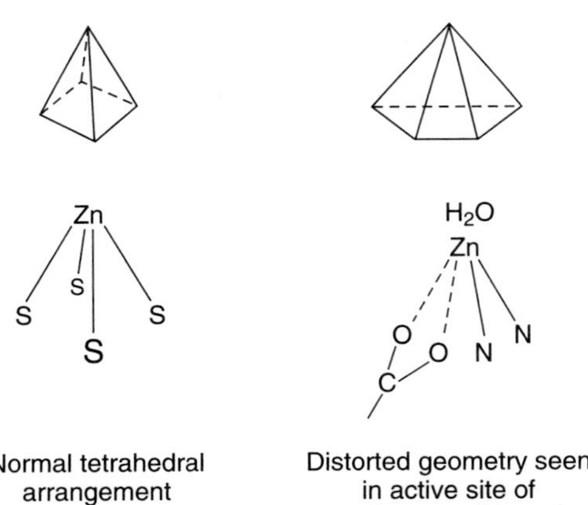

Figure 37-2 Distorted geometry of ligand binding is associated with the entatic state seen in the active site of enzymes. Zinc is shown bound to the enzyme via ligands to the sulfhydryl group of cysteine residues (*S*), the imidazole nitrogen of histidine residues (*N*), or the carboxylate group of glutamate residues (COO^-).

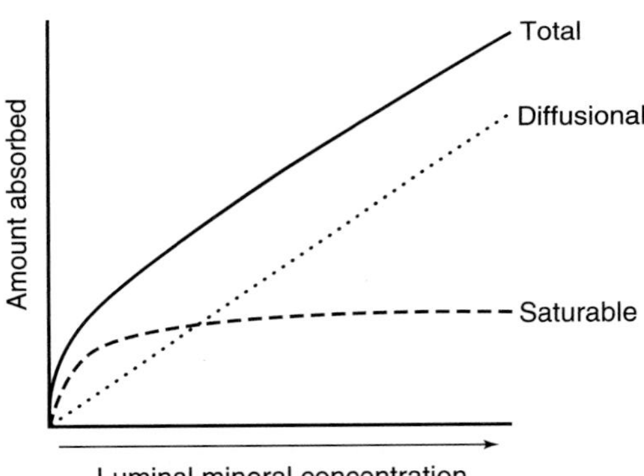

Figure 37-3 A generalized scheme of intestinal mineral absorption kinetics. Regulated intestinal mineral absorption is a combination of both diffusional processes *(dotted line)* and saturable processes *(dashed line)*. The diffusional component is defined by a linear relationship between the intestinal content of the mineral and the total amount of mineral absorbed. In contrast, the saturable component varies depending upon the mineral content of the intestine. At low mineral content, this component is very effective, and at high mineral content, the saturable component plateaus.

membrane through the cell and exiting at the basolateral membrane, is a carrier-mediated process. Paracellular transport occurs by simple diffusion as the concentration of zinc in the lumen exceeds the ability of the transcellular mechanism to transport zinc into the intestinal cell at its apical surface. Paracellular transport occurs as zinc diffuses through the tight junctions between intestinal cells. The model for zinc absorption is shown in Figure 37-4. As the transcellular mechanism becomes saturated with increasing zinc concentrations in the intestinal lumen, absorption by simple diffusion (paracellular transport) increasingly predominates.

Two zinc transporters that facilitate carrier-mediated zinc uptake into the intestinal cell have been identified, ZIP4 (Zrt/Irt-like protein 4) and ZNT5 (zinc transporter 5). Molecular studies of patients with the genetic disease acrodermatitis enteropathica (AE) have revealed that the gene for ZIP4, *SLC39A4*, is mutated in these individuals (Dufner-Beattie et al., 2003). This transporter protein is located at the apical surface of intestinal cells, and its presence is responsive to dietary zinc, increased with zinc deficiency, and decreased during zinc sufficiency (Kim et al., 2004).

The control for intestinal zinc transport is not fully understood. The mechanism is likely to be complex, as recent cellular studies suggest. Elegant cell culture studies using cells transfected with the mouse *SLC39A4* gene showed that, under normal zinc levels, the ZIP4 transporter recycled rapidly via endocytosis between the plasma membrane and an endosomal vesicular compartment (Kim et al., 2004). Under zinc-deficient culture conditions, more of the ZIP4 transporter remained at the plasma membrane while less was observed within the intracellular vesicular compartment. Conversely, when the cultured cells were exposed to an increasing concentration of zinc in the culture medium, less of the transporter was located at the plasma membrane, with a corresponding increase in the transporter within intracellular endosomal vesicles. Furthermore, the increased presence of the transporter at the plasma membrane corresponded with increased zinc uptake, with the converse also being true. Therefore, these current studies with ZIP4 agree with whole animal and small intestine cell culture studies performed earlier showing that zinc deficiency increases intestinal zinc transport and absorption. However, the zinc-dependent trigger for the translocation of the ZIP4 zinc

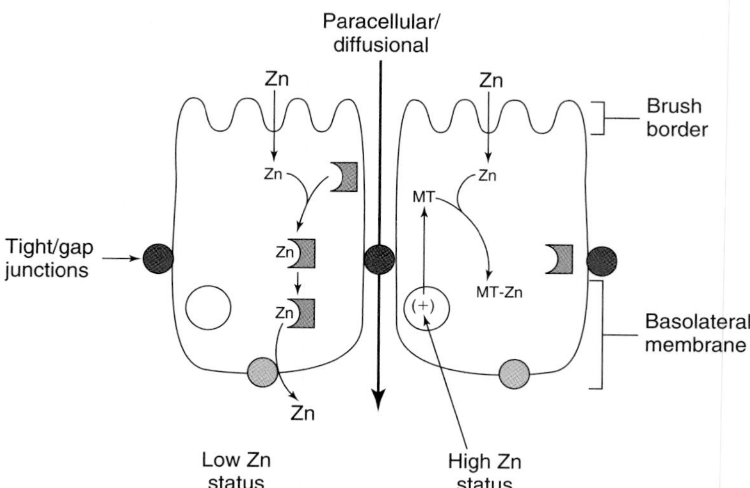

Figure 37-4 A proposed model for intestinal zinc absorption under conditions of high and low zinc status. In this model the diffusional component of transport is shown as movement of zinc between the cells (paracellular transport), and the regulated, saturable component is shown as the movement through the cells (transcellular transport). The right side of the figure illustrates how zinc absorption may be limited when zinc status is high by induction of metallothionein synthesis and the resulting increased binding of zinc by metallothionein (MT), which results in increased retention of zinc in the enterocyte.

transporter between the intracellular vesicles and the plasma membrane is not known at this time.

The mechanism of the intracellular transport of zinc from the apical to the basolateral intracellular surface for transport to the portal circulation is not known at this time. The extrusion of zinc from the enterocyte was previously thought to be by a carrier-dependent ATP-driven mechanism (e.g., a specific Zn^{2+}-ATPase), though its identity had not been established. However, another energy-independent transporter of the cation diffusion family of transporters, ZNT1, is now proposed to be responsible for cellular Zn^{2+} extrusion (McMahon and Cousins, 1998; Palmiter and Findley, 1995).

AE is caused by an autosomal recessive mutation and is characterized by symptoms normally associated with severe zinc deficiency. Symptoms include dermatitis, alopecia, poor growth, immune deficiencies, hypogonadism, night blindness, impaired taste, and diarrhea. Studies have shown that a primary defect in AE patients is reduced intestinal zinc absorption. Other studies have shown that cellular zinc uptake is reduced in intestinal biopsies and in cultured fibroblasts of AE patients (Grider and Young, 1996). The AE mutation has been mapped to chromosomal region 8q24.3. Several mutations within the AE gene (*SLC39A4*, which encodes ZIP4) have been identified. The mutations, found in genomic DNA from AE patients, include missense mutations and a premature termination codon. Several of the missense mutations have been studied thus far using transfected cell culture models; the mutations affect either the translocation of ZIP4 to the plasma membrane or its endocytosis from the plasma membrane (Wang et al., 2004). (The posttranslational regulation of trafficking between membrane compartments has also been shown for the copper transporting P-type ATPases ATP7A and ATP7B.)

Copper Absorption

As with zinc, manganese, and other trace elements, intestinal copper transport requires the following three steps:

1. Uptake from the intestinal lumen across the brush-border membrane
2. Intracellular transport to the basolateral membrane
3. Transport across the plasma membrane to the portal circulation

Two potential apical membrane copper transporters have been identified in intestinal absorptive cells: (1) the Ctr1 copper transporter, and (2) the divalent cation transporter 1 (DCT-1; also called Nramp2 or divalent metal transporter 1 [DMT-1]). Ctr1 transports monovalent copper (Cu^{1+}) (Lee et al., 2002a, 2002b). DCT-1 transports divalent iron, but can also transport divalent copper (Cu^{2+}) (Gunshin et al., 1997). Most of the dietary copper is in its cupric state (Cu^{2+}). It has been reported that reduction of copper by ascorbate inhibits intestinal copper absorption, although recent evidence using a cell culture model for the intestinal cell did not find any effect of ascorbate on copper uptake (Zerounian et al., 2003). It would appear that, in vivo, other unknown factors may be involved in the inhibition of Cu^{1+} intestinal absorption by ascorbate.

Once inside the cell, copper is bound by chaperones that carry copper to various copper-binding proteins, cuproenzymes, or ATP7A, a membrane-associated copper transporting ATPase. Atox1 is a cytosolic copper chaperone that delivers copper from Ctr1 to ATP7A located at the trans-Golgi network. The copper is then exported from the intestinal cell at its basolateral side by this copper transporting ATPase. Menkes' disease is caused by a mutation in the gene encoding for ATP7A, resulting in a lethal reduction in copper absorption (Tumer et al., 2003).

Inhibition of Intestinal Zinc and Copper Absorption by Metallothionein

At low zinc status, transcellular zinc absorption is at its most efficient; at high zinc status, zinc absorption is inhibited. Research suggests that this downregulation of zinc absorption is due to the production of metallothionein, a zinc-binding protein. Metallothionein is a low-molecular-weight protein (6.1 kDa) found in the cell cytosol, and it is produced in response to high levels of dietary zinc or copper, as well as toxic heavy metals such as cadmium (Cd^{2+}) and mercury (Hg^{2+}) (Cousins, 1985). It has been proposed that high levels of metallothionein in enterocytes act as a mucosal block by binding zinc and preventing its movement through the cell, thereby limiting absorption. The "blocked" metal is later lost from the body as the enterocyte is sloughed off into the intestine. Similarly, the induced production of metallothionein by copper may serve to downregulate copper absorption by this same mechanism. Functions for metallothionein in tissues other than the intestine have also been proposed (discussed in subsequent text).

Some studies have shown that high levels of zinc can inhibit intestinal copper absorption; this observation has been used to reduce copper absorption and help minimize the copper toxicity that is characteristic of Wilson's disease. The high zinc diet stimulates the production of metallothionein, which then causes a reduction in copper absorption by serving as a block to transcellular transport. In contrast, high levels of dietary copper do not reduce zinc absorption. One explanation for this latter observation is that high copper is handled differently than high zinc. Zinc is a much stronger inducer of intestinal metallothionein compared to copper (Leone et al., 1985). Copper may not reach the metal-regulatory element of the metallothionein gene as rapidly as zinc, when intake is excessive, because of its shuttling to various copper-binding protein compartments via chaperones. The primary cellular response to excess zinc, however, may be its induction of metallothionein expression and subsequent binding of zinc by intestinal metallothionein.

Bioavailability

Just as the biological roles of copper, zinc, and manganese are defined by their chemical interactions with ligands, so are the interactions of these metals with dietary components. These interactions can influence how well copper, zinc, or manganese is absorbed from the diet, but the luminal interactions leading to increased or decreased absorption are less well characterized than those for ligand interactions of copper, zinc, and manganese with enzymes (Lonnerdal and Sandstrom, 1995).

Chemical similarities with other nutrients may result in competition for common binding sites between related minerals. This could explain the inhibition of manganese absorption caused by high dietary iron, or the zinc–copper antagonism discussed previously. Binding of minerals to organic components of the diet in the lumen of the gastrointestinal tract can alter absorption. The classic example of this is the inhibitory effect that the phosphate-rich plant compound phytate (*myo*-inositol pentaphosphates and hexaphosphates) has on the absorption of zinc and many other minerals (e.g., copper and iron) from the diet (Torre et al., 1992). The presence of calcium and phytate together in the same meal enhances the inhibitory effect on mineral absorption due to the stabilization of phytate by calcium. Others have suggested that binding of zinc or copper to low-molecular-weight ligands such as amino acids (e.g., histidine) may enhance intestinal absorption, but it is not clear how this enhancement would occur. Although ascorbate enhances iron absorption, it inhibits copper absorption. The chemical effects of ascorbate on iron and copper are the same; ascorbate promotes the reduction of both metals (to Fe^{2+} and Cu^{1+}). This suggests that copper is optimally transported in the Cu^{2+} state. Dietary components can also influence other points of zinc or copper utilization. For example, high dietary molybdenum has been shown to increase urinary copper losses, and high dietary calcium increases exogenous zinc losses in the intestine.

TRANSPORT IN PLASMA AND TISSUE UPTAKE

Once absorbed, both copper and zinc are bound primarily to albumin in the plasma and transported to the liver.

Cellular Zinc Transporters

After reaching the liver, zinc is repackaged and released into the circulation bound to α_2-macroglobulin. At any given time, the relative distribution of zinc in the circulation is approximately 57% bound to albumin, 40% to α_2-macroglobulin, and 3% to low-molecular-weight ligands such as amino acids. There is evidence that the uptake of zinc into cells is regulated (note the discussion in the preceding text concerning the ZIP4 zinc transporter).

Several zinc transporter molecules have been identified (including ZIP1, ZIP4, and ZnT5), but none of these transporters appear to require energy for their function. In endothelial cells, albumin is taken up by endocytosis. This mechanism may provide for the majority of the internalization of zinc by cells because most zinc in the circulation is bound to albumin. A portion of this endocytosis occurs through nonclathrin-coated pits and may involve caveolae and/or lipid rafts. These caveolae are specialized plasma membrane compartments that contain an unusually high amount of cholesterol and sphingolipids. They are involved in numerous signal transduction pathways and may be involved in some aspect of zinc uptake. After endocytosis the albumin likely releases the zinc, allowing it to be transported across the endosomal membrane and into the cytosol. Once in the cytosol it binds to proteins within the zinc-binding protein pool, including metallothionein.

Recent discoveries have led to the identification of two families of zinc transporter proteins: (1) the ZRT/ IRT-like proteins (ZIP; *SLC39A* gene family), and (2) the cation diffusion facilitator family (CDF; *SLC30* gene family) (reviewed in Kambe et al., 2004). These transporters differ in several ways. The ZIP transporters that have been characterized thus far transport zinc into the cytosol, either into the cell from the extracellular milieu or into the cytosol from within intracellular membrane compartments. The CDF transporters exhibit the opposite function, facilitating zinc efflux from the cytosol to the outside of the cell or into intracellular membrane compartments. There are 86 ZIP family members found in fungi, plants, insects, nematodes, and mammals. Of the mammalian ZIP transporters, seven (genes or proteins) are actively being investigated for their role in zinc transport (ZIP1, ZIP2, ZIP3, ZIP4, LIV-1, BIGM103, and hKE4). Currently, nine CDF transporters have been identified, which are labeled ZNT1 through ZNT9 (Liuzzi and Cousins, 2004).

Both transporter families are transmembrane proteins. The ZIP family contains proteins exhibiting seven or eight transmembrane domains, with extracellular amino and carboxyl ends. The CDF family is made up mostly of proteins containing six transmembrane regions. Their amino and carboxyl ends are located intracellularly. The zinc transport/binding site for both families is an intracellular histidine-rich loop. However, this loop is located between transmembrane regions three and four in the ZIP family and between transmembrane regions four and five in the CDF family. One of the members of the CDF family, ZNT5/ZTL1, does not fit the general description of the other members of the CDF family. It has twelve transmembrane regions and has been implicated in extracellular zinc influx into intestinal cells (Cragg et al., 2002).

Copper and Ceruloplasmin

Once copper reaches the liver, it is incorporated into ceruloplasmin. Then the copper–ceruloplasmin complex is released into the circulation for delivery to peripheral tissues. Scientists have traditionally thought that ceruloplasmin is a critical protein in the metabolism and function of copper (Vulpe and Packman, 1995). It is a large glycoprotein of 132 kDa, which contains 6% to 7% carbohydrate and which can bind six atoms of copper; 90% to 95% of serum copper is bound to ceruloplasmin. Ceruloplasmin is produced in the liver, and its synthesis is regulated by copper as well as inflammatory mediators such as interleukin-1 (IL-1) and glucocorticoids. These and other factors associated with the acute-phase response are presumably responsible for the increase in serum copper and ceruloplasmin that occurs following acute inflammation or infection.

In cell culture studies, the mechanism of copper uptake into cells was through the binding of ceruloplasmin–copper to a cell-surface receptor (Percival and Harris, 1990). Whereas the circulating transferrin–iron complex is internalized after it binds to the transferrin receptor on the cell surface, copper is reduced and released from ceruloplasmin, at which point the copper can be taken up by the cell as the free metal through the Ctr1 copper transporter. Paradoxically, individuals who have a genetic mutation in the ceruloplasmin gene, leading to a total lack of ceruloplasmin in the serum (i.e., aceruloplasminemia), do not have overt symptoms of copper deficiency as one might predict from the cell culture studies (Harris et al., 1995). Instead, these individuals have altered iron metabolism. This raises questions regarding the biological role of ceruloplasmin in serum copper transport.

Other proteins are also involved in copper movement. Most, if not all, copper ions in cells are bound to superoxide dismutase (SOD) or other proteins. Studies in animals and cells have shown that a copper chaperone for SOD (CCS) is necessary for the insertion of copper into SOD. Rats fed copper-deficient diets displayed a dose-dependent increase in CCS expression in liver and erythrocytes (Bertinato et al., 2003).

Manganese Plasma Transport and Tissue Uptake

Manganese is handled slightly differently than are copper and zinc. Following absorption, manganese is thought to bind to α_2-macroglobulin for delivery to the liver. Because manganese can be oxidized to the Mn^{3+} state, it can bind to transferrin for subsequent delivery to other tissues. It is not clear, however, whether this system was intended to accommodate manganese or whether the binding is simply opportunistic. Regardless, this binding behavior suggests that manganese uptake into cells occurs by the same mechanism as iron uptake, by receptor-mediated endocytosis of the metal–transferrin complex.

STORAGE

When animals are fed experimental diets lacking copper, zinc, or manganese, their status rapidly declines. This suggests that there is not a storage pool of these minerals to be used during times of low intake or increased need (i.e., for the production of new metal-containing proteins and enzymes). For example, zinc can be localized in the bones under conditions of high zinc intake, but this zinc cannot be specifically mobilized to serve the needs of the organism under conditions of low zinc intake. When zinc or copper intake is high, metallothionein increases dramatically in liver, kidney, and/or intestine. Although metallothionein can avidly bind copper and zinc, the functional significance of this is unclear.

Metallothionein

The only serious candidate for a zinc storage protein is metallothionein. Since its discovery in 1960, experiments on the biological role of this protein have been a central feature of zinc research. Metallothionein is a low-molecular-weight protein comprising 61 amino acids, of which 20 residues are cysteine residues (Cousins, 1985). It is surprising that there are no disulfide bridges in metallothionein; all the thiol groups are involved in metal binding. Seven atoms of zinc or the related transition elements (cadmium, mercury, copper, and silver) have been found to bind to metallothionein in vitro. The metals are normally bound in two clusters, with one cluster binding four metal ions and the other binding three. Under normal physiological conditions, zinc is the primary metal bound to metallothionein. It is unlikely that a significant amount of metal-free metallothionein exists. There are multiple isoforms of metallothionein in mammalian tissues; four isoforms have been identified in mice, and at least 12 metallothionein genes have been identified in humans.

Metallothionein is rapidly induced in liver, kidney, pancreas, and/or intestine by exposure to high levels of heavy metals, particularly zinc and cadmium. Hepatic levels of metallothionein are also directly induced by glucocorticoids and the cytokine IL-6. This accounts for the redistribution of zinc from the plasma to the liver during the acute-phase response that occurs following bacterial infection or as a result of inflammatory conditions, such as rheumatoid arthritis and intense exercise. Hepatic metallothionein levels are also elevated in the newborn infant and may serve as a short-term depot for zinc during the initial days of life.

The transcription of the metallothionein genes is mediated through regulatory elements in the promoter region of the genes. Studies have elucidated how zinc promotes metallothionein gene transcription (Palmiter, 1994). Under low zinc conditions, metal-response element-binding transcription factor-1 (called MTF-1) is normally bound to a zinc-sensitive inhibitor (MTI). MTI dissociates from MTF-1 in the presence of zinc, thereby allowing MTF-1 to interact with the metal-response elements in the metallothionein promoter to activate transcription of the metallothionein gene.

Because metallothionein so avidly binds to zinc, researchers have tried to demonstrate a biological role for this protein in normal zinc homeostasis. This goal has been aided by the development of mice lacking or overexpressing the metallothionein genes. Transgenic mice that overexpress metallothionein I (the predominant form of the protein in mice) appear to resist dietary zinc deficiency compared with normal mice, which suggests that metallothionein functions as a repository for zinc (Dalton et al., 1996). In contrast, mice lacking the genes for metallothionein I and II (the forms found in intestine, liver, kidney, and most other cells except the brain) are born healthy and do not show any obvious symptoms of zinc deficiency when their mothers are fed a diet that contains adequate zinc (Kelly et al., 1996). However, kidney abnormalities are seen in newborn pups lacking metallothionein if their mothers are fed zinc-deficient diets while the pups are nursing. This suggests there may be a developmental role for metallothionein as a storage protein that protects the offspring when maternal zinc status is low.

Preliminary studies suggest that animals lacking metallothionein in the intestine do not reduce intestinal zinc absorption in response to high zinc status (Davis et al., 1996). This supports the proposed role of intestinal metallothionein in limiting the amount of zinc that leaves the enterocyte and enters the portal circulation. Finally, metallothionein "knockout" mice are excessively sensitive to cadmium toxicity, which supports the role of metallothionein as a heavy metal detoxification protein. Recent studies have shown that metallothionein is also essential for the redistribution of zinc from the plasma to the liver, which is characteristic of the acute-phase response.

Menkes' Syndrome and Wilson's Disease: Copper Transporting P-Type ATPases

Both Menkes' syndrome and Wilson's disease are genetic disturbances in copper metabolism (DiDonato and Sarkar, 1997; Danks, 1995). Menkes' syndrome is an X-linked recessive disorder that occurs at a rate greater than 1 in 300,000 live births and is usually fatal within 3 years after birth. It is characterized by low serum copper and ceruloplasmin levels and low copper levels in the liver and brain but markedly elevated cellular copper levels in the intestinal mucosa, muscle, spleen, and kidney. Other symptoms include abnormal ("steely") hair and progressive cerebral degeneration.

Wilson's disease has autosomal recessive inheritance and occurs with an incidence greater than 1 in 100,000 live births. The onset of Wilson's disease is much slower than that of Menkes' syndrome, and it is usually diagnosed during or after the third decade of life. As in Menkes' syndrome, serum ceruloplasmin levels are low in patients with Wilson's disease, but, in contrast to Menkes' syndrome, copper accumulates in the liver and brain. Patients with Wilson's disease appear to have a defect in the ability to excrete copper via the bile. Neurological damage and hepatic cirrhosis are end-stage effects of uncontrolled Wilson's disease. If diagnosed early, patients can be treated by reducing copper intake, undergoing chelation therapy (with D-penicillamine), and taking oral zinc supplements (which will increase intestinal metallothionein and reduce copper absorption).

These diseases are caused by mutations in the genes encoding two P-type ATPases, ATP7A (Menkes' syndrome) and ATP7B (Wilson's disease) (Lutsenko and Petris, 2002). The P-type ATPases are a family of cation-transporting proteins found in all organisms and consists of over 200 members. Copper transport by ATP7A and B requires the catalytic hydrolysis of ATP. ATP7A and B are related, but are two different proteins, exhibiting about 60% homology. The tissue distribution of these two transport proteins is different. ATP7A mRNA is found in all tissues except the liver, whereas ATP7B mRNA is highest in the liver, followed by the kidney, brain, placenta, heart, and lungs (Cox and Moore, 2002). Normally, increasing copper levels stimulates ATP7A, the Menkes' protein, to translocate from the *trans*-Golgi network to the plasma membrane. ATP7B, however, travels from the *trans*-Golgi network to intracellular vesicles and liver bile canaliculi with increasing copper levels. Therefore, their movement between compartments is post-translationally regulated in response to copper as has been shown for the ZIP4 zinc transporter. The various genetic mutations underlying Menkes' and Wilson's diseases may result in the presence of mutant ATP7A or B proteins that display different patterns of copper-dependent trafficking between the *trans*-Golgi and their functional compartments.

EXCRETION

Under normal circumstances, very little zinc, copper, or manganese is lost through the urine or through cutaneous losses; most of the losses are through the feces. Of the endogenous fecal loss, some is from the sloughing off of intestinal cells into the intestinal lumen and is considered nonspecific. However, when dietary zinc or copper intake is high and metallothionein levels are induced, this loss can be significant. The specific loss of copper and manganese through the gastrointestinal tract is via their secretion in the bile. The incorporation of manganese into bile is thought to be very rapid. When manganese is transported into the liver, it either rapidly enters the mitochondria (where it is incorporated into mitochondrial SOD) or is sequestered into lysosomes. Lysosomal manganese is then actively transported into the bile, and it is concentrated in the gallbladder to a concentration 150-fold greater than that seen in the plasma. Almost all copper excretion is via the bile, and biliary copper appears to be complexed in such a way as to make it unavailable for reabsorption in the intestine.

Zinc excretion in urine varies with zinc intake, but urinary zinc generally amounts to less than 10% of total excretion. Approximately 90% of zinc excretion is through the feces; the actual level of excretion via the intestinal route varies with dietary intake and with the zinc status of the individual. As a result, the fine-tuning of zinc balance is mainly through intestinal secretion and fecal excretion. Although bile and gastroduodenal secretions contribute to endogenous zinc excretion, pancreatic secretions are the major contributor to endogenous zinc losses. The zinc-containing fraction of pancreatic secretions is made up of zinc-dependent enzymes, including carboxypeptidase A and B. These enzymes can be digested, and most of the zinc from them can be reabsorbed.

SELECTED FUNCTIONS OF ZINC, COPPER, AND MANGANESE

The following sections detail a few of the interesting biological functions of copper, zinc, and manganese for which mechanisms have been proposed.

ZINC-FINGER PROTEINS AS GENE TRANSCRIPTION FACTORS

Since the 1980s, a nonenzymatic role for zinc in proteins has been shown to be important in the regulation of genes. Klug coined the term "zinc finger" to describe the folding pattern of amino acids around zinc that he observed in the transcription factor TFIIIA (Rhodes and Klug, 1993). In this model, zinc binding to certain transcription factors results in the formation of a loop, or "finger," in the protein that permits the folded region to bind DNA sequences in the promoter region of genes (Fig. 37-5). Therefore, without zinc, the transcription factor cannot bind DNA and stimulate transcription of a gene. The zinc-finger motif requires four amino acid residues as ligands (two cysteinyl and two histidyl residues) per mole of zinc. Despite the level of acceptance regarding the importance of zinc-finger proteins in biology, there are few proven instances of zinc fingers. Putative zinc-finger motifs have been observed in the primary sequences of various nuclear hormone receptors (e.g., the vitamin D receptor and thyroid hormone receptor) and various other transcription factors.

ZINC REGULATION OF GROWTH

A primary feature of severe zinc deficiency in young animals and in children is slow growth. The classic observation, made over 30 years ago, was that low-zinc, high-phytate, plant-based diets stunted growth of Iranian adolescents (Reinhold, 1971). More recently, researchers have shown that low-income Hispanic children who fall in the lower growth percentiles and infants with a nutritional pattern of failure to thrive

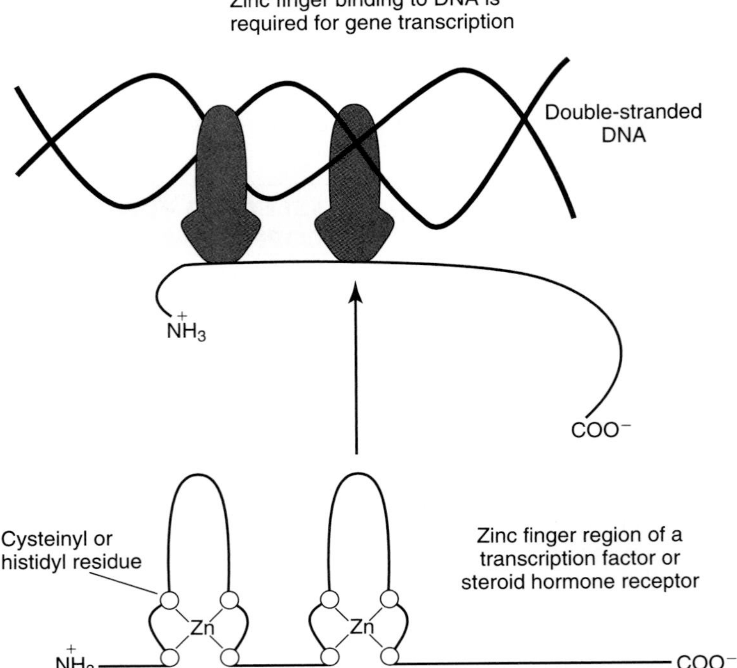

Figure 37-5 Zinc-finger proteins are important for binding of transcription factors to DNA. By binding to histidine and cysteine residues in transcription factors and nuclear hormone receptors, zinc introduces a finger-like secondary structure to the proteins. This structure allows the transcription factors to interact properly with response elements in the promoters of genes.

respond to zinc supplementation by growing. This suggests that mild zinc deficiency is one of the etiological factors contributing to these conditions.

Zinc deficiency appears to retard growth by disrupting the function of insulin-like growth factor I (IGF-I), the factor that mediates the cellular effects of growth hormone. Studies have shown that serum IGF-I levels are reduced in zinc-deficient animals (Roth and Kirchgessner, 1994). However, normalizing serum levels of IGF-I by infusing zinc-deficient rats with IGF-I did not increase either food intake or growth, which suggests that additional points of growth regulation are also impaired (Browning et al., 1998). One possible mechanism is that zinc deficiency causes a reduction in the cellular levels of the IGF-I receptor (Williamson et al., 1997). Although this observation is preliminary, it is consistent with the observation that the promoter for the IGF-I receptor can be activated by a promoter-specific transcription factor (Sp1) that contains a zinc-finger DNA–binding region.

IMMUNOREGULATION BY ZINC AND COPPER

Both zinc and copper deficiency impair immune function. Most of the work in this area has been conducted using mouse models. Studies in humans are more difficult because of the rarity of severe zinc or copper deficiency and the practical difficulties related to the identification of people with marginal zinc or copper deficiency. Nevertheless, in both animals and humans, zinc deficiency appears to reduce immune function because of an overall loss in the total numbers of lymphocytes (B and T cells) of the peripheral immune system (Walsh et al., 1994), whereas copper deficiency results in neutropenia (a lack of circulating neutrophils/granulocytes)

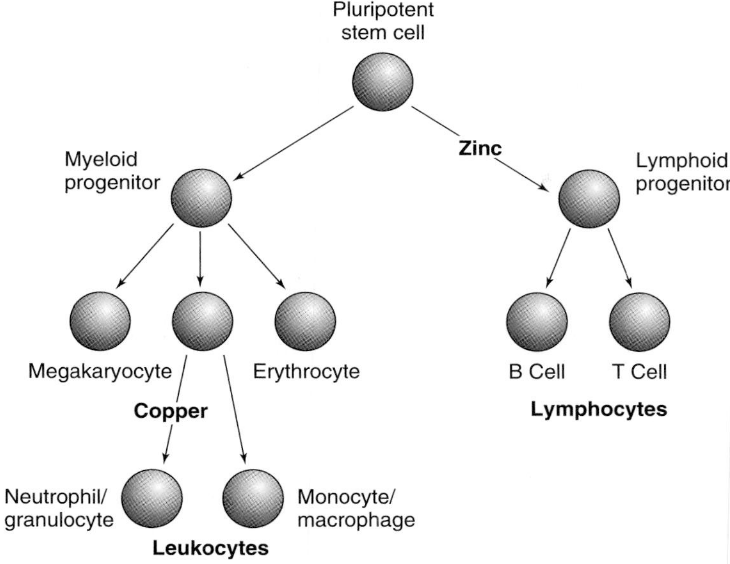

Figure 37-6 The putative sites of action for copper and zinc in immune cell differentiation. Severe copper deficiency results in reduced numbers of neutrophils, whereas severe zinc deficiency results in reduced numbers of T and B lymphocytes. This is partly due to impaired differentiation of these terminally differentiated cells from their precursors. The proposed points of action of copper and zinc on immune cell differentiation are shown in the figure.

(Percival, 1995), as well as lower numbers of T lymphocytes (Failla and Hopkins, 1997).

Preliminary evidence suggests that the loss of lymphocytes and neutrophils results from reduced production of new cells rather than from excessive or early death of existing cells. The effects that zinc deficiency has on the lymphocytes may result partially from atrophy of the thymus, an organ that controls the development of T lymphocytes, and the loss of the zinc-dependent hormone thymulin that is secreted by the thymus gland. In zinc deficiency, the proportion of T lymphocytes and B lymphocytes (and subsets of these cell types) and the functional capacity of the lymphocytes present in zinc-deficient animals appear to be normal. Addition of copper to cultures of HL-60 cells (a promyelocytic cell line) promotes differentiation of these cells toward the granulocyte–neutrophil phenotype by enhancing the progression of the cells from promyelocytes to myelocytes. Therefore, although both copper and zinc are important for optimal development of the immune system, their effects appear to be on different aspects of marrow stem cell differentiation (Fig. 37-6). Exactly how copper or zinc directly influences immune cell differentiation is not known.

Copper deficiency inhibits the proliferation of T cells (particularly the T helper, or CD4+, cells) in response to mitogens. More detailed studies show that the T-cell precursors can be activated and become competent during copper deficiency. Interleukin-2 (IL-2) mediates T-cell proliferation in response to mitogens, but copper-deficient cells do not make as much IL-2 as do cells from copper-adequate animals. It is not clear how copper deficiency alters the production of IL-2.

COPPER AND IRON METABOLISM

In addition to its proposed role as a plasma copper transport protein, ceruloplasmin also has an enzymatic function as a ferroxidase, oxidizing Fe^{2+} released from iron stores to Fe^{3+}, which can then bind to transferrin and be delivered to cells for use in processes such as heme synthesis (Fig. 37-7; see also Chapter 36). It also is possible that this ferroxidase function could be important in the plasma to help control the level of free Fe^{3+} and prevent it from initiating free-radical damage. Copper is proposed to

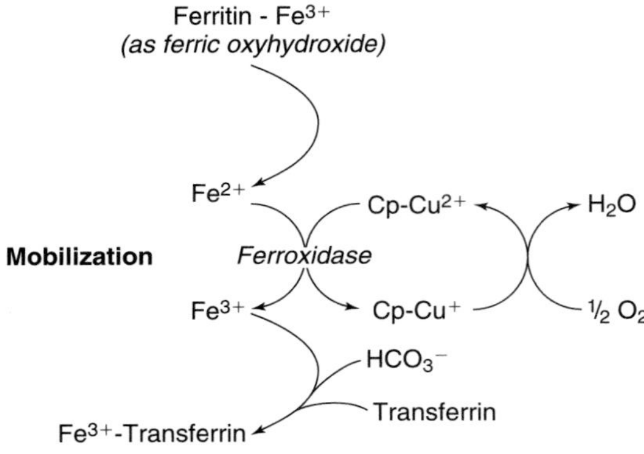

Figure 37-7 The proposed mechanism of the ferroxidase function of ceruloplasmin (*Cp*) in mobilizing stored iron.

function in the catalytic site of ceruloplasmin/ferroxidase, where it exchanges electrons with iron. This ferroxidase role of ceruloplasmin was first proposed following observations of anemia in severely copper-deficient animals, which was characterized by normal hepatic iron stores (Owen, 1973). The anemia could be reversed by dietary copper but not iron. Other data are inconsistent with the proposed ferroxidase function of ceruloplasmin. However, individuals have been identified who genetically lack the ability to produce ceruloplasmin and are thus aceruloplasminemic, and these persons also show signs of irregular iron metabolism with tissue deposition of iron and mild anemia, providing additional support for a role for ceruloplasmin in iron metabolism (Harris et al., 1995).

Clinical Correlation

Role of Ceruloplasmin in Iron Metabolism

Subsequent to the identification of the mutated gene responsible for Wilson's disease, it became possible to screen adult patients with neurological degeneration and low serum ceruloplasmin concentrations for molecular diagnosis of Wilson's disease. Wilson's disease is caused by defective coding for a putative copper-transporting ATPase located in hepatic membranes; this transport protein is required for copper trafficking into a common pool for biliary excretion and holoceruloplasmin biosynthesis. Failure to incorporate copper during ceruloplasmin biosynthesis results in unstable ceruloplasmin that lacks oxidase activity.

As patients were referred for molecular diagnosis, it became clear that some of the patients with low or absent ceruloplasmin did not have Wilson's disease. Further molecular genetic analysis of patients with non–Wilson's disease aceruloplasminemia revealed mutations in the ceruloplasmin gene that resulted in truncation of the open reading frame. Harris and colleagues (1995) described one of two sisters with undetectable ceruloplasmin. This patient was homozygous for a mutation in exon 7 of the ceruloplasmin gene. She had developed degeneration of the retina and basal ganglia during the fifth decade of life. Liver biopsy revealed a normal hepatic copper concentration but elevated iron stores. Indirect evidence for iron deposition in the basal ganglia of the brain was also obtained. The association of defects in ceruloplasmin synthesis with abnormalities in iron metabolism in this and other patients confirms an essential role of ceruloplasmin in human iron metabolism and supports a role of ceruloplasmin as a ferroxidase (Harris and Gitlin, 1996). However, the major problem in patients with aceruloplasminemia seems to be excessive iron deposition or storage, with much milder problems related to iron delivery or utilization. How a plasma protein can be involved in release of iron from tissue ferritin is not yet clear.

Clinical Correlation

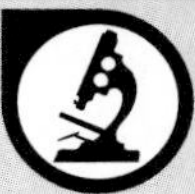

Role of Ceruloplasmin in Iron Metabolism—cont'd

Thinking Critically

1. Explain how a lack of ceruloplasmin could result in iron overload in liver and other tissues.
2. A low serum iron concentration and an elevated serum ferritin concentration are found in patients with defects in the ceruloplasmin gene. Anemia is seen in some but not all patients with defects in the ceruloplasmin gene. (a) Explain how each of these clinical/biochemical manifestations could result from a defect in ferroxidase activity. (b) Are these changes in measures of iron status similar to or different from the changes that would occur in iron deficiency anemia? (See Chapter 36 for more information about iron metabolism.)
3. Copper metabolism and transport seem to be relatively normal in patients with defects in ceruloplasmin synthesis. What might this tell us about the role of ceruloplasmin in copper transport in the body?

COPPER IN BONE AND VASCULAR FUNCTION

Copper deficiency results in abnormal bone metabolism and in skeletal abnormalities in most species. This is not due to abnormal calcium metabolism or mineralization of bone but occurs because the collagen matrix of bone is incompletely formed. The root cause of this defect is reduced activity of the copper-containing enzyme lysyl oxidase (Rucker et al., 1996). Lysyl oxidase is required for the removal of the ε–amino group of lysyl and hydroxylysyl residues with oxidation of the ε-carbon to an aldehyde, which results in the production of a variety of cross-linkages with amino acid residues in collagen. A loss of lysyl oxidase activity results in lower strength and stability of bone collagen.

The lack of this cross-linking by lysyl oxidase also affects elastin. Elastin is a protein that normally gives the aorta its needed flexibility. During copper deficiency the aorta is weakened and aortic rupture may occur. Additional cardiac abnormalities have been observed in association with copper deficiency; these include cardiac hypertrophy, altered electrocardiograms, abnormal mitochondrial structure, and reduced levels of ATP and phosphocreatine. It is not clear what aspect of copper deficiency causes these latter effects, but they are not thought to be attributable to reduced lysyl oxidase activity.

SUPEROXIDE DISMUTASE AND FREE RADICAL PROTECTION

Superoxide dismutases (SODs) are part of the body's natural defense against reactive oxygen species. Reactive oxygen species are free radicals that, if left uncontrolled, can damage DNA, proteins, and lipids within cells and can alter or inhibit cellular function (Noor et al., 2002; Halliwell, 1994). SODs catalyze the reaction by which superoxide is removed: $2O_2^{\dot{+}} + 2H^+ \rightarrow H_2O_2 + O_2$. The hydrogen peroxide generated is further metabolized by either catalase (an iron-containing enzyme) or glutathione peroxidase (a selenium-containing enzyme). Cytosolic Cu/Zn-SOD is made up of two identical subunits, each of which contains 1 atom of copper and 1 atom of zinc. Extracellular Cu/Zn-SOD is a secreted tetrameric glycoprotein that is related, but not identical, to the cytosolic form of Cu/Zn-SOD. The manganese-containing SOD catalyzes the same reaction as the Cu/Zn-SOD, but Mn-SOD is located in the mitochondria as opposed to the cytosol or extracellular fluids. In the active site of the enzymes, copper or manganese is alternately reduced and oxidized by superoxide to produce hydrogen peroxide. Therefore, the enzyme activity is completely inhibited in the absence of these minerals. In contrast, some Cu/Zn-SOD activity is retained when zinc is removed or replaced with other chemically similar metals (e.g., cadmium, mercury, or copper). Zinc may serve two functions: it may stabilize the native structure of the enzyme, and a zinc-histidyl-copper triad may act as a proton donor during the oxidation cycle of the enzyme.

The genetic overexpression of cytosolic Cu/Zn-SOD or Fe-dependent catalase in the fruit fly, an insect model of aging, prolongs life, presumably due to improved protection from free radical damage (Orr and Sohal, 1994). These types of studies have provided strong support for the free radical theory of aging. Experimental evidence shows that a reduction in cytosolic or extracellular Cu/Zn-SOD can also occur in animals fed zinc- or copper-deficient diets. This may have physiological consequences. For example, erythrocytes from copper-deficient animals with low cytosolic Cu/Zn-SOD levels are more susceptible to lipid peroxidation and hemolysis in vitro (Rock et al., 1995). In addition, young rats fed a copper-deficient diet have lower Cu/Zn-SOD activity in the lung and liver and have lower survival times when exposed to high-oxygen conditions. Collectively, these data suggest that dietary deficiencies of copper and zinc can have functional consequences related to reduced free radical defenses.

The mitochondria are the site of oxidative phosphorylation and are, therefore, a tremendous source of potentially hazardous reactive oxygen species and free radicals. Therefore, deficiency of manganese becomes a condition of superoxide radical poisoning, owing to the loss of Mn-SOD activity. This can have several identifiable consequences. First, researchers have identified abnormalities in cell function and ultrastructural abnormalities in mitochondria in manganese deficiency. The mitochondrial changes (elongation and reorientation of cristae, presence of vacuoles in the matrix, and separation of inner and outer mitochondrial membranes) are likely the result of observed increases in mitochondrial lipid peroxidation. Disruption of mitochondrial integrity may result in disturbed energy metabolism through disruption of oxidative phosphorylation. Manganese deficiency alters carbohydrate metabolism through the destruction of pancreatic β cells. This could account for the decreased glucose utilization, reduced pancreatic insulin, and lower insulin output from perfused pancreas observed in manganese-deficient animals. Although it is not clear how manganese contributes to pancreatic β cell abnormalities, researchers have proposed that free radical damage resulting from the lack of Mn-SOD activity is a factor.

MANGANESE IN CARTILAGE FORMATION

As with copper deficiency, skeletal abnormalities that are unrelated to impaired mineralization of bone are a characteristic of manganese deficiency. For example, in growing animals manganese deficiency results in an inhibition of endochondral osteogenesis at the growth plates/epiphyseal cartilages. This is caused by a reduction in the synthesis of proteoglycans such as chondroitin sulfate (the proteoglycan affected most by manganese deficiency) (Liu et al., 1994). Proteoglycans (glycosaminoglycan–protein complexes) are essential structural components of cartilage, which explains the sensitivity of the growth plate to manganese deficiency. Chondroitin sulfate synthesis is regulated by manganese at two sites. The polymerase responsible for the polymerization of UDP-*N*-acetylgalactosamine to UDP-glucuronic acid to form the glycosaminoglycan chain requires manganese. Galactotransferase, an enzyme that catalyzes the incorporation of galactose into a galactose–galactose–xylose trisaccharide, which is required for the linkage of the polysaccharide chain to the protein associated with it, is also a manganese-requiring enzyme. Other glycosyltransferases are also activated by manganese.

In the least severe stage of manganese deficiency, animals will give birth to viable offspring, but some of the young will exhibit ataxia and loss of equilibrium. This condition is the result of a structural defect in the development of the inner ear, resulting in impaired vestibular function. As with the bone defects noted earlier, these inner-ear structural defects are also the result of impaired cartilage development associated with reduced proteoglycan formation.

ASSESSMENT OF ZINC, COPPER, AND MANGANESE STATUS AND DEFICIENCY SYMPTOMS

STATUS ASSESSMENT

The "Holy Grail" of status assessment is the availability of a functional parameter that changes with the dietary deficiency of a required nutrient. Unfortunately, there are no reliable functional assessment tools for zinc, copper, or manganese. Researchers have examined a number of metal-dependent enzymes for their ability to serve as sensitive indicators of zinc (e.g., alkaline phosphatase, Cu/Zn-SOD, 5′ nucleotidase) and copper (e.g., Cu/Zn-SOD) status (Delves, 1985). Although some of these assays show promise, none has to date been proved useful. The remaining option is static assessment tools, such as mineral levels in serum, hair, and red or white blood cells.

In normal, healthy people, the plasma concentration of zinc does not appear to change except under conditions of extreme deficiency. Therefore, plasma or serum zinc concentration is an inadequate measure for assessment of more subtle changes in status. The plasma zinc level does fall significantly during pregnancy, but this decrease is associated with a fall in plasma albumin concentration and an expansion of maternal blood volume. These changes may be important to the development of the fetus and the viability of the pregnancy, and it is not clear that this decline in plasma zinc indicates inadequate zinc intake during pregnancy (Swanson and King, 1983). Serum copper and ceruloplasmin have shown some utility as measures of copper status, but these measures (as well as serum zinc) are very sensitive to acute inflammation. During acute inflammation, serum zinc levels fall and serum copper and ceruloplasmin levels increase, giving the false impression that zinc status is low and copper status is high. Hair mineral levels can be a useful crude measure of long-term mineral status, but hair mineral content is sensitive to contamination from the environment (e.g., shampoos and emissions). Erythrocyte or serum metallothionein levels have been evaluated as a measure of zinc status. Although extremes of zinc status can be assessed by this method, there is no indication that metallothionein concentration is useful for assessment of marginal zinc status. Lymphocyte zinc content has been shown to be more sensitive to marginal zinc intake in small, well-controlled studies. However, the association of lymphocyte zinc concentration with zinc intake has not been verified in larger groups, and the difficulty in isolating these white blood cells reduces the utility of this measure for assessing zinc status in the population. Finally, urinary excretion poorly reflects changes in intakes of zinc, copper, and manganese. Clearly, the development of reliable functional assessment tools is essential for establishing the true requirements for zinc, copper, and manganese and for defining the true health risks of inadequate intake of these minerals.

DEFICIENCY SYMPTOMS

Zinc

The symptoms of zinc deficiency have been observed in humans in populations consuming diets high in phytate and low in meat (e.g., the classic studies of zinc deficiency in Iranian children), as well as in subjects with acrodermatitis enteropathica (AE). As a result of its occurrence in humans, zinc deficiency has been studied extensively. Many symptoms of zinc deficiency have been characterized (Table 37-2), but the underlying biochemical defects responsible for most of them have not been found. For example, loss of appetite is one of the first signs associated with specific dietary zinc inadequacy. Although this clearly contributes to the growth depression seen in zinc-deficient children, the reason for the loss of appetite is not known. This is also true for the classic symptoms of zinc deficiency, such as loss of normal taste sensation, alopecia, hyperkeratinization of skin, and reproductive abnormalities. Because of the vast array of zinc-dependent enzymes, as well as the proposed importance of the zinc-finger structure in modulating the interaction between transcription factors and DNA, it is unlikely that a single root cause will be determined for many of these conditions.

Box 37-1

CHARACTERISTICS OF ZINC, COPPER, AND MANGANESE DEFICIENCY IN ANIMALS AND HUMANS

Zinc	Copper	Manganese
Loss of appetite	Anemia	Poor growth
Poor growth	Skeletal defects	Abnormal bone
Alopecia	Cardiac enlargement	Impaired glucose tolerance
Immune dysfunction	Altered pigmentation	Poor reproduction
Hypogonadism	Reproductive failure	Malformations in offspring
Poor wound healing	Lower aortic elasticity	
Impaired taste acuity	Neutropenia	

Copper

Experimental copper deficiency has helped us understand the role of copper in iron metabolism, immune function, and cartilage production. The symptoms listed for copper deficiency in Box 37-1 are all associated with either severe dietary copper deficiency or copper deficiency associated with the genetic condition called Wilson's disease. These conditions are rare in humans. In contrast, researchers have noted several symptoms (e.g., irregular heartbeat and impaired glucose utilization) that occur before the onset of severe deficiency and that may have more general relevance to human health. The degree of copper deficiency or low intake that leads to these milder symptoms is not clearly defined, but epidemiological evidence linking low serum copper levels to an elevated risk of cardiovascular disease suggests that marginal copper status may be of practical concern.

Manganese

Reduced growth is a general feature of manganese deficiency. Although food consumption does fall in manganese-deficient animals, it is not a prominent feature of the deficiency. As discussed earlier, some of the deficiency signs that have been observed for manganese can be linked to the loss of specific enzyme functions. In contrast, the cause of the disrupted reproductive ability (lower conception, increased spontaneous abortion, stillbirths, lower birth weights, defective ovulation, and testicular degeneration) observed in manganese-deficient animals is unknown. Similarly, although animal studies reveal a greater susceptibility to convulsions and electroencephalogram readings reminiscent of those for epileptics, the underlying basis for these phenomena is not clearly understood.

DIETARY REFERENCE INTAKES AND FOOD SOURCES OF ZINC, COPPER, AND MANGANESE

DIETARY REFERENCE INTAKES

The Institute of Medicine (IOM) published the dietary reference intakes (DRIs) for zinc, copper, and manganese in 2001 (IOM, 2001). These DRIs replaced the recommended dietary allowance (RDA) for zinc and the estimated safe and adequate daily dietary intakes for copper and manganese that had been set as part of the 1989 recommended dietary allowances.

Zinc

The adequate intake (AI) of zinc for infants from birth to 6 months of age was set as 2 mg/day. This value was based on the zinc intake of breast-fed infants, which declined from approximately 2.3 mg/day at 2 weeks to 1 mg/day at 6 months. The decline in intake with age is due to an unusually rapid physiological decline in the zinc concentration of human milk from approximately 4 mg/L at 2 weeks postpartum to 1.2 mg/L at 6 months postpartum. Factorial estimates of zinc requirements based on fractional absorption of dietary zinc and endogenous losses yielded a similar range of estimates for the zinc requirement—2.1 mg/day at 1 month and 1.54 mg/day at 5 months—as did measurements of intake. There is some evidence that the zinc content of human milk is growth-limiting for some infants after 4 months of age, so the AI was set near the upper end of the range.

Human milk alone is an inadequate source of zinc after the first 6 months. For older infants and children, a factorial apporach was used to arrive at the need for dietary zinc to replace losses and to support growth. In most cases, zinc losses were extrapoplated from measurements made in adults, and requirements for growth were based on an average zinc content of 20 μg/g wet weight of tissue. For infants 7 to 12 months of age, total zinc losses were estimated as 64 μg/kg/day and the requirement for growth as 260 μg/day based on accretion of 13 g new tissue per day. For children ages 1 through 3 years, total losses were estimated as 48 μg/kg/day, and the requirement for growth was estimated as 20 μg/g × 6 g/day. For children ages 4 to 8 years, total losses were estimated as 48 μg/kg/day and the requirement for growth as 20 μg /g × 7 g/day. For children 9 to 13 years of age, total losses were estimated as 48 μg/kg/day and the requirement for growth as 20 μg /g × 10 g/day. Using an estimated fractional absorption of zinc of 0.3 and reference weights for each of the groups, the estimated average requirements (EARs) were set as 2.5 mg/day for infants ages 7 to 12 months and for children from 1 to 3 years of age, as 4 mg/day for children from 4 to 8 years, as 7 mg/day for boys ages 9 to 13 years, and 8 mg/day for girls ages 9 to 13 years. In the absence of information about the standard deviation of the requirement, the RDA was set as equal to the EAR plus 20%.

A similar factorial approach was also used in setting the DRIs for adolescents, ages 14 through 18 years, but with addition of an estimate to allow for semen or menstrual losses of zinc and using a fractional absorption estimate of 0.4 derived from studies with men. The EAR and RDA, respectively, for adolescent boys are 8.5 and 11 mg zinc/day, and those for adolescent girls are 7.3 and 9 mg zinc/day.

The EAR of adults for zinc was also determined by factorial analysis. The average endogenous loss of zinc via all routes other than the intestine was calculated to be 1.27 mg/day for men and 1.0 mg/day for women. The minimum amount of absorbed zinc required to match endogenous zinc losses from the intestine was estimated as 2.57 mg/day for men and 2.3 mg/day for women. With fractional absorptions of 0.41 for men and 0.48 for women, the EARs were set as the amount of zinc required to replace the total calculated loss of zinc by men and women:

Men: $(1.27 + 2.57)/0.41 = 9.3$ mg/day

Women: $(1.0 + 2.3)/0.48 = 6.8$ mg/day

The RDA was set as the EAR + 20%: 11 mg/day for men and 8 mg/day for women. On the basis of the third National Health and Nutrition Examination Survey (NHANES III) dataset, zinc intake by adults in the United States ranges from about 5 mg/day to 25 mg/day. The median intake of zinc from food by adult men and women in the United States is approximately 13 mg/day for men and 9 mg/day for women. Thus, median intakes only slightly exceed the RDAs for zinc.

Additional zinc intake is recommended for pregnant and lactating women. The EAR was increased by 2.7 mg/day for pregnant women, based on accumulation of absorbed zinc by maternal and fetal tissues during the fourth quarter of pregnancy, and by 3.6 mg/day for lactating adult women, based on the net additional loss of absorbed zinc during lactation. The RDAs for pregnant and lactating adult women are 11 and 12 mg/day, respectively.

Copper

The recommended intakes of copper for infants reflect the mean copper intake of infants principally fed human milk. The AI for infants from 0 through 6 months of age is 0.20 mg/day (0.25 mg copper/L milk × 0.78 L/day). For infants from 7 to 12 months of age, the AI was based on copper intake from human milk (0.20 mg Cu/L milk × 0.6 L/day) plus an intake of 0.10 mg Cu/day from complementary foods, to yield a total of 0.22 mg /day. Because no data were available on which to base EARs for copper for children or adolescents, the EARs were estimated by extrapolating from the adult EAR (see subsequent text) using metabolic weight ($kg^{0.75}$) as the basis for the extrapolation.

The adult EAR for copper was established based on several studies of adult copper

RDAs Across the Life Cycle

	Zinc RDAs mg per Day	Copper RDAs mg per Day	Manganese AIs mg per Day
Infants			
0 to 0.5 yr	2.0 (AI)	0.20 (AI)	0.003
0.5 to 1 yr	3.0	0.22 (AI)	0.6
Children			
1 to 3 yr	3.0	0.34	1.2
4 to 8 yr	5.0	0.44	1.5
Males			
9 to 13 yr	8.0	0.70	1.9
14 to 18 yr	11.0	0.89	2.2
19 to > 70 yr	9.4	0.90	2.3
Females			
9 to 13 yr	8.0	0.70	1.6
14 to 18 yr	9.0	0.89	1.6
19 to >70 yr	8.0	0.90	1.8
Pregnant	11.0	1.00	2.0
Lactating	12.0	1.30	2.6

Data from Institute of Medicine (IOM) (2004) Dietary Reference Intakes for Vitamin A, Vitamin K, Arsenic, Boron, Chromium, Copper, Iodine, Iron, Manganese, Molybdenum, Nickel, Silicon, Vanadium, and Zinc. National Academy Press, Washington, DC.

requirements that used biochemical indicators of copper status. The indicators included the concentrations of plasma and platelet copper, serum ceroluplasmin concentration, and erythrocyte SOD activity. The EAR for copper in men and women is 0.7 mg/day. Factorial analysis, used to determine the minimum amount of dietary copper intake to replace obligatory losses, yielded a estimate similar to that of the EAR for copper, which supported the EAR based on the indicators for copper status. The RDA for copper is defined as the EAR + 2(CV), with the CV for copper being estimated as 15%. The RDA for both men and women is set at 0.9 mg/day. An increase in the EAR by 0.10 mg copper/day was recommended for pregnant women based on the amount of copper accumulated by the maternal and fetal tissues adjusted by an estimate of copper absorption. An increase in the EAR by 0.30 mg/day was recommended for lactating women based on the amount of copper secreted in human milk adjusted by an estimate of copper absorption. Copper bioavailability was considered to be 65% to 70%. After adding 30% (2 CVs) and rounding, the RDAs for adult women during pregnancy and lactation were set at 1.0 mg/day and 1.3 mg/day, respectively. Based on data from NHANES III (1988-1994), the median intake of copper from foods (not including supplements) by adults (ages 19 to 70 years) is 1.6 mg/day for men and 1.1 mg/day for women, which is higher than the RDAs for adults.

Manganese

To date, no functional criteria for manganese status have been established. Therefore, recommended intakes of manganese are set as adequate intakes for all age and sex groups. For infants, the AIs are based on the manganese intake of breast-fed infants from human milk and from complementary foods during the second half of the first year of life. Mean manganese concentration of human milk is approximately 4 μg/L at 1 month and 1.9 μg/L by 3 months postpartum. The AI for infants in the first 6 months of life is set as: 3.5 μg Mn/L × 0.78 L/day = 3 μg/day. This amount of manganese would be inadequate if complementary foods were not introduced into the diet of the infant. Based on average manganese intake by older infants of approximately 567 μg/day from complementary foods, the AI for infants that are 7 to 12 months of age is set as 600 μg/day or 0.6 mg/day. The AIs for children were set based on median manganese intake by children in the various age groups. These AIs range from 1.2 mg/day for children who are 1 to 3 years of age up to 2.2 mg/day for boys who are 14 to 18 years of age.

In adults, manganese balance has been observed to occur for a wide range of manganese intakes. Median intake of manganese in the United States is 2.25 mg/day for men and 1.74 mg/day for women (ages 19 to 70 years), based on the Total Diet Study (1991-1997). The AI for men was set at 2.3 mg/day, and that for women was set at 1.8 mg/day. An increment of 0.2 mg/day was added for pregnant women, based on a gain of 16 kg body weight, to give an AI of 2 mg/day. The AI for lactating women was set at 2.6 mg/day based on the higher median intake of manganese by lactating women.

FOOD SOURCES

Zinc

Red meats, organ meats (e.g., liver), and shellfish (e.g., oysters) are generally the best dietary sources for zinc. Whole grain cereals are rich sources of zinc, but refined grain products are poor sources because the zinc is found primarily in the bran and germ. Many breakfast cereals made from refined grain products are supplemented with zinc and other nutrients during production and therefore may be good sources of zinc. Nuts and legumes are also relatively good plant sources of zinc. In contrast, fruits and vegetables are generally low in zinc. Excessive intake of phytate-rich foods (e.g., some grains) is known to inhibit zinc bioavailability. Infant formulas are often supplemented with zinc, but this is up to the discretion of the producer.

Copper

As for zinc, shellfish, nuts, legumes, the bran and germ portions of grains, and liver are rich sources of copper (greater than 0.3 mg of copper per 100 g). Most meats, mushrooms,

Food Sources

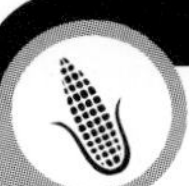

Food Sources of Zinc, Copper, and Manganese

Zinc

2.5 to 6.5 mg/3 oz serving crab
3 to 8 mg/3 oz beef or lamb
1.7 to 4 mg/3 oz pork, chicken, and turkey
0.9 to 4.6 mg/1 cup ready-to-eat cereals (unfortified)
15 to 23 mg/cup fortified cereals
0.7 to 1.5 mg/½ cup legumes, mature seeds (chickpeas, lentils, soybeans, limas, or kidney), cooked
1.2 to 1.8 mg/oz nuts, dry (pine nuts, cashews, or pecans)
2 mg/8 to oz container yogurt, plain
1.6 mg/½ cup ricotta cheese, part skim

Copper

3.7 mg/3 oz oysters
1.6 mg/3 oz lobster
0.3 to 0.6 mg/3 oz clams and crabs
0.3 to 0.6 mg/oz nuts (cashew, hazelnuts, walnuts)
0.1 to 0.4 mg/½ cup legumes, mature seeds (soybeans, lentils, kidney, or limas)
0.1 to 0.2 mg/½ cup green leafy vegetables (spinach, turnip greens, or kale), cooked
0.15 mg/½ cup tomatoes (stewed)
0.13 mg/½ cup potatoes, sweet potatoes, pumpkin
0.13 mg/½ cup raspberries, blackberries, raw

Manganese

0.7 to 1.7 mg/oz nuts (hazelnuts, pecans, or walnuts)
0.6 mg/oz peanuts, roasted
0.3 to 0.9 mg/½ cup legumes (chickpeas, limas, soybeans, or lentils)
0.9 mg/½ cup brown rice, cooked
0.7 mg/½ cup oatmeal, cooked
0.3 to 2.7 mg/cup ready-to-eat cereals
0.3 to 0.5 mg/6 oz tea
0.4 to 0.8 mg/½ cup leafy green vegetables (spinach, collards, or turnip greens)
0.3 to 0.5 mg/½ cup berries (raspberries, strawberries, or blueberries)

Data from U.S. Department of Agriculture/Agricultural Research Service (USDA/ARS) (2005) USDA Nutrient Database for Standard Reference, Release 18. USDA/ARS, Washington, DC. Retrieved November 15, 2005 from www.ars.usda.gov/ba/bhnrc/ndl/.

tomatoes, dried fruits, bananas, potatoes, and grapes have moderate amounts of copper (0.1 to 0.3 mg/100 g). Poor sources of copper are cow's milk and dairy products, chicken, and many fish, as well as fruits and vegetables other than those just listed.

Manganese

Manganese can be found in unrefined cereals, nuts, tea, and leafy vegetables, but refined grains, meats, seafood, and dairy products are poor sources.

TOXICITY OF ZINC, COPPER, AND MANGANESE

As a general rule, zinc, copper, and manganese are relatively nontoxic when consumed in the diet. Toxic exposure is most likely to result from accidental exposure, from environmental contamination, or from overconsumption of dietary supplements.

ZINC

Manifestations of overt toxicity will occur with long-term exposure to as little as 100 to 300 mg of zinc per day. The symptoms of zinc toxicity include induced copper deficiency (characterized by anemia and neutropenia), impaired immune function, and reduction of HDL cholesterol levels in some individuals. Extremely high zinc intake will cause vomiting, epigastric pain, lethargy, and fatigue. The most consistent adverse effect associated with excess zinc intake was reduced copper status, as measured by reduced erythrocyte Cu/Zn-SOD activity (IOM, 2001).

Because zinc intake in pharmacological amounts decreases copper absorption, the adverse effects of zinc supplements on copper metabolism (copper status) was used for establishing the tolerable upper intake level (UL) for zinc (IOM, 2001). The UL for zinc intake by adults was determined as the zinc intake that resulted in a reduction in erythrocyte Cu/Zn-SOD activity, a sensitive measure of copper status. The UL for zinc intake by adults is 40 mg/day, which includes zinc from foods, water, and supplements.

It was recently reported that taking zinc gluconate lozenges within 24 hours of the onset of cold symptoms reduces the duration of symptoms of the common cold (Mosssad et al., 1996). Although this is a potentially exciting finding, misuse of this product could result in zinc toxicity. To get the benefit of this product, users must take a lozenge containing 13.3 mg of zinc every 2 waking hours until the symptoms have been eliminated (4 to 7 days). This dose (greater than 150 mg/day) may have toxic effects, particularly if people attempt to use the lozenges prophylactically by consuming them throughout the cold and flu season.

COPPER

Copper toxicity in humans has not been studied extensively. Wilson's disease is a hereditary disease that causes copper accumulation in the liver and other organs and is an example of the damage excessive copper can cause. However, liver damage is rare for individuals with normal mechanisms for copper homeostasis when consuming up to 10 mg copper per day for 12 weeks (Pratt et al., 1985). There is a report of acute liver failure occurring in an individual consuming supplements containing 30 mg copper per day for 2 years, followed by the consumption of 60 mg of copper per day for 1 year (O'Donohue et al., 1993). Under conditions of chronic overconsumption of copper, toxicity occurs only when the capacity of the liver to bind and sequester copper is exceeded. The amount of dietary copper required to cause toxicity is not well established, but gastrointestinal discomfort has been seen with intakes of as little as 5 mg of copper per day. The consequences of copper toxicity are weakness, listlessness, and anorexia in the early stages, which can progress to coma, hepatic necrosis, vascular collapse, and death.

The IOM used liver damage as the critical endpoint for copper toxicity in setting the UL for copper at 10 mg/day (IOM, 2001). The UL was based on a no-observed-adverse-effect level of 10 mg/day, as observed in a study of adults who consumed this level of copper for 12 weeks. Consumption of higher levels of copper resulted in acute liver failure.

MANGANESE

Manganese is considered one of the least toxic minerals. Oral toxicity is extremely rare. However, airborne manganese from industrial and automobile emissions can have serious toxic effects if exposure is sufficiently high. Symptoms associated with manganese toxicity include pancreatitis and neurological disorders that are similar to those observed in patients with schizophrenia and Parkinson's disease. Manganese toxicity has been observed in children receiving long-term parenteral nutrition. In addition, the use of methylcyclopentadienyl manganese tricarbonyl as a gasoline additive in the United States has raised concerns that environmental exposure to manganese may increase in the future.

The UL for manganese intake from all sources was set at 11 mg/day (IOM, 2001). Available data indicate that individuals eating vegetarian and Western diets consume up to 11 mg/day of manganese. No adverse effects have been observed with the consumption of this level of manganese from the diet (Greger, 1999). Conversely, data from another study indicated that consumption of 15 mg/day of manganese for 25 days caused a significant increase in serum manganese concentration and, after 90 days, an increase in lymphocyte Mn-SOD activity (Davis and Greger, 1992). Therefore, the lowest-observed-adverse-effect level was established at 15 mg of manganese per day. The UL for manganese is the no-observed-adverse-effect level of 11 mg/day.

REFERENCES

Bertinato J, Iskandar M, L'Abbe MR (2003) Copper deficiency induces the upregulation of the copper chaperone for Cu/Zn superoxide dismutase in weanling rats. J Nutr 133:28-31.

Browning JD, MacDonald RS, Thornton WH, O'Dell BL (1998) Reduced food intake in zinc deficient rats is normalized by megestrol acetate but not by insulin-like growth factor-I. J Nutr 128:136-142.

Cousins RJ (1985) Absorption, transport, and hepatic metabolism of copper and zinc: special reference to metallothionein and ceruloplasmin. Physiol Rev 65:238-309.

Cox DW, Moore SDP (2002) Copper transporting P-type ATPases and human disease. J Bioenerg Biomemb 34:333-338.

Cragg RA, Christie GR, Phillips SR, Russ RM, Kury S, Mathers JC, Taylor PM, Ford D (2002) A novel zinc-regulated human zinc transporter, hZTL1, is localized to the enterocyte apical membrane. J Biol Chem 277:22789-22797.

Dalton T, Fu K, Palmiter RD, Andrews GK (1996) Transgenic mice that overexpress metallothionein-I resist dietary zinc deficiency. J Nutr 126:825-833.

Danks DM (1995) Disorders of copper transport. In: Scriver DR, Beaudet AL, Sly WS, Valle D (eds) The Metabolic and Molecular Bases of Inherited Disease, 7th ed. Vol. 2. McGraw-Hill, New York, pp 2211-2235.

Davis W, Chowrimootoo GF, Seymour CA (1996) Defective biliary copper excretion in Wilson's disease: the role of caeruloplasmin. Eur J Clin Invest 26:893-901.

Davis CD, Greger JL (1992). Longitudinal changes of manganese-dependent superoxide dismutase and other indexes of manganese and iron status in women. Am J Clin Nutr 55:747-752.

Delves HT (1985) Assessment of trace element status. Clin Endocrinol Metab 14:725-760.

DiDonato M, Sarkar B (1997) Copper transport and its alterations in Menkes and Wilson diseases. Biochim Biophys Acta 1360:3-16.

Dufner-Beattie J, Wang F, Kuo YM, Gitschier J, Eide D, Andrews GK (2003) The acrodermatitis enteropathica gene ZIP4 encodes a tissue-specific zinc-regulated zinc transporter in mice. J Biol Chem 278:33474-33481.

Failla ML, Hopkins RG (1997) Copper and immunocompetence. In: Fischer RWF, L' Abbe MR, Cockell KA, Gibson RS (eds) Trace Elements in Man and Animals—9: Proceedings of the Ninth International Symposium on Trace Elements in Man and Animals. NRC Research Press, Ottawa, Canada, pp 425-428.

Glusker JP (1991) Structural aspects of metal liganding to functional groups in proteins. Adv Protein Chem 42:1-76.

Greger JL (1999) Nutrition versus toxicology of manganese in humans: evaluation of potential biomarkers. Neurotoxicol 20:205-212.

Grider A, Young EM (1996) The acrodermatitis enteropathica mutation transiently affects zinc metabolism in human fibroblasts. J Nutr 126:219-224.

Gunshin H, Mackenzie B, Berger UV, Gunshin Y, Romero MF, Boron WF, Nussberger S, Gollan JL, Hediger MA (1997) Cloning and characterization of a mammalian proton-coupled metal-ion transporter. Nature 388:482-488.

Halliwell B (1994) Free radicals and antioxidants: a personal view. Nutr Rev 52:253-265.

Harris ZL, Gitlin JD (1996) Genetic and molecular basis for copper toxicity. Am J Clin Nutr 63:836S-841S.

Harris ZL, Takahashi Y, Miyajima H, Serizawa M, MacGillivray RT, Gitlin JD (1995) Aceruloplasminemia: molecular characterization of this disorder of iron metabolism. Proc Natl Acad Sci U S A 92:2539-2543.

Institute of Medicine (IOM) (2001) Dietary Reference Intakes for Vitamin A, Vitamin K, Arsenic, Boron, Chromium, Copper, Iodine, Iron, Manganese, Molybdenum, Nickel, Silicon, Vanadium, and Zinc. National Academy Press, Washington, DC.

Kambe T, Yamaguchi-Iwai Y, Sasaki R, Nagao M (2004) Overview of mammalian zinc transporters. Cell Mol Life Sci 61:49-68.

Kelly EJ, Quaife CJ, Froelick GJ, Palmiter RD (1996) Metallothionein I and II protect against zinc deficiency and zinc toxicity in mice. J Nutr 126:1782-1790.

Kim BE, Wang F, Dufner-Beattie J, Andrews GK, Eide DJ, Petris MJ (2004) Zn^{2+}-stimulated endocytosis of the mZIP4 zinc transporter regulates its location at the plasma membrane. J Biol Chem 279:4523-4530.

Lee J, Pena MMO, Nose Y, Thiele DJ (2002a) Biochemical characterization of the human copper transporter Ctr1. J Biol Chem 277:4380-4387.

Lee J, Petris MJ, Thiele DJ (2002b) Characterization of mouse embryonic cells deficient in the Ctr1 high affinity copper transporter. J Biol Chem 277:40253-40259.

Leone A, Pavlakis GN, Hamer DH (1985). Menkes' disease: abnormal metallothionein gene regulation in response to copper. Cell 40:301-309.

Liu AC, Heinrichs BS, Leach RM (1994) Influence of manganese deficiency on the characteristics of proteoglycans of avian epiphyseal growth plate cartilage. Poult Sci 73:663-669.

Liuzzi JP, Cousins RJ (2004) Mammalian zinc transporters. Annu Rev Nutr 24:151-172.

Lonnerdal B, Sandstrom B (1995) Factors influencing the uptake of metal ions from the digestive tract. In: Berthon G (ed) Handbook of Metal-Ligand Interactions in Biological Fluids. Vol. 1. Marcel Dekker, New York, pp 331-337.

Lutsenko S, Petris MJ (2002) Function and regulation of the mammalian copper-transporting ATPases: insights from biochemical and cell biological approaches. J Membrane Biol 191:1-12.

McMahon RJ, Cousins RJ (1998) Regulation of the zinc transporter ZnT-by dietary zinc. Proc Natl Acad Sci U S A 95:4841-4846.

Mossad SB, Macknin ML, Medendorp SV, Mason P (1996) Zinc gluconate lozenges for treating the common cold. A randomized, double-blind, placebo-controlled study. Ann Intern Med 125:81-88.

Noor R, Mittal S, Iqbal J (2002) Superoxide dismutase—applications and relevance to human diseases. Med Sci Monit 8:RA210-RA215.

O'Donohue J, Reid MA, Varghese A, Portmann B, Williams R (1993) Micronodular cirrhosis and acute liver failure due to chronic copper self-intoxication. Eur J Gastroenterol Hepatol 5:561-562.

Orr WC, Sohal RS (1994) Extension of life-span by overexpression of superoxide dismutase and catalase in *Drosophila melanogaster*. Science 263:1128-1130.

Owen CA (1973) Effects of iron on copper metabolism and copper on iron metabolism in rats. Am J Physiol 224:514-518.

Palmiter RD (1994) Regulation of metallothionein genes by heavy metals appears to be mediated by a zinc-sensitive inhibitor that interacts with a constitutively active transcription factor, MTF-1. Proc Natl Acad Sci U S A 91:1219-1223.

Palmiter RD, Findley SD (1995) Cloning and functional characterization of a mammalian zinc transporter that confers resistance to zinc. EMBO J 14:639-649.

Percival SS (1995) Neutropenia caused by copper deficiency: Possible mechanisms of action. Nutr Rev 53:59-66.

Percival SS, Harris ED (1990) Copper transport from ceruloplasmin: characterization of the cellular uptake mechanism. Am J Physiol 258:C140-C146.

Pratt WB, Omdahl JL, Sorenson JR (1985) Lack of effects of copper gluconate supplementation. Am J Clin Nutr 42:681-682.

Reinhold JG (1971) High phytate content of rural Iranian bread: a possible cause of human zinc deficiency. Am J Clin Nutr 24:1204-1206.

Rhodes D, Klug A (1993) Zinc fingers. Sci Am, February:56-65.

Rock E, Gueux E, Mazur A, Motta C, Rayssiguier Y (1995) Anemia in copper-deficient rats: Role of alterations in erythrocyte membrane fluidity and oxidative damage. Am J Physiol 269:C1245-C1249.

Roth HP, Kirchgessner M (1994) Influence of alimentary zinc deficiency on the concentration of growth hormone (GH), insulin-like growth factor I (IGF-I) and insulin in the serum of force-fed rats. Horm Metab Res 26:404-408.

Rucker RB, Romero-Chapman,N, Wong T, Lee J, Steinberg FM, McGee C, Clegg MS, Reiser K, Kosonen T, Uriu-Hare JY, Murphy J, Keen CL (1996) Modulation of lysyl oxidase by dietary copper in rats. J Nutr 126:51-60.

Schroeder HA, Balassa JJ, Tipton IH (1966) Essential trace metals in man: manganese. A study in homeostasis. J Chron Dis 19:545-571.

Swanson CA, King JC (1983) Reduced serum zinc concentrations during pregnancy. Obstet Gynecol 62:313-318.

Torre M, Rodriguez AR, Saura-Calixto F (1992) Effects of dietary fiber and phytic acid on mineral availability. Crit Rev Food Sci Nutr 30:1-22.

Tumer Z, Moller LB, Horn N (2003) Screening of 383 unrelated patients affected with Menkes disease and finding of 57 gross deletions in ATP7A. Hum Mutat 22:457-464.

U.S. Department of Agriculture/Agricultural Research Service (USDA/ARS) (2005) USDA Nutrient Database for Standard Reference, Release 18. USDA/ARS, Washington, DC. Retrieved November 15, 2005, from www.ars.usda.gov/ba/bhnrc/ndl/.

Vallee BL, Galdes A (1984) The metallobiochemistry of zinc enzymes. Adv Enzymol Relat Areas Mol Biol 56:283-430.

Vulpe CD, Packman S (1995) Cellular copper transport. Annu Rev Nutr 15:293-322.

Walsh CT, Sandstead HH, Prasad AS, Newbern PM, Fraker PJ (1994) Zinc: Health effects and research priorities for the 1990s. Environ Health Perspect 102:5-46.

Wang F, Kim BE, Dufner-Beattie J, Petris MJ, Andrews G, Eide DJ (2004) Acrodermatitis enteropathica mutations affect transport activity, localization and zinc-responsive trafficking of the mouse ZIP4 zinc transporter. Hum Mol Genet 13:563-571.

Williamson PS, Brown EC, Browning JD, Wollard LC, Thornton WH, O'Dell BL, MacDonald RS (1997) Decreased insulin-like growth factor-I (IGF-I) receptor concentration and IGF-I binding in small intestine of zinc-deficient rats. FASEB J 11:A194.

Zerounian NR, Redekosky C, Malpe R, Linder MC (2003) Regulation of copper absorption by copper availability in the Caco-2 cell intestinal model. Am J Physiol 284:G739-G747.

RECOMMENDED READINGS

Cousins RJ (1985) Absorption, transport, and hepatic metabolism of copper and zinc: special reference to metallothionein and ceruloplasmin. Physiol Rev 65:238-309.

Cox DW, Moore SDP (2002) Copper transporting P-type ATPases and human disease. J Bioenerg Biomemb 34:333-338.

Institute of Medicine (2001) Dietary Reference Intakes for Vitamin A, Vitamin K, Arsenic, Boron, Chromium, Copper, Iodine, Iron, Manganese, Molybdenum, Nickel, Silicon, Vanadium, and Zinc. National Academy Press, Washington, DC.

Hill CH, Matrone G (1970) Chemical parameters in the study of in vivo and in vitro interactions of transition elements. Fed Proc 29:1474-1481.

Kambe T, Yamaguchi-Iwai Y, Sasaki R, Nagao M (2004) Overview of mammalian zinc transporters. Cell Mol Life Sci 61:49-68.

Liuzzi JP, Cousins RJ (2004) Mammalian zinc transporters. Annu Rev Nutr 24:151-172.

Lutsenko S, Petris MJ (2002) Function and regulation of the mammalian copper-transporting ATPases: insights from biochemical and cell biological approaches. J Membr Biol 191:1-12.

Prohaska JR, Gybina AA (2004) Intracellular copper transport in mammals. J Nutr 134:1003-1006.

Vulpe CD, Packman S (1995) Cellular copper transport. Annu Rev Nutr 15:293-322.

Walsh CT, Sandstead HH, Prasad AS, Newbern PM, Fraker PJ (1994) Zinc: health effects and research priorities for the 1990s. Environ Health Perspect 102:5-46.

Chapter 38

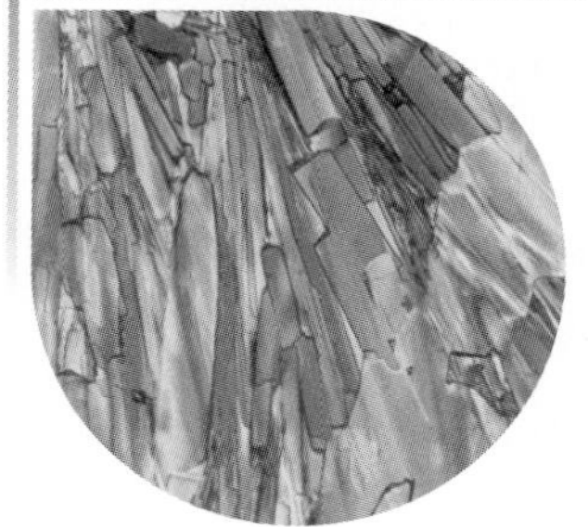

Iodine

Hedley C. Freake, PhD

OUTLINE

COMMON ABBREVIATIONS

IDD	iodine deficiency disorder
rT_3	reverse T_3
RXR	retinoid X receptor
T_3	3,5,3′-triiodothyronine
T_4	thyroxine
TR	thyroid hormone receptor
TRE	thyroid hormone response element
TRH	thyrotropin-releasing hormone
TSH	thyroid-stimulating hormone, thyrotropin

UNIQUENESS OF IODINE

Iodine is an extremely unusual and interesting nutrient from almost every perspective. For the chemist, it possesses the distinction of being the heaviest element required for human nutrition, with an atomic weight of 127. The iodide anion is also extremely large, with an ionic radius of 0.216 nm. Iodine is responsible for just a single function in the body, the synthesis of thyroid hormones. However, the multiple actions of thyroid hormones mean that iodine has an impact on a wide range of metabolic and developmental functions. The definition of those functions, and the unraveling of the molecular mechanisms that underlie them, have occupied numerous physiologists, biochemists, and molecular biologists for decades. Deficiency of iodine is common, and the consequences of that deficiency are so profound, particularly in the neonatal period, that this deficiency represents one of the largest public health problems in the world today (World Health Organization [WHO], 2001). The occurrence of iodine in soils is variable, so dietary deficiency depends almost entirely on where food sources are grown, rather than which are selected. Yet eradicating that deficiency is relatively simple, has been increasingly successful, and in many parts of the world has resulted in dramatic improvements in human function.

PRODUCTION AND METABOLISM OF THYROID HORMONES

USE OF IODINE: THYROID HORMONES

Inorganic iodine occurs predominantly in nature in the form of the anion iodide. The sole function of iodine in humans and other mammals is the synthesis of thyroid hormones. These iodinated derivatives of the amino acid tyrosine, shown in Figure 38-1, are thyroxine, or 3,5,3′,5′-tetraiodothyronine (T_4), and 3,5,3′-triiodothyronine (T_3). Because they are derived from amino acids, thyroid hormones are in the L-form. D-Isomers can be synthesized but have lower biological activity.

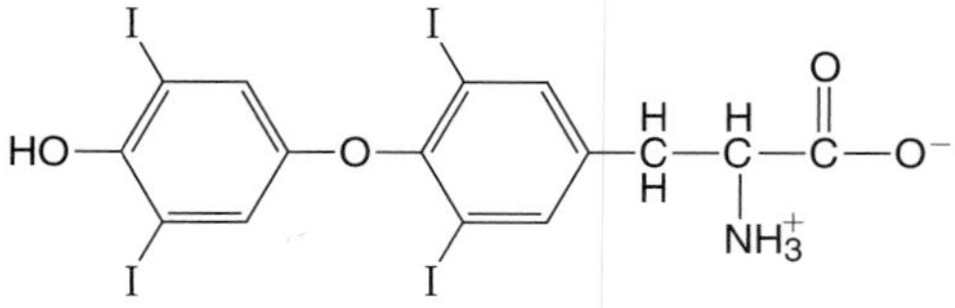

Thyroxine (T_4)

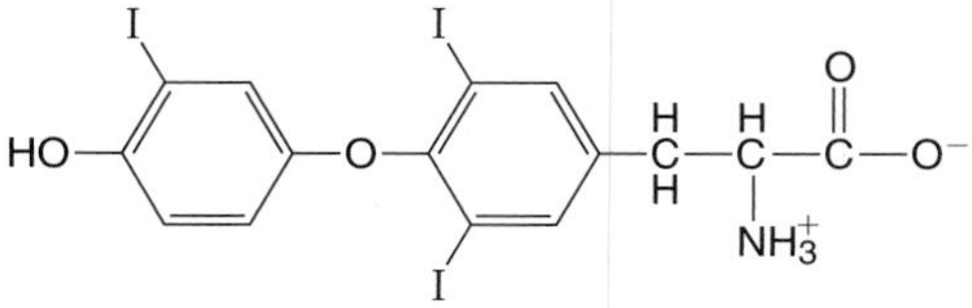

3,5,3′-Triiodothyronine (T_3)

Figure 38-1 Chemical structures of the thyroid hormones.

DIETARY SOURCES OF IODINE

Iodine is a reasonably abundant element, but its solubility leads to wide regional variations in its availability. The iodine content of soils is diminished by exposure to rain, snow, and glaciation, which leach out the mineral and deposit it in the oceans. Although iodine is volatilized from the sea and returns to land through rainwater, this does not make up for the long-term loss of iodine from older exposed soils. Iodine-deficient areas include mountainous regions, such as the Himalayas, Andes, and Alps, and also river deltas, such as the Ganges and the Yellow River, where frequent flooding has leached out the mineral (Hetzel and Maberly, 1986).

The iodine content of plants averages 1 mg/kg dry weight, but it may be only 1 % of that in plants grown in iodine-deficient areas. Its content in animal foods, including milk, reflects the amount found in the feeds supplied to the animals. Foods arising from the sea, such as fish and seaweed, provide a rich source. In more developed parts of the world, the food available to a particular community is usually drawn from a variety of geographical locations and thus, in aggregate, is less likely to be deficient in iodine. However, supplementation, particularly in the form of iodized salt as has been used in the United States and many other parts of the world, is the only reliable way to ensure an adequate dietary supply in low-iodine areas. This relatively simple public health program has reaped enormous benefits. A good example of this is Switzerland, where iodine deficiency, which once affected the majority of the population, has now been virtually eradicated. Iodine intakes may also be increased by the use of iodine-containing products at various points in the food production process. For example, iodates are used in bread making, and iodine-containing antiseptics are used in dairy facilities.

ABSORPTION, STORAGE, AND EXCRETION OF IODINE

Iodine may be found in different forms in foods, including iodide (I^-) and iodate (IO_3^-), the compound added to bread. Dietary iodine is reduced to iodide and absorbed efficiently along the length of the gastrointestinal tract.

The adult human body contains 15 to 20 mg of iodine, and about three fourths of this is found in the thyroid gland. This gland has a unique and powerful ability to take up iodide actively. Concentrations in the gland are 100-fold those in plasma under normal circumstances and can become still higher in iodine deficiency. Iodine accumulates to a much lesser extent in other tissues such as the salivary glands, stomach, and ovaries/testicles. The kidneys are the other principal site for iodine removal from the circulation. However, they are incapable of conserving the mineral, and hence the kidneys represent the main route for excretion. The amount of iodine found in urine is proportional to the plasma concentration and can be used as a convenient index of iodine status. Feces and sweat, together with secreted milk in lactating women, represent other routes of iodine loss from the body.

SYNTHESIS OF THYROID HORMONES

The process of thyroid hormone synthesis is illustrated in Figure 38-2. Iodine is actively transported into the thyroid gland, coupled to the action of Na^+,K^+-ATPase. It traverses the thyroid cells and enters the colloid space. The iodine is then oxidized by thyroid peroxidase, using hydrogen peroxide as a co-substrate, and the reactive intermediate is coupled to tyrosyl residues in the protein thyroglobulin. These then become monoidotyrosyl or diiodotyrosyl residues, depending on whether one or two iodine molecules are incorporated.

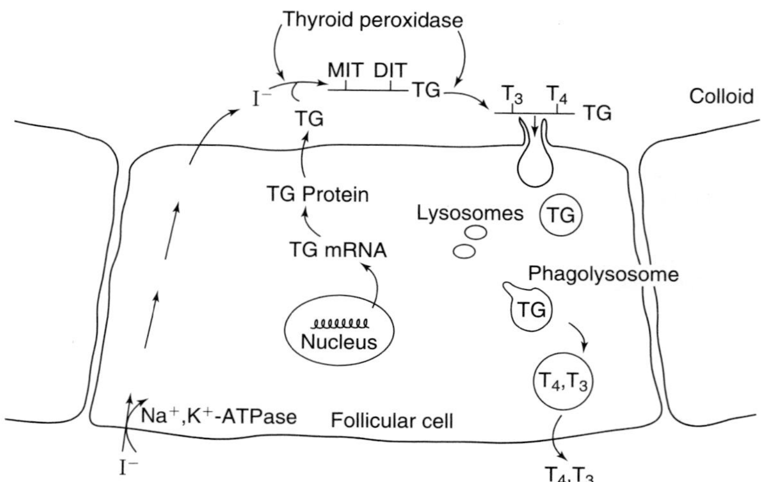

Figure 38-2 Synthesis of thyroid hormones. Iodide is pumped into the follicular cells of the thyroid gland. It diffuses across the cells and enters the colloid space, where it is incorporated into thyroglobulin (*TG*), leading to the synthesis of MIT and DIT (monoiodotyrosines and diiodotyrosines), which then condense to form thyroid hormones. The hormones, still within thyroglobulin, are stored in the colloid space. When stimulated by thyroid-stimulating hormone (*TSH*), the secretion pathway begins with the uptake of a droplet of colloid, which fuses with a lysosome to form a phagolysosome. The lysosomal enzymes degrade the thyroglobulin, leading to release of the thyroid hormones and their secretion from the cell.

Thyroglobulin is a very large glycoprotein and may constitute up to one half the protein in the thyroid gland. Only selected tyrosyl residues in this protein become iodinated. Monoiodotyrosyl or diiodotyrosyl residues within thyroglobulin condense with each other to form T_4 or T_3 residues. This reaction is also catalyzed by thyroid peroxidase. When the iodophenolic ring of one iodotyrosyl residue is condensed with another, the rest of the donor residue is left in the thyroglobulin chain in the form of a serine residue. Thyroid hormones are stored in the colloid space, still as a part of thyroglobulin.

For release of thyroid hormones, portions of colloid that contain iodinated thyroglobulin are taken into the follicular cells by pinocytosis. These droplets then fuse with lysosomes within the cells to form phagolysosomes, and the thyroglobulin within them is broken down by proteolytic enzymes. This results in the release of free thyroid hormones, which are able to diffuse out into the circulation. T_4 is the predominant form released, but a small amount of T_3 is also generated. The proportion of T_3 released appears to be increased under hypothyroid conditions by intrathyroidal deiodination of T_4.

Hypothyroidism can result not only from insufficient dietary iodine but also from the ingestion of goitrogens. These are present in some foods, notably the cruciferous family of vegetables (e.g., broccoli and cabbage) and also cassava and millet. Cassava and millet may be more important, as they are dietary staples eaten in large quantities by some populations. Cruciferous vegetables themselves are not likely to be eaten in sufficient quantities to cause concern. Goitrogens work either by competitively inhibiting iodine uptake by the thyroid gland or by blocking its incorporation into the tyrosyl residues of thyroglobulin and their subsequent condensation. Antithyroid drugs, such as propylthiouracil and methimazole, work by the latter mechanism and are used clinically in the treatment of hyperthyroidism.

CIRCULATION

Thyroid hormones are carried in the blood on three proteins: thyroid-binding globulin, thyroid-binding prealbumin, and albumin. The prealbumin is also known as transthyretin and functions with retinol-binding protein in retinol transport (see Chapter 30). More than 99% of both T_4 and T_3 circulate bound to these proteins, but T_4 is bound more tightly than T_3. It appears likely that only the small free fraction is available for tissue uptake, either to exert biological activity or for further metabolism. This tight binding means that thyroid hormones, particularly T_4, have relatively long plasma half-lives and also that there is a large plasma pool of thyroid hormones, which can become available to tissues after dissociation from the binding proteins. The T_4 plasma concentration in normal humans is approximately 100 nmol/L, which is 50- to 100-fold higher than that for T_3. The relative abundance of T_4 reflects both that T_4 is the primary product of the thyroid gland and that it has a longer plasma half-life than does T_3.

ACTIVATION

T_4, the predominant circulating thyroid hormone, is really a prohormone that requires deiodination at the 5′ position in the outer ring to generate the biologically active T_3. Deiodination serves not only to activate thyroid hormones but also as a deactivation pathway (Fig. 38-3). Removal of iodine from the inner ring of T_4 will result in the production of reverse T_3 (rT_3; 3,3′,5′-triiodothyronine), and similar processing of T_3 produces 3,3′-diiodothyronine, both of which are inactive metabolites.

A family of microsomal enzymes is responsible for deiodination (Bianco et al., 2002). The type I deiodinase is found in liver, kidney, and thyroid gland. It is found associated with the plasma membrane and is thought to contribute significantly to circulating T_3 concentrations. It can perform inner ring as well as outer ring deiodinations, and its preferred substrate is rT_3. Type I deiodinase activity is increased in hyperthyroidism and decreased in the hypothyroid state. These properties are consistent with a primary role for this deiodinase in the inactivation of T_4. It is also inhibited by propylthiouracil, giving a second site of action for this antithyroid drug.

The type II deiodinase, located in brain, pituitary, and brown adipose tissue, operates solely on the outer ring. It is located in the

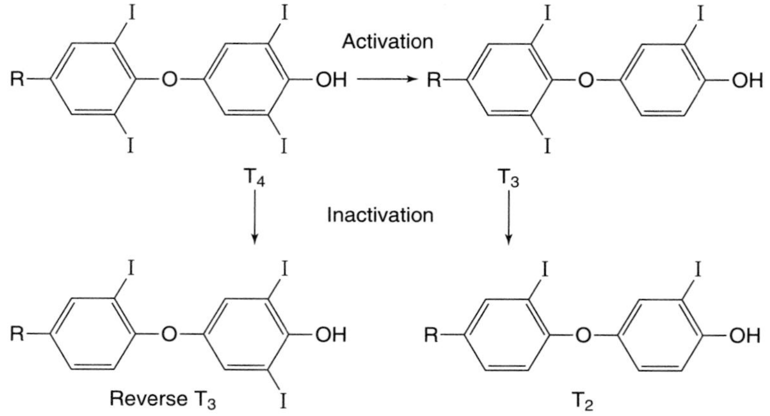

Figure 38-3 Deiodination pathways for thyroid hormones. The parent compound thyroxine (T_4) is activated by monodeiodination of the outer ring to form 3,5,3′-triiodothyronine (T_3). Either one of these may be inactivated by inner ring deiodination to form reverse T_3 or diiodothyronine (T_2).

endoplasmic reticulum and specifically functions to convert T_4 to T_3 for local use within these tissues. However, it is now appreciated that type II deiodinase can also contribute significantly to circulating levels of T_3 in plasma. In tissues containing the type II enzyme, thyroid hormone status will depend primarily on plasma levels of T_4 rather than T_3. The activity of this enzyme is increased in the hypothyroid state, which means that these tissues may be partially protected from the effects of hypothyroidism by this local production.

Type III deiodinase operates exclusively on the inner ring and therefore inactivates thyroid hormones. It has been found in brain and placenta and its activity is increased with elevation of thyroid hormone status.

Genes encoding all three enzymes have now been cloned in multiple species and this has allowed many insights into the functioning and regulation of this enzyme family (Bianco et al., 2002). Of particular interest is the discovery that all three enzymes contain the unusual amino acid selenocysteine at their active site. This amino acid is similar to cysteine, except that the sulfur is substituted by selenium. The nucleotide triplet UGA encodes this substitution, which is critical for the catalytic properties of the enzyme. Under most circumstances this triplet is read as a stop codon but other sequences within the deiodinase mRNAs override this coding and dictate the incorporation of selenocysteine. The limited number of proteins that incorporate selenium in this way, as well as further details of the underlying mechanisms are discussed further in Chapter 39. This linkage between thyroid hormone deiodination and selenium explains earlier work in rats, which showed that selenium deficiency reduced plasma T_3 and thereby impaired thyroid status. It also may explain some of the diversity seen in the spectrum of iodine deficiency disorders.

FURTHER METABOLISM AND EXCRETION

Removal of iodine from the inner ring is an irreversible degradative step. There are additional pathways of thyroid hormone metabolism. The phenolic hydroxyl group of the outer ring can be conjugated with glucuronate or sulfate. This occurs primarily in the liver, with glucuronidation being favored for T_4 and sulfation for T_3. These conjugates are then secreted into the bile and may be lost in the feces. However, a significant amount is likely to be hydrolyzed in the intestine, followed by reabsorption of the free thyroid hormones. Deamination or decarboxylation also occurs, resulting in carboxylate or amine analogs of the thyroid hormones, respectively. Although metabolic activity has been suggested for some of these analogs,

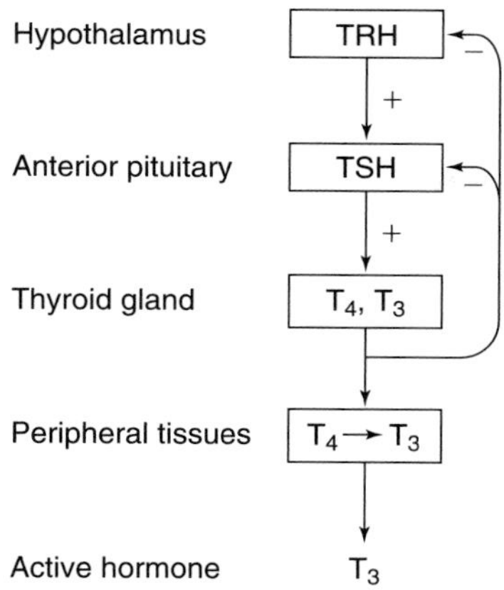

Figure 38-4 Feedback regulation of thyroid hormone status. *TRH,* Thyrotropin-releasing hormone; *TSH,* thyroid-stimulating hormone; T_4, thyroxine; T_3, 3,5,3′-triiodothyronine.

this seems unlikely because they are further degraded very quickly.

Any iodine produced by the peripheral metabolism of thyroid hormones will be either taken up by the thyroid gland and used for further synthesis or lost in the urine.

REGULATION OF THYROID HORMONE STATUS

From the preceding discussion it is apparent that thyroid hormone status can be modified at a number of different levels. The primary site may be output from the thyroid gland, but the rate of conversion of the prohormone to active T_3 is also important.

Under normal circumstances, circulating thyroid hormone levels are tightly regulated because of a negative feedback loop on their production (Fig. 38-4). Thyrotroph cells in the anterior pituitary produce thyrotropin, or thyroid-stimulating hormone (TSH), a glycoprotein that is a heterodimer of two subunits, which are encoded by separate genes. The α-subunit of TSH is similar to that of the gonadotropic pituitary hormones (luteinizing hormone and follicle-stimulating hormone), whereas the β-subunit is unique. TSH acts on the thyroid gland, primarily by a cyclic AMP–mediated mechanism, to stimulate iodine uptake and organification and also the release of thyroid hormones. T_4 travels back to the pituitary, where it is deiodinated by the type II enzyme. The T_3 that is produced operates at a transcriptional level to inhibit the production of both subunits of TSH, thereby completing the cycle. TSH is also under the control of the hypothalamic tripeptide thyrotropin-releasing hormone (TRH), which is responsible for basal production of TSH by the pituitary. It provides a mechanism by which thyroid status can be modulated at a central level, either positively (e.g., in response to cold) or negatively (e.g., in response to stress or illness). T_3 has also been shown to inhibit transcription of the TRH gene, showing that the negative feedback loop extends up to the hypothalamus.

This hypothalamic–pituitary–thyroid axis is responsible for producing the appropriate amounts of thyroid hormones, but thyroid status can also be regulated by altering the rate of T_4 to T_3 conversion. The deiodinase enzymes can be differentially regulated. This allows the possibility that tissues may differ in thyroid status, according to whether they depend on the type I or type II deiodinase for supply of T_3. For example, plasma T_3 is reduced by fasting and increased by carbohydrate feeding in humans, and these effects are achieved by altering the activity of the type I deiodinase. This response to decreased food availability helps conserve fuel by reducing metabolic rate. In particular, protein catabolism is minimized by a reduction in its T_3-stimulated turnover rate. However, because the type II enzyme is not affected by fasting, generation of T_3 in the brain and pituitary, and therefore T_3-dependent functions in those tissues, is maintained.

Although T_3 is the active thyroid hormone, thyroid status is usually better determined by measuring plasma T_4. This provides a more sensitive indicator of hypothyroidism (such as that resulting from iodine deficiency) than does plasma T_3. Circulating levels of T_3 may be maintained, even in the face of inadequate thyroid hormone production, both by increasing the proportion of T_3 produced by the thyroid gland and by stimulating peripheral conversion. Therefore, plasma T_3 values may be within the normal range, despite reduced levels of T_4. This compensation may occur at the expense of the brain, because brain derives T_3 from plasma T_4 by the type II deiodinase-catalyzed reaction.

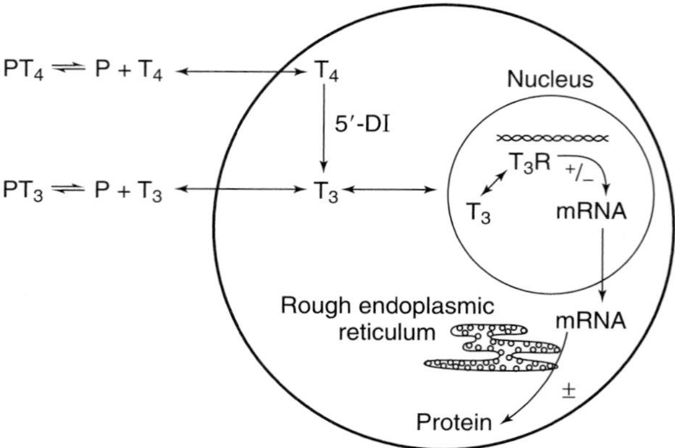

Figure 38-5 Outline of thyroid hormone action. Thyroid hormones circulate bound to plasma proteins (*P*), from which they must dissociate to enter the cell. Tissues containing the deiodinase enzyme (*5′DI*) convert T_4 to T_3. T_3 travels to the nucleus, where it is bound by specific receptor proteins (*R*). Together they interact with target genes, resulting in a change of their transcriptional rate. This results in altered mRNA levels, leading to different rates of protein synthesis and therefore different amounts of the protein products of the target genes, which ultimately produce the biological effect.

The body uses T_4 as its own indicator of thyroid status; as mentioned, TSH production in the pituitary is downregulated by T_3 that is locally produced from T_4. Measurement of plasma TSH is also widely used clinically as a sensitive indicator of thyroid status, because elevated levels indicate hypothyroidism. Plasma TSH concentrations are used to confirm normal thyroid status in newborn infants.

MECHANISM OF ACTION OF THYROID HORMONES

In recent years it has come to be accepted that most and perhaps all actions of thyroid hormones are mediated by effects within the nucleus. This mechanism is outlined in Figure 38-5. Following dissociation from plasma proteins, T_4 and T_3 enter the cell. The T_4 is deiodinated and T_3 enters the nucleus. There it is bound by specific nuclear receptor proteins, which are associated with a set of target genes. Hormone binding to these receptors alters these associations in a manner that leads to a change in the rate of transcription of the target genes. Changes in gene transcription, in turn, leads to changed amounts of messenger RNA (mRNA), which are translated to correspondingly different amounts of protein. Thereby the physiological state is altered.

NUCLEAR RECEPTORS

Enormous progress has been made in the last 20 years in understanding the mechanism of action of thyroid hormone on a molecular level (Yen, 2003a). An important starting point for these advances was the cloning in 1986 of complementary DNAs (cDNAs) encoding thyroid hormone receptors (TRs), from chick and human sources in two independent laboratories (Sap et al., 1986; Weinberger et al., 1986). The cDNAs for thyroid receptors were initially identified on the basis of their similarity to the genes encoding receptors for other nuclear acting hormones, namely estrogen and glucocorticoids.

Functional Regions of Receptors

The realization that TRs are part of a family of nuclear acting proteins has facilitated progress in understanding their mechanism of action, because analogies can be drawn with other members of the class (Aranda and Pascual, 2001). This family includes receptors not only for steroid hormones but also for retinoic acid, 1,25-dihydroxyvitamin D, fatty acids, steroids, and a host of other less well-known or uncharacterized ligands. These receptors have a modular structure (Fig. 38-6). They all have a carboxy-terminal region that binds to the ligand, and this region provides each

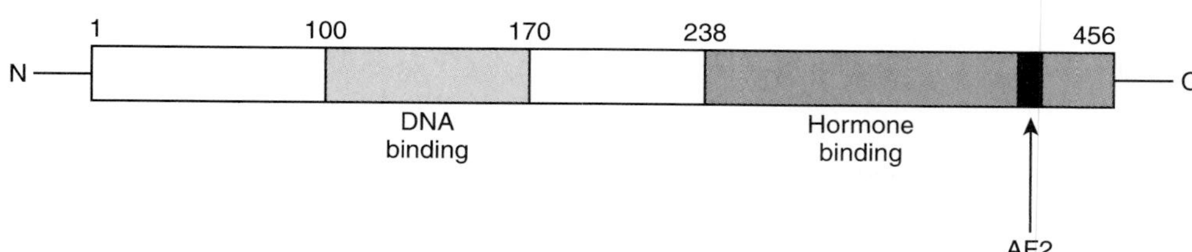

Figure 38-6 The modular structure of thyroid hormone receptors (TRs). In common with other members of the nuclear receptor family, the TRs have defined regions for DNA and hormone binding, separated by a hinge region. Sequences required for dimer formation have been described within both the DNA- and hormone-binding domains. The amino-terminal region does not appear to be required for function of TRs although in other nuclear receptors this region contains an activation domain. The activation function-2 (AF2) domain is required for interaction with coactivating proteins. Sites required for interaction with corepressors have been located elsewhere in the ligand binding domain as well as in the hinge region. The numbers shown represent amino acids in the human TRβ1 sequence.

receptor with its hormone ligand specificity. The area that is most highly conserved across the family is the DNA-binding region through which the receptors recognize and bind to their target genes. Regions that appear to be required for nuclear localization of the protein, that facilitate dimerization between receptors, or that are required for communicating the signal for altered transcription have also been described.

The DNA-binding region contains multiple cysteine residues, which do not vary in their relative location between different members of the receptor class. By analogy to other nuclear DNA-binding proteins, it was suggested that these receptors would use eight of these cysteine residues to chelate two atoms of zinc and that the mineral would then stabilize a receptor conformation appropriate for DNA binding. Much evidence in favor of this hypothesis has accumulated for various members of the receptor class, and it is generally accepted that they are zinc proteins (Vallee et al., 1991). As such, they are members of a large class of nuclear transcription factors that appear to utilize zinc. This allows for the theoretical possibility that zinc deficiency could lead to loss of zinc from nuclear receptor proteins and therefore inability to bind to DNA. To date, however, this prediction has been validated only with in vitro systems. The role of zinc as a component of nuclear proteins involved in the transcriptional process is discussed in Chapter 37.

Multiple Thyroid Hormone Receptors

The cloning of TRs has also served to complicate our understanding of their mechanism of action. It had been assumed previously that a single receptor was responsible for mediating T_3 action. Two thyroid hormone receptors were cloned in 1986, and, although they were derived from different species, they appeared to be generated from independent genes. The existence of two human thyroid hormone receptor (TR) genes (α on chromosome 17 and β on chromosome 3) has subsequently been confirmed. In addition, these two genes result in multiple protein products. There are two thyroid hormone β receptors: β1 that has a broad tissue distribution and β2 that appears to be restricted to the pituitary and certain areas of the brain. Multiple products derived from the α gene have also been described, although only one of them, α1, retains an intact hormone-binding region and, therefore, appears capable of performing a receptor function. Other forms may play important roles, however, and it has been suggested that they may antagonize T_3 action. In particular, the nonhormone-binding variant α2 is expressed at high levels in the brain and in the testis, and it has been suggested that this could explain the metabolic non-responsiveness of these tissues to T_3 in the adult (Lazar, 1993).

Response Elements in Target Genes

The TR must be capable of selecting the genes that it specifically regulates from among the background of the entire genome. This specificity is achieved by DNA sequences in the control regions of target genes, known as thyroid hormone response elements (TREs). A TRE consists of a hexanucleotide with the sequence AGGTCA, although some substitutions within that sequence are permissible. The TREs are usually found in pairs, although sometimes three or even more copies of this sequence are present. The same recognition motif is used by some other members of the nuclear receptor family, notably receptors for retinoic acid and vitamin D, which indicates that not only the recognition sequences but also their arrangement within the promoter are important for determining target gene specificity. It has, therefore, been suggested that a TRE consists of two repeats of the sequence AGGTCA with a four-nucleotide separation. Although such a sequence certainly is able to respond to the thyroid hormone–receptor complex, the sequences actually found within target genes frequently deviate from this. Therefore, despite considerable attention to this question, the exact requirements for a DNA sequence to confer responsiveness to thyroid hormone remain to be established.

Heterodimerization of Receptors

The fact that recognition motifs for TRs, as well as for other members of the nuclear receptor family, are found in pairs suggests that the receptors might bind to the response elements as dimers. This has proved to be the case, although for thyroid hormone heterodimers rather than homodimers appear to be the favored form. Retinoic acid has a naturally occurring isomer, 9-*cis*-retinoic acid, which has its own nuclear receptor, termed the RXR or retinoid X receptor. This is distinct from the receptor for all-*trans*-retinoic acid, the RAR. These retinoid receptors are discussed in detail in Chapter 30. Studies with in vitro systems have shown that, in the presence of T_3, heterodimers between TRs and RXRs bind more tightly to TREs and confer a more robust transcriptional response than do homodimers of TRs (Yen and Chin, 1994). RXRs heterodimerize in a similarly effective way with both RARs and vitamin D receptors. Three distinct RXR genes have been discovered, and each of these generates multiple isoforms of the receptor. Given the multiplicity of TRs, it appears reasonable to suppose that the combination of different receptor isoforms as heterodimerization partners would give a host of possibilities for achieving gene- and tissue-specific responses to thyroid hormone. The fact that a range of receptor heterodimers is available may also help explain why variations are observed in the response elements of target genes. The particular organization of a response element may favor a specific pair of TR/RXR isoforms.

EFFECTS ON TRANSCRIPTION

The occupation of TRs by T_3 leads to a change in the transcription rate of the target genes, although the precise way in which this occurs is not well understood. A depiction of the current model is shown in Figure 38-7. Studies in vitro have indicated that the TRs are bound to the TREs in both the presence and absence of hormone. Therefore, the hormone does not cause binding of the receptor to the target gene. Rather, T_3 binding to TR alters the interaction between this ligand-activated transcription factor and the proteins that constitute the basal transcriptional apparatus. Additional coregulatory proteins, called coactivators and corepressors, appear to mediate this linkage between the receptors and the transcriptional process (Aranda and Pascual, 2001). In the absence of ligand, the TR:RXR heterodimer, bound to the response element, is associated with corepressor proteins, which mediate an inhibitory interaction with the proteins of the basal transcriptional apparatus. Addition of hormone leads to dissociation of corepressors and recruitment of coactivators, which then switches on transcription. In this model, absence of hormone is not just a lack of stimulation of transcription but actually an inhibition. In addition to direct interaction of coregulatory molecules with the basal transcriptional apparatus, evidence has accumulated that acetylation of histones may play an important role. Co-repressor proteins associate not only with unliganded TR but also with proteins that are able to deacetylate histones. DNA can be wound more tightly around deacetylated histones and tends to be transcriptionally inactive. Therefore, at least a part

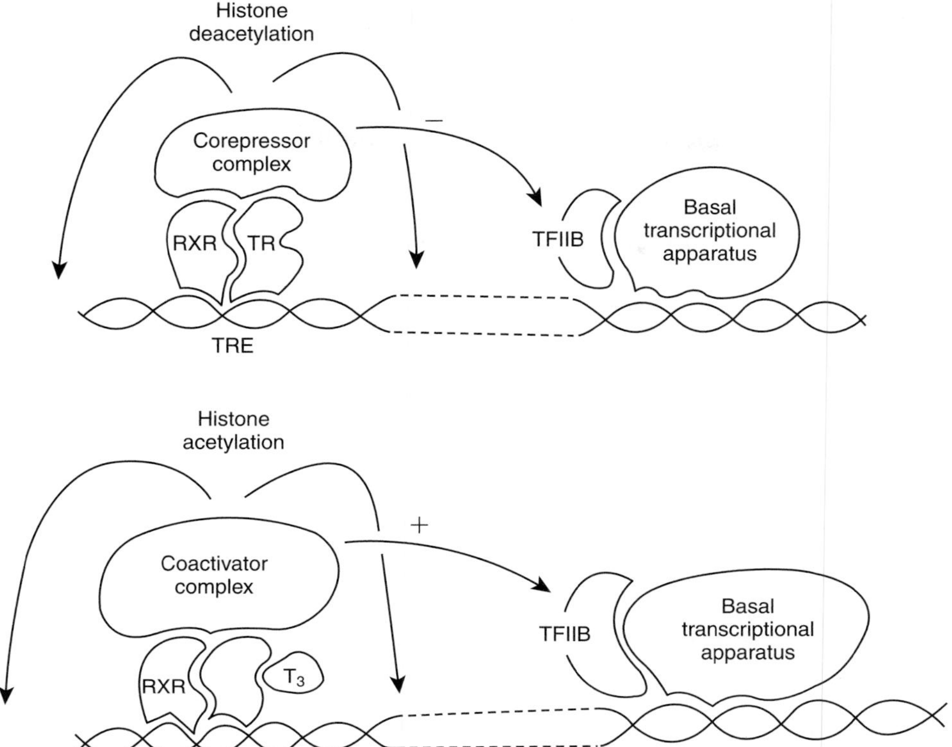

Figure 38-7 Thyroid hormone action in the nucleus. The efficient regulator of transcription that binds to the thyroid hormone response element (TRE) of target genes appears to be a heterodimer between a thyroid hormone receptor (TR) and a retinoid X receptor (RXR). In the absence of T_3, this dimer is associated with a co-repressor protein, which is part of a complex that has histone deacetylase activity. This complex also interacts with the basal transcriptional apparatus through one of its associated proteins, transcription factor IIB (TFIIB), and inhibits transcription. In the presence of T_3, a coactivating complex replaces the corepressor. This results in histone acetylation and initiation of transcription. A break is shown between the two portions of the DNA to indicate that TREs are often far upstream of the transcriptional start site, requiring folding of the DNA to bring the two regions together.

of the transcriptional inhibition in the absence of thyroid hormone may be explained by this mechanism. Coactivators, in contrast, are associated with histone acetylation, thereby opening up DNA structures and allowing transcription to occur.

Transcription can be either stimulated or inhibited by T_3, depending on the target gene. Although the majority of the actions described are stimulatory, the autoregulation of thyroid status itself is an example of negative transcriptional control. T_3 acts at the transcriptional level in the anterior pituitary gland to limit the production of TSH, which results in decreased production of thyroid hormones. Clearly negative regulation of gene transcription in response to T_3 must require a different relationship between TRs and coregulatory proteins from that described in the preceding text.

S14: A MODEL THYROID HORMONE–RESPONSIVE GENE

Several target genes for T_3 have been identified and have proved useful for understanding the physiology of thyroid hormone action as well as the molecular events occurring within the nucleus that initiate the biological effects. A partial listing of target genes is given in Box 38-1. The physiology of thyroid hormone action is described next. Here, one example of a thyroid

Clinical Correlation

Thyroid Hormone Resistance

Hereditary disorders, termed thyroid hormone resistance, have been described in which individuals appear hypothyroid despite normal or elevated circulating thyroid hormone levels and inappropriately normal or elevated TSH (Yen, 2003b). Whereas symptoms of hypothyroidism may vary both in extent and degree of severity, goiter, neurological deficits, and other developmental abnormalities are common. Families with this condition are located rarely, but they provide a useful opportunity to learn more of the mechanism of action of T_3.

Approximately 250 such families have been described, and when the genetic loci of thyroid hormone resistance have been determined, they have all been found in the carboxy-terminal, ligand-binding portion of the TRβ gene. These mutations result in a diminished ability of the receptors to bind T_3 and also in a decreased ability of the TRβ to mediate a transcriptional response to T_3 in various systems in vitro. The disorder is almost always heterozygous (i.e., the affected individuals also possess one normal β-receptor gene). This means that the mutant receptors must have a dominant negative activity (i.e., they can inhibit the transcriptional activation that would operate through the normal wild-type receptor). This might be predicted because mutations in the ligand-binding region leave the DNA-binding region of the TRβ unaffected. Therefore, the mutant receptors may block the access of biologically active receptors to TR-binding sites on their target genes. Occupation of the TRE by the mutant receptor will stabilize the corepressor complex on the promoter and inhibit its transcriptional activity. In addition, one family has been described that has complete deletion of both copies of the TRβ gene, yet only mild thyroid hormone resistance. Under this circumstance, no receptors will be bound to the TRE and so no co-repressor will be present either, allowing a basal level of gene transcription to occur. Therefore, possession of a single mutant TRβ gene is worse than no gene at all, emphasizing the dominant negative activity of these mutant receptors.

It is interesting that no germline mutations in TRα have been described in humans. There are two, quite opposite, potential explanations for this. Either mutations in TRα have insignificant effects on the phenotype so that they are not recognized or the effects are lethal to the embryo so that affected fetuses do not survive. However, at least in mice, deletion of both TRα and TRβ is not embryonically lethal, rendering the second possibility less likely.

Box 38-1

SELECTED TARGET GENES FOR THYROID HORMONES

Metabolic

Fatty acid synthase
Malic enzyme
Pyruvate kinase
Spot 14
Phosphoenolpyruvate carboxykinase

Cardiac

Myosin heavy chain
Calcium ATPase

Endocrine

Growth hormone
Thyroid-stimulating hormone (TSH)
Thyroid hormone receptor (TR, α and β)

Mitochondrial

Cytochrome c

Ion Transport

Na^+,K^+-ATPase

hormone–responsive gene will be taken to illustrate the regulatory mechanisms.

A key metabolic target for T_3 is the liver. In 1981, Oppenheimer, Towle, and coworkers sought to identify hepatic gene products that changed in abundance in response to thyroid status (Seelig et al., 1981). Nineteen such products were identified, some of which increased and some of which decreased with T_3 treatment. Attention was particularly focused on one product, called spot 14 or S14, and a cDNA clone coding for this product was isolated. The identity of the S14 protein was and still is unknown, but T_3 treatment results in a rapid and large induction in the expression of the mRNA. This stimulation occurs at the level of transcription and can be detected as soon as 10 minutes after intravenous T_3 injection into a hypothyroid rat. The *S14* gene clearly represents a direct target for T_3 action, and subsequent effort has been directed toward elucidating the steps involved in its transcriptional regulation.

The regions of DNA that contain the TRE and mediate the response to T_3 have been identified and are noteworthy because they are relatively far (2.5 to 2.8 kilobase pairs) from the transcriptional start site (Zilz et al., 1990). Other sites in the *S14* gene promoter have been found that mediate a positive transcriptional response to carbohydrate feeding or a negative response to polyunsaturated fatty acids. The carbohydrate response is particularly relevant here because it is synergistic with that to T_3. Induction of the *S14* gene by T_3 is also dependent on binding sites for other transcription factors that are much closer to the transcriptional start site, notably sites for binding of sterol regulatory element binding protein (SREBP) and nuclear factor-Y (NF-Y) (Jump et al., 2001).

Use of a specific antibody has demonstrated that the S14 protein is located within the nuclear compartment of the cell (Kinlaw et al., 1992). It has a zonal distribution in liver, being restricted to the perivenous area, the site of fatty acid synthesis. Overall, it appears that S14 acts within the nucleus to coordinate the regulation of a subset of genes involved in lipid metabolism. Supporting this idea is the demonstration that specifically blocking the production of S14 protein within cultured hepatocytes also removed the ability of the cells to increase lipogenesis in response to T_3 and glucose (Brown et al., 1997).

Most studies regarding the regulation of S14 have been limited to liver. The gene is expressed in several other tissues, in particular adipose tissue, and this distribution has supported a role for the protein in lipid metabolism. However, the responsiveness of *S14* gene expression to T_3 is quite tissue-specific. In contrast to liver, for example, lung and brain, which also actively synthesize fatty acids, do not alter either S14 expression or lipogenesis in response to T_3 (Blennemann et al., 1995). Identifying the elements of the *S14* promoter and the nuclear proteins that interact with them to dictate this cell-specific regulation of expression is an important area of research for both *S14* and other T_3-regulated genes.

NON-NUCLEAR PATHWAYS

The nuclear pathway for thyroid hormone action is now well established. Non-nuclear mechanisms have also been suggested, but evidence in their favor is much less complete and sometimes contradictory. The stimulatory effects of thyroid hormone on oxygen consumption are well known, and this knowledge led to the suggestion that they might act directly on mitochondria. Mitochondrial receptors for T_3 have been described, but such descriptions have been inconsistent. Although T_3 clearly affects mitochondrial structure and function, it appears likely that such actions are mediated by the nuclear transcriptional pathway described previously. Binding proteins that recognize thyroid hormones have also been identified in the plasma membrane and the cytoplasm. These may serve transport functions governing the delivery of T_3 to the nucleus, rather than initiating biological functions independent of nuclear receptors. The means whereby T_3, which is not very soluble and binds easily to proteins, enters the cell and reaches the nucleus are not clear. Although proof for a non-nuclear mechanism for thyroid hormone action is lacking, more complete evidence has accumulated in favor of such a non-nuclear pathway for some related ligands such as 1,25-dihydroxyvitamin D.

PHYSIOLOGICAL FUNCTIONS OF THYROID HORMONES

The physiological actions of T_3 can be divided into two components: metabolic and developmental. These actions are best known in terms of the regulation of basal energy expenditure on the one hand and the thyroid hormone requirement for normal brain development on the other. It is interesting to note that, although these actions of thyroid hormone have been known for decades and although the molecular mechanism of T_3 action within the nucleus has been increasingly well delineated, large gaps remain in our physiological understanding of how thyroid hormone regulates these processes.

REGULATION OF BASAL METABOLIC RATE

Thyroid hormone increases oxygen consumption in all warm-blooded animals. The effect is seen in the basal portion of metabolic rate (i.e., that measured in the postabsorptive, resting state). Basal or resting oxygen consumption is reduced about 30% in hypothyroid individuals and is increased 50% in hyperthyroidism (Freake and Oppenheimer, 1995). Thus overall, basal metabolism can be doubled by alterations in thyroid state. It is generally assumed that most tissues, with the exception of brain, spleen, and testis, respond to thyroid hormone by increasing oxygen consumption. However, this is based on measuring oxygen consumption in vitro in preparations of tissue taken from animals of different thyroid states. The extent to which such measurements correspond to metabolic activity of tissues of intact animals is clearly open to question.

There is a considerable lag time following administration of thyroid hormone before an increase in oxygen consumption can be detected. This delay is approximately 1 day and is consistent with the nuclear pathway for thyroid hormone action. Appearance of the physiological effects requires the transcription of mRNAs and the translation and accumulation of the relevant proteins, a process that is likely to take hours.

Efficiency of Energy Production

An early and attractive explanation for the stimulation of metabolic rate observed with thyroid hormone treatment was that the hormone acted directly on mitochondria to uncouple electron transport from ATP synthesis. Indeed, such effects could be demonstrated in vitro. However, this required very high concentrations of thyroid hormone and could not be reproduced at physiological levels. Thus, this concept was discarded. More recently, it has been revived, although in different forms. Treatment with thyroid hormone produces numerous effects on mitochondria (Freake and Oppenheimer, 1995). These include induction of several components of the electron transport chain; increased activity of the ADP translocator protein, which is responsible for the import of ADP into mitochondria and, therefore, necessary for oxidative phosphorylation; increases in mitochondrial membrane surface area; and changes in membrane lipid composition. Some investigators believe that a considerable portion of resting oxygen consumption can be attributed to the passive leak of protons back into mitochondria (Harper et al., 1993). The operation of the electron transport chain is coupled to the extrusion of protons from the inner mitochondrial space. The mitochondrial membrane contains proton ports, which allow their return coupled to the synthesis of ATP. However, in addition to these ports, it has been shown that the mitochondrial membrane itself is not completely impermeable to protons. Moreover, such thyroid-induced effects as increased membrane surface area or changed membrane lipid composition may enhance this permeability; this would result in increased oxygen consumption without altering ATP production, and thus enhance basal metabolic rate. In addition, in recent years a role for uncoupling proteins (UCPs) in thyroid thermogenesis has been suggested (Lanni et al., 2003). UCP allows the return of protons into the mitochondria without the synthesis of ATP. UCP was originally thought to be confined to brown adipose tissue, explaining the heat production of that specialized tissue. It is now appreciated that there are additional forms of this protein, coded by separate genes, found elsewhere in the body. Some of these UCPs are induced by thyroid hormone and therefore could contribute to its thermogenic effects.

Although efficiency of energy production may be decreased, these effects likely account for only a part of the thyroid hormone–dependent increase in metabolic rate. Treatment with T_3 not only results in increased amounts of respiratory chain components but also in a greater state of reduction of these components. This implies an enhanced delivery of reducing equivalents to the chain, which is equivalent to increased energy consumption. It has also been shown that T_3 increases the production of ATP, which must then be utilized at a faster rate. Otherwise respiration will be limited by a lack of ADP. Numerous ATP-consuming processes are enhanced by thyroid hormone and collectively account for the increased load on mitochondria.

Effects on Energy-Consuming Processes

A well-known effect of hyperthyroidism is increased heart rate (Klein, 1990). Cardiac size, stroke volume, and output are all increased. These changes may be partially attributed to direct transcriptional effects on cardiac genes, but the increased load on the heart also plays an important role. Increased oxygen consumption overall results in an enhanced requirement for oxygen supply and therefore blood flow.

A second target of thyroid hormone is the cell membrane Na^+,K^+-ATPase. This protein utilizes ATP to pump sodium out and potassium into cells, both against considerable concentration gradients. The expression of the gene encoding Na^+,K^+-ATPase is stimulated by thyroid hormone treatment, and earlier experiments suggested this could account for the major portion of increased oxygen consumption in some tissues. However, these experiments, which involved measurement of oxygen consumption in tissue preparations in vitro, have been criticized as nonphysiological. Subsequent studies in more intact systems have suggested a much more limited role for this protein, perhaps accounting for 5% to 10% of the enhanced oxygen consumption (Clausen et al., 1991).

Changes in heart rate and ion pumping provide only a partial explanation for the thyroid hormone–dependent increase in ATP consumption. Stimulation of fat, carbohydrate, and protein metabolism by T_3 also increases requirements for ATP, and these effects are discussed in the next section.

REGULATION OF MACRONUTRIENT METABOLISM

The nutritional significance of iodine and the thyroid hormones is magnified by the fact that T_3 regulates the metabolism of all the macronutrients. An unusual characteristic of this regulation is that it operates on both the anabolic and catabolic arms of these pathways. Although construction and destruction of macromolecules may appear to be wasteful, it is completely consistent with the central role of thyroid hormones to generate heat for the maintenance of body temperature.

Lipids

Thyroid hormone stimulates fatty acid synthesis by enhancing expression of the genes involved in this process. The principal target is liver, but smaller inductions also occur in other tissues. The target genes, which respond in a coordinated fashion, include acetyl CoA carboxylase and fatty acid synthase, which are directly responsible for assembling the carbon skeleton of palmitate, as well as enzymes of the hexose monophosphate shunt and malic enzyme, which generate the required reducing equivalents as NADPH. The esterification of fatty acids into triacylglycerols and phospholipids is also increased by T_3. (See Chapters 16 through 18 for details of lipid metabolism.)

This induction of lipid synthesis might surprise a clinician who would be more familiar with the reduced triacylglycerol stores associated with hyperthyroidism. Thyroid hormone also enhances lipolysis, probably by increasing the sensitivity of adipose cells to circulating catecholamines. The fatty acids released are also oxidized at an enhanced rate. This is because thyroid hormone also stimulates the expression of carnitine palmitoyltransferase, the protein that governs the entry of fatty acids into the mitochondria for β-oxidation. Many of these pathways of lipid metabolism are counter-regulated. For example, the activity of carnitine palmitoyltransferase is inhibited by malonyl CoA, the product of acetyl CoA carboxylase, which catalyzes the first step of fatty acid synthesis. Similarly, long-chain fatty acids, which are elevated in catabolic states, inhibit the activity of acetyl CoA carboxylase and therefore limit fatty acid synthesis. This counter-regulation is overcome by thyroid hormone by increasing the expression of the genes encoding these enzymes. The increased enzyme mass then allows greater flux through both pathways, despite the mutual inhibition.

A negative relationship between thyroid status and plasma cholesterol levels is another feature of thyroid disease well known to clinicians. Regulation of cholesterol metabolism is also an example of the double action of thyroid hormone. T_3 treatment increases the levels of mRNA encoding the hydroxymethylglutaryl CoA reductase enzyme, thereby increasing cholesterol synthesis. However, it also stimulates the biliary clearance of cholesterol; this effect predominates and results in the lower levels observed in the circulation. Beneficial effects of thyroid hormone on circulating cholesterol concentrations and also on weight loss have led to an active search for analogs that might activate these pathways while leaving heart rate unaffected (Webb, 2004).

Carbohydrates

Hyperthyroidism increases and hypothyroidism decreases substrate cycling through multiple pathways of glucose metabolism. Glycolysis is accelerated as well as gluconeogenesis in hyperthyroidism. Glycogen stores are depleted in the hyperthyroid state, which further emphasizes the importance of lipid stores to meet the energy demands under this condition. It seems reasonable to suppose that these effects are mediated by transcriptional regulation of the enzymes involved. Perhaps the best-investigated step in this context is phosphoenolpyruvate carboxykinase, which plays a key regulatory role in gluconeogenesis. Treatment with thyroid hormone stimulates transcription of this gene, at least in the rat, and a TRE has been identified in its promoter.

Proteins

Protein turnover is also sensitive to thyroid state. Less is known about T_3 regulation of these pathways in comparison with those involving the other macronutrients. Hyperthyroidism leads to a generalized increase in RNA synthesis in both cardiac and skeletal muscle, which in turn accelerates protein synthesis. However, muscle mass has been shown to be decreased in the thyrotoxic state, so that, as with lipid and carbohydrate metabolism, the overall effect of high T_3 is catabolic.

The pathways underlying the thermogenic effects of thyroid hormone are summarized in Figure 38-8. Many specifics, including the relative contributions of these various components and of different organ systems to the overall effect, remain to be determined. (Additional information on regulation of energy metabolism can be found in Chapters 21 through 23.)

REGULATION OF GROWTH AND DEVELOPMENT

It is quite clear in the rat that T_3 stimulates transcription of the growth hormone gene, and indeed this system has been widely used as a model for the regulation of gene expression by thyroid hormone. The situation is less clear in humans, and attempts to demonstrate responsiveness of the human growth hormone gene to T_3 have met with mixed results. However, it appears that growth hormone secretion is impaired in hypothyroid individuals, as is signaling through the insulin-like growth factor-1 pathway. Therefore, T_3 does appear to be necessary for normal growth hormone activity in humans. The effects of thyroid hormone on growth and development, at the level of a particular tissue or organ system, are the aggregate of direct T_3 effects and of those produced by growth hormone as well as by other secondary signals influenced by thyroid state.

Brain Development

The brain has traditionally represented a fascinating conundrum to investigators of thyroid hormone action. On the one hand, the devastating effects of a lack of thyroid hormones are all too apparent in the syndrome of cretinism (discussed in the next section). On the other hand, the brain is one of the few organs that do not appear to respond to thyroid hormone in terms of alterations in

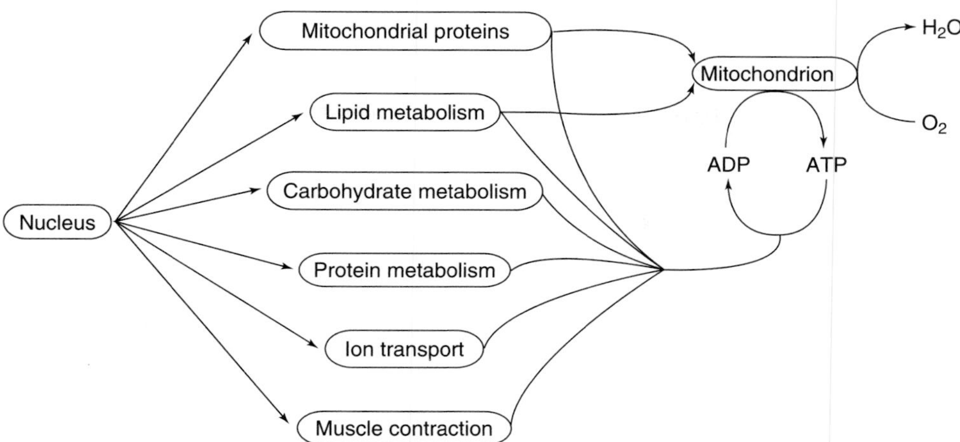

Figure 38-8 Mechanisms underlying the stimulation of oxygen consumption by thyroid hormone. T_3, acting via its nuclear receptors, regulates the levels of proteins required for the synthesis and breakdown of macronutrients, for ion transport, and for muscle contraction. Both the synthesis and operation of these proteins consume ATP and therefore stimulate respiration. Thyroid state also affects mitochondrial function by changing the membrane lipid composition and by altering the level of mitochondrial proteins encoded by both the mitochondrial and nuclear genomes. (*Modified from Freake HC, Oppenheimer JH [1995] Thermogenesis and thyroid function. Annu Rev Nutr 15:263-291. Copyright 1995 by Annual Reviews Inc.*)

metabolic rate. This illustrates the separation between the metabolic and developmental aspects of T_3 action. Also relevant here is the fact that brain growth and development are completed relatively early in the life span of the organism. In humans, it appears to be complete in the third year of life (Porterfield and Hendrich, 1993).

Much of the work looking at thyroid hormones and brain development has utilized rodents. This is appropriate as long as it is appreciated that the chronology of brain development in these animals differs from that in humans. Although, of course, the human time line is much longer than that of the rat, brain development in the rat occurs relatively late so that more neurogenesis occurs postnatally. In humans, most neuronal cell division is complete at birth. However, the development of these neurons, including axonal outgrowth and synaptogenesis, continues into the first 2 years of life, as does the production of glial cells and the process of myelinogenesis. These processes (i.e., the development of appropriate brain architecture and organization) are thyroid hormone–dependent. The effects are likely mediated by the nuclear pathway at the transcriptional level. A growing list of gene targets have been identified, including those encoding myelin basic protein, cytoskeletal components, and various growth factors (Bernal et al., 2003).

In humans, the fetal thyroid begins to function in the third month of gestation. Prior to that time, requirements for thyroid hormone are met by placental transport of maternally synthesized hormones (Porterfield and Hendrich, 1993). During the second and third trimesters, fetal requirements are met by a combination of fetal and maternal sources. Iodine deficiency compromises both maternal and fetal thyroid hormone synthesis. The significance of the maternal supply is indicated by comparing the consequences of iodine deficiency with those of congenital hypothyroidism. In the latter condition, the maternal iodine supply is intact and the neurological symptoms in the newborn infant are distinctly milder.

Receptors for thyroid hormone are present in fetal brain by the 10th week of gestation. It appears likely that thyroid hormone plays a role in brain development from this early point through the first 2 years of life. The consequences of deficiency at any particular time may not be reversible by later supplementation. The extent of the reversibility will depend on the timing and the severity of the deficiency. Although in some cases cretinism may not be prevented by supplementation as early as the second trimester, the effects of congenital hypothyroidism are at least partially alleviated by treatment postnatally. The routine screening of the thyroid status of neonates in the United States is useful because postnatal treatment with thyroid hormones can improve the status of these infants, even though as a group they still have learning difficulties.

Although it is clear that thyroid hormone is required for normal brain development, it is less certain whether it plays a role in the functioning of the mature brain. However, recent experiments with mice lacking various TRs have suggested a role for the receptor in modulating behavior (Bernal et al., 2003).

Developmental Effects on Other Tissues

Hypothyroidism leads to reduced muscle mass and delayed skeletal maturation (Brown et al., 1981). Lung maturation in the fetus has also been reported to be dependent on thyroid hormone. The effects of thyroid state on the heart have already been mentioned, in terms of their contribution to energy expenditure. Effects on muscle mass are mediated in part by differential effects of T_3 on the expression of the myosin heavy chain genes (Izumo et al., 1986). There are two myosin heavy chain genes, α and β, and T_3 stimulates transcription of the α form. Growth hormone also has important influences, and thus at least some of the consequences of hypothyroidism are likely to be mediated by lack of this trophic hormone.

IODINE DEFICIENCY

SCOPE OF THE PROBLEM

Iodine deficiency is classically recognized by the enlargement of the thyroid gland, known as goiter. An insufficient supply of iodine results in reduced accumulation of the mineral in the thyroid gland and diminished production of thyroid hormones. Lower plasma levels of T_4 lead to an increased production of TSH by the anterior pituitary gland. This stimulates many aspects of thyroid gland function, including the hyperplasia that leads to the goiter. This chronic stimulation of the thyroid gland also causes more efficient iodine uptake. This uptake can be measured clinically using a radioactive isotope of iodine, and radioactive iodine uptake has been used to assess iodine status. This has also been a cause of concern, since this iodine deficiency–induced accelerated uptake would lead to greater morbidity in the event of a nuclear accident and exposure to radioactive iodine.

Goiter is only one of many symptoms resulting from lack of iodide, and the broader term iodine deficiency disorders (IDDs) is now preferred. The WHO has now switched from assessing iodine deficiency in terms of goiter rate to the proportion of the population with urinary iodine level of less than 100 μg/L (WHO, 2001). Based on data for 2002, 35% of the world's population, or 2 billion people, were at risk for iodine deficiency (Table 38-1). Those afflicted were found in all regions of the world. In many parts of Europe, IDDs are still widespread. Of the 54 countries in which WHO data suggest

Table 38-1
Prevalence of Iodine Deficiency Disorders

WHO Region*	Proportion of Population (%) With Urinary Iodine <100 μg/L	Population (in millions) With Urinary Iodine <100 μg/L†
Africa	42.6	260.3
Americas	9.8	75.1
South East Asia	39.8	624.0
Europe	56.9	435.5
Eastern Mediterranean	54.1	228.5
Western Pacific	24.0	365.3
TOTAL	35.2	1,988.7

From World Health Organization (WHO) (2004) Summary Table: Proportion of Population with Insufficient Iodine Intake. WHO Global Database on Iodine Deficiency, 1993-2003. WHO, Geneva. Retrieved April 14, 2005, from the WHO website: www.who.int.
*Data from 192 WHO member states.
†Based on population estimates for the year 2002.

that iodine deficiency is a significant problem, fully 23 of them are in Europe, and the only region where a greater number of people is affected is South East Asia. For example, in Italy, although iodized salt is available, only 3% of households actually use it. Thus, IDD and goiters are widespread. In contrast, in Switzerland, which historically had very high goiter rates, 94% of households use iodized salt and the condition has now been eliminated.

CRETINISM

Although goiter may be the most obvious form of IDD, the effects on neurological development are the most important. Iodine deficiency is generally considered to be the most significant preventable cause of brain damage and mental retardation in the world today. The extent of the neurological impairment depends on the timing and severity of the iodine deficiency. One critical period is in the first trimester of pregnancy, when a lack of maternally supplied thyroid hormones at a time of very active fetal brain development has irreversible consequences. Severe effects of iodine lack are called cretinism and have classically been divided into two types: neurological and myxedematous. In the former, the neurological symptoms are severe and include mental retardation, deaf mutism, and spastic diplegia (paralysis) of the legs. Myxedematous or hypothyroid cretinism has less severe neurological symptoms, but those affected are more clinically hypothyroid and growth retarded. It has been suggested that concurrent selenium deficiency may at least in part explain these symptomatic differences. Selenium-dependent glutathione peroxidase is essential to protect the thyroid gland in the oxidative environment required for thyroid hormone synthesis. Selenium deficiency may, therefore, lead to the greater thyroid damage associated with myxedematous cretinism. It may also underlie the relative preservation of neurological function in these individuals. Although selenium is required for all three deiodinase enzymes, inhibition of deiodinases I and III will both preserve plasma T_4. This enhanced supply for the brain may allow sufficient T_3 production to prevent the more extreme symptoms.

OTHER CONSEQUENCES

In addition to the long-term consequence of cretinism, an insufficient supply of iodine during pregnancy is also associated with an increased occurrence of spontaneous abortions, stillbirths, and congenital abnormalities, as well as perinatal and infant mortality (Hetzel and Maberly, 1986). It is clear that profound iodine lack results in cretinism and that this damage is irreversible by later treatment with thyroid hormones. What is less apparent is the extent to which mild iodine deficiency causes much smaller decrements in neurological function and whether these may be reversible. In areas of iodine deficiency, iodine supplementation of mothers prior to conception results in children with improved cognitive performance relative to those given a placebo (Pharoah et al., 1971). In addition, comparison of children in communities that are similar other than in the amount of iodine available suggests that iodine deficiency may lead to developmental delays (Pharoah and Connolly, 1995). However these effects may all be due to fetal iodine deficiency.

Iodine deficiency after birth can result in hypothyroidism and goiter. Whether it also leads to impaired neurological function and, if so, whether these effects can be reversed by iodine supplementation is an open question. It used to be said that the adult brain was refractory to thyroid hormone treatment because animal studies had shown that brain was one of the few tissues in the body that did not increase oxygen consumption in response to administration of thyroid hormone. In addition, a number of morphological and biochemical parameters were identified that were sensitive to thyroid hormone in the neonatal period, but not at later times. However, with the rat as a model, some biochemical responses to thyroid hormone in adult brain have been identified and behavioral effects suggested (Bernal et al., 2003). If the adult brain is responsive, the possibility exists that milder consequences of thyroid insufficiency can be remedied at later ages.

OTHER THYROID ABNORMALITIES

Deficiencies of iodine are entirely manifested through abnormalities in thyroid hormone

Nutrition Insight

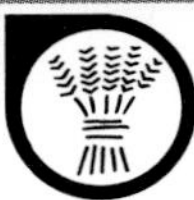

Please Pass the Iodine

Large areas of the northern United States have soil with low iodine, presumably because of mineral losses during the glaciation of the Ice Age. Therefore, iodine deficiency disorder (IDD) and goiter were endemic at the beginning of this century. The magnitude of this problem was noted at the time of World War I, when conscripts were turned away because they had goiters. Treatment with sodium iodide was shown to be effective. Therefore, both the cause and cure for the problem were apparent. The question was what was to be done or, more specifically, how could the iodine intake of large numbers of people be increased?

Many solutions were considered and rejected, including use of iodine-containing fertilizers, supplementing cows to increase the iodine content of milk, and iodination of public water supplies. Table salt, a product that is commonly eaten and that can be supplemented easily and cheaply, was selected as the vehicle for fortification. Iodization of salt began in 1924. The program was and is voluntary. Consequently, consumers had to be persuaded to buy the new fortified product. "Please Pass the Iodine" was a story that ran in the *Saturday Evening Post* at that time. In Michigan, where 40% of the population had goiters, a state-run education campaign was assisted by manufacturers and grocers and only iodized salt was sold. Four years later, the incidence of goiter had dropped to 10%, and it then declined further until 1951 when only 1.4% of schoolchildren in Michigan had goiters (Brush and Atland, 1952).

Acknowledgment is made to contributions of Linda Daube, M.S., in the preparation of this material.

metabolism and function. Situations are often seen clinically in which the latter are disordered in the face of normal iodine supply. Hypothyroidism can result from a primary defect in the thyroid gland itself, from a pituitary or hypothalamic dysfunction leading to insufficient stimulation of the gland by TSH, or from a peripheral resistance to thyroid hormone. The latter has usually been attributed to a defect in the receptor-signaling pathway, as described previously. The symptoms of hypothyroidism are fairly generalized, and most organ systems are affected. The symptoms include fatigue, cold intolerance, mental slowness, reduced cardiac function, and increased serum cholesterol. Increased serum TSH is a biochemical characteristic of thyroid hormone deficiency, and patients are treated with sufficient T_4 to return TSH levels to the normal range.

Hyperthyroidism is most often caused by Graves' disease, which results in a continuous stimulation of the thyroid gland and overproduction of thyroid hormones. This is an autoimmune disease, more often seen in women, caused by antibodies directed against the TSH receptor. Hyperthyroidism can also result from thyroid adenomas or thyroiditis. The symptoms include weight loss, increased heat production, tachycardia, muscular tremor, irritability, and nervousness, as well as exophthalmos (protrusion of the eyes) and enlargement of the thyroid. Treatment is by antithyroid drugs, radioactive iodine to cause necrosis of the thyroid cells, or surgical thyroidectomy. The latter two treatments can result in hypothyroidism, which may require that the patient be treated with thyroid hormone replacement.

PREVENTION

Iodine deficiencies can be combated by programs directed at the whole population or targeted at those particularly at risk. Iodization of salt represents a simple, inexpensive, and effective measure to supply iodine to a population, and there are numerous examples of it being used to eliminate IDD. Either potassium iodide or potassium iodate (which is more stable) can be used. However, the high prevalence of IDD in the face of the decades-old knowledge of how to prevent the condition shows that reality is more complex. The amount of iodized salt required is enormous, and its distribution to many of the communities at risk is very difficult. Most if not all populations in the world use salt and so have developed their own local means to produce it. The introduction of iodized salt, therefore, either means replacing the local product with potentially unacceptable, centrally produced iodized salt, or putting the technology in place to allow fortification on a local basis. Ensuring a stable and reliable supply of iodized salt may be very difficult or impossible using the latter approach. Despite these difficulties, the WHO now estimates that 68 % of the world's population consumes iodized salt. The fact that Europe, where logistical problems are likely to be relatively minor, constitutes the region with the lowest consumption rates (28 %) further emphasizes the potential success of this approach. Fortification of other foods has been attempted, often with success, but it is unlikely that fortification of other foods would have as widespread applicability as a salt supplementation program. However, milk has been suggested as an alternative vehicle in Europe, and this food already constitutes the principal dietary source of iodine in the United Kingdom.

Apart from iodized salt, the most common vehicle used for delivery of iodine is iodized oil (WHO, 2001). The fatty acids of the oil are chemically modified by iodination, and, once inside the body, the iodine is slowly released over a period of months to years. Injection of the oil is the usual route of administration; oral preparations, which are cheaper but less effective, are also available. These treatments are most often used in remote areas, where interactions with health services are rare and introduction of iodized salt is problematic. They permit the supply of iodine to those segments of the population who are particularly at risk (i.e., women of child-bearing age and infants and children).

Supplementation or restoration of an adequate diet to individuals who have had lifelong iodine deficiency can lead to thyrotoxicosis. The long-term stimulation of the thyroid gland can lead to its autonomous functioning; in other words, it continues to take up iodine and synthesize and secrete thyroid hormones even when adequate iodine is supplied and the stimulus of high TSH is removed. This complication, which is commonly seen in older adults in iodine-deficient regions, is easily treated with antithyroid drugs.

IODINE REQUIREMENTS AND DIETARY REFERENCE INTAKES

The IOM (2001) set the estimated average requirement (EAR) for iodine at 95 μg for both male and female adults; the recommended dietary allowance (RDA) for iodine was set as the EAR + 40 %, rounded to the nearest 50 μg, and is 150 μg for both male and female adults. These values for adults are based on measurements of radioiodine turnover in a range of studies. The EAR for pregnant women was increased by 65 μg/day based on thyroid iodine content of the newborn and iodine balance studies; therefore, the EAR and RDA for pregnant women are 160 and 220 μg/day of iodine, respectively. The EAR for lactating women is increased to allow for the average daily loss of iodine in human milk, approximately 114 μg/day; the EAR and RDA for lactating women are 209 and 290 μg/day of iodine, respectively. EARs and RDAs for children from 9 to 18 years of age were extrapolated down from adult data using metabolic body weight ($kg^{0.75}$); the EAR and RDA for children ages 9 to 13 years is 73 μg/day and 120 μg/day, respectively. For children ages 14 to 18 years, the EAR is 95 μg/day and the RDAs is 150 μg/day. EARs and RDAs for children from 1 to 8 years of age were based on balance study data; the EAR for this age-group is 65 μg/day and the RDA is 90 μg/day. Adequate intakes (AI) were estimated for infants; the AI for infants from 0 to 6 months of age was based on the average iodine intake from human milk (146 μg/L × 0.78 L/day) and the AI for 7- to 12-month-old infants was extrapolated from the value for younger infants. The AI for infants is 110 μg/day and 130 μg/day of iodine in the first and second half, respectively, of the first year of life. Interestingly, the AIs for infants are greater than the RDAs for 1- to 3- year- olds (90 μg/day). This is likely to reflect the different methodologies used to calculate these values, rather than a true difference in requirements.

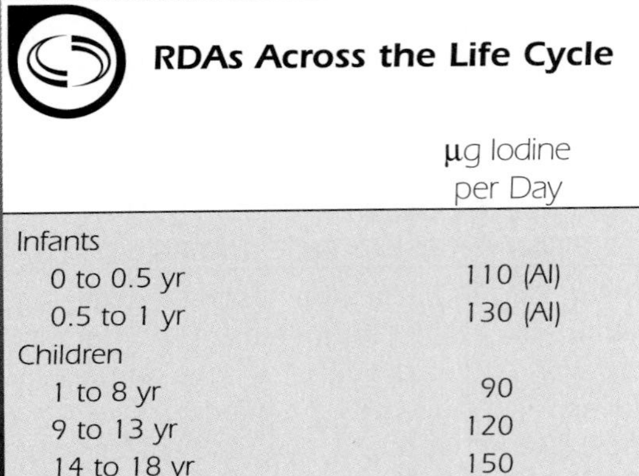

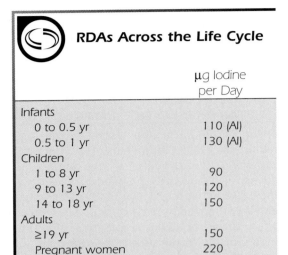

RDAs Across the Life Cycle

	μg Iodine per Day
Infants	
0 to 0.5 yr	110 (AI)
0.5 to 1 yr	130 (AI)
Children	
1 to 8 yr	90
9 to 13 yr	120
14 to 18 yr	150
Adults	
≥19 yr	150
Pregnant women	220
Lactating women	290

Data from Institute of Medicine (IOM) (2001). Iodine. In: Dietary Reference Intakes for Vitamin A, Vitamin K, Arsenic, Boron, Chromium, Copper, Iodine, Iron, Manganese, Molybdenum, Nickel, Silicon, Vanadium, and Zinc. National Academy Press, Washington, DC, pp 258-289.
AI, Adequate intake.

The iodine content of most food sources is low. Foods of marine origin have greater amounts of iodine because marine animals can concentrate iodine from seawater. Processed foods may contain enhanced levels of iodine due to the addition of iodized salt or other additives. Intakes in the United States are usually well in excess of these levels due to the use of iodized salt, which contains 76 μg of iodine per g, and also to the use of iodates in bread production (as dough improvers) and in dairy production (iodine-based antiseptics). The Total Diet Study (1991-1997) estimated a median iodine intake of 280 μg/day for adult men and 200 μg/day for adult women in the United States; the range of intake was from 43 μg/day (1st percentile for adult women) to 890 μg/day (99th percentile for adult men). A study of iodine concentration in milk of lactating women illustrates the effect of iodized salt intake: the median iodine concentration in milk of American women who consumed noniodized salt was 113 μg/L compared with 143 μg/L in women who consumed low amounts or iodized salt or to 270 μg/L for those who consumed high amounts of iodized salt (Gushurst et al., 1984).

Food Sources

Food Sources of Iodine

Rich Sources: Seafood (fish, shellfish, or seaweed)

~30 μg per 3 oz of shrimp
~100 to 140 mg per 3 oz of haddock or cod
~17 μg per 3 oz canned tuna

Variable Sources: Vegetables, Meats, Eggs

~60 μg per 1 medium baked potato
~35 μg per ½ cup navy beans
~30 μg per 1 large egg
~30 μg per 3 oz turkey breast
~8 μg per 3 oz ground beef

Fortified Foods: Iodized Salt

100 μg per 1 tsp salt

Adventitious Sources

Bread (iodates as dough improvers)
~35 μg per slice
Milk (iodine-based antiseptics)
~56 μg per 8 oz milk
~25 to 70 μg per ½ cup cottage cheese
~5 to 20 μg per 1 oz cheddar cheese

Data from U.S. Department of Agriculture/Agricultural Research Service (USDA/ARS) (2005) USDA Nutrient Database for Standard Reference, Release 18. USDA/ARS, Washington, DC. Retrieved November 17, 2005 from www.ars.usda.gov/ba/bhnrc/ndl/.

The IOM (2001) established an upper tolerable intake level (UL) for iodine. This was based on the amount of iodine that causes an elevated TSH concentration, which is an indicator for increased risk of developing hypothyroidism. The UL for adults is 1,100 μg/day of iodine. Those for children range from an UL of 200 μg/day of iodine for 1- to 3-year-old children up to 900 μg/day for adolescents.

REFERENCES

Aranda A, Pascual A (2001) Nuclear hormone receptors and gene expression. Physiol Rev 81:1269-1304.

Bernal J, Guadano-Ferraz A, Morte B (2003) Perspectives in the study of thyroid hormone action on brain development and function. Thyroid 13:1005-1012.

Bianco AC, Salvatore D, Gereben B, Berry MJ, Larsen PR (2002) Biochemistry, cellular and molecular biology, and physiological roles of the iodothyronine deiodinases. Endocrine Rev 23:38-89.

Blennemann B, Leahy P, Kim T-S, Freake, HC (1995) Tissue-specific regulation of lipogenic mRNAs by thyroid hormone. Mol Cell Endocrinol 110:1-8.

Brown JG, Bates PC, Holliday MA, Millward DJ (1981) Thyroid hormones and muscle protein turnover. Biochem J 194:771-782.

Brown SB, Maloney M, Kinlaw WB (1997) "Spot 14" protein functions at the pretranslational level in the regulation of hepatic metabolism by thyroid hormone and glucose. J Biol Chem 272: 2163-2166.

Brush BE, Altland JK (1952) Goiter prevention with iodized salt: Results of a thirty-year study. J Clin Endocrinol Metab 12:1380-1388.

Clausen T, Van Hardeveld C, Everts ME (1991) Significance of cation transport in control of energy metabolism and thermogenesis. Physiol Rev 71:733-774.

Freake HC, Oppenheimer JH (1995) Thermogenesis and thyroid function. Annu Rev Nutr 15: 263-291.

Gushurst CA, Mueller JA, Green JA, Sedor F (1984) Breast milk iodide: reassessment in the 1980s. Pediatrics 73:354-357.

Harper ME, Ballantyne JS, Leach M, Brand MD (1993) Effects of thyroid hormone on oxidative phosphorylation. Biochem Soc Trans 21:785-792.

Hetzel BS, Maberly GF (1986) Iodine. In: Mertz W (ed) Trace Elements in Human and Animal Nutrition. Academic Press, New York, pp 139-208.

Institute of Medicine (2001): Dietary Reference Intakes for Vitamin A, Vitamin K, Arsenic, Boron, Chromium, Copper, Iodine, Iron, Manganese, Molybdenum, Nickel, Silicon, Vanadium, and Zinc. National Academy Press, Washington, DC, pp 258-289.

Izumo S, Nadal-Ginard B, Mahdavi V (1986) All members of the MHC multigene family respond to thyroid hormone in a highly tissue-specific manner. Nature 231:557-560.

Jump DB, Thelen AP, Mater MK (2001) Functional interaction between sterol regulatory element-binding protein-1c, nuclear factor Y, and 3,5,3′-triiodothyronine nuclear receptors. J Biol Chem 276:34419-34427.

Kinlaw WB, Tron P, Friedmann AS (1992) Nuclear localization and hepatic zonation of rat "spot 14" protein: Immunochemical investigation employing anti-fusion protein antibodies. Endocrinology 131:3120-3122.

Klein I (1990) Thyroid hormone and the cardiovascular system. Am J Med 88:631-637.

Lanni A, Moreno M, Lombardi A, Goglia F (2003) Thyroid hormone and uncoupling proteins. FEBS Lett 543:5-10.

Lazar MA (1993) Thyroid hormone receptors: Multiple forms, multiple possibilities. Endocrinol Rev 14:184-193.

Pharoah POD, Buttfield IH, Hetzel BS (1971) Neurological damage to the fetus resulting from severe iodine deficiency during pregnancy. Lancet 1:398-410.

Pharoah POD, Connolly KJ (1995) Iodine and brain development. Dev Med Child Neurol 38:464-469.

Porterfield SP, Hendrich CE (1993) The role of thyroid hormones in prenatal and neonatal neurological development—current perspectives. Endocrinol Rev 14:94-106.

Sap J, Munoz A, Damm K, Goldberg Y, Ghsydael J. Leutz A, Beug H, Vennstrom B (1986) The c-erb-A protein is a high affinity receptor for thyroid hormone. Nature 324:635-640.

Seelig S, Liaw C, Towle HC, Oppenheimer JH (1981) Thyroid hormone attenuates and augments hepatic gene expression at a pretranslational level. Proc Natl Acad Sci U S A 78:4733-4737.

Vallee BL, Coleman JE, Auld DS (1991) Zinc fingers, zinc clusters, and zinc twists in DNA-binding protein domains. Proc Natl Acad Sci U S A 88:999-1003.

Webb P (2004) Selective activators of thyroid hormone receptors. Expert Opin Investig Drugs 13:489-500.

Weinberger C, Thompson CC, Ong ES, Lebo R, Gruol DJ, Evans RM (1986) The c-erb-A gene encodes a thyroid hormone receptor. Nature 324:641-646.

World Health Organization (WHO) (2001) Assessment of the Iodine Deficiency Disorders and Monitoring their Elimination. (Document WHO/NHD/01.1). WHO, Geneva.

World Health Organization (WHO) (2004) Iodine Status Worldwide: WHO Global Database on Iodine Deficiency (de Benoist B, Andersson, M, Egli I, Takkouche B, Allen H [eds]) WHO, Geneva.

Yen PM (2003a) Physiological and molecular basis of thyroid hormone action. Physiol Rev 81:1097-1142.

Yen PM (2003b) Molecular basis of resistance to thyroid hormone. Trends Endocrinol Metab 14:327-333.

Yen PM, Chin WW (1994) New advances in understanding the molecular mechanisms of thyroid hormone action. Trends Endocrinol Metab 5:65-72.

Zilz ND, Murray MB, Towle HC (1990) Identification of multiple thyroid hormone response elements located far upstream from the rat S14 promoter. J Biol Chem 265:8136-8143.

RECOMMENDED READINGS

Freake HC, Oppenheimer JH (1995) Thermogenesis and thyroid function. Annu Rev Nutr 15:263-291.

Hetzel BS, Maberly GF (1986) Iodine. In: Mertz W (ed) Trace Elements in Human and Animal Nutrition. Academic Press, New York, pp 139-208.

McNabb FMA (1992) Thyroid Hormones. Prentice-Hall, Englewood Cliffs, NJ.

Yen PM (2003) Physiological and molecular basis of thyroid hormone action. Physiol Rev 81:1097-1142.

RECOMMENDED WEBSITES

International Council for the Control of Iodine Deficiency Disorders

Links to website of ICCIDD formed in 1985 with support from UNICEF, WHO, and the Australian government.

www.people.virginia.edu/~jtd/iccidd/

World Health Organization

Links to WHO publications and data on iodine deficiency disease throughout the world.

http://www3.who.int/

Chapter 39

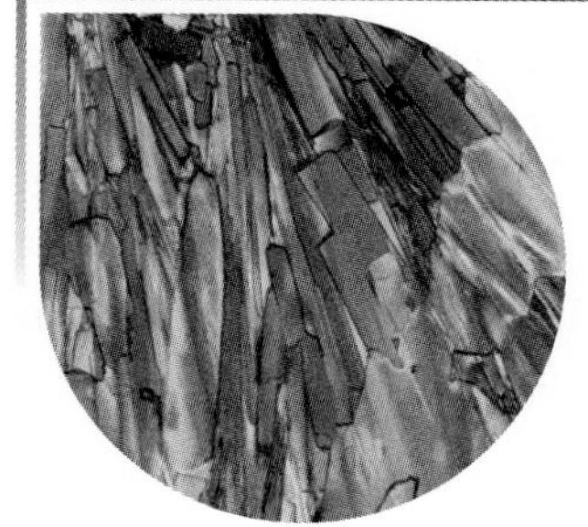

Selenium

Roger A. Sunde, PhD

OUTLINE

COMMON ABBREVIATIONS

Sec	selenocysteine
SECIS	selenocysteine insertion sequence
eEFsec	selenocysteine-specific eukaryotic elongation factor

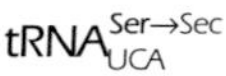

$tRNA^{Ser \rightarrow Sec}_{UCA}$ specific tRNA for selenocysteine with UCA anticodon that aligns with the UGA codon

U 1-letter amino acid symbol for selenocysteine

C 1-letter amino acid symbol for cysteine

CHEMISTRY OF SELENIUM

Selenium (Se) was discovered in 1817 by the Swedish chemist Jöns Jakob Berzelius in the flue dust of iron pyrite burners, and this new element was named after the Greek *selene* ("moon"). The remainder of the nineteenth century saw some limited use of selenium as CdSe in the ruby red coloring of glass. Selenium's notoriety as a toxic element emerged in the 1930s with the recognition that several forms of "loco diseases" in horses and cattle were caused by the ingestion of plants containing high levels of selenium. In 1943 a diet that contained 5 mg/kg selenium was reported to cause the development of neoplasms in rat liver, thus marking selenium as a carcinogenic agent. It was, therefore, surprising when Schwarz and Foltz (1957) reported that liver necrosis in rats could be prevented by inorganic selenium, leading to the demonstration that selenium was a nutritionally essential trace element. In the 1960s and 1970s epidemiological data and animal research began to demonstrate that selenium also possesses anticarcinogenic activity. In 1973 glutathione peroxidase-1 (GPX1) was discovered to be a selenoenzyme, and we now know that the human genome encodes 25 selenoproteins (Kryukov et al., 2003).

Selenium lies below oxygen and sulfur in the group VIa elements in the periodic table. Therefore, selenium has both metallic and nonmetallic properties, resulting in its unique chemistry and biochemistry. Its 34 electrons are distributed with 18 in the argon shell, 10 3d electrons, and 6 electrons in the 4s and

Nutrition Insight

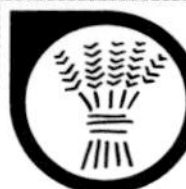

Selenium Geochemistry Influences Nutrition and Disease

Selenium is present in soils at both toxic and deficient levels. The origin of high-selenium soils is principally volcanic. Soil selenium in the Dakotas has been estimated to average as high as 0.1 g/cm^3 and to reach down to a thickness of 800 m. Rainfalls of less than 20 inches per year do not leach soil sufficiently, resulting in retention of the high soil concentrations of selenium. The hard wheat grown in these areas of the Great Plains gives rise to bread that is a good source of dietary selenium. These high-selenium areas also harbor plants that accumulate toxic levels of selenium, which caused the "loco diseases" (alkali disease, blind staggers) and other equine problems (loss of hair and hooves) that were reported in 1860 around Fort Randall in the Dakota Territory (Rosenfeld and Beath, 1964).

Toxic buildup of selenium in the Kesterson Reservoir of California is due to irrigation of Se-rich soils in the San Joaquin Valley. This reservoir, or wetland, was developed in the late 1970s to collect subsurface drainage from the tile drainage systems used to irrigate the agricultural land of the San Joaquin Valley. The problem of selenium buildup was identified when wildlife, especially birds, at the reservoir began dying in the early 1980s. Studies now indicate that existing concentrations of Se are toxic to birds because growing embryos in the eggs cannot excrete excess Se, whereas these levels of Se are not especially toxic to organisms that can homeostatically regulate Se status.

In contrast to areas with selenium-rich soils, lack of recent volcanic activity and low annual rainfall in some other regions of the country, such as Ohio and New York, have left some areas with soils that are deficient in selenium. Livestock in these selenium-deficient areas were formerly commonly afflicted by diseases that are now known to be due to selenium deficiency and which are now prevented by selenium supplementation.

4p orbitals. The 4s and 4p electrons, when lost, give rise to the common +6 and +4 oxidation states, whereas the addition of 2 electrons to the 4p orbitals completes the octet to yield the −2 oxidation state. The atomic weight of the naturally abundant isotope of selenium is 78.96, and 6 naturally occurring stable isotopes of selenium have potential for use as tracers.

Selenium's chemical properties (Cotton and Wilkinson, 1972) have a strong impact on selenium biology. First, the empty dπ orbitals of selenium can be filled by pπ electrons of oxygen, resulting in multiple "dπ-pπ bonds" similar to those of sulfur, thereby permitting the formation of more than four σ bonds to other atoms, as might occur during selenium-catalyzed enzyme reactions (Fig. 39-1). These dπ-pπ orbitals also confer unique electronic properties to selenium which facilitate novel reactions of selenoenzymes. Second, selenium and sulfur have similar radii, so that covalent sulfur and selenium compounds (C–S–X or C–Se–X) are not readily distinguished by enzymes based upon bond length. Third, selenium and sulfur also have similar chemical reactivity; genome sequencing of different

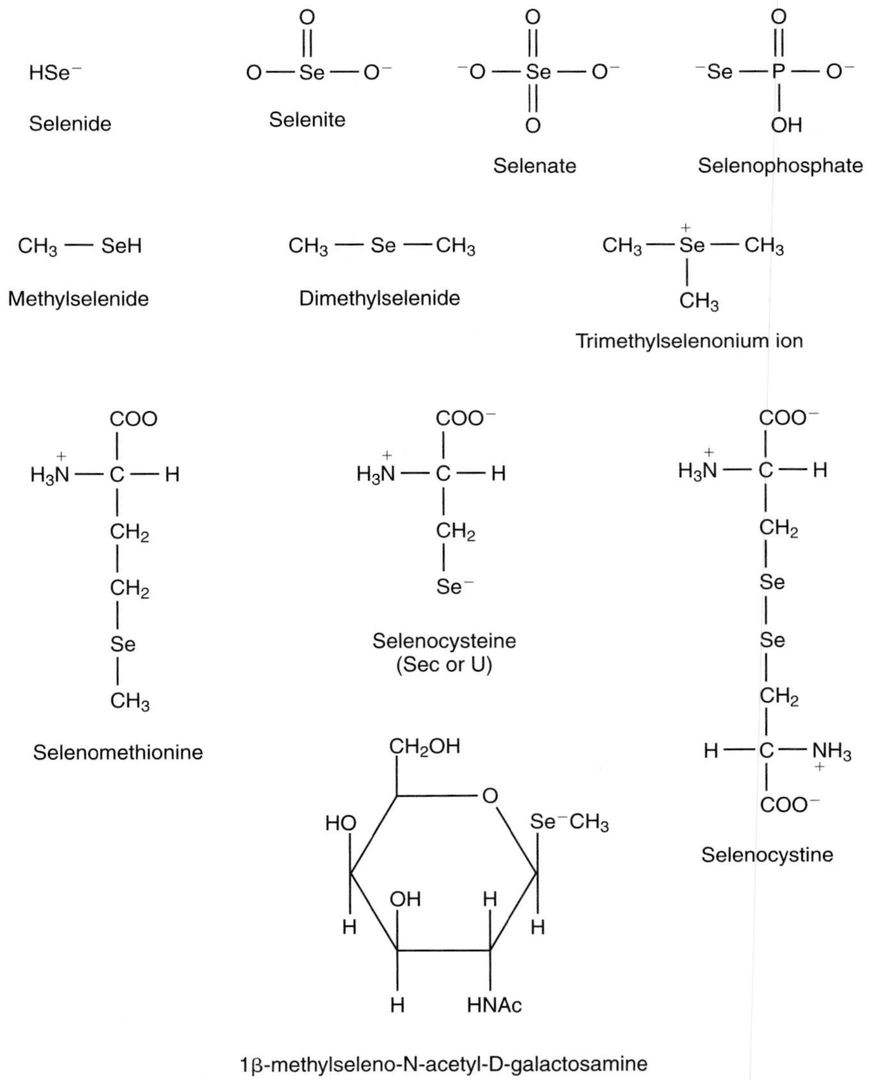

HSe^- Selenide

Selenite

Selenate

Selenophosphate

$CH_3—SeH$ Methylselenide

$CH_3—Se—CH_3$ Dimethylselenide

Trimethylselenonium ion

Selenomethionine

Selenocysteine (Sec or U)

Selenocystine

1β-methylseleno-N-acetyl-D-galactosamine

Figure 39-1 Structures of common selenium metabolites at physiological pH.

species is revealing that homologous genes of the selenoproteins are usually present in other organisms with cysteine encoded instead of selenocysteine (Sec).

Two aspects of selenium and sulfur chemistry differ significantly, however, thereby permitting ready separation of selenium and sulfur under physiological conditions. First, hydrogen selenide (H_2Se) is a much stronger acid than is hydrogen sulfide (H_2S). At physiological pH, the amino acid selenocysteine has a selenol pK_a of 5.24 and is predominantly deprotonated, whereas the cysteine thiol with a pK_a of 8.25 is largely protonated. Second, the reduction potentials of selenious and selenic acid are much greater than those of the analogous sulfur acids, so biological metabolism directs selenium toward reduction and sulfur toward oxidation.

SELENIUM DEFICIENCY AND ESSENTIALITY

The use of purified and semipurified diets led to the identification of selenium as a nutritionally essential mineral element. A water-soluble factor present in American brewer's yeast was found to prevent liver necrosis in rats fed a diet based on torula yeast as the protein source. Supplementation of this diet with cystine, vitamin E, or this water-soluble "factor 3" prevented liver necrosis in rats. This degenerative liver disease was distinct from fatty liver and liver cirrhosis and, if untreated, resulted in death in 21 to 28 days. In 1957 Schwarz and Foltz discovered that "factor 3" isolated from pig kidney contained selenium, and that a variety of inorganic as well as organic forms of selenium would prevent liver necrosis in rats. Selenium alone was later shown to be unconditionally essential for rats and chickens fed diets containing adequate levels of vitamin E and sulfur amino acids.

Clear-cut evidence for the essentiality of selenium in humans was not reported until two decades later. Human selenium deficiency in a New Zealand woman undergoing total parenteral nutrition (TPN) was first reported in 1979. The patient lived in a rural area with low-selenium soils; endemic white muscle disease in sheep was controlled by selenium dosing. Following surgery, the patient was given TPN. After 20 days she had dry, flaky skin; after 30 days she developed bilateral muscular discomfort and muscle pain. The patient's plasma selenium dropped to 9 μg/L after 30 days of TPN from a concentration of 25 μg/L immediately before the start of TPN. The muscle pain was sufficient to aggravate walking, and a generalized muscular wasting occurred. The patient was then infused intravenously with 100 μg/day of Se; within the next week muscle pain disappeared and she returned to full mobility. TPN-associated selenium deficiency in humans is not restricted solely to countries with low-selenium content in the soil. A similar TPN-induced case of muscle pain and cardiomyopathy leading to death has been reported in the United States. These cases were associated with very low levels of selenium in plasma and red blood cells, with low erythrocyte GPX1 activity, with elevated plasma marker enzymes indicative of tissue damage, and often with white nail beds.

Selenium deficiency is not simply a clinical curiosity. Just as with animal species consuming feed produced locally, humans linked solely to regional food production are potentially susceptible to nutrient deficiency disease. An endemic Se-responsive disease, Keshan disease, formerly affecting peasant populations in Se-deficient areas of China, was eradicated by an aggressive Se-supplementation program, but cessation of the program, following economic and dietary advances in the 1990s, has led to the reappearance of clustered cases of the disease in economically disadvantaged populations in these areas. A regional disease of unknown origin, called Kashin Beck disease, which continues to affect 8 million individuals in regions of northern China who eat corn-based diets, also has been hypothesized to have selenium deficiency as a contributing factor.

SELENIUM ABSORPTION, DISTRIBUTION, AND EXCRETION

Absorption of dietary selenium is highly efficient, and selenium is lost from the body primarily in the urine. Most of the selenium present in body tissues is present as Sec residues in selenoproteins.

Clinical Correlation

Keshan Disease

The dramatic impact of selenium deficiency in humans is revealed in the descriptions of Keshan disease, an endemic cardiomyopathy that occurred until the 1980s in China. Keshan disease affected primarily children younger than 15 years of age and women of child-bearing age. The prevalence rates prior to the start of selenium supplementation were on the order of 6.5 to 13.5 individuals per thousand, and the disease was primarily localized in the peasant populations in certain hilly and mountainous regions with low soil selenium. Urban inhabitants and families of managerial classes living in the same areas were unaffected owing to an improved diet with more animal products and with foods from a more diverse geographical range. The main pathological feature of Keshan disease is a multiple focal myocardial necrosis scattered throughout the heart muscle. Criteria for diagnosis include acute or chronic heart function insufficiency, heart enlargement, gallop rhythm or dysrhythmia, electrocardiographic (ECG) changes, and pulmonary edema. Subacute cases may also have facial edema.

The demonstration that selenium was essential for laboratory animals and livestock in the 1960s, and the observations that the cardiomyopathy associated with Keshan disease was similar to that observed in Se-deficient mice and swine suggested trials with selenium. Encouraging preliminary results indicated selenium might be preventive. All affected areas were found to be invariably poor in selenium, and a large-scale study was begun in 1974 with all children in 119 production teams in three communes (Chen et al., 1980). Half the children were given weekly sodium selenite tablets orally and the other half were given a placebo. Children 1 to 5 years old received 0.5 mg and children 6 to 9 years old received 1 mg of sodium selenite (0.23 and 0.46 mg of Se per week, respectively). A total of 46,033 children were in this study. In the first 2 years, there were 5.6 deaths per thousand in the control group versus 0.08 per thousand in the treatment group. Because of the effectiveness of selenium supplementation, the control group was omitted for the last 2 years of the study. Total cases in the selenium-treatment group were not immediately eliminated but progressively declined over the 4-year study period, suggesting that more than restoration of selenium status may be involved in the disease.

The average hair selenium in nonaffected sites was greater than 0.2 μg/g versus an average below 0.12 μg/g for all affected sites. GPX1 activity in the blood of peasant children was two thirds of that observed in staff children. The average daily selenium intake for women in these affected areas was estimated to be 12 μg/day, which is considerably lower than the New Zealand estimate of 20 μg/day necessary for maintenance of normal human health (Robinson and Thompson, 1983; Chen et al., 1980).

The disease was virtually eliminated by selenium supplementation programs, but those programs ceased as the overall economic condition in the areas improved. The result has been a reemergence of a handful of cases each year in impoverished populations in the same regions. The ineffectiveness of selenium to eradicate the disease completely in one season following selenium supplementation and a seasonal prevalence of the disease both suggest that other factors are involved. A cardiotoxic virus has been isolated from the hearts of individuals who died from Keshan disease, suggesting that a viral infection may be the underlying cause.

SELENIUM IN FOODS

The majority of selenium in most plants is in proteins as selenomethionine (see Fig. 39-1). In "selenium-accumulator" plants, however, selenium is accumulated as selenium analogs of metabolites of sulfur amino acids, such as selenocystathionine and methylselenocysteine. In contrast, the majority of selenium in products from animals fed usual levels of dietary selenium is present as selenoproteins and thus mostly as Sec. Only elemental selenium, dimethylselenide, and the mercury-selenium complex in tuna are forms of selenium that are basically not available for conversion to biologically active forms of selenium. In large part, concern about the particular dietary form of selenium is a moot academic point, because selenium absorption from most sources is very high; homeostasis at the organism level does not occur via regulation of absorption.

Inorganic selenium is commonly used to supplement animal feeds and to provide inexpensive selenium in vitamin-mineral supplements. The most common inorganic form of selenium used in animal supplements is sodium selenite (Na_2SeO_3); sodium selenate (Na_2SeO_4) is increasingly used because, without the free electron pair, selenate is far less likely than selenite to oxidize other components of the diet.

Intake of selenium varies widely depending on the selenium content of the soil in which foods are grown as well as on supplement use. The median dietary Se intake for adults in the United States is 146 and 98 μg/day for men and women, respectively (Institute of Medicine [IOM], 2000) (Fig. 39-2). Typical intakes from food are 20 μg/day in China, 35 μg/day in Finland and New Zealand, and 30 to 50 μg/day in Britain and Ireland.

SELENIUM ABSORPTION

In humans, both selenite and selenomethionine are highly available. Absorption from relatively large doses providing 200 μg of Se (~3 times the recommended intake) was estimated to be 84% for selenium provided as selenite and 98% for selenium provided as selenomethionine (Patterson et al., 1989). Under physiological conditions, selenium homeostasis is clearly not regulated by absorption, but rather urinary excretion is likely to be important for homeostasis (Burk, 1976). The enzymes and transporters responsible for absorption or movement of selenium across membranes are mostly unknown. Selenomethionine is actively transported by the same system that transports methionine.

SELENIUM EXCRETION

Under deficient to adequate conditions, we now know that selenium is excreted in the urine as monomethylated selenium in the form of a selenosugar, 1β-methylseleno-*N*-acetyl-D-galactosamine (Kobayashi et al., 2002). Both the size of the dose as well as the selenium status of an animal influences the form and amount of urinary selenium excretion. Methylseleno-*N*-acetyl-galactosamine is the usual major form of urinary selenium in rats given selenium at the required or slightly higher levels.

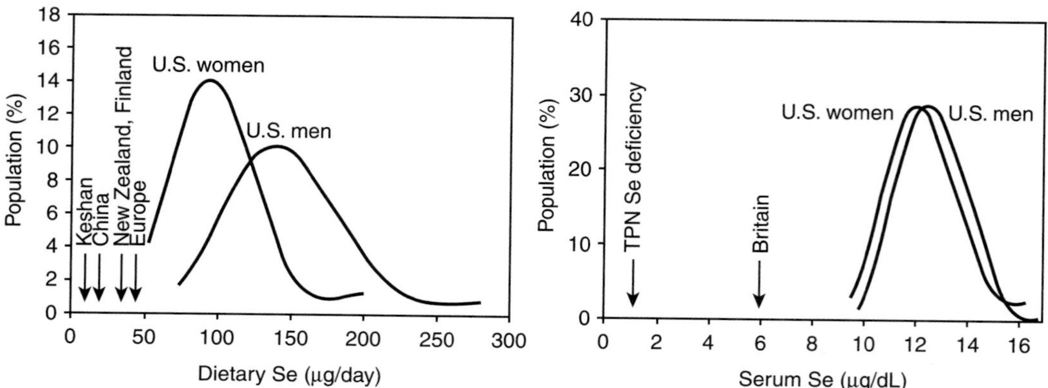

Figure 39-2 The distribution of dietary intakes of selenium *(left)* and serum selenium concentrations *(right)* for adults (31 to 50 years old) living in the United States. *Arrows* show reported levels in other countries, as discussed in the text. *(Data from third National Health and Nutrition Examination Survey [NHANES III, 1988-1994], as provided in Institute of Medicine [IOM] [2000] Dietary Reference Intakes for Vitamin C, Vitamin E, Selenium, and Carotenoids. National Academy Press, Washington, DC.)*

Trimethylselenonium constitutes only a small fraction of urinary selenium in rats given selenium at required levels. However, trimethylselenonium is the major urinary selenium form in animals ingesting supernutritional levels of selenium. When pharmacological doses of selenium were injected into rats, selenium was expired in the breath as dimethylselenide; 50% of the Se from selenite and 35% of that from selenomethionine were expired as dimethylselenide in the first 24 hours after rats were injected with 5 mg of Se per kg of body weight (McConnell and Roth, 1966).

It is probable that methylseleno-*N*-acetylgalactosamine is also the major urinary form of selenium in humans, because only 7% to 17% of urinary selenium is accounted for by the trimethylselenonium ion (Francesconi and Pannier, 2004). After 200 μg of selenium enriched with ^{74}Se tracer was administered to selenium-adequate adult subjects, 17% of tracer selenite and 11% of tracer selenomethionine appeared in the urine over the following 12 days (Patterson et al., 1989). Trace amounts of dimethylselenide, which has a garlic-like odor, may be detected in the breath of people ingesting high levels of selenium.

MODELS OF SELENIUM METABOLISM

Elegant studies using the radioactive tracer ^{75}Se or stable isotopes have been conducted in rats and humans to monitor selenium flux. Figure 39-3 shows a whole-body model of human selenium metabolism from selenite, based on stable isotope kinetic modeling in humans as well as information from other studies with humans and rats. The diagram illustrates the fate of 70 μg of Se as selenite over a 12-day period in a Se-adequate subject. The diagram consists of intestine, the major site of selenium absorption, and compartments for blood, liver/pancreas, kidney, and muscle (muscle represents muscle plus other tissues). An important aspect of this model is that plasma selenium is shown to consist of three distinctly different compartments: selenoprotein P (Sel-P), plasma glutathione peroxidase (GPX3), and a low-molecular-weight compartment of mainly hydrogen selenide (HSe^-).

In the model, selenium absorption is 84%, or 59 μg of Se, with 16% released in the feces. Biliary recycling returns an additional 32 μg to the intestine, and 12 μg (17%) of the dose is released in the urine over the first 12 days. The remaining absorbed selenium is incorporated into tissue selenoproteins as part of normal protein turnover, thereby displacing the original selenium, which mixes with the low-molecular-weight pool and is excreted, keeping the subject in selenium balance.

Intestinal selenite is most likely reduced to selenide during absorption, and red blood cells and other tissues also readily reduce selenite to selenide; thus selenide in the low-molecular-weight pool in plasma peaks about 2 hours after ingestion and disappears with a half-life of 20 minutes. The majority of this selenium is taken up by liver, incorporated into selenoprotein P (Sel-P), and secreted into the circulation. Plasma selenoprotein P concentration peaks at 10 hours, with a half-life of 3 hours. Kidney is the major source of GPX3 in humans, and GPX3 levels in plasma peak at 13 hours, with a half-life of 12 hours. Selenoprotein P is essential for normal distribution of selenium in the body and provides targeted delivery to the testes and brain (Burk and Hill, 2005). To date, specific uptake of GPX3 has not been demonstrated for any tissue. Therefore, the diagram shows distribution of selenoprotein P and GPX3 selenium directly to reticulocytes, muscle, and other tissues, although turnover of these species may occur in liver or kidney with passage of this selenium through the plasma selenide pool before its uptake by these other tissues.

TISSUE DISTRIBUTION OF SELENIUM

Estimates of total selenium content of humans, determined from cadavers, range between 13.0 and 20.3 mg (Schroeder et al., 1970). Metabolic stable isotope methodology models predict that total body selenium asymptomatically approaches 30 mg, but these studies are based on subjects dosed with 200 μg of Se as the tracer (Patterson et al., 1989). Individuals living in New Zealand or China, who have average selenium intakes considerably lower than 200 μg/day, would be presumed to have a much lower total body content of Se. Muscle, liver, blood, and kidneys contain 61% of the estimated total body selenium in humans; if skeleton is included, this increases to 91.5%.

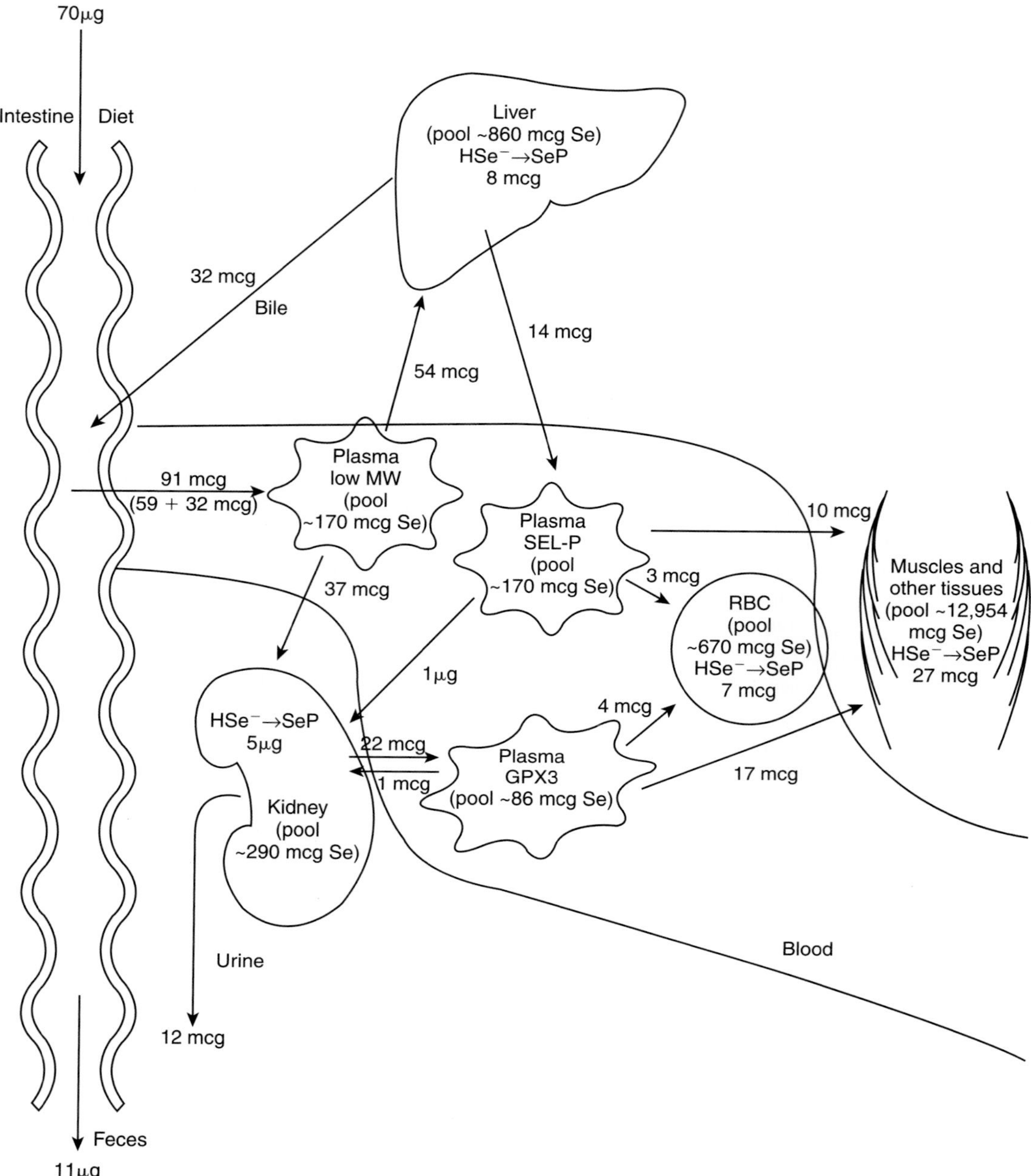

Figure 39-3 Whole-body model of human selenium metabolism. This model shows the following compartments: intestine, liver (plus pancreas), kidney, muscle plus other tissues, and blood, including a low-molecular-weight pool of selenium (HSe^-) and the selenoprotein P (SEL-P), GPX3, and red blood cell (RBC) pools. Pool values within compartments indicate the estimated pool sizes (in micrograms of Se). Values adjacent to *arrows* show the estimated flux between pools (in micrograms of Se) arising from ingestion of 70 μg of Se as selenite, as followed over the subsequent 12 days in a selenium-adequate human. Fluxes were estimated from the observed percentage absorption and excretion values and from fractional fluxes associated with plasma pools, as reported by Patterson and colleagues (1989) and described by Sunde (1997). Within liver, kidney, RBC, and muscle, $HSe^- \rightarrow SeP$ indicates the estimated incorporation of the ingested Se (in micrograms of Se) into tissue selenoproteins (SeP).

METABOLIC PATHWAYS OF SELENIUM

The intracellular metabolism of selenium is complex not only because this trace "metal" bonds covalently to carbon, but also because unique metabolic pathways are necessary to convert simple dietary forms of selenium into the form found in selenium-containing enzymes. These pathways include inorganic selenium metabolism, pathways of metabolism for low-molecular-weight organic selenium compounds, and the major pathways as well as several alternative pathways for incorporation of selenium into selenium-containing proteins or enzymes.

INORGANIC SELENIUM METABOLISM

Conversion of dietary selenate to selenite, shown in path (1) of Figure 39-4, is thought to involve adenosine phosphoselenate (APSe) or phosphoadenosine phosphoselenate (PAPSe)

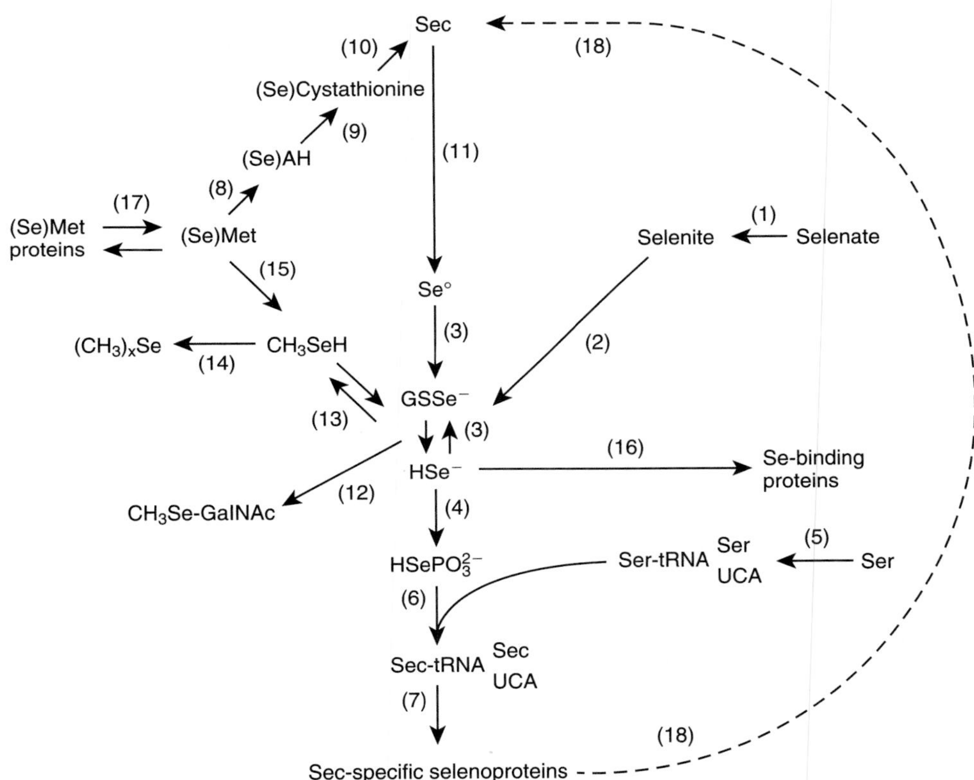

Figure 39-4 Metabolic pathways of selenium. Path *(1)*, selenate reduction to selenite via adenosine phosphoselenate (APSe) or phosphoadenosine phosphoselenate (PAPSe); path *(2)*, thioredoxin reductase reduction of selenite; path *(3)* glutathione (GSH)-dependent reduction; path *(4)*, selenophosphate synthase; path *(5)*, seryl-tRNA synthase; path *(6)*, selenocysteine synthase; path *(7)*, translational selenocysteine insertion, mediated by $tRNA^{Sec}$, SBP2, and eEFsec at the position specified by the UGA codon; path *(8)*, formation of adenosylselenomethionine and transmethylation resulting in formation of adenosylselenohomocysteine (SeAH); path *(9)*, cystathionine β-synthase; path *(10)*, cystathionine γ-lyase; path *(11)*, selenocysteine lyase; path *(12)*, synthesis of methylseleno-*N*-acetyl-galactosamine (CH_3Se-GalNAc) from selenide or glutathione selenopersulfide (GS-Se^-); path *(13)*, *S*-methyltransferase; path *(14)*, thioether *S*-methyltransferase; path *(15)*, transamination pathway resulting in methyl selenide; path *(16)*, selenide binding to proteins; path *(17)*, selenomethionine acylation of $tRNA^{Met}$ followed by incorporation at positions specified by an AUG codon; path *(18)*, release of Sec in proteolysis of selenoproteins.

intermediates. Selenite is reduced in an NADPH-dependent series of reactions to selenide (path [2]) by the Se-dependent enzyme thioredoxin reductase (Hatfield, 2001). Reduction to selenide can occur in intestinal cells or in red blood cells but also readily occurs in other cells. Reduction by glutathione and glutathione reductase may be important when selenium deficiency reduces thioredoxin reductase levels. Path (3) shows nonenzymatic reduction of Se to selenide via a glutathione selenopersulfide ($GS\text{-}Se^-$) intermediate. Selenide and ATP are the substrates for selenophosphate synthetase (path [4]), which produces selenophosphate, the activated selenium compound used for the transfer RNA (tRNA)–mediated synthesis of selenoproteins (paths [5], [6], [7]). In addition, selenide can bind nonenzymatically to proteins (path 16), which is likely to account for the acute toxicity of selenium.

CATABOLISM OF ORGANIC SELENIUM

Selenomethionine, like methionine, is not synthesized by higher animals. Selenomethionine is the common form of selenium in most plant-derived foods and is metabolized by the same enzymes responsible for methionine catabolism. Therefore, selenomethionine is activated to form adenosylselenomethionine (SeAM). SeAM, like adenosylmethionine, is an excellent methyl donor in mammalian systems and thus is converted to adenosylselenohomocysteine (SeAH) (path [8] in Fig. 39-3). SeAH in turn is a substrate for cystathionine β-synthase and cystathionine γ-lyase (paths [9] and [10] in Fig. 39-3) and thus is converted to Sec in mammalian tissues. Here the sulfur and selenium paths diverge.

Sec is degraded by Sec lyase, a selenium-specific enzyme that directly releases elemental selenium (path [11] in Fig. 39-3). The elemental selenium is reduced nonenzymatically to selenide (path [3]) by glutathione or other thiols. Selenide apparently is then converted to the methylseleno-*N*-acetyl-galactosamine (path [12]), the selenosugar that is the usual major urinary form of selenium under low-to-moderate dietary intakes of selenium (Kobayashi et al., 2002). This reaction may use glutathione selenopersulfide ($GS\text{-}Se^-$) as the actual substrate. Under high dietary intakes of selenium, methylation of selenide (path [13]) or further methylation steps (path [14]) result in dimethylselenide or trimethylselenonium ion. Methyl selenide or methylseleno-*N*-acetyl-galactosamine is also produced more directly from methionine via the enzymatic transamination and decarboxylation reactions (path [15]) of the methionine transamination pathway. Proteolysis of selenoproteins (path [18]) will release Sec. Sec must be metabolized through the selenide pool prior to reincorporation of its selenium into selenoproteins.

SELENIUM INCORPORATION INTO SELENOPROTEINS

Selenium incorporation into selenoproteins occurs cotranslationally during protein synthesis as the amino acid Sec (Hatfield, 2001). The cotranslational synthesis of Sec proceeds through several unusual intermediates and requires the following five unique gene products (four proteins and one tRNA):

1. Selenophosphate synthetase (SPS)
2. Selenocysteine insertion sequence (SECIS)–binding protein-2 (SBP2)
3. Eukaryotic selenocysteinyl-tRNA-specific elongation factor (eEFsec)
4. Selenocysteine synthase (SecS)
5. A Sec-specific tRNA ($tRNA_{UCA}^{Ser \rightarrow Sec}$), which is a unique tRNA

Two unique elements in the messenger RNA (mRNA) for the selenoprotein being synthesized are also required:

1. The UGA (uracil-guanine-adenine) codon
2. The SECIS (selenocysteine insertion sequence) element.

This process illustrates the importance of biochemistry and molecular biology in understanding the nutrition of a trace element. Although we now know much about the mammalian players in this process, the nature of many of the themes in Sec synthesis and incorporation were first established in bacteria.

THE SELENOCYSTEINE MOIETY

Experiments with GPX1 conducted just after it was shown to contain selenium revealed that this metalloenzyme was different from many other metalloproteins. Dialysis would not remove the trace element and dialysis with inorganic selenium would not restore GPX1 activity when hemolysates of red blood cells from selenium-deficient animals were incubated with selenite alone or with components of the selenite-reduction pathway. Pioneering studies on bacterial selenoproteins led to the identification of selenocysteine (Sec) as the chemical form of the selenium moiety in mammalian selenoproteins. Furthermore, this Sec is incorporated into the peptide backbone. The presence of Sec in bacteria, archaea, and eukaryotes indicates that this amino acid is of ancient origin. Because Sec is specifically incorporated into proteins during translation, it is considered the 21st amino acid required for protein synthesis. Sec is the three-letter code commonly used for selenocysteine, and U is used as the one-letter code in protein sequences. The codon for Sec is TGA (thymine-guanine-adenine) in DNA and UGA in mRNA, as shown in Figure 39-5 for GPX1. Intact Sec from the diet or from selenomethionine catabolism is not used for synthesis of selenoproteins. Instead, inorganic selenium in an activated form is used along with serine, which provides the carbon skeleton for Sec, and the reaction proceeds while the serine is esterified to a tRNA, as shown in Figure 39-6.

SELENOPHOSPHATE SYNTHETASE

Selenophosphate synthetase (SPS) catalyzes formation of the active selenium donor species from selenide and ATP, as shown in Figure 39-6. Humans have two *SPS* genes, with *SPS2* encoding a 448 amino acid protein with Sec at position 60. *SPS1*, however, is a paralog that encodes threonine in place of Sec; the gene product of *SPS1* may allow a modest amount of Sec to be synthesized even in Se-deficiency. The Se-dependent SPS2 enzyme allows expanded synthesis of Sec under Se-adequate conditions. Studies with the bacterial enzyme suggest that the reaction begins with ATP binding and formation of enzyme-phosphate and ADP intermediates. Subsequent addition of selenide forms selenophosphate ($HSePO_3^{2-}$) containing the γ-phosphate of ATP, and liberates inorganic phosphate and AMP. Selenophosphate is labile.

SELENOCYSTEINE $tRNA_{UCA}^{Ser \to Sec}$

Synthesis of selenoproteins requires a unique RNA gene product—the $tRNA_{UCA}^{Sec}$, which is more completely designated $tRNA_{UCA}^{Ser \to Sec}$ or more simply designated $tRNA^{Sec}$ (Fig. 39-7). The mammalian $tRNA_{UCA}^{Sec}$ has a UCA (uracil-cytosine-adenine) anticodon and has 90 nucleotides, compared with 76 nucleotides for all common tRNAs. The extra base pairs

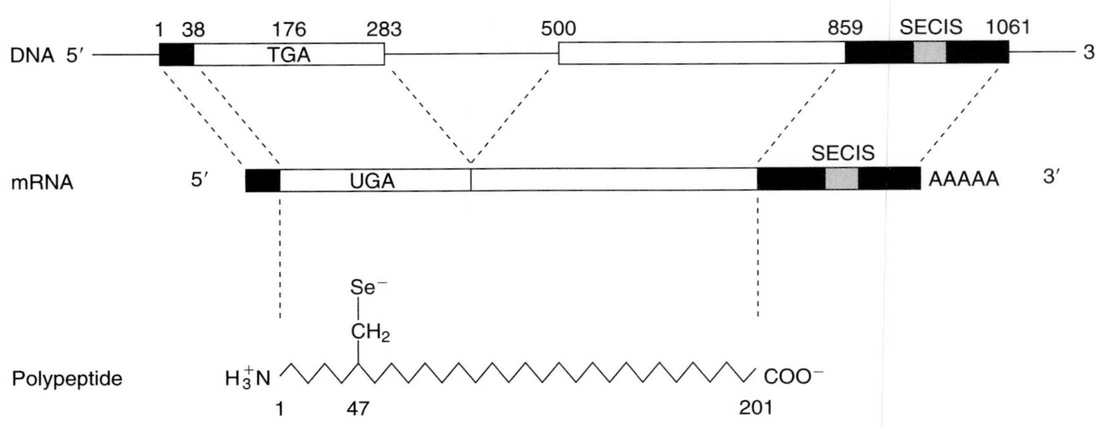

Figure 39-5 Diagrammatic alignment of the glutathione peroxidase-1 (*GPX1*) gene, GPX1 mRNA, and GPX1 protein. *Solid bars* indicate UTRs (untranslated regions), *gray bars* the SECIS (selenocysteine insertion sequence) element, and *open bars* indicate exons. Numbers indicate the position of the nucleotide base and amino acid residues in the genomic, message, and polypeptide sequences, respectively.

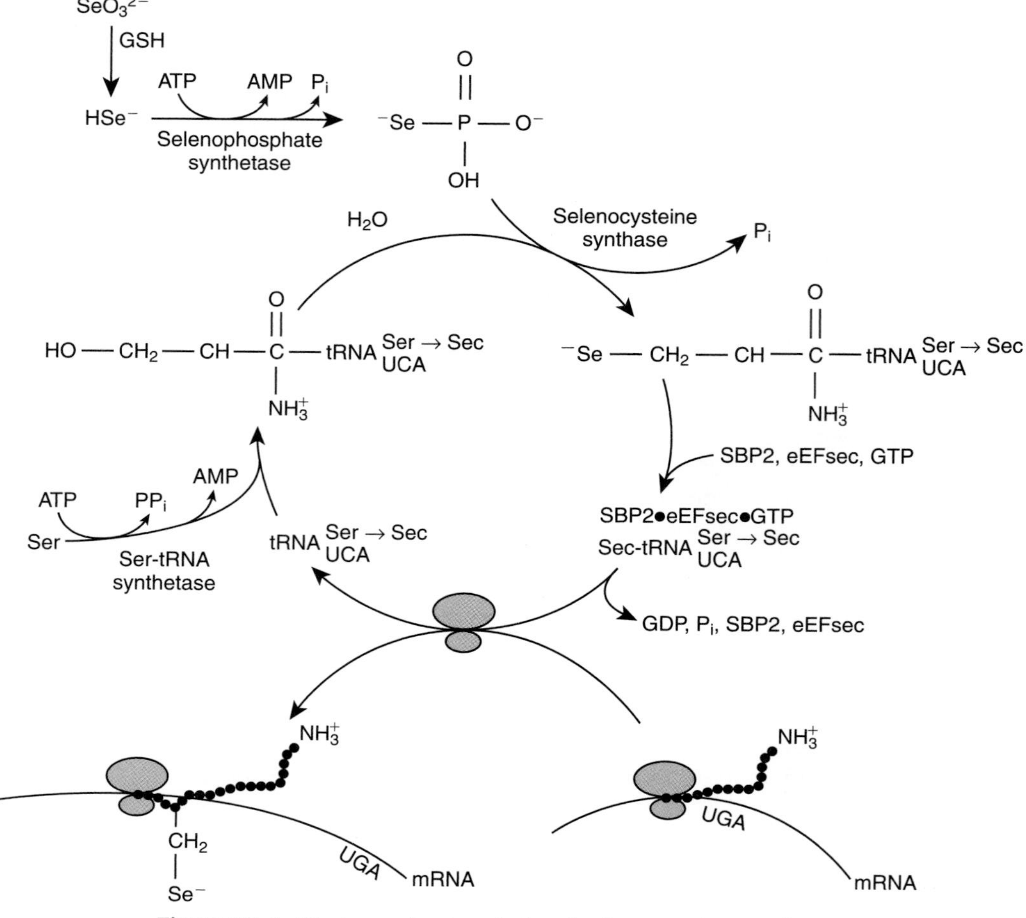

Figure 39-6 Diagram of cotranslational selenocysteine synthesis.

are in the acceptor stem of the tRNA (9 versus the usual 7 base pairs) and in a longer d-loop (with approximately 16 bases and 5 base pairs, compared with the usual 5 bases and no base pairs). Mammalian $tRNA^{Sec}_{UCA}$ undergoes maturation to two isoforms, which arise from the same gene but differ in that the modified uridine at the 5′ position of the UCA anticodon (i.e., 5-methylcarboxymethyl uridine, or mcm^5U) may or may not be methylated (i.e., 5-methylcarboxymethyl uridine-2′-*O*-methylribose, or mcm^5Um) (Hatfield, 2001).

Serine, from the same cellular pool used for protein synthesis, is esterified to the 3′ terminal adenosine (A) of the $tRNA^{Ser\rightarrow Sec}_{UCA}$ to form the corresponding seryl-tRNA, as shown in Figure 39-6. This reaction is catalyzed by cellular seryl-tRNA synthases, which apparently do not differentiate between the 76-nucleotide serine $tRNA^{Ser}$ and the 90-nucleotide $tRNA^{Ser\rightarrow Sec}_{UCA}$. The $tRNA^{Ser\rightarrow Sec}_{UCA}$ comprises only about 1% to 3% of the total seryl tRNAs in mammalian tissues.

SELENOCYSTEINE SYNTHASE

Sec is synthesized enzymatically from serine in a novel mechanism catalyzed by selenocysteine synthase. The reaction is specific for seryl-$tRNA^{Sec}$. The enzyme, which contains pyridoxal phosphate, catalyzes the dehydration of L-serine while attached to the tRNA to form aminoacrylyl-$tRNA^{Sec}$, followed by a C-2–C-3 addition of selenium via selenophosphate to form the Sec moiety still esterified to the $tRNA^{Sec}$, as shown in Figure 39-6. Consequently, three unique gene products (selenophosphate synthetase,

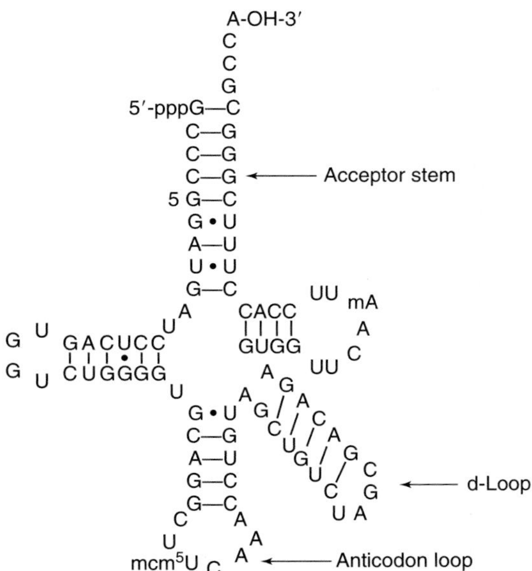

Figure 39-7 Eukaryotic tRNA$^{Ser \rightarrow Sec}_{UCA}$ consisting of 90 nucleotides. Methylation of the 5-methylcarboxymethyl uridine (mcm^{5}U) in the anticodon is present in some isoforms; 2′-*O*-methylation causes a change in the conformation of the tRNA. *(Modified from Amberg R, Urban C, Reuner B, Scharff P, Pomerantz SC, McCloskey JA, Gross HJ [1993] Editing does not exist for mammalian Sec tRNAs. Nucleic Acids Res 21:5583-5588, with permission from Oxford University Press.)*

selenocysteine synthase, and tRNA^{Sec}) are involved in synthesis of the direct precursor or Sec donor (Sec-tRNA^{Sec}) that is used in the translational incorporation of selenium into selenoproteins. Two additional unique proteins, SECIS-binding protein-2 and eukaryotic selenocysteinyl-tRNA-specific elongation factor, and two *cis*-acting mRNA elements are necessary for the actual synthesis of mammalian selenoproteins.

THE UGA CODON IN SELENOPROTEIN mRNA

The *GPX1* gene was the first selenoprotein gene to be cloned and sequenced (see Fig. 39-5). The gene, consisting of two exons, encodes a polypeptide of 201 amino acid residues. Most significantly, a TGA codon in the middle of the open reading frame of the first exon specifies the position of Sec. All characterized mammalian selenoproteins to date contain Sec that is encoded by TGA in the gene. This is also true for all Sec-containing bacterial and archaeal selenoproteins. Because UGA in the mRNA unambiguously serves as a termination codon for many mammalian proteins, it is obvious that a UGA alone is not sufficient to specify Sec incorporation into selenoproteins.

THE SELENOCYSTEINE INSERTION SEQUENCE ELEMENT IN SELENOPROTEIN mRNA

Studies on expression of cloned selenoproteins revealed that the 3′-UTR (3′-untranslated region) of the mRNA was necessary for UGA-encoded Sec incorporation. Berry and colleagues (1991) fused the coding region of 5′-deiodinase (DI1) and the 3′-UTR of GPX1 and used this chimeric construct to identify a consensus 87-base stem-loop element in rat DI1 or GPX1 3-′UTR that catalyzes the insertion of selenium into DI1. This element is called a eukaryotic SECIS element. A single SECIS is also present in the 3′-UTR of the mRNAs of all selenoproteins with the exception of selenoprotein P mRNA, which has two SECIS elements present in its 3′-UTR.

A model SECIS element is shown in Figure 39-8. The consensus SECIS element is a stem-loop structure with a variable apical loop consisting of 7 to 10 unpaired bases, including a consensus AA (adenine-adenine) sequence. A consensus AUGA (adenine-uracil-guanine-adenine) sequence is 5′ to the loop, and a consensus GA (guanine-adenine) sequence is located 3′ to the loop. This AUGA ... AA ... GA motif is critical, but base pair changes in the intervening stem do not affect efficacy for mediating selenium incorporation (Kryukov et al., 2003). In addition, a few mammalian SECIS elements contain a variant AUGA ... CC ... GA motif. The model SECIS element has two helical regions separated by an internal loop. The top helix ends in the consensus UGA and GA sequences and forms a quartet motif of non–Watson and Crick base pairs, which results in a greater than 90-degree kink in the stem-loop (Walczak et al., 1996). About half the mammalian SECIS elements have an additional stem extending from the apical loop. The specific secondary structure of the SECIS elements found in different selenoproteins

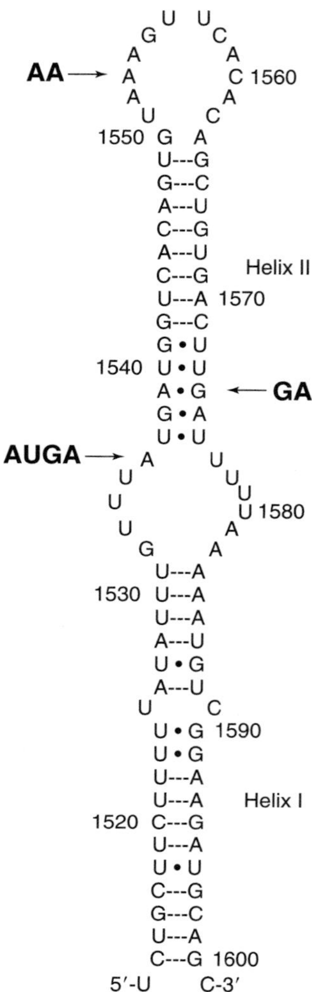

Figure 39-8 Selenocysteine insertion sequence (SECIS) elements. Eukaryotic SECIS element that resides in the 3′-UTR of rat DI1. The AUGA ... AA ... GA motif is indicated. *(Modified from Walczak R, Westhof E, Carbon P, Krol A [1996] A novel RNA structural motif in the Sec insertion element of eukaryotic selenoprotein mRNAs. RNA 2:367-379, with permission from Cambridge University Press.)*

may affect the rate of Sec insertion. The role of the two SECIS elements in selenoprotein P is unknown.

It should be noted that bacteria use a different SECIS element for recognition of UGA as a Sec codon. The prokaryotic SECIS (pSECIS) is a 38-nucleotide stem-loop element located in the open reading frame of the prokaryotic selenoprotein mRNA immediately following the UGA codon. The constraints of maintaining this secondary structure may limit the ability of bacterial genes to place Sec at the active site of enzymes. In contrast, selenoprotein genes in archaea have the SECIS element in the 3′-UTR as do those in eukaryotes.

EUKARYOTIC SECIS BINDING PROTEIN AND SELENOCYSTEINE-SPECIFIC ELONGATION FACTOR

In bacteria, a single elongation factor is required to bind the SECIS element and the Sec-tRNA. In eukaryotes and archaea, this role is split between two proteins. The search for a homolog to the bacterial elongation factor led to the discovery of the eukaryotic SECIS binding protein (SBP2). SBP2 binds to specific regions of the eSECIS (thought to be primarily in the AUGA/GA nucleotides in the stem). SBP2 does not share homology with elongation factors but rather with translation release factors and with ribosomal binding proteins.

In eukaryotes, a Sec-specific elongation factor (eEFsec) partners with SBP2 for incorporation of UGA-encoded Sec. In archaea, an unassigned elongation factor was shown to be specific for Sec-tRNA, and orthologs in mammalian genomes led to the identification of eEFsec. The eEFsec binds Sec-$tRNA^{Sec}$ but does not bind seryl-$tRNA^{Ser}$, thus preventing misincorporation of Ser in place of Sec. As do other elongation factors, eEFsec also binds GTP.

The selenoprotein mRNA, SBP2, eEFsec, Sec-tRNA, and GTP assemble in a complex on the ribosome for cotranslational Sec incorporation, as illustrated in Figure 39-9. The bases between the UGA and the SECIS element of the selenoprotein mRNA serve as a flexible tether. On eukaryotic ribosomes, the SPB2–eEFsec–GTP–Sec-$tRNA^{Sec}$ complex thus can orient the anticodon on the tRNA to interact with the approaching acceptor site (also called the aminoacyl site, or A-site) on the ribosome. Peptide bond formation is then catalyzed by peptidyltransferase, resulting in the formation of a peptide bond between Sec and the nascent polypeptide.

HUMAN SELENOPROTEINS

Early nutritional biochemists tracked down biochemical functions for selenium by focusing on differences between Se-adequate and

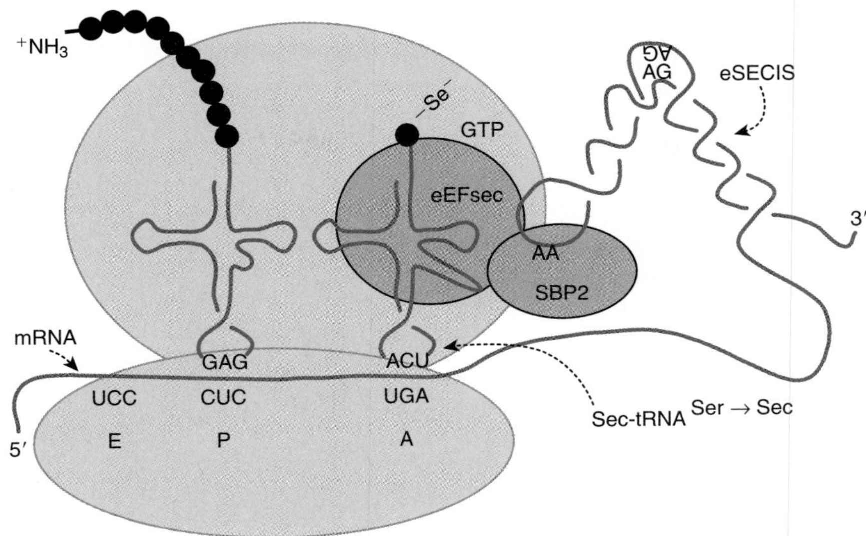

Figure 39-9 Model for the ribosomal mRNA–SBP2–eEFsec-GTP–Sec-tRNA$^{Ser \rightarrow Sec}_{UCA}$ complex. (See text for explanation.) *(Modified from Sunde RA [1997] Selenium. In: O'Dell BL, Sunde RA [eds] Handbook of Nutritionally Essential Mineral Elements. Marcel Dekker, New York, pp 493-556.)*

Se-deficient animals and by purifying and characterizing ^{75}Se-labeled proteins. The advent of gene sequencing brought serendipitous discovery of an unexpected selenoprotein when a cloned gene was sequenced and found to contain an in-frame UGA. Today, significant interaction between nutritional sciences and genomics has applied new knowledge on how selenoproteins are encoded and synthesized to facilitate bioinformatics-based screening of the human genome and other genomes for all selenoproteins using a SECIS-search protocol developed by Gladyshev (Kryukov et al., 2003). By using conserved SECIS elements, conserved secondary structure, and the thermodynamics of the SECIS elements, the human genome was screened for potential selenoproteins. The presence of SECIS elements in orthologous selenoprotein genes in rodents further helped to reduce this list of potential selenoproteins. Next, upstream genomic sequences were screened for open reading frames that contained in-frame TGA codons. Lastly, these predicted human selenoprotein genes were further screened for homologs in other species that contained cysteine rather than selenocysteine. The result was that the entire human "selenoproteome" has been identified (Kryukov et al., 2003); a list of human selenoproteins in given in Table 39-1.

The selenocysteine in almost all selenoproteins in eukaryotes, bacteria, and archaea is present in a motif involving cysteine (C), threonine (T), or serine (S). The majority of the selenoproteins appear to be enzymes, or to be derived from enzyme families, with the Sec (U) positioned as a substitution into a variant of the CxxC motif that is found in many redox proteins. In these enzymes, one of the cysteine residues serves as a nucleophilic attacking group, and almost all of the CxxC motifs precede an alpha helix that provides a platform for the catalytic site (Fomenko and Gladyshev, 2003).

The picture emerging from the evaluation of various genomes for selenoproteins reveals that selenoproteins have a scattered phylogenetic distribution; the majority of selenoproteins have homologs that contain cysteine instead of Sec. GPX6 is a selenoprotein in humans and swine, but a cysteine-containing protein in rodents; the rodent GPX6 mRNA contains a nonfunctional SECIS element. Therefore, the rodent proteome contains 24 selenoproteins, whereas both the human and porcine proteomes contain 25 selenoproteins.

Table 39-1
Human Selenoproteins

Abbreviation	Selenoprotein	Other Information
GPX1	Glutathione peroxidase-1	General cytosolic GPX
GPX2	Glutathione peroxidase-2	In gastrointestinal tract
GPX3	Glutathione peroxidase-3	In plasma, milk, and extracellular fluids
GPX4	Glutathione peroxidase-4	Phospholipid hydroperoxide PX
GPX6	Glutathione peroxidase-6	Oderant metabolizing protein
TRR1	Thioredoxin reductase-1	General cytosolic TRR
TRR2	Thioredoxin reductase-2	Mitochondial TRR
TRR3	Thioredoxin reductase-3	In testis
DI1	Iodothyronine 5′ deiodinase-1	In liver, kidney, and muscle
DI2	Iodothyronine 5′ deiodinase-2	In endocrine tissues
DI3	Iodothyronine 5 deiodinase-3	In fetal and endocrine tissues
SelP	Selenoprotein-P	In plasma
SelW	Selenoprotein-W	In muscle
Sep15	15-kDa Selenoprotein	Binds to UDP-glucose glucosyl transferase
SelR	Methionine-R-sulfoxide reductase (MsrB1)	
SPS2	Selenophosphate synthetase-2	
SelV	Selenoprotein-V	Paralog of SelW
SelT	Selenoprotein-T	Globular selenoprotein
SelH	Selenoprotein-H	Globular selenoprotein
SelM	Selenoprotein-M	In Golgi and ER, distant homolog of Sep15
SelO	Selenoprotein-O	Globular selenoprotein
SelN	Selenoprotein-N	Globular selenoprotein
SelI	Selenoprotein-I	Choline/ethanolamine phosphotransferase
SelK	Selenoprotein-K	Membrane protein
SelS	Selenoprotein-S	Membrane protein

Methionine *S*-sulfoxide reductase (MsrA) occurs as a selenoprotein in *Chlamydomonas reinhardtii*, a green algae, but contains cysteine in vertebrates. A novel selenoprotein family, named selenoprotein U, was recently identified in the puffer fish, but mammals, worms, and land plants contain the cysteine homolog. Humans contain three separate genes in the selenoprotein U family, but each encodes a cysteine-containing protein (Castellano et al., 2004).

No selenoproteins have yet been found in yeast and land plants. The yeast *Saccharomyces cerevisiae* and *Saccharomyces pombe* and the plant *Arabidopsis* genomes do not contain genes for selenoproteins or for any of the unique proteins associated with selenocysteine synthesis and insertion. Other species, such as *Caenorhabditis elegans* and *Drosophila melanogaster*, have only a few known selenoproteins (one and three, respectively, for *C. elegans* and *D. melanogaster*). Clearly, higher animals have more fully taken advantage of the unique chemical as well as biochemical and genetic aspects of selenium. A brief description of the 25 members of the human selenoproteome follows.

GLUTATHIONE PEROXIDASE-1

Most cells and blood plasma contain glutathione peroxidase (GPX) activity. GPX activities decrease in plasma and cells in selenium deficiency, and selenium supplementation restores these activities to normal. Although it was initially assumed that a single gene was responsible for GPX activities, careful biochemical studies have established distinct differences in the nature of the GPXs. We now know that there are at least six distinct members of the GPX family in higher animals (see Table 39-1).

Glutathione peroxidase (glutathione:H_2O_2 oxidoreductase) was discovered by Mills (1957) in a search for factors that protect erythrocytes against oxidative hemolysis. GPX1 is unique with respect to many other peroxidases because it is not inhibited by azide or cyanide, and hydroperoxides as well as H_2O_2 are substrates for the enzyme. The enzyme catalyzes the following reaction:

$$2\ GSH + ROOH \rightarrow GSSG + ROH + H_2O$$

GPX1 is specific for glutathione (GSH) as the donor substrate, and no other substrate results in more than 30% of the activity obtained with GSH as substrate. However, GPX1 is not at all specific for the acceptor substrate and thus destroys many organic hydroperoxides (ROOH) at rates very similar to those for H_2O_2. Only cholesterol-25-hydroperoxide, cholesterol-7α-hydroperoxide, and phospholipid hydroperoxides such as phosphatidyl choline hydroperoxide are poor substrates for GPX1. The enzyme reaction follows a ter-uni ping-pong mechanism as shown in the following equation. The intermediates, beginning with the deprotonated selenium Se^- in the Sec residue of the enzyme (E), are also indicated.

$$\begin{array}{ccccccc} & ROOH\downarrow \quad ROH\uparrow & & GSH\downarrow \quad HOH\uparrow & & GSH\downarrow \quad GSSG\uparrow & \\ \hline E\text{-}Se^- & & E\text{-}Se\text{-}OH & & E\text{-}Se\text{-}SG & & E\text{-}Se^- \end{array}$$

GPX1 is a tetrameric protein with four identical subunits, each with a molecular mass of approximately 23 kDa and each containing one Se atom. The Sec moiety is located at the end of an α-helix associated with two parallel β-sheets in a $\beta\alpha\beta$ structure. In GPXs, the Sec is present in a UxxT motif, which is a variation of the CxxC redox motif found in thioredoxins and isomerases (Fomenko and Gladyshev, 2003). The threonine (T) hydroxal may hydrogen-bond with the Se^- of the Sec (U) to stabilize the Se^- as the attacking group in the reaction. Charged amino acids within the active site apparently confer specificity for glutathione. Recombinant analogs of GPX1, with cysteine or serine replacing the Sec moiety, have been prepared; the analog with serine in place of Sec is completely without activity, whereas the cysteine mutant has 1/1,000 the activity of the wild type of enzyme, clearly demonstrating the biochemical essentiality of selenium. Knockout mice lacking the *GPX1* gene are without phenotype under unstressed conditions.

GLUTATHIONE PEROXIDASE-2 IN INTESTINE

GPX2 is also called GPX-GI because it is expressed in gastrointestinal cells as well as some other cell types. The mRNA for GPX2 is detected in human liver and colon, but not in kidney, heart, lung, placenta, or uterus. More than 70% of the total GPX activity in the rat small bowel is due to GPX2. The discovery of this second GPX might at first glance suggest that various GPX activities are redundant, but it appears that individual GPXs have somewhat unique niches. As with GPX1, the GPX2 knockout mouse is without phenotype, but double knockout mice lacking both GPX1 and GPX2 develop ileocolitis around the time of weaning (Esworthy et al., 2005).

GLUTATHIONE PEROXIDASE-3 IN PLASMA

Almost immediately after the discovery that GPX1 was a selenium-dependent enzyme, researchers observed that plasma GPX activity responds more quickly than GPX1 to selenium deficiency and to selenium resupplementation. We now know that plasma contains a distinct enzyme arising from the *GPX3* gene. The specific activity of the purified plasma GPX3, however, is only 10% of GPX1 specific activity. Screening of tissues for GPX3 mRNA suggests that the kidney is the major source of circulating GPX3. Human patients undergoing chronic dialysis due to renal failure have low levels of plasma GPX3 despite normal plasma selenium content. After renal transplantation, plasma GPX3 increases up to 200% of normal levels. GPX3 is a secreted enzyme, and therefore it is not surprising in hindsight that 90% of human milk GPX activity is precipitated by anti-GPX3 antibodies. The expression of GPX3 in milk may have evolved specifically to maintain milk selenium levels rather than to protect milk from peroxidation in the (short) trip from breast to infant stomach.

PHOSPHOLIPID HYDROPEROXIDE GLUTATHIONE PEROXIDASE

Phospholipid hydroperoxide glutathione peroxidase, or GPX4, is an intracellular selenoperoxidase, and it is active as a monomer. Its peroxide substrate specificity is broader than for the other glutathione peroxidases; the enzyme will reduce phospholipid hydroperoxides as well as cholesterol hydroperoxides, which are not substrates for GPX1 (Maiorino et al., 1990). GPX4 appears to be associated with cell membranes, suggesting that GPX4 may "roll along" intracellular surfaces of the plasma membrane and within the mitochondrial intermembrane space and act to protect membrane components by detoxifying hydroperoxides that would otherwise damage or impair membrane function. Knocking out GPX4 in mice is embryonically lethal (Yant et al., 2003).

Selenium has long been known to be an important nutrient with regard to reproduction, but the specific nature of this has been unclear. Studies of selenium-deficient sperm in rodents and in livestock found impaired motility and mid-piece breakage resulting in loss of flagella. GPX4 was found to be the selenoprotein associated with the high selenium content of the mitochondrial capsule in mammalian sperm (Ursini et al., 1999). This GPX4 is systematically inactivated in mature spermatozoa, and cannot be reactivated under biological conditions. GPX4 makes up at least 50% of structurally important material in the mid-piece of sperm. These findings indicate that the GPX4 enzyme changes its role from that of an enzyme to a structural protein as the spermatozoa matures, providing a unique example of an apparent enzyme that can be inactivated and oxidatively cross-linked to become a key structural protein.

OTHER GLUTATHIONE PEROXIDASES

GPX5 is an androgen-regulated epididymal secretory protein with about 67% identity to GPX1 but with cysteine located at the analogous position of Sec and without a functional SECIS element in its mRNA. GPX6 is an odorant-metabolizing protein that appears to be expressed only in Bowman's gland of the rodent olfactory system. GPX6 is a close homolog of plasma GPX3. GPX6 in humans and swine is a selenoprotein, but the orthologs in mice and rats contain Cys in place of Sec (Kryukov et al., 2003). GPX7 is another member of the GPX family that so far has only been found as a Cys homolog. The function of these GPX homologs is especially unclear, as enzymatic activity of Cys versus Sec homologs are expected to differ dramatically.

A non–selenium-dependent GPX activity found in the liver of selenium-deficient humans and animals is due to the activity of several of the glutathione *S*-transferases. Levels of glutathione *S*-transferases increased twofold in selenium-deficient liver, but only after liver GPX was fully depleted. This delayed response to selenium deficiency indicated that more than just loss of GPX was occurring, and this observation helped point the way to the discovery of additional mammalian selenoenzymes.

THIOREDOXIN REDUCTASE

The thioredoxin reductase family is another family of Se-dependent enzymes. They were identified by Tamura and Stadtman (1996) as selenoenzymes by purification of ^{75}Se-labeled proteins from cultured cells. Thioredoxin reductase regulates intracellular redox state, reduces small intracellular molecules, is needed for synthesis of deoxynucleotides, and may be important in cell cycling. Deletion of the thioredoxin gene is fetal-lethal, illustrating the importance of this enzyme system in biology. This NADPH-dependent flavoenzyme, found in animals, plants, and bacteria, transfers reducing equivalents from NADPH through a tightly bound flavin adenine dinucleotide (FAD) to a disulfide in the enzyme, and then to thioredoxin (Trx):

$$\text{NADPH} + \text{H}^+ + \text{Trx-S}_2 \rightarrow \text{NADP}^+ + \text{Trx-(SH)}_2$$

In bacteria, archaea, yeast, and plants, thioredoxin reductase has cysteine at the active site, but in mammals, three genes all encode thioredoxin reductase enzymes and all contain Sec as the penultimate amino acid with Sec adjacent to Cys in a CU motif. Thioredoxin reductase 1 is a cytosolic enzyme, thioredoxin reductase 2 is a mitochondrial enzyme, and thioredoxin reductase 3 is preferentially expressed in testis. Splicing variants further expand this complexity, including the potential for thioredoxin reductase to bind to and regulate the estrogen receptor (Damdimopoulos et al., 2004). In rats, thioredoxin reductase activity in liver and other tissues is less affected by selenium deficiency than is GPX1 activity but more affected than is the plasma selenoprotein P level. Loss of thioredoxin reductase activity may be important in the development of the signs and symptoms of selenium deficiency. Recent research indicates that thioredoxin reductase will reduce dehydroascorbic acid and that ascorbate levels are decreased in Se-deficient rat liver. This offers a new potential antioxidant role for a selenoprotein.

IODOTHYRONINE 5′-DEIODINASE

Iodothyronine 5′-deiodinase-1, often referred to in the literature as type I 5′-deiodinase (DI1), is the major enzyme that converts thyroxine (T_4) to triiodothyronine (T_3). Liver DI1 is responsible for the majority of the circulating plasma T_3 levels, but two additional deiodinase isozymes are also found in more specialized tissues. In the early 1990s, three research groups independently discovered that the deiodinases were selenoenzymes. John Arthur in Scotland observed elevated T_4 and reduced T_3 in selenium deficiency, and focused in on a new selenoprotein (Arthur et al., 1990). Concurrently, Dietrick Behne in Germany used ^{75}Se-labeling to discover a 28-kDa selenoprotein at high concentrations in thyroid, liver, and kidney (Behne et al., 1990). And in 1991, Marla Berry and Reid Larsen in Boston used expression cloning to isolate and sequence DI1 (Berry et al., 1991). These three approaches revealed that DI1 contains Sec. DI1 appears to function as a homodimer, with a molecular mass of approximately 55 kDa.

DI1 is localized in the membrane and co-purifies with microsomal (endoplasmic reticulum [ER]) markers from liver and with the basolateral membrane of kidney proximal convoluted tubule cells. A single transmembrane segment of the protein is located at the N-terminus of the protein and orients the catalytic portion toward the cytoplasm.

DI1 catalyzes both outer and inner ring deiodination of thyroxine, but the preferred reaction is removal of the outer ring 5′ iodine from either T_4 or reverse T_3 (rT_3) leading to T_3 or T_2, respectively. Formation of T_3 is thought to be the most important physiological role for DI1, but production of T_2 from rT_3 may also be of biological importance in the elimination of excess thyroid hormone from the circulation. DI1 contains a SxxU motif that is involved in catalysis in a manner analogous to the GPX1 reaction:

$$T_4 + 2\ GSH \rightarrow T_3 + GSSG + I^- + H^+$$

Reduced GSH is the likely physiological substrate, and thus the mechanism is best described as a ter-uni ping-pong mechanism similar to that for GPX1, which proceeds via formation of an enzyme-Se-I intermediate.

Although more than 90% of plasma T_3 is produced by DI1 in liver, kidney, and muscle, two additional deiodinases, deiodinase-2 (DI2) and deiodinase-3 (DI3), also contain selenium as Sec and arise from distinct genes. DI2 catalyzes the 5′-deiodination of the outer ring of T_4 and is found in brain, pituitary, brown adipose tissue, placenta, and skin. Its principal physiological role is for local, intracellular production of T_3.

DI3 catalyzes the 5-deiodination of the inner ring, resulting in inactivation. DI3 activity levels are highest in adult brain, skin, and placenta, and in fetal liver, muscle, brain, and central nervous system. The role of DI3 has been proposed as protecting fetal tissue from high levels of T_3 and T_4 during development by converting them to the inactive T_2 and rT_3, respectively.

This array of three deiodinases may confer additional regulation on iodine metabolism. In iodine deficiency, downregulation of DI1 conserves precious iodine by limiting DI1's conversion of T_4 to circulating T_3, thereby making the limited T_4 available for intracellular conversion by DI2 in important endocrine organs. Combined selenium and iodine deficiency may contribute to the etiology of endemic myxedematous cretinism in populations in Democratic Republic of Congo (Zaire); administration of selenium alone appears to aggravate this disease by restoring DI1 activity, leading to increased utilization of T_4 for production of plasma T_3, which in turn further reduces the concentration of T_4 substrate for DI2 in critical endocrine tissues. (See Chapter 38 for more discussion of iodine.)

PLASMA SELENOPROTEIN P

Selenoprotein P is an extracellular selenoprotein that is labeled rapidly with ^{75}Se within 3 to 4 hours after rats are injected with ^{75}Se (Burk and Hill, 2005). Mature selenoprotein P contains 360 amino acid residues with at least four glycosylation sites. Human plasma contains 5 to 6 mg selenoprotein P per liter, whereas rat plasma has 30 mg selenoprotein P per liter. The concentration of selenoprotein P mRNA is highest in liver, with smaller amounts in kidney, heart, testis, and some in lung, indicating that liver is the major source of selenoprotein P. Selenoprotein P contains about 40% of the plasma selenium in normal individuals, and the level of selenoprotein P decreases in patients with liver disease.

Unlike all other selenoprotein mRNAs, which contain one UGA, selenoprotein P mRNA in humans and rats contains 10 UGA codons along with two SECIS elements in the 3′-UTR. One UGA is present early in the mRNA, and the other nine UGAs are located in the coding region for the latter half of the protein. Interestingly, the zebrafish genome contains two selenoprotein P genes: one encoding a selenoprotein with a single Sec, which is analogous to the N-terminal portion of the mammalian selenoprotein P, and a second encoding a selenoprotein containing 17 Sec residues with 16 of the 17 Sec residues located in the C-terminal end of the protein. To date, selenoprotein P has only been identified in the genomes of vertebrates. Analysis of purified plasma selenoprotein P revealed that it contains 5 to 6 Se atoms/molecule, whereas the cDNA sequence has 10 TGA codons in the open reading frame and encodes a protein with 10 Se atoms per molecule. When selenium is limiting, early termination at the second or a later UGA in the mRNA reduces the selenium content of selenoprotein P and results in smaller circulating proteins.

The selenoprotein *P* gene has now been knocked out in mice (Burk and Hill, 2005). Deletion of selenoprotein P results in dramatic decreases in brain and testis selenium concentrations and increased urinary excretion of ingested Se, consistent with the role of selenoprotein P as a critical selenium transport protein. Hypothetical selenoprotein P receptors in brain, testis, and perhaps other organs thus could direct limiting selenium to these tissues. Mice lacking selenoprotein P develop a lack of coordination leading to paralysis and then death, indicating a critical role for selenium in neurological tissues, and further indicating the importance of delivering selenium to these tissues. Dietary administration of high levels of Se will prevent these conditions. Knockout mice also have low fertility, and the males cannot be used for breeding even when they are supplemented with high selenium diets. Studies in rats indicate that approximately 25% of whole-body selenium circulates through the plasma as selenoprotein P, presumably synthesized in the liver; this strongly suggests that the function of selenoprotein P is to deliver selenium to important tissues. In cells, selenoprotein P is degraded for use in synthesizing other selenoproteins.

The N-terminal Sec in selenoprotein P is present as a UxxC motif, suggesting that it may have a dual role as a redox protein and as a selenium transport protein, or that this protein has evolved from such proteins. Additional hypotheses include a role for selenoprotein P in disulfide exchange and a role for selenoprotein P associated with regions rich in histidine residues, which may potentiate interaction with membranes or function as a metal-binding motif.

Selenoprotein P concentrations in plasma of selenium-deficient Chinese populations are 10% to 20% of levels found in the United States population, showing that this protein reflects Se intake in human populations and may be associated with the onset of selenium deficiency disease. Immunohistochemical localization studies indicate that selenoprotein P coats both the luminal and the interstitial surfaces of the vascular system, except in brain where the blood-brain barrier apparently restricts access to brain interstitium. Burk and Hill (1994) have shown that injecting selenium-deficient rats with 50 μg of selenium rapidly protects against toxicity of the herbicide diquat and raises selenoprotein P levels with virtually no change in GPX1 activity 10 hours after injection, suggesting that selenoprotein P may function as an antioxidant protein in the interstitial space. Preliminary reports suggest that selenoprotein P may have peroxidase activity.

MUSCLE SELENOPROTEIN W

The search for a mammalian selenoprotein to explain white muscle disease in selenium-deficient sheep and cattle pointed in 1972 to a small selenoprotein that was lacking in lambs suffering from white muscle disease. This protein has now been purified and named selenoprotein W. It is interesting that purified selenoprotein W is often isolated with one tightly bound GSH. Human selenoprotein W encodes an 87-amino-acid polypeptide that includes a UGA-encoded Sec at residue 13. The Sec in selenoprotein W is present as CxxU. Selenoprotein W mRNA is abundant in muscle, skeletal muscle, and brain of primates and sheep, but not in rodent muscle (Hatfield, 2001). Selenoprotein W mRNA abundance in muscle of rats fed adequate levels of selenium (0.1 mg of Se/kg diet) increases fourfold greater than the abundance in selenium-deficient rats (Vendeland et al., 1995). The role of this low-molecular-weight protein in protecting muscle against white muscle disease is unknown, but it may be related to a redox function of selenoprotein W or GSH-selenoprotein W (Hatfield, 2001).

SELENOPROTEIN 15

A 15-kDa selenoprotein, selenoprotein 15, was initially purified from human T cells as a ^{75}Se-labeled protein (Hatfield, 2001). The gene for selenoprotein 15 is apparently universally expressed in mammalian cells and encodes a protein with an N-terminal signal peptide that directs this protein to the ER. In the ER, it associates with UDP-glucose glycoprotein glucosyl transferase. Therefore, it is speculated that selenoprotein 15 is involved in protein folding. The protein is differentially expressed in tumor cells, and single nucleotide polymorphisms (SNPs) in the selenoprotein 15 gene suggest that the allelic frequency may correlate with susceptibility to cancer. The Sec is present in a CxU motif in the protein (Hatfield, 2001).

SELENOPROTEIN R OR METHIONINE-R-SULFOXIDE REDUCTASE

Methionine sulfoxide is produced by oxidative attack of proteins, and, therefore, methionine-sulfoxide reductases are essential in coping with oxidative stress. Early bioinformatics identified selenoprotein R as a mammalian selenoprotein within an unknown function but found cysteine homologs that encoded a methionine-sulfoxide reductase. Biochemical characterization revealed that the selenoprotein gene encoded a small (12-kDa) selenoprotein that contains zinc and reduces methionine-R-sulfoxide but not methionine-S-sulfoxide. Selenoprotein R is now designated MsrB1 (Kim and Gladyshev, 2004). MsrB1 has Sec present in a UxxS motif. The mammalian genome codes for two other MsrB proteins, but both of these MsrBs contain cysteine rather than Sec, have lower catalytic activity, and are localized to mitochondria and ER. An additional human gene, MsrA, encodes a cysteine-containing enzyme that is specific for methionine-S-sulfoxide.

SELENOPHOSPHATE SYNTHETASE 2

As discussed in the preceding text, one of the mammalian selenophosphate synthetases, SPS2, is a Sec-containing selenoprotein. The Sec is present as a CxU motif. SPS2 seems to be involved in assimilating selenium from selenite reduction, whereas SPS1 appears to be associated with recycling selenium from Sec (Tamura et al., 2004). SPS1 has threonine at the active site in place of Sec.

SELENOPROTEINS V, T, H, M, AND O WITH CxxU MOTIFS

A number of selenoproteins of unknown function were discovered in the SECIS-search of the human genome. Selenoprotein V is a paralog of selenoprotein W and has a CxxU motif. In the mouse, expression of selenoprotein V mRNA is restricted to testis, where it occurs in the seminiferous tubules.

Selenoprotein T is a 182-amino-acid protein containing Sec in a CxxU motif. This globular protein has no known function.

Selenoprotein H was discovered in the human genome using the SECIS-search program and was subsequently shown to be a selenoprotein by transfecting the gene into mammalian cells and demonstrating ^{75}Se-labeling of the selenoprotein. Selenoprotein H is a globular selenoprotein with a CxxU motif.

The selenoprotein M gene was identified in a mammalian EST database as an open reading frame with an in-frame TGA. The Sec is present in a CxxU motif in the N-terminal portion of selenoprotein M. Identification of this new selenoprotein resulted in the discovery of a variant SECIS in the 3′-UTR, as mentioned previously, with an AUGA … CC … GA motif. Selenoprotein M is distantly homologous to selenoprotein 15, but the Sec motif (a CxxU) resembles selenoprotein W and selenoprotein T. The N-terminal protein contains a signal peptide that locates the selenoprotein to the Golgi and ER. Selenoprotein M mRNA is present in multiple organs, especially in brain, kidney, and uterus (Korotkov et al., 2002).

Selenoprotein O is another globular selenoprotein identified using the SECIS-search program. Selenoprotein O was verified as a selenoprotein by ^{75}Se-incorporation into the recombinantly expressed protein. Selenoprotein O is the largest human selenoprotein (669 residues) with a Sec located three residues from the C terminus in a CxxU motif. The SECIS also has the AUGA … CC … GA motif.

SELENOPROTEINS N AND I

Selenoproteins N and I were also identified by the SECIS-search of the human genome. Selenoprotein N is a selenoprotein with no homology to any known protein. Sec is present in the C-terminal half of selenoprotein N, with the Sec flanked by cysteine in a CU motif similar to that found in thioredoxin reductase. Selenoprotein I is homologous to human and yeast choline and ethanolamine phosphotransferases and has seven putative transmembrane domains. In human and mouse, the Sec is present in a SxU motif.

MEMBRANE SELENOPROTEINS K AND S

Selenoprotein K and selenoprotein S are unique because they are the first demonstrated membrane selenoproteins. Their localization was first predicted from their amino acid sequences, and subsequently these proteins were shown to localize at the plasma membrane when expressed in mammalian cells. Selenoprotein K and selenoprotein S mRNAs are found in a variety of mouse tissues (Kryukov et al., 2003). Selenoprotein K contains Sec as the third-to-last amino acid, and notably, there are no adjacent C, S, or T residues. Sec in selenoprotein S, is located as the penultimate amino acid residue, as in thioredoxin reductase, but in a SxxU motif.

Selenoprotein S gene expression is increased by glucose deprivation and/or disturbances in the ER that generally cause the accumulation of misfolded proteins. Therefore, selenoprotein S appears to be a novel member of the glucose-regulated protein family. Overexpression of selenoprotein S can significantly increase cell tolerance to oxidative stress, suggesting that selenoprotein S may have a role in regulating reactive oxygen species (Gao et al., 2004).

SELENIUM-BINDING PROTEINS

Several additional apparent "selenium-binding proteins," identified as ^{75}Se-labeled proteins, have been reported for proteins with known cDNA sequences that do not contain an in-frame UGA or a SECIS element in the 3′-UTR of the mRNA. Many of these reports now appear to be due to co-purification of the identified protein with trace levels of a contaminating selenoprotein of the same size. Nevertheless, selenide binding to proteins (path [16] of Fig. 39-4), such as the 130-kDa Cd/Se-binding protein found in plasma or the eukaryotic initiation factor-2α (eIF-2α) involved in initiation of translation, clearly indicates that the full nutritional impact of selenium is likely to be mediated by more than just the UGA-encoded selenoproteins.

SELENOMETHIONINE-CONTAINING PROTEINS

Selenomethionine from dietary sources can be incorporated nonspecifically into proteins because selenomethionine is an excellent analog for methionine in protein synthesis. Selenomethionine can be esterified to tRNA^{Met} at rates only slightly less favorable than that for methionine itself (K_m of 11 μmol/L for selenomethionine versus 7 μmol/L for methionine), and therefore dietary selenomethionine is readily incorporated into protein (path [17] of Fig. 39-4). Hemoglobin and plasma proteins can be major pools of blood selenium in human populations that obtain selenium primarily from plant-derived foods that are rich in selenomethionine.

BACTERIAL AND ARCHAEAL SELENOENZYMES

A number of selenoenzymes have been identified in microorganisms (Hatfield, 2001). The study of these selenoenzymes has led to the discovery of many unique aspects of selenium biochemistry. A recent adaptation of the SECISsearch to bacterial and archaeal genomes (Kryukov and Gladyshev, 2004) revealed that selenoproteins are encoded in approximately 20% of the completed bacterial genomes and approximately 14% of completed archaeal genomes. Most are redox proteins that use Sec to coordinate a redox-active metal, such as molybdenum, nickel, or tungsten for UxxC-motif–mediated redox catalysis. Identified genes include some bacterial formate dehydrogenases that were clustered with necessary Sec-insertion genes, suggesting an ancient origin of these Sec-dependent enzymes. Conversely, the numerous cases of Sec proteins with Cys-homologs suggest recent origin of selenoproteins from Cys-containing proteins. Only one bacterial Sec enzyme, glycine reductase (selenoprotein A) was found solely as a Sec-homolog. Bacterial selenoproteins that are homologs of mammalian selenoproteins include glutathione peroxidases, selenophosphate synthetase, selenoprotein W, and a Sec-containing thioredoxin reductase.

Selenium is also present in a readily dissociable form in some bacterial enzymes. In nicotinic acid hydroxylase, Se is associated with a molybdenum cofactor, perhaps in a terminal selenide (=Se) on the molybdenum. The Se in bacterial xanthine dehydrogenase, carbon monoxide dehydrogenase, and purine hydroxylase is thought to be present bound to cysteine in a selenotrisulfide (–S–Se–S–) or selenopersulfide (R–S–Se^-) form. Some bacteria also synthesize a selenium-substituted uridine found in tRNAs. These enzymes are likely to serve as models for additional new roles for selenium in higher organisms; examples might be enzymes using Sec as a ligand for nickel, and enzymes containing molybdenum–selenium cofactors that do not involve Sec.

SELENIUM REQUIREMENTS

Reviews of nutrient requirements explicitly recommend that additional research is needed to identify and use biochemical markers of nutrient status (IOM, 2000). A number of direct as well as indirect biological markers or biomarkers could be used to determine selenium requirements. Death and development of overt disease are obviously the most stringent as well as clear-cut. Growth and reproductive success are other practical biomarkers. Tissue selenium concentrations or levels of specific selenoenzymes or selenoproteins are biochemical assays that offer potential convenience and precision when shown to be relevant. Just as a series of parameters are often necessary to fully describe a curve, a series of biomarkers or parameters are needed to fully describe the nutritional status of an individual with regard to a specific nutrient. This is readily apparent in the case of selenium if one considers that some biochemical pools turn over rapidly (e.g., selenoprotein P) and thus reflect recent Se intakes, whereas other pools reflect average Se status over the life span of the molecules in the pool (e.g., erythrocytes), and still other pools most strongly reflect past Se status (perhaps Se in bone). These changes may also be influenced by regulation of the steady-state level of the protein; some selenoprotein mRNA levels are regulated by Se status but others are likely to be controlled by factors unrelated to Se status. For this discussion, parameter is defined as a measured concentration, rate, or level the value of which can vary with the nutrient status of the subject. The parameters that are most useful as biomarkers for assessment of selenium status or requirement remain to be established (IOM, 2000; Sunde, 1997; Sunde, 1994).

STUDIES OF SELENIUM REQUIREMENTS AND STATUS IN EXPERIMENTAL ANIMALS

Studies with experimental animals, especially the rat, provided the basis for understanding the nutritional biochemistry of selenium as well as the nutritional requirement for selenium. Although Schwarz and Foltz (1957) first estimated the selenium requirement for prevention of overt disease (prevention of weanling rats from dying from liver necrosis within 30 days) to be 0.05 to 0.1 mg of Se per kg diet, their studies were conducted with rats that were selenium-deficient at the beginning of the experiment and that were fed diets deficient in vitamin E and sulfur amino acids. It has since been established that less than 0.002 mg of Se per kg diet is sufficient to prevent overt disease in rats fed diets with adequate levels of vitamin E and other nutrients. Rats purchased commercially in 1971 and fed the Se-deficient diet of Schwarz, but with adequate sulfur amino acids and vitamin E, grew at 85% of the rate of animals supplemented with 0.1 mg of Se per kg diet. Supplementation with 0.05 mg of Se per kg diet or higher raised growth to equal that of animals supplemented with 0.1 mg of Se per kg diet. Experiments conducted with commercially available weanling rats in the 1990s, however, did not show major effects on growth from feeding similar selenium-deficient diets, and did not show impact on growth or disease from feeding crystalline amino acid diets containing 0.002 to 0.003 mg of Se per kg diet for 28 days (Sunde, 1997; Lei et al., 1995). Pups from selenium-deficient dams, however, grew at markedly lower rates when fed a selenium-deficient diet than when fed a diet with 0.1 mg of Se per kg, demonstrating that severe selenium deficiency does impair growth. These studies illustrate the value of body stores of a nutrient in maintenance of function during prolonged deficiency.

A number of efforts have been focused on establishing a biochemical parameter that is a useful measure of selenium status. Effects of selenium intake on erythrocyte GPX1 activity, plasma GPX3 activity, liver GPX1 activity, liver GPX4 activity, plasma selenoprotein P level, liver DI1 activity, and liver thioredoxin reductase (TRR1) activity have indicated that liver GPX1 decreases to the greatest extent in Se-deficient rats. As shown in Figure 39-10, hepatic GPX1 activity fell to undetectable levels when weanling (21-day-old) rats were fed a selenium-deficient diet for 21 days, whereas hepatic GPX4 decreased to only 41% of the level in selenium-adequate animals (Lei et al., 1995). The other selenoproteins that have been assessed also decreased with selenium deficiency, usually to levels in the range of 5% to 20% of the levels in selenium-adequate animals. The dietary level of selenium required to achieve maximal or plateau levels of various selenoproteins also varies for the different selenoproteins. Liver GPX1 does not reach a maximal level until about 0.1 mg of Se per kg diet, whereas liver GPX4 activity reaches a plateau by 0.05 mg of Se per kg diet (Lei et al., 1995) and liver TRR1 activity by 0.075 mg Se per kg diet (Hadley and Sunde, 2001). It is important to note that plasma GPX3 activity approximates its plateau level when the diet contains 0.07 mg of Se per kg (Weiss et al., 1996). Therefore, plasma GPX3 activity is a useful biomarker because it reflects a level of dietary Se that provides sufficient Se for maximal GPX4 synthesis but not for maximal GPX1 synthesis. A level of 0.1 mg of Se per kg diet is sufficient to obtain maximal concentrations of most selenoproteins; an exception is erythrocyte GPX1 activity (not shown in Fig. 39-10), which continues to increase in young rats with addition of Se beyond the level of 0.1 mg of Se per kg diet; erythrocyte GPX1 activity does plateau in longer experiments with rats (Sunde et al., 2005).

Tissue selenium levels are another possible measure of selenium nutritional status. Increases in dietary selenium levels between 0 and 0.1 mg of Se per kg diet increase erythrocyte selenium concentration in the rat, but the erythrocyte selenium concentration continues to increase at higher levels of dietary selenium, following a pattern similar to that observed for erythrocyte GPX1 activity. Although the blood or erythrocyte Se levels and/or erythrocyte GPX1 activity are convenient measures of Se status, they are not useful as markers for the purpose of setting Se requirements because they do not always become saturated at levels of intake that otherwise are clearly adequate or even in excess. Liver and kidney Se concentrations generally follow the same relative pattern as liver GPX1 activity, but after 0.1 mg of Se per kg diet, tissue Se concentration can further increase in a manner similar to that of erythrocyte Se, making tissue Se concentrations difficult to interpret. The presence of selenomethionine-containing proteins

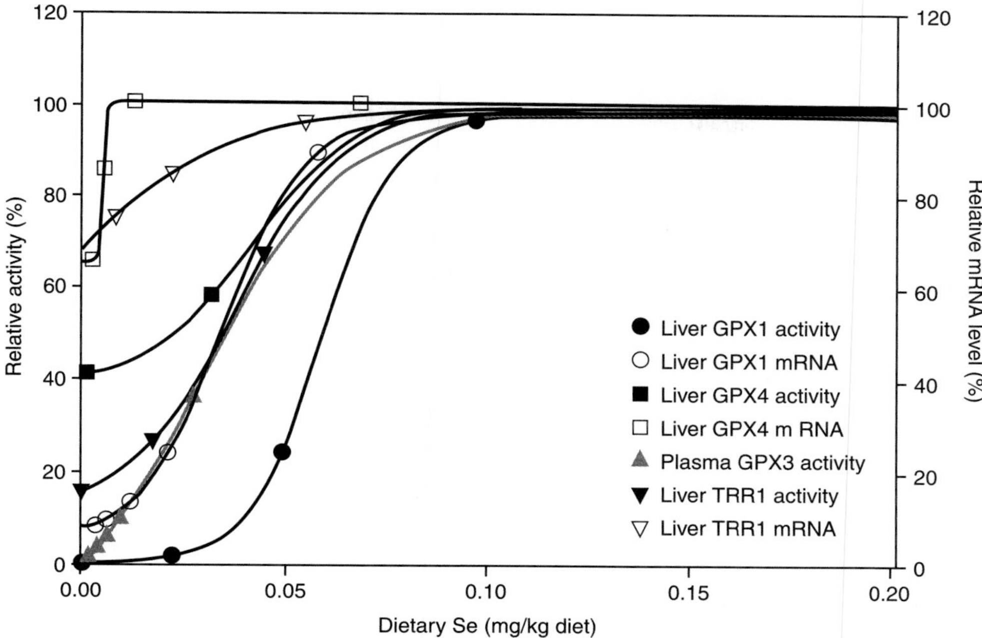

Figure 39-10 Effect of dietary selenium concentration on liver GPX1, GPX4 and thioredoxin reductase (TRR) activities and mRNA levels in male rats. Male weanling rats were fed graded levels of dietary Se from 0 to 0.2 mg/kg for 28 days, following which liver GPX1 activity, GPX1 mRNA level, GPX4 activity, GPX4 mRNA level, TRR1 activity, TRR1 mRNA level, and plasma GPX3 activity were determined. *(Data from Hadley KB, Sunde RA [2001] Selenium regulation of thioredoxin reductase activity and mRNA levels in rat liver. J Nutr Biochem 12:693-702; Lei XG, Evenson, JK, Thompson KM, Sunde RA [1995] Glutathione peroxidase and phospholipids hydroperoxide glutathione peroxidase are differentially regulated in rats by dietary selenium. J Nutr 125:1438-1446; and Weiss SL, Evenson JK, Thompson KM, Sunde RA [1997] Dietary selenium regulation of glutathione peroxidase-1 mRNA levels. RNA 4:816-827.)*

further complicates the use of tissue selenium concentration as a marker for functional selenium status.

The amount of dietary selenium required to produce maximal levels is different for the various parameters that have been studied. Responses for most occur within the range of 0.002 to 0.1 mg of Se per kg diet, but a few continue to increase with Se levels greater than 0.1 mg/kg. The selenium requirement for maximal response varies in the following order, from lowest to highest, for the different possible outcome parameters; growth < overt disease < GPX4 activity < TRR1 activity, GPX3 activity < GPX1 activity, liver Se, and erythrocyte Se (Hadley and Sunde, 2001). The choice of the appropriate parameter to use as the biochemical marker is clearly difficult at this point, but characterization of the molecular mechanisms that underlie these biochemical parameters should enable more precise determination of selenium requirements in the future.

Selenium requirements have been established for a wide variety of animals, and most current estimates of requirements are based on plasma, erythrocyte, or liver GPX activity. Unlike the requirements for almost all the other trace elements, the selenium requirement is virtually the same for all species, ranging from humans to laboratory animals to domestic animals to most poultry and even fish. The minimal selenium requirement for most species is 0.1 mg of Se per kg diet when based on dietary selenium levels necessary for maximal tissue levels of GPX1 activity. Specific molecular mechanisms must be maintaining the dietary requirement across this range of species. Some published recommendations for Se levels in the diets of various species, however, are higher than 0.1 mg of Se per kg diet because these recommendations include margins of safety or have been expanded to include unique situations in which additional dietary selenium seems to be protective.

HUMAN SELENIUM REQUIREMENTS

The current recommended dietary allowance (RDA) for selenium is one of two human dietary requirements for a mineral element that is based on a biochemical parameter (as opposed to dietary assessment or balance studies). This shows the fortuitousness of the discovery of GPX3 because balance studies are of little usefulness in determining selenium requirements due to the homeostatic mechanisms that regulate selenium balance. The current RDA for selenium is 55 μg/day for both men and women (IOM, 2000).

The 1989 RDA was set at 70 and 55 μg/day for North American men and women, respectively (National Research Council [NRC], 1989), based on an intake (40 μg Se per day) that maintained plasma GPX3 activity in adult Chinese men and with adjustments for body weight and addition of a 30% safety factor. Without the safety factor, this is equivalent to 0.10 mg of Se per kg diet. Comparison of dietary selenium intakes in adult Chinese people living in areas susceptible to Keshan disease with those of Chinese people living in areas seemingly protected from Keshan disease suggested a protective Se level of 21 μg/day for 65-kg men and 16 μg/day for 55-kg women (see Fig. 39-2). Estimated daily selenium intakes that were not associated with any selenium deficiency symptoms in the New Zealand population suggest that 33 and 23 μg/day are adequate for men and women, respectively. These and other studies demonstrate that daily selenium intakes less than the RDA are typical for much of the world's population and yet that selenium intakes that are half or less than half the RDA are not associated with any apparent adverse impact on health.

The World Health Organization ([WHO], 1996) used a new approach for setting selenium requirements that was not based on attainment of maximal glutathione peroxidase activity. WHO established a basal requirement of 21 and 16 μg of Se per day for men and women, respectively, based on the selenium intake of Chinese populations that were protected from Keshan disease, as the intake necessary to prevent pathological and clinical signs of selenium deficiency. They also defined a normative requirement that would maintain a desirable level of selenium storage and reserves; this was calculated by estimating the dietary intake needed to achieve two thirds of the maximal attainable activity of plasma GPX3 and was set at 26 μg of Se per day for a 65-kg man. Further adjustment for interindividual variation resulted in estimates of 40 μg of Se per day for adult men and 30 μg of Se per day for adult women as lower limits of the safe range of population mean intakes. These 1996 WHO requirements are therefore considerably less than the 1989 RDA recommendations but far more in line with typical Se consumption worldwide.

In 2000 the IOM released new dietary reference intakes (DRIs) for selenium. The IOM used data from two studies to establish an estimated average requirement (EAR) based on the amount of Se necessary to maximize plasma GPX3. In the first study, New Zealand subjects with basal selenium intake of 28 μg/day were supplemented with graded levels of selenium, provided as selenomethionine. Plasma glutathione peroxidase activity reached plateau levels between 2 and 8 weeks after supplementation. The study was complicated because the unsupplemented control group as well as the other groups showed considerable variability in plasma GPX3 activities such that only those for the group supplemented with 10 μg (total intake of 38 μg/day) were significantly different from the basal control values. Therefore, an EAR of 38 μg /day was indicated by this study. The second study, conducted with Chinese subjects in 1983, indicated that plateau plasma GPX3 activity was reached with a selenium intake of 41 μg/day which, after adjustment for American body weights, was judged to be 52 μg Se per day. The average of these two estimates, 45 μg/day, was chosen as the EAR. Using a coefficient of variation of 10%, the RDA for Se was set at 55 μg/day (45 μg/day + 20%) for both men and women of all ages.

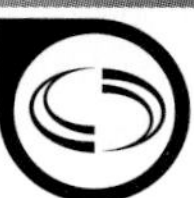

RDAs Across the Life Cycle

	μg Selenium per Day
Infants	
0 to 0.5 yr	15 (AI)
0.5 to 1 yr	20 (AI)
Children	
1 to 3 yr	20
4 to 8 yr	30
9 to 13 yr	40
14 to 18 yr	55
Adults	
19 to > 70 yr	55
Pregnant	60
Lactating	70

Data from Institute of Medicine (IOM) (2000) Dietary Reference Intakes for Vitamin C, Vitamin E, Selenium, and Carotenoids. National Academy Press, Washington, DC. *AI*, Adequate intake.

Food Sources

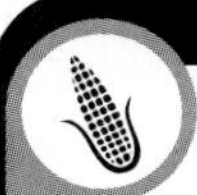

Food Sources of Selenium

Nuts and Seeds

540 μg per 1 oz Brazil nuts
25 μg per ¼ cup (~1 oz) sunflower seeds

Fish, Meat, and Poultry

65 μg per 3 oz canned tuna
30 to 65 μg per 3 oz fish (swordfish, flounder, sole, halibut, or cod)
20 to 40 μg per 3 oz mollusks (oysters, scallops, or clams)
35 μg per 3 oz crustaceans (crab or shrimp)
20 to 40 μg per 3 oz pork
20 to 35 μg per 3 oz beef
20 to 30 μg per 3 oz lamb
25 to 35 μg per 3 oz turkey
15 to 25 μg per 3 oz chicken

Grains and Cereals

20 μg per ½ cup couscous, cooked
15 μg per ½ cup spaghetti or macaroni, cooked
18 μg per waffle
10 μg per pancake
31 μg per 1 cup cream of wheat, cooked with water
19 μg per 1 cup oatmeal, cooked in water
22 μg per hard roll
11 to 14 μg per English muffin
10 μg per ½ cup brown rice, cooked
6 to 7 μg per ½ cup white rice, cooked

Dairy Products

18 μg per ½ cup ricotta cheese
8 to 12 μg per ½ cup cottage cheese

Miscellaneous

9 μg per ½ cup cooked mushrooms
6 μg per 1 large egg
5 to 7 μg per ½ cup beans, mature seeds (soy, pinto, or lima, cooked)
12 μg per cup soymilk

Data from U.S. Department of Agriculture/Agricultural Research Service (USDA/ARS) (2005) USDA Nutrient Database for Standard Reference, Release 18. USDA/ARS, Washington, DC. Retrieved November 15, 2005, from www.ars.usda.gov/ba/bhnrc/ndl/.

RDAs for children were extrapolated from the adult RDA. Recommendations for infants were based on the typical intake of selenium from human milk during the first 6 months (18 μg/L × 0.78 L/day ≅ 15 μg/day) and from human milk plus complementary foods during the second half of the first year of life (18 μg from milk + 11 μg from foods ≅ 20 μg/day). An incremental intake of selenium was recommended for pregnant and lactating women, resulting in an RDA of 60 μg/day for pregnant women and 70 μg/day for lactating women.

As mentioned in the preceding text, the selenium content of food varies greatly depending on the selenium content of the soil where the plant is grown or the animal is raised. Meat and seafood are good sources of selenium and contain both Sec in selenoproteins and selenomethionine incorporated in place of methionine in amounts that largely reflect the animal's intake of selenomethionine from plant sources. Wheat grown in the Great Plains of the United States, where the soil is rich in selenium, is a good source of selenium. Because of wide variation in the selenium content of foods depending on the region in which they are grown, food composition table values do not yield reliable estimates of actual intakes of individuals. Based on NHANES III, 1988-1994, median selenium intake in the United States is about 150 μg/day for adult men and 100 μg/day for adult women. The range of intakes (5th to 95th percentiles) are approximately 90 to 250 μg/day for men and 60 to 175 μg/day for women. Therefore, intakes of almost all adults are likely to be considerably higher than the RDA for selenium.

A more recent study has further carefully evaluated the human selenium requirement in Se-deficient subjects in China (Xia et al., 2005). These individuals were consuming an average of 9 μg Se per day for women and 11 μg Se per day for men and had plasma selenium values of 22 μg Se per liter (i.e., 18% of average plasma selenium levels of adults living in the United States). At baseline, plasma glutathione peroxidase values were 40% and plasma selenoprotein P levels were 23% of the average levels found in adults in the United States. These plasma parameters clearly documented that the subjects used in this study were initially Se-deficient. Subjects were supplemented with graded levels of selenium up to 66 μg Se per day as selenite or selenomethionine for 4 months. Full expression of plasma GXP3 was achieved with 37 μg Se per day as selenomethionine, consistent with earlier estimates, and therefore a total intake of 47 μg Se per day. Interestingly, a higher level of selenium from selenite supplementation, 66 μg Se per day, was required for plasma GXP3 to achieve plateau levels, clearly indicating a dramatic difference in the bioavailability of selenium from inorganic selenite versus selenomethionine in these subjects when supplements were provided as a single dietary pill per day. Plasma selenoprotein P levels were also very low but continued to increase with increasing dietary selenium at all levels of Se, indicating that an apparent plateau, as observed in the United States population, could not be achieved with 4 months of supplementation as done in this study. Because selenoprotein P appears to be a transport form of Se, it is not clear whether this indicates that selenium supplementation as high as 66 μg Se per day is suboptimal in these subjects, that these initially Se-deficient subjects were still not at steady-state, or that the selenoprotein P transport protein cannot be saturated at these levels of intake. Whatever the case, it is clear that supplementation in acutely Se-deficient individuals over the course of 120 days was not sufficient to raise Se levels to those observed in Americans habitually consuming an average of 98 to 145 μg of Se per day.

The basis for the selenium requirement in humans is clearly more solid than for many of the other nutrients, but a better understanding of the underlying biochemistry and molecular biology is necessary to ensure that the calculations and extrapolations are indeed reasonable. Well-understood biomarkers are needed so that we can reliably and safely make nutrient recommendations.

MECHANISM AND FUNCTION OF REGULATION OF GPX1 EXPRESSION BY SELENIUM

It makes sense that GPX1 activity declines when selenium is lacking, given that selenium is the integral cofactor necessary for activity, but what about the GPX1 protein and mRNA? When weanling rats are fed a selenium-deficient diet, GPX1 mRNA levels in liver fall to approximately one tenth of those found in selenium-adequate animals. In progressive selenium deficiency there is a coordinated dramatic exponential drop in GPX1 mRNA ($t_{1/2}$ = 3.2 days), as well as GPX1 activity ($t_{1/2}$ = 3.3 days) and GPX1 protein ($t_{1/2}$ = 5.0 days), suggesting that GPX1 is regulated at the level of mRNA (Sunde, 1990; Sunde et al., 1989).

As illustrated in Figure 39-10, in a study with male weanling rats, both liver GPX1 activity and GPX1 mRNA levels responded sigmoidally to increasing dietary selenium concentration, with the rise in GPX1 mRNA levels preceding the rise in GPX1 activity. It is important to note that further increases in selenium intake at levels greater than 0.1 mg of Se per kg diet had no additional effect on either liver GPX1 mRNA or GPX1 activity (Weiss et al., 1997). In female rats, which have more than 2.5 times the levels of liver GPX1 mRNA and activity found in male rats, the relationships of dietary selenium level to liver GPX1 activity and GPX1 mRNA (expressed as a percentage of the maximal level) are virtually identical to those in male rats, despite the increased need for Se incorporation into GPX1 (Weiss et al., 1996). Compared to GPX1 mRNA, the mRNA levels for a number of other selenoproteins are less markedly affected by low selenium intakes. GPX4 mRNA, selenoprotein P mRNA, and kidney GPX3 mRNA levels are little affected by low selenium intakes. Selenoprotein W mRNA and thioredoxin reductase mRNA are less affected by low selenium intake than is DI1 mRNA, and DI1 mRNA is less affected than is GPX1 mRNA. The more robust response of GPX1 over a range of selenium intakes suggests that GPX1 may play a unique physiological role.

Sunde and colleagues (2005) recently evaluated the selenium requirements of pregnant and lactating rats. Selenium response curves were determined for ten parameters on days 1, 12, and 18 of pregnancy and days 7 and 18 of lactation, similar to the curves shown in Figure 39-2. Growth, and mRNA levels for selenoprotein P, DI1, and GPX4 were not decreased by selenium deficiency. GPX4 activity required 0.05 mg of Se per kg diet for maximum activity, similar to the relationship observed in growing rats. Dietary selenium requirements for maximum plasma GPX3 activity decreased 33% in pregnancy, but returned in lactation to the growing-rat requirement. The selenium requirement for maximum GPX1 activity decreased 25% in pregnancy but not in lactation. This study showed that rat selenium requirements do not increase during pregnancy and lactation relative to requirements in growing rats. Unexpectedly, GPX1 mRNA and activity levels in selenium-adequate rats declined to <40% and 50% of non-pregnant selenium-adequate levels, respectively, during pregnancy and lactation. This study illustrates the importance of fully understanding biomarkers at all stages of the life cycle before interpreting a reduced biomarker levels as an indicator of nutrient deficiency.

All the GPXs can function as antioxidants, and this has long been assumed to be the role of GPX1. Sunde (1994) suggested that selenium regulation of *GPX1* gene expression is an important component of the function of GPX1 and that GPX1 has a second important function as a "biological selenium buffer." This hypothesis suggests that an important role of GPX1 in the liver, and perhaps other tissues, is to be part of the homeostatic mechanism. Upregulation of GPX1 expression when cellular selenium concentrations rise facilitates Se incorporation into GPX1 and thus keeps the concentration of free selenium at a rather fixed, low, and nontoxic level. The effect of this homeostatic regulation of GPX1 is to expand the range of dietary selenium intakes that do not cause a rise in intracellular free selenium, just as a buffer expands the capacity of a solution to absorb protons without a major change in pH. In turn, downregulation of GPX1 in times of selenium deficiency makes selenium available for other functions. This dynamic and homeostatic ability of GPX1 to regulate selenium metabolism is why Sunde (1994) described GPX1 as a biological selenium buffer, rather than as a "selenium store" or "selenium sink." The demonstration that GPX1 knockout mice, completely lacking GPX1, grow and reproduce normally (Spector et al., 1996) provides solid proof that this enzyme is not essential when mice are fed diets that contain a moderate level of selenium!

The mechanism for the regulation of GPX1 mRNA level in response to selenium status has now been established. Neither transcription of GPX1 mRNA nor translocation of GPX1 mRNA from the nucleus is affected by Se deficiency. Therefore, this regulation must occur posttranscriptionally. The location of the UGA within the first exon of GPX1 mRNA is important for the regulation of GPX1 mRNA stability by selenium status (Weiss and Sunde, 1998). The most logical mechanism is that the intracellular concentration of one particular selenium species (e.g., selenite, selenophosphate, or selenocysteinyl-tRNA) specifically regulates GPX1 mRNA stability in a manner analogous to iron regulation of transferrin receptor mRNA stability (see Chapter 36). In support of this idea, Sachdev and Sunde (2001) found that GPX1 mRNA in Se-deficient rat liver is modestly abundant, with about 2,500 and 5,000 copies per liver cell in male and female rats, respectively, as compared to 650 copies per cell for glyceraldehyde phosphate dehydrogenase mRNA. Remarkably, those levels increase to 19,000 and 27,000 copies of GPX1 mRNA per cell for male and female rats, respectively, with Se supplementation. This mechanism clearly can account for increased capacity to store Se in GPX1 in Se-adequate rats. This promises to be an exciting area for future research. The key nutrition concepts arising from this hypothesis are that there is a molecular regulatory mechanism that controls GPX1 mRNA level and GPX1 activity; that this process, like a "selenium thermostat," monitors selenium status; and, consequently, that changes in selenium parameters associated with this regulation can be used to determine selenium status and selenium requirements.

These concepts with respect to GPX1 expression can be used to analyze the underlying assumptions used by the WHO and the IOM in setting recommendations for selenium intake based on the response of plasma GPX3 activity to selenium supplementation. The rat model shows that setting requirements based on a second, noninvasive parameter, such as plasma GPX3 activity, could have sound scientific basis if it accurately reflects the cellular Se status (see Fig. 39-10). In the experiment summarized in Figure 39-10, a dietary level of 0.05 mg of Se per kg diet resulted in plasma GPX3 activity levels that were 67% of maximum (Lei et al., 1995). As discussed previously, 0.05 mg of Se per kg provides selenium at a rate sufficient to meet cellular needs for synthesis of selenoproteins such as GPX4, thioredoxin reductase, selenoprotein P, and selenoprotein W. At this level of dietary Se, liver GPX1 (the selenium buffer) will be at approximately 40% of maximum. If the dietary supply of selenium is increased and exceeds needs, the excess will promote GPX1 mRNA stability and then be incorporated into GPX1. If selenium intake is decreased, selenium from GPX1 turnover will be used for synthesis of other selenoproteins, and GPX1 levels will decrease.

Nutrition Insight

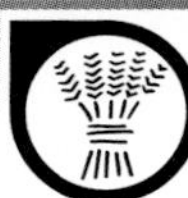

Selenium and Viral Resistance

Exciting studies by Beck (Beck et al., 2004) demonstrated that the nutritional status of the host can influence the genetic makeup of a virus and thus its infectivity. A virulent Coxsackie virus B3 (CVB3/20) that induces myocardial lesions in the hearts of mice was more virulent in Se-deficient than in Se-supplemented mice. Subsequent to viral infection, lesions occurred more quickly and more severely, and a higher virus titer was detected in heart and liver of selenium-deficient mice versus selenium-adequate mice. In addition, infection of mice with a cloned and sequenced benign endocarditic Coxsackie virus B3 (CVB3/0), which causes no pathology in the hearts of selenium-adequate mice, induced extensive cardiac pathology in selenium-deficient mice. In contrast, CVB3/0 virus recovered from the hearts of selenium-deficient mice and inoculated into selenium-adequate mice induced significant heart damage, suggesting that the mutation of the virus to a virulent genotype was predisposed by culturing in the selenium-deficient mice. Coxsackie virus has been isolated from patients who died from Keshan disease, suggesting a possible antiviral component to selenium's role in preventing human disease.

These studies with Coxsackie virus have now been expanded in mice to show similar effects of vitamin E deficiency, dietary excess of iron, or deletion of the *GPX1* gene. Furthermore, they also have demonstrated similar effects in mice infected with influenza virus. Additional examples of viral mutations in malnourished human populations suggest that this is not just a novel laboratory observation. Poor nutritional status of livestock or wild animals may play a role in the periodic emergence of new viral diseases as well as old viral diseases with new pathogenic properties (Beck et al., 2004).

Shisler and colleagues (1998) discovered that a human skin poxvirus, molluscum contagiosum, has acquired in its genome a complementary DNA sequence for mammalian GPX1. The discoverers propose that the poxvirus expresses the captured mammalian GPX1 as a countermeasure to the host's antiviral mechanisms, which include peroxidative stimulation of programmed cell death.

SELENIUM AND VITAMIN E

Vitamin E and selenium have been inexorably linked since the discovery that selenium would prevent liver necrosis. Early studies showed that combined selenium and vitamin E deficiency results in elevated levels of tissue malondialdehyde, which arises from the free radical attack on polyunsaturated fatty acids. A more-specific indicator of peroxidation is ethane and pentane evolution in the breath, which is due to the peroxidative breakdown of ω3 or ω6 unsaturated fatty acids, respectively. Ethane and pentane evolution is minimized by vitamin E alone, and it is partially reduced to 40% of the rate in doubly deficient rats by 0.2 mg of Se per kg diet.

F_2-Isoprostanes result from the nonenzymatic, free radical–catalyzed peroxidation of arachidonic acid in vivo; they are structurally similar to the F_2 prostaglandins. They are found esterified to phospholipids in tissues and are also found as free F_2-isoprostanes in plasma. Plasma F_2-isoprostanes in rats fed a diet deficient in vitamin E are two times control levels, whereas plasma F_2-isoprostanes in rats fed a diet deficient in both vitamin E and selenium are five times the level in animals fed an adequate control diet (Awad et al., 1994). Selenium deficiency alone is not associated with any excess production of F_2-isoprostanes. F_2-Isoprostanes present in phospholipids in various tissues also show similar results, with selenium deficiency exacerbating the effect of a vitamin E deficiency in most tissues but with selenium deficiency alone having no effect.

These studies suggest that vitamin E is the primary antioxidant molecule that intercepts and detoxifies damaging prooxidants before these species cause detectable damage. In general, selenium-dependent protective mechanisms appear to be an important "second arm" of the overall protective mechanism, although it is possible that selenium may play a more critical role than does vitamin E under certain conditions. The specific physiological roles of all the selenoproteins are still unknown, but it appears that selenium-dependent functions of GPX1 are not an essential component of the protective functions of selenium. The minimal role of GPX1 could be due to overlapping functions of the various GPXs or to no role for GPX1 in antioxidant function under normal conditions; GPX1 activity can fall to near-zero levels in selenium deficiency or in GPX1 knockout mice without appreciable tissue damage and with maintenance of substantial activities of other selenium-dependent enzymes. Circulating GPX3 or selenoprotein P in the plasma, GPX4 rolling along membranes of the ER or in the mitochondrial intermembrane space, thioredoxin reductase in cells, selenoprotein W in muscle, or another as yet undiscovered selenoprotein could be the major selenium-dependent antioxidant agent. Alternatively, a number of selenium-dependent antioxidant agents with somewhat overlapping functions may serve to defend the body against prooxidant species.

SELENIUM TOXICITY

The range of dietary selenium concentrations that is adequate and yet not toxic is very narrow. In rats, the minimum dietary requirement is 0.1 mg of Se per kg diet, and dietary levels greater than 2 mg are chronically toxic, resulting in a factor of 20 between the dietary selenium requirement and the lower end of the toxic range. In rats, hydrogen selenide is the most toxic form of selenium, and exposure to 0.02 mg of H_2Se per liter of air for 60 minutes results in death in 25 days. The relative toxicity of various low-molecular-weight selenium compounds is illustrated by the following LD_{50} or LD_{75} values (the lethal dose resulting in death of 50% to 75% of the animals) in rats given intraperitoneal injections (in mg of Se per kg body weight):

- Sodium selenite, 3.25 to 3.5
- DL-Selenocysteine, 4
- DL-Selenomethionine, 4.3
- Sodium selenate, 5.5 to 5.8
- Diselenodipropionic acid, 25 to 30
- Trimethylselenonium chloride, 49
- Dimethylselenide, 1,600

Long-term intake of dietary selenium at levels of 4 to 5 mg/kg diet are sufficient to cause growth inhibition and result in tissue damage as shown by elevated levels of

Nutrition Insight

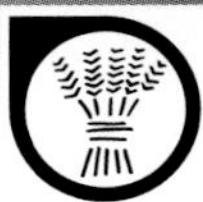

Selenium Intoxication

An interesting case of selenium intoxication in the United States occurred in 13 people who were taking over-the-counter dietary selenium supplements that had been improperly formulated. The pills contained 27.3 mg of Se per tablet (182 times higher than the amount specified on the label). Symptoms experienced by these individuals included nausea, abdominal pain, diarrhea, nail and hair changes, peripheral neuropathy, fatigue, and irritability. One individual took one tablet a day for a 2.5-month period despite these symptoms (Helzlsouer et al., 1985).

This incident has numerous lessons: it demonstrates that ingestion of nutrients above the requirement is not the benign process that the public and even physicians often assume; it demonstrates the need for quality control in the manufacturing of nutritional supplements; and it also illustrates how easily an individual's faith in the health-promoting aspects of supplements can overshadow a negative impact as well as a lack of benefit on health.

marker enzymes released into the plasma from damaged tissues. Liver toxicity and hyperplastic hepatocytes have been reported in rats receiving 0.5 to 2 mg of Se per kg diet for 30 months. Higher concentrations of Se between 4 and 16 mg/kg diet cause edema and poor hair quality, as well as shortened life spans. The biochemical mechanism underlying selenium toxicity is unknown.

Selenium toxicity in humans is initially associated with nausea, weakness, and diarrhea. With continuous intakes of excess selenium, these symptoms lead to loss of hair, changes in nail structure, lesions of the skin and nervous system, and mottling of the teeth. These toxicity symptoms are present with selenium intakes ranging from 3,200 to 6,700 μg/day. Milder symptoms of selenium toxicity include morphological changes in the fingernails of individuals consuming an average of 1,260 μg/day.

The high prevalence of selenosis in Enshi in southern China provided an opportunity to study individuals with high selenium intakes (Yang and Zhou, 1994). Hair loss and nail sloughing were observed with higher frequency in subjects with selenium intakes greater than 900 μg/day. Data from follow up of subjects after recovery from selenium poisioning were used to estimate a no-observed-adverse-effect level for selenium intake of 800 μg/day, which was associated with typical blood selenium levels of less than or equal to 1 mg/L (IOM, 2000; Yang and Zhou, 1994; Abernathy et al., 1993). Similarly, there was no evidence of selenium poisoning in a study of 142 subjects in seleniferous areas of South Dakota and Wyoming who were consuming as much as 724 μg of Se per day (Longnecker et al., 1991). The IOM (2000) set the tolerable upper intake level (UL) for selenium at 400 μg/day for adults.

The danger of selenium toxicity in the United States, however, is not just a question for Great Plains' residents and academic researchers. Increasing interest in anticancer nutriceuticals and in self-medication makes an improved biochemical marker of selenium toxicity an important research goal.

Acute Se toxicity, fatal or near-fatal, has occurred in a few cases due to ingestion of high Se-solutions such as gun blueing (containing selenious acid, nitric acid, and copper nitrate) or sheep drench. These cases usually involve consumption of gram quantities of Se and are typically followed by severe gastrointestinal and neurological disturbances, acute respiratory failure, myocardial infarction, and renal failure (IOM, 2000).

SELENIUM AND CANCER

The selenium and cancer story began in 1943 with the report that rats fed 10 mg of Se per kg diet for up to 24 months developed liver cell adenoma or low-grade carcinoma without metastasis (NRC, 1982). A repeat of this study 24 years later was not able to confirm these findings, but the stigma of selenium being a carcinogen has remained. Epidemiological studies conducted in the late 1960s and 1970s provided solid evidence of an inverse relationship between selenium intake and cancer mortality, as well as the incidence of leukemia and cancers of the colon, rectum, pancreas, breast, ovaries, prostate, bladder, lung, and skin. Therefore, it is clear that selenium is anticarcinogenic under at least some conditions.

In a number of systems, selenium supplementation at levels that are chronically toxic (2 to 5 mg of Se per kg diet) will decrease the tumor incidence in animals treated with chemical carcinogens such as 7,12-dimethylbenz[a]anthracene, in animals infected with virally transmitted spontaneous mammary tumors, or in animals given intraperitoneally injected ascites tumor cells. Selenium must be provided both during the initiation and promotional stages of tumor formation for maximal effectiveness. Near-maximal inhibition is obtained when selenium is provided 1 to 2 weeks after administration of the carcinogen, indicating that the major role of selenium may be to inhibit proliferation of tumors.

Excitement about selenium's anticarcinogenic role arose in the 1980s as a result of a retrospective study using prediagnostic serum selenium concentrations, which found that subjects in the lowest quintile of serum selenium concentration had risks for breast and several other cancers that were twice as high as for those for subjects in the highest quintile. This excitement, however, has been reduced because a number of case-control and prospective studies looking at tissue selenium concentrations and risk of breast cancer found no evidence of a protective effect of selenium.

A randomized trial with 1,312 patients who had histories of basal cell or squamous cell carcinomas of the skin, who were given either an oral supplement of 200 μg of Se per day or a placebo, did not demonstrate any significant effect of selenium supplementation on the incidence of new basal or squamous cell carcinoma of the skin. Selenium treatment, however, was associated with a statistically significant reduction in several secondary endpoints that were not the primary focus of the study; these included total mortality and lung cancer mortality, total cancer incidence, colon and rectal cancer incidence, and prostate cancer incidence. Total cancer incidence was 42% lower in the selenium group (Combs et al., 1997). Subsequent analysis has revealed that a significant reduction in cancer risk was confined to males and only for total cancer and prostate cancer but not for lung and colorectal cancer. These effects were only seen in subjects in the lowest two tertiles of plasma Se (less than 121.6 μg/L) at entry into the study; those males in the highest tertile had an elevated risk (Duffield-Lillico et al., 2002). In two randomized nutrition intervention trials conducted in a rural county in north central China, involving nearly 30,000 participants over 5 years, there was a small but significant reduction in total mortality in subjects receiving a combination of 15 mg of β-carotene, 50 μg of Se as selenized yeast, and 30 mg of α-tocopherol, whereas no appreciable effects were found for other supplements, including retinol, zinc, riboflavin, niacin, ascorbate, and molybdenum.

The IOM (2000) reviewed these and other reports, and concluded that these "studies are compatible with the possibility that intake of selenium above those needed to maximize selenoproteins have an anticancer effect in humans. These findings support the need for large-scale trials. They cannot, however, serve as the basis for determining dietary selenium requirements at this time" (IOM, 2000, p. 291). Although the story about selenium and cancer is not yet clear, studies such as these continue to stimulate interest in the role of selenium in human health.

REFERENCES

Abernathy CO, Cantilli R, Du JT, Levander OA (1993) Essentiality versus toxicity: some considerations in the risk assessment of essential trace elements. In: Saxena J (ed) Hazard Assessment of Chemicals. Taylor and Francis, Washington, DC.

Arthur JR, Nicol F, Beckett GJ (1990) Hepatic iodothyronine 5′-deiodinase. The role of selenium. Biochem J 272:537-540.

Awad JA, Morrow JD, Hill KE, Roberts LJ, Burk RF (1994) Detection and localization of lipid peroxidation in selenium- and vitamin E–deficient rats using F2-isoprostanes. J Nutr 124:810-816.

Beck MA, Handy J, Levander OA (2004) Host nutritional status: the neglected virulence factor. Trends Microbiol 12:417-423.

Behne D, Kyriakopoulos A, Meinhold H, Kohrle J (1990) Identification of type I iodothyronine 5′-deiodinase as a selenoenzyme. Biochem Biophys Res Commun 173:1143-1149.

Berry MJ, Banu L, Chen Y, Mandel SJ, Kieffer JD, Harney JW, Larsen PR (1991) Recognition of a UGA as a selenocysteine codon in Type I deiodinase requires sequences in the 3′ untranslated region. Nature (London) 353:273-276.

Berry MJ, Banu L, Larsen PR (1991) Type I iodothyronine deiodinase is a selenocysteine-containing enzyme. Nature 349:438-440.

Burk RF (1976) Selenium in man. In: Prasad AS (ed) Trace Elements in Human Health and Disease. Academic Press, New York, pp 105-133.

Burk RF, Hill KE (2005) Selenoprotein P: an extracellular protein with unique physical characteristics and a role in selenium homeostasis. Annu Rev Nutr 25:215-235.

Burk RF, Hill KE (1994) Selenoprotein P: a selenium-rich extracellular glycoprotein. J Nutr 124:1891-1897.

Castellano S, Novoselov SV, Kryukov GV, Lescure A, Blanco E, Krol A, Gladyshev VN, Guigo R (2004) Reconsidering the evolution of eukaryotic selenoproteins: a novel nonmammalian family with scattered phylogenetic distribution. EMBO Rep 5:71-77.

Chen X, Yang G, Chen J, Wen Z, Ge K (1980) Studies on the relations of selenium and Keshan Disease. Biol Trace Elem Res 2:91-107.

Combs GF Jr, Clark LC, Turnbull BW (1997) Reduction of cancer risk with an oral supplement of selenium. Biomed Environ Sci 10:227-234.

Cotton FA, Wilkinson G (1972) Advanced Inorganic Chemistry. John Wiley and Sons, New York, pp 421-457.

Damdimopoulos AE, Miranda-Vizuete A, Treuter E, Gustafsson J, Spyrou G (2004) An alternative splicing variant of the selenoprotein thioredoxin reductase is a modulator of estrogen signaling. J Biol Chem 279: 38721-38729.

Duffield-Lillico AJ, Reid ME, Turnbull BW, Combs GF, Jr., Slate EH, Fischbach LA, Marshall JR, Clark LC (2002) Baseline characteristics and the effect of selenium supplementation on cancer incidence in a randomized clinical trial: a summary report of the Nutritional Prevention of Cancer Trial. Cancer Epidemiol Biomarkers Prev 11:630-639.

Esworthy RS, Yang L, Frankel P, Chu F (2005) The role of epithelium-specific glutathione peroxidase, Gpx2, in prevention of intestinal inflammation in selenium-deficient mice. J Nutr 135:740-745.

Fomenko DE, Gladyshev VN (2003) Identity and functions of CxxC-derived motifs. Biochemistry 42:11214-11225.

Francesconi KA, Pannier F (2004) Selenium metabolites in urine: a critical overview of past work and current status. Clin Chem 50:2240-2253.

Gao Y, Feng H, Walder K, Bolton K, Sunderland T, Bishara N, Quick M, Kantham L, Collier G (2004) Regulation of the selenoprotein SelS by glucose deprivation and ER stress: SelS is a novel glucose-regulated protein. FEBS Lett 563:185-190.

Hadley KB, Sunde RA (2001) Selenium regulation of thioredoxin reductase activity and mRNA levels in rat liver. J Nutr Biochem 12:693-702.

Hatfield DL (2001) Selenium: Its Molecular Biology and Role in Human Health. Kluwer Academic Publishers, Norwood, MA.

Helzlsouer K, Jacobs R, Morris S (1985) Acute selenium intoxication in the United States (abstract). Fed Proc 44:1670.

Institute of Medicine (2000) Dietary Reference Intakes for Vitamin C, Vitamin E, Selenium, and Carotenoids. National Academy Press, Washington, DC.

Kim HY, Gladyshev VN (2004) Methionine sulfoxide reduction in mammals: characterization of methionine-R-sulfoxide reductase. Mol Biol Cell 15:1055-1064.

Kobayashi Y, Ogra Y, Ishiwata K, Takayama H, Aimi N, Suzuki KT (2002) Selenosugars are key and urinary metabolites for selenium excretion within the required to low-toxic range. Proc Natl Acad Sci U S A 99:15932-15936.

Korotkov KV, Novoselov SV, Hatfield DL, Gladyshev VN (2002) Mammalian selenoprotein in which selenocysteine (Sec) incorporation is supported by a new form of Sec insertion sequence element. Mol Cell Biol 22:1402-1411.

Kryukov GV, Castellano S, Novoselov SV, Lobanov AV, Zehtab O, Guigo R, Gladyshev VN (2003) Characterization of mammalian selenoproteins. Science 300:1439-1443.

Kryukov GV, Gladyshev VN (2004) The prokaryotic selenoproteome. EMBO Rep 5:538-543.

Lei XG, Evenson JK, Thompson KM, Sunde RA (1995) Glutathione peroxidase and phospholipid hydroperoxide glutathione peroxidase are differentially regulated in rats by dietary selenium. J Nutr 125:1438-1446.

Longnecker MP, Taylor PR, Levander OA, Howe M, Veillon C, McAdam PA, Patterson KY, Holden JM, Stampfer MJ, Morris JS, Willett WC (1991) Selenium in diet, blood, and toenails in relation to human health in a seleniferous area. Am J Clin Nutr 53:1288-1294.

Maiorino M, Gregolin C, Ursini F (1990) Phospholipid hydroperoxide glutathione peroxidase. Methods Enzymol 186:448-457.

McConnell KP, Roth DM (1966) Respiratory excretion of selenium. Proc Soc Exp Biol Med 123:919-921.

Mills GC (1957) Hemoglobin catabolism. I. Glutathione peroxidase, an erythrocyte enzyme which protects hemoglobin from oxidative breakdown. J Biol Chem 229:189-197.

National Research Council (1989) Recommended Dietary Allowances. National Academy Press, Washington, DC.

National Research Council (1982) Diet, Nutrition, and Cancer. National Academy Press, Washington, DC, pp 163-169.

Patterson BH, Levander OA, Helzlsouer K, McAdam PA, Lewis SA, Taylor PR, Veillon C, Zech LA (1989) Human selenite metabolism: a kinetic model. Am J Physiol 257:R556-R567.

Robinson MF, Thomson CD (1983) The role of selenium in the diet. Nutr Abst Rev 53:3-26.

Rosenfeld I, Beath OA (1964) Selenium: Geobotany, Biochemistry, Toxicity and Nutrition. Academic Press, New York.

Sachdev SW, Sunde RA (2001) Selenium regulation of transcript abundance and relative translational efficiency of glutathione peroxidase 1 and 4 in rat liver. Biochem J 357:851-858.

Schroeder HA, Frost DV, Balassa JJ (1970) Essential trace metals in man: selenium. J Chron Dis 23:227-243.

Schwarz K, Foltz CM (1957) Selenium as an integral part of factor 3 against dietary necrotic liver degeneration. J Am Chem Soc 79:3292-3293.

Shisler JL, Senkevich TG, Berry MJ, Moss B (1998) Ultraviolet-induced cell death blocked by a selenoprotein from a human dematotropic poxvirus. Science 279:102-105.

Spector A, Yang Y, Ho YS, Magnenat JL, Wang RR, Ma W, Li WC (1996) Variation in cellular glutathione peroxidase activity in lens epithelial cells, transgenics and knockouts does not significantly change the response to H_2O_2 stress. Exp Eye Res 62:521-540.

Sunde RA (1990) Molecular biology of selenoproteins. Annu Rev Nutr 10:451-474.

Sunde RA (1994) Intracellular glutathione peroxidases—structure, regulation and function. In: Burk RF (ed) Selenium in Biology and Human Health. Springer-Verlag, New York, pp 45-77.

Sunde RA (1997) Selenium. In: O'Dell BL, Sunde RA (eds) Handbook of Nutritionally Essential Mineral Elements. Marcel Dekker, New York, pp 493-556.

Sunde RA, Evenson JK, Thompson KM, Sachdev SW. (2005) Dietary selenium requirements based on glutathione peroxidase-1 activity and mRNA levels and other selenium parameters are not increased by pregnancy and lactation in rats. J Nutr 135:2144-50.

Sunde RA, Saedi MS, Knight SAB, Smith CG, Evenson JK (1989) Regulation of expression of glutathione peroxidase by selenium. In: Wendel A (ed) Selenium in Biology and Medicine. Springer-Verlag, Heidelberg, Germany, pp 8-13.

Tamura T, Stadtman TC (1996) A new selenoprotein from human lung adenocarcinoma cells: purification,properties, and thioredoxin reductase activity. Proc Natl Acad Sci U S A 93:1006-1011.

Tamura T, Yamamoto S, Takahata M, Sakaguchi H, Tanaka H, Stadtman TC, Inagaki K (2004) Selenophosphate synthetase genes from lung adenocarcinoma cells: Sps1 for recycling L-selenocysteine and Sps2 for selenite assimilation. Proc Natl Acad Sci U S A 101:16162-16167.

Ursini F, Heim S, Kiess M, Majorino M, Roveri A, Wissing J, Flohé L (1999) Dual function of the selenoprotein PHGPx during sperm maturation. Science 285:1393-1396.

Vendeland SC, Beilstein MA, Yeh JY, Ream W, Whanger PD (1995) Rat skeletal muscle selenoprotein W: cDNA clone and mRNA modulation by dietary selenium. Proc Natl Acad Sci U S A 92:8749-8753.

Walczak R, Westhof E, Carbon P, Krol A (1996) A novel RNA structural motif in the selenocysteine insertion element of eukaryotic selenoprotein mRNAs. RNA 2:367-379.

Weiss SL, Evenson JK, Thompson KM, Sunde RA (1996) The selenium requirement for glutathione peroxidase mRNA level is half of the selenium requirement for glutathione peroxidase activity in female rats. J Nutr 126:2260-2267.

Weiss SL, Evenson JK, Thompson KM, Sunde RA (1997) Dietary selenium regulation of glutathione peroxidase mRNA and other selenium-dependent parameters in male rats. J Nutr Biochem 8:85-91.

Weiss SL, Sunde RA (1998) Cis-acting elements are required for selenium regulation of glutathione peroxidase-1 mRNA levels. RNA 4:816-827.

World Health Organization (WHO) (1996) Selenium. In: Trace Elements in Human Nutrition and Health. WHO, Geneva, pp 105-122.

Xia Y, Hill KE, Byrne DW, Xu J, Burk RF (2005) Effectiveness of selenium supplements in a low-selenium area of China. Am J Clin Nutr 81:829-834.

Yang G-Q, Zhou R-H (1994) Further observations on the human maximum safe dietary selenium intake in a seleniferous area of China. J Trace Elem Electrolytes Health Dis 8:159-165.

Yant LJ, Ran Q, Rao L, Van Remmen H, Shibatani T, Belter JG, Motta L, Richardson A, Prolla TA (2003) The selenoprotein GPX4 is essential for mouse development and protects from radiation and oxidative damage insults. Free Radic Biol Med 34:496-502.

RECOMMENDED READINGS

Hatfield DL (2001) Selenium: Its Molecular Biology and Role in Human Health. Kluwer Academic Publishers, Norwood, MA.

Institute of Medicine (2000) Selenium. In: Dietary Reference Intakes for Vitamin C, Vitamin E, Selenium, and Carotenoids. National Academy Press, Washington, DC, pp 284-324.

Kryukov GV, Castellano S, Novoselov SV, Lobanov AV, Zehtab O, Guigo R, Gladyshev VN (2003) Characterization of mammalian selenoproteins. Science 300:1439-1443.

Sunde RA (1997) Selenium. In: O'Dell BL, Sunde RA (eds) Handbook of Nutritionally Essential Mineral Elements. Marcel Dekker, New York, pp 493-556.

Chapter 40

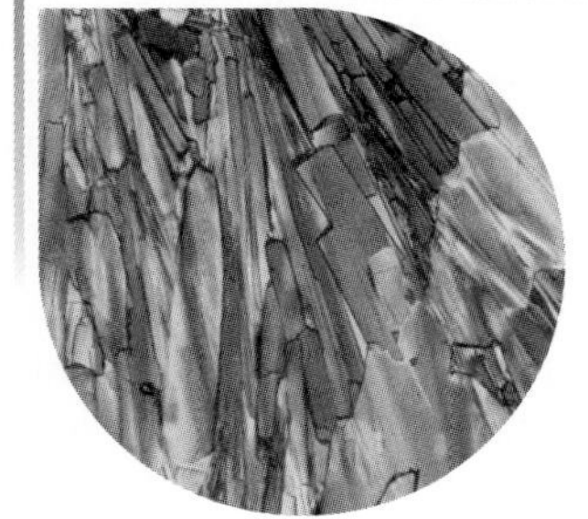

Fluoride

Gary M. Whitford, PhD, DMD

OUTLINE

OVERVIEW

Fluoride (F^-), the ionic form of the element fluorine, is the 13th most abundant element in the crust of the earth and has been found in all naturally occurring animate and inanimate materials. Because of its high affinity for divalent and trivalent cations, fluoride exists in the earth mainly in combination with calcium, magnesium, aluminum, and other metals. Similarly, the bulk of fluoride in the human body (about 99%) is associated with the skeleton and teeth.

Results from early studies with rodents suggested adverse effects on growth, reproduction, and hematopoiesis when the diet contained only traces of fluoride. Based on such findings, fluoride was classified as an essential element by the National Research Council in 1974. Subsequent studies were unable to confirm these effects. Although no longer considered essential, fluoride is regarded as beneficial, owing to its ability to prevent dental decay.

The behavior and effects of fluoride in biological systems differ in several important ways from those of other halogens. The ability of fluoride to bond with hydrogen to form a weak acid, HF ($pK_a = 3.4$), is unique among the halogens and accounts for several aspects of its physiology. Whereas other halogens are largely excluded from the intracellular fluids of soft tissues, the tissue-to-plasma concentration ratios of fluoride range from 0.5 to 0.9, except in adipose tissue and brain, in which the ratios are lower, and kidney, in which the ratio is higher. The rate at which fluoride is removed from the body by the kidneys is many times higher than the rates for excretion of the other halogens. Fluoride is concentrated in calcified tissues. As a general rule, approximately 50% of the fluoride absorbed by adults each day is deposited in calcified tissues, and the rest is excreted in the urine. Unlike iodide, fluoride does not accumulate in the thyroid gland. Fluoride, in high concentrations, has the ability to inhibit the activity of a wide variety of enzymes, and its potential to cause acute toxicity is relatively high. The ability of fluoride to stimulate new bone formation is unique among osteoactive agents. Its ability to inhibit the initiation and even reverse the progression of dental caries is also unique. The remainder of this chapter will develop some of these characteristics and actions in greater detail.

DENTAL FLUOROSIS AND DENTAL CARIES

Early in the twentieth century, Frederick McKay and other investigators drew attention to several regions in the southwestern United States where opacities and discoloration of the teeth were endemic. The identification of fluoride as the etiological factor involved the efforts of chemists, biologists, and epidemiologists during the following three decades. The condition, previously known by several descriptive names such as "Colorado brown stain," is now called dental fluorosis.

CHARACTERISTICS OF DENTAL FLUOROSIS

Dental fluorosis is a developmental disorder of the enamel that occurs only pre-eruptively (Fejerskov et al., 1977). After enamel mineralization is complete, no amount of fluoride intake (or of topically applied fluoride) can cause dental fluorosis. Dental fluorosis is classified as mild, moderate, or severe, with the degree of involvement being dependent on the amount of fluoride intake during tooth development. In the milder forms, the enamel has whitish, horizontal striations that may be localized to certain regions of the teeth, frequently the incisal thirds (biting edges) of the anterior teeth and cusps of the posterior teeth ("snow-capping"). Mild fluorosis is not easily noticed by the casual observer and requires some experience to recognize. The moderate and severe forms are characterized by graded degrees of brownish discoloration, sometimes with pitting of the enamel. Histologically, the enamel is more porous (i.e., less dense than normal enamel). The discoloration, which is due to diffusion of sulfur, iron, and other dietary pigments into the porous enamel, occurs slowly over time after the teeth have erupted. Chemically, the enamel has a relatively high protein content, which accounts for the porosity. Dental fluorosis is generally regarded as an aesthetic problem, not an adverse health effect. The enamel of the maxillary central incisors, which are the teeth most noticeable, appears to be most susceptible to fluorosis between 15 and 24 months of age for males and between 21 and 30 months of age for females—the time-period when the teeth are in the late secretory and early maturation stages of development (Evans and Darvell, 1995). Later developing teeth are most susceptible at later ages.

FLUORIDE INTAKE AND THE PREVALENCE OF DENTAL FLUOROSIS

An average daily fluoride intake of 0.05 mg/kg body weight (range 0.03 to 0.07 mg/kg) by children with developing teeth is associated with the milder forms of fluorosis in approximately 10% of the population. These levels of fluoride intake (average and range) are those found when the water fluoride concentration is optimal (about 1.0 ppm or 1.0 mg/L), and the water is the main source of fluoride intake. An average daily intake of 0.10 mg/kg is associated with a prevalence of mild fluorosis of about 50% in a population, with about 5% of the population exhibiting moderate fluorosis.

WATER FLUORIDATION AND DENTAL CARIES

The investigators who documented the relationship between fluoride concentrations in drinking water and dental fluorosis in the 1930s also recorded a striking effect on dental caries (Fig. 40-1). It was concluded that the consumption of water containing 1.0 ppm fluoride was associated with the near-maximum protection against dental caries and an acceptably low prevalence of the milder forms of dental fluorosis. This is how 1.0 ppm was established as the "optimum" concentration in drinking water. The optimum range is from 0.7 to 1.2 ppm, depending on the average regional temperature. The lower concentrations are recommended for warmer climates, where water intake tends to be higher.

The first study of controlled water fluoridation began on January 25, 1945, in Grand Rapids, Michigan. After 6.5 years, the caries experience among 4- to 6-year-old children in Grand Rapids was approximately 50% lower than in the control city of Muskegon, Michigan. Many subsequent studies confirmed this effect with caries reductions ranging from 20% to 80% and averaging approximately 50%. At present, community water supply systems with controlled fluoride concentrations serve more than 60% of the American population. Another 4% of the population lives in some 3340 communities with natural water fluoridation. Some of these water systems are equipped with defluoridating units because the natural concentrations are too high.

The difference in the prevalence of dental decay between American communities with and without water fluoridation is lower today than it was prior to 1970. A national survey conducted in 1979 to 1980 found a 33% lower prevalence among 5- to 17-year-old children who had always been exposed to fluoridated water compared with those who had never been exposed; a 1986-1987 survey found a

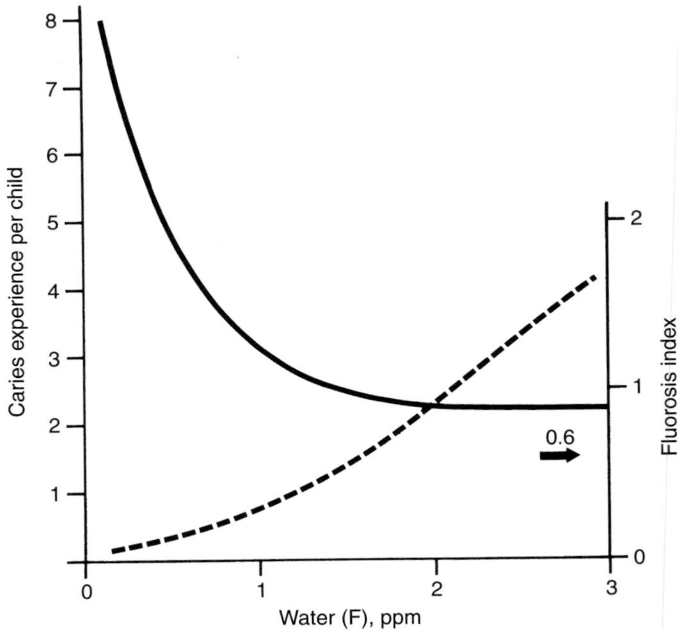

Figure 40-1 The relationships between caries experience *(solid line)* and the community dental fluorosis index *(dotted line)* and the fluoride concentration in drinking water as reported by Dean (1942). A total of 7,257 12- to 14-year-old children were examined. A fluorosis index value of 0.6, which occurred where the water fluoride concentration approached 2.0 ppm, was judged to represent the threshold for a problem of public health significance. (*From Whitford GM [1983] Fluorides: metabolism, mechanisms of action, and safety. Dental Hygiene 57:16-29. Copyright [1983] American Dental Hygienists' Association.)*

25% lower prevalence (Brunelle and Carlos, 1990). The widespread use of topical fluoride products and the "halo" effect, which is discussed in subsequent text, appear to largely account for the smaller differences.

TOPICAL FLUORIDE PRODUCTS

Several kinds of products designed for the topical application of fluoride to the teeth have become available since the mid-1960s. These include gels and solutions with high fluoride concentrations, which are applied in the dental office, and toothpastes and mouth rinses used at home. The fluoride concentrations in these products range from 230 ppm in the over-the-counter mouth rinses to 12,300 ppm in the professionally applied gels. Most toothpastes sold in the United States have a fluoride concentration in the 900 to 1,100 ppm (mg/kg) range. Clinical studies with toothpastes have resulted in caries reductions that ranged from 18% to 28%, with an average reduction close to 25%. When water fluoridation and fluoridated toothpastes are used together, the reductions in dental caries are roughly additive.

Three national epidemiological surveys conducted in 1971 to 1973 (National Center for Health Statistics), 1979 to 1980, and 1986 to 1987 (National Institute of Dental Research) revealed a progressive decline in tooth decay. Compared with the 1971 to 1973 data, there were 53% fewer affected tooth surfaces in the 1986-1987 survey. In 1979 through 1980, 36.6% of the 5- to 17-year-old children surveyed had no dental decay; in 1986 to 1987, the percentage had increased to 49.9%. It is generally agreed that the combination of water fluoridation and increased use of topical fluoride products has been responsible for these findings.

HOW FLUORIDE PREVENTS DENTAL CARIES

The main minerals of tooth enamel and dentin are various calcium phosphate salts, principally hydroxyapatite and hydroxyfluorapatite ($Ca_{10}(PO_4)_6(OH)_{2-n}F_n$; n = 0, 1 or 2). Fluoride-containing apatite is less soluble in acid than is hydroxyapatite that contains no fluoride. Dental caries are caused by the action of acid produced several times each day during the metabolism of carbohydrates by bacteria in dental plaque. The mechanisms by which fluoride prevents dental caries include the following:

- Increased resistance of enamel to acid attack
- Promotion of remineralization of incipient enamel lesions, which are initiated at the ultrastructural level several times daily according to the frequency of eating or drinking foods containing carbohydrates (Ten Cate, 1990)
- Increasing the deposition of minerals in plaque, which, especially under acidic conditions, provides mineral ions (calcium, phosphate, and fluoride) that retard demineralization and promote remineralization (Tatevossian, 1990)
- A reduction in the amount of acid produced through inhibition of bacterial enzymes (especially enolase) and glucose uptake (Hamilton, 1990)

These various mechanisms require frequent exposure to fluoride throughout life in order to maintain adequate concentrations of the ion in the dental plaque and enamel. The plaque and enamel receive fluoride from the blood via the saliva (saliva is a continuous source of fluoride except during sleep) and from water, food, and dental products (Whitford, 1996).

FLUORIDE INTAKE

The major sources of ingested fluoride are the diet, especially water and beverages made with fluoride-containing water, and dental products. The ingestion of fluoride from dental products may be intentional, as with dietary supplements, or unintentional, which occurs to varying degrees when toothpastes or mouth rinses are used.

RECOMMENDED FLUORIDE INTAKE

In setting the dietary reference intakes (DRIs), the Institute of Medicine (IOM, 1997) set adequate intakes (AIs) for fluoride across the life cycle. The AI is based on estimated intakes that have been shown to significantly reduce the occurrence of dental caries in a population without causing unwanted side effects, including moderate dental fluorosis. Except for infants

RDAs Across the Life Cycle

	mg Fluoride per Day
Infants	
0 to 0.5 yr	0.01
0.5 to 1 yr	0.5
Children	
1 to 3 yr	0.7
4 to 8 yr	1
9 to 13 yr	2
Males	
14 to 18 yr	3
19 to >70 yr	4
Females*	
14 to 18 yr	3
19 to >70 yr	3

*No additional intake recommended for pregnant and lactating women.
Data from Institute of Medicine (1997) Dietary Reference Intakes for Calcium, Phosphorus, Magnesium, Vitamin D, and Fluoride. National Academy Press, Washington, DC.

Table 40-1
Fluoride Concentrations in 12 Ready-to-Eat Food Classes Served to Hospital Patients in Rochester, NY, in 1982-1983

Food	Fluoride Concentration (mg/kg) Average	Range
Fruits	0.06	0.02 to 0.08
Meat, fish, poultry	0.22	0.04 to 0.51
Dairy products	0.25	0.02 to 0.82
Oils and fats	0.25	0.02 to 0.44
Leafy vegetables	0.27	0.08 to 0.70
Sugar and adjunct	0.28	0.02 to 0.78
Root vegetables	0.38	0.27 to 0.48
Grain and cereal products	0.42	0.08 to 2.01
Potatoes	0.49	0.21 to 0.84
Legume vegetables	0.53	0.49 to 0.57
Nonclassifiable*	0.59	0.29 to 0.87
Beverages	0.76	0.02 to 2.74

Data from Taves DR (1983) Dietary intake of fluoride: ashed (total fluoride) v. unashed (inorganic fluoride) analysis of individual foods. Br J Nutr 49:295-301.
*Nonclassifiable foods included certain soups, puddings, and other miscellaneous foods.
1.0 mg/kg = 1.0 ppm = 0.052 mmol/kg.

up to the age of 6 months, for whom intake from breast milk is regarded as adequate, the AI values are based on an average daily intake of 0.05 mg/kg body weight. No increase in the AI was recommended for pregnant or lactating women.

FLUORIDE CONCENTRATIONS IN FOODS

The fluoride concentration of most unprepared foods is less than 0.5 ppm (0.5 mg/kg). The concentrations occurring naturally in drinking water supplies in the United States range from 0.05 to 6 ppm; the great majority are considerably less than 1.0 ppm. The higher concentrations are mainly found in the southwestern United States. The concentrations in foods may increase or decrease depending on the fluoride concentration of the water used for cooking. Tea and marine fish (without bones) have higher concentrations that typically range from 1 to 6 ppm (1 to 6 mg/L or mg/kg).

Table 40-1 shows the average and range of fluoride concentrations of ready-to-eat foods fed to adult hospital patients in Rochester, New York (Taves, 1983). When preparation required the use of water (e.g., some beverages, juices, and boiled vegetables), the local water was used (1.0 ppm). It was estimated that the average daily intake of fluoride from this hospital diet was 1.8 mg, which is midway between the extreme average values of 1.2 and 2.4 mg/day determined in seven other studies of dietary fluoride intake conducted from 1958 to 1985 (Burt, 1992).

FLUORIDE INTAKE BY INFANTS AND YOUNG CHILDREN

Human milk, like cow's milk, has a low fluoride concentration (about 0.01 ppm). Therefore, a liter of milk provides not more than 0.01 mg of fluoride, an intake level that has been shown to result in a negative fluoride balance (total excretion > total intake) in infants, which indicates a net loss from calcifying tissues of fluoride that was acquired in utero (Ekstrand et al., 1984).

Prior to 1980, many American manufacturers of ready-to-feed infant formulas prepared their products using fluoridated water, which

Table 40-2
Average Dietary Fluoride Intake by U.S. Children as Reported in Five Studies Conducted From 1979 to 1988

		mg Fluoride/Day		mg Fluoride/kg Body Weight/Day	
Year	**Age**	**F**	**No F**	**F**	**No F**
1979	2 mo	0.63	0.05	0.13	0.01
	4 mo	0.68	0.10	0.10	0.02
	6 mo	0.76	0.15	0.09	0.02
1980	6 mo	0.21	0.35	0.03	0.04
	2 yr	0.61	0.32	0.05	0.03
1985	6 mo	0.42	0.23	0.05	0.03
	2 yr	0.62	0.21	0.05	0.02
1988	6 mo	0.4	0.2	0.05	0.03

Data from Burt BA (1992) The changing patterns of systemic fluoride intake. J Dent Res 71(Spec. Issue):1228-1237.
F, Foods processed and mixed with fluoridated water (>0.7 ppm); *No F,* foods not processed and mixed with fluoridated water (<0.4 ppm).

resulted in concentrations ranging from 0.6 to 1.2 ppm. However, a number of reports in the 1980s began to show an increase in the prevalence of dental fluorosis and raised concern about this practice. At a meeting sponsored by the American Dental Association, investigators discussed the possible relationship between infant formulas and fluorosis with the manufacturers, who then agreed to prepare their products with low-fluoride water (Pendrys and Stamm, 1990). Today ready-to-feed formulas manufactured in the United States have fluoride concentrations that range from 0.09 to 0.20 ppm (McKnight-Hanes et al., 1988). These provide 0.20 mg or less of fluoride with each liter consumed. The fluoride concentrations of prepared liquid concentrates and powdered formulas span a wide range (0.1 to 1.2 ppm), depending mainly on the water used in the home to reconstitute these products.

Of particular interest is fluoride intake by young children at risk of dental fluorosis. When drinking water containing 1.0 ppm fluoride is the major source of the ion, the average daily intake by young children is approximately 0.05 mg/kg. Table 40-2 shows the results of five studies of dietary fluoride intake by children up to 2 years of age (Burt, 1992). Data were obtained for diets prepared with or without fluoridated water. In 1979, daily fluoride intake by 2- to 6-month-old infants living in areas with fluoridated water ranged from 0.09 to 0.13 mg/kg. These levels of intake were well above the optimum range and due partly to high-fluoride formulas. The more recent studies found lower daily intakes that were remarkably similar and close to 0.05 mg/kg. Table 40-2 also shows lower intakes in areas with low water fluoride concentrations. Average daily dietary fluoride intakes by older children and adults are somewhat less than 0.05 mg/kg because intake does not keep up with body weight (Burt, 1992).

The diet, however, is not the only source of fluoride intake. In a more recent study, Levy and colleagues (2003) monitored fluoride intake from water, other beverages, selected foods, toothpastes, and dietary supplements by 785 children from birth up to 36 to 72 months of age. The drinking water fluoride concentrations of nearly all of the children were either less than 0.3 ppm or between 0.6 and 1.1 ppm. Table 40-3 shows the history of intake (mean, 10th and 90th percentiles) by these children over the course of the study. As shown in Table 40-3, the overall averages for the intakes of children at 6 months and at 2 years are close to the AI levels recommended by the IOM (0.05 mg/kg) and only slightly higher than those shown in Table 40-2 for children whose drinking water was fluoridated. The 90th percentile intake values, however, are substantially higher. These higher levels of intake occurred mainly for children whose drinking water contained 0.6 ppm or more of fluoride. During the second and third years of life when, as noted

Table 40-3
Estimated Total Daily Fluoride Intake by Children From Water, Other Beverages, Selected Foods, Toothpaste, and Dietary Supplements

Age (months)	10th Percentile		Mean (± SD)		90th Percentile	
	mg	mg/kg	mg	mg/kg	mg	mg/kg
6	0.05	0.007	0.47±0.39	0.060±0.050	1.01	0.127
12	0.10	0.011	0.42±0.33	0.042±0.034	0.84	0.086
24	0.28	0.022	0.70±0.43	0.055±0.035	1.23	0.098
36	0.32	0.022	0.79±0.45	0.054±0.032	1.33	0.090
48	0.31	0.018	0.80±0.49	0.047±0.030	1.36	0.080
60	0.28	0.015	0.76±0.46	0.040±0.025	1.34	0.070
72	0.28	0.012	0.74±0.47	0.034±0.021	1.34	0.060

Data from Levy SM, Warren JJ, Broffitt B (2003) Patterns of fluoride intake from 36 to 72 months of age. J Public Health Dent 63:211-220.

in the preceding text, the incisors appear to be at greatest risk of dental fluorosis, the 90th percentile values are consistent with the occurrence of scattered cases of moderate dental fluorosis. In the cohort studied by Levy and colleagues (2003), the most important sources of fluoride intake (in descending order) were toothpaste, beverages, and drinking water.

FLUORIDE INTAKE FROM DENTAL PRODUCTS

Unlike the situation that existed 35 or more years ago when the diet was the only important source of fluoride intake, fluoridated dental products now contribute significantly to intake by both children and adults. An important observation that drew attention to this fact was the increase in the prevalence of dental fluorosis in the United States (Leverett, 1982). The products that are used most frequently and contribute most to fluoride intake are toothpastes, mouth rinses, and dietary fluoride supplements.

When the toothbrush bristles are covered with toothpaste, a weight of approximately 1.0 g is used, which, in the case of a standard 1,000-ppm product, contains 1.0 mg of fluoride. Studies have shown that from 10% to nearly 100% of the amount used by individual children is swallowed. Among children younger than 6 years of age, the amount ingested is inversely related to age because of inadequate control of the swallowing reflex. The overall average is close to 30%, so that about 0.3 mg of fluoride is ingested with each brushing. This is equal to or more than the average total daily intake with the diet in nonfluoridated areas and about 50% of the dietary intake where the water is optimally fluoridated (see Table 40-2). Similar amounts of unintended fluoride intake have been documented when over-the-counter mouth rinses are used as recommended by the manufacturers.

Several studies have shown that the use of fluoridated toothpaste starting at an early age increases the risk of dental fluorosis (mostly the milder forms) by 2 to 10 fold (Burt, 1992). As a result of such findings, several workshops conducted since 1985 have produced several precautionary recommendations for children with developing teeth, including (1) parental supervision of brushing, (2) the use of pea-sized portions of toothpaste, (3) teaching how to rinse and empty the mouth at an early age, and (4) the production of products with lower concentrations of fluoride. Some United States manufacturers now market toothpastes for children, but so far the changes have been limited to flavors, appearance (e.g., sparkles), and colorful packaging because, unfortunately, the U.S. Food and Drug Administration requires the fluoride concentration to be between 900 and 1,100 ppm. Several European countries, however, market 250-ppm toothpastes for use by children. The effectiveness of these products in controlling dental caries is virtually the same as that of the 1,000-ppm products.

DIETARY FLUORIDE SUPPLEMENTS

Dietary fluoride supplements intended for use by children whose drinking water contains low fluoride concentrations became available in the United States in the 1960s. When taken as recommended, they have been shown to be nearly as effective as water fluoridation in the control of dental decay. The major disadvantages of fluoride supplements are their relatively high cost and the frequent lack of compliance with the dosage schedule.

Supplements have also been identified as a risk factor for dental fluorosis (Pendrys and Morse, 1995; Leverett, 1982). Because of this risk, a new dosage schedule was approved by the American Academy of Pediatrics and the American Dental Association in 1994 (Table 40-4). The new schedule contains the following four changes to the previously recommended dosing schedule:

1. The drinking water fluoride concentration above which supplements are not recommended was reduced from 0.7 ppm to 0.6 ppm.
2. Supplementation should begin at 6 months rather than at birth.
3. The dose for children between the ages of 3 and 6 years was reduced by 50%.
4. The upper age limit for taking supplements was increased from 13 to 16 years.

The second change was based on clinical studies that failed to clearly demonstrate the efficacy of supplementation prior to 6 months of age. The third and probably most important change was based on clinical and laboratory studies showing that the permanent anterior teeth are most susceptible to fluorosis during the second and third years of life.

Table 40-4

Supplemental Fluoride Dosage Schedule Recommended by the American Dental Association and the American Academy of Pediatrics Starting in 1994

	Drinking Water Fluoride Concentration (ppm)		
Age	**<0.3**	**0.3-0.6**	**>0.6**
6 mo to 3 years	0.25	0	0
3 to 6 years	0.50	0.25	0
6 to 16 years	1.00	0.50	0

Data from American Dental Association Council on Dental Therapeutics (1994) New fluoride guidelines proposed. J Am Dent Assoc 125:366.
Values are given in milligrams of fluoride per day (2.2 mg NaF = 1.0 mg F).

ESTIMATING TOTAL FLUORIDE INTAKE: COMPLICATING FACTORS

As shown in Table 40-2, the average dietary fluoride intake by young children since 1980 has remained relatively constant both in areas with and without water fluoridation. The literature indicates that intake with the diet has also been relatively constant among adults. Before the mid-1960s the diet accounted for nearly all fluoride intake so that total intake could be estimated rather easily. Today, however, the situation is considerably different. The variable intake associated with the use of dental products was discussed earlier. Other factors of current importance include (1) increased sales of bottled water, (2) the use of home water purification systems, and (3) the “halo” or “diffusion” effect.

Most bottled waters contain small amounts of fluoride (less than 0.2 ppm) but some, such as Vichy water from France, contain 5 ppm or more. Nearly two dozen brands bottled in the United States contain added fluoride in concentrations ranging from 0.5 to 1.0 ppm. If the fluoride is added by the manufacturer, the law requires that the label show the concentration, but this is not required if the fluoride occurs naturally. The popular filtration purification systems used in many homes today remove little or no fluoride from water, but fluoride is effectively removed by distillation or reverse osmosis systems. The halo effect refers to the distribution of foods and beverages prepared with fluoridated water to other communities where the water is not fluoridated. Dietary fluoride supplements are recommended for children in communities where the water supplies are low in fluoride, but, because of the halo effect, some children in these communities may already have sufficient fluoride intake. The ingestion of dietary supplements by such children increases their risk of dental fluorosis. Considering all of these variables, it is clear that some persons living in communities without water fluoridation can ingest as much or more fluoride as some persons in fluoridated communities.

FLUORIDE PHYSIOLOGY

Figure 40-2 shows the main features of fluoride metabolism, a subject covered in detail by Whitford (1996). The overall process is relatively uncomplicated because fluoride is not known to undergo biotransformation to form complex chemical compounds, each of which might have its own special metabolic characteristics.

FLUORIDE ABSORPTION

In the absence of high concentrations of calcium and certain other cations with which fluoride forms insoluble compounds that are poorly absorbed, 80% to 90% of ingested fluoride is absorbed. When taken with milk or other foods high in calcium, absorption is reduced to 50% to 70%. The average half-time for absorption is 30 minutes. Although the stomach is not structurally or functionally designed for absorption, as much as 40% of ingested fluoride can cross the gastric mucosa. The rate and extent of gastric absorption are directly related to the acidity of the stomach contents. This is due to the formation of a highly permeating weak acid, hydrogen fluoride (HF, $pK_a = 3.4$). Most of the fluoride not absorbed from the stomach will be absorbed from the upper intestine, where the pH of the contents appears to have little effect on fluoride absorption. Regardless of the site, there is no evidence for any absorptive mechanism other than diffusion.

FLUORIDE IN CALCIFIED TISSUES

Fluoride concentrations in plasma and most soft tissues are low and typically between 0.01 and 0.05 ppm. Approximately 99% of the fluoride in the body is contained in the skeleton and teeth, where it exists mainly as hydroxyfluorapatite. Fluoride concentrations in calcified tissues usually range from 600 to 1,500 ppm and depend on past intake and the age of the individual. Higher soft and hard tissue concentrations may occur in people who work in certain industries, such as phosphate fertilizer or aluminum processing factories, or who live in areas with unusually high fluoride concentrations in drinking water.

As indicated by the double arrows in Figure 40-2, fluoride is strongly, but not irreversibly, bound in calcified tissues. The skeleton has both rapidly exchangeable and slowly exchangeable fluoride pools. Fluoride in the latter pool is found firmly bound within the

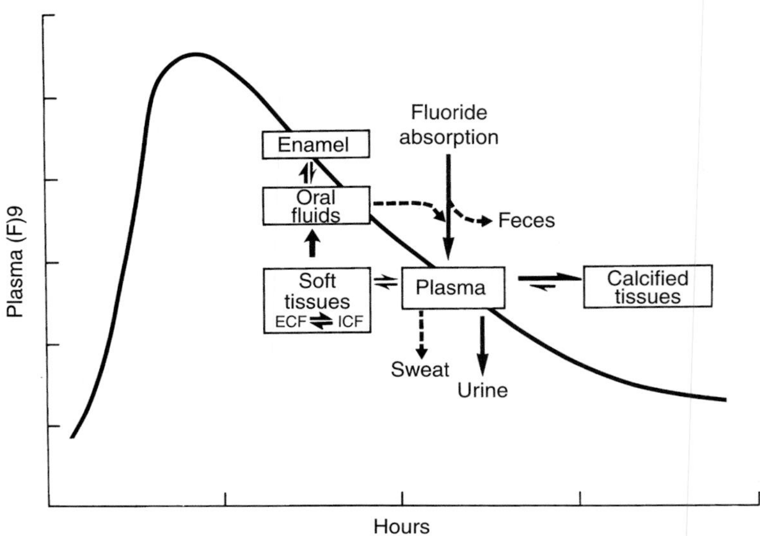

Figure 40-2 The major characteristics of fluoride metabolism and a typical curve showing plasma concentrations after ingestion of a small amount of fluoride. *(From Whitford GM [1990] The physiological and toxicological characteristics of fluoride. J Dent Res 69[Spec. Issue]: 539-549.)*

mineral latticework of mature calcified tissues. Fluoride is mobilized from this pool during the slow but continuous process of bone resorption by osteoclasts.

The rapidly exchangeable pool is located in the hydration shells on the surface of bone crystallites to which fluoride is attracted electrostatically. There appears to be a fixed ratio for the fluoride concentration in the hydration shell and the surrounding extracellular fluid. Therefore, when the plasma concentration increases, as after a meal, there is net uptake into the rapidly exchangeable pool. After approximately 30 minutes, when the plasma concentration is falling, net migration occurs of most of the fluoride back into the extracellular fluid. A small fraction of the fluoride, however, becomes associated with newly forming crystallites so that the skeletal concentration usually increases gradually throughout life. In the postabsorptive state when plasma concentrations are steady, there is little or no net fluoride uptake.

EXCRETION OF FLUORIDE

The excretion of fluoride occurs mainly via the kidneys. The fecal excretion of fluoride usually accounts for only 10% to 20% of daily intake. Even under extreme conditions of heat or exercise, only minor amounts of fluoride are excreted in sweat, which has a low fluoride concentration that is close to that of plasma (about 0.02 ppm). Therefore, a liter of sweat contains only approximately 0.02 mg of fluoride.

The renal handling of fluoride is characterized by free filtration through the glomerular capillaries, followed by a variable degree of tubular reabsorption. The renal clearance of fluoride, that is, the volume of plasma from which it is completely removed per unit time, is approximately 35 mL/min in healthy adults. Various studies found averages ranging from

Nutrition Insight

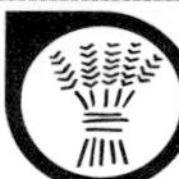

Prenatal Fluoride Supplementation Followed by Breast Feeding

Research on the benefits of prenatal fluoride supplementation for the deciduous teeth of the offspring has yielded conflicting results. A large and well-designed study (randomized and double-blind; Leverett et al., 1997) was unable to detect a statistically significant difference in dental caries between two groups of 5-year-old children whose mothers did or did not take fluoride supplements during pregnancy. Although no longer recommended by professional pediatric or dental organizations, some physicians and dentists still recommend that women take additional fluoride during pregnancy in the belief that it will make the deciduous teeth more resistant to dental caries. Much of the fluoride acquired by the fetal calcified tissues, however, could be lost if the infant is breast-fed.

Strong evidence for the mobilization of fluoride from the rapidly exchangeable pool came from a Swedish study (Ekstrand et al., 1984). Two groups of infants born to mothers residing in the same community were studied for several weeks. One group was fed human milk, which has a low fluoride concentration (~0.01 ppm). The other group was fed a formula reconstituted using the local drinking water that had a fluoride concentration of 1 ppm. The average daily fluoride intakes by the two groups were 10.6 and 861 μg, respectively. The average daily excretions (urinary plus fecal) were 32 and 383 μg. Therefore, the breast-fed infants were in a negative balance, whereas the formula-fed infants were in a strongly positive balance. These findings indicated that the higher fluoride intake was sufficient to maintain or increase the plasma concentrations established in utero and promote accumulation in calcifying tissues. The lower intake by the breast-fed infants, which would have resulted in gradually declining plasma concentrations, caused mobilization from the rapidly exchangeable pool.

Therefore, if it is assumed that prenatal fluoride supplementation of the mother has some beneficial effect on the deciduous teeth, it appears that the practice is rational only if the infant's postnatal fluoride intake is substantially greater than that provided by breast feeding.

27 to 42 mL/min but a much wider range among individuals (12 to 71 mL/min). The clearances in children are lower, but, when factored for body weight, they are practically the same as for adults. The efficiency with which the kidneys clear fluoride from the body is due to the relatively large hydrated radius of the ion that restricts its reabsorption from the renal tubular fluid back into the blood.

URINARY pH AND THE BALANCE OF FLUORIDE

Like absorption from the stomach, the reabsorption of fluoride from the renal tubular fluid is strongly dependent on pH and the diffusion of HF (Fig. 40-3). The fraction of fluoride that exists in the form of HF is directly related to the acidity of the renal tubular fluid. When the pH is high, say 7.4, only 0.01 % of the fluoride is in the form of HF and available for reabsorption. This results in a high clearance rate. When the pH is close to the physiologically possible lower limit (~4.0), nearly 20 % exists as HF. Under this condition, reabsorption is more rapid and the clearance rate is low.

The dependence of the renal clearance on urinary pH is a major factor in determining the metabolic balance (intake minus excretion) of fluoride. Urinary pH may be affected significantly by several conditions or factors, including certain diseases such as diabetes mellitus, renal tubular acidosis, the chronic obstructive pulmonary diseases, and some hormonal disorders; acidifying or alkalinizing drugs; altitude of residence; and composition of the diet. The latter factor is probably the most important in that it affects the urinary pH in all people.

SKELETAL DEVELOPMENT AND THE BALANCE OF FLUORIDE

At the beginning of this chapter, it was stated that about 50 % of the fluoride absorbed by adults each day is deposited in calcified tissues and the rest is excreted in the urine. This is only a rough generalization, however, as is indicated by the variability among individuals in the renal excretion of fluoride, as discussed in the preceding section. Another factor important in determining fluoride balance is the stage of skeletal development. The uptake

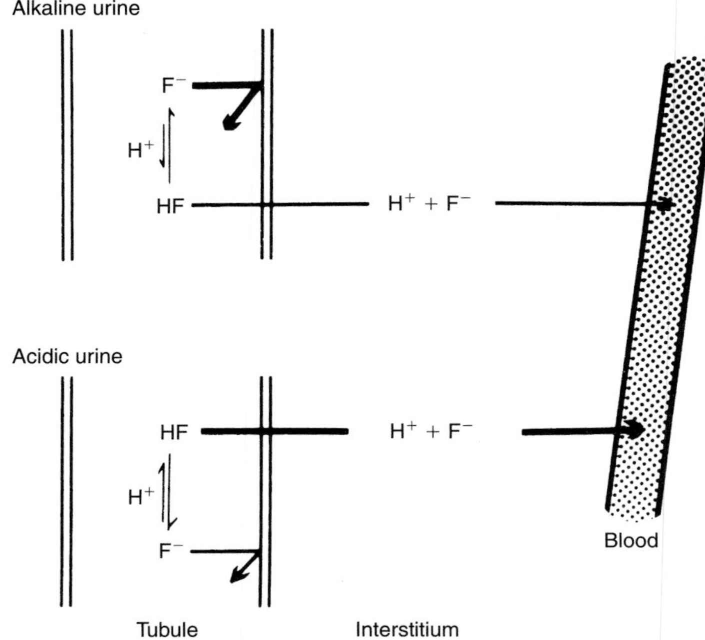

Figure 40-3 The mechanism for the reabsorption of fluoride from the kidney tubule. The tubular epithelium is virtually impermeable to ionic fluoride (F^-); it is easily permeated by the undissociated acid, HF, which lacks a charge. *(From Whitford GM [1990] The physiological and toxicological characteristics of fluoride. J Dent Res 69[Spec. Issue]:539-549.)*

of fluoride by calcified tissues is directly related to the total surface area of the crystallites. Developing crystallites are small in size, large in number, loosely organized, and heavily hydrated, and they have a large surface-to-volume ratio. Therefore, the fraction of absorbed fluoride that is retained in the body is inversely related to age during growth. A longitudinal study with growing dogs determined the retention (percentage of dose not excreted in the urine) of intravenously administered fluoride for nearly 20 months (Whitford, 1990). The results are shown in Figure 40-4. Shortly after the pups were weaned, only about 10%

Nutrition Insight

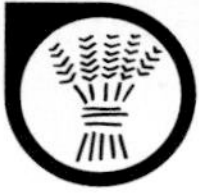

Urinary pH and the Balance of Fluoride

Many infants are fed either breast milk, which has a low acid load, or a cow's milk–based formula, which has a much higher acid load. The urinary pH of breast-fed infants ranges from the middle 6s to the lower 7s, whereas that of infants fed a cow's milk formula ranges from the lower 5s to the lower 6s (Moore et al., 1977). A diet consisting largely of vegetables and fruits (excluding cranberries, plums, and prunes) produces urinary pH values in the upper 6s and middle 7s, whereas a diet of meats and dairy products causes distinctly acidic pH values ranging from the upper 4s to the upper 5s.

Although data showing the effects of feeding infants human milk or cow's milk formulas are not available, it is likely that fluoride excretion is higher and balance is lower in breast-fed infants due to their higher urine pH. Research with young adults eating a vegetarian diet showed that the renal clearance of fluoride was significantly higher than when they were restricted to a meat and dairy product diet (Whitford and Weatherred, 1996). Compared with laboratory rats kept at sea level, rats residing at a simulated high altitude (hypobaric hypoxia) have a more acidic urine and significantly higher fluoride concentrations in plasma and calcified tissues. Therefore, several environmental and physiological variables can influence renal pH and the renal handling of fluoride sufficiently to alter fluoride retention and, potentially, its actions in the body.

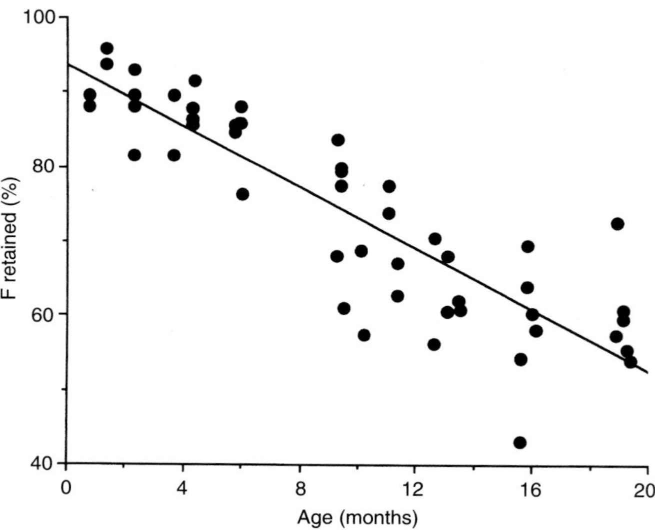

Figure 40-4 The inverse relationship between age and fluoride retention in growing dogs. *(From Whitford GM [1990] The physiological and toxicological characteristics of fluoride. J Dent Res 69[Spec. Issue]:539-549.)*

of the dose was excreted so that retention was close to 90%. Retention declined throughout the study and reached a final value close to 50%, which is the average for adult dogs several years of age. These findings are similar to those from studies with human infants and adults (Ekstrand et al., 1994). Although there are no data with which to judge, it is likely that in the later years of life, when bone resorption begins to exceed accretion, retention of fluoride falls to even lower levels.

ACUTE FLUORIDE TOXICITY

Life-threatening or fatal cases of acute fluoride toxicity are now extremely rare. Substantial amounts of fluoride in toothpastes, mouth rinses, or dietary supplements, however, are found in most American homes. Because of the suspected or actual overingestion of these products, especially by young children, several thousand calls to poison control centers are made each year.

SIGNS, SYMPTOMS, AND TREATMENT OF ACUTE FLUORIDE TOXICITY

Acute fluoride toxicity can develop with alarming rapidity. Nausea and vomiting almost always occur immediately after swallowing a large amount of fluoride and should be treated as initial signs of a potentially serious sequence of events. A variety of nonspecific signs and symptoms including excessive salivation and tearing, sweating, headache, diarrhea, and generalized weakness, may follow within minutes. Spasm of the extremities, tetany, and/or convulsions may develop if a potentially fatal dose has been swallowed. These effects will be accompanied by hypotension and possibly cardiac dysrhythmias, all of which are consequences of hyperkalemia and severe hypocalcemia. As renal function and respiration become depressed, a mixed metabolic and respiratory acidosis develops progressively and may end in coma.

Treatment on site and in the hospital is aimed at reducing absorption, promoting excretion, and supporting the vital signs. It should begin immediately. The oral administration of 1% calcium gluconate or calcium chloride reduces absorption. If calcium solutions are not available, milk may slow absorption. While these actions are being taken, the hospital should be advised that a case of acute fluoride poisoning is in progress so that preparations for appropriate treatment can be made before arrival.

DOSES PRODUCING SERIOUS SYSTEMIC TOXICITY

The "probably toxic dose" (PTD) is defined as the "minimum dose that could cause serious or life-threatening systemic signs and symptoms and that should trigger immediate therapeutic intervention and hospitalization" (Whitford, 1996, p. 118). Based on reasonably well-documented case reports, the PTD has been estimated at 5 mg fluoride per kg. One 3-year-old child died in an emergency room 3 hours after swallowing a fluoride solution in a dental office. The estimated dose was between 24 and 35 mg/kg. Another 3-year-old died in a hospital after swallowing about 200 1.0-mg fluoride tablets. In this case the dose was approximately 16 mg/kg. A third 27-month-old child died 5 days after swallowing an unknown number, but less than 100, of 0.5-mg fluoride tablets. The dose in this case was estimated to be slightly less than 5 mg/kg. In each of these cases, the child vomited almost immediately so that the absorbed dose was less than the ingested dose. The survival times after the doses were inversely related to the size of the doses. Based on these reports, it has been concluded that a fluoride dose of 15 mg/kg will probably cause death and that a dose of 5 mg/kg may be fatal. It should be noted that acute toxicity stemming from the ingestion of optimally fluoridated water (1 mg/L) is not possible because 5 L/kg of body weight would be required to reach the PTD.

The IOM (1997), in setting the DRIs for fluoride, established a tolerable upper intake level (UL) of 0.10 mg/kg/day (equating to 0.7 to 2.2 mg/day) for infants and children up to 8 years of age on the basis of minimizing the risk of dental fluorosis. The UL was set at 10 mg/day for children older than 8 years and adults. The UL for adults was based on studies of fluoride exposure from dietary sources or work environments (Hodge and Smith, 1977) that indicated 10 mg/day for 10 or more years carries only a small risk for an individual to develop preclinical or stage 1 skeletal fluorosis.

DENTAL PRODUCTS AS SOURCES OF HIGH FLUORIDE DOSES

During the first half of this century, sodium fluoride was a popular pesticide. Large amounts of it were stored in the kitchens of some homes and institutions. Being a finely divided white powder easily mistaken for powdered milk, flour, sodium bicarbonate, and similar products, there were numerous individual and several mass poisonings (Hodge and Smith, 1965). In 1941, for example, approximately 17 pounds of sodium fluoride was mistaken for powdered milk and used to prepare scrambled eggs at the Oregon State Hospital. There were 263 cases of poisoning, 47 of which were fatal. More than 600 deaths were due to fluoride ingestion in the United States between 1933 and 1965, which accounted for nearly 1% of all fatal poisonings during that period.

Other compounds have replaced sodium fluoride as a pesticide and fluoride-related fatalities are now rare. Owing to the presence of vitamins, dietary supplement tablets, and dental products containing fluoride in most American homes, however, the number of nonfatal cases has increased sharply. The American Association of Poison Control Centers reported that about 30,000 fluoride-related reports were made to U.S. Poison Control Centers annually from 1998 to 2002. Among these, approximately 2.5% of the cases were treated in a health facility each year. Toothpastes and mouth washes were involved in approximately 79% of the total number of reports each year. More than 90% of the cases involved young children. The "medical outcome" classification of the great majority of cases was "none" (transient and minor signs and symptoms), but 32 to 56 cases each year were classified in the more serious "moderate" and "major" categories, including eight "major" cases (long-term sequelae) and one death. The fatality was listed as a suicide due to acute ingestion of toothpaste by a 51-year-old person (Watson et al., 2003).

The PTD for a 1-year-old child of average weight (10 kg) is 50 mg. Each gram of conventional, 1,000-ppm toothpaste contains 1.0 mg of fluoride, so ingestion of 50 g (1.6 oz.) could cause serious toxicity. For an average 5- to 6-year-old (20 kg), the PTD is contained in 100 g of toothpaste. Most of the over-the-counter mouth rinses have a fluoride concentration of 230 ppm or 0.23 mg/mL. Therefore, the PTD for a 10-kg child is contained in 217 mL (7.3 oz.) of mouth rinse. These products should be stored out of the reach of small children, and their use should be supervised by an adult.

CHRONIC FLUORIDE TOXICITY

Perhaps because of its early use as a pesticide, fears and claims of harm surrounding the fluoridation of water, including a variety of allergic reactions, cancer, birth defects, and genetic disorders, were heard from the beginning. None of these claims has stood the test of controlled scientific research, as indicated in reviews by Kaminsky and colleagues (1990), the U.S. Public Health Service (1991), the National Research Council (1993), the U.K. National Health Service (NHS) Centre for Reviews and Dissemination (2000), and the Irish Forum on Fluoridation (2002). It was noted in some of these reports, however, that further epidemiological studies are required to determine whether an association exists between various levels of fluoride in the drinking water and bone fractures. This latter subject is currently receiving considerable research attention and deserves further discussion.

EFFECTS ON THE SKELETON

Chronic, Low-Level Intake

The 1993 report by the National Research Council concluded that the database on the possible relationship between fluoride exposure and the risk of bone fracture was limited and confusing. Some studies found no relationship, others found an increased risk, and still others found a decreased risk. Most of the studies were "ecological" in design; they compared fracture rates in areas with or without significant concentrations of fluoride in the drinking water, but did not gather information concerning previous fluoride intake or bone fluoride concentrations for individuals with or without fractures. Furthermore, most of the studies failed to control for variables known to increase the risk of bone fractures. The report recommended that "... additional studies of hip and other fractures be conducted in geographic areas with high and low concentrations in the drinking water, and that studies should use information from individuals rather than population groups" (National Research Council, 1993, p. 61). The recommendation of specified risk factors for individuals that should be evaluated in such studies including "... fluoride intake from drinking water and from all other sources, reproductive history, past and current hormonal status, intake of dietary and supplemental calcium and other cations, bone density, and other factors that might influence risk of fracture" (National Research Council, 1993, p. 61).

The report by the NHS Centre for Reviews and Dissemination (2000) critically evaluated 23 published studies dealing with the relationship between water fluoridation and the risk of bone fracture. Figure 8.1 (page 47) of the NHS report shows that most of the 95% confidence intervals in the 23 studies included a relative risk of 1.0, which means that the difference between fluoridated and nonfluoridated populations was not statistically significant. Among those that did not include a relative risk of 1.0, five suggested an increased risk of fracture in the fluoridated population, and four suggested a decreased risk of fracture. The report also noted that few of the studies controlled for all of the major variables known to influence the risk of fracture. It was concluded that "the best available evidence on the association of water fluoridation and bone fractures show no association" (NHS, 2000, p. 67).

Chronic, High-Level Intake: Skeletal Fluorosis

Skeletal fluorosis is a condition characterized by several stages of severity. The changes progress according to the amount and duration of fluoride intake, from the asymptomatic preclinical stage in which there is a slight increase in cortical bone density (osteosclerosis) detectable on X-ray films; through stage I in which bone density is further increased; through stage II in which there is further osteosclerosis, some stiffness and pain in the joints, and slight calcification of ligaments; and ultimately to crippling skeletal fluorosis in which irregular, bony outgrowths (exostoses) on previously smooth bone surfaces are present and marked calcification of ligaments limits joint mobility. Among adults with life-long exposure to optimally fluoridated water (about 1 mg/L), bone ash fluoride concentrations are usually less than 1,500 ppm, which are well below those associated with skeletal changes. Bone ash concentrations range from 3,500 to 5,500 ppm in the preclinical stage of skeletal fluorosis to over 9,000 ppm in the crippling stage. It may take 10 years or more of daily ingestion of approximately 20 mg of fluoride to reach the skeletal fluoride concentrations associated with crippling fluorosis. Only five cases of crippling fluorosis have been documented in the United States in the last 40 years. The U.S. Environmental Protection Agency (EPA) has set the MCL (maximum contaminant level) for fluoride in drinking water at 4 ppm to protect against the earliest signs of skeletal fluorosis.

Treatment of Osteoporosis

Based on its ability to increase bone mass, fluoride is used as an experimental drug in the treatment of osteoporosis (10 to 30 mg/day, usually for 3 to 5 years). Fluoride stimulates bone-forming cells (osteoblasts) to increase the production of several proteins, collectively called osteoid, some of which undergoes mineralization to form new bone. Although the literature contains conflicting reports concerning the effects of this treatment on bone strength, studies with a slow-release fluoride formulation have shown positive results (Pak et al., 1997).

REFERENCES

American Dental Association Council on Dental Therapeutics) (1994) New fluoride guidelines proposed. J Am Dent Assoc 125:366.

Brunelle JA, Carlos JP (1990) Recent trends in dental caries in U.S. children and the effect of water fluoridation. J Dent Res 69(Spec. Issue): 723-727.

Burt BA (1992) The changing patterns of systemic fluoride intake. J Dent Res 71(Spec. Issue): 1228-1237.

Dean HT (1942) The investigation of physiologic effects by the epidemiologic method. In: Moulton FR (ed) Fluorine and Dental Health. American Association for the Advancement of Science, Washington, DC, pp 23-31.

Ekstrand J, Hardell LI, Spak CJ (1984) Fluoride balance studies on infants in a 1-ppm-water-fluoride area. Caries Res 18:87-92.

Ekstrand J, Ziegler EE, Nelson SE, Fomon SJ (1994) Absorption and retention of dietary and supplemental fluoride by infants. Adv Dent Res 8:175-180.

Evans RW, Darvell BW (1995) Refining the estimate of the critical period for susceptibility to enamel fluorosis in human maxillary central incisors. J Public Health Dent 55:238-249.

Fejerskov O, Thylstrup A, Larsen MJ (1977) Clinical and structural features and possible pathogenic mechanisms of dental fluorosis. Scand J Dent Res 85:510-534.

Hamilton IR (1990) Biochemical effects of fluoride on oral bacteria. J Dent Res 69(Spec. Issue): 660-667.

Hodge HC, Smith FA (1965) Biological properties of inorganic fluorides. In: Simons JH, (ed) Fluorine Chemistry. Vol 4.Academic Press, New York, pp 1-42.

Hodge HC, Smith FA (1977) Occupational fluoride exposure. J Occup Med 19:12-39.

Institute of Medicine (1997) Dietary Reference Intakes for Calcium, Phosphorus, Magnesium, Vitamin D, and Fluoride. National Academy Press, Washington, DC.

Irish Forum on Fluoridation (2002) Irish Department of Health and Children. Government of Ireland, Dublin. Retrieved April 15, 2005, from www.doh.ie/publications/fluoridation/forum_final.html.

Kaminsky LS, Mahoney MC, Leach J, Melius J, Miller MJ (1990) Fluoride: benefits and risks of exposure. Crit Rev Oral Biol Med 1:261-281.

Leverett DH (1982) Fluoride and the changing prevalence of dental caries. Science 217:26-30.

Leverett DH, Adair SM, Vaughan BW, Proskin HM, Moss ME (1997) Randomized clinical trial of the effect of prenatal fluoride supplements in preventing dental caries. Caries Res 31:174-179.

Levy SM, Warren JJ, Broffitt B (2003) Patterns of fluoride intake from 36 to 72 months of age. J Public Health Dent 63:211-220.

McKnight-Hanes MC, Leverett DH, Adair SM (1988) Fluoride content of infant formulas: soy-based formulas as a potential factor in dental fluorosis. Pediatric Dent 10:189-194.

Moore A, Ansell C, Barrie H (1977) Metabolic acidosis and infant feeding. Brit Med J 1: 129-131.

National Research Council (NRC) (1993) Health Effects of Ingested Fluoride. National Academy Press, Washington, DC.

National Health Service (NHS) Centre for Reviews and Dissemination (2000) A Systematic Review of Water Fluoridation. Report 18. University of York, UK.

Pak CY, Sakhaee K, Rubin CD, Zerwekh M (1997) Sustained release of sodium fluoride in the management of established postmenopausal osteoporosis. Am J Med Sci 313:23-32.

Pendrys DG, Morse DE (1995) Fluoride supplement use by children in fluoridated communities. J Public Health Dent 55:160-164.

Pendrys DG, Stamm JW (1990) Relationship of total fluoride intake to beneficial effects and enamel fluorosis. J Dent Res 69(Spec. Issue):529-538.

Tatevossian A (1990) Fluoride in dental plaque and its effects. J Dent Res 69(Spec. Issue): 645-652.

Taves DR (1983) Dietary intake of fluoride: Ashed (total fluoride) v. unashed (inorganic fluoride) analysis of individual foods. Br J Nutr 49:295-301.

Ten Cate, JM (1990) In vitro studies on the effects of fluoride on de- and remineralization. J Dent Res 69(Spec. Issue):614-619.

U.S. Public Health Service (1991) Review of Fluoride: Benefits and Risks. U.S. Public Health Service, Dept. of Health and Human Services, Bethesda, MD.

Watson WA, Litovitz TL, Rodgers GC Jr, Klein-Schwartz W, Youniss J, Rose SR, Borys D, May ME (2003) 2002 annual report of the American Association of Poison Control Centers Toxic Exposure Surveillance System. Am J Emergency Med 21:353-421.

Whitford GM (1990) The physiological and toxicological characteristics of fluoride. J Dent Res 69(Spec. Issue):539-549.

Whitford GM (1996) The Metabolism and Toxicity of Fluoride, In: Myers HM (ed) Monographs in Oral Science, 2nd ed. No. 16. S. Karger, Basel, Switzerland.

Whitford GM, Weatherred TW (1996) Fluoride pharmacokinetics: effects of urinary pH changes induced by the diet. J Dent Res 75(Spec. Issue):354(Abs. 2695).

RECOMMENDED READINGS

Burt BA (1992) The changing pattern of systemic fluoride intake. J Dent Res 71:1228-1237.

Proceedings, Joint IADR/ORCA International Symposium on Fluorides (1990) Mechanisms of Action and Recommendations for Use. J Dent Res 69(Spec. Issue):505-835.

Whitford GM (1996) The Metabolism and Toxicity of Fluoride. In Myers HM (ed) Monographs in Oral Science 16, 2nd Edition. S. Karger, Basel.

Chapter 41

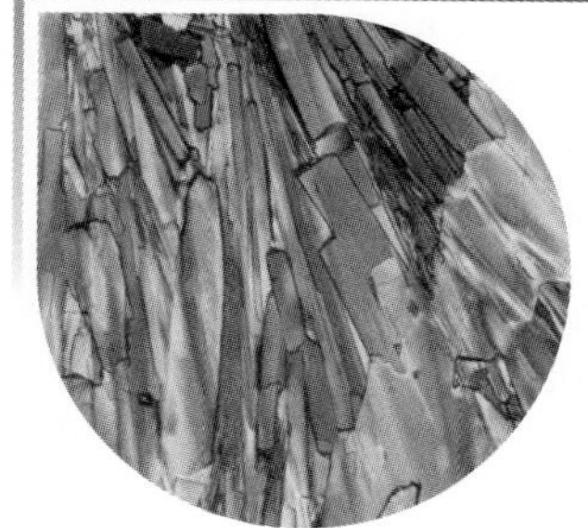

The Ultratrace Elements

Forrest H. Nielsen, PhD

OUTLINE

CHARACTERISTICS OF ULTRATRACE ELEMENTS

Trace minerals essential for health are those elements of the periodic table that occur in the body in microgram per gram of tissue amounts and are usually required by humans in amounts of milligrams per day. In 1980, the term ultratrace element began to appear in the nutritional literature; the definition for this term was an element that was required by animals in amounts of 50 ng or less per gram of diet. For humans, the term has been used recently to indicate elements with established, estimated, or suspected requirements quantified by micrograms per day. The term also has been applied to elements suggested to be essential but for which biochemical functions have not been defined.

The quality of the experimental evidence for nutritional essentiality varies widely for the ultratrace elements. The evidence for the essentiality of four ultratrace elements—cobalt, iodine, molybdenum, and selenium—is substantial and noncontroversial; specific biochemical functions have been defined for these elements. Iodine and selenium are recognized as elements of major nutritional importance and received their deserved attention in Chapters 38 and 39. Although cobalt is required in ultratrace amounts, it has to be in the form of vitamin B_{12}; therefore, cobalt as part of vitamin B_{12} was covered in Chapter 25. Very little nutritional attention is given to molybdenum because a deficiency has not been unequivocally identified in humans other than in an individual nourished by total parenteral nutrition or individuals with rare genetic defects that cause metabolic disturbances involving the functional roles of this element. Therefore, molybdenum is discussed in this chapter.

Boron and chromium have not been firmly established as nutritionally essential because they lack clearly defined essential biochemical functions. However, these elements probably should be considered nutritionally important ultratrace elements because numerous human studies have shown that they are bioactive food components that may influence health and disease by directly or indirectly producing beneficial functional outcomes. Animal studies indicate that several other elements (e.g., nickel, silicon, vanadium, and arsenic) may be essential or bioactive food components. Because of the lack of findings from controlled human studies, they will be only briefly summarized at the end of this chapter.

Individuals involved in professions providing nutritional guidance should be aware of the possible importance of the bioactive or possibly essential ultratrace elements in nutrition. The public is continuously exposed to health claims that appear in the popular media, pamphlets, and advertisements for several of these elements. Knowledge of the bases for these claims will help give informed guidance about usefulness of specific ultratrace elements in maintaining health and well-being to an inquirer, who usually has read some convincing statements that have been expertly prepared, as often is done by those interested in selling supplements. In addition, because some of the ultratrace elements have beneficial bioactive, if not essential, effects in humans, suggesting that diets providing abundant amounts of these elements may enhance health and well-being may be a justifiable action.

BORON

NUTRITIONAL AND PHYSIOLOGICAL SIGNIFICANCE

The foremost evidence for the nutritional essentiality of boron is that it is required by some animals to complete the life cycle. In particular, the lack of boron prevents the proper development of the embryo. Dietary boron deprivation of the African clawed frog (*Xenopus laevis)* resulted in necrotic eggs and a high frequency of abnormal gastrulation in the embryo. Abnormal gastrulation was characterized by bleeding yolk and exogastrulation, which suggested abnormal cell membrane structure or function (Fort et al., 2002). Boron deprivation of zebrafish resulted in a high rate of death during the zygote and cleavage periods before the formation of a blastula (Eckhert and Rowe, 1999). Pathological changes in the embryo before death included extensive blebbing and the extrusion of cytoplasm, which suggested membrane alterations.

Experiments with mammals have not shown that the life cycle can be interrupted by boron deprivation; that is, by impaired growth, development, or maturation such that procreation is prevented. However, substantial evidence exists for boron being a bioactive food component that is beneficial, if not required, for bone growth and maintenance, immune function, psychomotor skills, and cognitive function (Nielsen, 2001, 2000). Evidence that boron affects these processes in humans has come mainly from three studies. In two of these studies (Nielsen, 1994) men older than the age of 45 years, postmenopausal women, and postmenopausal women receiving hormone replacement therapy were fed a diet low in boron—approximately 0.25 mg/2,000 kcal for 63 days, and then were fed the same diet supplemented with 3 mg of boron per day for 49 days. These dietary intakes were near the low and high values in the range of dietary boron intakes (0.5 to 3.1 mg/day) that have been found in a limited number of surveys. Some of the effects of boron supplementation (after the boron-depletion period) that were found in these two experiments are listed in Table 41-1. In one experiment, copper was marginal and magnesium was inadequate; in the other experiment, both elements were adequate. The intakes of copper and magnesium apparently affected the response to the changes in dietary boron, as indicated by the footnotes to Table 41-1. Boron supplementation following the depletion period also enhanced or mimicked the effects of estrogen therapy

(Nielsen, 1994). Furthermore, boron supplementation after depletion yielded changes in encephalograms that suggested improved behavioral activation (e.g., less drowsiness) and mental alertness, improved psychomotor skills, and elicited improvements in the cognitive processes of attention and memory (Penland,1998). In the third study, perimenopausal women excreting an average of 1.1 and 3.0 mg boron per day during placebo and supplemental boron periods, respectively, had an increased number of total white blood cells, with an increased percentage of polymorphonuclear neutrophils and a decreased percentage of lymphocytes, during the boron supplementation period (Nielsen and Penland, 1999).

Table 41-1
Responses of Boron-Deprived Subjects to a 3-mg/Day Boron Supplement for 49 Days*

Metabolism Affected	Evidence for Effect
Macromineral	Increased serum 25-hydroxyvitamin D
	Decreased serum calcitonin†
Energy	Decreased serum glucose†
	Increased serum triacylglycerols‡
Nitrogen	Decreased blood urea nitrogen
	Decreased serum creatinine
Oxidative	Increased erythrocyte superoxide dismutase
	Increased serum ceruloplasmin
Erythropoiesis/ hematopoiesis	Increased blood hemoglobin‡
	Increased mean corpuscular hemoglobin content‡
	Decreased hematocrit‡
	Decreased platelet number‡
	Decreased red cell number‡

From Nielsen FH (1994) Biochemical and physiologic consequences of boron deprivation in humans. Environ Health Perspect 102(Suppl):59-63.
*Deprivation consisted of 0.25 mg/2,000 kcal of boron for 63 days. Subjects included men older than age of 45 years, postmenopausal women not on hormone replacement therapy, and postmenopausal women on estrogen therapy.
†Found when dietary copper and magnesium were inadequate.
‡Found when dietary copper and magnesium were adequate.

Processes affected by dietary boron in humans are also affected in animal models. In chicks, low dietary boron exacerbated the distortion of marrow sprouts (i.e., the location of calcified scaffold erosion and new bone formation) and the delay in initiation of cartilage calcification in bones during marginal vitamin D deficiency (Hunt, 1996). Low dietary boron also diminished bone strength characteristics in pigs (Armstrong et al., 2000) and induced abnormal limb development in frogs (Fort et al., 2000). In rats, boron enhanced the beneficial effects of 17β-estradiol on trabecular bone volume and plate density in tibias of ovariectomized rats (Sheng et al., 2001). Boron deprivation was found to influence brain electrical activity systematically in mature rats; electrocorticograms (a recording of voltage fluctuations of the cortical surface of the brain) showed that the principal effect was on the frequency distribution of electrical activity (Penland, 1994). Evidence that boron affects the inflammatory process or immune function in higher animals includes the finding that, in rats injected with antigen to induce arthritis, boron deprivation resulted in more swelling of the paws, higher circulating neutrophil concentrations, and lower concentrations of natural killer cells (Hunt and Idso, 1999). In addition, low dietary boron increased inflammation caused by the intradermal injection of phytohemagglutinin in pigs (Armstrong et al., 2001).

BIOCHEMICAL FORMS AND ACTIONS INVOLVED OR IMPLICATED IN PHYSIOLOGICAL ACTIONS

Boron exists in biological material mainly bound to oxygen. Therefore, boron biochemistry is essentially that of boric acid. Boron has three *L*-shell electrons available for bonding as in boric acid, but there is a tendency for boron to acquire an additional electron pair to fill the fourth orbital. Therefore, boric acid acts as a Lewis acid and accepts an electron pair from a base (H_2O) to form tetracovalent boron compounds such as $B(OH)_4^-$. Thus, the reaction:

$$B(OH)_3 + H_2O \rightarrow B(OH)_4^- + H^+$$

at the pH of blood (7.4) results in dilute aqueous boric acid solutions composed of $B(OH)_3$ and $B(OH)_4^-$. Because the pK_a of boric acid is 9.2, the abundance of these two species in blood should be 98.4% and 1.6%, respectively.

Boric acid forms ester complexes with hydroxyl groups of organic compounds; this preferably occurs when the hydroxyl groups are adjacent and *cis* (Hunt, 2002). Among the hydroxylated substances of biological interest with which boron forms complexes are adenosine 5′-phosphate, pyridoxine, riboflavin, dehydroascorbic acid, and pyridine nucleotides. Formation of these complexes may be biologically important because in vitro formation of these complexes results in the competitive inhibition of some enzymes. Because borate complexes have a lower pK_a than free boric acid, boron may be an inhibitor of enzymes at physiological pH by shifting the pK_a of enzyme inhibitor complexes dependent upon an ionizing group in the protein (Hunt, 2002). Although boron monoesters are easily hydrolyzed when exposed to aqueous solutions, boron esters may have biological action in a hydrophobic environment such as in the lipid portions of cell membranes. The added stabilization of hydrogen bonding between the hydroxyl bound to boron and the hydrogen of an imidazole or amino group allows complexes to be formed between boric acid and compounds that contain a single hydroxyl group. Through formation of this type of complex, borate ($B_4O_7^{2+}$) and boronic acid derivatives [$RB(OH)_2$] can form transition state analogs that inhibit the activity of some enzymes. For example, serine protease is inhibited when a tetrahedral complex is formed between the serine hydroxyl group and borate, with hydrogen bonding to an imidazole ring of an adjacent histidine adding stabilization.

Naturally occurring organoboron compounds identified to date contain boron bound to four oxygen groups or as more stable boron diesters. Among these compounds are several antibiotics including boromycin, an antibiotic synthesized by *Streptomyces antibioticus* that has the ability to encapsulate alkali metal cations and increase the permeability of the cytoplasmic membrane to potassium ions. Boromycin strongly inhibits the replication of isolated human immunodeficiency virus-1 (HIV-1) and apparently blocks the release of infectious particles from cells infected with this virus (Kohno et al., 1996).

Two hypotheses have been advanced for the biochemical function of boron in higher animals. It is emphasized that these are speculated, not confirmed, functions of boron. The hypotheses accommodate a large and varied response to boron deprivation and the known biochemistry of boron. One hypothesis is that boron has a role in cell membrane function or stability such that it influences the response to hormone action, transmembrane signaling, or transmembrane movement of regulatory cations or anions (Nielsen, 1994). This hypothesis is supported by the recent identification of a bacterial quorum-sensing signal molecule that is a furanosyl borate diester (Chen et al., 2002). Quorum-sensing is the cell-to-cell communication in bacteria that is accomplished through the exchange of extracellular signaling molecules called autoinducers. The boron autoinducer (AI-2) has been proposed to be a universal signal for interspecies communication among bacteria. AI-2 is synthesized from adenosylmethionine, which supplies the 2′-3′-*cis*-diol of a ribose moiety that binds boron well. Another group of biomolecules that contain ribose moieties, the diadenosine phosphates, has been characterized as novel boron binders (Ralston and Hunt, 2001). Diadenosine phosphates function as signal nucleotides associated with platelet aggregation and neuronal response (Hunt, 2002). Boron deprivation affects the aggregation of platelets obtained from rats, suggesting boron may play a role in diadenosine phosphate signaling (Nielsen et al., 2002).

The second hypothesis is based upon the knowledge that two classes of enzymes are competitively inhibited in vitro by borate or its derivatives and upon findings showing that dietary boron can alter the activity in vivo of a number of these enzymes. Therefore, it has been hypothesized that boron is a metabolic regulator; that is, boron controls a number of metabolic pathways by competitively inhibiting some key enzyme reactions (Hunt, 1994). The reactions inhibited may include oxidoreductases that require the boron-binding *cis*-hydroxyl-containing pyridine of flavin nucleotides as a cofactor. Perhaps boron regulates the inflammatory process by dampening the activity of NADP-requiring oxidoreductase, which is involved in the generation of reactive oxygen species during the respiratory burst in activated leukocytes (Hunt, 2002). Further evidence that boron affects the metabolism of reactive oxygen species includes increased red blood cell catalase activity in rats (Hunt and Idso, 1999), increased plasma 8-iso-prostaglandin $F_{2\alpha}$ in rats (Nielsen, 2004), and decreased erythrocyte superoxide dismutase activity in men and postmenopausal women (Nielsen, 1997) in response to boron deprivation.

DIETARY CONSIDERATIONS

Both intestinal absorption and urinary excretion of boron are very efficient. Boron is thought to be transported in the blood as $B(OH)_3$, and its concentration can be decreased or increased by apparent deficient and excessive intakes of boron, respectively. The highest concentrations of boron are found in fruits, fruit-based beverages, vegetables, legumes and nuts. Depending upon the source, water can contribute a major portion of dietary boron. Municipal drinking water in the United States contains about 0.005 to 2 mg boron per liter. Based on data from the third National Health and Nutrition Examination Survey (NHANES III; 1988-1994), the median boron intake from foods is 1.3 and 1.0 mg/day for adults (19 to 70 years of age) in the United States; estimates for adults of similar ages were 1.2 and 0.9 mg/day based on the Continuing Survey of Food Intakes by Individuals (CSFII,1994-1996) database. Intakes ranged from a low of approximately 0.33 mg/day to a high of 3.0 mg/day. Supplements, particularly "body-building supplements," can be a significant source of boron intake.

In the human studies described in the preceding text, subjects responded to boron supplementation (3 mg/day) following a boron-depletion period during which they consumed a diet supplying only about 0.25 mg of boron per 2,000 kcal for 63 days. Therefore, humans apparently receive benefit from a boron intake greater than 0.25 mg per day or have a dietary boron requirement greater than this amount. A World Health Organization Expert Consultation on Trace Elements in Human Nutrition (WHO, 1996) suggested that an acceptable safe range of population mean intakes for boron for adults could be 1 to 13 mg/day. The Institute of Medicine (IOM) of the National Academy of Science in the United States chose not to establish recommendations for daily boron intake because of the lack of a clear biological function for boron in humans and the limited evidence on which to base a recommendation (IOM, 2001).

The IOM did, however, set tolerable upper intake levels (ULs) for different age groups for boron. The ULs are based largely on animal studies using adverse reproductive and developmental effects as the critical endpoint. The UL for adults is 20 mg/day.

CHROMIUM

NUTRITIONAL AND PHYSIOLOGICAL SIGNIFICANCE

Approximately 45 years ago, trivalent chromium was reported to be the active component of the "glucose tolerance factor" that alleviated impaired glucose tolerance in rats fed torula yeast–sucrose diets (Schwarz and Mertz, 1959). At that time the generally accepted definition of essentiality was that a dietary deficiency of a substance had to consistently and adversely change a biological function from optimal, and this change had to be reversible or preventable by nutritional, not pharmacological, intakes of the substance. Because chromium apparently was needed for normal glucose tolerance, it was designated as an essential nutrient for higher animals. Essentiality for humans gained acceptance when it was reported that a human on long-term total parenteral nutrition containing a low amount of chromium developed impaired glucose tolerance, or high blood sugar with glucose spilling into the urine, and a resistance to insulin action; these abnormalities were reversed by supplementation with 250 μg of chromium per day for 2 weeks (Jeejeebhoy et al., 1977). Similar symptoms and benefits of chromium supplementation were observed in two other patients on TPN (Freund et al., 1979; Brown et al., 1986). Subsequently, a number of reports from numerous research groups described beneficial effects of chromium supplementation of subjects with varying degrees of glucose intolerance, ranging from hypoglycemia (low blood sugar) to insulin-dependent diabetes (Anderson, 1993; Anderson et al., 1997). Also, beneficial effects of chromium supplementation on blood lipid profiles were reported. These findings promoted the concept of chromium essentiality.

However, as the decades passed without a defined biochemical function for chromium, doubts arose about it being categorized as essential. These doubts were heightened by difficulties in inducement of consistent signs of chromium deficiency in experimental animals. Nutritional, metabolic, physiological, or hormonal stressors generally had to be employed to induce experimental animals to respond to chromium deprivation; in most cases, the responses were not remarkable. In addition, numerous studies in humans found no observable effect of chromium supplementation on lipid profiles, glucose tolerance, or diabetes. The development of the controversy about chromium essentiality has been reviewed by Vincent (2004, 2001). It is possible that chromodulin, a naturally occurring, bioactive peptide containing chromium, may be the biologically active form of chromium. Chromodulin was previously called low-molecular-weight Cr-binding substance (Davis and Vincent, 1997). It has been suggested that chromodulin is nothing more than a molecule for the detoxification and excretion of chromium (Stearns, 2000). However, Vincent (2004) recently provided substantial evidence for chromodulin having an insulin amplification role.

POSSIBLE BIOCHEMICAL FORMS AND PHYSIOLOGICAL ACTIONS

Cr^{3+} is the most stable oxidation state of chromium and most likely is the valence state of importance in biological systems. Cr^{+6}, which is a byproduct of manufacturing stainless steel, pigments, chromate chemicals, and other products, also is stable. However, Cr^{+6} would presumably be readily reduced to Cr^{+3} by reducing agents in foods or within the upper gastrointestinal tract. Estimates of Cr^{3+} absorption, based on metabolic balance studies or on urinary excretion from physiological intakes, range from 0.4% to 2.5%. Most ingested chromium is excreted unabsorbed in the feces. Most absorbed chromium is excreted rapidly in the urine. The highest levels of chromium in human tissues are found in liver, spleen, and bone. There is evidence that chromium absorption may be increased with resistance exercise. Cr^{3+} competes for one of the binding sites on transferrin, and most of the chromium in blood apparently is found bound to transferrin.

In aqueous solutions, Cr^{3+} complexes are relatively inert kinetically such that ligand-displacement reactions have half-times in the range of several hours. Therefore, chromium is unlikely to be involved as a metal catalyst at the active site of enzymes where the rate of exchange needs to be rapid. However, chromium may have a structural role such as in the tertiary structure of a protein or nucleic acid. In addition, chromium may bind ligands in the proper orientation to facilitate enzymatic catalysis; this apparently is the role for chromodulin.

Chromodulin is a mammalian oligopeptide with a mass of about 1.5 kDa that is composed of glycine, cysteine, aspartate, and glutamate and that binds four chromic ions tightly and cooperatively ($K_a \sim 10^{21}\ M^{-4}$) (Vincent, 2004, 2003). Apochromodulin, which is apparently the predominant form in vivo, can accept chromic ions from other biological molecules such as transferrin, which apparently can serve as a transporter of chromium (Clodfelder et al., 2001). Two potential functions for chromodulin have been described (Vincent, 2004). First, chromodulin may be involved in chromium detoxification because it carries chromium into the urine after a large dose is given. Second, chromodulin may provide a unique autoamplification system for insulin signaling. Chromodulin has been shown to activate the tyrosine kinase activity of insulin-activated insulin receptors. The binding of insulin to its receptor on an insulin-sensitive cell causes a conformational change resulting in the autophosphorylation of tyrosine residues on the internal side of the receptor. The receptor becomes an active tyrosine kinase that transmits the insulin signal into the cell. In response to insulin, chromium also moves into insulin-sensitive cells, which contain apochromodulin, to form holochromodulin. The holochromodulin then binds to the receptor to assist in maintaining it in an active form, thus amplifying the receptor's kinase activity. When blood insulin decreases, a change in the conformation of the insulin receptor causes a release of the holochromodulin from the cell to blood and excretion in the urine. Chromium is specifically needed by the oligopeptide for activity. Apochromodulin was inactive in stimulating insulin receptor kinase activity. Titration with chromic ions completely restored activity, whereas other transition metals known to be essential failed to restore activity (Vincent, 2004).

Ribonucleic acid (RNA) synthesis directed by free DNA in vitro has been shown to be enhanced by the binding of chromium to the template. Furthermore, chromium is concentrated in hepatic nuclei 48 hours after intraperitoneal injection of $CrCl_3$. The chromium is preferentially bound to DNA in chromatin and increases the number of initiation sites, which enhances RNA synthesis. Perhaps chromium, or a biologically active form of chromium, has a role in regulating gene expression of a critical substance in glucose metabolism.

Nutrition Insight

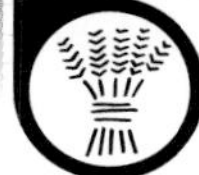

Use of Chromium Picolinate Supplements for Weight Reduction and Muscle Building

The general media and health-food or supplement industry, frequently with help from the scientific community, have reported on various nutrients in such a way that the American public is misguided, bewildered, or uncertain as to what to believe. Quite often, a nutrient bursts onto the scene and is touted everywhere as an aid to improving health or body image; shortly thereafter, findings are reported that dispute these claims. Promotion of chromium, especially as chromium picolinate, as an ergogenic aid or weight-loss inducer fits into this category.

The most compelling evidence that chromium picolinate can help build muscles has come from the laboratory of the scientist who patented the method to make this compound. Several studies reported subsequently have not confirmed that the use of chromium supplements, including the picolinate form, will bring forth the overzealously touted propitious effects on muscle accretion, strength gain, or athletic performance.

In addition to a number of studies indicating little or no effect of chromium picolinate supplements, studies used as a basis for claims that chromium picolinate promotes weight reduction and muscle building provide limited evidence to support the claims. For example, weight reduction claims are based on the conjecture that insulin action is affected by chromium so that glucose is less likely to be converted into fat and will suppress appetite. Only a few studies have shown that chromium picolinate supplementation results in reductions in body weight; these reductions have been small and questionable. In one study (Kaats et al., 1991), the average fat loss was 4.2 pounds, with an average 1.4-pound increase in fat-free mass over a 72-day period of chromium supplementation; this translates to a loss of only 2.8 pounds after 10 weeks of treatment. This amount of weight loss does not conform to the usual claims for chromium supplements. In another study (Kaats et al, 1992), the weight loss program was not limited to chromium supplementation; it included moderate caloric restriction and other dietary modifications. Therefore, although a respectable average weight loss of 15 pounds was achieved in 8 weeks in this study, the loss could not be attributed solely to the chromium picolinate supplement. These studies, coupled with a small fat loss with a weight-training program reported by the holder of the chromium picolinate patent and with hearsay and testimonial evidence, are the basis for the weight loss claims for chromium. In contrast to weight-loss claims,

Continued

Nutrition Insight

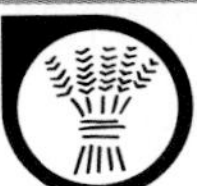

Use of Chromium Picolinate Supplements for Weight Reduction and Muscle Building—cont'd

most studies of participants in weight-training programs involving chromium picolinate supplementation gained weight. In other words, there are no data from well-controlled studies to support the astonishing weight-loss claims made for the use of chromium picolinate supplements.

Thinking Critically

1. One advertisement claims that a supplement containing chromium picolinate can "blast off" 49 pounds in only 29 days without exercising and with no problem in eating up to six times a day. Does this claim seem possible given what you know about energy metabolism? (See Chapters 21 and 22.)
2. It has been found that a supplement of 1,000 μg of chromium per day as chromium picolinate may reduce some of he abnormalities of diabetes. Should this intake of chromium be considered nutritional?

DIETARY CONSIDERATIONS

In the absence of a functional criterion for assessing chromium status, the IOM (2001) set adequate intakes (AIs) for chromium rather than estimated average requirements (EARs) and recommended dietary allowances (RDAs). On the basis of a limited number of chromium balance studies and determinations of dietary intakes of chromium by adults, the Food and Nutrition Board of the IOM determined that the mean chromium content of well-balanced daily diets was 13.4 μg/1,000 kcal (IOM, 2001). With use of this relationship between chromium and energy in the diet, AIs were set for children and adults. The AI for chromium was set at 35 and 25 μg/day for men and women, respectively, ages 19 to 50 years. Because of lower energy intakes, the AIs for men and women ages 51 to 70 years and older than 70 years were set at 30 μg/day and 20 μg/day. An increment of 5 μg/day was added for pregnant women, based on addition of 16 kg to the reference weight of the woman. For lactating women, an increment of 20 μg/day was added based on secretion of 0.2 μg/day in milk and the assumption that 1% of dietary chromium is absorbed. AIs for children were extrapolated from those for adults, ages 19 through 30 years, using metabolic weight ($kg^{0.75}$). Metabolic body weight was used as a base for extrapolation because the urinary excretion of chromium is increased with exercise. The AIs replaced the estimated safe and adequate daily dietary intake (ESADDI) of 50 to 200 μg/day set by the National Research Council as part of the 10th edition of the *Recommended Dietary Allowances* (NRC, 1989).

For infants, AIs were based on chromium intake from human milk (0.25 μg/L × 0.78 L/day) for newborns to 6-month-old infants, and on intake from human milk (0.25 μg/L × 0.60 L/day) plus complementary foods (5.36 μg/day) for 7- to 12-month-old infants. The AIs for infants in the first and second half of the first year of life are 0.2 μg/day and 5.5 μg/day, respectively. The mean concentrations of chromium in cow's milk and infant formulas (about 0.8 and 4.8 μg/L, respectively) are higher than that for human milk.

No national survey data are available on chromium intakes. Chromium is widely distributed throughout the food supply, but the chromium content of a food is highly variable among different lots of the same food and is subject to increases or decreases during food processing. Whole grains, pulses, some vegetables (e.g., broccoli and mushrooms), liver, processed meats, ready-to-eat cereals, spices, and beer are generally good sources. Dietary chromium content based on paired food or duplicate meal analyses for self-selected diets yielded mean chromium intakes of 22 to 48 μg/day for 10 adult men and 13 to 36 μg/day for

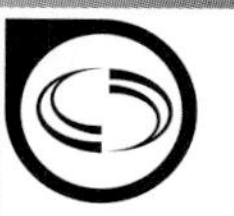

DRIs Across the Life Cycle

	AI µg Chromium per Day	RDA µg Molybdenum per Day
Infants		
0 to 0.5 yr		2 (AI)
0.5 to 1 yr		3 (AI)
Children		
1 to 3 yr	11	17
4 to 8 yr	15	22
Males,		
9 to 13 yr	25	34
14 to 18 yr	35	43
19 to 50 yr	35	45
>50 yr	30	45
Females		
9 to 13 yr	21	34
14 to 18 yr	24	43
19 to 50 yr	25	45
>50 yr	20	45
Pregnant	30	50
Lactating	45	50

NOTE: No RDA or AI has been established for boron.
Data from Institute of Medicine (2001) Dietary Reference Intakes for Vitamin A, Vitamin K, Arsenic, Boron, Chromium, Copper, Iodine, Iron, Manganese, Molybdenum, Nickel, Silicon, Vanadium, and Zinc. National Academy Press, Washington, DC.
AI, Adequate intake; *RDA*, recommended dietary allowance.

23 adult women (Anderson and Kozlovsky, 1985); these estimates are probably lower than normal intakes because of evidence that subjects decrease their energy intake when involved in a dietary collection or study. Based on NHANES III, 8 % of adults take supplements that contain chromium, and the average intake of supplemental chromium by these adults is 23 µg/day. The most popular form of supplemental chromium is chromium picolinate; other forms include chromium chloride, chromium nicotinate, and chromium histidine. Chromodulin mimetics are being proposed as a form for chromium supplementation. Few serious adverse effects have been reported as the result of excess intake of chromium from food.

Food Sources

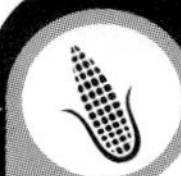

Good Food Sources of Boron, Chromium, and Molybdenum

Boron

Fruits
Leafy and cruciferous vegetables
Nuts
Legumes and pulses
Wine and cider

Chromium

Whole grain products, including some ready-to-eat bran cereals
Nuts and pulses
Organ meats (liver)

Molybdenum

Milk and milk products
Pulses or dried legumes
Organ meats (liver and kidney)
Cereals

No UL was set for dietary chromium (soluble Cr^{+3} salts) because of insufficient data and little evidence for adverse effects. It should be noted, however, that hexavalent chromium has a much higher level of toxicity and is classified as a human carcinogen, mutagen, and clastogen. Recently, it has been suggested that further study of long-term supplementation with chromium picolinate (Vincent, 2004) and chromodulin mimetics (Mulyani et al, 2004) is needed because of the possibility that the chromium in these compounds is converted into Cr^{+6} in vivo.

MOLYBDENUM

Molybdenum is an established essential element on the basis of a nutritional requirement for inorganic molybdenum for synthesis of a molybdenum cofactor that is required for the activity of sulfite oxidase, xanthine dehydrogenase, and aldehyde oxidase in mammals. The identification of inborn errors of metabolism that affected molybdenum cofactor synthesis provided the bulk of the evidence for molybdenum's classification as essential.

BIOCHEMICAL FORMS AND ACTIONS INVOLVED OR IMPLICATED IN PHYSIOLOGICAL ACTIONS

Molybdenum is a transition element that readily changes its oxidation state and can thus act as an electron transfer agent in oxidation–reduction reactions in which it cycles from Mo^{6+} to reduced states. This explains why molybdenum functions as an enzyme cofactor in all forms of life. Molybdenum is present at the active site in a small nonprotein cofactor containing a pterin nucleus in all known molybdoenzymes except nitrogenase (Johnson, 1997). More than 40% of the molybdenum not attached to an enzyme in the liver exists as this cofactor bound to the mitochondrial outer membrane. This form is transferred to an apomolybdoenzyme to make the holomolybdoenzyme (Rajagoplan, 1988). The molybdoenzymes in mammalian systems also contain Fe–S centers and flavin cofactors. Molybdoenzymes catalyze the hydroxylation of various substrates by using oxygen atoms from water. Aldehyde oxidase oxidizes and detoxifies various pyrimidines, purines, pteridines, and related compounds. Xanthine oxidase/dehydrogenase catalyzes the transformation of hypoxanthine to xanthine and of xanthine to uric acid. Hypoxanthine and xanthine are intermediates in the degradation of purines. Sulfite oxidase catalyzes the transformation of sulfite, formed mainly from cysteine catabolism, to sulfate.

ABSORPTION, TRANSPORT, AND EXCRETION

Turnlund and colleagues (1995b) conducted a study in four young men who were fed five amounts of molybdenum, ranging from 22 to 1,490 μg/day, for periods of 24 days each. No adverse effects were observed at any of the intakes. However, urinary excretion of uric acid was decreased and urinary xanthine excretion was increased in response to a load dose of adenosine monophosphate (AMP) when the men were adapted to the lowest level of molybdenum (22 μg/day); these findings indicate that xanthine oxidase activity was decreased by the low-molybdenum regimen. Using stable isotopes of molybdenum as tracers, Turnlund and colleagues (1995b) determined that molybdenum was efficiently absorbed, 88% to 93%, at all dietary molybdenum intakes, and absorption was most efficient at the highest level of dietary molybdenum. The amount and percentage of molybdenum excreted in the urine increased as dietary molybdenum increased, suggesting that molybdenum retention is regulated by urinary excretion.

MOLYBDENUM COFACTOR SYNTHESIS

The molybdenum cofactor is an unstable reduced pterin with a unique four-carbon side chain, which is synthesized by a complex pathway that requires the protein products encoded by at least four different genes (*MOCS1, MOCS2, MOCS3*, and *GEPH*). Both *MOCS1* (molybdenum cofactor synthesis-step 1) and *MOCS2* (molybdenum cofactor synthesis-step 2) are bicistronic genes, encoding two proteins in different open reading frames. The protein products are designated MOCS1A and B and MOCS2A and B and are required for synthesis of the organic moiety of the molybdenum cofactor; this moiety is called molybdopterin. Molybdopterin synthase (MOCS2A and B) must be activated by a sulfotransferase that is the product of *MOCS3*. *GEPH* encodes gephyrin, which is required during cofactor assembly for insertion of molybdenum. Gephyrin is a bifunctional protein that is essential for synaptic clustering of inhibitory neurotransmitter receptors in the central nervous system as well as the biosynthesis of the molybdenum cofactor in peripheral tissues. The steps in molybdenum cofactor formation are illustrated in Figure 41-1.

INBORN ERRORS IN MOLYBDENUM COFACTOR SYNTHESIS

Molybdenum cofactor deficiency is a rare inborn error of metabolism. Mutations that affect molybdenum cofactor synthesis result in the simultaneous loss of activity of all human molybdenum cofactor–dependent enzymes that in humans include sulfite oxidase, xanthine dehydrogenase, and aldehyde oxidase. Combined deficiency of these enzymes leads to a severe phenotype, which clinically is very similar to that observed in patients with the rarer isolated sulfite oxidase deficiency.

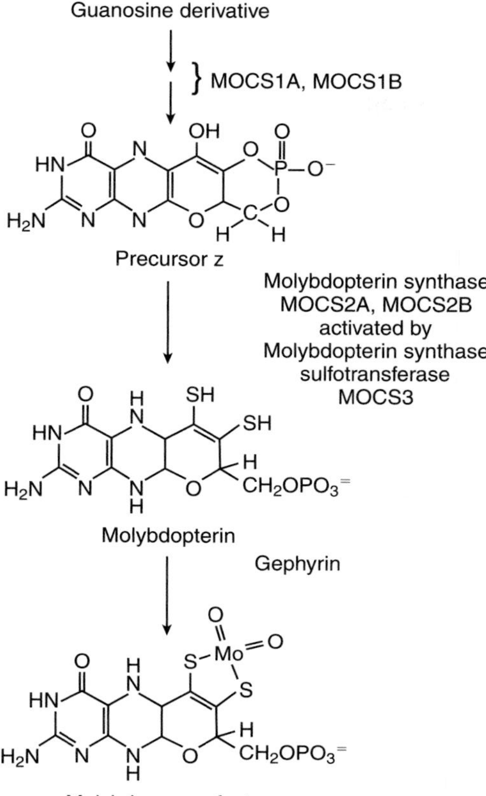

Figure 41-1 Pathway of molybdenum cofactor biosynthesis. The genes/proteins that are responsible for molybdenum cofactor synthesis are named MOCS for molybdenum cofactor synthesis and are numbered 1, 2 and 3. The gephyrin protein (encoded by *GEPH*) is necessary for insertion of molybdenum during cofactor assembly. *From Reis J, Johnson JL (2003) Mutations in the molybdenum cofactor biosynthetic genes MOCS1, MOCS2, and GEPH. Hum Mutat 21:570. Reprinted with permission of Wiley-Liss, Inc., a subsidiary of John Wiley & Sons, Inc.*

The two conditions can easily be distinguished by diminished uric acid levels and elevated xanthine concentrations in plasma and urine that result from the decreased xanthine dehydrogenase activity in the combined cofactor deficiency but not in isolated sulfite oxidase deficiency.

Diagnosis of molybdenum cofactor deficiency is usually made shortly after birth because of a failure to thrive and neonatal seizures that are often unresponsive to therapy. Biochemical findings include abnormal sulfur and purine metabolites in urine, such as elevated urinary sulfite and S-sulfocysteine, hypouricemia, and the detection of molybdoenzyme activity deficiency in fibroblasts. S-sulfonated transthyretin is currently being explored as a possible tool for laboratory diagnosis of sulfite oxidase deficiency; in one study the S-sulfonated transthyretin peak was less than 2% of total transthyretin in control sera but greater than 85% of total transthyretin in patients with molybdenum cofactor deficiency (Kishikawa et al., 2000). There currently is no effective therapy for molybdenum cofactor deficiency, and the prognosis is usually poor. The disease is associated with a pronounced and progressive loss of white matter in the brain. Mild cases of the disease have been reported, probably the result of a low level residual activity of the mutant protein. However, most recognized cases have been severe; most patients die in early childhood and some survive for only a few days.

Most disease-producing mutations have been identified in *MOCS1* and *MOCS2* (Reiss and Johnson, 2003). Mutations of *MOCS3* are very rare (Yamamoto et al., 2003; Ichida et al., 2001). A mutation in *GEPH* was recently identified in fibroblasts of a patient from a family with three deceased children who had all been diagnosed as molybdenum cofactor–deficient. (Reiss et al., 2001). Supplementation of the fibroblast culture medium with 1 mmol/L molybdate restored the normal phenotype, suggesting that molybdate supplementation might be of therapeutic benefit in patients with this more unusual form of the disease.

NUTRITIONAL REQUIREMENT FOR MOLYBDENUM

Although molybdenum is an established essential element, it is not of much practical concern in human nutrition. Reports of signs of nutritional molybdenum deficiency in humans are very few (Rajagopalan, 1988). As mentioned in the preceding text, mild biochemical signs of molybdenum deficiency were observed by Turnlund and colleagues (1995a) in men fed only 22 μg molybdenum per day for 24 days. In a separate study, the low molybdate diet was fed for 102 days; molybdenum balance was slightly positive from days 49 to 102 and no biochemical signs of deficiency were observed (Turnlund et al., 1995b). Preadolescent girls maintained positive balance on molybdenum intakes between 43 and 80 μg/day (Engel et al., 1967).

A convincing case of molybdenum deprivation was observed in a patient receiving prolonged parenteral nutrition therapy (Abumrad et al., 1981). Signs and symptoms exhibited by this patient, which were exacerbated by methionine administration, included high methionine and low uric acid levels in blood, high oxypurines and low uric acid in urine, and very low urinary sulfate excretion. This patient had mental disturbances that progressed to coma. Intravenous supplementation of the patient with ammonium molybdate improved the clinical condition, reversed the sulfur-handling defect, and normalized uric acid production.

Molybdenum deficiency signs also are difficult to induce in animals (Mills and Davis, 1987). In rats and chicks, excessive dietary tungsten was used to restrict molybdenum absorption and thus induce molybdenum deficiency signs, which included depressed activities of molybdoenzymes, disturbed uric acid metabolism, and increased susceptibility to sulfite toxicity.

DIETARY REFERENCE INTAKES FOR MOLYBDENUM

Although molybdenum apparently is normally of minor nutritional concern, it should not be ignored. Molybdenum may have beneficial effects when a person is stressed by high intakes of xenobiotics. Molybdenum hydroxylases apparently are as important as the microsomal monooxygenase systems in the metabolism of drugs and foreign compounds (Beedham, 1985). This may be the basis for a few reports suggesting that molybdenum may be anticarcinogenic.

Although molybdenum deficiency has not been observed in healthy people, dietary reference intakes (DRIs) have been set for molybdenum (IOM, 2001). An AI for infants was based on the molybdenum intake from human milk and set at 2 and 3 μg/day, respectively, for infants ages 0 to 6 months and 7 to 12 months. Human milk contains approximately 2 μg of molybdenum per liter, whereas cow's milk (~50 μg/L) and soymilk contain more. Based on the balance studies done by Turnlund and colleagues (1995b), which indicated adults could achieve molybdenum balance on an intake of 22 μg/day, the requirement was estimated to be 25 μg/day (22 μg/day plus 3 μg/day to allow for miscellaneous losses not measured in the study). Because some foods, such as soy, have lower bioavailability than the foods provided in the balance studies done by Turnlund and coworkers, the IOM used an average bioavailability of 75% to set an EAR of 34 μg/day for adults. The RDA was set as the EAR + 30% and is 45 μg/day for adults. DRIs for children were extrapolated from the adult value, using metabolic weight ($kg^{0.75}$) as the base for extrapolation. An increment of 5 μg per day to the RDA for pregnant women was based on a gain of 16 kg during pregnancy. The molybdenum RDA for lactating women was increased by 5 μg per day based on daily secretion of 1.6 μg molybdenum in the milk (2 μg/L × 0.78 L/day).

For most of the population, the diet is the most important source of molybdenum. Plant foods are the major sources of molybdenum in the diet, and their molybdenum content depends upon the content of the soil in which they are grown. Good food sources of molybdenum include legumes, grain products, and nuts. Two studies of molybdenum intake in the United States yielded average intakes ranging from 76 to 240 μg/day for adults (Pennington and Jones, 1987; Tsongas et al., 1980). Therefore, almost all diets should meet the RDA for molybdenum.

Molybdenum has relatively low toxicity. Although molybdenum is mainly obtained from the diet, ammonium tetrathiomolybdate is used as an experimental chelating agent for copper in patients with Wilson's disease. Based largely on animal studies, the IOM (2001) set the UL for molybdenum at 2,000 μg/day for adults.

PROSPECTIVE BIOACTIVE ULTRATRACE ELEMENTS: NICKEL, VANADIUM, SILICON, AND ARSENIC

Nickel, vanadium, silicon, and arsenic are bioactive in higher animals and are components of naturally occurring and biologically important molecules. Biological roles for these elements have been established in lower forms of life, which indicate that they may be essential or have beneficial bioactive actions in humans.

NICKEL

Nickel is generally acknowledged as being essential for plants and some bacteria. In these lower forms of life, nickel has been identified as an essential component of seven different enzymes: urease, hydrogenase, carbon monoxide dehydrogenase, methyl-coenzyme M reductase, Ni-superoxide dismutase, glyoxalase I, and acireductone dioxygenase (Pochapsky et al., 2002; Watt and Ludden, 1999). In the six different microbial enzymes known to contain nickel, the nature of the nickel-containing active center varies widely. Interestingly, the substrates or products for all these enzymes are dissolved gases: hydrogen, carbon monoxide, carbon dioxide, methane, oxygen, and ammonia. Although an essential biochemical function in higher animals has not been identified for nickel, deprivation studies show that it has beneficial, if not essential, functions in several experimental animal models. Nickel deprivation detrimentally affects vision, sperm production and motility, blood pressure, iron metabolism, and sodium homeostasis in animals (Yokoi et al., 2003; Nielsen et al., 2002). Yokoi and colleagues (2003) speculated that nickel may affect the function of cyclic nucleotide-gated channels.

Nickel appears to be a universal component of ureases (urea amidohydrolases). Nickel has been found in ureases from bacteria, mycoplasmata, fungi, yeasts, algae, higher plants, and invertebrates. Highly purified urease contains two Ni^{2+} ions per 97-kDa subunit; the two Ni^{2+} ions are coordinated in a tetrapyrrole complex. An elegant model has been proposed for the mechanism of urease action, which involves polarization of the urea carbonyl by one nickel ion to allow nucleophilic attack by an activated hydroxyl anion associated with the second nickel ion (Ragsdale, 2000).

The hydrogenases are an extremely heterogeneous group of enzymes that catalyze the simplest oxidation–reduction process of $H_2 \leftrightarrow 2H^+ + 2e^-$. Hydrogenases that contain nickel have been identified for more than 35 species of bacteria, including methanogenic, hydrogen-oxidizing, sulfate-reducing, phototrophic, and aerobic N_2-fixing bacteria. Nickel may be a common constituent of hydrogenases that function physiologically to oxidize rather than to evolve H_2. Nickel is redox active in hydrogenases and interacts with the substrate H_2. In hydrogenases Ni^{2+} is coordinately linked to S of three cysteine residues, one of which is also coordinated with an Fe atom (Mobley et al., 1995).

Carbon monoxide dehydrogenase, which oxidizes CO to CO_2, is a nickel enzyme found in acetogenic, methanogenic, phototrophic, and sulfate-reducing anaerobic bacteria (Thauer, 2001). In addition to oxidizing CO to CO_2, carbon monoxide dehydrogenase in acetogenic bacteria catalyzes the reduction of CO_2 to CO and the synthesis and degradation of acetyl CoA, and therefore can also be designated as an acetyl CoA synthase. Nickel CO dehydrogenase contains a novel Ni–4Fe–5S cluster in its active site. The Ni^{2+} is bound by four S atoms of cysteine residues and shares three of these S atoms with the four Fe atoms in the cluster.

Methyl-*S*-coenzyme M reductase is the terminal enzyme in the conversion of CO_2 to methane in methanogenic bacteria (Goenrich et al., 2004). This enzyme contains a Ni^{1+} porphyrinoid prosthetic group. During catalysis, the nickel is oxidized to Ni^{2+} or Ni^{3+}.

Nickel superoxide dismutase from *Streptomyces seoulensis* contains a Ni^{3+} ion coordinately bonded to the amino and amidazole groups of His-1, the amide and thiolate groups of Cys-2, and the thiolate of Cys-6 that is lost in the chemically reduced state, in an N-terminal active-site loop (His-Cys-X-X-Pro-Cys-Gly-X-Tyr) (Barondeau et al., 2004; Wuerges et al., 2004).

Glyoxalase I in *Escherichia coli* contains Ni^{2+}, which is coordinated by two water molecules, two histidine residues, and two glutamate residues (Davidson et al., 2001). Most glyoxalase enzymes, including human glyoxalase, are active with Zn^{2+}.

Acireductone dioxygenase in *Klebsiella pneumoniae* is a metalloenzyme that catalyzes two different reactions depending upon the metal ion bound in its active site (Pochapsky et al., 2002). When Ni^{2+} is bound the acireductone produced in the methionine salvage pathway and oxygen is converted into methylthiobutyric acid, formate, and carbon monoxide. Acireductone dioxygenase is a stable single

179-residue polypeptide. Nickel is bound by three histidine and one glutamate residue in the enzyme. When iron is bound to acireductone dioxygenase, acireductone is converted into ketoacid, the precursor of methionine, and formate.

In addition to its redox role, nickel apparently has a regulatory role in the expression of hydrogenase (Kim et al., 1991). Nickel may be required for the synthesis of the hydrogenase mRNA in *Bradyrhizobium japonicum*. For the hydrogenase gene to be expressed, O_2 and H_2 diffuse into the cell and affect the redox state of the nickel bound to a nickel-containing, DNA-binding protein, which in turn leads to transcriptional upregulation of expression of the hydrogenase gene.

Typical daily dietary intakes for nickel are 70 to 260 μg/day for adults in the United States and Canada. For individuals taking supplements, the average intake from supplements is 5 μg/day. Rich sources of nickel include chocolate, nuts, legumes, and grains. Absorption of dietary nickel is typically less than 10% of intake. In the plasma, most nickel is bound to albumin. The IOM (2001) did not set an RDA or AI for nickel because of lack of evidence for an essential function in humans. If a dietary requirement for nickel is found for humans, it most likely will be less than 100 μg/day.

The IOM (2001) did establish ULs for nickel based on levels that caused general systemic toxicity in rats. The UL is 1.0 mg/day for adults. The risk of adverse effects from excess intakes of nickel from food and supplements is low. Exposure to excess nickel via contaminated water or environmental exposure is of greater risk.

VANADIUM

There is no question that vanadium is a bioactive element. Its ability to selectively inhibit protein tyrosine phosphatases at submicromolar concentrations probably explains the broad range of effects vanadium has on cellular regulatory cascades. The mechanism by which vanadium inhibits protein tyrosine phosphatases has been suggested to involve the generation of H_2O_2 upon the conversion of the pentavalent V^{+5} anion, vanadate (VO_3^-), to the intracellular tetravalent V^{+4} anion, vanadyl (VO_2^+), which is catalyzed by NADPH oxidase. The vanadyl may then react with H_2O_2 to form peroxovanadate (Hulley and Davison, 2003). Peroxovanadate quickly and irreversibly oxidizes the active site cysteine to cysteic acid in protein tyrosine phosphatase. Protein tyrosine phosphatase inhibition apparently is the basis for vanadium having insulin-like actions at the cellular level and stimulating cellular proliferation and differentiation. The insulin-mimetic action of vanadium has resulted in an effort to develop vanadium compounds that could be therapeutic agents for diabetes (Marzban and McNeill, 2003). In addition to having effects at pharmacological intakes, vanadium may affect phosphorylation–dephosphorylation at physiological or nutritional intakes such that a regulatory cascade is altered. This may be the basis for observations of altered thyroid metabolism and depressed growth in rats deprived of vanadium (Nielsen, 1998). In goats, vanadium deprivation decreased the life span, increased the rate of spontaneous abortions, caused convulsions, and resulted in skeletal deformities in the forelegs (Anke et al., 1990).

A relationship between vanadium and H_2O_2 apparently exists in lower forms of life (algae, lichens, fungi, and bacteria) in which vanadium has functional roles (Eady, 1990; Wever and Krenn, 1990). Vanadium-dependent bromoperoxidases have been found in a number of marine brown algae, marine red algae, and a terrestial lichen. Vanadium-dependent iodoperoxidases have been detected in brown seaweeds, and a vanadium-dependent chloroperoxidase has been identified in the fungus *Curvularia inaequalis*. Haloperoxidases catalyze the oxidation of halide ions by hydrogen peroxide, thereby facilitating the formation of a carbon–halogen bond. The mechanism of action of vanadium in the haloperoxidases, as indicated by studies of the bromoperoxidases, is H_2O_2 reacting with vanadium as V^{5+} to form a dioxygen species that reacts with the halide to yield an oxidized halide species, which is the intermediate that forms the carbon–halogen bond.

No RDA or AI was set by the IOM (2001) for vanadium based on a lack of evidence for a requirement in humans. Based on animal experiments, any requirement for vanadium would be small; a daily dietary intake of 10 μg probably would meet any postulated requirement. Typical intake of vanadium from foods is 6 to 18 μg/day for adults, and intake from supplements averages about 9 μg/day for those who take supplements containing vanadyl sulfate or sodium metavanadate (Pennington and Jones, 1987). Good sources of vanadium include grains and grain products, sweeteners, infant cereals, mushrooms, parsley, and shellfish. Absorbed vanadate (V^{5+}, $H_2VO_4^-$) is converted to the vanadyl cation (V^{4+}, VO^{2+}), which can complex with ferritin and transferrin in the plasma. Based on evidence for renal toxicity in animals, the IOM (2001) set the UL for adults at 1,800 μg of vanadium per day. This is many times the normal intake from diet and supplements.

SILICON

Silicon is essential for lower forms of life (Carlisle, 1984). Silicon plays a structural role in diatoms, radiolarians, and some sponges. It may be needed by some higher plants, including rice. Diatoms, which are unicellular microscopic plants, have an absolute requirement for silicon as monomeric silicic acid for normal cell growth. The diatom, *Cylindrotheca fusiformis*, has five silicon transporter genes that tightly control silicon uptake and use in cell wall formation (Hildebrand et al., 1998). Silicon is bioactive or essential in higher animals because experiments with rats comparing low intakes with physiological intakes show that silicon affects collagen and glycosaminoglycan formation and is beneficial in promoting bone formation and wound healing (Seaborn and Nielsen, 1993). Recently, low intakes of silicon have been associated with an increased incidence of hip fracture (Reffitt et al., 2003; Jugdaohsingh et al., 2002).

The IOM (2001) judged that animal and human data are too limited to allow setting any DRIs for silicon. Based on the Total Diet Study (1991-1997), the median daily intakes of silicon were 15 and 22 mg/day for women and men (ages 19 to 70 years), respectively. The range of intakes (1st and 99th percentile intakes for all individuals) was 3.5 to 80 mg/day. Median intake from supplements by supplement users was 2 mg/day. The richest sources of silicon are unrefined grains of high fiber content and cereal products.

ARSENIC

Arsenic is unquestionably a bioactive element in higher animals and humans. However, the concept that arsenic has beneficial or essential activity at physiological intakes is not well accepted. Animal deprivation studies indicate that arsenic is beneficial to chickens, hamsters, goats, pigs, and rats (Uthus, 1992). Correlation-type findings suggest that arsenic is nutritionally important for humans (Nielsen, 2001, 1991). Decreased serum arsenic concentrations in patients undergoing hemodialysis were correlated to injuries of the central nervous system, vascular diseases, and cancer. In addition, it has been observed that the incidence of skin cancer is higher in areas where no arsenic is detected in drinking water than in areas where detectable amounts of arsenic are found in the water.

Humans have enzymes that are used specifically to methylate inorganic arsenic (Thomas et al., 2001). Methylation of arsenic takes place in the liver, following glutathione-dependent reduction of arsenate (As^{5+}) to arsenite (As^{3+}), and is catalyzed by an arsenite methyltransferase that utilizes *S*-adenosylmethionine as the methyl donor. The monomethylarsonate precursor formed from arsenite can be methylated again to form dimethylarsinate. In animals, the methylation of arsenic can be modified by changing glutathione, methionine, or choline status. Methylated arsenic compounds occur normally in all organisms. The end-products of methylation include arsenocholine, arsenobetaine, dimethylarsinic acid, and methylarsonic acid (Le, 2002). Except when high amounts of seafood are eaten, dimethylarsinic acid is the major form of arsenic found in human urine. Arsenolipids and arsenosugars are found in a variety of marine life.

The mechanism through which arsenic is bioactive most likely involves the utilization of labile methyl groups arising from methionine. By altering labile methyl group metabolism, arsenic affects the function of metabolically or genetically important molecules dependent on or regulated by methyl incorporation.

Absorption of arsenic from food is about 65% and absorption of inorganic arsenite or arsenate from water is about 90% of that ingested. Once absorbed, inorganic arsenic is transported to the liver where it is reduced and methylated. Both inorganic arsenic and various methylated forms are rapidly excreted in the urine. Based on the Total Diet Study (1991-1997), the median intake of arsenic from foods is 2.0 and 2.6 μg/day for women and men (ages 19 to 70 years), respectively. Sources of arsenic include fish, meat and poultry, grains and cereal products, grape juice, and spinach. The IOM (2001) did not set any DRIs for arsenic due to the lack of data supporting a biological role for arsenic in humans. Although no UL was set, high intakes of inorganic arsenic are clearly toxic. Organic forms of arsenic that occur naturally in foods have much lower toxicity than does inorganic arsenic.

ABSTRUSE ULTRATRACE ELEMENTS

The nutritional importance of the other ultratrace elements not specifically described in this chapter is quite limited and effectively summarized in Table 41-2. The evidence that these elements have beneficial effects or

Table 41-2
Abstruse Ultra Trace Elements of Possible Human Nutritional Significance Based Upon Animal Experimentation

Element	Reported Deficiency Signs	Apparent Deficient Dietary Intake	Other Apparent Beneficial or Physiological Actions	Typical Daily Dietary Intake and Dietary Sources for Humans
Aluminum (Al)	*Goat:* Increased spontaneous abortions, depressed growth, incoordination and weakness in hind legs, and decreased life expectancy *Chick:* Depressed growth	*Goat:* 162 μg/kg	Stimulates DNA synthesis in cell cultures; stimulates osteoblasts to form bone; enhances operant performance and food motivation of mice	2-10 mg Baked goods prepared with baking powder; processed cheese, grains, vegetables, tea
Bromine (Br)	*Goat:* Depressed growth, fertility, hematocrit, hemoglobin, and life expectancy; increased spontaneous abortions	*Goat:* 0.8 mg/kg	Substitutes for part of chloride requirement for chicks; alleviates growth retardation caused by hyperthyroidism in mice and iodine toxicity in chicks; insomnia associated with bromide deficit	2-8 mg Grains, nuts, fish
Cadmium (Cd)	*Rat:* Depressed growth *Goat:* Depressed growth	*Rat:* <4 μg/kg *Goat:* 20 μg/kg	Transforming growth factor activity; stimulates growth of cells in soft agar	10-20 μg Shellfish, grains grown on high-cadmium soils, leafy vegetables
Fluorine (F)	*Rat:* Depressed growth and incisor pigmentation *Goat:* Depressed growth and lifespan, histological changes in kidney and endocrine organs	*Rat:* 0.04-0.46 mg/kg *Goat:* <0.3 mg/kg	Stimulates bone formation; anti-osteoporotic; prevents tooth decay; prevents phosphorus induced nephrocalcinosis; alleviates depressed fertility, hematopoiesis and growth in iron-deficient rats and mice	1.4-3.4 mg with fluoridated water; 0.3-1.0 mg without fluoridation Fish, legumes, root vegetables, grain and cereal products, tea, fluoridated water

Table 41-2
Abstruse Ultra Trace Elements of Possible Human Nutritional Significance Based Upon Animal Experimentation—cont'd

Element	Reported Deficiency Signs	Apparent Deficient Dietary Intake	Other Apparent Beneficial or Physiological Actions	Typical Daily Dietary Intake and Dietary Sources for Humans
Germanium (Ge)	*Rat:* Altered bone and liver mineral composition, decreased tibial DNA	*Rat:* 0.7 mg/kg	Alleviates silicon deficiency signs, enhances immune response and has antitumor activity in experimental animals; improves bone strength and density in rats with experimental osteoporosis	0.4-3.4 mg Wheat bran, vegetables, leguminous seeds
Lead (Pb)	*Rat:* Depressed growth, anemia, disturbed iron metabolism, and altered liver lipid metabolism *Pig:* Depressed growth and elevated serum cholesterol, phospholipids and bile acids	*Rat:*18-45 μg/kg *Pig:* 30-32 μg/kg	Alleviates iron deficiency signs in young rats; activates a lead ribozyme	15-100 μg Seafood, plant foodstuffs grown under high-lead conditions
Lithium (Li)	*Goat:* Depressed fertility, birth weight, lifespan *Rat:* Depressed fertility, birth weight, litter size, and weaning weight	*Goat:* <1.5 mg/kg *Rat:* 0.6-15 μg/kg	Stimulates growth of some cultured cells; has insulinomimetic and immunomodulatory actions; low lithium status associated with violent crime, learning disability, and heart disease.	200-600 μg Eggs, meat, processed meat, fish, milk, milk products, potatoes, potatoes, vegetables (content varies with geographic origin)
Rubidium (Rb)	*Goat:* Depressed food intake, growth, and life expectancy, increased spontaneous abortions *Rat:* Altered tissue mineral concentrations	*Goat:* 180 μg/kg *Rat:* 0.54 mg/kg		1-5 mg Coffee, black tea, fruits, vegetables (especially asparagus), poultry, fish
Tin (Sn)	*Rat:* Depressed growth, response to sound and feed efficiency, altered heart, muscle, spleen, kidney and lung mineral composition, alopecia	*Rat:* 17 μg/kg	Influences heme oxygenase activity; associated with thymus immune function	1-40 mg Canned foods

NOTE: References for the material presented are given in a review by Nielsen (2001).

essential roles at physiological intakes is generally limited to a few gross observations in one or two species by one or two research groups. Moreover, some of the changes in deprivation studies were not very marked, not necessarily indicative of a suboptimal biological function, or obtained under less than satisfactory experimental conditions. Therefore, discussion of their nutritional or biochemical significance is judged to be premature at this time.

REFERENCES

Abumrad NN, Schneider AJ, Steel D, Rogers LS (1981) Amino acid intolerance during prolonged total parenteral nutrition reversed by molybdate therapy. Am J Clin Nutr 34:2551-2559.

Anderson RA (1993) Recent advances in the clinical and biochemical effects of chromium deficiency. In: Prasad AS (ed) Essential and Toxic Trace Elements in Human Health and Disease: An Update. Wiley-Liss, New York, pp 221-234.

Anderson RA, Cheng N, Bryden NA, Polansky MM, Cheng N, Chi J, Feng J (1997) Elevated intakes of supplemental chromium improve glucose and insulin variables in individuals with type 2 diabetes. Diabetes 46:1786-1791.

Anderson RA, Kozlovsky AS (1985) Chromium intake, absorption and excretion of subjects consuming self-selected diets. Am J Clin Nutr 41:1177-1183.

Anke M, Groppel B, Arnhold W, Langer M, Krause U (1990) The influence of the ultra trace element deficiency (Mo, Ni, As, Cd, V) on growth, reproduction performance and life expectancy. In: Tomita H (ed) Trace Elements in Clinical Medicine. Springer-Verlag, Tokyo, pp 361-376.

Armstrong TA, Spears JW, Crenshaw TD, Nielsen FH (2000) Boron supplementation of a semipurified diet for weanling pigs improves feed efficiency and bone strength characteristics and alters plasma lipid metabolites. J Nutr 139:2575-2581.

Armstrong TA, Spears JW, Lloyd KE (2001) Inflammatory response, growth, and thyroid hormone concentrations are affected by long-term boron supplementation in gilts. J Anim Sci 79:1549-1556.

Barondeau DP, Kassmann CJ, Bruns CK, Tainer JA, Getzoff ED (2004) Nickel superoxide dismutase structure and mechanism. Biochemistry 43:8038-8047.

Beedham C (1985) Molybdenum hydroxylases as drug-metabolizing enzymes. Drug Metab Rev 16:119-156.

Brown RO. Forloines-Lynn S, Cross RE, Heizer WD (1986) Chromium deficiency after long-term parenteral nutrition. Dig Dis Sci 31:661-664.

Carlisle EM (1984) Silicon. In: Friedlen E (ed) Biochemistry of the Essential Ultratrace Elements. Plenum Press, New York, pp 257-291.

Chen X, Schauder S, Potier N, Van Dorsselaer A, Pelczer I, Bassier BL, Hughson FM (2002) Structural identification of a bacterial quorum-sensing signal containing boron. Nature 415:545-549.

Clodfelder BJ, Emamaullee J, Hepburn DDD, Chakov NE, Nettles HS, Vincent JB (2001) The trail of chromium (III) in vivo from the blood to the urine: the roles of transferrin and chromodulin. J Biol Inorg Chem 6:608-617.

Davidson G, Clugston SL, Honek JF, Maroney MJ (2001) An XAS investigation of product and inhibitor complexes of Ni-containing GlxI from *Escherichia coli*: mechanistic implications. Biochemistry 40:4569-4582.

Davis CM, Vincent JB (1997) Chromium oligopeptide activates insulin receptor tyrosine kinase activity. Biochemistry 36:4382-4385.

Eady RR (1990) Vanadium nitrogenases. In: Chasteen ND (ed) Vanadium in Biological Systems. Kluwer Academic, Dordrecht, The Netherlands, pp 99-127.

Eckhert CD, Rowe RI (1999) Embryonic dysplasia and adult retinal dystrophy in boron deficient zebrafish. J Trace Elem Exp Med 12:213-219.

Engel RW, Price NO, Miller RF (1967) Copper, manganese, cobalt, and molybdenum balance in preadolescent girls. J Nutr 92:197-204.

Fort DJ, Stover EL, Rogers RL, Copley HF, Morgan LA, Foster ER (2000) Chronic boron or copper deficiency induces limb teratogenesis in *Xenopus*. Biol Trace Elem Res 77:173-187.

Fort DJ, Rogers RL, McLaughin DW, Sellers CM, Schlekat CL (2002) Impact of boron deficiency on *Xenopus laevis*. Biol Trace Elem Res 90:117-142.

Freund H, Atamian S, Fischer JE (1979) Chromium deficiency during total parenteral nutrition. J Am Med Assoc 241:496-498.

Goenrich M, Mahlert F, Duin EC, Bauer C, Jaun B, Thauer RK (2004) Probing the reactivity of Ni in the active site of methyl-coenzyme M reductase with substrate analogues. J Biol Inorg Chem 9:691-705.

Hildebrand M, Dahlin K, Volcani BE (1998) Characterization of a silicon transporter gene family in *Cylindrotheca fusiformis*: sequences, expression analysis, and identification of homologs in other diatoms. Mol Gen Genet 260:480-486.

Hulley P, Davison A (2003) Regulation of tyrosine phosphorylation cascades by phosphatases; what the actions of vanadium teach us. J Trace Elem Exp Med 16:281-290.

Hunt CD (2002) Boron-binding-biosubstances: a key to understanding the beneficial physiologic effects of dietary boron from prokaryotes to humans. In: Goldbach HE, Rerkasem B, Wimmer MA, Brown PH, Thellier M, Bell RW (eds) Boron in Plant and Animal Nutrition. Kluwer Academic/Plenum Publishers, New York, pp 21-36.

Hunt CD, Idso JP (1999) Dietary boron as a physiological regulator of the normal inflammatory response: a review and current research progress. J Trace Elem Exp Med 12:221-233.

Hunt CD (1996) Biochemical effects of physiologic amounts of dietary boron. J Trace Elem Exp Med 9:185-213.

Hunt CD (1994) The biochemical effects of physiologic amounts of dietary boron in animal nutrition models. Environ Health Perspect 102(Suppl):35-43.

Ichida K, Matsumura T, Sakuma R, Hosoya T, Nishino T (2001) Mutation of human molybdenum cofactor sulfurase gene is responsible for classical xanthinuria type II. Biochem Biophys Res Commun 282:1194-1200.

Institute of Medicine (2001) Dietary Reference Intakes for Vitamin A, Vitamin K, Arsenic, Boron, Chromium, Copper, Iodine, Iron, Manganese, Molybdenum, Nickel, Silicon, Vanadium, and Zinc. National Academy Press, Washington, DC.

Jeejeebhoy KN, Chu RC, Marliss EB, Greenberg GR, Bruce-Robertson A (1977) Chromium deficiency, glucose tolerance, and neuropathy reversed by chromium supplementation, in a patient receiving long-term total parenteral nutrition. Am J Clin Nutr 30:531-538.

Johnson JL (1997) Molybdenum. In: O'Dell BL, Sunde RA (eds) Handbook of Nutritionally Essential Mineral Elements. Marcel Dekker, New York, pp 413-438

Jugdaohsingh R, Anderson SHC, Tucker KL, Elliott H, Kiel DP, Thompson PH, Powell JJ (2002) Dietary silicon intake and absorption. Am J Clin Nutr 75:887-893.

Kaats GR, Ficher JA, Blum K (1991) The effects of chromium picolinate supplementation on body composition in different age groups. Am Aging Assoc Abstr 21:138.

Kaats GR, Wise JA, Blum K, Morin RJ, Adelman JA, Craig J, Croft HA (1992) The short-term therapeutic efficacy of treating obesity with a plan of improved nutrition and moderate caloric restriction. Curr Ther Res 51:261-274.

Kim H, Yu C, Maier RJ (1991) Common *cis*-acting region responsible for transcriptional regulation of *Bradyrhizobium japonicum* hydrogenase by nickel, oxygen, and hydrogen. J Bacteriol 173:3993-3999.

Kishikawa M, Nakanishi T, Shimizu A, Yoshino M (2000) Detection by mass spectrometry of highly increased amount of S-sulfonated transthyretin in serum from a patient with molybdenum cofactor deficiency. Pediatr Res 47:492-494.

Kohno J, Kawahata T, Otake T, Morimoto M, Mori H, Ueba N, Nishio M, Kinumaki A, Komatsubara S, Kawashima K (1996) Boromycin, an anti-HIV antibiotic. Biosci Biotechnol Biochem 60:1036-1037.

Le XC (2002) Arsenic speciation in the environment and humans. In: Frankenberger WT Jr (ed) Environmental Chemistry of Arsenic. Marcel Dekker, New York, pp 95-116.

Marzban L, McNeill JH (2003) Insulin-like actions of vanadium: potential as a therapeutic agent. J Trace Elem Exp Med 16:253-267.

Mills CF, Davis GK (1987) Molybdenum. In: Mertz W (ed) Trace Elements in Human and Animal Nutrition. Vol. 1. Academic Press, San Diego, pp 429-463..

Mobley HL, Island MD, Hausinger RP (1995) Molecular biology of microbial ureases. Microbiol Rev 59:451-480.

Mulyani I, Levina A, Lay PA (2004) Biomimetic oxidation of chromium (III): does the antidiabetic activity of chromium (III) involve carcinogenic chromium (VI)? Angew Chem Int Ed 43:4504.

National Research Council (NRC) (1989) Recommended Dietary Allowances, 10th ed. National Academy Press, Washington, DC.

Nielsen FH (2004) Boron status affects differences in blood immune cell populations in rats fed diets containing fish oil or safflower oil. In: Anke M, Flachowsky G, Kisters K, Müller R, Schafer U, Schenkel H, Seifert M, Stoeppler M (eds) Macro and Trace Elements. Vol. 2. Schubert-Verlag, Leipzig, pp 959-964.

Nielsen FH (2001) Boron, manganese, molybdenum, and other trace elements. In: Bowman BA,

Russell RM (eds) Present Knowledge of Nutrition, 8th ed. ILSI Press, Washington, DC, pp 384-400.

Nielsen FH (2000) The emergence of boron as nutritionally important throughout the life cycle. Nutr 16:512-514.

Nielsen FH (1998) The nutritional essentiality and physiological metabolism of vanadium in higher animals. In: Tracey AS, Crans DC (eds) Vanadium Compounds. Chemistry, Biochemistry, and Therapeutic Applications. American Chemical Society, Washington, DC, pp 297-307.

Nielsen FH (1997) Boron in animal and human nutrition. Plant Soil 193:199-208.

Nielsen FH (1994) Biochemical and physiologic consequences of boron deprivation in humans. Environ Health Perspect 102(Suppl):59-63.

Nielsen FH (1991) Nutritional requirements for boron, silicon, vanadium, nickel, and arsenic: Current knowledge and speculation. FASEB J 5:2661-2667.

Nielsen FH, Penland JG (1999) Boron supplementation of peri-menopausal women affects boron metabolism and indices associated with macromineral metabolism, hormonal status and immune function. J Trace Elem Exp Med 12:251-261.

Nielsen FH, Yokoi K, Uthus EO (2002) The essential role of nickel affects physiological functions regulated by the cyclic-GMP signal transduction system. In: Khassanova L, Collery PH, Maymard I, Khassanova Z, Etienne J-C (eds) Metal Ions in Biology and Medicine. Vol. 7. John Libbey Eurotext, Paris, pp 29-33.

Penland JG (1998) The importance of boron nutrition for brain and psychological function. Biol Trace Elem Res 66:299-317.

Penland JG (1994) Dietary boron, brain function, and cognitive performance. Environ Health Perspect 102(Suppl):65-72.

Pennington JAT, Jones JW (1987) Molybdenum, nickel, cobalt, vanadium, and strontium in total diets. J Am Diet Assoc 87:1644-1650.

Pochapsky TC, Pochapsky S, Ju T, Mo H, Al-Mjeni F, Maroney MJ (2002) Modeling and experiment yields the structure of acireductone dioxygenase from *Klebsiella pneumoniae*. Nat Struct Biol 9:966-972.

Ragsdale SW (2000) Nickel containing CO dehydrogenases and hydrogenases. Subcell Biochem 35:487-518.

Rajagopalan KV (1988) Molybdenum: an essential trace element in human nutrition. Annu Rev Nutr 8:401-427.

Ralston NVC, Hunt CD (2001) Diadenosine phosphates and S-adenosylmethionine: novel boron binding biomolecules detected by capillary electrophoresis. Biochim Biophys Acta 1527:20-30.

Reffitt DM, Ogston N, Jugdaohsingh R, Cheung HFJ, Evans BAJ, Thompson RPH, Powell JJ, Hampson GN (2003) Orthosilicic acid stimulates collagen type I synthesis and osteoblastic differentiation in human osteoblast-like cells in vitro. Bone 32:127-135.

Reiss J, Gross-Hardt S, Christensen E, Schmidt P, Mendel RR, Schwarz G (2001)A mutation in the gene for the neurotransmitter receptor-clustering protein gephyrin causes a novel form of molybdenum cofactor deficiency. Am J Hum Genet 68:208-213.

Reiss J, Johnson JL (2003) Mutations in the molybdenum cofactor biosynthetic genes MOCS1, MOCS2, and GEPH. Hum Mutat 21:569-576.

Schwarz K, Mertz W (1959) Chromium (III) and the glucose tolerance factor. Arch Biochem Biophys 85:292-295.

Seaborn CD, Nielsen FH (1993) Silicon: a nutritional beneficence for bones, brain and blood vessels? Nutr Today 28:13-18.

Sheng MH-C, Taper LJ, Veit H, Qian H, Ritchey SJ, Lau K-HW (2001) Dietary boron supplementation enhanced the action of estrogen, but not that of parathyroid hormone, to improve trabecular bone quality in ovariectomized rats. Biol Trace Elem Res 81:29-45.

Stearns DM (2000) Is chromium a trace essential metal? BioFactors 11:149-162.

Thauer RK (2001) Nickel to the fore. Science 293:1264-1265.

Thomas DJ, Styblo M, Lin S (2001) The cellular metabolism and systemic toxicity of arsenic. Toxicol Appl Pharmacol 176:127-144.

Tsongas TA, Meglen RR, Walravens PA, Chappell WR (1980) Molybdenum in the diet: an estimate of average daily intake in the United States. Am J Clin Nutr 33:1103-1107.

Turnlund JR, Keyes WR, Peiffer GL (1995a) Molybdenum absorption, excretion, and retention studied with stable isotopes in young men at five intakes of dietary molybdenum. Am J Clin Nutr 61:790-796.

Turnlund JR, Keyes WR, Peiffer GL, Chiang G (1995b) Molybdenum absorption, excretion, and retention studied with stable isotopes in young men during depletion and repletion. Am J Clin Nutr 61:1102-1109.

Uthus EO (1992) Evidence for arsenic essentiality. Environ Geochem Health 14:55-58.

Vincent JB (2004) Recent developments in the biochemistry of chromium (III). Biol Trace Elem Res 99:1-16.

Vincent JB (2003) Recent advances in the biochemistry of chromium (III). J Trace Elem Exp Med 16:227-236.

Vincent JB (2001) The bioinorganic chemistry of chromium (III). Polyhedron 20:1-26.

Watt RK, Ludden PW (1999) Nickel-binding proteins. Cell Mol Life Sci 56:604-625.

Wever R, Krenn BE (1990) Vanadium haloperoxidases. In: Chasteen ND (ed) Vanadium in Biological Systems. Kluwer Academic, Dordrecht, The Netherlands, pp 81-97.

World Health Organization (WHO) (1996) Trace Elements in Human Nutrition and Health. WHO, Geneva.

Wuerges J, Lee JW, Yim YI, Yim HS, Kang SO, Carugo KD (2004) Crystal structure of nickel-containing superoxide dismutase reveals another type of active site. Proc Natl Acad Sci U S A 101:8569-8574.

Yamamoto T, Moriwaki Y, Takahashi S, Tsutsumi Z, Tuneyoshi K, Matsui K, Cheng J, Hada T (2003) Identification of a new point mutation in the human molybdenum cofactor sulferase gene that is responsible for xanthinuria type II. Metabolism 52: 1501-1504.

Yokoi K, Uthus EO, Nielsen FH (2003) Nickel deficiency diminishes sperm quantity and movement in rats. Biol Trace Elem Res 93:141-153.

RECOMMENDED READINGS

O'Dell BL, Sunde RA (eds) (1997) Handbook of Nutritionally Essential Mineral Elements. Marcel Dekker, New York (Chapters 12-23).

Nielsen FH (2001) Boron, manganese, molybdenum, and other trace elements. In: Bowman BA, Russell RM (eds) Present Knowledge in Nutrition, 8th ed. ILSI Press, Washington, DC, pp 384-400.

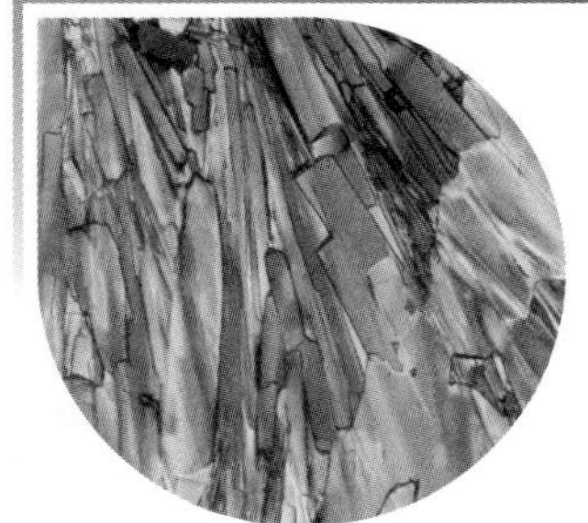

Index

Page numbers followed by b indicate boxed material; f, figures; t, tables.

B

F

J

K

L

M

N

S